DSM-IV-TR™
MENTAL DISORDERS

DIAGNOSIS, ETIOLOGY, AND TREATMENT

●FIRST
●TASMAN

DSM-IV-TR™
MENTAL DISORDERS

DIAGNOSIS, ETIOLOGY,
AND TREATMENT

Edited by
Michael B. First
Associate Professor of Clinical Psychiatry
Department of Psychiatry
Columbia University College of Physicians and Surgeons
New York, NY
USA

Allan Tasman
Professor and Chair
Department of Psychiatry and Behavioral Sciences
University of Louisville School of Medicine
Louisville, KY
USA

WILEY

Copyright © 2004 John Wiley & Sons, Ltd,
The Atrium,
Southern Gate,
Chichester,
West Sussex,
PO19 8SQ, England

Telephone (+44) 1243 779777
Email (for orders and customer service enquires): cs-books@wiley.co.uk
Visit our Home Page on www.wiley.co.uk or www.wiley.com

This publication is designed to provide accurate and authoritative information in regard to the subject matter
covered. It is sold on the understanding that the Publisher is not engaged in rendering professional services.
If professional advice or other expert assistance is required, the services of a competent professional should
be sought.

Other Wiley Editorial Offices

John Wiley & Sons, Inc., 111 River Street,
Hoboken, NJ 07030, USA

Jossey-Bass, 989 Market Street,
San Francisco, CA 94103-1741, USA

Wiley-VCH Verlag GmbH, Boschstr. 12,
D-69469 Weinheim, Germany

John Wiley & Sons Australia, Ltd, 33 Park Road,
Milton, Queensland, 4064, Australia

John Wiley & Sons (Asia) Pte Ltd, 2 Clementi Loop #02-01,
Jin Xing Distripark, Singapore 129809

John Wiley & Sons Canada Ltd, 22 Worcester Road,
Etobicoke, Ontario, Canada, M9W 1L1

Wiley also publishes its books in a variety of electronic formats. Some content that appears in print may not
be available in electronic books.

Library of Congress Cataloging-in-Publication Data

First, Michael B., 1956-
DSM-IV-TR mental disorders : diagnosis, etiology, and treatment/Michael B. First, Allan Tasman.
    p. ; cm.
"The factual content of the chapters in this book has been adapted from the 'Disorders' section of the second
edition of the two-volume Tasman, Kay, and Lieberman textbook, Psychiatry, which was published by John
Wiley & Sons in 2003"–Pref.
    Includes bibliographical references and index.
    ISBN 0-470-86089-8 (cloth : alk. paper)
    1. Mental illness–Diagnosis. 2. Mental illness–Classification. 3. Mental illness–Etiology.
    4. Mental illness–Treatment. [DNLM: 1. Mental Disorders–diagnosis. 2. Mental Disorders–therapy.
    3. Mental Disorders–physiopathology. WM 141 F527dg 2004] I. Tasman, Allan, 1947-
    II. Diagnostic and statistical manual of mental disorders. III. Psychiatry. IV. Title.

RC455.2.C4F573 2004
616.89′075–dc22   2003027340

British Library Cataloguing in Publication Data

A catalogue record for this book is available from the British Library

ISBN 0-470-86089-8

Typeset in 9.5/11.25pt Times-Roman by Laserwords Private Limited, Chennai, India
Printed and bound in Great Britain by William Clowes Ltd, Beccles, Suffolk.
This book is printed on acid-free paper responsibly manufactured from sustainable forestry
in which at least two trees are planted for each one used for paper production.

Dedications

To my mentors: Robert L. Spitzer, Allen Frances, and Harold A. Pincus

Michael

With love to Cathy, Josh, David, and Sarah

Allan

Table of Contents

Preface

The publication of DSM-III in 1980 revolutionized the field of mental health research and treatment. Among its many accomplishments (e.g. increased diagnostic reliability), it provided both a common language for naming, describing, and identifying the complete range of mental disorders seen in clinical practice, as well as providing an organizational plan that was embodied in the diagnostic groupings contained in the DSM-III classification (i.e., grouping together organic mental disorders, psychotic disorders, mood disorder, anxiety disorders, etc.). Although many aspects of the DSM-III system have been rightly criticized (e.g. use of criteria sets that imply the existence of distinct boundaries among disorders; the grouping together of obsessive-compulsive disorder, generalized anxiety disorder, and posttraumatic stress disorder within the same diagnostic class), its adoption of widely agreed upon categories has facilitated research, clinical practice, and education.

Using the DSM classification as a structural foundation, this book provides the reader with a comprehensive presentation of the diagnosis, etiology, and treatment of the various mental disorders identified in the DSM-IV-TR. It goes well beyond the bounds of the DSM-IV-TR itself, which primarily restricts its discussion to diagnostic and epidemiological information. Minimal information is provided in DSM-IV-TR regarding the etiology or pathophysiology of the mental disorders, which is only obliquely touched upon in the Familial Pattern and Associated Laboratory Features sections of the text, and no information whatsoever is provided about treatment. Thus, this textbook can be regarded as a sort of "DSM-IV-TR Plus" in that it contains a wealth of information about all three of these critically important domains.

The organization of the chapters in this book closely parallels the layout of disorders in the DSM-IV-TR. The amount of space allocated to each disorder in this book, however, varies according to its clinical importance. Thus, unlike DSM-IV-TR, in which all of the anxiety disorders are covered in the same chapter, the book splits up the major anxiety disorders among several different chapters. For the most part, each chapter in this book follows a consistent structure. The Diagnosis section for each disorder begins with introductory material describing the features of the disorder and includes information about assessment issues, comorbid conditions, and associated diagnostic, physical examination, and laboratory features. Additional subsections include Epidemiology (which includes prevalence, incidence, gender ratio, and other information derived from epidemiological studies), Course (which includes age at onset, prognosis, and outcome), and Differential Diagnosis. Since the precise etiology and pathophysiology of the vast majority of mental disorders remain unknown, the Etiology sections summarize what is known with regard to genetic factors, neurobiological factors, and psychological factors that may contribute to the development of the disorders. The Treatment sections summarize the available treatments for the disorders, and are often broken down into Somatic Treatments and Psychosocial Treatments for ease of reference.

The factual content of the chapters in this book has been adapted from the Disorders section of the second edition of the two-volume Tasman, Kay, and Lieberman textbook, *Psychiatry*, which was published by John Wiley & Sons in 2003. Jerry Kay and Jeff Lieberman, two of the co-editors of that two-volume set, deserve special thanks for their efforts in making that edition an outstanding reference. We would like also to acknowledge the excellent contributions made by the original authors of the Disorders chapters, and they are duly listed in the Acknowledgments. Two new chapters, covering Amphetamine-Related Disorders by Kevin Sevarino and Reactive Attachment Disorder by Brian Stafford and Charles Zeanah were developed specifically for this book, as no chapters covering these disorders were included in the original two-volume textbook.

We would also like to express our gratitude to Charlotte Brabants and Amelia Bennett at John Wiley & Sons for their help in the editing and production of this book. In addition, Joan Roberts in Allan Tasman's office provided invaluable help in the preparation of the manuscript.

MICHAEL B. FIRST

ALLAN TASMAN

April 2004

Acknowledgments

We would like to gratefully acknowledge the authors of those chapters in *Psychiatry* 2nd Edition from which material in this book was adapted.

Henry David Abraham	*Substance Abuse: Hallucinogen- and MDMA-Related Disorders*
Sonia Ancoli-Israel	*Sleep and Sleep-Wake Disorders*
Martin M. Antony	*Anxiety Disorders: Social and Specific Phobias*
Gordon J. G. Asmundson	*Anxiety Disorders: Panic Disorder With and Without Agoraphobia*
Thomas F. Babor	*Substance Abuse: Alcohol Use Disorders*
Mark S. Bauer	*Mood disorders: Bipolar (Manic-Depressive) Disorders*
Jean C. Beckham	*Anxiety Disorders: Traumatic Stress Disorders*
Olga Brawman-Mintzer	*Anxiety Disorders: Generalized Anxiety Disorder*
Alan Breier	*Schizophrenia and Other Psychoses*
Deborah L. Cabaniss	*Clinical Evaluation and Treatment Planning: A Multimodal Approach*
Irene Chatoor	*Childhood Disorders: Feeding and Other Disorders of Infancy or Early Childhood*
Edwin H. Cook	*Childhood Disorders: The Autism Spectrum Disorders*
Francine Cournos	*Clinical Evaluation and Treatment Planning: A Multimodal Approach*
Jonathan R. T. Davidson	*Anxiety Disorders: Traumatic Stress Disorders*
Christian R. Dolder	*Medication-Induced Movement Disorders*
Jane L. Eisen	*Obsessive-Compulsive Disorder*
Stuart Eisendrath	*Factitious Disorders*
Rif S. El-Mallakh	*Substance Abuse: Hallucinogen- and MDMA-Related Disorders*
Milton Erman	*Sleep and Sleep-Wake Disorders*
Susan J. Fiester	*Substance Abuse: Nicotine Dependence*
Anne Fleming	*Factitious Disorders*
Robert Freedman	*Psychiatric Pathophysiology: Overview*
Robert L. Frierson	*Delirium and Dementia*
Paul J. Fudala	*Substance Abuse: Opioid Use Disorder*
J. Christian Gillin	*Sleep and Sleep-Wake Disorders*
Reed D. Goldstein	*Mood Disorders: Depression*

Roland R. Griffiths	*Substance Abuse: Caffeine Use Disorders*
Amanda J. Gruber	*Substance Abuse: Cannabis-Related Disorders*
Alan M. Gruenberg	*Mood Disorders: Depression*
Jeffrey M. Halperin	*Childhood Disorders: Attention-Deficit and Disruptive Behavior Disorders*
John H. Halpern	*Substance Abuse: Hallucinogen- and MDMA-Related Disorders*
Carlos A. Hernandez-Avila	*Substance Abuse: Alcohol Use Disorders*
Dilip V. Jeste	*Medication-Induced Movement Disorders*
Charles Y. Jin	*Substance Abuse: Cocaine Use Disorders*
William M. Klykylo	*Childhood Disorders: Communication Disorders*
Thomas R. Kosten	*General Approaches to Substance and Polydrug Use Disorders*
Henry R. Kranzler	*Substance Abuse: Alcohol Use Disorders*
James L. Levenson	*Psychological Factors Affecting Medical Condition*
Bennett L. Leventhal	*Childhood Disorders: The Autism Spectrum Disorders*
Stephen B. Levine	*Sexual Disorders*
Walter Ling	*Substance Abuse: Sedative, Hypnotic, or Anxiolytic Use Disorders*
Joyce H. Lowinson	*Substance Abuse: Phencyclidine Use Disorders*
Christopher P. Lucas	*Childhood Disorders: Elimination Disorders and Childhood Anxiety Disorders*
R. Bruce Lydiard	*Anxiety Disorders: Generalized Anxiety Disorder*
Mario Maj	*Global Perspectives on Mental Health Services*
José R. Maldonado	*Dissociative Disorders*
John S. March	*Anxiety Disorders: Traumatic Stress Disorders*
Randi E. McCabe	*Anxiety Disorders: Social and Specific Phobias*
Elinore F. McCance-Katz	*Substance Abuse: Cocaine Use Disorders*
Laura F. McNicholas	*Substance Abuse: Opioid Use Disorders*
Robyn R. Miller	*Combined Therapies: Psychotherapy and Pharmacotherapy*
Jeannine Monnier	*Anxiety Disorders: Generalized Anxiety Disorder*
David P. Moore	*Mental Disorders due to a General Medical Condition*
Stephanie Mullins	*Personality Disorders*
Jeffrey H. Newcorn	*Childhood Disorders: Attention-Deficit and Disruptive Behavior Disorder; Adjustment Disorders*
Thomas Owley	*Childhood Disorders: The Autism Spectrum Disorders*
Jayendra K. Patel	*Schizophrenia and Other Psychoses*
Michele T. Pato	*Obsessive-Compulsive Disorder*
Teri Pearlstein	*Mood Disorders: Premenstrual Dysphoric Disorder*
Katharine A. Phillips	*Obsessive-Compulsive Disorder*
Debra A. Pinals	*Schizophrenia and Other Psychoses*
Harrison G. Pope, Jr	*Substance Abuse: Cannabis-Related Disorders*
Michelle B. Riba	*Combined Therapies: Psychotherapy and Pharmacotherapy*
Mark A. Riddle	*Childhood Disorders: Tic Disorders*
Neil Rosenberg	*Substance Abuse: Inhalant-Related Disorders*
Kurt P. Schulz	*Childhood Disorders: Attention-Deficit and Disruptive Behavior Disorders*

David Shaffer — *Childhood Disorders: Elimination Disorders and Childhood Anxiety Disorders*

Vanshdeep Sharma — *Childhood Disorders: Attention-Deficit and Disruptive Behavior Disorders*

Charles W. Sharp — *Substance Abuse: Inhalant-Related Disorders*

Larry B. Silver — *Childhood Disorders: Learning and Motor Skills Disorders*

Daphne Simeon — *Impulse Control Disorders*

David E. Smith — *Substance Abuse: Sedative, Hypnotic, or Anxiolytic Use Disorders*

David Spiegel — *Dissociative Disorders*

Eric C. Strain — *Substance Abuse: Caffeine Use Disorders*

James J. Strain — *Adjustment Disorders*

Scott Stroup — *Global Perspectives on Mental Health Services*

Ludwik S. Szymanski — *Childhood Disorders: Mental Retardation*

Steven Taylor — *Anxiety Disorders: Panic Disorder With and Without Agoraphobia*

Jane A. Ungemack — *Substance Abuse: Alcohol Use Disorders*

John T. Walkup — *Childhood Disorders: Tic Disorders*

B. Timothy Walsh — *Eating Disorders*

Donald R. Wesson — *Substance Abuse: Sedative, Hypnotic or Anxiolytic Use Disorders*

Thomas A. Widiger — *Personality Disorders*

Maija Wilska — *Childhood Disorders: Mental Retardation*

Ronald M. Winchel — *Impulse Control Disorders*

George E. Woody — *Substance Abuse: Opioid Use Disorder*

Yoram Yovell — *Impulse Control Disorders*

Sean H. Yutzy — *Somatoform Disorders*

Douglas Ziedonis — *Substance Abuse: Nicotine Dependence*

Stephen R. Zukin — *Substance Abuse: Phencyclidine Use Disorders*

Ilana Zylberman — *Substance Abuse: Phencyclidine Use Disorders*

1 Diagnosis

There is a natural human predilection to categorize and classify for simplifying and organizing the wide range of observable phenomena and experiences that one is confronted with, thus facilitating both their understanding and their predictability. Many (if not most) of the mental disorders that afflict contemporary individuals have occurred in antiquity. For example, the first recorded depiction of mental illness dates to 3000 B.C. Egypt, with a description of the syndrome senile dementia attributed to Prince Ptah-hotep (Mack et al. 1994). The current system for the diagnosis of mental disorders, the *Diagnostic and Statistical Manual of Mental Disorders*, Fourth Edition Text Revision (DSM-IV-TR) (American Psychiatric Association 2000), is just the latest example from the long and colorful history of psychiatric classification.

Goals of the DSM-IV-TR

Perhaps the most important goal of the DSM-IV-TR is to allow mental health practitioners and researchers to communicate more effectively with each other by establishing a convenient shorthand for describing the mental disorders that they see (First 1992). For example, telling a colleague that an individual whom you have just evaluated has major depressive disorder can convey a great deal of information in only a few words. First of all, it indicates that depressed mood or loss of interest is a central aspect of the presenting problem and that the depression is not the kind of "normal" mood fluctuation that lasts for only a few days but rather that it persists every day for an extended period of time, for at least 2 weeks. Furthermore, one can expect to find a number of additional symptoms occurring at the same time, like suicidal ideation and changes in appetite, sleep, energy, and psychomotor activity. Finally, information is also communicated about what is not to be found in this individual—specifically, that the depression is not caused by the direct physiological effects of alcohol, other drugs, medications, or a general medical condition; that substance use and general medical conditions have been ruled out as etiological factors; and that there is no history of schizophrenia or manic or hypomanic episodes.

DSM-IV-TR also facilitates the identification and management of mental disorders in both clinical and research settings. Most of the DSM-IV-TR diagnostic labels provide considerable and important predictive power. For example, making a diagnosis of bipolar disorder suggests the choice of treatment options (e.g., mood stabilizers), that a certain course may be likely (e.g., recurrent and episodic), and that there is an increased prevalence of this disorder in family members. By defining more or less homogeneous groups of individuals for study, DSM-IV-TR can also further efforts to understand the etiology of mental disorders. The classifications of the manual have been a reflection of, and a major contribution to, the development of an empirical science of psychiatry. DSM-IV-TR also plays an important role in education. In its organization of disorders into major classes, the system offers a structure for teaching phenomenology and differential diagnosis. DSM-IV-TR is also useful in psychoeducation by showing individuals suffering from symptoms of a mental disorder that their pattern of symptoms is not mysterious and unique but rather has been identified and studied in others.

Approaches to Psychiatric Classification

Etiological Versus Descriptive

Historically, there have been two fundamental approaches to formulating systems of psychiatric classification: etiological and descriptive (First 1994). Etiology-based classification systems organize categories around pathogenetic processes so that disorders corresponding to a particular category share the same underlying cause. Although such systems tend to have relatively few categories and therefore are easy to use, their ultimate value is constrained by the limited extent to which underlying etiological factors have been elucidated. For example, the sixteenth-century Swiss physician Paracelsus developed a classification system in which he divided psychotic presentations into three types of disorders on the basis of the presumed etiology. The first category, vesania, for disorders caused by poisons, is analogous to current-day substance-induced disorders. Insanity, for diseases caused by heredity, is analogous to modern disorders such as schizophrenia and bipolar disorder, which appear to have a strong familial component. His category of lunacy, which described a periodical condition influenced by the phases of the moon, has no analogous condition today because we know that the phases of the moon are not a direct cause of psychopathological conditions.

Because the etiological basis for most psychiatric conditions remains elusive, etiological classification systems tend to be based instead on a particular conceptualization of the process of mental disorders. Although such classifications may be heuristically useful to proponents of the particular conceptualization that forms the basis of the system, they are often considerably less useful for proponents of different etiological principles, which greatly limits their utility. For this reason, a descriptive approach to classification has proved to be of greater utility, given our current understanding. The descriptive approach aims to eschew particular etiological theories and instead relies on clinical descriptions of presenting symptoms. This approach, advanced by the work of the nineteenth-century psychiatrist Emil Kraepelin (1883), formed the basis for the system of classification of the *Diagnostic and Statistical Manual of Mental Disorders*, Third Edition (DSM-III) introduced in 1980. As a result, DSM-III and its successors, the *Diagnostic and Statistical Manual of Mental Disorders*, Third Edition, Revised (DSM-III-R), DSM-IV, and DSM-IV-TR, have proved to be useful in a variety of different settings and by psychiatrists of widely different backgrounds and conceptual orientations.

Syndrome Versus Symptom

Given that the manual lacks a specific etiological conceptualization, what is its organizing principle? The fundamental element is the syndrome, that is, a group or pattern of symptoms that appear together temporally in many individuals (First et al. 1992). It is assumed that these symptoms cluster together because they are associated in some clinically meaningful way, which perhaps may reflect a common etiological process, course, or treatment response. Alternatively, individual symptoms could have been emphasized as the fundamental conceptual entities so that a person's disorder would be classified by enumerating all of his or her relevant symptoms. In fact, historically, there have been classifications that have been symptom-based. For example, Boisser de Sauvages proposed a medical classification that arranged presenting symptoms into numerous classes, orders, and genera, comparable to the classification of plants and animals. This approach generated 2400 disorders, each of which was essentially a symptom.

Although it was hoped that the syndromes identified in the DSM represented relatively homogeneous subpopulations of patients, over the past 25 years since the publication of these definitions in DSM-III, the goal of discovering common etiologies for each of the DSM-defined syndromes has remained elusive. Epidemiologic and clinical studies have shown extremely high rates of comorbidities among the disorders, undermining the hypothesis that the syndromes represent distinct etiologies. Furthermore, epidemiologic studies have shown a high degree of short-term diagnostic instability for many disorders. With regard to treatment, lack of specificity in treatment response is the rule rather than the exception. The efficacy of many psychotropic medications cuts across the DSM-defined categories. For example, the selective serotonin reuptake inhibitors (SSRIs) have been demonstrated to be efficacious in a wide variety of disorders from many different sections of the DSM, including major depressive disorder, panic disorder, obsessive–compulsive disorder, dysthymic disorder, bulimia nervosa, social anxiety disorder, posttraumatic stress disorder, generalized anxiety disorder, hypochondriasis, body dysmorphic disorder, and borderline personality disorder. Results of twin studies have also contradicted the DSM assumption that separate syndromes have a different underlying genetic basis. For example, twin studies have shown that generalized anxiety disorder and major depressive disorder may share the same genetic risk factors (Kendler 1996), and evidence from molecular genetics research (Berrettini 2000) indicates that three of the putative susceptibility loci associated with DSM-defined bipolar disorder also contribute to the risk of DSM-defined schizophrenia.

Given these clear limitations in the syndromal approach, it is important that users of the DSM resist the temptation to reify the DSM diagnostic categories as if they were actual diseases. They are best viewed as clinical, useful constructs that are helpful in facilitating communication and recordkeeping, and in selecting treatment. As more information about the causes of mental disorders become evident over the next decades, it is more than likely that the syndromal approach will be replaced by a classification system that is more reflective of the underlying etiology and pathophysiology. A hypothetical example (Table 1-1) of what such a classification system might look like is described in the Neuroscience Research Agenda white paper that was prepared in advance of the starting work on DSM-V (Charney et al. 2002).

Table 1-1	Outline for a Possible Future Classification System

Axis I: Genotype
Identification of disease/symptom-related genes
Identification of resiliency/protective genes
Identification of genes related to therapeutic responses and side effects to specific psychotropic drugs

Axis II: Neurobiological Phenotype
Identification of intermediate phenotypes (neuroimaging, cognitive function, emotional regulation) related to genotype
Relates to targeted pharmacotherapy

Axis III: Behavioral Phenotype
The range and frequency of expressed behaviors associated with genotype, neurobiological phenotype, and environment
Relates to targeted therapies

Axis IV: Environmental Modifiers or Precipitants
Environmental factors that alter the behavioral and neurobiological phenotype

Axis V: Therapeutic Targets and Response

Source: Kupfer DJ, First MB, and Regier DA (2002) *A Research Agenda for DSM-V*. American Psychiatric Publishing, Washington, DC, p. 72.

Categorical Versus Dimensional

The diagnoses included in DSM-IV-TR are defined categorically, that is, diagnostic criteria are provided that indicate whether an individual's clinical presentation either meets or does not meet the diagnostic criteria for a particular disorder. This method of classification is similar to that used in other fields in medicine, namely, that a patient either has or does not have a particular diagnosis, like pneumonia, colon cancer, multiple sclerosis, and so on. This tendency to define illness in terms of categories is undoubtedly due to the fact that it is reflective of basic human thought processes, embodied by the use of nouns in everyday speech to indicate categories of "things" (e.g., chairs, tables, dogs, cats, etc.).

In principle, however, variation in the symptomatology can be represented by a set of dimensions rather than by multiple categories. An example of this in medicine is blood pressure, which is measured along a continuum from low to high. (It only becomes categorical when we apply the label "hypertension" to indicate that an individual has a significant elevated level of blood pressure that puts him or her at risk for developing serious illness.) Dimensional approaches to describing psychiatric symptomatology have been proposed as well. For example, Wittenborn and colleagues (1953) developed a multidimensional representation of the phenomena of psychotic illness nearly 50 years ago, and since then others have developed dimensional models to portray the symptomatology of depressive and anxiety disorders, personality disorders, schizophrenia, and even the entire range of psychopathology.

While a categorical approach to classification has important heuristic appeal, it may not represent the true state of things. Implicit in the categorical approach is an assumption that mental disorders are discrete entities, separated from one another and from normality, either by recognizably distinct combinations of symptoms or by demonstrably distinct etiologies. While this has been shown to be the case for a small number of conditions (e.g., Down syndrome, fragile X syndrome, phenylketonuria, Alzheimer's disease, Huntington's disease, and Creutzfeldt–Jakob disease), there is little evidence supporting the applicability of this model for most other psychiatric symptoms. Indeed, in the last 20 years, the categorical approach has been increasingly questioned as evidence has accumulated that the so-called categorical disorders like major depressive disorder and anxiety disorders, and schizophrenia and bipolar disorder seem to merge imperceptibly both into one another and into normality (Kendler and Gardner 1998) with no demonstrable natural boundaries.

Dimensional approaches do have some clear advantages. First of all, the commonly observed phenomena of excessive comorbidity (i.e., an individual receiving multiple, simultaneous DSM diagnoses) is arguably a direct result of having a categorical system with more than 250 categories. A dimensional approach, which would characterize an individual's psychopathology by indicating the extent of his or her psychiatric symptomatology across a number of dimensions, virtually eliminates apparent comorbidity. For example, consider an individual who presents with depression, anxiety, and social avoidance. Using the DSM-IV-TR categorical system, criteria might be met for three diagnoses (i.e., major depressive disorder, social phobia, and generalized anxiety disorder), thus warranting a diagnosis of all three disorders on Axis I. A dimensional approach may simply indicate that the person has "high scores" on the depression, anxiety, and social avoidance dimensions. Another advantage of the dimensional approach is that it avoids setting particular thresholds for distinguishing between pathology and normality. Rather than categorically saying that an individual has major depressive disorder, a dimensional approach might say that the person is high on the depression dimension.

There are a number of practical problems that potentially limit the utility of adopting a dimensional approach. First of all, clinicians are accustomed to thinking in terms of diagnostic categories, and the existing knowledge base about the presentation, etiology, epidemiology, course, prognosis, and treatment is based on these categories. Furthermore, decisions about the management of patients (e.g., whether to treat and with what type of treatment) are also much easier to make if the patient is thought of as having a particular disorder (with its associated prognostic and treatment implications) rather than as a profile of scores across a series of dimensions. It should be noted that, at least for personality disorders, current dissatisfaction with the categorical approach has led to proposals for research that might allow for the adoption of a dimensional approach to classifying personality functioning in DSM-V (First et al. 2002).

History of the DSM Classification System

DSM-I and DSM-II

The predecessors of DSM-IV-TR arose from the need to develop a classification system of mental disorders for statistical, epidemiological, and reporting purposes. The first official international classification of mental disorders, the sixth revision of the *International Classification of Diseases* (ICD-6), was considered unacceptable by most countries because of its heavy reliance on unproven etiological concepts. The *Diagnostic and Statistical Manual of Mental Disorders*, First Edition (DSM-I) was published in 1952 as an alternative to ICD-6 and included glossary definitions of the various disorders (American Psychiatric Association 1952). The *Diagnostic and Statistical Manual of Mental Disorders*, Second Edition (DSM-II) (American Psychiatric Association 1968) was published in 1968. Like DSM-I, DSM-II retained many etiological concepts (e.g., neuroses).

DSM-III

After reviewing early drafts of ICD-9 in the early 1970s, the American Psychiatric Association (1980) opted to develop DSM-III because of concerns that the international nature of the ICD-9 resulted in inconsistent terminology and definitions and that the subtyping was inadequate for clinical and research use. DSM-III represented a major paradigm shift from the etiologically based frameworks of DSM-I and DSM-II. It adopted a descriptive approach that was meant to facilitate communication among mental health professionals operating under various theoretical orientations that continue to flourish in psychiatry and psychology.

Two innovations were introduced in DSM-III. Each DSM-III disorder was defined by the use of explicit diagnostic criteria, which greatly improved the reliability of the system and provided researchers with well-defined categories for scientific study. DSM-III also included a multiaxial system for evaluation that facilitated the use of a biopsychosocial model of evaluation by separating (and thereby calling attention to) developmental and personality disorders (Axis II), physical conditions (Axis III), stressors (Axis IV), and level of adaptive functioning (Axis V) from the presenting diagnoses (Axis I).

DSM-III-R

Although DSM-III-R (American Psychiatric Association 1987), originally intended only as a fine-tuning to correct inconsistencies and problems identified after the publication of DSM-III (Boyd et al. 1987, Spitzer and Williams 1987), more substantive changes were made, many reflecting new evidence not available to the developers of DSM-III. Although the publication of DSM-III-R demonstrated that the system is self-correcting, DSM-III-R has been criticized as being too much of a change occurring too soon after the adoption of DSM-III.

DSM-IV

DSM-IV-TR was envisioned as a modification and refinement of previous editions of the manual rather than a radical reconceptualization (Frances et al. 1990). The most significant change in DSM-IV is in the process by which DSM-III-R was revised to produce DSM-IV (Widiger et al. 1991). Prior revision efforts were guided almost exclusively by expert consensus. Although these experts were certainly familiar with the then current state of knowledge about the psychiatric disorders, their decisions were subject to potential biases. In contrast, whenever possible, DSM-IV decisions were based on a systematic review of the then current empirical database.

The method used to establish an empirical basis for changes in DSM-IV was divided into three stages. As a first step, the approximately 150 questions most deserving consideration for DSM-IV were identified (Widiger et al. 1990). Each of these then received an extensive and systematic review of the literature to determine what evidence was available and what additional evidence would need to be collected to support possible changes. One obvious shortcoming of relying on the literature reviews was that many important questions arose that were not addressed by the published literature. The second stage of the process was to conduct a series of approximately 40 data reanalyses of previously compiled data sets to supplement the evidence available from published studies. Although useful in generating new criteria sets for DSM-IV, the data reanalyses were limited by the fact that the data were collected before the DSM-IV process. Therefore, a series of 12 focused field trials were conducted (Table 1-2). Each field trial drew subjects from at least five different sites (with a minimum of 50 patients per site) (Frances et al. 1991). The field trials served to test the performance characteristics of the proposed criteria sets and to compare them with the DSM-III, DSM-III-R, and ICD-10 criteria sets. A summary of the results of the empirical review process as well as the rationale for the changes in DSM-IV is published in the four-volume *DSM-IV Sourcebook* (Widiger et al. 1994, 1996, 1997, 1998).

The following example serves to illustrate this three-stage process. One of the main goals of the DSM-IV revision process was to improve the clinical utility of the criteria sets. In this regard, several of the DSM-III-R criteria sets had been identified as being particularly difficult to apply in clinical settings. One of the most cumbersome criteria sets was that for somatization disorder, which provided a list of 35 different unexplained physical symptoms, of which at least 13 were required for a diagnosis. A literature review was first conducted to investigate the performance characteristics of the DSM-III-R criteria set. It demonstrated, as expected, that the DSM-III-R definition was among the most reliable and valid in the manual. Any attempt to modify the criteria set would therefore have to result in

Table 1-2	DSM-IV Focused Field Trials

Schizophrenia
Mood disorders
Panic disorder
Mixed anxiety–depressive disorder
Obsessive–compulsive disorder
Posttraumatic stress disorder
Somatization disorder
Sleep disorders
Pervasive developmental disorders
Disruptive behavior disorders
Substance dependence
Antisocial personality disorder

a criteria set that defined the same group of individuals as did DSM-III-R and be comparably reliable. A more user-friendly criteria set was generated through the data reanalysis process. Data sets of individuals with somatization disorder were pooled, and different diagnostic algorithms were investigated. The resulting proposed criteria set required symptoms for a period of several years that occur in the following pattern: at least four pain symptoms, two gastrointestinal symptoms, one sexual symptom, and one conversion symptom. To ensure the generalizability of this proposed criteria set, a focused field trial was conducted that compared this simplified definition with the original DSM-III-R definition, along with DSM-III, ICD-10, and the historical definition of Briquet' syndrome. The field trial found that all of the definitions identified essentially the same group of individuals with comparable reliability, providing empirical support for the DSM-IV decision to replace the DSM-III-R criteria set for somatization disorder.

DSM-IV-TR

During the DSM-IV-TR revision process, some criticisms were voiced about the rapid pace of DSM revisions (Zimmerman et al. 1991), arguing that undertaking an extensive revision of the classification every 7 years was disruptive to researchers and was not necessarily justified by the pace of psychiatric research. DSM-IV was timed for publication in 1994 in order to coincide with the publication of ICD-10 in 1992. In the absence of any externally imposed time frame (given that there is no anticipated date for commencing work on ICD-11), it was decided that the interval between DSM-IV and the next revision would be greatly extended to at least 16 years (i.e., DSM-V will not come out until 2010, or perhaps later). One consequence of this is the effect on the currency of the DSM-IV text, which was based on a literature review that extended only to mid-1992. Thus, in order to maintain continued clinical utility and educational value, a revision of the DSM-IV text was begun in 1996 (First and Pincus 2002). Following the DSM-IV precedent of making changes only if supported by data (Widiger et al. 1991), changes to the text were made on the basis of a comprehensive review of the literature relevant to the text categories that was published since 1992. The text revision (American Psychiatric Association 2000), called *DSM-IV-TR* to distinguish it from DSM-IV, was published in June 2000.

DSM-V

In advance of starting work on DSM-V, which is not anticipated to commence until the middle of this decade, a preliminary DSM-V research-planning process has been initiated in order to (1) stimulate research that will enrich the empirical database prior to the start of the DSM-V revision process and (2) devise a research and analytic agenda that would facilitate the integration of findings from animal studies, genetics, neuroscience, epidemiology, clinical research, and cross-cultural and clinical services research, which will lead to the eventual development of an etiologically based scientifically sound classification system (Regier et al. 2002). Six work groups were given the task of producing white papers that would serve to summarize the current issues in each of six broad topic areas and then to recommend a research agenda. The six topic areas were (1) basic nomenclature issues; (2) the role of neuroscience and genetics; (3) developmental issues; (4) gaps in the DSM classification of personality and relational disorder; (5) the relationship between symptoms and disability; and (6) cross-cultural issues. The six white papers were published as a monograph in 2002 (Kupfer et al. 2002). Ten diagnosis-focused research conferences are also planned over the intervening years in order to identify issues and stimulate research that might be instrumental to the future DSM-V work groups' decisions.

Differential Diagnosis Using DSM-IV-TR

Differential diagnosis is defined in Stedman's medical dictionary (24th edition) as "the determination of which of two or more diseases with similar symptoms is the one from which the patient is suffering." This definition reflects the fact that many of the DSM-IV-TR diagnoses share symptoms in common and thus many diagnoses are possible, given a particular presenting symptom. For example, if an individual presents with depressed mood, possible DSM-IV-TR disorders that could account for the depressed mood include major depressive disorder and dysthymic disorder, of course (since depressed mood is the main defining feature of these disorders), as well as bipolar I or II disorder, currently depressed; schizoaffective disorder, depressive type; postpsychotic depression of schizophrenia, adjustment disorder with depressed mood, mood disorder due to a general medical condition, and substance-induced mood disorder. The task of differential diagnosis entails considering all of the possible diagnoses that could explain the presenting symptom, and then collecting additional information (from personal history, family history, mental status examination, and laboratory investigations) to allow a winnowing down of the list to a single "most likely" contender, which becomes the initial diagnosis leading to the initial treatment plan. Confirmation of the initial diagnosis often requires the passage of time so that the telltale features of the disorder's course of illness can play itself out.

DSM-IV-TR includes several features to assist in making a differential diagnosis. The descriptive text for each disorder contains a section called "Differential Diagnosis" that describes those disorders with similar features that must be considered and ruled out. In addition, DSM-IV-TR Appendix A contains six "Decision Trees for Differential Diagnosis." Each decision tree starts with a set of clinical features (i.e., symptoms due to the direct effects of a general medical condition, substance-induced symptoms, psychotic symptoms, mood symptoms, anxiety symptoms, and somatoform symptoms). When one of these features is a prominent part of the clinical presentation, the clinician should consult the relevant decision tree and follow the series of questions in order to consider and/or rule out the various disorders. We will describe each of the six decision trees in turn.

Decision Tree for Symptoms Due to a General Medical Condition

It is a crucial part of the evaluation of every individual presenting for treatment to consider the possibility that the symptom may be the direct physiological effect of a general medical condition (see Figure 1-1). In fact, psychiatric symptoms such as depression and anxiety may be the first harbinger of a not-yet diagnosed general medical illness. Determining that a general medical condition is the cause of the individual's psychiatric symptoms has clear treatment implications—successful treatment of the general medical condition often results in resolution of the psychiatric symptoms. However, making this determination is sometimes quite difficult for several reasons: (1) symptom of some psychiatric disorders and of many general medical conditions can be identical (e.g., fatigue, weight loss); (2) for some general medical conditions, the presenting symptom may be psychiatric (e.g., depression preceding neurological manifestations of a brain tumor); and (3) patients are often seen in settings that are primarily focused on the diagnosis and treatment of mental disorders in which there is a lower expectation for, or less familiarity with, general medical presentations.

It should be recognized that psychiatric symptoms can arise in the context of the person having a general medical condition but through a psychological mechanism, that is, the prognosis, management, or painful symptoms of a general medical condition can act as a stressor to trigger a psychiatric disorder, such as adjustment disorder or even major depressive disorder. That type of etiological relationship is not being covered in this tree. Other trees should be consulted on the basis of the psychiatric symptoms that occur in response to having the medical condition (e.g., if depressed mood is a result, consult the depression tree, Figure 1-4).

Two clues, albeit fallible ones, can help point the way toward suspecting that a psychiatric symptom is due to the direct physiological effects of a general medical condition on the central nervous system. The first clue involves the temporal relationship between the general medical condition and the course of the psychiatric symptoms. If the onset of the psychiatric symptoms generally follow the onset of the general medical condition, if the symptoms vary in severity with the severity of the medical condition, and if the symptoms resolve when the medical condition goes into remission, that would provide strong evidence that the two are causally related. However, even a close temporal relationship may not be helpful is distinguishing between a direct physiological cause versus a psychological cause, since both causal mechanisms might be expected to demonstrate a close temporal relationship. A second clue is when the psychiatric presentation is "atypical" in symptom pattern, age at onset, or course. For example, severe memory loss and marked weight loss accompanied by relatively mild depressed mood strongly suggests that an undiagnosed general medical condition may be responsible. Similarly, the first onset of a manic episode at age 75 should raise strong suspicions for a general medical etiology. Of course, atypicality by itself is not a sufficient indicator of a general medical etiology since atypicality is the rule, rather than the exception, when it comes to psychiatric presentations. In this cause, it should mainly serve as a "red flag," alerting you to the necessity of a careful medical evaluation.

Once a general medical etiology has been established, this decision tree is useful in determining which DSM-IV-TR disorder best fits the clinical picture. It should be noted, however, that not every psychiatric symptom arising from a general medical condition necessarily warrants a diagnosis of a mental disorder due to a general medical condition. Certainly, most individuals who are a bit anxious, sad, fatigued, or having sleepless nights because of a general medical condition do not have a mental disorder that would be covered in this decision tree. The disorders in this tree should be considered only when the psychiatric symptoms are sufficiently severe and/or prolonged to warrant independent clinical attention.

Decision Tree for Substance-induced Disorders

Substance-related disorders are frequently encountered in mental health, substance treatment, and primary care settings. Therefore, a substance-related disorder must be considered in every DSM-IV-TR differential diagnosis. In DSM-IV-TR, the term substance-related disorder refers to disorders associated with drugs of abuse, the side effects of medications, and toxin-induced states. There are two types of substance-related diagnoses in DSM-IV-TR: substance Use Disorders, which describes patterns of problematic substance use (i.e., substance Dependence and substance Abuse), and substance-induced disorders, which describe psychiatric symptoms that arise because of the direct physiological effects of the substance on the central nervous system (e.g., substance intoxication, substance-induced psychotic disorder). This decision tree (see Figure 1-2) is confined to the Substance-Induced Disorders that are listed in the right-hand column of the decision tree. However, since relatively high doses of substances are required in order to cause a substance-induced disorder and since individuals with problematic patterns of substance use are more likely to consume larger quantities of drugs (as compared to those without dependence or abuse), these conditions often occur in the context of a Substance Use Disorder. In such cases, both should be diagnosed. For example, an alcoholic who develops DT's in the hospital while awaiting elective surgery would get two diagnoses: alcohol dependence (a substance use disorder) and alcohol withdrawal delirium (a substance-induced disorder).

Since substance-induced disorders are characterized by psychopathology that can virtually mimic the appearance of the primary counterparts, they must *always* be considered in the differential diagnosis of every psychiatric condition. Determining whether

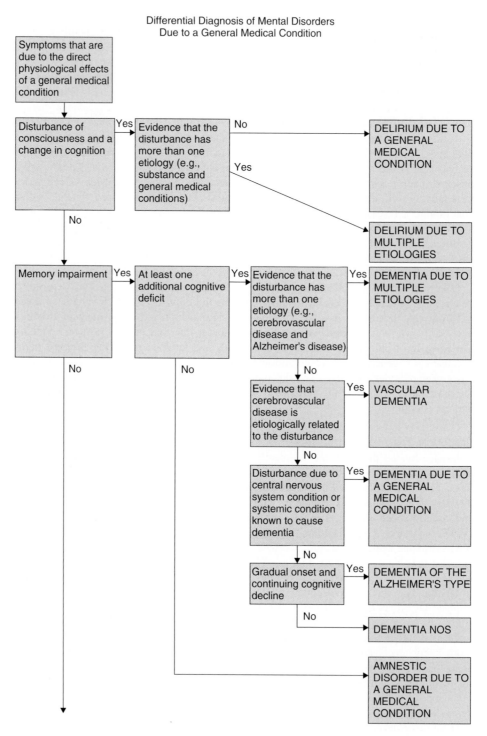

Figure 1-1 *Differential diagnosis of mental disorders due to a general medical condition. (Source: American Psychiatric Association (2000) Diagnostic and Statistical Manual of Mental Disorders, 4th ed., Text Rev. APA, Washington, DC, pp. 746–747.)*

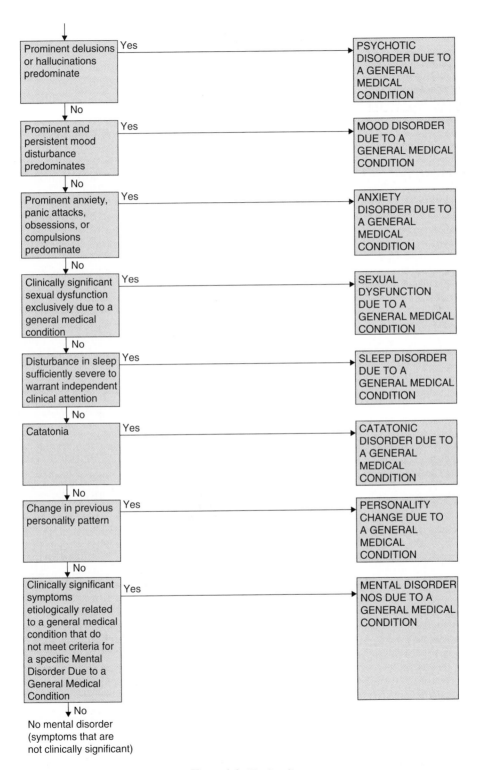

Figure 1-1 *(Continued)*

Differential Diagnosis of Substance-Induced Disorders
(Not Including Dependence and Abuse)

Figure 1-2 *Differential diagnosis of substance-induced disorders. (Source: American Psychiatric Association (2000) Diagnostic and Statistical Manual of Mental Disorders, 4th ed., Text Rev. APA, Washington, DC, pp. 748–749.)*

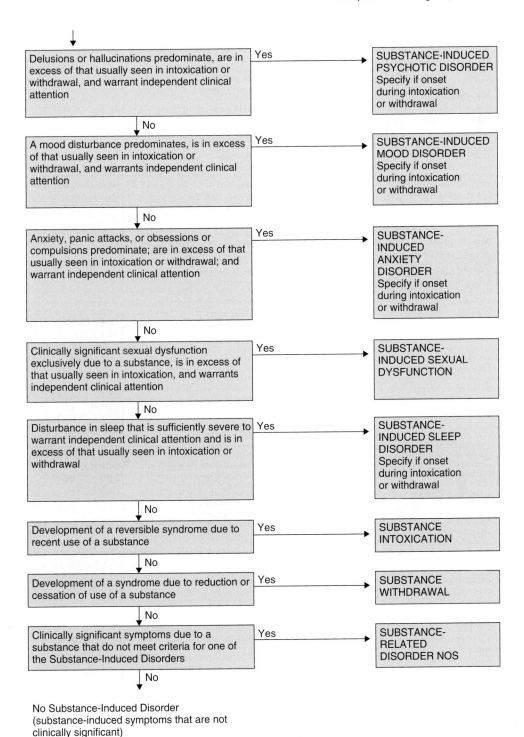

Figure 1-2 *(Continued)*

psychopathology is due to substance use can be difficult because, although substance use is widely ubiquitous and a wide variety of different substances can induce psychopathology, the mere co-occurrence between substance use and psychopathology does not necessarily imply a cause-and-effect relationship. There are three possible relationships between the substance and the comorbid psychiatric symptoms—discerning which of the three relation-ships applies determines the appropriate DSM-IV-TR diagnosis: (1) that the psychiatric symptoms are a direct result of the effects of the substance on the central nervous system (CNS) (in which case the diagnosis is a Substance-Induced Disorder); (2) that substance use is a consequence or associated feature of having a primary disorder, so that the individual can be seen as using the substance to "self-medicate" the psychiatric symptoms (in which case the diagnosis is a primary psychiatric disorder with accompanying substance use); or (3) that the substance use and psychiatric symptoms are independent. Most commonly the correct relationship can be discerned by examining the temporal relationship between the substance use and the psychiatric symptoms. If there is a period of time in which the person had psychiatric symptoms while abstinent from drugs, then that establishes the fact that the psychiatric symptoms constitute a primary psychiatric disorder. If, on the other hand, the individual experiences psychiatric symptoms ONLY when intoxicated or in withdrawal from drugs, then the diagnosis is most probably a substance-induced disorder.

As the structure of the tree illustrates, symptom-specific Substance-Induced presentations are diagnosed if the symptoms warrant independent clinical attention. Otherwise, a diagnosis of Substance Intoxication and Substance Withdrawal are made.

Decision Tree for Psychotic Disorders

Psychotic symptoms in DSM-IV-TR include delusions, hallucinations, disorganized speech, or grossly disorganized or catatonic behavior. The Psychotic Disorders decision tree (see Figure 1-3) should be consulted if any of these symptoms are part of the clinical presentation. The tree first determines whether the psychotic symptoms are "organic," that is, whether they are due to the direct physiological effects of a general medical condition or to the direct effects of a substance (including drugs of abuse, medications, and toxin exposure). If not, you have ruled out the secondary causes of psychosis and are left with a primary psychotic or mood disorder.

The next decision point (i.e., have there been symptoms of the active phase of schizophrenia present for at least one month) splits the tree into schizophrenia and related disorders (including schizophreniform and schizoaffective disorder) and other psychotic disorders (including delusional disorder and brief psychotic disorder). Within the schizophrenia branch, if a mood episode has been present, one is faced with the differential diagnosis between schizophrenia, schizoaffective disorder, and mood disorder with psychotic features. This decision is based on whether the psychotic symptoms occur concurrently with the mood episodes (if not, then schizophrenia is automatically diag-nosed) and whether the mood symptoms are a brief part of the total picture (if so, then it is schizophrenia again). Schizoaffective disorder and mood disorder with psychotic features are differentiated by whether the psychotic symptoms occur in the absence of prominent mood symptoms (if so, schizoaffective disorder is favored over mood disorder with psychotic features).

Decision Tree for Mood Disorders

Mood disturbance may be characterized by depressed, elevated, expansive, or irritable mood, and is one of the most common presenting symptoms in mental health settings (see Figure 1-4 for decision tree). As with the other decision trees in DSM-IV-TR, the first determination is whether the mood symptoms are either due to the direct physiological effects of a general medical condition or due to substance. Once these secondary causes of mood disturbance have been ruled out, the next consideration is to determine the type of current and past mood episodes (i.e., manic, hypomanic, major depressive, and mixed), since their pattern determines the specific DSM-IV-TR mood disorder diagnosis. After considering the presence of mood episodes, the decision tree goes on to determine whether the disorder is part of the bipolar spectrum versus a unipolar depressive disorder. If there has been *any* lifetime manic or mixed episodes, then the differential diagnosis includes bipolar I disorder, schizoaffective disorder, bipolar type, or bipolar disorder NOS. A pattern of hypomanic and major depressive episodes indicates a diagnosis of bipolar II disorder. Clinically significant symptoms of mania that do not meet criteria for bipolar I or bipolar II indicate a diagnosis of bipolar disorder NOS or cyclothymic disorder. On the unipolar side, a history of major depressive episodes indicates that the differential diagnosis includes major depressive disorder, schizoaffective disorder, or depressive disorder NOS (for major depressive episodes superimposed on a psychotic disorder). The remaining disorders in the unipolar differential include dysthymic disorder, adjustment Disorder with depressed mood, and depressive disorder NOS.

Decision Tree for Anxiety Disorder

Although the common presenting symptom in this tree is anxiety, whether these disorders are pathophysiologically related is a matter of debate. This tree includes panic disorder, the phobias, generalized anxiety disorder, obsessive–compulsive disorder, and reactions to severe trauma (see Figure 1-5). As with the decision trees for psychotic and mood disorders, the first step in the differential diagnosis is to consider whether the anxiety symptoms are either due to the direct physiological effects of a general medical condition or a substance. When the unexpected anxiety occurs in discrete episodes and is accompanied by certain somatic (e.g., palpitations, shortness of breath) and/or cognitive symptoms (e.g., fear of going crazy or having a heart attack), then the diagnosis is panic disorder. The remaining steps in this decision tree are determined by the focus of the anxiety (e.g., anxiety about separation from attachment figures suggests separation anxiety disorder), the form of the anxiety (e.g., whether it is associated with obsessions and/or compulsions) or the context (e.g., if it is associated with severe trauma). Clinically significant anxiety symptoms not meeting criteria for one of the specific disorders is diagnosed either as adjustment disorder if it represented a response to a stressor, or anxiety disorder not otherwise specified.

Decision Tree for Somatoform Disorders

The disorders covered in this tree are characterized by unexplained physical symptoms or by irrational fears about illness or physical appearance. (See Figure 1-6). There are three ways of understanding unexplained physical symptoms: (1) that the symptoms are accounted for by an underlying general medical condition that has not yet manifested itself with clearly discernable objective findings (e.g., multiple sclerosis); (2) that the physical symptoms are accounted for by a DSM-IV-TR disorder like conversion disorder; or (3) that the physical symptoms are intentionally being produced by the individual (e.g., factitious disorder). In determining whether an unexplained physical symptom is attributable to a Somatoform Disorder, the presence of a general medical condition must first be considered and ruled out. Contact with the individual's general medical physician is important as well as a thorough review of the individual's medical records and any available laboratory tests. Ultimately, the determination of whether a coexisting physical condition fully accounts for the individual's physical symptoms is inherently imperfect. Even if one determines that a general medical condition accounts for the individual's physical symptoms, psychological factors could still play an important role in the course of the illness and the individual's response to treatment.

Differential Diagnosis of Psychotic Disorders

```
┌─────────────────────────────────┐
│ Delusions, hallucinations,      │
│ disorganized speech, or grossly │
│ disorganized behavior           │
└─────────────────────────────────┘
                │
                ▼
┌─────────────────────────────────┐  Yes    ┌──────────────┐
│ Due to the direct physiological │────────▶│ PSYCHOTIC    │
│ effects of a general medical    │         │ DISORDER     │
│ condition                       │         │ DUE TO A     │
│                                 │         │ GENERAL      │
│                                 │         │ MEDICAL      │
│                                 │         │ CONDITION    │
└─────────────────────────────────┘         └──────────────┘
                │ No
                ▼
┌─────────────────────┐  Yes            ┌──────────────┐
│ Due to the direct   │────────────────▶│ SUBSTANCE-   │
│ physiological       │                 │ INDUCED      │
│ effects of a        │                 │ PSYCHOTIC    │
│ substance (e.g., a  │                 │ DISORDER     │
│ drug of abuse, a    │                 │              │
│ medication, or a    │                 │              │
│ toxin)              │                 │              │
└─────────────────────┘                 └──────────────┘
                │ No
                ▼
┌───────────────┐ Yes ┌──────────────┐ No
│ Symptoms of   │────▶│ Major        │──────┐
│ active phase  │     │ Depressive   │      │
│ of            │     │ or Manic     │      │
│ Schizophrenia,│     │ Episode      │      │
│ lasting at    │     │ concurrent   │      │
│ least 1 month │     │ with active- │      │
└───────────────┘     │ phase        │      │
        │ No          │ symptoms     │      │
        │             └──────────────┘      │
        │                   │ Yes           │
        │                   ▼               ▼
        │        ┌────────────┐ Yes ┌────────────┐ Yes ┌──────────┐
        │        │ Total      │────▶│ Duration   │────▶│ SCHIZO-  │
        │        │ duration   │     │ at least   │     │ PHRENIA  │
        │        │ of mood    │     │ 6 months   │     │          │
        │        │ episodes   │     │            │     │          │
        │        │ has been   │     │            │ No  │          │
        │        │ brief      │     │            │──┐  │          │
        │        │ relative   │     └────────────┘  │  └──────────┘
        │        │ to         │                     │
        │        │ duration   │                     ▼
        │        │ of active  │              ┌──────────────┐
        │        │ and        │              │ SCHIZO-      │
        │        │ residual   │              │ PHRENIFORM   │
        │        │ periods    │              │ DISORDER     │
        │        └────────────┘              └──────────────┘
        │               │ No
        │               ▼
        │        ┌──────────────┐ Yes         ┌──────────────┐
        │        │ At least 2   │────────────▶│ SCHIZO-      │
        │        │ weeks of     │             │ AFFECTIVE    │
        │        │ delusions or │             │ DISORDER     │
        │        │ hallucinations│ No         │              │
        │        │ in the       │──┐          └──────────────┘
        │        │ absence of   │  │
        │        │ prominent    │  │          ┌──────────────┐
        │        │ mood symptoms│  │          │ MOOD         │
        │        └──────────────┘  └─────────▶│ DISORDER     │
        │                                     │ WITH         │
        ▼                                     │ PSYCHOTIC    │
                                              │ FEATURES     │
                                              │ (see Mood    │
                                              │ Disorders    │
                                              │ tree)        │
                                              └──────────────┘
```

Figure 1-3 *Differential diagnosis of psychotic disorders. (Source: American Psychiatric Association (2000) Diagnostic and Statistical Manual of Mental Disorders, 4th ed., Text Rev. APA, Washington, DC, pp. 750–751.)*

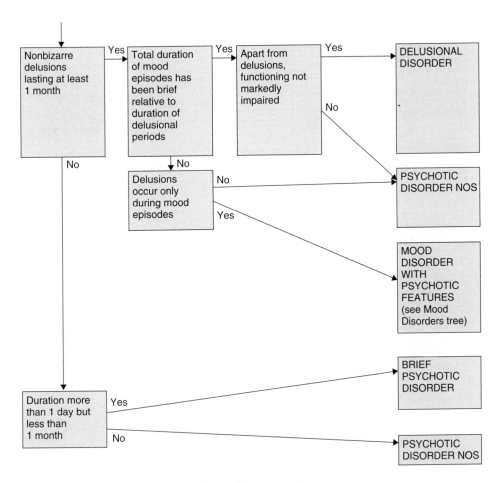

Figure 1-3 *(Continued)*

The differential diagnosis with factitious disorder and malingering rests on whether the individual is consciously feigning or producing the physical symptoms (i.e., the individual is aware that he or she is producing the symptoms). In contrast, unexplained physical complaints arising from conversion disorder or somatization disorder are experienced by the individual as happening to him or her, despite the fact that there is no physiological explanation available to account for them. The remaining disorders covered in this tree illustrate the hierarchical relationship among the various somatoform disorders in DSM-IV-TR. Somatization disorder is the most pervasive of the somatoform disorders and is characterized by multiple physical complaints occurring over years. Conversion disorder, pain disorder, and undifferentiated somatoform disorder cover more limited presentations and should not be diagnosed separately if criteria are met for somatization disorder. In body dysmorphic disorder and hypochondriasis, in contrast with the other somatoform disorders, the primary problem is distorted beliefs about the underlying explanation for unexplained physical symptoms or about one's physical appearance.

DSM-IV-TR Overview

The remainder of this chapter provides an overview of the DSM-IV-TR multiaxial system as well as a presentation of some of the organizational principles of the various diagnostic

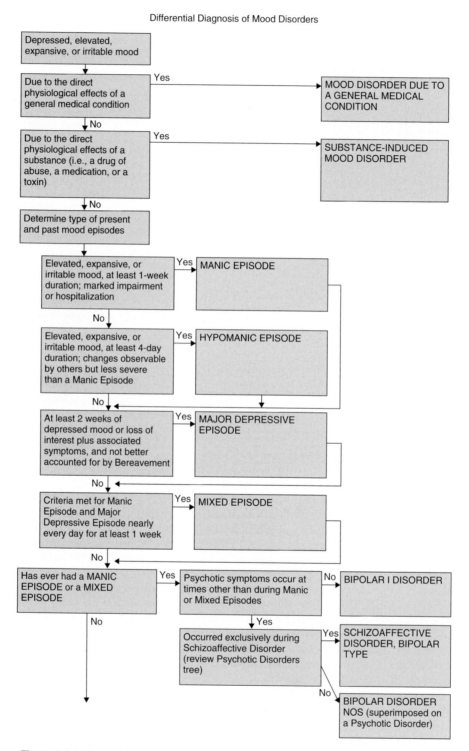

Differential Diagnosis of Mood Disorders

Figure 1-4 *Differential diagnosis of mood disorders. (Source: American Psychiatric Association (2000) Diagnostic and Statistical Manual of Mental Disorders, 4th ed., Text Rev. APA, Washington, DC, pp. 751–752.)*

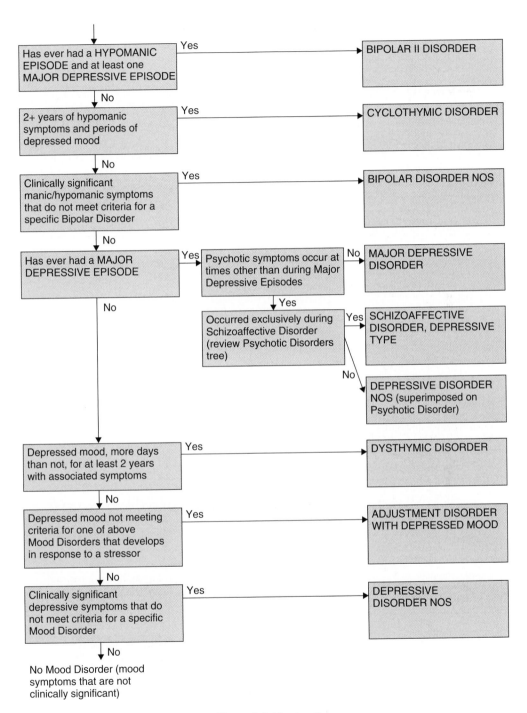

Figure 1-4 *(Continued)*

Differential Diagnosis of Anxiety Disorders

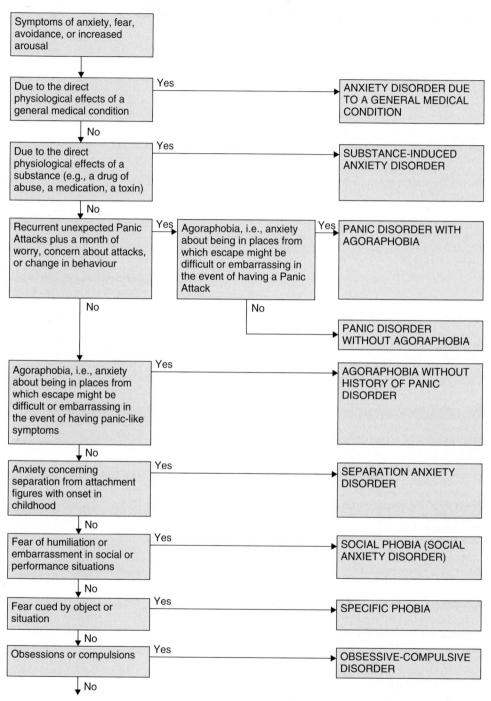

Figure 1-5 *Differential diagnosis of anxiety disorders. (Source: American Psychiatric Association (2000) Diagnostic and Statistical Manual of Mental Disorders, 4th ed., Text Rev. APA, Washington, DC, pp. 753–754.)*

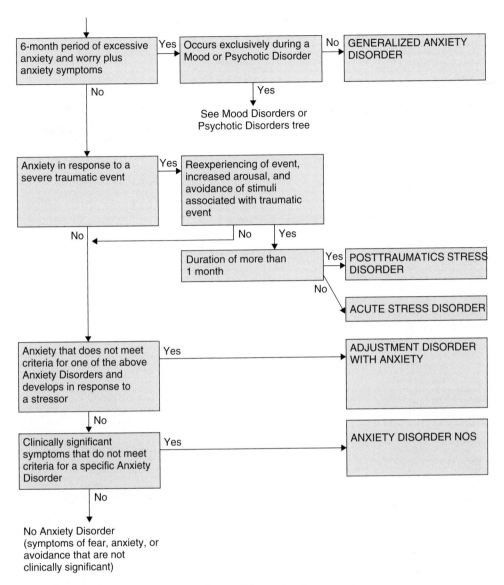

Figure 1-5 *(Continued)*

groupings included in the DSM-IV-TR classification. The chapters in this book are organized according to their presentation in the DSM-IV-TR classification and provide detailed information regarding the diagnosis, etiology and pathophysiology, epidemiology, course, and treatment of these DSM-IV-TR disorders.

DSM-IV-TR Multiaxial System

The multiaxial system was first introduced by DSM-III (Williams 1987) in order to encourage the clinician to focus his or her attention during the evaluation process on issues above and beyond the psychiatric diagnosis. Use of the multiaxial system requires that information be noted on each of the five different axes, each axis devoted to a different

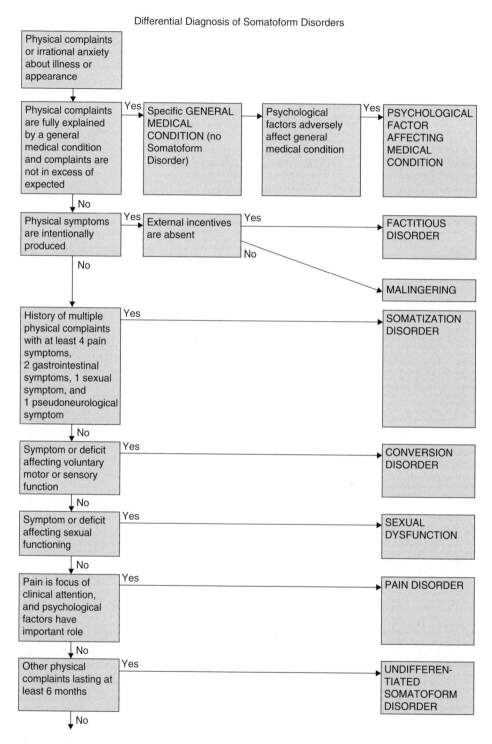

Figure 1-6 *Differential diagnosis of somatoform disorders. (Source: American Psychiatric Association (2000) Diagnostic and Statistical Manual of Mental Disorders, 4th ed., Text Rev. APA, Washington, DC, pp. 755–756.)*

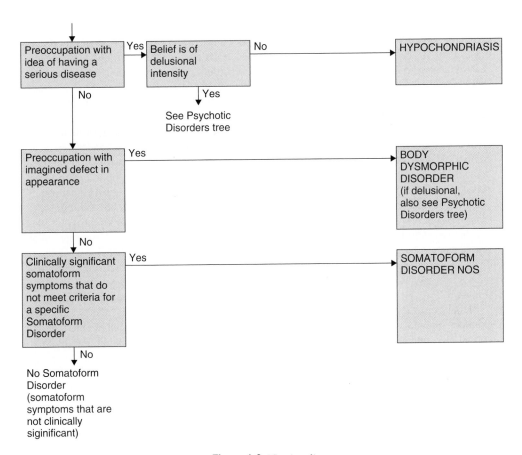

Figure 1-6 *(Continued)*

aspect of the evaluation process. Axes I, II, and III are the diagnostic axes that divide up the diagnostic pie into three separate domains. Axis I is for "clinical syndromes and disorders," an admittedly confusing name since Axis II and Axis III also include clinical disorders. The most accurate name for Axis I is "diagnoses not coded on Axis II and Axis III," since Axis II and Axis III were carved out of Axis I specifically to draw attention to certain disorders that clinicians were more likely to overlook.

That said, Axis II is designated for coding personality disorders and traits and mental retardation. There have been many recent criticisms of the coding of personality disorders on Axis II. Critics correctly point out that there is no firm conceptual basis for this division. Although disorders on Axis II tend to be lifelong and pervasive, a number of disorders on Axis I (e.g., schizophrenia, autistic disorder, dysthymic disorder) fit this description as well. Others have made the incorrect assumption that categories on Axis II are unresponsive to medication treatment, which is at odds with more recent evidence that medications are often helpful in the treatment of personality disorders. The fact is that the Axis I/Axis II division is strictly pragmatic. It was introduced in DSM-III as a way of drawing attention to a set of disorders that were thought not to be given adequate attention by mental health professionals. First introduced in DSM-III, Axis II was designed to draw attention to certain disorders that were thought to be overshadowed in the face of the more florid Axis I presentations. In DSM-III, Axis II was reserved for personality disorders in adults and specific developmental disorders in children. In DSM-III-R, all of the developmental disorders (i.e., mental retardation, pervasive developmental disorders, specific developmental disorders) were coded on Axis II along with the personality disorders. In DSM-IV-TR, Axis II was modified once again so that only personality disorders and traits and mental retardation remain on Axis II. Certainly the placement of personality disorders on a separate axis has increased both their clinical visibility and their importance as a subject for research studies. Whether the Axis I/Axis II division has finally outlived its usefulness remains a topic of heated debate and will be revisited during the DSM-V deliberations.

Axis III, like Axis II, is intended to encourage clinicians to pay special attention to conditions that they tend to overlook, in this case, clinically relevant general medical conditions. The concept of "clinically relevant" is intended to be broad. For example, it would be appropriate to list hypertension on Axis III even if its only relationship to an Axis I disorder is its impact on the options for the choice of antidepressant medication.

Psychosocial stressors are well known to play an important role in the etiology, maintenance, and management of a number of mental disorders. Axis IV provides the psychiatrist with the opportunity to list clinically relevant psychosocial and environmental problems (e.g., homelessness, poverty, divorce). To facilitate a comprehensive evaluation of such problems, DSM-IV-TR includes a psychosocial and environmental checklist that allows the psychiatrist to indicate which types of problems are present and relevant (Figure 1-7).

Mental disorders differentially impact on the individual's level of functioning. For example, one individual with schizophrenia may function quite well, being able to live in the community, marry and have a family, and maintain a steady job, whereas another individual with schizophrenia may function quite poorly, requiring chronic institutionalization. Since both of these individuals have symptoms that meet the diagnostic criteria for schizophrenia, their important differences in functioning are not captured by the clinical diagnosis alone. Some of the differences in functioning may be due to different symptom profiles or symptom severities. Other differences may be related to resilience factors or different

Check:

___ Problems with primary support group (childhood, adult, parent–child). Specify: _____

___ Problems related to the social environment. Specify: _____

___ Educational problems. Specify: _____

___ Occupational problems. Specify: _____

___ Housing problems. Specify: _____

___ Economic problems. Specify: _____

___ Problems with access to health care services. Specify: _____

___ Problems related to interaction with the legal system/crime. Specify: _____

___ Other psychosocial problems. Specify: _____

Figure 1-7 *DSM-IV-TR Axis IV: psychosocial and environmental checklist. (Source: Modified from American Psychiatric Association (2000) Diagnostic and Statistical Manual of Mental Disorders, 4th ed., Text Rev. APA, Washington, DC, p. 36.)*

Global Assessment of Functioning (GAF) Scale

Consider psychological, social and occupational functioning on a hypothetical continuum of mental health-illness. Do not include impairment in functioning due to physical (or environmental) limitations.

Code **(Note: Use intermediate codes when appropriate, e.g., 45,68,72.)**

100 | **Superior functioning in a wide range of activities, life's problems never seem to get out of hand, is sought out by others because of many positive qualities.**
91 | **No symptoms.**

90 | **Absent or minimal symptoms** (e.g., mild anxiety before an examination), **good functioning in all areas, interested and involved in a wide range of activities, socially effective, generally satisfied with life, no more than everyday problems or concerns** (e.g., an occasional argument with family
81 | members).

80 | **If symptoms are present, they are transient and expectable reactions to psychosocial stressors** (e.g., difficulty concentrating after family argument); **no more than slight impairment in social, occupational, or school functioning**
71 | (e.g., temporarily falling behind in school work).

70 | **Some mild symptoms** (e.g., depressed mood and mild insomnia) **OR some difficulty in social, occupational, or school functioning** (e.g., occasional truancy, or theft within the household), **but generally functioning pretty**
61 | **well, has some meaningful interpersonal relationships.**

60 | **Moderate symptoms** (e.g., flat affect and circumstantial speech, occasional panic attacks) **OR moderate difficulty in social, occupational, or school**
51 | **functioning** (e.g., few friends, conflicts with peers or coworkers).

50 | **Serious symptoms** (e.g., suicidal ideation, severe obsessional rituals, frequent shoplifting) **OR any serious impairment in social, occupational, or school**
41 | **functioning** (e.g., no friends, unable to keep a job).

40 | **Some impairment in reality testing or communication** (e.g., speech is at times illogical, obscure, or irrelevant) **OR major impairment in several areas, such as work or school, family relations, judgment, thinking, or mood** (e.g., depressed man avoids friends, neglects family, and is unable to work; child frequently beats up
31 | younger children, is defiant at home, and is failing at school).

30 | **Behavior is considerably influenced by delusions or hallucinations OR serious impairment in communication or judgment** (e.g., sometimes incoherent, acts grossly inappropriately, suicidal preoccupation) **OR inability to function in almost**
21 | **all areas** (e.g., stays in bed all day; no job, home or friends).

20 | **Some danger of hurting self or others** (e.g., suicide attempts without clear expectation of death, frequently violent, manic excitement) **OR occasionally fails to maintain minimal personal hygiene** (e.g., smears feces) **OR gross impairment in**
11 | **communication** (e.g., largely incoherent or mute).

10 | **Persistent danger of severely hurting self or others** (e.g., recurrent violence) **OR persistent inability to maintain minimal personal hygiene OR serious suicidal**
1 | **act with clear expectation of death.**

0 | Inadequate information

Figure 1-8 *DSM-IV-TR Axis V: Global Assessment of Functioning Scale. (Source: American Psychiatric Association (2000) Diagnostic and Statistical Manual of Mental Disorders, 4th ed., Text Rev. APA, Washington, DC, p. 34.)*

levels of psychosocial support. Whatever the reason, the DSM-IV-TR multiaxial system provides the clinician with the ability to indicate the individual's overall level of functioning in addition to the diagnosis on Axis V, using the Global Assessment of Functioning (GAF) Scale (Figure 1-8). This GAF Scale has been criticized because it is not actually

Table 1-3	Example of DSM-IV-TR Multiaxial Evaluation*
Axis I	296.23 Major depressive disorder, single episode, severe but without psychotic features, with postpartum onset.
	307.51 Bulimia nervosa
Axis II	301.6 Dependent personality disorder
	Frequent use of denial
Axis III	Rheumatoid arthritis
Axis IV	Partner relational problem
Axis V	GAF = 35 (current)

* GAF, Global Assessment of Functioning Scale score.

a "pure" measure of an individual's ability to function since it incorporates symptom severity into the scale, for example, level 41 to 50 is for serious symptoms (e.g., suicidal ideation, severe obsessional rituals, frequent shoplifting) or any serious impairment in social, occupational, or school functioning (e.g., no friends, unable to keep a job). For this reason, the DSM-IV-TR includes a scale (the Social and Occupational Functioning Scale [SOFAS]) that relies exclusively on functioning in its appendix of Criteria Sets and Axes Provided for Further Study (American Psychiatric Association 2000, pp. 817–818). An example of a DSM-IV-TR multiaxial evaluation for a hypothetical individual with depression is shown in Table 1-3.

DSM-IV-TR Classification and Diagnostic Codes

The "DSM-IV-TR Classification of Mental Disorders" refers to the comprehensive listing of the official diagnostic codes, categories, subtypes, and specifiers (see below). It is divided into various "diagnostic classes" that group disorders together on the basis of common presenting symptoms (e.g., mood disorders, anxiety disorders), typical age at onset (e.g., disorders usually first diagnosed in infancy, childhood, and adolescence), and etiology (e.g., substance-related disorders, mental disorders due to a general medical condition).

The diagnostic codes listed in the DSM-IV-TR are derived from the *International Classification of Diseases*, Ninth Revision, Clinical Modification (ICD-9-CM), the official coding system for reporting morbidity and mortality in the United States. That is the reason the codes go from 290.00 to 319.00; they are actually derived from the mental disorders section of a much larger coding system for all medical disorders that extend from 001 to 999. Clinicians working in the United States are required to use ICD-9-CM in order to get reimbursement from both government agencies (e.g., Medicare and Medicaid) and private insurers. To insure that users of the DSM-IV-TR are able to meet this requirement without doing any cumbersome code conversions, the DSM-IV-TR contains the current ICD-9-CM codes. Because the ICD-9-CM codes are updated on a yearly basis (i.e., every October 1), the DSM-IV-TR codes have to be similarly updated as changes to the codes in the ICD-9-CM mental disorder section occur. Although these changes have been relatively infrequent, they have necessitated some changes to the DSM-IV-TR codes. In 2007 or 2008, it is expected that the US government will adopt ICD-10-CM as the official system for coding medical diagnosis and thus, the DSM-IV-TR codes will have to be revised once again to reflect these rather substantial changes. We anticipate that a DSM-IV-CR (code revision) will be published to coincide with national adoption of ICD-10-CM.

DSM-IV-TR CLASSIFICATION

NOS = Not Otherwise Specified.

An x appearing in a diagnostic code indicates that a specific code number is required.

An ellipsis (...) is used in the names of certain disorders to indicate that the name of a specific mental disorder or general medical condition should be inserted when recording the name (e.g., 293.0 Delirium Due to Hypothyroidism).

If criteria are currently met, one of the following severity specifiers may be noted after the diagnosis:

Mild
Moderate
Severe

If criteria are no longer met, one of the following specifiers may be noted:

In Partial Remission
In Full Remission
Prior History

Disorders Usually First Diagnosed in Infancy, Childhood, or Adolescence

Mental Retardation
Note: *These are coded on Axis II.*

317   Mild Mental Retardation
318.0   Moderate Mental Retardation
318.1   Severe Mental Retardation
318.2   Profound Mental Retardation
319   Mental Retardation, Severity Unspecified

Learning Disorders
315.00   Reading Disorder
315.1   Mathematics Disorder
315.2   Disorder of Written Expression
315.9   Learning Disorder NOS

Motor Skills Disorder
315.4   Developmental Coordination Disorder

Communication Disorders
315.31   Expressive Language Disorder
315.32   Mixed Receptive–Expressive Language Disorder
315.39   Phonological Disorder
307.0   Stuttering
307.9   Communication Disorder NOS

Pervasive Developmental Disorders
299.00   Autistic Disorder
299.80   Rett's Disorder

299.10	Childhood Disintegrative Disorder
299.80	Asperger's Disorder
299.80	Pervasive Developmental Disorder NOS

Attention-Deficit and Disruptive Behavior Disorders

314.xx	Attention-Deficit/Hyperactivity Disorder
.01	Combined Type
.00	Predominantly Inattentive Type
.01	Predominantly Hyperactive-Impulsive Type
314.9	Attention-Deficit/Hyperactivity Disorder NOS
312.xx	Conduct Disorder
.81	Childhood-Onset Type
.82	Adolescent-Onset Type
.89	Unspecified Onset
313.81	Oppositional-Defiant Disorder
312.9	Disruptive Behavior Disorder NOS

Feeding and Eating Disorders of Infancy or Early Childhood

307.52	Pica
307.53	Rumination Disorder
307.59	Feeding Disorder of Infancy or Early Childhood

Tic Disorders

307.23	Tourette's Disorder
307.22	Chronic Motor or Vocal Tic Disorder
307.21	Transient Tic Disorder
	Specify if: Single Episode/Recurrent
307.20	Tic Disorder NOS

Elimination Disorders

—.—	Encopresis
787.6	With Constipation and Overflow Incontinence
307.7	Without Constipation and Overflow Incontinence
307.6	Enuresis (Not Due to a General Medical Condition)
	Specify type: Nocturnal Only/Diurnal Only/Nocturnal and Diurnal

Other Disorders of Infancy, Childhood, or Adolescence

309.21	Separation Anxiety Disorder
	Specify if: Early Onset
313.23	Selective Mutism
313.89	Reactive Attachment Disorder of Infancy or Early Childhood
	Specify type: Inhibited Type/Disinhibited Type
307.3	Stereotypic Movement Disorder
	Specify if: With Self-Injurious Behavior
313.9	Disorder of Infancy, Childhood, or Adolescence NOS

Delirium, Dementia, and Amnestic and Other Cognitive Disorders

Delirium

293.0   Delirium Due to ... [*Indicate the General Medical Condition*]

—.—   Substance Intoxication Delirium (*refer to Substance-Related Disorders for substance-specific codes*)

—.—   Substance Withdrawal Delirium (*refer to Substance-Related Disorders for substance-specific codes*)

—.—   Delirium Due to Multiple Etiologies (*code each of the specific etiologies*)

780.09   Delirium NOS

Dementia

294.xx   Dementia of the Alzheimer's Type, With Early Onset (*also code 331.0 Alzheimer's disease on Axis III*)

   .10   Without Behavioral Disturbance
   .11   With Behavioral Disturbance

294.xx   Dementia of the Alzheimer's Type, With Late Onset (*also code 331.0 Alzheimer's disease on Axis III*)

   .10   Without Behavioral Disturbance
   .11   With Behavioral Disturbance

290.xx   Vascular Dementia

   .40   Uncomplicated
   .41   With Delirium
   .42   With Delusions
   .43   With Depressed Mood
          Specify if: With Behavioral Disturbance

Code presence or absence of a behavioral disturbance in the fifth digit for Dementia Due to a General Medical Condition:

294.10 = Without Behavioral Disturbance
294.11 = With Behavioral Disturbance

294.1x   Dementia Due to HIV Disease (*also code 042 HIV on Axis III*)

294.1x   Dementia Due to Head Trauma (*also code 854.00 head injury on Axis III*)

294.1x   Dementia Due to Parkinson's Disease (*also code 331.82 Dementia with Lewy Bodies on Axis III*)

294.1x   Dementia Due to Huntington's Disease (*also code 333.4 Huntington's disease on Axis III*)

294.1x   Dementia Due to Pick's Disease (*also code 331.11 Pick's disease on Axis III*)

294.1x   Dementia Due to Creutzfeldt–Jakob Disease (*also code 046.1 Creutzfeldt–Jakob disease on Axis III*)

294.1x   Dementia Due to ... [*Indicate the General Medical Condition not listed above*] (*also code the general medical condition on Axis III*)

—.—   Substance-Induced Persisting Dementia (*refer to Substance-Related Disorders for substance-specific codes*)

—.—   Dementia Due to Multiple Etiologies (*code each of the specific etiologies*)

294.8   Dementia NOS

Amnestic Disorders
294.0   Amnestic Disorder Due to . . . [*Indicate the General Medical Condition*]
         Specify if: Transient/Chronic
—.—   Substance-Induced Persisting Amnestic Disorder (*refer to Substance-Related Disorders for substance-specific codes*)
294.8   Amnestic Disorder NOS

Other Cognitive Disorders
294.9   Cognitive Disorder NOS

Mental Disorders Due to a General Medical Condition Not Elsewhere Classified
293.89   Catatonic Disorder Due to . . . [*Indicate the General Medical Condition*]
310.1   Personality Change Due to . . . [*Indicate the General Medical Condition*]
         Specify type: Labile Type/Disinhibited Type/Aggressive Type/Apathetic Type/Paranoid Type/Other Type/Combined Type/Unspecified Type
293.9   Mental Disorder NOS Due to. . . [*Indicate the General Medical Condition*]

Substance-Related Disorders
The following specifiers apply to Substance Dependence as noted:
         [a]With Physiological Dependence/Without Physiological Dependence
         [b]Early Full Remission/Early Partial Remission Sustained Full Remission/Sustained Partial Remission
         [c]In a Controlled Environment
         [d]On Agonist Therapy/

The following specifiers apply to Substance-Induced Disorders as noted:
         [I]With Onset During Intoxication/[W]With Onset During Withdrawal

Alcohol-Related Disorders

Alcohol Use Disorders
303.90   Alcohol Dependence[a,b,c]
305.00   Alcohol Abuse

Alcohol-Induced Disorders
303.00   Alcohol Intoxication
291.81   Alcohol Withdrawal
         Specify if: With Perceptual Disturbances
291.0   Alcohol Intoxication Delirium
291.0   Alcohol Withdrawal Delirium
291.2   Alcohol-Induced Persisting Dementia
291.1   Alcohol-Induced Persisting Amnestic Disorder
291.x   Alcohol-Induced Psychotic Disorder
  .5   With Delusions[I,W]
  .3   With Hallucinations[I,W]
291.89   Alcohol-Induced Mood Disorder[I,W]
291.89   Alcohol-Induced Anxiety Disorder[I,W]
291.89   Alcohol-Induced Sexual Dysfunction[I]

291.89	Alcohol-Induced Sleep Disorder[I,W]
291.9	Alcohol-Related Disorder NOS

Amphetamine (or Amphetamine-like)-Related Disorders

Amphetamine Use Disorders
304.40	Amphetamine Dependence[a,b,c]
305.70	Amphetamine Abuse

Amphetamine-Induced Disorders
292.89	Amphetamine Intoxication
	Specify if: With Perceptual Disturbances
292.0	Amphetamine Withdrawal
292.81	Amphetamine Intoxication Delirium
292.xx	Amphetamine-Induced Psychotic Disorder
.11	With Delusions[I]
.12	With Hallucinations[I]
292.84	Amphetamine-Induced Mood Disorder[I,W]
292.89	Amphetamine-Induced Anxiety Disorder[I]
292.89	Amphetamine-Induced Sexual Dysfunction[I]
292.89	Amphetamine-Induced Sleep Disorder[I,W]
292.9	Amphetamine-Related Disorder NOS

Caffeine-Related Disorders

Caffeine-Induced Disorders
305.90	Caffeine Intoxication
292.89	Caffeine-Induced Anxiety Disorder[I]
292.89	Caffeine-Induced Sleep Disorder[I]
292.9	Caffeine-Related Disorder NOS

Cannabis-Related Disorders

Cannabis Use Disorders
304.30	Cannabis Dependence[a,b,c]
305.20	Cannabis Abuse

Cannabis-Induced Disorders
292.89	Cannabis Intoxication
	Specify if: With Perceptual Disturbances
292.81	Cannabis Intoxication Delirium
292.xx	Cannabis-Induced Psychotic Disorder
.11	With Delusions[I]
.12	With Hallucinations[I]
292.89	Cannabis-Induced Anxiety Disorder[I]
292.9	Cannabis-Related Disorder NOS

Cocaine-Related Disorders

Cocaine Use Disorders
304.20   Cocaine Dependence[a,b,c]
305.60   Cocaine Abuse

Cocaine-Induced Disorders
292.89   Cocaine Intoxication
          Specify if: With Perceptual Disturbances
292.0   Cocaine Withdrawal
292.81   Cocaine Intoxication Delirium
292.xx   Cocaine-Induced Psychotic Disorder
  .11   With Delusions[I]
  .12   With Hallucinations[I]
292.84   Cocaine-Induced Mood Disorder[I,W]
292.89   Cocaine-Induced Anxiety Disorder[I,W]
292.89   Cocaine-Induced Sexual Dysfunction[I]
292.89   Cocaine-Induced Sleep Disorder[I,W]
292.9   Cocaine-Related Disorder NOS

Hallucinogen-Related Disorders

Hallucinogen Use Disorders
304.50   Hallucinogen Dependence[b,c]
305.30   Hallucinogen Abuse

Hallucinogen-Induced Disorders
292.89   Hallucinogen Intoxication
292.89   Hallucinogen Persisting Perception Disorder (Flashbacks)
292.81   Hallucinogen Intoxication Delirium
292.xx   Hallucinogen-Induced Psychotic Disorder
  .11   With Delusions[I]
  .12   With Hallucinations[I]
292.84   Hallucinogen-Induced Mood Disorder[I]
292.89   Hallucinogen-Induced Anxiety Disorder[I]
292.9   Hallucinogen-Related Disorder NOS

Inhalant-Related Disorders

Inhalant Use Disorders
304.60   Inhalant Dependence[b,c]
305.90   Inhalant Abuse

Inhalant-Induced Disorders
292.89   Inhalant Intoxication
292.81   Inhalant Intoxication Delirium
292.82   Inhalant-Induced Persisting Dementia
292.xx   Inhalant-Induced Psychotic Disorder
  .11   With Delusions[I]

.12   With Hallucinations[I]
292.84 Inhalant-Induced Mood Disorder[I]
292.89 Inhalant-Induced Anxiety Disorder[I]
292.9   Inhalant-Related Disorder NOS

Nicotine-Related Disorders

Nicotine Use Disorder
305.1   Nicotine Dependence[a,b]

Nicotine-Induced Disorder
292.0   Nicotine Withdrawal
292.9   Nicotine-Related Disorder NOS

Opioid-Related Disorders

Opioid Use Disorders
304.00 Opioid Dependence[a,b,c,d]
305.50 Opioid Abuse

Opioid-Induced Disorders
292.89 Opioid Intoxication
        Specify if: With Perceptual Disturbances
292.0   Opioid Withdrawal
292.81 Opioid Intoxication Delirium
292.xx Opioid-Induced Psychotic Disorder
   .11 With Delusions[I]
   .12 With Hallucinations[I]
292.84 Opioid-Induced Mood Disorder[I]
292.89 Opioid-Induced Sexual Dysfunction[I]
292.89 Opioid-Induced Sleep Disorder[I,W]
292.9   Opioid-Related Disorder NOS

Phencyclidine (or Phencyclidine-like)-Related Disorders

Phencyclidine Use Disorders
304.60 Phencyclidine Dependence[b,c]
305.90 Phencyclidine Abuse

Phencyclidine-Induced Disorders
292.89 Phencyclidine Intoxication
        Specify if: With Perceptual Disturbances
292.81 Phencyclidine Intoxication Delirium
292.xx Phencyclidine-Induced Psychotic Disorder
   .11 With Delusions[I]
   .12 With Hallucinations[I]
292.84 Phencyclidine-Induced Mood Disorder[I]
292.89 Phencyclidine-Induced Anxiety Disorder[I]
292.9   Phencyclidine-Related Disorder NOS

Sedative-, Hypnotic-, Oranxiolytic-Related Disorders

Sedative, Hypnotic, or Anxiolytic Use Disorders
304.10   Sedative, Hypnotic, or Anxiolytic Dependence[a,b,c]
305.40   Sedative, Hypnotic, or Anxiolytic Abuse

Sedative-, Hypnotic-, or Anxiolytic-Induced Disorders
292.89   Sedative, Hypnotic, or Anxiolytic Intoxication
292.0   Sedative, Hypnotic, or Anxiolytic Withdrawal
          Specify if: With Perceptual Disturbances
292.81   Sedative, Hypnotic, or Anxiolytic Intoxication Delirium
292.81   Sedative, Hypnotic, or Anxiolytic Withdrawal Delirium
292.82   Sedative-, Hypnotic-, or Anxiolytic-Induced Persisting Dementia
292.83   Sedative-, Hypnotic-, or Anxiolytic-Induced Persisting Amnestic Disorder
292.xx   Sedative-, Hypnotic-, or Anxiolytic-Induced Psychotic Disorder
    .11   With Delusions[I,W]
    .12   With Hallucinations[I,W]
292.84   Sedative-, Hypnotic-, or Anxiolytic-Induced Mood Disorder[I,W]
292.89   Sedative-, Hypnotic-, or Anxiolytic-Induced Anxiety Disorder[W]
292.89   Sedative-, Hypnotic-, or Anxiolytic-Induced Sexual Dysfunction[I]
292.89   Sedative-, Hypnotic-, or Anxiolytic-Induced Sleep Disorder[I,W]
292.9   Sedative-, Hypnotic-, or Anxiolytic-Related Disorder NOS

Polysubstance-Related Disorder
304.80   Polysubstance Dependence[a,b,c,d]

Other (or Unknown) Substance-Related Disorders

Other (or Unknown) Substance Use Disorders
304.90   Other (or Unknown) Substance Dependence[a,b,c,d]
305.90   Other (or Unknown) Substance Abuse

Other (or Unknown) Substance-Induced Disorders
292.89   Other (or Unknown) Substance Intoxication
          Specify if: With Perceptual Disturbances
292.0   Other (or Unknown) Substance Withdrawal
          Specify if: With Perceptual Disturbances
292.81   Other (or Unknown) Substance-Induced Delirium
292.82   Other (or Unknown) Substance-Induced Persisting Dementia
292.83   Other (or Unknown) Substance-Induced Persisting Amnestic Disorder
292.xx   Other (or Unknown) Substance-Induced Psychotic Disorder
    .11   With Delusions[I,W]
    .12   With Hallucinations[I,W]
292.84   Other (or Unknown) Substance-Induced Mood Disorder[I,W]
292.89   Other (or Unknown) Substance-Induced Anxiety Disorder[I,W]
292.89   Other (or Unknown) Substance-Induced Sexual Dysfunction[I]
292.89   Other (or Unknown) Substance-Induced Sleep Disorder[I,W]
292.9   Other (or Unknown) Substance-Related Disorder NOS

Schizophrenia and Other Psychotic Disorders
295.xx   Schizophrenia

The following Classification of Longitudinal Course applies to all subtypes of
    Schizophrenia.
Episodic With Interepisode Residual Symptoms (*specify if*: With Prominent Negative
    Symptoms)/Episodic With No Interepisode Residual Symptoms/Continuous (*specify if*:
    With Prominent Negative Symptoms)
Single Episode In Partial Remission (*specify if*: With Prominent Negative
    Symptoms)/Single Episode In Full Remission
Other or Unspecified Pattern

.30	Paranoid Type
.10	Disorganized Type
.20	Catatonic Type
.90	Undifferentiated Type
.60	Residual Type

295.40   Schizophreniform Disorder
          Specify if: Without Good Prognostic Features/With Good Prognostic Features
295.70   Schizoaffective Disorder
          Specify type: Bipolar Type/Depressive Type
297.1   Delusional Disorder
          Specify type: Erotomanic Type/Grandiose Type/Jealous Type/Persecutory
              Type/Somatic Type/Mixed Type/Unspecified Type
298.8   Brief Psychotic Disorder
          Specify if: With Marked Stressor(s)/Without Marked Stressor(s)/With
              Postpartum Onset
297.3   Shared Psychotic Disorder
293.xx   Psychotic Disorder Due to... [*Indicate the General Medical Condition*]
    .81   With Delusions
    .82   With Hallucinations
—.—   Substance-Induced Psychotic Disorder (*refer to Substance-Related Disorders*
              for substance-specific codes)
          Specify if: With Onset During Intoxication/With Onset During Withdrawal
298.9   Psychotic Disorder NOS

Mood Disorders
Code current state of Major Depressive Disorder or Bipolar I Disorder in fifth digit:

1 = Mild
2 = Moderate
3 = Severe Without Psychotic Features
4 = Severe With Psychotic Features
      Specify: Mood-Congruent Psychotic Features/Mood-Incongruent Psychotic Features
5 = In Partial Remission
6 = In Full Remission
0 = Unspecified

The following specifiers apply (for current or most recent episode) to Mood Disorders as noted:

[a]Severity/Psychotic/Remission Specifiers/[b]Chronic/[c]With Catatonic Features/[d]With Melancholic Features/[e]With Atypical Features/[f]With Postpartum Onset

The following specifiers apply to Mood Disorders as noted:

[g]With or Without Full Interepisode Recovery/[h]With Seasonal Pattern/[i]With Rapid Cycling

Depressive Disorders

296.xx   Major Depressive Disorder,
.2x   Single Episode[a,b,c,d,e,f]
.3x   Recurrent[a,b,c,d,e,f,g,h]
300.4   Dysthymic Disorder
          Specify if: Early Onset/Late Onset
          Specify: With Atypical Features
311   Depressive Disorder NOS

Bipolar Disorders

296.xx   Bipolar I Disorder,
.0x   Single Manic Episode[a,c,f]
          Specify if: Mixed
.40   Most Recent Episode Hypomanic[g,h,i]
.4x   Most Recent Episode Manic[a,c,f,g,h,i]
.6x   Most Recent Episode Mixed[a,c,f,g,h,i]
.5x   Most Recent Episode Depressed[a,b,c,d,e,f,g,h,i]
.7   Most Recent Episode Unspecified[g,h,i]
296.89   Bipolar II Disorder[a,b,c,d,e,f,g,h,i]
          Specify (current or most recent episode): Hypomanic/Depressed
301.13   Cyclothymic Disorder
296.80   Bipolar Disorder NOS
293.83   Mood Disorder Due to... [*Indicate the General Medical Condition*]
          Specify type: With Depressive Features/With Major Depressive-like Episode/With Manic Features/With Mixed Features
—.—   Substance-Induced Mood Disorder (*refer to Substance-Related Disorders for substance-specific codes*)
          Specify type: With Depressive Features/With Manic Features/With Mixed Features
          Specify if: With Onset During Intoxication/With Onset During Withdrawal
296.90   Mood Disorder NOS

Anxiety Disorders

300.01   Panic Disorder Without Agoraphobia
300.21   Panic Disorder With Agoraphobia
300.22   Agoraphobia Without History of Panic Disorder
300.29   Specific Phobia
          Specify type: Animal Type/Natural Environment Type/Blood-Injection-Injury Type/Situational Type/Other Type

300.23	Social Phobia
	Specify if: Generalized
300.3	Obsessive–Compulsive Disorder
	Specify if: With Poor Insight
309.81	Posttraumatic Stress Disorder
	Specify if: Acute/Chronic
	Specify if: With Delayed Onset
308.3	Acute Stress Disorder
300.02	Generalized Anxiety Disorder
293.89	Anxiety Disorder Due to... [*Indicate the General Medical Condition*]
	Specify if: With Generalized Anxiety/ With Panic Attacks/With Obsessive–Compulsive Symptoms
—.—	Substance-Induced Anxiety Disorder (*refer to Substance-Related Disorders for substance-specific codes*)
	Specify if: With Generalized Anxiety/ With Panic Attacks/With Obsessive–Compulsive Symptoms/With Phobic Symptoms
	Specify if: With Onset During Intoxication/With Onset During Withdrawal
300.00	Anxiety Disorder NOS

Somatoform Disorders

300.81	Somatization Disorder
300.82	Undifferentiated Somatoform Disorder
300.11	Conversion Disorder
	Specify type: With Motor Symptom or Deficit/With Sensory Symptom or Deficit/With Seizures or Convulsions/With Mixed Presentation
307.xx	Pain Disorder
.80	Associated With Psychological Factors
.89	Associated With Both Psychological Factors and a General Medical Condition
	Specify if: Acute/Chronic
300.7	Hypochondriasis
	Specify if: With Poor Insight
300.7	Body Dysmorphic Disorder
300.82	Somatoform Disorder NOS

Factitious Disorders

300.xx	Factitious Disorder
.16	With Predominantly Psychological signs and Symptoms
.19	With Predominantly Physical Signs and Symptoms
.19	With Combined Psychological and Physical Signs and Symptoms
300.19	Factitious Disorder NOS

Dissociative Disorders

300.12	Dissociative Amnesia
300.13	Dissociative Fugue
300.14	Dissociative Identity Disorder
300.6	Depersonalization Disorder
300.15	Dissociative Disorder NOS

Sexual and Gender Identity Disorders

Sexual Dysfunctions
The following specifiers apply to all primary Sexual Dysfunctions:

Lifelong Type/Acquired Type Generalized Type/Situational Type Due to Psychological Factors/Due to Combined Factors

Sexual Desire Disorders
302.71   Hypoactive Sexual Desire Disorder
302.79   Sexual Aversion Disorder

Sexual Arousal Disorders
302.72   Female Sexual Arousal Disorder
302.72   Male Erectile Disorder

Orgasmic Disorders
302.73   Female Orgasmic Disorder
302.74   Male Orgasmic Disorder
302.75   Premature Ejaculation

Sexual Pain Disorders
302.76   Dyspareunia (Not Due to a General Medical Condition)
306.51   Vaginismus (Not Due to a General Medical Condition)

Sexual Dysfunction Due to a General Medical Condition
625.8   Female Hypoactive Sexual Desire Disorder Due to... [*Indicate the General Medical Condition*]
608.89   Male Hypoactive Sexual Desire Disorder Due to... [*Indicate the General Medical Condition*]
607.84   Male Erectile Disorder Due to... [*Indicate the General Medical Condition*]
625.0   Female Dyspareunia Due to... [*Indicate the General Medical Condition*]
608.89   Male Dyspareunia Due to... [*Indicate the General Medical Condition*]
625.8   Other Female Sexual Dysfunction Due to... [*Indicate the General Medical Condition*]
608.89   Other Male Sexual Dysfunction Due to... [*Indicate the General Medical Condition*]
—.—   Substance-Induced Sexual Dysfunction (*refer to Substance-Related Disorders for substance-specific codes*)
          Specify if: With Impaired Desire/With Impaired Arousal/With Impaired Orgasm/With Sexual Pain
          Specify if: With Onset During Intoxication
302.70   Sexual Dysfunction NOS

Paraphilias
302.4   Exhibitionism
302.81   Fetishism

302.89   Frotteurism
302.2   Pedophilia
            Specify if: Sexually Attracted to Males/Sexually Attracted to Females/Sexually
            Attracted to Both
            Specify if: Limited to Incest
            Specify type: Exclusive Type/Nonexclusive Type
302.83   Sexual Masochism
302.84   Sexual Sadism
302.3   Transvestic Fetishism
            Specify if: With Gender Dysphoria
302.82   Voyeurism
302.9   Paraphilia NOS

Gender Identity Disorders
302.xx   Gender Identity Disorder
  .6   in Children
  .85   in Adolescents or Adults
            Specify if: Sexually Attracted to Males/Sexually Attracted to Females/Sexually
            Attracted to Both/Sexually Attracted to Neither
302.6   Gender Identity Disorder NOS
302.9   Sexual Disorder NOS

Eating Disorders
307.1   Anorexia Nervosa
            Specify type: Restricting Type; Binge-Eating/Purging Type
307.51   Bulimia Nervosa
            Specify type: Purging Type/Nonpurging Type
307.50   Eating Disorder NOS

Sleep Disorders

Primary Sleep Disorders

Dyssomnias
307.42   Primary Insomnia
307.44   Primary Hypersomnia
            Specify if: Recurrent
347   Narcolepsy
780.59   Breathing-Related Sleep Disorder
307.45   Circadian Rhythm Sleep Disorder
            Specify type: Delayed Sleep Phase Type/Jet Lag Type/Shift Work
            Type/Unspecified Type
307.47   Dyssomnia NOS

Parasomnias
307.47   Nightmare Disorder
307.46   Sleep Terror Disorder
307.46   Sleepwalking Disorder
307.47   Parasomnia NOS

Sleep Disorders Related to Another Mental Disorder

307.42   Insomnia Related to. . . [*Indicate the Axis I or Axis II Disorder*]
307.44   Hypersomnia Related to. . . [*Indicate the Axis I or Axis II Disorder*]

Other Sleep Disorders

780.xx   Sleep Disorder Due to. . . [*Indicate the General Medical Condition*]
  .52   Insomnia Type
  .54   Hypersomnia Type
  .59   Parasomnia Type
  .59   Mixed Type
—.—   Substance-Induced Sleep Disorder (*refer to Substance-Related Disorders for substance-specific codes*)
       Specify type: Insomnia Type/Hypersomnia Type/Parasomnia Type/ Mixed Type
       Specify if: With Onset During Intoxication/With Onset During Withdrawal

Impulse Control Disorders Not Elsewhere Classified

312.34   Intermittent Explosive Disorder
312.32   Kleptomania
312.33   Pyromania
312.31   Pathological Gambling
312.39   Trichotillomania
312.30   Impulse-Control Disorder NOS

Adjustment Disorders

309.xx   Adjustment Disorder
  .0   With Depressed Mood
  .24   With Anxiety
  .28   With Mixed Anxiety and Depressed Mood
  .3   With Disturbance of Conduct
  .4   With Mixed Disturbance of Emotions and Conduct
  .9   Unspecified
       Specify if: Acute/Chronic

Personality Disorders

Note: *These are coded on Axis II*

301.0   Paranoid Personality Disorder
301.20   Schizoid Personality Disorder
301.22   Schizotypal Personality Disorder
301.7   Antisocial Personality Disorder
301.83   Borderline Personality Disorder
301.50   Histrionic Personality Disorder
301.81   Narcissistic Personality Disorder
301.82   Avoidant Personality Disorder
301.6   Dependent Personality Disorder
301.4   Obsessive–Compulsive Personality Disorder
301.9   Personality Disorder NOS

Other Conditions That May Be a Focus of Clinical Attention

Psychological Factors Affecting Medical Condition

316   ... [*Specified Psychological Factor*]
             Affecting... [*Indicate the General Medical Condition*]

Choose name based on nature of factors:

Mental Disorder Affecting Medical Condition
Psychological Symptoms Affecting Medical Condition
Personality Traits or Coping Style Affecting Medical Condition
Maladaptive Health Behaviors Affecting Medical Condition
Stress-Related Physiological Response Affecting Medical Condition
Other or Unspecified Psychological Factors Affecting Medical Condition

Medication-Induced Movement Disorders

332.1   Neuroleptic-Induced Parkinsonism
333.92   Neuroleptic Malignant Syndrome
333.7   Neuroleptic-Induced Acute Dystonia
333.99   Neuroleptic-Induced Acute Akathisia
333.82   Neuroleptic-Induced Tardive Dyskinesia
333.1   Medication-Induced Postural Tremor
333.90   Medication-Induced Movement Disorder NOS

Other Medication-Induced Disorder

995.2   Adverse Effects of Medication NOS

Relational Problems

V61.9   Relational Problem Related to a Mental Disorder or General Medical Condition
V61.20   Parent–Child Relational Problem
V61.10   Partner Relational Problem
V61.8   Sibling Relational Problem
V62.81   Relational Problem NOS

Problems Related to Abuse or Neglect

V61.21   Physical Abuse of Child (*code 995.54 if focus of attention is on victim*)
V61.21   Sexual Abuse of Child (*code 995.53 if focus of attention is on victim*)
V61.21   Neglect of Child (*code 995.52 if focus of attention is on victim*)
—.—   Physical Abuse of Adult
V61.12   (if by partner)
V62.83   (if by person other than partner) (*code 995.83 if focus of attention is on victim*)
—.—   Sexual Abuse of Adult
V61.12   (if by partner)
V62.83   (if by person other than partner) (*code 995.83 if focus of attention is on victim*)

Additional Conditions That may be a Focus of Clinical Attention

V15.81   Noncompliance With Treatment
V65.2   Malingering
V71.01   Adult Antisocial Behavior
V71.02   Child or Adolescent Antisocial Behavior
V62.89   Borderline Intellectual Functioning

Note: *This is coded on Axis II*

780.93	Age-Related Cognitive Decline
V62.82	Bereavement
V62.3	Academic Problem
V62.2	Occupational Problem
313.82	Identity Problem
V62.89	Religious or Spiritual Problem
V62.4	Acculturation Problem
V62.89	Phase of Life Problem

Additional Codes

300.9	Unspecified Mental Disorder (nonpsychotic)
V71.09	No Diagnosis or Condition on Axis I
799.9	Diagnosis or Condition Deferred on Axis I
V71.09	No Diagnosis on Axis II
799.9	Diagnosis Deferred on Axis II

Multiaxial System

Axis I	Clinical Disorders
	Other Conditions That May Be a Focus of Clinical Attention
Axis II	Personality Disorders
	Mental Retardation
Axis III	General Medical Conditions
Axis IV	Psychosocial and Environmental Problems
Axis V	Global Assessment of Functioning

Disorders Usually First Diagnosed in Infancy, Childhood, or Adolescence

The classification begins with disorders usually first diagnosed in infancy, childhood, or adolescence. The provision for a separate section for so-called childhood disorders is only for convenience. Although most individuals with these disorders present for clinical attention during childhood or adolescence, it is not uncommon for some of these conditions to be diagnosed for the first time in adulthood (e.g., attention-deficit/hyperactivity disorder). Moreover, many disorders included in other sections of the DSM-IV-TR have an onset during childhood (e.g., major depressive disorder). Thus, a clinician evaluating a child or adolescent should not only focus on those disorders listed in this section but also consider disorders from throughout the DSM-IV-TR. Similarly, when evaluating an adult, the clinician should also consider the disorders in this section since many of them persist into adulthood (e.g., stuttering, learning disorders, tic disorders).

The first set of disorders included in this diagnostic class (mental retardation, learning and motor skills disorders, and communication disorders) is covered in detail in Chapters 4, 5, and 6, respectively. While these are not, strictly speaking, regarded as mental disorders, they are included in the DSM-IV-TR to facilitate differential diagnosis and to increase recognition of these conditions among mental health professionals. Autism and other pervasive developmental disorders are discussed in Chapter 7 and are characterized by gross qualitative impairment in social relatedness, in language, and in repertoire of interests and activities. Disorders covered include autistic disorder, Asperger's disorder, Rett's disorder, and childhood disintegrative disorder. Attention-deficit/hyperactivity disorder and other disruptive behavior disorders (Chapter 8) are grouped together because they are all characterized (at least in their childhood presentations) by disruptive behavior. The chapter on feeding disorders (Chapter 9) includes both the DSM-IV-TR categories of pica, rumination disorder, and feeding disorder of infancy and early childhood (also known as *failure to thrive*). Tic disorders (Chapter 10) and elimination and other disorders of infancy and early childhood (Chapter 12) conclude the childhood section.

Delirium, Dementia, Amnestic Disorder, and Other Cognitive Disorders

In DSM-III-R, delirium, dementia, amnestic disorder, and other cognitive disorders were included in a section called *organic mental disorders*, which contained disorders that were due to either a general medical condition or substance use. In DSM-IV-TR, the term organic was eliminated because of the implication that disorders not included in that section (e.g., schizophrenia, bipolar disorder) did not have an organic component (Spitzer et al. 1992). In fact, virtually all mental disorders have both psychological and biological components, and to designate some disorders as organic and the remaining disorders as nonorganic reflected a reductionistic mind–body dualism that is at odds with our understanding of the multifactorial nature of the etiological underpinnings of disorders.

DSM-IV-TR replaced each unitary organic mental disorder (e.g., organic mood disorder) with its two component parts: mood disorder due to a general medical condition and substance-induced mood disorder. Because of their central roles in the differential diagnosis of cognitive impairment, delirium, dementia, and amnestic disorder are contained within the same diagnostic class in DSM-IV-TR and are discussed in Chapter 13.

Whereas both delirium and dementia are characterized by multiple cognitive impairments, delirium is distinguished by the presence of clouding of consciousness, which is manifested by an inability to appropriately maintain or shift attention. DSM-IV-TR includes three types of delirium: delirium due to a general medical condition, substance-induced delirium, and delirium due to multiple etiologies.

Dementia is characterized by clinically significant cognitive impairment in memory that is accompanied by impairment in one or more other areas of cognitive functioning (e.g., language, executive functioning). DSM-IV-TR includes several types of dementia based on etiology, including dementia of the Alzheimer's type, vascular dementia, a variety of dementia due to general medical and neurological conditions (e.g., human immunodeficiency virus infection, Parkinson's disease), substance-induced persisting dementia, and dementia due to multiple etiologies.

In contrast to dementia, amnestic disorder is characterized by clinically significant memory impairment occurring in the absence of other significant impairments in cognitive functioning. DSM-IV-TR includes amnestic disorder due to a general medical condition and substance-induced persisting amnestic disease.

Mental Disorders Due to a General Medical Condition Not Elsewhere Classified

This diagnostic class includes all of the specific mental disorders due to a general medical condition and is discussed in Chapter 14. In DSM-IV-TR, most of the mental disorders due to a general medical condition have been distributed throughout the various diagnostic classes alongside their "nonorganic" counterparts in the classification. For example, mood disorder due to a general medical condition and substance-induced mood disorder are included in the mood disorders section of DSM-IV-TR. Two specific types of mental disorders due to a general medical condition (i.e., catatonic disorder due to a general medical condition and personality change due to a general medical condition) are physically included in this diagnostic class.

Substance-Related Disorders

Substance-related disorders in DSM-IV-TR are more than just disorders related to taking drugs of abuse. They also include medication side effects and the consequences of toxin exposure. Two types of substance-related disorders are included in DSM-IV-TR: substance use disorders (dependence and abuse), which describe the maladaptive nature of the pattern of substance use; and substance-induced disorders, which cover psychopathological processes caused by the direct effects of substances on the central nervous system. Criteria sets for substance dependence, substance abuse, substance intoxication, and substance withdrawal that apply across all drug classes are included before the substance-specific sections of DSM-IV-TR. A discussion of these so-called generic criteria that apply to all substance-related disorders is covered in Chapter 15. Detailed discussions of each of the DSM-IV-TR drug classes are covered in Chapters 16 to 26.

Schizophrenia and Other Psychotic Disorders

The title of this diagnostic class is potentially misleading for two reasons: (1) there are other disorders that have psychotic features that are not included in this diagnostic class (e.g., mood disorders with psychotic features, delirium) and (2) it may incorrectly imply that the other psychotic disorders included in this section are related in some way to schizophrenia (which is only true for schizophreniform disorder and possibly schizoaffective disorder). Instead, what ties together all of the disorders in this diagnostic class is the presence of prominent psychotic symptoms. Included here are schizophrenia, schizophreniform disorder, schizoaffective disorder, delusional disorder, shared psychotic disorder, and brief psychotic disorder, each of which is discussed in varying detail in Chapter 27.

It should be noted that the definition of the term *psychosis* has been used in different ways historically and is not even used consistently across the various categories in the DSM-IV-TR. The most restrictive definition of psychosis (used in substance-induced psychotic disorder) requires a break in reality testing such that the person has delusions or hallucinations with no insight into the fact that the delusions or hallucinations are caused by taking drugs. A somewhat less restrictive definition of psychosis (not used in DSM-IV-TR but advocated by some members of the DSM-IV Psychotic Disorders Workgroup as more appropriate for substance-induced psychosis) includes hallucinations or delusions even if the person has insight into their origin (e.g., it would include an individual who was hallucinating after taking phencyclidine [PCP] even if he were aware that the hallucinations were due to the PCP). A much broader definition of psychosis (utilized in the definition of schizophrenia, schizophreniform, and brief psychotic disorder) goes beyond delusions and hallucinations to include grossly disorganized speech and catatonic or grossly disorganized behavior as evidence for psychosis. Finally, the term psychosis was in the past used most broadly to refer to any condition that caused serious functional impairment (e.g., "affective psychosis" is used in ICD-9 to refer to major mood disorders). This definition is not used in DSM-IV-TR.

Mood Disorders

This diagnostic class includes disorders in which the predominant disturbance is in the individual's mood. Although the term *mood* is broadly defined to include depression, euphoria, anger, and anxiety, the DSM-IV-TR generally restricts mood disturbances to depressed, elevated, or irritable mood.

The mood disorders section begins with the criteria for mood episodes (major depressive episode, manic episode, hypomanic episode, mixed episode), which are the building blocks for the episodic mood disorders. The codable mood disorders come next and are divided into the depressive disorders (i.e., major depressive disorder and dysthymic disorder, described in Chapter 28) and the bipolar disorders (i.e., bipolar I disorder, bipolar II disorder, and cyclothymic disorder, described in Chapter 30). Finally, the many specifiers that provide important treatment-relevant information close this section. Several so-called *subthreshold mood disorders* (i.e., they are characterized by depression but fall short of meeting the diagnostic criteria for either major depressive disorder or dysthymic disorder) are included in DSM-IV-TR appendix B, for Criteria Sets and Axes Provided for Further Study. These include minor depressive disorder, brief recurrent depressive disorder, mixed anxiety depressive disorder, postpsychotic depressive disorder of schizophrenia (all briefly described in Chapter 30), and premenstrual dysphoric disorder (described in detail in Chapter 29).

Anxiety Disorders

The common element joining these disparate categories together is the fact that the anxiety is a prominent part of their clinical presentation. This grouping has been criticized because of evidence suggesting that at least some of the disorders are likely to be etiologically distinct from the others. Most particularly, obsessive–compulsive disorder and posttraumatic stress disorder seem to share little in common with the other anxiety disorders. In fact, separate diagnostic classes for stress-related disorders (that would also include adjustment disorders and perhaps dissociative disorders) and for obsessive–compulsive spectrum disorders (which might also include trichotillomania, tic disorders, hypochondriasis, body dysmorphic disorder, and other disorders characterized by compulsive behavior) have been proposed.

Detailed discussions of the various anxiety disorders are covered in Chapters 31 to 35 in this section of the textbook.

Somatoform Disorders

This diagnostic class includes disorders in which the defining feature is a physical complaint or bodily concern that is not better accounted for by a general medical condition or another mental disorder. These disorders (which are discussed in detail in Chapter 36) can be divided into three groups on the basis of the focus of the individual's concerns: (1) focus on the physical symptoms themselves (somatization disorder, undifferentiated somatoform disorder, pain disorder, and conversion disorder); (2) focus on the belief that one has a serious physical illness (hypochondriasis); and (3) focus on the belief that one has a defect in physical appearance (body dysmorphic disorder).

Factitious Disorders

This diagnostic class contains only one disorder: factitious disorder, which describes presentations in which the individual intentionally produces or feigns physical or psychological symptoms in order to fulfill a psychological need to assume the sick role. It is discussed in detail in Chapter 37. Factitious disorder should always be distinguished from malingering, in which the individual similarly pretends to have physical or psychological symptoms. The difference is that in malingering, the person's motivation is to achieve some external gain (e.g., disability benefits, lessening of criminal responsibility, shelter for the night). For this reason, unlike factitious disorder, malingering is not considered a mental disorder.

Dissociative Disorders

The common element in this group of disorders is the symptom of dissociation that is defined as a disruption in the usually integrated functions of consciousness, memory, identity, and perception. Four specific disorders are included (dissociative amnesia, dissociative fugue, dissociative identity disorder, and depersonalization disorder) and are discussed in detail in Chapter 38.

Sexual and Gender Identity Disorders

This diagnostic class contains three relatively disparate types of disorders, linked together only by virtue of their involvement in human sexuality. Sexual dysfunctions refer to disturbances in sexual desire or functioning, paraphilias refer to unusual sexual preferences that interfere with functioning (or in the case of preferences that involve harm to others like pedophilia, merely acting on those preferences), and gender identity disorder refers to a serious conflict between one's internal identity of maleness and femaleness (gender identity) and one's anatomical sexual characteristics. These categories are discussed in detail in Chapter 39.

Eating Disorders

Although the name of this diagnostic class focuses on the fact that the disorders in this section are characterized by abnormal eating behavior (refusal to maintain adequate body weight in the case of anorexia nervosa and discrete episodes of uncontrolled eating of excessively large amounts of food in the case of bulimia nervosa), of near equal importance is the individual's pathological overemphasis on body image. A third category, which is being actively researched but has not been officially added to the DSM-IV-TR, is binge-eating disorder (included in the appendix of Criteria Sets and Axes Provided for Further Study). Like bulimia nervosa, individuals with binge-eating disorder have frequent episodes of binge-eating. However, unlike bulimia nervosa, these individuals do not do anything significant to counteract the effects of their binge-eating (i.e., they do not purge, use laxatives or diet pills, or excessively exercise). All three disorders are described in Chapter 40.

Sleep Disorders

Sleep disorders are grouped into four sections on the basis of presumed etiology (primary, related to another mental disorder, due to a general medical condition, and substance induced). Two types of primary sleep disorders are included in DSM-IV-TR: dyssomnias (problems in regulation of amount and quality of sleep) and parasomnias (events that occur during sleep). The dyssomnias include primary insomnia, primary hypersomnia, circadian rhythm sleep disorder, narcolepsy, and breathing-related sleep disorder, whereas the parasomnias include nightmare disorder, sleep terror disorder, and sleepwalking disorder. Sleep disorders are described in detail in Chapter 41.

Impulse Control Disorders Not Elsewhere Classified

As is suggested by the title of this diagnostic grouping, no one diagnostic class in DSM-IV-TR comprehensively includes all of the impulse control disorders. A number of disorders characterized by impulse control problems are classified elsewhere (e.g., conduct disorder, attention-deficit/hyperactivity disorder, oppositional-defiant disorder, delirium, dementia, substance-related disorders, schizophrenia and other psychotic disorders, mood disorders, antisocial and borderline personality disorders). What ties together the disorders in this class is that they present with clinically significant impulsive behavior and that they are not better accounted for by one of the mental disorders included in other parts of DSM-IV-TR. Five such disorders are included here: intermittent explosive disorder, pathological gambling, pyromania, kleptomania, and trichotillomania. These are discussed in Chapter 42.

Adjustment Disorders

All DSM-IV-TR categories (except NOS categories) take priority over adjustment disorder. This category is intended to apply for maladaptive reactions to psychosocial stressors that do not meet the criteria for any specific DSM-IV-TR disorder. These are discussed in Chapter 43.

Personality Disorders

This diagnostic class is for personality patterns that significantly deviate from the expectations of the person's culture, are pervasive, and lead to significant impairment or distress. Ten specific personality disorders are included in DSM-IV-TR: paranoid personality disorder (pervasive distrust and suspiciousness of others), schizoid personality disorder (detachment from social relationships and a restricted expression of emotions), schizotypal personality disorder (acute discomfort with close relationships, perceptual distortions, and eccentricities of behavior), antisocial personality disorder (disregard for the rights of others), borderline personality disorder (instability of personal relationships, instability of self-image, and marked impulsivity), histrionic personality disorder (extensive emotionality and attention seeking), narcissistic personality disorder (grandiosity, need for admiration, and lack of empathy), avoidant personality disorder (social inhibition, feelings of inadequacy, and hypersensitivity to negative evaluation), dependent personality disorder (excessive need to be taken care of), and obsessive–compulsive personality disorder (preoccupation with orderliness, perfectionism, and mental and personal control at the expense of flexibility, openness, and efficiency). These are discussed in detail in Chapter 44.

Other Conditions That May Be a Focus of Clinical Attention

This section of DSM-IV-TR is for problems that are not mental disorders but that may be a focus of attention for treatment by a mental health professional. *Psychological factors affecting medical condition* are intended to allow the psychiatrist to note the presence of psychological factors (e.g., Axis I or II disorder) that adversely affect the course of a general medical condition, including factors that interfere with treatment and factors that constitute health risks to the individual. This condition is described in Chapter 45. Six specific *medication-induced movement disorders*, discussed in Chapter 46, are also included because of their importance in treatment and differential diagnosis; five are related to neuroleptic administration and one (medication-induced postural tremor) is most often associated with the use of lithium carbonate. Although these are best considered medical conditions, by DSM-IV-TR convention they are coded on Axis I.

Table 1-4	Criteria Sets and Axes Provided for Further Study
Postconcussional disorder	
Mild cognitive disorder	
Caffeine withdrawal	
Postpsychotic depression of schizophrenia	
Simple deteriorative disorder	
Minor depressive disorder	
Recurrent brief depressive disorder	
Premenstrual dysphoric disorder	
Mixed anxiety–depressive disorder	
Factitious disorder by proxy	
Dissociative trance disorder binge-eating disorder	
Depressive personality disorder	
Passive–aggressive personality disorder (negativistic personality disorder)	
Defensive Functioning Scale	
Global Assessment of Relational Functioning Scale	
Social and Occupational Functioning Assessment Scale	

Source: Data from American Psychiatric Association (1994) *Diagnostic and Statistical Manual of Mental Disorders*, 4th ed. APA, Washington, DC.

Appendix Categories

DSM-IV-TR aims to be on the trailing edge rather than the cutting edge of research (Pincus et al. 1992). A new category was considered for inclusion only if there was a substantial research literature behind it. Although there were proposals for more than 100 new categories to be introduced into DSM-IV, only a handful of new categories were added. Text and criteria for another 17 proposed categories have been included in a DSM-IV-TR appendix, Criteria Sets and Axes Provided for Further Study (Table 1-4). These criteria sets have been included to provide a common language for researchers and psychiatrists who are interested in further investigating their potential utility and validity.

References

American Psychiatric Association (1952) *Diagnostic and Statistical Manual of Mental Disorders.* APA, Washington, DC.

American Psychiatric Association (1968) *Diagnostic and Statistical Manual of Mental Disorders,* 2nd ed. APA, Washington, DC.

American Psychiatric Association (1980) *Diagnostic and Statistical Manual of Mental Disorders,* 3rd ed. APA, Washington, DC.

American Psychiatric Association (1987) *Diagnostic and Statistical Manual of Mental Disorders,* 3rd ed., Rev. APA, Washington, DC.

American Psychiatric Association (1994) *Diagnostic and Statistical Manual of Mental Disorders,* 4th ed. APA, Washington, DC.

American Psychiatric Association (2000) *Diagnostic and Statistical Manual of Mental Disorders,* 4th ed., Text Rev. APA, Washington, DC.

Berrettini WH (2000) Are schizophrenic and bipolar disorders related? A review of family and molecular studies. *Biol Psychiatr* **48**(6), 531–538.

Boyd JH, Burke JD, Gruenberg E, et al. (1987) The exclusion criteria of DSM-III, a study of the co-occurrence of hierarchy-free syndromes. In *Diagnosis and Classification in Psychiatry. A Critical Appraisal of DSM-III,* Tischler GL (ed). Cambridge University Press, New York, pp. 403–424.

Charney DS, Barlow DH, Botteron K, et al. (2002) Neuroscience research agenda to guide development of a pathophysiologically based classification system. In *A Research Agenda for DSM-V,* Kupfer DJ, First MB, and Regier DA (eds). American Psychiatric Publishing, Washington, DC, pp. 31–83.

First MB (1992) Trends in psychiatric classification: DSM-III-R to DSM-IV. *Psychiatr Hung* **7**, 539–546.

First MB (1994) Principles of disease classification and diagnostic criteria. In *Headache Classification and Epidemiology,* Olesen J (ed). Raven Press, New York, pp. 17–26.

First MB and Pincus HA (2002) The DSM-IV Text Rev. Rationale and potential impact on clinical practice. *Psychiatr Serv* **53**(3), 288–292.

First MB, Bell CC, Cuthbert B, et al. (2002) Personality disorders and relational disorders: A research agenda for addressing crucial gaps in DSM. In *A Research Agenda for DSM-V,* Kupfer DJ, First MB, and Regier DA (eds). American Psychiatric Publishing, Washington, DC, pp. 123–200.

First MB, Frances A, and Widiger TA (1992) DSM-IV and behavioral assessment. *Behav Assess* **14**, 297–306.

Frances A, Davis W, Kline M, et al. (1991) The DSM-IV field trials: Moving towards an empirically-derived classification. *Eur Psychiatr* **6**, 307–314.

Frances A, Pincus HA, Widiger TA, et al. (1990) DSM-IV: work in progress. *Am J Psychiatry* **147**, 1439–1448.

Kendler KS (1996) Major depression and generalised anxiety disorder: same genes, (partly) different environments—revisited. *Br J Psychiatry* **168**(Suppl. 30),, 68–75.

Kendler KS and Gardner CO (1998) Boundaries of major depression: an evaluation of DSM-IV criteria. *Am J Psychiatry* **155**, 172–177.

Kraepelin E (1883) *Compendium der Psychiatrie: Zum Gebrauche Adur Studirende und Aerzte.* Verlag von Ambr, Abel, Leipzig.

Kupfer DJ, First MB, and Regier DA (2002) *A Research Agenda for DSM-V.* American Psychiatric Publishing, Washington, DC.

Mack AH, Forman L, Brown R, et al. (1994) A brief history of psychiatric classification. From the ancients to DSM-IV. *Psychiatr Clin N Am* **17**, 515–523.

Pincus HA, Frances A, Wakefield-Davis W, et al. (1992) DSM-IV and the new diagnostic categories: Holding the line on proliferation. *Am J Psychiatry* **149**, 112–117.

Regier DA, Narrow WE, First MB, et al. (2002) The APA classification of mental disorders: future perspectives. *Psychopathology* **35**(2–3), 166–170.

Spitzer RL and Williams JBW (1987) Revising DSM-III, the process and major issues. In *Diagnosis and Classification in Psychiatry. A Critical Appraisal of DSM-III,* Tischler GL (ed). Cambridge University Press, New York.

Spitzer RL, First MB, Williams JBW, et al. (1992) Now is the time to retire the term "organic mental disorders". *Am J Psychiatry* **149**, 240–244.

Widiger T, Frances A, Pincus H, et al. (1990) DSM-IV literature reviews: Rationale, process, limitations. *J Psychopathol Behav Assess* **12**, 189–202.

Widiger T, Frances A, Pincus H, et al. (1991) Toward a more empirical diagnostic system. *Can Psychol* **32**, 174–176.

Widiger TA, Frances A, Pincus H, et al. (eds) (1994) *DSM-IV Sourcebook*, Vol. 1. American Psychiatric Association, Washington, DC.

Widiger TA, Frances A, Pincus H, et al. (eds) (1996) *DSM-IV Sourcebook*, Vol. 2. American Psychiatric Association, Washington, DC.

Widiger TA, Frances A, Pincus H, et al. (eds) (1997) *DSM-IV Sourcebook*, Vol. 3. American Psychiatric Association, Washington, DC.

Widiger TA, Frances A, Pincus H, et al. (eds) (1998) *DSM-IV Sourcebook*, Vol. 4. American Psychiatric Association, Washington, DC.

Williams JBW (1987) Multiaxial diagnosis. In *An Annotated Bibliography of DSM-III*, Skodol AE and Spitzer RL (eds). American Psychiatric Press, Washington, DC, pp. 31–36.

Wittenborn JR, Holzberg JD, and Simon B (1953) Symptom correlates for descriptive diagnosis. *Genet Psychol Monogr* **47**, 237–301.

Zimmerman M, Jampala VC, Sierles FS, et al. (1991) DSM-IV: A nosology sold before its time? *Am J Psychiatry* **148**(4), 463–467.

2 ● Etiology

The search for the etiology and pathophysiology of mental disorders has its origins in Western medicine in the physicians of ancient Greece. Hippocrates and his school coined the term *melancholia* to indicate the role of black bile in severe depression. They also described *hysteria*, the first link identified between personality disorder and human sexuality. Our modern terms *dysthymia*, *cyclothymia*, and *euthymia* commemorate Hippocrates' hypothesis that the thymus regulates mood. Parallel developments in other cultures have also linked bodily function with mental behavior. The chakras of Buddhism, for example, linked autonomic ganglia and behavior.

Rene Descartes postulated a distinction between the physical body and the spiritual mind. However, Cartesian dualism did not impede a steady progression of physicians from seeking biological mechanisms of behavioral abnormalities. Freud (1886), for example, attempted to describe pathology in terms of neuronal energy in his psychoeconomic model, which proposed that symptoms arise from the overflow of such energies. In his "Project for a Scientific Psychology," he envisioned a full resolution of brain and behavioral analyses of psychopathology. The search for mechanisms has not always been scientifically rigorous or uniformly helpful to individuals suffering from a mental disorder. For example, the psychosurgery movement, which advocated frontal lobotomies, was based on a mechanistic view of the role of frontal lobes in obsessional symptoms and postulated the interruption of frontal circuits as the appropriate therapeutic modality (Valenstein 1990).

As in all fields of medicine, serendipitous observation has contributed much to the understanding of psychopathology at both the basic and clinical levels. The observation that chlorpromazine changed the intensity of psychotic symptoms led to the discovery of the role of dopamine in psychosis in an attempt to explain the mechanism of the drug's action. Psychiatrists investigating explanations for the drug's action have contributed to the understanding of the role of receptors in the brain, initially for dopamine and eventually for entire families of neurotransmitters (Snyder 1981).

Thus, the search for mechanisms of psychopathology is part of a long-held desire by humans to understand how their own behavior is generated. The search is clearly in its infancy, as the complexity of the brain is unparalleled in the rest of human biology. However, observations of psychopathology continue to be an impetus for understanding the brain and how its mechanisms can be responsible for deviance from its normal functioning.

The etiology sections of each chapter consider possible etiological and pathophysiological mechanisms of the various DSM-IV-TR mental disorders. Basic questions include how symptoms arise from brain dysfunction, the role of genes and environment in these dysfunctions, and their amenability to correction with pharmaceuticals and other treatments. There is no set of Koch's postulates to tell investigators or clinicians how adequate their explanations might be. Until very recently, since most treatments were discovered and validated empirically, there was little impact of these theories on clinical practice. Today, modern pharmaceutical discovery is heavily guided by neurochemical theories of psychopathology. For example, the serotonin reuptake inhibitors were synthesized because of the theory that older antidepressant drugs acted by blocking serotonin reuptake into presynaptic nerve terminals (Stahl 1993). Another example is the use of antiepileptic drugs to treat bipolar disorder, an intervention that was derived from observations of the similarity of the clinical course of bipolar disorder with the time course of experimental epileptogenesis in animal models. Both conditions seemed to have a similar pattern of increasing severity after repeated episodes (Post et al. 1991).

Theories of human psychopathology as neuronal dysfunction rely heavily on animal model research because of the strong prohibition against invading the human brain for research and for most diagnostic purposes. The validity of animal models for human behavioral illnesses is only partial because most of the symptoms are mental and, therefore, not observable with any degree of reliability in most laboratory animals. Several new technological developments are likely to revolutionize the field in the next several decades. First, dramatic improvements in human brain imaging are occurring, which increase the prospect of actually observing pathophysiological behavior in the living human brain. Second, the recognition that the largest proportion of risk for mental illness is genetic, accompanied by the elucidation of the human genome, means that much of psychopathology can be reduced to testable questions involving human genes. Because genes can be sampled noninvasively, many such questions can be proposed and then directly verified or rejected by sequencing DNA from appropriate genes.

However, the genetic revolution has not as yet yielded the fruits for psychiatric research that it has in other illnesses, particularly those that arise from a single gene. Instead, there appear to be multiple signals, with many populations showing several moderately positive chromosomal loci that appear to convey risk for illness. A number of the loci that are positive in schizophrenia are also positive in bipolar disorder and vice versa (Baron 2001). Few of these loci have been resolved into abnormalities in the function of specific genes. Genetic studies have also not produced evidence to support common theories of psychopathology: the dopamine theories of schizophrenia and addiction, the serotonin theory of depression, the noradrenergic theory of mania, or the cholinergic theory of dementia. From an optimist's standpoint, these findings mean that there is a great deal of new information to be uncovered, so that our understanding of psychopathology is likely to deepen. Furthermore, the involvement of multiple genes has the corollary that genetic abnormalities are likely quite common in our population if several are required to produce relatively common illnesses such as schizophrenia and bipolar illness (Freedman et al. 2001). Thus, many psychopathological mechanisms are likely to be normal biological variants that become pathological in individuals who have accumulated several such variants, along with additional environmental factors ranging from developmental brain problems to head injury to psychosocial stressors. Finally, the overlap between illnesses in their genetic predisposition suggests that psychopathological research may revise yet again the diagnostic classification of mental illness.

The role of genetic factors also prompts reexamination of the time course of illness. Although it is conceivable that a genetic factor might be entirely silent until the onset of psychopathology in adulthood, most brain genes are active throughout the life cycle. Although we conceive of many neuronal functions in terms of their role in signaling, most neurotransmitters and receptors have important roles in the migration of neurons and their formation of connections. Indeed, the brain seems to be able to construct itself from the same set of genes that it will later use for its operation. For many genes, expression is highest during fetal brain development, suggesting that their role in development is their most critical function. For clinicians interested in prevention and early treatment, the critical period may well be the second trimester when brain growth is maximal. A similar conclusion has been reached by epidemiological studies that have demonstrated that nongenetic influences such as poor maternal nutrition, stress, or infection may significantly affect the risk of illness (Hulshoff Pol et al. 2000). Primary preventive efforts will likely increase the attention paid to the role of genetic and environmental factors like psychopathological mechanisms on brain development. Beyond the fetal period, children who carry genetic risk and its neuronal concomitants may present with subclinical symptoms of illness long before the first episode of serious decompensation. Elements of psychopathology that relate these first subclinical symptoms to the eventual onset of recognized illness include attentional and behavioral disturbances in a wide variety of illnesses such as schizophrenia, affective disorder, and substance abuse (Erlenmeyer-Kimling 2001). As the child passes into puberty, the interaction of the genetic predisposition with changes in the brain caused by puberty itself introduces other elements of psychopathology. For example, the normal loss of gray matter in adolescence appears to be accelerated in schizophrenia (Thompson et al. 2001). Each development stage thus casts a different light on the mechanism of psychopathology and also affords new possibilities for therapeutic intervention.

A final reason for studying the mechanisms of psychopathology is to inform individuals undergoing treatment, their families, and society of the causes of mental illness. At some time in the course of their illness, most patients and families need some explanation of what has happened and why. Sometimes the explanation is as simplistic as "a chemical imbalance," while at other times, patients and families may request brain imaging so that they can see the possible psychopathology or request genetic analyses to calculate genetic risk. Many individuals presenting for treatment want to know if blood tests can confirm if they are truly ill because the symptoms appear, even to themselves, to be a sort of personal weakness. Sometimes the explanation is potentially destructive. The labeling of mothers as "schizophrenogenic" is the classic example. Careful reading of the sections on etiology and pathophysiology may help clinicians deliver a clear message without resorting to pseudoscience. The process of helping someone confront the nature of their mental disability is a duty and privilege granted to mental health clinicians. Society, which all too frequently stigmatizes mentally ill individuals and their families, can better deal with issues like antistigma campaigns and laws to guarantee parity in access to treatment if the public is properly informed about the mechanisms of psychopathology.

References

Baron M (2001) Genetics of schizophrenia and the new millennium: progress and pitfalls. *Am J Hum Genet* **68**, 299–312.

Erlenmeyer-Kimling L (2001) Early neurobehavioral deficits as phenotypic indicators of the schizophrenia genotype and predictors of later psychosis. *Am Med Genet* **105**, 23–24.

Freedman R, Leonard S, Olincy A, et al. (2001) Evidence for the multigenic inheritance of schizophrenia. *Am J Med Genet* **105**, 794–800.

Freud S (1886) Project for a scientific psychology. In *The Standard Edition of the Complete Psychological Works of Sigmund Freud (1966)*, Vol. 1, Strachey J (trans). Hogarth Press, London, pp. 283–410.

Hulshoff Pol HE, Hoek HW, Susser E, et al. (2000) Prenatal exposure to famine and brain morphology in schizophrenia. *Am J Psychiatry* **157**, 1170–1172.

Post RM, Altshuler LL, Ketter TA, et al. (1991) Antiepileptic drugs in affective illness. Clinical and theoretical implications. *Adv Neurol* **55**, 239–277.

Snyder SH (1981) Dopamine receptors, neuroleptics, and schizophrenia. *Am J Psychiatry* **138**, 460–464.

Stahl SM (1993) Serotonergic mechanisms and the new antidepressants. *Psychol Med* **23**, 281–285.

Thompson PM, Vidal C, Giedd JN, et al. (2001) Mapping adolescent brain change reveals dynamic wave of accelerated gray matter loss in very early-onset schizophrenia. *Proc Natl Acad Sci U S A* **98**, 11650–11655.

Valenstein ES (1990) The prefrontal area and psychosurgery. *Prog Brain Res* **85**, 539–533.

3 Treatment

Good treatment planning can flow only from an appropriate evaluation, and the type of evaluation done may differ depending on a variety of factors. More detailed information about specific evaluation methods and disease-related diagnosis and evaluation issues can be found in the general diagnosis chapter and chapters covering each disease entity.

The complete psychiatric evaluation consists of the clinical interview; physical examination, including neurological assessment; laboratory testing; and, as appropriate, neuropsychological testing, structured interviews, and brain imaging. The results of the evaluation are then used to assess risk, reach tentative and, if possible, definitive diagnoses, and complete initial and comprehensive treatment plans. Clearly, the length, the detail, and the order of the evaluation need to be modified when it is conducted in different settings. The clinician needs to assess the goals of the interview, the patient's tolerance for questioning, and the time available. Table 3-1 shows the variation of the psychiatric evaluation with the type of setting.

When all information has been gathered and organized, it may be possible to reach definitive diagnoses, but sometimes this must await further evaluation and the development of the comprehensive treatment plan.

Initial Treatment Plan

The initial treatment plan follows the case formulation, which has already established the nature of the current problem and a tentative diagnosis. The plan distinguishes between what must be accomplished now and what is postponed for the future. Treatment planning works best when it follows the biopsychosocial model.

Somatic Intervention

This includes an immediate response to any life-threatening medical conditions and a plan for the treatment of other less acute general medical conditions, including those that may contribute to an altered mental status. Prescription of psychotropic medications in accordance with the tentative diagnosis is the most common biological intervention.

Psychosocial Intervention

This includes immediate plans to prevent violent or suicidal behavior and addresses adverse external circumstances. An overall strategy must be developed that is both realistic and responsive to the patient's situation. Developing this strategy requires an awareness of the social support systems available to the individual; the financial resources of the individual; the availability of services in the area; the need to contact other agencies, such as child welfare or the police; and the need to ensure child care for dependent children.

Initial Disposition

The primary task of the initial disposition is to select the most appropriate level of care after completion of the psychiatric evaluation. Disposition is primarily focused on immediate goals. After referral, the patient and the treatment team develop longer-term goals.

Table 3-1	Psychiatric Evaluation and Treatment Planning		
Setting	**Psychiatric Interview and Mental Status Examination (MSE)**	**Physical or Neurological Examination, Laboratory Assessments, Brain Imaging**	**Treatment Planning**
Emergency room	Most often lengthy and extensive, except as limited by patient's ability or willingness to communicate.	Physical examination is often performed; other tests and examinations are ordered as indicated.	Primary focus is on disposition.
Psychiatric inpatient unit	Extensive, but complete information may be obtained in a series of interviews over time.	Physical and neurological examinations and laboratory tests are always performed. Other tests and examinations are ordered as indicated.	Comprehensive and formal plans are developed.
Consultation liaison service	Depth of interview is highly variable depending on reasons for referral and patient's medical condition. An attempt is made to obtain a complete MSE.	Most medical information is obtained from the chart. Psychiatric consultant may request further assessment.	Recommendations focus on reasons for referral and are made to the primary treatment team.
Outpatient office or clinic	Urgency of situation is assessed. In nonurgent situations, the initial interview usually focuses on the chief complaint and MSE.	Medical information is obtained as needed, usually by referral to a general practitioner or specialist.	Planning may be formal or informal, depending on applicable regulatory and reimbursement requirements.
Third-party interviews (e.g., for court, disability determinations)	Interview addresses the reason for referral and may be narrowly focused, but contains a complete MSE.	Assessments are ordered according to the purpose of the interview.	Not usually relevant except for recommendations pertaining to the purpose of the interview.

Hospitalization

The first decision in any disposition plan is whether hospitalization is required to ensure safety. There are times when an individual presents with such severe risk of harm to self or others that hospitalization seems essential. In other cases, the patient could be managed outside the hospital, depending on the availability of other supports. This might include a family who can stay with the patient or a crisis team in the community that is able to treat the individual at home. The more comprehensive the system of available services, the easier it is to avoid hospitalization. Because hospitalization is associated with extreme disruption of usual life activities and in and of itself can have many adverse consequences, plans to avoid hospitalization are usually appropriate as long as they do not compromise safety.

Day Programs, Crisis Residences, and Supervised Housing

These interventions provide ongoing supervision but at a lower level than that available within the hospital. They are most often used to treat individuals with alcohol and substance-use disorders or severe mental illness. Crisis housing can be useful when a patient cannot safely return home, when caregivers need respite, and when the individual is homeless. Other forms of supervised housing usually have a waiting period and may not be immediately available.

There are many different types of and names for daylong programming, including partial hospitalization, day treatment, psychiatric rehabilitation, and psychosocial clubs. Depending on the nature of the program, it may provide stabilization, daily medication, training in social and vocational skills, and treatment of alcohol and substance-use problems. Long-term day programs should generally be avoided if a patient is functioning successfully in a daytime role, such as in a job or as a homemaker. In these instances, referral to a day program may promote a lower level of functioning than the individual is capable of.

Outpatient Medication and Psychotherapy

The most common referral after psychiatric evaluation is to psychotherapy and/or medication management. In office-based settings, the clinician decides whether she or he has the time and expertise to treat the patient and makes referrals to other practitioners as appropriate. Hospital staff usually have a broad overview of community resources and refer accordingly. There are high rates of dropout when patients are sent from one setting to another. These can be reduced by providing introductions to the treatment setting and/or conducting follow-up to ensure that the referral has been successful.

Comprehensive Treatment Planning

The psychiatric evaluation usually continues beyond the initial disposition. The providers assuming responsibility for the patient, who may be inpatient staff, outpatient staff, mental health staff, or private practitioners, complete the evaluation and take responsibility for developing the comprehensive treatment plan. This plan covers the entire array of concerns that affect the course of the individual's psychiatric problems. In hospital settings, the initial treatment plan is usually completed within 24 to 72 hours after admission, followed by comprehensive treatment plan after more extensive evaluation.

The comprehensive treatment plan usually includes more definitive diagnoses and a well-formulated management plan with central goals and objectives. For severely ill or hospitalized patients, every area is usually covered (Table 3-2). It is best for the patient and, as appropriate, for the family to have input into the plan. The comprehensive treatment plan guides and coordinates the direction of all treatment for an extended time, usually months, and is periodically reviewed and updated. For more focal problems (e.g., phobias, sexual dysfunctions) and more limited interventions (e.g., brief interpersonal, cognitive, and behavioral therapies in office-based practices), the comprehensive treatment plan may focus on only a few of the possible areas.

Integrated Treatment

The advent of effective medications to treat mental disorders has revolutionized modern psychiatry, yet the provision of pharmacological treatment in combination with psycho-therapy was initially met with adversarial reactions by both biological psychiatrists and by psychiatrists favoring psychotherapeutic treatment approaches to the treatment of mental illness. The rationale for combining treatment modalities is based on the idea that the strengths of each modality are promoted, while the weaknesses are minimized, producing results that are better than with either modality alone (Hollon and Fawcett 1995).

Integrated, or combined treatment, does not yet appear to be completely supported through an evidence-based model mainly because of the lack of a substantial research base in this area, at least in terms of symptom reduction. This is partly due to the methodological issues in setting up the necessary types of studies, including the difficulty in setting up studies with sufficient number of subjects to detect small advantages between two efficacious treatments (Hollon and Fawcett 2001). There appears, however, to be a consensus that combined treatment does not appear to be contraindicated in any patient population (Hollon and Fawcett 1995, Paykel 1995, Rounsaville et al. 1981), unless either single modality is contraindicated or in the existence of medical conditions that need to be addressed prior to implementation of psychopharmacotherapy or psychotherapy (Hollon and Fawcett 2001). Hollon and Fawcett (1995) have outlined four ways in which combined treatment may prove

Table 3-2	Areas Covered by Comprehensive Treatment Plan

Mental health
   Diagnoses on five axes
   Psychiatric management, including medications
Physical health
   Medical diagnoses
   Medical management, including medications
Personal strengths and assets
Rehabilitation needs
   Educational
   Occupational
   Social
   Activities of daily living skills
   Use of leisure time
Living arrangements
Social supports and family involvement
Finances
   Personal finances
   Insurance coverage
   Eligibility for social service benefits
Legal or forensic issues
Central goals and objectives
Listing of treatment team members
Evidence of participation by patient and, as appropriate, family members and others
Criteria for discharge from treatment

advantageous over either treatment alone: increase the magnitude, probability, or breadth of clinical response, and increase the acceptability to the patient of either modality. In general, they feel that there is adequate literature to support the statement that combined treatment enhances the breadth of clinical response. It is within this context that clinical practice guidelines published by the Agency for Health Care Policy and Research support the use of combined treatment in depressive disorders (Depression Guideline Panel 1993).

Benefits of Integrated Treatment

Various authors discuss the potential benefits of employing pharmacotherapy within a psychotherapeutic context (Klerman 1991, Kay 2001). Pharmacotherapy has been noted to have a quicker onset of action on acute symptoms than most psychotherapies, perhaps with the exclusion of cognitive therapy (Hollon and Fawcett 2001). It is felt that this rapid dampening of symptoms may enhance the individual's ability to more productively participate in therapy by a variety of mechanisms. These have been described cogently by Klerman (1985, 1991) and include enhancing the individual's self-esteem, creating a safe environment in which emotions are more freely discussed, reducing the stigma of seeking mental health care through a positive placebo effect, improving cognition (verbalization and abreaction), and functioning as a transitional object during breaks in therapy, among others.

The benefits of employing psychotherapy within a primarily psychopharmacologic relationship have also been described. Empirical evidence exists across the spectrum of mental health disorders to support the following hypothesized benefits of adding psychotherapy to medications. It decreases the incidence of illness relapse (Hogarty et al. 1986) as well as symptom relapse upon medication discontinuation (Wiborg and Dahl 1996, Spiegel et al. 1994). It fosters the individual's ability to utilize healthy coping strategies, addresses issues that are not typically targeted by psychopharmacologic treatment such as dysfunctional relationship patterns or negative self-appraisals due to traumatic past events, and enhances psychotropic compliance (Paykel 1995).

Split Treatment

Although multimodal, or integrated, treatment may be an optimal treatment choice, resources to provide it in most parts of the world, including the United States, may be inadequate. The psychiatrists may not be in a position to directly provide all components of care, and various clinicians may be responsible for each component of treatment. This approach may be called *split treatment*. A key aspect of split treatment is how complex and difficult such treatment is for the clinicians, the patient, and the patient's family. Unless one works in a clinic or an organized setting where relationships between clinicians are well delineated (e.g., one psychiatrist works with a specific group of nonmedical therapists), much thought must go into managing safe and effective split treatment.

It may be helpful to think of split therapy having a beginning, a middle course, and an end. In order to avoid or minimize the pitfalls associated with split treatment, the following clinical suggestions are provided as organizing principles for its three stages (Rand 1999, Tasman and Riba 2000):

Beginning of Treatment

- Communication is key to providing excellent care in split treatment. At the beginning, both clinicians should obtain a signed release-of-information form from the patient. Communication must be regular and frequent between the clinicians, and the individual should be made aware of these discussions. The forms of regular communication should be decided at the onset—routine telephone calls, faxes, emails, follow-up letters, and the like. The patient should not be a messenger between the clinicians.
- Issues of confidentiality should be discussed and reviewed at the beginning of treatment. Confidentiality should not be used as a cover to hide from taking the time to make telephone calls, to send copies of evaluations and follow-up notes, to send emails or faxes, or to have joint sessions with both the clinicians and the patient.
- Diagnostic impressions should be independently arrived at, then discussed and agreed upon. If there is a difference of opinion, an understanding must be reached before treatment proceeds.
- The clinicians must work with each other and with the patient to determine the treatment plan. The treatment plan should specify how often each of the clinicians expects to see the patient and what process to pursue if the patient does not follow up or if there is a missed appointment. If the patient wishes to end either the therapy, the medications, or both, it has to be understood that all parties will discuss this important decision. It is desirable for a written contract to be drawn up between the clinicians and the patient so that all parties understand what the agreement for services will entail. Included in the contract should be a delineation of the clinicians' roles and responsibilities as well as those of the patient.
- Clinician's vacation schedules and other on call and coverage issues must be discussed regularly and documented. The patient needs to know whom to call in an emergency. At the beginning of split treatment, both the clinicians and the patient should be aware of their respective beliefs regarding medication and psychotherapy.
- There must be a discussion about what type of care would be optimal for the patient and if there are barriers to such care. The patient should be informed of this review; if possible, he or she should participate in it.
- The clinicians should discuss their professional backgrounds and training with each other at the beginning of the individual's treatment. Issues such as licensure, ethics, violations, malpractice claims, hospital privileges, coverage of professional liability insurance, participation on managed care panels, and commitment to split treatment should all be made clear.

- The clinicians need to agree on who will communicate with third parties regarding the patient's care. Further, each clinician should know the individual's mental health benefits and means of payment. There needs to be an agreement by all parties as to the use of such benefits.
- The clinicians need to understand how best to interface with the individual's family or significant others.
- If the patient has health providers other than the psychiatrist and the therapist (e.g., primary care physician, cardiologist, physical therapist, etc.), it should be decided which clinician will be the designated communicator or coordinator with those other providers.
- At the beginning of treatment, there should be a review of how each clinician will assess and manage the patient's thoughts regarding or attempts at suicide, homicide, violence, and domestic abuse.
- It should be made clear to the patient what symptoms or types of issues should be brought to the attention of which clinician.
- It is helpful for the clinicians to decide how problems will be handled as the need arises.
- The clinicians should discuss differences in fee schedules, cancellation policies, length of visits, and frequency of visits.

Middle Course

- Special attention must be paid to transference and countertransference in this type of system of care. Disparaging and negative remarks made by the patient concerning either clinician, therapy, or medication must be understood and managed in the context of this complex type of treatment.
- Clinicians should review how many cases of split treatment they have in their practices and whether or not this is a safe mix. Factors to consider include the clinical complexity of the cases, how busy the practice is, the influence of third-party payers and the hassle factor, the number of different clinicians one is working with, the psychiatric disorders of one's patients, and so on. It may be prudent to determine the risks involved in having a large patient population in split treatment and to weed the number of such individuals down to an acceptable level. Further, clinicians should minimize the number of collaborators, since it is virtually impossible to keep track of a large number of clinicians' credentials, vacation schedules, communication patterns, and so on.
- Adherence to medications and to psychotherapy should be addressed equally.
- Treatment plans should be regularly reviewed and updated between the clinicians and the patient.
- Use of the individual's mental health benefits should be regularly reviewed and discussed between the clinicians and the patient when appropriate.
- There must be an agreement that either clinician can terminate the split therapy but that the patient must be provided adequate and appropriate warning and referrals to other clinicians. In other words, the patient cannot be abandoned.

Ending Split Treatment

- After reviewing the treatment plan, both the clinicians and the patient will decide together on the goals that have been met or have not been realized and the best time for termination. They should decide how to stagger the discontinuation of therapy and of medication.
- It is important to consider how to manage follow-up and recurrence of symptoms.

The clinicians must have a system for giving each other feedback on the care each is providing to the patient. Ideally, after the treatment is complete, the clinicians should review any aspects of the case that could have been managed or handled differently and the patient should be part of this evaluation process as a way of assuring continuous quality improvement. Most importantly, throughout all stages of the split treatment process, clinicians need to respect both the patient and each other's professional understanding.

Although the challenges of split treatment are great, there are many reasons for clinicians and patients to try to surmount the obstacles. Good communication patterns between clinicians and many of the suggestions noted here may be guideposts on the path toward successful split treatment.

Global Perspectives on Treatment

Both industrialized and later developing countries have one thing in common—their mental health resources are grossly inadequate. There are striking differences across countries, but there is a worldwide shortage of mental health personnel, services, and other resources for the prevention and treatment of mental disorders. In virtually every country, in spite of the high prevalence of mental illness and the human and economic burden of these disorders, mental health services are inferior to general health services.

There is, however, room for modest optimism about mental health care and the fate of persons with mental disorders. The WHO (2001) and the US Surgeon General (US Department of Health and Human Services 1999) have recently published reports that highlight the importance of mental health and make reasonable suggestions for making progress.

The World Health Report 2001 (WHO 2001) made 10 overall recommendations for countries to improve mental health, as follows: (1) provide mental health treatment in primary care settings; (2) make psychotropic drugs available; (3) give care in the community; (4) educate the public about mental illnesses; (5) educate communities, families, and consumers; (6) establish national mental health policies, programs, and legislation; (7) develop human resources not only to create more specialists but also to help general and allied health providers to recognize and treat mental illnesses; (8) link with other sectors, including the general health sector and traditional healers who can serve as case finders, referrers, counselors, and monitors; (9) monitor community mental health, and (10) support more research.

Some of these recommendations are not feasible or are extremely low priority for developing countries struggling to cope with extreme poverty, inadequate nutrition, the consequences of war, and acute communicable diseases. Mental health services are suboptimal worldwide except for a few model programs.

The most widely promoted strategy for improving the treatment of persons with mental disorders worldwide is the integration of mental health care into primary care settings. This is a practical approach because most countries have an existing primary care system even though these vary widely within and between countries. There is considerable evidence that primary health workers can be trained to recognize, treat, and refer common mental disorders, but that long-term success will depend upon ongoing guidance, support, and monitoring from secondary and tertiary care centers. Links between primary care clinicians and traditional healers who are commonly consulted in many countries are also desirable so that the strengths of each may be optimized. Although effective, affordable, and humane treatments and systems are attainable, only incremental and modest progress toward these goals is likely in the near future.

References

Depression Guideline Panel (1993) *Depression in Primary Care, Vol. 2: Treatment of Major Depression* (Clinical Practice Guideline No. 5; AHCPR Publ No. 93-0551). US Department of Health and Human Services, Public Health Service, Agency for Health Care Policy and Research, Rockville, MD.

Hogarty G, Anderson CM, Reiss DJ, et al. (1986) Family education, social skills training, and maintenance chemotherapy in the aftercare of schizophrenia. *Arch Gen Psychiatry* **43**, 633–642.

Hollon SD and Fawcett J (1995) Combined medication and psychotherapy. In *Treatments of Psychiatric Disorders*, Vol. 1, 2nd ed., Gabbard GO (ed). American Psychiatric Press, Washington, DC, pp. 1222–1236.

Hollon SD and Fawcett J (2001) Combined medication and psychotherapy. In *Treatments of Psychiatric Disorders*, Vol. 1 and 2, 3rd ed., Gabbard GO (ed-in-chief). American Psychiatric Press, Washington, DC.

Kay J (2001) Integrated treatment: an overview. In *Integrated Treatment for Psychiatric Disorders: Review of Psychiatry*, Vol. 20, Kay J (ed). American Psychiatric Press, Washington, DC, pp. 1–29.

Klerman GL (1985) Trends in utilization of mental health services. *Med Care* **23**, 584.

Klerman GL (1991) Ideologic conflicts. In *Integrating Pharmacotherapy and Psychotherapy*, Beitman BB and Klerman G (eds). American Psychiatric Press, Washington, DC, pp. 3–20.

Paykel ES (1995) Psychotherapy, medication combinations, and compliance. *J Clin Psychiatry* **56**(Suppl. 1), 24–30.

Rand EH (1999) Guidelines to maximize the process of collaborative treatment. In *Psychopharmacology and Psychotherapy: A Collaborative Approach*, Riba MB and Balon R (eds). American Psychiatric Press, Washington, DC, pp. 353–380.

Rounsaville BJ, Klerman GL, and Weissman MM (1981) Do psychotherapy and pharmacotherapy of depression conflict. *Arch Gen Psychiatry* **38**, 24–29.

Spiegel DA, Bruce TJ, Gregg SF, et al. (1994) Does cognitive–behavior therapy assist slow-taper alprazolam discontinuation in panic disorder. *Am J Psychiatry* **151**, 876–881.

Tasman A and Riba MB (2000) Psychological management in psychopharmacologic treatment. In *Psychiatric Drugs*, Lieberman J and Tasman A (eds). W. B. Saunders, Philadelphia, PA, pp. 242–249.

US Department of Health and Human Services (1999) *Mental Health: A Report of Surgeon General US Department of Health and Human Services, Substance Abuse and Mental Health Services Administration/Center for Mental Health Services*. National Institute of Health, Rockville (Available online at: www.surgeongeneral.gov/library/mental-health/home.html).

Wiborg IM and Dahl AA (1996) Does brief dynamic psychotherapy reduce the relapse rate of panic disorder. *Arch Gen Psychiatry* **53**, 689–694.

World Health Organization (2001) *The World Health Report 2001. Mental Health: New Understanding, New Hope*. World Health Organization, Geneva.

4 Childhood Disorders: Mental Retardation

Diagnosis

Some common misconceptions about mental retardation are that it is a specific and lifelong disorder with a unique personality pattern and that comorbid mental disorders existing with mental retardation are different from those encountered in other individuals. Although mental retardation is listed as a mental disorder in the *Diagnostic and Statistical Manual of Mental Disorders*, Fourth Edition, Text Revision (DSM-IV-TR) (American Psychiatric Association 2000), it is not a unique nosological entity. Instead, a diagnosis of mental retardation refers to the level of a person's intellectual and adaptive functioning below a cutoff point that is not even natural but is arbitrarily chosen in relation to the average level of functioning of the population at large. Its chief function is administrative, defining a group of persons who are in need of support and educational services. Thus, mental retardation does not have a single cause, mechanism, course, or prognosis. It has to be differentiated from the diagnosis (if known) of the underlying medical condition.

The American Association on Mental Retardation (AAMR) has published over the years 10 definitions of mental retardation. The most recent definition published in 2002 in the 10th edition of the manual on definition, classification, and system of supports of the American Association on Mental Retardation is as follows: "Mental retardation is a disability characterized by significant limitations both in intellectual functioning and in adaptive behavior as expressed in conceptual, social, and practical adaptive skills. This disability originates before age 18 years." Significant limitation in intellectual functioning is defined as at least 2 standard deviations below the mean for the assessment instrument. The standard error of measurement for the instrument (usually between 3 and 5 points) should be taken into consideration. Persons with mental retardation can be classified in various ways, such as by IQ levels, or by the intensity of supports required by them, depending on the purpose for which the diagnosis is used. Significant limitation in adaptive behavior is defined as performance of at least 2 standard deviations below the mean on an instrument normed on the general population. The AAMR manual emphasizes the requirement for detailed assessment of individuals and their needs in all relevant domains, including psychological and emotional, and is by far the most modern and comprehensive available.

DSM-IV-TR defines mental retardation in a manner generally compatible with the AAMR definition. (See DSM-IV-TR diagnostic criteria on page 62). Mental retardation is coded on Axis II, as conceptually, it fits more with personality disorders listed on this axis than with the other mental illnesses listed on Axis I. It was also expected that placement on Axis II would encourage clinicians to diagnose both mental retardation and mental disorders when faced with a person who has such comorbidity, rather than subsume both under the diagnosis of mental retardation.

⊣ DSM-IV-TR Criteria

317-319 Mental Retardation

A. Significantly subaverage intellectual functioning: an IQ of approximately 70 or below on an individually administered IQ test (for infants, a clinical judgment of significantly subaverage intellectual functioning).

B. Concurrent deficits or impairments in present adaptive functioning (i.e., the person's effectiveness in meeting the standards expected for his or her cultural group) in atleast two of the following areas: communication, self-care, home living, social/interpersonal skills, use of community resources, self-direction, functional academic skills, work, leisure, health, and safety.

C. The onset is before age 18 years.

Severity	Approximate IQ Range	Code
Mild	50–55 to approx. 70	317
Moderate	35–40 to approx. 50–55	318
Severe	20–25 to approx. 35–40	318.1
Profound	Below 20–25	318.2
Unspecified		319

Reprinted with permission from the Diagnostic and Statistical Manual of Mental Disorders, Fourth Edition, Text Revision. Copyright 2000 American Psychiatric Association.

The clinical presentation of persons with mental retardation is influenced by multiple factors, which can be grossly divided into biological (such as syndromes underlying the retardation), psychological (the level of the person's intellectual and adaptive functioning), and environmental (such as cultural expectations and services received).

The more severe the mental retardation, the earlier the child will come to medical attention, because the developmental delay will be obvious earlier, and associated physical impairments will be more prevalent. Conversely, children with mild mental retardation may not be diagnosed until they reach school age, when they fail in academic learning. If the sociocultural environment does not value and stress early academic learning and early education is not available, mild mental retardation might go undetected, especially if the person has relatively good adaptive skills. A false-positive diagnosis of mental retardation can also occur, especially if psychological tests are not sensitive to cultural background, and there is a language barrier between the child and the tester.

The importance of the earliest diagnosis possible cannot be overstated because the prognosis will be much better if the intervention that results from the diagnostic knowledge is begun as early as possible.

The American Association on Mental Retardation has published in 2002 a new edition of its manual *Mental Retardation: Definition, Classification and Systems of Supports.* Several dimensions of mental retardation are described, which might also serve as an outline for its assessment:

Dimension I: Intellectual abilities.

Dimension II: Adaptive behavior (Conceptual, social, and practical skills).
Assessment of the above dimensions is essentially ascertaining that the respective criteria for the diagnosis of mental retardation are met. The intellectual functioning is assessed in individual testing with one of the standardized intelligence tests appropriate for the person's cultural, linguistic, and social background, and communication skills. An appropriate amount of time and a suitable environment should be provided because many persons with mental retardation may be less than cooperative, having been tested many times before and viewing the tests as proof of their inadequacy. Even "nontestable" persons can be adequately assessed through prolonged observations, partial test completion, detailed history taking, and patience. Similar principles apply to the assessment of adaptive functioning. Standardized tests and scales, such as the Vineland Adaptive Behavior Scales and the American Association on Mental Retardation Adaptive Behavior Scales as well as history and direct observations are used.

Dimension III: Participation, interactions, and social roles.

Dimension IV: Health (physical health, mental health, etiological factors). This is described in the later sections of this chapter.

Dimension V: Context (environments and culture).
This is a comprehensive description of the person's current environment: its nature, strengths, and weaknesses, supports for the person's development and well-being, (including factors such as poverty, family and its attitudes, availability of education, and other services).

In all aspects of the assessment, attention should be paid both to the strengths as well as to the weaknesses and the impairments.

Biomedical causes of mental retardation have their origin in genetic or external factors or injury causing structural or functional disturbances of the central nervous system (CNS). The structural changes may or may not be recognizable by available clinical techniques, such as neuroimaging, computed tomography, magnetic resonance imaging (MRI), positron emission tomography, and single-photon emission computed tomography. Special staining methods have revealed changes in dendrites and synapses (hypoconnection) in some retardation syndromes (Huttenlocher 1991). As medical technology becomes more sophisticated, it is hoped that it will be possible to recognize the biological causes in an increasing number of individuals with mental retardation.

Mental retardation associated with syndromes and disorders with obvious phenotypical features is usually recognized earliest, such as in the case of Down syndrome. The diagnosis is then confirmed by chromosomal or other appropriate laboratory studies. If there was a suspicion of a family's risk for a genetic disorder before the birth (such as through prior genetic counseling), appropriate studies are performed in the neonatal period. Some cases of congenital mental retardation (e.g., phenylketonuria (PKU)) are discovered in the course of routine neonatal screening. Newborns with perinatal risk factors like prematurity and asphyxia should be followed up closely for later manifestations of developmental delay. Other children might come to medical attention because of a delay in achieving developmental milestones or regression in a previously normal developmental pattern. Finally, many children with mental retardation will be referred for diagnostic assessment when they reach school age because of failure in academic learning.

Elements of Biomedical Assessment

First Stage Workup

The scheme for assessing the etiology of mental retardation is summarized in Figure 4-1. This workup has been used by Finnish physicians for 20 years (Wilska and Kaski 1999, 2001), and will be described in detail here.

History

Obtaining a detailed history is most important. The family history, especially occurrence in the family of similar cases, congenital anomalies, severe mental illness, and consanguinity should be explored. The risk of recessively inherited diseases increases if there has been intermarriage between the parents' families in earlier generations. Drawing the family tree is helpful. The gestational, birth and neonatal, as well as developmental history is also most important. The presence of an appropriate relationship between weight, length, and head circumference at birth must be assessed as well as their relationship to the gestational age to evaluate possible intrauterine growth retardation, microcephaly, and so on. All events that may have affected CNS development during childhood as well as developmental milestones must be recorded.

Physical Examination

This is essential and should also focus on searching for physical phenotypical manifestations of various mental retardation–associated syndromes and dysmorphic features different from familial phenotype. Neurological examination and growth measurements are part of physical examination.

Diagnostic Studies

There is frequent discussion as to which diagnostic/laboratory studies should be performed routinely. The Consensus Conference for Evaluation of Mental Retardation recommended, in addition to previously mentioned history taking and physical examination, the following: banded karyotype and fragile X studies by DNA method for both males and females with unexplained mental retardation. These studies are essential if the family history is positive or if the physical and behavioral phenotypes are without major findings. Neuroimaging, preferably MRI, is to be performed if the individual has neurologic symptoms, cranial abnormalities, microcephaly, or macrocephaly (Curry et al. 1997).

After this basic workup, the probable cause or at least timing of the injury should become apparent, thus allowing discussion with the family concerning possible inheritance. Sometimes the history alone might provide this information, but even then a detailed physical examination for signs indicative of abnormal prenatal development is necessary. If there are congenital anomalies or more than three dysmorphic features, special genetic studies, like FISH (fluorescent *in situ* hybridization) and/or DNA studies, should be done with the collaboration of the geneticist. If there is a suspicion of a progressive brain disease, consultations of the neurologist, neurological ophthalmologist and geneticist are needed. In such cases, biopsies of muscle, skin, and rectum are often helpful.

The "etiological tree" seen in Figure 4-1 was created during a process of reorganizing the ICD-10 diagnoses according to the timing of the injury to CNS. This illustration functions as a reference for those who want to understand this "time and cause" approach to the etiology of functional disturbances of the CNS. It can also be used in teaching and genetic counseling of the families.

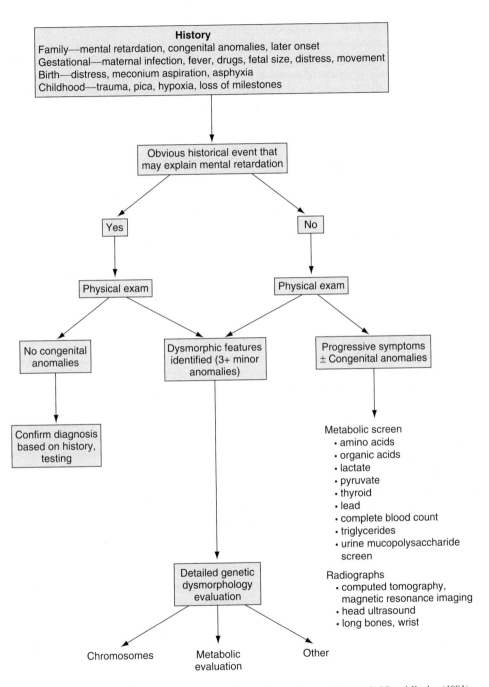

Figure 4-1 *Diagnostic approach to mental retardation of all ages. (Source: Szymanski LS and Kaplan (1991) Mental retardation. In Textbook of Child and Adolescent Psychiatry, Wiener JM (ed). American Psychiatric Press, Washington, DC, p. 157.)*

Prenatal Diagnosis

Prenatal diagnostic methods are increasingly available. Amniocentesis with chromosomal studies is usually recommended for women 35 years or older. Prenatal diagnostic studies should be made available to everyone requesting them and should be used if there is a known risk for a genetic or congenital problem. Even if the parents do not plan a therapeutic abortion, if the results are positive for a certain disorder, they will be able to prepare for the birth of a child with special needs and to marshal support.

The currently available techniques include amniocentesis (useful in diagnosing chromosomal and metabolic disorders), chorionic villus sampling (for chromosomal and molecular genetic studies), and maternal serum alpha-fetoprotein screening (for neural tube defects). Ultrasound scanning is often performed around the 20th week of gestation to screen for major malformations. Carrier screening, which is increasingly available for certain recessive disorders, should be offered to all persons in high-risk populations, such as Ashkenazi Jews (for Tay–Sachs disease). Careful counseling is necessary to help the prospective parents decide on all available options if they are found to be positive for the particular trait.

Epidemiology

The results of epidemiological studies of mental retardation depend on two major factors: the definition of mental retardation that is used and how the results are ascertained. There have been various models for estimating the prevalence of mental retardation. A model based on IQ score alone used the expected statistical distribution of intelligence levels. The past definition based only on an IQ that was 1 standard deviation or greater below the mean implied that almost 15% of the population could be classified as having mental retardation. With the introduction of the diagnostic criterion of impairment in adaptive behavior and an IQ cutoff at 2 standard deviations below the mean (approximately 70), the prevalence of mental retardation was commonly thought to be 3% of the population. More recent population-based studies, using multiple methods of ascertainment and a current definition of mental retardation, suggest that the prevalence might be closer to 1%. In the study of McLaren and Bryson (1987), the prevalence of mild mental retardation was 0.37 to 0.59%, whereas the prevalence of moderate, severe, and profound retardation was 0.3 to 0.4%. When age is considered, the highest prevalence is in the school-age group, when the child cannot meet the expectations of academic learning. The United States Department of Education indicated the prevalence of mental retardation among school-age children (6–17 years of age) to be 1.14%, with variations reported by different states (Massey and McDermott 1995). Conversely, some persons who are diagnosed with mild mental retardation when of school age lose that diagnosis in adulthood when their good adaptive skills are more relevant than their academic achievement.

Course

The development of an individual with mental retardation depends on the type and the extent of the underlying disorder, the associated disabilities and disorders, environmental factors (such as general health, education, treatment, and other services), and psychological factors (cognitive abilities, comorbid psychopathological conditions). Some general principles concerning the developmental trajectories of various mental retardation–associated disorders and syndromes are seen in Figure 4-2.

Life expectancy depends on a number of factors already discussed. Persons with profound mental retardation with multiple disabilities and an inability to ambulate or self-feed have a much shorter life expectancy according to an extensive study conducted in California (Eyman et al. 1990).

When a medical patient is a person with mental retardation, even ordinary ailments may be difficult to diagnose (and may become life threatening), as the person may be unable to describe the complaints because of communication difficulties. Physical pain and other discomforts are often communicated by these individuals through their behavior, such as aggression or self-injurious behavior (SIB), leading to a psychiatric referral while the

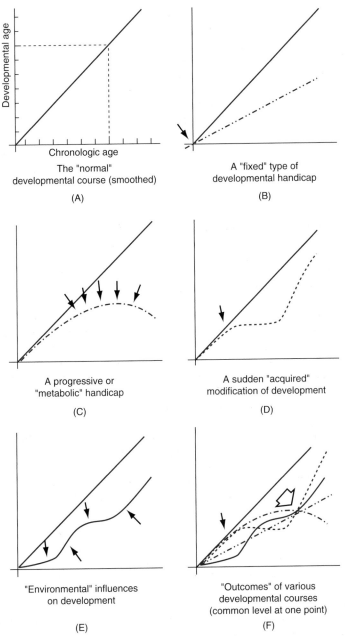

Figure 4-2 *Schematic representation of patterns of developmental disorders (arrows refer to the point of insult): (A) normal developmental course; (B) fixed, nonprogressive type of developmental disorder; (C) metabolic type of disorder of development in which the manifestations of the underlying process (e.g., Tay–Sachs disease) occur after birth and evolve into a progressively deteriorating course; (D) acquired developmental disorder: the curve represents normal development up to a point of insult (arrow) to the CNS; (E) environmental disorder of development: a fluctuating course, with periods of stress (downward arrows) and periods of nurturance or positive intervention, or both (upward arrows); (F) outcomes: the convergence (arrow) of the various developmental courses represents the point at which the physician becomes aware of the developmental disorder. (Source: Szymanski LS, Rubin LL, and Tarjan G (1989) Mental retardation. In American Psychiatric Press Review of Psychiatry, Vol. 8, Tasman A, Hales RE, and Frances AJ (eds). American Psychiatric Press, Washington, DC, p. 227.)*

physical disorder remains undiagnosed. Many syndromes predispose the person to certain health problems that have to be anticipated. Illnesses typical of Down syndrome have been discussed earlier. Nonambulatory persons are at risk for both respiratory and urinary tract infections. Gastroesophageal reflux is common and often leads to aspiration and anemia.

Differential Diagnosis

The diagnosis of mental retardation itself should be relatively straightforward as it reflects the current level of intellectual and adaptive functioning. Some persons with learning disorders or communication disorders might appear to have a low level of functioning, but appropriate psychological and communication testing will demonstrate that the impairment is in the development of specific skills and is not generalized. Dementia can be diagnosed at any age, whereas mental retardation is diagnosed only if the onset is before age 18 years. However, both disorders might be diagnosed in persons younger than age 18. It is often asked how one differentiates between mental retardation and autistic disorder. Actually, such a question is erroneous because these disorders are not mutually exclusive; in fact, most persons with autism also have mental retardation. An uncomplicated mental retardation is not associated with qualitative impairment in social interaction and communication, which is diagnostic of autistic disorder.

Etiology

Intellectual abilities depend to a great degree on the integrity of the CNS. A variety of biomedical causes can disrupt this integrity and start the process leading to mental retardation. It should be kept in mind, however, that the term mental retardation describes the overall level of functioning, encompassing current intellectual and adaptive skills. These, in turn, are shaped by other factors besides CNS integrity, such as the individual's general state of health and associated disabilities, environmental factors (such as nurturing, learning opportunities, supports), and psychological factors (such as the person's self-image, psychopathological characteristics, motivation). Thus, a biomedical cause, whether genetic or acquired, may be a primary cause that will start the process of developmental delay but will not necessarily be the only factor responsible for the functional outcome, which will depend on the synergistic or cumulative effects of all factors involved. It is important to know as much as possible about the "primary" cause for a number of reasons:

- Treatment possibilities, which can include early institution of diet in phenylketonuria (PKU) and thyroid hormone supplementation in congenital hypothyroidism.
- Prevention, such as primary prevention of the recurrence of the same condition using, for example, parental education to prevent fetal alcohol syndrome (FAS) and enabling genetic counseling for the family.
- Early recognition and treatment of complications known to be associated with the particular mental retardation syndrome, such as hypothyroidism in Down syndrome.
- Research on causation and prevention.
- Assessment of epidemiology, which is important in public policy (planning for services) as well as in prevention.
- Understanding of prognosis in association with a particular disorder.
- Support for the family and other caregivers by dispelling misconceptions and anxieties related to uncertainty about the cause.

For these reasons, it is important for physicians, including psychiatrists, to ascertain whether the persons with mental retardation to whom they provide care have had adequate and up-to-date etiological assessments that reflect current medical knowledge.

The prevalence of diagnosable (using current techniques) biomedical causes of mental retardation varies with the degree of the disability. When the retardation is severe, a prenatal cause can be identified in 59 to 73% of individuals, but in mild mental retardation, such a cause can be identified in only 23 to 43% of individuals (Table 4-1).

Table 4-1	**Causes of Mental Retardation by Time of Insult to the Central Nervous System: Literature Summary**				
Study	**Cohort (*n*; age)**	**% of Study Population***			
		Prenatal	**Perinatal**	**Postnatal**	**Unknown**
	Studies of persons with severe mental retardation				
Gustavson et al. (1997a)	121; 5–16 yr	73	10	5	12
Gustavson et al. (1997a)	161; 5–16 yr	68	8	2	22
McQueen et al. (1986)	221; 7–10 yr	59	10	4	27
	Studies of persons with mild mental retardation				
Blomquist et al. (1981)	171; school age	43	7	7	43
Hagberg et al. (1981)	91; school age	23	18	2	55

* The percentages are of subjects in each study in whom the retardation was thought to be owing to causation at the pre-, peri-, or postnatal period, respectively, or the cause could not be found.

Table 4-2	**Etiological Classification of Mental Retardation Based on the Timing and Type of the Central Nervous System Insult*†**	
Division and Group	**Percent**	**Examples**
Prenatal: Genetic Disorders	32	
Chromosomal aberrations		Trisomy 21, trisomy 13 m cri du chat syndromes
Malformations due to microdeletions		Angelman's and Prader–Willi syndromes, William's syndrome, Rubinstein–Taybi syndrome
Monogenic mutations		Tuberous sclerosis, metabolic disorders, fragile-X syndrome
Multifactorial mental retardation		"Familial" mental retardation
Malformations, Cause Unknown	8	
Malformations of the CNS		Holoprosencephaly, lissencephaly, neural tube defects
Multiple malformation syndromes		de Lange's syndrome, Sotos' syndrome
Prenatal: Disorders due to External Causes	12	
Maternal infections		Rubella and HIV, cytomegalovirus, and *Toxoplasma* infections
Toxins		Fetal alcohol syndrome, fetal hydantoin syndrome
Toxemia, placental insufficiency		IUGR, prematurity
Other		Radiation, trauma
Perinatal Causes	11	
Infections		Meningitis, herpes
Delivery problems		Asphyxia, trauma
Other		Hypoglycemia, hyperbilirubinemia
Postnatal Causes	8	
Infections		Meningitis, encephalitis
Toxins		Lead poisoning
Other CNS disorders		Cerebrovascular accidents, tumors, traumas
Psychosocial problems		
Unknown Causes	25	

* These data are based on the Finnish National Board of Social Welfare registry of persons, with mental retardation, who were receiving special services in the 1980s. There were about 19,000 persons in that registry. In about 4%, no etiological information was recorded (unpublished data).
† CNS, central nervous system; HIV, human immunodeficiency virus; IUGR, intrauterine growth retardation.

The classification of causes of MR used in this chapter reflects both the timing and the type of the causative process, which will affect the development and function of the CNS (Table 4-2) (Wilska and Kaski 1999).

Prenatal Causes: Genetic Disorders

Prenatal genetic disorders are characterized by changes in the genetic material that may or may not have been inherited from the parents.

Chromosomal Aberrations

Down Syndrome This syndrome is the best-known example of prenatal genetic disorders. In the large majority of cases, it is caused by trisomy 21, in which the extra chromosome 21 in the egg or sperm cell results from the nondisjunction in the meiotic stage. When such a gamete becomes fertilized, the fetus will have an extra chromosome 21 in all cells for a total of 47 chromosomes. In cases of Down syndrome caused by translocation, there are 46 chromosomes. However, chromosomal material from 47 chromosomes is present because an extra chromosome 21 is attached (translocated) to another chromosome, usually chromosome 14 [designated as t(14;21)]. In about half the translocation cases, a parent (usually the mother) has a balanced translocation: 45 chromosomes with t(14;21). If a child has translocation Down syndrome, the parents should be examined for the presence of a balanced translocation. This is important in genetic counseling because when the mother or father has a t(14;21) translocation, there is a 1 in 10 or a 1 in 20 chance, respectively, of having a child with Down syndrome. In another variant, mosaicism, some cells have 47 chromosomes, and others have 46 because of an error in one of the first cell divisions of the fertilized egg. The characteristic phenotype of Down syndrome is basically the same in trisomy 21 and in translocation.

The main features are upward-slanted palpebral fissures, a low nasal bridge with epicanthal folds, a flat nasal bridge, a small mouth and ears, a single palmar crease (simian crease), short and wide palms, and a characteristic dermatoglyphic pattern. Considerable hypotonia and a tendency toward respiratory problems are common. The level of retardation varies from severe to mild with a mean IQ of approximately 50. The severity of symptoms in the mosaic form varies, and children with normal intelligence have been described. The global incidence of Down syndrome is 1 in 700 live births, but it rises with maternal age to about 1 in 40 live births in mothers older than 40 years of age. Children with Down syndrome, adorable and affectionate, used to be described as "Prince Charming." However, various behavioral problems and psychopathological conditions can occur, including autistic disorder. Early diagnosis and intervention, including physical therapy and developmental stimulation, are essential to enable these children to reach their developmental potential.

Many structural and functional anomalies cause individuals with Down syndrome to be at risk for associated health problems. It is important to be aware of this to enable early diagnosis and treatment as well as prevention (Hayes and Batshaw 1993, Cunniff et al. 2001). There is an increased risk for congenital heart defects (in 40–50% of persons), gastrointestinal atresias (in 12%), Hirschprung disease (<1%), and leukemia (<1%). Hearing loss, mostly conductive, secondary to otitis media (75%), needs attention lest it impedes speech development. Respiratory and ear infections are common, partially secondary to anatomical features, partially due to deficient cellular immunity. Obstructive sleep apnea is seen frequently among persons with Down syndrome. Eye problems are common, including congenital cataracts (in 1–3% of children, and increasing with age up to 15%) (Hayes and Batshaw 1993). There are also accommodation problems and severe refractive errors requiring corrective glasses (in 50%). Gluten intolerance is diagnosed in 4 to 20% of individuals with Down syndrome and should be kept in mind in cases of gastrointestinal problems. Atlanto–axial instability is seen in 10% and may cause problems in contact sports or intratracheal intubation. Hypothyroidism may be congenital or may develop later, the incidence increasing with age. It may cause "reversible dementia," which is treatable with thyroid hormone replacement. Therefore, annual thyroid function screening is recommended. The Committee on Genetics of the American Academy of Pediatrics has recently published guidelines concerning health supervision for children with Down syndrome (Cunniff et al. 2001).

It has been well documented that persons with Down syndrome have neuropathological changes of Alzheimer's dementia often in a relatively early age. Amyloid plaques involved in this disease are found in them, as a rule, after 40 years of age, probably because of the increased dose of the gene for beta-amyloid that is on chromosome 21 (Wisniewski et al. 1985). The neuropathological changes usually are not accompanied by clinical symptoms of dementia until the fifth or sixth decade of life. This phenomenon is due to the fact that the effect of ApoE4 allele is not as strong among the individuals with Down syndrome as in normal population. In addition, they have ApoE2 allele protecting them from the development of dementia (Prasher et al. 1997).

The quality of life (QOL) and the life expectancy for individuals with Down syndrome has improved markedly during the recent decades owing to improved living conditions, availability of antibiotics, and possibilities for surgical correction of anomalies, especially heart defects.

Deletions   A loss of part of a chromosome that can be visualized under a microscope is called a *deletion*. The best-known example is *cri du chat* syndrome, which is characterized by a high-pitched voice and is caused by a deletion in chromosome 5p3. It should be noted that most fetuses with chromosomal aberrations are not viable. About 40 to 50% of spontaneously aborted fetuses have a chromosomal anomaly. In fact, only two of ten fetuses with Down syndrome are born alive.

Malformation Syndromes Due to Microdeletions

A new method of using DNA probes and FISH, in which the chromosomes are treated with specific fluorescent dyes to reveal deviant genes, has brought new light to many of the malformation syndromes previously classified as being of unknown origin. The same submicroscopic deletions (microdeletions) of DNA have been reported in chromosome 15q11–12 in the *Prader–Willi syndrome* and *Angelman syndrome*, despite the fact that these syndromes have different phenotypes. Persons with Angelman syndrome are severely retarded, unable to speak, atactic, have a large mouth, and characteristically are constantly laughing. The Prader–Willi babies are hypotonic, and have small hands and feet. They are mildly to moderately retarded. Prader–Willi syndrome results when the microdeletion is in the chromosome of paternal origin, and the Angelman syndrome results when it is of maternal origin (Bregman and Hoop 1991, Knoll et al. 1993). About 70% of the individuals with these syndromes have *de novo* deletions without recurrence risk in the family. The rest have several complicated genetic patterns that need advanced techniques for diagnostic assessment. Persons with the Prader–Willi syndrome develop, after having been poor feeders as babies, an excessive appetite and indiscriminate eating habits that lead often to severe obesity. Because this syndrome has no clear pathognomonic features, it may remain undiagnosed and such individuals might even be referred for psychiatric treatment because of an eating disorder. Obviously, psychological factors are not the primary cause here, but supportive psychotherapy might be helpful. The treatment is based on behavioral modification and imposing strict environmental limits on food intake as well as necessary educational and habilitative programming. Initially, it was found that one of four persons with the *Rubinstein–Taybi syndrome* had a microdeletion in chromosome 16p13.3 (Breuning et al. 1993). Since then, even smaller percentages of deletion have been found among individuals with this syndrome diagnosed clinically. What the connection is between this deletion and the phenotype is not known at the present time. The aortic stenosis in *Williams syndrome* has been linked to the elastin gene on chromosome 7. Microdeletion in this location has been documented in up to 90% of the cases (Ewart et al. 1993). The phenotype of the Williams syndrome includes short stature, aortic stenosis or other congenital heart defects, and hypercalcemia in childhood. The facial appearance is characteristic and may include periorbital fullness, a long philtrum, full lips with open mouth, a stellate iris pattern, and early graying of hair. The behavioral phenotype may also be characteristic and includes an outgoing personality and overwhelming talkativeness that might even tax the caregivers' patience. The symptoms vary, however, and even autistic disorder and aggressiveness have been found in these individuals.

Velocardiofacial syndrome (VCFS), also called *Shprinzen* or *CATCH 22 syndrome*, has been recognized by cleft palate (at least submucosal), congenital heart or major vascular anomaly, high nasal bridge, and overfolding of earlobe. Persons with this syndrome have mild developmental delay/learning disabilities and are at significant risk for psychiatric disorders including attention deficit/hyperactivity disorder (ADHD) and psychosis. With FISH method, it has been possible to demonstrate microdeletion at the 22q11.2 site. The prevalence of VCFS is estimated to be 1 in 2000 live births.

Table 4-3	Examples of Various Malformation Syndromes Connected with Mental Retardation*
Syndrome	**Features**
Chromosomal aberrations	
Trisomy 21: Down syndrome	See text
Trisomy 13 syndrome	IQ < 50; growth retardation; polydactyly; holoprosencephaly; ear, eye, and scalp defects; CHD
Deletion 5p: *cri du chat* syndrome	IQ 20–50, growth retardation, microcephaly, catlike cry, hypertelorism, epicanthus
Malformation syndromes due to microdeletions	
Prader–Willi syndrome	IQ 20–80, almond-shaped eyes, small hands and feet, cryptorchidism, hypotonia, obesity
Angelman's (happy puppet) syndrome	IQ < 50, ataxia, seizures, microbrachycephaly, large mouth, prognathism, jerky gait
Williams' syndrome	IQ 40–80, long philtrum, prominent lips, supravalvular aortic stenosis, loquacious, "cocktail party manners," hypercalcemia in infancy
Rubinstein–Taybi syndrome	IQ 20–85; growth retardation; beaked, long nose; broad thumbs; narrow palate
Malformation syndromes of unknown cause	
De Lange's syndrome	IQ < 50, growth retardation, microcephaly, hirsutism, synophrys, anteverted nostrils
Sotos' syndrome	Sometimes mental retardation, large size, macrocephaly, prognathism, downward-slanting palpebral fissures
Prenatal infections	
Congenital rubella pigmentation	± Mental retardation, microcephaly, hearing loss, cataracts, CHD, microphthalmia, retinal
Toxoplasmosis	± Mental retardation hydrocephalus microcephaly, chorioretinitis, cataracts, intracranial calcifications, hepatosplenomegaly
Toxic agents	
Fetal hydantoin syndrome	± Mental retardation, growth retardation, short nose, hypertelorism, cleft lip, CHD

* CHD, Congenital heart disease.
Source: Data from Jones KL (1988) Smith's Recognizable Patterns of Human Malformation, 4th ed. W. B. Saunders, Philadelphia.

These syndromes had previously been classified as malformation syndromes of unknown origin (see later in the chapter), but because of the described findings of microdeletions, they are now placed in a separate category between chromosomal aberrations and monogenic mutations (Tables 4-2 and 4-3).

Monogenic Mutations

A mutation in a gene results in the production of a faulty protein (usually an enzyme) coded for by this gene. This, in turn, adversely influences the organism's development, producing a disorder specific to the mutation. The inheritance might be dominant or recessive, but the actual effect of the faulty gene also depends on the penetrance and expressivity.

Disorders with Autosomal Dominant Inheritance
Tuberous sclerosis is an example of the disorders in this group, which might be associated with mental retardation. It is caused by a mutation in a gene affecting the formation of the ectodermal layer of the embryo. Because the skin and the CNS develop from this layer, abnormalities are seen in both. The skin lesions include angiofibromas in the form of macules on the cheeks (*adenoma sebaceum*), with a butterfly-like distribution, especially after puberty. *Café au lait* spots or nonpigmented ash leaf–shaped areas are also found. Mental retardation, epilepsy, and calcifications in the brain are seen, as are tumors. Epileptic seizures often begin as infantile spasms, which should alert the physician to look for other symptoms of this disorder. If tuberous sclerosis is diagnosed, both parents should be examined carefully because the mutation is inherited in about 28% of cases. Because of the dominant inheritance, the risk of recurrence is 50% for each pregnancy. The expression of this gene mutation varies from small skin discolorations (which may indicate a carrier state) to multiple disabling conditions. It is a relatively rare disorder (with a prevalence of 1 in 30 000 to 1 in 50 000 live births), but it may be found in about 0.5% of persons with severe mental retardation.

Disorders with Autosomal Recessive Inheritance
Most metabolic disorders belong to this category. They are caused by single mutated genes that disturb the metabolism by deficient enzyme activity. The risk of healthy carrier parents having an affected child is 25% for each pregnancy. The diagnosis is made by detection of abnormal metabolic products in the urine, blood, or tissues and/or by low or absent enzyme activity. When there is high clinical suspicion and the possibility of gene detection, direct DNA techniques might be used. The metabolism of amino acids, carbohydrates, lipids, and mucopolysaccharides is affected in different disorders. A few examples of inborn errors of metabolism are given in Table 4-4. PKU is the best known and the most common of the metabolic disorders, with a prevalence of about 1 in 10 000 live births. The enzymatic defect is diminished activity of phenylalanine hydroxylase, which leads to a high serum phenylalanine level affecting, among other things, myelination of the CNS. It was described in 1934 by Folling in 10 children with mental retardation, hypertonia, and hyperreflexia, with a musty odor in urine and sweat. Seizures and tremors are common, as are eczema and psychotic manifestations. The clinical symptoms can be prevented by use of a low-phenylalanine diet soon after birth. In most developed countries, all newborns are screened for PKU. Increasingly, a lifelong low-phenylalanine diet is recommended to prevent later deterioration in cognitive functions. Women with PKU who were successfully treated do not have clinical manifestations themselves but still have phenylalanine blood levels high enough to cause brain damage to a fetus if they become pregnant. To avoid this, they should start to follow the diet again before they become pregnant.

The phenylalanine hydroxylase gene has been mapped to 12q22–24.1. Prenatal diagnosis and carrier detection are possible.

Table 4-4	Examples of Inborn Errors of Metabolism Causing Mental Retardation*			
Disorder	Enzyme Defect	Onset/Life Expectancy	Clinical Features	Laboratory Diagnosis/Treatment
Aminoacidurias				
PKU	Phenylalanine hydroxylase	I/A	If not on diet: vomiting, musty odor, eczema, seizures, tremors, psychosis	U: ferric chloride test; gene locus 12q22–24; diet: low in phenylalanine
Homocystinuria	Cystathionine β-synthetase	I/A	Seizures, venous thromboses→cerebrovascular accidents, Marfan's habitus, malar flush, lens subluxation, often MR	U: cyanide-nitroprusside test
Lysosomal disorders				
Glycoproteinoses				
Mannosidosis	Mannosidase	6–36 mo/A	Coarse facial features, short stature, skeletal changes, hepatosplenomegaly, loose joints, hearing loss, ataxia	U: oligosaccharides
I-cell disease	Multiple lysosomal hydrolases	I/2–8 yr	Early facial feature coarsening, short stature, stiffness of joints, gum hyperplasia	U: sialyl oligosaccharides
Mucopolysaccharidoses				
MPS I (Hurler's)	L-Iduronidase	I/10 yr	Early facial feature coarsening, hepatosplenomegaly, growth failure, corneal clouding, skeletal changes	U: heparan sulfate, dermatan sulfate
MPS II (Hunter's)	Iduronidate sulfatase	I/15 yr	Symptoms milder and progression slower than in MPS I	U: heparan sulfate, dermatan sulfate
Sphingolipidoses				
Tay–Sachs (GM$_2$)	GM$_2$ ganglioside–N-acetylhexosaminidase	3–6 mo/2–3 yr	Hypotonia→rigidity, macularcherry red spot→blindness, seizures, hyperacusis	Serum hexosaminidase assay
Metachromatic leukodystrophy	Arylsulfatase A deficiency	1–4 yr/10–15 yr	Gait disturbance, ataxia, motor incoordination	U: metachromatic cells, sulfatase A assay; sural nerve biopsy

* All disorders cause mental retardation except that in homocystinuria it does not occur in every case. Dietary treatment benefits patients with PKU and galactosemia. Prenatal diagnosis is available for all disorders. Inheritance is autosomal recessive, except for MPS II and Lesch–Nyhan which are X-linked. I, Infancy; A, adulthood; U, urinary; MR, mental retardation.
Source: Adapted from Nelhaus G, Stumpf DA, and Moe PG (1984) Neurologic and muscular disorders. In *Current Pediatric Diagnosis and Treatment*, 8th ed., Kempe CH, Silver HK, and O'Brien D (eds). Large Medical Publications, Los Altos, CA, pp. 628–711; Robinson A, Goodman SI, and O'Brian D (1984) Neurologic and muscular disorders. In *Current Pediatric Diagnosis and Treatment*, 8th ed., Kempe CH, Silver HK, and O'Brien D (eds). Lange Medical Publications, Los Altos, CA, pp. 992–1030. Copyright 1984 Appleton & Lange.

The incidence of PKU varies among populations. In the United States, it is 1 in 8000 live births among whites and about 1 in 50 000 live births among African-Americans.

X-Linked Mental Retardation
Fragile X syndrome (fraX) is the most common inherited form of mental retardation and, after Down syndrome, its most common genetic form. It is X-linked, with dominant inheritance, and the penetrance is lower in females. Because of a constriction at the location Xq27.3, it appears as if the chromosome is fragile and a part of it is breaking off. Demonstrating this phenomenon requires a folate-poor cell

culture medium. Fragile X syndrome was first reported by Lubs (1969) and was connected to the clinical syndrome by Harvey in 1977 (Harvey et al. 1977). It has been studied more consistently since the early 1980s when the connection with folate-poor medium was identified. The prevalence was thought to be as high as 1/1000 in males, but reexamination of the individuals suspected of this disorder by the means of DNA technique gave a more realistic figure of 1/4000 in males (Turner et al. 1996).

The genetic defect involved in the fragile X-linked mental retardation has been traced to the *FMR1* gene, an unstable region, where there is a mutation consisting of repeats of the triplet nucleotide CGG (cytosine and guanine). The normal X chromosome has only 6 to 50 copies of this triplet; asymptomatic carrier females or males have 50 to 200 copies (premutation), and affected males have over 200 copies (full mutation). Half the children born to carrier women receive the X chromosome with the mutated *FMR1* gene. It may remain as a premutation (in 20%) or increase to a full mutation (triplet repeat expansion), which causes mental retardation in males. Only a full mutation is associated with clinical symptoms but only about half of females with a full mutation have cognitive deficits. Methylation of fully mutated gene causes inactivation of FMR-protein (FMRP), which is the basic defect in the fragile X syndrome (Tassone et al. 1999). The range of the triplet repeats can be demonstrated by the Southern Blot Technique, which is now used for the diagnosis of fragile X syndrome and the carrier state. An excellent review of the fragile X syndrome has been provided by Sutherland, one of the pioneers in the research of this condition (Sutherland et al. 1993).

About 20% of the sons of carrier females with a premutation have normal intelligence and phenotype but are carriers; these sons transmit the premutation to all their daughters who, through the expansion mechanism, might produce affected children. Fragile X syndrome is thought to occur in 1 in 1200 newborn boys and in 1 in 2400 newborn girls.

Prepubertal boys with this syndrome look quite normal. They are often restless and hyperactive and have a short attention span. Their developmental milestones, especially speech development, are delayed. After puberty, the characteristic phenotypical features may appear. They include an oblong face, prominent ears and jaw, and macroorchidism. Most have moderate mental retardation, but it is severe in others. Male carriers do not have mental retardation. Females with fragile X syndrome who have the full mutation and are symptomatic usually have learning disabilities or mild mental retardation. Behavioral symptoms have been described in these individuals—hyperactivity and social withdrawal in about 50% and depression in about 25% (Mandel et al. 1992).

Males with fragile X syndrome were initially thought to be at high risk for autistic disorder because of a frequent behavioral pattern that included avoidance of eye contact, echolalia, abnormal staccato speech, stereotypic motor behavior, and unusual responses to sensory stimuli. They are usually able to relate to others, however, and most of them do not have enough symptoms to fulfill the diagnostic criteria for autistic disorder.

The Rett syndrome is found in females only and has been thought to be X-linked. The DSM-IV-TR includes Rett syndrome in the pervasive developmental disorders (PDD) category. Girls with this syndrome have normal development through the first five months of life. Between that age and about 4 years, head growth decelerates. Between 5 and 30 months of age, there is a loss of purposeful hand movements, and the characteristic "hand-washing" mannerism appears. Other symptoms include ataxia, tremor, poorly coordinated gait, teeth grinding, hyperventilation, and often seizure disorder. The deterioration is rapid at the beginning but slows later. Some skills may even be regained occasionally (Hagberg et al. 1983).

The basic cause of Rett syndrome has been the target of extensive research since 1980s. It has been postulated that the mutated gene probably was on the X chromosome because only girls with Rett syndrome were reported. The mutation was thought to be lethal for male fetuses. Females who have a normal second X chromosome survive. The mutation was found to be in the X-linked MECP2 encoding methyl-CpG-binding protein 2 (Amir et al. 1999). This protein is necessary in differentiation of tissues during organogenesis. This mutation is seen in over 90% of cases. In addition, 30 families with more than one affected female have been studied. This mutation was seen in only five of them, and other mutations that were found were "nonsense" or "missense" (Webb and Latif 2001). In this group also, a few boys were seen with atypical, milder symptoms.

Multifactorial Mental Retardation

More than half the individuals with mild mental retardation have no other disability. Their speech development in childhood is delayed, and at school age, they might be described as immature. Some of their first-degree relatives have a history of educational problems. A history of mental illness is also common in these families. The environmental factors and the family's socioeconomic situation are often suboptimal. However, with improvement in medical technologies, detailed assessment of such children has disclosed that biological factors could have contributed to the genesis of mental retardation. In a study of British children with mild mental retardation, genetic factors were estimated to be present in 20% and other biological factors were seen in an additional 37%. In almost 40% of the cases with a background of biological factors, the families also had a history of school problems. Thus, in these children, environmental and socioeconomic as well as genetic and biological factors are probably involved (Lamont and Dennis 1988, Hagberg et al. 1981). This form of mental retardation has variously been called nonorganic, familial, cultural–familial, or retardation owing to psychosocial disadvantage. Our understanding of the basic pathological features of this entity is vague. It is certain that many individuals with mental retardation have been labeled with these terms because of lack of a better alternative.

Prenatal Causes: Malformations and Malformation Syndromes of Unknown Cause

Various congenital (present at the time of birth but not necessarily genetic) structural malformations or anomalies are placed in this category. They usually occur during organogenesis of the embryo and are seen in about 3% of newborns. Up to 40% of persons with mental retardation of unknown cause have three or more major or minor anomalies.

Major malformations result from an intrinsic error in organogenesis, an example of which is cleft lip. Minor malformations or dysmorphic features, such as epicanthal folds and simian palmar creases, do not cause functional problems, but they are a sign of disturbance in organogenesis. Deformation is defined as an abnormality of a body part caused by mechanical compression, such as club foot. Disruption is destruction of a previously normal structure. These should not be considered malformations because their origin is extrinsic and they usually occur later than malformations (Graham 1992).

Malformations may occur as single entities or in more or less defined combinations or syndromes that carry a specific name. With medical diagnostic advances, when the causation and pathogenesis of many of these syndromes are identified, they are better classified in another category. A good example is Down syndrome, which includes a number of malformations. With the elucidation of its genetic mechanism, it is now placed in the category of genetic disorders (chromosomal aberrations). Angelman and Williams syndromes, formerly classified as malformation syndromes of unknown origin, belong now to microdeletions, a subgroup of genetic causation.

Malformations of the Central Nervous System

The development of the CNS begins at the third and fourth weeks of gestation when the neural plate twists itself into a neural tube; development and maturation continue several years after birth.

The CNS malformations may be connected with genetic abnormalities or may be caused by external insults and are then classified accordingly. Those with unknown causes are classified in this group.

Holoprosencephaly is connected with midfacial anomalies and may occur as part of other syndromes, for example, trisomy 13. *Anencephaly* originates from day 26 of gestation. *Microcephaly* may be connected with chromosomal anomalies; may have autosomal dominant, recessive, or X-linked inheritance; and may result from arrested brain growth caused by factors such as prenatal and neonatal viral infections as well as intracranial hemorrhage. Disturbances during the cell migration that occurs from 7 to 24 weeks of gestation may result in cortical gyrus anomalies—*lissencephaly* (nongyral cortex) and *pachygyria* (broad gyri). These may also be connected with chromosomal deletions. An example is the *Miller–Dieker syndrome* with multiple major and minor anomalies. Agenesis of the *corpus callosum* also originates from a disturbance of cell migration and is connected with many syndromes. Occasionally, it is also seen on neuroimaging studies of nonsymptomatic individuals. Hydrocephalus (enlargement of ventricles with increased cerebrospinal fluid volume) may be the result of an unknown malformation, but it can also have X-linked inheritance, develop in connection with meningomyelocele, or result from pre-, neo-, or postnatal infection, tumors, and other causes.

Neural tube defects are examples of severe CNS malformations known to be multifactorial—partly genetic and partly extrinsic in origin. Their incidence is between 1 and 2 in 1000 births (Graham 1992). They have assumed a new importance because it has been shown that they might be preventable to a large extent by vitamin (folic acid) supplementation before conception and in early pregnancy (Czeizel and Dudas 1992). They range from anencephaly (which results in a nonviable child) to an asymptomatic, usually undiagnosed, occult *spina bifida*. *Meningomyelocele* is a neural tube defect characterized by various neurological deficits, depending on the level of involvement of the spinal cord. It is often associated with other CNS malformations, especially hydrocephalus, that may result in mental retardation. However, there are severely disabled individuals with meningomyelocele who have intact intelligence.

Malformation Syndromes of Unknown Origin

An estimated 50% or more of the malformation syndromes have no known cause. Many of these syndromes are known by the name of their discoverer (see Table 4-4). In clinical practice, however, one often encounters malformation syndromes that have not been formally described and named; these are sometimes called *private syndromes*. With improved genetic techniques, the cause of many of these malformations will certainly be delineated.

External Prenatal Causes

External prenatal causes include the deleterious effects of identifiable external factors on the developing fetus. These external prenatal causes are estimated to be responsible for 6 to 15% of mental retardation cases (McQueen et al. 1986, Blomquist et al. 1981).

Maternal Infections

Viral infections in the mother can interfere with organogenesis, and the earlier in pregnancy they occur, the more severe their effect will be, as exemplified by *congenital rubella*. Rubella infection during the first month of pregnancy affects the organogenesis of 50% of embryos. Infection in the third month of pregnancy still disturbs the development of 15% of fetuses. Various systems are affected, and as a result, symptoms and impairments may vary and include mental retardation, microcephaly, hearing and vision impairment, congenital heart disease, and behavior problems. Fortunately, the incidence of congenital rubella has greatly decreased because of the availability of immunization for prospective mothers.

Congenital cytomegalovirus infection may result in microcephaly, sensorineural hearing loss, and psychomotor retardation. Antibodies against cytomegalovirus are found in about 80% of adults. Depending on the population, primary infections occur during 2 to 5% of pregnancies. Cytomegalovirus inclusion bodies are seen in urine specimens of newborns who were infected prenatally.

Congenital toxoplasmosis may result in significant problems in about 20% of infected infants (hydrocephalus, microcephaly, psychomotor retardation, vision and hearing impairment) and in milder developmental problems later in life.

Congenital human immunodeficiency virus infection has been increasing in importance. In a German study of 41 children born to human immunodeficiency virus–positive mothers, neurological symptoms were described at 1 to 7 years of age (Schmitt et al. 1991). Human immunodeficiency virus encephalopathy was characterized by microcephaly, progressive neurological deterioration, mental retardation, cerebellar symptoms, and behavioral changes. Prophylactic intravenous immunoglobulin therapy with and without zidovudine was often able to prevent regression. Improvement was seen with zidovudine treatment.

Toxic Substances

The most important of the teratogenic substances is ethanol, which is the cause of *fetal alcohol syndrome* (FAS). The prevalence of this syndrome varies around the world, but its occurrence in industrialized countries is estimated to be about 1 in 1000 newborns. When used heavily during pregnancy, alcohol causes abnormalities in three main categories: (1) dysmorphic features, which originate in the period of organogenesis; (2) pre- and postnatal growth retardation, including microcephaly; and (3) CNS dysfunction, including mild to moderate mental retardation, delay in motor development, hyperactivity, and attention deficit. The severity of the symptoms is related to the amount of alcohol ingested (Coles 1993). In a milder condition, called *fetal alcohol effects* (FAE), only two of the three main features are seen. Poor academic achievement and behavior problems are typical for these children. Social environmental factors during the early years have an important role in the outcome.

Some "prescription drugs" may have various teratogenic effects. *Fetal hydantoin syndrome* (FHS) has long been known, and alternative drugs are recommended for seizure control in pregnant women.

Toxemia of Pregnancy and Placental Insufficiency

Intrauterine growth retardation has many causes, the most important being maternal toxemia with its consequences, ending in insult to the CNS (Figure 4-3). Prematurity may be of maternal or fetal origin. When it is connected with fetal developmental deviations, the prognosis depends on the infant's general condition. Prematurity and especially intrauterine growth retardation predispose to many perinatal complications, which may result in insult to the CNS and developmental problems.

Perinatal Causes

The period referred to is 1 week before birth to 4 weeks after birth.

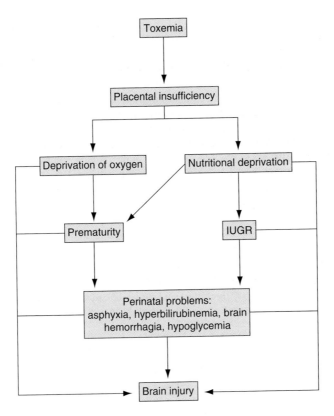

Figure 4-3 *Toxemia of pregnancy and its consequences.*

Infections

During the neonatal period, the most important infection from the point of view of its developmental sequelae is herpes simplex type 2. The neonate is infected during the delivery and may develop encephalitis within two weeks. Early treatment with acyclovir may alleviate the otherwise poor outcome—microcephaly, profound mental retardation, and neurological deficits. Neonatal bacterial infections might result in sepsis and meningitis, which in turn may cause hydrocephalus.

Delivery Problems

During delivery, asphyxia is the most important factor causing an insult to the CNS. It leads to cell death, which might be demonstrated with neuroimaging techniques as leukomalacia. Premature infants and those with intrauterine growth retardation are at special risk for damage to the cortex or the thalamus, which, in addition to affecting intelligence, causes various symptoms of CP and seizure disorder, depending on the location of the pathological condition. It is important to know that asphyxia does not cause mental retardation alone.

Neurological symptoms during the neonatal period have a strong association with prenatal developmental deviations and later with neurological integrity as well as with intellectual level. For these reasons, infants with perinatal problems need a thorough examination for dysmorphic features and close follow-up because multiple disabilities might become evident later in life.

Other Perinatal Problems

Retinopathy of prematurity (formerly referred to as *retrolental fibroplasia*) was seen frequently when the use of 100% oxygen in neonates was common, resulting in blindness. It is often associated with other CNS damage, mental retardation, and other developmental problems. Extremely low-birth-weight infants are at risk for intracranial hemorrhage as well as hypoglycemia resulting from a lack of hepatic glycogen storage. These neonatal problems may have results similar to those of asphyxia. Hyperbilirubinemia may result from increased destruction of red cells (e.g., hemolysis owing to maternal–child blood group incompatibility) or decreased excretion of bilirubin (e.g., owing to an immaturity of liver function). The brain damage that may ensue results in manifestations of various degrees, including CP, sensorineural hearing loss, and mental retardation.

Postnatal Causes

Infections

Bacterial and viral infections of the brain during childhood may cause meningitis and encephalitis and result in permanent damage. The number of these complications has decreased because of improved treatment and the availability of immunizations such as that for measles.

Toxic Substances

Lead poisoning is still an important cause of mental retardation in the United States. The most frequent source of lead is pica—ingestion of flaking old lead-based paint. Other sources of lead are certain fruit tree sprays, leaded gasoline, some glazed pottery, and fumes from burning automobile batteries. Gastrointestinal symptoms dominate in acute poisoning. Headache may be associated with increased intracranial pressure, which may even lead to coma. Late manifestations include developmental retardation, ataxia, seizures, and personality changes.

Other Postnatal Causes

Among childhood malignancies, brain tumors are second in frequency after leukemias. Of these, 70 to 80 are gliomas, symptoms of which depend mostly on the location. Some are benign and treatable but most have deleterious effects resulting in various neuropsychiatric symptoms depending on their location and extent. In addition, treatment such as surgery and radiation might affect the integrity and function of the brain. Traffic accidents, drowning, and other traumas are the most common causes of death during childhood. Even greater is the number of children who become disabled. Near-drowning is often devastating, but even in these cases, improvement of functional capacity may be achieved by rehabilitation because of the ability of the developing brain to recover.

Psychosocial Problems

The developmental level of a growing individual depends on the integrity of the CNS and on environmental and psychological factors. The importance of environmental stimulation for child development has been appreciated since research on children in institutions showed that development was severely affected in a depriving environment, even if there was adequate physical care. Poverty predisposes the child to many developmental risks, such as teenage pregnancies, malnutrition, abuse, poor medical care, and deprivation. Severe maternal mental illness is another risk factor. Mothers with severe and chronic illness might have difficulty in providing adequate care and stimulation. Children of mothers who have schizophrenia are at risk for the development of cognitive deficits (although these may not be secondary to maternal illness but may represent a genetically determined predisposition to schizophrenia). Psychotic illness in a child has been shown to be associated with a decline in cognitive abilities.

Unknown Causes

Despite detailed assessment, no cause can be identified in about 30% of cases of severe mental retardation and in 50% of cases of mild mental retardation (McLaren and Bryson 1987). This, of course, reflects the inadequacy of diagnostic techniques rather than a lack of causation.

Treatment

Mental retardation is a functional disability: thus, the goal of treatment should be to reduce or eliminate the disability. There are three aspects to the treatment:

1. Treatment of the underlying disorder that is causative of mental retardation (e.g., PKU).
2. Treatment of the comorbid disorders that add to the functional disability, whether physical or mental.
3. Interventions targeted at the functional disability of the mental retardation itself: educational, habilitative, and supportive approaches depending on the person's individualized needs.

The current approach to the services for persons with mental retardation is based on the following principles:

- The *normalization principle* (Nirje 1969), which refers to "making available to the mentally retarded patterns and conditions of everyday life that are as close as possible to the norms and patterns of the mainstream of society." This has largely evolved into the *principle of inclusion*, which is usually interpreted as an active effort to include persons with mental retardation in all normal aspects and opportunities of society's life, through providing them with supports necessary for success. The ultimate goal is to eventually end segregated services and education and provide persons with mental retardation with the necessary, specialized support services in regular educational, living, and work settings.
- The *right to community living*, which confers the right to live with a family, preferably one's own or a substitute one if necessary (foster or adoptive). This includes moving individuals living in large residential facilities to as normal a setting as possible, for example, community residences, supervised apartments, and foster homes. Furthermore, children are not to be institutionalized, regardless of the level of retardation, and, generally, neither are adults. However, some children are still placed in special residential schools (usually private) for specific reasons, typically medical or behavioral needs that require specialized treatment. Historically, a majority of persons with mental retardation lived at home and no more than 10% were in institutions at any point. However, institutions played a disproportionate role in attitudes to their care. At their peak in 1967, there were 194,650 persons living in them: this number dropped to 52,801 in 1998. In 2000, there were eight states that closed all their large residential facilities. In contrast, the number of persons living in small (less than six persons) residences in the community increased dramatically (Braddock et al. 2000).
- *Education and training for all children* to a maximum possible extent, regardless of their disability and the degree of the disability, by including them full time in an age-appropriate regular classroom. This educational program is individualized according to the child's needs. Services of special educators and therapists, as necessary, are also provided in these programs. This has to be distinguished from mainstreaming, which

refers to placement in special classes in regular schools but with participation in some activities of regular classes.
- *Employment of adults in the community* according to their abilities is another aspect of inclusion. The current trend is to employ them in competitive job markets with supports, such as vocational training and supports by job coaches. However, many individuals, especially with severe degrees of disability, are still placed in sheltered workshops or occupational–recreational day programs.
- *Use of normal community services and facilities* (shopping, banking, transportation, recreation) through training and ongoing supports.
- *Advocacy and appropriate protective measures*, for example, against inappropriate use of pharmacological and behavioral measures as substitutes for active education and treatment, inclusion in research programs without proper, truly informed consent, and general exploitation and abuse.

Prevention of Mental Retardation

Primary Prevention   The goal of primary prevention is to prevent mental retardation from arising in the first place. To be effective, it should encompass medical, public health, educational, and other measures. Examples include, immunizations to prevent congenital rubella, measles (encephalitis), and Rh mother–child incompatibility; measures to prevent lead poisoning and teenage pregnancies; provision of prenatal vitamin supplementation (to prevent neural tube defects); better neonatal care; measures to prevent substance abuse in pregnancy and childhood trauma (e.g., the use of infant car seats), and early intervention and enrichment programs for children at psychosocial risk. It is a question of personal values whether prenatal diagnosis and elective termination of pregnancy (e.g., if Down syndrome is found) would be called primary prevention, as childbirth rather than the disorder is prevented.

Secondary Prevention   Secondary prevention includes measures to recognize conditions that can lead to mental retardation as early as possible and to treat them to prevent retardation. Examples include the early diagnosis and treatment of PKU and other metabolic conditions and congenital hypothyroidism.

Tertiary Prevention   Tertiary prevention could be called habilitation as well (Rowitz 1986) because it aims to attain a functional level that is as good as possible in the presence of mental retardation. It includes both biomedical and sociocultural measures, such as early intervention for disabled infants, proper education, multifaceted family support, and prevention or early treatment of comorbid disorders that could reduce functioning, both medical and mental.

Prevention of Psychosocial Dysfunction   An essential part of tertiary prevention consists of preventing psychosocial dysfunction because mental disorders are an important cause of maladaptation in persons with mental retardation (Szymanski 1987). This category can also be subdivided. *Primary prevention* includes proper education and employment and opportunities to achieve in life so that the person can develop a sense of self-worth and self-esteem; training in social skills and sexuality; and provision of appropriate social supports and recreation. *Secondary prevention* includes early diagnosis and treatment of emerging mental disorders rather than a focus on behavioral crisis intervention only. *Tertiary prevention* includes good psychiatric care and habilitation as well as a proper milieu when a person has a chronic mental illness (including substance abuse) that requires continuous care. In all situations, prevention has to include measures directed at both the person and the environment (caregivers, services, public policies).

Overall Goals of Psychiatric Treatment of Persons with Mental Retardation

The most common mistake made by mental health clinicians treating persons with mental retardation is to consider suppression (usually with medications) of single problems (as a rule disruptive behaviors) as the only goal of treatment. This approach used to be the rule in the past when people with mental retardation were not expected to achieve any measure of independence and keeping them docile was the goal. Lately, such approaches are reemerging, partly related to the pressure from insurers to achieve a fast and inexpensive symptomatic improvement, even if short lived. Fortunately, in the past three decades, the quality of life (QOL) has been assuming a central role as the goal of treatment in the mental retardation field. Numerous scales to measure the QOL have been designed, usually focused on concrete indicators related to factors such as services or health and typically reflecting the view of the caregivers. More recently, the importance of the subjective aspects of QOL have been stressed: the individual's subjective feeling of contentment, well-being, and satisfaction with his or her own life as opposed to the caregiver's satisfaction. In other words, personal happiness of the person with mental retardation is now stressed as a goal of habilitation as well as specific treatment (Szymanski 2000). The measurement of the latter is not easy with nonverbal persons, or even with verbal ones, considering their tendency to answer in a way to please the questioner. Thus, both self report from the individual and observations by trained team of professionals are needed. A sense of positive self-image is an essential part of feeling happiness for persons with mental retardation, as for everyone else. This is often difficult for the former to acquire, because of the awareness of being "different" from others, at least in terms of many abilities, and because of frequent rejection and teasing.

The goal of any form of psychiatric treatment of persons with mental retardation is to contribute to this sense of satisfaction with one's own life, or happiness, in the context of a comprehensive treatment program. Suppression of behaviors inconvenient to caregivers is not enough, especially if they are a response to an inadequate habilitation program and the treatment (usually medications) is used in lieu of such a program. Furthermore, medications may suppress a person's functioning through side effects such as drowsiness. The mental health clinician should not assume that "nonpsychiatric" problems are taken care of by someone else, but should take an active part in the team's assessment of various factors contributing to the clinical presentation, as well as the person's need for various supports. This is not to say that the psychiatrist should be in charge of behavioral modification or vocational rehabilitation, but that these approaches should be closely coordinated with specific psychiatric treatments and should be targeted toward the common therapeutic goal.

Principles of the Use of Psychotropic Drugs

This outline is based largely on an excellent review of Kalachnik and coworkers, Rinck (1998), as well as on the American Academy of Child and Adolescent Psychiatry (1999), and the Health Care Financing Administration (1997).

Purpose of Drug Use

These drugs are used to treat a diagnosed mental disorder toward the goal of maximizing a person's quality of life. They should not be used merely to suppress a single, objectionable behavior without regard to the effect on a person's global adjustment, functioning, and quality of life. They cannot be used as punishment, for staff convenience (such as in understaffed facilities), in lieu of appropriate habilitative programs (if such is unavailable), or in dosages that interfere with such programs and with a person's quality of life (Rinck 1998, page 52).

Context of Drug Use

These drugs are always used as part of a comprehensive, treatment/habilitation program designed and supervised by an interdisciplinary team of which the psychiatric clinician is an integral part. They should not be prescribed merely in brief "psychopharmacology consultation" or "medication review," in isolation from other aspects of the treatment.

Prerequisites for Drug Use

1. Comprehensive psychiatric diagnostic assessment resulting in a psychiatric diagnosis.
2. Presence of a comprehensive treatment plan and evidence that less-intrusive measures have not been effective (such as behavior modification, psychotherapies, milieu supports, etc.).
3. Comprehensive evaluation to rule out medical conditions that could have caused the presenting symptoms.
4. Existence of a reliable system to collect behavioral data individualized to the particular individual that measures occurrence of symptoms considered an index of the person's mental disorder. This should also provide reliable baseline data and functional analysis of behavior that would assess the influence of immediate and more remote antecedents and consequences of the individual's behaviors and other symptoms.
5. Satisfaction of all relevant regulatory and legal requirements, especially obtaining informed consent of the individual with mental retardation and/or legal guardian.

Follow-up on Drug Effectiveness

1. The members of the interdisciplinary treatment team should follow the individual's progress regularly (at least quarterly), based on changes in individualized index behaviors, symptoms, general adjustment, functioning, and well being. Presence of side effects and their findings should be communicated among the members of the team. Behavioral changes should be documented by reliable data. The follow-up should include a direct psychiatric interview and/or observation of the individual. The implementation of all aspects of the treatment program and not just the medications should be monitored and adjusted as needed to insure that medications are not used in lieu of, but concurrently with, a habilitation program.
2. The medication should be tried at an effective dose for an adequate period of time. If there is no clear evidence of effectiveness it should be discontinued appropriately. It should be kept in mind that "ups and downs" are to be expected, such as in reaction to environmental and physical stressors common in the lives of these individuals. Medication effectiveness should therefore be judged by a pattern evident over a reasonable period of time and not by one-point observations. For the same reason, preset dosage schedules linking dosage changes to specific frequencies of index behaviors are impractical. Multiple medications should be tried only if there is evidence that a combination is known to be more effective than a single medication.

Dosages and Discontinuation

1. The optimal dosage is the lowest one that achieves the best compromise between improving the individual's quality of life and side effects.
2. A trial of dose reduction and possibly discontinuation should be regularly considered but should be implemented only if not contraindicated clinically. Discontinuation, if attempted, should be gradual, and it may need a prolonged period depending on the type of medication and expected withdrawal effects. It is essential that all involved caregivers be aware of the possibility of such effects and be ready to deal with them, rather than

demand immediate cessation of the discontinuation trial (this is particularly important with antipsychotics).

3. As-needed (prn) use of the medication is best avoided to prevent unnecessary use, or limited to clear situations, such as premedication prior to medical tests if stressful for the individual.

Monitoring Side Effects

Side effects should be monitored regularly through direct examination (especially important with nonverbal persons), laboratory tests, tardive dyskinesia examination, and so on, as appropriate for the particular drug. Possible drug interactions should be monitored, as these individuals are often on multiple medications.

Review of Classes of Psychotropic Drugs

Only issues specific to persons with mental retardation are discussed here.

Neuroleptics (Antipsychotics)

The use of antipsychotic drugs in persons with mental retardation is the same as that for the general population—primarily for the treatment of psychosis, sometimes for Tourette's disorder, and as an emergency treatment of dangerous behavior. The problem with persons with mental retardation, as described above, is in making the correct diagnosis of psychosis, especially schizophrenia. Perhaps because of the difficulty (or ignorance) of making a more specific diagnosis, antipsychotic agents have been used for "off-label" indications, such as aggression, destructiveness, SIB, and any disruptive behavior. While these medications may sometimes be effective in these cases, success cannot be reliably predicted. If the drug is effective in alleviating such behaviors, it does not necessarily mean that the individual had a psychotic disorder. The recognition of side effects might be difficult in persons with limited language, and extended observation by trained staff may be necessary. Drowsiness might have an adverse effect on learning and on general level of activity. A common mistake is to confuse akathisia, especially upon withdrawal, with reemergence of behavior problems and to make the disorder worse by increasing the dose. Many adults with mental retardation have been on older antipsychotics for years, often for no clear reason. Many of these individuals have side effects such as Parkinsonian symptoms, and tardive dyskinesia (that might appear only upon discontinuation trial). Because of a higher tendency to cause adverse effects (to which this population might be more susceptible), these drugs (thioridazine in particular) are being discontinued and, if necessary, changed to newer, second generation antipsychotics. The latter are, of course, not free from side effects and new types of side effects may yet emerge. Weight gain, especially from olanzapine and clozapine, might be particularly severe and troublesome. The discontinuation of antipsychotic medications should be gradual and slow to minimize side effects from withdrawal, including behavior problems such as irritability, insomnia, SIB, and aggression (Gualtieri et al. 1986). Clonidine might be helpful for these symptoms.

There are case reports of successful use of clozapine in persons with mental retardation and schizophrenia or bipolar disorder who did not respond to other agents. The need for weekly blood tests may be a problem in less than cooperative persons.

Antidepressants

The principal uses of antidepressant medications, as in the general population, include treatment of depression as well as anxiety, panic, and obsessive compulsive disorder (OCD) (Sovner et al. 1998). Selective serotonin reuptake inhibitors (SSRIs) are now first-line drugs because of favorable effectiveness/side effect profile. Tricyclic antidepressants, principally desipramine, were used in the treatment of ADHD if stimulants and clonidine were not effective, but there has been concern about cardiotoxic side effects. Precipitation of excitement, mania, and seizures by antidepressants might be a problem, and careful prior diagnostic assessment and follow-up are necessary. There are a few studies, mostly case reports, that have suggested that selective serotonin reuptake inhibitors might be helpful in reducing self-stimulatory, ritualistic, and self-injurious behaviors, although the improvement might be short-lived. In some cases where antidepressants are effective in reducing aggressive behavior, there is the possibility that they actually might help the underlying depression that has led to the aggression.

Antianxiety Drugs

Benzodiazepines have been used for alleviation of anxiety, but their side effects, such as paradoxical rage reactions, adverse effects on cognition, and serious withdrawal symptoms argue against their chronic use, and a trial of an SSRI might be preferable. Occasional use might be helpful in emergency situations in which extreme anxiety is present as well as in preparation for anxiety-inducing medical procedures. The usefulness of buspirone, a nonsedating anxiolytic, with short half-life in persons with combined anxiety and aggression or SIB, has been suggested by one study. Benzodiazepines are still used for the treatment of generalized anxiety and panic disorders, but usually only when there is no response to antidepressants. There is still a fair amount of combined use of neuroleptics and anxiolytics, especially in institutionalized persons with a history of aggression. However, this may lead to significant CNS depression, and benzodiazepine use might actually lead to disinhibition (Werry 1998). Therefore, prolonged use of anxiolytics to control undesirable behaviors is generally not recommended (Werry 1998).

As with other medications, comprehensive diagnostic assessment is a prerequisite to the use of anxiolytics. In particular, environmental anxiety-provoking factors have to be ruled out and, if present, have to be dealt with in addition to pharmacological means if these are used.

Mood Stabilizers

The use of these agents in persons with and without mental retardation is similar. Lithium carbonate, the original mood stabilizer, was shown to be effective for bipolar disorders in persons with mental retardation during the 1970s. However, it has considerable side effects and managing them may be difficult in persons who might be less than cooperative. It has been supplanted increasingly by anticonvulsants, including carbamazepine, valproic acid, as well as newer ones, like gabapentin and lamotrigine. Currently, the primary use is in the treatment of mania and for augmentation of antidepressants. There are also studies that indicate the effectiveness in some individuals with implusive aggressive behavior (Craft et al. 1987). Some clinical experiences indicate that the prognosis might be better in the presence of mood lability and an abnormal electroencephalogram. As seizures are frequently associated with mental retardation, these drugs offer a parsimonious way of managing both seizures and behavioral symptoms.

Stimulants

As in persons without mental retardation, drugs such as methylphenidate and dextroamphetamine are effective in the treatment of ADHD (Arnold et al. 1998). They have been studied primarily in children and adolescents with mild mental retardation or PDD. Their effectiveness in persons with significant retardation is less certain. Tics are one side effect of methylphenidate: if the individual is engaging in self-stimulatory behaviors, videotaping might provide a record for later reference regarding whether additional tics have emerged. The diagnosis of ADHD in this population may not be easy, especially in persons with significant mental retardation, as the symptoms have to be assessed in the context of the developmental level.

Other Psychotropic Agents

Propranolol and other beta-adrenergic blockers have been used following earlier reports on the beneficial effects in rage attacks associated with a definite pathological brain condition (Williams et al. 1982). They have been tried extensively in all kinds of aggressive behavior, often with mixed or poor results. Depression might be a side effect of these agents, leading to reduction in the person's functioning, even if the aggressive behaviors might appear to improve, because of apathy induced by the drug. They may be also effective in the treatment of anxiety, especially its somatic symptoms, and for akathisia related to neuroleptic drugs.

Clonidine, a presynaptic alpha-2-adrenergic agonist also used as an antihypertensive, is commonly used in the treatment of ADHD in children without mental retardation, and more recently for children with PDD; there have been case reports of its effectiveness in persons with fragile-X (Hagerman et al. 1998). While tics are not a side effect, drowsiness, hypotension, bradycardia, and skin rash (from patch) might be troublesome. It has also been reported to be effective in some cases of akathisia related to neuroleptic drug withdrawal (Sovner 1995).

Naltrexone, an oral antagonist of endogenous opioid receptors, has been tried in a number of studies in cases of severe SIB, following some case reports of earlier successes with a similar agent, naloxone, which had to be administered parenterally. It appears that it is effective in 35 to 70% of cases, at least for a short time (Sandman et al. 1998).

Other Treatments

For many years, there have been reports of beneficial effects of a variety of treatments, especially in children with PDDs, Down syndrome, and fragile X syndrome. These treatments include various nutritional supplements, vitamin supplements (such as megavitamins, various combinations of vitamins, minerals and enzymes, B_6, B_6 with magnesium, folic acid, etc.), restriction diets (such as diets without certain food additives, gluten, casein, yeast), and so on. Often, these approaches generate considerable excitement both in families and researchers. However, as a rule, they are based on anecdotal reports or studies with methodological problems, results of which are not replicated in well-designed studies (American Academy of Child and Adolescent Psychiatry 1999, Singh et al. 1998). However, one should bear in mind that persons with developmental disabilities, especially PDDs, may have very unusual eating habits resulting in restricted diets. Therefore, in such cases a nutritional consultation is advisable. If a deficiency is found, an appropriate supplementation and correction of dietary habits is, of course, needed. One example is zinc deficiency associated with pica, which was shown to disappear or decrease after treatment with 100 mg of chelated zinc for 2 weeks (Lofts et al. 1990).

Electroconvulsive therapy has fallen into disuse in this population as the result of past inappropriate uses and strict, current regulations. Occasional case reports of its successful use can still be found in the literature.

Psychosocial Interventions

Programmatic and Educational Approaches

The goal of these interventions is to provide a proper living and programmatic environment. For instance, certain persons easily become overstimulated, anxious, and disruptive in noisy and confused large workshops; arranging for a smaller and quieter workroom is preferable to a prescription for a neuroleptic. The vocational and educational program should be individualized and should focus on developing the person's strengths and providing an opportunity for success. In turn, this will lead to results such as an improvement in self-image. Many persons with severe mental retardation are placed in prevocational training indefinitely, for example, screwing or unscrewing nuts and bolts, although no one expects them to ever be employed on an assembly line. They often engage in a struggle with caregivers because of their noncompliance and may resort to aggression, which leads to removal for a "time out" and thus avoidance of a boring task. Creating a more suitable task—even such as making rounds of the workshop to collect or deliver materials—might be more interesting and appropriate. Functional analysis of behavior is an invaluable guide to these interventions. As discussed previously, such approaches should be explored prior to resorting to the use of medications for disruptive behaviors.

Psychotherapies

Individual and group psychotherapies had already been used in persons with mental retardation in the 1930s (Stacey and DeMartino 1957), and there have also been recent case reports on its success. Psychotherapy in this population is not different in nature from psychotherapy in persons with average intelligence and is similar to treating children, inasmuch as in both cases, the techniques and the therapist have to adapt to the developmental needs of the individual. The treatment should be driven by the individual's needs and responses and not by the therapist's theoretical orientation. Detailed techniques that can be used have been described (Szymanski 1980a, Szymanski and Rosefsky 1980). The indications are the presence of concerns and conflicts, especially about oneself; impairments in interpersonal skills; or other mental disturbances that are known to improve through psychotherapy. The prerequisites include communication skills permitting a meaningful interchange with the therapist, an ability to develop even a minimal relationship, and the availability of a trained, experienced, and unprejudiced therapist who is comfortable working in a team setting. From applicable literature, Reiss and Benson (1985) summarized the guidelines for psychotherapy in this population, which include the following:

1. Appropriate goals should be set and should be reconciled with the expectations of the caregivers, the therapist, and the individual with mental retardation. Common goals include improvement in self-image and impulse control, learning to express feelings in a socially appropriate manner, and understanding in a constructive manner one's own disabilities and strengths.
2. Verbal techniques should be adapted to the individual's language and cognitive level, and nonverbal ones should be age-appropriate.
3. Limits and directiveness should be used as needed: nondirective therapy might lead to the individual's confusion.
4. The therapist has to be active (supportive but not paternalistic), has to use herself or himself liberally as a treatment tool, and has to be able to focus on the immediate reality rather than just intellectualize. A mix of techniques, for example, cognitive psychotherapy and behavior modification, may be required.
5. As in all treatment modalities, the therapist should be involved in all aspects of the individual's program and should collaborate with other providers and with the family.

Group psychotherapy might be particularly effective in helping individuals with mental retardation handle issues related to the understanding of their own disability and learn social skills because of the peer support the group offers (Szymanski and Rosefsky 1980). In general, therapy should be seen as a cognitive learning process, using the therapist's support and leading individuals to the acquisition of understanding and necessary skills, both of concrete behaviors and of handling one's own emotions. Group psychotherapy should be differentiated from group counseling, which is usually educational in nature, focused on a specific subject (e.g., sexuality education), and does not have to be conducted by a mental health professional with a therapeutic goal and plan.

Behavioral Treatment

Detailed functional analysis is a prerequisite. This treatment should optimally use rewards that should be age-appropriate, preferably social, and the frequency of rewarding should be adapted to a person's cognitive level, so that he or she can understand why they are given. Consistency and generalization among different settings are essential. Thus, if such techniques are successfully used at the school, the family or other caregivers should be trained to use them at home as well. The focus should not be on elimination of objectionable behaviors only, but on teaching appropriate replacement behaviors. Aversive techniques involving active punishment (electric shocks, spraying of noxious substances into a person's face) are not used except in a few controversial settings. There is a professional consensus that these techniques should not be used at all, or used only when all other techniques have failed and the individual's behavior poses severe danger to herself or himself or to others (such as intractable SIB). Even then, these techniques should be used only if proved effective and for a limited time.

Comparison of DSM-IV/ICD-10 Diagnostic Criteria

The method of defining the levels of severity differ slightly between the two systems. The ICD-10 Diagnostic Criteria for Research define the levels using exact cutoff scores: Mild is defined as 50 to 69, Moderate is defined as 35 to 49, Severe is defined as 20 to 34, and Profound is defined as below 20. In contrast, DSM-IV-TR provides somewhat greater flexibility in relating severity to a given IQ score by defining severity levels using overlapping scores (i.e., mild is 50 to 55, moderate is 35–40 to 50–55, severe is 20–25 to 35–40, and profound is below 20–25). Within the overlapping range, the severity is determined by the level of adaptive functioning.

References

American Academy of Child and Adolescent Psychiatry (1999) Practice parameters for the assessment and treatment of children, adolescents and adults with mental retardation and comorbid mental disorders. *J Am Acad Child Adolesc Psychiatry* **38**(Suppl.), 12.

American Psychiatric Association (2000) *Diagnostic and Statistical Manual of Mental Disorders*, 4th ed., Text Rev. APA, Washington, DC.

Amir RE, Van den Veyver IB, Wan M, et al. (1999) Rett syndrome is caused by mutations in X-linked MECP2, encoding methyl-CpG-binding protein 2. *Nat Genet* **23**, 185–188.

Arnold LE, Gadow K, Pearson DA, et al. (1998) Stimulants. In *Psychotropic Medications and Developmental Disabilities: The International Consensus Handbook*, Reiss S and Aman MG (eds). Ohio State University Nisonger Center, pp. 229–257.

Blomquist HK, Gustavson K-H, and Holmgren G (1981) Mild mental retardation in a northern Swedish county. *J Ment Defic Res* **25**, 169–185.

Braddock D, Hemp R, Parish S, et al. (2000) *The State of the States in Developmental Disabilities: 2000 Study Summary*. Department of Disability and Human Development, University of Illinois, Chicago.

Bregman JD and Hodapp RM (1991) Current developments in the understanding of mental retardation, Part I: biological and phenomenological perspectives. *J Am Acad Child Adolesc Psychiatry* **30**, 707–719.

Breuning MH, Dauwerse HG, Fugazza G, et al. (1993) Rubinstein-Taybi syndrome caused by submicroscopic deletions within 16p13.3. *Am J Hum Genet* **52**, 249–254.

Coles CD (1993) Impact of prenatal alcohol exposure on the newborn and the child. In *Clinical Obstetrics and Gynecology: Toxic Exposure in Pregnancy*, Vol. 2, Woods JR and Rubin MC (eds). JB Lippincott, Philadelphia, pp. 36, 255–266.

Craft M, Ismail IA, Krishnamurti D, et al. (1987) Lithium in the treatment of aggression in mentally handicapped patients. A double-blind trial. *Br J Psychiatry* **150**, 685–689.

Cunniff C (chairperson), Frias JL, Kaye C, et al. (2001) Health supervision for children with Down syndrome. *Pediatrics* **107**, 442–449.

Curry CJ, Stevenson RE, Aughton D, et al. (1997) Evaluation of mental retardation: recommendations of a consensus conference. *Am J Med Genet* **72**, 468–477.

Czeizel A and Dudas I (1992) Prevention of the first occurrence of neural tube defects by periconceptional vitamin supplementation. *N Engl J Med* **327**, 1832–1836.

Ewart AK, Morris CA, Atkinson D, et al. (1993) Hemizygosity at the elastin locus in a developmental disorder, Williams syndrome. *Nat Genet* **5**, 11–16.

Eyman RK, Grossman HJ, Chaney RH, et al. (1990) The life expectancy of profoundly handicapped people with mental retardation. *N Engl J Med* **323**, 584–589.

Graham JM (1992) Congenital anomalies. In *Developmental-Behavioral Pediatrics*, 2nd ed., Levine MD, Carey WB, and Crocker AC (eds). W. B. Saunders, Philadelphia, pp. 229–243.

Gualtieri CT, Schroeder SR, Hicks RE, et al. (1986) Tardive dyskinesia in young mentally retarded individuals. *Arch Gen Psychiatry* **43**, 335–340.

Gustavson KH, Hagberg B, Hagberg G, et al. (1977a) Severe mental retardation in a Swedish county. II. Etiologic and pathogenic aspects of children born 1959–1970. *Neuropaëdiatrie* **8**, 293–304.

Gustavson KH, Holmgren G, Jonsell G, et al. (1977b) Severe mental retardation in children in a northern Swedish county. *J Ment Defic Res* **21**, 161–180.

Hagberg B, Aicardi J, Dias K, et al. (1983) A progressive syndrome of autism, dementia, ataxia, and loss of purposeful hand use in girls: Rett's syndrome: Report of 35 cases. *Ann Neurol* **14**, 471–479.

Hagberg B, Hagberg G, Lewerth A, et al. (1981) Mild mental retardation in Swedish school children. II. Etiologic and pathogenetic aspects. *Acta Paediatr Scand* **70**, 445–452.

Hagerman R, Bregman JD, and Tirosh E (1998) Clonidine. In *Psychotropic Medications and Developmental Disabilities: The International Consensus Handbook*, Reiss S and Aman MG (eds). Ohio State University Nisonger Center, pp. 259–269.

Harvey J, Judge C, and Wiener S (1977) Familial X-linked mental retardation with X chromosome abnormality. *J Med Genet* **14**, 46–50.

Hayes A and Batshaw ML (1993) Down syndrome. *Pediatr Clin N Am* **40**, 523–535.

Health Care Financing Administration (1997) *Psychopharmacological Medications: Safety Precautions for Persons with Developmental Disabilities.* Health Care Financing Administration, Washington, DC.

Huttenlocher PR (1991) Dendritic and synaptic pathology in mental retardation. *Pediatr Neurol* **7**, 79–85.

Jones KL (1988) *Smith's Recognizable Patterns of Human Malformation*, 4th ed. W. B. Saunders, Philadelphia.

Knoll JHM, Wagstaff J, and Lalande M (1993) Cytogenetic and molecular studies in the Prader-Willi and Angelman syndromes: an overview. *Am J Med Genet* **46**, 2–6.

Lamont LA and Dennis NR (1988) Aetiology of mild mental retardation. *Arch Dis Child* **63**, 1032–1038.

Lofts RH, Schroeder SR, and Maier RH (1990) Effects of serum zinc supplementation on pica behavior of persons with mental retardation. *Am J Ment Retard* **95**, 103–109.

Lubs HA (1969) A marker X chromosome. *Am J Hum Genet* **21**, 231–244.

Mandel J-L, Hagerman R, Froster U, et al. (1992) Conference report. fifth international workshop on the fragile X and X-linked mental retardation. *Am J Med Genet* **43**, 5–27.

Massey PS and McDermott S (1995) State-specific rates of mental retardation—United States, 1993. *MMWR* **45**, 61–65.

McLaren J and Bryson SE (1987) Review of recent epidemiological studies of mental retardation: prevalence, associated disorders, and etiology. *Am J Ment Retard* **92**, 243–254.

McQueen PC, Spence MW, Garner JB, et al. (1987) Prevalence of major mental retardation and associated disabilities in the Canadian maritime provinces. *Am J Ment Defic* **91**, 460–466.

McQueen PC, Spence MW, Winsor EJT, et al. (1986) Causal origins of major mental handicap in the Canadian maritime provinces. *Dev Med Child Neurol* **28**, 697–707.

Nelhaus G, Stumpf DA, and Moe PG (1984) Neurologic and muscular disorders. In *Current Pediatric Diagnosis and Treatment*, 8th ed., Kempe CH, Silver HK, and O'Brien D (eds). Large Medical Publications, Los Altos, CA, pp. 628–711.

Nirje B (1969) A Scandinavian visitor looks at US institutions. In *Changing Patterns in Residential Services for the Mentally Retarded*, Wolfensberger W and Kugel R (eds). President's Committee on Mental Retardation, Washington, DC, pp. 51–58.

Prasher VP, Chowdhury TA, Rowe BR, et al. (1997) ApoE genotype and Alzheimer's disease in adults with Down syndrome: meta-analysis. *Am J Ment Retard* **102**, 103–110.

Reiss S (1990) Prevalence of dual-diagnosis in community-based day programs in the Chicago metropolitan area. *Am J Ment Retard* **94**, 578–585.

Reiss S (1992) Assessment of a man with dual diagnosis. *Ment Retard* **30**, 1–6.

Reiss S (1994) *Handbook of Challenging Behavior: Mental Health Aspects of Mental Retardation.* IDS Publishing, Worthington, OH.

Reiss S and Benson BA (1985) Psychosocial correlates of depression in mentally retarded adults: Minimal social support and stigmatization. *Am J Ment Defic* **89**, 331–337.

Rinck C (1998) Epidemiology and psychoactive medication. In *Psychotropic Medications and Developmental Disabilities: The International Consensus Handbook*, Reiss S and Aman MG (eds). Ohio State University Nisonger Center, pp. 31–44.

Robinson A, Goodman SI, and O'Brian D (1984) Neurologic and muscular disorders. In *Current Pediatric Diagnosis and Treatment*, 8th ed., Kempe CH, Silver HK, and O'Brien D (eds). Large Medical Publications, Los Altos, CA, pp. 992–1030.

Rowitz L (1986) Multiprofessional perspectives on prevention (editorial). *Ment Retard* **24**, 1–3.

Sandman CA, Thompson T, Barrett RP, et al. (1998) Opiate blockers. In *Psychotropic Medications and Developmental Disabilities: The International Consensus Handbook*, Reiss S and Aman MG (eds). Ohio State University Nisonger Center, pp. 291–302.

Schmitt B, Seeger J, Kreuz W, et al. (1991) Central nervous system involvement of children with HIV infection. *Dev Med Child Neurol* **33**, 535–540.

Singh NN, Ellis CR, Mulick JA, et al. (1998) Vitamin, mineral and dietary treatments. In *Psychotropic Medications and Developmental Disabilities: The International Consensus Handbook*, Reiss S and Aman MG (eds). Ohio State University Nisonger Center, pp. 311–320.

Sovner R (1995) Thioridazine withdrawal-induce behavioral deterioration treated with clonidine: two case reports. *Ment Retard* **33**, 221–225.

Sovner R, Pary RJ, Dosen A, et al. (1998) Antidepressant drugs. In *Psychotropic Medications and Developmental Disabilities: The International Consensus Handbook*, Reiss S and Aman MG (eds). Ohio State University Nisonger Center, pp. 179–200.

Stacey CL and DeMartino MF (eds). (1957) *Counseling and Psychotherapy with the Mentally Retarded*. Free Press, Glencoe, IL.

Sutherland GR, Mulley JC, and Richards RI (1993) Fragile X syndrome: the most common cause of familial intellectual handicap. *Med J Aust* **158**, 482–485.

Szymanski LS (1980a) Individual psychotherapy with retarded persons. In *Emotional Disorders of Mentally Retarded Persons*, Szymanski LS and Tanguay PE (eds). University Park Press, Baltimore, pp. 131–147.

Szymanski LS (1987) Prevention of psychosocial dysfunction in persons with mental retardation. *Ment Retard* **25**, 215–218.

Szymanski LS (2000) Happiness as a treatment goal. *Ment Retard* **105**, 352–362.

Szymanski LS and Kaplan LC (1991) Mental retardation. In *Textbook of Child and Adolescent Psychiatry*, Wiener JM (ed) American Psychiatric Press, Washington, DC, p. 157.

Szymanski LS and Rosefsky QB (1980) Group psychotherapy with retarded persons. In *Emotional Disorders of Mentally Retarded Persons*, Szymanski LS and Tanguay PE (eds). University Park Press, Baltimore, pp. 174–194.

Szymanski LS, Rubin LL, and Tarjan G (1989) Mental retardation. In *American Psychiatric Press Review of Psychiatry*, Vol. 8, Tasman A, Hales RE, and Frances AJ (eds). American Psychiatric Press, Washington, DC, p. 227.

Tassone F, Hagerman RJ, Ikle DN, et al. (1999) FMRP expression as potential prognostic indicator in fragile X syndrome. *Am J Med Genet* **84**, 250–261.

Turner G, Webb S, Wake S, et al. (1996) Prevalence of fragile X syndrome. *Am J Med Genet* **64**, 196–197.

Webb T and Latif F (2001) Rett syndrome and the MECP2 gene (Review). *J Med Genet* **38**, 217–223.

Werry JS (1998) Anxiolytics and sedatives. In *Psychotropic Medications and Developmental Disabilities: The International Consensus Handbook*, Reiss S and Aman MG (eds). Ohio State University Nisonger Center, pp. 201–214.

Williams DT, Mehl R, Yudofsky S, et al. (1982) The effects of propranolol on uncontrolled rage outbursts in children and adolescents with organic brain dysfunction. *J Am Acad Child Psychiatry* **21**, 129–135.

Wilska M and Kaski M (1999) Aetiology of intellectual disability—The Finnish classification: development of a method to incorporate WHO ICD-10 coding. *J Intellect Disabil Res* **43**, 242–250.

Wilska ML and Kaski MK (2001) Why and how to assess the aetiological diagnosis of children with intellectual disability/mental retardation and other neurodevelopmental disorders: description of the Finnish approach. *Eur J Paediatr Neurol* **5**, 7–13.

Wisniewski KE, Wisniewski HM, and Wen GY (1985) Occurrence of neuropathological changes and dementia of Alzheimer's disease in Down's syndrome. *Ann Neurol* **17**, 278–282.

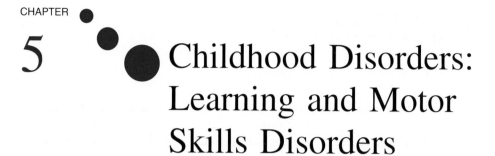

CHAPTER

5 Childhood Disorders: Learning and Motor Skills Disorders

Diagnosis

It is important to understand the diagnostic criteria used in DSM-IV-TR as well as the criteria used by school systems. In clinical practice, the clinician usually needs to help the family in getting the school system to identify the child or adolescent as having a disability and to provide the necessary services. Thus, the clinician must know and understand the educational criteria.

The research of the past 30 years on neurologically based learning disorders stressed not the specific skill disorder but the underlying processing problems. The psychological and educational diagnostic tests used, clarify areas of learning abilities and learning disabilities covering the four phases of processing (Table 5-1). Thus, although one assesses for problems with reading, mathematics, or writing, it is important in the diagnostic process also to explore the underlying processing problems that result in these skill disorders.

The criteria in DSM-IV-TR for establishing the diagnosis of a learning disorder are on pages 93 and 94. For each of these diagnostic categories, the criteria in DSM-IV-TR is that if a general medical (e.g., neurological) condition or sensory deficit is present, the disorder should be coded on Axis III.

Table 5-1	Areas of Psychological Processing That Affect Learning	
Area of Processing	**Examples**
Input	Visual or auditory perception
Integration	Sequencing, abstracting, organization
Memory	Short-term, rote, long-term
Output	Language, motor

DSM-IV-TR Diagnostic Criteria

315.00 Reading Disorder

A. Reading achievement, as measured by individually administered standardized tests of reading accuracy or comprehension, is substantially below that expected, given the person's chronological age, measured intelligence, and age-appropriate education.
B. The disturbance in criterion A significantly interferes with academic achievement or activities of daily living that require reading skills.
C. If a sensory deficit is present, the reading difficulties are in excess of those usually associated with it.

Reprinted with permission from the Diagnostic and Statistical Manual of Mental Disorders, Fourth Edition, Text Revision. Copyright 2000 American Psychiatric Association.

DSM-IV-TR Diagnostic Criteria

315.1 Mathematics Disorder

A. Mathematical ability, as measured by individually administered standardized tests, is substantially below that expected, given the person's chronological age, measured intelligence, and age-appropriate education.
B. The disturbance in criterion A significantly interferes with academic achievement or activities of daily living that require mathematical ability.
C. If a sensory deficit is present, the difficulties in mathematical ability are in excess of those usually associated with it.

Reprinted with permission from the Diagnostic and Statistical Manual of Mental Disorders, Fourth Edition, Text Revision. Copyright 2000 American Psychiatric Association.

DSM-IV-TR Diagnostic Criteria

315.2 Disorder of Written Expression

A. Writing skills, as measured by individually administered standardized tests (or functional assessments of writing skills), are substantially below those expected, given the person's chronological age, measured intelligence, and age-appropriate education.
B. The disturbance in criterion A significantly interferes with academic achievement or activities of daily living that require the composition of written texts (e.g., writing grammatically correct sentences and organized paragraphs).

C. If a sensory deficit is present, the difficulties in writing skills are in excess of those usually associated with it.

Within the motor skills disorder section of DSM-IV-TR, there is only one disorder listed, developmental coordination disorder (see below). If a general medical (e.g., neurological) condition or sensory deficit is present, the developmental coordination disorder is to be coded on Axis III.

DSM-IV-TR Diagnostic Criteria

315.2 Developmental Coordination Disorder

A. Performance in daily activities that require motor coordination is substantially below that expected, given the person's chronological age and measured intelligence. This may be manifested by marked delays in achieving motor milestones (e.g., walking, crawling, sitting), dropping things, *clumsiness*, poor performance in sports, or poor handwriting.
B. The disturbance in criterion A significantly interferes with academic achievement or activities of daily living.
C. The disturbance is not due to a general medical condition (e.g., cerebral palsy, hemiplegia, or muscular dystrophy) and does not meet criteria for a pervasive developmental disorder.
D. If mental retardation is present, the motor difficulties are in excess of those usually associated with it.

The most recent USA federal guidelines for determining whether a student in a public school is eligible for special programs for learning disabilities list four criteria (Silver and Hagin 1992):

1. Documented evidence indicating that general education has been attempted and found to be ineffective in meeting the student's educational needs.
2. Evidence of a disorder in one or more of the basic psychological processes required for learning. A psychological process is a set of mental operations that transform, access, or manipulate information. The disorder is relatively enduring and limits ability to perform specific academic or developmental learning tasks. It may be manifested differently at different developmental levels.
3. Evidence of academic achievement significantly below the student's level of intellectual function (a difference of 1.5 to 1.75 standard deviations between achievement and intellectual functioning is considered significant) on basic reading skills, reading comprehension, mathematical calculation, mathematical reasoning, or written expression.

4. Evidence that the learning problems are not due primarily to other handicapping conditions (i.e., impairment of visual acuity or auditory acuity, physical impairment, emotional handicap, mental retardation, cultural differences, or environmental deprivation).

The presence of a central nervous system processing deficit is essential for the diagnosis of a learning disability. A child might meet the discrepancy criteria, but without central processing deficits in functions required for learning, he or she is not considered to have a learning disability. The question of the significant discrepancy between potential and actual achievement determines eligibility for services. Different school systems use different models for determining the extent of discrepancy (Silver and Hagin 1992, 1993).

If a child or adolescent is experiencing academic difficulty, she or he would normally be referred to the special education professionals within the school system. However, the student with academic difficulties often presents with emotional or behavior problems and is more likely to be referred to a mental health professional. It is critical to understand this potential referral bias. This mental health professional must clarify whether the observed emotional, social, or family problems are causing the academic difficulties or whether they are a consequence of the academic difficulties and the resulting frustrations and failures experienced by the individual, the teacher, and the parents (Silver 1989, 1993b, 1998, Bender 1987, Hunt and Cohen 1984, Valletutti 1983).

The evaluation of a child or adolescent with academic difficulties and emotional or behavior problems includes a comprehensive assessment of the presenting emotional, behavior, social, or family problems as well as a mental status examination. The clinician should obtain information from the child or adolescent, parents, teachers, and other education professionals to help clarify whether there might be a learning disorder or a motor skills disorder and whether further psychological or educational studies are needed. Descriptions by teachers, parents, and the child or adolescent being evaluated will give the clinician clues that there might be one of the learning disorders or a motor skills disorder.

Children who experience problems in reading typically have difficulty in decoding the letter–sound associations involved in phonic analysis (Rourke and Strang 1983). As a result, they may read in a disjointed manner, knowing a few words on sight and stumbling across other unfamiliar words. If they have difficulty with visual tracking, they may skip words or lines. If comprehension is a problem, they report that they have to read material over and over before they understand.

Children with mathematical difficulties may have problems learning math concepts or retaining this information. They may make careless mistakes when doing calculations. Math is a written language in that one is graded on what is put on paper. Thus, problems with visual–spatial tasks or with sequencing might interfere with producing on paper what is known. A problem may not be completed or steps skipped. They might have difficulty shifting from one operation to the next and, as a result, add when they should subtract. A visual–spatial difficulty might result in misaligned columns or rows, or decimals put in the wrong place.

Children who have difficulties with writing may have a problem with handwriting. They grasp the pencil or pen differently and tightly. They write slowly, and their hands get tired. Often, they prefer printing rather than cursive writing. Most also have problems with the language of writing. They have difficulty with spelling, often spelling phonetically. They may have difficulty with grammar, punctuation, and capitalization (Poplin et al. 1980).

Many if not most students with a learning disorder also have difficulties with memory or organization. The child or adolescent with a memory problem has difficulty following multistep directions or reads a chapter in a book but forgets what was read. Others might have sequencing problems, performing instructions out of order. In speaking or writing, the facts may come out but in the wrong sequence. Students with organizational difficulties may not be able to organize their life (notebook, locker, desk, bedroom); they forget things or lose things; they have difficulty with time planning; or they have difficulty using parts of information from a whole concept or putting parts of information together into a whole concept.

Children and adolescents with a developmental coordination disorder may show evidence of gross motor or fine motor difficulties. The gross motor problems might result in difficulty with walking, running, jumping, or climbing. The fine motor problems may result in difficulty with buttoning, zipping, tying, holding a pencil or pen or crayon, arts and crafts activities, or handwriting. Both gross and fine motor difficulties may result in the individual performing poorly in certain sports activities.

The evaluation of cognitive, academic, and neuropsychological functioning is critical to any assessment of learning problems. Results of this psychoeducational assessment will indicate the parameters of the individual's academic and cognitive liabilities while identifying her or his assets. In some instances, borderline cognitive development or mental retardation may be the primary explanation for learning difficulties. Developmental delays are particularly evident with a preschool child; rapid and uneven developmental changes can lead to considerable variability in findings derived by measures of intellectual functioning. If any of the clinical evaluations yield results suggestive of a learning disorder, a more involved psychoeducational assessment is needed. An appropriate psychoeducational evaluation will reveal the magnitude of the child's learning difficulties as well as the nature of the child's cognitive assets and deficits. From this understanding, appropriate interventions can be designed and special accommodations can be initiated.

A family evaluation must include an assessment of the parents and of the entire family. A judgment is made on the order in which these assessments are best done. The first clinical question is whether the family is functional or dysfunctional. If the family is largely functional, there may be normal parenting issues that may be contributing to the child's difficulty. If there is no evidence of a psychopathological process within the family, alternative explanations should be considered for the learning disorder, which do not relate to family issues.

Learning problems are attributed to cognitive deficits or behavior problems in the child or adolescent. Environmental factors involving the school or community, however, can also contribute to academic difficulties. Thus, the clinician should be aware of how social, cultural, or institutional structures can influence learning. In many instances, such an awareness is developed over time and in the process of conducting a clinical practice. Data collection within this context is accomplished through formal and informal observations of the system and the cultural milieu. Through ongoing interactions with the community and the school system, a clinician may develop an appreciation for the community values and the general programmatic resources provided by the school. With this understanding as a backdrop, one can conduct a more direct assessment of how specific environmental or school considerations can affect a given individual.

Individuals with a learning disorder or a motor skills disorder might have other mental disorders or a related neurological disorder. They might also have social problems.

It is not uncommon for children and adolescents with learning disorders or a motor skills disorder to also have a diagnosable mental disorder. For many, these psychological problems are secondary to the frustrations and failures experienced because these disabilities were not identified or were inadequately treated. For others, these conditions may be another reflection of a dysfunctional nervous system. The presenting behavioral or emotional issues might be the individual's characterological style for coping with a dysfunctional nervous system.

Studies of youths diagnosed as having a conduct disorder or young adults diagnosed as having a personality disorder, especially the borderline type, show that about one-third have unrecognized or recognized and poorly treated learning disabilities (learning disorders) (Hunt and Cohen 1984, Forness 1981, Rutter et al. 1970). Similar findings have been observed with adolescent boys in detention centers (Berman and Siegal 1976, Keilitz et al. 1979, Lewis et al. 1979, Lewis and Balla 1980, Mauser 1974, Robbins et al. 1983, Hazel and Schumaker 1988).

The learning disabilities that result in learning disorders or motor skills disorder may directly contribute to peer problems by interfering with success in doing activities required to interact with certain age groups (e.g., visual perception and visual–motor problems interfering with ability to quickly do such eye–hand activities as catching, hitting, or throwing a ball).

Many children and adolescents with learning disorders have difficulty learning social skills and being socially competent (Hazel and Schumaker 1988). These individuals do not pick up such social cues as facial expressions, tone of voice, or body language and therefore do not adapt their behaviors appropriately. Rourke (1987, 1988, 1989), Rourke and Fuerst (1991) using the definition of learning disabilities, identified a specific subtype of learning disabilities, called nonverbal learning disabilities. These students do not have difficulties with interpersonal interactions found in pervasive developmental disorders. This pattern of learning disabilities includes deficits in tactile perception, visual perception, complex psychomotor tasks, and accommodation to novel material as well as difficulty in simple motor skills, auditory perception, and mastery of rote material. A small subset of these students show difficulty in social and emotional functioning that includes a predisposition toward adolescent and adult depression and suicide risk (Rourke and Fuerst 1991).

The first neurologically based disorder recognized as frequently associated with a learning disability (learning disorder) was attention-deficit/hyperactivity disorder (ADHD) (Silver 1981, Halperin et al. 1984). Studies suggest that there is a continuum of disorders associated with neurological dysfunction that are often found together. Thus, when one is diagnosed, the others must be considered in the diagnostic process.

The related theme with these possibly comorbid neurologically based disorders appears to be that if something has an impact on the developing brain during pregnancy or during the critical early months of life, the effects will depend on which areas of the brain are involved and when and for how long the impact took place. This impact might be based on a familial pattern and be directed by the genetic code or might relate to subtle shifts or changes in specific amino acids at the level of the genome. In most cases, the cause or type of impact is not known.

Some studies suggest that other disorders might be part of this continuum of brain dysfunctions. Each might reflect the brain's difficulty in modulating the many stimulant and inhibitory functions involved with cognitive, language, and motor functioning. For some, the problems relate to integrating and modulating the sensory inputs needed to coordinate body movement and motor planning activities; this clinical problem is called a sensory integrative disorder. If the dysfunctional areas relate to certain modulating tasks, the clinical picture might include motor or vocal tics, and the problem is called a chronic motor tic disorder or Tourette's disorder; or the clinical picture might include obsessive thoughts or compulsive behaviors and be called an obsessive–compulsive disorder.

The early statistical data supporting the concept of a continuum of neurological dysfunctions are growing. For individuals with learning disabilities, 20 to 25% have ADHD (Silver 1981, Lewis and Balla 1980). Between 70 and 80% of individuals with ADHD have a learning disability (Silver 1981). About 60% of individuals with Tourette's disorder have a learning disability (Silver 1981, Halperin et al. 1984). Further, 50% of individuals with Tourette's disorder have ADHD (Comings 1990, Comings and Comings 1987, 1988, Hagin et al. 1982, Hagin and Kugler 1988). Fifty percent of individuals with Tourette's disorder have obsessive–compulsive disorder (Frankel et al. 1986, Pauls et al. 1990, Pitman et al. 1987).

Epidemiology

The true prevalence of these disorders is not known, because of the many case definitions used in different studies and in diverse settings. There remains controversy about which definition to use. The Centers for Disease Control and Prevention (1987) attempted to establish the prevalence of learning disabilities. These researchers concluded that because the definition and the diagnostic criteria have not been fully standardized, consistency in the design of prevalence studies has not been maintained. Thus, accurate analyses of data over time are not possible. In the absence of good prevalence data, they concluded that between 5 and 10% was a reasonable estimate of the percentage of persons affected by learning disabilities.

In DSM-IV-TR, prevalence figures are noted for each of the learning disorders and the motor skill disorders. The prevalence of reading disorder in the United States is estimated at 4% of school-age children. It is estimated that 1% of school-age children have a mathematics disorder. No data are noted for disorder of written expression. The prevalence of developmental coordination disorder is estimated to be as high as 6% for children in the age range of 5 to 11 years.

Studies consistently note an increased prevalence of learning disabilities in boys. The ratio ranges from 3 : 1 to 5 : 1 and higher (Ackerman et al. 1983, Finucci and Childs 1981, Rutter et al. 1976). Some studies suggest that this increased prevalence in boys may, in part, be explained by referral bias. Because they are more likely to act out, boys are more likely to be referred for study (Berry et al. 1985). Girls appear to tolerate deficits in reading and spelling skills more easily than boys do, showing less antipathy to reading and less emotional impact (Finucci and Childs 1981). Johnson and Blalock (1987) found no specific cognitive differences or patterns of problems between the sexes.

Furthermore, recent studies suggest that there may be no sexual differences in the prevalence of learning disabilities (Shaywitz et al. 1990, 1992) and that apparent differences may be secondary to possible bias of the assessment test used. Some tests were standardized on males only and might identify more male than female students with learning disabilities. In these studies, all children in a specific grade were evaluated for a possible learning disability. These data were compared with the school system data, based on the number of children identified and serviced. The school-identified population showed a 3 : 1 ratio of boys to girls. The true data based on assessing all children showed a ratio of 1 : 1.

Differential Diagnosis

The presenting problem is academic difficulty. The differential diagnostic process must clarify the reason for the academic difficulty. A *decision tree* for academic difficulties developed by Silver and Ostrander is useful for exploring all of the possible reasons for such difficulties (see Figure 5-1). Three principal areas of inquiry concerning the factors contributing to the student's learning difficulties are explored. The first involves considerations that are related to the child's or adolescent's psychiatric, medical, or psychoeducational status. The second area of inquiry is family functioning. The third area to explore involves the environmental and cultural context in which the student functions.

Difficulties in academic performance of children or adolescents can be related to a range of psychiatric, medical, or cognitive factors. To best determine the primary source of academic difficulties, the evaluation should involve a comprehensive examination of these areas. The psychiatric evaluation should clarify whether there is a psychopathological process. If one is present, it is useful first to determine whether the problems relate to a disruptive behavior disorder or to another mental disorder. In particular, the disruptive behavior disorders have high comorbidity with academic difficulties. A full assessment should clarify whether a disruptive behavior disorder is causing the difficulty with academic performance or is secondary to this difficulty. Disruptive behavior disorders can result in the

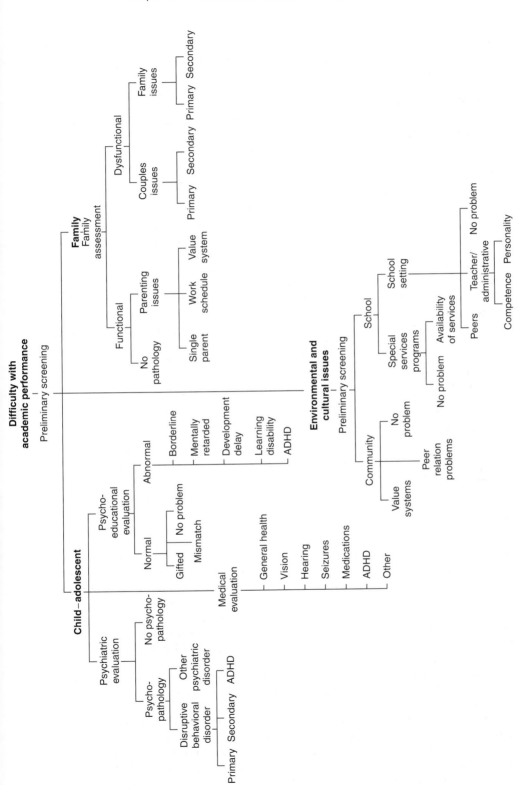

Figure 5-1 *Academic underachievement and the clinical decision-making process. ADHD, Attention-deficit/hyperactivity disorder. (Source: Reprinted from Child Adolesc Psychiatr Clin N Am* **2**, *Ostrander Clinical observations suggesting a learning disability, 249–263, Copyright 1993 with permission from Elsevier.)*

student being unavailable for learning or being so disruptive as to require his/her removal from traditional learning environments. The frustration and failures caused by a learning disorder can be manifested by a disruptive behavior disorder. In some cases, the disruptive behavior disorder coexists with the learning disorder and the relation is less clear. Children and adolescents with ADHD have particular difficulty maintaining attention, and possibly with processing information. As a result, the same variables that have an impact on their attention also have an impact on their ability to learn. In such instances, they may have a learning disorder and ADHD.

Internalizing disorders such as depression or anxiety may result in an uncharacteristic disinterest in or avoidance of school expectations. If one of the internalizing disorders is present, it is important to clarify whether it is secondary or primary to the academic difficulty. Cognitive and language deficits as well as social skills deficits are often associated with learning disorders and can contribute to a dysphoric or anxious presentation.

The medical evaluation is necessary to explore the influence of health factors on the individual's availability and ability to learn. Problems in acquiring academic content can be significantly affected by most visual or hearing deficits. Generally poor health can influence the stamina, motivation, and concentration needed to focus adequately on academic demands. Medications used for any purpose might cause sedation or other side effects that may affect the child's ability to learn. Early developmental insults can result in global or focal deficits in neurological development. Undiagnosed seizures, especially *petit mal* and partial complex seizures, can result in difficulties in general cognitive functioning, specific deficits in memory, and problems with attention.

Etiology

Earlier research focused on the concept of brain damage (Knobloch and Pasamanick 1959, Towbin 1971). Subtle central nervous system damage may result from circulatory, toxic metabolic, or other forms of insult to the fetal nervous system during a critical period of prenatal development, perinatal stresses to the brain, or stress to the nervous system during the critical early years of life (e.g., trauma, fever, inflammation). There may be a spectrum of disorders caused by prenatal, perinatal, and postnatal brain damage. Depending on location, extent of damage, time of life, and developmental stage at the time of damage, the stress might cause fetal or neonatal death, cerebral palsy, epilepsy, or mental retardation. The less severe forms might produce a variety of learning disorders.

More of the later research focused on physiological changes rather than on structural changes, that is, on the types of impacts that might affect the developing nervous system, causing areas of the brain to "wire itself" differently than expected. Galaburda and colleagues (Papez 1937, Galaburda et al. 1985), doing microscopic studies of brains of individuals known to have learning disabilities, showed a consistent pattern of cortical cells that maintained an earlier developmental stage of migration and development, suggesting that something had an impact on the brain during development, halting or slowing down the normal developmental stages. Some of the factors studied as possibly contributing to the stress that results in neurological dysfunction are maternal cigarette smoking during pregnancy, convulsions during pregnancy, low fetal heart rate during the second stage of labor, lower placental weight, breech presentations, and chorionitis. Also noted, is a history of maternal alcohol consumption (two to three drinks daily) during pregnancy.

Research has also focused on the genetic basis for these disorders. Several studies have shown a familial pattern in approximately 40 to 50% of children with learning disabilities (Silver 1971, Morrison and Stewart 1971, Cantwell 1975). In longitudinal studies of twins, identical pairs are more likely than fraternal pairs to be concordant for academic difficulties (McCarty and McCarty 1969). These studies support the possibility that this is a heterogeneous disorder.

Recent research in reading disorders shows an inability to segment the written word into the underlying phonologic components (Shaywitz 1996, Talial 1985). This deficit in phonological awareness impairs decoding, preventing word identification. This basic deficit in what is essentially a lower-order linguistic function blocks access to higher-order linguistic processes and impairs the child's ability to gain meaning from text. Thus, the child has difficulty with reading fluency and text comprehension. It is not uncommon to find a spelling disability associated with a reading disorder because spelling requires the same phonologic skills as reading.

Studies of the brain using functional magnetic resonance imaging clearly shows a difference in brain function between individuals who have no reading problems and those with a reading disorder. Brain activation patterns differ significantly between groups of individuals with a reading disability and those without, showing relative underactivation in posterior regions (Wernicke's area, the angular gyrus, and striate cortex) and related overactivation in an anterior region (inferior frontal gyrus). These results are seen as confirming that the impairment in reading disorders is phonologic in nature and these brain activation patterns may provide neural proof for this impairment (Shaywitz et al. 1998).

Research in disorders of written expression focus on the need for immediate and automatic carrying out of most of the lower-level mental activities required for skilled writing. These lower-level mental activities guide handwriting, spelling, word choice, and the construction of sentences that conform to the conventions of written language. Lower-level mental activities also guide the construction of textural connections, specifically, spacing and punctuations. The writer's attention can then focus on the content, organization, and clarity of the task. One can shift attention between levels of mental processing without losing control of the flow of the text. Difficulties with lower-level mental activities appear to be the source of the problem in expressive writing disorders (Torgeson 1982).

Research on mathematics achievement suggest that there may be four primary factors involved: language, conceptual, visual–spatial, and memory (Bryan and Pearl 1979). In addition, knowing how to use the correct strategy is important (NAS 2000a). Proficiency in mathematics requires more than computational skills. The difficulty might be in an inability to develop a systematic plan for problem solution. Memory is essential to the ability to do mathematics. One must retain basic number facts. In addition, it is necessary to remember specific equations or other steps necessary to solve a problem. Once a problem is started, students must remember where they are in the process as they proceed from step to step.

Recent findings suggest a possible connection between environmental toxins and the increased incidence of developmental, learning, and behavioral problems (Physicians for Social Responsibility 2000). The National Academy of Science released two studies (NAS 2000a,b) on general developmental and specific neurologic toxins. US companies reported to the Environmental Protection Agency (EPA) that in 1998, they released a total of 1.2 billion pounds of chemicals into the nation's air and water that have the potential to affect the way a child's body and brain develops. More than half (53%) of these are known or suspected to be developmental or neurologic toxins. There is great concern about the impact of these environmental toxins on the increased incidence of learning and attentional disorders.

Treatment

Treatment is directed at the underlying disabilities by use of educational interventions. Psychological interventions are also directed at any existing emotional, social, or family difficulties. In addition, social skills training may be helpful.

Somatic Treatments

No medication has been found to be effective for treating the learning disorders or motor skills disorder. If the individual with these disorders also has ADHD, it is important that medication be used to minimize the hyperactivity, distractibility, or impulsivity so that the student can be available for learning.

Educational Interventions

The goal of special educational interventions is to help children and adolescents overcome or compensate for their learning disorders or motor skills disorder so that they can succeed in school. These efforts involve remedial and compensatory approaches and use a multisensory approach that facilitates building on all areas of strength while compensating for any areas of weakness. These efforts are to be provided in as close to a regular classroom setting as possible. It is essential that the classroom teacher knows how to adapt the classroom, curriculum, and teaching style to best accommodate each student's areas of difficulty.

Educational Interventions for Reading Disorders

The process of reading involves two tasks, decoding or word recognition and reading comprehension. Decoding refers to the act of transcribing a printed word into speech. Comprehension refers to the process of interpreting the message or meaning of the text. Decoding is unique to reading and different from the recognition of words in speech; however, the linguistic skills that subserve reading comprehension are the same for both reading and listening (Gough and Tunmer 1986).

Most students with a reading disorder have difficulty (which is sometimes extreme) acquiring the knowledge and skills essential for rapid automatic decoding. Reading comprehension, thus, is limited by weak decoding skills. Because spelling uses the same knowledge as word recognition, it is also frequently impaired.

Direct instruction in reading (and spelling and writing) is considered to be the essential treatment for a student with a reading disorder. These efforts are provided by a person trained to use appropriate remedial methods. These methods emphasize explicit instruction in letter–sound associations. Instruction is described as multisensory. Children see a letter and hear its name and sound; they trace the letter, saying its name and sound; and then they write the letter, repeating its name and sound. Sounds and letters are blended to form words. Reading, spelling, and writing are taught simultaneously. Instruction involves extended practice and is supplemented by speech segmentation training and study skills instructions. Parents are asked to read to their children to enhance appreciation of reading and to give the children access to knowledge normally obtained by reading.

Learning disorders, specifically reading disorders, are not cured. With appropriate interventions, children and adolescents with reading disorders learn to read and spell at a slower rate than do normally developing individuals. It is essential for these students to learn compensatory skills and for the classroom teachers to provide essential accommodations.

Educational Interventions for Mathematics Disorders

Children and adolescents with a mathematics disorder may have a wide range of symptoms, including delays in the acquisition of basic spatial and number concepts, problems learning and using number words and number facts or writing numbers correctly (and in correct alignment when doing computations), and difficulty in applying arithmetic skills when solving everyday problems (Fleischner and Garnett 1993, Kose 1992). Because mathematics achievement is highly dependent on the quality of instruction offered to students, it may be that a significant number of those students who are coded as having a learning disability by the school system in fact do not have intrinsic mathematics disorders, but rather have not had appropriate instruction (Carnine 1991).

Specific interventions focus on the underlying difficulties. Some students have problems related to acquiring the conceptual underpinnings of the subject; some have problems related to procedural learning, recall of discrete information, and self-monitoring. Remedial efforts must take into account the student's areas of learning abilities and learning disabilities.

Educational Interventions for Disorders of Written Expression Reading requires the ability to decode letters into sounds and blend these sounds into words. Writing requires outflow of the language or sounds in the brain back into graphic symbols. Thus, reading and writing problems are frequently seen together.

It is helpful to distinguish between a fine motor problem that results in difficulty with the mechanics of writing and a language-based learning disability that results in problems with the language of writing (Uhry and Shepherd 1993). Individuals with a disorder of written expression might have a fine motor problem but always have a language-based disorder, resulting in difficulty with spelling, grammar, punctuation, capitalization, or composition.

Poor spelling might be the first indicator of a writing disorder. By third or fourth grade, additional writing problems are apparent. Children with a writing disorder exhibit grammatical and punctuation errors at the sentence level. Paragraphs are poorly organized. In later grades, taking notes is difficult. It is nearly impossible for these students to analyze a rapidly paced lecture and to write at the same time.

Treatment for a writing disorder might involve a skills approach or a holistic approach. Skills programs are often used with younger children and focus on letter–sound associations, with emphasis on reading and spelling (Cox 1984, Slingerland 1971). Children may be asked to listen carefully for the sounds in words and then to represent these sounds with written letters, saying each letter aloud as it is written.

The holistic approach to writing begins with the student's ideas. It involves a series of highly structured steps for narrowing ideas to one topic, writing a first draft, reading it aloud to an audience of peers, and then refining organization and language. The final step involves working on mechanics in preparation for "publishing" a draft for peers to read.

Most efforts combine these two approaches (Uhry and Shepherd 1993). Children with a writing disorder need direct, sequential instructions in letter–sound associations and in spelling rules as well as in sentence structure and the connections between sentences and paragraphs that make text cohesive. Even with good remedial interventions, writing requires enormous effort because this disorder is not cured and must be compensated for, and this compensation must continue into adulthood. Appropriate accommodations, such as using a computer, may be needed throughout the individual's education and career.

Educational Interventions for Developmental Coordination Disorders The approaches for helping children and adolescents with this disorder focus on academic skills, life skills, or athletic skills. That is, the focus of intervention might be on specific skills needed for school (e.g., handwriting), on dressing and other life skills (e.g., buttoning, zipping, tying, eating), or on skills needed to do better in sports (e.g., catching, hitting, throwing, running).

Occupational therapists work in all of these areas using sensory integrative approaches involving visual, visual–motor, gross motor, fine motor, proprioceptive, and vestibular stimulation and strengthening to improve functioning. Within school systems, the special education professional may work on handwriting, and the adaptive physical education teacher may work on physical education-related activities.

Psychotherapeutic Interventions
Learning disorders affect all aspects of the child's or adolescent's life. The same processing problems that interfere with reading, writing, mathematics, and language may interfere with communicating with peers and family, with success in sports and activities, and with such daily life skills as dressing oneself or cutting food (Silver 1993b).

Lack of success in school can lead to a poor self-image and low self-esteem (Black 1974, Bryan and Pearl 1979, Rogers and Saklofske 1985, Shaw et al. 1982). These individuals might feel that they have minimal control over their life and compensate by trying to be in more control (Silver 1993c). Some individuals may become anxious or depressed, or a disruptive behavior disorder may develop.

Genetic and family studies show that in about 40% of children and adolescents with learning disabilities (learning disorders), there is a familial pattern (Johnson 1988). Thus, from an early identification perspective, each sibling must be considered as possibly having a learning disorder. Also, there is a 40% likelihood that one of the parents may also have a learning disorder. This parent may not have known of this problem. If this is true, the parent, for the first time, may be able to understand a lifetime of difficulties or underachievement. Further, when the psychiatrist offers suggestions for this parent, the parent's areas of difficulty must be considered. Do not ask a mother to be more organized when she has been just as disorganized as her child all her life.

Some children or adolescents may need specific individual, behavioral, group, or family therapy. If so, it is critical that the therapist understands the impact that the learning disorder has had on the individual and how these disabilities might affect the process of therapy (Silver 1993a). As noted earlier, many students with a learning disorder have difficulties with peers and social skills problems. Social skills training might be helpful.

Once the diagnosis is established, it is critical that the clinician explains to the individual and to the parents what the problems are, focusing not only on the areas of learning difficulties but also on the areas of learning strengths.

Parents must understand this information so that they can develop a better understanding of their child or adolescent (Silver 1998). Mental health professionals working with these children and adolescents must understand the concept of learning disabilities (learning disorders) well enough to teach the individual and family members what the areas of disabilities and abilities are, as well as the effects these disabilities have had on peer, family, and school activities.

The child or adolescent needs to begin to understand and to rethink concepts of self. Parents begin to modify their images of this child or adolescent and modify their responses and behaviors. Siblings may gain a new understanding of the problems in the family.

If the presenting behavior problems are not serious, it may be best first to provide family education and to give some time to see how this new knowledge affects the family. Concurrently, the parents are taught how to advocate for the necessary services within the school system. It may be that once the academic issues are addressed and the family begins to change, the behavior problems will diminish and no further help will be needed.

The next step is family counseling. Parents are taught how to use their knowledge of their son's or daughter's strengths and weaknesses to modify family patterns; select appropriate chores; choose appropriate activities, sports, and camps; and address stresses within the family (Silver 1998). Once taught the necessary knowledge about the child or adolescent and the concepts of intervention, families can often move ahead, creatively working out their own problems (Silver 1998).

For some children and adolescents, individual behavioral therapy or psychotherapy may be indicated to help them develop new strategies for interacting with peers, parents, and teachers.

Because this form of therapy requires listening and talking, it is important for the therapist to know whether the individual has a disability in these areas. If so, the therapist has to develop ways of accommodating these problems if therapy is to progress. If a speech and language therapist is working with the individual, she or he might offer suggestions.

The initial phases of family therapy might focus on helping the identified individual regain control over his or her behavior and helping the parents retake control of the family. A behavioral management approach is often the first intervention.

The model of family therapy used will depend on the needs of the family and the orientation of the therapist. For the child or adolescent with these disorders, it is important to keep in mind the impact of these disabilities on the individual and the family. It is also important to keep in mind the impact these disabilities might have on this individual's ability to participate in the family therapy. As with individual therapy, if the individual has difficulties with language or with other disabilities, he or she might have difficulty participating in the family therapy sessions. Accommodations will be necessary.

Children and adolescents with these disorders often have problems with peer relationships (Hazel and Schumaker 1998, Rourke 1988). There appears to be an association between poor peer relationships and a high risk for later psychological problems (Cowen et al. 1973) as well as dissatisfaction and loneliness (Asher and Wheeler 1985). Poor childhood social skills and peer acceptance have been related to adjustment problems in adulthood (Gresham and Elliott 1989, Wiener et al. 1990). Thus, it is important to address these problems early.

The specific learning disabilities may be interfering with success in sports or other peer activities. In addition, many of these individuals have difficulty reading social cues or learning social skills (Hazel and Schumaker 1998). It is not understood why these problems exist; however, they are not uncommon. Social skills training can be helpful.

Such interventions attempt to enhance social–cognitive skills and are directed at altering specific behavior patterns (Dodge 1989, McIntosh et al. 1991). Social–cognitive approaches are based on those cognitive processes that are related to competent, prosocial behavior. Targets of intervention are directed toward the underlying cognitive variables that are linked to positive peer acceptance.

The enhancement of social–cognitive skills typically involves three kinds of skill development: (1) accurate interpretation of social situations; (2) effective use of social behaviors in interactions with others; and (3) the evaluation of one's own performance and the ability to make adjustments, depending on the environmental context.

The first step in developing these skills typically requires the clinician to provide verbal instructions concerning the relevant skills (e.g., conversational skills). The skills are then modeled by the clinician. It is also important to discuss and emphasize positive outcomes associated with these skills. In the process, the clinician must confront and restructure thoughts that may inhibit the desired behaviors. The child is then required to rehearse the skills in simulated conditions, with the clinician providing reinforcement and corrective feedback as warranted. Generalization is stressed through homework assignments whereby skills are attempted in the natural environment and classroom (Dodge 1989, McIntosh et al. 1991).

Comparison of DSM-IV-TR/ICD-10 Diagnostic Criteria

In ICD-10, DSM-IV-TR Reading Disorder is referred to as "Specific Reading Disorder" and DSM-IV-TR Mathematics Disorders as "Specific Disorder of Arithmetic Skills." For both of these learning skills disorders, the ICD-10 Diagnostic Criteria for Research suggest that the cutoff be 2 standard deviations below the expected level of reading achievement and mathematics achievement respectively. In contrast, DSM-IV-TR does not specify a score cutoff, instead recommending that the score be "substantially below that expected, given the person's chronological age, measured intelligence, and age-appropriate education". Furthermore, in contrast to DSM-IV-TR, which permits both to be diagnosed if present, ICD-10 Reading Disorder takes precedence over Mathematics Disorder so that if criteria are met for both, only Reading Disorder is diagnosed.

ICD-10 does not include a Disorder of Written Expression (as in DSM-IV-TR), but instead includes a Specific Spelling Disorder. DSM-IV-TR includes spelling problems as part of the definition of Disorder of Written Expression but requires writing problems in addition to spelling in order to warrant this diagnosis.

Finally, DSM-IV-TR Coordination Disorder is referred to as "Specific Developmental Disorder of motor function" in ICD-10. Furthermore, the ICD-10 Diagnostic Criteria for Research suggest that the cutoff be two standard deviations below the expected level on a standardized test of fine or gross motor coordination.

References

Ackerman P, Dykman R, and Oglesby D (1983) Sex and group differences in reading and attention disordered children with and without hyperkinesis. *J Learn Disabil* **16**, 407–415.

Asher SR and Wheeler V (1985) Children's loneliness: a comparison of rejected and neglected peer status. *J Consult Clin Psychol* **53**, 500–505.

Bender WN (1987) Secondary personality and behavioral problems in adolescents with learning disabilities. *J Learn Disabil* **20**, 280–285.

Berman A and Siegal A (1976) Adaptive and learning skills in delinquent boys. *J Learn Disabil* **9**, 583–590.

Berry CA, Shaywitz SE, and Shaywitz BA (1985) Girls with attention deficit disorder: a silent minority? A report on behavioral and cognitive characteristics. *Pediatrics* **76**, 801–809.

Black FW (1974) Self-concept as related to achievement and age in learning disabled children. *Child Dev* **45**, 1137–1140.

Bryan T and Pearl R (1979) Self-concept and locus of control of learning disabled children. *J Clin Child Psychol* **8**, 223–226.

Cantwell DP (1975) Genetic studies of hyperactive children. In *Genetic Research in Psychiatry*, Fiere R, Rosenthal D, and Brill H (eds). The Johns Hopkins University Press, Baltimore, pp. 273–280.

Carnine D (1991) Reforming mathematics instruction: the role of curriculum materials. *Behav Educ* **1**, 37–57.

Centers for Disease Control and prevention (1987) *Assessment of the Number and Characteristics of Persons Affected by Learning Disabilities*, Interagency Committee on Learning Disabilities, A Report to the US Congress. US Department of Health and Human Services, Washington, DC, pp. 107–123.

Comings DE (1990) *Tourette Syndrome and Human Behavior*. Hope Press, Durante, CA.

Comings DE and Comings BG (1987) A controlled study of Tourette syndrome I–VII. *Am J Hum Genet* **41**, 701–866.

Comings DE and Comings BG (1988) Tourette syndrome and attention deficit disorder. In *Tourette's Syndrome and Tic Disorders: Understanding and Treatment*, Cohen DJ, Bruun RD, and Leckman JF (eds). John Wiley, New York, pp. 19–35.

Cowen EL, Rederson A, Babigan H, et al. (1973) Long-term follow-up of early detected vulnerable children. *J Consult Clin Psychol* **41**, 438–446.

Cox A (1984) *Structures and Techniques: Multisensory Teaching of Basic Language Skills*. Educators Publishing Service, Cambridge, MA.

Dodge KA (1989) Problems in social relationships. In *Treatment of Childhood Disorders*, Mash EJ and Barkley RA (eds). Guilford Press, New York, pp. 222–244.

Finucci JM and Childs B (1981) Are there really more dyslexic boys than girls. In *Sex Differences in Dyslexia*, Ansara A, Geshwind N, Galaburda A, et al. (eds). Orton Dyslexia Society, Towson, MD, pp. 1–9.

Fleischner JE and Garnett K (1993) Math disorders. *Child Adolesc Psychiatr Clin N Am* **2**, 221–231.

Forness SB (1981) *Recent Concepts in Dyslexia: Implications for Diagnosis and Remediation*, ERIC Exceptional Child Education Reports. VA.

Frankel M, Cummings JL, Robertson MM, et al. (1986) Obsessions and compulsions in Gilles de la Tourette's syndrome. *Neurology* **36**, 378–382.

Galaburda AM, Sherman GF, Rosen GD, et al. (1985) Developmental dyslexia: four consecutive patients with cortical anomalies. *Ann Neurol* **18**, 222–233.

Gough PB and Tunmer WE (1986) Decoding reading and reading disability. *Remed Spec Educ* **7**, 6–10.

Gresham FM and Elliott SN (1989) Social skills assessment technology for LD students. *Learn Disabil Q* **12**, 141–152.

Hagin RA, Beecher R, Pagano G, et al. (1982) Effects of Tourette syndrome on learning. In *Gilles de la Tourette Syndrome*, Friedhoff AJ and Chase TN (eds). Raven Press, New York.

Hagin RA and Kugler J (1988) School problems associated with Tourette's syndrome. In *Tourette's Syndrome and Tic Disorders: Clinical Understanding and Treatment*, Cohen DJ, Bruun RD, and Leckman JF (eds). John Wiley, New York.

Halperin JM, Gittelman R, Klein DF, et al. (1984) Reading-disabled hyperactive children: a distinct subgroup of attention deficit disorder with hyperactivity. *J Abnorm Child Psychol* **12**, 1–14.

Hazel JS and Schumaker JB (1988) Social skills and learning disabilities: current issues and recommendations for future research. In *Learning Disabilities: Proceedings of the National Conference*, Kavanagh JF and Truss TJ (eds). York Press, Parkton, MD, pp. 293–344.

Hunt RD and Cohen DJ (1984) Psychiatric aspects of learning difficulties. *Pediatr Clin N Am* **31**, 471–497.

Johnson DJ (1988) Review of research on specific reading, writing, and mathematics disorders. In *Learning Disabilities: Proceedings of the National Conference*, Kavanagh JF and Truss TJ (eds). York Press, Parkton, MD, pp. 79–163.

Johnson D and Blalock J (eds) (1987) *Adults with Learning Disabilities: Clinical Studies*. Grune & Stratton, New York.

Keilitz I, Zaremba BA, and Broder PK (1979) The link between learning disabilities and juvenile delinquency. *Learn Disabil Q* **2**, 2–11.

Knobloch H and Pasamanick B (1959) The syndrome of minimal cerebral damage in infancy. *JAMA* **70**, 1384–1387.

Kosc L (1992) Developmental dyscalculia. *J Learn Disabil* **7**, 165–178.

Lewis D and Balla D (1980) Psychiatric correlates of severe reading disabilities in an incarcerated delinquent population. *J Am Acad Child Psychiatr* **19**, 611–622.

Lewis D, Shanok SS, and Pincus JH (1979) Juvenile male sexual assaulters. *Am J Psychiatr* **136**, 1194–1196.

Mauser AJ (1974) Learning disabilities and delinquent youth. *Acad Ther* **9**, 389–402.

McCarty JJ and McCarty DJ (1969) *Learning Disabilities*. Allyn & Bacon, Boston.

McIntosh R, Vaughn S, and Zaragaza N (1991) A review of social interventions for students with learning disabilities. *J Learn Disabil* **24**, 451–458.

Morrison JR and Stewart MA (1971) A family study of the hyperactive child syndrome. *Biol Psychiatr* **3**, 189–195.

National Academy of Science (2000a) *Scientific Frontiers in Developmental Toxicology and Risk Assessment*. National Academy of Science, Washington, DC.

National Academy of Science (2000b) *Toxicological Effects of Methylmercury*. National Academy of Science, Washington, DC.

Ostrander R (1993) Clinical observations suggesting a learning disability. *Child Adolesc Psychiatr Clin N Am* **2**, 249–263.

Papez JW (1937) A proposed mechanism of emotion. *Arch Neurol Psychiatr* **38**, 725–743.

Pauls DC, Pakstis A, Kurlan R, et al. (1990) Segregation and linkage analysis of Tourette's syndrome and related disorders. *J Am Acad Child Adolesc Psychiatr* **29**, 195–203.

Physicians for Social Responsibility (2000) *In Harm's Way: Toxic Threats to Child Development*. Greater Boston Physicians for Social Responsibility, Boston.

Pitman RK, Gren RC, Jenicke MA, et al. (1987) Clinical comparison of Tourette's disorder and obsessive–compulsive disorder. *Am J Psychiatr* **144**, 1166–1171.

Poplin M and Gray R, et al. (1980) A comparison of components of written expression abilities in learning disabled and non-learning disabled students at three grade levels. *Learn Disabil Q* **3**, 46–53.

Robbins DM, Beck JC, Pries R, et al. (1983) Learning disability and neuropsychological impairment in adjudicated, unincarcerated male delinquents. *J Am Acad Child Psychiatr* **22**, 40–46.

Rogers H and Saklofske DH (1985) Self-concepts, locus of control and performance expectations of learning disabled students. *J Learn Disabil* **18**, 244–267.

Rourke BP (1987) Syndrome of nonverbal learning disabilities: the final common pathway of white-matter disease/dysfunction. *Clin Neuropsychol* **1**, 209–234.

Rourke BP (1988) Socioemotional disturbances of learning disabled children. *J Consult Clin Psychol* **56**, 801–810.

Rourke BP (1989) *Nonverbal Learning Disabilities: The Syndrome and the Model*. Guilford Press, New York.

Rourke BP and Fuerst DR (1991) *Learning Disabilities and Psychosocial Functioning: A Neuropsychological Perspective*. Guilford Press, New York.

Rourke BP and Strang JD (1983) Subtypes of reading and arithmetical disabilities: a neuropsychological analysis. In *Developmental Neuropsychiatry*, Rutter M (ed). Guilford Press, New York, pp. 473–488.

Rutter M, Tizard J, and Whitmore K (1970) *Education in Health and Behavior*. Longman, London.

Rutter M, Tizard J, Yule W, et al. (1976) Research report Isle of Wight studies, 1964–1974. *Psychol Med* **6**, 313–332.

Shaw L, Levine MD, and Belfer M (1982) Developmental double jeopardy: a study of clumsiness and self-esteem in children with learning problems. *Dev Behav Pediatr* **3**, 191–196.

Shaywitz SE (1996) Dyslexia. *Sci Am* **275**, 98–104.

Shaywitz SE, Shaywitz BA, Fletcher JM, et al. (1990) Prevalence of reading disability in boys and girls: results of the connecticut longitudinal study. *JAMA* **265**, 998–1002.

Shaywitz SE, Shaywitz BA, and Fletcher JM (1992) The yale center for the study of learning and attentional disorders. *Learn Disabil* **3**, 1–12.

Shaywitz SE, Shaywitz BA, Pugh UR, et al. (1998) Functional disruption in the organization of the brain for reading in dyslexia. *Proc Natl Acad Sci U S A* **95**, 2636–2641.

Silver LB (1971) Familial patterns in children with neurologically-based learning disabilities. *J Learn Disabil* **4**, 349–358.

Silver LB (1981) The relationship between learning disabilities, hyperactivity, distractibility, and behavioral problems. *J Am Acad Child Psychiatr* **20**, 385–397.

Silver LB (1989) Psychological and family problems associated with learning disabilities: assessment and intervention. *J Am Acad Child Adolesc Psychiatr* **28**, 319–325.

Silver LB (1993a) Psychological interventions and therapies for children and adolescents with learning disabilities. *Child Adolesc Psychiatr Clin N Am* **2**, 323–337.

Silver LB (1993b) The secondary emotional, social, and family problems found with children and adolescents with learning disabilities. *Child Adolesc Psychiatr Clin N Am* **2**, 295–308.

Silver LB (1993c) Introduction and overview to the clinical concepts of learning disabilities. *Child Adolesc Psychiatr Clin N Am* **2**, 181–192.

Silver LB (1998) The misunderstood child. *A Guide for Parents of Children with Learning Disabilities*, 3rd ed. Random House/Times Books, New York.

Silver AA and Hagin RA (1992) *Disorders of Learning in Childhood*. John Wiley, New York, pp. 23–42.

Silver AA and Hagin RA (1993) The educational diagnostic process. *Child Adolesc Psychiatr Clin N Am* **2**, 265–281.

Slingerland BH (1971) *A Multi-sensory Approach to Language Arts for Specific Language Disability Children: A Guide for Primary Teachers*, Books 1–3. Educators Publishing Service, Cambridge, MA.

Talial P (1985) Neuropsychological foundations of specific developmental disorders (language, reading, articulation). *Psychiatry* **3**, 1–10.

Torgeson J (1982) The learning disabled child as an inactive learner: educational implications. *Top Learn Disabil* **2**, 45–52.

Towbin A (1971) Organic causes of minimal brain dysfunction. Perinatal origin of minimal cerebral lesions. *JAMA* **217**, 1207–1209.

Uhry JK and Shepherd MJ (1993) Writing disorder. *Child Adolesc Psychiatr Clin N Am* **2**, 209–219.

Valletutti P (1983) The social and emotional problems of children with learning disabilities. *Learn Disabil* **2**, 17–29.

Wiener J, Harris PJ, and Shirer C (1990) Achievement and social behavioral correlations of peer status in LD children. *Learn Disabil Q* **13**, 114–126.

6   Childhood Disorders: Communication Disorders

The disorders of communication have traditionally been insufficiently familiar to mental health professionals despite the fact that clinical practice is founded upon communication. A knowledge of these disorders is especially of crucial importance in the care of children, since they are deeply interwoven in all aspects of normal development, psychopathology, and the functions of daily life. This section includes both disorders of speech, the oral representation of language, and of language itself. The disorders included in this section are expressive language disorder, mixed receptive–expressive language disorders, phonological disorder, stuttering, and communication disorder not otherwise specified (CDNOS). These disorders share many common features, as noted in Table 6-1. Selective mutism is not regarded as a disorder of communication *per se*, and is included among other disorders of childhood (see Chapter 11).

Assessment of Communication Disorders

It is essential that the mental health professional seeing children is familiar with the expected milestones of speech and language development. This knowledge forms the basis for effective observation in a clinical setting (see Figure 6-1 for diagnostic decision tree). The clinician should ask the parents or guardians about the child's speech and language, both in terms of development and in terms of current function. Paul (1982) and Gulley-Smith (1998) provide detailed outlines for this, but much can be learned from even a few questions: Does the child seem to hear and understand what is being said? Does the child require visual prompts? Does the child in fact use spoken language to communicate? How long and complicated are his sentences? Does the child "make sense" to outsiders? Can he/she be clearly understood even by strangers? Which sounds does the child find difficult? Does the child use unusual volume, pitch, or nasality? Does he/she observe the rules of conversation? Parent–child communication should also be observed.

Table 6-1	Features Common to All Communication Disorders

Inadequate development of some aspect of communication
Absence (in developmental types) of any demonstrable causes of physical disorder, neurological
    disorder, global mental retardation, or severe environmental deprivation
Onset in childhood
Long duration
Clinical features resembling the functional levels of younger normal children
Impairments in adaptive functioning, especially in school
Tendency to occur in families
Predisposition toward boys
Multiple presumed etiological factors
Increased prevalence in younger age range
Diagnosis requiring a range of standardized techniques
Tendency toward certain specific associated problems, such as attention-deficit/hyperactivity disorder
Wide range of subtypes and severity

Source: Reprinted from *Psychiatric Disorders in Children and Adolescents*, Baker L, Specific communication disorders, 257–270, Copyright 1990 with permission from Elsevier.

Children must be assessed in an environment that fosters verbal communication and observed in a variety of interactions because their speech and language vary so much over time in quantity and quality. For younger children, this may best be done in the context of a play situation. Rutter (1987) recommends that the clinician assesses *inner language*, comprehension, production, phonation, and pragmatics. "Inner language" means symbolization, which may be observed in a younger child by the child's representational use of play materials. For example, a block could be a house or a vehicle. "Comprehension" is assessed through conversation and the use of developmentally appropriate questions and commands, especially with nonverbal augments or prompts. The clinician should note how well a child can follow and draw inferences from a conversation. "Production" refers to speech, its fluency, and intelligibility. "Phonation" refers to the utterance of vocal sounds produced by the larynx. "Pragmatics" are those aspects of language that render it useful for social communication beyond the most concrete level. Does the child appreciate the nuances of his/her partner's conversation, as for example, when they signal beginnings and endings of conversations, topic changes, or the child's turn to talk?

Pragmatic language involves nonverbal elements. Deficiencies in this area impair abstraction and may render the individual almost "robotlike." In all cases, observations should be made in as relaxed a fashion as possible, avoiding interrogation or rote exercises. If a child fails to communicate a given item, necessary help including nonverbal prompts should be offered, so that the child has the experience of success. A sense of failure will stifle communication.

In school settings, all of the phenomena seen in a clinical interview may also be pursued. Children with communication disorders often feel challenged by the demands of the classroom and may limit or withdraw from conversation entirely. Thus, the task-oriented group setting of the classroom may not elicit a child's best communication. It may, however, demonstrate the practical effectiveness of the child's everyday efforts. At the same time, teachers sometimes have more individual conversations with children than even their parents do, and their experiences may make them the first adults to detect communication problems. In many areas, young children receive some type of formal communication screening in school. Therefore, teacher input is essential in the evaluation of these children.

The need for a clinician to be aware of normal developmental expectations has been cited. In settings as geographically and culturally diverse as the English-speaking countries, special sensitivity must be exercised for the range of dialects and conversational styles encountered. English is spoken with an extraordinary range of accents, even within each

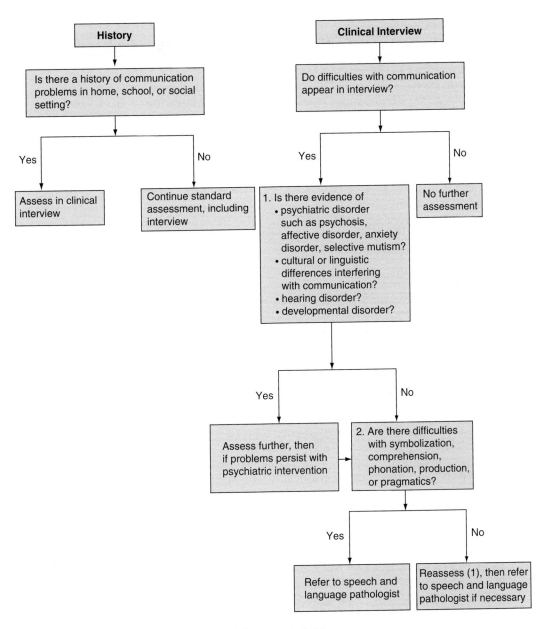

Figure 6-1 *Diagnostic decision tree.*

dialect group. It is essential that one should not pathologize a difference in intonation into a phonological disorder (PD), or of dialect into an expressive language disorder (ELD). Many American children grow up in multilingual environments and may speak with a synthesis of grammar and vocabulary, especially during their preschool years. Finally, children of minority groups who have suffered social discrimination and children who live in physically dangerous environments may necessarily be cautious and less forthcoming with language; this may be adaptive in some cases and not a disorder at all.

Epidemiology

Past reports of prevalence and incidence of communication disorders have been complicated by variations in setting, case-finding, and diagnostic criteria. Numbers from 1 to 13% have been posited for the prevalence of language disorders, and numbers as high as 32% for speech disorders (Baker 1990). Acquired language disorders are reported to be less common than the developmental types. Overall, between 3 and 7% of all children were suspected of having a developmental ELD. Mixed receptive–expressive language disorder is less common but may still be seen in as many as 3% of school-age children. Speech disorders are similarly common but become less frequent with age. Phonological disorder (PD) occurs in approximately 2% of six- and seven-year-olds, but this prevalence falls to 0.5% by age 17. Stuttering occurs in approximately 1% of children aged 10 and younger, declining modestly to 0.8% in later adolescence. All of the developmental communication disorders have a male to female predominance; that of stuttering is as high as 3 : 1. By contrast, no gender influences have been reported in the nondevelopmental (i.e., acquired) language disorders. In all, the prevalence of these disturbances is comparable in magnitude to many other common psychiatric disorders of childhood.

Comorbidity

Clinician should be acutely concerned with the comorbidity of all these disorders with many mental disorders. In their seminal work, Cantwell and Baker (1991) demonstrate that approximately half of the children with a speech or language disorder have some other definable Axis I clinical disorder. Similarly, among children with a psychiatric diagnosis made first, there is a remarkably increased likelihood of speech and language disorders, which often go undetected (Cohen et al. 1993). Typical are the studies of Beitchman (1985) who found more than four times the prevalence of psychiatric illness in kindergartners with communication disorders compared to nondisordered children. Some studies also suggest that mental disorders are associated with greater severity of communication problems. For example, in Cantwell and Baker's (1991) population of 302 children with a psychiatric diagnosis as well as a speech and language disorder, the subjects were more likely to have multiple or more severe language disorders than were speech- and language-disordered children who were psychiatrically well. Furthermore, language and phonologic disorders are frequently concurrent in the same individuals. Unfortunately, language disorders too often are unsuspected by parents and professionals alike.

It should come as no surprise that children with communication disorders, and especially with language disorders, are academically vulnerable. Education, as we know it, especially for younger children, is largely based upon language. Bashir and Scavuzzo (1992) suggest that these children's vulnerability arises from the persistence of these disorders in the face of the continuing need for language in school. Moreover, even if a language disorder has been remediated, children may have failed in the meantime; and it is immensely hard for many children in many schools to succeed again, once they have failed for any reason. A further complication is the comorbidity of language disorder in these children. In all, some 50 to 75% of children with language disorders will have persistent academic problems (Aram and Hall 1989). They tend to learn less at any given time and learn more slowly than their peers (Shaywitz 1989). These children need ongoing comprehensive special educational services and regular reevaluation of their educational needs. Children with phonological disorder (PD) may also have persistent problems. These are generally less severe than those with language-disordered children, unless both types of disorders are present. Lewis and Fairbairn (1992) reported mild but persistent problems with reading and spelling in individuals with phonological disorder, even into young adulthood. Subjects tended to steadily improve over time, however. Although most of the subjects and all the adolescents and adults were considered normal speakers, they tended to show subtle phonological problems on specialized tests. Again, children with an associated language disorder fared less well.

The relationship of socioeconomic status (SES) with the occurrence of communication disorders is not altogether certain. Many studies indicate a positive correlation between communication disorders and low SES, but other work suggests that this correlation is weak at best. The need for clinicians to avoid regarding variations in accent and dialect as pathological has been cited. Very little empirical literature on cultural variations in communication therapy is extant. McCrary (1992) and others have pointed out the need for cultural sensitivity in treatment, citing the efforts of ASLHA in this area.

Diagnosis of Expressive Language Disorder and Mixed Receptive–Expressive Language Disorder

Expressive language disorder denotes an impairment in the development of expressive language (see DSM-IV-TR diagnostic criteria below). Its diagnosis requires the use of one or more standardized assessment measures that are individually administered. When appropriate instruments are unavailable, as for example, in the case of a member of a population for which no instrument has been standardized, this diagnosis may be made through a thorough functional investigation of an individual's language ability. Individuals with this disorder have expressive language scores well below those obtained from measures of nonverbal intelligence and of receptive language. DSM-IV-TR does not require any particular degree of discrepancy in scores.

▬ DSM-IV-TR Diagnostic Criteria ▬

315.31 Expressive Language Disorder

A. The scores obtained from standardized individually administered measures of expressive language development are substantially below those obtained from standardized measures of both nonverbal intellectual capacity and receptive language development. The disturbance may be manifest clinically by symptoms that include having a markedly limited vocabulary, making errors in tense, or having difficulty recalling words or producing sentences with developmentally appropriate length or complexity.

B. The difficulties with expressive language interfere with academic or occupational achievement or with social communication.

C. Criteria are not met for mixed receptive–expressive language disorder or a pervasive developmental disorder.

D. If mental retardation, a speech–motor or sensory deficit, or environmental deprivation is present, the language difficulties are in excess of those usually associated with these problems.

Reprinted with permission from the Diagnostic and Statistical Manual of Mental Disorders, Fourth Edition, Text Revision. Copyright 2000 American Psychiatric Association.

The presence of a test score by itself does not define the condition: the affected individual must have clinical symptoms that might include disturbances of vocabulary, grammar (e.g., tenses), or syntax (e.g., sentence length or complexity). The diagnosis of this condition also requires that the individual having it experiences social, academic, or occupational difficulties directly related to the condition. The presence of a mixed receptive–expressive language disorder (MRELD) or a pervasive developmental disorder (PDD) supersedes this diagnosis, and it is not made in their presence. Similarly, it may not be made in the presence of mental retardation, motor or sensory deficits, or environmental observation, unless the expressive language difficulties experienced are beyond what would be expected for individuals with these conditions. This condition may be acquired, as from a medical condition affecting the central nervous system (CNS), or it may be developmental, in the sense of arising early in life without known origin.

The manifestations of Expressive Language Disorder vary with age and severity. Vocabulary, word-finding, sentence length, variety of expression, and grammatical complexity may all be reduced. Most children with this disorder demonstrate a slower than expected rate of language development, associated with the developmental subtype. Often auxiliary words or prepositions are omitted, resulting in a telegraphic sort of speech: "He was going to school" becomes "He going school." Word order of essential importance in English may be garbled: "Him like too me" for "I like him too." Words or phrases may be repeated to the degree that speech may be echolalic, perseverative, or both. Conversation may be tangential with sudden inappropriate changes of topic, or conversely, perseveration. Pragmatic difficulties, such as in initiating or terminating conversations, and much avoidance of conversation are also frequently seen. Because of these problems these children are frequently regarded as socially inappropriate or inept, and at times may be suspected of having a formal thought disorder. These children frequently have associated learning problems because of their difficulty in responding verbally to exercises. They may have motor coordination problems and various other neurodevelopmental abnormalities documented upon neurological examination, EEG, or neuroimaging, although no consistent patterns are seen.

The inclusion of Mixed Receptive–Expressive Language Disorder in DSM-IV represented the most significant change from previous classification systems, which posited the existence of receptive language disorders in a solitary form. The existence of this category reflects the clinical observation that receptive language disorders in children seldom, if ever, can occur without concurrent (and perhaps resultant) problems with expression (see DSM-IV-TR diagnostic criteria on page 115). DSM-IV-TR notes that this is in direct contrast with such entities as Wernicke's aphasia in adults, which affects reception alone. Children with these conditions have significant measurable deficits in standardized individual assessments, of both receptive and expressive language, compared to their similarly assessed nonverbal intelligence. These deficiencies may occur in both verbal and sign language, interfere with social, academic, and occupational function, and by definition in DSM-IV-TR, do not occur in the presence of a PDD. This condition may be acquired from some CNS injury or may be purely developmental. In the latter case, affected individuals exhibit a persistent pattern of delayed language development, in which speech develops late and advances slowly. Children with this disorder may manifest any and all of the symptoms of ELD. They also have difficulty with various aspects of receptive language, including misunderstanding of individual words or whole statements and deficits in auditory processing skills (sound discrimination and association, recall, storage, and sequencing).

DSM-IV-TR Diagnostic Criteria

315.31 Mixed Receptive–Expressive Language Disorder

A. The scores obtained from a battery of standardized individually administered measures of both receptive and expressive language development are substantially below those obtained from standardized measures of both nonverbal intellectual capacity. Symptoms include those for expressive language disorder as well as difficulty understanding words, sentences, or specific types of words, such as spatial terms.

B. The difficulties with receptive and expressive language significantly interfere with academic or occupational achievement or with social communication.

C. Criteria are not met for a pervasive developmental disorder.

D. If mental retardation, a speech–motor or sensory deficit, or environmental deprivation is present, the language difficulties are in excess of those usually associated with these problems.

Reprinted with permission from the Diagnostic and Statistical Manual of Mental Disorders, Fourth Edition, Text Revision. Copyright 2000 American Psychiatric Association.

Children with Mixed Receptive–Expressive Language Disorder may have all the problems of ELD. In addition, they do not understand all that they hear. The deficits may be mild or severe, and at times deceptively subtle, since children with this disorder may conceal them or avoid interaction. All areas and levels of language comprehension may be disturbed. Thus, the child may not understand speech that is rapid, certain words or categories of words such as abstract quantities, or types of statements, such as conditional clauses. This may cause these children to seem not to hear or attend, or to misbehave by not following commands correctly. At times, when conversation is redirected to them in a slower or more concise fashion, they may understand and respond belatedly, and thereby be accused of willful avoidance. More severely impaired children may not understand the rules of syntax or word order, and thus may be unable to distinguish between subjects and objects or questions and declarations. Often, in more severe cases, disabilities may be multiple and pervasive, affecting processing, recall, and association. Children with this disorder may fail to understand pragmatic or social conventions of language. For example, they may fail to comprehend the verbal and nonverbal signals that accompany a change of topic or the end of a conversation. Such deficits have immense social consequences. They may even cause the child to be misidentified as having a pervasive developmental disorder. A very severe acquired language disorder is seen in Landau–Kleffner syndrome (acquired epileptic aphasia), accompanied by seizures and other CNS dysfunctions, and usually occurring between ages 3 and 9.

Phonological disorder is especially common among children with these disorders. In addition, many of these children may present at least some manifestations of learning disorders. Other conditions that are broadly considered as neurodevelopmental are also noted in these children, such as motor delays, coordination disorders, and enuresis. The extent of these associations, while apparently considerable, is difficult to quantify because of methodologic variations in the literature. The combination of these disorders and the stress they create frequently lead to adjustment disorders and social withdrawal. Cantwell and Baker (1991) found that the most common psychiatric disorder among children with communication disorders overall was attention-deficit/hyperactivity disorder (ADHD), representing 19% of their sample of 600 children referred for a communication evaluation. The combination of language and disruptive behavior disorders appears to be associated with greater severity of impairment in both disorders. Some authors have speculated that ADHD may be concordant with a putative entity known as central auditory processing disorder (CAPD), which refers to deficits in the processing of audible signals and which can be subsumed under the DSM-IV-TR language disorders. A total concordance is unlikely, but Riccio and associates (1994) suggest that 50% of children with CAPD also have ADHD. Ongoing work in neuroimaging and brain activity measurement may be expected to delineate this area more fully.

Course

Contrary to some popular beliefs, language disorders do not always spontaneously resolve, nor do children always "grow out of it." In general, the course of these disorders is lengthy, and the more severe disorders are usually more persistent. Language disorders of the developmental type are generally recognized gradually as children grow up; the less severe cases were identified later in childhood or adolescence. Language disorders acquired secondary to other medical illnesses tend to occur more precipitously and can appear at any age. In the case of ELD, DSM-IV-TR reports that most children with this condition acquire more or less normal language abilities by late adolescence, but that subtle deficits may persist. The prognosis is worse in the case of MRELD, and only a minority of these children are free from some communication problems in adulthood. Even when their communication skills seem grossly normal, subtle deficits may persist, and they may go on to manifest learning disorders. The prognosis for individuals with acquired language disorders must be assessed according to the severity of injury or medical illness, as well as the premorbid state of the child, in each case.

Differential Diagnosis

These disorders are distinguished from each other by the presence or absence of receptive problems. Children with autism may have any or all of the characteristics of the language disorders. However, they have many additional problems including the use of language in a restricted and often stereotypic fashion rather than for communicative purposes. They also have difficulties with a wider range of interactions with persons and objects in their environment, and exhibit a restricted range of behaviors. The language impairments of mental retardation, oral–motor deficits, or environmental deprivation are not diagnosed in this category unless they are well in excess of what is expected. Language impairment due to environmental deprivation tends to improve dramatically with environmental improvement. Sensory deficits, especially hearing impairment, may restrict language development. Any indication of potential hearing impairment, no matter how tenuous, should prompt a referral for an audiologic evaluation. Obviously, hearing and language disorders can and do coexist. Some children develop an acquired aphasia as a complication of general medical illness. This condition is usually temporary; only if it persists beyond the acute course of the medical illness is a language disorder diagnosed.

Diagnosis of Phonological Disorder and Stuttering

Phonological Disorder was formerly known as articulation or developmental articulation disorder. It is characterized by an individual's failure to use speech sounds appropriate for one's developmental level and dialect (see DSM-IV-TR diagnostic criteria below). The affected individual may substitute one sound for another (e.g., /l/ for /r/), omit certain sounds entirely, or exhibit other errors in organization, use, or production of sounds. By definition in DSM-IV-TR these difficulties interfere with social, academic, or occupational functions. The symptoms may occur during development without discernible cause or they may be related to CNS, motor, or sensory dysfunction, or to environmental deprivation. In the latter cases, speech difficulties must be in excess of those usually associated with the particular problem for the diagnosis to be made. This condition ranges in severity from very mild problems to severe disorders, which render speech totally unintelligible.

DSM-IV-TR Diagnostic Criteria

315.39 Phonological Disorder

A. Failure to use developmentally expected speech sounds that are appropriate for age and dialect (e.g., errors in sound production, use, representation, or organization such as, but not limited to, substitutions of one sound for another [use of /t/ for target /k/ sound] or omissions of sounds such as final consonants).
B. The difficulties in speech sound production interfere with academic or occupational achievement or with social communication.
C. If mental retardation, a speech–motor or sensory deficit, or environmental deprivation is present, the speech difficulties are in excess of those usually associated with these problems.

Reprinted with permission from the Diagnostic and Statistical Manual of Mental Disorders, Fourth Edition, Text Revision. Copyright 2000 American Psychiatric Association.

Outside of DSM-IV-TR, the term *phonology* often refers to rules governing the combination of sounds into syllables and words. In this case, a phonologic disorder may refer to a type of disorder characterized by difficulty in generating sound combinations, according to these criteria.

This category, which subsumed the DSM-III-R articulation disorder, is characterized by persistent errors in the production of speech. These include omission, substitution, or distortion of sounds. Omissions include single or multiple sounds: "I go o coo o the but" (I go to school on the bus) or "I re a boo" (I read a book). Substitutions include w/l, t/s, w/r, and d/g: "I taw a wittle wed wadio. It pwayed dood music." A common distortion is lisping. A frontal lisp leads to an /s/ sound resembling /th/. A lateral lisp, with sound coming from the sides of the mouth, leads to a "slushy" /s/ sound: "Shuffering shnakes!" Defects in the order of sounds or insertions of extraneous sounds may also be heard: "catht" for "cats." The occurrence of these errors is persistent but not constant. Baker (1990) points out that "conditioning factors" such as the location within a word, or the rate or length of a statement may determine whether a phonologic error is produced. Only some sounds are usually affected, as for example, in lisping the misarticulation of sibilants. Some articulation errors are expected in early childhood, especially involving sounds that are usually mastered at a later age (in English /l/, /r/, /s/, /z/, /th/, /ch/); these errors are not regarded as pathological unless they persist and result in adverse consequences to the individual. It is estimated that 90% or more of children have mastered the more difficult sounds by age 6 to 8.

Stuttering is one of the most commonly recognized disorders of speech. Some occurrence of the symptoms of stuttering is normal in the earlier stages of development, and the condition is properly diagnosed only when the symptoms are perceived to be in excess of what is developmentally expected. Similarly, since occasional symptoms appear in the speech of nearly all persons, the diagnosis is not made unless the disturbances interfere with social, academic, or occupational functioning. The condition may be associated with motoric or sensory deficits; when this is the case, the diagnosis is made only when symptoms exceed those expected with these problems. The characteristic symptoms of stuttering, as shown in the DSM-IV-TR criteria for stuttering are disturbances in fluency (such as repetitions of sounds, syllables or words, interjections, and circumlocutions) and in time patterning (sound prolongations, broken words, and blocking). "Cluttering," the disturbance in rate and length of speech noted in DSM-III-R, is subsumed in DSM-IV-TR under CDNOS, or ELD.

DSM-IV-TR Diagnostic Criteria

370.0 Stuttering

A. Disturbance in the normal fluency and time patterning of speech (inappropriate for the individual's age), characterized by frequent occurrences of one or more of the following:

(1) sound and syllable repetitions
(2) sound prolongations
(3) interjections
(4) broken words (e.g., pauses within a word)
(5) audible or silent blocking (filled or unfilled pauses in speech)
(6) circumlocutions (word substitutions to avoid problematic words)
(7) words produced with an excess of physical tension
(8) monosyllabic whole-word repetitions (e.g., "I-I-I-I see him")

B. The disturbance in fluency interferes with academic or occupational achievement or with social communication.
C. If a speech–motor or sensory deficit is present, the speech difficulties are in excess of those usually associated with these problems.

The familiar symptoms of this disorder are noted in criterion A. Stuttering is the communication disorder most easily recognized by both the lay public and physicians. It varies in severity among individuals. It may be more or less evident in different situations and may vary over time. It is typically most severe when the affected child is stressed or anxious, and especially when communication is expected. Children who stutter can sing or talk to themselves without difficulty. Because of its often gradual onset, children are at first frequently not aware of its presence. Over time they may become more anxious and withdraw from conversation as the degree of social discrimination they experience increases. Stuttering may be accompanied by various movements, which may seem either to express or discharge anxiety, such as blinking, grimacing, or hyperventilation. Sometimes, children who stutter may attempt to stop momentarily by slowing down or pausing in their speech, but this is frequently unsuccessful and leads to an exacerbation. Thus, a pattern of habitual fear and avoidance emerges.

Children with PD may present with clearly associated causal factors such as anatomic malformations, neurological diseases, or cognitive disorders, though most do not. They do have a higher prevalence of language disorders with all their associated problems, than do normal controls. Even if they are free of language disorders they are still more likely to have ADHD, though probably not as commonly as do children with language disorders. Children with PD, especially when associated with stuttering or hyperactivity, are prone to social discrimination and isolation with subsequent consequences.

There is much less literature extant that addresses the comorbidity of stuttering compared to other communication disorders. Other communication disorders are more frequently reported in those with stuttering rather than in normal controls. Stuttering is frequently accompanied by many linguistic mechanisms and social maneuvers to avoid its manifestation. Conversely, it appears more frequently and intensely in affected individuals when they experience anxiety or stress. The literature is replete with anecdotal and biographical accounts of the social and occupational discrimination, disappointment, and low self-esteem faced by persons with this condition. The negative stereotype of stutterers in society is well documented. They have been mocked in drama and cinema (including cartoons) for centuries, and are all too often regarded as being intellectually impaired.

Course

The course of PD is much more encouraging than those of other communication disorders. Milder cases may not be discovered until the child starts school. These cases often recover spontaneously, especially if the child does not encounter adverse psychosocial consequences because of his speech. Severe cases associated with anatomic malformations may at times require surgical intervention, and its course and outcome depend upon the results of the surgery. Between these two extremes are children who gradually improve, often to the point of total remission, and whose improvement may be accelerated by speech therapy.

Stuttering usually appears in early childhood, as early as 2 years of age and frequently has its onset around age 5. The onset of stuttering is typically regarded as gradual, with repetition of initial consonants or first words or phrases heard in the beginning. However, a study by Yairi and colleagues (1993) suggested that often early stuttering takes on a moderate to severe form, and that identification of problems in this period has been affected by parents' tendency to postpone professional consultation. Children are generally not aware of this condition in themselves until it is pointed out to them by others. The disorder can wax and wane during childhood. By early adolescence it abates spontaneously in some cases, and from 60 to 80% of individuals eventually recover totally or to a major extent. DSM-IV-TR asserts that spontaneous recovery typically occurs before age 16. Stuttering may persist into adulthood often leading to adverse social and occupational consequences.

Differential Diagnosis

These conditions should be distinguished from the normal dysfluencies that occur among young children. For example, misarticulation of some sounds, such as /l/, /r/, /s/, /z/, /th/, and /ch/, is common among preschoolers and resolves with age. As with the language disorders, these diagnoses are given in the case of motor or sensory deficit, mental retardation, or environmental deprivation only if the disorder is much more severe than expected in these conditions. Problems limited to voice alone are included under CDNOS.

Diagnosis of Communication Disorder not Otherwise Specified

This category includes disorders that do not meet criteria for other specific communication disorders or do so incompletely. DSM-IV-TR cites voice disorders of pitch, loudness, quality, tone, or resonance, as an example. It is used to describe disorders that do not fit the criteria for any of the other communication disorders and is generally used only to describe voice disorders. These are disorders of pitch, intonation, volume, or resonance. Hyponasality is one example of a voice disorder as characterized by the "adenoidal" speech that brought many children to surgery in an earlier era. Hypernasality, secondary to velopharyngeal insufficiency, may be associated with serious voice problems. Air escapes into the nasal cavity resulting in nasal air emission, snorting, or a nasal grimace during speech.

Etiology of Communication Disorders

Genetic Factors

Many clinicians believe that communication disorders tend to "run in families," but the extent to which this is true is unclear. No clear mechanisms of transmission have been elucidated, but a number of instances of family aggregation have been reported. At least one of these (Gopnik and Crago 1991) suggested the presence of a single dominant autosomal gene. Tomblin (1989) reported increased concordance of language disorders among siblings. An increasing number of family studies now suggest that these disorders are familial. Prominent among these is the twins early development study (TEDS) in the United Kingdom (Plomin and Dale 2000). These reports cannot absolutely prove any genetic hypothesis; however, they are provocative and suggestive of a polygenetic basis. Plomin, (2001) in an authoritative review, suggests that the application of a quantitative trait loci (QTL) model may elucidate the variable pattern of transmission and presentation of these disorders. This area of inquiry is complicated not only by methodologic issues but also by larger controversies over the degree to which specific features of language, such as grammar, arise from a "preprogrammed" genetic base. The recent work of Baker (2001) influenced by the model of Chomsky (1988) suggests that grammar in all language may be a product of an innate and limited series of "hard-wired" options.

A genetic basis for stuttering has been proposed for many years. The Yale Family study of stuttering (YFSS) suggested that 15% of first-degree relatives of stutterers are affected at some time in their lives (Kidd 1983). A concordance of 77% in identical twins and 32% in fraternal twins has also been reported (Howie 1981). These reports were subsequently confirmed by other studies (Yairi et al. 1996, Andrews et al. 1991).

Biological Factors

Baker (1990) and others propose that communication disorders arise from at least three interrelated sets of factors: neurophysiologic (including structural), cognitive–perceptual, and environmental. The great majority of children with communication disorders give no evidence of specific CNS damage. Thus, in these children minimal or subclinical damage has been postulated. The relative frequency of "soft" neurological signs and lateral dominance problems in this population provokes this speculation. However, at this time no clear neurophysiologic mechanisms or pathology can be correlated with these disorders, despite the appeal of this model to many physicians. Some interesting findings are emerging however. For example, recent reports of magnetic resonance imaging (MRI) studies in stuttering (Foundas et al. 2001) have suggested anatomical differences in Broca's and

Wernicke's areas of the left cerebral cortex in affected subjects. In a minority of children with communication disorders, a neuropathologic cause is painfully apparent. Localizable brain damage may arise from trauma, infection, vascular disease, or neoplasm. Perinatal factors such as prematurity, low birth weight, and asphyxia have also been implicated. A number of toxic agents have been associated with communication disorders, particularly lead. Recently, concerns have been raised about prenatal alcohol exposure (Abkarian 1992) and also about the physical sequelae of abuse and neglect (Law and Conway 1992).

Developmental and Psychological Factors

These hypotheses relate communication disorders to various deficits in the reception, acquisition, processing, storage, or recall of different elements of communication. Work in this area has largely been pursued through a multidisciplinary model addressing children with "developmental" communication disorders. Perceptual hypotheses posit that speech or language develops improperly because of a failure of input, that is a failure of the child to perceive or process communicated information. Without proper input proper communication cannot come about. At times, a related model of perceptual immaturity has also been proposed. This model has undeniable intuitive appeal, but does not by itself explain why language development may not "catch up" despite age and maturation (Table 6-2). More purely cognitive hypotheses have also been proposed. Their details are beyond the scope of this chapter, but they implicate deficits in symbolization, categorizing, hierarchical processing, and related areas. The concordance between communication and learning disorders supports these hypotheses. However, not all children with communication disorders have cognitive deficits. Some authors (Friel-Patti 1992, Helmuth 2001) propose that there are certain language-specific abilities; this notion is invigorated by the phenomenology of Williams syndrome, in which affected individuals may have good language skills in the presence of mental retardation. The special phenomenology of stuttering suggests the

Table 6-2	Hypotheses About Influencing Factors in Communication Disorders	
Types of Hypotheses	**Specific Hypotheses**	
Neurological impairments	Specific localizable brain damage	
	Subclinical (minimal) brain damage	
Perceptual deficits	Deficits in auditory discrimination	
	Deficits in auditory attention	
	Deficits in auditory figure-ground	
	Deficits in auditory memory	
	Deficits in auditory–visual association	
	Deficits in the processing of specific linguistic units	
Cognitive deficits	Deficits in symbolic or concept development	
	Deficits in anticipatory imagery	
	Deficits in sorting or categorizing	
	Deficits in hierarchical processing	
Environmental factors	Inadequate parent–child interaction	
	Socioeconomic factors (large family size, lower social class, late birth order, and environmental deprivation)	
	Medical factors (e.g., prematurity, history of recurrent otitis media)	
Multifactorial etiology	Combinations of all of the above	

Source: Reprinted from *Psychiatric Disorders in Children and Adolescents*, Baker L, Specific communication disorders, 257–270, Copyright 1990 with permission from Elsevier.

possibility of dyssynchrony between phonation and articulation, as reported by Perkins (2001).

Inadequate or pathologic parent–child interaction has also been associated with the rate of language acquisition, though not so clearly with eventual outcome. Other socioeconomic variables such as class, family size, income, and birth order all clearly affect the amount of verbal interaction children receive and have also been implicated. Some authors (Law and Conway 1992) have attempted to elucidate specific effects upon language of child abuse, mainly in regard to syntactic form, but this is speculative at best. No definitive relationship between any psychosocial factor and the type or severity of communication disorder has been established. In the past, various psychodynamic etiologies have been proposed for stuttering; these have been more stigmatizing than illuminating. The association between the exacerbation of stuttering and stress is well known, however. Work in this area (as in others) has frequently confounded predisposing, triggering, and maintaining factors (Schulze and Johannsen 1991).

Review of these influences reveals a considerable amount of overlap, with potentially complex interrelationships of causality and concurrence. Clinical observation seldom if ever suggests a unitary causality of communication disorders in individuals presenting for treatment. Thus, these conditions in most children are ultimately described as multifactorial. The clinician should be aware that many or all of the factors cited may be present in any communication-disordered child, and may have complex effects on communication as well as on other aspects of the child's life.

Treatment of Communication Disorders

Speech and language therapy typically has three major goals: the development and improvement of communication skills with concurrent remediation of deficits, the development of alternative or augmentative communication strategies where required, and the social habilitation of the individual in regard to communication. Thus, a very great range of approaches and components must be employed in treating children with communication disorders. The speech and language pathologist (SLP) plays the most direct role in treatment of these conditions: this role is illustrated by the diagnostic treatment tree (Figure 6-2). SLPs may employ an exceedingly wide range of techniques with children. Their work, not unlike medical psychotherapy, requires both science and art. As in child psychotherapy, the participation of parents is necessary. Parent–infant work involves demonstration and modeling of language-stimulation techniques. Individual therapy can usually be begun by 3 years of age, and early initiation of therapy is frequently recommended. Individual sessions can include traditional exercises along with seemingly less structured but nonetheless carefully directed verbal and play interactions. A lay observer of a session might recognize exercises of the "Peter-piper-picked-a-peck" type as therapeutic. However, the same session might also include periods of seemingly free play or undirected conversation that in fact subtly model and direct the child in the skills of speech and language. Group therapy can also be used especially in the development of language skills applied to a social context, but it should not be regarded as a low-budget substitute for individual treatment. In any treatment regimen, constant monitoring and regular reassessment are necessary as is ongoing support to parents who must reinforce the treatment at home. Similarly, regular reconsultation with other professionals from the multidisciplinary team may be required. The treatment of stuttering has provoked special interest in recent years, particularly as its adverse consequences in adulthood have been recognized. Approaches to this problem address both the mechanics of speech and associated attitudinal and affective patterns. Guitar (1985) notes that therapists attempt to modify speech rhythm and speed, leading subjects to regularize rhythm, and as a temporary measure, prolong their speech. Thus, these children might be heard speaking in a slow, drawn-out,

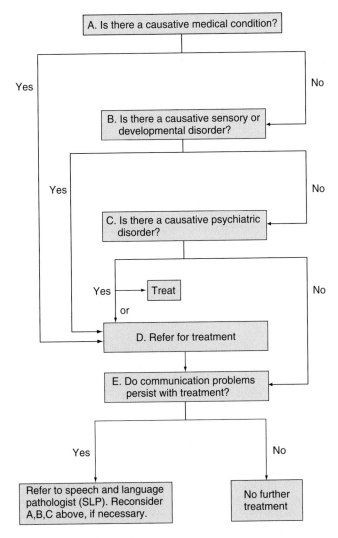

Figure 6-2 *Diagnostic treatment tree.*

singsong fashion. Much attention is also directed to respiration, airflow, and "gentle" onset of phonation.

Drug therapy for this disorder remains at best controversial. Individual and family psychotherapy may be a useful augment in reducing the stress these children encounter. The literature on the outcome of treatment for stuttering is somewhat more complete than for the other communication disorders, since symptoms of this disorder can be readily quantified by electronic and other means. Success rates for various treatments of up to 70% have been reported, though with varying follow-up periods and relapse rates (Guitar 1985). Some speech and language pathologists specialize in the treatment of this disorder (Rafuse 1994).

The mental health professional may have a major role in the treatment of communication disorders. These children and their families may present for psychotherapy or other treatment for disorders based on or related to communication problems. Thus, the clinician may, in the first place, be a case finder or a case manager, facilitating the evaluation and treatment of these disorders by a multidisciplinary team. The demonstrated psychiatric comorbidity of these disorders will necessitate the clinician's involvement on many levels, both as a clinician primarily treating a child, and as a therapist, counselor, and agent of advice and support for the entire family. Psychotherapy does not directly address language disorders, although older literature has cited improvement in stuttering following family and individual treatment. The psychotherapist must, in any event, be sensitive to the manner in which communication disorders can affect or interfere with the therapeutic process. Nonverbal augments or prompts should be sensitively provided to children who need them.

The role of psychotropic medication in the management of these disorders is mainly limited to the treatment of comorbid psychiatric problems according to standard practices. From time to time, some interest in the use of drugs, specifically for these conditions has arisen. In the 1960s and 1970s, some reports of haloperidol treatment for stuttering emerged. However, enthusiasm was tempered by recognition of this agent's side effects (Andrews and Dozsa 1977), and it is very seldom used for this condition today.

Outcome studies of communication therapy, especially for the language disorders, have often been complicated by multiple theories of language development, diagnostic and methodologic variations, lack of standardization of therapeutic techniques, and comorbidity. Thus, the literature in this area is relatively sparse and not always conclusive. Like the outcome of psychotherapy, this is a difficult area to study. Nonresponse to initial treatment may be common, requiring patience and persistence. It is important to note in assessing these issues that, even when communication therapy does not lead to apparent improvements in language beyond developmental improvements, it may still facilitate the child's use of extant language for environmental- and self-control (Goldstein and Hockenberger 1991).

Comparison of DSM-IV/ICD-10 Diagnostic Criteria

Regarding expressive language disorder, the ICD-10 Diagnostic Criteria for Research suggest specific cutoffs for the expressive language scores: 2 standard deviations below the expected level and one standard deviation below nonverbal IQ. Furthermore, in contrast to DSM-IV-TR, the diagnosis cannot be made if there are any neurological, sensory, or physical impairments that directly affect the use of spoken language or if there is mental retardation.

For DSM-IV-TR mixed receptive–expressive language disorder, the corresponding ICD-10 disorder is "receptive language disorder." In contrast to DSM-IV-TR, which specifies both expressive and receptive language difficulties because these generally occur together, the ICD-10 definition only mentions deviations in language comprehension. Like with expressive language disorder, the ICD-10 Diagnostic Criteria for Research suggest a cutoff of receptive language scores of 2 standard deviations below the expected level and 1 standard deviation below nonverbal IQ. Furthermore, in contrast to DSM-IV-TR, the diagnosis cannot be made if there are any neurological, sensory, or physical impairments that directly affect receptive language or if there is mental retardation.

As compared to DSM-IV-TR phonological disorder, in which no mention is made of assessment using standardized tests, the ICD-10 Diagnostic Criteria for Research suggest that articulation skills, as assessed on standardized tests, are 2 standard deviations below the expected level and 1 standard deviation below nonverbal IQ. Furthermore, in contrast to DSM-IV-TR, the diagnosis cannot be made if there are any neurological, sensory, or physical impairments that directly affect receptive language or if there is mental retardation.

Regarding stuttering, in contrast to DSM-IV-TR, which establishes clinical significance based on interference with academic or occupational achievement or with social communication, the ICD-10 Diagnostic Criteria for Research establish clinical significance by requiring a minimum duration of at least three months.

References

Abkarian GG (1992) Communication effects of prenatal alcohol exposure. *J Commun Disord* **25**, 221–240.

Andrews G and Dozsa M (1977) Haloperidol and the treatment of stuttering. *J Fluency Dis* **2**, 217–224.

Andrews G, Morris-Yates A, and Howie P (1991) Genetic factors in stuttering confirmed. *Arch Gen Psychiatry* **48**, 1034–1035.

Aram DM and Hall NE (1989) Longitudinal follow-up of children with preschool communication disorders: treatment implications. *School Psychol Rev* **18**(4), 487–501.

Baker L (1990) Specific communication disorders. In *Psychiatric Disorders in Children and Adolescents*, Garfinkel BD, Carlson GA, and Weller EB (eds). W. B. Saunders, Philadelphia, pp. 257–270.

Baker MC (2001) *The Atoms of Language: The Mind's Secret Rules of Grammar*. Basic Books, New York.

Bashir AS and Scavuzzo A (1992) Children with language disorders: natural history and academic success. *J Learn Disabil* **25**(1), 53–65.

Beitchman JH (1985) Speech and language impairment and psychiatric risk: toward a model of neurodevelopmental immaturity. *Psychiatr Clin N Am* **8**, 721–735.

Cantwell DP and Baker L (1991) *Psychiatric and Developmental Disorders in Children with Communication Disorder*. American Psychiatric Press, Washington, DC.

Chomsky N (1988) *Language and Problems of Knowledge*. The MIT Press, Cambridge, MA.

Cohen NJ, Davine M, Horodezky N, et al. (1993) Unsuspected language impairment in psychiatrically disturbed children: prevalence and language and behavioral characteristics. *J Am Acad Child Adolesc Psychiatry* **32**(3), 595–603.

Foundas AL, Bollich AM, Corey DM, et al. (2001) Anomalous anatomy of speech-language areas in adults with persistent developmental stuttering. *Neurology* **57**(2), 207–215.

Friel-Patti S (1992) Research in language disorders: What do we know and where are we going?. *Folia Phoniatr* **44**, 126–142.

Goldstein H and Hockenberger EH (1991) Significant progress in child language intervention: an 11-year retrospective. *Res Dev Disabil* **12**, 401–424.

Gopnik M and Crago MB (1991) Familial aggregation of a developmental language disorder. *Cognition* **39**, 1–50.

Guitar B (1985) Stammering and stuttering. In *The Clinical Guide to Child Psychiatry*, Shaffer D, Ehrhardt AA, and Greenhill L (eds). Free Press, New York, pp. 97–109.

Gulley-Smith P (1998) Learning and communication disorders. In *Clinical Child Psychiatry*, Klykylo WM, Kay J, and Rube D (eds). W. B. Saunders, Philadelphia, pp. 326–336.

Helmuth L (2001) From the mouths (and hands) of babes. *Science* **293**, 1758–1759.

Howie P (1981) Concordance for stuttering in monozygotic and dizygotic twin pairs. *J Speech Hear Res* **5**, 343–348.

Kidd K (1983) Genetic aspects of speech and language disorders. In *Genetic Aspects of Speech and Language Disorders*, Ludlow C and Cooper J (eds). Academic Press, New York, pp. 197–213.

Law J and Conway J (1992) Effect of abuse and neglect on the development of speech and language. *Dev Med Child Neurol* **34**(11), 943–948.

Lewis BA and Fairbairn L (1992) Residual effects of preschool phonology disorders in grade school, adolescence, and adulthood. *J Speech Hear Res* **35**, 819–831.

McCrary MB (1992) Urban multicultural trauma patients. *ASLHA* **34**(4), 37–40, 42.

Paul R (1982) Communication development and its disorders: a psycholinguistic perspective. *Schizophr Bull* **8**, 287–290.

Perkins WH (2001) Stuttering: a matter of bad timing. *Science* **294**, 786.

Plomin R (2001) Genetic factors contributing to learning and language delays and disabilities. *Child Adolesc Psychiatr Clin N Am* **10**(2), 259–277.

Plomin R and Dale PS (2000) Speech and language impairments in children: causes, characteristics, intervention, and outcome. In *Speech and Language Impairments in Children*, Bishop DVM and Leonard BE (eds). Psychology Press, Hove, East Coast Sussex, pp. 35–51.

Rafuse J (1994) Early intervention, intensive therapy can help people who stutter. *Can Med Assoc J* **150**(5), 754–755.

Riccio CA, Hynd GW, Morris MJ, et al. (1994) Comorbidity of central auditory processing disorder and attention-deficit hyperactivity disorder. *J Am Acad Child Adolesc Psychiatry* **33**(6), 849–857.

Rutter M (1987) Assessment objectives and principles. In *Language Development and Disorders*, Yule W and Rutter M (eds). JB Lippincott, Philadelphia.

Schulze H and Johannsen HS (1991) Importance of parent–child interaction in the genesis of stuttering. *Folia Phoniatr* **43**, 133–143.

Shaywitz SE (1989) Developmental changes in learning and behavior: results of the Connecticut longitudinal study. Paper Presented at the Fifth Annual Conference on Learning Disorders. Cambridge, MA.

Tomblin JB (1989) Familial concentration of developmental language impairment. *J Speech Hear Disord* **54**, 287–295.

Yairi E, Ambrose N, and Cox N (1996) Genetics of stuttering: a critical review. *J Speech Lang Hear Res* **39**, 771–784.

Yairi E, Ambrose NG, and Niermann R (1993) The early months of stuttering: a developmental study. *J Speech Hear Res* **36**, 521–528.

7 Childhood Disorders: Pervasive Developmental Disorders

The pervasive developmental disorders (PDDs) have been more recently conceptualized as the autism spectrum disorders (ASDs) in order to recognize the commonality of these conditions with the paradigmatic disorder, autistic disorder. The ASDs are a group of neurodevelopmental syndromes characterized by disturbances in social interactions, language and communication, and the presence of stereotyped behaviors and interests. Diagnoses subsumed under the category of the ASDs (and PDDs) include Autistic Disorder (see DSM-IV-TR diagnostic criteria below), Rett's Disorder (see DSM-IV-TR diagnostic criteria on page 128), Childhood Disintegrative Disorder (see criteria on page 129), Asperger's Disorder (see DSM-IV-TR diagnostic criteria on page 129), and Pervasive Developmental Disorder Not Otherwise Specified (PDDNOS). A comparison of the definitions of the ASDs is shown in Table 7-1.

DSM-IV-TR Diagnostic Criteria

299.00 Autistic Disorder

A. A total of six (or more) items from (1), (2), and (3), with at least two from (1) and one each from (2) and (3):

   (1) qualitative impairment in social interaction as manifested by at least two of the following:

   (a) marked impairment in the use of multiple nonverbal behaviors such as eye-to-eye gaze, facial expression, body postures, and gestures to regulate social interaction

   (b) failure to develop peer relationships appropriate to developmental level

   (c) a lack of spontaneous seeking to share enjoyment, interests, or achievements with other people (e.g., by a lack of showing, bringing, or pointing out objects of interest)

     (d) lack of social or emotional reciprocity

(2) qualitative impairments in communication manifested by at least one of the following:

     (a) delay in, or total lack of, the development of spoken language (not accompanied by an attempt to compensate through alternative modes of communication such as gesture or mime)

     (b) in individuals with adequate speech, marked impairment in the ability to initiate or sustain a conversation with others

     (c) stereotyped and repetitive use of language or idiosyncratic language

     (d) lack of varied, spontaneous make-believe play or social imitative play appropriate to developmental level

(3) restricted repetitive and stereotyped patterns of behavior, interests, and activities, as manifested by at least one of the following:

     (a) encompassing preoccupation with one or more stereotyped and restricted patterns of interest that is abnormal in either intensity or focus

     (b) apparently inflexible adherence to specific, nonfunctional routines or rituals

     (c) stereotyped and repetitive motor mannerisms (e.g., hand or finger flapping or twisting, or complex whole-body movements)

     (d) persistent preoccupation with parts of objects

B. Delays or abnormal functioning in at least one of the following areas, with onset before age 3 years: (1) social interaction, (2) language as used in social communication, or (3) symbolic or imaginative play.

C. The disturbance is not better accounted for by Rett's disorder or childhood disintegrative disorder.

Reprinted with permission from the Diagnostic and Statistical Manual of Mental Disorders, Fourth Edition, Text Revision. Copyright 2000 American Psychiatric Association.

DSM-IV-TR Diagnostic Criteria

299.80 Rett's Disorder

A. All of the following:

(1) apparently normal prenatal and perinatal development
(2) apparently normal psychomotor development through the first 5 months after birth
(3) normal head circumference at birth.

B. Onset of all of the following after the period of normal development:

(1) deceleration of head growth between ages 5 and 48 months
(2) loss of previously acquired purposeful hand skills between ages 5 and 30 months with the subsequent development of stereotyped hand movements (e.g., hand wringing or hand washing)
(3) loss of social engagement early in the course (although often social interaction develops later)
(4) appearance of poorly coordinated gait or trunk movements

(5) severely impaired expressive and receptive language development with severe psychomotor retardation.

DSM-IV-TR Diagnostic Criteria

299.10 Childhood Disintegrative Disorder

A. Apparently normal development for at least the first 2 years after birth as manifested by the presence of age-appropriate verbal and nonverbal communication, social relationships, play, and adaptive behavior.
B. Clinically significant loss of previously acquired skills (before age 10 years) in at least two of the following areas:

(1) expressive or receptive language
(2) social skills or adaptive behavior
(3) bowel or bladder control
(4) play
(5) motor skills

C. Abnormalities of functioning in at least two of the following areas:

(1) qualitative impairment in social interaction (e.g., impairment in nonverbal behaviors, failure to develop peer relationships, lack of social or emotional reciprocity)
(2) qualitative impairments in communication (e.g., delay or lack of spoken language, inability to initiate or sustain a conversation, stereotyped and repetitive use of language, lack of varied make-believe play)
(3) restricted, repetitive, and stereotyped patterns of behavior, interests, and activities, including motor stereotypies and mannerisms

D. The disturbance is not better accounted for by another specific pervasive developmental disorder or by schizophrenia.

DSM-IV-TR Diagnostic Criteria

299.80 Asperger's Disorder

A. Qualitative impairment in social interaction, as manifested by at least two of the following:

(1) marked impairment in the use of multiple nonverbal behaviors such as eye-to-eye gaze, facial expression, body postures, and gestures to regulate social interaction
(2) failure to develop peer relationships appropriate to developmental level

    (3) a lack of spontaneous seeking to share enjoyment, interests, or achievements with other people (e.g., by a lack of showing, bringing, or pointing out objects of interest to other people)

    (4) lack of social or emotional reciprocity

B. Restricted repetitive and stereotyped patterns of behavior, interests, and activities, as manifested by at least one of the following:

    (1) encompassing preoccupation with one or more stereotyped and restricted patterns of interest that is abnormal in either intensity or focus

    (2) apparently inflexible adherence to specific, nonfunctional routines or rituals

    (3) stereotyped and repetitive motor mannerisms (e.g., hand or finger flapping or twisting, or complex whole-body movements)

    (4) persistent preoccupation with parts of objects

C. The disturbance causes clinically significant impairment in social, occupational, or other important areas of functioning.

D. There is no clinically significant general delay in language (e.g., single words used by age 2 years, communicative phrases used by age 3 years).

E. There is no clinically significant delay in cognitive development or in the development of age-appropriate self-help skills, adaptive behavior (other than in social interaction), and curiosity about the environment in childhood.

F. Criteria are not met for another specific pervasive developmental disorder or schizophrenia.

More recently, the ASDs have been conceptualized as a spectrum of conditions that are related by the common features of the disorders: difficulties in social interactions and use of language, and restricted interests and repetitive behaviors. The term spectrum implies that there are phenomenological commonalities to these disorders that justify that they are grouped, but that component symptoms in each syndrome vary in severity (Tager-Flusberg et al. 2001). Despite the enormous heterogeneity evident in this area, there is increasing evidence that conceptualizing these disorders as a spectrum is useful and valid (Folstein and Mankoski 2000).

Diagnosis

ASDs are notoriously heterogeneous in their presentation: there may be variability in the particular symptoms manifested in any individual at a given point in time and there may be significant levels of comorbidity. Nonetheless, autism has been consistently one of the most reliably diagnosed disorders of childhood. Accurate diagnosis requires that the clinician looks for the particular symptoms and signs that characterize it: peculiar and deficient modes of social interaction, deficits in communication, and the focused behaviors and interests.

Many consider the disturbance of social development, including difficulty in developing meaningful attachments and interpersonal reciprocity, to be the central impairment in ASD (Lord et al. 2000a, Rutter 1985). There is definitely variation in the clinical presentation. For instance, while many children with ASD will seem aloof and unattached to their parents, many will display age-appropriate separation anxiety. Typically, a child with autistic disorder has abnormal patterns of eye contact and facial expression. When compared with normal children, children with autism fail to consistently maintain eye contact or vary facial

Table 7-1	Comparison of Domains of Diagnostic Criteria for Pervasive Developmental Disorders				
	Autistic Disorder	**Rett's Disorder**	**Childhood Disintegrative Disorder**	**Asperger's Disorder**	**Pervasive Developmental Disorder NOS**
Age at onset	Delays or abnormal functioning in social interaction, language, or play by age 3 years.	Apparently normal prenatal development. Apparently normal motor development for first 5 months. Deceleration of head growth between ages 5 and 48 months	Apparently normal development for at least the first 2 years. Clinically significant loss of previously acquired skills before 10 years of age	No clinically significant delay in language, cognitive development, or development of age-appropriate self-help skills, adaptive behavior, and curiosity about the environment in childhood	Category used in cases of pervasive impairment in social interaction and communication, with presence of stereotyped behaviors or interests when criteria are not met for a specific disorder
Social interaction	Qualitative impairment in social interaction, as manifested by at least two of the following: • Marked impairment in the use of multiple nonverbal behaviors (e.g., eye-to-eye gaze) • Failure to develop peer relationships appropriate to developmental level • Lack of spontaneous seeking to share enjoyment with other people • Lack of social or emotional reciprocity	Loss of social engagement early in the course (although often social interaction develops later)	Same as autistic disorder along with loss of social skills (previously acquired)	Same as autistic disorder	
Communication	Qualitative impairments of communication as manifested by at least one of the following: • Delay in, or total lack of, the development of spoken language	Severely impaired expressive and receptive language development and severe psychomotor retardation	Same as autistic disorder along with loss of expressive or receptive language previously acquired	No clinically significant delay in language	

(continued overleaf)

Table 7-1 (continued)

	Autistic Disorder	Rett's Disorder	Childhood Disintegrative Disorder	Asperger's Disorder	Pervasive Developmental Disorder NOS
	• Marked impairment in initiating or sustaining a conversation with others, in individuals with adequate speech • Stereotyped and repetitive use of language or idiosyncratic language • Lack of varied, spontaneous make-believe, or imitative play				
Behavior	Restricted, repetitive, and stereotyped patterns of behavior, as manifested by one of the following: • Preoccupation with one or more stereotyped or restricted patterns of interest • Adherence to nonfunctional routines or rituals • Stereotyped and repetitive motor mannerisms • Persistent preoccupation with parts of objects	Loss of previously acquired purposeful hand movement. Appearance of poorly coordinated gait or trunk movements	Same as autistic disorder along with loss of bowel or bladder control, play, motor skills previously acquired	Same as autistic disorder	
Exclusions	Disturbance not better accounted for by Rett's disorder or childhood disintegrative disorder		Disturbance not better accounted for by another PDD or schizophrenia	Criteria are not met for another PDD or schizophrenia	

Source: Adapted from American Psychiatric Association (2000) Diagnostic and Statistical Manual of Mental Disorders, 4th ed.-Text Revision APA, Washington, DC.

expression to establish social contact (Willemsen-Swinkels et al. 1998). These children seem to have considerable difficulty in effectively coordinating social cues (Carter et al. 1998, Lord 1984). They have difficulty demonstrating empathy or perceiving or anticipating others' moods or responses (Bacon et al. 1998). The child with ASD often acts in a socially inappropriate manner or lacks the social responsiveness needed to succeed in social settings, leading to difficulty in the development of close, meaningful relationships (Hobson and Lee 1998, Libby et al. 1997). Some children with ASD eventually develop warm, friendly relationships with family while their relationships with peers lag behind considerably, and these deficits typically persist across time (Njardvik et al. 1999).

Another area of difficulty is in the acquisition and proper use of language for communication. It is estimated that only about half of the children with autistic disorder develop functional speech. This is not merely a delay in development of speech; speech patterns may be deviant and idiosyncratic compared with normal children. If autistic children do begin to speak, their babble is frequently decreased in quantity and lacking in vocal experimentation (Bartak et al. 1975, Lord et al. 1997). When children with autistic disorder do acquire some speech, it is often peculiar and lacking in social perspective (Tager-Flusberg and Anderson 1991). Some children with autistic disorder are even loquacious, although their speech tends to be repetitive and self-directed rather than aimed at maintaining a reciprocal dialogue. People with autistic disorder commonly make use of stereotyped speech, including immediate and delayed echolalia, pronoun reversal, and neologisms (Volden and Lord 1991). Speech usage is often idiosyncratic, may consist of concrete and poorly constructed grammar, may not be used to convey social meaning, and is often literal, lacking in inference, and lacking in imagination (Happe 1993). The delivery of speech is frequently abnormal with atypical tone, pitch, and cadence. Paradoxically, children with autistic disorder often have echolalia, in which prosody and other aspects of speech are frequently imitated verbatim.

Individuals with autistic disorder routinely engage in unusual patterns of behavior. Most people with ASD also resist or have significant difficulty with new experiences or transitions. They are commonly resistant to changes in their environment. They often repeatedly perform stereotyped motor acts such as hand clapping or flapping, or peculiar finger movements. These movements frequently occur at the periphery of their vision near their own face. Some children with autistic disorder engage in self-injurious behaviors including biting or striking themselves or banging their heads. This is most likely to occur with severe or profound mental retardation but is also seen in children with autistic disorder without mental retardation. Their play only occasionally involves traditional toys, and objects may be used in ways other than intended (for instance, a doll is used as a hammer), and there is a paucity of make-believe play. Individuals with autistic disorder seem to have unusual sensitivity to some sensory experiences, particularly, specific sounds.

Other problems in autistic disorder and other PDDs include impairment in "joint attention," the sharing or mutual focus on an object or event by two or more people, and the ability to shift attention when the social situation calls for it (Kasari et al. 1990, Mundy and Sigman 1989). Many children with ASD also have symptoms of hyperactivity and difficulty sustaining attention, but these should be distinguished from the joint attentional dysfunction found in all individuals with autistic disorder. Examples of joint attention include social exchanges that require pointing, referential gaze, and gestures showing interest.

Asperger's disorder and autistic disorder, as classically described, share many common features. Asperger remarked that the children he studied began to speak at about the same time as other children did and eventually gained a full complement of language and syntax. However, he noted their unusual use of pronouns, continuous repetition of certain words or phrases, and exhaustive focus of speech on particular topics. Asperger also described that these children had difficulty in social reciprocity, engaged in repetitive play, and focused on certain interests excessively (Asperger 1944). Thus, the predominant differentiating feature between autistic disorder and Asperger's disorder is that those with Asperger's disorder did not have a delay in general (i.e., nonsocial) language development.

Individuals with Asperger's disorder may be recognized as impaired at a later age. Asperger's disorder was formally recognized as a separate PDD in DSM-IV. Much work is needed to further characterize this disorder.

Rett's disorder is a developmental disorder that preferentially strikes girls and differs substantially from autistic disorder past the toddler stage (see DSM-IV-TR diagnostic criteria page 128). The disorder was first described by Rett when 22 individuals were reported to be affected in 1966 (Rett 1966). Typically, a child with Rett's disorder has an uneventful prenatal and perinatal course that continues through at least the first 6 months. With the onset of the classic form of the disease, there is deceleration of head growth, usually between 5 months and 4 years of age. In toddlerhood, the manifestations can be similar to autistic disorder in which there is frequently impairment in language and social development, along with presence of stereotyped motor movements. In particular, there is a loss of acquired language, restricted interest in social contact or interactions, and the start of hand-wringing, clapping, or tapping in the midline of the body. This type of activity begins after purposeful hand movement is lost. Serious psychomotor retardation as well as receptive and expressive language impairments sets in. Between the ages of 1 and 4 years, truncal apraxia and gait apraxia typically ensue (Hagberg et al. 1985). Since the vast majority of Rett's disorder cases have mutations in *MECP2*, it has been possible to confirm that many variants of Rett's disorder, including those with preserved ambulation and preserved speech, are due to mutations in the same gene (Amir et al. 1999, Kim and Cook 2000).

Childhood disintegrative disorder and autistic disorder have some similarities in that they both involve deficits in social interaction and communication as well as repetitive behaviors. However, the symptoms of childhood disintegrative disorder appear abruptly or in the period of a few months' time after 2 years or more of normal development. There is generally no prior serious illness or insult, although a few cases have been linked to certain brain ailments such as measles, encephalitis, leukodystrophies, or other diseases. With the onset of childhood disintegrative disorder, the child loses previously mastered cognitive, language, and motor skills and regresses to such a degree that there is loss of bowel and bladder control (Volkmar and Cohen 1989). Children with childhood disintegrative disorder tend to lose abilities that would normally allow them to take care of themselves, and their motor activity contains fewer complex, repetitive behaviors than autistic disorder. Some children with this disorder experience regression that occurs for a time and then becomes stable. Another group of children has a poorer outcome, with the onset of focal neurological findings and seizures in the face of a worsening course and greater motor impairment (Corbett and Harris 1977). The majority of children with this disorder deteriorate to a severe level of mental retardation; a few retain selected abilities in specific areas. Differential diagnosis of childhood disintegrative disorder requires obtaining a particularly thorough developmental history, history of course of illness, and an extensive neurological evaluation and testing.

PDDNOS (also known as atypical autism) should be reserved for cases in which there are qualitative impairments in reciprocal social development, and either communication or imaginative and flexible interests are met, but not the full criteria for a specific PDD. It is important in the education of parents, teachers, and colleagues to be clear that PDDNOS is closely related to autistic disorder, because many families have been given diagnoses of both autistic disorder and PDDNOS and have the mistaken impression that this represents strong diagnostic disagreement between clinicians.

Autistic disorder and the other PDDs are complex clinical syndromes. It is likely there are multiple causes and perhaps even multiple additional syndromes that will eventually be subsumed under these diagnostic categories. However, it is clear that ASDs are a group of syndromes that reflect substantial impairment in related areas of functioning and that these problems tend to follow a consistent and stable natural history.

The diagnosis of ASD first involves completing a comprehensive psychiatric examination (Table 7-2). The clinician should obtain a full developmental history, including all information regarding pregnancy and delivery. While questioning about neonatal development, particular attention should be paid to social, communicative, and motor milestones. The clinician needs to understand fully the child's adaptive skills, including what tasks can be undertaken independently, including grooming skills, feeding skills, and the ability to self-initiate. There should be a sense of the child's vocabulary, receptive and expressive language skills, articulation, and pragmatic communication. A full medical history should be obtained, and should include queries regarding any hearing or vision problems, any history of seizures, and information regarding the use of any medications.

In terms of direct observation, the child with ASD poses some unique challenges. Because of his or her dislike of novelty, the first visit to the clinician's office is sometimes an anxiety-provoking undertaking. It is not unusual (and is in fact helpful diagnostically) to allow a child with ASD to extensively explore the clinician's office, looking under desks or opening drawers, in an attempt to become familiar with the surroundings. Some children will appear shy and self-absorbed. Because of this problem with novelty, it is ideal if the clinician can arrange an opportunity to see the child in another environment in addition to the office. Observation of the child interacting with the parents and siblings is helpful in understanding modes of interaction and social skills. If the child is having difficulty, it is usually preferable, especially on the first visit, to allow the parents to intervene. This will allow the clinician to see how (effectively) the family responds to this distress, and how the child responds to the efforts of caregivers to soothe the child. During observation, the clinician needs to assess social interaction, communication, unusual behaviors, and all other information in the context of developmental level.

A full physical examination should be undertaken. In addition to the standard comprehensive examination, the clinician should observe for dysmorphic features and unusual dermatologic lesions. The clinician must maintain a high suspicion for seizures in this population, both when taking the history and during the examination. A full neurological

Table 7-2	Suggested Workup for Children and Adults with Autistic Disorder or Other Pervasive Developmental Disorders

History
    Particular attention to
        Developmental phases of language, social interactions, play
        Family history of psychiatric and neurological disease
Physical examination
    Thorough physical examination including a search for
        Neurological problems
        Cardiac problems
        Congenital anomalies
        Skin lesions or abnormalities
        Dysmorphology
Psychological evaluation
    Autism Diagnostic Interview-Revised
    Autism Diagnostic Observation Schedule
    Cognitive testing (e.g., Differential Abilities Scales)
    Vineland Adaptive Behavior Scales
Speech and language evaluation
Audiological evaluation
Visual acuity evaluation

examination should be done with an emphasis on looking at motor impairments like hypotonia and apraxia. A Wood's light examination for hypopigmented lesions consistent with tuberous sclerosis should be done.

There are no diagnostic laboratory tests for ASD. What laboratory tests are ordered as a part of an initial workup is dependent on history and examination results. If the child has not had routine labs (blood count, liver function tests, thyroid, lead level, etc.) done, these should be completed, as with any child. Children with mental retardation or dysmorphology should have chromosomal analysis performed. Fluorescent *in situ* hybridization (FISH) studies for possible interstitial duplication of 15q11–13 should be suggested after consultation with the family. Fragile X testing should also be considered. There should be a low threshold for ordering an electroencephalogram (EEG), and one should always be ordered in the context of unusual movements, regressive behavior, regressive loss of previously acquired sleep, or in the face of unusually poor sleep. Structural brain imaging (i.e., MRI) should be done only if the physical examination or history suggests that a treatable lesion is present. Done routinely, these scans have a very low clinical yield, are quite expensive, and in this population often require anesthesia, a seemingly unnecessary risk. Consultative services should be utilized as needed, and this often means the involvement of pediatric neurologists and geneticists. Difficulties with motor development will often mean a referral to an occupational or physical therapist. Children with Rett's syndrome will often require referral to neurologists, and developmental pediatricians.

All children with autism require a careful language assessment that may include hearing testing and assessment of expressive and receptive, verbal and nonverbal language. Speech and language therapists trained to work with this population are an essential part of the assessment team.

Children with ASD should have a neuropsychological assessment at the time of initial assessment and at periodic intervals thereafter. The initial evaluation helps establish the diagnosis and a baseline level of functioning. Additionally, it can be utilized to make the appropriate adjustments in the child's educational plan. The later evaluations serve to chart progress, evaluate the success of (pharmacological, behavioral, and academic) interventions, and to assess for possible regression in particular areas. The evaluations should be undertaken with a neuropsychologist who is familiar with ASD and with the instruments being utilized. For cognitive assessment, both verbal and nonverbal cognitive levels must be assessed. When appropriate, achievement testing as well as the use of an appropriate standard, structured assessment of adaptive behaviors should be considered.

While there are many rating scales and structured interviews to assist in making the diagnosis of ASD, the current gold standard in diagnostic assessment is the autism diagnostic observation schedule-generic (ADOS-G) (Lord et al. 2000b), a standardized observation of social and communicative behavior performed directly with the child for more than 20 to 40 minutes. This is often given with the autism diagnostic inventory-revised (ADI-R) (Lord et al. 1994), which is a comprehensive, clinician-administered interview of the child's primary caregiver and covers most developmental and behavioral aspects of autism. The ADI/ADOS combination is now established as a reliable and valid method for making the diagnosis of ASD.

Epidemiology

Large scale epidemiologic studies of early childhood onset neuropsychiatric disorder simply have not been undertaken, thus making prevalence rates of many pediatric onset disorders relatively obscure. It is also worth noting that disorders that are relatively uncommon pose particular problems when it comes to the ascertainment of prevalence rates. Disorders with low prevalence require large sample sizes, and differences in prevalence, as a function of research methodology (case definition, case-finding procedures, participation rates), may be magnified as each identified case carries more statistical weight. Autistic disorder is no exception.

In addition, a number of historical and phenomenological problems make epidemiological estimation of autistic disorder particularly challenging. As described above, there has been enormous change in the operational definitions and criteria used to diagnose ASD over the past 50 years. This has led to more diagnostic precision, but the concept of ASD as a spectrum has also recently led to the inclusion of many subjects that would not previously have been included under the classic definition of autistic disorder. Increased awareness of ASD through laudable efforts at better education of mental health workers, pediatricians, and school personnel has led to better (and earlier) identification of the core symptoms that had previously gone undiagnosed (Filipek et al. 1999).

All of the factors described above would tend to lead to an apparent increase in prevalence, and that has been the trend in epidemiological surveys (Fombonne 1999). Early surveys from the 1970s found estimates from 0.7 per 10 000 (Treffert 1970) to 4.8 per 10 000 (Wing et al. 1976). More recent studies have ranged from 4.9 per 10 000 (Fombonne et al. 1997) to 21 per 10 000 (Honda et al. 1996). Combining the most recent surveys from 1989 to 1998, Fombonne (1999) determined the current rate of ASD to be approximately 7.2 per 10 000. This was most recently amended by Chakrabarti and Fombonne (2001) to 20 per 10 000. While there is no definitive way to know what accounts for the rise in ASD (and an increase due to, for instance, an environmental insult cannot be ruled out), the current informed consensus is that this increased prevalence rate reflects better recognition and detection together with more inclusive diagnostic definitions.

There is a significant difference in prevalence of ASD with respect to gender, with boys being affected more than girls in a 4 : 1 ratio (Fombonne 1999, Ritvo et al. 1989). The exception is Rett's disorder, which is found almost exclusively in females. Interestingly, the gender ratio in ASD increases to about 6 : 1 when cases with mental retardation are excluded, and decreases to approximately 1.7 : 1 when only cases with moderate to severe mental retardation are considered (Fombonne 1999). The reasons for this difference in gender ratio in relation to intellectual functioning are not known.

The prevalence rates of ASD do not appear to be influenced by immigrant status or socioeconomic status. (Fombonne 1999, Tsai et al. 1982, Wing 1980).

With the exception of childhood disintegrative disorder (in which all affected children are mentally retarded) (Kurita et al. 1992), there is wide individual variability in intellectual functioning in ASD (Siegel et al. 1996, Volkmar et al. 1994). Only about 20 to 25% of children with ASD have an IQ over 70, with 30 to 35% having mild to moderate mental retardation, and 40 to 45% having severe to profound mental retardation (Fombonne 1999). However, with more intensive case-finding (i.e., less dependence on mental retardation for referral), the number of children with ASD who have an IQ over 70 may be as high as 50%. Follow-up studies suggest that IQ levels tend to be constant from the time of diagnosis (when over 5 years old at the time of diagnosis) and are stable over time (Freeman et al. 1985), and thus are thought to be important predictors of outcome (Venter et al. 1992). Particular cognitive deficits are seen in language, abstraction, sequencing, and coding operations, while visual–spatial skills are often a relative strength (Lord et al. 1997, Rutter 1983).

Course

While children with ASD can usually be diagnosed between 2 and 4 years of age, there is wide variability in the age of diagnosis between one case and the next (Lord 1995). Retrospective analysis of some children reveals deficits in the first year of life (Osterling and Dawson 1994), while those with less severe symptoms may not be diagnosed until their first years of school or, in the case of higher functioning persons with ASD, even later (Nordin and Gillberg 1998). It is not uncommon (15–22%) for deterioration in functioning with the onset of puberty, characterized by mood lability, aggressiveness, and hyperactivity (Gillberg et al. 1982). Gillberg and Schaumann (1981) have also suggested that low IQ, female sex, epilepsy, and family history of mood difficulties may be risk factors for this pubertal deterioration. Others have reported that some individuals with ASD improve during their teen years (Kanner et al. 1972, Kobayashi et al. 1992).

Episodes of depression are common for individuals with ASD in their teens, especially among those with Asperger's syndrome. It has been hypothesized that this may be a function of these individuals' better recognition of their social inadequacies. This may also lead to subsequent demoralization and dysphoria (Tantam 1988, Wing 1981).

Epilepsy presents in a bimodal fashion, with many children first experiencing seizures before starting school, and another group having their onset at the time of puberty; overall, 25 to 30% of individuals will experience seizures before the age of 30 (Volkmar and Nelson 1990). It should be noted that there is an inverse correlation between the incidence of seizures and cognitive level (Olsson et al. 1988). Given that the estimates of seizures in ASD were based on studies of clinical populations, ascertainment could be biased toward lower functioning individuals with ASD, thus making the overall prevalence rate of epilepsy in these studies higher than what might be expected in an epidemiologic sample.

Long-term follow-up studies predict a poor or very poor long-term outcome for up to 75% of cases, and a good outcome (using social life, and school or vocational functioning as outcome measures) in only 5 to 15% of cases (Gillberg and Steffenburg 1987, Nordin and Gillberg 1998). It appears that IQ is the best predictor of outcome (Gillberg 1991). There is wide variability in final outcome, with most individuals with low IQs unable to live independently, and with many high-functioning individuals able to work (sometimes very successfully) and live independently, as well as raise children (Szatmari et al. 1989).

Differential Diagnosis

Although there may initially be some difficulty in differentiating ASD from other syndromes (Table 7-3), especially in the context of considerable comorbidity, the diagnosis usually becomes clear with careful differentiation. Mental retardation commonly occurs in ASD, and children with mental retardation may present with stereotyped movements or obsessiveness. However, the child with mental retardation and not with ASD will have social and communicative skills commensurate with their level of overall development.

Differentiating ASD from childhood schizophrenia is not usually difficult. The onset of psychosis in childhood is extraordinarily rare; and, hallucinations and delusions are not a part of the ASD picture. It is important not to diagnose some of the atypical features in ASD as psychotic and equally important to recognize that verbal individuals with ASD

Table 7-3	Differential Diagnosis of Autistic Disorder and Other Pervasive Developmental Disorders

Developmental language disorder
Mental retardation
Acquired epileptic aphasia (Landau-Kleffner's syndrome)
Fragile X syndrome
Schizophrenia
Selective mutism
Psychosocial deprivation
Hearing impairment
Visual impairment
Traumatic brain injury
Dementia
Metabolic disorders (inborn errors of metabolism, e.g., phenylketonuria)

have impaired language that should not be confused with schizophrenia. One should also recognize that onset of symptoms before age 3 is almost never consistent with schizophrenia. Selective mutism can be differentiated by the child's ability to interact normally in some environments.

Children exposed to severe neglect can sometimes present with symptoms that look like ASD, but these symptoms will usually show dramatic improvement when the child is in a more appropriate environment.

Perhaps the most difficult differentiation is in a child with severe obsessive–compulsive disorder (OCD) who also has unusual interests and is somewhat rigid in terms of being inflexible to changes in routines or transitions to a new activity. It is even further complicated if attentional problems coexist. In these cases, it is important to emphasize the social difficulties of children with ASD; even if the child with OCD is difficult interpersonally, his or her ability to maintain eye contact, interpret social situations and emotions, and otherwise interact socially is relatively preserved.

Etiology

Currently, the precise etiology and pathogenesis of ASDs are unknown. Strong evidence for genetic bases for the disorders, along with the advent of sophisticated genetic techniques, has led to a shift toward looking for the genetic underpinnings in the disorder. Most contemporary etiological theories strongly suggest a genetic or other early neurodevelopmental disruption with overt clinical manifestations potentially modified by social or environmental experiences.

Genetics

The evidence for a genetic basis to the etiology of autistic disorder is strong. ASD has a relatively low prevalence of approximately 2 per 1000 (Chakrabarti and Fombonne 2001), yet the recurrence risk to siblings is 4 to 5% (Ritvo et al. 1989). Concordance in monozygotic twin pairs has ranged from 60 to 90%, while dizygotic twin pairs in these studies have generally found a concordance similar to that found in siblings of affected children (Cook 2001). Even these concordance numbers are likely underestimates of the genetic contribution, since many pairs discordant for autistic disorder were concordant for another ASD. When considered as a spectrum disorder, twin studies suggest that at least 92% of monozygotic twin pairs are concordant for at least milder but similar deficits in the social and communication realms (compared to a 10% rate in these studies for dizygotic twin pairs) (Bailey et al. 1995, 1998).

ASD is currently thought to be a complex genetic disorder. In complex disorders, no single gene is sufficient to produce the phenotype; a number of susceptibility genes of varying strengths are necessary for full phenotypic expression. The varying strength of the contributions of different loci is likely also to be responsible for the genetic heterogeneity that characterizes ASD. In ASD, findings so far suggest a disease process with greater than 10, and perhaps as many as 100 loci (Risch et al. 1999). Finding the genes responsible for the phenotypic expression of any complex genetic disorder is a difficult task.

Chromosomal abnormalities have provided some clues as to where some of these susceptibility genes may be (Table 7-4). The most common chromosomal abnormality associated with ASD has been in a region of chromosome 15 (15q11–13). These abnormalities usually involve either an interstitial duplication or a supernumerary pseudodicentric chromosome (an extra chromosome with two centromeres; "pseudo" refers to the fact that only one centromere can be active) (Baker et al. 1994, Cook et al. 1997a).

Linkage studies have been accumulating evidence for particular loci that may be involved in ASD. There is evidence of linkage in several polymorphisms in the area of chromosome 15 noted above, including the gamma-aminobutyric acid receptor subunit gene (*GABRB3*)

Table 7-4	Chromosomal Abnormalities Associated with Autistic Disorder or Other Pervasive Developmental Disorders
	Fragile X syndrome (trinucleotide expansion at Xq27.3) Down's syndrome (trisomy 21) Prader–Willi syndrome (deletion or maternal isodisomy of chromosome 15) Marker chromosome Duplication of 15q11–13

(Shao et al. 2002), and transmission disequilibrium for markers in *GABRB3* has also been found (Buxbaum et al. 2002, Cook 1998, Martin et al. 2000). One group's findings suggest that the strongest evidence thus far seems to implicate linkage on chromosomal regions at 2q, 7q, 16p, and 17q (International Molecular Genetic Study of Autism Consortium 2001). The highest single point lod score in the IMGSAC study was at the intron *2VNTR* in the serotonin transporter gene. Family based association studies have looked at polymorphic variants of the serotonin transporter promoter region (*5HTTLPR*). One study found an association with the short variant (Cook et al. 1997b), another with preferential transmission of the long variant (Klauck et al. 1997), while some have not replicated either finding (Maestrini et al. 1999). Most recently, evidence of transmission disequilibrium was found to peak at another region of the serotonin transporter gene, supporting evidence of involvement of the gene, but not specifically the *5HTTLPR* variant (Kim et al. 2002).

There has been significant progress in terms of identifying the genetic basis of Rett's syndrome. Mutations in the gene (*MECP2*) encoding X-linked methyl-CpG-binding protein 2 (MeCP2) have been identified as the cause of more than 80% of classic cases of Rett's syndrome (Amir et al. 1999, Buyse et al. 2000).

Biological Factors

Although a number of neurotransmitter systems have been implicated as possibly being involved in ASD, there have consistently been findings of dysfunction in the serotonin system. Serotonin dysfunction has been implicated as a possible factor in the genesis of autistic disorder since the finding of significantly elevated whole blood 5-HT in these individuals (Schain and Freedman 1961). Hyperserotonemia is a robust finding in autistic disorder and has been consistently replicated (Abramson et al. 1989, Chugani et al. 1999b, Cook et al. 1990, Kuperman et al. 1985, Leboyer et al. 1999, Leventhal et al. 1990).

Interestingly, hyperserotonemia in autistic disorder appears to have a familial component; that is, in keeping with a genetic model. Several studies have shown that whole blood serotonin levels have a positive correlation between probands with autism and their parents and siblings (Abramson et al. 1989, Cook et al. 1990, Kuperman et al. 1985, Leboyer et al. 1999, Leventhal et al. 1990). Additionally, individuals with autism who have siblings with autism have higher platelet serotonin than autistic subjects without an autistic sibling (Piven et al. 1991), suggesting that hyperserotonemia may be an indicator of autism with a higher risk of sibling recurrence (Cook and Leventhal 1996).

It is clear that it is serotonin within platelets that is responsible for the findings of increased whole blood hyperserotonemia. More than 99% of whole blood serotonin is contained in platelets, and platelet-poor plasma ultrafiltrate serotonin levels are not elevated in subjects with hyperserotonemia (Cook et al. 1988). This suggests that individuals with autism exhibit either increased serotonergic uptake in platelets, or decreased serotonergic release from platelets, leading to an increased steady state level of serotonin in platelets (Cook and Leventhal 1996). There is evidence for a positive correlation between platelet serotonin levels and the rate of platelet serotonin transport (Cook et al. 1993).

Since the first autopsy studies in ASD in the early 1980s, a number of neuroanatomic differences in ASD have been reported. However, at this time there is no established gross or microscopic neuropathology associated with ASD.

Some investigators have found evidence for differences in the hippocampus and amygdala. Bauman and Kemper (1985), while noting no gross abnormalities in their study of the brains of six autistic individuals, noted increased cell packing and diminished neuronal size in the hippocampus and some nuclei in the amygdala. They also found decreased complexity and extent of dendritic arbors in hippocampal pyramidal cells. They speculated that such lesions might produce changes in behavior similar to those with Klüver Bucy Syndrome (hyperexploratory behavior, severe impairment of social interaction) and some cases of limbic injuries leading to memory loss (and a subsequent "rigidly specific habit memory system"). Others (Bachevalier 1994, Brothers 1989) have suggested that such changes might result in difficulty in assigning affective significance to social stimuli.

Another commonly reported neuroanatomical finding in ASD has been related to cerebellar structures. A number of investigators have noted loss of cerebellar Purkinje cells (Ritvo et al. 1986, Williams et al. 1980) as well as changes in neurons of the deep cerebellar nuclei (Kemper and Bauman 1998). Such findings have led to the hypothesis that such lesions could affect selective attention, in particular leading to stimulus overselectivity and difficulties in shifting attention (Courchesne et al. 1994).

Positron-emission tomography scans revealed increased generalized metabolism in one study (Rumsey et al. 1985), but a number of subsequent studies did not show this change (DeVolder et al. 1987, Herold et al. 1988), while another revealed decreased metabolism in some subcortical structures (thalamus, putamen) (Buchsbaum et al. 1992). Haznedar and colleagues (1997) found reductions in portions of the right anterior cingulate during a word list learning task, and Schifter (1994) found hypometabolism in many brain regions during a resting state PET scan of autistic children with both mental retardation and seizure disorders. Chugani and colleagues (1996) conducted PET scans on children with infantile spasms, and found that 10 of 14 children that had bitemporal hypometabolism met criteria for ASD at a later follow-up. Using PET and functional magnetic resonance imaging, Muller and colleagues (1998) showed that a small group of high-functioning ASD adults had reversal of the usual left hemisphere dominance when listening to sentences.

Chugani and colleagues (1997) scanned autistic children utilizing an analog of tryptophan to act as a tracer in order to look at serotonin synthesis in the brain. They found asymmetries in serotonin synthesis in many of the autistic subjects. In a later study, again scanning with this tracer, they also found that the global cerebral serotonin synthesis capacity of ASD children tended to increase with age (versus control subjects that show a steady decrease with age toward adult levels) (Chugani et al. 1999a). Similar methods using a tracer to look at dopamine storage and metabolism have revealed that accumulation of this tracer was significantly reduced in the anterior medial prefrontal cortex compared to controls (Ernst et al. 1997).

There have been numerous attempts to use static and functional neuroimaging techniques to clarify the neuropathologic etiologies of ASD. However, to date, small sample size problems in establishing proper controls and technical difficulties associated with scanning individuals with autism have all contributed to a general lack of conclusive findings in this area of research.

The Role of MMR Vaccinations

Some have suggested that there is a variant of ASD called *autistic enterocolitis* that involves developmental regression and gastrointestinal symptoms, and that this variant is a consequence of measles–mumps–rubella (MMR) immunization (Wakefield and Montgomery 2000). This hypothesis, which has been postulated to account for the rise in the number of cases of ASD, suggests that there are specific biological findings in these children that result from a persistent measles viral infection. If such a hypothesis were found to be true, it would have important implications for future research into the neurobiological underpinnings of ASD; alternatively, the public health consequences of not immunizing children and thereby losing the herd immunity currently in place could be potentially disastrous. For these reasons, this issue has generated considerable controversy. A full discussion of these issues is beyond the scope of this review and can be accessed elsewhere (Fombonne and Chakrabarti 2001). At the current time, investigations into this hypothesis have found no relationship between MMR vaccinations and the development of ASD; this lack of evidence argues against changes in MMR vaccination programs.

Treatment

Developing a comprehensive individual intervention program for a child with ASD is a daunting task for the child's parents (Figure 7-1). Each child is unique, with a different set of difficulties as well as strengths. The child's primary physician must work with the parents to help make this task less overwhelming. This usually means maintaining a tempered optimism about the future and providing encouragement without being unrealistic. The physician can anticipate being asked about a wide array of alternative treatments being offered in the community, which vary enormously in their claims, in the integrity of those making the claims, and in their ultimate safety and utility. The physician who immediately and pejoratively dismisses these alternatives as useless is not helpful to the child or his family (the exception being dangerous or cost-prohibitive prospective treatments). Rather, it is helpful to listen and then educate the family, at a level commensurate with their sophistication, about how to analyze and interpret claims and the science underlying these treatments. Most parents are able to incorporate information about the need for

Identification of developmental delay by caretaker

↓↓
↓↓

Evaluation by pediatrician

↓↓
↓↓ Referral for specialty testing
↓↓

ADOS, ADI, measures of intellectual functioning and daily functioning, full physical, history, and labs

↓↓
↓↓ Autism spectrum disorder established
↓↓

Initiation of treatment includes:

1. Implementing changes in the child's academic program including relevant changes in the curriculum in order to tailor it to the child's specific needs, as well as probable speech, occupational, and physical therapy.

2. The use of behavioral programs in order to improve social and communication difficulties as well as address negative behaviors.

3. Examination of any symptoms that may be potential target symptoms for a pharmacological intervention.

Figure 7-1 *An example of the typical progression from identification, to evaluation, to treatment of a child with ASD (ADOS, Autism Diagnostic Observation Schedule; ADI, Autism Diagnostic Inventory).*

Table 7-5	Goals for Treatment

Advancement of normal development, particularly regarding cognition, language, and socialization
Promotion of learning and problem solving
Reduction of behaviors that impede learning
Assistance of families coping with autistic disorder
Treatment of comorbid psychiatric disorders

controlled studies, replication, and the importance of information being published in peer-reviewed journals.

Autistic disorder is recognized as a chronic disorder with a changing course requiring a long-term course of treatment that includes the necessity of intervention with various treatments at different times. At the present time, most treatments for the ASDs are symptom directed. Thus, treatments of the other ASDs are the same as those used in autistic disorder because similar types of symptoms are targeted for treatment in each of these disorders. Given that there is no current cure for autistic disorder or the other ASDs goals of treatment should encompass the short-term and long-term needs of the individual and his or her family (Table 7-5). Rutter (1985) defined goals for treatment in terms of four quintessential aims including

1. the advancement of normal development, particularly regarding cognition, language, and socialization;
2. the promotion of learning and problem solving;
3. the reduction of behaviors that impede the learning process;
4. the assistance of families coping with autism.

These goals are broad in nature; therefore, it is key to separate these goals into immediate and long-term needs for each individual with ASD. Each goal requires a distinct scheme of its own.

Every attempt should be made to achieve treatment goals in a community-based environment since institutionalization may hinder a child's ability to learn means of functioning and adapting in typical social settings. Community-based treatment can usually be maintained, except in times of extreme stress or need, during which time a child (and family) might benefit from respite care or brief hospitalization. Effective treatment often entails setting appropriate expectations for the child and adjusting the child's environment to foster success.

Psychological Treatments

Because the autistic individual often requires diverse treatments and services simultaneously, the role of the primary physician is to be the coordinator of services. Frequent visits with the child and the child's caretakers initially allow the physician to assess the individual needs of the child while establishing a therapeutic alliance. An effective approach often calls for the services of a number of professionals working in a multidisciplinary fashion. This group may include psychiatrists, pediatricians, pediatric neurologists, psychologists, special educators, speech and language therapists, social workers, and other specialized therapists (Table 7-6).

There is significant controversy over what particular forms of therapy are best for children with ASD. Some of this controversy is a result of claims of children making dramatic improvements with some of these therapies. For instance, Lovaas (1996) has at times suggested that children receiving his specific form of intensive, behavioral treatment may even "recover" (which they define as having a normal IQ and being mainstreamed in school),

Table 7-6	Summary of Treatment Principles

Psychosocial Interventions

Educational
  Curricula that target communication
  Behavioral techniques
  Structured milieu
  Vocational training and placement: other specialized interventions such as
    speech and language therapy, physical therapy, and occupational therapy
Social skills training
Individual psychotherapy for high-functioning individuals

Medical Interventions

Cohesive physician–patient relationship
Supportive measures with families coping with autistic disorder
Behavioral treatment
Pharmacotherapy to address problem signs and symptoms

although there has been significant criticism of these studies in terms of subject selection and research design; empirical investigations of this method, while showing statistically significant improvement in many areas, have not suggested that these children "leave" the autistic spectrum (Sheinkopf and Siegel 1998).

Another form of behavioral intervention is applied behavioral analysis (ABA). This intervention uses careful assessment of adaptive and maladaptive behaviors and the design of specific interventions to address each of these individual behaviors. The most successful interventions use a variety of positive reinforcement schedules to enhance the desired behaviors and extinguish undesirable behaviors. Discrete trial training, an operant conditioning model, is particularly useful in this regard. Generalization of skills from the behavioral training environment to other settings is a key to success. When carefully applied, ABA has shown consistent usefulness in controlled trials (Rosenwasser and Axelrod 2001). Children receiving ABA have shown significant improvement in a number of areas, including IQ, visual–spatial skills, language, and academics (Smith 2001).

A prerequisite to putting a behavioral plan in place with a child with ASD is to identify the problem behaviors. These behaviors often include interfering repetitive actions, self-injurious behaviors, or aggression. While there is little difficulty in identifying these highly visible behaviors, what is much more difficult is (1) determining the antecedents to these behaviors and (2) knowing what constitutes an appropriate reaction to these behaviors on the part of the caregiver. To determine the antecedent is often extraordinarily difficult, since it is often not apparent as to what exactly happened in the environment that stimulated the behavior. This is particularly true if the behavior is chronic and has developed some autonomous function (i.e., no longer a stimulus–response event). To make things more complicated, it could be internal perception or the meaning of what happened in a child with autism (poor language and socially nonresponsive) that may have initiated the behavior (Howlin 1998).

Durand and Carr (1991) attempted to determine the function of problem behaviors in children with ASD. They concluded that most behaviors could be classified as

1. a need for help,
2. a desire to escape a stressful situation,
3. a desire to obtain an object,
4. an attempt to protest unwanted events,
5. an attempt to obtain stimulation or attention.

There are scales available to help caretakers determine the primary functions behind typical problem behaviors (Sturmey et al. 1996). Despite the notorious difficulty in determining the function of a problem behavior in these children (Emerson and Bromley 1995), if the function(s) can be identified, a behavioral intervention will likely be successful in diminishing the atypical, maladaptive behavior and enhance overall adaptation and behavioral functioning (Durand and Carr 1991).

Children with ASD often engage in rituals and routines. The precise reasons for the presence of these behaviors in ASD remain unclear, but they often appear to be an attempt to relieve anxiety and/or to exert control over their environment. The key to success is a gradual shaping of the behavior rather than dramatic expectations and harsh consequences. One should begin intervention by evaluating possible, underlying stimuli or predisposing factors for the behavior. Strategies include determining when, where, and for how long an activity can take place. Additional strategies include making environmental changes that reduce anxiety and even ignoring behaviors that do not create undue problems (Howlin 1998). Adjunct pharmacological intervention is often helpful.

Up to 50% of children with ASD will not acquire useful language (Lord et al. 1994). For those with some but not fully intact language skills, speech therapy is an important part of therapeutic and academic planning. An emphasis on the social use of language is often helpful, and when the child can articulate some of his or her needs, there is often a reduction in problem behaviors.

Longitudinal studies indicate that children who have not acquired useful language by the age of 7 usually have long-standing verbal communication difficulties. For these children, it is often helpful to devise an alternative means of communication. Some children can learn sign language, although there is great variability in how much each child is able to learn, difficulties with generalizing to environments other than where signs are learned, and the fact that signs continue to be used mostly to satisfy needs rather than being utilized in a spontaneous social sense. Additionally, it seems to be best to continue to pair signs with appropriate vocalizations, however limited. Alternatively (or additionally), the use of augmentative communication systems may be helpful. These can include computers that "speak" either typed language or when a particular key or image is touched. The use of picture exchange communication system (PECS) (Erdmann et al. 1996) may also be quite useful. PECS involves the use of photographs or line drawings on cards. The child then points out or hands the appropriate card or cards to another person in order to effect communication. Once again, children are encouraged to use verbalization, when possible, in conjunction with sharing the cards. Irrespective of the technique used, establishing a consistent method of communication is central to the treatment of individuals with ASD.

Problems with social interactions, especially reciprocal social interactions, are common to every person with ASD. Children and adults with ASD lack many of the innate and learned social skills that most people simply take for granted. Maintaining appropriate interpersonal distance, spontaneously initiating conversation, participating in reciprocal social exchange, and other facets of complex social interaction are not easily incorporated in the routine behaviors and activities of individuals with ASDs. Subtlety and changing complexity of social interaction as well as the innateness of many social skills is a central part of daily life and a key to successful adaptation for typically functioning individuals. Helping individuals with ASDs address these challenges is difficult but also critical for enhancing overall functioning.

Weiss and Harris (2001) reviewed strategies and therapies for improving social functioning for individuals with ASDs. They emphasize the need for these children to be involved and learn from their peers. Odom and Strain (1986) identified the following three primary techniques that can be effectively utilized:

1. **Establish proximity**

   Proximity refers to the fact that it is very helpful to have the child with ASD near other children in the environment. The mere proximity increases the likelihood of interaction and imitation as well as positive social reinforcement. There is empirical evidence that such proximity is actually helpful (Roeyers 1996).

2. **Use prompts and reinforcement**

   The use of prompts relates to having specific cues to use previously learned behaviors in social settings (e.g., "Raise your hand if you have a question"). Attention to reinforcement means that even a less than fully competent attempt at appropriate social behavior, even if it is a response to a prompt, gets clear and effective reinforcement when it occurs (e.g., calling on the child promptly when he raises his hand to ask a question and also saying "You did a good job when you raised your hand to ask the question"). Teaching such prompting and reinforcement should be for everyone who interacts with the individual with ASD.

3. **Encourage peer initiation**

   It is helpful to train peers who are likely to interact with the child or adult with ASD in techniques for initiating social contact. For many individuals, this means explaining the disability and dealing with fears or biases. For others, it may mean encouraging them to persist in their attempts at engagement, even in the face of limited, inappropriate, or inadequate responses. Persistence usually leads to familiarity and eventually to some level of social engagement.

While these techniques have also shown positive results, there still appears to be a paucity of social initiation on the part of the ASD children, and it is unclear whether these techniques can teach behaviors that will readily generalize to other environments (Roeyers 1996). The need for increased social initiation has been recognized (Oke and Schreibman 1990) and sessions concentrated on teaching initiation have had some success (Taylor et al. 1998, Taylor and Harris 1995, Zanolli et al. 1996).

Considering the many needs of the child with ASD, academic resources and placement naturally emerge as important components to the child's overall treatment. The reasons for this are manifold. First and foremost, schools are where children go to acquire social skills and acquaintances, as well as academic skills. Secondly, schools often have a variety of skilled professionals who are trained to provide necessary services for the individual with ASD. And, finally, in the United States, all public schools have a statutory obligation to provide all children (even those with disabilities) with a free and appropriate education in the least restrictive environment. Thus, schools often become the base and the requisite individualized educational plan (IEP) becomes the road map of interventions for children with ASD.

Somatic Treatments

At this time, there are no pharmacological agents with US Food and Drug Administration (FDA) approved labeling specific for the treatment of autistic disorder or other PDDs in either children or adults. This is all the more problematic because many of the symptoms commonly seen in autistic disorder and other PDDs (rituals, aggressive behavior, and hyperactivity) are also commonly seen in children, adolescents, and adults with mental retardation but without a PDD. Some of the pharmacological strategies for the treatment of autistic disorder have been extrapolated from studies of related conditions, largely in adults, including attention-deficit/hyperactivity disorder and OCD. While there may not be FDA-approved treatments, there are treatment options available. However, clinicians and families should be reminded before any treatment is initiated that (1) current treatments target symptoms (2) current treatments do not target a specific etiological mechanism for ASD (3) anecdotal reports do not establish efficacy, effectiveness, or safety for any treatment (4) controlled, double-blind trials (preferably with replication) are the contemporary standard for determining if a treatment is safe and appropriate (5) all treatments have side effects.

Before specific pharmacological agents are discussed, it must be stressed that one should not use psychopharmacological agents with the expectation that they will cure children with autistic disorder. Although this seems obvious, one should realize that many parents and teachers of children with autistic disorder expect medication to eliminate core social, cognitive, and communication dysfunction. There is no pharmacological substitute for appropriate educational, behavioral, psychotherapeutic, vocational, and recreational programming. It is essential to remember and to remind parents, teachers, and others that medication should always be seen as an adjunct to these core interventions that address the developmental challenges associated with these disorders. The clinician providing the medication should reiterate this message to the parents and others involved in the child's treatment by consistently reminding them of the specific behavioral targets of the medication, and assessing the effectiveness of the medication in the context of change in these behavioral symptoms, and how the pharmacotherapy facilitates the other interventions.

Because many individuals with autistic disorder and other PDDs have impairments in language and social communication, the use of rating scales becomes an essential part of the treatment. Standard rating scales not only provide the pharmacotherapist with a framework in which to assess response to medication but they also provide a relatively easy and straightforward way to collect standard information about the individual's functioning in a variety of settings. Although rating scales and instruments are available for several target symptoms of interest, such as attention and concentration deficits, impulsivity, and hyperactivity, the Aberrant Behavior Checklist—Community Version (Aman 1994) has the advantage of asking questions that cover these areas for most individuals with ASD. We have found this instrument to be especially sensitive to clinical changes in the critical symptoms of hyperactivity and irritability (Jaselskis et al. 1992). Although rating scales cannot replace careful clinical examination of the individuals and interviews with parents and teachers, they may be graphed next to dosages of medications to assist in treatment planning in response to the individual's clinical condition. This is often not only helpful in making clinical decisions but also gives families and service providers a concrete sense of how a treatment is progressing. This enhances compliance and other aspects of a successful treatment.

The use of medications to treat autistic disorder and other ASDs appears to have significant potential as an adjunct to educational, environmental, and social interventions. It is a reasonable goal for the pharmacotherapist to adopt the judicious use of psychopharmacological agents to assist in alleviating symptoms that have been found to respond to pharmacological intervention (Table 7-7). This focus on facilitating adaptation requires attention to five important principles:

1. Environmental manipulations, including behavioral treatment, may be as effective as, if not more effective than, medication for selected symptomatic treatment.
2. It is essential that the living arrangement for the individual must ensure safe and consistent administration and monitoring of the medication to be used.

Table 7-7	Summary of Pharmacotherapy Principles
Psychosocial interventions should accompany medication treatment.	
The individual's living arrangement must ensure safe, consistent administration of medications.	
Maintain a high index of suspicion for comorbid disorders, and treat these appropriately.	
Establish a means of monitoring effects of medications on symptoms over time.	
Assess the risk/benefit ratio of starting medications and educate the patient and family about these.	

Table 7-8	Psychopharmacological Approach to Presenting Symptoms in Pervasive Developmental Disorders

Rituals, Compulsions, Irritability
Potent serotonin transporter inhibitors
  Selective serotonin reuptake inhibitor
    Fluoxetine 5–80 mg/d in a single dose
    Paroxetine 2.5–50 mg/d in one or two divided doses
    Sertraline 25–200 mg/d in one or two divided doses
    Fluvoxamine 25–300 mg/d in two or three divided doses
    Citalopram 5–40 mg/d in a single or two divided doses
  Tricyclic antidepressants
    Clomipramine 25–250 mg/d in one or two divided doses

Hyperactivity, Distractibility, Impulsivity
Stimulant medications
  Methylphenidate 5–60 mg/d in three to five divided doses
  Dextroamphetamine 5–60 mg/d in three to five divided doses
  Pemoline 37.5–112.5 mg/d in a single dose
Clonidine 0.05–0.3 mg/d in one to three divided doses or by transdermal skin patch
Naltrexone 0.5–2.0 mg/kg/d in a single dose

Aggression, Irritability
Sympatholytics
  Propranolol 20–400 mg/d in three to four divided doses
  Nadolol 40–400 mg/d in a single dose
Anticonvulsants
  Carbamazepine to a blood level of 4–12 ng/mL
  Valproate to a blood level of 50–100 ng/mL
Lithium to a serum level of 0.8–1.2 mEq/L
Neuroleptics
Naltrexone 0.5–2.0 mg/kg/d in a single dose

3. Individuals with autistic disorder and other ASDs often have other DSM-IV-TR Axis I disorders. If a comorbid DSM-IV-TR Axis I disorder is present, standard treatment for that disorder should be initiated first.

4. Medication should be selected on the basis of potential effects on target symptoms and there should be an established way of specifically monitoring the response to the treatment over time.

5. A careful assessment of the risk/benefit ratio must be made before initiating treatment and, to the extent possible, the individual's caretakers and the individual must understand the risks and benefits of the treatment.

This class of agents includes selective serotonin reuptake inhibitors (SSRIs) (fluoxetine, sertraline, paroxetine, fluvoxamine, and citalopram) as well as the less selective but potent clomipramine, a tricyclic antidepressant (Table 7-8).

Potent Serotonin Transporter Inhibitors This group of medications is most effective when insistence on routines or rituals are present to the point of manifest anxiety or aggression in response to interruption of the routines or rituals (Awad 1996, Brodkin et al. 1997, Cook et al. 1992, Gordon et al. 1993, McDougle et al. 1998a, Posey et al. 1999), or after the onset of another disorder such as major depressive disorder or OCD (Ghaziuddin et al. 1991). The common side effects associated with SSRIs are motor restlessness, insomnia, elation, irritability, and decreased appetite, each of which may occur alone or, more often, together. Because many of these symptoms may be present in the often cyclical natural course of ASD before the medication is initiated, the emergence of new symptoms, a different quality of the symptoms, and occurrence of these symptoms in a new cluster are clues that the symptoms are side effects of medication rather than part of the natural course of the disorder (Cook et al. 1992).

Stimulants   Small but significant reductions in inattention and hyperactivity ratings may be seen in children with autistic disorder in response to stimulants such as methylphenidate (Quintana et al. 1995), dextroamphetamine, and pemoline. In a placebo-controlled crossover study, 8 of 13 subjects showed a reduction of at least 50% on methylphenidate (Handen et al. 2000). However, stereotypies may worsen, so drug trials must always be assessed to determine whether the therapeutic effects outweigh side effects. A key distinction in assessing attentional problems of children with ASD is the distinction between poor sustained attention (characteristic of children with attention-deficit/hyperactivity disorder) and poor joint attention (characteristic of children with autistic disorder). Problems in joint attention require educational and behavioral interventions or treatment of rituals with a potent serotonin transporter inhibitor. Problems in maintenance of attention of the type seen in attention-deficit/hyperactivity disorder are more likely to respond to stimulants.

Sympatholytics   The α2-adrenergic receptor agonist clonidine reduced irritability as well as hyperactivity and impulsivity in two double-blind, placebo-controlled trials (Fankhauser et al. 1992, Jaselskis et al. 1992). However, tolerance developed several months after initiation of the treatment in each child who was treated long-term (Jaselskis et al. 1992). Tolerance was not prevented by transdermal skin patch administration of the drug. However, tolerance may have been reduced in several cases by administering clonidine in the morning and then 6 to 8 hours later with a 16- to 18-hour interval between the last dose of one day and the first dose of the next day. If tolerance does develop, the dose should not be increased because tolerance to sedation does not occur, and sedation may lead to increased aggression due to disinhibition or decreased cognitive control of impulses. Adrenergic receptor antagonists, such as propranolol and nadolol, have not been tested in double-blind trials in ASD. However, open trials have reported the use of these medications in the treatment of aggression and impulsivity in developmental disorders (Williams et al. 1982) including autistic disorder (Ratey et al. 1987).

Typical Neuroleptics   Because they were among the first modern psychopharmacological agents, typical neuroleptics have been among the most extensively studied drugs in autistic disorder. Trifluoperazine, thioridazine, haloperidol, and pimozide have been studied in double-blind, controlled trials lasting from 2 to 6 months. Reduction of fidgetiness, interpersonal withdrawal, speech deviance, and stereotypies has been documented in response to these treatments (Anderson et al. 1984, 1989, Campbell et al. 1976, Cohen et al. 1980, Ernst et al. 1992, Fish et al. 1966, Naruse et al. 1982, Perry et al. 1989). However, individuals with autistic disorder are as vulnerable to potentially irreversible tardive dyskinesia as any other group of young children with a mental disorder (Campbell et al. 1988, Wilmut et al. 1997). Owing to the often earlier age at initiation of pharmacotherapy, individuals with ASD treated with typical neuroleptics may be at higher risk because of the potential increased lifetime exposure of medication. These medications also have significant additional side effects of varying sorts and severity that should significantly limit their routine use in the care of individuals with ASD, especially as first-line treatments.

Atypical Neuroleptics   Because of the positive response of many children with autistic disorder to typical neuroleptics, similar medications with reduced risk of tardive dyskinesia must be considered. In addition, atypical neuroleptics are often effective in treating the negative symptoms of schizophrenia, which seem similar to several of the social deficits in autistic disorder. Both risperidone and olanzapine have shown promise in open label trials in reducing hyperactivity, impulsivity, aggressiveness, and obsessive preoccupations (Barber et al. 1998, Malone et al. 2001, Masi et al. 2001, McDougle et al. 1997, Potenza et al. 1999, Unis et al. 1997). A double-blind, placebo-controlled study found risperidone to be more effective than placebo in the treatment of repetitive behavior, aggression, and irritability (McDougle et al. 1998b). Other studies are being conducted at the time of this writing but they have not yet stood the test of careful peer review and scrutiny. However, it seems clear that atypical neuroleptics will likely play a role for the treatment of carefully selected individuals with severe symptoms of ASD.

Anticonvulsants   Because 25 to 33% of individuals with autistic disorder have seizures, the psychopharmacological management of individuals with autistic disorder or other ASD must take into consideration the past or current history of epilepsy and the potential role of anticonvulsants (Volkmar and Nelson 1990). Unfortunately, very few studies have been undertaken in this area. In an open trial of divalproex, 10 of 14 individuals responded favorably, showing improvements in affective stability, impulsivity, and aggression (Hollander et al. 2001). The anticonvulsant class to be avoided, when possible, is the category comprising barbiturates (e.g., phenobarbital). Because barbiturates have been associated with hyperactivity, depression, and cognitive impairment, they should be changed to an alternative drug, depending on the seizure type (Brent et al. 1987, Vining et al. 1987). In addition, phenytoin (Dilantin) is sedating and causes hypertrophy of the gums and hirsutism, which may contribute to the social challenges for people with autistic disorder. Carbamazepine and valproate may have positive psychotropic effects, particularly when cyclical irritability, insomnia, and hyperactivity are present. Several children with autistic disorder were treated with valproic acid after electroencephalographical abnormalities were found. These children had an improvement in behavioral symptoms associated with autistic disorder after valproate treatment (Plioplys 1994).

Naltrexone   The opiate antagonist, naltrexone, was suggested as a specific treatment for autistic disorder. However, double-blind trials have demonstrated that naltrexone has little efficacy in treating the core social and cognitive symptoms of autistic disorder (Campbell et al. 1993). While the use of naltrexone as a specific treatment for autistic disorder no longer seems to be likely, it may have a role in the treatment of self-injurious behavior, although the controlled data are equivocal (Campbell et al. 1993, Willemsen-Swinkels et al. 1995). Controlled trials have shown a modest reduction in symptoms of hyperactivity and restlessness sometimes associated with autistic disorder (Campbell et al. 1993, Feldman et al. 1999, Herman et al. 1993, Willemsen-Swinkels et al. 1999, 1996). Potential side effects include nausea and vomiting. Controlled trials in autistic disorder have not shown liver dysfunction or other physical side effects. Naltrexone may have an adverse effect on the outcome of Rett's disorder based on a relatively large, randomized, double-blind, placebo-controlled trial (Percy et al. 1994).

Lithium   Adolescents and adults with autistic disorder often exhibit symptoms in a cyclic manner and so there is much interest in how these individuals might respond to agents typically used in bipolar disorder. A single open trial of lithium revealed no significant improvement in symptoms in individuals with autistic disorder without bipolar disorder (Campbell et al. 1972).

Anxiolytics   Benzodiazepines have not been studied systematically in children and adolescents with autistic disorder. However, their use in reducing anxiety in short-term treatment, such as before dental procedures, is similar to their use in management of anxiety in people without a PDD. One open label study has found a decrease in anxiety and irritability in individuals receiving the anxiolytic buspirone (Buitelaar et al. 1998).

Glutamatergic Agents   Interest in these agents has been sparked by the hypothesis that ASDs may be a disorder of hypoglutaminergic activity (Carlsson 1998). In a double-blind, placebo-controlled study of the glutamatergic antagonist amantadine hydrochloride, there were substantial improvements in clinician-rated hyperactivity and irritability, although parental reports did not reach statistical significance (which may have been partially due to a strong placebo response) (King et al. 2001). Further study of this medication and consideration of this hypothesis is warranted.

Pyridoxine and Dietary Supplements   Pyridoxine, the water-soluble essential vitamin B_6, has been used extensively as a pharmacological treatment in autistic disorder. In the doses used for autistic disorder, it is not being used as a cofactor for normally regulated enzyme function or as a vitamin; rather, it is used to modulate the function of neurotransmitter enzymes, such as tryptophan hydroxylase and tyrosine hydroxylase. While Martineau and associates (1988) showed modest improvements in about 30% of children, recent reviews have concluded that there are little data to support the claim that vitamin B_6 improves developmental course (Kleijnen and Knipschild 1991, Pfeiffer et al. 1995).

Fenfluramine   Although fenfluramine originally showed promise in the treatment of autistic disorder and associated cognitive dysfunction (Geller et al. 1982), double-blind controlled trials did not confirm an improvement in cognitive function or a reduction in core autistic symptoms (Aman and Kern 1989, Leventhal et al. 1993). However, much like naltrexone, fenfluramine may reduce hyperactivity and impulsivity commonly present in autistic disorder and other developmental disorders (Aman et al. 1991). The potential changes in neurochemical regulation after long-term administration (Leventhal et al. 1993), which may represent neurotoxic effects (Schuster et al. 1986) and potential for acquired cardiac valvular disease, suggest that fenfluramine no longer be used in autistic disorder.

Secretin   A case series of three autistic individuals who showed improvement in core symptoms after receiving the gastrointestinal hormone secretin (Horvath et al. 1998), led to a series of studies on this substance as a possible treatment for ASD. The results have been disappointing, with all studies done so far (Chez et al. 2000, Coniglio et al. 2001, Dunn-Geier et al. 2000, Owley et al. 2001, Roberts et al. 2001, Sandler et al. 1999) showing the substance to be no more useful than placebo. These studies, along with the negative studies that followed initial excitement following open label studies of naltrexone and fenfluramine, point to the necessity of performing double-blind, placebo-controlled studies of any putative treatments to ensure safety and to establish effectiveness.

Comparison of DSM-IV-TR/ICD-10 Diagnostic Criteria
The DSM-IV-TR and ICD-10 item sets and diagnostic algorithms for autistic disorder are almost identical. However, the ICD-10 exclusion criterion is considerably more broad, requiring that a number of other disorders should be considered instead (e.g., early onset schizophrenia, mental retardation with an associated emotional or behavioral disorder). In ICD-10, this disorder is referred to as childhood autism.

The DSM-IV-TR and ICD-10 item sets and diagnostic algorithms for Rett's disorder and Asperger's disorder are almost identical. In ICD-10, these disorders are referred to as Rett's syndrome and Asperger's syndrome respectively.

Regarding childhood disintegrative disorder, the DSM-IV-TR and ICD-10 item sets and diagnostic algorithms are identical except for the C criterion, in which ICD-10 also allows for a "general loss of interest in objects and the environment." In ICD-10, this disorder is referred to as other childhood disintegrative disorder.

References

Abramson RK, Wright HH, Carpenter R, et al. (1989) Elevated blood serotonin in autistic probands and their first-degree relatives. *J Autism Dev Disord* **19**, 397–407.

Aman M (1994) *Aberrant Behavior Checklist—Community.* Slosson Educational Publications, East Aurora, New York.

Aman MG and Kern RA (1989) Review of fenfluramine in the treatment of the developmental disabilities. *J Am Acad Child Adolesc Psychiatry* **28**, 549–565.

Aman MG, Kern RA, Arnold LE, et al. (1991) Fenfluramine and mental retardation. *J Am Acad Child Adolesc Psychiatry* **30**, 507–508.

Amir RE, Van den Veyver IB, Wan M, et al. (1999) Rett syndrome is caused by mutations in X-linked MECP2, encoding methyl-CpG-binding protein 2. *Nat Genet* **23**, 185–188.

Anderson LT, Campbell M, Adams P, et al. (1989) The effects of haloperidol on discrimination learning and behavioral symptoms in autistic children. *J Autism Dev Disord* **9**, 227–239.

Anderson LT, Campbell M, Grega DM, et al. (1984) Haloperidol in the treatment of infantile autism: effects on learning and behavioral symptoms. *Am J Psychiatry* **141**, 1195–1202.

Asperger H (1944) Die "Autistischen Psychopathen" kindesalter. *Arch Psychiatr Nervenkr* **117**, 76–136.

Awad GA (1996) The use of selective serotonin reuptake inhibitors in young children with pervasive developmental disorders: some clinical observations. *Can J Psychiatry* **41**, 361–366.

Bachevalier J (1994) Medial temporal lobe structures and autism: a review of clinical and experimental findings. *Neuropsychologia* **32**, 627–648.

Bacon AL, Fein D, Morris R, et al. (1998) The responses of autistic children to the distress of others. *J Autism Dev Disord* **28**, 129–142.

Bailey A, Le Couteur A, Gottesman I, et al. (1995) Autism as a strongly genetic disorder: evidence from a British twin study. *Psychol Med* **25**, 63–78.

Bailey A, Luthert P, Dean A, et al. (1998) A clinicopathological study of autism. *Brain* **121**, 889–905.

Baker P, Piven J, Schwartz S, et al. (1994) Duplication of chromosome 15q11–13 in two individuals with autistic disorder. *J Autism Dev Disord* **24**, 529–535.

Barber J, Cross I, Douglas F, et al. (1998) Neurofibromatosis pseudogene amplification underlies euchromatic cytogenetic duplications and triplications of proximal 15q. *Hum Genet* **103**, 600–607.

Bartak L, Rutter M, and Cox A (1975) A comparative study of infantile autism and specific developmental receptive language disorder. I: The children. *Br J Psychiatry* **126**, 127–145.

Bauman M and Kemper TL (1985) Histoanatomic observations of the brain in early infantile autism. *Neurology* **35**, 866–874.

Brent DA, Crumrine PK, Varma RR, et al. (1987) Phenobarbital treatment and major depressive disorder in children with epilepsy. *Pediatrics* **80**, 909–917.

Brodkin ES, McDougle CJ, Naylor ST, et al. (1997) Clomipramine in adults with pervasive developmental disorders: a prospective open-label investigation. *J Child Adolesc Psychopharmacol* **7**, 109–121.

Brothers L (1989) A biological perspective on empathy. *Am J Psychiatry* **146**, 10–19.

Buchsbaum MS, Siegel BV Jr., Wu JC, et al. (1992) Brief report: attention performance in autism and regional brain metabolic rate assessed by positron emission tomography. *J Autism Dev Disord* **22**, 115–125.

Buitelaar JK, Willemsen-Swinkels S, and Van Engeland H (1998) Naltrexone in children with autism. *J Am Acad Child Adolesc Psychiatry* **37**, 800–802.

Buxbaum J, Silverman J, Smith C, et al. (2002) Association between a GABRB3 polymorphism and autism. *Mol Psychiatry* **7**(3), 311–316.

Buyse IM, Fang P, Hoon KT, et al. (2000) Diagnostic testing for Rett syndrome by DHPLC and direct sequencing analysis of the MECP2 gene: identification of several novel mutations and polymorphisms. *Am J Hum Genet* **67**(6), 1428–1436.

Campbell M, Adams P, Perry R, et al. (1988) Tardive and withdrawal dyskinesia in autistic children: a prospective study. *Psychopharm Bull* **24**, 251–255.

Campbell M, Anderson L, Small A, et al. (1993) Naltrexone in autistic children: behavioral symptoms and attentional learning. *J Am Acad Child Adolesc Psychiatry* **32**, 1283–1291.

Campbell M, Anderson LT, Meier M, et al. (1976) A comparison of haloperidol and behavior therapy and their interaction in autistic children. *J Am Acad Child Psychiatry* **17**, 640–655.

Campbell M, Fish B, Korein J, et al. (1972) Lithium and chlorpromazine: a controlled crossover study of hyperactive severely disturbed young children. *J Autism Child Schizophr* **2**, 234–263.

Carlsson ML (1998) Hypothesis: Is infantile autism a hypoglutamatergic disorder? Relevance of glutamate—serotonin interactions for pharmacotherapy. *J Neural Transm* **105**, 525–535.

Carter AS, Volkmar FR, Sparrow SS, et al. (1998) The Vineland adaptive behavior scales: supplementary norms for individuals with autism. *J Autism Dev Disord* **28**, 287–302.

Chakrabarti S and Fombonne E (2001) Pervasive developmental disorders in preschool children. *J Am Med Assoc* **285**, 3093–3099.

Chez MG, Buchanan CP, Bagan BT, et al. (2000) Secretin and autism: a two-part clinical investigation. *J Autism Dev Disord* **30**, 87–94.

Chugani DC, Muzik O, Behen M, et al. (1999a) Developmental changes in brain serotonin synthesis capacity in autistic and nonautistic children. *Ann Neurol* **45**, 287–95.

Chugani DC, Muzik O, Rothermel R, et al. (1997) Altered serotonin synthesis in the dentatothalamocortical pathway in autistic boys. *Ann Neurol* **42**, 666–669.

Chugani DC, Sundram BS, Behen M, et al. (1999b) Evidence of altered energy metabolism in autistic children. *Prog Neuropsychopharmacol Biol Psychiatry* **23**, 635–641.

Chugani HT, Da Silva E, and Chugani DC (1996) Infantile spasms: III. Prognostic implications of bitemporal hypometabolism on positron emission tomography. *Ann Neurol* **39**, 643–649.

Cohen IL, Campbell M, Posner D, et al. (1980) Behavioral effects of haloperidol in young autistic children. An objective analysis using a within subject reversal design. *J Am Acad Child Psychiatry* **19**, 665–677.

Coniglio SJ, Lewis JD, Lang C, et al. (2001) A randomized, double-blind, placebo-controlled trial of single-dose intravenous secretin as treatment for children with autism. *J Pediatr* **138**, 649–655.

Cook E (1998) Genetics of autism. *Ment Retard Dev Disabil Res Rev* **4**, 113–120.

Cook E, Arora R, Anderson G, et al. (1993) Platelet serotonin studies in hyperserotonemic relatives of children with autistic disorder. *Life Sci* **52**, 2005–2015.

Cook E and Leventhal B (1996) The serotonin system in autism. *Curr Opin Pediatr* **8**, 348–354.

Cook E, Lindgren V, Leventhal B, et al. (1997a) Autism or atypical autism in maternally but not paternally derived proximal 15q duplication. *Am J Hum Genet* **60**, 928–934.

Cook EH (2001) Genetics of autism. *Child Adolesc Psychiatr Clin N Am* **10**, 333–350.

Cook EH Jr., Courchesne R, Lord C, et al. (1997b) Evidence of linkage between the serotonin transporter and autistic disorder. *Mol Psychiatry* **2**, 247–250.

Cook EH Jr., Rowlett R, Jaselskis C, et al. (1992) Fluoxetine treatment of children and adults with autistic disorder and mental retardation. *J Am Acad Child Adolesc Psychiatry* **31**, 739–745.

Cook EH, Leventhal BL, and Freedman DX (1988) Free serotonin in plasma: autistic children and their first-degree relatives. *Biol Psychiatry* **24**, 488–491.

Cook EH, Leventhal BL, Heller W, et al. (1990) Autistic children and their first-degree relatives: relationships between serotonin and norepinephrine levels and intelligence. *J Neuropsychiatr Clin Neurosci* **2**, 268–274.

Corbett J and Harris R (1977) Progressive disintegrative psychosis of childhood. *J Child Psychol Psychiatry* **18**, 211–219.

Courchesne E, Townsend J, and Saitoh O (1994) The brain in infantile autism: posterior fossa structures are abnormal. *Neurology* **44**, 214–223.

DeVolder A, Bol A, Michel C, et al. (1987) Brain glucose metabolism in children with the autistic syndrome: positron tomography analysis. *Brain Dev* **9**, 581–587.

Dunn-Geier J, Ho HH, Auersperg E, et al. (2000) Effect of secretin on children with autism: a randomized controlled trial. *Dev Med Child Neurol* **42**, 796–802.

Durand VM and Carr EG (1991) Functional communication training to reduce challenging behavior: maintenance and application in new settings. *J Appl Behav Anal* **24**, 251–264.

Emerson E and Bromley J (1995) The form and function of challenging behaviors. *J Intellect Disabil Res* **39**, 388–398.

Erdmann J, Shimron-Abarbanell D, Rietschel M, et al. (1996) Systematic screening for mutations in the human serotonin-2A (5-HT$_{2A}$) receptor gene: identification of two naturally occurring receptor variants and association analysis in schizophrenia. *Hum Genet* **97**, 614–619.

Ernst M, Magee HJ, Gonzalez NM, et al. (1992) Pimozide in autistic children. *Psychopharmacol Bull* **28**, 187–191.

Ernst M, Zametkin AJ, Matochik JA, et al. (1997) Low medial prefrontal dopaminergic activity in autistic children [letter]. *Lancet* **350**, 638.

Fankhauser MP, Karumanchi VC, German ML, et al. (1992) A double-blind, placebo-controlled study of the efficacy of transdermal clonidine in autism. *J Clin Psychiatry* **53**, 77–82.

Feldman HM, Kolmen BK, and Gonzaga AM (1999) Naltrexone and communication skills in young children with autism. *J Am Acad Child Adolesc Psychiatry* **38**, 587–593.

Filipek PA, Accardo PJ, Baranek GT, et al. (1999) The screening and diagnosis of autistic spectrum disorders. *J Autism Dev Disord* **29**, 439–484.

Fish B, Shapiro T, and Campbell M (1966) Long-term prognosis and the response of schizophrenic children to drug therapy: a controlled study of trifluoperazine. *Am J Psychiatry* **123**, 32–39.

Folstein SE and Mankoski RE (2000) Chromosome 7q: Where autism meets language disorder? *Am J Hum Genet* **67**, 278–281.

Fombonne E (1999) The epidemiology of autism: a review. *Psychol Med* **29**, 769–786.

Fombonne E and Chakrabarti S (2001) No evidence for a new variant of measles–mumps–rubella-induced autism. *Pediatrics* **108**, E58.

Fombonne E, Du Mazaubrun C, Cans C, et al. (1997) Autism and associated medical disorders in a French epidemiological survey. *J Am Acad Child Adolesc Psychiatry* **36**, 1561–1569.

Freeman BJ, Ritvo ER, Needleman R, et al. (1985) The stability of cognitive and linguistic parameters in autism: a five-year prospective study. *J Am Acad Child Adolesc Psychiatry* **24**, 459–464.

Geller E, Ritvo ER, Freeman BJ, et al. (1982) Preliminary observations on the effect of fenfluramine on blood serotonin and symptoms in three autistic boys. *N Engl J Med* **307**, 165–169.

Ghaziuddin M, Tsai L, and Ghaziuddin N (1991) Fluoxetine in autism with depression. *J Am Acad Child Adolesc Psychiatry* **30**, 508–509.

Gillberg C (1991) Outcome in autism and autistic-like conditions. *J Am Acad Child Adolesc Psychiatry* **30**, 375–382.

Gillberg C and Schaumann H (1981) Infantile autism and puberty. *J Autism Dev Disord* **11**, 365–371.

Gillberg C and Steffenburg S (1987) Outcome and prognostic factors in infantile autism and similar conditions: a population-based study of 46 cases followed through puberty. *J Autism Dev Disord* **17**, 273–287.

Gillberg C, Trygstad O, and Foss I (1982) Childhood psychosis and urinary excretion of peptides and protein-associated peptide complexes. *J Autism Dev Disord* **12**, 229–241.

Gordon C, State R, Nelson J, et al. (1993) A double-blind comparison of clomipramine, desipramine, and placebo in the treatment of autistic disorder. *Arch Gen Psychiatry* **50**, 441–447.

Hagberg B, Goutieres F, Hanefeld F, et al. (1985) Rett syndrome: criteria for inclusion and exclusion. *Brain Dev* **7**, 372–373.

Handen BL, Johnson CR, and Lubetsky M (2000) Efficacy of methylphenidate among children with autism and symptoms of attention-deficit hyperactivity disorder. *J Autism Dev Disord* **30**, 245–255.

Happe FG (1993) Communicative competence and theory of mind in autism: a test of relevance theory. *Cognition* **48**, 101–119.

Haznedar MM, Buchsbaum MS, Metzger M, et al. (1997) Anterior cingulate gyrus volume and glucose metabolism in autistic disorder. *Am J Psychiatry* **154**, 1047–1050.

Herman B, Asleson G, and Papero P (1993) Acute and chronic naltrexone decreases the hyperactivity of autism. *Soc Neurosci Abstr* **19**, (Part 2), 1785.

Herold S, Frackowiak RSJ, Le Couteur A, et al. (1988) Cerebral blood flow and metabolism of oxygen and glucose in young autistic adults. *Psychol Med* **18**, 823–831.

Hobson RP and Lee A (1998) Hello and goodbye: a study of social engagement in autism. *J Autism Dev Disord* **28**, 117–127.

Hollander E, Dolgoff-Kaspar R, Cartwright C, et al. (2001) An open trial of divalproex sodium in autism spectrum disorders. *J Clin Psychiatry* **62**, 530–534.

Honda H, Shimizu Y, Misumi K, et al. (1996) Cumulative incidence and prevalence of childhood autism in children of Japan. *Br J Psychiatry* **169**, 228–235.

Horvath K, Stefanatos G, Sokolski KN, et al. (1998) Improved social and language skills after secretin administration in patients with autistic spectrum disorders. *J Assoc Acad Minor Phys* **9**, 9–15.

Howlin P (1998) Practitioner review: psychological and educational treatments for autism. *J Child Psychol Psychiatry* **39**, 307–322.

International Molecular Genetic Study of Autism Consortium (2001) A genome wide screen for autism: strong evidence for linkage to chromosomes 2q, 7q and 16p. *Am J Hum Genet* **69**, 570–581.

Jaselskis CA, Cook EH, Fletcher KE, et al. (1992) Clonidine treatment of hyperactive and impulsive children with autistic disorder. *J Clin Psychopharm* **12**, 322–327.

Kanner L, Rodriguez A, and Ashenden B (1972) How far can autistic children go in matters of social adaptation. *J Autism Child Schizophr* **2**, 9–33.

Kasari C, Sigman M, Mundy P, et al. (1990) Affective sharing in the context of joint attention interactions of normal, autistic, and mentally retarded children. *J Autism Dev Disord* **20**, 87–94.

Kemper TL and Bauman M (1998) Neuropathology of infantile autism. *J Neuropathol Exp Neurol* **57**, 645–652.

Kim SJ and Cook EH Jr. (2000) Novel de novo nonsense mutation of MECP2 in a patient with Rett syndrome. *Hum Mutat (Online)* **15**, 382–383.

Kim S-J, Cox N, Courchesne R, et al. (2002) Transmission disequilibrium mapping in the serotonin transporter gene (SLC6A4) region in autistic disorder. *Mol Psychiatry* **7**(3), 278–288.

King B, Wright D, Handen B, et al. (2001) A double-blind, placebo-controlled study of amantidine hydrochloride in the treatment of children with autistic disorder. *J Am Acad Child Adolesc Psychiatry* **40**, 658–665.

Klauck SM, Poustka F, Benner A, et al. (1997) Serotonin transporter (5-HTT) gene variants associated with autism? *Hum Mol Genet* **6**, 2233–2238.

Kleijnen J and Knipschild P (1991) Niacin and vitamin B[6] in mental functioning: a review of controlled trials in humans. *Biol Psychiatry* **29**, 931–941.

Kobayashi R, Murata T, and Yoshinaga K (1992) A follow-up study of 201 children with autism in Kyushu and Yamaguchi areas, Japan. *J Autism Dev Disord* **22**, 395–411.

Kuperman S, Beeghly JH, Burns TL, et al. (1985) Serotonin relationships of autistic probands and their first-degree relatives. *J Am Acad Child Psychiatry* **24**, 186–190.

Kurita H, Kita M, and Miyake Y (1992) A comparative study of development and symptoms among disintegrative psychosis and infantile autism with and without speech loss. *J Autism Dev Disord* **22**, 175–188.

Leboyer M, Philippe A, Bouvard M, et al. (1999) Whole blood serotonin and plasma beta-endorphin in autistic probands and their first-degree relatives. *Biol Psychiatry* **45**, 158–163.

Leventhal BL, Cook EH Jr., Morford M, (1990) Relationships of whole blood serotonin and plasma norepinephrine within families. *J Autism Dev Disord* **20**, 499–511.

Leventhal BL, Cook EH Jr., Morford M, (1993) Clinical and neurochemical effects of fenfluramine in children with autism. *J Neuropsychiatr Clin Neurosci* **5**, 307–315.

Libby S, Powell S, Messer D, et al. (1997) Imitation of pretend play acts by children with autism and Down syndrome. *J Autism Dev Disord* **27**, 365–383.

Lord C (1984) The development of peer relations in children with autism. In *Applied Developmental Psychology*, Vol. 1, Morrison F, Lord C, and Keating D (eds). Academic Press, New York, pp. 165–229.

Lord C (1995) Follow-up of two-year-olds referred for possible autism. *J Child Psychol Psychiatry* **36**, 1365–1382.

Lord C, Cook E, Leventhal B, et al. (2000a) Autism spectrum disorders. *Neuron* **28**, 355–364.

Lord C, Pickles A, McLennan J, et al. (1997) Diagnosing autism: analyses of data from the autism diagnostic interview. *J Autism Dev Disord* **27**, 501–517.

Lord C, Risi S, Lambrecht L, et al. (2000b) The autism diagnostic observation schedule-generic: a standard measure of social and communication deficits associated with the spectrum of autism. *J Autism Dev Disord* **30**, 205–223.

Lord C, Rutter M, and Le Couteur A (1994) Autism diagnostic interview—revised: a revised version of a diagnostic interview for caregivers of individuals with possible pervasive developmental disorders. *J Autism Dev Disord* **24**, 659–685.

Lovaas OI (1996) The UCLA young autism model of service delivery. In *Behavioral Interventions for Young Children with Autism*, Maurice C (ed). Austin, TX.

Maestrini E, Lai C, Marlow A, et al. (1999) Serotonin transporter (5-HTT) and gamma-aminobutyric acid receptor subunit beta 3 (GABRB3) gene polymorphisms are not associated with autism in the IMGSA families. *Am J Med Genet* **88**, 492–496.

Malone RP, Cater J, Sheikh RM, et al. (2001) Olanzapine versus haloperidol in children with autistic disorder: an open pilot study. *J Am Acad Child Adolesc Psychiatry* **40**, 887–894.

Martin ER, Menold MM, Wolpert CM, et al. (2000) Analysis of linkage disequilibrium in γ-aminobutyric acid receptor subunit genes in autistic disorder. *Am J Med Genet (Neuropsychiatr Genet)* **96**, 43–48.

Martineau J, Barthelemy C, Cheliakine C, et al. (1988) Brief report: an open middle-term study of combined vitamin B^6–magnesium in a subgroup of autistic children selected on their sensitivity to this treatment. *J Autism Dev Disord* **18**, 435–447.

Masi G, Cosenza A, Mucci M, et al. (2001) Open trial of risperidone in 24 young children with pervasive developmental disorders. *J Am Acad Child Adolesc Psychiatry* **40**, 1206–1214.

McDougle CJ, Epperson CN, Price LH, et al. (1998a) Evidence for linkage disequilibrium between serotonin transporter protein gene (SLC6A4) and obsessive compulsive disorder. *Mol Psychiatry* **3**, 270–273.

McDougle CJ, Holmes JP, Bronson MR, et al. (1997) Risperidone treatment of children and adolescents with pervasive developmental disorders: a prospective open-label study. *J Am Acad Child Adolesc Psychiatry* **36**, 685–693.

McDougle CJ, Holmes JP, Carlson DC, et al. (1998b) A double-blind, placebo-controlled study of risperidone in adults with autistic disorder and other pervasive developmental disorders. *Arch Gen Psychiatry* **55**, 633–641.

Muller RA, Chugani DC, Behen ME, et al. (1998) Impairment of dentato-thalamo-cortical pathway in autistic men: language activation data from positron emission tomography. *Neurosci Lett* **245**, 1–4.

Mundy P and Sigman M (1989) The theoretical implications of joint-attention deficits in autism. *Dev Psychopathol* **1**, 173–183.

Naruse H, Nagahata M, Nakane Y, et al. (1982) A multi-center double-blind trial of pimozide (Orap), haloperidol and placebo in children with behavioral disorders, using crossover design. *Acta Paedopsychiatry* **48**, 173–184.

Njardvik U, Matson JL, and Cherry KE (1999) A comparison of social skills in adults with autistic disorder, pervasive developmental disorder not otherwise specified, and mental retardation. *J Autism Dev Disord* **29**, 287–295.

Nordin V and Gillberg C (1998) The long-term course of autistic disorders: update on follow-up studies. *Acta Psychiatr Scand* **97**, 99–108.

Odom SL and Strain PS (1986) A comparison of peer-initiation and teacher–antecedent interventions for promoting reciprocal social interaction of autistic preschoolers. *J Appl Behav Anal* **19**, 59–71.

Oke NJ and Schreibman L (1990) Training social initiations to a high-functioning autistic child: assessment of collateral behavior change and generalization in a case study. *J Autism Dev Disord* **20**, 479–497.

Olsson L, Steffenburg S, and Gillberg C (1988) Epilepsy in autism and autistic-like conditions: a population-based study. *Arch Neurol* **45**, 666–668.

Osterling J and Dawson G (1994) Early recognition of children with autism: a study of first birthday home videotapes. *J Autism Dev Disord* **24**, 247–257.

Owley T, McMahon W, Cook EH, et al. (2001) Multi-site, double-blind, placebo-controlled trial of porcine secretin in autism. *J Am Acad Child Adolesc Psychiatry* **40**, 1293–1299.

Percy AK, Glaze DG, Schultz RJ, et al. (1994) Rett syndrome: controlled study of an oral opiate antagonist, naltrexone. *Ann Neurol* **35**, 464–470.

Perry R, Campbell M, Adams P, et al. (1989) Long-term efficacy of haloperidol in autistic children: continuous versus discontinuous drug administration. *J Am Acad Child Adolesc Psychiatry* **28**, 87–92.

Pfeiffer SI, Norton J, Nelson L, et al. (1995) Efficacy of vitamin B^6 and magnesium in the treatment of autism: a methodology review and summary of outcomes. *J Autism Dev Disord* **25**, 481–493.

Piven J, Tsai G, Nehme E, et al. (1991) Platelet serotonin, a possible marker for familial autism. *J Autism Dev Disord* **21**, 51–59.

Plioplys A (1994) Autism: electroencephalographic abnormalities and clinical improvement with valproic acid. *Arch Pediatr Adolesc Med* **148**, 220–222.

Posey DJ, Walsh KH, Wilson GA, et al. (1999) Risperidone in the treatment of two very young children with autism. *J Child Adolesc Psychopharmacol* **9**, 273–276.

Potenza MN, Holmes JP, Kanes SJ, et al. (1999) Olanzapine treatment of children, adolescents, and adults with pervasive developmental disorders: an open-label pilot study. *J Clin Psychopharmacol* **19**, 37–44.

Quintana H, Birmaher B, Stedge D, et al. (1995) Use of methylphenidate in the treatment of children with autistic disorder. *J Autism Dev Disord* **25**, 283–294.

Ratey J, Bemporad J, Sorgi P, et al. (1987) Brief report: open trial effects of beta-blockers on speech and social behaviors in 8 autistic adults. *J Autism Dev Disord* **17**, 439–446.

Rett A (1966) On an until now unknown disease of a congenital metabolic disorder. *Krankenschwester* **19**, 121–122.

Risch N, Spiker D, Lotspeich L, et al. (1999) A genomic screen of autism: evidence for a multilocus etiology. *Am J Hum Genet* **65**, 493–507.

Ritvo E, Jorde L, Mason-Brothers A, et al. (1989) The UCLA-University of Utah epidemiologic survey of autism: recurrence risk estimates and genetic counseling. *Am J Psychiatry* **146**, 1032–1036.

Ritvo ER, Freeman BJ, Scheibel AB, et al. (1986) Lower Purkinje cell counts in the cerebella of four autistic subjects: initial findings of the UCLA- NSAC autopsy research report. *Am J Psychiatry* **143**, 862–866.

Roberts W, Weaver L, Brian J, et al. (2001) Repeated doses of porcine secretin in the treatment of autism: a randomized, placebo-controlled trial. *Pediatrics* **107**, E71.

Roeyers H (1996) The influence of nonhandicapped peers on the social interactions of children with a pervasive development disorder. *J Autism Dev Disord* **26**, 303–320.

Rosenwasser B and Axelrod S (2001) The contributions of applied behavior analysis to the education of people with autism. *Behav Modif* **25**(5), 671–677.

Rumsey JM, Duara R, Grady C, et al. (1985) Brain metabolism in autism: resting cerebral glucose utilization rates as measured with positron emission tomography. *Arch Gen Psychiatry* **42**, 448–455.

Rutter M (1983) Cognitive deficits in the pathogenesis of autism. *J Child Psychol Psychiatry* **24**, 513–532.

Rutter M (1985) Infantile autism. In *The Clinical Guide to Child Psychiatry*, Shaffer D, Ehrhardt AA, and Greenhill LL (eds). Free Press, New York, pp. 48–78.

Sandler AD, Sutton KA, DeWeese J, et al. (1999) Lack of benefit of a single dose of synthetic human secretin in the treatment of autism and pervasive developmental disorder. *N Engl J Med* **341**, 1801–1806.

Schain RJ and Freedman DX (1961) Studies on 5-hydroxyindole metabolism in autistic and other mentally retarded children. *J Pediatr* **58**, 315–320.

Schifter T, Hoffman JM Jr., Hatten H, et al. (1994) Neuroimaging in infantile autism. *J Child Neurol* **9**, 155–161.

Schuster CR, Lewis M, and Seiden LS (1986) Fenfluramine: neurotoxicity. *Psychopharm Bull* **22**, 148–151.

Shao Y, Wolpert C, Raiford K, et al. (2002) Genomic screen and follow-up analysis for autistic disorder. *Am J Med Genet (Neuropsychiatr Genet)* **114**, 99–105.

Sheinkopf SJ and Siegel B (1998) Home-based behavioral treatment of young children with autism. *J Autism Dev Disord* **28**(1), 15–23.

Siegel BW, Freedman J, Vaal MJ, et al. (1996) Activities of novel aryloxyalkylimidazolines on rat 5-HT$_{2A}$ and 5-HT$_{2C}$ receptors. *Eur J Pharmacol* **296**, 307–318.

Smith T, Groen AD, and Wynn JW (2001) Randomized trial of early intervention for children with pervasive developmental disorder. *Am J Ment Retard* **105**(4), 269–285.

Sturmey P, Jamieson J, Burcham J, et al. (1996) The factor structure of the Reiss screen for maladaptive behaviors in institutional and community populations. *Res Dev Disabil* **17**, 285–291.

Szatmari P, Offord D, and Boyle M (1989) Ontario child health study: prevalence of attention deficit disorder with hyperactivity. *J Child Psychol Psychiatry* **30**, 205–217.

Tager-Flusberg H and Anderson M (1991) The development of contingent discourse ability in autistic children. *J Child Psychol Psychiatry* **32**, 1123–1134.

Tager-Flusberg H, Joseph R, and Folstein S (2001) Current directions in research on autism. *Ment Retard Dev Disabil Res Rev* **7**, 21–29.

Tantam D (1988) Lifelong eccentricity and social isolation. II: Asperger's syndrome or schizoid personality disorder? *Br J Psychiatry* **153**, 783–791.

Taylor A, Pickering K, Lord C, et al. (1998) *Mixed and Multilevel Models for Longitudinal Data: Growth Curve Models of Language Development Statistical Analysis Of Medical Data: New Developments*. Oxford University Press, New York, pp. 127–145.

Taylor BA and Harris SL (1995) Teaching children with autism to seek information: acquisition of novel information and generalization of responding. *J Appl Behav Anal* **28**, 3–14.

Treffert DA (1970) Epidemiology of infantile autism. *Arch Gen Psychiatry* **22**, 431–438.

Tsai L, Jacoby C, Stewart M, et al. (1982) Unfavourable L-R asymmetries of the brain and autism: a question of methodology. *Br J Psychiatry* **140**, 312–319.

Unis A, Cook E, Vincent J, et al. (1997) Platelet serotonin measures in adolescents with conduct disorder. *Biol Psychiatry* **42**, 553–559.

Venter A, Lord C, and Schopler E (1992) A follow-up study of high-functioning autistic children. *J Child Psychol Psychiatry* **33**, 489–507.

Vining EPG, Mellits D, Dorsen MM, et al. (1987) Psychologic and behavioral effects of antiepileptic drugs in children: a double-blind comparison between phenobarbital and valproic acid. *Pediatrics* **80**, 165–174.

Volden J and Lord C (1991) Neologisms and abnormal functional usage of language in autistic speakers. *J Autism Dev Disord* **21**, 1–22.

Volkmar F and Cohen D (1989) Disintegrative disorder or "late onset" autism. *J Child Psychol Psychiatry* **30**, 717–724.

Volkmar F, Klin A, Siegel B, et al. (1994) Field trial for autistic disorder in DSM-IV. *Am J Psychiatry* **151**, 1361–1367.

Volkmar FR and Nelson DS (1990) Seizure disorders in autism. *J Am Acad Child Adolesc Psychiatry* **29**, 127–129.

Wakefield AJ and Montgomery SM (2000) Measles, mumps, rubella vaccine: through a glass, darkly. *Adverse Drug React Toxicol Rev* **19**, 265–283; discussion 284–292.

Weiss MJ and Harris SL (2001) Teaching social skills to people with autism. *Behav Modif* **25**, 785–802.

Willemsen-Swinkels SH, Buitelaar JK, van Berckelaer-Onnes IA, et al. (1999) Brief report: six months continuation treatment in naltrexone- responsive children with autism: an open-label case-control design. *J Autism Dev Disord* **29**, 167–169.

Willemsen-Swinkels SH, Buitelaar JK, Weijnen FG, et al. (1998) Timing of social gaze behavior in children with a pervasive developmental disorder. *J Autism Dev Disord* **28**, 199–210.

Willemsen-Swinkels SHN, Buitelaar JK, and Van Engeland H (1996) The effects of chronic naltrexone treatment in young autistic children: a double-blind placebo-controlled crossover study. *Biol Psychiatry* **39**, 1023–1031.

Willemsen-Swinkels SHN, Buitelaar JK, Weijnen FG, et al. (1995) Placebo-controlled acute dosage naltrexone study in young autistic children. *Psychiatr Res* **58**, 203–215.

Williams DT, Mehl R, Yudofsky S, et al. (1982) The effect of propranolol on uncontrolled rage outbursts in children and adolescents with organic brain dysfunction. *J Am Acad Child Adolesc Psychiatry* **21**, 129–135.

Williams RS, Hauser SL, Purpura DP, et al. (1980) Autism and mental retardation: neuropathologic studies performed in four retarded persons with autistic behavior. *Arch Neurol* **37**, 749–753.

Wilmut I, Schnieke AE, McWhir J, et al. (1997) Viable offspring derived from fetal and adult mammalian cells. *Nature* **385**, 810–813.

Wing L (1980) Childhood autism and social class: a question of selection? *Br J Psychiatry* **137**, 410–417.

Wing L (1981) Asperger's syndrome: a clinical account. *Psychol Med* **11**, 115–129.

Wing L, Yeates SR, Brierley LM, et al. (1976) The prevalence of early childhood autism: comparison of administrative and epidemiological studies. *Psychol Med* **6**, 89–100.

Zanolli K, Daggett J, and Adams T (1996) Teaching preschool age autistic children to make spontaneous initiations to peers using priming. *J Autism Dev Disord* **26**, 407–422.

8 Childhood Disorders: Attention-Deficit and Disruptive Behavior Disorders

Diagnosis

Attention-deficit/hyperactivity disorder (ADHD), conduct disorder (CD), and oppositional defiant disorder (ODD) form the attention-deficit and disruptive behavior disorders (AD-DBDs) in DSM-IV-TR. As a group, these are the most common disorders of childhood and among the most researched areas of childhood psychopathology. There is also an increasing recognition that these disorders continue into adulthood. Since the advent of DSM-III diagnostic criteria for each of the three disorders have been evolving although the core features have not changed substantially. In DSM-IV-TR, ADHD is defined as a persistent pattern of inattention and/or hyperactivity–impulsivity that is more frequently displayed and more severe than is typically observed in individuals at a comparable level of development (see DSM-IV-TR diagnostic criteria below). Three subtypes of ADHD are identified: (1) a predominantly hyperactive–impulsive type, (2) a predominantly inattentive type, and (3) a combined type. In order to qualify for the diagnosis, at least some of the symptoms must have been present and caused impairment before age 7 years. Additionally, some symptoms causing impairment in social or academic/occupational functioning must be evident in more than one setting. ADHD can be diagnosed in individuals of all ages, although it is sometimes difficult to establish the childhood onset of symptoms in older individuals.

DSM-IV-TR Diagnostic Criteria

314.0x Attention-Deficit/Hyperactivity Disorder

A. Either (1) or (2)

(1) Six (or more) of the following symptoms of "inattention" have persisted for at least 6 months to a degree that is maladaptive and inconsistent with developmental level:

Inattention

    (a) often fails to give close attention to details or makes careless mistakes in schoolwork, work, or other activities.

    (b) often has difficulty sustaining attention in tasks or play activities.

    (c) often does not seem to listen when spoken to directly.

    (d) often does not follow through on instructions and fails to finish schoolwork, chores, or duties in the workplace.

    (e) often has difficulty organizing tasks and activities.

    (f) often avoids, dislikes, or is reluctant to engage in tasks that require sustained mental effort.

    (g) often loses things necessary for tasks or activities.

    (h) is often easily distracted by extraneous stimuli.

    (i) is often forgetful in daily activities.

(2) Six (or more) of the following symptoms of "hyperactivity–impulsivity" have persisted for at least 6 months to a degree that is maladaptive and inconsistent with developmental level:

Hyperactivity

    (a) often fidgets with hands or feet or squirms in seat.

    (b) often leaves seat in classroom or in other situations in which remaining seated is expected.

    (c) often runs about or climbs excessively in situations in which it is inappropriate (in adolescents or adults, may be limited to subjective feelings of restlessness).

    (d) often has difficulty playing or engaging in leisure activities quietly.

    (e) is often "on the go" or often acts as if "driven by a motor."

    (f) often talks excessively.

Impulsivity

    (g) often blurts out answers before questions have been completed.

    (h) often has difficulty awaiting turn.

    (i) often interrupts or intrudes on others.

B. Some hyperactive–impulsive or inattentive symptoms that caused impairment were present before age 7 years.

C. Some impairment from the symptoms is present in two or more settings (e.g., at school [work] and at home).

D. There must be clear evidence of clinically significant impairment in social, academic, or occupational functioning.

E. The symptoms do not occur exclusively during the course of a Pervasive Developmental Disorder, Schizophrenia, or other Psychotic Disorder and are not better accounted for by another mental disorder (e.g., Mood Disorder, Anxiety Disorder, Dissociative Disorder, or a Personality Disorder).

Code based on type:

314.01 Attention-Deficit/Hyperactivity Disorder, Combined Type: if both Criteria A1 and A2 are met for the past 6 months;

314.00 Attention-Deficit/Hyperactivity Disorder, Predominantly Inattentive Type: if Criterion A1 is met but Criterion A2 is not met for the past 6 months;

314.01 Attention-Deficit/Hyperactivity Disorder, Predominantly Hyperactive-Impulsive Type: if Criterion A2 is met but Criterion A1 is not met for the past 6 months.

Coding note: For individuals (especially adolescents and adults) who currently have symptoms that no longer meet full criteria, "In Partial Remission" should be specified

Reprinted with permission from the Diagnostic and Statistical Manual of Mental Disorders, Fourth Edition, Text Revision. Copyright 2000 American Psychiatric Association.

The essential feature of CD is a repetitive and persistent pattern of behavior in which the basic rights of others or major age-appropriate societal norms or rules are violated (see DSM-IV-TR diagnostic criteria below). From a list of 15 symptoms, at least three must be present during the past year, with at least one present in the last 6 months. Similar to ADHD, symptoms of CD are seen in multiple settings and cause significant impairment in functioning. Adults with conduct problems, whose behavior does not meet criteria for antisocial personality disorder, may have symptoms that meet criteria for CD and thus qualify for the diagnosis. Subtypes of CD are determined on the basis of age of onset. The childhood-onset subtype is diagnosed in children who show at least one of the behaviors before the age of 10 years, while the adolescent-onset subtype is characterized by the absence of any CD behaviors before 10 years of age.

DSM-IV-TR Diagnostic Criteria

312.8x Conduct Disorder

A. A repetitive and persistent pattern of behavior in which the basic rights of others or major age-appropriate societal norms or rules are violated, as manifested by the presence of three (or more) of the following criteria in the past 12 months, with at least one criterion present in the past 6 months.

Aggression to people and animals

   (1) often bullies, threatens, or intimidates others.
   (2) often initiates physical fights.
   (3) has used a weapon that can cause serious physical harm to others.
   (4) has been physically cruel to people.
   (5) has been physically cruel to animals.
   (6) has stolen while confronting a victim.
   (7) has forced someone into sexual activity.

Destruction of property

(1) has deliberately engaged in fire setting with the intention of causing serious damage.
(2) has deliberately destroyed others' property.

Deceitfulness or theft

(1) has broken into someone else's house, building or car.
(2) often lies to obtain goods or favors or to avoid obligations.
(3) has stolen items of nontrival value without confronting a victim.

Serious violations of rules

(1) often stays out at night despite parental prohibitions, beginning before age 13 years.
(2) has run away from home overnight at least twice while living in parental or parental surrogate home.
(3) is often truant from school, beginning before age 13 years.

B. The disturbance in behavior causes clinically significant impairment in social, academic or occupational functioning.
C. If the individual is age 18 years or older, criteria are not met for Antisocial Personality Disorder.

Code based on age at onset:

312.81 Conduct Disorder, Childhood-Onset Type: onset of at least one criterion characteristic of Conduct Disorder prior to age 10 years

312.82 Conduct Disorder, Adolescent-Onset Type: absence of any criteria characteristic of Conduct Disorder prior to age 10 years

312.89 Conduct Disorder, Unspecified Onset: age at onset is not known

Specify severity:

Mild: few if any conduct problems in excess of those required to make the diagnosis and conduct problems cause only minor harm to others (e.g., lying, truancy, staying out after dark without permission)

Moderate: number of conduct problems and effect on others intermediate between "mild" and "severe" (e.g., stealing without confronting a victim, vandalism)

Severe: many conduct problems in excess of those required to make the diagnosis or conduct problems cause considerable harm to others (e.g., forced sex, physical cruelty, use of a weapon, stealing while confronting a victim, breaking and entering)

The essential feature of ODD is a recurrent pattern of negativistic, defiant, disobedient, and hostile behavior toward authority figures that persists for at least 6 months (see DSM-IV-TR diagnostic criteria on page 162). The predecessor of ODD, oppositional disorder (OD) was first described in DSM-III, but it was not grouped with either ADHD or CD. It was a diagnosis given to those children whose behavior was principally oppositional.

In DSM-III-R, the disorder was broadened to include minor conduct problems and was renamed ODD. The definition was changed only slightly in DSM-IV with the elimination of one symptom and the addition of an impairment criterion, based on results from the field trials.

▬ DSM-IV-TR Diagnostic Criteria ▬

313.81 Oppositional Defiant Disorder

A. A pattern of negativistic, hostile, and defiant behavior lasting at least 6 months, during which four (or more) of the following are present:

   (1) often loses temper.
   (2) often argues with adults.
   (3) often actively defies or refuses to comply with adults' requests or rules.
   (4) often deliberately annoys people.
   (5) often blames others for his or her mistakes or misbehavior.
   (6) is often touchy or easily annoyed by others.
   (7) is often angry and resentful.
   (8) is often spiteful or vindictive.

Note: Consider a criterion met only if the behavior occurs more frequently than is typically observed in individuals of comparable age and developmental level.

B. The disturbance in behavior causes clinically significant impairment in social, academic, or occupational functioning.
C. The behaviors do not occur exclusively during the course of a Psychotic or Mood Disorder.
D. Criteria are not met for Conduct Disorder, and, if the individual is age 18 years or older, criteria are not met for Antisocial Personality Disorder

---

Reprinted with permission from the Diagnostic and Statistical Manual of Mental Disorders, Fourth Edition, Text Revision. Copyright 2000 American Psychiatric Association.

The rationale for grouping ADHD, CD, and ODD is that similar areas of difficulty are present in children with these disorders. Academic difficulties, poor social skills, and overrepresentation of boys are among the shared characteristics (Werry et al. 1987). Further, the three disorders demonstrate a commonality of core symptoms, with impulsivity being prominent in all three conditions. Not surprisingly, there is a high degree of comorbidity among the three disorders. In part related to this, there has been extensive debate as to whether these conditions are truly distinct from each other. While there is now a consensus that ADHD and CD are separable diagnoses (Szatmari et al. 1989) with distinct correlates and outcome (Hinshaw 1987), the relationship of ODD to both disorders is less clear. Subsequent research has indicated that ODD is at least partially distinct not only from ADHD (Waldman and Lilienfeld 1991) but from CD as well (Lahey et al. 1992, Loeber 1991, Loeber et al. 1991b). Furthermore, the impairment criterion added in DSM-IV helps demarcate the boundary of ODD from normalcy.

The clinical evaluation of a child with possible AD-DBD requires a multisource, multimethod approach (Gresham 1985). In addition to clinical interviews of parents and children, supplemental information may be obtained from school reports, rating scales completed by teachers and parents, neuropsychological test data and direct observations of the child. In addition, several structured and semistructured interviews are available, although these tend to be used primarily in research settings. Generally, adults are considered to be the best informants of disruptive behaviors, although children and adolescents may provide important data regarding internalizing symptoms and some infrequent behavior problems, such as antisocial acts (American Academy of Child and Adolescent Psychiatry 1997, Barkley et al. 1991a, Loeber et al. 1991a).

Rating scales facilitate the systematic acquisition of information about the child's behavior in different settings in a cost-effective manner. Most are standardized and provide scores that are norm referenced by age and gender. The systematic use of these instruments ensures that a complete set of specific behaviors is assessed at different points in time, enabling comparisons over the course of treatment. The high rates of comorbidity in this group of disorders make the use of rating scales essential.

There is an ever-growing number of rating scales, but the most commonly used are the Conners (1998a,b), and the Achenbach (1991a,b) scales, which are available in parent and teacher versions and possess solid normative bases. The Conners Teachers Rating Scale—Revised (CTRS-R) is a 28-item scale that is normed for children from 3 to 17 years of age. It differentiates hyperactive children from normal children, clinically referred nonhyperactive children and learning disabled children (Breen and Barkley 1988, Horn et al. 1989), and is sensitive to medication effects (Barkley et al. 1988). The Conners Parent Rating Scale (CPRS-R) contains 48 items. Data support the scale's ability to differentiate groups of ADHD children from normals, as well as its sensitivity to treatment effects. The child behavior checklist (CBCL) is a 138-item parent report questionnaire and is useful with children from ages 4 to 16 years. This instrument assesses a broad range of behavior problems and competencies and generates T-scores for two broadband factors (i.e., internalizing and externalizing). The CBCL is also available in a more recently developed Teacher Report Form (Achenbach 1991b), which is similar to the parent form and applicable for children aged 4 to 18 years (Breen and Altepeter 1990).

Rating scales have several limitations, and diagnoses should not be made on the bases of these data alone. Interviews with children and their parents form the core of the clinical evaluation. In clinical practice, interviews usually follow a loosely structured format with a flexible approach that allows for the in-depth exploration of relevant clinical information. It is essential that the interviewer directly enquires about all symptoms of ADHD and common comorbidities, and therefore some structured questioning is usually required.

Psychological and cognitive test performance is generally not required to determine the presence of an AD-DBD. Nevertheless, because the AD-DBDs are frequently associated with learning problems, neuropsychological testing may be indicated, particularly when assessment of cognitive functioning is required. Information from a neuropsychological and/or educational evaluation can often be used to supplement the clinical evaluation by providing an understanding of the individual child's level of cognitive and attentional functioning, as well as screening for suspected mental retardation or learning disabilities.

Objective measures of activity level, such as stabilometric chairs, wrist actometers and solid state actigraphs have also been used in the assessment of ADHD. Although these devices provide a judgment-free assessment of activity level, their validity, as assessed by correlations with ratings of behavior, has been inconsistent. At the present time, it is suggested that these measures are not used to diagnose clinical syndromes (Halperin et al. 1994a).

Several studies have used direct behavioral observation in the assessment of the AD-DBDs, but this procedure is not a part of routine clinical practice. Various standardized methods have been used, both in a structured playroom and in a school setting. In a structured playroom setting, measures include counting the number of times a child crosses grids marked on the floor, recording the number of toys touched, the amount of time played with each toy and the amount of time the child spends focused on a particular task (Roberts 1990). In the school setting, typical measures include monitoring the amount of time the child spends on-task, remains in his/her seat, and so on (Abikoff et al. 1980). These observational measures have consistently been found to differentiate ADHD children from normals, although their utility in discriminating among clinical groups is less clear (Barkley 1991).

At the present time, there are no laboratory measures that can serve as diagnostic tools for AD-DBDs. Similarly, findings from neuroimaging studies have neither been consistent enough nor specific enough to warrant their use as diagnostic tools.

Many children with AD-DBDs have impaired social skills and consequently experience difficulties with peer relationships. The level of hyperactivity, age of onset of aggression, and the developmental level of the child, all affect the extent of peer rejection experienced (Pope et al. 1989). Other indicators of social impairment may include the number of times a child is suspended or expelled from school and the number of police contacts (Walker et al. 1991). Information regarding social adjustment is crucial in treatment planning, since increased impairment in social and school function is predictive of poor outcome.

Parent–child interactions also play a role in the maintenance of disruptive behaviors, poor social skills, the presence of internalizing symptoms, and response to treatment. It has been noted that reductions in negative and ineffective parenting practices at home mediate improvement in children's social skills in the school setting (Hinshaw et al. 2000). However, improvement in the child's behavior was only achieved when changes in parenting practices were fairly robust.

There is a high rate of comorbidity among the three disorders that comprise the AD-DBD group and several other diagnostic categories (Jensen et al. 1988, Kovacs et al. 1988, Livingston et al. 1990, Woolston et al. 1989). Among the AD-DBDs, approximately 90% of children with CD would also meet the criteria for ODD. Furthermore, 40% of children with ADHD also have ODD and 40% of children with ODD have ADHD. In terms of the comorbidity of the AD-DBD group with other diagnostic categories, it has been estimated that 15 to 20% of children with ADHD have comorbid mood disorders (Barkley et al. 1991b, Biederman et al. 1991a,c), 20 to 25% have anxiety disorders (Biederman et al. 1991b,c, Pliszka 1992) and 6 to 20% have learning disabilities (Forness et al. 1992). However, when a broader definition of academic underachievement is used, the rates show a wide variability from a low of 10% to as high as 90% (Cantwell and Baker 1991, Hinshaw et al. 1992, McGee and Share 1988, Semrud–Clikeman et al. 1992). Other conditions which may occur comorbidly with the AD-DBDs include Tourette's disorder (TD) (Pauls et al. 1986, Comings and Comings 1984, 1987), drug and alcohol abuse or dependence (Alterman et al. 1984, Eyre et al. 1982, Wood et al. 1983), and mental retardation (Hunt and Cohen 1988, Koller et al. 1983).

Epidemiology

Studies examining prevalence rates of the AD-DBDs in community samples are characterized by considerable variability, although rates are generally high. Methodological differences, the use of different systems of classification, and variability in the definition of caseness employed by different researchers make these discrepant findings difficult to interpret (Bauermeister et al. 1994, Szatmari 1992). While DSM-IV-TR estimates the prevalence rates for ADHD to range from 2 to 7% in school-age children (Costello et al. 1988), rates as high as 17.1% have been reported in community surveys (Cohen et al. 1993). Rates for CD have been estimated to be as low as 0.9% (Esser et al. 1990) for school-age children but as high as 8.7% in adolescents (Kashani et al. 1987). The overall prevalence of ODD varies across studies from 5.7% (Anderson et al. 1987) to 9.9% (Bird et al. 1988).

In school-age children, boys have higher rates than girls for all three disorders (Anderson et al. 1987, Costello et al. 1988, Esser et al. 1990, Kashani et al. 1987). In clinic settings, the ratio of boys to girls is about 9 : 1, but in community samples, this decreases to approximately 3 : 1 (Gaub and Carlson 1997, Gershon 2002, Lahey et al. 1994). Furthermore, teachers tend to identify fewer girls than boys as having ADHD symptoms. The combined type of ADHD is the most common subtype in both genders. However, in the predominantly hyperactive–impulsive subtype of ADHD, the male-to-female ratio is approximately 4 : 1 (Gershon 2002), while in the predominantly inattentive subtype the ratio falls to 2 : 1 (Lahey et al. 1994, Wolraich et al. 1996). In general, prevalence declines with age, but follow-up studies of children and adolescents indicate that the disorder frequently persists into adulthood. Longitudinal studies have reported rates of childhood cases that persist into adulthood to range from 4 to 75% (Fischer 1997, Hechtman 1992, Mannuzza et al. 1993). These highly variable rates may be accounted for by methodological differences. Factors that appear to predict the persistence of ADHD into adulthood include a positive family history for ADHD and the presence of psychiatric comorbidity, particularly aggression.

Course

Some behaviors characteristic of the AD-DBDs are observable as early as the preschool years. Hyperactive behaviors such as "moves too much during sleep" have been reported as early as age one and a half years, followed by the appearance of "difficulty playing quietly" and "excessive climbing/running" by age 3 years (Loeber et al. 1992). Attentional problems are usually reported after hyperactivity. However, it is likely that these problems are present from early on but are not reported until the child enters school, when there are increased environmental and cognitive demands. Hyperactivity and attentional problems emerge gradually (Campbell 1985) and may overlap with the emergence of oppositional behaviors, giving the appearance of a simultaneous, rather than a sequential, onset. It is now recognized that while hyperactivity and, to a lesser extent, attentional problems show a gradual decline through adolescence and adulthood, many individuals with ADHD continue to have attentional, behavioral and emotional problems well into adolescence and adulthood (Klein and Mannuzza 1991, Lambert et al. 1987, Satterfield et al. 1982, Weiss et al. 1985). Typically, adults with ADHD are less overtly overactive, although they may retain a subjective sense of restlessness. Impairment in these adults is more often a result of inattention, disorganization, and impulsive behavior.

The developmental course of oppositional behaviors shows greater variability. During the preschool years, transient oppositional behavior is very common. However, when the oppositionality is of a persistent nature and lasts beyond the preschool years, the escalation to more disruptive behaviors is more likely. Research data suggest two possible developmental trajectories. In most oppositional children, who are usually not physically aggressive, oppositional behaviors peak around age 8 years and decline beyond that (Loeber et al. 1991b, 1992). In a second group of children, delinquent behaviors (Loeber 1990, Loeber and Schmaling 1985) follow the onset of oppositional behaviors. Early physical aggression is a key predictor of this latter trajectory, with physically aggressive children being more likely to progress from early oppositional behaviors to more severe and disabling conduct problems. Coexistent ADHD tends to speed this escalation to more severe conduct problems and the development of antisocial personality disorder in adulthood.

Generally, conduct problems first appear in middle childhood. The progression of conduct problems is from rule violations, such as poor school attendance, to aggression toward animals and people. In males, the progression to more serious forms of conduct problems, such as rape or mugging, generally emerge after age 13 years (Loeber 1990). A different group of children show conduct problems for the first time during adolescence, without preexisting oppositional or aggressive behaviors. This latter group tends to have disorders that are transient and nonaggressive in nature (Loeber 1990, Loeber et al. 1993, Lucas 1992, Moffit 1990). When CD is seen in adolescence for the first time, the problems tend to diminish by adulthood. However, if CD is present from middle childhood, there is a much greater degree of persistence of aggression through adulthood and often a history of arrests and/or incarceration.

Considerable data indicate that a subgroup of hyperactive children show high rates of delinquency and substance abuse during adolescence, and this continues into adulthood (Farrington 1990). However, it is likely because of the comorbidity with CD or bipolar disorder that higher rates of substance abuse are found in adolescents with ADHD (Babor et al. 1992, Barkley et al. 1990, Biederman et al. 1997). Families of these children tend to be less stable, have higher divorce rates, and move more frequently. First-degree relatives have been found to have higher rates of antisocial behaviors, substance abuse, and depression (Biederman et al. 1987, Cadoret and Stewart 1991, Lahey et al. 1988). The difficulties experienced by these adolescents and adults include poor self-esteem, difficulty in interpersonal relationships, difficulties in holding on to jobs, as well as assault and armed robbery in a minority of cases (Hechtman et al. 1981). Individuals with childhood symptoms representing both ADHD and CD are overrepresented in this latter group.

Differential Diagnosis

Proper differential diagnosis of ADHD, CD, and ODD requires not only discrimination among the three disorders but also from a wide range of other psychiatric, developmental, and medical conditions. Among the AD-DBDs, the relationship between ADHD and CD has been the most studied. It is now generally accepted that the two disorders can be differentiated despite the high degree of overlap, both in terms of symptom presentation and co-occurrence within individuals. ADHD can be conceptualized as a cognitive/developmental disorder, with an earlier age of onset than CD. ADHD children more frequently show deficits on measures of attentional and cognitive function, have increased motor activity and greater neurodevelopmental abnormalities (Werry et al. 1987). In contrast, CD children tend to be characterized by higher levels of aggression and greater familial dysfunction.

A significant proportion of children present with symptoms of both ADHD and CD, and both conditions should be diagnosed when this occurs. Comorbid ADHD and CD are consistently reported to be more disabling than either disorder alone. These children retain the difficulties found in both disorders and tend to show increased levels of aggressive behaviors at an early age, which remain remarkably persistent. This is in contrast to the more typical episodic course seen in children who have CD alone (Carlson and Rapoport 1989, Moffit 1990, Szatmari et al. 1989, Werry et al. 1987). Finally, children with comorbid ADHD and CD appear to have a poorer long-term outcome than either disorder alone.

The relationship of ADHD to ODD is less well studied. However, it does appear that among children with ADHD, those who are most hyperactive/impulsive are at greatest risk for developing ODD. Despite the high degree of comorbidity, it is possible to distinguish between the two disorders. ODD symptoms, such as "loses temper," "actively defies," and "swears," are less characteristic of children with ADHD (Waldman and Lilienfeld 1991). In general, the onset of ODD symptoms peaks by age 8 years and shows a declining course thereafter. On the other hand, hyperactivity and attentional problems appear at a much earlier age (Jensen et al. 1988, Moffit 1990) and often persist, although the levels of inattentiveness and/or hyperactivity often decrease with age.

The relationship of ODD and CD is more complex. The question has been raised as to whether these diagnoses constitute different levels of severity of a single phenomenon, or whether they should be viewed as distinct. A diagnosis of CD supersedes ODD since approximately 90% of children with CD would also meet the criteria for ODD. Although the majority of ODD children will not develop CD (Lahey et al. 1992), in some cases ODD appears to represent a developmental precursor of CD. In cases where ODD precedes CD, the onset of CD is typically before age 10 years (childhood-onset CD). In children who have the onset of CD after age 10 years, symptoms of ODD and ADHD are usually not present during early childhood. It has been shown that children with ODD demonstrate lower degrees of impairment and are more socially competent as compared to children with CD (Rey et al. 1988). Furthermore, children with CD come from less-advantaged families, and have greater conflict with school and judicial systems as compared to children with ODD. Family adversity scores in children with ODD are usually intermediate between those of children with CD and normal children (Lahey et al. 1992, Schachar and Wachsmuth 1990b).

Mood and anxiety disorders, learning disorders, mental retardation, pervasive developmental disorders, organic mental disorders, and psychotic disorders may all present with impairment of attention, as well as hyperactive/impulsive behaviors. The diagnosis of ADHD in DSM-IV-TR requires that the symptoms of inattention/cognitive disorganization and impulsivity/hyperactivity are not better accounted for by one of the above conditions. Differentiating ADHD from bipolar disorder in childhood is complicated by the low base rate of bipolar disorder and the variability in clinical presentation. Even though there are phenomenological similarities between the two disorders, there is little evidence to suggest that most children with externalizing symptoms are at risk for bipolar disorder. A positive family history of bipolar disorder is especially helpful in diagnosing bipolar disorder in children (Carlson and Weintraub 1993). In addition, a variety of medical conditions such as epilepsy, Tourette's disorder, thyroid disease, postinfectious and/or post-traumatic encephalopathy, and sensory impairments can present with symptoms similar to ADHD and must also be considered. Finally, many medications that are prescribed to children can mimic ADHD symptomatology. Examples include anticonvulsants (e.g., pheno-barbital), antihistamines, decongestants, bronchodilators (e.g., theophylline), and systemic steroids.

Etiology

There is no single etiology for any of the AD-DBDs (Barkley 1990, Taylor 1986); it is likely that each of these disorders is heterogeneous. Nevertheless, a variety of studies using neurochemical markers, family-genetic analyses, patterns of comorbidity, and family studies have begun to delineate more homogenous groups.

Biological Factors

Attention-Deficit Hyperactivity Disorder (ADHD)

Although the specific nature of the pathophysiology in ADHD has remained elusive, recent advances in research methodology and technology have provided some clues to the neurobiological correlates of the disorder. This research has focused on neural circuits centered in the prefrontal cortex and striatum, as well as on the brain stem catecholamine systems that innervate these circuits. Emerging data from neuroimaging studies suggest that impairments in these prefrontal–striatal regions play a central role in the pathophysiology of ADHD.

Morphological studies using magnetic resonance imaging (MRI) have identified subtle anomalies in the prefrontal cortex and basal ganglia unique to ADHD. Findings of smaller right prefrontal cortex, as well as smaller caudate nucleus and globus pallidus, in children with ADHD (Castellanos et al. 1996a) suggest that ADHD may be associated with fewer prefrontal corticostriatal fibers and less pallidal feedback to prefrontal regions. In addition, reduced area in the corresponding anterior genu region of the corpus callosum in children with ADHD (Hynd et al. 1991) indicates the presence of fewer interhemispheric fibers in prefrontal regions. Anomalies have also been found in ADHD in regions that project to the prefrontal cortex, including in the parietal–occipital region (i.e., reduced white matter; Filipek et al. 1997) and the cerebellum (i.e., smaller posterior vermis; Mostofsky et al. 1998). The latter findings raise the possibility that brain anomalies in ADHD extend beyond the prefrontal cortex and striatum to the posterior and subcortical regions that innervate these frontal circuits.

Functional neuroimaging studies have provided additional evidence of prefrontal–striatal impairment in ADHD. Studies with single photon emission computerized tomography (SPECT) and positron emission tomography (PET) have reported lower basal activity in the prefrontal cortex and striatum of children (Amen and Carmichael 1997, Lou et al. 1989) and adults (Zametkin et al. 1990), but not adolescents with ADHD (Zametkin et al. 1993). More recent studies employing functional MRI (fMRI) have tentatively linked altered prefrontal–striatal activation with deficits in inhibitory control. Reduced striatal activation during response inhibition tasks has been consistently reported in children and adolescents with ADHD (Vaidya et al. 1998, Rubia et al. 1999, 2001). However, prefrontal activation during the same tasks was enhanced in children with ADHD (Vaidya et al. 1998), but reduced in adolescents with the disorder (Rubia et al. 1999, 2001). Normal age-related declines in prefrontal activation may account for the disparate findings.

The prefrontal cortex and striatum are highly sensitive to catecholaminergic input from brainstem nuclei, including noradrenaline (NA) from the locus coeruleus, and dopamine (DA) from the ventral tegmental area and substantia nigra (Goldman-Rakic 1987). The fact that virtually all medications that are efficacious in ADHD affect NA and DA transmission strongly suggest that perturbations of these catecholamine inputs play a significant role in the pathophysiology of ADHD. Yet, a plethora of studies of catecholamine function in ADHD have yielded highly inconsistent findings (Zametkin and Rapoport 1987). Only more recent studies that used central indices of catecholamine function or that examined more homogeneous subgroups of children with ADHD have provided evidence of DA and NA dysfunction associated with ADHD. For example, cerebrospinal (CSF) levels of the DA metabolite homovanillic acid were positively correlated with ratings of hyperactivity and stimulant response in boys with ADHD (Castellanos et al. 1996a, Kruesi et al. 1990). Further, dividing boys with ADHD based on the presence or absence of reading disabilities revealed differences in plasma levels of the NA metabolite 3-methoxy-4-hydroxy-phenylglycol (MHPG) that correlated with differences in clinical characteristics (Halperin et al. 1997a).

A promising recent development has been the use of PET and SPECT imaging in combination with DA-selective radiotracers to examine localized DA function *in vivo*. These studies have revealed preliminary evidence of increased striatal DA transporter binding in adults with ADHD (Dougherty et al. 1999, Krause et al. 2000) and altered DA synthesis in the prefrontal cortex and right midbrain of children and adults with ADHD (Ernst et al. 1998, 1999). These data point to localized DA deficits in the nigrostriatal and mesocortical fiber systems in ADHD. Similar evidence of NA dysfunction in ADHD awaits the development of NA-selective radiotracers.

Conduct Disorder (CD)

The neurobiologic basis of CD has focused primarily on the neurochemical substrates of aggressive behaviors. An early body of literature pointed to a role for reduced noradrenergic function. Several studies found negative correlations between plasma and CSF concentrations of MHPG and aggression and conduct problems (Kruesi et al. 1990, Rogeness et al. 1987). Children with CD were also reported to exhibit low activity of the enzyme dopamine-beta-hydroxylase (Rogeness et al. 1987), which converts DA into NA. These data suggest that NA dysfunction may play a role in aggression through its involvement in the regulation of behavioral arousal.

More recent research has focused on the role of central serotonergic (5-HT) function in aggression and antisocial behavior (Markowitz and Coccaro 1995). Aggressive and antisocial adults have consistently been shown to have reduced CSF levels of 5-HT metabolites (Markowitz and Coccaro 1995, Stanley et al. 2000) and blunted responses to 5-HT challenge agents (Markowitz and Coccaro 1995, O'Keane et al. 1992). However, extrapolation of these data to aggressive children or children with CD has proven difficult. Among seven studies that examined central 5-HT function in aggressive children, only one found decreased 5-HT (Castellanos et al. 1996a), three reported increased 5-HT (Castellanos et al. 1994, Halperin et al. 1994b, Pine et al. 1997), and three found no group differences (Stoff et al. 1992, Halperin et al. 1997c, Schulz et al. 2001). Thus, the relationship between 5-HT and aggression in children is not characterized by the simple inverse relationship found in adults. Nevertheless, reduced central 5-HT function is associated with numerous risk factors for persistence in aggressive children, including affective lability (Newcorn et al. 1996), adverse child-rearing practices (Pine et al. 1997), and parental history of aggression (Halperin et al. 1997b). In view of the link between reduced 5-HT and aggression in adults, and given the fact that only about half of aggressive children progress to violence as adults, these data raise the possibility that reduced central 5-HT function may itself constitute a risk factor for persistence in aggressive children. However, this hypothesis has never been directly tested.

Genetic Factors

Several parallel lines of research indicate a substantial genetic contribution to the etiology of the AD-DBDs (Biederman et al. 1992, Sherman et al. 1997, Slutske et al. 1997). These data support the familial transmission of ADHD and CD and suggest that these disorders may share common familial vulnerabilities (Biederman et al. 1992). Estimates of heritability range from 60 to 80% for ADHD (Sherman et al. 1997) and from 30 to 70% for CD (Slutske et al. 1997).

Newer molecular genetic studies have identified a number of individual genes as potential candidate genes in the AD-DBDs. Evidence of altered DA activity in ADHD has focused on the search for candidate genes among DA system genes, including the DA D2 (DRD2; Comings et al. 1991), DA D4 (DRD4; Swanson et al. 1998), and DA D5 (DRD5; Daly et al. 1999) receptor genes, and the DA transporter gene (DAT1; Daly et al. 1999). However, the evidence is strongest linking ADHD with the 7-repeat allele of DRD4 (Swanson et al. 1998), which mediates a blunted intracellular response to DA, and the 10-repeat allele of DAT1 (Daly et al. 1999), which is linked to elevated DA reuptake. Preliminary data have also linked the 10-repeat allele of DAT1 with poor response to methylphenidate (Winsberg and Comings 1999), which acts primarily by inhibiting the DA transporter in the striatum.

The role of specific genes in CD has not been determined, but several 5-HT system genes have been identified as candidates for study in aggression. These include the genes encoding the enzymes tryptophan hydroxylase (TPH; Manuck et al. 1999) and monoamine oxidase A (MAOA; Manuck et al. 2000), which are involved in the synthesis and metabolism of 5-HT, respectively. However, these genes likely code for behavioral traits that constitute risk factors for aggression (i.e., impulsivity) rather than for the behavioral phenotype of aggression and CD.

Environmental Factors

Paradoxically, twin studies have provided some of the strongest evidence implicating environmental factors in the etiology of the AD-DBDs (Sherman et al. 1997, Slutske et al. 1997). These studies indicate that a moderate-to-significant proportion of the susceptibility to AD-DBDs is accounted for by nonshared factors (i.e., factors that differ between twins). Nonshared factors have their greatest effect in CD (Slutske et al. 1997) and are less important contributors to ADHD (Sherman et al. 1997). Examples of nonshared factors include low verbal intelligence (Farrington 1989), poor school performance, difficult temperament-inflated self-esteem (Baumeister et al. 1996), impulsivity (White et al. 1994), and biological events such as perinatal insults and head trauma. Among the most salient risk factors for CD is the presence of early ODD and ADHD (Hinshaw 1987).

Shared family, peer, and neighborhood risk factors also play a role in the etiology of ODD and CD, and to a lesser degree of ADHD. These so-called adversity factors include large sibships, families that have experienced separation, single-parent households (Capaldi and Patterson 1996), child neglect (Smith and Thornberry 1995), parental conflict (McCord 1979), and poverty. Parental child-rearing practices, such as harsh physical discipline and poor supervision, have also been implicated in ODD and CD (Frick et al. 1992). However, the most salient familial risk factor for CD is parental criminality (Frick et al. 1992), which likely has both environmental and genetic components. Delinquent peer membership and repeated victimization by peers also add to the etiology of CD and aggression. Finally, residing in a neighborhood with high rates of crime, poverty, and/or unemployment is associated with an earlier onset of CD (Farrington and Loeber 2000). These factors seem to operate in an additive fashion, with the probability of CD increasing linearly with the aggregation of risk factors (Rutter et al. 1975).

Treatment

Successful treatment planning in children with AD-DBDs requires consideration of not only the core symptomatology but also of family and social factors and comorbidity with other disorders. Given the heterogeneity of the three disorders that make up the AD-DBDs, the wide-ranging effects of the disruptive behaviors, the high rates of comorbidity, and the presence of associated features such as learning disabilities, multimodal treatments (i.e., psychopharmacologic and psychosocial) are almost always warranted. Nevertheless, good response can be achieved with either treatment alone in certain instances (e.g., medication treatment for uncomplicated ADHD or ADHD + ODD; psychosocial treatment for ADHD + anxiety disorder) (MTA Cooperative Group 1999a,b). A diagnosis of ODD without any comorbid condition will usually be responsive to behavioral intervention without medication. However, one should always attempt to rule out the possibility that ADHD is also present. Similarly, treatment of children with CD without comorbidity usually involves psychosocial interventions with the possibility of augmenting treatment with one of several pharmacological agents. In contrast, comorbid ADHD + CD almost always requires medication, and medication response is augmented if psychosocial treatment is offered concomitantly (Jensen et al. 2001).

Somatic Treatments

Psychostimulants   It is well established that psychostimulants are extremely effective in treating a wide range of disruptive behaviors (Klein et al. 1997) above and beyond their effects on ADHD. Nevertheless, ADHD remains the primary indication for the use of these medications. Methylphenidate (MPH), dextroamphetamine (DEX), mixture of amphetamine salts (MAS) (which is a mixture of several amphetamine compounds, 75% of which is DEX) and pemoline have all been shown to be effective in treating ADHD. Of these, MPH is the most often prescribed and accounts for approximately 60% of stimulant use in the United States (Goodman and Nachman 2000). MAS has become a popular alternative to MPH, and despite slight differences in mechanism of action, profiles of response and adverse effects (see below), there are no strong data to indicate that any one stimulant preparation is substantially more effective or better tolerated than any other (Arnold 2000).

The stimulants produce significant improvement in attention, hyperactivity, impulse control, and aggressiveness, leading to better organization of behavior, task completion, and self-regulation. There is a fairly robust improvement in social skills, as evidenced by peer ratings (Whalen et al. 1989) and parent and teacher ratings of social function (Smith et al. 1998, Winsberg et al. 1982). There is also improvement in academic productivity, although change in actual academic performance has been more difficult to demonstrate. Although most data with stimulants have been obtained in samples of school-age children with ADHD, there is increasing recognition that stimulants can be used successfully across the lifespan.

The decision to prescribe psychostimulant medication is best undertaken following a comprehensive assessment, with full consideration given to the range of pharmacologic and nonpharmacologic treatment options that are available. Several of the rating scales used in assessment (e.g., the Conners questionnaires) are sensitive to medication effects and can be used to monitor adequacy of dose and maintenance of medication effects. Prior to a trial with any of the stimulants, baseline data should be obtained, including general medical status, and more specific evaluations of height, weight, blood pressure, and a complete blood count. In the case of pemoline, baseline liver function tests should be obtained as well, because of the possibility of severe liver toxicity, which can lead to significant morbidity or even death. Although this is a very rare event, a recent black box warning from the FDA has substantially reduced the use of this medication (Safer et al. 2001).

The past several years have seen a veritable explosion in the number of stimulant treatment options for individuals with ADHD. Most of the attention has been focused on development of sustained release preparations, which eliminate the need to take medication several times over the course of the day and to provide a more consistent profile of delivery. This has the added benefit of decreasing the need for in-school dosing and along with it the potential for stigmatization of children with ADHD and diversion of medication.

The decision regarding which stimulant to select is best determined by considering properties intrinsic to the different medications—such as duration of activity and adverse effect profile—as well as the individual circumstances of the individual (e.g., when is peak medication level needed most, what is the individual's lifestyle, etc.). Practitioners who favor MPH as the first stimulant option would point to its favorable adverse effect profile. Insomnia and appetite suppression are often present but are possibly less intense than with DEX (Arnold 2000). Growth retardation may also be less of a concern with MPH than DEX, but the entire question of growth retardation following stimulant administration is controversial, and disputed by some authors (Spencer et al. 1996). Those who favor MAS as the first choice for treatment would point to reports of slightly higher efficacy based on the findings of two recent studies (Pliszka et al. 2000a, Faraone et al. 2001). However, these studies did not provide optimal titration of both medications equally. Regardless of one's view regarding the first choice stimulant, and although the different stimulants work on average about as well as one another, nonresponders to one medication may respond well to another, since their mechanisms of action are not identical. Therefore, if there is not adequate response to one stimulant medication, another should be tried (Elia 1993).

Increasingly, MPH is given in its long-acting forms as a first-line approach. The usual starting dose for Concerta (12-hour formulation) is 18 mg, which is equivalent to 5-mg IR-MPH administered three times daily (Pelham et al. 2001, Wolraich et al. 2001). Doses can be increased by 18 mg at a time. There is now also the option to give a 27-mg dose. As of this writing, Metadate CD (8-hour formulation) is only available as a 20-mg formulation (i.e., equivalent to 10-mg IR b.i.d.); Ritalin LA (8-hour formulation) will soon be available in 20-mg, 30-mg, and 40-mg formulations. The older sustained release preparation (i.e., MPH-SR) is also still available in both branded and generic forms. Immediate-release (IR) MPH can also be used as a primary therapeutic agent, given in either b.i.d. or t.i.d. dosing schedules; however, its niche increasingly is to supplement the longer-acting preparations, either to achieve more rapid onset of effect or to extend duration of action. When IR-MPH is used as a primary option, the usual starting dose is 5 mg. The dose is then increased in 5-mg increments. When a t.i.d. dosing schedule is used, the third dose is sometimes sculpted to half the morning or noon dose to prevent insomnia. Three-times-daily dosing is particularly helpful for providing coverage during homework time and providing an opportunity for children to interact with parents and peers while experiencing the beneficial effects of medication (Stein et al. 1996). Doses are usually given at 4-hour intervals, since the half-life is 2 to 2 1/2 hours, and peak activity is seen by 1 1/2 to 2 1/2 hours. The upper recommended dose for MPH is 60 mg, although use of higher doses may be required in certain cases and has achieved a certain degree of recognition among experts in the field (American Academy of Pediatrics 2001, Greenhill et al. 2002).

MAS and DEX can often be administered in a manner similar to MPH and also come in a variety of IR and extended release formulations. Adderall XR (MAS) is the only amphetamine preparation formulated to act for 12 hours (Grcevich 2001). Brand Adderall or generic MAS are also available in a shorter acting form that lasts approximately 5 to 6 hours (Swanson et al. 1998). DEX is available in both a spansule, with duration of activity comparable to the shorter acting MAS, and an IR preparation, which lasts approximately 4 hours. A recent study found that DEX spansule and MAS have comparable efficacy and duration (James et al. 2001). DEX and MAS are more potent than MPH, so the initial starting dose and upper dose limit are lower. The recommended dosage range for DEX is 2.5 to 40 mg. Although DEX has a somewhat longer half-life than MPH, a t.i.d. schedule is still often required.

Pemoline had been a popular stimulant option prior to the development of the longer-acting formulations of MPH and MAS and before the possibility for severe liver toxicity was carefully reviewed and publicized. It is now relegated to a second- or third-tier option. Advantages of pemoline include its long duration of action (half-life of 12 hours) and the possibility that it has a lower abuse potential (class V rather than class II schedule). Because of its long half-life, pemoline can be given once daily. The smallest pemoline dose is 18.75 mg, and the recommended upper limit is 112.5 mg/day.

Adverse effects (AE) of stimulants are generally mild, but occasionally can become problematic. The most commonly observed AEs include headache, abdominal pain, decreased appetite (with or without weight loss), and initial insomnia. There are slight increases in pulse and BP, which are not very meaningful at the group level (Findling et al. 2001), but can take on greater significance for particular individuals. Affective changes, including blunted affect, irritability and mood lability can also be seen, either at peak dose or when the dose wears off. Use of longer-acting psychostimulants tends to minimize mood lability and other AEs that are often considered to be a reflection of the on–off effects that are more frequently seen with IR preparations. Motor or vocal tics can develop or, more often, can be exacerbated (Borcherding et al. 1990). However, there has been a convergence of evidence that stimulant treatment does not necessarily exacerbate tics (Castellanos et al. 1997, Gadow et al. 1999, Law and Schachar 1999) and even some suggestions that these conditions are relatively independent (Coffey et al. 2000, Spencer et al. 2001). There has been some concern that stimulants can precipitate psychotic symptoms such as hallucinations (Cherland and Fitzpatrick 1999), although this is very rare and almost always seen as a reflection of excessive dosing or use in individuals with disorders other than ADHD (e.g., psychotic disorders).

Atomoxetine (Strattera) Atomoxetine is a new medication with highly potent and selective activity to block the noradrenergic transporter. It is structurally distinct from both the stimulants and the tricyclic antidepressants and is the first nonstimulant medication labeled for the treatment of ADHD. Atomoxetine has been studied extensively in both children and adults, and initial efficacy data have begun to appear in the literature. Atomoxetine was shown to be effective in reducing both inattentive and hyperactive/impulsive symptoms over a 9-week period in a sample of children and adolescents (Michelson et al. 2001). Doses of 0.5 mg/kg, 1.2 mg/kg, and 1.8 mg/kg were studied. All doses had treatment effects that were different from placebo, with treatment effects seen at the first postmedication treatment visit, but the highest degree of improvement was found in the 1.2 mg/kg and the 1.8 mg/kg groups. The medication also produced a change in functional measures as well as ADHD symptoms, with the greatest degree of change in the 1.8 mg/kg group. In a small pilot study, efficacy was relatively comparable to MPH, although that study was not powered to detect differences across treatments (Kratochvil et al. 2001).

Atomoxetine can be administered on either a twice-daily or once-daily schedule, despite the fact that its half-life in the overwhelming majority of individuals is 4 hours. Despite this fact, therapeutic benefit seems to be maintained over the full day. Adverse effects with atomoxetine have been relatively mild, with decreased appetite and a small increase in pulse and BP being the two most consistent findings. Because it is not a stimulant, and because its effects are highly selective for NA and not DA, atomoxetine is thought to not have abuse potential.

Tricylic Antidepressants The noradrenergic tricyclic antidepressants, principally imipramine and desipramine, have been the most extensively studied and, until the mid-1990s, were the most often prescribed nonstimulant medication for individuals with ADHD. For desipramine, doses between 2.5 and 5 mg/kg/day have been recommended (Biederman et al. 1989). In the case of both of these medications, cardiac side effects are of concern and premedication workup must include at least an EKG. Tachycardia and postural hypotension are commonly seen but are not often problematic. Prolongation of the PR and QT intervals may be a greater source of concern and should be reviewed with a pediatric cardiologist. The decision to prescribe tricyclics for ADHD children must be made with the knowledge that several sudden deaths have been reported in children taking desipramine (Popper 1997, Riddle et al. 1991). Although it has been argued that data do not support the conclusion and that tricyclics have a high degree of cardiovascular toxicity in children (Biederman 1991), proper informed consent should be obtained. It should also be noted that neither imipramine nor desipramine is FDA approved for the treatment of ADHD children.

Other Antidepressants Bupropion and venlafaxine are chemically unrelated to other known antidepressants. Both have been studied for their potential utility in the AD-DBDs. Investigations of bupropion in ADHD have demonstrated the effectiveness of the medication compared with placebo (Conners et al. 1996, Simeon et al. 1986) but not as effective as stimulants (Casat et al. 1987, 1989). In contrast to this latter finding, others have found bupropion to be as effective as methylphenidate (Barrickman et al. 1995). While the efficacy of bupropion in ADHD has been established, the equivalence of its response to stimulant treatments remains unclear.

There are similar but more preliminary data indicating that venlafaxine might be useful for ADHD (Popper 1997). Significant improvements in attention, concentration, and other cognitive functions have been reported in volunteers (Saletu et al. 1992). Open label studies of adults with ADHD also found venlafaxine to be effective. The most common side effects reported were nausea and sedation (Adler et al. 1995, Findling et al. 1996, Hedges et al. 1995). An open label study in 8- to 17-year-old subjects found significant reductions in impulsivity and hyperactivity as rated by parents (Olvera et al. 1996). However, double-blind, placebo-controlled trials have not yet been conducted.

Monoamine Oxidase Inhibitors (MAOIs) MAOIs are nonspecific enhancers of monoamine neurotransmission. One study examined their possible role in ADHD, and that was primarily to test a heuristic model rather than a treatment approach. In that study, tranylcypromine was found to be as effective as DEX (Zametkin et al. 1985). However, its use in children and adolescents is impractical, given the likelihood of dietary indiscretions. In addition, Deprenyl has demonstrated positive results in children with ADHD and TD (Jankovic 1993, Feigin et al. 1996), but these have not been replicated in a controlled trial in adults with ADHD (Ernst et al. 1996).

Serotonin Reuptake Inhibitors Clomipramine, a mixed noradrenergic and seroton-ergic agonist, and fluoxetine, a selective serotonin reuptake inhibitor (SSRI), have been used in the treatment of children with ADHD. In one study, clomipramine was found to decrease scores related to aggressiveness and poor impulse control (Garfinkel et al. 1983). Two open studies found that fluoxetine is effective in the treatment of children with ADHD with or without comorbid mood disorder (Barrickman et al. 1991, Gammon and Brown 1993). Although there have been no studies using SSRIs in ADHD and comorbid CD/ODD, these medications are of some interest in light of recent findings implicating serotonergic mechanisms in aggression and reported utility of fluoxetine in treating adults with impulsive aggression (Coccaro and Kavoussi 1997). At present, there are no controlled trials to support the efficacy of the SSRIs for the core symptoms of ADHD, and their role in treating comorbid ADHD and CD/ODD is inferential only (Emslie et al. 1997).

Alpha-2-adrenergic Agonists Since the mid-1980s, there has been considerable interest in the use of alpha-2-adrenergic agonists in the treatment of ADHD and aggression (Hunt et al. 1985, 1991). Initial studies were conducted with clonidine, but the more specific alpha-2 agent guanfacine has recently been the focus of investigation. The alpha-2 agonists are reportedly most effective in treating symptoms of hyperactivity, impulsivity, and aggression for children with ADHD. Effects on attentional symptoms have been less clear, although a recent study found that guanfacine treatment was associated with improved ratings and CPT measures of attention (Scahill et al. 2001). Because of their role in treating overarousal and aggression, the alpha-2 agonists seem ideally suited for use in children with comorbid ODD/CD/aggression. They have been effective in treating individuals suffering from ADHD who either have diagnosed tic disorders (Steingard et al. 1993), or are at increased risk to develop them, such as those children with a positive family history of tics. This is particularly important since as many as 40 to 60% of individuals with Tourette's syndrome seen in psychiatric settings also have ADHD (Biederman et al. 1991c), and many of these individuals have significant behavior problems. Although the alpha-2 agonists may be less effective than stimulants in the treatment of ADHD, they may be particularly useful in individuals whose tics worsen on a stimulant medication. These agonists have also been used in combination with a stimulant. However, there have been safety considerations involving this combination. These primarily involve the possibility of additive risk of rebound hypertension of alpha-2 agonists with the mild increase in pulse and blood pressure from stimulants.

Clonidine has been the most often studied of the alpha-2s, although the empirical database for both clonidine and guanfacine remains quite small. Clonidine has a gradual onset of action that may be related to the time required for receptor downregulation (Hunt et al. 1991). The usual dose ranges from 0.05 to 0.3 mg/day, often in a three-times-a-day dosing schedule. One of the advantages is that it can be used to treat the initial insomnia, which sometimes results from late afternoon stimulant use (Rubinstein et al. 1994). Clonidine is available in both tablet form and a depot skin patch preparation. The latter provides sustained coverage for one week, and may be particularly useful for treating children with ADHD, whose behavior is characterized by a variable pattern of extreme lability, especially in the early morning, before stimulants and oral clonidine take effect. Guanfacine comes only in an oral preparation. Guanfacine tablets are of 1.0 mg strength, so care must be taken to not confuse the different doses for clonidine and guanfacine. Since guanfacine has a somewhat longer half-life than clonidine, it can often be given in a two- or three-times-a-day dosing schedule.

The most common side effect of the alpha-2 medications is sedation, although this tends to decrease after several weeks (Hunt et al. 1985). Dry mouth, nausea, and photophobia are among the other adverse effects reported. At high doses, hypotension and dizziness are also possible. The skin patch often causes local pruritic dermatitis. Glucose tolerance may decrease, especially in those at risk for diabetes. It is important to carefully evaluate cardiovascular function when using the alpha-2 agonists, especially when used in combination with stimulant treatment as noted earlier. Additionally, there have been reports of sudden death in three cases treated with the combination of clonidine and methylphenidate, although a review of this situation by the FDA concluded that these unfortunate events were not attributable to the combination (Fenichel 1995). However, careful monitoring is required. Since clonidine is not FDA approved for use in ADHD, informed consent should clearly indicate that this is an "off-label" treatment.

Other Agents   A variety of other pharmacotherapeutic agents have been utilized in the treatment of aggression and episodic dyscontrol, although efficacy in children with comorbid ADHD and CD has not yet been demonstrated. Among these medications, lithium has been the best studied. Lithium has been found to be effective in well-designed studies of aggressive children (Campbell et al. 1984), impulsive–aggressive adolescents and young adult delinquents, although there are some questions regarding the magnitude of effect (Campbell et al. 1995). Antiepileptic medications have also been used in the treatment of behavior problems characterized by aggressiveness and impulsivity. Carbamazepine is considered an effective treatment for aggression in children (Kafantaris et al. 1992), but more recent findings have tempered the initial enthusiasm (Cueva et al. 1996). Sodium valproate is another antiepileptic shown to be effective in the treatment of chronic temper outbursts and mood lability (Donovan et al. 1997, 2000). Although valproate has been used for the treatment of aggressive individuals for over a decade, very few published reports have used a controlled design (Hollander et al. 2001). A number of newer antiepileptic medications are currently being investigated for use in children suffering from mood disorders. However, their usefulness in treating aggressiveness in children with AD-DBDs is unclear. Finally, beta-adrenergic blockers such as propranolol have also been found to be useful in treating aggression, but require further evaluation in children and adolescents (Campbell et al. 1992).

Neuroleptic medications have also been used in treatment of the AD-DBDs, principally to treat children with severe behavioral problems characterized by aggression and combativeness. Although older neuroleptics such as chlorpromazine, thioridazine, and halperidol are FDA approved for the treatment of severe behavior problems in children, they are infrequently used at present. Recently, there has been more interest in the atypical neuroleptic risperidone. In a double-blind placebo-controlled study, risperidone was found to be superior to placebo in ameliorating aggression in youths with CD (Findling et al. 2000).

During the course of the last few years, there has been a remarkable increase in the number of medications that are used in the treatment of ADHD and CD. It is important to keep in mind that the majority of the medications are not approved by the FDA for specific use in ADHD and/or CD and as such their use for these two disorders continues to be "off-label". An additional complication is that, in general, prescribing practices tend to vary among different settings and even among different physicians in the same setting. Consequently, less-than-optimal treatment is likely to result in inadequate or partial improvement, as demonstrated in the community standard group of the multimodal treatment study of children with ADHD (i.e., MTA), which is discussed in more detail below. In order to reduce this variability in treatment practices, there have been attempts recently to develop treatment algorithms. The purpose of such algorithms is to integrate relevant research findings and clinical experience in the development of medication decision trees. Recently, an expert panel has reported on the development and implementation of an algorithm for the treatment of ADHD and its common comorbid conditions (Pliszka et al. 2000b,c).

Psychosocial Treatments A variety of psychosocial therapies have been found to be useful for treating children with AD-DBD. Among the systematically studied psychosocial interventions are home-based interventions/parent training, classroom-based behavior modifications, social skills training and intensive summer treatment programs. Since family, peer, and school interactions are important in the morbidity and maintenance of these disorders, it is important to utilize psychosocial treatments to target each of these areas. In contrast to these more structured techniques, individual play therapy with children is generally ineffective in decreasing problem behaviors of the AD-DBDs (Kazdin 1987).

Behavior therapy (BT) relies primarily on training parents and/or teachers to be the agents of change. The focus is on decreasing the frequency of problematic behaviors and/or increasing the rate of desirable behaviors. Parent management training is one of the most common techniques and consists of group and individual sessions with parents in order to offer psychoeducational intervention and to teach the principles and implementation of behavioral programs. Consultation with classroom teachers to set up parallel behavioral programs in the school is also an important adjunct to this treatment.

Another aspect of BT is contingency management (CM), which is implemented directly with the child in the setting in which the problem behaviors occur. CM programs use both reward procedures and negative consequences, such as time-out and response cost or "punishments" (Hinshaw et al. 1992, Barkley 1990). In some situations, maintenance of appropriate behavior following withdrawal of contingencies is better for a negative consequence than for a reward (Sullivan and O'Leary 1989). Similarly to BT, CM approaches are extremely labor-intensive, and questions regarding their generalizability remain.

Cognitive–behavioral approaches (CBT) are based on the premise that the difficulties experienced by children with AD-DBDs are a result of deficient self-control and problem-solving skills, or that changes in these domains of function can override other deficits. Examples of CBT include training in self-monitoring, anger control, and self-reinforcement. Although initial studies utilizing CBT approaches generated promise on the basis of the findings of enhanced generalization and maintenance of appropriate behaviors (Kazdin et al. 1989), the initial enthusiasm has been tempered by other findings reporting marginal success (Abikoff 1991). However, some CBT procedures, such as anger control, have shown more consistent success (Hinshaw et al. 1992, Whalen and Henker 1991).

Despite their potential benefits, difficulties encountered with psychosocial interventions are that short-term gains are often limited to the period that the programs are actually in effect. Furthermore, a substantial number of children, particularly those with the most severe presentation and with greatest psychosocial adversity, fail to show improvement. Additional problems in implementation include the unwillingness of many teachers to use behavioral programs and the fact that as many as half the parents discontinue parent training. Finally, the fact that these interventions are labor-intensive and reported long-term improvements have been modest make these therapies of limited value when used alone (Abikoff 1991, Abikoff and Klein 1992, Hinshaw et al. 1992, Pelham and Hinshaw 1992, Pelham 1999). However, it is important to note that in the MTA study, the presence of anxiety (as reported by parents on the DISC interview) moderated the outcome of treatment, such that psychosocial interventions were more efficacious than medication alone in children with ADHD who also had symptoms of anxiety (March et al. 2000).

Combined Treatments

The multimodal treatment study of children with ADHD (MTA) was a landmark multisite clinical trial, conducted at six performance sites across the US and Canada, that examined the comparative response to 14 months of medication and psychosocial treatments, administered alone or together, in 579 seven- to nine-year-old children with combined subtype ADHD. The principal objectives of the study were to determine the relative effectiveness of the three active treatments in comparison to one another, and in comparison with community standard care (Arnold et al. 1997a,b).

Results of the 14-month intent-to-treat analyses indicated that, for ADHD symptoms, treatments that included medication performed better than other treatments in reducing ADHD symptoms (MTA Cooperative Group 1999a). For non-ADHD symptoms, only combined treatment was statistically superior to the community standard care, although it was not different from the medication group. However, composite measures of treatment response indicated that the combined treatment group did relatively better than the medication-only group, but with a small overall effect size. There were few moderators of treatment outcome; factors such as age, gender, and comorbid CD/ODD had little impact. However, children with comorbid ADHD and anxiety disorders tended to have a relatively better response to the psychosocial treatment administered alone as compared to those without comorbid anxiety. Medication was as effective in treating comorbid ADHD and anxiety as it was in the group with ADHD only (MTA Cooperative Group 1999b, March et al. 2000). Lower effectiveness was seen in the community standard group, despite the fact that two-thirds of the community-treated children received medication at some time over the 14-month period of the study.

Impact of Comorbidity on Treatment

Studies of stimulant treatment have shown that ADHD children with and without aggression respond equally well to MPH treatment in terms of ADHD symptoms (Barkley et al. 1989, Klorman et al. 1988, Livingston et al. 1992). Treatment of comorbid ADHD and CD/ODD in the MTA study was superior when medication was used, although the best outcome was seen with combined treatment (Jensen et al. 2001).

A large body of research has addressed the question of whether stimulant medication improves learning and academic achievement in children with AD-DBD (Hinshaw et al. 1992, Swanson et al. 1991). While earlier studies suggested that stimulant treatment did not lead to improvement in academic achievement (Barkley 1990), more recent investigations have indicated a favorable response in children with ADHD on a variety of cognitive measures in both classroom and laboratory settings (Douglas et al. 1986, Pelham et al. 1985, Rapport et al. 1985). While it is now clear that stimulant treatment can improve performance on a wide array of cognitive measures, treatment of comorbid learning disabilities requires direct, nonpharmacological, academic interventions.

It is not yet clear whether the optimal dosage of stimulant medication required for treating ADHD children varies as a function of comorbidity. It has been argued (Swanson et al. 1991) that titrating medication to a higher dose in the presence of comorbid externalizing disorders could have a detrimental effect on learning, since generally lower doses are required to produce a change in attentional function than behavioral function. Nevertheless, others have found that a dose as high as 0.7 mg/kg of MPH leads to improvements on several cognitive measures, most notably reading (Kupietz et al. 1988, Richardson et al. 1988). Still other studies have evaluated a variety of doses, with no clear pattern emerging.

In contrast to studies in children with ADHD who are aggressive, studies of stimulant response in ADHD children with comorbid anxiety have produced somewhat inconsistent findings. Earlier investigations reported that children with comorbid ADHD and anxiety have a less robust response to stimulant medication, along with a higher incidence of adverse effects when compared with children with ADHD who did not also have an anxiety disorder (Pliszka 1989, Tannock and Schachar 1992). However, more recent studies have found that medication is equally effective in comorbid ADHD and anxiety disorders (Diamond et al. 1999, MTA Cooperative Group 1999a). Other studies have found that children with ADHD and anxiety respond as well as those without comorbid anxiety, to the antidepressant DMI (Biederman et al. 1993a).

Comparison of DSM-IV-TR/ICD-10 Diagnostic Criteria

For attention-deficit/hyperactivity disorder, the item set chosen for the ICD-10 Diagnostic Criteria for Research is almost identical to the items in the DSM-IV-TR criteria set but the algorithm is quite different resulting in a more narrowly defined ICD-10 category. Specifically, whereas the DSM-IV-TR algorithm requires either six inattention items or six hyperactive/impulsive items, the ICD-10 Diagnostic Criteria for Research requires at least six inattention items, at least three hyperactive items, and at least one impulsive item. Instead of subtyping the disorder on the basis of the predominant type, ICD-10 subspecifies the condition whether criteria are also met for a CD.

Although formatted quite differently, the DSM-IV-TR and ICD-10 item sets and diagnostic algorithms for CD are almost identical. Although ICD-10 provides a list of 23 items (in contrast with the 15 included in the DSM-IV-TR criteria for CD, only the last 15 items count towards a diagnosis of CD. Although the first 8 items on the CD list are identical to the DSM-IV-TR items for OD, ICD-10 ODD can be considerably more severe because up to 2 of the items can be drawn from the 15 items that comprise the CD item set.

References

Abikoff H (1991) Cognitive training in ADHD children: less to it than meets the eye. *J Learn Disabil* **24**, 205–209.

Abikoff H and Klein RG (1992) Attention-deficit hyperactivity and conduct disorder: comorbidity and implications for treatment. *J Consult Clin Psychol* **60**, 681–682.

Abikoff H, Gittelman R, and Klein DF (1980) Classroom observation code for hyperactive children: a replication of validity. *J Consult Clin Psychol* **48**, 555–565.

Achenbach TM (1991a) *Integrative Guide for the 1991 CBCL/4-18, YSR, and TRF profiles.* Department of Psychiatry, University of Vermont, Burlington, VT.

Achenbach TM (1991b) *Manual for the Teacher's Report Form and 1991 Profile.* University of Vermont, Department of Psychiatry, Burlington, VT.

Adler LA, Resnick S, Kunz M, et al. (1995) Open-label trial of venlafaxine in adults with attention-deficit disorder. *Psychopharmacol Bull* **31**, 785–788.

Alterman AI, Tarter RE, Baughman TG, et al. (1984) Differentiation of alcoholics high and low in childhood hyperactivity. *Drug Alcohol Depend* **15**, 111.

Amen DG and Carmichael BD (1997) High-resolution brain SPECT imaging in ADHD. *Ann Clin Psychiatry* **9**, 81–86.

American Academy of Child and Adolescent Psychiatry (1997) Practice parameters for the assessment and treatment of children, adolescents, and adults with attention-deficit/hyperactivity disorder. *J Am Acad Child Adolesc Psychiatry* **36**, 85S–121S.

American Academy of Pediatrics (2001) Clinical practice guideline: treatment of the school-aged child with attention-deficit/hyperactivity disorder. *Pediatrics* **108**, 1033–1344.

Anderson JC, Williams S, McGee R, et al. (1987) DSM-III disorders in preadolescent children: prevalence in a large sample from the general population. *Arch Gen Psychiatry* **44**, 69–76.

Arnold L (2000) Methylphenidate vs. amphetamine: comparative review. *J Atten Disord* **3**, 200–211.

Arnold LE, Abikoff HB, Cantwell DP, et al. (1997a) National institute of mental health collaborative multimodal treatment study of children with ADHD (the MTA). Design challenges and choices. *Arch Gen Psychiatry* **54**, 865–870.

Arnold LE, Abikoff HB, Cantwell DP, et al. (1997b) NIMH collaborative multimodal treatment study of children with ADHD (MTA): design, methodology, and protocol evolution. *J Atten Disord* **2**, 141–158.

Babor TF, Hofmann M, DelBoca FK, et al. (1992) Types of alcoholics. I. Evidence for an empirically derived typology based on indicators of vulnerability and severity. *Arch Gen Psychiatry* **49**, 599–608.

Barkley RA (1990) *Attention-deficit Hyperactivity Disorder: A Handbook for Diagnosis and Treatment*. Guilford Press, New York.

Barkley RA (1991) The ecological validity of laboratory and analogue assessment methods of ADHD symptoms. *J Abnorm Child Psychol* **19**, 149–178.

Barkley RA, Anastopolous AD, Guevremont DC, et al. (1991a) Adolescents with ADHD: patterns of behavioral adjustment, academic functioning and treatment utilization. *J Am Acad Child Adolesc Psychiatry* **30**, 752–761.

Barkley RA, Fischer M, Edelbrock CS, et al. (1990) The adolescent outcome of hyperactive children diagnosed by research criteria: I. An 8-year prospective follow-up study. *J Am Acad Child Adolesc Psychiatry* **29**, 546–557.

Barkley RA, Fischer M, Edelbrock C, et al. (1991b) The adolescent outcome of hyperactive children diagnosed by research criteria. III. Mother–child interactions, family conflicts and maternal psychopathology. *J Child Psychol Psychiatr Allied Disc* **32**, 233–255.

Barkley RA, Fischer M, Newbt R, et al. (1988) Development of a multi-method clinical protocol for assessing stimulant drug responses in ADHD children. *J Clin Child Psychol* **17**, 14–24.

Barkley RA, McMurray MB, Edelbrock CS, et al. (1989) The response of aggressive and nonaggressive ADHD children to two doses of methylphenidate. *J Am Acad Child Adolesc Psychiatry* **28**, 873–881.

Barrickman L, Noyes R, Kuperman S, et al. (1991) Treatment of ADHD with fluoxetine: a preliminary trial. *J Am Acad Child and Adolesc Psychiatry* **30**, 762–767.

Barrickman LL, Perry PJ, Allen AJ, et al. (1995) Bupropion versus methylphenidate in the treatment of attention-deficit hyperactivity disorder. *J Am Acad Child Adolesc Psychiatry* **34**, 649–657.

Bauermeister JJ, Canino G, and Bird H (1994) Epidemiology of disruptive behavior disorders. *Child Adolesc Psychiatr Clin N Am* **3**, 177–194.

Baumeister RF, Smart L, and Boden JM (1996) Relation of threatened egotism to violence and aggression: the dark side of high self-esteem. *Psychol Bull* **103**, 5–33.

Biederman J (1991) Sudden death in children treated with a tricyclic antidepressant. *J Am Acad Child Adolesc Psychiatry* **30**, 495–498.

Biederman J, Baldessarini RJ, Wright V, et al. (1989) A double-blind placebo controlled study of desipramine in the treatment of ADD I. Efficacy. *J Am Acad Child Adolesc Psychiatry* **28**, 777–784.

Biederman J, Baldessarini RJ, Wright V, et al. (1993a) A double blind placebo-controlled study of desipramine in the treatment of attention deficit disorder. III. Lack of impact of comorbidity and family history factors on clinical response. *J Am Acad Child Adolesc Psychiatry* **32**, 199–204.

Biederman J, Faraone SV, Keenan K, et al. (1991a) Evidence of familial association between attention deficit disorder and major affective disorders. *Arch Gen Psychiatry* **48**, 633–642.

Biederman J, Faraone SV, Keenan K, et al. (1991b) Familial association between attention deficit disorder (ADD) and anxiety disorder. *Am J Psychiatry* **148**, 251–256.

Biederman J, Faraone SV, Keenan K, et al. (1992) Further evidence for family-genetic risk factors in attention-deficit hyperactivity disorder. Patterns of comorbidity in probands and relatives in psychiatrically and pediatrically referred samples. *Arch Gen Psychiatry* **49**, 728–738.

Biederman J, Munir K, and Knee D (1987) Conduct and oppositional disorder in clinically referred children with attention deficit disorder: A controlled family study. *J Am Acad Child Adolesc Psychiatry* **26**, 724–727.

Biederman J, Newcorn J, and Sprich S (1991c) Comorbidity of attention-deficit hyperactivity disorder with conduct, depressive, anxiety, and other disorders. *Am J Psychiatry* **148**, 564–577.

Biederman J, Wilens T, Mick E, et al. (1997) Is ADHD a risk factor for psychoactive substance use disorders? Findings from a four-year prospective follow-up study. *J Am Acad Child Adolesc Psychiatry* **36**, 21–29.

Bird HR, Canino G, Rubio–Stipec M, et al. (1988) Estimates of the prevalence of childhood maladjustment in a community survey in Puerto Rico: the use of combined measures. *Arch Gen Psychiatry* **45**, 1120–1126.

Borcherding BG, Keysor CS, Rapoport JL, et al. (1990) Motor/vocal tics and compulsive behaviors on stimulant drugs: is there a common vulnerability. *Psychiatr Res* **33**, 83–94.

Breen MJ and Altepeter TS (1990) Evaluating disruptive behavior disorders: child behavior questionnaires, laboratory measurements and observations. In *Disruptive Behavior Disorders in Children*, Breen MJ and Altepeter TS (eds). Guilford Press, New York, pp. 65–113.

Breen MJ and Barkley RA (1988) Child psychopathology and parenting stress in girls and boys having attention deficit disorder with hyperactivity. *J Pediatr Psychol* **2**, 265–280.

Cadoret JR and Stewart MA (1991) An adoption study of attention-deficit hyperactivity/aggression and their relationship to adult antisocial personality. *Compr Psychiatry* **32**, 73–82.

Campbell SB (1985) Hyperactivity in preschoolers: correlates and prognostic implications. *Clin Psychol Rev* **5**, 405–428.

Campbell M, Adams PB, Small AM, et al. (1995) Lithium in hospitalized aggressive children with conduct disorder: a double-blind and placebo-controlled study. *J Am Acad Child Adolesc Psychiatry* **34**, 445–453.

Campbell M, Gonzalez NM, and Silva RR (1992) The pharmacotherapy of conduct disorders and rage outbursts. *Psychiatr Clin N Am* **15**, 69–85.

Campbell M, Small AM, Green WH, et al. (1984) Behavioral efficacy of haloperidol and lithium carbonate. *Arch Gen Psychiatry* **41**, 650–656.

Cantwell DP and Baker L (1991) Association between attention-deficit-hyperactivity disorder and learning disorders. *J Learn Disabil* **24**, 88–95.

Capaldi DM and Patterson GR (1996) Can violent offenders be distinguished from frequent offenders? Prediction from childhood to adolescence. *J Res Crime Delinq* **33**, 206–231.

Carlson GA and Rapoport MD (1989) Diagnostic classification issues in attention-deficit hyperactivity disorder. *Psychiatr Ann* **19**, 576–583.

Carlson GA and Weintraub S (1993) Childhood behavior problems and bipolar disorder—relationship or coincidence. *J Affect Disord* **28**, 143–153.

Casat CD, Pleasants DZ, Schroeder DH, et al. (1989) Bupropion in children with attention deficit disorder. *Psychopharmacol Bull* **25**, 198–201.

Casat CD, Pleasants DZ, and Van Wyck Fleet J (1987) A double-blind trial of bupropion in children with attention deficit disorder. *Psychopharmacol Bull* **23**, 120–122.

Castellanos FX, Elia J, Kruesi MJ, et al. (1996a) Cerebrospinal fluid homovanillic acid predicts behavioral response to stimulants in 45 boys with attention-deficit/hyperactivity disorder. *Neuropsychopharmacology* **14**, 125–137.

Castellanos FX, Elia J, Kruesi MJP, et al. (1994) Cerebrospinal fluid monoamine metabolites in boys with attention-deficit hyperactivity disorder. *Psychiatr Res* **52**, 305–316.

Castellanos FX, Giedd JN, Elia J, et al. (1997) Controlled stimulant treatment of ADHD and comorbid Tourette's syndrome: effects of stimulant and dose. *J Am Acad Child Adolesc Psychiatry* **36**, 589–596.

Cherland E and Fitzpatrick R (1999) Psychotic side effects of psychostimulants: a 5-year review. *Can J Psychiatry* **44**, 811–813.

Coccaro EF and Kavoussi RJ (1997) Fluoxetine and impulsive aggressive behavior in personality-disordered subjects. *Arch Gen Psychiatry* **54**, 1081–1088.

Coffey RJ, Biederman J, Geller DA, et al. (2000) Distinguishing illness severity from tic severity in children and adolescents with Tourette's disorder. *J Am Acad Child Adolesc Psychiatry* **39**, 56–61.

Cohen P, Cohen J, Kasen S, et al. (1993) An epidemiological study of disorders in late childhood and adolescence. I. Age- and gender-specific prevalence. *J Child Psychol Psychiatry* **34**, 851–867.

Comings DE and Comings BG (1984) Tourette syndrome and attention-deficit disorder with hyperactivity: are they genetically related. *J Am Acad Child Adolesc Psychiatry* **23**, 138–146.

Comings DE and Comings BG (1987) A controlled study of Tourette syndrome. I. Attention deficit disorder, learning disorders, and school problems. *Am J Hum Genet* **41**, 701–741.

Comings DE, Comings BG, Muhleman D, et al. (1991) The dopamine D_2 receptor locus as a modifying gene in neuropsychiatric disorders. *J Am Med Assoc* **266**, 1793–1800.

Conners CK, Casat CD, Gualtieri CT, et al. (1996) Bupropion hydrochloride in attention deficit disorder with hyperactivity. *J Am Acad Child Adolesc Psychiatry* **35**, 1314–1321.

Conners CK, Sitarenios G, Parker JDA, et al. (1998a) The Revised Conners' Parent Rating Scale (CPRS-R): factor structure, reliability, and criterion validity. *J Abnorm Child Psychol* **26**, 257–268.

Conners CK, Sitarenios G, Parker JDA, et al. (1998b) Revision and restandardization of the Conners teacher rating scale (CTRS-R): factor structure, reliability, and criterion validity. *J Abnorm Child Psychol* **26**, 279–291.

Costello EJ, Costello AJ, Edelbrock C, et al. (1988) Psychiatric disorders in pediatric primary care. *Arch Gen Psychiatry* **45**, 1107–1116.

Cueva JE, Overall JE, Small AM, et al. (1996) Carbamezapine in aggressive children with conduct disorder: a double-blind and placebo-controlled study. *J Am Acad Child Adolesc Psychiatry* **35**, 480–490.

Daly G, Hawi Z, Fitzgerald M, et al. (1999) Mapping susceptibility loci in attention-deficit hyperactivity disorder: preferential transmission of parental alleles at DAT1, DBH and DRD5 to affected children. *Mol Psychiatry* **4**, 192–196.

Diamond IR, Tannock R, and Schachar RJ (1999) Response to methylphenidate in children with ADHD and comorbid anxiety. *J Am Acad Child Adolesc Psychiatry* **38**, 402–409.

Donovan SJ, Stewart JW, Nunes EV, et al. (2000) Divalproex treatment for youth with explosive temper and mood lability: a double-blind, placebo-controlled crossover design. *Am J Psychiatry* **157**, 818–820.

Donovan SJ, Susser ES, Nunes EV, et al. (1997) Divalproex treatment of disruptive adolescents: a report of 10 cases. *J Clin Psychiatry* **58**, 12–15.

Dougherty DD, Bonab AA, Spencer TJ, et al. (1999) Dopamine transporter density in patients with attention-deficit hyperactivity disorder. *Lancet* **354**, 2132–2133.

Douglas VI, Barr RG, O'Neil ME, et al. (1986) Short-term effects of methylphenidate on the cognitive, learning and academic performance of children with attention deficit disorder in the laboratory and classroom. *J Child Psychol Psychiatry* **27**, 191–211.

Elia J (1993) Drug treatment for hyperactive children: therapeutic guidelines. *Drugs* **46**, 863–871.

Emslie GJ, Rush AJ, Weinberg WA, et al. (1997) A double-blind, randomized, placebo-controlled trial of fluoxetine in children and adolescents with depression. *Arch Gen Psychiatry* **54**, 1031–1037.

Ernst M, Liebenauer LL, Jons PH, et al. (1996) Selegiline in adults with attention-deficit hyperactivity disorder: clinical efficacy and safety. *Psychopharmacol Bull* **32**, 327–334.

Ernst M, Zametkin AJ, Matochik JA, et al. (1998) DOPA decarboxylase activity in attention-deficit hyperactivity disorder adults. A [fluorine-18]fluorodopa positron emission tomographic study. *J Neurosci* **18**, 5901–5907.

Ernst M, Zametkin AJ, Matochil JA, et al. (1999) High midbrain [^{18}F]DOPA accumulation in children with attention-deficit hyperactivity disorder. *Am J Psychiatry* **156**, 1209–1215.

Esser G, Schmidt MH, and Woerner W (1990) Epidemiology and course of psychiatric disorders in school-age children—results of a longitudinal study. *J Child Psychol Psychiatry* **32**, 243–263.

Eyre SL, Rousaville BJ, and Kleber HD (1982) History of childhood hyperactivity in a clinical population of opiate addicts. *J Nerv Ment Disord* **170**, 522–529.

Faraone SV, Plizska SR, Olvera RL, et al. (2001) Efficacy of Adderall and methylphenidate in attention-deficit hyperactivity disorder: a reanalysis using drug–placebo and drug–drug response curve methodology. *J Child Adolesc Psychopharmacol* **11**, 171–178.

Farrington DP (1989) Early predictors of adolescent aggression and adult violence. *Viol Victim* **4**, 79–100.

Farrington DP (1990) Long-term criminal outcomes of hyperactivity-impulsivity-attention-deficit (HIA) and conduct problems in childhood. In *Straight and Devious Pathways from Childhood to Adulthood*, Robins LN and Rutter M (eds). Cambridge University Press, New York, pp. 62–81.

Farrington DP and Loeber R (2000) Epidemiology of juvenile violence. *Child Adolesc Psychiatr Clin N Am* **9**, 733–748.

Feigin A, Kurlan R, McDermott MP, et al. (1996) A controlled trial of deprenyl in children with Tourette's syndrome and attention-deficit hyperactivity disorder. *Neurology* **46**, 965–968.

Fenichel RR (1995) Combining methylphenidate and clonidine: the role of postmarketing surveillance. *J Child Adolesc Psychopharmacol* **5**, 155–156.

Filipek PA, Semrud-Clikeman M, Steingard RJ, et al. (1997) Volumetric MRI analysis comparing subjects having attention-deficit hyperactivity disorder with normal controls. *Neurology* **48**, 589–601.

Findling RL, McNamara NK, Branicky LA, et al. (2000) A double-blind pilot study of risperidone in the treatment of conduct disorder. *J Am Acad Child Adolesc Psychiatry* **39**, 509–516.

Findling RL, Schwartz MA, Flannery DJ, et al. (1996) Venlafaxine in adults with attention-deficit/hyperactivity disorder: an open clinical trial. *J Clin Psychiatry* **57**, 184–189.

Findling RL, Short EJ, and Manos MJ (2001) Short-term cardiovascular effects of methylphenidate and adderall. *J Am Acad Child Adolesc Psychiatry* **40**, 525–529.

Fischer M (1997) Persistence of ADHD into adulthood: it depends on whom you ask. *ADHD Rep* **5**, 8–10.

Forness SR, Swanson JM, Cantwell DP, et al. (1992) Stimulant medication and reading performance: follow-up on sustained dose in ADHD boys with and without conduct disorders. *J Learn Disabil* **25**, 115–123.

Frick PJ, Lahey BB, Loeber R, et al. (1992) Familial risk factors to oppositional defiant disorder and conduct disorder: parental psychopathology and maternal parenting. *J Consult Clin Psychol* **60**, 49–55.

Gadow KD, Sverd J, Sparfkin J, et al. (1999) Long-term methylphenidate therapy in children with comorbid attention-deficit hyperactivity disorder and chronic multiple tic disorder. *Arch Gen Psychiatry* **56**, 330–336.

Gammon GD and Brown TE (1993) Fluoxetine and methylphenidate in combination for treatment of attention deficit disorder and comorbid depressive disorder. *J Child Adolesc Psychopharmacol* **3**, 1–10.

Garfinkel BD, Wender PH, Sloman L, et al. (1983) Tricyclic antidepressant and methylphenidate treatment of attention deficit disorder in children. *J Am Acad Child Adolesc Psychiatry* **22**, 343–348.

Gaub M and Carlson CL (1997) Gender differences in ADHD: a meta-analysis and critical review. *J Am Acad Child Adolesc Psychiatry* **36**, 1036–1045.

Gershon J (2002) A meta-analytic review of gender differences in ADHD. *J Atten Disord* **5**, 143–154.

Goldman-Rakic PS (1987) Circuitry of the primate prefrontal cortex and the regulation of behavior by representational memory. In *Handbook of Physiology, the Nervous System, Higher Functions of the Brain*, Vol. 5, Plum F (ed). American Physiological Society, Bethesda, MD, pp. 373–417.

Goodman M and Nachman G (2000) *Industry Overview. The ADHD Market: It's Time to Pay Attention*. Morgan Stanley Dean Witter, New York.

Grcevich S (2001) SLI381: a long-acting psychostimulant preparation for the treatment of attention-deficit hyperactivity disorder. *Expert Opin Invest Drugs* **10**, 2003–2011.

Greenhill LL, Pliszka S, Dulcan MK, et al. (2002) Practice parameter for the use of stimulant medications in the treatment of children, adolescents, and adults. *J Am Acad Child Adolesc Psychiatry* **41**, 26S–49S.

Gresham FM (1985) Behavior disorder assessment: conceptual, definitional and practical considerations. *School Psychol Rev* **14**, 495–509.

Halperin JM, McKay KE, Matier K, et al. (1994a) Attention, response inhibition and activity level in children: developmental neuropsychological perspectives. *Adv Child Neuropsychol* **2**, 1–54.

Halperin JM, Newcorn JH, Koda VH, et al. (1997a) Noradrenergic mechanisms in ADHD children with and without reading disabilities: a replication and extension. *J Am Acad Child Adolesc Psychiatry* **36**, 1688–1697.

Halperin JM, Newcorn JH, Kopstein I, et al. (1997b) Serotonin, aggression, and parental psychopathology in children with attention-deficit hyperactivity disorder. *J Am Acad Child Adolesc Psychiatry* **36**, 1391–1398.

Halperin JM, Newcorn JH, Schwartz ST, et al. (1997c) Age-related changes in the association between serotonergic function and aggression in boys with ADHD. *Biol Psychiatry* **41**, 682–689.

Halperin JM, Sharma V, Siever LJ, et al. (1994b) Serotonergic function in aggressive and nonaggressive boys with attention-deficit hyperactivity disorder. *Am J Psychiatry* **151**, 243–248.

Hechtman L (1992) Long-term outcome in attention-deficit hyperactivity disorder. *Psychiatr Clin N Am* 1, 553–565.

Hechtman L, Weiss G, Perlman T, et al. (1981) Hyperactives as young adults: various clinical outcomes. *Adolesc Psychiatr* **9**, 295–306.

Hedges D, Reimherr FW, Rogers A, et al. (1995) An open trial of venlafaxine in adult patients with attention-deficit hyperactivity disorder. *Psychopharmacol Bull* **31**, 779–783.

Hinshaw SP (1987) On the distinction between attentional-deficits/hyperactivity and conduct problems/aggression in child psychopathology. *Psychol Bull* **101**, 443–463.

Hinshaw SP (1992) Academic underachievement, attention-deficits, and aggression: comorbidity and implications for intervention. *J Consult Clin Psychol* **60**, 893–903.

Hinshaw SP, Heller T, and McHale JP (1992) Covert antisocial behavior in boys with attention-deficit hyperactivity disorder: External validation and effects of methylphenidate. *J Consult Clin Psychol* **60**, 274–281.

Hinshaw SP, Owens EB, Wells KC, et al. (2000) Family processes and treatment outcome in the MTA: negative/ineffective parenting practices in relation to multimodal treatment. *J Abnorm Child Psychol* **28**, 555–568.

Hollander E, Allen A, Lopez RP, et al. (2001) A preliminary double-blind, placebo-controlled trial of divalproex sodium in borderline personality disorder. *J Clin Psychiatry* **62**, 199–203.

Horn HF, Wagner AE, and Ialongo N (1989) Sex differences in school-aged children with pervasive attention-deficit hyperactivity disorder. *J Abnorm Child Psychol* **17**, 109–125.

Hunt RD and Cohen DJ (1988) Attentional and neurochemical components of mental retardation: new methods for an old problem. In *Mental Retardation and Mental Health: lassification, Diagnosis, Treatment Services*, Stark JA, Menolascino FJ, Albarelli MH, et al. (eds). Springer-Verlag, New York.

Hunt RD, Lau S, and Ryu J (1991) Alternative therapies for ADHD. In *Ritalin: Theory and Patient Management*, Greenhill LL and Osman BB (eds). Mary Ann Liebert, New York, pp. 75–95.

Hunt RD, Minderaa RB, and Cohen DJ (1985) The therapeutic effect of clonidine in attention deficit disorder with hyperactivity: report of a double-blind, placebo-controlled crossover study. *J Am Acad Child Adolesc Psychiatry* **24**, 617–629.

Hynd GW, Semrud-Clikeman M, Lorys AR, et al. (1991) Corpus callosum morphology in attention deficit-hyperactivity disorder: morphometric analysis of MRI. *J Learn Disabil* **24**, 141–146.

James RS, Sharp WS, Bastain TM, et al. (2001) Double-blind, placebo-controlled study of single-dose amphetamine formulations in ADHD. *J Am Acad Child Adolesc Psychiatry* **40**, 1268–1276.

Jankovic J (1993) Deprenyl in attention-deficit associated with Tourette's syndrome. *Arch Neurol* **50**, 286–288.

Jensen JB, Burke N, and Garfinkel BD (1988) Depression and symptoms of attention-deficit disorder with hyperactivity. *J Am Acad Child Adolesc Psychiatry* **27**, 742–747.

Jensen PS, Hinshaw SP, Kraemer HC, et al. (2001) ADHD comorbidity findings from the MTA study: comparing comorbid subgroups. *J Am Acad Child Adolesc Psychiatry* **40**, 147–158.

Kafantaris V, Campbell M, and Padron–Gayol MV (1992) Carbamazepine in hospitalized aggressive conduct disorder children: an open pilot study. *Psychopharmacol Bull* **28**, 193–199.

Kashani JH, Beck NC, Hoeper EW, et al. (1987) Psychiatric disorders in a community sample of adolescents. *Am J Psychiatry* **144**, 584–589.

Kazdin AE (1987) Treatment of antisocial behavior in children: current status and future directions. *Psychol Bull* **102**, 187–203.

Kazdin AE, Bass D, Siegel T, et al. (1989) Cognitive–behavioral therapy and relationship therapy in the treatment of children referred antisocial behavior. *J Consult Clin Psychol* **57**, 522–535.

Klein RG and Mannuzza S (1991) Long-term outcome of hyperactive children: a review. *J Am Acad Child Adolesc Psychiatry* **30**, 383–387.

Klein RG, Abikoff H, Klass E, et al. (1997) Clinical efficacy of methylphenidate in conduct disorder with and without attention-deficit hyperactivity disorder. *Arch Gen Psychiatry* **54**, 1073–1080.

Klorman R, Brumaghim JT, Salzman LF, et al. (1988) Effects of methylphenidate on attention-deficit hyperactivity disorder with and without aggressive/noncompliant features. *J Abnorm Psychol* **97**, 413–422.

Koller H, Richardson SA, and Katz M (1983) Behavior disturbance since childhood among a 5-year birth cohort of all mentally retarded young adults in a city. *Am J Ment Def* **87**, 386–395.

Kovacs M, Paulauskas S, Gatsonis C, et al. (1988) Depressive disorders in childhood. III. A longitudinal study of comorbidity with and risk for conduct disorders. *J Affect Disord* **15**, 205–217.

Kratochvil CJ, Bohac D, Harrington M, et al. (2001) An open-label trial of tomoxetine in pediatric attention-deficit hyperactivity disorder. *J Child Adolesc Psychopharmacol* **11**, 167–170.

Krause K-H, Dresel SH, Krause J, et al. (2000) Increased striatal dopamine transporter in adult patients with attention-deficit hyperactivity disorder: effects of methylphenidate as measured by single photon emission computed tomography. *Neurosci Lett* **285**, 107–110.

Kruesi MJ, Rapoport JL, Hamburger SD, et al. (1990) Cerebrospinal fluid monoamine metabolites, aggression, and impulsivity in disruptive behavior disorders of children and adolescents. *Arch Gen Psychiatry* **47**, 419–426.

Kupietz SS, Winsberg BG, and Richardson E (1988) Effects of methylphenidate dosage in hyperactive reading-disabled children: I. Behavior and cognitive performance effects. *J Am Acad Child Adolesc Psychiatry* **27**, 70–77.

Lahey B, Applegate B, McBurnett K, et al. (1994) DSM-IV field trials for attention-deficit hyperactivity disorder in children and adolescents. *Am J Psychiatry* **151**, 1673–1685.

Lahey BB, Loeber R, Quay HC, et al. (1992) Oppositional defiant and conduct disorders: issues to be resolved for DSM-IV. *J Am Acad Child Adolesc Psychiatry* **31**, 539–546.

Lahey BB, Piacentini J, McBurnett MS, et al. (1988) Psychopathology in the parents of children with conduct disorder and hyperactivity. *J Am Acad Child Adolesc Psychiatry* **27**, 163–170.

Lambert N, Hartsaugh C, and Sassone D (1987) Persistance of hyperactivity symptoms from childhood to adolescence and associated outcomes. *Am J Orthopsychiatry* **57**, 22–32.

Law SF and Schachar RJ (1999) Do typical clinical doses of methylphenidate cause tics in children treated for attention-deficit hyperactivity disorder. *J Am Acad Child Adolesc Psychiatry* **38**, 944–945.

Livingston R, Dykman RA, and Ackerman PT (1990) The frequency and the significance of additional self-reported psychiatric diagnoses in children with attention-deficit disorder. *J Abnorm Child Psychol* **19**, 465–478.

Livingston RL, Dykman RA, and Ackerman PT (1992) Psychiatric comorbidity and response to two doses of methylphenidate in children with attention-deficit disorder. *J Child Adolesc Psychopharmacol* **2**, 115.

Loeber R (1990) Developmental and risk factors of juvenile antisocial behavior and delinquency. *Clin Psychol Rev* **10**, 1–41.

Loeber R (1991) Oppositional defiant disorder and conduct disorder. *Hosp Comm Psychiatry* **42**, 1099–1100.

Loeber R and Schmaling KB (1985) The utility of differentiating between mixed and pure forms of antisocial child behavior. *J Abnorm Child Psychol* **13**, 315–336.

Loeber R, Green SM, Lahey BB, et al. (1991a) Differences and similarities between children, mothers and teachers as informants on disruptive child behavior. *J Abnorm Child Psychol* **19**, 75–95.

Loeber R, Green SM, Lahey BB, et al. (1992) Developmental sequences in the age of onset of disruptive child behaviors. *J Child Fam Stud* **1**, 21–41.

Loeber R, Lahey BB, and Thomas C (1991b) Diagnostic conundrum of oppositional defiant disorder and conduct disorder. *J Abnorm Psychol* **100**, 379–390.

Loeber R, Wung P, Keenan K, et al. (1993) Developmental pathways in disruptive child behavior. *Dev Psychopathol* **5**, 103–133.

Lou HC, Henriksen L, and Bruhn P (1989) Striatal dysfunction in attention deficit and hyperkinetic disorder. *Arch Neurol* **46**, 48–52.

Lucas CP (1992) Attention deficit disorders and hyperactivity. *Curr Opin Psychiatry* **5**, 518–522.

Mannuzza S, Klein RG, Bessler A, et al. (1993) Adult outcome of hyperactive boys: educational achievement, occupational rank and psychiatric status. *Arch Gen Psychiatry* **50**, 565–576.

Manuck SB, Flory JD, Ferrell RE, et al. (1999) Aggression and anger-related traits associated with polymorphism of the tryptophan hydroxylase gene. *Biol Psychiatry* **45**, 603–614.

Manuck SB, Flory JD, Ferrell RE, et al. (2000) A regulatory polymorphism of the monoamine oxidase-A gene may be associated with variability in aggression, impulsivity, and central nervous system serotonergic responsivity. *Psychiatr Res* **95**, 9–23.

March JS, Swanson JM, Arnold LE, et al. (2000) Anxiety as a predictor and outcome variable in the multimodal treatment study of children with ADHD (MTA). *J Abnorm Child Psychol* **28**, 527–541.

Markowitz PI and Coccaro EF (1995) Biological studies of impulsivity aggression, and suicidal behavior. In *Impulsivity and Aggression*, Hollander E and Stein D (eds). John Wiley, Chichester, pp. 71–91.

McCord J (1979) Some child-rearing antecedents of criminal behavior in adult men. *J Pers Soc Psychol* **9**, 1477–1486.

McGee R and Share DL (1988) Attention deficit disorder-hyperactivity and academic failure: which comes first and what should be treated. *J Am Acad Child Adolesc Psychiatry* **27**, 318–325.

Michelson D, Faries D, Wernicke J, et al. (2001) Atomoxetine in the treatment of children and adolescents with attention-deficit/hyperactivity disorder: a randomized, placebo-controlled, dose-response study. *Pediatrics* **108**, E83.

Moffit TE (1990) Juvenile delinquency and attention-deficit disorder: boys' developmental trajectories from age 3 to 5. *Child Dev* **61**, 893–910.

Mostofsky SH, Reiss AL, Lockhart P, et al. (1998) Evaluation of cerebellar size in attention-deficit hyperactivity disorder. *J Child Neurol* **13**, 434–439.

MTA Cooperative Group (1999a) A 14-month randomized clinical trial of treatment strategies for attention-deficit/hyperactivity disorder: the multimodal treatment study of children with ADHD. *Arch Gen Psychiatry* **56**, 1073–1086.

MTA Cooperative Group (1999b) Moderators and mediators of treatment response for children with attention-deficit/hyperactivity disorder: the multimodal treatment study of children with attention-deficit/hyperactivity disorder. *Arch Gen Psychiatry* **56**, 1088–1096.

Newcorn JH, McKay KE, Loeber R, et al. (1996) Emotionality and serotonergic function in aggressive and nonaggressive ADHD children. In *Scientific Proceedings of the 43rd Annual Meeting of the American Academy of Child and Adolescent Psychiatry*, Schwab-Stone ME (ed). Philadelphia, PA, p. 94.

O'Keane V, Moloney E, O'Neill H, et al. (1992) Blunted prolactin responses to d-fenfluramine in sociopathy: evidence for subsensitivity of central serotonergic function. *Br J Psychiatry* **160**, 643–646.

Olvera RL, Piszka SR, Luh J, et al. (1996) An open trial of venlafaxine in the treatment of attention-deficit/hyperactivity disorder in children and adolescents. *J Child Adolesc Psychopharmacol* **6**, 241–250.

Pauls DL, Hurst CR, Kruger SD, et al. (1986) Gilles de la Tourette's syndrome and attention deficit disorder with hyperactivity: evidence against a genetic relationship. *Arch Gen Psychiatry* **43**, 1177–1179.

Pelham WE (1999) The NIMH multimodal treatment study for attention-deficit hyperactivity disorder: just say yes to drugs alone. *Can J Psychiatry* **44**(10), 981–90.

Pelham WE and Hinshaw SP (1992) Behavioral intervention for attention-deficit hyperactivity disorder. In *Handbook of Clinical Behavior Therapy*, Turner SM, Calhoun KS, and Adams HE (eds). John Wiley, New York, pp. 259–283.

Pelham WE, Bender ME, Caddell JM, et al. (1985) The dose-response effects of methylphenidate on classroom academic and social behavior in children with attention deficit disorder. *Arch Gen Psychiatry* **42**, 948–952.

Pelham WE, Gnagy EM, Burrows–MacLean L, et al. (2001) Once-a-day concerta methylphenidate versus three-times-daily methylphenidate in laboratory and natural settings. *Pediatrics* **107**, E105.

Pine DS, Coplan JD, Wasserman GA, et al. (1997) Neuroendocrine response to fenfluramine challenge in boys. *Arch Gen Psychiatry* **54**, 839–846.

Pliszka SR (1989) Effect of anxiety on cognition, behavior, and stimulant response in ADHD. *J Am Acad Child Adolesc Psychiatry* **28**, 882–887.

Pliszka SR (1992) Comorbidity of attention-deficit hyperactivity disorder and overanxious disorder. *J Am Acad Child Adolesc Psychiatry* **31**, 197–203.

Pliszka SR, Browne RG, Olvera RL, et al. (2000a) A double-blind, placebo-controlled study of Adderall and methylphenidate in the treatment of attention-deficit/hyperactivity disorder. *J Am Acad Child Adolesc Psychiatry* **39**, 619–626.

Pliszka SR, Greenhill LL, Crismon ML, et al. (2000b) The Texas children's medication algorithm project: report of the Texas consensus conference panel on medication treatment of childhood attention-deficit/hyperactivity disorder. Part I. Attention-deficit/hyperactivity disorder. *J Am Acad Child Adolesc Psychiatry* **39**, 908–919.

Pliszka SR, Greenhill LL, Crismon ML, et al. (2000c) The Texas children's medication algorithm project: report of the Texas consensus conference panel on medication treatment of childhood attention-deficit/hyperactivity disorder. Part II. Tactics. Attention-deficit/hyperactivity disorder. *J Am Acad Child Adolesc Psychiatry* **39**, 920–927.

Pope AW, Bierman KL, and Mumma GH (1989) Relations between hyperactive and aggressive behavior and peer relations at three elementary grade levels. *J Abnorm Child Psychol* **17**, 253–267.

Popper CW (1997) Antidepressants in the treatment of attention-deficit/hyperactivity disorder. *J Clin Psychiatry* **58**(Suppl. 14), 14–29.

Rapport MD, Stoner G, DuPaul GJ, et al. (1985) Methylphenidate in hyperactive children: differential effects of dose on academic, learning and social behavior. *J Abnorm Child Psychol* **13**, 227–243.

Rey JM, Bashir MR, Schwarz M, et al. (1988) Oppositional disorder: fact or fiction? *J Am Acad Child Adolesc Psychiatry* **27**, 157–162.

Richardson E, Kupietz SS, Winsberg BG, et al. (1988) Effects of methylphenidate dosage in hyperactive reading-disabled children. II. Reading achievement. *J Am Acad Child Adolesc Psychiatry* **27**, 78–87.

Riddle MA, Nelson JC, Kleinman CS, et al. (1991) Sudden death in children receiving Norpramin: a review of three reported cases and commentary. *J Am Acad Child Adolesc Psychiatry* **30**, 104–108.

Roberts MA (1990) A behavioral observation method for differentiating hyperactive and aggressive boys. *J Abnorm Child Psychol* **18**, 131–142.

Rogeness GA, Javors MA, Maas JW, et al. (1987) Plasma dopamine-b-hydroxylase, HVA, MHPG, and conduct disorder in emotionally disturbed boys. *Biol Psychiatry* **22**, 1158–1162.

Rubia K, Overmeyer S, Taylor E, et al. (1999) Hypofrontality in attention-deficit hyperactivity disorder during higher-order motor control: a study with functional MRI. *Am J Psychiatry* **156**, 891–896.

Rubia K, Taylor E, Smith AB, et al. (2001) Neuropsychological analyses of impulsiveness in childhood hyperactivity. *Br J Psychiatry* **179**, 138–143.

Rubinstein S, Silver LB, and Licamele WL (1994) Clonidine for stimulant-related sleep problems. *J Am Acad Child Adolesc Psychiatry* **33**, 281–282.

Rutter M, Cox A, Tupling C, et al. (1975) Attainment and adjustment in two geographical areas, Vol. 1. The prevalence of psychiatric disorders. *Br J Psychiatry* **126**, 493–509.

Safer DJ, Zito JM, and Gardner JF (2001) Pemoline hepatotoxicity and postmarketing surveillance. *J Am Acad Child Adolesc Psychiatry* **40**, 622–629.

Saletu B, Grunberger J, Anderer P, et al. (1992) Pharmacodynamics of venlafaxine evaluated by EEG brain mapping, psychometry and psychophysiology. *Br J Clin Pharmacol* **33**, 589–601.

Satterfield J, Hoppe C, and Schell A (1982) Prospective study of delinquency in 110 adolescent boys with attention deficit disorder and 89 normal adolescent boys. *Am J Psychiatry* **139**, 797–798.

Scahill L, Chappell PB, Kim YS, et al. (2001) A placebo-controlled study of guanfacine in the treatment of children with tic disorders and attention-deficit hyperactivity disorder. *Am J Psychiatry* **158**, 1067–1074.

Schachar R and Wachsmuth R (1990b) Hyperactivity and parental psychopathology. *J Child Psychol Psychiatry* **31**, 381–392.

Schulz KP, Newcorn JH, McKay KE, et al. (2001) Relationship between central serotonergic function and aggression in prepubertal boys: effect of age and attention-deficit/hyperactivity disorder. *Psychiatr Res* **101**, 1–10.

Semrud–Clikeman M, Biederman J, Sprich–Buckminster S, et al. (1992) Comorbidity between ADDH and learning disability: a review and report in a clinically referred sample. *J Am Acad Child Adolesc Psychiatry* **31**, 439–448.

Sherman D, Iacono W, and McGue M (1997) Attention-deficit hyperactivity disorder dimensions: a twin study of inattention and impulsivity-hyperactivity. *J Am Acad Child Adolesc Psychiatry* **36**, 745–753.

Simeon JG, Ferguson HB, and Van Wyck Fleet J (1986) Bupropion effects in attention deficit and conduct disorders. *Can J Psychiatry* **31**, 581–585.

Slutske WS, Heath AC, Dinwiddie SH, et al. (1997) Modeling genetic and environmental influences in the etiology of conduct disorder: a study of 2,682 adult twin pairs. *J Abnorm Psychol* **106**, 266–279.

Smith BH, Pelham WE, Evans S, et al. (1998) Dosage effects of methylphenidate on the social behavior of adolescents diagnosed with attention-deficit hyperactivity disorder. *Exp Clin Psychopharmacol* **6**, 187–204.

Smith C and Thornberry TP (1995) The relationship between child maltreatment and adolescent involvement in delinquency. *Criminology* **33**, 451–477.

Spencer TJ, Biederman J, Faraone S, et al. (2001) Impact of tic disorders on ADHD outcome across the life cycle: Findings from a large group of adults with and without ADHD. *Am J Psychiatry* **158**, 611–617.

Spencer TJ, Biederman J, Harding M, et al. (1996) Growth deficits in ADHD children revisited: evidence for disorder-associated growth delays. *J Am Acad Child Adolesc Psychiatry* **35**, 1460–1469.

Spencer T, Biederman J, Wilens T, et al. (2001) Efficacy of a mixed amphetamine salts compound in adults with attention-deficit/hyperactivity disorder. *Arch Gen Psychiatry* **58**, 775–782.

Stanley B, Molcho A, Stanley M, et al. (2000) Association of aggressive behavior with altered serotonergic function in patients who are not suicidal. *Am J Psychiatry* **157**, 609–614.

Stein MA, Blondis TA, Schnitzer ER, et al. (1996) Methylphenidate dosing: twice daily versus three times daily. *Pediatrics* **98**, 748–756.

Steingard R, Biederman J, Spencer T, et al. (1993) Comparison of clonidine response in the treatment of attention-deficit hyperactivity disorder with and without comorbid tics. *J Am Acad Child Adolesc Psychiatry* **32**, 350–353.

Stoff DM, Pasatiempo AP, Yeung JH, et al. (1992) Neuroendocrine responses to challenge with dl-fenfluramine and aggression in disruptive behavior disorders of children and adolescents. *Psychiatr Res* **43**, 263–276.

Sullivan MA and O'Leary SG (1989) Differential maintenance following reward and cost token programs with children. *Behav Ther* **21**, 139–151.

Swanson JM, Cantwell D, Lerner M, et al. (1991) Effects of stimulant medication on learning in children with ADHD. *J Learn Disabil* **24**, 219–230.

Swanson JM, Sunohara GA, Kennedy JL, et al. (1998) Association of the dopamine receptor D_4 (DRD4) gene with a refined phenotype of attention-deficit hyperactivity disorder (ADHD): a family-based approach. *Mol Psychiatry* **3**, 38–41.

Swanson JM, Wigal S, Greenhill LL, et al. (1998) Analog classroom assessment of Adderall in children with ADHD. *J Am Acad Child Adolesc Psychiatry* **37**, 519–526.

Szatmari P (1992) The epidemiology of attention-deficit hyperactivity disorders. *Child Adolesc Psychiatr Clin N Am* **1**, 361–371.

Szatmari P, Boyle M, and Offord DR (1989) ADDH and conduct disorder: degree of diagnostic overlap and differences among correlates. *J Am Acad Child Adolesc Psychiatry* **28**, 865–872.

Tannock R and Schachar R (1992) Is ADHD with comorbid overanxious disorder different from ADHD? Paper presentation in the symposium: comorbidity of ADHD. Discriminating Features and Methodologic Problems at the *39th Annual Meeting of the American Academy of Child and Adolescent Psychiatry*.

Taylor EA (1986) Childhood hyperactivity. *Br J Psychiatry* **149**, 562–573.

The Medical Letter (1984) Sustained-release methylphenidate. *The Med Lett Drugs Therapeut* **26**, 97–98.

The Medical Letter (2000) A new long-acting methylphenidate (Concerta). *The Med Lett Drugs Therapeut* **42**, 80–81.

The Medical Letter (2001) Another long-acting methylphenidate (Metadate CD). *The Med Lett Drugs Therapeut* **43**, 83–84.

Vaidya CJ, Austin G, Kirkorian G, et al. (1998) Selective effects of methylphenidate in attention-deficit hyperactivity disorder: a functional magnetic resonance study. *Proc Nat Acad Sci U S A* **95**, 14494–14499.

Waldman ID and Lilienfeld SO (1991) Diagnostic efficiency of symptoms for oppositional defiant disorder and attention-deficit hyperactivity disorder. *J Consult Clin Psychol* **59**, 732–738.

Walker JL, Lahey BB, Russo MF, et al. (1991) Anxiety, inhibition and conduct disorder in children. I. Relations to social impairment. *J Am Acad Child Adolesc Psychiatry* **30**, 187–191.

Weiss G, Hechtman L, Milroy T, et al. (1985) Psychiatric status of hyperactives as adults: a controlled prospective 15-year follow-up of 63 hyperactive children. *J Am Acad Child Adolesc Psychiatry* **24**, 211–220.

Werry JS, Reeves JC, and Elkind GS (1987) Attention deficit, conduct, oppositional, and anxiety disorders in children. I. A review of research on differentiating characteristics. *J Am Acad Child Adolesc Psychiatry* **26**, 133–143.

Whalen CK and Henker B (1991) Therapies for hyperactive children: comparisons, combinations, and compromises. *J Consult Clin Psychol* **59**, 126–137.

Whalen CK, Henker B, Buhrmeister D, et al. (1989) Does stimulation medication improve peer status of hyperactive children. *J Consult Clin Psychol* **57**, 545–549.

White J, Moffitt TE, Caspi A, et al. (1994) Measuring impulsivity and examining its relation to delinquency. *J Abnorm Psychol* **103**, 192–205.

Winsberg BG and Comings DE (1999) Association of the dopamine transporter gene (DAT1) with poor methylphenidate response. *J Am Acad Child Adolesc Psychiatry* **38**, 1474–1477.

Winsberg BG, Kupietz SS, Sverg J, et al. (1982) Methylphenidate oral dose plasma concentrations and behavioral response in children. *Psychopharmacology (Berl)* **76**, 329–332.

Wolraich MI, Greenhill LL, Pelham W, et al. (2001) Randomized, controlled trial of oros methylphenidate once a day in children with attention-deficit/hyperactivity disorder. *Pediatrics* **108**, 883–892.

Wolraich M, Hannah J, Pinnock T, et al. (1996) Comparison of diagnostic criteria for attention-deficit hyperactivity disorder in a country-wide sample. *J Am Acad Child Adolesc Psychiatry* **35**, 319–324.

Wood D, Wender PH, and Rheimherr FW (1983) The prevalence of attention deficit disorder, residual type, or minimal brain dysfunction, in a population of male alcoholic patients. *Am J Psychiatry* **140**, 95–98.

Woolston JL, Rosenthal SL, Riddle M, et al. (1989) Childhood comorbidity of anxiety/affective disorders and behavior disorder. *J Am Acad Child Adolesc Psychiatry* **28**, 707–713.

Zametkin AJ and Rapoport JL (1987) Neurobiology of attention-deficit disorder with hyperactivity: where have we come in 50 years. *J Am Acad Child Adolesc Psychiatry* **26**, 676–686.

Zametkin AJ, Liebenauer LL, Fitzgerald GA, et al. (1993) Brain metabolism in teenagers with attention-deficit hyperactivity disorder. *Arch Gen Psychiatry* **50**, 333–340.

Zametkin AJ, Nordahl TE, Gross M, et al. (1990) Cerebral glucose metabolism in adults with hyperactivity of childhood onset. *New Engl J Med* **323**, 1361–1366.

Zametkin AJ, Rapoport JL, Murphy DL, et al. (1985) Treatment of hyperactive children with monoamine oxidase inhibitors. I. Clinical efficacy. *Arch Gen Psychiatry* **42**, 962–996.

9 Childhood Disorders: Feeding and Eating Disorders of Infancy or Early Childhood

FEEDING DISORDER OF INFANCY OR EARLY CHILDHOOD

Diagnosis

In the literature, the term "feeding disorder" generally encompasses a variety of conditions ranging from problem behaviors during feeding—poor appetite, food refusal, food selectivity, food avoidance, and pica to rumination and vomiting (Benoit 1993). The term "feeding disorder" is generally used to emphasize the dyadic nature of eating problems in infants and young children (Budd et al. 1992).

Feeding Disorder of Infancy or Early Childhood is defined in the DSM-IV-TR as a persistent failure to eat adequately with significant failure to gain weight or a significant loss of weight over a period of at least 1 month (see DSM-IV-TR diagnostic criteria on page 188). This general definition of feeding disorder in DSM-IV-TR does not take into account the heterogeneity of feeding and growth problems in infants and its implication for treatment.

Some authors have used various diagnostic methods and assigned different labels to address the heterogeneity of feeding problems associated with failure to thrive (Sanders et al. 1993, Singer et al. 1991, Woolston 1983). The pediatric literature has focused primarily on failure to thrive as a diagnostic label. The term "failure to thrive" describes infants and young children who demonstrate failure in physical growth, often associated with delay of social and motor development. Research has used an awkward and, in many cases, not useful dichotomy, namely, the differentiation of organic from nonorganic failure to thrive. Nonorganic failure to thrive is commonly thought to reflect a failure or relative absence of adequate maternal care and warmth (Caldwell 1971, Patton and Gardner 1962, Reinhart 1979). Several authors have suggested a third category of failure to thrive for infants who present with a combination of organic and nonorganic factors in the etiology of their growth disturbance (Homer and Ludwig 1981, Casey et al. 1984).

DSM-IV-TR Diagnostic Criteria

307.59 Feeding Disorder of Infancy or Early Childhood

A. Feeding disturbance as manifested by persistent failure to eat adequately with significant failure to gain weight or significant loss of weight over at least 1 month.
B. The disturbance is not due to an associated gastrointestinal or other general medical condition (e.g., esophageal reflux).
C. The disturbance is not better accounted for by another mental disorder (e.g., rumination disorder) or by lack of available food.
D. The onset is before age 6 years.

Reprinted with permission from the Diagnostic and Statistical Manual of Mental Disorders, Fourth Edition, Text Revision. Copyright 2000 American Psychiatric Association.

Because of the diversity of feeding disorders associated with failure to thrive and the lack of a subclassification of feeding disorder as defined in DSM-IV-TR, Chatoor proposed a classification of feeding disorders based on the definition of psychiatric disorders suggested by Wing (1973, 1979), which is used in this chapter. Three developmental feeding disorders are described as (1) feeding disorder of state regulation, (2) feeding disorder of poor mother–infant reciprocity, and (3) feeding disorder of separation (infantile anorexia). In addition, two feeding disorders are described that are not linked to specific developmental stages: (1) sensory food aversions, a common feeding disorder that becomes evident during the introduction of different milks, baby food, or table food with various tastes and consistencies, and (2) posttraumatic feeding disorder, which is characterized by an acute disruption in the regulation of eating and can occur at various ages and stages of feeding development.

Feeding Disorder of State Regulation In this condition, the infant has difficulty reaching and maintaining a calm state of alertness for feeding, either being too sleepy or too agitated or distressed to feed. Young infants who present with feeding difficulties and growth failure dating to the postnatal period need to be considered for the diagnosis of a feeding disorder of state regulation. The evaluation should begin by obtaining a history of the mother's pregnancy and delivery and a report of the infant's history of feeding, development, and medical illnesses that might contribute to the feeding problems. In addition, the mother's functioning and her social support system need to be explored. Most important, the mother and her infant should be observed during feeding and during play to assess the infant's special characteristics, the infant's regulation of state and feeding behavior, and the mother's ability to read the infant's signals and to respond to them in a contingent way.

In a study of mother–infant interactions during feeding, Chatoor and colleagues (1997) observed that mothers and infants with feeding disorders of state regulation (homeostasis) showed less dyadic reciprocity compared to a control group of well-feeding mother–infant dyads.

The information from the infant's and the mother's histories and the observation of the mother–infant dyad will determine which factors contribute to the difficulties in the infant's regulation of feeding. Because medical problems (e.g., cardiac or pulmonary disease) may contribute to the feeding problems, their impact on the feeding relationship of mother and infant needs to be considered.

Feeding Disorder of Poor Caregiver–Infant Reciprocity   Children with this condition show a lack of developmentally appropriate signs of social reciprocity with the primary caregiver during feeding, leading to significant growth deficiency. This feeding disorder has been referred to in the early literature as maternal deprivation (Patton and Gardner 1963), deprivation dwarfism (Silver and Finkelstein 1967), and psychosocial deprivation (Caldwell 1971). The growth failure and developmental delay of these infants were considered a consequence of a continuum of neglect and/or maltreatment of the child leading to insecure attachment to the caregiver. In DSM-III, this disorder was defined as reactive attachment disorder of infancy associated with failure to thrive. However, DSM-IV has changed the definition of reactive attachment disorder to encompass only the problems in relatedness of young children. In previous publications, Chatoor referred to this feeding disorder as "feeding disorder of attachment." However, because of the difficulty of assessing attachment in infants under 1 year of age, feeding disorder of poor caregiver–infant reciprocity was chosen as diagnostic label to capture the lack of engagement between mother and infant in this feeding disorder.

Most of these infants are not brought for pediatric well-baby care but present to the emergency department because of an acute illness, when their poor nutritional state draws the attention of pediatricians. Because of their severe failure to thrive, these infants frequently require hospitalization. During the hospitalization, the psychiatric consultant is usually called in to assist in the diagnosis and treatment of the infant's growth and developmental problems. The evaluation should include an assessment of the infant's feeding, developmental, and health history, including any changes in the infant's behavior during the hospitalization. In addition, the mother's pregnancy, delivery, family situation, and social support need to be thoroughly explored. A mental status examination of the mother should be performed to rule out severe psychiatric illness, particularly whether she suffers from depression or is abusing alcohol or drugs.

Many of these mothers are elusive and avoidant of any contact with professionals. Consequently, the observation of mother–infant interactions may have to be obtained indirectly, through the report of other professionals who admitted the infant to the hospital. In a study of mother–infant interactions in infants with three types of developmental feeding disorders and matched control groups of well-feeding infants, Chatoor and colleagues (1997) observed that those with a feeding disorder of poor mother–infant reciprocity (feeding disorder of attachment) were characterized by poor dyadic reciprocity between mother and infant and by noncontingency of the mothers to their infants' cues.

Another important part of the assessment involves the direct observation and examination of these infants. Infants with feeding disorders of poor mother–infant reciprocity characteristically feed poorly, avoid eye contact, and are weak in the first few days of hospitalization. When picked up, they might scissor their legs and hold up their arms in a surrender posture to balance their heads, which seem too heavy for their little weak bodies. They usually do not cuddle like healthy well-fed infants, rather they keep their legs drawn up or appear hypotonic, like rag dolls. However, these infants appear to blossom under the tender care of a primary care nurse who engages with them during feeding and plays with them. They become increasingly responsive, begin to smile, feed hungrily, and gain weight. These striking changes in behavior of these young infants when they are fed and attended to by a nurturing caretaker are characteristic of a feeding disorder of poor mother–infant reciprocity and differentiate these infants from infants with organic problems that have resulted in growth failure and developmental delays. The infants with organic failure to thrive usually respond best to their mothers and do not show the avoidance of eye contact and general withdrawal so characteristic of infants with this feeding disorder.

Infantile Anorexia In this condition, the infant refuses to eat adequate amounts of food for at least 1 month, leading to significant growth deficiency. The onset of the food refusal under 3 years of age is most commonly during the transition to spoon- and self-feeding. Furthermore, the infant does not communicate hunger signals, lacks interest in food, but shows strong interest in exploration and/or interaction with the caregiver. Infants with this infantile anorexia are usually referred for a psychiatric evaluation due to food refusal and growth failure. The infants' food refusal usually becomes of concern between 6 months and 3 years, most commonly between 9 and 18 months of age, during the transition to spoon- and self-feeding. However, some parents report that even during the first few months of life, these infants were easily distracted by external stimuli and became disinterested in feeding. Then, the mothers were able to compensate for the infants' poor feeding by feeding them more frequently. However, by the end of the first year when infants are transitioned to spoon- and self-feeding, these infants take only a few bites and want to get out of the high chair to play. Most parents report that these infants hardly show any signals of hunger and seem more interested in exploring and playing rather than eating. Usually, the parents become increasingly worried about their infants' poor food intake and try to increase their infants' eating by coaxing, distracting, offering different food, feeding during play, feeding at night, threatening, and even force-feeding their infants. However, most parents report that these methods worked only temporarily, if at all, and that their infants continued to eat poorly in spite of all their efforts.

The diagnostic evaluation of this feeding disorder should include the infant's feeding, developmental, and health history, and the observation of mother and infant during feeding. In addition to the infant's history, the mother's perception of her infant's temperament, her family situation, her childhood background, and her own eating habits and attitude toward limit setting need to be explored.

Sensory Food Aversions In this disorder, the infant consistently refuses to eat specific foods with specific tastes, textures, and/or smells. Sensory food aversions occur along a spectrum of severity. Some children refuse to eat only a few types of food, making it possible for the parents to accommodate the child's food preferences. Others may refuse most foods, disrupt family meals, and cause serious parental concern about the children's nutrition. The diagnosis of a feeding disorder should only be made if the food selectivity results in nutritional deficiencies, and/or has led to oral motor delay.

It is also important to know that many children with sensory food aversions experience hypersensitivities in other sensory areas as well. Parents may report that the children do not like to touch food, have difficulty walking on sand or grass, refuse to wear socks or certain fabrics, or object to labels in their clothing. Many of these children are also hypersensitive to odors and sounds.

The evaluation of infants and young children with sensory food aversions should address how many foods the child consistently refuses and how many foods he or she usually accepts. A nutritional assessment needs to look not only at the anthropometric measures of the child to rule out acute and/or chronic malnutrition, but needs to address whether the child may lack adequate intake of vitamins, zinc, iron, and/or protein. In addition, an oral motor assessment needs to determine whether the child has fallen behind in this area of development. Delayed oral motor development will limit the kind of foods the child should be offered in order to prevent choking, and may be associated with a delay in speech development. In addition, the parents' food preferences during childhood and adulthood should be explored to assess whether the parents may be limited in the variety of foods they offer their child.

Posttraumatic Feeding Disorder   These children refuse to eat any solid food after they have experienced an episode of choking. This disorder is characterized by the infant's consistent refusal to either drink from the bottle or to eat any solid foods, and in most severe cases, by the infant's refusal to eat at all. Depending on the mode of feeding that the infants appear to associate with the traumatic event(s), some refuse to eat solids, but will continue to drink from the bottle; whereas others may refuse to drink from the bottle, but are willing to eat solids. Some infants may put baby food in their mouths, but then spit out any food that has any little lumps in it. Most infants get stuck in these food patterns and may lose weight or lack certain nutrients because of their limited diet.

Reminders of the traumatic event(s), (e.g., the bottle, the bib, or the high chair) may cause intense distress for some infants, whereby they become fearful when they are positioned for feedings and/or presented with feeding utensils and food. They resist being fed by crying, arching, and refusing to open their mouths. If food is placed in their mouths, they intensely resist swallowing. They may gag or vomit, let the food drop out, actively spit the food out, or store the food in their cheeks and spit it out later. The fear of eating seems to override any awareness of hunger. Therefore, infants who refuse all foods, including liquids and solids, require acute intervention due to dehydration and starvation.

In addition to a thorough history about the onset of the infant's food refusal and the medical and developmental history, the observation of the infant and mother during feeding is critical for understanding this feeding disorder and differentiating it from infantile anorexia and from sensory food aversions. It is helpful to ask the mother to bring a variety of foods, including those that the infant refuses and those that he or she accepts. Infants with a posttraumatic feeding disorder characteristically appear engaged and comfortable with their mothers as long as the feared food is out of sight. Some infants begin to show distress when they are placed in the high chair and they struggle to get away. In less severe cases, the infant might allow the food to go into the mouth but then spit it out and show distress only when urged to swallow. This anticipatory fear of food differentiates infants with a posttraumatic feeding disorder from anorectic infants, whose food refusal appears random and related to issues of control in the relationship with the mothers. Toddlers with sensory aversions to certain types of food might also show distress when urged to eat these foods. However, their mothers do not remember a traumatic event that seemed to trigger the food refusal behaviors.

Epidemiology

It is estimated that up to 25% of otherwise normally developing infants and up to 80% of those with developmental handicaps have feeding problems (Chatoor et al. 1994, Lindberg et al. 1991, Reilly et al. 1999). These common feeding difficulties include the infant's food refusal, eating "too little" or "too much," restricted food preferences, delay in self-feeding, objectionable mealtime behaviors, and bizarre food habits (Satter 1990). Dahl and Sundelin

(1986) reported that 1 to 2% of infants under 1 year of age demonstrated severe food refusal and poor growth.

Course

Few studies have investigated the natural history of feeding disorders. Dahl and Sundelin (1992) reported that those infants who at 3 to 12 months of age were identified for refusal to eat for at least 4 weeks with no apparent medical cause had significantly more problems in eating patterns, behavior, and growth, and were more susceptible to infection than the control infants at 2 years of age. At 4 years of age, 17 of the 24 children with early refusal to eat (71%) were reported by the parents as still having feeding problems. A study by Marchi and Cohen (1990), who observed a sample of more than 800 children for a 10-year period from early childhood to late childhood–adolescence, found that feeding problems in young children were stable over time. This study establishes the connection between feeding problems in early childhood and eating disorders later in adolescence.

Etiology

Feeding Disorder of Sensory Regulation   Both infant and maternal characteristics appear to contribute to the difficulties in the regulation of feeding. After birth, the infant needs to establish regular rhythms of sleep and wakefulness, and of feeding and elimination. In order to feed successfully, the infant needs to reach a state of calm alertness. However, some infants may be too irritable or too difficult to awaken for feedings. Other infants may tire quickly or become distracted during feeding and terminate feedings without taking in adequate amounts of milk to grow. Some mothers learn to compensate for these vulnerabilities by adjusting the environment and the degree of stimulation of the infant during feeding. However, other mothers become anxious, fatigued, or depressed, and consequently they inadvertently intensify the feeding difficulties of their infants.

Feeding Disorder of Poor Caregiver-Infant Reciprocity   Much has been written about mothers whose infants fail to thrive and appear to have a disorder of reciprocity. They are frequently described as suffering from character disorder, affective illness, alcohol abuse, and drug abuse (Fischhoff et al. 1971, Evans et al. 1972, Fosson and Wilson 1987, Polan et al. 1991). Glaser and coworkers (1968) suggested that the highest risk exists when the mother's needs take precedence over those of the infant. Fraiberg and colleagues (1975) suggested that difficulties of these mothers in nurturing their infants stem from the unmet needs of the mothers during their own childhood.

Family problems and distressed marital relationships have been reported in a number of noncontrolled and controlled studies of failure to thrive (Crittenden 1987, Benoit et al. 1989, Drotar and Eckerle 1989, Mitchell et al. 1980, Stewart 1973). Some authors also reported that mothers of infants with failure to thrive were more often abused by their partners or parents than were mothers of thriving infants (Crittenden 1987, Benoit et al. 1989, Drotar and Eckerle 1989, Mitchell et al. 1980, Stewart 1973, Weston and Colloton 1993). In addition, socially adverse living conditions, poverty, and unemployment are reported to be more prevalent in these families of infants with failure to thrive (Altemeier et al. 1985, Drotar and Malone 1982, Hufton and Oates 1977).

The growth failure of these infants with poor caregiver–infant reciprocity appears to be a critical manifestation of a failed relationship between a mother and her infant during the first year of life, when the foundation for mutual engagement and attachment is usually laid. A transgenerational pattern of insecure attachment appears to be at the root of the mother's difficulty to engage with her infant and leads to a lack of emotional and physical nurturance of the infant.

Infantile Anorexia Chatoor and colleagues (2000) tested a transactional model for the understanding of infantile anorexia by which certain characteristics of the infant combine with certain vulnerabilities in the mother to bring out negative responses and conflict in their interactions. They also found that infants with infantile anorexia were rated higher by their mothers on temperament difficulty, irregularity of feeding and sleeping patterns, negativity, dependence, and unstoppable behaviors than healthy eaters were by their mothers. The mothers of children with infantile anorexia were found to demonstrate more attachment insecurity to their own parents. The mothers' attachment insecurity frequently stemmed from extremes of parental discipline in the form of parental overcontrol or emotional unavailability while they were growing up. The infants' temperament characteristics, their mothers' insecure attachment to their own parents, and the mothers' drive to be thin themselves correlated significantly with mother–infant conflict during feeding (Chatoor et al. 2000). In addition, the more difficult the infants were considered to be by their mothers, and the more conflict mothers and infants displayed during feeding, the more malnourished the infants were.

It is helpful to look at infantile anorexia from a developmental perspective. Between 9 and 18 months of age, the general developmental task of separation and individuation takes on special significance in the feeding relationship. Issues of autonomy versus dependency must be worked out in the dyad, particularly during the transition to self-feeding. The mother and her infant need to negotiate who is going to put the spoon into the infant's mouth. In other words, the mother needs to figure out why the infant refuses to open his or her mouth, whether the infant wants to feed himself/herself or is satiated. If the mother is able to read the infant's signals correctly and responds contingently, the infant will learn to differentiate physiological feelings of hunger and fullness from emotional experiences such as anger, frustration, or the wish for attention. In this case, the infant's food intake will be internally regulated through physiological cues of hunger and satiety. On the other hand, if the mother is insecure in how to interpret the infant's cues and responds in a noncontingent way (offers the bottle when the infant is emotionally distressed or distracts the infant with a toy to slip food into the infant's mouth when the infant does not want to eat), the infant will learn to associate feeding with negative or positive emotional experiences. In the latter case, the infant's eating will be externally controlled through the infant's emotional experiences with the caretaker. Consequently, infants who are irregular and whose cues are difficult to read, and mothers who are insecure in how to interpret their infants' cues and respond in an inconsistent and noncontingent way, will develop conflict during feeding, and the infant will fail to develop internal regulation of eating.

Sensory Food Aversion Empirical studies have not explored the origins of selective food refusal in infants and toddlers. However, research with older children and adults has found that food preferences are related to taste sensitivities; for example, some individuals avoid particular foods because they find their taste and/or odor too aversive (Anliker et al. 1991, Bauer et al. 2000, Tepper and Nurse 1997). Some studies have documented that parents and their biological children can share taste sensitivities, and various models of heritability have been suggested, for instance, incomplete penetrance (Das 1958), multilocus and multiallele models (Morton et al. 1981), and a two locus model (Olson et al. 1989).

Posttraumatic Feeding Disorder Although it is difficult to say what the inner experience of a young infant might be, the affective and behavioral expressions of infants provide a window to their inner life. In a study of infants diagnosed with posttraumatic feeding disorder, also including a control group of healthy eaters and a group of anorectic infants matched by age, sex, race, and socioeconomic background, Chatoor and colleagues

(2001) observed conflict in mother–infant interactions during feeding in both feeding-disordered groups. However, only those subjects with a posttraumatic feeding disorder demonstrated intense preoral and intraoral feeding resistance. They appeared distressed, cried and pushed the food away in anticipation of being fed, and kept solid food in their cheeks or spat it out if the mothers were able to place any food in their mouths. The mothers usually reported that these defensive behaviors started abruptly after the infant experienced severe vomiting, gagging, or choking or underwent invasive manipulation of the oropharynx (e.g., insertion of feeding and endotracheal tubes or vigorous suctioning).

It appears that these infants associate painful or frightening experiences with feeding and then experience intense anxiety when they are exposed to food. Interestingly, several mothers reported that not only the infants' feeding but also their sleep was greatly disrupted after the traumatic events. The infants became more fretful during the day and woke up frequently during the night crying and appearing fearful.

Treatment

Treatment begins with the first contact with the infant and his or her caregivers. The establishment of a therapeutic alliance with the caregivers is critical to any successful treatment. The diagnostic evaluation needs to identify the specific dynamics of each feeding disorder in order to develop a specific treatment plan. This is discussed in more detail for each feeding disorder.

Feeding Disorder of Sensory Regulation Treatment of these infants needs to be individualized. It is necessary to take maternal as well as infant factors that have interfered with feeding into consideration. Treatment can be directed toward the infant, toward the mother, and toward the mother–infant interaction. In severe cases, if the infant's growth is seriously impaired, nasogastric tube feeding might have to be used to supplement oral feedings in an infant who tires quickly. This will allow an anxious mother to relax because her infant is getting adequate nutrition to grow. Subsequently, a more relaxed mother can tune into her infant more readily and break the cycle of dyadic escalation of tension during feedings.

On the other hand, the intervention might have to be directed primarily toward the mother to treat her anxiety, fatigue, or depression to enable her to be more effective in dealing with her infant. In addition, most mothers can be helped by assisting them in problem solving in how to facilitate a feeding environment that provides the optimal amount of stimulation for their vulnerable infants. Infants who are irritable and easily overloaded with stimulation should be fed in the quietest room in the house away from the telephone and other distractions. Videotaping the feeding and observing the tape together with the mother can heighten her awareness of the infant's reactions during feeding and enhance her ability to read the infant's cues. The therapist can then engage the mother in a dialogue on how to respond to the infant's cues most effectively. Because of the complexity of the factors that may contribute to this feeding disorder, the therapist needs to use a flexible approach when addressing both partners in the feeding relationship.

Feeding Disorder of Poor Caregiver–Infant Reciprocity Various treatment approaches have been proposed, ranging from home-based interventions to hospitalization in severe cases. In an intervention study that compared three treatment approaches (short-term assistance with social and economic problems, family centered intervention, and parent intervention), Sturm and Drotar (1989) found that none of the treatment methods was superior to the other in outcome. In a controlled prospective study of infants with failure to thrive by Black and coworkers (1994), infants were randomly assigned to treatment in a multidisciplinary feeding and nutrition clinic or to a home-based intervention by trained lay visitors. Children in both types of intervention improved their growth pattern; however, the mothers in the home-based intervention created a more child-focused home environment for their children with failure to thrive. Because of the complexity of the issues involved in the etiology of nonorganic failure to thrive, most psychiatrists and researchers suggest that multiple and case-specific interventions may be required.

During the hospitalization, a number of infant-directed interventions can be carried out while a more in-depth evaluation of the mother and the mother–infant relationship takes place. It is most important to assign a primary care nurse who can be warm and nurturing to woo the infant into a mutual relationship. Improvement of the infant's health and affective availability can then be used to engage the mother with her infant and in the treatment process. The mother's ability to engage her infant and to participate in the treatment process has to be at the core of the treatment plan. Ayoub and Milner (1985) reported that the degree of parental awareness and cooperation was predictive of outcome for failure to thrive.

Because these mothers frequently present with a variety of psychological and social disturbances, their problems need to be explored while nutritional, emotional, and developmental rehabilitation goes on with the infant. Many of these mothers have experienced neglect or abuse during their own childhoods and are, therefore, distrustful and avoidant of professionals. It is important to look for and identify any positive behavior a mother shows toward her infant and to use it as a building block to bolster her competence and interest in her infant. As Fraiberg and colleagues (1975) pointed out, nurturance of the mother is the first critical step in the treatment to facilitate her potential to nurture her infant. Not only does the mother need to be taken into consideration, but the family, in its relationship to the mother–infant pair and its social and economic support, also needs to be considered. As Drotar and Sturm (1987) pointed out, the family can serve as a stress-buffering or stress-producing system. The hospitalization of the infant provides a critical time to assess whether the infant needs to be placed in alternative care. In some situations of severe neglect or associated abuse, the case needs to be reported to protective services, which at times can be instrumental in mobilizing the family or in finding foster care.

Discharge from the hospital is a critical time when all services need to be in place to ensure appropriate follow-through of the treatment plan for these vulnerable infants. The treatment plan needs to be individualized for each mother–infant pair to make use of all the resources that can support their relationship. For some infants, daycare in a nurturing environment will give the mother an opportunity to pursue some of her own interests and needs as well as to make the time with her infant more special and enjoyable. Visits by a home care nurse or regular treatment sessions in the home by a social worker, as suggested by Fraiberg and colleagues (1975), are some of the alternatives to consider because many of these mothers struggle with coming to therapy in an office setting. Because of the complexity of the problems involved in the etiology of this feeding disorder, a flexible multidisciplinary approach that is coordinated by the primary therapist is usually most effective for both partners in the feeding relationship.

Infantile Anorexia The psychotherapeutic intervention is based on the developmental psychopathological model of infantile anorexia as outlined in the section on etiology. The major goal of the intervention is to "facilitate internal regulation of eating" by the infant. The intervention consists of three components:

1. Assess and then explain the infant's special temperamental characteristics and developmental conflicts to the mother to help her understand the lack of expected hunger cues and the infant's struggle for control during the feeding situation.
2. Explore the mother's upbringing and the effect it has had on the parenting of her infant to help the mother understand her conflicts and difficulties in regard to limit setting.

3. Explain the concept of internal versus external regulation of eating. Help the mother to develop mealtime routines that facilitate the infant's awareness of hunger, leading to internal regulation of eating, improved food intake, and growth. In addition, coach the parents to set limits to the infant's behaviors that interfere with eating. These feeding guidelines include:

   a. Schedule meals and snacks at regular 3- to 4-hour intervals and do not allow the infant to snack or drink from the bottle or breast in between.
   b. Limit meal duration to 30 minutes.
   c. Praise the infant for self-feeding but stay emotionally neutral whether the infant eats little or a lot.
   d. Do not use distracting toys or television during feedings.
   e. Eliminate desserts or sweets as a reward at the end of the meal; rather integrate them into regular meals and snacks.
   f. Put the infant in "time-out" for inappropriate behaviors during feeding (e.g., throwing the spoon or food, climbing out of the high chair).

These three steps in the treatment are best accomplished in three sessions lasting 2 to 3 hours each and grouped close together within a two- to three-week period. The intensity of this brief intervention facilitates a close therapeutic alliance between the therapist and the mother and gives the mother the opportunity to experience the support she needs to make major changes in her interactions with her infant.

This initial intensive phase of the intervention can be followed up by a telephone call and by a few visits spaced 3 to 4 weeks apart. It is helpful for the mother to have time and space to practice the new feeding guidelines and, at the same time, it is important for her to have the opportunity to check in with the therapist to clarify any questions or doubts she might have. Once the mother changes her rules with the infant, some infants adapt quickly and change their eating behavior within days, whereas others can be resistant and take weeks and months before they become fully aware of their hunger cues. The longer interval between appointments allows the mother the time to work with the infant on these changes without feeling pressured.

Thus far, only the mother and the infant have been taken into consideration. However, frequently the father, a childcare worker, or a relative is also involved in the infant's feeding. The intervention focuses primarily on the mother because in infantile anorexia, the mother's feeding relationship with the infant is seen as central. Nevertheless, the other relationships should not be overlooked.

Giving the mother the choice as to who in the family (or anyone else) should be included in the therapeutic process, and at what point, is part of putting the mother in control. Because many of these mothers have felt helpless as children and ineffective as parents, the empowerment of the mother is critical to the success of the treatment.

Sensory Food Aversion The research by Birch (1998) and colleagues (1982, 1990) indicates that in young infants (4–7 months of age), a few repeated exposures to new foods enhance the infants' acceptance not only of that food but also of other similar foods. However, this changes in the second year of life, when the acceptance of new foods only increased significantly after 10 or more exposures to those same foods. In addition, these authors found that novel flavors became more preferred after repeated pairing with high caloric carbohydrates versus low caloric carbohydrates.

When translating these research findings into clinical practice, it is useful to introduce a variety of foods during the first year of life when infants, in general, are less discriminating in their food preferences. However, if infants show strong aversive reactions (e.g., gagging or vomiting) early on when offered a certain food, it is advisable to give up on that particular food and not offer it again. If the infant shows a less severe reaction (e.g., grimaces or wants to spit out a new food), it is also best to stop offering the new food during that feeding, but introduce it again after a few days in a small amount and paired with some other food that the infant likes. It is important to increase the amounts of the new food very gradually until the infant appears comfortable with it.

For toddlers, the challenge remains how to keep them interested in trying new foods after they have had aversive experiences with some foods. Birch and colleagues (1982) have demonstrated that coercive techniques, for example, threatening children to sit at the table until they finish eating everything on their plate or depriving them of certain privileges, have a significant negative effect. On the other hand, toddlers are very responsive to modeling by their parents. Toddlers are more willing to try a new food if they can observe their parents eating it without being offered. If they ask for their parents' food, it is best to give them only a small amount while saying that they can have more if they like the food. If the parents stay neutral as to whether the toddler likes the food or not, toddlers remain neutral as well and do not appear to become scared of trying new foods. However, once children fear to try new foods, their diet becomes more and more limited and, by 3 years of age, most young children are not swayed by what their parents eat. Some young children like to imitate their peers and may be willing to eat new foods in a preschool setting; however, others become anxious in social situations and try to avoid eating with others.

Posttraumatic Feeding Disorder   Because of the complexity of many of these cases, a multidisciplinary team (consisting of a pediatrician or gastroenterologist, a psychiatrist or psychologist, a social worker, an occupational therapist or hearing and speech specialist, a nutritionist, and a specially trained nurse to serve as team coordinators) is best equipped to meet all the needs of these infants and their parents.

Before any psychiatric treatment can be successfully initiated, the medical and nutritional needs of the infant need to be addressed. In severe cases of total food refusal, it is important to act quickly to maintain the infant's hydration. The medical and psychiatric team members must work together to assess whether temporary nasogastric tube feedings are indicated or whether plans for a gastrostomy should be made. Unfortunately, the repeated insertion of nasogastric feeding tubes can intensify a posttraumatic feeding disorder, and an infant in a labile medical condition can take months if not years to recover. In less severe cases (if the infant drinks milk but refuses all solid food or, in a reverse case, refuses the bottle but accepts baby food from the spoon), the nutritional impact of a limited diet as such needs to be assessed and plans for nutritional supplementation need to be made before the psychiatric treatment is undertaken. Otherwise, the parents will be too anxious to engage in the treatment process.

The psychiatric treatment of this feeding disorder involves a desensitization of the infant to overcome the anticipatory anxiety about eating and return to internal regulation of eating in response to hunger and satiety. It is most important to help the parents understand the dynamics of a posttraumatic feeding disorder so that they can recognize the infant's anticipatory anxiety and become active participants in the treatment. After identification of triggers of anticipatory anxiety (e.g., the sight of the high chair, the bottle, or certain types of food), a desensitization by gradual exposure can be initiated as proposed by Chatoor and colleagues (1987), or a more rapid desensitization through more intensive behavioral techniques as described by Benoit and colleagues (Benoit and Coolbear 1998, Benoit et al. 2000) can be implemented.

With both techniques, it is important to have a professional assess the infant's oral motor coordination because many infants who refuse to eat for extended periods fall behind in their oral motor development due to lack of practice. Consequently, a 2-year-old may have the oral motor skills of a 1-year-old and will not be able to handle the chunky foods that require chewing. The rapid introduction of table food to a child who has delayed oral motor skills may lead to choking, thereby creating a setback to the desensitization process.

During the desensitization process, the infant has to be reinforced for swallowing the food. This behavioral manipulation of the infant's eating frequently leads to external regulation of eating in response to the reinforcers. Once the infant has become comfortable with eating, it is important to phase out these external reinforcers to allow the infant to regain internal regulation of eating in response to hunger and fullness. This can be a difficult transition because many infants gain control over their parent's emotions by eating or not eating. The techniques described under infantile anorexia—the implementation of the feeding guidelines contained in step 3—can be helpful in making this transition.

As summarized in Figure 9-1, each of these five feeding disorders presents with specific symptom patterns and characteristic mother–infant interactions that help diagnose and differentiate the various feeding disorders. The correct diagnosis is critical because a treatment that is helpful for one feeding disorder may be ineffective or even worsen another feeding disorder. These treatments are based primarily on clinical experience, and further empirical research is needed to establish which treatments are most effective for each feeding disorder.

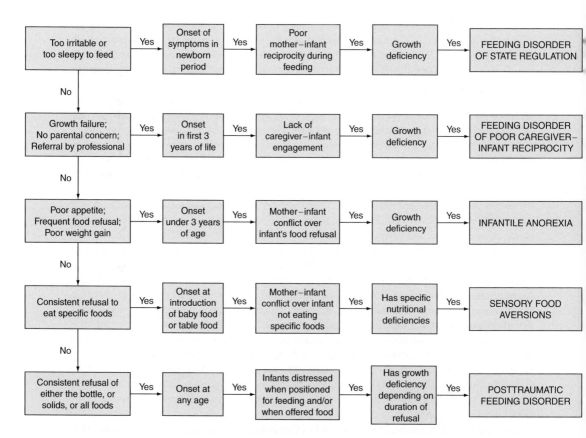

Figure 9-1 *Diagnostic decision tree for differential diagnosis of feeding disorders of infancy or early childhood.*

RUMINATION DISORDER

Diagnosis

Infants with Rumination disorder repeatedly regurgitate and rechew food for a period of at least 1 month following a period of normal functioning (see DSM-IV-TR diagnostic criteria below). Most frequently, infants who ruminate come to the attention of professionals because of "frequent vomiting" and weight loss. Some infants ruminate primarily during the transition to sleep when left alone, and their ruminatory activity might not be readily observed. However, these infants are frequently found in a puddle of vomitus, which should raise suspicion of rumination. Other infants can be observed to posture with the back arched, to put the thumb or whole hand into the mouth, or to suck on the tongue rhythmically to initiate the regurgitation of food. Most of the regurgitated food is initially vomited, but gradually the infant appears to learn to hold more of the food in the mouth to rechew and reswallow. "Experienced" ruminators appear to be able to bring up food through repeated tongue movements. They learn to rechew and reswallow the food without losing any of it. Their rumination can be inferred only from the movements of their cheeks and foul oral odor because of the frequent regurgitation.

DSM-IV-TR Diagnostic Criteria

307.53 Rumination Disorder

A. Repeated regurgitation and rechewing of food for a period of at least 1 month following a period of normal functioning.
B. The behavior is not due to an associated gastrointestinal or other general medical condition (e.g., esophageal reflux).
C. The behavior does not occur exclusively during the course of anorexia nervosa or bulimia nervosa. If the symptoms occur exclusively during the course of mental retardation or a pervasive developmental disorder, they are sufficiently severe to warrant independent clinical attention.

Reprinted with permission from the Diagnostic and Statistical Manual of Mental Disorders, Fourth Edition, Text Revision. Copyright 2000 American Psychiatric Association.

In addition to taking a thorough medical history, it is important to explore the onset of vomiting and the social context under which the symptoms developed. An acute medical illness or a stressor in the parents' life is frequently associated with the onset of vomiting. Some parents have noticed that the infant insists on putting his or her hand in the mouth, which makes the regurgitation worse, but most parents consider the infant's regurgitation vomiting and look for a physical explanation.

When exploring the stressors in the mother–infant relationship, one needs to be careful neither to alienate the mother nor to add additional stress to the relationship. It is best to observe the infant in various situations with the mother, with other caretakers, and alone in the crib during the transition to sleep. These observations will help in understanding how severe the rumination is, whether it is situational or pervasive. Some infants ruminate only when left alone or when stressed in a relationship; others appear so "addicted" to the rumination that they ruminate continuously after being fed, and they become distressed if interrupted in their ruminatory activity. In addition to assessing the rumination in the infant, the mother–infant relationship and the mother's life circumstances need to be evaluated because the mother's ability to soothe and to stimulate her infant is critical for successful intervention.

Epidemiology

Rumination disorder appears to be uncommon. It seems to occur more often in boys than in girls (Mayes et al. 1988) and also in individuals with mental retardation (Malcolm et al. 1997).

Course

The onset of rumination is frequently in the first year of life except in individuals with developmental delays, in whom the disorder may occur during later years. Rumination has also been reported to occur in adults with normal intelligence and in association with bulimia nervosa (Malcolm et al. 1997, Fairburn and Cooper 1984, Larocca 1988). In some infants and children, the disorder is believed to remit spontaneously (Reis 1994). However, electrolyte imbalance, weight loss, dehydration, and death have been reported to result from rumination, and rumination should always be taken seriously (Sajwaj and Agras 1974).

Etiology

Various etiological mechanisms have been proposed. Several authors have attributed rumination to an unsatisfactory mother–infant relationship (Flanagan 1977, Lourie 1954, Sheinbein 1975), including neglect or lack of stimulation, and sometimes to stressful life situations of the parent. Others have considered rumination a learned behavior that is maintained by special attention by the caregivers to the child's rumination and, consequently, the rumination has to be unlearned by counterconditioning (Lavigne et al. 1981, Winton and Singh 1983). Herbst and associates (1971) considered rumination one of the symptoms of gastroesophageal reflux. Through special radiographical techniques, they observed that the classic sucking movements of the tongue occurred after the entire esophagus was remarkably distended with refluxed barium. On the basis of their experiences with two adult women with a lifetime history of rumination, Blinder and colleagues (1986) postulated that opiate receptor insensitivity or reduced endorphinergic transmission may be implicated in rumination. Chatoor and coworkers (1984a) proposed a biopsychosocial model for the understanding of rumination. Rumination can be seen along a continuum: an infant may have gastrointestinal disease, such as hiatal hernia or reflux, and little psychiatric illness in the mother–infant relationship at one end of the spectrum; or the converse, an infant might have no reflux and severe psychiatric illness in the mother–infant relationship at the other end of the spectrum. Reflux or a temporary illness associated with vomiting frequently precedes the rumination. At some point, the infant seems to learn to initiate vomiting and turn it into rumination to achieve self-regulation. It appears that in circumstances in which the infant fails to elicit or loses either caring attention or tension-relieving responses from the caretaker, the infant resorts to rumination as a means of self-soothing and relief of tension. Once the infant has discovered rumination as a means of self-regulation, the rumination appears to develop into a habit that is difficult to break, like other habit disorders (e.g., head banging or hair pulling).

Treatment

Diverse theories of etiology have resulted in various proposed methods of treatment. Besides surgical intervention to prevent reflux and the early use of mechanical restraints, treatment has been primarily behavioral or psychodynamic or a combination of both.

On the basis of the assumption that rumination is a learned habit reinforced by increased attention for regurgitation, unlearning by counterconditioning has been suggested. Some authors have used electric shock after other methods had failed (Bright and Whaley 1968, Lang and Melamed 1969, Linscheid and Cunningham 1977). A number of alternative procedures of punishment, such as aversive taste stimuli (lemon juice or hot sauce), have been developed (Sajwaj and Agras 1974, Becker et al. 1978). Lavigne and colleagues (1981) have pointed to the difficulties of the use of aversive taste stimuli as punishment. Frequently, the infants are out of reach of the caretakers when they ruminate; consequently, the use of lemon juice or hot sauce is inconsistent, and this delays learning. Some infants appear to become adapted to these aversive taste stimuli. These authors suggest scolding the infant by shouting "No," placing the infant down, and leaving the room for 2 minutes immediately on initiation of rumination by the infant. If the infant is not ruminating on the caretaker's return, he or she is to be picked up, washed, and played with as a reward.

Whitehead and associates (1985) made a distinction between two behavioral causes of rumination: (1) reward learning through increased attention for regurgitation and (2) social deprivation. Whereas punishment with time-out may be necessary for the first type, these authors consider holding the child for 10 to 15 minutes before, during, and after meals as the treatment of choice for the second type. Richmond and Eddy (1958) were early proponents of a psychodynamic approach based on the assumption that rumination results from a disturbance in the mother–infant relationship. Mothers of ruminating infants were frequently found to be overwhelmed by their personal lives, which made them unavailable or tense in their relationship with their infants. Psychotherapy for the mother (Menking and Wagnitz 1969, Sauvage et al. 1985) and environmental changes that produce enhanced mothering (Franco et al. 1993) have been proposed.

Before embarking on treatment, Chatoor and coworkers (1984a) suggested looking at each child and the child's mother individually. The diagnostic evaluation needs to determine whether the infant's rumination is situational or pervasive, whether the infant has learned to ruminate because of little stimulation and gratification from the mother, or whether the rumination serves the infant as a way of relieving tension in a stressed mother–infant relationship. After an understanding of the mother's situation has been gained, treatment is best individualized by use of a combination of psychodynamic and behavioral interventions to enhance the mother–infant relationship in general, and to address the symptom of rumination in particular.

Pica

Diagnosis

Young children with this disorder typically eat plaster, paper, paint, cloth, hair, insects, animal droppings, sand, pebbles, and dirt (see DSM-IV-TR diagnostic criteria below). Because mouthing of objects is still common in toddlers between 1 and 2 years, the diagnosis of pica should be made only if the behavior is persistent and inappropriate for the child's developmental level. The diagnosis of pica should be explored in children with accidental poisoning, with lead intoxication, or with worm infestation. Young children with signs of malnutrition or iron deficiency should also be considered for the diagnosis of pica.

▄ DSM-IV-TR Diagnostic Criteria

307.52 Pica

A. Persistent eating of nonnutritive substances for a period of at least 1 month.
B. The eating of nonnutritive substances is inappropriate to the developmental level.

C. The eating behavior is not part of a culturally sanctioned practice.
D. If the eating behavior occurs exclusively during the course of another mental disorder (e.g., mental retardation, pervasive developmental disorder, schizophrenia), it is sufficiently severe to warrant independent clinical attention.

The assessment should include the history of the child's development, in general, and feeding in particular. Special attention should be given to other oral activities (e.g., thumb sucking or nail biting) that the child may use for self-soothing and relief of tension. In addition, the home environment and the parents' relationship with each other and with the child need to be explored to assess the parents' availability to nurture and supervise the child. Above all, mother and child should be observed during a meal and during play to gain a better understanding of their relationship and how the symptoms of pica can be understood in the context of that relationship.

If the diagnosis of pica is established, it is critical that the child undergo a thorough physical examination to rule out any of the complications associated with this disorder, such as nutritional deficiencies (especially iron deficiency), lead poisoning, intestinal infections (toxoplasmosis or intestinal parasites), or gastrointestinal bezoars (Sayetta 1986, Glickman et al. 1979).

Epidemiology

Pica is described as a common, but commonly missed problem by Rose and colleagues (2000). The onset of pica is usually during the toddler age between 12 and 24 months. Because infants commonly mouth objects, it is difficult to make the diagnosis in young infants. In a survey of 12- to 36-month-old toddlers in a pediatric clinic with a population representing a broad spectrum of races and socioeconomic backgrounds, Chatoor and associates (1994) reported that 22% of the mothers observed their children putting nonnutritive substances in their mouths. There was an almost linear decline of this behavior with age; 75% of 12-month-old infants were reported to put nonfood objects in their mouths, compared with an average of 15% of 2- to 3-year-old toddlers who engaged in this behavior. Most of these toddlers (88%) were good eaters, and their mothers had little concern about their growth. Estimates of the prevalence of pica among institutionalized mentally retarded individuals range from 10 to 33% (Danford and Huber 1982, McAlpine and Singh 1986).

The clinical profile of 108 children aged 1.5 to 10 years who practiced pica was compared with that of 50 children of the same age range without pica by Robinson and coworkers (1990). Of the children with pica, 85% were younger than 5 years; 29% were 1.5 to 2 years of age. The male/female ratio was 1 : 1.4. The most common form of pica was geophagia (eating of clay, dirt, or sand). The family history for pica was positive in 41% of the patients. The authors concluded that these children with pica were more susceptible to malnutrition, anemia, diarrhea or constipation, and worm infestation. Millican and colleagues (1962), who surveyed the prevalence of pica in three groups of children aged 1 to 6 years, reported that pica occurred in 32% of an African-American low-income group and in 10% of a white middle- and upper-class population; it was highest (55%) in a group of children hospitalized for accidental poisoning. Millican and colleagues (1962) observed that 63% of mothers with children with pica had pica themselves, and Gutelius and coworkers (1962) reported that 87% of children with pica had either mothers or siblings with pica.

Course

In many instances, the disorder is believed to be self-limited and to remit spontaneously after a few months. However, Millican and coworkers (1962) pointed to the seriousness of the developmental impact of the disorder in some children. The younger children were somewhat retarded in the use of their speech and showed conflicts about their dependency needs and aggressive feelings. Half of the adolescents evidenced some degree of depression; several had dependent or borderline personality disorders, engaged in other forms of disturbed oral activities (e.g., thumb sucking, nail biting), and used tobacco, alcohol, or drugs. Marchi and Cohen (1990) demonstrated a strong relationship between pica in childhood and symptoms of bulimia nervosa in adolescence.

Etiology

Various theories have been proposed to explain the phenomenon of pica. Organic, psychodynamic, socioeconomic, and cultural factors have been implicated in the cause of this disorder. Some authors have suggested that inadequate dietary intake of iron and calcium leading to abnormal cravings may induce pica (Crosby 1976, Johnson and Tenuta 1979, Federman et al. 1997). Reports that iron deficiency (Woods and Wessinger 1970) and a low-calcium diet (Jacobson and Snowdon 1976) induce pica in animals have supported this hypothesis. Other authors have implicated psychosocial stress, maternal deprivation, parental neglect and abuse, and disorganized and impoverished family situations in the etiology of pica (Lourie 1977, Madden et al. 1980, Singhi et al. 1981). In certain population groups, cultural acceptance of pica has been considered an important factor in the etiology of this disorder as well (Danford 1982, Forsyth and Benoit 1989, Vermeer and Frate 1979).

Millican and colleagues (1979) proposed a multifactorial etiology, whereby constitutional, developmental, familial, socioeconomic, and cultural factors interact with each other. These authors noted that the children who engaged in pica had experienced frequent separations from one or both parents followed by replacement of rapidly changing, inadequate caretakers who seemed to encourage oral gratification in response to the child's distress. They observed that these children showed a high degree of other oral activities (e.g., thumb sucking or nail biting) and also interpreted the pica behavior of these young children as a distorted form of seeking gratification caused by the lack of parental availability and nurture.

Treatment

In treating pica, one must consider the various factors that appear to contribute to the development of pica as well as its complications. It is important to treat the child medically while addressing the psychosocial needs of the child's family as well. The mothers need to be made aware of the dangers of pica and should be enlisted in providing a childproof environment. This might include removing lead from paint in old substandard housing units or instituting anthelmintic therapy for family pets (Sayetta 1986). Lourie (1977) proposed a psychoeducational treatment approach that, in addition to teaching the mothers the dangers of pica, would also provide social support to help them become more available to their children. Other investigators have used aversive and nonaversive behavioral therapy (Danford and Huber 1982), physical restraints (Singh and Bakker 1984), environmental enrichment with group or individual play (Madden et al. 1980), and time-out and overcorrection (Foxx and Martin 1975) to treat this disorder.

Comparison of DSM-IV-TR/ICD-10 Diagnostic Criteria

In contrast to DSM-IV-TR, which allows the diagnosis of Pica to be made in the presence of other mental disorders, if it is sufficiently severe to warrant independent clinical attention, the ICD-10 Diagnostic Criteria for Research for Pica exclude this diagnosis in the presence of any other mental disorder (except mental retardation). ICD-10 does not have a separate category for rumination disorder. Instead, it includes this DSM-IV-TR category within its definition of Feeding Disorder of Infancy and Childhood, which combines rumination with the persistent failure to eat adequately.

References

Altemeier WA, O'Connor SM, Sherrod KB, et al. (1985) Prospective study of antecedents for nonorganic failure to thrive. *J Pediatr* **106**, 360–365.

Anliker JA, Bartoshuk L, Ferris AM, et al. (1991) Children's food preferences and genetic sensitivity to the bitter taste of 6-n-propylthiouracil (PROP). *Am J Clin Nutr* **54**, 316–320.

Ayoub C and Milner J (1985) Failure to thrive: parental indicators, types, and outcomes. *Child Abuse Neglect* **9**, 491–499.

Bauer D, Santi AG, and Utermohlen V (2000) How individual differences in taste input impact smell and flavor perception. In *An Example of a Complex Process*, International Conference on Complex Systems, Nashua, NH.

Becker J, Turner S, and Sajwaj JL (1978) Multiple behavioral effects of the use of lemon juice with a ruminating toddler-age child. *Behav Modif* **2**, 267–278.

Benoit D (1993) Phenomenology and treatment of failure to thrive. *Child Adolesc Psychiatr Clin N Am* **2**, 61–73.

Benoit D and Coolbear J (1998) Posttraumatic feeding disorders in infancy: behaviors predicting treatment outcome. *Inf Ment Health J* **19**, 409–421.

Benoit D, Wang EE, and Zlotkin SH (2000) Discontinuation of enterostomy tube feeding by behavioral treatment in early childhood: a randomized control trial. *J Pediatr* **137**, 498–503.

Benoit D, Zeanah CH, and Barton ML (1989) Maternal attachment disturbances in failure to thrive. *Inf Ment Health J* **10**, 185–202.

Birch LL (1998) Psychological influences on the childhood diet. *J Nutr* **128**, S407–S410.

Birch LL, Birch D, Marlin D, et al. (1982) Effects of instrumental eating on children's food preferences. *Appetite* **3**, 125–134.

Birch LL, McPhee L, Steinberg L, et al. (1990) Conditioned flavor preferences in young children. *Physiol Behav* **47**, 501–505.

Black M, Hutcheson J, Dubowitz H, et al. (1994) Parenting style and developmental status among children with nonorganic failure to thrive. *J Pediatr Psychol* **19**, 689–707.

Blinder BJ, Bain N, and Simpson R (1986) Evidence for an opioid neurotransmission mechanism in adult rumination. *Am J Psychiatry* **143**, 225.

Bright GO and Whaley DL (1968) Suppression of regurgitation and rumination with aversive agents. *Mich Ment Health Res Bull* **2**, 17–20.

Budd KS, McGraw TE, Fabisz R, et al. (1992) Psychosocial concomitant of children's feeding disorders. *J Pediatr Psychol* **17**, 91–94.

Caldwell BM (1971) The effects of psychosocial deprivation on human development in infancy. In *Annual Progress in Child Psychiatry and Child Development*, Chess S and Thomas A (eds). Brunner & Mazel, New York, pp. 3–22.

Casey PH, Bradley R, and Wortham B (1984) Social and nonsocial home environments and infants with nonorganic failure to thrive. *Pediatrics* **73**, 348–353.

Chatoor I, Dickson L, and Einhorn A (1984a) Rumination: etiology and treatment. *Pediatr Ann* **13**, 924–929.

Chatoor I, Ganiban J, Harrison J, et al. (2001) The observation of feeding in the diagnosis of posttraumatic feeding disorder of infancy. *J Am Acad Child Adolesc Psychiatry* **40**, 595–602.

Chatoor I, Ganiban J, Hirsch R, et al. (2000) Maternal characteristics and toddler temperament in infantile anorexia. *J Am Acad Child Adolesc Psychiatry* **39**, 743–751.

Chatoor I, Getson P, Menvielle E, et al. (1997) A feeding scale for research and clinical practice to assess mother–infant interactions in the first three years of life. *Inf Ment Health J* **18**, 76–91.

Chatoor I, Hamburger E, Fullard R, et al. (1994) *In Scientific Proceedings of the Annual Meeting of the American Academy of Child and Adolescent Psychiatry*, Vol. 10. New York, p. 50.

Chatoor I, Kerzner B, Menvielle E, et al. (1987) A multidisciplinary team approach to complex feeding disorders in technology dependent infants, Presented at the Fifth Biennial National Training Institute. Washington, DC.

Crittenden PM (1987) Nonorganic failure to thrive: deprivation or distortion. *Inf Ment Health J* **8**, 51–64.

Crosby WH (1976) Pica: a compulsion caused by iron deficiency. *Br J Haematol* **34**, 341–342.

Dahl M and Sundelin C (1986) Early feeding problems in an affluent society: I. Categories and clinical signs. *Acta Paediatr Scand* **75**, 370–379.

Dahl M and Sundelin C (1992) Feeding problems in an affluent society: follow-up at 4 years of age in children with early refusal to eat. *Acta Paediatr Scand* **81**, 575–579.

Danford DE (1982) Pica and nutrition. *Ann Rev Nutr* **2**, 303–322.

Danford DE and Huber AM (1982) Pica among mentally retarded adults. *Am J Ment Defic* **87**, 141–146.

Das SR (1958) Inheritance of the PTC taste character in man: an analysis of 126 Rarhi Brahmin families of West Bengal. *Ann Hum Genet* **22**, 200–212.

Drotar D and Eckerle D (1989) The family environment in nonorganic failure to thrive: a controlled study. *J Pediatr Psychol* **14**, 245–257.

Drotar D and Malone C (1982) Family-oriented intervention in failure to thrive. In *Birth Interaction and Attachment*, Vol. 6, Klaus M and Robertson MO (eds). Johnson & Johnson Pediatric Round Table, Skillman, NJ, pp. 104–112.

Drotar D and Sturm LA (1987) Parental influences in nonorganic failure to thrive: implications for psychosocial management. *Inf Ment Health J* **8**, 37–50.

Evans SL, Reinhart JB, and Succop RA (1972) Failure to thrive: a study of 45 children and their families. *J Am Acad Child Psychiatry* **11**, 440–457.

Fairburn CG and Cooper PJ (1984) Rumination in bulimia nervosa. *Br Med J* **288**, 826–827.

Federman DG, Kirsner RS, and Liang Federman GS (1997) Pica: are you hungry for the facts? *Conn Med* **61**, 207–209.

Fischhoff J, Whitten CF, and Pettit MG (1971) A psychiatric study of mothers of infants with growth failure secondary to maternal deprivation. *J Pediatr* **79**, 209–215.

Flanagan CH (1977) Rumination in infancy: past and present. *J Am Acad Child Psychiatry* **16**, 140–149.

Forsyth CJ and Benoit GM (1989) "Rare ole dirty snacks": some research notes on dirt eating. *Dev Behav* **10**, 61–68.

Fosson A and Wilson J (1987) Family interactions surrounding feedings of infants with nonorganic failure to thrive. *Clin Pediatr* **26**, 518–523.

Foxx RM and Martin ED (1975) Treatment of scavenging behavior (coprophagy and pica) by overcorrection. *Behav Res Ther* **13**, 153–162.

Fraiberg S, Anderson E, and Shapiro U (1975) Ghosts in the nursery. *J Am Acad Child Psychiatry* **14**, 387–421.

Franco K, Campbell N, Tamburrino M, et al. (1993) Rumination: the eating disorder of infancy. *Child Psychiatr Hum Dev* **24**, 91–97.

Glaser HH, Heagarty MC, Bullard DM, et al. (1968) Physical and psychological development of children with early failure to thrive. *J Pediatr* **73**, 690–698.

Glickman LT, Cypress RH, Crumrine PK, et al. (1979) Toxocara infection and epilepsy in children. *J Pediatr* **94**, 75–78.

Gutelius MF, Millican FK, Layman EM, et al. (1962) Children with pica: treatment of pica with iron given intramuscularly. *Pediatrics* **29**, 1018–1023.

Herbst J, Friedland GW, and Zboraliski FF (1971) Hiatal hernia and rumination in infants and children. *J Pediatr* **78**, 261–265.

Homer C and Ludwig S (1981) Categorization of etiology of failure to thrive. *Am J Dis Child* **135**, 848–851.

Hufton IW and Oates RK (1977) Nonorganic failure to thrive: a long-term follow-up. *Pediatrics* **59**, 73–77.

Jacobson JL and Snowdon CT (1976) Increased lead ingestion in calcium deficient monkeys. *Nature* **162**, 51–52.

Johnson NE and Tenuta K (1979) Diets and lead blood levels of children who practice pica. *Environ Res* **18**, 369–376.

Lang PJ and Melamed BG (1969) Avoidance conditioning therapy of an infant with chronic ruminative vomiting. *J Abnorm Psychol* **74**, 1–8.

Larocca FE (1988) Rumination in patients with eating disorders. *Am J Psychiatry* **145**, 1610.

Lavigne JV, Burns WJ, and Cotter PD (1981) Rumination in infancy: recent behavioral approaches. *Int J Eating Disord* **1**, 7082.

Lindberg L, Bohlin G, and Hagekull B (1991) Early feeding problems in a normal population. *Int J Eating Disord* **10**, 395–405.

Linscheid TR and Cunningham CE (1977) A controlled demonstration of the effectiveness of electric shock in the elimination of chronic infant rumination. *J Appl Behav Anal* **10**, 500.

Lourie RS (1954) Experience with therapy of psychosomatic problems in infants. In *Psychopathology of Children*, Hoch PH and Zubin J (eds). Grune & Stratton, New York.

Lourie RS (1977) Pica and lead poisoning. *Am J Orthopsychiatry* **41**, 697–699.

Madden NA, Russo DC, and Michael FC (1980) Environmental influences on mouthing in children with lead intoxication. *J Pediatr Psychol* **5**, 207–216.

Malcolm A, Thumshirn MB, Camilleri M, et al. (1997) Rumination syndrome. *Mayo Clin Proc* **72**, 646–652.

Marchi M and Cohen P (1990) Early childhood eating behaviors and adolescent eating disorders. *J Am Acad Child Adolesc Psychiatry* **29**, 112–117.

Mayes SD, Humphrey FJ, Handford HA, et al. (1988) Rumination disorder: differential diagnosis. *J Am Acad Child Adolesc Psychiatry* **27**, 300–302.

McAlpine C and Singh NN (1986) Pica in institutionalized mentally retarded persons. *J Ment Defic Res* **30**, 171–178.

Menking M and Wagnitz JG (1969) Rumination: a near fatal psychiatric disease of infancy. *New Engl J Med* **280**, 802–804.

Millican FK, Dublin CC, and Lourie RS (1979) Pica. In *Basic Handbook of Child Psychiatry*, Vol. II, Noshpitz JD (ed). Basic Books, New York, pp. 660–666.

Millican FK, Lourie RS, Layman EM, et al. (1962) The prevalence of ingestion and mouthing of nonedible substances by children. *Clin Proc Children's Hosp DC* **18**, 207–214.

Mitchell W, Gorrell R, and Greenberg R (1980) Failure to thrive: a study in a primary care setting. *Pediatrics* **65**, 971–977.

Morton CC, Cantor RM, Cory LA, et al. (1981) A genetic analysis of taste threshold for phenylthiocarbamide. *Acta Genet Med Geme (Roma)* **30**, 51–57.

Olson JM, Boehnke M, Neiswanger K, et al. (1989) Alternative genetic models for the inheritance of the phenylthiocarbamide (PTC) taste deficiency. *Genet Epidemiol* **6**, 423–434.

Patton RG and Gardner LL (1962) Influence of family environment on growth: the syndrome of "maternal deprivation". *Pediatrics* **12**, 957–962.

Patton RG and Gardner LL (1963) *Growth Failure in Maternal Deprivation*, Thomas Charles C (ed). Springfield, IL.

Polan HJ, Leon A, Kaplan MD, et al. (1991) Disturbances of affect expression in failure to thrive. *J Am Acad Child Adolesc Psychiatry* **30**, 897–903.

Reilly SM, Skuse DH, Wolke D, et al. (1999) Oral-motor dysfunction of children who fail to thrive: organic or nonorganic. *Dev Med Child Neurol* **42**, 115–122.

Reinhart JB (1979) Failure to thrive. In *Basic Handbook of Child Psychiatry*, Vol. 2, Noshpitz JD (ed). Basic Books, New York, pp. 593–599.

Reis S (1994) Rumination in two developmentally normal children: case report and review of the literature. *J Fam Pract* **38**, 521–523.

Richmond JB and Eddy E (1958) Rumination. *Pediatrics* **22**, 49–55.

Robinson BA, Tolan W, and Golding-Beecher O (1990) Childhood pica: some aspects of the clinical profile in Manchester, Jamaica. *W Ind Med J* **39**, 20–26.

Rose EA, Porcerelli JH, and Neale AV (2000) Pica: common but commonly missed. *J Am Board Fam Pract* **13**, 353–358.

Sajwaj JL and Agras SL (1974) Lemon-juice therapy: the control of life-threatening rumination in a 6-month-old infant. *J Appl Behav Anal* **7**, 557–563.

Sanders MR, Patel RK, LeGrice B, et al. (1993) Children with persistent feeding difficulties: an observational analysis of the feeding interactions of problem and nonproblem eaters. *Health Psychol* **12**, 64–73.

Satter E (1990) The feeding relationship: problems and interventions. *J Pediatr* **12**, 115–120.

Sauvage D, Leddet I, Hameury L, et al. (1985) Infantile rumination: diagnosis and follow-up study of 20 cases. *J Am Acad Child Psychiatry* **24**, 197–203.

Sayetta RB (1986) Pica: an overview. *Am Fam Physician* **33**, 181–185.

Sheinbein M (1975) Treatment for the hospitalized infantile ruminator: programmed brief social reinforcers. *Clin Pediatr* **14**, 719–724.

Silver HK and Finkelstein M (1967) Deprivation dwarfism. *J Pediatr* **70**, 317–324.

Singer LT, Nofer JA, Benson-Szekely LJ, et al. (1991) Behavioral assessment and management of food refusal in children with cystic fibrosis. *J Dev Behav Pediatr* **12**, 115–120.

Singh NN and Bakker LW (1984) Suppression of pica by overcorrection and physical restraint: a comparative analysis. *J Aut Dev Disord* **14**, 331–341.

Singhi S, Singhi P, and Adwani GB (1981) Role of psychosocial stress in the case of pica. *Clin Pediatr* **20**, 783–785.

Stewart RF (1973) The family that fails to thrive. In *Family Health Care*, Hymovich DP and Barnard MU (eds). McGraw-Hill, New York, pp. 341–364.

Sturm LA and Drotar D (1989) Prediction of weight for height following intervention in 3-year-old children with early histories of nonorganic failure to thrive. *Child Abuse Neglect* **13**, 19–27.

Tepper BJ and Nurse RJ (1997) Fat perception is related to PROP taster status. *Physiol Behav* **61**, 949–954.

Vermeer DE and Frate DA (1979) Geophagia in rural Mississippi: environmental factors and cultural contexts and nutritional implications. *Am J Clin Nutr* **32**, 2129–2135.

Weston J and Colloton M (1993) A legacy of violence in nonorganic failure to thrive. *Child Abuse Neglect* **17**, 709–714.

Whitehead WE, Drescher VM, Morill-Corbin E, et al. (1985) Rumination syndrome in children treated by increased holding. *J Pediatr Gastroenterol Nutr* **4**, 550–556.

Wing JK (1973) International variations in psychiatric diagnosis. *Triangle* **13**, 31–36.

Wing JK (1979) The concept of disease in psychiatry. *J R Soc Med* **72**, 316–321.

Winton ASW and Singh NN (1983) Rumination in pediatric populations: a behavioral analysis. *J Am Acad Child Adolesc Psychiatry* **22**, 269–275.

Woods SC and Wessinger RS (1970) Pagophagia in the albino rat. *Science* **169**, 1334–1336.

Woolston JL (1983) Eating disorders in infancy and early childhood. *J Am Acad Child Adolesc Psychiatry* **22**, 114–121.

10 ● ● Childhood Disorders: Tic Disorders

It has been more than 100 years since Gilles de la Tourette first described the *maladie de tic* that now bears his name, Gilles de la Tourette syndrome (Tourette's disorder). In the past 30 years, efforts to increase awareness of Tourette's disorder and the other tic disorders, improve diagnostic accuracy, decrease stigma, and stimulate research have largely been successful. The tic disorders are much less rare than previously thought. Persons with tics, especially children, are able to live active, productive lives with less overt stigma, and the research in Tourette's disorder has become a model for research in other neuropsychiatric disorders. Current research efforts need continued support, but the next phase of the challenge is to develop a deeper understanding of the etiology and treatment of these often-complex disorders. In spite of significant scientific advances, clinical understanding and treatment approaches are sometimes inadequate for the difficult clinical problems that some of these individuals present with (Singer and Walkup 1991, Chase et al. 1992, Lombroso et al. 1995).

Diagnosis

Tourette's disorder is the most notable of the tic disorders. The cardinal features of Tourette's disorder and the other tic disorders are motor and vocal tics. Motor tics are usually brief, rapid, and stereotyped movements, but can also be slower, more rhythmical, or even dystonic in nature. Simple motor tics are movements of individual muscle groups and include brief movements such as eye blinking, head shaking, and shoulder shrugging. Complex motor tics involve multiple muscle groups, such as a simultaneous eye deviation, head turn, and shoulder shrug. Some complex tics appear more purposeful, such as stereotyped hopping, touching, rubbing, or obscene gestures (copropraxia). Vocal tics are usually brief, staccato-like sounds, but can also be words or phrases. Simple vocal tics, often caused by the forceful movement of air through the nose and mouth, include sniffing, throat clearing, grunting, or barking-type sounds. Complex vocal tics usually include words, phrases, or the repetition of one's own words (palilalia) or the words of others (echolalia). Coprolalia (repetition of obscene phrases), often incorrectly considered essential for the diagnosis of Tourette's disorder, is an uncommon symptom with only 2 to 6% of Tourette's disorder cases so affected (Robertson 1989).

Tics most often begin early in childhood, wax and wane in severity, and change in character and quality over time. Tics are exacerbated by excitement and tension, and can attenuate during periods of focused, productive activity and sleep. Tics are involuntary, yet because they are briefly suppressible or can be triggered by environmental stimuli (e.g., mimicking another person's movement, speech, or behavior), they may appear as volitional acts. Individuals with a tic disorder describe tension developing if a tic is resisted, which only subsides by completion of the tic. In some individuals, tics are preceded or provoked by a thought or physical sensation referred to as a premonitory urge (Leckman et al. 1993a).

There are four diagnostic categories included in the tic disorders section in DSM-IV-TR: (1) tourette's disorder (see DSM-IV-TR diagnostic criteria below); (2) chronic motor or vocal tic disorder (CT) (see DSM-IV-TR diagnostic criteria below); (3) transient tic disorder (see DSM-IV-TR diagnostic criteria on page 210); and (4) tic disorder not otherwise specified, which is a residual category for tic disorders not meeting the duration or age criteria of the other categories. In general, diagnostic decisions are based on whether both motor and phonic tics are present, duration of time affected with tics, age at onset, and the lack of another medical cause for the tics. Other diagnostic schemas have been developed for research purposes such as genetic and epidemiological studies and include special diagnostic modifiers (The Tourette Syndrome Classification Study Group 1993). For example, tic disorders that are not witnessed by a knowledgeable observer are deemed tic disorders *by history;* the modifiers *probable* and *definite* are added as estimates of diagnostic confidence of a tic disorder diagnosis.

DSM-IV-TR Diagnostic Criteria

307.23 Tourette's Disorder

A. Both multiple motor and one or more vocal tics have been present at some time during the illness, although not necessarily concurrently. (A *tic* is a sudden, rapid, recurrent, nonrhythmic, stereotyped motor movement or vocalization.)
B. The tics occur many times a day (usually in bouts) nearly everyday or intermittently throughout a period of more than 1 year, and during this period, there was never a tic-free period of more than 3 consecutive months.
C. The disturbance causes marked distress or significant impairment in social, occupational, or other important areas of functioning.
D. The onset is before age 18 years.
E. The disturbance is not due to the direct physiological effects of a substance (e.g., stimulants) or a general medical condition (e.g., Huntington's disease or postviral encephalitis).

Reprinted with permission from the Diagnostic and Statistical Manual of Mental Disorders, Fourth Edition, Text Revision. Copyright 2000 American Psychiatric Association.

DSM-IV-TR Diagnostic Criteria

307.22 Chronic Motor or Vocal Tic Disorder

A. Single or multiple motor or vocal tics (i.e., sudden, rapid, recurrent, nonrhythmic, stereotyped motor movements or vocalizations), but not both, have been present at some time during the illness.

B. The tics occur many times a day nearly everyday or intermittently throughout a period of more than 1 year, and during this period, there was never a tic-free period of more than 3 consecutive months.
C. The disturbance causes marked distress or significant impairment in social, occupational, or other important areas of functioning.
D. The onset is before age 18 years.
E. The disturbance is not due to the direct physiological effects of a substance (e.g., stimulants) or a general medical condition (e.g., Huntington's disease or postviral encephalitis).
F. Criteria have never been met for Tourette's disorder.

DSM-IV-TR Diagnostic Criteria

307.21 Transient Tic Disorder

A. Single or multiple motor and/or vocal tics (i.e., sudden, rapid, recurrent, nonrhythmic, stereotyped motor movements or vocalizations).
B. The tics occur many times a day, nearly everyday for at least 4 weeks, but for no longer than 12 consecutive months.
C. The disturbance causes marked distress or significant impairment in social, occupational, or other important areas of functioning.
D. The onset is before age 18 years.
E. The disturbance is not due to the direct physiological effects of a substance (e.g., stimulants) or a general medical condition (e.g., Huntington's disease or postviral encephalitis).
F. Criteria have never been met for Tourette's disorder or chronic motor or vocal tic disorder.

Specify if:
Single episode or **recurrent**

Before the 1980s, only people with the most severe and clinically obvious tics were diagnosed with Tourette's disorder. The majority of these individuals were adults who pursued care and were correctly diagnosed only when their tic symptoms were disabling and when classic symptoms such as coprolalia were present. Adults with milder tics generally did not pursue care and may have been stigmatized without the awareness of the cause of their movements. Children with tics were not identified at all or were identified as having other behavioral or psychiatric difficulties. Increasingly, as medical professionals and the public became more knowledgeable about tic disorders, mental health professionals began to see children at younger ages and with milder symptoms. Today, mental health professionals sometimes become involved even when the tics themselves are not obvious or even disabling. In today's clinical practice, the challenge is often not the treatment of the tics but identification of co-occurring and often more disabling psychiatric, behavioral, family, and school problems.

Clinical assessment of the tic disorders begins with identification of the specific movements and sounds. It is also important to identify the severity of and impairment caused by the tics. A number of structured and semistructured instruments are available for the identification of tics and the rating of tic severity (Kurlan and McDermott 1993). However, most of these instruments, such as the Yale Global Tic Severity Scale, are dependent on a clinical interview to collect descriptive data on the tics and resulting impairment (Leckman et al. 1989). Knowledge of the basic clinical parameters of tics and the course of illness dictates the evaluation. Questioning individuals with tics and their families about the presence of simple and complex movements in muscle groups from head to toe is a good beginning. Because vocal tics usually follow the development of motor tics, questions about the presence of simple sounds are next. Inquiring about the presence of complex vocal tics completes the tic inventory. It is helpful to elucidate other aspects of tic severity, such as the absolute number of tics; the frequency, forcefulness, and intrusiveness of the symptoms; the ability of the individual to successfully suppress the tics; and how noticeable the tics are to others. It is also important to know whether premonitory sensory or cognitive experiences are a component of specific tics because these intrusive experiences may disrupt functioning more than the tics themselves. Although the waxing and waning nature of the tics and the replacement of one tic with another do not directly affect severity, identifying the characteristic course of illness is important for diagnostic confidence.

Last, it is important to assess the impairment due to the tics themselves. Whereas tic severity is frequently correlated with overall impairment, it is not uncommon to identify individuals in whom tic severity and impairment are not correlated (Singer and Rosenberg 1989). Individuals who experience more impairment than their tic symptoms apparently warrant are a particular clinical challenge. A number of clinical features of tics are associated with impairment:

- Large, disruptive, or painful motor movements
- Vocalizations that call attention to the individual
- Premonitory sensations or cognitions that intrude into consciousness
- Tics that are socially unacceptable

Whereas tic severity and impairment are often correlated, many individuals with mild tics are most impaired by the comorbid conditions attention-deficit/hyperactivity disorder (ADHD), obsessive compulsive disorder (OCD), and learning disorders (see next section). An adequate assessment of these conditions is part of any comprehensive evaluation. The methods of assessment of these conditions are similar to those used in individuals without Tourette's disorder. The only exception is the assessment of tic-related obsessive–compulsive symptoms, for example, touching, tapping, rubbing, "evening up," repeating actions, stereotypical self-mutilation, staring, echolalia, and palilalia. Although these symptoms are often omitted from the traditional psychiatric and neurological review of symptoms, tic-related obsessions and compulsions should always be part of the routine evaluation of individuals with tics, OCD, or ADHD. Similarly, an evaluation of the child's school placement, intellectual capacities, and learning strengths and weaknesses is essential.

It is standard for any psychiatric evaluation to rule out all other psychiatric disorders. In complex cases of Tourette's disorder, the multitude of behavioral and emotional symptoms can be formulated in a number of different ways. Behavioral and emotional problems can be seen as components of the Tourette's disorder diathesis, as a reaction to having a chronic disorder, or as part of an independent psychiatric disorder that is complicating the clinical picture. Clinical formulations that oversimplify and do not consider the presence of multiple independent disorders may lead to incorrectly attributing unrelated symptoms to Tourette's disorder and may result in diagnostic imprecision and treatment failures. It is important to identify all possible psychiatric disorders in individuals with Tourette's disorder so that the hierarchy of disabling conditions can be identified and treatment initiated accordingly. Positive family history of another psychiatric disorder (e.g., major depressive disorder or panic disorder) may provide clues to the possible psychiatric disorder complicating the presentation of an individual with Tourette's disorder.

Psychosocial issues can play a role in tic severity and in overall adaptation and impairment. Assessment of family, peer, and school support for the youngster (adequate protection) along with assessment for the presence of opportunities to be intellectually, physically, and socially challenged is important. The balance between protection and challenge in children is critical for long-term development. An environment that is too protective decreases opportunities for building skills. An environment that is too challenging can lead to frustration, anger, and maladaptive coping.

Tic assessment requires a careful evaluation of observable tic symptoms. Interestingly, the absence of tic symptoms during an evaluation, in spite of the parent's or child's report, is not uncommon and should not necessarily lead to clinical doubt. Occasionally, an additional clinical observer (e.g., nurse or medical student) may identify tics more readily than the psychiatrist conducting the evaluation. Other than the observation of tics in the interview, there are no pathognomonic physical examination findings. Individuals with Tourette's disorder have been noted to have nonfocal and nonspecific subtle neurological findings ("soft" signs). If tic suppression with neuroleptic agents is considered, a more structured method of documenting the complex movements that are part of the pretreatment baseline evaluation is useful for following the progression of the disease and for subsequent assessment for neuroleptic-induced movements.

No specific laboratory or imaging tests are helpful in making the diagnosis or in assessing an individual with Tourette's disorder. Laboratory assessment is most often done as part of a routine health screen or in anticipation of medication interventions. Currently, laboratory testing for PANDAS (Pediatric Autoimmune Neuropsychiatric Disorders Associated with Streptococcal Infection) and group A beta-hemolytic streptococcal infections (e.g., throat culture, antistreptolysin titer, and screening for antineuronal antibodies) is experimental unless there are clinical signs and symptoms of acute infection.

Frequently Co-occurring Symptoms and Disorders

There is considerable evidence that there is a broad array of co-occurring clinical problems in clinically ascertained subjects with Tourette's disorder. These co-occurring problems can be more disabling than tics and are often the reason people with tics come to clinical attention. The nature and range of these problems is broad and includes problems with mood, impulse control, obsessive–compulsive behaviors, anxiety, attention and learning problems, and conduct problems. In some individuals, these problems reach diagnosable proportions, but in many others, they are less severe and do not fulfill diagnostic criteria. The most common co-occurring disorders are ADHD (50–60%) and OCD (30–70%). The exact relationship of these problems to Tourette's disorder is controversial.

Attention-Deficit/Hyperactivity Disorder   Upward of 50% of clinically ascertained children and adolescents with Tourette's disorder may be affected with problems of attention, concentration, activity level, or impulse control (Comings and Comings 1987, Pauls et al. 1986). In community-based epidemiological samples of subjects with Tourette's disorder, the estimated frequency of ADHD is lower (8–41%) than in clinic populations (Caine et al. 1988, Apter et al. 1993).

Obsessive–Compulsive Symptoms   Obsessions and compulsions are stereotyped, persistent, and intrusive thoughts and behaviors that are experienced as senseless. Because these thoughts and behaviors can be common in the general population, persons are considered "disordered" only when the obsessions or compulsions become severe, disabling, or time-consuming. Obsessions that are commonly seen in OCD include fears of contamination, fears of harm coming to oneself or others, scrupulosity, fear of losing control of one's impulses, counting, fear of losing things, fear of being unable to remember, or experiencing images of terrible things happening. Compulsions commonly seen in OCD include repeated or stereotyped washing and grooming rituals; repeated checking of locks, switches, or doors; and repetition of other senseless rituals.

Differences in clinical phenomenology have been noted in studies of obsessions and compulsions in individuals with Tourette's disorder compared with individuals with OCD (without Tourette's disorder) (George et al. 1993) (Table 10-1). Individuals with Tourette's disorder have greater concern with physical symmetry, evenness, and exactness, which are often described as "just right" phenomena (Leckman et al. 1993b), and concerns with impulse control. In contrast, individuals with OCD have more frequent concerns regarding contamination and more cleaning and grooming rituals than do individuals with Tourette's disorder. Also, the absolute number of independent concerns appears to be greater in individuals with Tourette's disorder than in individuals with OCD. Individuals with OCD more often have a single concern around which their symptoms coalesce, such as contamination. In contrast, individuals with Tourette's disorder may have multiple concerns, such as symmetry, violent or sexual images or urges, worries about losing control, or counting. Some investigators have argued that the obsessions and compulsions in Tourette's disorders are more sensory–motor in character, whereas those in OCD are more cognitive and affective (Miguel et al. 1993).

Whereas most cases of Tourette's disorder currently presenting for care are children, there are adults who seek a clinical evaluation as a result of having a child diagnosed with Tourette's disorder or learning about Tourette's disorder in the media. Often, these

Table 10-1	Obsessions and Compulsions Characteristic of Obsessive–Compulsive Disorder and Tourette's Disorder	
	Obsessive–Compulsive Disorder	**Tourette's Disorder**
Obsessions	Contamination Dirt and germs Body wastes Environmental	"Just right" phenomena Symmetry Blurting out obscenity Saying the right thing Violent images Sexual thoughts Embarrassment
Compulsions	Cleaning	Touching Blinking Repeating Self-injurious behavior Hoarding Counting Ordering

Source: Adapted from George MS, Trimble MR, Ring HA, et al. (1993) Obsessions in obsessive–compulsive disorder with and without Gilles de la Tourette's syndrome. *Am J Psychiatr* **150**, 93–97. Copyright 1993 American Psychiatric Association. Reprinted by permission.

adults have been able to function in spite of their tics. Others may have been given an incorrect diagnosis for their tic disorder or may have been in treatment for co-occurring psychiatric problems without any awareness of the relationship of those problems to the tic disorder. Even though these adults have not previously been diagnosed with a tic disorder, most are aware of their tics and may have experienced the psychosocial stigma commonly associated with a tic disorder. For these adults, a new diagnosis of Tourette's disorder may be psychologically complicated. The relief provided by knowing their diagnosis may be mixed with new questions about Tourette's disorder and its potential impact on their lives.

Epidemiology

Tourette's disorder has historically been viewed as a rare condition. Tic disorders, in contrast, are much more common. With the availability of improved epidemiological studies and more clearly defined diagnostic criteria, better estimates of the prevalence of Tourette's disorder and tic disorders are possible, but methodological issues in published studies remain. Tic disorders appear to be common ($>1:100$), whereas Tourette's disorder is less common ($5:10,000$), but perhaps not as rare as previously thought (Shapiro et al. 1988, Lucas et al. 1982, Caine et al. 1988, Apter et al. 1993).

In general, tic disorders are more common in children than adults, and people with mild tic disorders are much more common than those with severe, complex symptoms. Also, people with tic disorders may present for clinical attention with tics, but tics may not end up as the focus of clinical attention, as comorbid conditions are often more impairing than the tics themselves. Given these realities, the numbers of adults with persistent and severely impairing tics that warrant tic-suppressing medication is probably very small and may still be considered rare. A similar pattern is seen in children, with fewer children presenting with severe tics warranting tic suppression than children with mild to moderate tics and comorbid psychiatric disorders. Perhaps the most common are those children with transient tics that are not impairing and without comorbid conditions. This last group of children may never come to clinical attention.

Course

In Tourette's disorder, tic symptoms usually begin in childhood; mean age at onset is 7 years. The first tic may develop during the teenage years, but this is unusual. Motor tics of the eyes and face are the most common and the earliest presenting symptoms. In many individuals, the motor tics remain isolated in the face. When motor tics do progress, there is a tendency for additional tics to present sequentially from the head and face to the neck, shoulders, trunk, and extremities. Vocal tics tend to follow the development of motor tics. Complex tics of both types tend to follow the development of simple tics. Longitudinal studies suggest that tic severity is greatest in most individuals during the latency and early teenage years. Most individuals experience a decline in tic severity as they get older (Leckman et al. 1998) and only a small percentage of individuals (10%) experience a severe or deteriorating course (Bruun and Budman 1992).

The course of ADHD symptoms in persons with Tourette's disorder is similar to that in children without Tourette's disorder. ADHD symptoms usually begin earlier than the tic symptoms. Symptoms of hyperactivity attenuate before puberty, whereas problems with attention and concentration may continue into adulthood.

Obsessive–compulsive symptoms in persons with Tourette's disorder generally begin somewhat later than ADHD and tics, and may actually progress differentially from tic symptoms. Tic symptoms tend to improve into adulthood; obsessive–compulsive symptoms may actually increase in severity. Long-term studies of the course of obsessive–compulsive symptoms in persons with Tourette's disorder have not been done.

Table 10-2	Differential Diagnosis of Tics

Simple, rapid movements
   Myoclonus
   Chorea
   Seizures
Simple, sustained movements
   Dystonia
   Athetosis
Complex or sustained movements
   Mannerisms
   Stereotypies
   Restless legs

Source: Jankovic J (1992) Diagnosis and classification of tics and Tourette syndrome. *Adv Neurol* **58**, 7–14.

Differential Diagnosis

Tics have many characteristics that differentiate them from the other movement disorders (Jankovic 1992) (Table 10-2). Perhaps most important to "ruling in" tics as a diagnostic possibility is the childhood history of simple motor tics in the face. Other movement disorders do not have a similar pattern of movement onset or location. There are atypical presentations of tic disorders that may resemble other movement disorders, but these would be unusual and would probably require a consultation with a movement disorders expert.

Movement disorders such as chorea and dystonia are continuous movements and can be distinguished from tics, which are intermittent. Paroxysmal dyskinesias, although episodic, are more often characterized by choreiform and dystonic movements, which are different from tics. Myoclonic movements and exaggerated startle responses are also intermittent movements but are usually large-muscle movements that occur in response to a person-specific stimulus. Complex tics can be more difficult to differentiate from other complex movements such as mannerisms, gestures, or stereotypies. In a person with clear-cut motor tics, it may be difficult to differentiate a complex motor tic from a "camouflaged" tic (making a simple tic appear to be a purposeful action, e.g., an upward hand movement that the person turns into a hair smoothing gesture), mannerism, gesture, or stereotypy. Mannerisms or gestures are often not impairing; stereotypies tend to occur exclusively in children and adults with developmental disabilities and mental retardation (Jankovic 1992).

It is also possible to have a tic disorder and another movement disorder. For example, tic movements can co-occur with dystonia. Similarly, it is not uncommon in tertiary referral centers to see developmentally disabled children and adults with both tics and stereotypies.

Etiology

Genetics

Comparison of the concordance rates for Tourette's disorder in monozygotic and dizygotic twins identifies Tourette's disorder as an inherited condition. The twin studies, however, are unable to identify a particular mode of genetic transmission or the breadth of the clinical phenotype. To answer these questions, other research methods are required. Segregation analyses of family study data have been used to identify the pattern of genetic transmission and alternative phenotypes of the Tourette's disorder genetic diathesis. Despite the common conception of Tourette's disorder as an autosomal dominant disorder, this assumption is probably incorrect as more recent studies suggest a complex pattern of inheritance that includes multiple genes and environmental factors. Linkage studies of Tourette's disorder based on the assumption of Tourette's disorder as an autosomal dominant condition have been undertaken but to date have not been successful. Candidate gene studies based on the neurotransmitter hypotheses of the etiology of Tourette's disorder have also not been successful in identifying the Tourette's disorder gene(s). Recently, a large, federally funded sibpairs study of Tourette's disorder has published encouraging results.

Evidence from twin studies suggests an important role for both genetic and nongenetic factors in the development of Tourette's disorder. Two large twin studies (Price et al. 1985, Hyde et al. 1992) and a follow-up study (Walkup et al. 1987) showed high concordance rates in monozygotic twins for Tourette's disorder (both twins have Tourette's disorder) and for tic disorders (one twin has Tourette's disorder, the other has tics but not Tourette's disorder) (Table 10-3). In both the studies, the concordance rate for Tourette's disorder in monozygotic twins was more than 50%. When the concordance rates were calculated for the presence of any tic disorder, they approached 100%. By comparing the concordance rates of monozygotic twins with dizygotic twins, one can separate the role of genetic factors from other environmental factors. In the one study in which such a comparison was done, the concordance rate for Tourette's disorder in monozygotic twins was significantly higher than the concordance rate in dizygotic twins (Price et al. 1985), further suggesting a powerful role for genetics in Tourette's disorder.

There have been a number of family studies of Tourette's disorder (Comings and Comings 1987, LaBuda and Pauls 1993, Pauls and Leckman 1986, Eappen et al. 1993, Pauls et al. 1991). Although there are several studies suggesting Tourette's disorder being related to an autosomal dominant single major gene, more recent studies suggest that the condition has a more complex pattern of inheritance (Walkup 1996).

The results of the family and twin studies and the availability for research purposes of several large kindreds with multiple affected individuals stimulated great interest in genetic linkage studies. Despite a number of linkage efforts, no Tourette's disorder gene has been indentified (Conneally and Housman 1993).

Pursuing linkage at a specific site on the genome through the use of a candidate gene is another method for identifying the genetic locus of a given disorder. The choice of a candidate gene is often related to hypotheses regarding the candidate gene and the etiology of a given disorder. In Tourette's disorder, genes involved in the dopamine, serotonin and noradrenergic system have been perceived as ideal candidate genes because of the role of these medications in the treatment of Tourette's disorder and its comorbid conditions. To date, many candidate gene studies have been completed. The vast majority of candidate gene studies have not found an association (Heutnik et al. 1993). In those positive studies,

Table 10-3	Concordance Rates for Tics and Tourette's Disorder in Twins*	
Study	**Tourette's Disorder/Tourette's Disorder**	**Tourette's Disorder/Tic3**
Price et al. (1985)		
MZ twins $N = 30$	53% (16/30)	77% (23/30)
DZ twins $N = 13$	8% (1/13)	23% (3/13)
Walkup et al.[†] (1987)		
MZ twins $N = 18$	88% (16/18)	100% (18/18)
Hyde et al. (1992)		
MZ twins $N = 16$	56% (9/16)	94% (15/16)

* MZ, Monozygotic; DZ, Dizygotic.
[†] Follow-up study of Price and coworkers (1985), $N = 30$.

the candidate gene accounts for only a small portion of the risk and none of these studies have been replicated (Grice et al. 1996).

In the first Tourette's disorder sibpair study, approximately 100 sibpairs were assessed and two sites were identified with maximum likelihood scores (MLS) of >2 (>99/100 chance of being true). These sites identified were on chromosome 4q and 8p (The Tourette Syndrome Association International Consortium for Genetics 1999). Although these results are suggestive that Tourette's disorder genetic material may be in these regions, the level of certainty required for genetic studies is usually much higher. MLS scores of >3 (999/1000 chances of being true) are considered a minimum, but higher MLS scores >4 are associated with more confidence that a specific site actually contains specific genetic material. Subsequent to these findings, the Consortium has reviewed previous linkage and candidate gene studies as well as initiated new candidate gene and fine mapping approaches to look inside the regions identified through the sibpairs study. Given the lack of definitive findings in the first 100 sibpairs, plans are under way to collect an additional 200 to 300 sibpairs to enhance the power to identify multiple genes and gene of smaller effect.

Phenotypic Relationship with Other Disorders

Research efforts to understand the relationship of Tourette's disorder to other disorders have yielded conflicting results. Some studies support a broad Tourette's disorder phenotype that include commonly co-occurring comorbid conditions, whereas others identify a more circumscribed phenotype and define Tourette's disorder consistent with DSM-IV-TR diagnosis—impairing multiple motor and vocal tics of 1-year duration. The outcome of this controversy has implications for treatment, and also for the definition of what Tourette's disorder is.

For clinical purposes, it is recommended that clinicians use a narrow conceptualization of Tourette's disorder and describe other problems as they may or may not occur. In this way, each individual will carry diagnoses or problems that can be specifically described and appropriately addressed.

In the available research studies, there is general agreement that chronic vocal or motor tics are a milder form of Tourette's disorder and that some forms of OCD are an alternative expression of the Tourette's disorder genetic diathesis (LaBuda and Pauls 1993). ADHD is very common in clinically ascertained subjects with Tourette's disorder, but may not be as uniformly present in community samples of people with Tourette's disorder. Within the literature, there are two major hypotheses regarding the relationship of Tourette's disorder to co-occurring disorders.

(1) The putative Tourette's disorder gene is responsible for Tourette's disorder, CT, OCD, and some forms of ADHD in Tourette's disorder probands and their families. Other disorders that commonly co-occur in Tourette's disorder subjects are not associated with Tourette's disorder and are not part of the Tourette's disorder phenotype. The co-occurrence of these other disorders with Tourette's disorder reflects either ascertainment bias in the sample or the development of disorders secondary to living with Tourette's disorder.

The work of Pauls and colleagues best represents this viewpoint. After their seminal work identifying the genetic relationship of Tourette's disorder to CT and OCD (Pauls and Leckman 1986), this research group has undertaken efforts to identify the relationship of Tourette's disorder to other disorders commonly seen in individuals with Tourette's disorder. Pauls and colleagues (1993) found that first-degree relatives of probands with Tourette's disorder are at increased risk for ADHD. The results were interpreted as follows. ADHD in the absence of tics is not a variant expression of the Tourette's disorder gene. If the disorders do co-occur, and ADHD develops before Tourette's disorder, then ADHD is independent of Tourette's disorder. If ADHD develops after Tourette's disorder, then it is likely that the ADHD is secondary to Tourette's disorder.

Similar methods were used in a study of the co-occurrence of phobias, generalized anxiety disorder, panic disorder, and major depressive disorder in probands with Tourette's disorder and their families (Pauls et al. 1994). The elevated rates of affective and anxiety disorders in probands and their families compared with control subjects were primarily because of the presence of these disorders in subjects affected with OCD. Rates of affective and anxiety disorders were not elevated in relatives unaffected by Tourette's disorder, CT, or OCD, suggesting that affective and anxiety disorders were not alternative expressions of the Tourette's disorder gene but were related to OCD.

(2) The putative Tourette's disorder gene is responsible for Tourette's disorder and for the frequently associated psychiatric and behavioral problems seen in Tourette's disorder subjects.

The work of Comings and Comings (1987) best represents this view. They posited in a series of papers that a Tourette's disorder genetic factor is the underlying cause of Tourette's disorder and the comorbid conditions seen in individuals with Tourette's disorder. The results suggest that a number of disorders including ADHD, learning disorders (LDs), obsessive–compulsive behaviors, disruptive behavior disorders, affective disorders including mania, major anxiety disorders, addictive disorders, and a variety of impulse-control problems are associated with Tourette's disorder. In this sense, Tourette's disorder is considered a spectrum disorder similar to other psychiatric disorders (e.g., affective spectrum disorders) that appear to overlap clinically or to have genetic or pathophysiological similarities (Comings 1995). These investigators further suggest that the putative Tourette's disorder gene is the major etiological factor causing the disturbances of serotonin and dopamine that underlie all these psychiatric conditions even when they are not seen in association with Tourette's disorder.

Biological Factors

In Tourette's disorder, the complex clinical presentation suggests several neuroanatomical sites of disease as well as neurochemical substrates. Most speculation regarding the sites of neurological dysfunction in the tic disorders have focused on the basal ganglia and their interconnections with the frontal cortex and limbic system. Abnormalities in these structures could readily cause the wide variety of motor, sensory–motor, cognitive, and affective symptoms seen in individuals with Tourette's disorder. The complex phenotypic presentation seen in Tourette's disorder could also be produced by a neurochemical abnormality at various locations within this circuitry (Singer and Walkup 1991).

Increasingly sophisticated imaging methods, such as volumetric magnetic resonance imaging (MRI) and functional neuroimaging, have identified subtle abnormalities in the basal ganglia and its interconnections with cortical and limbic regions of the brain.

Two volumetric magnetic resonance studies identified the absence of the usual left–right asymmetry in the basal ganglia (i.e., larger left-sided basal ganglia structures in unaffected right-handed individuals), leading to speculation of hypoplasia or atrophy of the left basal ganglia in Tourette's disorder (Singer et al. 1993, Peterson et al. 1993). Other functional neuroimaging studies, such as single-photon emission computed tomography, have identified decreased blood flow to the basal ganglia (Hall et al. 1991), specifically the left lenticular region (Riddle et al. 1991). Positron emission tomography identified similar decrements of glucose use in the basal ganglia (Stoetter et al. 1992). Other studies have identified more specific areas of dysfunction. Areas associated with increased functioning in Tourette's disorder include the midbrain, lateral premotor and supplemental motor cortexes (Eidelberg et al. 1997), and areas associated with sensorimotor, executive, and paralimbic functioning (Stern et al. 2000). Areas associated with decrease functioning include the circuitry involving the caudate and thalamus, and their interconnections with the cortical and limbic areas (Eidelberg et al. 1997).

A number of neurochemical abnormalities have been proposed in Tourette's disorder in large part on the basis of responsiveness of symptoms to specific pharmacological agents. Tic suppression with dopamine blockers such as haloperidol and beta-adrenergic agonists such as clonidine have implicated the dopamine–acetylcholine and adrenergic systems, respectively. The serotonin system has been implicated because of the association of Tourette's disorder with OCD and the positive therapeutic effect of serotonin reuptake inhibitors in OCD. Reports of abnormalities in the opioid system are also intriguing. In general, the specific role of various neurochemicals and related receptors in Tourette's disorder is unclear. It is possible that they have a primary role or may be a secondary effect of another abnormality.

Much of the support for the role of dopaminergic overactivity in Tourette's disorder comes from studies of pharmacological agents that affect tic severity. Agents that diminish dopaminergic activity decrease tic severity in most individuals with Tourette's disorder. Conversely, agents that enhance dopaminergic activity (e.g., psychostimulants) have been associated with increases in tic severity. Speculation regarding the mechanism of dopaminergic overactivity in Tourette's disorder focuses on either dopamine excess or dopamine receptor supersensitivity. There is no direct support for dopamine excess in Tourette's disorder. However, the positive response of tics to dopamine receptor-blocking agents and early reports of low concentrations in the cerebrospinal fluid of homovanillic acid, the major dopamine metabolite, are suggestive of dopamine receptor supersensitivity (Singer et al. 1982).

There are few definitive studies on the role of other neurochemical systems in Tourette's disorder. The *serotoninergic system* has been implicated (Anderson et al. 1992) on the basis of postmortem brain studies that demonstrate trends toward decreases in levels of serotonin, its precursor tryptophan, and its primary metabolite 5-hydroxyindoleacetic acid, in subcortical regions (Anderson et al. 1992) in spite of normal levels in the cerebral cortex (Singer et al. 1990). These findings, in conjunction with presumably normal serotoninergic innervation, suggest abnormalities of the metabolism of serotonin and its precursor tryptophan (Anderson et al. 1992).

The *opioid system* has a role in movement control and is localized within the basal ganglia. A preliminary postmortem brain study identified a decrease in levels of the opioid dynorphin A in striatal fibers projecting to the globus pallidus (Haber et al. 1986). The finding of decreased dynorphin in brain tissue has not been replicated and is difficult to reconcile with a report of elevated cerebrospinal fluid dynorphin A concentrations in individuals with Tourette's disorder compared with control subjects (Leckman et al. 1988). The effectiveness of opiate antagonists in the treatment of individuals with Tourette's disorder is mixed; some investigators report improvement (Sandyk 1985), and others report few responders (Erenberg and Lederman 1989).

In several reports (Kiessling et al. 1993, Swedo et al. 1994), the development of tics as well as obsessive–compulsive symptoms in children and adolescents has been associated in time with group A beta-hemolytic streptococcal infection. The underlying mechanism is proposed to be similar to that involved in the development of Sydenham's chorea, in which antibodies developed in the course of infection cross-react with basal ganglia tissues, resulting in the characteristic choreiform movement disorder of Sydenham's. In Sydenham's chorea, there was often a time lag of 1 to 9 months between acute infection and the development of the characteristic movement disorder. Individuals with Tourette's disorder and OCD were described as having increases in tics and obsessive–compulsive symptoms in association with a recent history of a streptococcal infection or elevated antistrep antibodies.

Case reports have also described subjects with an abrupt onset or an exacerbation in symptoms occurring in parallel with antibody increases and with MRI changes in caudate size (Leonard et al. 1997). These cases have been given the acronym PANDAS (Swedo et al. 1998). These preliminary findings link the development of a movement disorder and psychiatric symptoms to an infectious agent and autoimmune processes, and suggest new and alternative treatments including the potential for vaccines for Tourette's disorder and OCD.

Environmental Factors

Whereas the evidence for a genetic etiology of Tourette's disorder is compelling, there is also evidence that environmental factors may play a role in tic symptom expression. To date, studies have not identified any specific factors that cause Tourette's disorder, yet it is increasingly clear that environmental factors have an impact on tic severity and, perhaps, even on the types of symptoms expressed. Clinical wisdom suggests that tic severity increases in response to stressful (e.g., examinations) or exciting life experiences (e.g., amusement parks). It is also not uncommon for persons with Tourette's disorder to be able to identify a particular environmental stimulus that initiated either a bout of symptoms or a new tic symptom.

Psychosocial and Developmental Factors

Psychosocial issues do not play a large etiological role in the development of the tic disorders; however, psychosocial issues do play a major role in adaptation and impairment in Tourette's disorder and are often the focus of treatment and rehabilitative efforts. Clinical work that involves the family, friends, school, and workplace is often the bedrock of treatment in an individual with Tourette's disorder. Many of the psychosocial issues in Tourette's disorder are not unique but are shared by other neuropsychiatric disorders.

For children with Tourette's disorder, the onset of symptoms occurs early in development and directly affects family life and relationships with peers and schoolmates. The diagnostic label of Tourette's disorder can be helpful for understanding the nature of a youngster's problems and can communicate the need to protect the youngster from excessive adversity. The diagnostic label can, however, be a problem. There is a tension between protecting a child with Tourette's disorder from adversity and ensuring that the child encounters and masters life's challenges. If the diagnostic label of Tourette's disorder offers too much protection, a child may run the risk of not developing a strong and complex identity adequate for the rigors of adult life. Today's children with Tourette's disorder will need to function at their highest level as adults in spite of having Tourette's disorder symptoms. Support from parents for mastering the challenges of development is key to long-term functioning of children with Tourette's disorder.

The transition to adulthood is difficult enough for most young people, but young adults with Tourette's disorder have a particular challenge. The transition to adulthood often occurs when an important component of their early experience and identity (i.e., Tourette's disorder) begins to show some improvement. Young adults most vulnerable during this transition are those who, as a result of their Tourette's disorder, did not develop the foundations of an adult identity as a child. These adults often face the rigors of adult life without the necessary skills to manage, but also without the presence of tic symptoms of sufficient severity to explain their impairment (see section on course of illness).

Today's adult with Tourette's disorder belongs to a different cohort than today's child with Tourette's disorder. As a result, they also have different needs. Most adults with

Tourette's disorder were not diagnosed in childhood. They did not have the "protection" of the diagnosis and often experienced significant confusion, isolation, and discrimination. Some adults with Tourette's disorder have significant anger, resentment, and distrust related to their early life experiences including ineffective treatments, which can have an impact on current functioning. Many adults who appear to function well in spite of their Tourette's disorder may be doing so at an emotional cost.

Treatment

The initiation of treatment can be a delicate process, given the difficulties individuals with tics and their families experience before finding appropriate care. Most families are frightened about their child's having a neuropsychiatric disorder and envision a grim prognosis. After the evaluation is completed, often in the first session, general education of the individual and family about the course of the tic disorder is essential (Table 10-4). Most children and families are relieved to hear that the majority of persons with tics have consistent improvement in tic severity as they move through their teenage years and into adulthood. They are also pleased to hear that tic symptoms are not inherently impairing. In this regard, it is often helpful to cite examples of sports personalities or other public figures who have identified themselves as having Tourette's disorder and are doing well both personally and professionally.

Once issues regarding the tics are discussed and clarified, the focus shifts to the presence of comorbid conditions. Identifying whether ADHD, LD, and OCD are present is especially important because they are often the more common impairing conditions in these children. Yet the transition to addressing the co-occurring problems is often not easy. Individuals, families, and mental health professionals are usually focused on the tic symptoms. Tics are more readily apparent and relatively easy to suppress with medications, whereas the co-occurring conditions, especially if they are internalizing disorders, are easy to overlook. One of the major pitfalls of treatment of individuals with Tourette's disorder is to pursue tic suppression to the exclusion of the treatment of other co-occurring conditions that are present and possibly more impairing.

It is also possible that other psychiatric disorders that are not traditionally thought to be part of the tic disorders will co-occur in individuals with Tourette's disorder. Psychoeducation regarding the role of comorbid conditions in the individual's current presentation is useful for targeting treatment (Table 10-5).

Creating the hierarchy of the most impairing conditions is the next major step in treatment. Most clinicians, as part of their formulation, create some clinical hierarchy; yet in Tourette's disorder, with the multitude of often-complex problems, it is essential that a conscious effort be made to formulate, organize, and create hierarchies for treatment. For example, children with moderate tics and separation anxiety with school refusal should be considered for a treatment with selective serotonin reuptake inhibitor (SSRI) for their separation anxiety rather than neuroleptics for tic suppression (The Research Unit on Pediatric Psychopharmacology Anxiety Study Group 2001). It is possible that with successful treatment of the anxiety disorder, the individual may also experience a reduction in tic severity.

Table 10-4	Goals of Treatment
Educate the patient and family about tic disorders.	
Define the co-occurring disorders.	
Create a hierarchy of the clinically impairing conditions.	
Treat the impairing conditions using somatic, psychological, and rehabilitative approaches.	
Aid in creating a supportive yet challenging psychosocial milieu.	

Table 10-5	Complex Clinical Presentations in Tourette's Disorder
Tics + ADHD + OCD + LD + major depressive disorder	
Tics + ADHD + OCD + LD + separation anxiety disorder	
Tics + ADHD + OCD + LD + panic disorder	
Tics + ADHD + OCD + LD + bipolar disorder	
Tics + ADHD + OCD + LD + autism–pervasive developmental disorder	
Tics + ADHD + OCD + LD + substance abuse	
Tics + ADHD + OCD + LD + conduct disorder	
Tics + ADHD + OCD + LD + personality disorders	

Somatic Treatments

This section focuses on the basic strategies for tic suppression and treatment of the common co-occurring disorders. Particular emphasis is placed on the complexities of clinical treatment.

The goal of pharmacological treatment is the reduction of tic severity, not necessarily the elimination of tics. Haloperidol has been used effectively to suppress motor and phonic tics for more than 30 years. Since that time, a number of other neuroleptic agents have also been identified as useful in tic suppression, including fluphenazine and pimozide. In Europe, the substituted benzamides, sulpiride and tiapride, and the nonneuroleptic tetrabenazine have also been shown to be useful. As new neuroleptic agents become available, clinical trials for tic suppression invariably occur. Preliminary results with risperidone have been mixed, whereas trials with clozapine are more uniformly negative (Chappel et al. 1995). The major drawback with neuroleptic agents is the frequent and significant side effects, which often preclude continued use of the medication.

There are continuing efforts to identify tic-suppressing agents with tolerable side effects. Most frequently cited in this regard are the alpha-adrenergic agonists clonidine and guanfacine. Both of these agents were developed as antihypertensives. These agents do not appear to be uniformly effective in tic suppression, but they can be effective for some individuals without significant side effects. Both clonidine and guanfacine also appear to be useful for some of the symptoms of ADHD, which makes these agents a reasonable first choice for those individuals with both Tourette's disorder and ADHD.

Haloperidol Haloperidol is a high-potency neuroleptic that preferentially blocks dopamine D_2 receptors. Historically, haloperidol has been the most frequently used medication for tic suppression. It is effective in a clear majority of individuals, although relatively few individuals are willing to tolerate the side effects to obtain the tic-suppressing benefits. Neuroleptics are often effective at low doses, and low doses minimize side effects. For haloperidol, doses in the range of 0.5 to 2.0 mg/day are usually adequate. Starting dosages are low (0.25–0.5 mg/day), with small increases in dose (0.25–0.5 mg/day) every 5 to 7 days. Most often the medication is given at bedtime, but with low doses, some individuals may require twice-a-day dosing for good tic control.

Side effects with all neuroleptics are common and are the reason that neuroleptics are not used by the majority of individuals with Tourette's disorder. Side effects include those traditionally seen with neuroleptics, such as sedation, acute dystonic reactions, extrapyramidal symptoms including akathisia, weight gain, cognitive dulling, and the common anticholinergic side effects. There have also been reports of subtle, difficult-to-recognize side effects with neuroleptics, including clinical depression, separation anxiety, panic attacks, and school avoidance (Bruun 1988).

Dosage reduction is the most prudent response to side effects, although the addition of medications such as benztropine for the extrapyramidal symptoms can be useful. Dosage reduction in those children with Tourette's disorder who have been administered neuroleptics long-term may be complicated by withdrawal dyskinesias and significant tic worsening or rebound. Withdrawal dyskinesias are choreoathetoid movements of the orofacial region, trunk, and extremities that appear after neuroleptic discontinuation or dosage reduction and tend to resolve in 1 to 3 months. Tic worsening even above pretreatment baseline level (i.e., rebound) can last up to 1 to 3 months after discontinuation or dosage reduction. Tardive dyskinesia, which is similar in character to withdrawal dyskinesia, most often develops during the course of treatment or is "unmasked" with dosage reductions. Rarely have cases of tardive dyskinesia been reported to occur in individuals with Tourette's disorder.

Fluphenazine Whereas fluphenazine has never undergone controlled trials, clinical experience suggests that it has somewhat fewer side effects than haloperidol. Fluphenazine has both dopamine D_1 and D_2 receptor-blocking activity, and the side effect profile is similar to that of haloperidol. Approaches to treatment are also similar, that is, treatment begins with low doses and slow upward dosage adjustments, while benefits are balanced with side effects. Fluphenazine is slightly less potent than haloperidol so that starting doses are somewhat higher (0.5–1 mg/day), as are treatment doses (3–5 mg/day).

Pimozide Pimozide is a potent and specific blocker of dopamine D_2 receptors. Its side effect profile is generally similar to that of the other neuroleptics, although it has fewer sedative and extrapyramidal side effects than haloperidol. In contrast to either haloperidol or fluphenazine, pimozide has calcium channel blocking properties that affect cardiac conduction, as evidenced by changes in the electrocardiogram. The coadministration of other medications that affect cardiac conduction, such as the tricyclic antidepressants (TCAs), is generally contraindicated. Baseline and follow-up electrocardiograms are important for adequate management of individuals. Beginning treatment with a dose of 1 mg/day is prudent, although with pimozide's long half-life, every-other-day dosing can be used to decrease the effective daily dose. Increases of up to 1 mg/day can occur every 5 to 7 days until symptoms are controlled. Most individuals experience clinical benefit with few side effects with doses of 1 to 4 mg/day. Higher doses can be associated with more side effects. In a comparison of pimozide, haloperidol, and no drug in individuals with Tourette's disorder and ADHD, pimozide at 1 to 4 mg/day was useful in decreasing tics and improving some aspects of cognition that are commonly impaired in ADHD (Sallee and Rock 1994). The potential to have impact on both Tourette's disorder and ADHD symptoms with a single drug is a clear advantage that pimozide may have over other neuroleptics.

Sulpiride and Tiapride Both of these agents are substituted benzamides available only in Europe. Like pimozide, they are unique in their combination of relatively specific dopamine D_2 receptor-blocking activity and the potential for reduced risk of extrapyramidal symptoms and tardive dyskinesia. Both agents have demonstrated efficacy in tic suppression (Eggers et al. 1988, Robertson et al. 1990). It is unlikely that these agents will become available in the United States.

Atypical Neuroleptics The atypical neuroleptics appear to have replaced the standard neuroleptics as the mainstay of treatment for the psychotic disorders. Given the potentially lower risk for tardive dyskinesia with these agents, their efficacy has been assessed for tic suppression in individuals with Tourette's disorder. To date, there are only small controlled or open trials to guide the clinician in the use of these agents. Clozapine does not appear to be effective as a tic-suppressing agent and its hematogological side effects preclude its use. Risperidone has been effective in reducing tic symptoms severity in one controlled trial (Dion et al. 2002) and may have the added benefit of augmenting SSRIs in treating tic-related OCD.

Olanzapine in low doses does not appear to have the same tic-suppressing power as the typical neuroleptics, which may be related to olanzapine's relatively weak dopamine D_2 blocking activity. Studies of quetiapine have not been conducted to date. The side effects, especially weight gain, have dampened the enthusiasm for the atypicals risperidone, olanzapine, and quetiapine. In one of the larger placebo-controlled trials ($N = 56$) of the new neuroleptics, ziprasidone was found to be effective in reducing tic symptoms. The mean dose was low 28 ± 10 mg/day. There were few side effects including a low incidence of weight gain. Concern regarding the impact of ziprasidone on cardiac conduction times, especially QTc, was not supported in this trial (Gilbert et al. 2000).

Clonidine and Guanfacine   There is a long history of the use of the alpha-adrenergic agonist clonidine for suppression of tics and ADHD symptoms. Whereas controlled trials have shown that some individuals benefit with symptom reduction, the overall effect of clonidine for tic suppression and ADHD is more modest than that achieved with the "gold standards" (haloperidol and the stimulants, respectively) for these conditions (Goetz 1993). Given clonidine's mild side effect profile, it is often the first drug used for tic suppression, especially in those children with Tourette's disorder and ADHD. Treatment is initiated at 0.025 mg/day and increased in increments of 0.025 to 0.05 mg/day every 3 to 5 days or as side effects (sedation) allow. Usual effective treatment doses are in the range of 0.1 to 0.3 mg/day and are given in divided doses (4–6 hours apart). Higher doses are associated with side effects, primarily sedation, and are not necessarily more effective. The onset of action is slower for tic suppression (3–6 weeks) than for ADHD symptoms. Side effects, in addition to sedation, include irritability, headaches, decreased salivation, and hypotension and dizziness at higher doses. Interestingly, owing to clonidine's short half-life, some individuals experience mild withdrawal symptoms between doses. More severe rebound in autonomic activity and tics can occur if the medication is discontinued abruptly (Leckman et al. 1986). Some individuals find that clonidine in the transdermal patch form provides a more stable clinical effect and avoid multiple doses each day. Children are usually stabilized on oral doses before they are switched to the patch. A rash at the site of the patch is a common, but manageable, complication of the treatment.

Guanfacine is an alpha-2-adrenergic agonist that potentially offers greater benefit than clonidine because of differences in site of action, side effects, and duration of action. In nonhuman primates, guanfacine appears to bind preferentially with alpha-2-adrenergic receptors in prefrontal cortical regions associated with attentional and organizational functions (Arnsten et al. 1988). On the basis of these animal models, it is hypothesized that guanfacine is likely to have a greater impact on attention without the significant sedation associated with the nonselective alpha-2-adrenergic agonist clonidine. Guanfacine's long half-life offers the advantage of twice-a-day dosing, which is more convenient than the multiple dosing required with clonidine. In a randomized, placebo-controlled trial ($N = 31$) of children with tics and ADHD, guanfacine in doses up to 0.3 mg/day had an average 31% reduction in tic severity compared to no reduction on placebo. Clinically, the effect on tics is less than would be expected on neuroleptics (Scahill et al. 2001).

Benzodiazepines   Benzodiazepines can be useful in decreasing comorbid anxiety in individuals with Tourette's disorder. In addition, clonazepam appears also to be useful in selected individuals for tic reduction. Often, doses of 3 to 6 mg/day may be necessary for tic reduction. Because sedation is a significant side effect at these dosages, an extended titration phase of 3 to 6 months may be necessary. Similarly, a slow taper is required to avoid withdrawal symptoms (Goetz 1992).

Pergolide Agonist activity on presynaptic dopamine neurons results in decreased dopamine release and may therefore result in decreased tic severity in people with Tourette's disorder. To exploit this finding, a number of small open trials of dopamine agonists and a small controlled trial of pergolide ($N = 24$) have been conducted. Pergolide, a mixed D_1–D_2–D_3 dopamine agonist often used for restless leg syndrome, was found to be superior to placebo in reducing tic severity and was associated with few adverse events (Gilbert et al. 2000). Doses used were low, as higher doses may be associated with dopamine agonist effects postsynaptically.

Baclofen Baclofen, a muscle relaxant, is GABA-B receptor agonist that acts presynaptically to inhibit the release of excitatory amino acids such as glutamate. In a small placebo-controlled crossover trial ($N = 10$), baclofen 20 mg t.i.d. was not found to be effective in reducing tic severity but did appear to have an effect on tic-related impairment (Singer et al. 2001).

Psychosocial Treatments

Published studies of behavioral approaches to tic suppression are few but show some promise (Piacentini and Chang 2001). The behavioral technique shown to be most effective is habit reversal training. For Tourette's disorder, habit reversal training is the use of a competing muscle contraction or behavioral response that opposes the tic movement. This method is usually combined with relaxation training, self-monitoring, awareness training, and positive reinforcement. In the few published studies of habit reversal training, there were marked overall reductions in tic frequency. Treatment averaged 20 training sessions during an 8- to 11-month period. Marked tic reduction was noted at 3 to 4 months. Interestingly, urges or sensations experienced before the tic movements also decreased with behavioral treatment (Azrin and Peterson 1990).

There are no published systematic studies of psychosocial interventions for individuals with Tourette's disorder. Most treatment efforts are based on a combination of traditional psychosocial interventions and clinical judgment.

Perhaps the most useful psychosocial and educational intervention is to make the individual aware of the Tourette Syndrome Association, both national and local chapters. This and other self-help groups can be useful as a source of support and education for individuals with tics, families, and mental health professionals.

Individual psychotherapy can be useful for support, development of awareness, or for addressing personal and interpersonal problems more effectively. Family therapy can be useful when families have problems adjusting, functioning, and communicating. Although most families do well, some families have difficulties understanding the involuntary nature of tics and may punish their children for their tics, even after diagnosis and education. Alternatively, some families have more behavior difficulties with their children after diagnosis than before. Many parents of children with Tourette's disorder inadvertently lower general behavior expectations because of confusion about what behaviors are tics and what behaviors are not tics. Sometimes parents decrease behavior expectations for their children because of the parents' desire not to add any additional stress to the youngster's life. Also, with confusion in the field regarding the scope of problems in Tourette's disorder, some parents see all maladaptive behaviors as involuntary and do not hold their children responsible for their behaviors. For children with Tourette's disorder to do well, they need support from their family to develop effective self-control in areas not affected by Tourette's disorder so that optimal adaptation can occur.

In newly diagnosed adults, psychotherapy oriented toward adequate adjustment to the diagnosis is important but not always easy. Adults frequently experience a mixture of relief to finally be diagnosed, with anger and resentment related to their past experiences with discrimination or inadequate medical care. Severely affected adults may also need psychotherapy to deal with the psychological and psychosocial difficulties related to having a chronic illness.

For children, active intervention at school is essential to create a supportive yet challenging academic and social environment. Efforts to educate teachers, principals, and other students can result in increased awareness of Tourette's disorder and tolerance for the child's symptoms.

Many young adults are finding Tourette's disorder support and social groups important for interpersonal contact and continued adult development. Efforts to keep people with Tourette's disorder working are important, as are rehabilitation efforts for those who are not working. Finding housing and obtaining disability or public assistance may be necessary for the most disabled individuals with Tourette's disorder.

Genetic Counseling

One question commonly asked by young adults with Tourette's disorder is their risk for having a child with Tourette's disorder. Given the fact that many who present for clinical attention with Tourette's disorder have comorbid conditions, genetic counseling of people with Tourette's syndrome should include not only the risk for Tourette's disorder but also the risk for other neuropsychiatric problems such as ADHD or OCD that may be part of the young person's history. In addition, because the base rate of neuropsychiatric disorders is high, it is not uncommon for spouses of people with Tourette's disorder to have a neuropsychiatric disorder. In providing counseling to these couples, it is important that genetic counseling be conducted not just about Tourette's syndrome but also about the other conditions that occur as part of the young couple's history.

Treatment-Refractory Cases

Perhaps the most important "treatment" in individuals with severe incapacitating tics is a full clinical reevaluation to assess the adequacy of previous evaluations and treatment efforts. It is not uncommon for treatment-refractory individuals to have had inadequate evaluations and treatment trials.

Two alternative treatment strategies are available for truly treatment-refractory tics. When a single tic or a few tics are refractory and impairing, the injection of botulinum toxin into the specific muscle group can be helpful. This strategy is most useful for painful, dystonic tics. Treatment has a long duration of action, but the effect does decrease in 2 to 4 months, and repeated injections may be necessary. Specific side effects are few, other than weakness in the affected muscle. Some individuals reported the loss of the premonitory sensation with their botulinum toxin treatment. For the mental health clinician it is essential to work with a neurologist experienced in using botulinum toxin (Jankovic 1994).

There have been reports in the literature and the media concerning the use of neurosurgical approaches for the treatment of refractory tics. To date, the optimal size and location of the surgical treatment lesions are not known. There are no well-controlled trials, although some data are available from individuals with OCD and tics who were treated for OCD. In these individuals, the impact on tic severity was mixed (Baer et al. 1994). Because these approaches are particularly controversial, it is important, before considering neurosurgical approaches, to complete a detailed and exhaustive reevaluation to determine whether all other treatment options are exhausted. It is also important that individuals who pursue neurosurgical approaches consider centers of clinical excellence in which controlled treatment trials are ongoing. It would be optimal if the outcome of all cases treated in this manner could be available for review in the scientific literature so that conclusions based on outcome can be drawn from these complex cases.

Comparison of DSM-IV-TR/ICD-10 Diagnostic Criteria
The ICD-10 and DSM-IV-TR criteria sets for the tic disorders are almost identical.

References

Anderson GM, Pollack ES, Chatterjee D, et al. (1992) Postmortem analysis of subcortical monoamines and amino acids in Tourette syndrome. *Adv Neurol* **58**, 123–134.

Apter A, Pauls DL, Bleich A, et al. (1993) An epidemiologic study of Gilles de la Tourette's syndrome in Israel. *Arch Gen Psychiatry* **50**, 734–738.

Arnsten AFT, Cai JX, and Goldman-Rakic PS (1988) The alpha-2 adrenergic agonist, guanfacine, improves memory in aged monkeys without sedative or hypotensive side effects: evidence for alpha-2 receptor subtypes. *J Neurosci* **8**, 4287–4298.

Azrin NH and Peterson AL (1990) Treatment of Tourette syndrome by habit reversal: a waiting list control group comparison. *Behav Ther* **21**, 305–318.

Baer L (1994) Factor analysis of symptom subtypes of obsessive–compulsive disorder and their relation to personality and tic disorders. *J Clin Psychiatry* **55**(Suppl.), 18–23.

Baer L, Rauch SL, and Jenike MA (1994) Cingulotomy in a case of concomitant obsessive–compulsive disorder and Tourette's syndrome. *Arch Gen Psychiatry* **51**, 73–74.

Bruun RD (1988) Subtle and under recognized side effects of neuroleptic treatment in children with Tourette's disorder. *Am J Psychiatry* **145**, 621–624.

Bruun RD and Budman CL (1992) The natural history of Tourette syndrome. *Adv Neurol* **58**, 1–6.

Caine ED, McBride MC, Chiverton P, et al. (1988) Tourette's syndrome in Monroe county school children. *Neurology* **38**, 472–475.

Chappel PB, Leckman JF, and Riddle MA (1995) The pharmacologic treatment of tic disorders. *Child Adolesc Psychiatr Clin N Am* **4**, 197–216.

Chase TN, Friedhoff AJ, and Cohen DJ (1992) Tourette syndrome: genetics, neurobiology and treatment. *Adv Neurol* **58** 341–362.

Comings DE (1995) Tourette's syndrome: a behavioral spectrum disorder. *Adv Neurol* **65**, 293–303.

Comings DE and Comings BG (1987) A controlled study of Tourette syndrome: I–VII. *Am J Hum Genet* **41**, 701–866.

Conneally PM and Housman D (chairs) (1993) Ninth Genetic Workshop on Tourette Syndrome sponsored by the Tourette Syndrome Association. Rotterdam, Netherlands.

Dion Y, Annable L, Sandor P, et al. (2002) Risperidone in the treatment of Tourette syndrome: a double-blind, placebo-controlled trial. *J Clin Psychopharmacol* **22**(1), 31–39.

Eappen V, Pauls DL, and Robertson MM (1993) Evidence for autosomal dominant transmission in Tourette's syndrome—United Kingdom Cohort Study. *Br J Psychiatry* **162**, 593–596.

Eggers CH, Rothenberger A, and Berghaus U (1988) Clinical and neurobiological findings in children suffering from tic disease following treatment with tiapride. *Eur Arch Psychiatr Neurol Sci* **237**, 223–229.

Eidelberg D, Moeller JR, Antonini A, et al. (1997) The metabolic anatomy of Tourette's syndrome. *Neurology* **48**(4), 927–934.

Erenberg G and Lederman RJ (1989) Naltrexone in the treatment of Tourette's syndrome. *Neurology* **39**(Suppl. 1), 232–329.

George MS, Trimble MR, Ring HA, et al. (1993) Obsessions in obsessive–compulsive disorder with and without Gilles de la Tourette's syndrome. *Am J Psychiatry* **150**, 93–97.

Gilbert DL, Sethuraman G, Sine L, et al. (2000) Tourette's syndrome improvement with pergolide in a randomized, double-blind, crossover trial. *Neurology* **54**(6), 1310–1315.

Goetz CG (1992) Clonidine and clonazepam. *Adv Neurol* **58**, 245–251.

Goetz CG (1993) Clonidine. In *Handbook of Tourette's Syndrome and Related Tic and Behavioral Disorders*, Kurlan R (ed). Marcel Dekker, New York, pp. 377–388.

Grice DE, Leckman JF, Pauls DL, et al. (1996) Linkage disequilibrium between an allele at the dopamine D_4 receptor locus and Tourette syndrome, by the transmission-disequilibrium test. *Am J Hum Genet* **59**(3), 644–652.

Haber SN, Kowall NW, Vonsattel JP, et al. (1986) Gilles de la Tourette's syndrome: a postmortem neuropathological and immunohistochemical study. *J Neurol Sci* **75**, 225–241.

Hall M, Costa DC, Shields J, et al. (1991) Brain perfusion patterns with Tc^{99m} HMPAO-SPECT in patients with Gilles de la Tourette syndrome—short report. In *Nuclear Medicine: The State of the Art of Nuclear Medicine in Europe*, Schmidt HAE and van der Schoot JB (eds). Schattauer, Stuttgart, pp. 243–245.

Heutnik P, Breedveld GJ, Niemeijer MF (1993) In *Progress in gene location*, Kurlan R (ed). New York, pp. 317–335.

Hyde TM, Aaronson BA, and Randolf C (1992) Relationship of birthweight to the phenotypic expression of Gilles de la Tourette's syndrome in monozygotic twins. *Neurology* **42**, 652–658.

Jankovic J (1992) Diagnosis and classification of tics and Tourette syndrome. *Adv Neurol* **58**, 7–14.

Jankovic J (1994) Botulinum toxin treatment of tics. In *Therapy with Botulinum Toxin*, Jankovic J (ed). Marcel Dekker, New York, pp. 503–509.

Kiessling LS, Marcotte AC, and Culpepper L (1993) Antineuronal antibodies in movement disorders. *Pediatrics* **92**(1), 39–43.

Kurlan R and McDermott MP (1993) Rating tic severity. In *Handbook of Tourette's Syndrome and Related Tic and Behavioral Disorders*, Kurlan R (ed). Marcel Dekker, New York, pp. 199–220.

LaBuda MC and Pauls DL (1993) Gilles de la Tourette syndrome. In *Molecular Basis of Neurology*, Conneally PM (ed). Blackwell Scientific, Boston, pp. 199–214.

Leckman JF, Ort S, Caruso KA, et al. (1986) Rebound phenomena in Tourette's syndrome after abrupt withdrawal of clonidine. Behavioral, cardiovascular, and neurochemical effects. *Arch Gen Psychiatry* **43**, 1168–1176.

Leckman JF, Riddle MA, Berrettini WH, et al. (1988) Elevated CSF dynorphin A[1–8] in Tourette's syndrome. *Life Sci* **43**, 2015–2023.

Leckman JF, Riddle MA, Hardin MT, et al. (1989) The Yale global tic severity scale: initial testing of a clinician-rated scale of tic severity. *J Am Acad Child Adolesc Psychiatry* **28**, 566–573.

Leckman JF, Walker DE, and Cohen DJ (1993a) Premonitory urges in Tourette's syndrome. *Am J Psychiatry* **150**, 98–102.

Leckman JF, Walker DE, Goodman WK, et al. (1993b) "Just right" perceptions associated with compulsive behaviors in Tourette's syndrome. *Am J Psychiatry* **151**, 675–680.

Leckman JF, Zhang H, Vitale A, et al. (1998) Course of tic severity in Tourette syndrome: the first two decades. *Pediatrics* **102**(1, Pt 1), 14–19.

Leonard HL, March J, Rickler KC, et al. (1997) Pharmacology of the selective serotonin reuptake inhibitors in children and adolescents. *J Am Acad Child Adolesc Psychiatry* **36**(6), 725–736.

Lombroso PJ, Scahill LD, Chappell PB, et al. (1995) Tourette's syndrome: a multigenerational, neuropsychiatric disorder. *Adv Neurol* **65**, 305–318.

Lucas AR, Beard CM, Rajput AH, et al. (1982) Tourette syndrome in Rochester, Minnesota, 1968–1979. *Adv Neurol* **35**, 267–269.

Miguel EC, Coffey BJ, Baer L, et al. (1993) Phenomenology of intentional repetitive behaviors in obsessive–compulsive disorder and Tourette's syndrome. *J Clin Psychiatry* **56**, 246–255.

Pauls DL and Leckman JF (1986) The inheritance of Gilles de la Tourette's syndrome and associated behaviors: evidence for autosomal dominant transmission. *N Engl J Med* **315**, 993–997.

Pauls DL, Hurst CR, Kruger SD, et al. (1986) Gilles de la Tourette's syndrome and attention deficit disorder with hyperactivity: evidence against a genetic relationship. *Arch Gen Psychiatry* **43**, 1177–1179.

Pauls DL, Leckman JF, and Cohen DJ (1993) The familial relationship between Gilles de la Tourette's syndrome, attention deficit disorder, learning disabilities, and speech disorders and stuttering. *J Am Acad Child Adolesc Psychiatry* **32**, 1044–1050.

Pauls DL, Leckman JF, and Cohen DJ (1994) Evidence against a genetic relationship between Gilles de la Tourette's syndrome, and anxiety, depression, panic and phobic disorders. *Br J Psychiatry* **164**, 215–221.

Pauls DL, Raymond CL, Leckman JL, et al. (1991) A family study of Tourette's syndrome. *Am J Hum Genet* **48**, 154–163.

Peterson BS, Riddle MA, Cohen DJ, et al. (1993) Reduced basal ganglia volumes in Tourette's syndrome using 3-dimensional reconstruction techniques from magnetic resonance images. *Neurology* **43**, 941–949.

Piacentini J and Chang S (2001) Behavioral treatments for Tourette syndrome and tic disorders: state of the art. *Adv Neurol* **85**, 319–331.

Price RA, Kidd K, Cohen DJ, et al. (1985) A twin study of Tourette syndrome. *Arch Gen Psychiatry* **42**, 815–820.

Riddle MA, Rasmussen AR, Woods SW, et al. (1991) SPECT imaging of cerebral blood flow in Tourette syndrome. *Adv Neurol* **58**, 207–211.

Robertson MM (1989) The Gilles de la Tourette syndrome: the current status. *Br J Psychiatry* **154**, 147–169.

Robertson MM, Schnieden V, and Lees AJ (1990) Management of Gilles de la Tourette syndrome using sulpiride. *Clin Neuropharmacol* **3**, 229–235.

Sallee FR and Rock CM (1994) Effects of pimozide on cognition in children with Tourette syndrome: interaction with comorbid attention deficit hyperactivity disorder. *Acta Psychiatr Scand* **90**, 4–9.

Sandyk R (1985) The effects of naloxone in Tourette's syndrome. *Ann Neurol* **18**, 367–368.

Scahill L, Chappell PB, Kim YS, et al. (2001) A placebo-controlled study of guanfacine in the treatment of children with tic disorders and attention-deficit hyperactivity disorder. *Am J Psychiatry* **158**(7), 1067–1074.

Shapiro AK, Shapiro ES, Young JG, et al. (1988) *Gilles de la Tourette Syndrome*, 2nd ed. Raven Press, New York.

Singer HS and Rosenberg LA (1989) The development of behavioral and emotional problems in Tourette syndrome. *Pediatr Neurol* **5**, 41–44.

Singer HS and Walkup JT (1991) Tourette syndrome and other tic disorders: diagnosis, pathophysiology, and treatment. *Medicine (Baltimore)* **70**, 15–32.

Singer HS, Butler IJ, Tune LE, et al. (1982) Dopaminergic dysfunction in Tourette syndrome. *Ann Neurol* **12**, 361–366.

Singer HS, Hahn I-H, Krowiak E, et al. (1990) Tourette syndrome: a neurochemical analysis of postmortem cortical brain tissue. *Ann Neurol* **27**, 443–446.

Singer HS, Reiss AL, Brown J, et al. (1993) Volumetric MRI changes in the basal ganglia of children with Tourette's syndrome. *Neurology* **43**, 950–956.

Singer HS, Wendlandt J, Krieger M, et al. (2001) Baclofen treatment in Tourette syndrome: a double-blind, placebo-controlled, crossover trial. *Neurology* **56**(5), 599–604.

Stern E, Silbersweig DA, Chee KY, et al. (2000) A functional neuroanatomy of tics in Tourette syndrome. *Arch Gen Psychiatry* **57**(8), 741–748.

Stoetter B, Braun AR, Randolf C, et al. (1992) Functional neuroanatomy of Tourette syndrome: limbic motor interactions studied with FDG PET. *Adv Neurol* **58**, 213–226.

Swedo SE, Leonard HL, Garvey M, et al. (1998) Pediatric autoimmune neuropsychiatric disorders associated with streptococcal infections: clinical description of the first 50 cases. *Am J Psychiatry* **155**(2), 264–271.

Swedo SE, Leonard HL, and Kiessling LS (1994) Speculations on antineuronal antibody-mediated neuropsychiatric disorders of childhood. *Pediatrics* **93**(2), 323–326.

The Research Unit on Pediatric Psychopharmacology Anxiety Study Group (2001) Fluvoxamine for the treatment of anxiety disorders in children and adolescents. *N Engl J Med* **344**(17), 1279–1285.

The Tourette Syndrome Association International Consortium for Genetics (1999) A complete genome screen in sib pairs affected by Gilles de la Tourette syndrome. *Am J Hum Genet* **65**(5), 1428–1436.

The Tourette Syndrome Classification Study Group (1993) Definitions and classifications of tic disorder. *Arch Neurol* **50**, 1013–1016.

Walkup JT, LaBuda MC, Singer HS, et al. (1996) Family study and segregation analysis of Tourette syndrome: evidence for a mixed model of inheritance. *Am J Hum Genet* **59**(3), 684–693.

Walkup JT, Price RA, Resnick S, et al. (1987) Non-genetic factors associated with the expression of Tourette syndrome. Scientific Proceedings of the Annual Meeting of the American Academy of Child and Adolescent Psychiatry. Washington, DC.

11 ● Childhood Disorders: Elimination Disorders and Childhood Anxiety Disorders

ENURESIS

Diagnosis

Functional enuresis is defined as the intentional or involuntary passage of urine in bed or clothes in the absence of any identified physical abnormality in children older than 4 years of age (APA 2000) (see DSM-IV-TR diagnostic criteria). Although there is no good evidence that the condition is primarily psychogenic, it is often associated with psychiatric disorder, and enuretic children are frequently referred to mental health services for treatment.

DSM-IV-TR Diagnostic Criteria

307.6 Enuresis (Not Due to a Medical Condition)

A. Repeated voiding of urine into bed or clothes (whether involuntary or intentional).
B. The behavior is clinically significant as manifested by either a frequency of twice a week for at least 3 consecutive months or the presence of clinically significant distress or impairment in social, academic (occupational), or other important areas of functioning.
C. Chronological age is at least 5 years (or equivalent developmental level).
D. The behavior is not due exclusively to the direct physiological effect of a substance (e.g., a diuretic) or a general medical condition (e.g., diabetes, spina bifida, a seizure disorder).

Specify type:

Nocturnal only: passage of urine only during nighttime sleep

Diurnal only: passage of urine during waking hours

Nocturnal and diurnal: a combination of the two subtypes above

Reprinted with permission from the Diagnostic and Statistical Manual of Mental Disorders, Fourth Edition, Text Revision. Copyright 2000 American Psychiatric Association.

Information on the frequency, periodicity, and duration of symptoms is needed to make the diagnosis and distinguish functional enuresis from sporadic seizure-associated enuresis. If there is diurnal enuresis, an additional treatment plan is required. A family history of enuresis increases the likelihood of a diagnosis of functional enuresis and may explain the later age at which the children are presented for treatment. Projective identification by the affected parent—whereby the parent does not separate their own feelings about having had the diagnosis with the current experience of their affected child—may further hinder treatment. For subjects with secondary enuresis, the precipitating factors should be elicited, although such efforts often represent an attempt to assign a meaning after the event.

The child's views and any misconceptions that he or she may have about the enuresis, its causes, and its treatment should be fully explored. Asking the child for three wishes may help determine whether the enuresis is a concern to the child. This may unmask marked embarrassment or guilt from behind a facade of denial about the problem, and can be educational for parents who believe their children could stop wetting "if only they wanted to or tried harder." Pictures drawn by the child that describe how the child views himself or herself when enuresis is a problem and when it is not is appropriate for younger children, and can graphically illustrate the misery experienced by children with enuresis.

All children should have a routine physical examination, with particular emphasis placed on the detection of congenital malformations, that are possibly indicative of urogenital abnormalities. A midstream specimen of urine should be examined for the presence of infection. Radiological or further medical investigation is indicated only in the presence of infected urine, enuresis with symptoms suggestive of recurrent urinary tract infection (UTI) (frequency, urgency, and dysuria), or polyuria.

Course

The acquisition of urinary continence at night is the end stage of a fairly consistent developmental sequence. Bowel control during sleep marks the beginning of this process and is followed by bowel control during waking hours. Bladder control during the day occurs soon after and finally, after a variable interval, nighttime bladder control is achieved. Most children achieve this final stage by the age of 36 months. With increasing age, the likelihood of spontaneous recovery from enuresis becomes less (Oppel et al. 1968), so that, for instance, 40% of 2-year-olds with enuresis become dry in the next year and 20% of enuretic 3-year-olds become dry before age 4 years but only 6% of enuretic 4-year-olds become dry in the following year. The chronic nature of the condition is further shown in the study by Rutter and colleagues (Rutter et al. 1973), in which only 1.5% of 5-year-old bed wetters became dry during the next 2 years.

Nocturnal enuresis is as common in boys as in girls until the age of 5 years, but by age 11 years, boys outnumber girls 2 : 1 (Oppel et al. 1968, Rutter et al. 1973, Essen and Peckham 1976). Not until the age of 8 years do boys achieve the same levels of nighttime continence that are seen in girls by the age of 5 years (Verhulst et al. 1985). This appears to

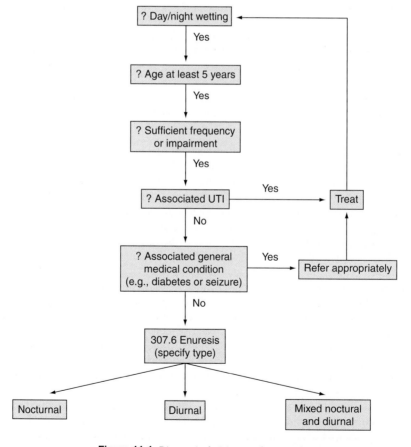

Figure 11-1 *Diagnostic decision tree for enuresis.*

be due to slower physiological maturation in boys. In addition, the increased incidence of secondary enuresis (occurring after an initial 1-year period of acquired continence) in boys further affects the sex ratio seen in later childhood. Daytime enuresis occurs more commonly in girls (Blomfield and Douglas 1956, Hallgren and Enuresis 1956, Jarvelin et al. 1988) and is associated with higher rates of psychiatric disturbance (Rutter et al. 1973).

Differential Diagnosis

The presence or absence of conditions often seen in association with enuresis, such as developmental delay, UTI, constipation, and comorbid psychiatric disorder, should be assessed and ruled out as appropriate (Figure 11-1). Other causes of nocturnal incontinence should be excluded, for example, those leading to polyuria (diabetes mellitus, renal disease, diabetes insipidus) and, rarely, nocturnal epilepsy.

Etiology

Identifying a cause for enuresis is not a simple task despite numerous descriptions of correlations or associations between enuresis and a wide variety of biological and psychosocial factors.

Biological factors described include a structural pathological condition or infection of the urinary tract (or both), low functional bladder capacity, abnormal antidiuretic hormone secretion, abnormal depth of sleep, genetic predisposition, and developmental delay. Evidence has also been found for sympathetic hyperactivity (Dundaroz et al. 2001) and delayed organ maturation as seen by delay in ossification (Dundaroz et al. 2001).

Structural causes for enuresis should be considered as the exception rather than the rule (Sorotzkin 1984). Furthermore, because treating the infection rarely stops the bed-wetting, UTI is probably a result rather than a cause of enuresis (Forsythe and Redmond 1974). Although low functional capacity may predispose the child to enuresis, successful behavioral treatment does not appear to increase that capacity. It seems rather that, in treated individuals, the sensation of a full (small) bladder promotes waking to pass urine so that enuresis does not occur (Fielding 1980). Reduction of nocturnal secretion of anti diuretic hormone (ADH) has been described in a small number of children with enuresis (Norgaard et al. 1985, Rittig et al. 1989). Although it is widely believed by parents that children who have enuresis at night sleep more deeply and are especially difficult to wake, this subjective opinion was not supported by Boyd's study (Boyd 1960) that compared the time it took to awaken normal children and children with enuresis.

The evidence for some genetic predisposition is strong. Approximately 70% of children with nocturnal enuresis have a first-degree relative who also has or has had nocturnal enuresis (Bakwin 1961). Twin studies have shown greater monozygotic (68%) than dizygotic (36%) concordance (Bakwin 1971). An association between enuresis and early delays in motor, language, and social development has been noted in both the prospective community samples (Essen and Peckham 1976, Fergusson et al. 1986) and a large retrospective study of clinical subjects (Steinhausen and Gobel 1989). Genetic factors are probably the most important in the etiology of nocturnal enuresis, but somatic and psychosocial environmental factors have a major modulatory effect. Most commonly, nocturnal enuresis is inherited via an autosomal dominant mode of transmission with high penetrance (90%). However, a third of all cases are sporadic, and the difference between sporadic and familial forms is not known. Four gene loci associated with nocturnal enuresis have been identified but the existence of others is presumed (locus heterogeneity) (von Gontard et al. 2001). Many psychosocial correlates have also been described, including delayed toilet training, low socioeconomic class, stress events, and other child psychiatric disorders.

Psychiatric disorder occurs more frequently in enuretic children than in other children, although there have been no specific types of psychiatric disorder identified in children with enuresis (Mikkelsen and Rapoport 1980). However, there is little evidence that enuresis is a symptom of underlying disorder because psychotherapy is ineffective in reducing enuresis (Werry and Cohrssen 1965), anxiolytic drugs have no antienuretic effect, tricyclic antidepressants exert their therapeutic effect independent of the child's mood (Blackwell et al.), and purely symptomatic therapies, such as the bell and pad, are equally effective in disturbed and nondisturbed children (Young and Morgan 1973).

Treatment of Nocturnal Enuresis

Questions that are useful in obtaining information for treatment planning include "Why is this a problem?" and "Why does this need treatment now?" because these factors may influence the choice of treatment (is a rapid effect needed?) or point to other pressures or restrictions on therapy. It is important to inquire about previous management strategies—for example, fluid restriction, night lifting (getting the child out of bed to take to the toilet, in an often semiasleep state), rewards, and punishments—used at home. Parents often come with the assertion that they have tried everything and that nothing has helped. Examining the reasons for the failure of simple strategies is useful for ensuring that more sophisticated treatments do not befall the same fate. Practical management for nocturnal enuresis is presented in Table 11-1.

Table 11-1	Practical Management of Nocturnal Enuresis
Stage 1	**Assessment**
	Obtain history: frequency, periodicity, and duration of wetting.
	Why is this a problem? Why now?
	Mental status: views and misconceptions (parent and child).
	Discover reasons for previous failure or failures.
	Perform routine physical examination (any minor congenital abnormalities?).
	Midstream specimen of urine must be obtained.
	Radiology and further physical investigation is needed only if symptoms or evidence of urinary tract infection (dysuria and frequency or positive culture results) or polyuria.
Stage 2	**Advice**
	Education that enuresis is common and not deliberate.
	Aim to reduce punitive behavior.
	Transmit optimism: however, anticipate disappointment at no instant cure.
	Preview the stepwise recovery and warn of the possibility of relapse.
Stage 3	**Baseline**
	Use star chart.
	Focus on positive achievements (be creative).
	Examine the effect of simple interventions (e.g., lifting)
Stage 4	**Night Alarm**
	First-line management unless important to obtain rapid short-term effect.
	Demonstrate night-alarm equipment in the office.
	Telephone follow-up within a few days of commencing therapy.
	Or
	Drug Therapy
	If rapid suppression of wetting is needed (e.g., before vacation or camp, to defuse aggressive or hostile situation between child and parents and siblings).
	When family has proved incapable of using the equipment.
	After failure or multiple relapses.
	Medication of choice: DDAVP, (Desmopressin) 20–40 µg at night

About 10% of children have a reduction in the number of wet nights after a single visit to a clinician in which the only intervention was the recording of baseline wetting frequency and simple reassurance (Shaffer et al. 1968). Such reassurance should make clear that enuresis is a biological condition that is made worse by stress and that may be associated in a noncausal way with other psychiatric disorders. Younger children can be told that their problem is shared by many others of the same age. The excellent prognosis for individuals who comply with therapy should be stressed. Recording the frequency of enuresis can be achieved by using a simple star chart. This is most effective if performed by the child, who records each dry night with a star. The completed chart is then shown to the parents on a daily basis, and they can provide appropriate praise and reinforcement.

Waking and Fluid Restriction

Although systematic studies have failed to show any effect of these interventions with enuretic inpatients, it may be that these strategies work for the majority of enuretic children who are not referred for treatment. If waking does appear to reduce the number of wet nights from baseline, a more systematic application may be indicated.

Surgery

On the basis of the premise that enuresis is causally associated with outflow-tract obstruction, various surgical procedures have been advocated. Reported positive treatment effects are slight (no controlled studies exist), and there remains a significant potential for adverse effects (urinary incontinence, epididymitis, and aspermia).

Pharmacotherapy

Although it has been repeatedly demonstrated that temporary suppression rather than cure of enuresis is the usual outcome of drug therapy, it remains the most widely prescribed treatment in the United States (Foxman et al. 1986). Four classes of drugs have principally been employed: synthetic antidiuretic hormones, tricyclic antidepressants, stimulants, and anticholinergic agents.

Synthetic Antidiuretic Hormone

A number of randomized double-blind placebo-controlled trials have shown that the synthetic vasopeptide DDAVP (desmopressin) is effective in enuresis (Dimson 1986, Miller and Klauber 1990). The drug is usually administered intranasally, although oral preparations of equal efficacy have been developed (equivalent oral dose is 10 times the intranasal dose). It has been shown (Miller et al. 1989) that almost 50% of children are able to stop wetting completely with a single nightly dose of 20 to 40 mcg of DDAVP given intranasally. A further 40% are afforded a significant reduction in the frequency of enuresis with this treatment. As with tricyclic antidepressants, however, when treatment is stopped, the vast majority of individuals relapse. (Leebeek-Groenewegen et al. 2001) Side effects of this medication include nasal pain and congestion, headache, nausea, and abdominal pain. Serious problems of water intoxication, hyponatremia, and seizures are rare. It is important to be aware that intranasal absorption is reduced when the child has a cold or allergic rhinitis. The mode of action of desmopressin is unknown. It may reduce the production of nighttime urine to an amount less than the (low) functional volume of the enuretic bladder, thereby eliminating the urge to micturate. It is uncertain whether desmopressin administration is correcting a natural deficiency of vasopressin or is exerting a true pharmacological effect. With regard to identifying those most likely to respond to DDAVP treatment, it has been found (Kruse et al. 2001) that those most likely to be permanently dry with desmopressin treatment are older children who respond to lower dose (20 mcg) desmopressin and who do not wet frequently.

Tricyclic Antidepressants   The short-term effectiveness of imipramine and other related antidepressants has also been demonstrated via many randomized double-blind placebo-controlled trials (Shaffer et al. 1968, Rapoport et al. 1980, Simeon et al. 1981). Imipramine reduces the frequency of enuresis in about 85% of bed wetters and eliminates enuresis in about 30% of these individuals. Nighttime doses of 1 to 2.5 mg/kg are usually effective (Jorgensen et al. 1980), and a therapeutic effect is usually evident in the first week of treatment. Relapse after withdrawal of medication is almost inevitable, so that 3 months after the cessation of tricyclic antidepressants, nearly all children will again have enuresis at pretreatment levels (Shaffer et al. 1968). Side effects are common and include dry mouth, dizziness, postural hypotension, headache, and constipation. Toxicity after accidental ingestion or overdose is a serious consideration, causing cardiac effects, including arrhythmias and conduction defects, convulsions, hallucinations, and ataxia. Concern has been expressed about the possibility of sudden death (presumably caused by arrhythmia) in children taking tricyclic drugs. The mode of action for tricyclic antidepressants is unclear. It does not appear to depend on their antidepressant properties because response is unrelated to the presence or absence of mood symptoms. One observation is that tricyclic agents seem to increase functional bladder volumes (Shaffer et al. 1979), possibly resulting from noradrenergic reuptake inhibition (Rapoport et al. 1980).

Stimulant Medication   Sympathomimetic stimulants such as dexamphetamine have been used to reduce the depth of sleep in children with enuresis but because there is no evidence that enuresis is related to abnormally deep sleep, their lack of effectiveness in stopping bed-wetting is no surprise (McConaghy 1969).

Anticholinergic Drugs   Drugs such as propantheline, oxybutynin, and terodiline can reduce the frequency of voiding in individuals with neurogenic bladders, reduce urgency, and increase functional bladder capacity. There is no evidence, however, that these anticholinergic drugs are effective in bed-wetting, although they may have a role in diurnal enuresis (Wallace and Forsythe 1969, Elmer et al. 1988). Side effects are frequent and include dry mouth, blurred vision, headache, nausea, and constipation (Baigrie et al. 1988).

Psychosocial Treatments

The original night alarm used two electrodes separated by a device (e.g., bedding) connected to an alarm. When the child wet the bed, the urine completed the electrical circuit, sounded the alarm, and the child awoke. All current night-alarm systems are merely refinements on this original design. A vibrating pad beneath the pillow can be used instead of a bell or buzzer, or the electrodes can be incorporated into a single unit or can be miniaturized so that they can be attached to night (or day) clothing. With treatment, full cessation of enuresis can be expected in 80% of cases. Reported cure rates (defined as a minimum of 14 consecutive dry nights) have ranged from 50% to 100% (Forsythe and Butler 1989, Butler 1991).

The main problem with this form of enuretic treatment, however, is that cure is usually achieved only within the second month of treatment (Kolvin et al. 1972). This factor may influence clinicians to prescribe pharmacological treatments that, although are more immediately gratifying, do not offer any real prospect of cure. It has been suggested that adjuvant therapy with methamphetamine (Young and Turner 1965) or desmopressin (Bollard and Nettlebeck 1981) will reduce the amount of time before continence is achieved. Using a louder auditory stimulus (Finley and Wansley 1977) or using the body-worn alarm (Butler et al. 1990) may also improve the speed of treatment response. Factors associated with delayed acquisition of continence include failure of the child to wake with the alarm, maternal anxiety, and a disturbed home environment, although no influence has been seen regarding the age of the child or the initial wetting frequency (Young and Morgan 1973, Dische et al. 1983).

A further consequence of the delayed response to a night alarm is that families fail to persist with the treatment and may abandon the treatment too soon. Premature termination can occur in as many as 48% of cases (Turner et al. 1970), and is more common in families that have made little previous effort to treat the problem, in families that are negative or intolerant of bed-wetting, and in children who have other behavioral problems (Wagner and Johnson 1988). Aspects of treatment that may also reduce compliance with the alarm include failure to understand or follow the instructions, failure of the child to awaken, and frequent false alarms (Turner et al. 1970). Relapse after successful treatment, if it occurs, will usually take place within the first 6 months after cessation of treatment. It is reported that approximately one-third of children relapse (Doleys et al. 1977); however, no clear predictors of relapse have been identified (Fielding 1985).

The mode of action of the night alarm can be explained using theories of classical or operant conditioning. In classical conditioning, bladder distention or a sense of the need to pass urine becomes associated with the auditory signal, leading to the conditioned response of waking. Operant conditioning theories would view the alarm as a punishment to be avoided and may explain why individuals still become dry when the alarm is placed in the bed but is not switched on (Deleon and Mandell 1966). Social learning is also important because the night alarm and associated systematic recording may help the family focus on dry nights and provide contingent rewards (praise).

Table 11-2 presents various remedies for night-alarm problems.

Ultrasonic Bladder Volume Alarm   Although the traditional enuresis alarm has good potential for a permanent cure, the child is mostly wet during treatment. Furthermore, the moisture alarm requires that the child make the somewhat remote association between the alarm event and a full bladder after the bladder has emptied. In an exploratory study (Pretlow 1999), a new approach to treating nocturnal enuresis was investigated using a miniature bladder-volume measurement instrument during sleep. In this, an alarm sounded when bladder volume reached 80% of the typical enuretic volume. On the basis of preliminary results, bladder-volume tracking seems to be a promising treatment for nocturnal enuresis in that it prevents the enuretic event, appears to facilitate a permanent cure, and is noninvasive.

Acupuncture   The efficacy of traditional Chinese acupuncture has been studied (Serel et al. 2001) in a small ($n = 50$) clinical sample. It was reported that within 6 months, 86%

Table 11-2	Problem Solving for the Night Alarm *If...*
Bell "does not work"	Check position, connections, and batteries. If using separating sheet, check that it is porous. Check that child is not turning off equipment. Place alarm out of easy reach.
Child does not wake	Make alarm louder. Parent should wake child.
Child does not become dry	Ensure compliance. Ensure that child responds promptly. Use adjuvant DDAVP or dextroamphetamine. Ensure that child has role (e.g., change own bedsheets) after alarm.
False alarms	Ensure that separating sheet is big enough, not soiled, and will insulate. Use thicker nightclothes.
Relapse	Repeat treatment. Consider overlearning after response to re-treatment.

of children were completely dry and a further 10% of children were dry on at least 80% of nights. Relapse rates appeared better than with psychopharmacologic agents.

Treatment of Diurnal Enuresis

Daytime enuresis, although it can occur together with nighttime enuresis, has a different pattern of associations, and responds to different methods of treatment. It is much more likely to be associated with urinary tract abnormalities, including UTI, and to be comorbid with other psychiatric disorders. As a result, a more detailed and focused medical and psychiatric evaluation is indicated. Urine should be checked repeatedly for infection, and the threshold for ordering ultrasonographical visualization of the urological system should be low. The history may make it apparent that the daytime wetting is situation specific. For example, school-based enuresis in a child who is too timid to ask to use the bathroom could be alleviated by the teacher tactfully reminding the child to go to the bathroom at regular intervals.

Observation of children with diurnal enuresis (Fielding et al. 1978) has established that they do experience an urge to pass urine before micturition but that either this urge is ignored or the warning comes too late to be of any use because of an "irritable bladder." Therefore, treatment strategies are based on establishing a pattern of toileting before the times that diurnal enuresis is likely to occur (usually between 12 noon and 5 PM), and using positive reinforcement to promote regular use of the bathroom (Berg et al. 1982).

Portable systems that can be worn on the body and use a sensor in the underwear as well as an alarm that can be worn on the wrist have been developed. Halliday and associates (Halliday et al. 1987) studied two versions of this apparatus—one in which the alarm sounding was contingent on the sensor's detecting wetness in the underwear and another in which the alarm merely went off at predetermined intervals. Interestingly, success rates (two thirds of children were cured and mostly maintained continence for a full 2-year follow-up period) showed no significant differences between the wetness alarm and the simple timed alarm. A simple therapeutic alternative, therefore, is to buy the child a digital watch with a count-down alarm timer.

Unlike nocturnal enuresis, drug treatment with tricyclic antidepressants, such as imipramine, is ineffective (Meadow and Berg 1982), whereas the use of anticholinergic agents such as oxybutynin and terodiline shows a therapeutic impact on the frequency of daytime enuresis (Baigrie et al. 1988, Pfaundler 1904).

ENCOPRESIS

Diagnosis

Encopresis is usually defined as the intentional or involuntary passage of stool in inappropriate places in the absence of any identified physical abnormality in children older than 4 years (see DSM-IV-TR diagnostic criteria).

DSM-IV-TR Diagnostic Criteria

Encopresis

A. Repeated passage of feces into inappropriate places (e.g., clothing or floor) whether involuntary or intentional.
B. At least one such event a month for at least 3 months.
C. Chronological age is at least 4 years (or equivalent developmental level).

D. The behavior is not due exclusively to the direct physiological effect of a substance (e.g., laxatives) or a general medical condition except through a mechanism involving constipation.

Code as follows:

787.6 Encopresis, with constipation and overflow incontinence: there is evidence of constipation on physical examination or by history.

307.7 Encopresis, without constipation and overflow incontinence: there is no evidence of constipation on physical examination or by history.

Reprinted with permission from the Diagnostic and Statistical Manual of Mental Disorders, Fourth Edition, Text Revision. Copyright 2000 American Psychiatric Association.

The distinction is drawn between encopresis with constipation (retention with overflow) and encopresis without constipation. Other classification schemes include making a primary–secondary distinction (based on having a 1-year period of continence), or soiling with fluid or normal feces.

Less than one-third of children in the United States have completed toilet training by the age of 2 years (Steubens and Silber 1974), with a mean age of 27.7 months (Brazelton 1962). Bowel control is usually achieved before bladder control. The age cutoff for "normality" is set at 4 years, the age at which 95% of children have acquired fecal continence (Stein and Susser 1967). As with urinary continence, girls achieve bowel control earlier than boys do.

Although the diagnosis can rarely be confused with other less odoriferous conditions, the main efforts during the diagnostic process are to establish the presence or absence of constipation and, to a lesser extent, distinguish continuous (primary) from discontinuous (secondary) soiling (Figure 11-2). Three types of identifiable encopresis in children have been identified: (1) it is known that the child can control defecation, but she or he chooses to defecate in inappropriate places; (2) there is true failure to gain bowel control, and the child is unaware of or unable to control soiling; and (3) soiling is due to excessively fluid feces, whether from constipation and overflow, physical disease, or anxiety. In practice, there is frequently an overlap among types or progression from one to another. Unlike enuresis, fecal soiling rarely occurs at night or during sleep, and if present, is indicative of a poor prognosis (Levine 1982).

In the first group, in which bowel control has been established, the stool may be soft or normal (but different from fluid-type feces seen in overflow). Soiling due to acute stress events (e.g., the birth of a sibling, a change of school, or parental separation) is usually brief once the stress has abated, given a stable home environment and sensible management. In more severe pathological family situations, including punitive management or frank physical or sexual abuse (Boon 1991), the feces may be deposited in places designed to cause anger or irritation or there may be associated smearing of feces on furniture and walls. Other covert aggressive antisocial acts may be evident, with considerable denial by the child of the magnitude or seriousness of the problem.

In the second group, in which there is failure to learn bowel control, a nonfluid stool is deposited fairly randomly in clothes, at home, and at school. There may be conditions such as mental retardation or specific developmental delay, spina bifida, or cerebral palsy that impair the ability to recognize the need to defecate, and the appropriate skills needed to defer this function until a socially appropriate time and location. In the absence of low IQ or pathological physical condition, individuals with encopresis have been reported as having associated enuresis, academic skills problems, and antisocial behavior. They present to pediatricians primarily, and are usually younger (age 4 to 6 years) than other encopretic individuals.

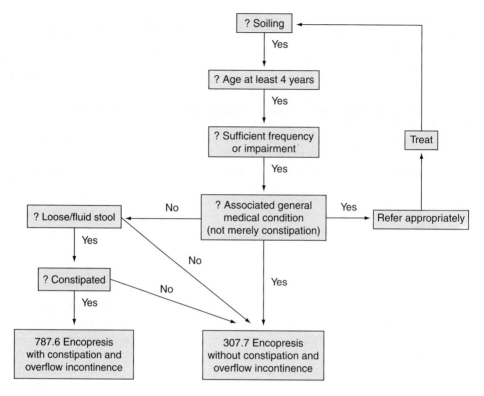

Figure 11-2 *Diagnostic decision for encopresis.*

It is thought that this type of soiling is considerably more common in socially disadvantaged, disorganized multiproblem families (Anthony 1957, Berg and Jones 1964, Easson 1960) because of faulty or inconsistent training or stresses during the sensitive period of training.

In the third group, excessively fluid feces are passed, which may result from conditions that cause true diarrhea (e.g., ulcerative colitis) or, much more frequently, from constipation with overflow causing spurious diarrhea. A history of retention, either willful or in response to pain, is prominent in the early days of this form of encopresis, although later it may be less apparent because of fecal overflow. Behavior such as squatting on the heels to prevent defecation or marked anxiety about the prospect of using the toilet (although rarely amounting to true phobic avoidance) may be described.

Having identified the presence of encopretic behavior and formed some idea of the type of encopresis (primary, secondary, retentive, or a combination), the remaining task is to discover the presence and extent of any associated conditions, both medical and psychological. The comprehensive assessment process should include a medical evaluation, psychiatric and family interviews, and a systematic behavioral recording.

The medical evaluation comprises a history, review of systems, physical examination, and appropriate hematological and radiological tests. Although the vast majority of individuals with encopresis are medically normal, a small proportion have pathological features of etiological significance. Physical causes of encopresis without retention include inflammatory bowel disease (e.g., ulcerative colitis, Crohn's disease), central nervous system disorders, sensory disorders of the anorectal region, or pelvic floor muscles (e.g., spina bifida, cerebral palsy). Organic causes of encopresis with retention include Hirschsprung's disease (aganglionosis in intermuscular and submucous plexuses of the large bowel extending proximally from the anus), neurogenic megacolon, hypothyroidism, hypercalcemia, chronic codeine or laxative usage, anorectal stenosis, and fissure (Fleisher 1976). It should also be remembered that these conditions rarely have their first presentation with encopresis alone.

The physical assessment should include an abdominal and rectal examination, although a plain abdominal radiograph is the most reliable way to determine the presence of fecal impaction. Anorectal manometry should be considered in the investigation of children with severe constipation and chronic soiling, especially those in whom Hirschsprung's disease is suspected (Clayden and Agnarsson 1991).

Psychiatric and family interviews should include a developmental history and a behavioral history of encopresis (antecedents, behavior, and consequences). Specific areas of stress, acute or chronic, affecting the child or family, or both, should be discovered. Associated psychopathological conditions are more commonly found in the older child, in secondary encopresis, and when soiling occurs not only in clothes. Anxiety surrounding toileting may indicate pot phobia, coercive toileting, or a history of painful defecation. A history should be obtained of the parents' previous attempts at treatment, together with previously prescribed therapy, so that reasons for previous failure can be identified and anticipated in future treatment planning.

Epidemiology

The overall prevalence of encopresis in 7- and 8-year-old children has been shown to be 1.5%, with boys (2.3%) affected more commonly than girls (0.7%). There was a steadily increasing likelihood of continence with increasing age, until by age 16 years the reported prevalence was almost zero (Bellman 1966). Rutter and coworkers (Rutter et al. 1970) reported a rate of 1% in 10- to 12-year-old children, with a strong (5 : 1) male/female ratio. Retrospective study of clinic-referred encopretic children has shown that 40% of cases are primary (true failure to gain control), with a mean age of 6.7 years, and 60% of cases are secondary, with a mean age of 8 years (Levine 1975). Eighty percent of the children were constipated, with no difference in this feature seen between primary and secondary subtypes.

Etiology

No clear single causative pathway has been established. The constipated–nonconstipated distinction does, however, generate some specificity in terms of associations that may be important etiologically. Within the first year of life, children can show a tendency toward constipation (Levine 1982), with concordance for constipation being six times more frequent in monozygotic than in dizygotic twins (Bakwin 1971). Fecal retention and reduced stool frequency between 12 and 24 months of age can predict later encopresis (Levine 1975). Encopretic children with constipation and overflow are found to have rectal and colonic distention, massive impaction with hard feces, and a number of specific abnormalities of anorectal physiology. These abnormalities, which may be primary or secondary to constipation, include elevated anal resting tone, decreased anorectal motility and weakness of the internal anal sphincter (Loening-Baucke and Younoszai 1982), and dysfunction of the external anal sphincter, for example, contraction during defecation (Wald et al. 1986, Loening-Baucke et al. 1987).

Encopresis may occur after an acute episode of constipation following illness or a change in diet (Pettei et al.). In addition to the pain and discomfort caused by attempts to pass an extremely hard stool, a number of specific painful perianal conditions such as anal fissure can lead to stool withholding and later fecal soiling. Stressful events such as the birth of a sibling or attending a new school have been associated with up to 25% of cases of secondary encopresis (Levine 1975). In nonretentive encopresis, the main theories center on faulty toilet training. Stress during the training period, coercive toileting leading to anxiety and "pot phobia," and failure to learn or to have been taught the appropriate behavior

(Anthony 1957, Berg and Jones 1964) have all been implicated. True fecal urgency, which may have a physiological or pathological basis, may also be important in a small proportion of cases (Woodmansey 1967).

Treatment

Practical management for encopresis is presented in Table 11-3. The principal approach to treatment is predicated on the results of the evaluation and the clinical category assigned. This differentiates between the need to establish a regular toileting procedure in children in whom there has been a failure to learn this social behavior and the need to address a psychiatric disorder, parent–child relationship difficulties, or other stresses in the child who exhibits loss of this previously acquired skill in association with these factors. In both cases, analysis of the soiling behavior may identify reinforcing factors important in maintaining dysfunction. Detection of significant constipation will, in addition, provide an indication for adjuvant laxative therapy.

Table 11-3	Practical Management of Encopresis
Stage 1	**Assessment**
	Whether primary or secondary.
	Is there physical cause?
	Presence or absence of constipation.
	Presence or absence of acute stress.
	Presence or absence of psychiatric disorder including phobic symptoms or smearing.
	ABC (antecedents, behavior, consequences) of encopresis including secondary gain.
	Discover reasons for previous failure or failures.
Stage 2	**Advice**
	Education regarding diet, constipation, and toileting.
	Aim to reduce punitive or coercive behavior.
	Transmit optimism; however, anticipate disappointment at no instant cure.
	Preview the stepwise recovery and warn of the possibility of relapse.
Stage 3	**Toileting**
	Baseline observation using star chart.
	Focus on positive achievements, e.g., toileting, rather than soiling.
	High-fiber diet (try bran in soup, milk shakes).
	Toilet after meals, 15 minutes maximum.
	Check that adequately rising intra-abdominal pressure is present.
	Graded exposure scheme if "pot phobic."
	with
	Laxatives
	Indicated if physical examination or abdominal radiograph shows fecal loading.
	Medication of choice: Senokot syrup (senna) up to 10 mL b.i.d., lactulose syrup up to 30 mL (20 mg) b.i.d.
	Dosage will be reduced over time; titrate with bowel frequency.
	Enemas
	Microenema (e.g., bisacodyl, 30 mL) if the bowel is excessively loaded with rock-like feces.
Stage 4	**Biofeedback**
	Consider after relapse or failure to respond to toileting or laxatives.

Behavioral Treatments

Behavioral therapy is the mainstay of treatment for encopresis. In the younger child who has been toilet trained, this focuses on practical elimination skills, for example, visiting the toilet after each meal, staying there for a maximum of 15 minutes, using muscles to increase intra-abdominal pressure, and cleaning oneself adequately afterward. Parents or caretakers, or both, need to be educated in making the toilet a pleasant place to visit and should stay with the younger child, giving encouragement and praise for appropriate effort. Systematic recording of positive toileting behavior, not necessarily being clean (depending on the level of baseline behavior), should be performed with a personal star chart.

Removing the child's and family's attention from the encopresis alone and onto noticing, recording, and rewarding positive behavior often defuses tension and hostility and provides the opportunity for therapeutic improvement. Identifying and eliminating sources of secondary gain, whereby soiling is reinforced by parental (or other individuals) actions and attention, even if negative or punitive, make positive efforts more fruitful. Formal therapy, either individual or family based, is indicated in only a minority of individuals with an associated psychiatric disorder, marked behavioral disturbance (e.g., smearing, other aggressive soiling), or clear remediable family or social stresses.

Physical Treatments

In children with retention, leading to constipation and overflow, medical management is nearly always required, although it is usually done with oral laxatives or microenemas alone. The use of more intrusive and invasive colonic and rectal washout or surgical disimpaction procedures is nearly always the result of the clinician's impatience rather than the true clinical need. Uncontrolled studies of combined treatment with behavioral therapy and laxatives reported marked improvement in symptoms (not cure) in approximately 70 to 80% of individuals with encopresis (Levine and Bakow 1976).

Biofeedback Therapy

The finding that some children with treatment-resistant retentive encopresis involuntarily contract the muscles of the pelvic floor and the external anal sphincter, effectively impeding passage of stool (Loening-Baucke and Cruickshank 1986), has led to efforts to use biofeedback in such instances. Although it has been reported that as few as six sessions of biofeedback therapy can lead to a significant reduction in symptom frequency for as many as 86% of previously treatment-resistant children (Loening-Baucke 1995), this has been challenged by van Ginkel et al., who showed (van Ginkel et al. 2001) that anorectal manometry offered no additional advantage over conventional therapy (dietary advice, diary, toilet training, oral laxatives, and enemas) in chronic constipation/encopresis. It is possible, however, that biofeedback is principally of benefit to nonretentive chronic soilers (van Ginkel et al. 2000).

SEPARATION ANXIETY DISORDER

Diagnosis

Separation anxiety disorder (SAD) is typified by developmentally inappropriate and excessive anxiety concerning separation from home or attachment figures (see DSM-IV-TR diagnostic criteria on page 244).

DSM-IV-TR Diagnostic Criteria

309.21 Separation Anxiety Disorder

A. Developmentally inappropriate and excessive anxiety concerning separation from home or from those to whom the individual is attached, as evidenced by three (or more) of the following:

  (1) recurrent excessive distress when separation from home or major attachment figures occurs or is anticipated
  (2) persistent and excessive worry about losing, or about possible harm befalling major attachment figures
  (3) persistent and excessive worry that an untoward event will lead to separation from a major attachment figure (e.g., getting lost or being kidnapped)
  (4) persistent reluctance or refusal to go to school or elsewhere because of fear of separation
  (5) persistently and excessively fearful or reluctant to be alone, or without major attachment figures at home, or without significant adults in other settings
  (6) persistent reluctance or refusal to go to sleep without being near a major attachment figure or to sleep away from home
  (7) repeated nightmares involving the theme of separation
  (8) repeated complaints of physical symptoms (such as headaches, stomachaches, nausea, or vomiting) when separation from major attachment figures occurs or is anticipated

B. The duration of the disturbance is at least 4 weeks.
C. The onset is before age 18 years.
D. The disturbance causes clinically significant distress or impairment in social, academic (occupational), or other important areas of functioning.
E. The disturbance does not occur exclusively during the course of a pervasive developmental disorder, schizophrenia, or other psychotic disorder and, in adolescents and adults, is not better accounted for by panic disorder with agoraphobia.

Specify if:

Early Onset: if onset occurs before age 6 years.

The assessment strategy will depend upon the child's age, symptom profile, the sources of available information, and the purpose of the assessment. Separation anxiety is normal at some ages, and is maximal around 14 months of age (Crowell et al. 1990). The most prevalent symptoms in young children (aged 5–8) are worry about losing, or about possible harm to an attachment figure, and reluctance or refusal to go to school. Children aged 9–12 most frequently reported recurrent excessive distress when separated from home or attachment figures, whereas adolescents (aged 13–16 years) had physical symptoms on school days. More symptoms were reported with decreasing age.

Other anxiety disorders must be distinguished from separation anxiety disorder. In contrast to SAD where the anxiety is focused on separation issues, in Generalized anxiety disorder (GAD) the anxiety is more free floating, less situation specific, and occurs independent of separation from the primary attachment figure. Children with social phobia will display a fear of social situations in which they may be the object of public scrutiny. This anxiety may be ameliorated by the presence of a familiar person but will not occur exclusively when the attachment figure is absent, as with separation anxiety.

School refusal has long been associated with separation anxiety disorder, though this relationship holds mainly for younger children when school nonattendance is most closely linked to fear of separation, whereas in adolescents fear of school and social-evaluative situations is more typical. It is important in the assessment of school nonattendance, a frequent impairment associated with SAD, to distinguish anxiety-related school refusal from conduct disorder–related truancy. Typically the school-refusing child will stay at home or with parents, whereas the truanting child will go off with peers. In the presence of school refusal, a useful approach (Kearney and Silverman 1999) is to attempt to categorize the behavior as fulfilling one of the following four functions: (1) avoidance of stimuli-provoking specific fearfulness or anxiety (e.g., separation); (2) escape from aversive social or evaluative situations (e.g., social phobia); (3) attention-getting behavior (e.g., physical complaints/tantrums); or (4) positive tangible reinforcement (e.g., parental collusion).

Epidemiology

The community prevalence of SAD is generally estimated to be around 4% in children and young adolescents; it decreases in prevalence from childhood through adolescence (Moreau et al.). Amongst clinically referred subjects (aged 5–18) with anxiety disorders, separation anxiety disorder was found (Last et al. 1992) to be the most frequently occurring disorder, with a lifetime prevalence of 44.7%. Separation anxiety, particularly in younger samples, is found more frequently in girls than in boys—ratio as high as 2.5 : 1 (Anderson et al. 1987).

Course

The age of onset has been reported to be 4–7 years of age, with earlier onset being associated with clinical status and comorbidity (Biederman et al. 1997, Keller et al. 1992). In a 3–4-year prospective study (Last et al. 1996) of subjects with anxiety disorders, 29% of children had separation anxiety disorder (21% had SAD as their primary diagnosis at baseline). On follow-up, 92% of children previously diagnosed with SAD no longer had symptoms that met full criteria for SAD, although 25% had developed a new disorder, most frequently a depressive disorder. Finding that 50% of adult individuals with panic disorder had experienced separation anxiety during childhood, it has been hypothesized (Gittleman and Klein 1984) that separation anxiety may be a childhood precursor to adult panic disorder and agoraphobia. Evidence supporting this link is uneven since most studies are retrospective, focus on separation anxiety symptoms rather than the full disorder and/or fail to include an appropriate control group.

Etiology

Sensitivity to suffocation cues, important in the carbon dioxide (CO_2) challenge paradigm in panic disorder and respiratory response may differentiate children with anxiety disorder, and separation anxiety in particular from children without an anxiety disorder (Pine et al. 1998). Inhalation of air containing raised CO_2 concentration results in increased catecholamine release throughout the body and perceived anxiety. This response appears mediated via the locus ceruleus, a group of norepinephrine-containing neurons originating in the pons, and projecting to all major brain areas. The locus ceruleus forms part of the reticular activating system (RAS), and functions to regulate noradrenergic tone and activity. Hypothalamic and thalamic nuclei also play a role in the perception of and response to external threats. They act by transmitting arousal information from the RAS to limbic and cortical areas involved in sensory integration and perception. The thalamus is thought to have a role in the perception of anxiety, whereas the hypothalamic nuclei mediate the response by the neuroendocrine system. Experiments in rhesus monkeys inducing separation anxiety suggest roles for both the locus ceruleus/noradrenergic system as well as the hypothalamic pituitary axis (HPA) (Chrousos and Gold 1992). Urinary cortisol has been shown to be raised (indicative of HPA overactivity) in infants aged 1 year who demonstrated extreme distress when separated from their primary attachment figure (Tennes et al. 1977).

Separation anxiety, when developmentally appropriate, is seen via attachment theory as an adaptive response that infants use to enhance proximity to their caregivers (Bowlby 1973). In this, when the infant has adequate proximity to the caregiver in a given context, attachment behaviors (separation anxiety symptoms) subside and are replaced by alternate behaviors. On the basis of their response to various experimental paradigms, infants can be categorized into having different types of attachment. Although the nosology of attachment has varied, the most frequently described type of pathological attachment is known as *insecure attachment*. Excessive distress on separation evinced by insecurely attached infants appears to be the earliest manifestation of separation anxiety disorder, but this pattern is not specific in that it can be the precursor of other types of anxiety (e.g., social phobia/avoidant disorder, panic disorder) in childhood (Manassis et al. 1995) and adolescence.

Treatment

Following a good behavioral and functional analysis, the most frequently employed clinical approach to the treatment of separation anxiety and school refusal is behavioral. The principles of systematic desensitization to feared objects or situations will be employed, gradually increasing the amount of separation that can be tolerated in a graduated fashion. Systematic desensitization usually has three components. Firstly a response, incompatible with anxiety (often progressive muscular relaxation, but can be imagery or breathing exercises) is taught. The second component is the collaborative construction of a hierarchy of feared situations. These will range from the very mild (producing mild disquiet) to the most anxiety provoking (avoided at all costs!). It is important to include a great deal of specificity in describing these situations including the duration spent in the feared situation, the degree to which others are present, the distance from home/attachment figure etc. After ranking these feared situations, the final component of treatment is the regular progression of exposure to feared situations whilst employing anxiety management techniques. It is important that the child is allowed to exercise some control over the speed with which the new settings are experienced. The avoidance of reinforcement of unwanted behaviors and the promotion of fear-coping strategies is similarly important.

In the particular example of school refusal associated with separation anxiety, it is important to encourage an early return to school so that secondary impairments (academic failure and social isolation) are minimized. Generally, if the period of absence has been less than 2 months then return is very often successful, longer than this is frequently associated with much greater difficulty negotiating adequate attendance.

In older subjects, cognitive approaches may be more successful than the primary behavior strategies usually employed with younger children. Cognitive approaches postulate that the child's maladaptive thoughts, beliefs and attitudes (schema) cause or maintain the experience of anxiety. Treatment consists of identifying negative self-statements ("I can't ever do this"), or external beliefs ("If I'm not there my mom won't be able to cope") and replacing them with more adaptive beliefs.

Pharmacological treatment studies of separation anxiety have tended to focus on samples with school-refusal behavior and various comorbidities. A recent study (2001) of 128 children with anxiety disorders (social phobia, separation anxiety disorder, and/or generalized anxiety disorder) aged 6 to 17 years who failed to respond to an initial 3 weeks of psychological treatment were then randomly assigned to a double-blind, placebo-controlled trial of fluvoxamine, up to a maximum of 300 mg per day, for 8 weeks. Children randomized to fluvoxamine showed significantly greater drops in anxiety disorder symptoms compared to placebo ($P < 0.001$). Pure cases of separation anxiety were very hard to find in this clinical sample, but therapeutic effect was seen in all symptom areas. Considering safety and efficacy, the SSRIs appear to be the first-line treatment for separation anxiety disorder, but more studies are needed to confirm the preliminary results. Tricyclic antidepressants and benzodiazepines may be considered when the child has not responded to SSRIs or when adverse effects have exceeded benefits.

In practice, however, clinicians often combine drug and psychosocial treatments, capitalizing on differences in dose-response and time-response parameters. There is some evidence that treatments can be additive (each treatment having unique benefits) or synergistic (the benefit of the combination is greater that the additive combination). Alternatively, when combining drug and psychosocial treatments, a lower dose of one or both may be possible, with a resultant decrease in expense, inconvenience, or adverse events. Drug effects are often seen sooner than those due to exposure-based therapy, though it is hoped that the slower to emerge benefits of therapy may be more long lasting.

SELECTIVE MUTISM

Diagnosis

The essential feature of selective mutism is the persistent failure to speak in specific social situations (e.g., school, or with peers) where speaking is expected, despite speaking in other situations (e.g., home) (see DSM-IV-TR diagnostic criteria). Previously referred to as Elective Mutism, in DSM-III the condition was renamed Selective Mutism, so as to be less judgmental (doesn't speak rather than chooses not to speak).

DSM-IV-TR Diagnostic Criteria

313.23 Selective Mutism

A. Consistent failure to speak in specific social situations (in which there is an expectation for speaking, e.g., at school) despite speaking in other situations.
B. The disturbance interferes with educational or occupational achievement or with social communication.
C. The duration of the disturbance is at least 1 month (not limited to the first month of school).
D. The failure to speak is not due to a lack of knowledge of, or comfort with, the spoken language required in the social situation.
E. The disturbance is not better accounted for by a communication disorder (e.g., stuttering) and does not occur exclusively during the course of a pervasive developmental disorder, schizophrenia, or other psychotic disorder.

Prior to making a diagnosis of selective mutism, a comprehensive evaluation should be conducted to rule out other explanations for mutism and to assess important comorbid factors. For obvious reasons, the parental interview will form the mainstay of evaluation, but as discussed below direct observation (and interview if possible) of the child can afford important diagnostic information.

It is important to obtain information about the nature of the onset (insidious or sudden), any uncharacteristic features (i.e., not talking to family members, abrupt cessation of speech in one setting, absence of communication in all settings) suggestive of other neurological or psychiatric disorders (e.g., pervasive developmental disorders, acquired aphasias), and any history of neurological insult/injury, developmental delays or atypical language and/or speech. The assessment should also include the degree to which nonverbal communication or non-face-to-face communication is possible, the presence of anxiety symptoms in areas other than speaking, social and behavioral inhibition, medical history including ear infections, and hearing deficiencies. Parents will be able to give information on where and to whom the child will speak, the child's speech and language complexity at home, articulation problems, use of nonverbal communication (gestures etc.), any history of speech and language delays, and the possible importance of bilingualism (where primary language is not English). It can be useful to have the parents provide an audiotape of the child speaking at home.

The child evaluation can assess the presence of anxiety and social inhibition (willingness to communicate through gesture or drawing). Physical examination of oral sensory and motor ability may provide evidence of neurological problems (i.e., drooling, asymmetry, orofacial weakness, abnormal gag reflex, impaired sucking or swallowing). Specialist audiometry (pure tone and speech stimuli as well as tympanometry and acoustic reflex testing) may provide evidence of hearing and/or middle ear problems that can have a significant effect on speech and language development. Cognitive abilities may be difficult to assess, but the performance section of the WISC-R (Wechsler 1974) or Raven's Progressive Matrices (Raven 1976) as well as the Peabody Picture Vocabulary Test (Dunn and Dunn 1981) may be useful in the nonverbal child.

Epidemiology

The prevalence is usually reported as 0.6 to 7 per 1000 (Brown and Lloyd 1975, Fundudis et al. 1979), with higher incidence in females rather than males (Hayden 1980). When subjects failing to speak in the first few weeks of school (a DSM-IV-TR requirement) are excluded rates do not exceed 2 per 1000. Onset is usually in the preschool years, but the peak age of presentation and diagnosis is between 6 and 8 years (Dow et al. 1995). A high incidence of insidious onset of refusal to speak with anyone except family members is reported. The other typical picture is one of acute onset of mutism on starting school (Hayden 1980, Kolvin and Fundudis 1981).

Etiology

Three basic theories have been proposed to explain the etiology of selective mutism: children who are negative, oppositional, and controlling; traumatized children; and children who have severe anxiety, chiefly social phobia. Although early psychodynamic theorists (Hayden 1980) described an enmeshed relationship between mother and child, the father being distant and ineffectual, and a conflicted relationship between the parents' the only two controlled studies of selective mutism did not find family functioning worse compared to the families of other emotionally disturbed children (Kolvin and Fundudis 1981, Wilkins 1985). Associated features include a history of delayed speech and articulation problems, and possibly increased incidence of enuresis and/or encopresis (Dow et al. 1995, Kolvin and Fundudis 1981, Wilkins 1985). There may be a family history of general shyness, or of elevated levels of anxiety in the parents (Hayden 1980, Kolvin and Fundudis 1981).

Treatment

Treatment has long been regarded as difficult and prognosis poor. Approaches have included behavioral therapy, family therapy, speech therapy, and more recently pharmacological agents (Cline and Baldwin 1994). Unfortunately, most published studies are single case reports, with very few controlled studies.

Behavioral treatment focuses on mutism as a means of getting attention and/or escaping from anxiety. A controlled study (Calhoun and Koenig 1973) of eight subjects with random assignment to treatment (teacher & peer reinforcement of verbal behavior) or control showed significant increases in mean number of vocalizations after 5 weeks of treatment. These gains were not, however, maintained at 12-month follow-up. Other techniques have included graded exposure, shaping, and modeling. The goal of a treatment program should be to decrease the anxiety associated with speaking whilst encouraging the child to interact verbally.

Regarding pharmacotherapy, early success with phenelzine in a 7-year-old girl with mutism and shyness (Golwyn and Weinstock 1990) led to the use of SSRI medication in cases of selective mutism with associated anxiety (principally social phobia). Successful case reports were followed by open and controlled studies using fluoxetine. An open trial of 21 children using a mean dose of 28.1 mg/day showed improvement in 76% of cases (Dummit et al. 1996). A placebo-controlled double-blind study showed mixed results, though both groups remained highly symptomatic. More chronic (>14 weeks) treatment was recommended (Black and Uhde 1994).

References

Anderson JC, Williams S, McGee R, et al. (1987) DSM III disorders in preadolescent children: Prevalence in a large sample from a general population. *Arch Gen Psychiatry* **44**, 69–76.

Anthony EJ (1957) An experimental approach to the psychopathology of childhood: Encopresis. *Br J Med Psychol* **30**, 146–175.

Baigrie RJ, Kelleher JP, Fawcett DP, et al. (1988) Oxybutynin: Is it safe? *Br J Urol* **62**, 319–322.

Bakwin H (1961) Enuresis in children. *J Pediatr* **58**, 806–819.

Bakwin H (1971) Enuresis in twins. *Am J Dis Child* **121**, 222–225.

Bakwin H (1971) Enuresis in twins. *Am J Dis Child* **121**, 222–225.

Bellman M (1966) Studies on encopresis. *Acta Paediatr Scand* (Suppl. 170), 1+.

Berg I and Jones KV (1964) Functional fecal incontinence in children. *Arch Dis Child* **39**, 465–472.

Berg I, Forsythe I, and McGuire R (1982) Response of bed-wetting to the enuresis alarm. Influence of psychiatric disturbance and maximum functional bladder capacity. *Arch Dis Child* **57**, 394–396.

Black B and Uhde TW (1994) Treatment of elective mutism with fluoxetine: A double-blind placebo-controlled study. *J Am Acad Child Adolesc Psychiatry* **33**, 1000–1006.

Blomfield JM and Douglas JWB (1956) Bed-wetting-prevalence among children aged 4–7 years. *Lancet* **1**, 850–852.

Bollard J and Nettlebeck T (1981) A comparison of dry bed training and standard urine-alarm conditioning treatment of childhood bed-wetting. *Behav Res Ther* **19**, 215–226.

Boon F (1991) Encopresis and sexual assault. *J Am Acad Child Adolesc Psychiatry* **30**, 479–482.

Bowlby JK (1973) *Attachment and Loss: Attachment*. Basic Books, New York.

Boyd MM (1960) The depth of sleep in enuretic school children and in non-enuretic controls. *J Psychosom Res* **44**, 274–281.

Brazelton TB (1962) A child-oriented approach to toilet training. *Pediatrics* **29**, 121–128.

Brown JB and Lloyd H (1975) A controlled study of children not speaking at school. *J Assoc Workers Maladjusted Child* **3**, 49–63.

Butler RJ (1991) Establishment of working definitions in nocturnal enuresis. *Arch Dis Child* **66**, 267–271.

Butler RJ, Forsythe WI, and Robertson J (1990) The body worn alarm in treatment of childhood enuresis. *Br J Child Psychiatry* **44**, 237–241.

Calhoun J and Koenig KP (1973) Classroom modification of elective mutism. *Behav Ther* **4**, 700–702.

Chrousos GP and Gold PW (1992) The concepts of stress and stress system disorders: Overview of physical and behavioral homeostasis. *JAMA* **267**, 1244–1252.

Clayden G and Agnarsson U (1991) *Constipation in Childhood*. University Press, Oxford.

Cline T and Baldwin S (1994) *Selective Mutism*. Whurr Publishers, London.

Crowell JA and Watus E (1990) Separation anxiety. In *Handbook of Developmental psychopathology*, Lewis M and Miller S (eds). Plenum press, New York, pp. 209–218.

Deleon G and Mandell W (1966) A comparison of conditioning and psychotherapy in the treatment of enuresis. *J Clin Psychol* **22**, 326–330.

Dimson SB (1986) DDAVP and urine osmolality in refractory enuresis. *Arch Dis Child* **61**, 1104–1107.

Dische S, Yule W, Corbett J, et al. (1983) Childhood nocturnal enuresis: Factors associated with outcome of treatment with an enuresis alarm. *Dev Med Child Neurol* **25**, 67–81.

Doleys DM, McWhorter MS, Williams SC, et al. (1977) Encopresis: its treatment and relation to nocturnal enuresis. *Behav Ther* **8**, 77–82.

Dundaroz MR, Denli M, Uzun M, et al. (2001) Analysis of heart rate variability in children with primary nocturnal enuresis. *Int Urol Nephrol* **32**(3), 393–397.

Dunn LM and Dunn LM (1981) *Peabody Picture Vocabulary Test-Revised*. American Guidance Services, Circle Pines, MN.

Easson RI (1960) Encopresis-psychogenic soiling. *Can Med Assoc J* **82**, 624–628.

Elmer M, Norgaard JP, Djurhuus JC, et al. (1988) Terodiline in the treatment of diurnal enuresis in children. *Scand J Primary Health Care* **6**, 119–124.

Essen J and Peckham C (1976) Nocturnal enuresis in childhood. *Dev Med Child Neurol* **18**, 577–589.

Fergusson DM, Horwood LJ, and Shannon FT (1986) Factors related to the age of attainment of nocturnal bladder control: An 8 year longitudinal study. *Pediatrics* **78**, 884–890.

Fielding D (1980) The response of day and night wetting children and children who wet only at night to retention control training and the enuresis alarm. *Behav Res Ther* **18**, 305–317.

Fielding D (1985) Factors associated with drop out, relapse and failure in conditioning treatment of nocturnal enuresis. *Behav Psychother* **13**, 174–185.

Fielding D, Berg I, and Bell S (1978) An observational study of posture and limb movements of children who wet by day and at night. *Dev Med Child Neurol* **20**, 453–461.

Finley WW and Wansley RA (1977) Auditory intensity as a variable in the conditioning treatment of enuresis nocturna. *Behav Res Ther* **15**, 181–185.

Fleisher D (1976) Diagnosis and treatment of disorders of defecation in children. *Pediatr Ann* **5**, 700–722.

Forsythe WI and Butler RJ (1989) Fifty years of enuretic alarms. *Arch Dis Child* **64**, 879–885.

Forsythe WI and Redmond A (1974) Enuresis and spontaneous cure rate. A study of 1129 enuretics. *Arch Dis Child* **49**, 259–263.

Foxman B, Valdez RB, and Brook RH (1986) Childhood enuresis: prevalence, perceived impact and prescribed treatments. *Pediatrics* **77**, 482–487.

Gittleman R and Klein DF (1984) Relationship between separation anxiety and panic and agoraphobia disorders. *Psychopathology* **17**, 56–65.

Golwyn DH and Weinstock RC (1990) Phenelzine treatment of elective mutism: a case report. *J Clin Psychiatry* **51**, 384–385.

Hallgren B and Enuresis I (1956) A study with reference to the morbidity risk and symptomatology. *Acta Psychiatr Neurol Scand* **31**, 379–403.

Halliday S, Meadow SR, and Berg I (1987) Successful management of daytime enuresis using alarm procedures: a randomly controlled trial. *Arch Dis Child* **62**, 132–137.

Hayden TL (1980) Classification of elective mutism. *J Am Acad Child Adolesc Psychiatry* **19**, 118–133.

Jarvelin MR, Vikevainen-Tervonen L, Moilanen I, et al. (1988) Enuresis in seven-year-old children. *Acta Paediatr Scand* **77**, 148–153.

Jorgensen OS, Lober M, Christiansen J, et al. (1980) Plasma concentration and clinical effect in imipramine treatment of childhood enuresis. *Clin Pharmacokinet* **5**, 386–393.

Kearney CA and Silverman WK (1999) Functionally-based prescriptive and non-prescriptive treatment for children and adolescents with school refusal behavior. *Behav Ther* **30**, 673–695.

Kolvin I and Fundudis T (1981) Elective mute children: psychological development and background factors. *J Child Psychol Psychiatry* **22**, 219–232.

Kolvin I, Taunch J, Currah J, et al. (1972) Enuresis: a descriptive analysis and a controlled trial. *Dev Med Child Neurol* **14**, 715–726.

Kruse S, Hellstrom AL, Hanson E, et al. The Swedish Enuresis Trial (SWEET) Group (2001) Treatment of primary monosymptomatic nocturnal enuresis with desmopressin: predictive factors. *Bju Int* **88**(6), 572–576.

Leebeek-Groenewegen A, Blom J, Sukhai R, et al. (2001) Efficacy of desmopressin combined with alarm therapy for monosymptomatic nocturnal enuresis. *J Urol* **166**(6), 2456–2458.

Levine MD (1975) Children with encopresis: a descriptive analysis. *Pediatrics* **56**, 412–416.

Levine MD (1982) Encopresis, its potential evaluation and alleviation. *Med Clin North Am* **29**, 315–330.

Levine MD and Bakow H (1976) Children with encopresis: a study of treatment outcome. *Pediatrics* **50**, 845–852.

Loening-Baucke V (1995) Biofeedback treatment for chronic constipation and encopresis in childhood: Long-term outcome. *Pediatrics* **96**, 105–110.

Loening-Baucke VA and Cruickshank BM (1986) Abnormal defecation dynamics in chronically constipated children with encopresis. *J Pediatr* **108**, 562–566.

Loening-Baucke VA and Younoszai MK (1982) Abnormal anal sphincter response in chronically constipated children. *J Pediatr* **100**, 213–218.

Loening-Baucke VA, Cruickshank B, and Savage C (1987) Defecation dynamics and behavior profiles in encopretic children. *Pediatrics* **80**, 672–679.

Meadow R and Berg I (1982) Controlled trial of imipramine in diurnal enuresis. *Arch Dis Child* **57**, 714–716.

McConaghy N (1969) A controlled trial of imipramine, amphetamine, pad and bell, conditioning and random awakening in the treatment of nocturnal enuresis. *Med J Aust* **2**, 237–239.

Mikkelsen EJ and Rapoport JL (1980) Enuresis: psychopathology sleep stage and drug response. *Urol Clin North Am* **7**, 361–377.

Miller K and Klauber GT (1990) Desmopressin acetate in children with severe primary nocturnal enuresis. *Clin Ther* **12**, 357–366.

Miller K, Goldberg S, and Atkin B (1989) Nocturnal enuresis: experience with long-term use of intranasally administered desmopressin. *J Pediatr* **14**, 723–726.

Norgaard JP, Pederson EB, and Djurhuus JC (1985) Diurnal antidiuretic hormone levels in enuretics. *J Urol* **134**, 1029–1031.

Oppel WC, Harper PA, and Rider RV (1968) Social, psychological and neurological factors associated with enuresis. *Pediatrics* **42**, 627–641.

Pfaundler M (1904) Demonstration eines Apparates zur selbstätig Signalisieursang stattgehabter Bettnassung. *Verh Ges Kinderheilk* **21**, 219–220.

Pretlow RA (1999) Treatment of nocturnal enuresis with an ultrasound bladder volume controlled alarm device. *J Urol* **162**, 1224–1228.

Rapoport JL, Mikkelsen EJ, Zavardil A, et al. (1980) Childhood enuresis II: Psychopathology, tricyclic concentration in plasma, and antienuretic effect. *Arch Gen Psychiatry* **37**, 1146–1152.

Raven JC (1976) *The Colored Progressive Matrices*. HK Lewis, London.

Rittig S, Knudsen U, Norgaard J, et al. (1989) Abnormal diurnal rhythm of plasma vasopressin and urinary output in patients with enuresis. *Am J Physiol* **256**, 664–671.

Rutter M, Tizard J, and Whitmore K (eds) (1970) *Education, Health and Behavior*, Longman, London.

Rutter ML, Yule W, and Graham PJ (1973) Enuresis and behavioral deviance: some epidemiological considerations. In *Bladder Control and Enuresis. Clinics in Developmental Medicine*, Kolvin I, MacKeith R, and Meadow SR (eds), Nos. 48/49. Heinemann/Spastics International Medical Publications, London, pp. 137–147.

Serel TA, Perk H, Koyuncuoglu HR, et al. (2001) Deniz: Acupuncture therapy in the management of persistent primary nocturnal enuresis–preliminary results. *Scand J Urol Nephrol* **35**(1), 40–43.

Shaffer D, Costello AJ, and Hill JD (1968) Control of enuresis with imipramine. *Arch Dis Child* **43**, 665–671.

Shaffer D, Stephenson JD, and Thomas DV (1979) Some effects of imipramine on micturition and their relevance to their antienuretic activity. *Neuropharmacology* **18**, 33–37.

Simeon J, Maguire J, and Lawrence S (1981) Maprotiline effects in children with enuresis and behavioral disorders. *Prog Neuropsychopharmacol* **5**, 495–498.

Sorotzkin B (1984) Nocturnal enuresis: current perspectives. *Clin Psychol Rev* **4**, 293–316.

Stein Z and Susser M (1967) Social factors in the development of sphincter control. *Dev Med Child Neurol* **9**, 692–700.

Steinhausen HC and Gobel D (1989) Enuresis in child psychiatric clinic patients. *J Am Acad Child Adolesc Psychiatry* **28**, 279–281.

Steubens JA and Silber DL (1974) Parental expectations vs. outcome in toilet training. *Pediatrics* **54**, 493–495.

Turner R, Young G, and Rachman S (1970) Treatment of nocturnal enuresis by conditioning techniques. *Behav Res Ther* **8**, 367–381.

van Ginkel R, Benninga MA, Blommaart PJ, et al. (2000) Lack of benefit of laxatives as adjunctive therapy for functional nonretentive fecal soiling in children. *J Pediatrics* **137**(6), 808–813.

van Ginkel R, Buller HA, Boeckxstaens GE, et al. (2001) The effect of anorectal manometry on the outcome of treatment in severe childhood constipation: a randomized, controlled trial. *Pediatrics* **108**(1), E9.

Verhulst FC, Van Der Lee JH, Akkerhuis GW, et al. (1985) The prevalence of nocturnal enuresis: do DSM-III criteria need to be changed? A brief research report. *J Child Psychiatry* **26**, 989–993.

von Gontard A, Schaumburg H, Hollmann E, et al. (2001) The genetics of enuresis: a review. *J Urol* **166**(6), 2438–2443.

Wagner WG and Johnson JT (1988) Childhood nocturnal enuresis: the prediction of premature withdrawal from behavioral conditioning. *J Abnorm Child Psychol* **16**, 687–692.

Wald A, Chandra R, Chiponis D, et al. (1986) Anorectal function and continence mechanisms in childhood encopresis. *J Paediatr Gastroenterol Nutr* **5**, 346–351.

Wallace IR and Forsythe WI (1969) The treatment of enuresis. A controlled clinical trial of propantheline, propantheline and phenobarbitone, and placebo. *Br J Clin Pract* **23**, 207–210.

Wechsler D (1974) *Manual for the Wechsler Intelligence Scale for Children Revised*. The Psychological Corporation, New York.

Werry JS and Cohrssen J (1965) Enuresis: an etiologic and therapeutic study. *J Pediatr* **67**, 423–431.

Wilkins R (1985) A comparison of elective mutism and emotional disorders in children. *Br J Psychiatry* **146**, 198–203.

Woodmansey AC (1967) Emotion and the motions: an inquiry into the causes and prevention of functional disorders of defecation. *Br J Med Psychol* **40**, 207–223.

Young GC and Morgan RTT (1973) Rapidity of response to the treatment of enuresis. *Dev Med Child Neurol* **15**, 488–496.

Young GC and Turner RK (1965) CNS stimulant drugs and conditioning treatment of nocturnal enuresis. *Behav Res Ther* **3**, 93–101.

12 Childhood Disorders: Reactive Attachment Disorder of Infancy or Early Childhood

Brian S. Stafford
Charles H. Zeanah, Jr

REACTIVE ATTACHMENT DISORDER

Diagnosis

DSM-IV-TR defines reactive attachment disorder (RAD) as markedly disturbed and developmentally inappropriate social relatedness in most contexts, beginning before age 5 years, as evidenced by either restricted or indiscriminate social interaction (see DSM-IV-TR diagnostic criteria below). The abnormal relatedness cannot strictly be accounted for by developmental delay or by autism. In addition, evidence of pathogenic care such as institutionalization, emotional or physical neglect, or multiple changes in primary caregivers is evident. The diagnosis means to imply that the child's attachment relationships are impaired in reaction to "pathogenic caregiving." The socially aberrant behaviors are evident across social contexts.

DSM-IV-TR Diagnostic Criteria

313.89 Reactive Attachment Disorder of Infancy or Early Childhood

A. Markedly disturbed and developmentally inappropriate social relatedness in most contexts, beginning before age 5 years, as evidenced by either (1) or (2)''

(1) persistent failure to initiate or respond in a developmentally appropriate fashion to most social interactions, as manifested by excessive inhibited, hypervigilant, or highly ambivalent and contradictory responses (e.g., the child may respond to caregivers with a mixture of approach, avoidance, and resistance to comforting, or may exhibit frozen watchfulness).

(2) diffuse attachments as manifest by indiscriminate sociability with marked inability to exhibit appropriate selective attachments (e.g., excessive familiarity with strangers or lack of selectivity in choice of attachment figures).

B. The disturbance in Criterion A is not accounted for solely by developmental delay (as in Mental Retardation) and does not meet current criteria for a Pervasive Developmental Disorder.

C. Pathogenic care as evidenced by at least one of the following:

(1) persistent disregard of the child's basic emotional needs for comfort, stimulation, and affection

(2) persistent disregard of the child's basic physical needs

(3) repeated changes of primary caregiver that prevent formation of stable attachments (e.g., frequent changes in foster care).

D. There is a presumption that the care in Criterion C is responsible for the disturbed behavior in Criterion A (e.g., the disturbance in Criterion A began following the pathogenic care in Criterion C).

Reactive Attachment Disorder has two subtypes: the inhibited/emotionally withdrawn subtype and the disinhibited/indiscriminately social subtype. The inhibited subtype is marked by emotional withdrawal, failure of social and emotional reciprocity, and lack of seeking or responding to comforting when distressed. Attachment behaviors, such as seeking and accepting comfort, showing and responding to affection, relying on caregivers for help, and cooperating with caregivers are absent or markedly restricted. In addition, exploratory behavior is limited owing to the absence of a preferred attachment figure. These children may also demonstrate problems of emotion regulation that range from affective blunting to withdrawal, to "frozen watchfulness". This subtype has been described in institutionalized children (Tizard and Rees 1975, Smyke et al. 2002) and in abused or neglected children (Boris et al. 1998, Boris et al. 2000, Zeanah et al. 2001).

The disinhibited/indiscriminately social subtype is characterized by more interaction with caregivers; however, there is failure to demonstrate selectivity in interacting with others. Stranger wariness, which appears as early as 7 months of age and remains apparent for several years, is absent. Children with this subtype may approach strangers without expected social wariness around unfamiliar adults, may seek comfort or help from a stranger, and may demonstrate a variety of social relatedness problems that depend upon accurately reading social cues and understanding interpersonal boundaries. This subtype has been demonstrated in maltreated children (Zeanah et al. 2001), institutionalized children (Tizard and Rees 1975, Zeanah et al. 2001, Zeanah et al. 2002), and children adopted out of institutions (Chisholm 1998, O'Connor and Rutter 2001).

By definition, the disorder is a consequence of or reaction to early and profoundly pathologic caregiving. Since someone other than the early primary caregiver often brings the child in for evaluation, the history of early social development can be unavailable, lacking in detail, or contradictory (Hinshaw-Fuselier et al. 1999, Zeanah et al. 1993). Despite these challenges, inquiries from all potential sources (e.g., pediatric records, Child Protective Service documents, etc.) to elicit or document a history of pathogenic caregiving should be made. DSM-IV-TR has operationalized these etiologic factors in Criterion C as: (1) persistent disregard of the child's basic emotional needs; (2) persistent disregard of the child's basic physical needs; (3) repeated changes of primary caregiver that prevent formation of stable attachments.

Documentation of pathogenic caregiving does not automatically ensure a diagnosis of RAD since not all children who experience abuse or profound deprivation develop attachment-disordered behavior. In fact, O'Connor and colleagues (2000) found that 70% of children exposed to profound deprivation for more than 2 years did not exhibit marked or severe attachment-disordered behavior at age 6 years. There are preliminary data of note that suggest a dose-response between duration of deprivation and disturbances in attachment behavior, specifically indiscriminate behavior (O'Connor et al. 2003). Current criteria require documentation of etiology (i.e., pathogenic care); failure to do so precludes diagnosis and may be a limitation of the current criteria.

The disturbed social behavior that characterizes RAD should be evident by report or observation across most social contexts and relationships. Obviously, self-report in young children is less likely to be obtained or elicit relevant clinical information; therefore, caregiver report is essential. Observation of the child in the clinic interacting with relative strangers as well as in naturalistic settings are quite valuable (Zeanah et al. 1997, Stafford et al. 2003). Specialized structured clinical interviews and semistructured observational assessments may be helpful in eliciting disturbances in sociability related to attachment (Boris et al. 1999).

The current diagnostic requirement is that marked disturbances in social behavior are apparent before the age of 5 years. There is no research evidence to support this upper limit, although the literature on maternal deprivation, maltreatment, and institutionalization suggests that earlier insults to social development and attachment result in persistent and pervasive defects in social competence. The diagnosis, currently, can also be applied as early as the first month of life, since no lower age limit exists. This may be a vestige of the DSM-III criteria, which described RAD more as a syndrome of failure to thrive than as an attachment disorder. Given that the onset of focused attachment occurs around 7 to 9 months of age, it is hypothetically possible that a child could be diagnosed with reactive attachment disorder before it is developmentally possible for the child to have a focused attachment. This issue needs to be addressed in future modifications of the criteria.

A variety of impairments are associated with RAD. By definition, children with the disorder are socially impaired, either withdrawn and detached or socially disinhibited and indiscriminating. Long-term impairments in peer relationships are associated with indiscriminate behavior at age 4 and 8 years (Hodges and Tizard 1989). In addition, cognitive delays often arise in the same contexts of deprivation that give rise to signs of RAD (Zeanah 1996, Zeanah 2000).

Although there are few studies of comorbidity with RAD, much is known about associated conditions with institutionalization, abuse, and neglect (see Zeanah 2000). Medical abnormalities include malnutrition, a variety of serious medical problems (Johnson 1992), and physical and brain growth deficiencies (Aronson and Johnson 1999) have been noted in institutionalized infants adopted out to the United States and Canada. Other developmental abnormalities include cognitive problems (O'Connor 1998, Morrison 1995), speech and language delays (Albers 1997, Smyke et al. 2002), stereotypies (Cermak 1997, Smyke et al. 2002), and other social and behavioral abnormalities (Fisher 1997, O'Connor 1999).

The cognitive deficits are most likely an associated feature related to malnutrition, deprivation, and inadequate stimulation but remarkably improve when those risk factors are addressed within the context of an appropriate caregiving environment (O'Connor 1999, O'Connor 2000, Zeanah et al. 2003). Speech and language delays range from poor articulation to echolalia and are likely related to lack of exposure to linguistic stimuli; these features typically improve with intervention. The course of stereotypies is unknown, but likely improves as language development improves (Smyke 2002).

Other behavioral abnormalities that may mimic mental disorders include a quasi-autistic syndrome (Federici 1999, Rutter 1999, Shin 1999, Mukkades et al. 2000) that appears to arise as a result of institutionalization rather than genetic or intrinsic neurobiological abnormalities. Although symptomatically virtually indistinguishable from classic autism, this institutional syndrome does not show male predominance, is not associated with enlarged head circumference, and generally shows marked improvement after the child is placed with a family.

Externalizing behavior disorders also have been noted, especially a syndrome of inattention and overactivity (Kreppner et al. 2001, Roy et al. in press). What is unclear is whether this syndrome of inattention/overactivity is distinguishable from more conventional attention-deficit/hyperactivity disorder (ADHD).

Epidemiology

There are limited data available on the prevalence of RAD. DSM-IV-TR suggests that the disorder appears to be uncommon. This is most likely true in the general population; in certain populations, however, where pathogenic care is more likely to occur, such as extreme poverty, family violence, or in institutional care, the diagnosis is much less rare. In a validation study of the criteria in a sample of children less than 4 years old with documented abuse and neglect (Boris et al. 1998), as many as one-third met criteria for an alternative classification of attachment disorder. In two studies of young children in institutions, in which there was limited opportunity to form selective attachments to caregivers, 50 to 65% of the children developed clinical signs of RAD (Tizard and Rees 1975, Smyke et al. 2002). In a retrospective chart review of 94 abused and neglected children admitted to an intervention program, more than a third met criteria for RAD (Zeanah et al. 2000).

To date, no gender or ethnic differences have been described. No evidence of gender differences have appeared (Chisholm 1998, Shin 1999, O'Connor and Rutter 2000, Smyke et al. 2002).

The lack of data about prevalence of the diagnosis in both the general population and in high-risk environments underscores the importance of developing research and clinical methods with procedural validity for defining and assessing attachment disorder (Zeanah et al. 2000, Stafford et al. 2003).

Course

To date, there have been no investigations on the course of RAD as defined by DSM-IV-TR criteria. Still, some data relevant to understanding the course of RAD have appeared.

The inhibited/emotionally withdrawn pattern of RAD appears to be incompatible with having a preferred attachment relationship. Once the caregiving environment improves, the inhibited/emotionally withdrawn behavior appears to improve. For example, although the inhibited/emotionally withdrawn subtype is clearly evident in institutionalized children (Smyke et al. 2002), this subtype is not apparent in children adopted out of institutions (Chisholm 1998, O'Connor and Rutter 2000). This suggests that this form of the disorder resolves if the child is placed in a more "normalized" or less pathological caregiving setting and develops an attachment to a caregiver (O'Connor and Rutter 2000). To date, no direct tests of this conclusion have appeared, but studies underway should be able to provide a more direct test.

The course of the disinhibited/indiscriminately social subtype appears to be quite different. In contrast to inhibited/emotionally withdrawn attachment, disinhibited/indiscriminately social attachment disorder is more likely to persist even when the caregiving environment is improved, and the child develops an attachment relationship (Chisholm 1998, Hodges and Tizard 1989, O'Connor et al. 2003, O'Connor and Rutter 2000). In addition, peer relational problems have been documented in adolescents who as younger children exhibited indiscriminate sociability (Hodges and Tizard 1989), suggesting that this subtype is associated with increased risk for long-term deficiencies in the capacity for social relationships.

Differential Diagnosis
Several conditions of early childhood may have symptoms that overlap with RAD and cause diagnostic confusion.

Mental Retardation (MR)
Young children with RAD often have significant developmental delays, and the same deprivation that causes RAD also increases risk for developmental delays. Infants and toddlers with mental retardation may not develop attachments that are consistent with their age, but they should be consistent with their developmental level. Thus, it is important to assess the cognitive level of children who appear indiscriminate to be sure that they are not merely delayed in the development of selectivity as evidenced by the absence of stranger wariness and separation anxiety. A developmental screen and adjustment for the child's overall mental age should suffice.

Pervasive Developmental Disorders (PDD)
Although deficits in reciprocal social interaction are at the core of autism and *Pervasive Developmental Disorders* (PDD) and are observed early in life, children with these disorders do form selective attachments, although they may be deviant (Capps et al. 1994). Also complicating this picture is that these children also have cognitive delay and stereotypies, conditions that are frequently associated with institutionalization or profound neglect (see below). If the psychosocial and caregiving environment is deemed adequate and there is no history of pathologic caregiving, the social disturbance is likely a social deficit in the child rather than reactive to the caregiving environment. In this case, PDD will be the most likely diagnosis. Changes in the caregiving environment will not result in improved social or attachment behaviors and may worsen the child's condition because of loss of an attachment figure.

In addition, in most cases, although cognitive and language delays may be apparent in both socially deprived children and children with PDD, there is no reason to expect the pattern of restricted interest and activities associated with PDD in children with RAD. Instead, one may expect children with the inhibited/emotionally withdrawn pattern to exhibit a pervasive social and emotional withdrawal. Furthermore, there is no reason to expect a selective deficit in symbolization in RAD; instead, one would expect expressive and receptive language and pretend play to be roughly at the same level as overall cognitive level (e.g., as assessed by developmental tests such as the Bayley scores).

Posttraumatic Stress Disorder (PTSD)
Children who have been abused or witnessed violence may show fear, clinging, or withdrawal from caregivers (Hinshaw-Fuselier et al. 1999), symptoms that may be consistent with the hyperarousal and avoidant clusters of a toddler's posttraumatic symptomatology (Scheeringa et al. 2001). These symptoms overlap with the inhibited, hypervigilant, or highly ambivalent and contradictory responses defined by DSM-IV-TR criteria. To be certain, abuse and exposure to

domestic violence is "pathogenic caregiving," but it is uncertain whether these symptoms should primarily be considered as Posttraumatic Stress Disorder (PTSD) or RAD, inhibited/emotionally withdrawn type. If in question, the clinician should inquire into and observe for reexperiencing symptoms (posttraumatic play, play reenactment, nightmares, dissociation, distress on exposure), and increased arousal (sleep disturbances, impaired concentration, hypervigilance, and exaggerated startle) (Scheeringa et al. 1995). At this point, however, there is no reason not to diagnose both conditions if evidence for both exists.

Failure to Thrive (FTT)   The DSM-III conceptualization of RAD included growth failure and lack of social responsivity as central features, and confusion about this initial overlap continues in the literature (APA Textbook of Clinical Psychiatry, 4th ed). The link between failure-to-thrive and RAD was eliminated in DSM-III-R. Hence, in early infancy, lack of eye tracking or responsive smiling by 2 months of age, and failure to reach out to be picked up by 6 months of age should be noted as aberrant social behaviors but not diagnosed as RAD, inhibited type. Some children who do have *Failure to Thrive* (FTT) share risk factors with children who do develop RAD, but no follow-up studies of these infants have looked for evidence of RAD (Coolbear and Benoit 1999). If the child demonstrates psychosocial dwarfism and social inhibition or indiscriminateness, both diagnoses would be appropriate.

Conduct Disorder   There has been much confusion in older children and adolescents about RAD and psychopathy (Zeanah 2000). In fact, it is unclear if RAD is identifiable in middle childhood and adolescence, and if so, what its manifestations are. The possibilities are as follows: (1) RAD resolves itself in early childhood or soon after transition to middle childhood, (2) RAD has different and yet-to-be-defined characteristics in middle childhood and adolescence, or (3) RAD is a pathway into another kind of disorder, such as disruptive behavior disorders. Some of the confusion appears to derive from the problem that children with disruptive behavior disorders often have troubled relationships with their caregivers, thus leading to an assumption that symptoms and signs of aggression, oppositionality, and anger are, in fact, disorders of attachment. In many cases, the emphasis on oppositionality, aggression, and lack of empathy suggests something other than RAD, perhaps a unique developmental path to oppositional defiant disorder or early conduct disorder.

Attention-Deficit Hyperactivity Disorder   Young children with RAD, disinhibited type, demonstrate a persistent pattern of socially impulsive behavior. These behaviors must be distinguished from the impulsivity that characterizes ADHD. Complicating the distinction is evidence that a syndrome of inattention and overactivity may develop in the context of institutionalization (Goldfarb 1945, Kreppner et al. 2003, Roy et al. in press, Tizard and Hodges 1978, Vorria et al. 1998). A recent study demonstrates that inattention/overactivity (I/O) is directly correlated with duration of deprivation and may constitute an institutional-deprivation syndrome that may or may not present a different clinical picture than ordinary varieties of ADHD (Kreppner et al. 2003).

Although ADHD and the disinhibited type of RAD may be associated with social impulsivity, there is no reason to expect children with disinhibited RAD to manifest inattention or hyperactivity. If, on the other hand, the child meets criteria for both disorders, both diagnoses should be assigned.

No gender effects were noted as girls had the same incidence as boys and were therefore not protected by their gender status (Kreppner et al. 2003). The findings do suggest that the phenomena of inattention and overactivity "can arise through several developmental routes and should not be used on their own to infer a particular diagnosis" (page 525). It is unknown if this I/O syndrome responds to stimulants, alpha agonists, or other treatments for ADHD, but it does appear to cause impairment (Kreppner et al. 2001).

Etiology

RAD is one of the few mental disorders that includes etiology as part of the diagnostic criteria. Still, the critical elements of grossly pathogenic care that contribute to the onset of this disorder are unclear, as are the neurobiologic substrate that may also predispose an infant to disorder. Further, it is unclear why the same caregiving environments, those characterized by extremes of neglect, produce both the inhibited/emotionally withdrawn pattern and the disinhibited/indiscriminately social pattern.

A transactional model of development has emerged to explain the diverse outcomes from maltreatment (Cicchetti 1987). Intrinsic individual factors, such as temperament, colic, and physical anomalies may increase the likelihood that a child will be neglected or victimized, at least within the context of an adverse caregiving environment. These factors are likely not to be linearly related to specific outcomes. For example, a difficult temperament may increase the likelihood of being maltreated in an environment characterized by domestic violence, substance abuse, and parental psychopathology, while in an institutional context this temperament may elicit care from the few available caregivers.

To date, there is little understanding of the neurobiology of normative attachment in humans. Even less is understood about the pathophysiology of RAD. Largely on the basis of animal work, speculation about circuitry involving the amygdala and the orbito-prefrontal cortex has been advanced (Schore 2000), but there are insufficient human data available yet to confirm or refute this speculation. Electrophysiological studies have demonstrated reduced power and increased EEG coherence in institutionalized young children in Romania, but no results are yet available indicating how these effects relate to signs of RAD (Marshall and Fox 2002, Zeanah et al. in press).

Treatment

By definition, attachment disorders are encountered in children who have not experienced an opportunity to form lasting secure relationships. Common scenarios include children raised in institutions, placed in multiple foster care homes, or who have had extremely disturbed experiences of care with a single caregiver. Intervention, therefore, should take into account the totality of the child's prior experience, current placement, and other significant relationships.

The first consideration is the child's current health and safety. Maltreatment of children under 4 years of age is associated with significant morbidity and mortality; therefore, involvement of child protective services is frequently warranted. The child should be assessed by a pediatrician for sequelae of malnutrition, substandard health care, and abuse. Given the extreme comorbidity with cognitive and speech delay, the child should also be referred to early intervention services.

Once these issues have been addressed, the nurturing environment should be evaluated and supported to help the current caregivers provide an appropriately nurturing and stimulating environment. If the child currently resides in a dangerous or destructive caregiving environment, an assessment of parental fitness may be warranted. Removal of the child is mandated if the child has sustained life-threatening injuries or is in imminent jeopardy. While the placement of the child in foster care necessarily disrupts the child's relationship with the primary caregiver, safety must be the first priority.

After placement in care, approaches to determining whether reunification is possible, or whether the child should be freed for adoption should be implemented. While the placement of the child in foster care necessarily creates a disruption (Rosenfeld et al. 1997), clinical approaches designed to minimize harm to the child in this context have been advocated

(Larrieu and Zeanah in press, Smyke et al. in press). These approaches emphasize building new attachment relationships and helping the child transition from one setting to the next gradually. Throughout, it is necessary to maintain a focus on the child's best interest while determining whether reunification or termination of parental rights and adoption is indicated.

Owing to the multiple needs of children in foster care and their caregivers, coordination and integration of services for the child, biological parents, and foster parents is critical. Appropriate mental health, substance use, and other supportive services programs should be made available to the caregivers. Critical for all caregivers is the desire to value the baby as an individual and the ability to appropriately respond to the child's bids for comfort, safety, and autonomy.

Educational instruction about developmental capacities, temperamental characteristics, and appropriate interpretations and responses to a child's negative emotion may be indicated. Focusing on improving the parent's ability to respond as a "secure base" from which the child can explore his environment and a "safe-haven" to return to when distressed can be accomplished through focusing on the parent's behavioral interaction with the child, the parent's perception of the child's intentional bids, or a combination of the two. Barriers to the caregiver's emotional availability may be addressed in individual therapy focused on the parent's own experience of care and its influence on their own provision of care.

Long-term intervention is frequently necessary and a successful intervention should address crisis intervention, developmental guidance, and infant/toddler–parent psychotherapy in which the child is present. If working with parents who are providing the improved nurturing environment—foster parents and adoptive parents—the clinician should focus on similar aspects as above and also on "goodness-of-fit" and should assess the parent's motivation to care for this child, the parent's perceptions of the child and their derivations, and the parent's fears about the impact of the child's early environment.

Pharmacotherapy
There are no reported case reports of psychopharmacological management of either the inhibited/emotionally withdrawn or disinhibited/ indiscriminately social subtypes of RAD, nor is there reason to expect these signs and symptoms to respond to psychopharmacological intervention. Indeed, given the apparent responsiveness of these disorders in young children to environmental enhancement, clinicians should resort to pharmacological approaches only after environmental approaches have not worked and then only for specifically targeted associated symptomatology.

Alternative Coercive Psychosocial Treatments
Several alternative treatments of attachment, such as "coercive holding therapies," "rebirthing therapies," and similar "rage reduction therapies," have resulted in the well-publicized death of as many as 6 children (AACAP in press). Parents of these children were following the advice of holding therapists, or allowing the therapists to coerce their children into rageful outbursts, followed by tragically misguided or frankly sadistic parental responses. It is more than likely that these cases represent early onset conduct disorders with a history of early pathologic caregiving rather than RAD. These nonconventional treatments may be called *attachment therapies*, but are not drawn from either attachment theory or research and appear to run the risk of retraumatizing already traumatized children. Further research about the long-term outcomes of maltreated children who demonstrate aggression, oppositionality, and lack of empathy and their response to intervention is necessary.

Comparison of DSM-IV-TR/ICD-10 Diagnostic Criteria
The DSM-IV-TR Reactive Attachment Disorder has two subtypes (inhibited type and disinhibited type) that roughly correspond to the two ICD-10 categories, reactive attachment

disorder of childhood and disinhibited attachment disorder of childhood. The ICD-10 categories are probably much more inclusive because they do not specify that disturbed behavior be the result of pathogenic care.

References

Albers LH, Johnson DE, Hostteter HK, et al. (1997) Health of children adopted from the former Soviet Union and Eastern Europe. *JAMA* **278**, 922–924.

AACAP Work Group on Quality Issues (Boris NW and Zeanah CH principal authors) (in press). Practice parameters for the assessment and treatment of children and adolescents with reactive attachment disorder of infancy and early childhood. *J Am Acad Child Adolesc Psychiatry*.

Boris N and Zeanah CH (2000) Reactive attachment disorder of infancy and early childhood. In Kaplan HI and Sadock BJ (eds). *Comprehensive Textbook of Psychiatry VII*, New York: Williams and Wilkins, pp. 2729–2735.

Boris NW, Aoki Y, and Zeanah CH (1999) The development of infant–parent attachment: considerations for assessment. *Infants Young Child* **11**, 1–10.

Boris NW, Hinshaw-Fuselier SS, Smyke AT, et al. (in press). Comparing criteria for attachment disorders: establishing reliability and validity in high-risk samples. *J Am Acad Child Adolesc Psychiatry*.

Boris NW, Wheeler E, Heller SS, et al. (2000) Attachment and developmental psychopathology. *Psychiatry* **63**, 75–84.

Boris N, Zeanah CH, Larrieu J, et al. (1998) Attachment disorders in infancy and early childhood: A preliminary study of diagnostic criteria. *Am J Psychiatry* **155**, 295–297.

Capps L, Sigman M, and Mundy P (1994) Attachment security in children with autism. *Dev Psychopathol* **6**, 249–262.

Cermak SA and Danhauer LA (1997) Sensory processing in the post-institutionalized child. *Am J Occup Ther* **51**, 500–507.

Chisholm K (1998) A three year follow-up of attachment and indiscriminate friendliness in children adopted from Romanian orphanages. *Child Dev* **69**, 1092–1106.

Coolbear J and Benoit D (1999) Failure to thrive: risk for clinical disturbance of attachment? *Infant Ment Health J* **20**, 87–104.

Federici RS (1999) Neuropsychological evaluation and rehabilitation of the post-institutionalized child. *Presented to the Conference for Children and Residential Care*, Stockholm, Sweden, May, 1999.

Fisher L, Ames EE, Chisholm K, et al. (1997) Problems reported by parents of Romanian orphans adopted to British Columbia. *Int J Behav Dev* **20**, 67–82.

Goldfarb W (1945) Effects of psychological deprivation in infancy and subsequent stimulation. *Am J Psychiatry* **102**, 18–33.

Hinshaw-Fuselier S, Boris N, and Zeanah CH (1999) Reactive attachment disorder in maltreated twins. *Infant Ment Health J* **20**, 42–59.

Hodges J and Tizard B (1989) Social and family relationships of ex-institutional adolescents. *J Child Psychol Psychiatry Allied Disciplines* **30**, 77–97.

Johnson DE (1992) The health of children adopted out of Romania. *JAMA* **268**, 3446–3451.

Kreppner JM, O'Connor TTG, Rutter M, and the English and Romanian Adoptees Study Team (2001) Can inattention/overactivity be an institutional deprivation syndrome? *J Abnorm Child Psychol* **29**, 513–528.

Larrieu JA and Zeanah CH (2003). Treating infant–parent relationships in the context of maltreatment: An integrated, systems approach. In Sameroff A, McDonough S, and Rosenblum K (eds). *Treatment of Infant–parent Relationship Disturbances*, Guilford Press, New York, pp. 243–264.

Marshall P and Fox N (2002 April) Electroencephalographic abnormalities in institutionalized children. *Paper Presented to the International Society on Infant Studies*, Montreal.

Morrison SJ, Ames EW, and Chisholm K (1995) The development of children adopted from Romanian orphanages. *Merrill-Palmer Quarterly* **41**, 411–430.

Mukkades NM, Bilge S, Alyanak B, et al. (2000) Clinical characteristics and treatment responses in cases diagnosed as reactive attachment disorder. *Child Psychiatr Hum Dev* **30**, 273–287.

O'Connor TG (2001) Attachment disorders of infancy and childhood. In *Child and Adolescent Psychiatry: Modern Approaches*, 4th ed., Rutter M and Taylor E (eds). Blackwell, London, pp. 776–792.

O'Connor T and Zeanah CH (2003). Attachment disorders: assessment strategies and treatment approaches. *Attach Hum Dev* **5**, 223–244.

O'Connor TG, Bredenkamp D, Rutter M, and the English and Romanian Adoptees study team (1999) Attachment disturbances and disorders in children exposed to early severe deprivation. *Infant Ment Health J* **20**, 10–29.

O'Connor TG, Rutter M, and the English and Romanian Adoptees study team (2000) Attachment disorder behavior following early severe deprivation: extension and longitudinal follow-up. *J Am Acad Child Adolesc Psychiatry* **39**, 703–712.

Rosenfeld AA, Pilowsky DJ, Fine P, Thorpe M, Fein E, Simms MD, Halfon N, Irwin M, Alfaro J, Salesky R, and Nickman S (1997) Foster care: an update. *J Am Acad Child Adolesc Psychiatry* **36**, 448–457.

Roy P, Rutter M, and Pickles A (in press). Institutional care: associations between overactivity and lack of selectivity in social relationships. *J Child Psychol Psychiatry Allied Disciplines*.

Rutter M, Anderson-Wood L, Beckett C, Bredenkamp D, Castle J, Groothues C, Keaveney L, Lord C, and O'Connot TG (1999) Quasi-autistic patterns following severe early global privation. *J Child Psychol Psychiatry* **40**, 537–549.

Scheeringa MS and Zeanah MD (1995) Symptom differences in traumatized infants and young children. *Infant Ment Health J* **16**, 259–270.

Scheeringa M, Peebles C, Cook C, et al. (2001) Towards establishing the procedural, criterion, and discriminant validity of PTSD in early childhood. *J Am Acad Child Adolesc Psychiatry* **40**, 52–60.

Schore AN (2000) The effects of early relational trauma on right brain development, affect regulation, and infant mental health. *Infant Ment Health J* **22**, 201–269.

Shin Y, Lee K, Min S, et al. (1999) A Korean syndrome of attachment disturbance mimicking symptoms of pervasive developmental disorder. *Infant Ment Health J* **20**, 60–76.

Smyke AT, Dumitrescu A, and Zeanah CH (2002) Disturbances of attachment in young children: I. The continuum of caretaking casualty. *J Am Acad Child Adolesc Psychiatry* **41**, 972–982.

Smyke A, Wajda-Johnston V, and Zeanah CH (in press). Working with young children in foster care. In *Traumatized Children*, Osofsky JD (ed). Wiley & Sons, New York.

Stafford B, Zeanah CH, and Scheeringa M (2003) Exploring psychopathology in early childhood: PTSD and attachment disorders in DC: 0–3 and DSM-IV. *Infant Ment Health J* **24**, 398–409.

Tizard B and Hodges J (1978) The effect of institutional rearing on the development of 8-year-old children. *J Child Psychol Psychiatry Allied Disciplines* **19**, 99–118.

Tizard B and Rees J (1975) The effect of early institutional rearing on the behavioral problems and affectional relationships of four-year-old children. *J Child Psychol Psychiatry* **27**, 61–73.

Vorria P, Rutter M, Pickles A, et al. (1998) A comparative study of Greek children in long-term residential group care and in two-parent families: I. Social, emotional, and behavioural differences. *J Child Psychol Psychiatry* **39**(2), 225–236.

Zeanah CH (1996) Beyond insecurity: a re-conceptualization of attachment disorders of infancy. *J Consul Clin Psychol* **64**, 42–52.

Zeanah CH (2000) Disturbances of attachment in young children adopted from institutions. *J Dev Behav Pediatr* **21**, 230–236.

Zeanah CH and Boris NW (2000) Disturbances and disorders of attachment in early childhood. In *Handbook of Infant Mental Health*, 2nd ed., Zeanah CH (ed). Guilford Press, New York, pp. 353–368.

Zeanah CH and Fox NA (2004) Temperament and attachment disorders. *J Clin Child Psychol* **33**, 32–41.

Zeanah CH and Smyke AT (2002) Clinical disturbances of attachment in early childhood. In *Emotional Regulation: Infancy And Early Childhood*, Zuckerman B, Lieberman A, and Fox N (eds). Johnson & Johnson Pediatric Institute, pp. 139–151.

Zeanah CH, Heller S, Smyke A, et al. (2001) Disorders of attachment in abused/neglected toddlers. *Paper Presented at the Biennial Meeting of the Society for Research in Child Development*, Minneapolis, MN.

Zeanah CH, Boris NW, Bakshi, S, et al. (2000) Disorders of attachment. In *WAIMH Handbook of Infant Mental Health*, Osofsky J and Fitzgerald H (eds). Wiley, New York, pp. 91–122.

Zeanah CH, Boris N, and Lieberman A (2000) Attachment disorders of infancy. In *Handbook of Developmental Psychopathology*, 2nd ed., Sameroff A, Lewis M, and Miller SM (eds). Kluwer Academic/Plenum Publishers, New York, pp. 293–307.

Zeanah CH, Boris N, and Scheeringa M (1997) Psychopathology in infancy. *J Child Psychol Psychiatry Allied Disciplines* **38**, 81–99.

Zeanah CH, Mammen O, and Liberman A (1993) Disorders of attachment. In Zeanah CH (ed) *Handbook of Infant Mental Health*. Guilford Press, New York, pp. 332–349.

Zeanah CH, Smyke AT, and Dumitrescu A (2002) Disturbances of attachment in young children: II. Indiscriminate behavior and institutional care. *J Am Acad Child Adolesc Psychiatry* **41**, 983–989.

Zeanah CH, Smyke A, Koga A, et al. (2003) Attachment in institutionalized children. *Paper Presented at the Biennial Meeting of the Society for Research in Child Development*, Tampa, FL.

13 Delirium, Dementia, and Amnestic Disorders

This chapter reviews delirium, dementia, and amnestic disorders. Traditionally, these conditions have been classified as organic brain disorders to distinguish them from such diseases as schizophrenia, mania, and major depressive disorder, the so-called functional disorders. With the publication of the DSM-IV, the distinction between functional and organic disorders was eliminated. Significant research into the neurobiological aspects of mental disorders and the utilization of sophisticated neurodiagnostic tests such as positron emission tomographic scanning in individuals with schizophrenia led to the inescapable conclusion that every psychiatric condition has a biological component. Thus, the term functional became obsolete and even misleading.

The conditions formerly called organic are classified in DSM-IV-TR into three groups: (1) delirium, dementia, and amnestic and other cognitive disorders; (2) mental disorders due to a general medical condition (covered in Chapter 14 of this book); and (3) substance-related disorders (covered in Chapter 15 in this book). Delirium, dementia, and amnestic disorders are classified as cognitive because they feature impairment in such parameters as memory, language, or attention as a cardinal symptom. Each of these three major cognitive disorders is subdivided into categories that ascribe the etiology of the disorder to a general medical condition, the persisting effects of a substance, or multiple etiologies. A "not otherwise specified" category is included for each disorder.

DELIRIUM

The disorders in the Delirium section share a common symptom presentation of a disturbance in consciousness and cognition, but are differentiated (as in DSM-IV-TR) on the basis of etiology (i.e., Delirium Due to a General Medical Condition, Substance-Induced Delirium, and Delirium Due to Multiple Etiologies). Information regarding the diagnosis, etiology, and treatment of delirium regardless of its specific etiology are presented first, followed by brief sections on Delirium Due to a General Medical Condition, Medication-induced Delirium, Substance Intoxication Delirium, Substance-Withdrawal Delirium, and Delirium Due to Multiple Etiologies.

Diagnosis

Delirium (also known as *acute confusional state, toxic metabolic encephalopathy*) is the behavioral response to widespread disturbances in cerebral metabolism (Lipowski 1983, 1987, 1989, 1990, Engel and Roman 1959). The term delirium is derived from the Latin for "off the track," and some have labeled the condition *reversible madness* (Lipowski 1983, 1989, Tobias et al. 1988). Like dementia, delirium is not a disease but a syndrome with many possible causes that result in a similar constellation of symptoms (the diagnostic criteria for the "syndrome" of delirium are listed as Criteria A, B, and C (see below).

DSM-IV-TR Diagnostic Criteria

293.0 Delirium due to. . . [Indicate the General Medical Condition]

A. Disturbance of consciousness (i.e., reduced clarity of awareness of the environment) with reduced ability to focus, sustain, or shift attention.
B. A change in cognition (such as memory deficit, disorientation, language disturbance) or the development of a perceptual disturbance that is not better accounted for by a preexisting, established, or evolving dementia.

C. The disturbance develops over a short period of time (usually hours to days) and tends to fluctuate during the course of the day.

D. There is evidence from the history, physical examination, or laboratory findings that the disturbance is caused by the direct physiological consequences of a general medical condition.

Coding note: If delirium is superimposed on a preexisting dementia of the Alzheimer's type or vascular dementia, indicate the delirium by coding the appropriate subtype of the dementia, for example, 290.3 dementia of the Alzheimer's type, with late onset, with delirium.

Coding note: Include the name of the general medical condition on Axis I, for example., 293.0 delirium due to hepatic encephalopathy; also code the general medical condition on Axis III.

Reprinted with permission from the Diagnostic and Statistical Manual of Mental Disorders, Fourth Edition, Text Revision. Copyright 2000 American Psychiatric Association.

According to DSM-IV-TR, the primary feature of delirium is a diminished clarity of awareness of the environment. Symptoms of delirium are characteristically global, of acute onset, fluctuating, and of relatively brief duration. In most cases of delirium, an often overlooked prodrome of altered sleep patterns, unexplained fatigue, fluctuating mood, sleep phobia, restlessness, anxiety, and nightmares occur. A review of nursing notes for the days before the recognized onset of delirium often illustrates early warning signs of the condition.

Several investigators have divided the clinical features of delirium into abnormalities of (1) arousal, (2) language and cognition, (3) perception, (4) orientation, (5) mood, (6) sleep and wakefulness, and (7) neurological functioning (Kaplan et al. 1994).

The state of arousal in individuals who are delirious may be increased or decreased. Some individuals exhibit marked restlessness, heightened startle, hypervigilance, and increased alertness. This pattern is often seen in states of withdrawal from depressive substances (e.g., alcohol) or intoxication by stimulants (phencyclidine, amphetamine, lysergic acid diethylamide). Individuals with increased arousal often have such concomitant autonomic signs as pallor, sweating, tachycardia, mydriasis, hyperthermia, piloerection, and gastrointestinal distress. These individuals often require sedation with neuroleptics or benzodiazepines. Hypoactive arousal states such as those occasionally seen in hepatic encephalopathy and hypercapnia are often initially perceived as depressed or demented states. The clinical course of delirium in any particular individual may include both increased and decreased arousal states. Many such individuals display daytime sedation with nocturnal agitation and behavioral problems (sundowning).

Individuals with delirium frequently have abnormal production and comprehension of speech. Nonsensical rambling and incoherent speech may occur. Other individuals may be completely mute. Memory may be impaired, especially primary and secondary memory. Remote memory may be preserved, although the individual may have difficulty distinguishing the present from the distant past (Kaplan et al. 1994).

Perceptual abnormalities in delirium represent an inability to discriminate sensory stimuli and to integrate current perceptions with past experiences (Lipowski 1983, 1987, 1989, 1990, Engel and Roman 1959, Tobias et al. 1988, Massie et al. 1983, Theobald 1987). Consequently, individuals tend to personalize events, conversations, and so forth that do not directly pertain to them, become obsessed with irrelevant stimuli, and misinterpret objects in their environment (Lipowski 1983, 1987, 1989, 1990, Engel and Roman 1959, Tobias et al. 1988). The misinterpretations generally take the form of auditory and visual illusions. Individuals with auditory illusions, for example, might hear the sound of leaves rustling and perceive it as someone whispering about them. This intepretation may result in paranoia and sleep phobia.. Typical visual illusions are that intravenous tubing is a snake or worm crawling into the skin, or that a respirator is a truck or farm vehicle about to collide with the individual. The former auditory illusion may lead to tactile hallucinations, but the most common hallucinations in delirium are visual and auditory.

Orientation is often abnormal in delirium. Disorientation, in particular, seems to follow a fluctuating course, with individuals unable to answer questions about orientation in the morning, yet fully oriented by the afternoon. Orientation to time, place, person, and situation should be evaluated in the individual who is delirious. Generally, orientation to time is the sphere most likely impaired, with orientation to person usually preserved. Orientation to significant people (parents, children) should also be tested. Disorientation to self is rare and indicates significant impairment. The examiner should always reorient the individuals who do not perform well in any portion of the orientation testing of the mental status examination, and serial testing of orientation on subsequent days is important.

Individuals with delirium are susceptible to rapid fluctuations in mood. Unprovoked anger and rage reactions occasionally occur and may lead to attacks on hospital staff. Fear is a common emotion and may lead to increased vigilance and an unwillingness to sleep because of increased vulnerability during somnolence. Apathy, such as that seen in hepatic encephalopathy, depression, use of certain medications (e.g., sulfamethoxazole (Bactrim)), and frontal lobe syndromes, is common as is euphoria secondary to medications (e.g., corticosteroids, DDC, zidovudine) and drugs of abuse (phencyclidine, inhalants).

Sleeping patterns of individuals who are delirious are usually abnormal. During the day, they can be hypersomnolent, often falling asleep in midsentence, whereas at night they are combative and restless. Sleep is generally fragmented, and vivid nightmares are common. Some individuals may become hypervigilant and develop a sleep phobia because of concern that something untoward may occur while they sleep.

Neurological symptoms often occur in delirium. These include dysphagia as seen after a CVA, tremor, asterixis (hepatic encephalopathy, hypoxia, uremia), poor coordination, gait apraxia, frontal release signs (grasp, suck), choreiform movements, seizures, Babinski's sign, and dysarthria. Focal neurological signs occur less frequently.

The appropriate workup of individuals who are delirious includes a complete physical status, mental status, and neurological examination. History taking from the individual, any available family, previous physicians, an old chart, and the individual's current nurse is essential. Previous delirious states, etiologies identified in the past, and interventions that proved effective should be elucidated. Appropriate evaluation of the delirious individual is reviewed in Figure 13-1.

Epidemiology

The overall prevalence of delirium in the community is low, but delirium is common among individuals who are hospitalized. Lipowski (Saito 1987) reported studies of elderly patients and suggested that about 40% of them admitted to general medical wards showed signs of delirium at some point during the hospitalization. Because of the increasing numbers of elderly in this country and the influence of life-extending technology, the population of hospitalized elderly is rising; and so is the prevalence of delirium. The intensive care unit, geriatric psychiatry ward, emergency department, alcohol treatment units, and oncology wards have particularly high rates of delirium (Korvath et al. 1989). Massie and colleagues (Lipowski 1987) reported that 85% of terminally ill patients studied had symptoms that met criteria for delirium, as did 100% of postcardiotomy patients in a study by Theobald

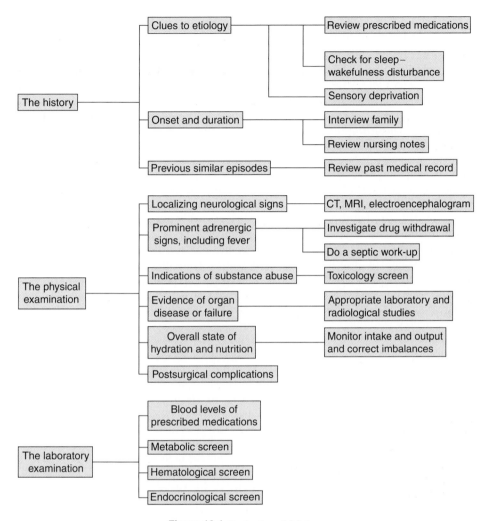

Figure 13-1 *Evaluation of delirium.*

(Lipowski 1989). Overall, it is estimated that 10% of hospitalized individuals are delirious at any particular point in time (Korvath et al. 1989).

Course

After elimination of the cause of the delirium, the symptoms gradually recede within 3 to 7 days. Some symptoms in certain populations may take weeks to resolve. The age of the individual and the period of time during which the individual was delirious affect the symptom resolution time (Kaplan et al. 1994). In general, the individual has a spotty memory for events that occurred during delirium. These remembrances are reinforced by comments from the staff ("You're not as confused today"), or the presence of a sitter, or use of wrist restraints. Such individuals should be reassured that they were not responsible for their behavior while delirious, and that no one hates or resents them for the behavior they may have exhibited. Individuals with underlying dementia show residual cognitive impairment after resolution of delirium, and it has been suggested that a delirium may merge into a dementia (Kaplan et al. 1994).

In general, the mortality and morbidity of any serious disease are doubled if delirium ensues (Korvath et al. 1989). The risk of dying after a delirious episode is greatest in the first 2 years after the illness, with a higher risk of death from heart disease and cancer in women and from pneumonia in men (Francis et al. 1990). Overall, the 3-month mortality rate for persons who have an episode of delirium is about 28%, and the 1-year mortality rate for such individuals may be as high as 50% (Kaplan et al. 1994).

Differential Diagnosis

Delirium must be differentiated from dementia because the two conditions may have different prognoses (Lipowski 1982, 1983). In contrast with the changes in dementia, those in delirium have an acute onset (Lipowski 1987). The symptoms in dementia tend to be relatively stable over time, whereas clinical features of delirium display wide fluctuation with periods of relative lucidity. Clouding of consciousness is an essential feature of delirium, but demented individuals are usually alert. Attention and orientation are more commonly disturbed in delirium, although the latter can become impaired in advanced dementia. Perception abnormalities, alterations in the sleep–wakefulness cycle, and abnormalities of speech are more common in delirium. Most important, a delirium is more likely to be reversible than is a dementia. Delirium and dementia can occur simultaneously; in fact, the presence of dementia is a risk factor for delirium. Some studies suggest that about 30% of individuals who are hospitalized with dementia have a superimposed delirium.

Delirium must often be differentiated from psychotic states related to such conditions as schizophrenia or mania and factitious disorders with psychological symptoms or malingering. Generally, the psychotic features of schizophrenia are more constant and better organized than are those in delirium, and individuals with schizophrenia seldom have the clouding of consciousness seen in delirium. The "psychosis" of individuals with factitious disorder or malingering is inconsistent, and these persons do not exhibit many of the associated features of delirium. Apathetic and lethargic individuals with delirium may occasionally resemble depressed individuals, but tests such as electroencephalogram (EEG) distinguish between the two. The EEG demonstrates diffuse slowing in most delirious states, except for the low-amplitude, fast activity EEG pattern seen in alcohol withdrawal (Lipowski 1987, Obrecht et al. 1979, Pro and Wells 1977, Brenner 1985). The EEG in a functional depression or psychosis is normal.

Etiology

Acetylcholine (ACh) is the primary neurotransmitter believed to be involved in delirium, and the primary neuroanatomical site involved is the reticular formation (Korvath et al. 1989). Thus, one of the frequent causes of delirium is the use of drugs with high anticholingeric potential. As the principal site of regulation of arousal and attention, the reticular formation and its neuroanatomical connections play a major role in the symptoms of delirium. The major pathway involved in delirium is the dorsal-tegmental pathway projecting from the mesencephalic reticular formation to the tectum and the thalamus (Kaplan et al. 1994).

Predisposing factors in the development of delirium include old age, young age (children), previous brain damage, prior episodes of delirium, malnutrition, sensory impairment (especially vision), and alcohol dependence.

The specific causes of delirium are summarized in Table 13-1. Information regarding the specific causes of delirium is included in the next sections.

Delirium Due to a General Medical Condition

The DSM-IV-TR diagnostic criteria for Delirium Due to a General Medical Condition are given on page 264. The causes of Delirium Due to a General Medical Condition may lie in

Table 13-1	Causes of Delirium

Medication effect or interaction
Substance intoxication or withdrawal
Infection
Head injury
Metabolic disarray
    Acid–base imbalance
    Dehydration
    Malnutrition
    Electrolyte imbalance
    Blood glucose abnormality
    Carbon dioxide narcosis
    Uremic encephalopathy
    Hepatic encephalopathy
Cerebrovascular insufficiency
    Congestive heart failure
    Hypovolemia
    Arrhythmias
    Severe anemia
    Transient ischemia
    Acute CVA
Endocrine dysfunction
Postoperative states
    Postcardiotomy delirium
Environmental factors
    Intensive care unit psychosis
Sleep deprivation

intracranial processes, extracranial ones, or a combination of the two. The most common etiological factors are as follows (Francis et al. 1990).

Infection Induced Infection is a common cause of delirium among individuals who are hospitalized and typically, infected patients will display abnormalities in hematology and serology. Bacteremic septicemia (especially that caused by gram-negative bacteria), pneumonia, encephalitis, and meningitis are common offenders. The elderly are particularly susceptible to delirium secondary to urinary tract infections.

Metabolic and Endocrine Disturbances Metabolic causes of delirium include hypoglycemia, electrolyte disturbances, and vitamin deficiency states. The most common endocrine causes are hyperfunction and hypofunction of the thyroid, adrenal, pancreas, pituitary, and parathyroid. Metabolic causes may involve consequences of diseases of particular organs, such as hepatic encephalopathy resulting from liver disease, uremic encephalopathy and postdialysis delirium resulting from kidney dysfunction, and carbon dioxide macrosis and hypoxia resulting from lung disease. The metabolic disturbance or endocrinopathy must be known to induce changes in mental status and must be confirmed by laboratory determinations or physical examination, and the temporal course of the confusion should coincide with the disturbance (Francis et al. 1990). In some individuals, particularly the elderly, brain injured, and demented, there may be a significant lag time between correction of metabolic parameters and improvement in mental state.

Low-Perfusion States Any condition that decreases effective cerebral perfusion can cause delirium. Common offenders are hypovolemia, congestive heart failure and other causes of decreased stroke volume such as arrhythmias, and anemia, which decreases oxygen binding. Maintenance of fluid balance and strict measuring of intake and output are essential in delirious states.

Intracranial Causes   Intracranial causes of delirium include head trauma, especially involving loss of consciousness, postconcussive states, and hemorrhage; brain infections; neoplasms; and such vascular abnormalities as CVAs, subarachnoid hemorrhage, transient ischemic attacks, and hypertensive encephalopathy.

Postoperative States   Postoperative causes of delirium may include infection, atelectasis, lingering effects of anesthesia, thrombotic and embolic phenomena, and adverse reactions to postoperative analgesia. General surgery in an elderly patient has been reported to be followed by delirium in 10 to 14% of cases and may reach 50% after surgery for hip fracture (Lipowski 1989).

Sensory and Environmental Changes   Many clinicians underestimate the disorienting potential of an unfamiliar environment. The elderly are especially prone to develop environment-related confusion in the hospital. Individuals with preexisting dementia, who may have learned to compensate for cognitive deficits at home, often become delirious once hospitalized. In addition, the nature of the intensive care unit often lends itself to periods of high sensory stimulation (as during a "code") or low sensory input, as occurs at night (Lipowski 1975, Kaufman 1990a). Often, individuals use external events such as dispensing medication, mealtimes, presence of housekeeping staff, and physicians' rounds to mark the passage of time. These parameters are often absent at night, leading to increased rates of confusion during nighttime hours (Cameron 1941). Often, manipulating the individual's environment (see section on treatment) or removing the individual from the intensive care unit can be therapeutic.

Medication-Induced Delirium

The list of medications that can produce the delirious state is extensive (Table 13-2). The more common ones include such antihypertensives as methyldopa and reserpine, histamine (H_2) receptor antagonists (cimetidine), corticosteroids, antidepressants, narcotics (especially opioid) and nonsteroidal analgesics, lithium carbonate, digitalis, baclofen (Lioresal), anticonvulsants, antiarrhythmics, colchicine, bronchodilators, benzodiazepines, sedative-hypnotics, and anticholinergics. Of the narcotic analgesics, meperidine can produce an agitated delirium with tremors, seizures, and myoclonus (Slaby and Erle 1993, Eisendrath et al. 1987). These

Table 13-2	Selected Drugs Associated with Delirium
Antihypertensives	Indomethacin
Amphotericin B	Ketamine
Antispasmodics	Levodopa
Antituberculous agents	Lidocaine
Baclofen	Lithium
Barbiturates	Meperidine
Cimetidine	Morphine
Corticosteroids	Procainamide
Colchicine	Pentamidine
Contrast media	Tricyclic antidepressants
Digitalis	Zalcitabine (DDC)
Ephedrine	Zidovudine (AZT)

features are attributed to its active metabolite normeperidine, which has potent stimulant and anticholingeric properties and accumulates with repeated intravenous dosing (Slaby and Erle 1993, Eisendrath et al. 1987). In general, adverse effects of narcotics are more common in those who have never received such agents before (the narcotically naive) or who have a history of a similar response to narcotics.

Lithium-induced delirium occurs at blood levels greater than 1.5 mEq/L and is associated with early features of lethargy, stuttering, and muscle fasciculations (Blass et al. 1988). The delirium may take as long as 2 weeks to resolve even after lithium has been discontinued, and other neurological signs such as stupor and seizures commonly occur. Maintenance of fluid and electrolyte balance is essential in lithium-induced delirium. Facilitation of excretion with such agents as aminophylline and acetazolamide helps, but hemodialysis is often required (Kaplan et al. 1994).

Principles to remember in cases of drug-induced delirium include the facts that (1) blood levels of possibly offending agents are helpful and should be obtained, but many persons can become delirious at therapeutic levels of the drug, (2) drug-induced delirium may be the result of drug interactions and polypharmacy and not the result of a single agent, (3) over-the-counter medications and preparations (e.g., agents containing caffeine or phenylpropanolamine) should also be considered, and (4) delirium can be caused by the combination of drugs of abuse and prescribed medications (e.g., cocaine and dopaminergic antidepressants).

Substance Intoxication Delirium

The DSM-IV-TR diagnostic criteria for Substance Intoxication Delirium are given below. The list of drugs of abuse that can produce delirium is extensive. Some such agents have enjoyed a resurgence after years of declining usage. These include lysergic acid diethylamide, psilocybin (hallucinogenic mushrooms), heroin, and amphetamines. Other agents include barbiturates, cannabis (especially dependent on setting, experience of the user, and whether it is laced with phencyclidine ("superweed" or heroin), jimsonweed (highly anticholingeric), and mescaline. In cases in which intravenous use of drugs is suspected, HIV spectrum illness must be ruled out as an etiological agent for delirium.

DSM-IV-TR Diagnostic Criteria

Substance Intoxication Delirium

A. Disturbance of consciousness (i.e., reduced clarity of awareness of the environment) with reduced ability to focus, sustain, or shift attention.

B. A change in cognition (such as memory deficit, disorientation, language disturbance) or the development of a perceptual disturbance that is not better accounted for by a preexisting, established, or evolving dementia.

C. The disturbance develops over a short period of time (usually hours to days) and tends to fluctuate during the course of the day.

D. There is evidence from the history, physical examination, or laboratory findings of either (1) or (2):

(1) the symptoms in Criteria A and B developed during substance intoxication

(2) medication use is etiologically related to the disturbance

Note: This diagnosis should be made instead of a diagnosis of substance intoxication only when the cognitive symptoms are in excess of those usually associated with the intoxication syndrome and when the symptoms are sufficiently severe to warrant independent clinical attention.

Note: The diagnosis should be recorded as substance-induced delirium if related to medication use.

Code: [specific substance] intoxication delirium:

(291.0 alcohol; 292.81 amphetamine [or amphetamine-like substance]; 292.81 cannabis; 292.81 cocaine; 292.81 hallucinogen; 292.81 inhalant; 292.81 opioid; 292.81 phencyclidine [or phencyclidine-like substance]; 292.81 sedative, hypnotic, or anxiolytic; 292.81 other [or unknown] substance [e.g., cimetidine, digitalis, benztropine])

Reprinted with permission from the Diagnostic and Statistical Manual of Mental Disorders, Fourth Edition, Text Revision. Copyright 2000 American Psychiatric Association.

The physical examination of an individual with suspected illicit drug-induced delirium may reveal sclerosed veins, "pop" scars caused by subcutaneous injection of agents, pale and atrophic nasal mucosa resulting from intranasal use of cocaine, injected conjunctiva, and pupillary changes. Toxicological screens are helpful but may not be available on an emergency basis.

Substance-Withdrawal Delirium

The DSM-IV-TR diagnostic criteria for Substance-Withdrawal Delirium are given below. Alcohol and certain sedating drugs can produce a withdrawal delirium when their use is abruptly discontinued or significantly reduced. Withdrawal delirium requires a history of use of a potentially addicting agent for a sufficient amount of time to produce dependence. It is associated with such typical physical findings as abnormal vital signs, pupillary changes, tremor, diaphoresis, nausea and vomiting, and diarrhea. Individuals generally complain of abdominal and leg cramps, insomnia, nightmares, chills, hallucinations (especially visual), and a general feeling of "wanting to jump out of my skin."

DSM-IV-TR Diagnostic Criteria

Substance Withdrawal Delirium

A. Disturbance of consciousness (i.e., reduced clarity of awareness of the environment) with reduced ability to focus, sustain, or shift attention.
B. A change in cognition (such as memory deficit, disorientation, language disturbance) or the development of a perceptual disturbance that is not better accounted for by a preexisting, established, or evolving dementia.
C. The disturbance develops over a short period of time (usually hours to days) and tends to fluctuate during the course of the day.
D. There is evidence from the history, physical examination, or laboratory findings that the symptoms in Criteria A and B developed during, or shortly after, a withdrawal syndrome.

Note: This diagnosis should be made instead of a diagnosis of substance withdrawal only when the cognitive symptoms are in excess of those usually associated with the withdrawal syndrome and when the symptoms are sufficiently severe to warrant independent clinical attention.

Code: [specific substance] withdrawal delirium:

(291.0 alcohol; 292.81 sedative, hypnotic, or anxiolytic; 292.81 other [or unknown] substance)

Some varieties of drug withdrawal, although uncomfortable, are not life threatening (e.g., opioid withdrawal). Others such as alcohol withdrawal delirium are potentially fatal. Withdrawal delirium is much more common among individuals who are hospitalized than among individuals living in the community. The incidence of delirium tremens, for example, is found in 1% of all alcoholics, but in 5% of hospitalized alcohol abusers. Improvement of the delirium occurs when the offending agent is reintroduced or a cross-sensitive drug (e.g., a benzodiazepine for alcohol withdrawal) is employed.

Delirium Due to Multiple Etiologies

In many individuals with delirium, there are often multiple simultaneous causal factors involved. In some cases, multiple general medical conditions may impact the central nervous system (CNS) in such a way as to lead to a delirium. For example, an individual with hepatic encephalopathy who falls and hits his head may develop a delirium attributable to the combined effects of both general medical conditions. Similarly, the combined effects of a medical condition coupled with the effects of medications used to treat that condition may cause a delirium. In such situations, the diagnosis Delirium Due to Multiple Etiologies is given (see DSM-IV-TR diagnostic criteria given below).

DSM-IV-TR Diagnostic Criteria

Delirium Due to Multiple Etiologies

A. Disturbance of consciousness (i.e., reduced clarity of awareness of the environment) with reduced ability to focus, sustain, or shift attention.
B. A change in cognition (such as memory deficit, disorientation, language disturbance) or the development of a perceptual disturbance that is not better accounted for by a preexisting, established, or evolving dementia.
C. The disturbance develops over a short period of time (usually hours to days) and tends to fluctuate during the course of the day.
D. There is evidence from the history, physical examination, or laboratory findings that the delirium has more than one etiology (e.g., more than one etiological general medical condition, a general medical condition plus Substance Intoxication or medication side effect).

Coding note: Use multiple codes reflecting specific delirium and specific etiologies, e.g., 293.0 Delirium Due to Viral Encephalitis; 291.0 Alcohol Withdrawal Delirium

Treatment

Once delirium has been diagnosed, the etiological agent must be identified and treated. For the elderly, the first step generally involves discontinuing or reducing the dosage of potentially offending medications. Some delirious states can be reversed with medication, as in the case of physostigmine administration for anticholinergic delirium. However, most responses are not as immediate, and attention must be directed toward protecting the individual from unintentional self-harm, managing agitated and psychotic behavior, and manipulating the environment to minimize additional impairment. Supportive therapy should include fluid and electrolyte maintenance and provision of adequate nutrition. Reorienting the individual is essential and is best accomplished in a well-lit room with a window, a clock, and a visible wall calendar. Familiar objects from home such as a stuffed animal, a favorite blanket, or a few photographs are helpful. Individuals who respond incorrectly to questions of orientation should be provided with the correct answers. Because these individuals often see many consultants, physicians should introduce themselves and state their purpose for coming at every visit. Physicians must take into account that impairments of vision and hearing can produce confusional states, and the provision of appropriate prosthetic devices may be beneficial. Around-the-clock accompaniment by hospital-provided "sitters" or family members may be required (see Table 13-3).

Despite these conservative interventions, the delirious individual often requires pharmacological intervention. The liaison psychiatrist is the most appropriate person to recommend such treatment. The drug of choice for agitated delirious individuals has traditionally been haloperidol (Haldol) (Gelfand et al. 1992). It is particularly beneficial when given by the intravenous route and some authors have reported using dosages as high as 260 mg/day without adverse effect (Gelfand et al. 1992, Steinhart 1983, Adams 1988, Tesar et al. 1985, Fernandez et al. 1988, Carter 1986). Extrapyramidal symptoms may be less common with haloperidol administered intravenously as opposed to oral and intramuscular administration (Menza et al. 1987). In general, doses in the range of 0.5 to 5 mg intravenously are used, with the frequency of administration depending on a variety of factors including the individual's age. An electrocardiogram should be obtained before administering haloperidol. If the QT interval is greater than 450, use of intravenous haloperidol can precipitate an abnormal cardiac rhythm known as *Torsades de pointes* (Glassman and Bigger 2001, Moss 1993, Kriwisky et al. 1990). Lorazepam has also been proven effective in doses of 0.5 to 2 mg intravenously. Some authors have suggested that haloperidol and lorazepam act synergistically when given to the agitated individual who is delirious (Menza et al. 1987). If the delirium is secondary to drug or alcohol abuse, benzodiazepines or clonidine should be used. For individuals who are mildly agitated or amenable to taking medications by mouth, oral haloperidol or lorazepam is appropriate. Recent studies have advocated the use of newer atypical antipsychotics for management of behavior and psychotic features in delirium (Torres et al. 2001, Glassman and Bigger 2001, Moss 1993, Kriwisky et al.

Table 13-3	Managing the Delirious Individual

Identify and correct the underlying cause.
Protect the patient from unintentional self-harm.
Stabilize the level of sensory input.
Reorient patient as often as possible.
Employ objects from the patient's home environment.
Provide supportive therapy (fever control, hydration).
Streamline medications.
Correct sleep deprivation.
Manage behavior with appropriate pharmacotherapy.
Address postdelirium guilt and shame for behavior that occurred during confusion.

1990, Tran et al. 1997, Sipahimalani and Massand 1997, 1998, Graver 2000). Such agents as quetiapine, olanzapine, risperdal, and ziprasidone have been used successfully to treat delirium. Newer agents may have lower incidences of dystonias and dyskinesias, but still carry the risk of QT interval prolongation, particularly in individuals with electrolyte abnormalities (Glassman and Bigger 2001). Quetiapine and olanzapine are quite sedating, and occasionally a combination of bedtime olanzapine and "as needed" haloperidol is utilized. Olanzapine may raise blood glucose levels and precipitate weight gain, and is available as a Zydis preparation, which is absorbed through the oral mucosa and can therefore be given to individuals who are unable to take medications by mouth (Osser et al. 1999, Bettinger et al. 2000). A parenteral form of ziprasidone is also available. Whatever antipsychotic is chosen, the individual should be carefully monitored for muscle rigidity, unexplained fever, tremor, and other warning signs of neuroleptic side effects.

DEMENTIA

The disorders in the Dementia section are characterized by the development of multiple cognitive deficits (including memory impairment) but are differentiated (as in DSM-IV-TR) on the basis of etiology (i.e., Dementia of the Alzheimer's Type, Dementia of the Alzheimer Type, Dementia Due to Pick's Disease, Dementia Due to Parkinson's Disease, Dementia Due to Huntington's Disease, Vascular Dementia, Dementia Due to HIV Disease, Dementia Due to Head Trauma, Dementia Due to Other General Medical Conditions, Substance-Induced Persisting Dementia, and Dementia Due to Multiple Etiologies). Information regarding the diagnosis of dementia regardless of its specific etiology is presented first, followed by sections on the various specific causes of dementia.

Diagnosis

Dementia is defined in DSM-IV-TR as a series of disorders characterized by the development of multiple cognitive deficits (including memory impairment) that are due to the direct physiological effects of a general medical condition, the persisting effects of a substance, or multiple etiologies (e.g., the combined effects of a metabolic and a degenerative disorder) (American Psychiatric Association 1994). (See DSM-IV-TR diagnostic criteria A and B below.) The disorders constituting the dementias share a common symptom presentation and are identified and classified on the basis of etiology. The cognitive deficits exhibited in these disorders must be of significant severity to interfere with either occupational functioning or the individual's usual social activities or relationships. In addition, the observed deficits must represent a decline from a higher level of function and not be the consequence of a delirium. A delirium can be superimposed on a dementia, however, and both can be diagnosed if the dementia is observed when the delirium is not in evidence. Dementia is typically chronic and occurs in the presence of a clear sensorium. If clouding of consciousness occurs, the diagnosis of delirium should be considered. Essential to the diagnosis of dementia is the presence of cognitive deficits that include memory impairment and at least one of the following abnormalities of cognition: aphasia, agnosia, apraxia, or a disturbance in executive function (American Psychiatric Association 1994).

DSM-IV-TR Diagnostic Criteria

294.1x Dementia of the Alzheimer Type

A. The development of multiple cognitive deficits manifested by both

(1) memory impairment (impaired ability to learn new information or to recall previously learned information)
(2) one (or more) of the following cognitive disturbances:

    (a) aphasia (language disturbance)
    (b) apraxia (impaired ability to carry out motor activities despite intact motor function)
    (c) agnosia (failure to recognize or identify objects despite intact sensory function)
    (d) disturbance in executive functioning (i.e., planning, organizing, sequencing, abstracting)

B. The cognitive deficits in criteria A1 and A2 each cause significant impairment in social or occupational functioning and represent a significant decline from a previous level of functioning.
C. The course is characterized by gradual onset and continuing cognitive decline.
D. The cognitive deficits in criteria A1 and A2 are not due to any of the following:

(1) other central nervous system conditions that cause progressive deficits in memory and cognition (e.g., cerebrovascular disease, Parkinson's disease, Huntington's disease, subdural hematoma, normal-pressure hydrocephalus, brain tumor)
(2) systemic conditions that are known to cause dementia (e.g., hypothyroidism, vitamin B_{12} or folic acid deficiency, niacin deficiency, hypercalcemia, neurosyphilis, HIV infection)
(3) substance-induced conditions

E. The deficits do not occur exclusively during the course of a delirium.
F. The disturbance is not better accounted for by another Axis I disorder (e.g., major depressive disorder, schizophrenia).

Code based on presence or absence of a clinically significant behavioral disturbance:

294.10 Without Behavioral Disturbance: if the cognitive disturbance is not accompanied by any clinically significant behavioral disturbance.

294.11 With Behavioral Disturbance: if the cognitive disturbance is accompanied by a clinically significant behavioral disturbance (e.g., wandering, agitation).

Specify subtype:

With Early Onset: if onset is at age 65 years or below

With Late Onset: if onset is after age 65 years

Coding note: Also code 331.0 Alzheimer's disease on Axis III. Indicate other prominent clinical features related to the Alzheimer's disease on Axis I (e.g., 293.83 Mood Disorder Due to Alzheimer's Disease, With Depressive Features, and 310.1 Personality Change Due to Alzheimer's Disease, Aggressive Type Code based on type of onset and predominant features.

Memory function is divided into three compartments that can easily be evaluated during a mental status examination. These are immediate recall (primary memory), recent (secondary) memory, and remote (tertiary) memory. Primary memory is characterized by a limited capacity, rapid accessibility, and a duration of seconds to a minute (Karp 1984). The anatomic site of destruction of primary memory is the reticular activating system, and the principal activity of the primary memory is the registration of new information. Primary memory is generally tested by asking the individual to repeat immediately a series of numbers in the order given. For instance, if the examiner mentions the numbers 1-2-3, the individual should be able to repeat them in the same order. This loss of ability to register new information accounts in part for the confusion and frustration the demented individual feels when confronted with unexpected changes in daily routine.

Secondary memory has a much larger capacity than primary memory, a duration of minutes to years, and relatively slow accessibility. The anatomic site of dysfunction for secondary memory is the limbic system, and individuals with a lesion in this area may have little difficulty repeating digits immediately, but show rapid decay of these new memories. In minutes, the individual with limbic involvement may be totally unable to recall the digits or even remember that a test has been administered (Karp 1984). Thus, secondary memory represents the retention and recall of information that has been previously registered by primary memory. Clinically, secondary memory is tested by having the individual repeat three objects after having been distracted (usually by the examiner's continuation of the Mental Status Examination) for 3 to 5 minutes. Like primary memory, secondary recall is often impaired in dementia. Often, if the examiner gives the demented individual a clue (such as "one of the objects you missed was a color"), the individual correctly identifies the object. If this occurs, the memory testing should be scored as "3 out of 3 with a clue," which is considered to be a slight impairment. Giving clues to the demented individual with a primary memory loss is pointless, because the memories were never registered. Wernicke–Korsakoff syndrome is an example of a condition in which primary memory may be intact while secondary recall is impaired.

Tertiary (remote) memory has a capacity that is probably unlimited, and such memories are often permanently retained. Access to tertiary memories is slow, and the anatomical dysfunction in tertiary memory loss is in the association cortex (Karp 1984). In the early stages of dementia, tertiary memory is generally intact. It is tested by instructing the individual to remember personal information or past material. The personal significance of the information often influences the individual's ability to remember it. For example, a woman who worked for many years as a seamstress might remember many details related to that occupation, but could not recall the names of past presidents or three large cities in the United States. Thus, an individual's inability to remember highly significant past material is an ominous finding. Collateral data from informants is essential in the proper assessment of memory function. In summary, primary and secondary memories are most likely to be impaired in dementia, with tertiary memory often spared until late in the course of the disease.

In addition to defects in memory, individuals with dementia often exhibit impairments in language, recognition, object naming, and motor skills. Aphasia is an abnormality of language that often occurs in vascular dementias involving the dominant hemisphere. Because this hemisphere controls verbal, written, and sign language, these individuals may have significant problems interacting with people in their environment. Individuals with dementia and aphasia may exhibit paucity of speech, poor articulation, and a telegraphic pattern of speech (nonfluent, Broca's aphasia). This form of aphasia generally involves the middle cerebral artery with resultant paresis of the right arm and lower face (Henderson 1990). Despite faulty communication skills, individuals having dementia with nonfluent aphasia have normal comprehension and awareness of their language impairment. As a result, such individuals often present with significant depression, anxiety, and frustration.

By contrast, individuals having dementia with fluent (Wernicke's) aphasia may be quite verbose and articulate, but much of the language is nonsensical and rife with such paraphasias as neologisms and clang (rhyming) associations. Whereas nonfluent aphasias are usually associated with discrete lesions, fluent aphasia can result from such diffuse conditions as dementia of the Alzheimer type. More commonly, fluent aphasias occur in conjunction with vascular dementia secondary to temporal or parietal lobe CVA. Because the demented individuals with fluent aphasia have impaired comprehension, they may seem apathetic and unconcerned with their language deficits if they are, in fact, aware of them at all. They do not generally display the emotional distress of individuals with dementia and nonfluent aphasia (Table 13-4).

Individuals with dementia may also lose their ability to recognize. Agnosia is a feature of a dominant hemisphere lesion and involves altered perception in which, despite normal sensations, intellect, and language, the individual cannot recognize objects. This is in contrast to aphasia in which the individual with dementia may not be able to name objects, but can recognize them (Berg et al. 1994). The type of agnosia depends on the area of the sensory cortex that is involved. Some demented individuals with severe visual agnosia cannot name objects presented, match them to samples, or point to objects named by the examiner. Other individuals may present with auditory agnosia and may be unable to localize or distinguish such sounds as the ringing of a telephone. A minority of demented individuals may exhibit astereognosis, or the inability to identify an object by palpation.

Demented individuals may also lose their ability to carry out selected motor activities despite intact motor abilities, sensory function, and comprehension of the assigned task (apraxia). Affected individuals cannot perform such activities as brushing their teeth, chewing food, or waving good-bye when asked to do so (Kaufman 1990a). The two most common forms of apraxia in demented individuals are ideational and gait apraxia. Ideational apraxia is the inability to perform motor activities that require sequential steps and results from a lesion involving both frontal lobes or the complete cerebrum. Gait apraxia, often seen in such conditions as normal-pressure hydrocephalus, is the inability to perform various motions of ambulation. It also results from conditions that diffusely affect the cerebrum.

Impairment of executive function is the ability to think abstractly, plan, initiate, and end complex behavior. On Mental Status Examination, individuals with dementia display problems coping with new tasks. Activities such as subtracting serial sevens may be impaired.

In addition to the diagnostic features already mentioned, individuals with dementia display other identifying features that often prove problematic. Poor insight and judgment are common in dementia and often cause individuals to engage in potentially dangerous activities or make unrealistic and grandiose plans for the future. Visual–spatial functioning may be impaired, and if individuals have the ability to construct a plan and carry it

Table 13-4	Classification of Aphasias		
Type	**Language**	**Comprehension**	**Motor**
Wernicke's (receptive)	Impaired Articulate Paraphasias	Impaired	Normal
Broca's (expressive)	Nonfluent Sparse Telegraphic Inarticulate	Intact	Right hemiparesis
Global	Nonfluent Mute	Impaired	Variable right hemiplegia

out, suicide attempts can occur. More common is unintentional self-harm resulting from carelessness, undue familiarity with strangers, and disregard for the accepted rules of conduct. Emotional lability, as seen in pseudobulbar palsy after cerebral injury, can be particularly frustrating for caregivers, as are occasional psychotic features such as delusions and hallucinations. Changes in their environment and daily routine can be particularly distressing for demented individuals, and their frustration can be manifested by violent behavior.

The mental status examination, in conjunction with a complete medical history from the individual and informants and an adequate physical examination, is essential in the evaluation and differential diagnosis of dementia (Table 13-5). The findings on the mental status examination vary depending on the etiology of the dementia. In general, symptoms seen on the mental status examination, whatever the etiology, are related to the location and extent of brain injury, individual adaptation to the dysfunction, premorbid coping skills and psychopathology, and concurrent medical illness (Slaby and Erle 1993).

Disturbance of memory, especially primary and secondary memory, is the most significant abnormality. Confabulation may be present as the individual attempts to minimize the memory impairment. Disorientation and altered levels of consciousness may occur, but are generally not seen in the early stages of dementia uncomplicated by delirium. Affect may be affected as in the masked facies of Parkinson's disease and the expansive affect and labile mood of pseudobulbar palsy after cerebral injury. The affect of individuals with hepatic encephalopathy is often described as blunted and apathetic. Lack of inhibition leading to such behavior as exposing oneself is common, and some conditions such as tertiary syphilis and untoward effects of some medication can precipitate mania.

The physical examination may offer clues to the etiology of the dementia; however, in the elderly, one must be aware of the normal changes associated with aging and differentiate them from signs of dementia. Often, the specific physical examination findings indicate the area of the central nervous system affected by the etiological process. Parietal lobe dysfunction is suggested by such symptoms as astereognosis, constructional apraxia, anosognosia, and problems with two-point discrimination (Kaufman 1990a). The dominant hemisphere parietal lobe is also involved in Gerstmann's syndrome, which includes agraphia, acalculia, finger agnosia, and right–left confusion.

Table 13-5	Evaluation of Dementia

Medical history and physical examination
Family interview
Routine laboratory
   Chemistry (SMA 20)
   Urinalysis
   Hematology (complete blood count)
Other routine tests
   Chest radiography
   Electrocardiography
Specialized laboratory
   Thyroid functions
   VDRL (fluorescent treponemal antibody screen if indicated)
   Drug screen
   Vitamin B_{12} and folate levels
   Cerebrospinal fluid analysis (if indicated)
   HIV testing (if indicated)
Other studies
   Computed tomography or magnetic resonance imaging
   Electroencephalography

Reflex changes such as hyperactive deep tendon reflexes, Babinski's reflex, and hyperactive jaw jerk are indicative of cerebral injury. However, primitive reflexes such as the palmar–mental reflex (tested by repeatedly scratching the base of the individual's thumb, with a positive response being slight downward movement of the lower lip and jaw) that occurs in 60% of normal elderly people, and the snout reflex, seen in a third of elderly individuals, are not diagnostically reliable for dementia (Wolfson and Katzman 1983).

Ocular findings such as nystagmus (as in brain stem lesions), ophthalmoplegia (Wernicke–Korsakoff syndrome), anisocoria, papilledema (hypertensive encephalopathy), cortical blindness (Anton's syndrome), visual field losses (CVA hemianopia), Kayser–Fleischer rings (Wilson's disease), and Argyll Robertson pupils (syphilis, diabetic neuropathy) can offer valuable clues to the etiology of the cognitive deficit (Victor and Adams 1974).

Movement disorders including tremors (Parkinson's disease, drug intoxication, cerebellar dysfunction, Wilson's disease), chorea (Huntington's disease, other basal ganglia lesions), myoclonus (subacute sclerosing panencephalitis, Creutzfeldt–Jakob disease, Alzheimer's disease, anoxia), and asterixis (hepatic disease, uremia, hypoxia, carbon dioxide retention) should be noted.

Gait disturbances, principally apraxia (normal-pressure hydrocephalus, inhalant abuse, cerebellar dysfunction) and peripheral neuropathy (Korsakoff's syndrome, neurosyphilis, heavy metal intoxication, solvent abuse, isoniazid or phenytoin toxicity, vitamin deficiencies, and HIV spectrum illnesses), are also common in dementia. Extrapyramidal symptoms in the absence of antipsychotics may indicate substance abuse, especially phencyclidine abuse, or basal ganglia disease. Although the many and varied physical findings of dementia are too numerous to mention here in any detail, it should be obvious that the physical examination is an invaluable tool in the assessment of dementia (Table 13-6).

Epidemiology

The prevalence of dementias is not precisely known. Estimates vary depending on the age range of the population studied and whether the individuals sampled were in the general community, acute care facilities, or long-term nursing institutions. A review of 47 surveys of dementia conducted between 1934 and 1985 indicated that the prevalence of dementia increased exponentially by age, doubling every 5 years up to age 95 years, and that this condition was equally distributed among men and women, with Alzheimer's dementia (AD) much more common in women (Slaby and Erle 1993). A National Institute of Mental Health Multisite Epidemiological Catchment Area study revealed a 6-month prevalence rate for mild dementia of 11.5 to 18.4% for persons older than 65 years living in the community (Kallmann 1989). The rate for severe dementia was higher for the institutionalized elderly: 15% of the elderly in retirement communities, 30% of nursing home residents, and 54% of the elderly in state hospitals (Cummings and Benson 1983).

Studies suggest that the fastest growing segment of the US population consists of persons older than the age of 85 years, 15% of whom are demented (Henderson 1990). Half of the US population currently lives to the age of 75 years and one quarter lives to the age of 85 (Berg et al. 1994). A study of 2000 consecutive admissions to a general medical hospital revealed that 9% were demented and, among those, 41% were also delirious on admission (Erkinjuntii et al. 1986). The cost of providing care for demented individuals exceeds $100 billion annually (about 10% of all health care expenditures), and the average cost to families in 1990 was $18,000 a year (Berg et al. 1994).

Course

The course of a particular dementia is influenced by its etiology. Although historically the dementias have been considered progressive and irreversible, there is, in fact, significant

Table 13-6	Physical Signs Associated with Dementia or Delirium
Physical Sign	**Condition**
Myoclonus	Creutzfeldt–Jakob disease
	Subacute sclerosing panencephalitis
	Postanoxia
	Alzheimer's disease (10%)
	AIDS dementia
	Uremia
	Penicillin intoxication
	Meperidine toxicity
Asterixis	Hepatic encephalopathy
	Uremia
	Hypoxia
Chorea	Huntington's disease
	Wilson's disease
	Hypocalcemia
	Hypothyroidism
	Hepatic encephalopathy
	Oral contraceptives
	Systemic lupus erythematosus
	Carbon monoxide poisoning
	Toxoplasmosis
	Pertussis, diphtheria
Peripheral neuropathy	Wernicke–Korsakoff syndrome
	Neurosyphilis
	Heavy metal intoxication
	Organic solvent exposure
	Vitamin B_{12} deficiency
	Medications: isoniazid, phenytoin

variation in the course of individual dementias. The disorder can be progressive, static, or remitting (American Psychiatric Association 1994). In addition to the etiology, factors that influence the course of the dementia include (1) the time span between the onset and the initiation of prescribed treatment, (2) the degree of reversibility of the particular dementia, (3) the presence of comorbid mental disorders, and (4) the level of psychosocial support. The previous distinction between treatable and untreatable dementias has been replaced by the concepts of reversible, irreversible, and arrestable dementias. Most reversible cases of dementia are associated with shorter duration of symptoms, mild cognitive impairment, and superimposed delirium. Specifically, the dementias caused by drugs, depression, and metabolic disorders are most likely to be reversible. Other conditions such as normal-pressure hydrocephalus, subdural hematomas, and tertiary syphilis are more commonly arrestable.

Although potentially reversible dementias should be aggressively investigated, in reality, only 8% of dementias are partially reversible and about 3% are fully reversible (Kaufman 1990b). There is some evidence to suggest that early treatment of demented individuals, particularly those with Alzheimer's type, with such agents as donepezil (Aricept), which acts as an inhibitor of acetylcholinesterase, and galanthamine (Reminyl) may slow down the rate of progression of the dementia.

Differential Diagnosis

Memory impairment occurs in a variety of conditions including delirium, amnestic disorders, and depression (American Psychiatric Association 1994). In delirium, the onset of altered

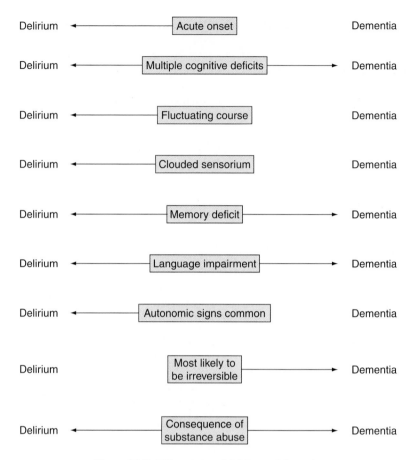

Figure 13-2 *Differentiation of delirium and dementia.*

memory is acute and the pattern typically fluctuates (waxing and waning) with increased proclivity for confusion during the night. Delirium is more likely to feature autonomic hyperactivity and alterations in level of consciousness. In some cases, a dementia can have a superimposed delirium (Figure 13-2).

Individuals with major depressive disorder often complain of lapses in memory and judgment, poor concentration, and seemingly diminished intellectual capacity. Often, these symptoms are mistakenly diagnosed as dementia, especially in elderly individuals. A thorough medical history and mental status examination focusing on such symptoms as hopelessness, crying episodes, and unrealistic guilt, in conjunction with a family history of depression, can be diagnostically beneficial. The term *pseudodementia* has been used to denote cognitive impairment secondary to a functional mental disorder, most commonly depression (Korvath et al. 1989). In comparison with demented individuals, those with depressive pseudodementia exhibit better insight regarding their cognitive dysfunction, are more likely to give "I don't know" answers, and may exhibit neurovegetative signs of depression. Pharmacological treatment of the depression should improve the cognitive dysfunction as well. Because of the rapid onset of their antidepressant action, the use of psychostimulants (e.g., methylphenidate, dextroamphetamine) to differentiate between dementia and pseudodementia has been advocated by some authors (Frierson et al. 1991). Some authors have proposed abandonment of the term pseudodementia, suggesting that most individuals so diagnosed have both genuine dementia and a superimposed affective disorder (Figure 13-3).

Amnestic disorder also presents with a significant memory deficit, but without the other associated features such as aphasia, agnosia, and apraxia. If cognitive impairment occurs only in the context of drug use, substance intoxication or substance withdrawal is the appropriate diagnosis. Although mental retardation implies below-average intellect and

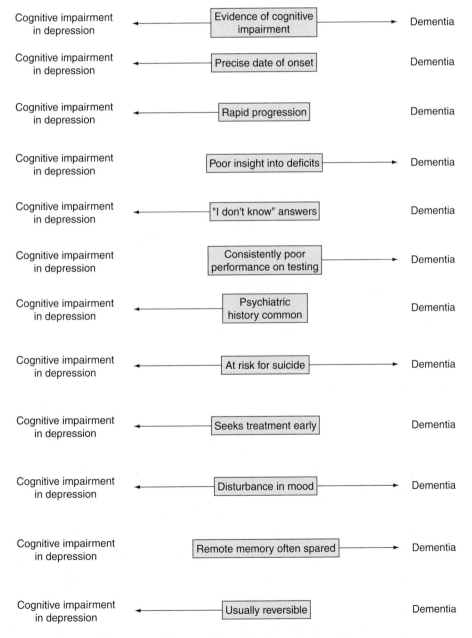

Figure 13-3 *Differential diagnosis of dementia and cognitive impairment in depression.*

subsequent impairment in other areas of function, the onset is before 18 years of age and abnormalities of memory do not always occur. Mental retardation must be considered in the differential diagnosis of dementias of childhood and adolescence along with such disorders as Wilson's disease (hepatolenticular degeneration), lead intoxication, subacute sclerosing panencephalitis, HIV spectrum disorders, and substance abuse, particularly abuse of inhalants. If an individual develops dementia before age 18 years and has an IQ in the mentally retarded range (i.e., below 70), an additional diagnosis of mental retardation may be justified.

Individuals with schizophrenia may also exhibit a variety of cognitive abnormalities, but this condition also has an early onset—a distinctive constellation of other symptoms (e.g., delusions, hallucinations, disorganized speech), and does not result from a medical condition or the persisting effects of a substance. Factitious disorder and malingering must be distinguished from dementia. The individual with factitious disorder and psychological symptoms may have some apparent cognitive deficits reminiscent of a dementia.

Dementia must also be distinguished from age-related cognitive decline (also known as benign senescence). Only when such changes exceed the level of altered function to be expected for the individual's age is the diagnosis of dementia warranted (American Psychiatric Association 1994).

DEMENTIA OF THE ALZHEIMER TYPE

Diagnosis

The course and clinical features of Dementia of the Alzheimer's Type (DAT) parallel those discussed for dementia in general. Typically, the early course of DAT is difficult to ascertain because the individual is usually an unreliable informant, and the early signs may be so subtle as to go unnoticed even by the individual's closest associates (Karp 1984). These early features include impaired memory, difficulty with problem-solving, preoccupation with long past events, decreased spontaneity, and an inability to respond to the environment with the individual's usual speed and accuracy (Karp 1984). Individuals may forget names, misplace household items, or forget what they were about to do. Often the individuals have insight into these memory deficits and occasionally convey their concerns to family members. Such responses as "You're just getting older," and "I do that sometimes myself" are common from these family members and as a result the individual becomes depressed, which can further affect cognitive functioning. Anomia, or difficulty with word finding, is common in this middle stage of Alzheimer's disease. Eventually the individual develops schemes, word associations, and excuses ("I never was very good in math") to assist in retention and cover up deficits. The individual may also employ family members as a surrogate memory (Karp 1984).

Because memory loss is usually most obvious for newly acquired material, the individual tries to avoid unfamiliar activities. Typically, the individual is seen by the clinician when confusion, aggression, wandering, or some other socially undesirable behavior ensues. At that time, disorders of perception and language may appear. The individual often turns to a spouse to answer questions posed during the history taking. By this time, the affected individual has lost insight into his or her dementia and abandons attempts to compensate for memory loss (Karp 1984). Finally, in the late stage of Alzheimer's disease, physical and cognitive effects are marked. Disorders of gait, extremity paresis and paralysis, seizures, peripheral neuropathy, extrapyramidal signs, and urinary incontinence are seen, and the individual is often no longer ambulatory. The aimless wandering of the middle stage has been replaced by a mute, bedridden state and decorticate posture. Myoclonus occasionally occurs. Significantly, affective disturbances remain a distinct possibility throughout the course of the illness. Alzheimer's disease progresses at a slow pace for 8 to 10 years to a state of complete helplessness.

The role of laboratory determinations in the evaluation for AD is to exclude other causes of dementia, especially those that may prove reversible or arrestable. Before death, AD is largely a diagnosis of exclusion. Throughout the course of this disorder, laboratory values are essentially normal. Some nonspecific changes may occur, but electroencephalography and lumbar puncture are not diagnostic. As the disease progresses, computed tomography (CT) and magnetic resonance imaging (MRI) may show atrophy in the cerebral cortex and hydrocephalus *ex vacuo*. MRI may show nonspecific alteration of white matter (leukoariosis), and eventually EEG shows diffuse-background slowing. Pneumoencephalography has demonstrated enlarged ventricles and widening of cortical sulci in Alzheimer's disease, and positron emission tomography in the later stages shows decreased cerebral oxygen and glucose metabolism in the frontal lobes. At present, in the workup of an individual with a slowly progressive dementia, a good family history, physical examination, and laboratory and radiographic tests to rule out other causes of dementia, are the most effective tools in the diagnosis of Alzheimer's disease.

Epidemiology

Alzheimer's disease is the most common cause of dementia, accounting for 55 to 65% of all cases (Korvath et al. 1989). There were fewer than 3 million cases diagnosed in the United States in 1980, but the Census Bureau predicted that there will be more than 10 million American citizens with Alzheimer's disease by the year 2050 (Evans 1990). Prevalence of the disease doubles with every 5 years between the ages of 65 and 85 years (Katzman and Kawas 1994).

Some authors separate Alzheimer's disease into senile and presenile forms, but the two disorders represent the same pathological process (Berg et al. 1994). Significantly, however, early-onset (that is, onset before the age of 65) Alzheimer's disease is associated with a more rapid course than later-onset disease (Lezak 1983).

Alzheimer's disease affects women three times as often as men, for unknown reasons (Bachman et al. 1992). Furthermore, at least one study suggests that dementia, including Alzheimer's, is more common in black than in white American women (Heyman et al. 1991). Comparison of population studies in diverse countries shows strikingly similar prevalence rates (Katzman and Kawas 1994).

Etiology

The etiology and pathogenesis of Alzheimer's disease are unknown. Multiple agents and pathways are likely involved in this disorder (Markesbery and Ehmann 1994). Many hypotheses have been proposed regarding the cause and progression of Alzheimer's disease including genetic factors, slow or unconventional viruses, defective membrane metabolism, endogenous toxins, autoimmune disorders, and neurotoxicity of such trace elements as aluminum and mercury (Markesbery and Ehmann 1994).

The brains of individuals with Alzheimer's disease contain many senile plaques, neurofibrillary tangles, and Hirano's bodies (Berg et al. 1994). There is degeneration of nerve cells, but the significant atrophy seen on neurodiagnostic examination may be more the result of shrinkage of neurons and loss of dendritic spines than of actual neuronal loss (Wolf 1980). The atrophy is most apparent in the associational cortex areas, and early decay on the primary motor and sensory areas are relatively spared. Neurochemically, the brains of individuals with Alzheimer's disease exhibit significant cholinergic abnormalities (Kaufman 1990b). There is a profound decrease in acetylcholine (ACh) in almost all individuals as well as decreased immunological activity of somatostatin- and corticotropin-releasing factors

(Kaufman 1990b). The enzyme required for ACh synthesis, choline acetyltransferase, is also greatly reduced. Other studies suggest involvement of noradrenergic and serotonergic systems in later-onset disease and diminished gamma-aminobutyric acid (GABA) (Kaufman 1990b). Although the involvement of cholinergic transmission along the hippocampus and nucleus basalis is essential to the ability to learn new information, it seems that many of the symptoms of Alzheimer's disease are not explainable solely on the basis of cholinergic abnormalities. Thus, investigators have examined a number of other potential etiological or contributory agents.

Some researchers have investigated the role of beta-amyloid protein in Alzheimer's disease, and some assert that this material, a significant component of all plaques, is a major contributor to the neurodegenerative changes in the disease as both an initiator and a promoter of the disease (Cotman and Pike 1994). Supporting this assertion are genetic studies of families with inheritable forms of presenile dementia, which show that disease occurrence is linked to mutations involving beta-amyloid-related systems (Kidd 1963). Other investigators have focused on the neurofibrillary tangles and the identification of a major component of its helical filament, the tau protein (Kidd 1963, Wisniewski et al. 1976). Specifically, these researchers analyzed the possibility that modification of tau protein, predominantly by phosphorylation, is an important feature of AD (Delacourte and Defossez 1986, Grundke-Igbal et al. 1986, Nukina and Ihara 1986).

Risk Factors

Longitudinal studies have revealed the importance of family history as a risk factor; however, no consistent genetic pattern has been established (Korvath et al. 1989). For Alzheimer's alone, the probability of developing dementia if a first-degree relative (parent or sibling) is afflicted is four times greater than that of the general population, and if two or more first-degree relatives have the disease the risk is increased eightfold compared with a normal sample of US citizens (Katzman and Kawas 1994). Among monozygotic twins 43% are concordant for the disorder, compared with only 8% of dizygotic twins (Berg et al. 1994).

Apolipoprotein (APO) E4 allele as a major genetic susceptibility risk factor has been confirmed by numerous studies (Katzman 1994). Corder and colleagues (1993) studied 234 members of 42 families with late-onset AD. Of 95 affected members, 80% had the E4 allele compared with 26% in the general population (Corder et al. 1993). Furthermore, in these families, 91% of those homozygous for E4 had developed Alzheimer's disease by 80 years of age—evidence that the APO E E4 allele is causing these familial cases (Corder et al. 1993). In a study of 176 autopsy specimens of confirmed AD, Schmechel and coworkers in 1993 found that 65% of individuals carried at least one APO E E4 gene (Katzman 1994). Examination of all such studies indicates that between 25 and 40% of AD cases can be attributable to this marker, making its presence one of the most common risk factors yet discovered for AD (Katzman 1994, Corder et al. 1993).

In addition to age, gender, and family history, the presence of Down syndrome, a history of head trauma, and a low level of education have been proposed as risk factors. Most studies concur that individuals with trisomy 21 develop the features of AD by age 35 years; however, studies have looked at the possibility that families with a member who has AD are more likely to produce offspring with Down syndrome and have had inconclusive results (Burger and Vogel 1973). Significant head injury, as either a single incident or a chronic occurrence as in sports injuries, increases the risk of developing Alzheimer's by a factor of 2 (Katzman and Kawas 1994). An uneducated person older than 75 years is about twice as likely to develop dementia as one who has 8 years or more schooling, leading to the speculation that the cognitive processes involved in obtaining an education may be partially protective (Katzman and Kawas 1994). Risk factors found in some but not all studies include myocardial ischemia in the elderly, having a child at 40 years or older, and exposure to aluminum (Katzman and Kawas 1994). For a more detailed examination of risk factors in AD, please see *Alzheimer's Disease* (Terry et al. 1994).

Treatment

The two principles of management in AD are to treat what is treatable without aggravating existing symptoms and to support caregivers who are also victims of this disease. Despite the significant decrease in ACh and choline acetyltransferase in Alzheimer's disease, treatments based on the cholinergic hypothesis have been unsuccessful (Kaufman 1990a). With the goal of increasing the central nervous system concentrations of ACh, precursors of ACh including choline and lecithin have been tried as well as centrally acting anticholinesterases, such as physostigmine and tetrahydroacridine, with the hope of decreasing ACh metabolism (Kaufman 1990b). ACh agonists such as areocholine, oxotremorine, and bethanechol have been investigated, and release of ACh has been stimulated from cerebral neurons by using piracetam (a cyclic relative of GABA) and nafronyl oxalate (Praxilene) (Kaufman 1990b). These pharmacological interventions have yielded inconsistent results and been largely ineffective.

Despite lackluster effects of physostigmine, a second cholinesterase inhibitor has shown promise (Mohs et al. 1985). Tetrahydroaminoacridine (tacrine) produced significant cognitive improvement in 16 of 17 individuals with AD in an early study (Summers et al. 1986). Subsequent studies have been less impressive, but significant improvement in a number of scales measuring cognitive performance illustrated the benefit of this agent for some individuals. Side effects, particularly hepatic and cholinergic, were noted; however, in 1993 the US Food and Drug Administration (USFDA) approved of tacrine for the treatment of AD (Thal 1994). Donepezil (Aricept), an inhibitor of acetylcholinesterase, has also been utilized in an attempt to enhance cholinergic function by inhibiting its breakdown. This agent must be given early in the course of the dementia.

The N-methyl-D-aspartate (NMDA) receptor, a glutamate receptor subtype, has important effects in learning and memory. Stimulation by the excitatory amino acid glutamate results in long-term potentiation of neuronal activity basic to memory formation (Cotman et al. 1988). There appears to be a decrease in cerebral cortcial and hippocampal NMDA receptors in Alzheimer's disease. Memantine (1-amino-3,5-dimethyladamantane) is a moderate affinity noncompetitive NMDA receptor antagonist approved in the US in 2003 for the treatment of dementia. A recent randomized, placebo-controlled trial showed that memantine 20 mg/day improved cognition consistently across different cognitive scales without side effects in numerous individuals with mild to moderate vascular dementia (Orgogozo et al. 2002). A multicenter study of 252 individuals showed reduced clinical deterioration in moderate to severe Alzheimer's disease (Reisberg et al. 2003). A postmarketing surveillance study conducted among German physicians who treated dementia patients with memantine in combination with an anticholinesterase inhibior (mainly Aricept) suggests that this combination is safe and well-tolerated (Hartmann and Mobius, 2003).

Depression is often associated with AD. If antidepressant medication is to be used, low doses (about one-third to one-half of the usual initial dose) are advised and only agents with minimal anticholinergic activity should be employed. Appropriate choices would be the selective serotonin reuptake inhibitors such as paroxetine (Paxil), fluoxetine (Prozac), sertraline (Zoloft), and citalopram (Celexa). Although sertraline and citalopram are least likely to cause drug–drug interactions, even these agents have the potential to increase confusion in Alzheimer's individuals. Agents such as trazodone (Desyrel) and mirtazapine (Remeron) have occasionally been employed because of their sedating properties. If tricyclic antidepressants are used, the secondary amines (e.g., desipramine, nortriptyline) are recommended over the tertiary ones (e.g., amitriptyline, doxepin). Careful attention to the possible side effects of these agents, particularly orthostatic hypotension, lowering of the seizure threshold, excessive fatigue, urinary retention, constipation, confusion, and accelerated memory impairment, is suggested. Most clinicians now feel that tricyclic antidepressants are inappropriate for this population.

Anxiety and psychosis, particularly paranoid delusions, are common in AD. Benzodiazepines can be disinhibiting in such individuals and may exacerbate confusion and should be avoided if possible. If minor tranquilizers are required, agents with a shorter duration of action (e.g., lorazepam, oxazepam) are preferred. Antipsychotic medications with high anticholinergic potential (e.g., thioridazine, chlorpromazine) may also affect memory adversely. While these agents have been favored in the past because of their tendency to produce sedation, newer agents such as olanzapine (zyprexa), risperidone (risperdal), quetiapine (Seroquel) and ziprasidone (geodon), have been reported to have lower incidences of neuroleptic-related side effects (Torres et al. 2001, Teste et al. 2000, Lerner et al. 2000). Haloperidol has less anticholinergic activity but has a greater tendency toward extrapyramidal effects.

The appropriate management of AD entails more than psychopharmacological intervention. Other elements of the treatment plan should be environmental manipulation and support for the family. In the attempt to maintain individuals with Alzheimer's disease in their homes for as long as possible, some adjustments of their environment are important. Written daily reminders can be helpful in the performance of daily activities. Prominent clocks, calendars, and windows are important. An effort should be made to minimize changes in the individual's daily activities and environment. Repeated demonstrations of how to lock doors and windows and operate appliances are helpful and arranging for rapid dialing of essential telephone numbers can be useful. Maintaining adequate hydration, nutrition, exercise, and cleanliness is essential.

The family of the individual with Alzheimer's disease is also a victim of the disease. Family members must watch the gradual deterioration of the individual and accept that a significant part of their own lives must be devoted to the care of the individual. Difficult decisions about institutionalization and termination of life support are distinct possibilities, and the patients often turn their anger and paranoia toward the caregiver. Education is a valuable treatment tool for families. Information about the disease and peer support are available through Alzheimer's associations, and many such agencies provide family members with a companion for the individual with AD to allow the family some time away. (The National Alzheimer's Education and Referral Service can be accessed by calling 1-800-621-0379.) For these reasons, family members are at risk for depression, anxiety disorders, insomnia, and a variety of other psychological manifestations. Should these occur, they should be promptly treated.

VASCULAR DEMENTIA

Diagnosis

Vascular dementia usually results from multiple CVAs or one significant CVA. It is generally considered the second most common cause of dementia after Alzheimer's disease, accounting for about 10% of all cases (Kaufman 1990b, Korvath et al. 1989). Men are twice as likely as women to be diagnosed with this condition (Torres et al. 2001). Vascular dementia is characterized by a stepwise progression of cognitive deterioration with accompanying lateralizing signs. (See DSM-IV-TR diagnostic criteria below.) It is always associated with evidence of systemic hypertension and usually involves renal and cardiac abnormalities. Risk factors for the development of a vascular dementia include those generally associated with obstructive coronary artery disease, including obesity, hypercholesterolemia, smoking, hypertension, stress, and lack of exercise. The actual incidence of vascular dementia has decreased somewhat with better standards of care, improved diagnostic techniques, and lifestyle changes.

DSM-IV-TR Diagnostic Criteria

290.4x Vascular Dementia

A. The development of multiple cognitive deficits manifested by both

(1) memory impairment (impaired ability to learn new information or to recall previously learned information)

(2) one (or more) of the following cognitive disturbances:

(a) aphasia (language disturbance)

(b) apraxia (impaired ability to carry out motor activities despite intact motor function)

(c) agnosia (failure to recognize or identify objects despite intact sensory function)

(d) disturbance in executive functioning (i.e., planning, organizing, sequencing, abstracting)

B. The cognitive deficits in criteria A1 and A2 each cause significant impairment in social or occupational functioning and represent a significant decline from a previous level of functioning.

C. Focal neurological signs and symptoms (e.g., exaggeration of deep tendon reflexes, extensor plantar response, pseudobulbar palsy, gait abnormalities, weakness of an extremity) or laboratory evidence indicative of cerebrovascular disease (e.g., multiple infarctions involving cortex and underlying white matter) that are judged to be etiologically related to the disturbance.

D. The deficits do not occur exclusively during the course of a delirium.

Code based on predominant features:

290.41 With Delirium: if delirium is superimposed on the dementia

290.42 With Delusions: if delusions are the predominant feature

390.43 With Depressed Mood: if depressed mood (including presentations that meet full symptom criteria for a major depressive episode) is the predominant feature. A separate diagnosis of mood disorder due to a general medical condition is not given.

209.40 Uncomplicated: if none of the above predominates in the current clinical presentation

Specify if:

With behavioral disturbance

Coding note: Also code cerebrovascular condition on Axis III.

Vascular dementia is characterized by the early appearance of localizing neurological signs. Spasticity, hemiparesis, ataxia, and pseudobulbar palsy are common. Pseudobulbar palsy is associated with injury to the frontal lobes and results in impairment of the corticobulbar tracts. It is characterized by extreme emotional lability, abnormal speech cadence, dysphagia, hyperactive jaw jerk, hyperactive deep tendon reflexes, and Babinski's reflex.

CT, MRI, and gross specimens show cerebral atrophy and infarctions, with the radiological procedures showing multiple lucencies and the gross specimens revealing distinct white- matter lesions (Kaufman 1990b, Hershey et al. 1987). The EEG is abnormal but nonspecific, and positron emission tomography reveals hypometabolic areas (Kaufman 1990b). Vascular dementia is differentiated from AD on the basis of its mode of progression, early appearance of neurological signs, and radiographical evidence of cerebral ischemia.

Treatment

Primary prevention and secondary prevention are important in the treatment of cerebrovascular disorders. Lifestyle changes are effective in arresting the progress of the disease; however, no known pharmacological treatment can reverse the effects of a completed stroke (Korvath et al. 1989). Such interventions as anticoagulants for frequent transient ischemic attacks after a hemorrhagic lesion have been investigated but excluded; aspirin for decreasing platelet aggregation, and surgical removal of obstructing plaques probably do not reverse the mental state (Korvath et al. 1989).

Depression occurs in 50 to 60% of individuals with CVAs and responds to traditional antidepressants. Tricyclic antidepressants, such as amitriptyline, in less than antidepressant doses, improve both CVA depression and pseudobulbar palsy. Physical rehabilitation is essential and often results in an improvement in mood and outlook.

DEMENTIA DUE TO HIV DISEASE

Diagnosis

Acquired Immunodeficiency Syndrome (AIDS) was first described in the United States in 1979. In the developed countries, the death rate from AIDS has been on the decline since the advent of new medication regimens utilizing traditional antiretrovirals and the newer protease inhibitors. These medication cocktails have also decreased the incidence of AIDS–dementia complex, so that physicians are now more likely to see AIDS-related delirium secondary to infection, metabolic disarray, and medication rather than traditional AIDS dementia. In the truest sense, AIDS is not a disease but an increased susceptibility to a variety of diseases caused by loss of immunocompetence. It results from infection with HIV, a retrovirus that attaches to the CD4 molecule on the surface of the T4 (thymus-derived) lymphocyte. Then, using reverse transcriptase, the virus reverses the usual sequence of genetic information and becomes integrated into the host cell's DNA (Kaufman 1990b). The ultimate result is destruction of the T4 cell, replication of the virus, a defect in cell-mediated immunity, and the development of various opportunistic infections and neoplasms.

The epidemiology of HIV spectrum diseases has changed significantly in the 16 years since its identification. Initially, homosexual and bisexual men with multiple partners were the highest-risk group. Intravenous drug abusers and recipients of tainted blood products were soon added to high-risk groups. In the 1990s, the number of new infections among homosexual men decreased significantly and rates for women, intravenous drug abusers who shared contaminated needles, and infants born to infected mothers increased significantly. Intravenous drug abusers, regardless of sexual orientation, represent the fastest growing population of the newly infected people. Conversely, instances of transmission by blood products have decreased since the development of laboratory testing for HIV antibodies. The CDC has now established a reactive HIV antibody screen, presence of an opportunistic condition, and a CD4$^+$ cell count of 200 or less (normal being 1000–1500) as criteria for the diagnosis of AIDS.

AIDS is now best considered as part of the spectrum of HIV infection (Wilson et al. 1991). There are four stages of infection.

Stage 1: Acute Infection: Most infected persons remember no signs or symptoms at the time of the initial infection. The acute syndrome follows infection by 4 to 6 weeks and is characterized by fevers, rigors, muscle aches, maculopapular rash, diarrhea, and abdominal cramps. These symptoms, often mistaken for those of influenza, resolve spontaneously after 2 to 3 weeks.

Stage 2: Asymptomatic carrier: This stage follows the acute infection. The infected individual is without symptoms for a variable amount of time. The mean symptom-free period has increased significantly since the disease was first identified and is now about 10 years. Most of the estimated 2 million infected Americans are at this stage. Even though these individuals are asymptomatic, they are carriers of the disease and can infect others.

Stage 3: Generalized adenopathy: In older terminology, this stage was referred to as the AIDS-related complex. It is characterized by palpable lymph nodes that persist for longer than 3 months. These nodes must be outside the inguinal area and due to no other condition except HIV.

Stage 4: Other diseases:
1. Constitutional symptoms such as lingering fever, wasting syndromes, and intractable diarrhea.
2. Secondary infections including *P. carinii* pneumonia, cytomegalovirus retinitis, parasitic colitis, and oral esophageal thrush.
3. Secondary neoplasms such as Kaposi's sarcoma and B-cell lymphomas.
4. Neurological diseases (AIDS dementia complex).

Thus, the diagnosis of AIDS is made when an infected individual develops either a CD4$^+$ cell count of less than 200 or a certain condition listed in the stages (Kallmann 1989, Wilson et al. 1991).

Initially, the behavioral abnormalities observed in HIV-positive individuals were attributed to the emotional reaction to the disease. Subsequent investigations demonstrated that neurological complications occur in 40 to 45% of individuals with AIDS, and in about 10% of cases, neurological signs are the first feature of the disease (Berg et al. 1994, Pajeau and Roman 1992). The neurological signs present in AIDS are believed to be related to both the direct effects of the virus on cells (such as macrophages) that enter the central nervous system and the neurological conditions that opportunistically affect these individuals. Ho and colleagues (1987) reported that 90% of the brains of the individuals affected by AIDS examined showed neuropathological abnormalities. AIDS dementia must be considered in the differential diagnosis of dementia in older individuals, because about 10% of AIDS individuals are older than 50 years of age (Berg et al. 1994, Scharnhorst 1992).

Individuals with AIDS dementia present with impairments of cognitive, behavioral, and motor systems. The cognitive disorders include memory impairment, confusion, and poor concentration. Behavioral features include apathy, reclusivity, anhedonia, depression, delusions, and hallucinations. Motor symptoms include incoordination, lower extremity paresis, unsteadiness, and difficulty with fine motor movements like handwriting and buttoning clothes (Berg et al. 1994, Kaufman 1990b). As the disease progresses, parkinsonism and myoclonus develop. Localizing signs such as tremors, focal seizures, abnormal reflexes, and hemiparesis can result. The protozoan *Toxoplasma gondii* commonly infects the central nervous system and can be diagnosed by CT or by increased toxoplasmosis antibody titers

(Kaufman 1990b). Discrete cerebral lesions are also produced by fungi such as *Candida* and *Aspergillus, Mycobacterium tuberculosis*, and viruses such as cytomegalovirus and papovavirus. Papovavirus causes progressive multifocal leukoencephalopathy (Kaufman 1990b). Tertiary syphilis has increased significantly since the advent of AIDS, and neoplasms such as lymphomas, metastatic Kaposi's sarcoma, and gliomas are also causes of AIDS dementia.

Many confounding factors can increase cognitive dysfunction in AIDS, including a high incidence of drug and alcohol abuse; medications such as histamine H_2 receptor antagonists (cimetidine), corticosteroids, narcotics, and antiviral drugs (e.g., zidovudine [formerly azidothymidine, AZT]) that increase confusion; and coexistent depression (Table 13-7).

The CT scan shows cerebral atrophy and MRI reveals nonspecific white-matter abnormalities (Kaufman 1990b). Neoplasms and lesions such as toxoplasmosis are also visible. Lumbar puncture reveals a pleocytosis and elevated protein levels, and autopsy demonstrates an atrophic brain with demyelination, multinuclear giant cells, and gliosis of the cerebral cortex (Kaufman 1990b).

Treatment

The increase in life span of individuals affected by HIV is directly related to improvements in treating the opportunistic conditions that occur. Aerosol pentamidine as prophylaxis for *P. carinii* pneumonia and ganciclovir for cytomegalovirus retinitis are examples of effective intervention. The use of antiviral agents has generated some controversy. Zidovudine, the first antiviral treatment for AIDS approved by the FDA increased or stabilized CD4$^+$ cell concentrations in early studies. Later investigations revealed that zidovudine has a narrow window of effectiveness and may not be appropriate immediately after such exposure as a needle stick. Studies suggest that administration of zidovudine to HIV-positive individuals during pregnancy, intravenously during delivery, and to the neonate for 6 weeks after birth

Table 13-7	Neuropsychiatric Effects of AIDS-related Drugs	
Drug	**Use**	**Effect**
Ketoconazole (Nizoral)	Antifungal	Severe depression Suicidality (rare)
Foscarnet	Cytomegalovirus retinitis Herpes	Depression Confusion
Ganciclovir	Cytomegalovirus retinitis	Anxiety Psychosis
Bactrim	*Pneumocystis* pneumonia	Hallucinations Depression Apathy
Pentamidine	*Pneumocystis* pneumonia	Delirium Hallucinations
Interferon alpha	Cancer	Depression
Rifampin	Tuberculosis	Delirium Behavioral changes
Isoniazid	Tuberculosis	Memory disturbance Psychosis
Dronabinol (Marinol)	Appetite stimulant Wasting syndrome Nausea	Depression Anxiety Psychosis Euphoria
Zalcitabine (DDC)	Antiviral	Psychosis Amnesia Confusion Depersonalization Depression Mania Suicidality Mood swings
Didanosine	Antiviral	Anxiety
Zidovudine (AZT)	Antiviral	Confusion, mania Depression, anxiety

can decrease the percentage of infants who seroconvert from 30% to as low as 10%. Subsequent antiviral agents such as dideoxyinosine and dideoxycytidine (DDC) have been associated with painful neuropathy and pancreatic disorders. DDC in particular can produce serious neuropsychiatric complications. Combined therapy with two antiviral agents may be more effective than single-drug therapy. Many pharmaceutical companies are combining two antivirals into a single pill, and the development of protease inhibitor agents such as indinavir (Crixivan) and nelfinavir (Viracept) have been especially effective in retarding the progression of the disease.

The treatment of neuropsychiatric disorders in AIDS involves utilizing agents that are least likely to interfere with other medications prescribed, or to exacerbate the symptoms of the disease. AIDS-related depression has responded well to the selective serotonin reuptake inhibitors (SSRIs) and to psychostimulants. Some HIV drugs can have interactions with SSRIs, particularly ritonavir (Norvir) and the SSRIs themselves, especially paroxetine and fluoxetine can interact with other agents the individual with HIV may have been prescribed, such as antiarrhythmics, benzodiazepines, and anticonvulsants by inhibiting the cytochrome P-450 enzyme system. Some individuals have suggested that citalopram is less likely to inhibit this enzyme system. Careful attention to drug–drug interactions, using lower starting doses of certain psychiatric drugs, and monitoring of blood levels of affected medications are recommended. Among the psychostimulants, methylphenidate is preferred to dextroamphetamine because of the latter's tendency to produce dyskinesias. Use of stimulants for treating individuals with a history of substance abuse is not recommended. Anticholingeric agents have a number of side effects such as mydriasis, decreased gastrointestinal motility, and postural hypotension. However, low dose tricyclic antidepressants are often used for their sedative, analgesic, and appetite stimulant properties. Most antidepressants and some mood stabilizers and antipsychotics can cause bone marrow suppression, so they should be used with care, and hematologic parameters should be routinely monitored. Lithium carbonate, which produces a leukocytosis, may be of benefit in recurrent unipolar and treatment-resistant depression, but may potentiate AIDS-related diarrhea. Many of the drugs used to treat AIDS-related conditions may produce untoward psychiatric effects. Depression has been well documented as a side effect of indinavir (Crixivan), and nelfinavir (Viracept) has been associated with anxiety, depression, mood lability, and even suicidality. St. John's Wort may decrease the concentration of many of the protease inhibitors and is therefore contraindicated in individuals taking these agents.

In summary, AIDS dementia is best treated by identifying the associated medical condition, instituting appropriate therapy, and managing behavior in the interim.

DEMENTIA DUE TO OTHER GENERAL MEDICAL CONDITIONS

See DSM-IV-TR diagnostic criteria for Dementia Due to a General Medical Condition below.

DSM-IV-TR Diagnostic Criteria

294.1x Dementia Due to Other General Medical Conditions

A. The development of multiple cognitive deficits manifested by both

  (1) memory impairment (impaired ability to learn new information or to recall previously learned information)

(2) one (or more) of the following cognitive disturbances:

   (a) aphasia (language disturbance)
   (b) apraxia (impaired ability to carry out motor activities despite intact motor function)
   (c) agnosia (failure to recognize or identify objects despite intact sensory function)
   (d) disturbance in executive functioning (i.e., planning, organizing, sequencing, abstracting)

B. The cognitive deficits in criteria A1 and A2 each cause significant impairment in social or occupational functioning and represent a significant decline from a previous level of functioning.
C. There is evidence from the history, physical examination, or laboratory findings that the disturbance is the direct physiological consequence of one of the general medical conditions listed below.
D. The deficits do not occur exclusively during the course of a delirium.

Code based on presence or absence of a clinically significant behavioral disturbance:

294.10 Without Behavioral Disturbance: if the cognitive disturbance is not accompanied by any clinically significant behavioral disturbance.

294.11 With Behavioral Disturbance: if the cognitive disturbance is accompanied by a clinically significant behavioral disturbance (e.g., wandering, agitation). 294.9 Dementia due to HIV Disease

Coding note: Also code the general medical condition on Axis III (e.g., 042 HIV infection, 854.00 head injury, 331.82 Dementia with Lewy Bodies, 333.4 Huntington's disease, 331.11 Pick's disease, 046.1 Creutzfeldt-Jakob disease; see Appendix G in DSM-IV-TR for additional codes)

Dementia due to Pick's Disease   Pick's disease is a rare form of progressive dementia clinically indistinguishable from Alzheimer's disease. It is about one-fifth as common as AD (Nolan et al. 1991). Pick's disease occurs in the sixth and seventh decades of life and has a duration that varies from 2 to 15 years. It has a strong familial tendency but a definite genetic pattern has not been established (Kaufman 1990b). ACh levels are reduced. The pathology of Pick's disease involves prominent changes (e.g., sclerosis, atrophy) in the frontal and temporal lobes. The parietal and occipital lobes are spared. Alzheimer himself noted the argentophilic (staining silver) intraneuronal inclusion in Pick's bodies.

The clinical features of Pick's disease are quite similar to those of Alzheimer's disease, and since neither condition is curable, an elaborate differential diagnosis is unnecessary. Because of parietal sparing, features such as apraxia and agnosia are less common in Pick's disease, and visual–spatial ability, often impaired in Alzheimer's disease, is preserved (Kaufman 1990b). Given the prominent changes in the frontal lobe, disinhibited behavior, loss of social constraints, and lack of concern about appearance and matters of personal hygiene occur relatively early in Pick's disease. Such speech disorders as echolalia and logorrhea are common, and individuals with Pick's disease are more likely to develop Klüver–Bucy syndrome (orality, hyperphagia, hypersexuality, placidity) indicative of damage to the temporal lobes (Torres et al. 2001). Significant memory impairment may occur relatively late in the course, and eventually the individual becomes listless, mute, and ultimately decerebrate and comatose. Like Alzheimer's disease, the treatment of Pick's disease is symptomatic.

Dementia Due to Parkinson's Disease   Although dementia rarely occurs as an initial symptom of Parkinson's disease, it is found in nearly 40% of such individuals older than 70 years of age (Kaplan et al. 1994). The prevalence in persons over 60 is 1%. The disease results from loss of dopamine production in the basal ganglia, and can be idiopathic or postencephalitic. Usually, the individual is 50 years of age or older, and unlike Alzheimer's and Pick's dementias, this disease occurs slightly more often in men (Berg et al. 1994). Dementia most commonly occurs in cases of Parkinson's disease in which the decline has been rapid and response to anticholinergics has been poor.

The pathology of Parkinson's disease involves depigmentation of the so-called pigmented nuclei of the brain (*locus coeruleus, substantia nigra*). These nuclei then contain eosinophilic Lewy bodies. As in Alzheimer's disease, the cerebral cortex of many of these individuals contains many senile plaques and neurofibrillary tangles, loss of neurons, and decreased concentrations of choline acetyltransferase (Kaufman 1990). Individuals with parkinsonian dementia also have reduced choline acetyltransferase in the cerebral cortex and substantia nigra (Kaufman 1990c).

The clinical features of Parkinson's disease are well described, with the cardinal triad being tremor, rigidity, and bradykinesia. Associated features include postural instability, a festinating gait, micrographia, seborrhea, urinary changes, constipation, hypophonia, and an expressionless facial countenance. The tremor in Parkinson's disease has a regular rate and is most prominent when the individual is sitting with arms supported; it has therefore been described as intention tremors. Paranoid delusions and visual hallucinations may occur, but auditory hallucinations are rare. Antipsychotics with low incidence of extrapyramidal symptoms such as quetiapine, olanzapine, and ziprasidone are recommended. The pharmacological treatment of Parkinson's disease involves the use of a number of types of medication. These include selegiline (Eldepryl), a selective monoamine oxidase inhibitor, levodopa, other dopamine agonists (pramipexole [Mirapex], bromocriptine, pergolide mesylate [Permax], amantadine), and various anticholinergic agents (e.g., benztropine). Selegiline should not be given to individuals on antidepressant medication as there is a risk that dopaminergic agents may activate psychosis or mania and that anticholinergic drugs may increase confusion. When discontinuing levodopa after a long course of treatment, the drug should be tapered so as to prevent a discontinuation syndrome similar in nature to the neuroleptic malignant syndrome. Some medications (metoclopramide, droperidol, several antipsychotics) may produce parkinsonian features such as masked facies, sparsity of speech, and tremor, and in those cases, the appropriate course of treatment is to discontinue the offending medication (Mamo et al. 2002). Several researchers are looking into the possibility of using embryonic stem cells implants as treatment for Parkinson's disease and several other conditions.

Dementia Due to Huntington's Disease   Dementia is also a characteristic of Huntington's disease, an autosomal, dominant, inheritable condition localized to chromosome 4. Unfortunately, this condition does not become apparent until age 35 to 45 years, usually after childbearing has occurred. Fifty percent of offspring are affected. There is also a juvenile form of the disease. Huntington's disease affects about 4 in 100,000 people, making it a significant cause of dementia in middle-aged adults (Teste et al. 2000). The pathology of Huntington's disease involves selective destruction in the caudate and putamen (Teste et al. 2000). In the caudate nuclei, GABA concentrations are reduced to 50% of normal

(Teste et al. 2000). The frontal lobes of the cerebral cortex are also involved, but GABA and choline acetyltransferase concentrations in the cortex are normal.

The most noticeable clinical feature of Huntington's disease is the movement disorder, which involves both choreiform movements (frequent movements that cause a jerking motion of the body) and athetosis (slow writhing movements). In the juvenile form of Huntington's disease, which represents about 3% of all cases, the chorea is replaced by dystonia, akinesia, and rigidity, and the course of the disease is more rapid than in the adult form (Teste et al. 2000). In the early stages of the disease, the chorea is not as noticeable and may be disguised by the individual by making the movements seem purposeful.

The dementia typically begins 1 year before or 1 year after the chorea and, unlike individuals with other dementias, individuals with Huntington's disease are often well aware of their deteriorating mentation. This may be a factor in the high rates of suicide and alcoholism associated with this condition. Although attempts have been made to increase ACh and GABA concentrations in these individuals, such pharmacological interventions have been unsuccessful, and the dementia is untreatable. Genetic counseling is indicated.

Subacute Sclerosing Panencephalitis   Subacute sclerosing panencephalitis is an infectious cause of dementia that usually appears in childhood. The average age at onset is 10 years, and most individuals are male and live in rural areas (Kaufman 1990b, Ziber et al. 1983). It is diagnosed on the basis of periodic complexes on the EEG and an elevated measles titer in the cerebrospinal fluid (CSF). The CT scan shows cerebral atrophy and dilated ventricles. Myoclonus and dementia are prominent features. It has been postulated that a mutant measles virus is the infectious agent, on the basis of the high CSF measles antibody titer and the fact that the disease is virtually nonexistent in children who have been vaccinated for measles (Kaplan et al. 1994). Affected individuals show an insidious onset of impairment of cognition usually preceded by behavioral problems.

Creutzfeldt–Jakob Disease   Dating from original descriptions by Creutzfeldt in 1920 and Jakob in 1921, this disease has received intense scientific scrutiny (Karp 1984). The primary features of Creutzfeldt–Jakob disease are dementia, basal ganglia and cerebellar dysfunction, myoclonus, upper motor neuron lesions, and rapid progression to stupor, coma, and death in a matter of months. The disease generally affects people 65 years of age or older, with a duration of 1 month to 6 years and an average life span of 15 months after the onset of the disease (Karp 1984).

The clinical and pathological features of Creutzfeldt–Jakob have been produced experimentally by injecting animals with brain tissue from affected adults. The agent of transmission is believed to be a prion-containing protein (not DNA or RNA). These prions have been detected in the cerebral cortex of autopsy specimens of both individuals with Creutzfeldt–Jakob disease and victims of kuru, a fatal disease transmitted by cannibalism (Kaplan et al. 1994, Prusiner 1987). Slow viruses have also been implicated as infectious agents in kuru. Creutzfeldt–Jakob has been accidentally transferred to humans by corneal and pituitary gland transplantation, electroencephalogram electrodes (Marzewski et al. 1988, Rappaport and Graham 1987), and ingesting meat infected with the disease (mad cow disease).

The memory loss in Creutzfeldt–Jakob disease involves all phases of memory, with recent (secondary) memory being the most impaired. Personality changes, immature behavior, and paranoia are early signs, and virtually every aspect of brain functioning can be involved. Motor disorders including rigidity, incoordination, paresis, and ataxia usually follow. As with subacute sclerosing panencephalitis, the EEG in Creutzfeldt–Jakob disease shows periodic complexes and biopsy specimens that reveal a characteristic spongiform encephalopathy and occasional amyloid plaques (Kaufman 1990b).

Neurosyphilis During the late 19th century, neurosyphilis was responsible for a significant number of admissions to psychiatric hospitals (Kaufman 1990b). The condition had decreased in incidence after the causative agent (*Treponema pallidum*) was identified and penicillin treatment became readily available. The rise of AIDS in the 1980s and 1990s has led to an increase in the number of diagnosed cases of neurosyphilis (Kaufman 1990b). Infection with *T. pallidum* is generally divided into four stages (Summergrad et al. 1993):

1. Primary syphilis occurs 3 to 6 weeks after contact with the organism. The symptoms include a chancre at the site and regional lymphadenopathy. Affected persons are infectious.
2. Secondary syphilis begins 6 to 8 weeks after the primary stage. It is manifested by a maculopapular rash over the trunk and especially over the soles of the feet and palms. The person is constitutionally ill with fever and adenopathy. Occasionally, secondary syphilis is asymptomatic in the last few weeks.
3. Latent syphilis presents with a normal examination and seropositivity. If individuals with latent syphilis continue to have a normal CSF profile 2 years after diagnosis, they are at low risk for neurosyphilis.
4. Late syphilis consists of ongoing inflammatory disease most likely in the aorta or nervous system (neurosyphilis), the latter occurring in about 10% of individuals. The neurosyphilis of the late stage can consist of (1) asymptomatic neurosyphilis, (2) meningovascular syphilis, and (3) parenchymal neurosyphilis that has two forms. One form of parenchymal neurosyphilis consists of general paresis, which occurs about 20 years after infection and includes cognitive impairment, myoclonus, dysarthria, personality changes, irritability, psychosis, grandiosity, and mania (Summergrad et al. 1993, Ross et al. 1990). Untreated general paresis leaves the individual a helpless invalid. The second form of parenchymal neurosyphilis is *tabes dorsalis* with onset 25 to 30 years after initial infection. Tabes features loss of position and vibratory sense, areflexia in lower extremities, chronic pain, ataxia, and incontinence (Summergrad et al. 1993).

The original screening test for syphilis is the venereal disease research laboratory (VDRL) test. This test has a significant false-positive rate, especially in the elderly and in individuals with addictions and autoimmune disorders (Kaufman 1990b). The VDRL test may revert to negative after a number of years, and 20 to 30% of individuals in the stage of late syphilis have a negative (nonreactive) VDRL result. A more specific test is the fluorescent treponemal antibody screen, which is positive 95% of the time in neurosyphilis. The false-positive rate for the fluorescent treponemal antibody screen is extremely low, and reversion to a nonreactive state is unlikely. In addition to a positive VDRL result, the CSF in individuals with neurosyphilis generally shows pleocytosis.

Dementia, secondary to neurosyphilis, produces various physical findings in advanced cases. These may include dysarthria, Babinski's reflex, tremor, Argyll Robertson pupils, myelitis, and optic atrophy. Although notorious, delusions of grandeur in neurosyphilis are rare. A reactive CSF VDRL result or a positive serum fluorescent treponemal antibody result in an individual with neurological symptoms who cannot document treatment should be treated with appropriate therapy. Penicillin often improves cognitive deficits and corrects CSF abnormalities, but complete recovery is rare.

Dementia Due to Head Trauma Head trauma is the leading cause of brain injury for children and young adults (Berg et al. 1994). It is estimated that more than 7 million head injuries and 500,000 hospital admissions related to the same cause occur in the United States annually (Berg et al. 1994, Bond 1986). Traumatic head injuries result in concussions, contusions, or open head injuries, and the physical examination often reveals such features as blood behind the tympanic membranes (Battle's sign), infraorbital ecchymosis, and pupillary abnormalities (Berg et al. 1994). The psychiatric manifestations of an acute brain injury are generally classified as a delirium or an amnestic disorder; however, head trauma-induced delirious states often merge into a chronic dementia. Episodes of repeated head trauma, as in *dementia pugilistica* (punchdrunk syndrome), can lead to permanent changes in cognition and thus are appropriately classified as demented states. The punchdrunk syndrome is seen in aging boxers and includes dysarthric speech, emotional lability, slowed thought, and impulsivity (Berg et al. 1994, Kaufman 1990b, Jordan 1987, Mawdsley and Fergusen 1953). A single head injury may result in a postconcussional syndrome with resultant memory impairment, alterations in mood and personality, hyperacusis, headaches, easy fatigability, anxiety, belligerent behavior, and dizziness. Alcohol abuse, postural hypotension, and gait disturbances are often associated with head injuries that result in dementia.

Normal-Pressure Hydrocephalus   Normal-pressure hydrocephalus is generally considered the fifth leading cause of dementia after Alzheimer's, vascular, alcohol-related, and AIDS dementias. Long considered reversible but often merely arrestable, normal-pressure hydrocephalus is a syndrome consisting of dementia, urinary incontinence, and gait apraxia (Kaufman 1990b, Fisher 1982, Benson et al. 1970). It results from subarachnoid hemorrhage, meningitis, or trauma that impedes CSF absorption (Kaufman 1990b).

Unlike other dementias, the dementia caused by normal-pressure hydrocephalus has physical effects that often overshadow the mental effects (Karp 1984). Psychomotor retardation, marked gait disturbances, and, in severe cases, complete incontinence of urine occur (Karp 1984). A cisternogram is often helpful in the diagnosis, and CT and MRI show ventricular dilatation without cerebral atrophy. CSF analysis reveals a normal opening pressure, and glucose and protein determinations are within the normal range. The hydrocephalus can be relieved by insertion of a shunt into the lateral ventricle to drain CSF into the chest or the abdominal cavity, where it is absorbed. Clinical improvement with shunting approaches 50% with a neurosurgical complication rate of 13 to 25% (Kaufman 1990b, Black 1980). Infection remains the most common complication.

Wilson's Disease   Hepatolenticular degeneration (Wilson's disease) is an inherited autosomal recessive condition associated with dementia, hepatic dysfunction, and a movement disorder. Localized to chromosome 13, this disorder features copper deposits in the liver, brain, and cornea (Kaufman 1990b, Chung et al. 1986, Cartwright 1978). Symptoms begin in adolescence to the early twenties and cases are often seen in younger children (Berg et al. 1994, Saito 1987). Wilson's disease should be considered along with Huntington's disease, AIDS dementia, substance abuse dementia, head trauma, and subacute sclerosing panencephalitis in the differential diagnosis of dementia that presents in adolescence and early adulthood. Personality, mood, and thought disorders are common, and physical findings include a wing-beating tremor, rigidity, akinesia, dystonia, and the pathognomonic Kayser–Fleischer ring around the cornea (Kaufman 1990b, Starosta-Rubinstein et al. 1987). Wilson's disease can mimic other conditions including Huntington's disease, Parkinson's disease, atypical psychosis, and neuroleptic-induced dystonia (Berg et al. 1994). Slit-lamp ocular examination, abnormal liver function tests, and markedly decreased serum ceruloplasmin levels are diagnostic. Chelating agents such as penicillamine, if administered early, can reverse central nervous system and nonneurological findings in about 50% of cases (Berg et al. 1994, Kaufman 1990b).

Other Medical Conditions   In addition to the conditions mentioned previously, other medical illnesses can be associated with dementia. These include endocrine disorders (hypothyroidism, hypoparathyroidism), chronic metabolic conditions (hypocalcemia, hypoglycemia), nutritional deficiencies (thiamine, niacin, vitamin B_{12}), structural lesions (brain tumors, subdural hematomas), and multiple sclerosis (Mortell 1946, Peterson 1968, Plum et al. 1962).

SUBSTANCE-INDUCED PERSISTING DEMENTIA

Diagnosis

In instances in which the features of dementia result from central nervous system effects of a medication, toxin, or drug of abuse (including alcohol), the diagnosis of dementia due to the persisting effects of a substance should be made (American Psychiatric Association 1994). (See DSM-IV-TR diagnostic criteria on page 299.) The most common dementias in this category are those associated with alcohol abuse, accounting for about 10% of all dementias (Korvath et al. 1989). The diagnosis of alcohol persisting dementia requires that the cognitive changes persist after the cessation of alcohol use and are not the result of changes in mentation associated with early abstinence, amnestic episodes (blackouts), or Wernicke–Korsakoff syndrome. In addition to various nutritional deficiencies and the toxic effects of alcohol itself, alcohol abusers are more prone to develop dementia as a result of head trauma and chronic hepatic encephalopathy.

DSM-IV-TR Diagnostic Criteria

Substance-Induced Persisting Dementia

A. The development of multiple cognitive deficits manifested by both

    (1) memory impairment (impaired ability to learn new information or to recall previously learned information)

    (2) one (or more) of the following cognitive disturbances:

        (a) aphasia (language disturbance)

        (b) apraxia (impaired ability to carry out motor activities despite intact motor function)

        (c) agnosia (failure to recognize or identify objects despite intact sensory function)

        (d) disturbance in executive functioning (i.e., planning, organizing, sequencing, abstracting)

B. The cognitive deficits in criteria A1 and A2 each cause significant impairment in social or occupational functioning and represent a significant decline from a previous level of functioning.

C. The deficits do not occur exclusively during the course of a delirium and persist beyond the usual duration of substance intoxication or withdrawal.

D. There is evidence from the history, physical examination, or laboratory findings that the deficits are etiologically related to the persisting effects of substance use (e.g., a drug of abuse, a medication).

Code: [specific substance]–induced persisting dementia:

(291.2 alcohol; 292.82 inhalant; 292.82 sedative, hypnotic, or anxiolytic; 292.82 other [or unknown] substance)

Severe alcohol dependence is the third leading cause of dementia. Alcohol-induced dementia is a relatively late occurrence, generally following 15 to 20 years of heavy drinking (Korvath et al. 1989). Dementia is more common in individuals with alcoholism who are malnourished. The CT scan shows cortical atrophy and ventricular dilatation after about 10 years with neuronal loss, pigmentary degeneration, and glial proliferation (Korvath et al. 1989). The frontal lobes are the most affected, followed by parietal and temporal areas (Korvath et al. 1989). The amount of deterioration is related to age, number of episodes of heavy drinking, and total amount of alcohol consumed over time.

Alcohol-induced dementia, secondary to the toxic effects of alcohol, develops insidiously and often presents initially with changes in personality. Increasing memory loss, worsening cognitive processing, and concrete thinking follow. The dementia may be affected by periodic superimposed delirious states including those caused by recurrent use of alcohol and cross-sensitive drugs, respiratory disease related to smoking, central nervous system hemorrhage secondary to trauma, chronic hypoxia related to recurrent seizure activity, folic acid deficiency, and higher rates of some neoplasms among those with alcoholism (Table 13-8).

Many other agents can produce dementia as a result of their persisting effects. Exposure to such heavy metals as mercury and bromide, chronic contact with various insecticides, and use of various classes of drugs of abuse may produce dementia. In particular, the abuse of organic solvents (inhalants) has been associated with neurological changes (Annan 1981, Byrne and Kirby 1990, Errebo-Knudson and Olsen 1986, Grabski 1961, Knox and Nelson 1966) (see Chapter 22). The inhalants are generally classified as anesthetics (halothane, chloroform, ether, nitrous oxide), solvents (gasoline, paint thinner, antifreeze, kerosene, carbon tetrachloride), aerosols (insecticides, deodorants, hair sprays), and nitrites (amyl nitrite). The solvent category is particularly toxic to the brain. In addition, acute anoxia may result from the common practice of inhaling a substance with a plastic bag around the head. Such neurological findings as peripheral neuropathy, paresis, paresthesias, areflexia, seizures, signs of cerebellar damage, and Babinski's sign are common. Although the cerebellum is often involved, any area of the cerebral cortex may be affected (Grabski 1961) (Table 13-9).

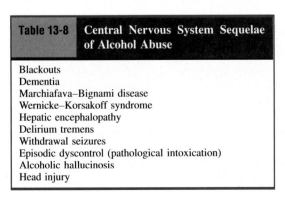

Table 13-8	Central Nervous System Sequelae of Alcohol Abuse

Blackouts
Dementia
Marchiafava–Bignami disease
Wernicke–Korsakoff syndrome
Hepatic encephalopathy
Delirium tremens
Withdrawal seizures
Episodic dyscontrol (pathological intoxication)
Alcoholic hallucinosis
Head injury

Table 13-9	Neurological Effects of Selected Inhalants	
Agent	**Use**	**Effect**
n-Hexane	Organic solvent	Peripheral neuropathy
Methyl butyl ketone	Paint thinner	Polyneuropathy
Toluene	Paint thinner	Cognitive dysfunction
		Cerebellar ataxia
		Optic neuropathy
		Sensorineural hearing loss
		Dementia
Trichloroethylene	Metal degreasing Extracting oils	Trigeminal neuropathy
Methylene chloride	Paint stripping Aerosol propellant	Carbon monoxide poisoning
		Hypoxic encephalopathy
1,1,1-trichloroethane	Solvent Industrial degreasing	Cerebral hypoxia

Treatment

The presence of dementia makes the treatment of alcoholism or other drug dependence more difficult. Most treatment programs depend on education about substance abuse, working the 12 steps, some degree of sociability, and such relatively abstract concepts as secondary gratification and a higher power. Such treatment programs are often reluctant to engage in the painstaking repetition that individuals with substance-induced persisting dementia often require. These individuals may become frustrated in peer support groups such as Alcoholics Anonymous. Despite these obstacles, individuals with alcoholism who complete a treatment program and remain sober do have some improvement in their mental state. There is an initial improvement that peaks at 3 to 4 weeks, followed by a slow but steady improvement detected at 6 to 8 months. In general, the presence of a cognitive deficit (dementia) dictates an alcohol treatment program that is behavior-based, concrete, structured, supportive, and repetitive.

DEMENTIA DUE TO MULTIPLE ETIOLOGIES

Dementia may have more than one cause in a particular individual. Certain types of dementia tend to occur together, including alcohol persisting dementia and dementia caused by head trauma, vascular dementia and dementia of the Alzheimer type, and alcohol persisting dementia and a nutritional dementia. For the purpose of DSM-IV-TR diagnosis, all conditions contributing to the dementia should be diagnosed by coding the various types of dementia on Axis I, for example alcohol persisting dementia and dementia due to head trauma (see DSM-IV-TR diagnostic criteria below).

DSM-IV-TR Diagnostic Criteria

Dementia due to Multiple Etiologies

A. The development of multiple cognitive deficits manifested by both

    (1) memory impairment (impaired ability to learn new information or to recall previously learned information)

    (2) one (or more) of the following cognitive disturbances:

    (3) aphasia (language disturbance)

(4) apraxia (impaired ability to carry out motor activities despite intact motor function)

(5) agnosia (failure to recognize or identify objects despite intact sensory function)

(6) disturbance in executive functioning (i.e., planning, organizing, sequencing, abstracting)

B. The cognitive deficits in criteria A1 and A2 each cause significant impairment in social or occupational functioning and represent a significant decline from a previous level of functioning.

C. There is evidence from the history, physical examination, or laboratory findings that the disturbance has more than one etiology (e.g., head trauma plus chronic alcohol use, dementia of the Alzheimer's type with the subsequent development of vascular dementia).

D. The deficits do not occur exclusively during the course of a delirium.

Coding note: Use multiple codes based on specific dementias and specific etiologies, e.g., 294.10 Dementia of the Alzheimer's Type, With Late Onset, Without Behavioral Disturbance; 290.40 Vascular Dementia, Uncomplicated.

Reprinted with permission from the Diagnostic and Statistical Manual of Mental Disorders, Fourth Edition, Text Revision. Copyright 2000 American Psychiatric Association.

AMNESTIC DISORDERS

Diagnosis

The amnestic disorders are characterized by a disturbance in memory related to the direct effects of a general medical condition (see DSM-IV-TR diagnostic criteria) or the persisting effects of a substance below. The impairment should interfere with social and occupational functioning and represent a significant decline from the previous level of functioning. The amnestic disorders are differentiated on the basis of the etiology of the memory loss. These disorders should not be diagnosed if the memory deficit is a feature of a dissociative disorder, is associated with dementia, or occurs in the presence of clouded sensorium, as individuals with amnestic disorder have impaired ability to learn new information (anterograde amnesia) or cannot remember material previously learned (retrograde amnesia). Memory for the event that produced the deficit (e.g., a head injury in a motor vehicle accident) may also be impaired (Torres et al. 2001, Garquonine 1991). Remote recall (tertiary memory) is generally good, so individuals may be able to accurately relate incidents that occurred during childhood but not remember what they had for breakfast. As illustrated by such conditions as thiamine amnestic syndrome, immediate memory is often preserved. In some instances, disorientation to time and place may occur, but disorientation to person is unusual.

DSM-IV-TR Diagnostic Criteria

294.0 Amnestic Disorder due to. . . [Indicate the General Medical Condition]

A. The development of memory impairment as manifested by impairment in the ability to learn new information or the inability to recall previously learned information.

B. The memory disturbance causes significant impairment in social or occupational functioning and represents a significant decline from a previous level of functioning.

C. The memory disturbance does not occur exclusively during the course of a delirium or a dementia.

D. There is evidence from the history, physical examination, or laboratory findings that the disturbance is the direct physiological consequence of a general medical condition (including physical trauma).

Specify if:

Transient: if memory impairment lasts for 1 month or less

Chronic: if memory impairment lasts for more than 1 month

Coding note: Include the name of the general medical condition on Axis I, e.g., 294.0 amnestic disorder due to head trauma; also code the general medical condition on Axis III.

DSM-IV-TR Diagnostic Criteria

Substance-Induced Persisting Amnestic Disorder

A. The development of memory impairment as manifested by impairment in the ability to learn new information or the inability to recall previously learned information.

B. The memory disturbance causes significant impairment in social or occupational functioning and represents a significant decline from a previous level of functioning.

C. The memory disturbance does not occur exclusively during the course of a delirium or a dementia and persists beyond the usual duration of substance intoxication or withdrawal.

D. There is evidence from the history, physical examination, or laboratory findings that the memory disturbance is etiologically related to the persisting effects of substance use (e.g., a drug of abuse, a medication).

Code: [specific substance]–induced persisting amnestic disorder:

(291.1 alcohol; 292.83 sedative, hypnotic, or anxiolytic; 292.83 other [or unknown] substance)

The onset of the amnesia is determined by the precipitant and may be acute as in head injury or insidious as in poor nutritional states (Nolan et al. 1991). DSM-IV-TR characterizes short-duration amnestic disorder as lasting less than 1 month and long-duration disorder lasting 1 month or longer. Often, individuals lack insight into the memory deficit and vehemently insist that their inaccurate responses on a Mental Status Examination are correct.

Epidemiology

The exact prevalence and incidence of the amnestic disorders are unknown (Kaplan et al. 1994). Memory disturbances related to specific conditions such as alcohol dependence and head trauma have been studied and these appear to be the two most common causes of amnestic disorders. Kaplan and coworkers (Torres et al. 2001) reported that in the hospital setting, the incidence of alcohol-induced amnestic disorders is decreasing, while that of amnestic disorders secondary to head trauma is on the rise (Korvath et al. 1989). This may be related to rigorous efforts by hospital personnel to decrease the incidence of iatrogenic amnestic disorder by giving thiamine before glucose is administered to an individual with chronic alcohol dependence and nutritional deficiencies.

Differential Diagnosis

Amnestic disorders must be differentiated from the less disruptive changes in memory that occur in normal aging, the memory impairment that is accompanied by other cognitive deficits in dementia, the amnesia that might occur with clouded consciousness in delirium, the stress-induced impairment in recall seen in dissociative disorders, and the inconsistent amnestic deficits seen in factitious disorder and malingering.

Etiology

Amnesia results from generally bilateral damage to the areas of the brain involved in memory. The areas and structures so involved include the dorsomedial and midline thalamic nuclei, temporal lobe-associated structures such as the hippocampus, amygdala, and mamillary bodies (Korvath et al. 1989, Kaplan et al. 1994). The left hemisphere may be more important than the right in the occurrence of memory disorders. Frontal lobe involvement may be responsible for such commonly seen symptoms as apathy and confabulation (Korvath et al. 1989, Kaplan et al. 1994).

The specific causes of amnestic disorders include (1) systemic medical conditions such as thiamine deficiency; (2) brain conditions, including seizures, cerebral neoplasms, head injury, hypoxia, carbon monoxide poisoning, surgical ablation of temporal lobes, electroconvulsive therapy, and multiple sclerosis; (3) altered blood flow in the vertebral vascular system, as in transient global amnesia; and (4) effects of a substance (drug or alcohol use and exposure to toxins) (Torres et al. 2001, Hodges and Warlow 1990, Melo et al. 1992, Fisher and Adams 1964).

Conditions that affect the temporal lobes such as herpes infection and Klüver–Bucy syndrome can produce amnesia. Among drugs that can cause amnestic disorders, triazolam (Halcion) has received the most attention, but all benzodiazepines can produce memory impairment, with the dose utilized being the determining factor (Kirk et al. 1990) (Table 13-10).

Selected Amnestic Disorders

Blackouts   Blackouts are periods of amnesia for events that occur during heavy drinking (Tarter and Schneider 1976). Typically, a person awakens the morning after consumption and does not remember what happened the night before. Unlike delirium tremens, which is related to chronicity of alcohol abuse, blackouts are more a measure of the amount of alcohol consumed at any one time. Thus, blackouts are common in binge pattern drinkers and may occur the first time a person ingests a large amount of alcohol. Blackouts are generally

Table 13-10	Causes of Amnestic Disorders

Types simplex encephalopathy
Substance-induced (alcohol) blackouts
Wernicke–Korsakoff syndrome
Multiple sclerosis
Klüver–Bucy syndrome
Electroconvulsive therapy
Seizures
Head trauma
Carbon monoxide poisoning
Metabolic
   Hypoxia
   Hypoglycemia
Medications
   Triazolam
   Barbiturates (thiopental sodium)
   Diltiazem (Cardizem)
   Zalcitabine (DDC)
Cerebrovascular disorders

transient phenomena, but some individuals may continue to have blackouts for weeks even after they have stopped using alcohol. These memory lapses are similar to blackouts experienced while using alcohol. With continued sobriety, the blackouts should end, but information forgotten during past blackouts is never remembered. Blackouts may also be produced by agents with cross-sensitivity to alcohol, such as benzodiazepines. Blackouts should not be confused with alcohol-induced dementia, which presents with cortical atrophy on CT scans, associated features of dementia, and a usually irreversible course.

Korsakoff's Syndrome   Korsakoff's syndrome is an amnestic disorder caused by thiamine deficiency. Although generally associated with alcohol abuse, it can occur in other malnourished states such as marasmus, gastric carcinoma, and HIV spectrum disease (Reulen et al. 1985, Victor 1987). This syndrome is usually associated with Wernicke's encephalopathy, which involves ophthalmoplegia, ataxia, and confusion. Korsakoff's syndrome is often associated with a neuropathy and occurs in about 85% of untreated individuals with Wernicke's disease (Kaplan et al. 1994). Complete recovery from Korsakoff's syndrome is rare.

Head Injury   Head injuries can produce a wide variety of neurological and mental disorders even in the absence of radiological evidence of structural damage. Delirium, dementia, mood disturbances, behavioral disinhibition, alterations of personality, and amnestic disorders may result (Torres et al. 2001). Amnesia in head injury is for events preceding the incident and the incident itself, leading some clinicians to consider these individuals as having factitious disorders or being malingerers. The eventual duration of the amnesia is related to the degree of memory recovery that occurs in the first few days after the injury (Torres et al. 2001, Garquonine 1991, Saneda and Corrigan 1992). Amnesia after head injury has become a popular plot device in novels and motion pictures, many of which are depictions that erroneously suggest that a second blow to the head is curative.

Treatment

As in delirium and dementia, the primary goal in the amnestic disorders is to discover and treat the underlying cause. Because some of these causes of amnestic disorder are associated with dangerous self-damaging behavior (e.g., suicide attempts by hanging, carbon monoxide poisoning, deliberate motor vehicle accidents, self-inflicted gunshot wounds to the head, and chronic alcohol abuse), some form of psychiatric management is often necessary. In the hospital, continuous reorientation by means of verbal redirection, clocks, and calendars can allay the individual's fears. Supportive individual psychotherapy and family counseling are beneficial.

Comparison of DSM-IV-TR/ICD-10 Diagnostic Criteria

The overall construct of delirium is similar in DSM-IV-TR and ICD-10 (i.e., a disturbance in consciousness and cognition with an acute onset and fluctuating course). The ICD-10 Diagnostic Criteria for Research include some additional items: impairment in short-term memory with intact long-term memory, disorientation, psychomotor disturbances and problems with sleep. ICD-10 does not include the DSM-IV-TR category delirium due to multiple etiologies.

Similarly, the overall construct of dementia is similar in DSM-IV-TR and ICD-10 (i.e., memory impairment plus a decline in other cognitive abilities). The ICD-10 Diagnostic Criteria for Research are more narrowly defined in several ways: the minimum duration of the disturbance is 6 months as compared with DSM-IV-TR, which does not specify any minimum duration. Required cognitive deficits, in addition to memory loss, are restricted to a deterioration in judgment and thinking (as opposed to DSM-IV-TR, which requires any one of aphasia, apraxia, agnosia, or disturbance in executive functioning); and there must also be a "decline in emotional control or motivation or a change in social behavior."

Like DSM-IV-TR, ICD-10 includes two subtypes of dementia of the Alzheimer's type: early-onset and late-onset. However, in contrast to DSM-IV-TR, the ICD-10 Diagnostic Criteria for Research for these subtypes also specify characteristic course features and types of deficits: early-onset cases must have a "relatively rapid onset and progression" and a characteristic type of cognitive impairment (e.g., aphasia), whereas late-onset cases have a very slow and gradual onset with a predominance of memory impairment over other intellectual deficits. In ICD-10, this disorder is referred to as *Dementia in Alzheimer's Disease*.

For vascular dementia, the ICD-10 Diagnostic Criteria for Research are more narrowly defined than the DSM-IV-TR criteria in that ICD-10 specifies that the deficits in higher cognitive functions are unevenly distributed and that there be both clinical *and* laboratory evidence of focal brain damage. Furthermore, ICD-10 subspecifies vascular dementia basis on acute onset, multi-infarct, subcortical, and mixed cortical and subcortical.

For amnestic disorder, the ICD-10 Diagnostic Criteria for Research are more narrowly defined than the criteria in DSM-IV-TR by virtue of requiring both an impaired ability to learn new information *and* a reduced ability to recall past experiences, as well as a requirement that immediate recall be preserved. In ICD-10, this disorder is referred to as *Organic Amnestic Syndrome*.

References

Adams F (1988) Emergency intravenous sedation of delirious medically ill patients. *J Clin Psychol* **48**(Suppl.), 22–27.

American Psychiatric Association (1994) *Diagnostic and Statistical Manual of Mental Disorders*, 4th ed. APA, Washington, DC, pp. 123–174.

Annau Z (1981) The neurobehavioral toxicity of trichloroethylene. *Neurobehav Toxicol Teratol* **3**, 417–424.

Bachman DL, Wolf PA, Linn R, et al. (1992) Prevalence of dementia of probable presenile dementia of the Alzheimer type in the Farmingham study. *Neurology* **42**, 115–119.

Benson DF, LeMay M, Patten DH, et al. (1970) Diagnosis of normal pressure hydrocephalus. *New Engl J Med* **283**, 609–615.

Berg R, Franzen M, and Wedding D (1994) *Neurological disorders. In Screening for Brain Impairment*, 2nd ed. Springer-Verlag, New York.

Bettinger TL, Mendelson SC, Dorson PG, et al. (2000) Olanzapine-induced glucose dysregulation. *Ann Pharmacother* **34**, 865–867.

Black PM (1980) Idiopathic normal-pressure hydrocephalus: Result of shunting in 62 individuals. *J Neurosurg* **52**, 371–377.

Blass J, Gleason P, Brush DPD, et al. (1988) Thiamine and Alzheimer's disease. *Arch Neurol* **45**, 833–835.

Bond MR (1986) Neurobehavioral sequelae of closed head injury. In *Neuropsychological Assessment of Neuropsychiatric Disorders*, Adams G and Adams KM (eds). Oxford University Press, New York.

Brenner RP (1985) The electroencephalogram in altered states of consciousness. *Neurol Clin* **3**, 615–631.

Burger PC and Vogel FS (1973) The development of the pathologic changes of Alzheimer's disease and senile dementia in patients with Down's syndrome. *Am J Pathol* **73**, 457–476.

Byrne A and Kirby B (1990) The neurotoxicity of inhaled toluene (letter). *Can J Psychiatr* **35**, 282.

Cameron DE (1941) Studies in senile nocturnal delirium. *Psychiatr Q* **15**, 47–53.

Carter JG (1986) Intravenous haloperidol in the treatment of acute psychosis. *Am J Psychiatr* **143**, 1316–1317.

Cartwright GE (1978) Diagnosis of treatable Wilson's disease. *New Engl J Med* **298**, 1347–1350.

Chung YS, Ravi SD, and Borge GF (1986) Psychosis in Wilson's disease. *Psychosomatics* **27**, 65–66.

Corder EH, Saunder AM, Strittmatten WJ, et al. (1993) Gene dose of apolipoprotein E type 4 allele and the risk of Alzheimer's disease in late onset families. *Science* **261**, 921–923.

Cotman CW, Monaghan DT, and Ganong AH (1988) Excitatoryamino acid neurotransmission: NMDA receptors and Hebb-type synaptic plasticity. *Annu Rev Neurosci* **11**, 61–80.

Cotman CW and Pike CJ (1994) Beta amyloid and its contributions to neurodegeneration in Alzheimer's disease. In *Alzheimer's Disease*, Terry RD, Katzman R, and Bick KL (eds). Raven Press, New York, pp. 305–317.

Cummings JL and Benson DF (1983) *Dementia: A Clinical Approach*. Butterworth, Boston.

Delacourte A and Defossez A (1986) Alzheimer's disease: Tau proteins, the promoting factors of microtubule assembly are major components of paired helical filaments. *J Neurosci* **76**, 173–186.

Eisendrath SJ, Goldman B, Douglas J, et al. (1987) Meperidine-induced delirium. *Am J Psychiatr* **144**, 1062–1065.

Engel GL and Roman J (1959) Delirium: A syndrome of cerebral insufficiency. *J Chronic Dis* **9**, 260–277.

Erkinjuntii T, Wikstrom J, Paolo J, et al. (1986) Evaluation of 2000 consecutive admissions. *Arch Intern Med* **146**, 1923–1926.

Errebo-Knudson EO and Olsen F (1986) Organic solvents and presenile dementia (the painter's syndrome): A critical review of the Danish literature. *Sci Total Environ* **48**, 45–67.

Evans DA (1990) Estimated prevalence of Alzheimer's disease in the United States. *Milbank Q* **68**, 276–289.

Fernandez F, Holmes VF, Adams F, et al. (1988) Treatment of severe, refractory agitation with a haloperidol drip. *J Clin Psychol* **49**, 239–241.

Fisher CM (1982) Hydrocephalus as a cause of gait disturbance in the elderly. *Neurology* **32**, 1358–1363.

Fisher CM and Adams RD (1964) Transient global amnesia. *Acta Neurol Scand* **39**, 605–608.

Francis J, Martin D, and Kapoor W (1990) A prospective study of delirium in hospitalized elderly. *JAMA* **263**, 1097–1101.

Frierson RL, Wey JJ, and Tabler JB (1991) Psychostimulants for depression in the medically ill. *Am Fam Phys* **43**, 163–170.

Garquonine PG (1991) Learning in post-traumatic amnesia following extremely severe closed head injury. *Brain Inj* **5**, 169–174.

Gelfand SB, Indelicato J, and Benjamin J (1992) Using intravenous Haldol to control delirium. *Hosp Comm Psychiatr* **43**, 215.

Glassman A and Bigger J (2001) Antipsychotic drugs: Prolonged Qtc interval, torsades de pointes, and sudden death. *Am J Psychiatr* **158**, 1774–1782.

Grabski DA (1961) Toluene sniffing producing cerebellar degeneration. *Am J Psychiatr* **118**, 461–462.

Graver DL (2000) Review of Quetiapine side effects. *J Clin Psychiatr* **61**, 31–33.

Grundke-Igbal I, Igbal K, Quinlan M, et al. (1986) Microtubule-associated protein tau: A component of paired helical filaments. *J Biol Chem* **261**, 6084–6089.

Hartmann S and Mobius HJ (2003) Tolerability of memantine in combination with cholinesterase inhibitors in dementia therapy. *Int Clin Psychopharmacol* **18**(2), 81–85.

Henderson AS (1990) Epidemiology of dementia disorders. *Adv Neurol* **51**, 15–25.

Hershey LA, Modic MT, Greenough PG, et al. (1987) Magnetic resonance imaging in vascular dementia. *Neurology* **37**, 29–36.

Heyman A, Fillenbaum G, Prosnitz B, et al. (1991) Estimated prevalence of dementia among elderly black and white community residents. *Arch Neurol* **48**, 594–599.

Ho D, Bredesen DE, Vinters HV, et al. (1987) AIDS dementia complex. *Ann Intern Med* **2**, 400–409.

Hodges JR and Warlow CP (1990) The etiology of transient global amnesia: A case-control study of 114 cases with prospective follow-up. *Brain* **113**, 639–657.

Jordan BD (1987) Neurologic aspects of boxing. *Arch Neurol* **44**, 453–459.

Kallmann MH (1989) Mental status assessment in the elderly. *Prim Care* **16**, 329–347.

Kaplan H, Sadock B, and Grebb J (1994) *Kaplan and Sadock's Synopsis of Psychiatry*, 7th ed. Williams & Wilkins, Baltimore.

Karp H (1984) Dementia in adults. In *Clinical Neurology*, Vol. 3, Baker AB and Baker LH (eds). Harper & Row, New York, pp. 1–32.

Katzman R (1994) Apolipoprotein E4 as the major genetic susceptibility factor for Alzheimer's disease. In *Alzheimer's Disease*, Terry RD, Katzman R, and Bick KL (eds). Raven Press, New York, pp. 455–457.

Katzman R and Kawas C (1994) Epidemiology of dementia and Alzheimer's disease. In *Alzheimer's Disease*, Terry RD, Katzman R, and Bick KL (eds). Raven Press, New York, pp. 105–123.

Kaufman D (1990a) Aphasia and related disorders. In *Clinical Neurology for Psychiatrists*. W. B. Saunders, Philadelphia, pp. 146–171.

Kaufman D (1990b) Dementia. In *Clinical Neurology for Psychiatrists*. W. B. Saunders, Philadelphia, pp. 107–146.

Kaufman DM (1990c) Involuntary movement disorders. In *Clinical Neurology for Psychiatrists*, 3rd ed. W. B. Saunders, Philadelphia, pp. 358–410.

Kidd M (1963) Paired helical filaments in electron microscopy of Alzheimer's disease. *Nature* **197**, 192–193.

Kirk T, Roache JD, and Griffiths RR (1990) Dose-response evaluation of the amnestic effects of triazolam and pentobarbital in normal subjects. *J Clin Psychopharmacol* **10**, 160–167.

Knox JW and Nelson JR (1966) Permanent encephalopathy from toluene inhalation. *New Engl J Med* **275**, 1494–1496.

Korvath T, Siever L, Mohs R, et al. (1989) Organic mental syndromes and disorders. In *Comprehensive Textbook of Psychiatry V*, Vol. I, Kaplan H and Sadock B (eds). Williams & Wilkins, Baltimore, pp. 599–642.

Kriwisky M, Perry G, Tarchitsky D, et al. (1990) Haloperidol-induced torsades de pointes. *Chest* **94**, 482–484.

Lerner D, Schuetz L, Holland S, et al. (2000) Low dose Risperidone for the irritable medically ill patient. *Psychosomatics* **41**, 69–71.

Lezak MD (1983) *Neuropsychological Assessment*, 2nd ed. Oxford University Press, New York.

Lipowski ZJ (1975) Sensory and information inputs overload: Behavioral effects. *Comp Psychiatr* **16**, 199–221.

Lipowski ZJ (1982) Differentiating delirium from dementia in the elderly. *Clin Gerontol* **1**, 3–10.

Lipowski ZJ (1983) Transient cognitive disorders (delirium, acute confusional states) in the elderly. *Am J Psychiatr* **140**, 1426–1436.

Lipowski ZJ (1987) Delirium (acute confusional states). *JAMA* **258**, 1789–1792.

Lipowski ZJ (1989) Delirium in the elderly patient. *New Engl J Med* **320**, 578–582.

Lipowski ZJ (1990) *Delirium: Acute Confusional States*. Oxford University Press, New York.

Markesbery WR and Ehmann WD (1994) Brain trace elements in Alzheimer's disease. In *Alzheimer's Disease*, Terry RD, Katzman R, and Bick KL (eds). Raven Press, New York.

Marzewski DJ, Towfighi J, Harrington MG, et al. (1988) Creutzfeldt-Jakob disease following pituitary-derived human growth hormone therapy: A new American case. *Neurology* **38**, 1131–1133.

Massie M, Holland J, and Glass E (1983) Delirium in terminally ill cancer patients. *Am J Psychiatr* **140**, 1048–1050.

Mawdsley C and Fergusen FR (1953) Neurologic disease in boxers. *Lancet* **2**, 795–801.

Melo TP, Ferro JM, and Ferro H (1992) Transient global amnesia: A case control study. *Brain* **115**, 261–270.

Menza MA, Murray GB, Holmes VF, et al. (1987) Decreased extrapyramidal symptoms with intravenous Haldol. *J Clin Psychol* **48**, 278–280.

Mohs RC, Davis BM, Johns CA, et al. (1985) Oral physostigmine in treatment of patients with Alzheimer's disease. *Am J Psychiatr* **142**, 28–33.

Mortell EJ (1946) Idiopathic hypoparathyroidism with mental deterioration: Effect of treatment of intellectual function. *J Clin Endocrinol* **6**, 266–271.

Moss AJ (1993) Measurement of the QT interval and the risk associated with Qtc interval prolongation: A review. *Am J Cardiol* **72**, 23B–25B.

Nolan K, Black R, Langberg J, et al. (1991) A trial of thiamine in Alzheimer's disease. *Arch Neurol* **48**, 81–83.

Nukina N and Ihara Y (1986) One of the antigenic determinants of paired helical filaments is related to tau protein. *J Biochem (Tokyo)* **99**, 1541–1544.

Obrecht R, Okhomina FOA, and Scott DF (1979) Value of EEG in acute confusional states. *J Neurol Neurosurg Psychiatr* **42**, 75–77.

Orgogozo JM, Rigaud AS, Stoffler A, et al. (2002) Efficacy and safety of memantine in patients with mild to moderate vascular dementia: a randomized, placebo-controlled trial (MMM 300). *Stroke* **33**, 1834–1839.

Osser DN, Najarjan DM, and Dufresne RL (1999) Olanzapine increases weight and serum triglyceride levels. *J Clin Psychiatr* **60**, 767–770.

Pajeau AK and Roman G (1992) HIV encephalopathy and dementia. *Psychiatr Clin N Am* **15**, 455–466.

Peterson P (1968) Psychiatric disorders in primary hyperparathyroidism. *J Clin Endocrinol* **28**, 1491–1496.

Plum F, Posner JB, and Hain RF (1962) Delayed neurological deterioration after anoxia. *Arch Intern Med* **110**, 18–25.

Pro JD and Wells CE (1977) The use of the electroencephalogram in the diagnosis of delirium. *Dis Nerv Syst* **38**, 804–808.

Prusiner SB (1987) Prions and neurodegenerative diseases. *New Engl J Medicine* **317**, 1571.

Rappaport EB and Graham DJ (1987) Pituitary growth hormone from human cadavers: Neurologic disease in 10 recipients. *Neurology* **37**, 1211–1213.

Reisberg B, Doody R, Storffler A, et al. (2003) Memantine in moderate-to-severe Alzheimer's disease. *N Engl J Med* **348**(14), 1333–1341.

Reulen JB, Girard DE, and Cooney TG (1985) Wernicke's encephalopathy. *New Engl J Med* **312**, 1035–1039.

Ross R, Smith G, and Guggenheim F (1990) Neurosyphilis and organic mood syndrome: A forgotten diagnosis. *Psychosomatics* **31**, 448–450.

Saito T (1987) Presenting symptoms and natural history of Wilson's disease. *Eur J Pediatr* **146**, 261–265.

Saneda DL and Corrigan JD (1992) Predicting clearing of post-traumatic amnesia following closed head injury. *Brain Inj* **6**, 167–170.

Scharnhorst S (1992) AIDS dementia complex in the elderly: Diagnosis and management. *Nurse Pract* **17**, 41–43.

Sipahimalani A and Massand P (1997) Use of risperidone in delirium: Case reports. *Ann Clin Psychiatr* **9**, 105–107.

Sipahimalani A and Massand P (1998) Olanzapine in the treatment of delirium. *Psychosomatics* **39**, 422–429.

Slaby AE and Erle SR (1993) Dementia and delirium. In *Psychiatric Care of the Medical Patient*, Stoudemire A (ed). Oxford University Press, New York, pp. 415–455.

Starosta-Rubinstein S, Young AB, Kluin K, et al. (1987) Clinical assessment of 31 patients with Wilson's disease. *Arch Neurol* **44**, 365–370.

Steinhart MJ (1983) The use of haloperidol in geriatric patients with organic mental disorder. *Curr Ther Res* **33**, 132–143.

Summergrad P, Rauch S, and Neal RR (1993) Human immunodeficiency virus and other infectious disorders affecting the central nervous system. In *Psychiatric Care of the Medical Patient*, Stoudemire A and Fogel BS (eds). Oxford University Press, New York.

Summers WK, Majorski LV, March GM, et al. (1986) Oral tetrahydroaminoacridine in long term treatment of senile dementia, Alzheimer type. *New Engl J Med* **315**, 1241–1245.

Tarter RE and Schneider DU (1976) Blackouts: Relationship with memory capacity and alcoholism history. *Arch Gen Psychiatr* **33**, 1492–1495.

Terry RD, Katzman R, and Bick KL (eds) (1994) *Alzheimer's Disease*. Raven Press, New York, pp. 65–74.

Tesar GE, Marray GB, and Cassen NH (1985) Use of intravenous Haldol in the treatment of agitated cardiac patients. *J. Clin Psychopharmacol* **5**, 344–347.

Teste D, Okamoto A, Napolitano J, et al. (2000) Low incidence of persistent tardive dyskinesia in elderly patients treated with Risperidone. *Am J Psychiatr* **157**, 1150–1155.

Thal L (1994) Clinical trials in Alzheimer's disease. In *Alzheimer's Disease*, Terry RD, Katzman R, and Bick KL (eds). Raven Press, New York, pp. 431–445.

Theobald D (1987) Delirium: Definition, evaluation, and management in the critically ill patient. *Indiana Med* **80**, 526–528.

Tobias CR, Turms DM, and Lippmann SB (1988) Psychiatric disorders in the elderly: Psychopharmacologic management. *Postgrad Med* **83**, 313–319.

Torres R, Mittal D, and Kennedy R (2001) Use of quetiapine in delirium. *Psychosomatics* **42**, 347–349.

Tran P, Hamilton S, Kuntz A, et al. (1997) Double-blind comparison of olanzapine versus risperidone in the treatment of schizophrenia and other psychotic disorders. *J Clin Psychopharmacol* **17**, 417–418.

Victor M (1987) *The Wernicke–Korsakoff Syndrome*, 2nd ed. FA Davis, Philadelphia.

Victor M and Adams RD (1974) Common disturbances of vision, ocular movement, and hearing. In *Harrison's Principles of Internal Medicine*, Vol. I, 7th ed. Wintrobe MM, Thron GW, and Adams RD (eds). McGraw-Hill, New York, pp. 100–110.

Wilson JD, Braunwald E, Isselbacher KJ, et al. (1991) Acquired immune deficiency syndrome (AIDS). In *Harrison's Principles of Internal Medicine, Companion Handbook*, 12th ed. Wilson JD, Braunwald E, Isselbacher KJ, et al. (eds). McGraw-Hill, New York, pp. 474–477.

Wisniewski HM, Narang HK, and Terry RD (1976) Neurofibrillary tangles of paired helical filaments. *J Neurol Sci* **27**, 173–181.

Wolf JK (1980) *Practical Clinical Neurology*. Medical Examination Publishing, Garden City, NY.

Wolfson LI and Katzman R (1983) The neurological consultation at age 80. In *Neurology of Aging*, Katzman R and Terry RD (eds). FA Davis, Philadelphia, pp. 221–244.

Ziber N, Rannon L, Alter M, et al. (1983) Measles, measles vaccination, and risk of subacute sclerosing panencephalitis (SSPE). *Neurology* **33**, 1558–1564.

14 Mental Disorders Due to a General Medical Condition

This chapter describes disorders characterized by mental symptoms, which occur due to direct physiological effect of a general medical condition. In evaluating individuals with mental symptoms of any sort, one of the first questions to ask is whether those symptoms are occurring as part of a primary mental disorder or are caused by a general medical condition, and Figure 14-1 presents a decision tree designed to help in making this decision. The first step is to review the history, physical examination, and laboratory tests to see if there is evidence for the presence of a general medical condition that could plausibly cause the mental symptoms in question. In making this determination, one looks not only for a temporal correlation (e.g., the onset of a psychosis shortly after starting or increasing the dose of a medication), but also keeps in mind well-documented associations between certain mental symptoms (e.g., depression) and certain general medical conditions (e.g., Cushing's syndrome). If it appears, at this point, that the mental symptoms could indeed be occurring secondary to a general medical condition, the next step involves determining whether these symptoms could be better accounted for by a primary mental disorder. For example, consider the case of a 45-year-old man with a history of recurrent major depressive disorder, currently euthymic, who begins a course of steroids for asthma and then, within a week, becomes depressed. The steroids are stopped but the depression continues. In this case, if the depression had cleared shortly after stopping the steroids, one might make the case that the depression occurred secondary to the steroid treatment; the persistence of the symptoms, however, argues strongly that this depression represents rather a recurrence of the major depressive disorder.

Once it appears that the mental symptoms in question could directly result from a general medical condition and could not be better accounted for by a primary mental disorder, then it remains to classify these symptoms into one of the specific types noted in Figure 14-1. There is also, at the end of the decision tree, a residual category for "unspecified" mental symptoms, and in this chapter, two such syndromes, not uncommonly found in consultation-liaison work, are included, namely pseudobulbar palsy and the Klüver–Bucy syndrome.

In caring for individuals with mental disorders due to a general medical condition, the question arises as to whether symptomatic treatment for these mental symptoms should be offered. Figure 14-2 provides a general treatment algorithm designed to help answer this question. First, one must determine whether the mental symptoms demand *emergent* treatment. Consider, for example, a postictal psychosis characterized by delusions of persecution, which prompt the individual to become assaultive: here, even though the condition itself will eventually resolve spontaneously, symptomatic treatment of the psychosis is required to protect the individual or others. In cases in which the mental symptoms do not present an emergency, one looks to whether the underlying general medical condition is treatable or not. For example, in the case of psychosis due to Huntington's disease, as the underlying condition is not treatable, one generally proceeds directly to symptomatic treatment. In cases in which the underlying condition is treatable, one must

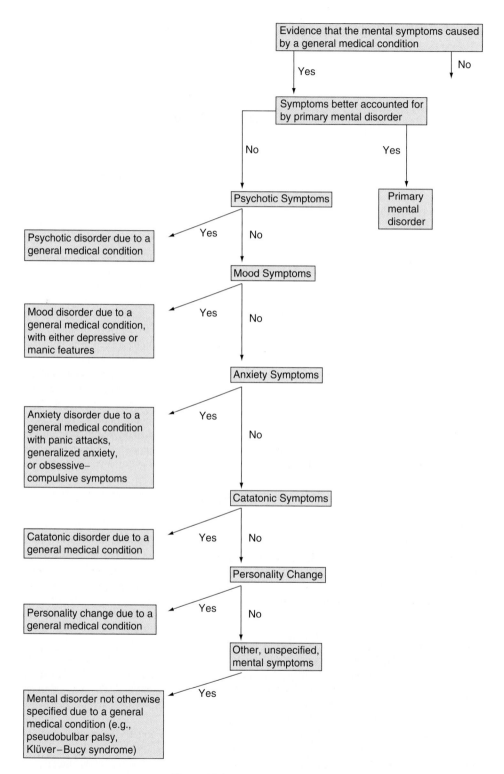

Figure 14-1 *Diagnostic decision tree.*

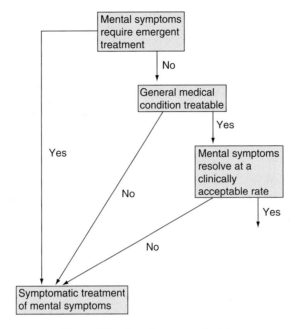

Figure 14-2 *General treatment algorithm.*

make a judgment as to whether, with treatment of the underlying general medical condition, the mental symptoms will resolve at a clinically acceptable rate. Consider, for example, an individual with anxiety due to hyperthyroidism who has just begun treatment with an antithyroid drug. In such a case, the decision as to whether to offer a benzodiazepine as symptomatic treatment for the anxiety depends not only on the severity and tolerability of the anxiety but also on the expected time required for the antithyroid drug to resolve the hyperthyroidism: here, clearly, considerable clinical judgment is required.

PSYCHOTIC DISORDER DUE TO A GENERAL MEDICAL CONDITION

Diagnosis

A psychotic disorder due to a general medical condition is characterized clinically by hallucinations or delusions occurring in a clear sensorium, without any associated decrement in intellectual abilities (see DSM-IV-TR diagnostic criteria below). Furthermore, one must be able to demonstrate, by history, physical examination or laboratory findings, that the psychosis is occurring on the basis of a general medical condition.

DSM-IV-TR Diagnostic Criteria

293.xx Psychotic Disorder Due to ... [Indicate the General Medical Condition]

A. Prominent hallucinations or delusions.
B. There is evidence from the history, physical examination, or laboratory findings that the disturbance is the direct physiological consequence of a general medical condition.

C. The disturbance is not better accounted for by another mental disorder.

D. The disturbance does not occur exclusively during the course of a delirium.

Code based on predominant symptom:

.81 With Delusions: if delusions are the predominant symptom

.82 With Hallucinations: if hallucinations are the predominant symptom

Coding note: Include the name of the general medical condition on Axis I. e.g., 293.81 Psychotic Disorder Due to Malignant Lung Neoplasm. With Delusions: also code the general medical condition on Axis III (see Appendix G for codes).

Coding note: If delusions are part of Vascular Dementia, indicate the delusions by coding the appropriate subtype, e.g., 290.42 Vascular Dementia, With Delusions

Reprinted with permission from the Diagnostic and Statistical Manual of Mental Disorders, Fourth Edition, Text Revision. Copyright 2000 American Psychiatric Association.

Psychotic disorder due to a general medical condition is a disorder that by definition occurs in a clear sensorium, without any associated decrement in intellectual abilities; both delirium and dementia are commonly accompanied by hallucinations and delusions, but these conditions are clearly distinguished from psychotic disorder due to a general medical condition by the presence of confusion or significant intellectual deficits. When these features are present, one should proceed to the differential for delirium and dementia described in the preceding chapter of this book.

In most cases, a thorough history and physical examination will disclose evidence of the underlying cause of the psychosis in question. In those cases, however, in which the individual's symptomatology is atypical for one of the primary causes of psychosis (e.g., schizophrenia), yet the history and physical examination fail to disclose clear evidence for another cause, a "laboratory screen," as listed in Table 14-1, may be appropriate. Clearly, one does not order all these tests at once, but begins with those most likely, given the overall clinical picture, to be the most informative.

Epidemiology

The overwhelming majority of individuals with a chronic psychosis have one of the primary disorders, that is, schizophrenia, schizoaffective disorder, or delusional disorder; secondary causes of psychosis are relatively uncommon.

Table 14-1	A "Laboratory Screen" for Secondary Psychosis

Serum or urine drug screen
Testosterone level (reduced in anabolic steroid abusers)
Red blood cell mean corpuscular volume (elevated in alcoholism and many cases of B_{12} deficiency)
Liver transaminases (elevated in alcoholism)
HIV testing
FTA
B_{12} levels (or, for increased sensitivity, plasma methylmalonic acid, and homocysteine levels)
ANA
Antithyroid antibodies (present in Hashimoto's encephalopathy)
Thyroid profile with TSH
Cortisol and ACTH levels and 24-hour urine for free cortisol
Copper and ceruloplasmin levels
MRI
EEG
Lumbar puncture

Course

The course of the psychosis is determined by the underlying cause. For example, whereas a psychosis occurring secondary to a medication, such as a dopaminergic drug, generally clears within days of discontinuation of the drug, the psychosis due to a chronic condition, such as Huntington's disease, is likewise chronic.

Etiology

Of all the causes of psychosis, the most commonly encountered are the three primary psychiatric disorders, namely, schizophrenia, schizoaffective disorder, and delusional disorder, each of these being covered in Chapter 27. Table 14-2 lists the various secondary causes of psychosis dividing them into those occurring *secondary to precipitants* (e.g., medications), those occurring *secondary to diseases with distinctive features* (e.g., the chorea of Huntington's disease), and finally a group occurring *secondary to miscellaneous causes* (e.g., cerebral tumors).

Psychosis occurring *secondary to precipitants* is perhaps the most common form of secondary psychosis. Among the various possible precipitants, substances are perhaps the most common, but these are covered in the various chapters on specific substances known to cause psychotic symptoms, like stimulants, hallucinogens, phencyclidine, cannabis, and alcohol. After drugs of abuse, various medications are the next most common precipitants, and of the medications listed in Table 14-1, the most problematic are the neuroleptics themselves. It appears that in a very small minority of individuals treated chronically with neuroleptics, a "supersensitivity psychosis" (or, as it has also been called, on analogy with tardive dyskinesia, "tardive psychosis") may occur. Making such a diagnosis in the case of individuals with schizophrenia may be difficult, as one may well say that any increase in psychotic symptoms, rather than evidence for a supersensitivity psychosis, may merely represent an exacerbation of the schizophrenia; in the case of individuals treated with antipsychotics for other conditions (e.g., Tourette's syndrome), however, the appearance of a psychosis is far more suggestive, as it could not be accounted for on the basis of the disease for which the neuroleptic was prescribed. Dopaminergic drugs capable of causing a psychosis include levodopa itself (Celesia and Barr 1970, Fenelon et al. 2000, Moskovitz et al. 1978), and such direct-acting dopamine agonists as bromocriptine and lergotrile (Serby et al. 1978). The other medications noted in Table 14-1 very rarely cause a psychosis.

Of the various encephalitidies that may have a psychosis as a sequela, the most classic is encephalitis lethargica (von Economo's disease), a disease which, though no longer occurring in epidemic form, may still be seen sporadically.

Of the psychoses *secondary to diseases with distinctive features*, the psychoses of epilepsy are by far the most important, and these may be ictal, postictal, or interictal. Ictal psychoses represent complex partial seizures and are immediately suggested by their exquisitely paroxysmal onset. Postictal psychoses are typically preceded by a "flurry" of grand mal or complex partial seizures and, importantly, are separated from the last of this "flurry" of seizures by a "lucid" interval lasting from hours to days. Interictal psychoses appear in one of two forms, namely, the psychosis of forced normalization and the chronic interictal psychosis. The psychosis of forced normalization appears when anticonvulsants have not only stopped seizures but also have essentially "normalized" the EEG; a disappearance of the psychosis with the resumption of seizure activity secures the diagnosis. The chronic interictal psychosis, often characterized by delusions of persecution and of reference and auditory hallucinations, appears subacutely, over weeks or months, in individuals with long-standing, uncontrolled grand mal or complex partial seizures.

Table 14-2	Causes of Psychosis due to a General Medical Condition

Secondary to Precipitants
Medications
　Neuroleptics (supersensitivity psychosis) (Chouinard and Jones 1980, Steiner et al. 1990)
　Dopaminergic drugs
　Disulfiram (Bicknell and Moore 1960)
　Sympathomimetics (Lambert 1987)
　Bupropion (Golden et al. 1985)
　Fluoxetine (Mandalos and Szarek 1990)
　Baclofen (upon discontinuation) (Swigar and Bowers 1986)

Other precipitants
　Postencephalitic psychosis
　Posthead trauma (Buckley et al. 1993, Hillbom 1951, Nasrallah et al. 1981)

Secondary to Diseases with Distinctive Features
Associated with epilepsy
　Ictal psychosis (Ellis and Lee 1978, Wells 1975)
　Postictal psychosis (Kanner et al. 1996, Lancman et al. 1994, Logsdail and Toone 1988, Savard et al. 1991, DeGreef et al. 1995)
　Psychosis of forced normalization (Pakainis et al. 1987)
　Chronic interictal psychosis (Kristensen and Sindrup 1979, Perez and Trimble 1980, Slater and Beard 1963a,b)
Encephalitic onset
　Herpes simplex encephalitis (Drachman and Adams 1962, Johnson et al. 1972, Williams and Lerner 1978, Wilson 1976)
　Encephalitis lethargica (Kirby and Davis 1921, Meninger 1926, Sands 1928)
　Infectious mononucleosis (Raymond and Williams 1948)

With other specific features:
　Huntington's disease (chorea) (Bolt 1970, Heathfield 1967)
　Sydenham's chorea (Hammes 1992)
　Chorea gravidarum (Beresford and Graham 1950, Wilson and Preece 1932)
　Manganism (parkinsonism) (Abd El Naby and Hassanein 1965)
　Creutzfeldt–Jakob disease (myoclonus) (Brown et al. 1984)
　Hashimoto's encephalopathy (myoclonus) (Cohen et al. 1996)
　Wilson's disease (various abnormal involuntary movements) (Beard 1959, Jackson and Zimmerman 1919)
　AIDS (thrush, *Pneumocystis* pneumonia) (Bulrich et al. 1988, Harris et al. 1991)
　Systemic lupus erythematosus (arthralgia, rash, pericarditis, pleurisy) (Devinsky et al. 1989, Johnson and Richardson 1968, Lim et al. 1988, Miguel et al. 1994)
　Hyperthyroidism (tremor, tachycardia) (Hodgson et al. 1992, Ingham and Nielsen 1931)
　Hypothyroidism (cold intolerance, voice change, constipation, hair loss, myxedema) (Asher 1949, Reed and Bland 1977, Karnosh and Stout 1935)
　Cushing's syndrome ("Cushingoid" habitus, e.g., "moon" facies) (Trethowan and Cobb 1952, Hertz et al. 1955)
　Adrenocortical insufficiency (abdominal complaints and dizziness) (Cleghorn 1951, McFarland 1963)
　Hepatic porphyria (abdominal pain) (Hirsch and Dunsworth 1955, Mandoki and Sumner 1994)
　Autosomal dominant cerebellar ataxia (Chandler and Bebin 1956)
　Dentatorubropallidoluysian atrophy (ataxia) (Adachi et al. 2001)
　Prader–Willi syndrome (massive obesity) (Clarke 1993)

Secondary to Miscellaneous Causes
　Cerebral tumors
　Cerebral infarction
　Multiple sclerosis (Fontaine et al. 1994, Geocaris 1957, Langworthy et al. 1941, Mathews 1979, Parker 1956)
　Neurosyphilis (Rothschild 1940, Schube 1934)
　Vitamin B_{12} deficiency (Smith 1929, Evans et al. 1983)
　Metachromatic leukodystrophy (Hyde et al. 1992, Muller et al. 1969)
　Subacute sclerosing panencephalitis (Cape et al. 1973, Salib 1988)
　Fahr's syndrome (Chabot et al. 2001, Francis and Freeman 1984)
　Thalamic degeneration (Deymeer et al. 1989)
　Velo–cardio–facial syndrome (Bassett and Chow 1999, Murphy et al. 1999)

Encephalitic psychoses are suggested by typical "encephalitic" features such as headache, lethargy, and fever. Prompt diagnosis is critical, especially in the case of herpes simplex encephalitis, given its treatability.

The other specific features listed in Table 14-1 are fairly straightforward. In the past, the differential between Huntington's disease and schizophrenia complicated by tardive dyskinesia was difficult; today, the availability of genetic testing has greatly simplified this diagnostic task.

Of the *miscellaneous causes* capable of causing psychosis, cerebral tumors are perhaps the most important, with psychosis being noted with tumors of the frontal lobe (Strauss and Keschner 1935), *corpus callosum* (Murthy et al. 1997), and temporal lobe (Gal 1958, Keschner et al. 1936, Malamud 1967, Strobos 1953, Tucker et al. 1986). Suggestive clinical evidence for such a cause includes prominent headache, seizures, or certain focal signs, such as aphasia. Cerebral infarction is likewise an important cause, and is suggested not only by accompanying focal signs but also by its acute onset; infarction of the frontal lobe (Hall and Young 1992), temporoparietal area (Peroutka et al. 1982, Thompson and Nielsen 1949), and thalamus (Feinberg and Rapcsak 1989) have all been implicated. Neurosyphilis should never be forgotten as a differential possibility in cases of psychosis of obscure origin, and an FTA (Fluorescent Treponemal Antibody) is appropriate in such cases. Vitamin B_{12} deficiency, likewise, should be borne in mind, especially as this may present with psychosis without any evidence of spinal cord or hematologic involvement. The remaining disorders listed in Table 14-1 are extremely rare causes of psychosis, and represent the "zebras" of this differential listing. Among these "zebras", however, one is of particular interest, namely, velo–cardio–facial syndrome. This genetic disorder, characterized by cleft palate, cardiovascular malformations and dysmorphic facies (micrognathia and prominent nose), and, often, mental retardation, also appears, in a substantial minority of cases, to cause a psychosis phenotypically very similar to that caused by schizophrenia.

Treatment

Treatment, if possible, is directed at the underlying cause. In those cases in which such treatment is unavailable or ineffective, or in which control of the psychosis is emergently required, neuroleptics are indicated. Although conventional neuroleptics, such as haloperidol, have long been used successfully, newer atypical agents, such as olanzapine or risperidone, may be better tolerated. In general, it is best to start with a low dose (e.g., 2.5 mg of haloperidol, 5 mg olanzapine or 1 mg of risperidone) with gradual incremental increases, if necessary.

MOOD DISORDER DUE TO A GENERAL MEDICAL CONDITION WITH DEPRESSIVE FEATURES

Diagnosis

A mood disorder secondary to a general medical condition with depressive features is characterized by a prominent and persistent depressed mood or loss of interest, and by the presence of evidence, from the history, physical examination or laboratory tests, of a general medical condition capable of causing such a disturbance (see DSM-IV-TR diagnostic criteria on page 318). Although other depressive symptoms (e.g., lack of energy, sleep disturbance, appetite change, or psychomotor change) may be present, they are not necessary for the diagnosis.

DSM-IV-TR Diagnostic Criteria

293.83 Mood Disorder Due to ... [Indicate the General Medical Condition]

A. A prominent and persistent disturbance in mood predominates in the clinical picture, and is characterized by either (or both) of the following:

    (1) depressed mood or markedly diminished interest or pleasure in all, or almost all, activities.
    (2) elevated, expansive, or irritable mood.

B. There is evidence from the history, physical examination, or laboratory findings that the disturbance is the direct physiological consequence of a general medical condition.
C. The disturbance is not better accounted for by another mental disorder (e.g., Adjustment Disorder With Depressed Mood in response to the stress of having a general medical condition).
D. The disturbance does not occur exclusively during the course of a delirium.
E. The symptoms cause clinically significant distress or impairment in social, occupational, or other important areas of functioning.

Specify type:

With Depressive Features: if the predominant mood is depressed but the full criteria are not met for a Major Depressive Episode

With Major Depressive-like Episode: if the full criteria are met (except Criterion D) for a Major Depressive Episode

With Manic Features: if the predominant mood is elevated, euphoric, or irritable

With Mixed Features: if the symptoms of both mania and depression are present but neither predominates

Coding note: Include the name of the general medical condition on Axis I. e.g., 293.83 Mood Disorder Due to Hypothyroidism. With Depressive Features: also code the general medical condition on Axis III (see Appendix G for codes).

Coding note: If depressive symptoms occur as part of a preexisting Vascular Dementia, indicate the depressive symptoms by coding the appropriate subtype, i.e., 290.43 Vascular Dementia, With Depressed Mood

Epidemiology

Depression is the most common of psychiatric symptoms and although the vast majority of cases of depression occur as part of one of the primary depressive disorders (most commonly major depressive disorder), depressions due to a general medical condition, in certain settings, should nevertheless, by virtue of their frequency in that setting, receive prime diagnostic consideration. Examples include treatment with ACTH or prednisone as in multiple sclerosis or collagen–vascular diseases and cases of cerebral infarction involving the left frontal area.

Course

Most medication-induced depressions begin to clear within days of discontinuation of the offending medication; depression as part of withdrawal from stimulants or anabolic steroids clears within days or weeks, and from anticholinergics, within days. Poststroke depression, as noted above, typically remits within a year. The course of depression secondary to head trauma or whiplash is generally prolonged, though quite variable. Most of the other conditions or disorders in the list are chronic, and depression occurring secondary to them likewise tends to be chronic; exceptions include depression in multiple sclerosis, which may have a relapsing and remitting course (Dalos et al. 1983), corresponding to the appearance and disappearance of appropriately situated plaques.

Etiology

The overwhelming majority of cases of depression occur as part of one of the primary mood disorders, including major depressive disorder, dysthymic disorder, bipolar disorder, cyclothymic disorder, or premenstrual dysphoric disorder, all of which are covered elsewhere in this text. The various secondary causes of depression are listed in Table 14-3.

In utilizing Table 14-3, the first question to ask is whether the depression could be *secondary to precipitants*. Of the various possible precipitants, substances of abuse (e.g., as seen in alcoholism or during stimulant withdrawal) are very common causes, and these are discussed in their respective chapters. Medications are particularly important; however, it must be borne in mind that most individuals are able to take the medications listed in Table 14-3 without untoward effect. Consequently, before ascribing a depression to any medication, it is critical to demonstrate that the depression did not begin before the medication was begun, and, ideally, to demonstrate that the depression resolved after the medication was discontinued. Anticholinergic withdrawal may occur within days after abrupt discontinuation of highly anticholinergic medications, such as benzotropine or certain tricyclic antidepressants, and is characterized by depressed mood, malaise, insomnia and gastrointestinal symptoms such as nausea, vomiting, abdominal cramping and diarrhea. Poststroke depression is not uncommon, and may be more likely when the anterior portion of the left frontal lobe is involved; although spontaneous remission within a year is the rule (Astrom et al. 1993, Robinson et al. 1987), depressive symptoms, in the meantime, may be quite severe (Lipsey et al. 1986). Both head trauma and whiplash injuries may be followed by depressive symptoms in close to half of all the cases.

Depression may occur *secondary to diseases with distinctive features*, and keeping such features in mind whenever evaluating depressed individuals will lead to a gratifying number of diagnostic "pick-ups." These features are noted in Table 14-3, and are for the most part self-explanatory; depression associated with epilepsy, however, may merit some further discussion. Ictal depressions are, in fact, simple partial seizures whose symptomatology is for the most part restricted to affective changes. The diagnosis of ictal depression is suggested by the paroxysmal onset of depression (literally over seconds); although such simple partial seizures may last only minutes, longer durations, up to months, have also been reported. Interictal depressions, rather than occurring secondary to paroxysmal electrical activity within the brain, occur as a result of long-lasting changes in neuronal activity, perhaps related to "kindling" within the limbic system, in individuals with chronically recurrent seizures, either grand mal or, more especially, complex partial (Indaco et al. 1992, Perini et al. 1996). Such interictal depressions are of gradual onset and are chronic.

Depression *occurring as part of certain neurodegenerative or dementing disorders* is immediately suggested by the presence of other symptoms of these disorders, such as dementia or distinctive physical findings, for example, Parkinsonism.

Table 14-3	Causes of Depression due to a General Medical Condition

Secondary to Precipitants
Medications
    Propranolol (Petrie et al. 1982, Pollack et al. 1985)
    Interferon (Neilley et al. 1996)
    ACTH (Falk et al. 1979)
    Prednisone (Wolkowitz et al. 1990)
    Reserpine (Jensen 1959, Quetsch et al. 1959)
    Alpha-methyldopa (DeMuth 1983)
    Nifedipine (Hullett et al. 1988)
    Ranitidine (Billings and Stein 1986)
    Bismuth subsalicylate (Supino-Viterbo et al. 1977)
    Pimozide (Bloch et al. 1997)
    Subdermal estrogen/progestin (Wagner 1998, Wagner and Berenson 1994)

Anticholinergic withdrawal ("cholinergic rebound") (Dilsaver et al. 1983)
Poststroke depression (Robinson et al. 1984, Vataja et al. 2001)
Head trauma (Federoff et al. 1992)
Whiplash (Ettlin et al. 1992)

Secondary to Diseases with Distinctive Features
Hypothyroidism (hair loss, dry skin, voice change) (Tonks 1964, Whybrow et al. 1969, Nickel and
    Frame 1958)
Hyperthyroidism (weight loss with *increased* appetite, tachycardia, and, in the elderly, atrial
    fibrillation or congestive heart failure) (Trzepacz et al. 1988)
Cushing's syndrome (moon facies, hirsutism, acne, "buffalo hump", and abdominal striae)
    (Haskett 1985)
Chronic adrenocortical insufficiency (nausea, vomiting, abdominal pain, and postural dizziness)
    (Varadaraj and Cooper 1986)
Obstructive sleep apnea (severe snoring) (Millman et al. 1989)
Multiple sclerosis (various focal findings) (Rabins et al. 1986)
Down syndrome (Collacott et al. 1992)

Epilepsy
    Ictal depression (Weill 1955, 1956, 1959, Williams 1956)
    Chronic interictal depression (Mendez et al. 1986)

Occurring as Part of Certain Neurodegenerative or Dementing Disorders
Alzheimer's disease (Burns et al. 1990, Starkstein et al. 1997)
Multi-infarct dementia (Cummings et al. 1987)
Diffuse Lewy body disease (Klatka et al. 1996)
Parkinson's disease (Mayeux et al. 1986, Starkstein et al. 1990)
Fahr's syndrome (Slyter 1979, Trautner et al. 1988)
Tertiary neurosyphilis (Storm-Mathisen 1969)
Limbic encephalitis (Corsellis 1968)

Miscellaneous or Rare Causes
Cerebral tumors (Ironside and Guttmacher 1929)
Hydrocephalus (Jones 1993, Pujol et al. 1989)
Pancreatic cancer (Pujol et al. 1989, Fras and Pearson 1967)
New-variant Creutzfeldt–Jakob disease (Zeidler et al. 1997a,b)
Hyperparathyroidism (Karpati and Frame 1964)
Systemic lupus erythematosus (Ainiala et al. 2001, Dennis et al. 1992)
Pernicious anemia (Fraser 1960)
Pellagra (Hardwick 1943)
Lead encephalopathy (Schottenfeld and Cullen 1984)
Hyperaldosteronism (Malinow and Lion 1979)

The *miscellaneous or rare causes* represent, for the most part, the "zebras" in the differential for depression, and should be considered when, despite a thorough investigation, the diagnosis of a particular case of depression remains unclear.

Treatment

Treatment efforts should be directed at relieving, if possible, the underlying cause. When this is not possible, antidepressants should be considered. Controlled studies have demonstrated the effectiveness of both nortriptyline (Robinson et al. 2000) and citalopram (Anderson et al. 1994) for poststroke depression, and nortriptyline for depression seen in Parkinson's disease (Anderson et al. 1980). For other secondary depressions, citalopram is probably a good choice, given its benign side-effect profile and notable lack of drug–drug interactions; nortriptyline should be used with caution in individuals with cardiac conduction defects (as it may prolong conduction time) and in those at risk for seizures as in head trauma (Wroblewski et al. 1990) as this agent may also lower the seizure threshold.

MOOD DISORDER DUE TO A GENERAL MEDICAL CONDITION WITH MANIC FEATURES

Diagnosis

Mood disorder due to a general medical condition with manic features is characterized by a prominent and persistently elevated, expansive, or irritable mood which, on the basis of the history, physical, or laboratory examinations can be attributed to an underlying general medical condition (see DSM-IV-TR diagnostic criteria on page 318). Other manic symptoms, such as increased energy, decreased need for sleep, hyperactivity, distractibility, pressured speech, and flight of ideas, may or may not be present.

As a rule, it is very rare for mania to constitute the initial presentation of any of the disease or disorders listed in Table 14-4; thus, other evidence of their presence will become evident during the routine history and physical examination. Exceptions to the rule include neurosyphilis (Binder and Dickman 1980), vitamin B_{12} deficiency (Goggans 1984), and Creutzfeldt–Jakob disease (Lendvai et al. 1999); however, in all these cases continued observation will eventually disclose the appearance of other evidence suggestive of the correct diagnosis.

Epidemiology

Relative to cases of primary mania (e.g., bipolar disorder), secondary mania is relatively rare. In certain settings, however, secondary mania may be so common as to merit a "top" position on the differential diagnosis; a prime example would be when prednisone is used in high doses, as in the treatment of multiple sclerosis or rheumatoid arthritis.

Course

Most cases of medication-induced mania begin to clear in a matter of days; for other causes, the course of the mania generally reflects the course of the underlying disease.

Etiology

The vast majority of cases of sustained, elevated, or irritable mood occur as part of four primary disorders, namely, bipolar I disorder, bipolar II disorder, cyclothymic disorder, and schizoaffective disorder (bipolar type). Cases of elevated or irritable mood secondary to other causes (e.g., secondary to treatment with corticosteroids) are much less common. Table 14-4 lists secondary causes of elevated or irritable mood, with these causes divided into categories designed to facilitate the task of differential diagnosis.

In utilizing Table 14-4, the first step is to determine whether the mania could be *secondary to precipitants*. Substance-induced mood disorder related to drugs of abuse is covered in the relevant substance-related disorders chapters in this textbook. Of the precipitating factors listed in Table 14-4, medications are the most common offenders. However, before

Table 14-4	Causes of Mania due to a General Medical Condition

Secondary to Precipitants
  Medications
    Corticosteroids or adrenocorticoptrophic hormone (Minden et al. 1988)
    Levodopa (Celesia and Barr 1970)
    Zidovudine (Wright et al. 1989)
    Oral contraceptives (Sale and Kalucy 1981)
    Isoniazid (Chaturvedi and Upadhyaya 1988)
    Buspirone (Price and Bielfeld 1989)
    Procyclidine (Coid and Strang 1982)
    Procarbazine (Mann and Hutchinson 1967)
    Propafenone (Jack 1985)
    Baclofen, upon discontinuation after long-term use (Kirubakaren et al. 1984)
    Reserpine upon discontinuation after long-term use (Kent and Wilber 1982)
    Methyldopa upon discontinuation after long-term use (Labbatte and Holzgang 1989)

  Closed head injury (Jorge et al. 1993a)
  Hemodialysis (Cooper 1967)
  Encephalitis (Hohman 1921, Moskovich et al. 1995)
  Aspartame (Walton 1986)
  Metrizamide (Kwentus et al. 1984)

Secondary to Diseases with Distinctive Features
  Hyperthyroidism (proptosis, tremor, tachycardia) (Trzepacz et al. 1988)
  Cushing's syndrome (moon facies, hirsutism, acne, "buffalo hump", abdominal striae) (Haskett 1985)
  Multiple sclerosis (various focal findings) (Rabins et al. 1986)
  Cerebral infarction (sudden onset with associated localizing signs)
  Sydenham's chorea (Reaser 1940)
  Chorea gravidarum (Wilson and Preece 1932)
  Hepatic encephalopathy (asterixis, delirium) (Murphy et al. 1948)
  Uremia (asterixis, delirium) (El-Mallakh et al. 1987)

  Epilepsy
    Ictal mania (Mulder and Daly 1952)
    Postictal mania (Kanemoto et al. 1996)

Occurring as part of Certain Neurodegenerative or Dementing Diseases
  Alzheimer's disease (Burns et al. 1990)
  Neurosyphilis (Storm-Mathisen 1969)
  Huntington's disease (Bolt 1970)
  Creutzfeldt–Jakob disease (Lendvai et al. 1999)

Miscellaneous or Rare Causes
  Cerebral tumors
  Systemic lupus erythematosus (Johnson and Richardson 1968)
  Vitamin B_{12} deficiency (Coggaus 1984)
  Metachromatic leukodystrophy (Besson 1980)
  Adrenoleukodystrophy (Weller et al. 1992)
  Tuberous sclerosis (Khanna and Borde 1989)

attributing the mania to one of these medications, it is critical to demonstrate that the mania occurred only after initiation of that medication; ideally, one would also want to show that the mania spontaneously resolved subsequent to the medication's discontinuation. Of the medications listed, corticosteroids, such as prednisone, are likely to cause mania, with the likelihood increasing in direct proportion to dose: in one study (Wolkowitz et al. 1990), 80 mg of prednisone produced mania within five days in 75% of subjects. Levodopa is the next most likely cause, and in the case of levodopa the induced mania may be so pleasurable that some individuals have ended up abusing the drug (Giovannoni et al. 2000). Anabolic steroid abuse may cause an irritable mania, and such a syndrome occurring in "bulked up" individuals should prompt a search for other clinical evidence of abuse, such as gynecomastia and testicular atrophy (Pope and Katz 1994). Closed head injury may be followed by mania either directly upon emergence from postcoma delirium (Bakchine 1989, Bracken 1987), or after an interval of months (Clark and Davison 1987, Nizamie et al. 1988). Hemodialysis may cause mania, and in one case (Jack et al. 1983) mania occurred as the presenting sign of an eventual dialysis dementia. Encephalitis may cause mania, as, for example, in postinfectious encephalomyelitis (Moskovich et al. 1995, Paskavitz et al. 1995), with the correct diagnosis eventually being suggested by more typical signs such as delirium or seizures. Encephalitis lethargica (Von Economo's disease; European Sleeping Sickness) may also be at fault, with the diagnosis suggested by classic signs such as sleep reversal or oculomotor paralyses (Hohman 1921). Aspartame taken in very high dose caused mania and a seizure in one individual (Walton 1986), and metrizamide myelography prompted mania in another (Kwentus et al. 1984).

Mania occurring *secondary to disease with distinctive features* is immediately suggested by these features, as listed in Table 14-4. Some elaboration may be in order regarding mania secondary to cerebral infarction. This cause, of course, is suggested by the sudden onset of the clinical disturbance, with the mania being accompanied by various other more or less localizing signs; what is most remarkable here is the variety of structures that, if infarcted, may be followed by mania. Thus, mania has been noted with infarction of the midbrain (Blackwell 1991, Kulisevsky et al. 1995), thalamus (either on the right side [Cummings and Mendez 1984, Bogousslavsky et al. 1988, Kulisevsky et al. 1993], or bilaterally [McGilchrist et al. 1993, Gentilini et al. 1987]), anterior limb of the internal capsule and adjacent caudate on the right (Starkstein et al. 1990), and subcortical white matter or cortical infarction on the right in the frontoparietal (Jampala and Abrams 1983, Starkstein et al. 1988), or temporal (Starkstein et al. 1988) areas. Mania associated with epilepsy may also deserve additional comment. Ictal mania is characterized by its paroxysmal onset, over seconds, and the diagnosis of postictal mania is suggested when mania occurs shortly after a "flurry" of grand mal or complex partial seizures.

Mania *occurring as part of certain neurodegenerative or dementing diseases* is suggested, in general, by a concurrent dementia, and in most cases the mania plays only a minor role in the overall clinical pictures. Neurosyphilis, however, is an exception to this rule, for in individuals with general paresis of the insane (dementia paralytica) mania may dominate the picture.

Of the *miscellaneous or rare causes* of mania, cerebral tumors are the most important to keep in mind, with mania being noted with tumors of the midbrain (Greenberg and Brown 1985), tumors compressing the hypothalamus (e.g., a craniopharyngioma [Malamud 1967]), or a pituitary adenoma (Alpers 1940), and tumors of the right thalamus (Stern and Dancey 1942), right cingulate gyrus (Angelini et al. 1980), or one or both frontal lobes (Gross and Herridge 1988).

Treatment

Treatment, if possible, is directed at the underlying cause. In cases where such etiologic treatment is not possible, or not rapidly effective enough, pharmacologic measures are in order. Mood stabilizers, such as lithium or divalproex used in a fashion similar to that for the treatment of mania occurring in bipolar disorder, are commonly used: both lithium (Siegal 1978) and divalproex (Abbas and Styra 1994) are effective in the prophylaxis of mania occurring secondary to prednisone; case reports also support the use of lithium for mania secondary to zidovudine (O'Dowd and McKegney 1988) and divalproex for mania secondary to closed head injury. As between lithium and divalproex, in cases where there is a risk for seizures (e.g., head injury, encephalitis, stroke, or tumors), divalproex clearly is preferable.

In cases where emergent treatment is required, before lithium or divalproex could have a chance to become effective, oral or intramuscular lorazepam or haloperidol (in doses of 2 mg and 5 mg, respectively) may be utilized, again much as in the treatment of mania in bipolar disorder.

ANXIETY DISORDER DUE TO A GENERAL MEDICAL CONDITION WITH PANIC ATTACKS OR WITH GENERALIZED ANXIETY

Diagnosis

Pathologic anxiety secondary to a general medical condition may occur in the form of well-circumscribed and transient panic attacks or in a generalized, more chronic form (see DSM-IV-TR diagnostic criteria below). As the differential diagnoses for these two forms of anxiety are quite different, it is critical to clearly distinguish among them.

DSM-IV-TR Diagnostic Criteria

293.89 Anxiety Disorder Due to … [Indicate the General Medical Condition]

A. Prominent anxiety, Panic Attacks, or obsessions or compulsions predominate in the clinical picture.
B. There is evidence from the history, physical examination, or laboratory findings that the disturbance is the direct physiological consequence of a general medical condition.
C. The disturbance is not better accounted for by another mental disorder (e.g., Adjustment Disorder With Anxiety in which the stressor is a serious general medical condition).
D. The disturbance does not occur exclusively during the course of a delirium.
E. The disturbance causes clinically significant distress or impairment in social, occupational, or other important areas of functioning.

Specify if:

With Generalized Anxiety: if excessive anxiety or worry about a number of events or activities predominates in the clinical presentation

With Panic Attacks: if Panic Attacks (see p. 395) predominate in the clinical presentation

With Obsessive–Compulsive Symptoms: if obsessions or compulsions predominate in the clinical presentation

Coding note: Include the name of the general medical condition on Axis I, e.g., 293.89 Anxiety Disorder Due to Pheochromocytoma. With Generalized Anxiety; also code the general medical condition on Axis III (see Appendix G for codes).

Panic attacks have an acute or paroxysmal onset, and are characterized by typically intense anxiety or fear which is accompanied by various "autonomic" signs and symptoms, such as tremor, diaphoresis, and palpitations. Symptoms rapidly crescendo over seconds or minutes and in most cases the attack will clear anywhere from within minutes up to a half-hour. Although attacks tend to be similar to one another in the same individual, there is substantial inter-individual variability in the symptoms seen.

Generalized anxiety tends to be of subacute or gradual onset, and may last for long periods of time, anywhere from days to months, depending on the underlying cause. Here, some individuals, rather than complaining of feeling anxious *per se*, may complain of being worried, tense, or ill at ease. Autonomic symptoms tend not to be as severe or prominent as those seen in panic attacks: shakiness, palpitations (or tachycardia), and diaphoresis are perhaps most common.

Epidemiology
Although epidemiologic studies are lacking, the clinical impression is that anxiety secondary to a general medical condition is common.

Course
This is determined by the underlying cause.

Etiology
Panic attacks are most commonly seen in one of the primary anxiety disorders, namely, panic disorder, agoraphobia, specific phobia, social phobia, obsessive–compulsive disorder, or posttraumatic stress disorder, all of which are covered elsewhere in this book. The causes of secondary panic attacks are listed in Table 14-5. Substance-induced anxiety disorder related to drugs of abuse (e.g., cannabis, LSD) is covered in the relevant substance-related disorders chapters in this textbook. Partial seizures and paraoxysmal atrial tachycardia are both characterized by their exquisitely paroxysmal onset, over a second or two; in addition, paroxysmal atrial tachycardia is distinguished by the prominence of the tachycardia and by an ability, in many cases, to terminate the attack with a Valsalva maneuver. Hypoglycemia is often suspected as a cause of anxiety, but before the diagnosis is accepted, one must demonstrate the presence of "Whipple's triad": hypoglycemia (blood glucose ≤ 45 mg/dL), typical symptoms, and the relief of those symptoms with glucose. Angina or acute myocardial infarction can present with a panic attack, with the diagnosis being suggested by the clinical setting, for example, multiple cardiac risk factors. A pulmonary embolus, at the moment of its lodgment in a pulmonary artery, may also present with a panic attack, and again here the correct diagnosis is suggested by the clinical setting, for example, situations, such as prolonged immobilization, which favor deep venous thrombosis. Acute asthmatic attacks are suggested by wheezing, and pheochromocytoma by associated hypertension. Individuals with Parkinson's disease treated with levodopa may experience panic attacks during "off" periods.

Generalized anxiety is most commonly seen in the primary mental disorder, generalized anxiety disorder, and is discussed in Chapter 35. The secondary causes of generalized anxiety are listed in Table 14-6. Sympathomimetics and theophylline, as used in asthma and chronic obstructive pulmonary disease (COPD) are frequent causes, as are many of the antidepressants. Hyperthyroidism is suggested by heat intolerance and proptosis, and Cushing's syndrome by the typical Cushingoid habitus (i.e., moon facies, hirsutism, acne, "buffalo hump," and abdominal striae). Hypocalcemia may be suggested by a history of seizures or tetany. Both COPD and congestive heart failure are suggested by marked dyspnea. Stroke and severe head trauma may be followed by chronic anxiety, but this is seen in only a minority of these individuals.

Table 14-5	Causes of Panic Attacks due to a General Medical Condition

Partial seizures (Biraben et al. 2001)
Paroxysmal atrial tachycardia
Hypoglycemia
Angina or acute myocardial infarction
Pulmonary embolus
Acute asthmatic attack
Pheochromocytoma (Starkman et al. 1985)
Parkinson's disease (Vazquez et al. 1993)

Table 14-6	Causes of Generalized Anxiety due to a General Medical Condition

Sympathomimetics
Theophylline
Various antidepressants (tricyclics, SSRIs, etc.)
Hyperthyroidism (MacCrimmon et al. 1979)
Cushing's syndrome (Kelly 1996)
Hypocalcemia (Lawlor 1988)
Chronic obstructive pulmonary disease
Congestive heart failure
Poststroke (Castillo et al. 1993, 1995, Starkstein et al. 1990)
Posthead trauma (Fann et al. 1995, Jorge et al. 1993b)

Treatment

Treatment is directed at the underlying cause, and this is sufficient for all cases of secondary panic attacks and most cases of secondary generalized anxiety; exceptions include poststroke and post–head trauma anxiety, and in these cases benzodiazepines have been used with success.

ANXIETY DISORDER DUE TO A GENERAL MEDICAL CONDITION WITH OBSESSIVE–COMPULSIVE SYMPTOMS

Diagnosis

Obsessions consist of unwanted, and generally anxiety-provoking, thoughts, images or ideas, which repeatedly come to mind despite attempts to stop them. Allied to this are compulsions that consist of anxious urges to do or undo things, urges which, if resisted, are followed by rapidly increasing anxiety that can often only be relieved by giving into the compulsion to act. The acts themselves that the individuals feel compelled to perform are often linked to an apprehension on the individuals' part that they have done something that they ought not to have done or have left undone something that they ought to have done. Thus, one may feel compelled to repeatedly subject the hands to washing to be sure that all germs have been removed, or to repeatedly go back and check on the gas to be sure that it had been turned off.

Epidemiology

Secondary obsessions and compulsions are relatively rare.

Table 14-7	Causes of Obsessions and Compulsions due to a General Medical Condition

Postencephalitic (Mulder et al. 1951, Jelliffe 1929)
Postanoxic (Escalona et al. 1997, LaPlane et al. 1984, 1989)
Postclosed head injury (Hillbom 1960, McKeon et al. 1984)
Clozapine (Baker et al. 1992)
Sydenham's chorea (Swedo et al. 1989, Swedo et al. 1993)
Huntington's disease (Anderson et al. 2001)
Simple partial seizures (Kroll and Drummond 1993, Mendez et al. 1996)
Infarction of the basal ganglia or right parietal lobe (Giroud et al. 1997, Simpson and Baldwin 1995)
Fahr's syndrome (Lopez-Villegas et al. 1996)

Course

Although the course of obsessions and compulsions due to fixed lesions, such as those seen with head trauma or cerebral infarction tends to be chronic, some spontaneous recovery may be anticipated over the following months to a year.

Etiology

In the vast majority of cases, obsessions and compulsions occur as part of certain primary mental disorders, including obsessive–compulsive disorder, depression, schizophrenia, and Tourette's syndrome. Those rare instances where obsessions and compulsions are secondary to a general medical condition or medication are listed in Table 14-7.

In most cases, these causes of secondary obsessions or compulsions are readily discerned, as for example, a history of encephalitis, anoxia, closed head injury, or treatment with clozapine. Sydenham's chorea is immediately suggested by the appearance of chorea; however, it must be borne in mind that obsessions and compulsions may constitute the presentation of Sydenham's chorea, with the appearance of chorea being delayed for days (Swedo et al. 1989). Ictal obsessions or compulsions, constituting the sole clinical manifestation of a simple partial seizure, may, in themselves, be indistinguishable from the obsessions and compulsions seen in obsessive–compulsive disorder, but are suggested by a history of other seizure types, for example, complex partial or grand mal seizures. Infarction of the basal ganglia or parietal lobe is suggested by the subacute onset of obsessions or compulsions accompanied by "neighborhood" symptoms such as abnormal movements or unilateral sensory changes. Fahr's syndrome, unlike the foregoing, may be an elusive diagnosis, only suggested perhaps when CT imaging incidentally reveals calcification of the basal ganglia.

Treatment

When treatment of the underlying cause is not possible, a trial of an SSRI, as used for obsessive–compulsive disorder, might be appropriate.

CATATONIC DISORDER DUE TO A GENERAL MEDICAL CONDITION

Diagnosis

Catatonia can develop as a result of the direct effects of a general medical condition on the central nervous system (see DSM-IV-TR diagnostic criteria on page 328). Catatonia exists in two subtypes, namely, stuporous catatonia (also known as the akinetic or "retarded" subtype) and excited catatonia, and each will be described in turn.

DSM-IV-TR Diagnostic Criteria

293.89 Catatonic Disorder Due to. . . [Indicate the General Medical Condition]

A. The presence of catatonia as manifested by motoric immobility, excessive motor activity (that is apparently purposeless and not influenced by external stimuli), extreme negativism or mutism, peculiarities of voluntary movement, or echolalia or echopraxia.

B. There is evidence from the history, physical examination, or laboratory findings that the disturbance is the direct physiological consequence of a general medical condition.

C. The disturbance is not better accounted for by another mental disorder (e.g., a Manic Episode).

D. The disturbance does not occur exclusively during the course of a delirium.

Coding note: Include the name of the general medical condition on Axis I. e.g., 293.89 Catatonic Disorder Due to Hepatic Encephalopathy: also code the general medical condition on Axis III (see Appendix G for codes).

Stuporous catatonia is characterized by varying combinations of mutism, immobility, and waxy flexibility; associated features include posturing, negativism, automatic obedience, and "echo" phenomena. Mutism ranges from complete to partial: some individuals may mumble or perhaps utter brief, often incomprehensible, phrases. Immobility, likewise, ranges in severity: some individuals may lie in bed for long periods, neither moving, blinking or even swallowing; others may make brief movements, perhaps to pull at a piece of clothing or to assume a different posture. Waxy flexibility, also known by its Latin name, *cerea flexibilitas*, is characterized by a more or less severe "lead pipe" rigidity combined with a remarkable tendency for the limbs to stay in whatever position they are placed, regardless of whether the individual is asked to maintain that position or not. Posturing is said to occur when individuals spontaneously assume more or less bizarre postures, which are then maintained: one individual crouched low with his arm wrapped over his head, another stood with one arm raised high and the other stuffed inside his belt. Negativism entails a mulish, intractable, and automatic resistance to whatever is expected, and may be either "passive" or "active." Passively negativistic individuals simply fail to do what is asked or expected: if clothes are laid out they will not dress; if asked to eat or take pills, their lips remain frozen shut. Active negativism manifests in doing the opposite of what is expected: if asked to come into the office, the individual may back into the hallway or if asked to open the eyes wide to allow for easier examination, they may cramp the eyes closed. Automatic obedience, as may be suspected, represents the opposite of negativism, with affected individuals doing exactly what they are told, even if this places them in danger. Echo phenomena represent a kind of automatic obedience: in echolalia individuals simply repeat what they hear and in echopraxia they mimic the gestures and activity of the examiner. It should be noted that in negativism, automatic obedience, and echo phenomena there is nothing natural or fluid about the individual's behavior. To the contrary, movements are often awkward, wooden, and tinged with the bizarre.

Excited catatonia manifests with varying degrees of bizarre, frenzied, and purposeless behavior. Such individuals typically keep to themselves: one marched in place, all the while chanting and gesticulating; another tore at his hair and clothing, broke plates in a corner then crawled under the bed where he muttered and thrashed his arms.

Epidemiology
Stuporous catatonia due to a general medical condition overall is, in general, a rare condition.

Course
This is determined by the course of the underlying cause.

Differential Diagnosis
Stuporous catatonia must be distinguished from akinetic mutism and from stupor of other causes. Akinetic mutes (Cairns et al. 1941) appear quite similar to immobile and mute catatonics; they, however, lack such signs as waxy flexibility, posturing, and negativism, all of which are typically seen in catatonia. Stupor of other causes is readily distinguished from catatonic stupor by the salient fact that catatonics remain alert, in stark contrast with the somnolence or decreased level of consciousness seen in all other forms of stupor.

Excited catatonia must be distinguished from mania. Mania is typified by hyperactivity, which at times may be quite frenzied: the difference with catatonia is that individuals with mania want to be involved, whereas those with catatonia keep to themselves; as Kraepelin (Bear et al. 1982) noted, in catatonia "the excitement, even when extremely violent, frequently takes place within the *smallest space. . . .* The patients have not as a rule any tendency to influence their surroundings, but their restlessness exhausts itself in wholly aimless activity. . . . "

Etiology
Stuporous catatonia, in the majority of cases, occurs as part of such primary mental disorders as schizophrenia or a depressive episode of either major depressive or bipolar disorder. The causes of catatonia due to a general medical condition or medications are listed in Table 14-8.

Stuporous catatonia occurring in association with epilepsy is often suggested by a history of grand mal or complex partial seizures. Ictal catatonia is further suggested by its exquisitely paroxysmal onset, and postictal catatonia by an immediately preceding "flurry" of grand mal or complex partial seizures. Psychosis of forced normalization is an interictal condition distinguished by the appearance of symptoms subsequent to effective control of seizures. The chronic interictal psychosis is also, as suggested by the name, an interictal condition, which however, appears not after seizures are controlled but rather in the setting of ongoing, chronic uncontrolled epilepsy. Of medications capable of causing catatonia, neuroleptics are by far the most common. Viral encephalitis is suggested by concurrent fever and headache: herpes simplex encephalitis should always be considered in such cases, given its treatability; further it must be kept in mind that although encephalitis lethargica no longer occurs in epidemics, sporadic cases still do occur. Focal lesions capable of causing catatonia are typically found in the medial or inferior portions of the frontal lobes. The miscellaneous conditions listed are all quite rare causes of catatonia.

Excited catatonia, in the vast majority of cases, is caused by either schizophrenia or bipolar disorder (during a manic episode); only rarely is it seen because of a general medical condition, as for example, a viral encephalitis.

Table 14-8	Causes of Catatonia due to a General Medical Condition

Stuporous Catatonia
  Associated with epilepsy
    Ictal catatonia (Engel et al. 1978, Gomez et al. 1982, Lim et al. 1986, Shah and Kaplan 1980)
    Postictal catatonia (Logsdail 1988)
    Psychosis of forced normalization (Pakainis et al. 1987)
    Chronic interictal psychosis (Kristensen and Sindrup 1979, Slater and Beard 1963a, 1963b)
  Medication
    Neuroleptics (Gelenberg and Mandel 1977)
    Disulfiram (Reisberg 1978, Weddington et al. 1980)
    Benzodiazepine withdrawal (Rosebush and Mazurek 1996)
  Viral encephalitis (Abrams and Taylor 1976, Kim and Perlstein 1970, Misra and Hay 1971)
    Herpes simplex encephalitis (Raskin and Frank 1974)
    Encephalitis lethargica (Kirby and Davis 1921)
  Focal lesions, especially of the frontal lobes (Belfer and d'Autremont 1971, Thompson 1970)
  Miscellaneous conditions
    Hepatic encephalopathy (Jaffe 1967)
    Limbic encephalitis (Tandon et al. 1988)
    Systemic lupus erythematosus (Lanham et al. 1985, Mac and Pardo 1983)
    Lyme disease, in stage III (Pfister et al. 1993)
    Subacute sclerosing panencephalitis, in stage I (Koehler and Jakumeit 1976)
    Tay–Sachs disease (Rosebush et al. 1995)
    Thrombotic thrombocytopenic purpura (Read 1983)

Excited Catatonia
  Viral encephalitis (Penn et al. 1972)

Treatment

In addition to treating, if possible, the underlying cause, catatonia may be symptomatically relieved by lorazepam given parenterally in a dose of 2 mg; in severe cases wherein lorazepam is not sufficiently effective and the individual is at immediate risk, consideration should be given to emergency ECT, which is typically dramatically effective, generally bringing relief after but a few treatments.

PERSONALITY CHANGE DUE TO A GENERAL MEDICAL CONDITION

Diagnosis

The personality of an adult represents a coalescence of various personality traits present in childhood and adolescence, and is generally quite enduring and resistant to change. Thus, the appearance of a significant change in an adult's personality is an ominous clinical sign and indicates the presence of intracranial pathology. Individuals themselves may not be aware of the change. However, to others, who have known the individual over time, the change is often quite obvious. Such observers often note that the individual is "not himself" anymore.

In most cases, the change is nonspecific in nature: there may be either a gross exaggeration of hitherto minor aspects of the individual's personality or the appearance of a personality trait quite uncharacteristic for the individual. Traits commonly seen in a personality change, as noted in DSM-IV-TR, include lability, disinhibition, aggressiveness, apathy, or suspiciousness (see DSM-IV-TR diagnostic criteria on page 331).

DSM-IV-TR Diagnostic Criteria

310.1 Personality Change Due to . . . [Indicate the General Medical Condition]

A. A persistent personality disturbance that represents a change from the individual's previous characteristic personality pattern. (In children, the disturbance involves a marked deviation from normal development or a significant change in the child's usual behavior patterns lasting at least 1 year).

B. There is evidence from the history, physical examination, or laboratory findings that the disturbance is the direct physiological consequence of a general medical condition.

C. The disturbance is not better accounted for by another mental disorder (including other Mental Disorders Due to a General Medical Condition).

D. The disturbance does not occur exclusively during the course of a delirium.

E. The disturbance causes clinically significant distress or impairment in social, occupational, or other important areas of functioning.

Specify type:

Labile Type: if the predominant feature is affective lability

Disinhibited Type: if the predominant feature is poor impulse control as evidenced by sexual indiscretions, etc.

Aggressive Type: if the predominant feature is aggressive behavior

Apathetic Type: if the predominant feature is marked apathy and indifference

Paranoid Type: if the predominant feature is suspiciousness or paranoid ideation

Other Type: if the predominant feature is not one of the above, e.g., personality change associated with a seizure disorder

Combined Type: if more than one feature predominates in the clinical picture

Unspecified Type

Coding note: Include the name of the general medical condition on Axis I, e.g., 310.1 Personality Change Due to Temporal Lobe Epilepsy: also code the general medical condition on Axis III (see Appendix G for codes).

In addition to these nonspecific changes, there are two specific syndromes which, though not listed in DSM-IV-TR, are well described in the literature, namely, the *frontal lobe syndrome* and the *interictal personality syndrome* (also known as the "Geschwind syndrome").

The *frontal lobe syndrome* is characterized by a variable mixture of disinhibition, affective changes, perseveration, and abulia. Disinhibition manifests with an overall coarsening of behavior. Attention to manners and social nuances is lost: individuals may eat with gluttony, make coarse and crude jokes, and may engage in unwelcome and inappropriate sexual behavior, perhaps by propositioning much younger individuals or masturbating in public. Affective changes tend toward a silly, noninfectious euphoria; depression, however, may also be seen. Perseveration presents with a tendency to persist in whatever task is currently at hand, and individuals may repeatedly button and unbutton clothing, open and close a drawer or ask the same question again and again. Abulia is characterized by an absence of desires, urges, or interests, and such individuals, being undisturbed by such phenomena, may be content to sit placidly for indefinite periods of time. Importantly, such abulic individuals are not depressed, nor are they incapable of activity. Indeed, with active supervision they may be able to complete tasks; however, once supervision stops, so too do the individuals, as they lapse back into quietude.

The *interictal personality syndrome*, a controversial entity (Bear et al. 1982, Rodin and Schmaltz 1984) is said to occur as a complication of long-standing uncontrolled epilepsy, with repeated grand mal or complex partial seizures. The cardinal characteristic of this syndrome is what is known as "viscosity," (Waxman and Geschwind 1975) or, somewhat more colloquially, "stickiness." Here, individuals seem unable to let go or diverge from the current emotion or train of thought: existing effects persist long after the situation that occasioned them, and a given train of thought tends to extend itself indefinitely into a long-winded and verbose circumstantiality or tangentiality. This viscosity of thought may also appear in written expression as individuals display "hypergraphia," producing long and rambling letters or diaries (Hermann et al. 1988). The inability to "let go" may even extend to such simple acts as shaking hands, such that others may literally have to extract their hand to end the handshake. The content of the individual's viscous speech and writing generally also changes, and tends toward mystical or abstruse philosophical speculations. Finally, there is also a tendency to hyposexuality, with an overall decrease in libido (Blumer 1970, Blumer and Walker 1967).

Epidemiology

Personality change is common, and is especially frequent after closed head injury and as a prodrome to the dementia occurring with such neurodegenerative disorders as Pick's disease, fronto-temporal dementia, and Alzheimer's disease.

Course

This is determined by the underlying cause; in the case of the interictal personality syndrome, it appears that symptoms persist even if seizure control is obtained.

Differential Diagnosis

Personality change must be clearly distinguished from a personality disorder. The personality disorders (e.g., antisocial personality disorder, borderline personality disorder), all in Chapter 44, do not represent a change in the individual's personality but rather have been present in a lifelong fashion. In gathering a history of an individual with a personality change, one finds a more or less distinct time when the "change" occurred; by contrast, in evaluating an individual with a personality disorder, one can trace the personality traits in question in a more or less seamless fashion back into adolescence, or earlier.

The frontal lobe syndrome, at times, may present further diagnostic questions, raising the possibility of either mania, when euphoria is prominent, or depression, when abulia is at the forefront. Mania is distinguished by the quality of the euphoria, which tends to be full and infectious in contrast with the silly, shallow, and noninfectious euphoria of the frontal lobe syndrome. Depression may be distinguished by the quality of the individuals' experience: depressed individuals definitely feel something, whether it be a depressed mood or simply a weighty sense of oppression. By contrast, the individual with abulia generally feels nothing: the "mental horizon" is clear and undisturbed by any dysphoria or unpleasantness. MRI scanning is diagnostic in most cases, and where this is uninformative, further testing is dictated by one's clinical suspicions (e.g., HIV testing).

The interictal personality syndrome must be distinguished from a personality change occurring secondary to a slowly growing tumor of the temporal lobe. In some cases, very small tumors, which may escape detection by routine MRI scanning, may cause epilepsy, and then, with continued growth, also cause a personality change. Thus, in the case of an individual with epilepsy who develops a personality change, the diagnosis of the interictal personality syndrome should not be made until a tumor has been ruled out by repeat MRI scanning.

Etiology

A personality change is not uncommonly seen as the prodrome to schizophrenia; however, in such cases the eventual appearance of the typical psychosis will indicate the correct diagnosis.

Personality change of the nonspecific or of the frontal lobe type, as noted in Table 14-9, may occur *secondary to precipitants* (e.g., closed head injury), *secondary to cerebral tumors* (especially those of the frontal or temporal lobes) or *as part of certain neurodegenerative or dementing disorders*. Finally, there is a group of *miscellaneous causes*. In Table 14-9, those disorders or diseases that are particularly prone to cause a personality change of the frontal lobe type are indicated by an asterisk. The interictal personality syndrome occurs only in the setting of chronic repeated grand mal or complex partial seizures, and may represent microanatomic changes in the limbic system which have been "kindled" by the repeated seizures (Adamec and Stark-Adamec 1983, Bear 1979).

In the case of personality change occurring *secondary to precipitants*, the etiology is fairly obvious; an exception might be cerebral infarction, but here the acute onset and the presence of "neighborhood" symptoms are suggestive. In addition to infarction of the frontal lobe, personality change has also been noted with infarction of the caudate nucleus (Mendez et al. 1989, Petty et al. 1996) and of the thalamus (Sandson et al. 1991).

Personality change occurring s*econdary to cerebral tumors* may not be accompanied by any distinctive features, and indeed a personality change may be the only clinical evidence of a tumor for a prolonged period of time.

Personality change *occurring as part of certain neurodegenerative or dementing disorders* deserves special mention, for in many instances the underlying disorder may present with a personality change—this is particularly the case with Pick's disease, fronto-temporal dementia, and Alzheimer's disease. The inclusion of amyotrophic lateral sclerosis here may be surprising to some, but it is very clear that, albeit in a small minority, cerebral symptoms may not only dominate the early course of amyotrophic lateral sclerosis (ALS) but may also constitute the presentation of the disease. In the case of the other neurodegenerative disorders (i.e., progressive supranuclear palsy, cortico–basal ganglionic degeneration, multiple system atrophy, Huntington's disease and Wilson's disease), a personality change, if present, is typically accompanied by abnormal involuntary movements of one sort or other, such as parkinsonism, ataxia, or chorea. The lacunar syndrome, occurring secondary to multiple lacunar infarctions affecting the thalamus, internal capsule, or basal ganglia, deserves special mention as it very commonly causes a personality change of the frontal lobe type by interrupting the connections between the thalamus or basal ganglia and the frontal lobe. Normal pressure hydrocephalus is an important diagnosis to keep in mind, as the condition is treatable. Other suggestive symptoms include a broad-based shuffling gait and urinary urgency or incontinence. AIDS should be suspected whenever a personality change is accompanied by clinical phenomena suggestive of immunodeficiency, such as thrush. Neurosyphilis may present with a personality change characterized by slovenliness and disinhibition. Creutzfeldt–Jakob disease may also present with a personality change, and this appears particularly likely with the "new variant" type, the eventual appearance of myoclonus suggests the correct diagnosis.

Table 14-9	Causes of Personality Change of the Nonspecific or Frontal Lobe Type

Secondary to Precipitants
 Closed head injury (Brooks et al. 1986, Max et al. 2001, Oder et al. 1992, Roberts 1976, Thomsen 1984)
 Head trauma with subdural hematoma (Cameron 1978)
 Postviral encephalitis (Friedman and Allen 1969, McGrath et al. 1997)
 Gunshot wounds (Lebensohn 1947, Lishman 1973)
 Cerebral infarction

Secondary to Cerebral Tumors
 Frontal lobe* (Avery 1971, Frazier 1936, Hunter et al. 1968, Williamson 1896)
 Corpus callosum* (in its anterior part) (Alpers and Grant 1931, Beling and Martland 1919, Moersch 1925)
 Temporal lobe (Keschner et al. 1936, Strobos 1953)

Occurring as Part of Certain Neurodegenerative or Dementing Disorders
 Pick's disease* (Litvan et al. 1997, Mendez et al. 1993)
 Fronto-temporal dementia* (Brun et al. 1994, Heutink et al. 1997, Neary et al. 1993)
 Alzheimer's disease* (Mega et al. 1996, Petry et al. 1988)
 Amyotrophic lateral sclerosis* (Cavalleri and De Renzi 1994, Massman et al. 1996, Neary et al. 1990, Peavy et al.
  1992)
 Progressive supranuclear palsy* (Venry et al. 1996)
 Cortico-basal ganglionic degeneration* (Bergeron et al. 1996)
 Multiple system atrophy* (Critchley and Greenfield 1948, Robbins et al. 1992)
 Huntington's disease (Pflanz et al. 1991)
 Wilson's disease (Bridgman and Smyth 1994, Dening and Berrios 1989, Starosta-Rubinstein et al. 1987, Walshe and
  Yealland 1992)
 Lacunar syndrome* (Ishii et al. 1986)
 Normal pressure hydrocephalus (Rice and Gendelman 1973)
 AIDS (Navia et al. 1986)
 Neurosyphilis (Storm-Mathisen 1969)
 Creutzfeldt–Jakob disease (Brown et al. 1994, Roos et al. 1973)

Miscellaneous Causes
 Granulomatous angiitis (Koo and Massey 1988)
 Vitamin B_{12} deficiency (Lindenbaum et al. 1988)
 Limbic encephalitis (Alamowitch et al. 1997)
 Metachromatic leukodystrophy (Hageman et al. 1995)
 Adrenoleukodystrophy (Schaumburg et al. 1975)
 Mercury intoxication (O'Carroll et al. 1995)
 Manganism (Abd El Naby and Hassanein 1965)

* Particularly likely to cause a frontal lobe syndrome.

The *miscellaneous causes* represent the diagnostic "zebras" in the differential for personality change. Of them two deserve comment, given their treatability: granulomatous angiitis is suggested by prominent headache, and vitamin B_{12} deficiency by the presence of macrocytosis or a sensory polyneuropathy.

Treatment

Treatment, if possible, is directed at the underlying cause. Mood stabilizers (i.e., lithium, carbamazepine, or divalproex) may be helpful for lability, impulsivity, and irritability; propranolol, in high dose, may also have some effect on irritability. Neuroleptics (e.g., olanzapine, risperidone, and haloperidol) may be helpful when suspiciousness or disinhibition are prominent. Antidepressants (e.g., an SSRI) may relieve depressive symptoms. Regardless of which agent is chosen, it is prudent, given the general medical condition of many of these individuals, to "start low and go slow." In many cases, some degree of supervision will be required.

MENTAL DISORDER NOT OTHERWISE SPECIFIED DUE TO A GENERAL MEDICAL CONDITION

This is a residual category in DSM-IV-TR for those clinical situations in which the mental disorder occurring secondary to a general medical condition does not fall into one of the specific categories described earlier. Of these various disorders, two are worthy of detailed description, namely, pseudobulbar palsy and the Klüver–Bucy syndrome. Both disorders are commonly seen in dementia clinics, and their occurrence often prompts a request for psychiatric consultation.

Pseudobulbar Palsy When fully developed, this syndrome is characterized by emotional incontinence (also known as "pathological laughing and crying"), dysarthria, dysphagia, a brisk jaw-jerk and gag reflex, and difficulty in protruding the tongue (Langsworthy and Hesser 1940).

The most remarkable aspect of the syndrome is the emotional incontinence. Here, individuals experience uncontrollable paroxysms of laughter or crying, often in response to minor stimuli, such as the approach of the physician to the bedside (Lieberman and Benson 1977). Importantly, despite the strength of these outbursts, individuals do not experience any corresponding sense of mirth or sadness. Some may attempt to stop the emotional display, only to become acutely distressed at their inability to do so. One individual, who experienced "gales of laughter" whenever he attempted to speak, "felt foolish and ashamed, and had tears in his eyes because he could not 'control the laughter.' " (Davison and Kelman 1939). Some may go out of their way to avoid having these paroxysms. In one case, described by Wilson (1924), the individual "used to walk about the hospital with his eyes glued to the ground (because) if he so much as raised them to meet anyone else's gaze he was immediately overcome by compulsory laughter, which sometimes lasted for 4 or 5 minutes."

Pseudobulbar palsy results from bilateral interruption of corticobulbar fibers (Besson et al. 1991); with this interruption occurring anywhere from the cortex (Davison and Kelman 1939, Wilson 1924) through the centrum semiovale (Ishii et al. 1986) to the internal capsule (Colman 1894) and down to the midbrain and pons (Asfora et al. 1989). Thus "released" from upper motor neuron control, the bulbar nuclei act reflexively, creating, in a sense, a kind of "spasticity" of emotional display. The various disorders capable of causing such a bilateral interruption are listed in Table 14-10.

Table 14-10	Causes of Pseudobulbar Palsy

Vascular Disorders
 Large vessel cortical infarctions (Wilson 1924)
 Subcortical lacunar infarctions (Ishii et al. 1986)
 Binswanger's disease (Caplan and Schoene 1978)
 CADASIL (Bergmann et al. 1996)

Certain Neurodegenerative Disorders
 Amyotrophic lateral sclerosis (Ironside 1956, Ziegler 1930)
 Progressive supranuclear palsy (Menza et al. 1995)
 Alzheimer's disease (Starkstein et al. 1995)

Miscellaneous Causes
 Cerebral tumors
 Closed head injury
 Multiple sclerosis (Feinstein et al. 1997)
 Behcet's syndrome (Motomura et al. 1980)

Vascular disorders are by far the most common cause of bilateral interruption of the corticobulbar tracts, as may be seen with infarctions of the cortex or with lacunar infarctions in the corona radiata or internal capsule. Although in some cases it appears that the syndrome occurs after only one stroke, further investigation typically reveals evidence of a preexisting lesion on the contralateral side, a lesion which had been clinically "silent" (Besson et al. 1991). Other vascular causes include Binswanger's disease, characterized by diffuse white matter damage in the centrum semiovale, and CADASIL (Cerebral Autosomal Dominant Arteriopathy with Subcortical Infarcts and Leukoencephalopathy), characterized by both subcortical infarctions and a widespread leukoencephalopathy.

Of the *neurodegenerative disorders* associated with pseudobulbar palsy, the most prominent is amyotrophic lateral sclerosis, wherein approximately one half of individuals are eventually so affected (Gallagher 1989).

Of the *miscellaneous causes*, cerebral tumors, which bilaterally compress or invade the brainstem (Achari and Colover 1976, Cantu and Drew 1966, Shafqat et al. 1998), are particularly important.

The diagnosis should be suspected whenever individuals present with exaggerated and uncontrollable emotional displays. Lability of affect, as may be seen in mania, is ruled out by the fact that the labile individual, while displaying the affect, also experiences a congruent emotional feeling; by contrast, in emotional incontinence the individual often feels nothing, except perhaps consternation at the unmotivated and uncontrollable emotional display. Inappropriate affect, as may be seen in schizophrenia, is similar to emotional incontinence in that individuals with schizophrenia may not experience any corresponding feeling; in schizophrenia, however, one sees other accompanying symptoms, such as mannerisms, hallucinations, and delusions, symptoms that are absent in pseudobulbar palsy. "Emotionalism," as may be seen after strokes, may suggest the diagnosis, especially given the clinical setting; however here, as with lability, individuals also experience a concurrent feeling that is congruent with the emotional display.

Findings on the neurologic examination are also helpful. Bilateral interruption of corticobulbar tracts, as noted above, typically leads to cranial nerve dysfunction with dysarthria, dysphagia, and brisk jaw-jerk and gag reflexes. Given the proximity of the corticospinal tracts, one often also finds evidence of long-tract damage, such as hemiplegia or Babinski signs.

MRI scanning is generally diagnostic in cases secondary to vascular lesions, tumors, and multiple sclerosis. Amyotrophic lateral sclerosis is suggested by the gradual progression of upper and lower motor neuron signs and symptoms; progressive supranuclear palsy by the presence of parkinsonism and supranuclear gaze palsy, and Alzheimer's disease by the long history of a gradually progressive dementia.

Pseudobulbar palsy is not uncommon: as noted above, it is found in almost half of the individuals with amyotrophic lateral sclerosis (Gallagher 1989). It may also be seen in a much smaller, but still clinically significant, proportion of individuals with vascular lesions (Besson et al. 1991), Alzheimer's disease (Starkstein et al. 1995), and multiple sclerosis (Feinstein et al. 1997).

In addition to treating, if possible, the underlying cause, various medications may be used to reduce the severity of the emotional incontinence, including tricyclics and SSRIs. Among the tricyclics, both amitriptyline (in doses of 50–75 mg) (Schiffer et al. 1985) and nortriptyline (in doses up to 100 mg) are effective, with nortriptyline generally better tolerated. Of the SSRIs, citalopram, in a dose of 20 mg, was effective, and there are also case reports of the effectiveness of paroxetine, sertraline, and fluoxetine (Seliger and Hornstein 1989). Overall, it is probably best to begin with an SSRI, and to hold nortriptyline in reserve.

Kluver–Bucy syndrome   In 1939, Klüver and Bucy (1939) noted some striking behavioral changes in monkeys which had been subjected to bilateral temporal lobectomy, and in so doing described the syndrome that now bears their names. Specifically, they described five characteristics which they named "hypermetamorphosis," "psychic blindness," "oral tendencies," "emotional changes," and "changes in sexual behavior." Given that this nomenclature is somewhat idiosyncratic to these authors, some concrete examples, taken from their article, may enable the reader to gain a sense of the syndrome as it appeared in the monkeys.

The hypermetamorphosis of these animals was manifested by "an excessive tendency to take notice of and to attend and react to every visual stimulus ... (and) to contact every object as soon as possible." Furthermore, this interest in things was indiscriminate: being psychically "blind," the animals would approach objects "no matter whether they are very large or very small, dead or alive, edible or inedible, moving or stationary ... (they) seem to be just as eager to examine the tongue of a hissing snake, the mouth of a cat, faeces, a wire cage or a wagon as a piece of bread." Once in contact with an object, the "oral tendencies" often became apparent in that the monkeys typically put "the object into the mouth, biting gently, chewing, licking, touching with the lips, and smelling (it)." Should another, perhaps dangerous, animal have been approached, the "emotional changes" immediately became apparent, in that the monkeys failed to show any "emotional reactions ... generally associated with anger and fear"; indeed, "after being attacked and bitten by another animal (they) may approach this animal again and again in an attempt to examine it." Finally, and in addition to all the foregoing changes, there were "changes in sexual behavior" manifested by an overall "increase in sexual activity" that was "blind", and could manifest with increased masturbation or an indiscriminant approach to others, regardless of their sex.

Over time, changes in the original nomenclature used to describe the syndrome have been made so as to facilitate clinical practice. Thus, although the term hypermetamorphosis has survived, "psychic blindness" has fallen into disfavor and most authors speak of a kind of "agnosia." The "oral tendencies" are now referred to as hyperorality, and the "emotional changes" as "emotional placidity." Finally, the varied "changes in sexual behavior" are now simply referred to as hypersexuality. Thus, the full syndrome is characterized by hypermetamorphosis, agnosia (albeit of a peculiar kind), hyperorality, emotional placidity, and hypersexuality. Some examples of the syndrome in humans follow:

The first example demonstrates hypersexuality, hyperorality, agnosia, and emotional placidity. The individual was a 31-year-old woman, who, after recovering from a herpes simplex encephalitis, "made inappropriate sexual advances to female attendants, both manually and orally. At home, she was constantly chewing and swallowing, and all objects within reach were placed in her mouth ... including toilet paper and faeces... Her affect was characterized by passivity and a pet-like compliance with those attending her" (Lilly et al. 1983).

The second example provides examples of hypermetamorphosis, hyperorality, agnosia, and hypersexuality. The individual, a 58-year-old man who had suffered from Alzheimer's disease for 6 years, "spent much of his time examining ordinary objects such as the doorstep, ashtrays, or spots on the floor. He placed many objects in his mouth and occasionally ate soil from plant containers ... he rubbed his genitals so frequently that he developed an excoriation on the shaft of his penis" (Lilly et al. 1983).

Finally, there is the case of a 46-year-old man, who, during a complex partial seizure, "was observed grabbing for objects on his bedside table, and he masturbated in front of the nursing staff. He also placed objects in his mouth, chewed on tissue paper, and attempted to drink from his urine container" (Nakada et al. 1984). Here, there are hypermetamorphosis, hypersexuality, hyperorality, and agnosia.

Table 14-11	Causes of the Klüver–Bucy Syndrome

Secondary to Precipitants
  Bilateral temporal lobectomy (Terzian and Dalle Ore 1955)
  Head trauma with bilateral damage to temporal lobes (Lilly et al. 1983)
  Herpes simplex encephalitis (Greenwood et al. 1983, Marlowe et al. 1975, Shoji et al. 1979)
  Status epilepticus (Mendez and Foti 1997)
  Heat stroke (Pitt et al. 1995)

Occurring as Part of Certain Neurodegenerative Disorders
  Pick's disease (Cummings and Duchen 1981)
  Fronto-temporal dementia (Heutink et al. 1997)
  Alzheimer's disease (Mendez et al. 1993, Teri et al. 1988)

Miscellaneous Causes
  Ictal (Nakada et al. 1984)
  Postictal (Anson and Kuhlman 1993)
  Adrenoleukodystrophy (Powers et al. 1980)

The various causes of the Klüver–Bucy syndrome are listed in Table 14-11; in each case, bilateral damage or dysfunction of the temporal lobes has occurred. The mechanism of such bilateral damage in the case of precipitants is fairly straightforward. The neurodegenerative disorders listed have a predilection for the temporal lobes, and this is particularly the case in Pick's disease and fronto-temporal dementia. Indeed, the appearance of the Klüver–Bucy syndrome early in the course of a dementia is a significant diagnostic clue to one of these two disorders; in the case of Alzheimer's disease, the syndrome, if it does occur, is generally seen only late in the course. Of the miscellaneous causes, an ictal Klüver–Bucy syndrome is suggested by its exquisitely paroxysmal onset and by the occurrence of other symptoms typical for a complex partial seizure, such as confusion, and a postictal Klüver–Bucy syndrome by the history of an immediately preceding generalized seizure. Adrenoleukodystrophy, the last in the list, is an extremely rare cause of the Klüver–Bucy syndrome.

The treatment of Klüver–Bucy syndrome involves treatment of the underlying cause, if possible. In chronic cases, neuroleptics have been reported to be helpful; there are, however, no controlled studies.

Comparison of DSM-IV-TR/ICD-10 Diagnostic Criteria

The DSM-IV-TR category Psychotic Disorder Due to a General Medical Condition is referred to in ICD-10 as "organic hallucinosis" or "organic delusional disorder" depending on the type of presenting symptom.

In contrast to DSM-IV-TR, which requires clinically significant mood symptoms of any type, the ICD-10 Diagnostic Criteria for Research for Mood Disorder due to a General Medical Condition require that the full symptomatic and duration criteria be met for a hypomanic, manic, or major depressive episode. This disorder is referred in ICD-10 as "organic mood disorder." Also in contrast to DSM-IV-TR, which requires anxiety symptoms of any type, the ICD-10 Diagnostic Criteria for Research for Anxiety Disorder Due to a General Medical Condition require that the clinical picture meet full symptomatic and duration criteria for panic disorder or generalized anxiety disorder.

For catatonic disorder due to a general medical condition, the ICD-10 Diagnostic Criteria for Research are more narrowly defined than the criteria in DSM-IV-TR by virtue of requiring both catatonic stupor/negativism and excitement and that there be a rapid alternation of stupor and excitement. In ICD-10, this disorder is referred to as "organic catatonic disorder."

The DSM-IV-TR category of Personality Change Due to a General Medical Condition corresponds to two ICD-10 categories: "organic personality disorder" and "organic emotionally labile disorder." The ICD-10 Diagnostic Criteria for Research for Organic Personality Disorder are probably more narrowly defined in that "at least three" features characteristic of a personality change are required.

References

Abbas A and Styra R (1994) Valproate prophylaxis against steroid-induced psychosis. *Can J Psychiatry* **39**, 188–189.

Abd El Naby S and Hassanein M (1965) Neuropsychiatric manifestations of chronic manganese poisoning. *J Neurol Neurosurg Psychiatry* **28**, 282–288.

Abrams R and Taylor MA (1976) Catatonia: a prospective clinical study. *Arch Gen Psychiatry* **33**, 579–581.

Achari AN and Colover J (1976) Posterior fossa tumors with pathological laughter. *JAMA* **235**, 1469–1471.

Adachi N, Arima K, Asada T, et al. (2001) Dentatorubral-pallidoluysian atrophy (DRPLA) presenting with psychosis. *J Neuropsychiatry Clin Neurosci* **13**, 258–260.

Adamec DE and Stark-Adamec C (1983) Limbic kindling in animal behavior: implications for human psychopathology associated with complex partial seizures. *Biol Psychiatry* **18**, 269–274.

Ainiala H, Loukkola J, Peltola J, et al. (2001) The prevalence of neuropsychiatric syndromes in systemic lupus erythematosus. *Neurology* **57**, 496–500.

Alamowitch S, Graus F, Uchuya M, et al. (1997) Limbic encephalitis and small cell lung cancer: clinical and immunological features. *Brain* **120**, 923–928.

Alpers BJ (1940) Personality and emotional disorders associated with hypothalamic lesions. In *Association for Research in Nervous and Mental Disease*, Vol. 20, *The Hypothalamus and Central Levels of Autonomic Function*, Fulton JF, Ranson SW, and Frantz AM (eds). Williams & Wilkins, Baltimore.

Alpers BJ and Grant FC (1931) The clinical syndrome of the corpus callosum. *Arch Neurol Psychiatry* **25**, 67–86.

Anderson J, Aabro E, Gulmann N, et al. (1980) Anti-depressive treatment in Parkinson's disease: a controlled trial of the effect of nortriptyline in patients with Parkinson's disease treated with l-dopa. *Acta Neurol Scand* **62**, 210–219.

Anderson KE, Louis ED, Stern Y, et al. (2001) Cognitive correlates of obsessive and compulsive symptoms in Huntington's disease. *Am J Psychiatry* **158**, 799–801.

Anderson G, Vestergaard K, and Lauritzen L (1994) Effective treatment of poststroke depression with the selective serotonin reuptake inhibitor citalopram. *Stroke* **25**, 1099–1104.

Angelini L, Mazzuchi A, Picciotto F, et al. (1980) Focal lesion of the right cingulum: a case report in a child. *J Neurol Neurosurg Psychiatry* **43**, 355–357.

Anson JA and Kuhlman DT (1993) Post-ictal Klüver–Bucy syndrome after temporal lobectomy. *J Neurol Neurosurg Psychiatry* **56**, 311–313.

Asfora WT, DeSalles AAF, Masamitsu ABE, et al. (1989) Is the syndrome of pathological laughing and crying a manifestation of pseudobulbar palsy? *J Neurol Neurosurg Psychiatry* **52**, 523–525.

Asher R (1949) Myxoedematous madness. *Br Med J* **2**, 555–562.

Astrom M, Adolfsson R, and Asplund K (1993) Major depression in stroke patients: a 3-year longitudinal study. *Stroke* **24**, 976–982.

Avery TL (1971) Seven cases of frontal tumor with psychiatric presentation. *Br J Psychiatry* **119**, 19–23.

Bakchine S, Lacomblez L, Beloit N, et al. (1989) Manic-like state after bilateral orbitofrontal and right temporoparietal injury: efficacy of clonidine. *Neurology* **39**, 777–781.

Baker RW, Chengappa R, Baird JW, et al. (1992) Emergence of obsessive–compulsive symptoms during treatment with clozapine. *J Clin Psychiatry* **53**, 439–442.

Bassett AS and Chow EW (1999) 22q11 deletion syndrome: a genetic subtype of schizophrenia. *Biol Psychiatry* **46**, 882–891.

Bear DM (1979) Temporal lobe epilepsy: a syndrome of sensory–limbic hyperconnection. *Cortex* **15**, 357–369.

Bear D, Levin K, Blumer D, et al. (1982) Interictal behavior in hospitalized temporal lobe epileptics: relationship to idiopathic psychiatric syndrome. *J Neurol Neurosurg Psychiatry* **45**, 481–488.

Beard AW (1959) The association of hepatolenticular degeneration with schizophrenia. *Acta Psychiatr Neurol Scand* **34**, 411–428.

Belfer ML and d'Autremont CC (1971) Catatonia-like symptomatology. *Arch Gen Psychiatry* **24**, 119–120.

Beling CC and Martland HS (1919) A case of tumor of the corpus callosum and frontal lobes. *J Nerv Ment Dis* **50**, 425–432.

Beresford OD and Graham AM (1950) Chorea gravidarum. *J Obstet Gynecol Br Emp* **57**, 616–625.

Bergeron C, Pollanen MS, Weyer L, et al. (1996) Unusual clinical presentation of cortico-basal ganglionic degeneration. *Ann Neurol* **40**, 893–900.

Bergmann M, Ebke M, Yuam Y, et al. (1996) Cerebral autosomal dominant arteriopathy with subcortical infarcts and leukoencephalopathy (CADASIL): a morphological study of a German family. *Acta Neuropathol* **92**, 341–350.

Besson G, Bogousslavsky J, Regli F, et al. (1991) Acute pseudobulbar or suprabulbar palsy. *Arch Neurol* **48**, 501–507.

Besson JAO (1980) A diagnostic pointer to adult metachromatic leukodystrophy. *Br J Psychiatry* **137**, 186–187.

Bicknell JN and Moore RA (1960) Psychological meaning of disulfiram (Antabuse) therapy. *Arch Gen Psychiatry* **2**, 661–668.

Billings RF and Stein MB (1986) Depression associated with ranitidine. *Am J Psychiatry* **143**, 915–916.

Binder RL and Dickman WA (1980) Psychiatric manifestations of neurosyphilis in middle-aged patients. *Am J Psychiatry* **137**, 741–742.

Biraben A, Taussig D, Thomas P, et al. (2001) Fear as the main feature of epileptic seizures. *J Neurol Neurosurg Psychiatry* **70**, 186–191.

Blackwell MJ (1991) Rapid-cycling manic–depressive illness following subarachnoid hemorrhage. *Br J Psychiatry* **159**, 279–280.

Bloch M, Stager S, Braun A, et al. (1997) Pimozide-induced depression in men who stutter. *J Clin Psychiatry* **58**, 433–436.

Blumer D (1970) Hypersexual episodes in temporal lobe epilepsy. *Am J Psychiatry* **126**, 1099–1106.

Blumer D and Walker AE (1967) Sexual behavior in temporal lobe epilepsy. *Arch Neurol* **16**, 37–43.

Bogousslavsky J, Ferrazzini M, Regli F, et al. (1988) Manic delirium and frontal-like syndrome with paramedian infarction of the right thalamus. *J Neurol Neurosurg Psychiatry* **51**, 116–119.

Bolt JMW (1970) Huntington's chorea in the west of Scotland. *Br J Psychiatry* **116**, 259–270.

Bracken P (1987) Mania following head injury. *Br J Psychiatry* **150**, 690–692.

Bridgman O and Smyth FS (1994) Progressive lenticular degeneration. *J Nerv Ment Dis* **99**, 534–543.

Brooks N, Campsie L, Symington C, et al. (1986) The five year outcome of severe blunt head injury: a relatives view. *J Neurol Neurosurg Psychiatry* **49**, 764–770.

Brown P, Gibbs CJ, Rodgers-Johnson P, et al. (1994) Human spongiform encephalopathy: the national institutes of health series of 300 cases of experimentally transmitted disease. *Ann Neurol* **35**, 513–529.

Brown P, Rodgers-Johnson P, Cathala F, et al. (1984) Creutzfeldt–Jakob disease of long duration: clinicopathological characteristics, transmissibility, and differential diagnosis. *Ann Neurol* **16**, 295–304.

Brun A, Englund B, Gustafson L, et al. (1994) Clinical and neuropathological criteria for fronto-temporal dementia. *J Neurol Neurosurg Psychiatry* **57**, 416–418.

Buckley P, Stack JP, Madigan C, et al. (1993) Magnetic resonance imaging of schizophrenia-like psychoses associated with cerebral trauma: clinicopathological correlates. *Am J Psychiatry* **150**, 146–148.

Bulrich N, Cooper DA, and Freed A (1988) HIV infection associated with symptoms indistinguishable from functional psychosis. *Br J Psychiatry* **152**, 649–653.

Burns A, Jacoby R, and Levy R (1990) Psychiatric phenomena in Alzheimer's disease. III: Disorders of mood. *Br J Psychiatry* **157**, 81–86.

Cairns H, Oldfield RC, Pennybacker JB, et al. (1941) Akinetic mutism with an epidermoid cyst of the 3rd ventricle. *Brain* **64**, 273–290.

Cameron MM (1978) Chronic subdural haematoma: a review of 114 cases. *J Neurol Neurosurg Psychiatry* **41**, 834–839.

Cantu RC and Drew JH (1966) Pathological laughing and crying associated with a tumor ventral to the pons. *J Neurosurg* **24**, 1024–1026.

Cape CA, Martinez AJ, Robertson JJ, et al. (1973) Adult onset of subacute sclerosing panencephalitis. *Arch Neurol* **28**, 124–127.

Caplan LR and Schoene WC (1978) Clinical features of subcortical arteriosclerotic encephalopathy (Binswanger disease). *Neurology* **28**, 1206–1215.

Castillo CS, Schultz SK, and Robinson RG (1995) Clinical correlates of early-onset and late-onset poststroke generalized anxiety. *Am J Psychiatry* **152**, 1174–1179.

Castillo CS, Starkstein SE, Federoff JP, et al. (1993) Generalized anxiety disorder after stroke. *J Nerv Ment Dis* **181**, 100–106.

Cavalleri F and De Renzi E (1994) Amyotrophic lateral sclerosis with dementia. *Acta Neurol Scand* **89**, 391–394.

Celesia GG and Barr AN (1970) Psychosis and other psychiatric manifestations of levodopa therapy. *Arch Neurol* **23**, 193–200.

Chabot B, Roulland C, and Dollfus S (2001) Schizophrenia and familial idiopathic basal ganglia calcification: a case report. *Psychol Med* **31**, 741–747.

Chandler JH and Bebin J (1956) Hereditary cerebellar ataxia: Olivo-pontocerebellar type. *Neurology* **6**, 187–195.

Chaturvedi SK and Upadhyaya M (1988) Secondary mania in a patient receiving isonicotinic acid hydrazide and pyridoxine: case report. *Can J Psychiatry* **33**, 675–676.

Chouinard G and Jones BD (1980) Neuroleptic-induced supersensitivity psychosis. *Am J Psychiatry* **137**, 16–21.

Clark AF and Davison K (1987) Mania following head injury: a report of two cases and a review of the literature. *Br J Psychiatry* **150**, 841–844.

Clarke DJ (1993) Prader–Willi syndrome and psychoses. *Br J Psychiatry* **163**, 680–684.

Cleghorn RA (1951) Adrenal cortical insufficiency: psychological and neurological observations. *Can Med Assoc J* **65**, 445–457.

Cohen L, Mouly S, Tassan P, et al. (1996) A woman with a relapsing psychosis who got better with prednisone. *Lancet* **347**, 1228.

Coid J and Strang J (1982) Mania secondary to procyclidine ("Kemadrin") abuse. *Br J Psychiatry* **141**, 81–84.

Collacott RA, Cooper S-A, and McGrother C (1992) Differential rates of psychiatric disorder in adults with Down's syndrome compared with other mentally handicapped adults. *Br J Psychiatry* **161**, 671–674.

Colman WS (1894) A case of pseudo-bulbar paralysis, due to lesions in each internal capsule; degeneration of direct and crossed pyramidal tracts. *Brain* **17**, 88–89.

Cooper AJ (1967) Hypomanic psychosis precipitated by hemodialysis. *Compr Psychiatry* **8**, 168–172.

Corsellis JAN, Goldberg GJ, and Norton AR (1968) "Limbic encephalitis" and its association with carcinoma. *Brain* **91**, 481–496.

Critchley M and Greenfield JG (1948) Olivo-ponto-cerebellar atrophy. *Brain* **71**, 343–364.

Cummings JL and Duchen LW (1981) Klüver–Bucy syndrome in Pick disease: clinical and pathologic correlations. *Neurology* **31**, 1415–1422.

Cummings JL and Mendez MF (1984) Secondary mania with focal cerebrovascular disease. *Am J Psychiatry* **141**, 1084–1087.

Cummings JL, Miller B, Hill MA, et al. (1987) Neuropsychiatric aspects of multi-infarct dementia and dementia of the Alzheimer-type. *Arch Neurol* **44**, 389–393.

Dalos NP, Rabins PV, Brooks BR, et al. (1983) Disease activity and emotional state in multiple sclerosis. *Ann Neurol* **13**, 573–577.

Davison C and Kelman H (1939) Pathologic laughing and crying. *Arch Neurol Psychiatry* **42**, 595–643.

DeGreef G, Barr WB, Lieberman JA, et al. (1995) Postictal and chronic psychoses in patients with temporal lobe epilepsy. *Am J Psychiatry* **152**, 224–231.

DeMuth GW (1983) Alpha-methyldopa and depression: a clinical study and review of the literature. *Am J Psychiatry* **140**, 534–538.

Dening TR and Berrios GE (1989) Wilson's disease: psychiatric symptoms in 195 cases. *Arch Gen Psychiatry* **46**, 1126–1134.

Dennis MS, Byrne EJ, Hopkinson N, et al. (1992) Neuropsychiatric systemic lupus erythematosus in elderly people: a case series. *J Neurol Neurosurg Psychiatry* **55**, 1157–1161.

Devinsky O, Petito CK, and Alonso DR (1989) Clinical and neuropathological findings in systemic lupus erythematosus: the role of vasculitis, heart emboli and thrombotic thrombocytopenic purpura. *Ann Neurol* **23**, 380–384.

Deymeer F, Smith TW, DeGirolami U, et al. (1989) Thalamic dementia and motor neuron disease. *Neurology* **39**, 58–61.

Dilsaver SC, Feinberg M, and Greden JF (1983) Antidepressant withdrawal symptoms treated with anticholinergic agents. *Am J Psychiatry* **140**, 249–251.

Drachman DA and Adams RD (1962) Herpes simplex and acute inclusion body encephalitis. *Arch Neurol* **7**, 45–63.

Ellis JM and Lee SI (1978) Acute prolonged confusion in later life as an ictal state. *Epilepsia* **19**, 119–128.

El-Mallakh RS, Shrader SA, and Widger E (1987) Single case study: Mania as a manifestation of end-stage renal disease. *J Nerv Ment Dis* **175**, 243–245.

Engel J, Ludwig BI, and Fetell M (1978) Prolonged partial complex status epilepticus: EEG and behavioral observations. *Neurology* **28**, 863–869.

Escalona PR, Adair JC, Roberts BB, et al. (1997) Obsessive–compulsive disorder following bilateral globus pallidus infarction. *Biol Psychiatry* **42**, 410–412.

Ettlin TM, Kischka U, Reichmann S, et al. (1992) Cerebral symptoms after whiplash injury of the neck: a prospective clinical and neuropsychological study of whiplash injury. *J Neurol Neurosurg Psychiatry* **55**, 943–948.

Evans DL, Edelsohn GA, and Golden RN (1983) Organic psychosis without anemia or spinal cord symptoms in patients with vitamin B_{12} deficiency. *Am J Psychiatry* **140**, 218–221.

Falk WE, Mahnke MD, and Poskanzer MD (1979) Lithium prophylaxis of corticotrophin-induced psychosis. *JAMA* **241**, 1011–1012.

Fann KR, Katon WJ, Uomoto JM, et al. (1995) Psychiatric disorders and functional disability in outpatients with traumatic brain injuries. *Am J Psychiatry* **152**, 1493–1499.

Federoff PJ, Starkstein SE, Forrester AW, et al. (1992) Depression in patients with acute traumatic brain injury. *Am J Psychiatry* **149**, 918–923.

Feinberg WM and Rapcsak SZ (1989) "Peduncular hallucinosis" following paramedian thalamic infarction. *Neurology* **39**, 1535–1536.

Feinstein A, Feinstein K, Gray T, et al. (1997) Prevalence and neurobehavioral correlates of pathological laughing and crying in multiple sclerosis. *Arch Neurol* **54**, 1116–1121.

Fenelon G, Mathieux F, Huon R, et al. (2000) Hallucinations in Parkinson's disease: prevalence, phenomenology and risk factors. *Brain* **123**, 733–745.

Fontaine B, Seilhean D, Tourbah A, et al. (1994) Dementia in two histologically confirmed cases of multiple sclerosis: one case with related dementia and one case associated with psychiatric symptoms. *J Neurol Neurosurg Psychiatry* **57**, 353–359.

Francis A and Freeman H (1984) Psychiatric abnormality and brain calcification over four generations. *J Nerv Ment Dis* **172**, 166–170.

Fras I and Pearson JS (1967) Comparison of psychiatric symptoms in carcinoma of the pancreas with those in some other intra-abdominal neoplasms. *Am J Psychiatry* **123**, 1553–1562.

Fraser TN (1960) Cerebral manifestations of Addisonian pernicious anemia. *Lancet* **2**, 458–459.

Frazier CH (1936) Tumor involving the frontal lobe alone: a symptomatic survey of one hundred and five verified cases. *Arch Neurol Psychiatry* **35**, 525–571.

Friedman HM and Allen H (1969) Chronic effects of complete limbic lobe destruction in man. *Neurology* **19**, 679–690.

Gal P (1958) Mental symptoms in cases of tumor of the temporal lobe. *Am J Psychiatry* **115**, 157–160.

Gallagher JP (1989) Pathologic laughter and crying in ALS: a search for their origin. *Acta Neurol Scand* **80**, 114–117.

Gelenberg AJ and Mandel MR (1977) Catatonic reactions to high-potency neuroleptic drugs. *Arch Gen Psychiatry* **34**, 945–950.

Gentilini M, De Renzi E, and Crisi G (1987) Bilateral paramedian thalamic artery infarcts: Report of eight cases. *J Neurol Neurosurg Psychiatry* **50**, 900–909.

Geocaris K (1957) Psychotic episodes heralding the diagnosis of multiple sclerosis. *Bull Mayo Clin* **21**, 107–116.

Giovannoni G, O'Sullivan JD, Turner K, et al. (2000) Hedonistic homeostatic dysregulation in patients with Parkinson's disease on dopamine replacement therapies. *J Neurol Neurosurg Psychiatry* **68**, 423–428.

Giroud M, Lemesle M, Madiner G, et al. (1997) Unilateral lenticular infarcts: radiological and clinical syndromes, etiology and prognosis. *J Neurol Neurosurg Psychiatry* **63**, 611–615.

Goggans FC (1984) A case of mania secondary to vitamin B_{12} deficiency. *Am J Psychiatry* **141**, 300–301.

Golden RN, James SP, Sherer MA, et al. (1985) Psychoses associated with bupropion treatment. *Am J Psychiatry* **142**, 1459–1462.

Gomez EA, Comstock BJ, and Rosario A (1982) Organic versus functional etiology in catatonia: case report. *J Clin Psychiatry* **43**, 200–201.

Greenberg DB and Brown GL (1985) Single case study: Mania resulting from brain stem tumor. *J Nerv Ment Dis* **173**, 434–436.

Greenwood R, Bhalla A, Gordon A, et al. (1983) Behavior disturbances during recovery from herpes simplex encephalitis. *J Neurol Neurosurg Psychiatry* **46**, 809–817.

Hageman ATM, Gabreels FJM, de Jong JGN, et al. (1995) Clinical symptoms of adult metachromatic leukodystrophy and arylsulfatase a pseudodeficiency. *Arch Neurol* **52**, 408–413.

Hall DP and Young SA (1992) Frontal lobe cerebral aneurysm rupture presenting as psychosis. *J Neurol Neurosurg Psychiatry* **55**, 1207–1208.

Hammes EM (1992) Psychoses associated with Sydenham's chorea. *J Am Med Assoc* **79**, 804–807.

Hardwick SW (1943) Pellagra in psychiatric patients: twelve recent cases. *Lancet* **2**, 43–45.

Harris MJ, Jeste DV, Gleghorn A, et al. (1991) New-onset psychosis in HIV-infected patients. *J Clin Psychiatry* **52**, 369–376.

Haskett RF (1985) Diagnostic categorization of psychiatric disturbance in Cushing's syndrome. *Am J Psychiatry* **142**, 911–916.

Heathfield KW (1967) Huntington's chorea. Investigation into the prevalence of this disease in the area covered by the North East metropolitan regional hospital board. *Brain* **90**, 203–232.

Hermann BP, Whitman S, Wyler AR, et al. (1988) The neurological, psychosocial and demographic correlates of hypergraphia in patients with epilepsy. *J Neurol Neurosurg Psychiatry* **51**, 203–208.

Hertz PE, Nadas E, and Wojtkowski H (1955) Case report: Cushing's syndrome and its management. *Am J Psychiatry* **112**, 144–145.

Heutink P, Stevens M, Rizzu P, et al. (1997) Hereditary fronto-temporal dementia is linked to chromosome 17q21–q22: a genetic and clinicopathological study of three Dutch families. *Ann Neurol* **41**, 150–159.

Hillbom E (1960) After-effects of brain injuries. *Acta Psychiatr Scand* **142**(Suppl.), 1–195.

Hillbom S (1951) Schizophrenia-like psychoses after brain trauma. *Acta Psychiatr Neurol Scand* **60**(Suppl.), 36–47.

Hirsch S and Dunsworth FA (1955) An interesting case of porphyria. *Am J Psychiatry* **111**, 703.

Hodgson RE, Murray D, and Woods MR (1992) Othello's syndrome and hyperthyroidism. *J Nerv Ment Dis* **180**, 663–664.

Hohman LB (1921) Epidemic encephalitis (lethargic encephalitis): its psychotic manifestations with a report of twenty-three cases. *Arch Neurol Psychiatry* **6**, 295–333.

Hullett FJ, Potkin SG, Levy AB, et al. (1988) Depression associated with nifedipine-induced calcium channel blockade. *Am J Psychiatry* **145**, 1277–1279.

Hunter R, Blackwood W, and Bull J (1968) Three cases of frontal meningiomas presenting psychiatrically. *Br Med J* **3**, 9–16.

Hyde TM, Ziegler JL, and Weinberger DR (1992) Psychiatric disturbances in metachromatic leukodystrophy: insights into the neurobiology of psychosis. *Arch Neurol* **49**, 401–406.

Indaco A, Carrieri PB, Nappi C, et al. (1992) Interictal depression in epilepsy. *Epilepsy Res* **12**, 45–50.

Ingham SD and Nielsen JM (1931) Thyroid psychosis: difficulties in diagnosis. *J Nerv Ment Dis* **74**, 271–277.

Ironside R (1956) Disorders of laughter due to brain lesions. *Brain* **79**, 589–609.

Ironside R and Guttmacher M (1929) The corpus callosum and its tumors. *Brain* **52**, 442–483.

Ishii N, Nishihara Y, and Imamura T (1986) Why do frontal lobe symptoms predominate in vascular dementia with lacunes? *Neurology* **36**, 340–345.

Jack RA (1985) A case of mania secondary to propafenone. *J Clin Psychiatry* **46**, 104–105.

Jack RA, Rivers-Bulkeley NT, and Rabin PL (1983) Single case study: secondary mania as a presentation of progressive dialysis encephalopathy. *J Nerv Ment Dis* **171**, 193–195.

Jackson JA and Zimmerman SL (1919) A case of pseudosclerosis associated with a psychosis. *J Nerv Ment Dis* **49**, 5–13.

Jaffe N (1967) Catatonia and hepatic dysfunction. *Dis Nerv Syst* **28**, 606–608.

Jampala VC and Abrams R (1983) Mania secondary to left and right hemisphere damage. *Am J Psychiatry* **140**, 1197–1199.

Jelliffe SE (1929) Oculogyric crises as compulsion phenomena in postencephalitis: their occurrence, phenomenology and meaning. *J Nerv Ment Dis* **69**, 59–68, 165–184, 278–297, 415–426, 531–551, 666–679.

Jensen K (1959) Depression in patients treated with reserpine for arterial hypertension. *Acta Psychiatr Neurol Scand* **34**, 195–204.

Johnson RI and Richardson EP (1968) The neurological manifestations of systemic lupus erythematosus. *Medicine* **47**, 337–369.

Johnson KP, Rosenthal MS, and Lerner PI (1972) Herpes simplex encephalitis. *Arch Neurol* **27**, 103–108.

Jones AM Jones AM (1993b) Psychiatric presentation of a third ventricular colloid cyst in a mentally handicapped woman. *Br J Psychiatry* **163**, 677–678.

Jorge RE, Robinson RG, Starkstein SE, et al. (1993a) Secondary mania following traumatic brain injury. *Am J Psychiatry* **150**, 916–921.

Jorge RE, Robinson RG, Starkstein SE, et al. (1993b) Depression and anxiety following traumatic brain injury. *J Neuropsychiatry Clin Neurosci* **5**, 369–374.

Kanemoto K, Kawasaki J, and Kawai I (1996) Postictal psychosis: a comparison with acute interictal and chronic psychoses. *Epilepsia* **37**, 551.

Kanner AM, Stagno S, Kotagal P, et al. (1996) Postictal psychiatric events during prolonged video-electro-encephalographic monitoring studies. *Arch Neurol* **53**, 258–263.

Karnosh LJ and Stout RE (1935) Psychoses of myxedema. *Am J Psychiatry* **91**, 1263–1274.

Karpati G and Frame B (1964) Neuropsychiatric disorders in primary hyperparathyroidism: clinical analysis with review of the literature. *Arch Neurol* **10**, 387–397.

Kelly WF (1996) Psychiatric aspects of Cushing's syndrome. *Q J Med* **89**, 543–551.

Kent TA and Wilber RD (1982) Single case study: reserpine withdrawal psychosis: the possible role of denerevation supersensitivity of receptors. *J Nerv Ment Dis* **170**, 502–504.

Keschner M, Bender MB, and Strauss I (1936) Mental symptoms in cases of tumor of the temporal lobe. *Arch Neurol Psychiatry* **35**, 572–596.

Khanna R and Borde M (1989) Mania in a five-year-old child with tuberous sclerosis. *Br J Psychiatry* **155**, 117–119.

Kim CH and Perlstein MA (1970) Encephalitis with catatonic schizophrenic symptoms. *Ill Med J* **138**, 503–507.

Kirby GH and Davis TK (1921) Psychiatric aspects of epidemic encephalitis. *Arch Neurol Psychiatry* **5**, 491–551.

Kirubakaren V, Mayfield D, and Rengachary S (1984) Dyskinesia and psychosis in a patient following baclofen withdrawal. *Am J Psychiatry* **141**, 692–693.

Klatka LA, Louis ED, and Schiffer RB (1996) Psychiatric features in diffuse Lewy body disease: a clinicopathologic study using Alzheimer's disease and Parkinson's disease comparison groups. *Neurology* **47**, 1148–1152.

Klüver H and Bucy PC (1939) Preliminary analysis of functions of the temporal lobes in monkeys. *Arch Neurol Psychiatry* **42**, 979–1000.

Koehler J and Jakumeit U (1976) Subacute sclerosing panencephalitis presenting as Leonhard's speech-prompt catatonia. *Br J Psychiatry* **129**, 29–31.

Koo EH and Massey EW (1988) Granulomatous angiitis of the central nervous system: protean manifestations and response to treatment. *J Neurol Neurosurg Psychiatry* **51**, 1126–1133.

Kristensen O and Sindrup EH (1979) Psychomotor epilepsy and psychosis, III: Social and psychological correlates. *Acta Psychiatr Scand* **59**, 1–9.

Kroll L and Drummond LM (1993) Temporal lobe epilepsy and obsessive–compulsive symptoms. *J Nerv Ment Dis* **181**, 457–458.

Kulisevsky J, Asuncion A, and Berthier ML (1995) Bipolar affective disorder and unilateral parkinsonism after a brain stem infarction. *Mov Disord* **10**, 799–802.

Kulisevsky J, Berthier ML, and Pujol J (1993) Hemiballismus and secondary mania following right thalamic infarction. *Neurology* **43**, 1422–1424.

Kwentus JA, Silverman JJ, and Sprague M (1984) Manic syndrome after metrizamide myelography. *Am J Psychiatry* **141**, 700–702.

Labbate LA and Holzgang AJ (1989) Holzgang AJ: Manic syndrome after discontinuation of methyldopa. *Am J Psychiatry* **146**, 1075–1076.

Lambert MT (1987) Paranoid psychoses after abuse of proprietary cold remedies. *Br J Psychiatry* **151**, 548–550.

Lancman ME, Craven WJ, Asconape JJ, et al. (1994) Clinical management of recurrent postictal psychosis. *J Epilepsy* **7**, 47–51.

Langsworthy OR and Hesser FH (1940) Syndrome of pseudobulbar palsy. *Arch Int Med* **65**, 106–121.

Langworthy OR, Kolb LC, and Androp S (1941) Disturbances of behavior in patients with disseminated sclerosis. *Am J Psychiatry* **98**, 243–249.

Lanham JG, Brown MM, and Hughes GRV (1985) Cerebral systemic lupus erythematosus presenting with catatonia. *Postgrad Med J* **61**, 329–330.

LaPlane D, Baulac M, Widlocher D, et al. (1984) Pure psychic akinesia with bilateral lesion of basal ganglia. *J Neurol Neurosurg Psychiatry* **47**, 377–385.

LaPlane D, Levasseur M, Pillon B, et al. (1989) Obsessive–compulsive and other behavioral changes with bilateral basal ganglia lesions. *Brain* **112**, 699–725.

Lawlor BA (1988) Hypocalcemia, hypoparathyroidism, and organic anxiety syndrome. *J Clin Psychiatry* **49**, 317–318.

Lebensohn ZM (1947) Self-inflicted bullet wound of frontal lobes in a depression with recovery. *Am J Psychiatry* **98**, 56–62.

Lendvai I, Saravay SM, and Steinberg MD (1999) Creutzfeldt–Jakob disease presenting as secondary mania. *Psychosomatics* **40**, 524–525.

Lieberman A and Benson DF (1977) Control of emotional expression in pseudobulbar palsy. *Arch Neurol* **34**, 717–719.

Lilly R, Cummings JL, Benson DF, et al. (1983) The human Klüver–Bucy syndrome. *Neurology* **33**, 1141–1145.

Lim L, Ron MA, Ormerod IEC, et al. (1988) Psychiatric and neurological manifestations in systemic lupus erythematosus. *Q J Med* **66**, 27–38.

Lim J, Yagnik P, Schraeder P, et al. (1986) Ictal catatonia as a manifestation of nonconvulsive status epilepticus. *J Neurol Neurosurg Psychiatry* **49**, 833–836.

Lindenbaum J, Healton EB, Savage DG, et al. (1988) Neuropsychiatric disorders caused by cobalamin deficiency in the absence of anemia or macrocytosis. *N Engl J Med* **318**, 1720–1728.

Lipsey JR, Spencer WC, Rabins PV, et al. (1986) Phenomenological comparison of poststroke depression and functional depression. *Am J Psychiatry* **143**, 527–529.

Lishman WA (1973) The psychiatric sequelae of head injury: a review. *Psychol Med* **3**, 304–318.

Litvan I, Agid Y, Sastrj N, et al. (1997) What are the obstacles for an accurate clinical diagnosis of Pick's disease? *Neurology* **49**, 62–69.

Logsdail SJ and Toone BK (1988) Postictal psychoses: a clinical and phenomenological description. *Br J Psychiatry* **152**, 246–252.

Lopez-Villegas D, Kulisevsky J, Deus J, et al. (1996) Neuropsychological alterations in patients with computed tomography-detected basal ganglia calcification. *Arch Neurol* **53**, 251–256.

Mac DS and Pardo MP (1983) Systemic lupus erythematosus and catatonia: a case report. *J Clin Psychiatry* **44**, 155–156.

MacCrimmon DJ, Wallace JE, Goldberg WM, et al. (1979) Emotional disturbances and cognitive deficits in hyperthyroidism. *Psychosom Med* **41**, 331–340.

Malamud N (1967) Psychiatric disorders with intracranial tumors of limbic system. *Arch Neurol* **17**, 113–123.

Malinow KC and Lion JR (1979) Hyperaldosteronism (Conn's disease) presenting as depression. *J Clin Psychiatry* **40**, 358–359.

Mandalos GE and Szarek BL (1990) Dose-related paranoid reaction associated with fluoxetine. *J Nerv Ment Dis* **178**, 57–58.

Mandoki MW and Sumner GS (1994) Psychiatric manifestations of hereditary coproporphyria in a child. *J Nerv Ment Dis* **182**, 117–118.

Mann AM and Hutchinson JL (1967) Manic reaction associated with procarbazine hydrochloride therapy of Hodgkin's disease. *Can Med Assoc J* **97**, 1350–1353.

Marlowe WB, Mancall EL, and Thomas TJ (1975) Complete Klüver–Bucy syndrome in man. *Cortex* **11**, 53–59.

Massman PJ, Sims J, Cooke N, et al. (1996) Prevalence and correlates of neuropsychological deficits in amyotrophic lateral sclerosis. *J Neurol Neurosurg psychiatry* **61**, 450–455.

Mathews WB (1979) Multiple sclerosis presenting with acute remitting psychiatric symptoms. *J Neurol Neurosurg Psychiatry* **42**, 859–863.

Max JE, Robertson BAM, and Lansing AE (2001) The phenomenology of personality change due to traumatic brain injury in children and adolescents. *J Neuropsychiatry Clin Neurosci* **13**, 161–170.

Mayeux R, Stern Y, Williams JBW, et al. (1986) Clinical and biochemical features of depression in Parkinson's disease. *Am J Psychiatry* **143**, 756–759.

McFarland HR (1963) Addison's disease and related psychoses. *Compr Psychiatry* **4**, 90–95.

McGilchrist I, Goldstein LH, Jadresic D, et al. (1993) Thalamo-frontal psychosis. *Br J Psychiatry* **163**, 113–115.

McGrath N, Anderson NE, Croxson MC, et al. (1997) Herpes simplex encephalitis treated with acyclovir: diagnosis and long-term outcome. *J Neurol Neurosurg Psychiatry* **63**, 321–326.

McKeon J, McGuffin P, and Robinson P (1984) Obsessive–compulsive neurosis following head injury. A report of four cases. *Br J Psychiatry* **144**, 190–192.

Mega MS, Cummings JL, Fiorello T, et al. (1996) The spectrum of behavioral changes in Alzheimer's disease. *Neurology* **46**, 130–135.

Mendez MF, Adams NL, and Lewandowski KS (1989) Neurobehavioral changes associated with caudate lesions. *Neurology* **39**, 349–354.

Mendez MF, Cherrier MM, and Perryman KM (1996) Epileptic forced thinking from left frontal lesions. *Neurology* **47**, 79–83.

Mendez MF, Cummings JL, and Benson DF (1986) Depression in epilepsy. Significance and phenomenology. *Arch Neurol* **43**, 766–770.

Mendez MF and Foti DJ (1997) Lethal hyperoral behavior from the Klüver–Bucy syndrome. *J Neurol Neurosurg Psychiatry* **62**, 293–294.

Mendez MF, Selwood A, Mastri AR, et al. (1993) Pick's disease versus Alzheimer's disease: a comparison of clinical characteristics. *Neurology* **43**, 289–292.

Meninger KA (1926) Influenza and schizophrenia. *Am J Psychiatry* **82**, 469–529.

Menza MA, Cocchiola J, and Golbe LI (1995) Psychiatric symptoms in progressive supranuclear palsy. *Psychosomatics* **36**, 550–554.

Miguel EC, Rodriguez Pereira RM, de Braganca Pereira CA, et al. (1994) Psychiatric manifestations of systemic lupus erythematosus: clinical features, symptoms and signs of central nervous system activity in 43 patients. *Medicine* **73**, 224–232.

Millman RP, Fogel BS, McNamara ME, et al. (1989) Depression as a manifestation of obstructive sleep apnea: reversal with nasal continuous positive airway pressure. *J Clin Psychiatry* **50**, 348–351.

Minden SL, Orav J, and Schildkraut JJ (1988) Hypomanic reactions to ACTH and prednisone treatment for multiple sclerosis. *Neurology* **38**, 1631–1634.

Misra PC and Hay GG (1971) Encephalitis presenting as acute schizophrenia. *Br Med J* **1**, 532–533.

Moersch FP (1925) Psychic manifestations in cases of brain tumors. *Am J Psychiatry* **81**, 707–724.

Moskovich DG, Singh MB, Eva FJ, et al. (1995) Acute disseminated encephalomyelitis presenting as an acute psychotic state. *J Nerv Ment Dis* **183**, 116–117.

Motomura S, Tabira T, and Kuroiwa Y (1980) A clinical comparative study of multiple sclerosis and neuro-Behcet's syndrome. *J Neurol Neurosurg Psychiatry* **43**, 210–213.

Mulder DW and Daly D (1952) Psychiatric symptoms associated with lesions of temporal lobe. *J Am Med Assoc* **150**, 173–176.

Mulder DW, Parrott M, and Thaler M (1951) Sequelae of western equine encephalitis. *Neurology* **1**, 318–327.

Muller D, Pilz H, and Ter Meulen V (1969) Studies on adult metachromatic leukodystrophy. I. Clinical, morphological and histochemical observations in two cases. *J Neurol Sci* **9**, 567–584.

Murphy TL, Chalmers TC, Eckhardt RD, et al. (1948) Hepatic coma: clinical and laboratory observations on 40 patients. *N Engl J Med* **239**, 605–612.

Murphy KC, Jones LA, and Owen MJ (1999) High rates of schizophrenia in adults with velo–cardio–facial syndrome. *Arch Gen Psychiatry* **56**, 940–945.

Murthy P, Jayakumar PN, and Sampat S (1997) Of insects and eggs: a case report. *J Neurol Neurosurg Psychiatry* **63**, 522–523.

Nakada T, Lee H, Kwee IL, et al. (1984) Epileptic Klüver–Bucy syndrome: case report. *J Clin Psychiatry* **45**, 87–88.

Nasrallah HA, Fowler RC, and Judd LL (1981) Schizophrenia-like illness following head injury. *Psychosomatics* **22**, 359–361.

Navia BA, Jordan BD, and Price RW (1986) The AIDS dementia complex: I. Clinical features. *Ann Neurol* **19**, 517–524.

Neary D, Snowden JS, Mann DMA, et al. (1990) Frontal lobe dementia and motor neuron disease. *J Neurol Neurosurg Psychiatry* **53**, 23–32.

Neary D, Snowden JS, and Mann DMA (1993) Familial progressive atrophy: its relationship to other forms of lobar atrophy. *J Neurol Neurosurg Psychiatry* **56**, 1122–1125.

Neilley LK, Goodin DD, Goodkin DE, et al. (1996) Side effect profile of interferon-1b in MS: results of an open-label trial. *Neurology* **46**, 552–554.

Nickel SN and Frame B (1958) Neurologic manifestations of myxedema. *Neurology* **8**, 511–517.

Nizamie SH, Nizamie A, Borde M, et al. (1988) Mania following head injury: case reports and neuropsychological findings. *Acta Psychiatr Scand* **77**, 637–639.

O'Carroll RE, Masterton G, Dougall N, et al. (1995) The neuropsychiatric sequelae of mercury poisoning: the Mad Hatter's disease revisited. *Br J Psychiatry* **167**, 95–98.

Oder W, Goldenberg G, Spatt J, et al. (1992) Behavioral and psychosocial sequelae of severe closed head injury and regional cerebral blood flow: a SPECT study. *J Neurol Neurosurg Psychiatry* **55**, 475–480.

O'Dowd MA and McKegney FP (1988) Manic syndrome associated with zidovudine. *JAMA* **260**, 3587–3588.

Pakainis A, Drake ME, John K, et al. (1987) Forced normalization: acute psychosis after seizure control in seven patients. *Arch Neurol* **44**, 289–292.

Parker N (1956) Disseminated sclerosis presenting as schizophrenia. *Med J Aust* **1**, 405–407.

Paskavitz JF, Anderson CA, Filley CM, et al. (1995) Acute arcuate fiber demyelinating encephalopathy following Epstein–Barr virus infection. *Ann Neurol* **38**, 127–131.

Peavy GM, Herzog AG, Rubin NP, et al. (1992) Neuropsychological aspects of dementia with motor neuron disease: a report of two cases. *Neurology* **42**, 1004–1008.

Penn H, Racy J, Lapham L, et al. (1972) Catatonic behavior, viral encephalopathy, and death: the problem of fatal catatonia. *Arch Gen Psychiatry* **27**, 758–761.

Perez NM and Trimble MR (1980) Epileptic psychosis–diagnostic comparison with process schizophrenia. *Br J Psychiatry* **137**, 245–249.

Perini GI, Tosin C, Carraro C, et al. (1996) Interictal mood and personality disorders in temporal lobe epilepsy and juvenile myoclonic epilepsy. *J Neurol Neurosurg Psychiatry* **61**, 601–605.

Peroutka SJ, Sohmer BH, Kumer AJ, et al. (1982) Hallucinations and delusions following a right temporo-parietal–occipital infarction. *Johns Hopkins Med J* **151**, 181–185.

Petrie WM, Maffucci RJ, and Woosley RL (1982) Propranolol and depression. *Am J Psychiatry* **139**, 93–94.

Petry S, Cummings JL, Hill MA, et al. (1988) Personality alterations in dementia of the Alzheimer type. *Arch Neurol* **45**, 187–1190.

Petty RG, Bonner D, Mouratoglou V, et al. (1996) Acute frontal lobe syndrome and dyscontrol associated with bilateral caudate nucleus infarctions. *Br J Psychiatry* **168**, 237–240.

Pfister H-W, Preac-Mursic V, Wilske B, et al. (1993) Catatonic syndrome in acute severe encephalitis due to *Borrelia burgdorferi* infection. *Neurology* **43**, 433–435.

Pflanz S, Besson JAO, Ebmeier KP, et al. (1991) The clinical manifestations of mental disorder in Huntington's disease: a retrospective case record study of disease progression. *Acta Psychiatr Scand* **83**, 53–60.

Pitt DC, Kriel RL, Wagner NC, et al. (1995) Klüver–Bucy syndrome following heat stroke in a 12-year-old girl. *Pediatr Neurol* **13**, 73–76.

Pollack MH, Rosenbaum JF, and Cassem NH (1985) Brief communication: propranolol and depression revisited: three cases and a review. *J Nerv Ment Dis* **173**, 118–119.

Pope HG and Katz DL (1994) Psychiatric and medical effects of anabolic-androgenic steroid use: a controlled study of 160 athletes. *Arch Gen Psychiatry* **51**, 375–382.

Powers JM, Schaumburg HH, and Gaffney CL (1980) Klüver–Bucy syndrome caused by adrenoleukodystrophy. *Neurology* **30**, 1131–1132.

Price WA and Bielfeld M (1989) Buspirone-induced mania. *J Clin Psychopharmacol* **9**, 150–151.

Pujol J, Leal S, Fluvia X, et al. (1989) Psychiatric aspects of normal pressure hydrocephalus. *Br J Psychiatry* **154**(Suppl. 4), 77–80.

Quetsch RM, Achor RWP, Litin EM, et al. (1959) Depressive reactions in hypertensive patients. *Circulation* **19**, 366–375.

Rabins PV, Brooks BR, O'Connell P, et al. (1986) Structural brain correlates of emotional disorder in multiple sclerosis. *Brain* **109**, 585–597.

Raskin DE and Frank SW (1974) Herpes encephalitis with catatonic stupor. *Arch Gen Psychiatry* **31**, 544–546.

Raymond RW and Williams RL (1948) Infectious mononucleosis with psychosis. *N Engl J Med* **239**, 542–544.

Read SL (1983) Catatonia in thrombotic thrombocytopenic purpura. *J Clin Psychiatry* **44**, 343–344.

Reaser EF (1940) Chorea of infectious origin. *South Med J* **33**, 1324–1328.

Reed K and Bland RC (1977) Masked "myxedema madness". *Acta Psychiatr Scand* **56**, 421–426.

Reisberg B (1978) Single case study: Catatonia associated with disulfiram therapy. *J Nerv Ment Dis* **166**, 607–609.

Rice E and Gendelman S (1973) Psychiatric aspects of normal pressure hydrocephalus. *JAMA* **223**, 409–412.

Robbins TW, Jones M, Lange TW, et al. (1992) Cognitive performance in multiple system atrophy. *Brain* **115**, 271–291.

Roberts AH (1976) Sequelae of closed head injuries. *Proc R Soc Med* **69**, 137–141.

Robinson RG, Bolduc P, and Price TR (1987) A two year longitudinal study of poststroke depression: diagnosis and outcome at one and two year follow-up. *Stroke* **18**, 837–843.

Robinson RG, Kubos KL, Starr LB, et al. (1984) Mood disorders in stroke patients. *Brain* **107**, 81–93.

Robinson RG, Schultz SK, Castillo C, et al. (2000) Nortriptyline versus fluoxetine in the treatment of depression and in short-term recovery after stroke: a placebo-controlled, double-blind study. *Am J Psychiatry* **157**, 351–359.

Rodin E and Schmaltz S (1984) The Bear–Fedio personality inventory and temporal lobe epilepsy. *Neurology* **34**, 591–596.

Roos R, Cajdusek DC, and Gibbs CJ (1973) The clinical characteristics of transmissible Creutzfeldt–Jakob disease. *Brain* **96**, 1–20.

Rosebush PI, MacQueen GM, Clarke JTR, et al. (1995) Late-onset Tay–Sachs disease presenting as catatonic schizophrenia: diagnostic and treatment issues. *J Clin Psychiatry* **56**, 347–353.

Rosebush PI and Mazurek MF (1996) Catatonia after benzodiazepine withdrawal. *J Clin Psychopharmacol* **16**, 315–319.

Rothschild D (1940) Dementia paralytica accompanied by manic–depressive and schizophrenic psychoses. *Am J Psychiatry* **96**, 1043–1060.

Sale A and Kalucy P (1981) Psychosis associated with oral contraceptive-induced chorea. *Med J Aust* **1**, 79–80.

Salib EA (1988) Subacute sclerosing panencephalitis (SSPE) presenting at the age of 21 as a schizophrenia-like state with bizarre dysmorphophobic features. *Br J Psychiatry* **152**, 709–710.

Sands IJ (1928) The acute psychiatric type of epidemic encephalitis. *Am J Psychiatry* **84**, 975–987.

Sandson TA, Daffner KR, Carvalho PA, et al. (1991) Frontal lobe dysfunction following infarction of the left-sided medial thalamus. *Arch Neurol* **48**, 1300–1303.

Savard G, Andermann F, Olivier A, et al. (1991) Postictal psychoses after partial complex seizures: a multiple case study. *Epilepsia* **32**, 225–231.

Schaumburg HH, Powers JM, Raine CS, et al. (1975) Adrenoleukodystrophy: a clinical and pathological study of 17 cases. *Arch Neurol* **32**, 577–591.

Schiffer RB, Herndon RM, and Rudick RA (1985) Treatment of pathologic laughing and weeping with amitriptyline. *N Engl J Med* **312**, 1480–1482.

Schottenfeld RS and Cullen MR (1984) Organic affective illness associated with lead intoxication. *Am J Psychiatry* **141**, 1425–1426.

Schube PG (1934) Emotional states of general paresis. *Am J Psychiatry* **91**, 625–638.

Seliger GM and Hornstein A (1989) Serotonin, fluoxetine and pseudobulbar affect. *Neurology* **39**, 1400.

Serby M, Angrist B, and Lieberman A (1978) Mental disturbances during bromocriptine and lergotrile treatment of Parkinson's disease. *Am J Psychiatry* **135**, 1227–1229.

Shafqat S, Elkind MSV, Chiocca EA, et al. (1998) Petroclival meningioma presenting with pathological laughter. *Neurology* 1918–1919.

Shah P and Kaplan SL (1980) Catatonic symptoms in a child with epilepsy. *Am J Psychiatry* **137**, 738–739.

Shoji H, Teramoto H, Satowa S, et al. (1979) Partial Klüver–Bucy syndrome following probable herpes simplex encephalitis. *J Neurol* **221**, 163–167.

Siegal FP (1978) Lithium for steroid-induced psychosis. *N Engl J Med* **299**, 155–156.

Simpson S and Baldwin B (1995) Neuropsychiatry and SPECT of an acute obsessive–compulsive syndrome patient. *Br J Psychiatry* **166**, 390–392.

Slater E and Beard AW (1963a) The schizophrenia-like psychoses of epilepsy. *Br J Psychiatry* **109**, 95–112.

Slater E and Beard AW (1963b) The schizophrenia-like psychoses of epilepsy. *Br J Psychiatry* **109**, 143–150.

Slyter H (1979) Idiopathic hypoparathyroidism presenting as dementia. *Neurology* **29**, 393–394.

Smith LH (1929) Mental and neurologic changes in pernicious anemia. *Arch Neurol Psychiatry* **22**, 551–557.

Starkman MN, Zelnick TC, Nesse RM, et al. (1985) Anxiety in patients with pheochromocytomas. *Arch Int Med* **145**, 248–252.

Starkstein SE, Boston JD, and Robinson RG (1988) Mechanism of mania after brain injury: 12 cases reports and review of the literature. *J Nerv Ment Dis* **176**, 87–100.

Starkstein SE, Chemerinski E, Sabe L, et al. (1997) Prospective longitudinal study of depression and anosognosia in Alzheimer's disease. *Br J Psychiatry* **171**, 47–52.

Starkstein SE, Cohen BS, Federoff P, et al. (1990) Relationship between anxiety disorders and depressive disorders in patients with cerebrovascular injury. *Arch Gen Psychiatry* **47**, 785–789.

Starkstein SE, Mayberg HS, Berthier ML, et al. (1990) Mania after brain injury: Neuroradiological and metabolic findings. *Ann Neurol* **27**, 652–659.

Starkstein SE, Migliorelli R, Teson A, et al. (1995) Prevalence and clinical correlates of pathological affective display in Alzheimer's disease. *J Neurol Neurosurg Psychiatry* **59**, 55–60.

Starkstein SE, Preziosi TJ, Bolduc PL, et al. (1990) Depression in Parkinson's disease. *J Nerv Ment Dis* **178**, 27–31.

Starosta-Rubinstein S, Young AB, Kluin K, et al. (1987) Clinical assessment of 31 patients with Wilson's disease: correlations with structural changes on magnetic resonance imaging. *Arch Neurol* **44**, 365–370.

Steiner W, Laporta M, and Chouinard G (1990) Neuroleptic-induced supersensitivity psychosis in patients with bipolar affective disorder. *Acta Psychiatr Scand* **81**, 437–440.

Stern K and Dancey TE (1942) Glioma of the diencephalon in a manic patient. *Am J Psychiatry* **98**, 716–719.

Storm-Mathisen A (1969) General paresis: a follow-up study of 203 patients. *Acta Psychiatr Scand* **45**, 118–132.

Strauss I and Keschner M (1935) Mental symptoms in cases of tumor of the frontal lobe. *Arch Neurol Psychiatry* **33**, 986–1007.

Strobos RRJ (1953) Tumors of the temporal lobe. *Neurology* **3**, 752–760.

Supino-Viterbo V, Sicard C, Risvegliato M, et al. (1977) Toxic encephalopathy due to ingestion of bismuth salts: clinical and EEG studies of 45 patients. *J Neurol Neurosurg Psychiatry* **40**, 748–752.

Swedo SE, Leonard HL, Schapiro MB, et al. (1993) Physical and psychological symptoms in St. Vitus' dance. *Pediatrics* **91**, 706–713.

Swedo SE, Rapoport JL, Cheslow DL, et al. (1989) High prevalence of obsessive–compulsive symptoms in patients with Sydenham's chorea. *Am J Psychiatry* **146**, 246–249.

Swigar ME and Bowers MB (1986) Baclofen withdrawal and neuropsychiatric symptoms: a case report and review of other case literature. *Compr Psychiatry* **27**, 394–400.

Tandon R, Walden M, and Falcon S (1988) Catatonia as a manifestation of paraneoplastic encephalopathy. *J Clin Psychiatry* **49**, 121–122.

Teri L, Larson EB, and Reifler BV (1988) Behavioral disturbances in dementia of the Alzheimer's type. *J Am Ger Soc* **36**, 1–6.

Terzian H and Dalle Ore G (1955) Syndrome of Klüver and Bucy: reproduced in man by bilateral removal of the temporal lobes. *Neurology* **5**, 373–380.

Thompson GN and Nielsen JM (1949) The organic paranoid syndrome. *J Nerv Ment Dis* **110**, 478–496.

Thomsen IV (1984) Late outcome of very severe blunt head trauma: a 10 to 15 year second follow-up. *J Neurol Neurosurg Psychiatry* **47**, 260–268.

Tonks CM (1964) Mental illness in hypothyroid patients. *Br J Psychiatry* **110**, 706–710.

Trautner RJ, Cummings JL, Read SL, et al. (1988) Idiopathic basal ganglia calcification and organic mood disorders. *Am J Psychiatry* **145**, 350–353.

Trethowan WH and Cobb S (1952) Neuropsychiatric aspects of Cushing's syndrome. *Arch Neurol Psychiatry* **67**, 283–309.

Trzepacz P, McCue M, Klein I, et al. (1988) A psychiatric and neuropsychological study of patients with untreated Grave's disease. *Gen Hosp Psychiatry* **10**, 49–55.

Tucker GJ, Price TRP, Johnson VB, et al. (1986) Phenomenology of temporal lobe dysfunction: a link to atypical psychosis: a series of cases. *J Nerv Ment Dis* **174**, 348–356.

Varadaraj R and Cooper AJ (1986) Addison's disease presenting with psychiatric features. *Am J Psychiatry* **143**, 553–554.

Vataja R, Pohjasvaara T, Leppavuori A, et al. (2001) Magnetic resonance imaging correlates after ischemic stroke. *Arch Gen Psychiatry* **58**, 925–931.

Vazquez A, Jimenez-Jimenez FJ, Garcia-Ruiz P, et al. (1993) "Panic attacks" in Parkinson's disease. *Acta Neurol Scand* **87**, 14–18.

Wagner KD (1998) Major depression and anxiety disorders associated with Norplant. *J Clin Psychiatry* **57**, 152–157.

Wagner KD and Berenson AB (1994) Norplant-associated major depression and panic disorder. *J Clin Psychiatry* **55**, 478–480.

Walshe JM and Yealland M (1992) Wilson's disease: the problem of delayed diagnosis. *J Neurol Neurosurg Psychiatry* **55**, 692–696.

Walton RG (1986) Seizure and mania after high intake of aspartame. *Psychosomatics* **27**, 218–220.

Waxman SG and Geschwind N (1975) The interictal behavior syndrome of temporal lobe epilepsy. *Arch Gen Psychiatry* **32**, 1580–1586.

Weddington MW, Marks RC, and Verghese JP (1980) Disulfiram encephalopathy as a cause of the catatonic syndrome. *Am J Psychiatry* **137**, 1217–1219.

Weill AA (1955) Depressive reactions associated with temporal lobe–uncinate seizures. *J Nerv Ment Dis* **121**, 505–510.

Weill AA (1956) Ictal depression and anxiety in temporal lobe disorders. *Am J Psychiatry* **113**, 149–157.

Weill AA (1959) Ictal emotions in temporal lobe dysfunction. *Arch Neurol* **1**, 101–111.

Weller M, Liedtke W, Petersen D, et al. (1992) Very-late-onset adrenoleukodystrophy: possible precipitation of demyelination of cerebral contusion. *Neurology* **42**, 367–370.

Wells CE (1975) Transient ictal psychosis. *Arch Gen Psychiatry* **32**, 1201–1203.

Whybrow PC, Prange AJ, and Treadway CR (1969) Mental changes accompanying thyroid gland dysfunction: a reappraisal using objective psychological measurement. *Arch Gen Psychiatry* **20**, 48–63.

Williams D (1956) The structure of emotions reflected in epileptic experiences. *Brain* **79**, 29–67.

Williams BB and Lerner AM (1978) Some previously unrecognized features of herpes simplex encephalitis. *Neurology* **28**, 1193–1196.

Williamson RT (1896) On the symptomatology of gross lesions (tumours and abscesses) involving the pre-frontal regions of the brain. *Brain* **19**, 346–365.

Wilson LG (1976) Viral encephalopathy mimicking functional psychosis. *Am J Psychiatry* **133**, 165–170.

Wilson P and Preece M (1932) Chorea gravidarum. *Arch Int Med* **49**, 671–697.

Wilson P and Preece M (1932) Chorea gravidarum. *Arch Int Med* **49**, 471–533.

Wilson SAK (1924) Some problems in neurology. No. II. Pathological laughing and crying. *J Neurol Psychopathol* **4**, 299–333.

Wolkowitz OM, Rubinow D, Doran AR, et al. (1990) Prednisone effects on neurochemistry and behavior. *Arch Gen Psychiatry* **47**, 963–968.

Wright JM, Sachdev PS, Perkins RJ, et al. (1989) Zidovudine related mania. *Med J Aust* **150**, 339–341.

Wroblewski BA, McColgan K, Smith K, et al. (1990) The incidence of seizures during tricyclic antidepressant drug treatment in a brain-injured population. *J Clin Psychopharmacol* **10**, 124–125.

Zeidler M, Johnstone EC, Bamber RWK, et al. (1997a) New variant Creutzfeldt–Jakob disease: psychiatric features. *Lancet* **350**, 908–910.

Zeidler M, Stewart GE, Barraclough CR, et al. (1997b) New variant Creutzfeldt–Jakob disease: neurological features and diagnostic tests. *Lancet* **350**, 903–907.

Ziegler LH (1930) Psychosis associated with myxedema. *J Neurol Psychopathol* **11**, 20–27.

15 Substance-Related Disorders: General Approaches to Substance and Polysubstance Use Disorders/Other Substance Use Disorders

This chapter provides an overview of the substance-use disorders (SUDs) (those disorders that represent maladaptive pattern of substance use, i.e., substance abuse and dependence), and the substance-induced disorders (those disorders that represent psychiatric symptoms that result from the direct effects of a substance on the central nervous system, i.e., substance intoxication, substance withdrawal, and the other specific substance-induced mental disorders). Included are their definition in the DSM-IV-TR; the general epidemiological features of substance abuse and dependence; their pathophysiological characteristics; and the clinical issues of diagnosis and treatment. Many of the general principles outlined in this chapter are elaborated on in later chapters with regard to specific abused substances. Note that the DSM-IV-TR diagnostic criteria sets included in this chapter are *generic* in that they potentially apply across all of the classes of substances included in DSM-IV-TR. In fact, only some of the generic criteria sets apply to each of the classes of substance (e.g., there is no Nicotine Abuse and no Opioid-Induced Mood Disorders). Please refer to Table 15-1 for a cross-listing of which substance-related diagnoses apply to each class of substance. Polysubstance dependence and some substances

Table 15-1   DSM-IV-TR Substance Diagnoses Associated with class of substance

	Dependence	Abuse	Intoxication	Withdrawal	Intoxication Delirium	Withdrawal Delirium	Dementia	Amnestic Disorder	Psychotic Disorders	Mood Disorders	Anxiety Disorders	Sexual Dysfunctions	Sleep Disorders
Alcohol	X	X	X	X	I	W	P	P	I/W	I/W	I/W	I	I/W
Amphetamines	X	X	X	X	I				I	I/W	I	I	I/W
Caffeine			X								I		I
Cannabis	X	X	X		I				I		I		
Cocaine	X	X	X	X	I				I	I/W	I/W	I	I/W
Hallucinogens	X	X	X		I				I*	I	I		
Inhalants	X	X	X		I		P		I	I	I		
Nicotine	X			X									
Opioids	X	X	X	X	I				I	I		I	I/W
Phencyclidine	X	X	X		I				I	I	I		
Sedatives, hypnotics, or anxiolytics	X	X	X	X	I	W	P	P	I/W	I/W	W	I	I/W
Polysubstance	X												
Other	X	X	X	X	I	W	P	P	I/W	I/W	I/W	I	I/W

*Also Hallucinogen Persisting Perception Disorder (Flashbacks).

Note: X, I, W, I/W, or P indicates that the category is recognized in DSM-IV-TR. In addition, I indicates that the specifier With Onset During Intoxication may be noted for the category (except for Intoxication Delirium); W indicates that the specifier With Onset During Withdrawal may be noted for the category (except for Withdrawal Delirium); and I/W indicates that either With Onset During Intoxication or With During Withdrawal may be noted for the category. P indicates that the disorder is persisting.

that do not clearly meet standards for abuse and dependence (e.g., steroids) are covered in this chapter.

Diagnosis

Substance Dependence The definition of substance dependence is based on the dependence syndrome of Griffith Edwards (Edwards and Gross 1976). Although this syndrome originally had 10 criteria, the DSM-IV-TR criteria for dependence have been reduced to 7, including tolerance and withdrawal (the first 2 criteria) and a pattern of compulsive use (criteria 3 through 7) (see DSM-IV-TR diagnostic criteria below). The severity of dependence can be indicated by the number of criteria met (from a minimum of 3 to a maximum of 7) and by whether or not physiological dependence occurs (i.e., whether there is tolerance or withdrawal), because physiological dependence is associated with a higher risk for immediate general medical problems and a higher relapse rate. The five criteria indicating compulsive use alone may define substance dependence if at least three occur at any time in the same 12-month period. Physiological dependence is much more likely with some drugs, such as opioids and alcohol, and is infrequent with other classes of drugs, such as hallucinogens.

DSM-IV-TR Diagnostic Criteria

Substance Dependence

A maladaptive pattern of substance use, leading to clinically significant impairment or distress, as manifested by three (or more) of the following, occurring at any time in the same 12-month period:

(1) tolerance, as defined by either of the following:

    (a) a need for markedly increased amounts of the substance to achieve intoxication or desired effect

    (b) markedly diminished effect with continued use of the same amount of the substance

(2) withdrawal, as manifested by either of the following:

    (a) the characteristic withdrawal syndrome for the substance (refer to criteria A and B of the criteria sets for withdrawal from the specific substances)

    (b) the same (or a closely related) substance is taken to relieve or avoid withdrawal symptoms

(3) the substance is often taken in larger amounts or over a longer period than was intended

(4) there is a persistent desire or unsuccessful effort to cut down or control substance use

(5) a great deal of time is spent in activities necessary to obtain the substance (e.g., visiting multiple doctors or driving long distances), use the substance (e.g., chain-smoking), or recover from its effects

(6) important social, occupational, or recreational activities are given up or reduced because of substance use

(7) the substance use is continued despite knowledge of having a persistent or recurrent physical or psychological problem that is likely to have been caused or exacerbated by the substance (e.g., current cocaine use despite recognition of cocaine-induced depression, or continued drinking despite recognition that an ulcer was made worse by alcohol consumption)

Specify if:

With physiological dependence: evidence of tolerance or withdrawal (i.e., either item 1 or 2 is present)

Without physiological dependence: no evidence of tolerance or withdrawal (i.e., neither item 1 nor 2 is present)

Course specifiers (see text for definitions):

Early full remission

Early partial remission

Sustained full remission

Sustained partial remission

On agonist therapy

In a controlled environment

Reprinted with permission from the Diagnostic and Statistical Manual of Mental Disorders, Fourth Edition, Text Revision. Copyright 2000 American Psychiatric Association.

Treatment-seeking opioid users are likely to meet most of the dependence syndrome criteria and therefore their pattern of use is at the high end of severity. Cannabis users, in contrast, are likely to meet relatively few dependence syndrome criteria and therefore their pattern of use is of a lesser degree of severity. Individuals with alcohol or cocaine dependence tend to demonstrate a much wider variability in the number of dependence criteria met, with the proportion of individuals having relatively low levels of dependence approximately equal to those having extremely high levels of dependence. Thus, the severity of substance dependence is variable depending on the type of drug abused. Some substances such as steroid abuse are of research interest but have not been clearly identified as producing the acute reinforcement or dependence and withdrawal symptoms that characterize the abuse of other substances. The heavy use of anabolic steroids by body builders, with the associated possible medical complications, has raised important public health issues, however.

Substance Abuse   Substance abuse is a maladaptive pattern of substance use leading to significant adverse consequences manifested by psychosocial, medical, or legal problems or use in situations in which it is physically hazardous occurring within a 12-month period. Since a diagnosis of substance dependence preempts a diagnosis of abuse, tolerance, withdrawal, and compulsive use are generally not present in individuals with a diagnosis of substance abuse (see DSM-IV-TR diagnostic criteria below).

DSM-IV-TR Diagnostic Criteria

Substance Abuse

A. A maladaptive pattern of substance use leading to clinically significant impairment or distress, as manifested by one (or more) of the following, occurring within a 12-month period:

   (1) recurrent substance use resulting in a failure to fulfill major role obligations at work, school, or home (e.g., repeated absences or poor work performance related

to substance use; substance-related absences, suspensions, or expulsions from school; neglect of children or household)
(2) recurrent substance use in situations in which it is physically hazardous (e.g., driving an automobile or operating a machine when impaired by substance use)
(3) recurrent substance-related legal problems (e.g., arrests for substance-related disorderly conduct)
(4) continued substance use despite having persistent or recurrent social or interpersonal problems caused or exacerbated by the effects of the substance (e.g., arguments with spouse about consequences of intoxication, physical fights)

B. The symptoms have never met the criteria for substance dependence for this class of substance.

Reprinted with permission from the Diagnostic and Statistical Manual of Mental Disorders, Fourth Edition, Text Revision. Copyright 2000 American Psychiatric Association.

Substance Intoxication Substance intoxication is a reversible substance-specific syndrome with maladaptive behavioral or psychological changes developing during or shortly after using the substance (see DSM-IV-TR diagnostic criteria below). It does not apply to nicotine. Recent use can be documented by history or toxicological screening of body fluids (urine or blood). Different substances may produce similar or identical syndromes and, in polydrug users, intoxication may involve a complex mixture of disturbed perceptions, judgment, and behavior that can vary in severity and duration according to the setting in which the substances were taken. Physiological intoxication is not in and of itself necessarily maladaptive and would not justify a diagnosis of the DSM-IV-TR category substance intoxication. For example, caffeine-induced tachycardia with no maladaptive behavior does not meet the criteria for substance intoxication.

DSM-IV-TR Diagnostic Criteria

Substance Intoxication

A. The development of a reversible substance-specific syndrome due to recent ingestion of (or exposure to) a substance. Note: Different substances may produce similar or identical syndromes.
B. Clinically significant maladaptive behavioral or psychological changes that are due to the effect of the substance on the central nervous system (e.g., belligerence, mood lability, cognitive impairment, impaired judgment, impaired social or occupational functioning) and develop during or shortly after use of the substance.
C. The symptoms are not due to a general medical condition and are not better accounted for by another mental disorder.

Reprinted with permission from the Diagnostic and Statistical Manual of Mental Disorders, Fourth Edition, Text Revision. Copyright 2000 American Psychiatric Association.

Substance Withdrawal Substance withdrawal is a syndrome due to cessation of, or reduction in, heavy and prolonged substance use (see DSM-IV-TR diagnostic criteria on page 354). It causes clinically significant impairment or distress and is usually associated with substance dependence. Most often, the symptoms of withdrawal are the opposite of intoxication with that substance. The withdrawal syndrome usually lasts several days to 2 weeks.

DSM-IV-TR Diagnostic Criteria

Substance Withdrawal

A. The development of a substance-specific syndrome due to the cessation of (or reduction in) substance use that has been heavy and prolonged.
B. The substance-specific syndrome causes clinically significant distress or impairment in social, occupational, or other important areas of functioning.
C. The symptoms are not due to a general medical condition and are not better accounted for by another mental disorder.

Reprinted with permission from the Diagnostic and Statistical Manual of Mental Disorders, Fourth Edition, Text Revision. Copyright 2000 American Psychiatric Association.

Other Substance-Induced Disorders Not infrequently, substance intoxication and substance withdrawal are characterized by psychopathology that mimics the other disorders contained in the rest of DSM-IV-TR. When this occurs, if the symptoms are in excess of those usually associated with the intoxication or withdrawal syndrome, and if they are sufficiently severe to warrant independent clinical attention, a specific substance-induced mental disorder should be diagnosed. For example, since dysphoric mood is commonly seen as a result of Cocaine Withdrawal, the mere presence of depression after stopping cocaine would not ordinarily warrant a diagnosis of Cocaine-Induced Mood Disorder; typically a diagnosis of Cocaine Withdrawal would suffice. However, if the depressed mood is especially severe and prolonged and is associated with suicidal ideation, then a diagnosis of Cocaine-Induced Mood Disorder would make clinical sense.

DSM-IV-TR includes nine substance-induced disorders. Seven of these (Substance Intoxication Delirium and Substance Withdrawal Delirium, Substance-Induced Psychotic Disorder, (see DSM-IV-TR diagnostic criteria on page 355) Substance-Induced Mood Disorder (see DSM-IV-TR diagnostic criteria on page 356) Substance-Induced Anxiety Disorder, (see DSM-IV-TR diagnostic criteria on page 357) Substance-Induced Sexual Dysfunction, (see DSM-IV-TR diagnostic criteria on page 358) and Substance-Induced Sleep Disorder (see DSM-IV-TR diagnostic criteria on page 359)) represent disorders that begin during acute intoxication or withdrawal and subside within 4 weeks of stopping the substance. A specifier is available to indicate whether the substance-induced disorder had its onset during intoxication or withdrawal (see Table 15-1 to determine which classes of substances lead to psychopathology during intoxication vs withdrawal). To facilitate differential diagnosis, these disorders have been placed in the DSM-IV-TR within the diagnostic groupings with which they share phenomenology (e.g., Substance-Induced Anxiety Disorder is included within the Anxiety Disorder section of DSM-IV-TR). Two of them (Substance-Induced Persisting Dementia and Substance-Induced Persisting Amnestic Disorder) represent psychopathology resulting from more or less permanent damage to the central nervous system, a consequence of prolonged periods of heavy substance use.

Diagnostic Criteria

Substance-Induced Psychotic Disorder

A. Prominent hallucinations or delusions. Note: Do not include hallucinations if the person has insight that they are substance induced.

B. There is evidence from the history, physical examination, or laboratory findings of either (1) or (2):

   (1) the symptoms in Criterion A developed during, or within a month of, Substance Intoxication or Withdrawal

   (2) medication use is etiologically related to the disturbance

C. The disturbance is not better accounted for by a Psychotic Disorder that is not substance induced. Evidence that the symptoms are better accounted for by a Psychotic Disorder that is not substance induced might include the following: the symptoms precede the onset of the substance use (or medication use); the symptoms persist for a substantial period of time (e.g., about a month) after the cessation of acute withdrawal or severe intoxication, or are substantially in excess of what would be expected given the type or amount of the substance used or the duration of use; or there is other evidence that suggests the existence of an independent non-substance-induced Psychotic Disorder (e.g., a history of recurrent non-substance-related episodes).

D. The disturbance does not occur exclusively during the course of a delirium.

Note: This diagnosis should be made instead of a diagnosis of Substance Intoxication or Substance Withdrawal only when the symptoms are in excess of those usually associated with the intoxication or withdrawal syndrome and when the symptoms are sufficiently severe to warrant independent clinical attention.

Code [Specific Substance]–Induced Psychotic Disorder:
291.5 Alcohol, With Delusions; 291.3 Alcohol, With Hallucinations; 292.11 Amphetamine [or Amphetamine-Like Substance], With Delusions; 292.12 Amphetamine [or Amphetamine-Like Substance], With Hallucinations;292.11 Cannabis, With Delusions; 292.12 Cannabis, With Hallucinations; 292.11 Cocaine, With Delusions; 292.12 Cocaine, With Hallucinations; 292.11 Hallucinogen, With Delusions; 292.12 Hallucinogen, With Hallucinations; 292.11 Inhalant, With Delusions; 292.12 Inhalant, With Hallucinations; 292.11 Opioid, With Delusions; 292.12 Opioid, With Hallucinations; 292.11 Phencyclidine [or Phencyclidine-Like Substance], With Delusions; 292.12 Phencyclidine [or Phencyclidine-Like Substance], With Hallucinations; 292.11 Sedative, Hypnotic, or Anxiolytic, With Delusions; 292.12 Sedative, Hypnotic, or Anxiolytic, With Hallucinations; 292.11 Other [or Unknown] Substance, With Delusions; 292.12 Other [or Unknown] Substance, With Hallucinations)

Specify if (see table for applicability by substance):

With Onset During Intoxication: if criteria are met for Intoxication with the substance and the symptoms develop during the intoxication syndrome

With Onset During Withdrawal: if criteria are met for Withdrawal from the substance and the symptoms develop during, or shortly after, a withdrawal syndrome

Diagnostic Criteria

Substance-Induced Mood Disorder

A. A prominent and persistent disturbance in mood predominates in the clinical picture and is characterized by either (or both) of the following:

(1) depressed mood or markedly diminished interest or pleasure in all, or almost all, activities
(2) elevated, expansive, or irritable mood

B. There is evidence from the history, physical examination, or laboratory findings of either (1) or (2):

(1) the symptoms in Criterion A developed during, or within a month of, Substance Intoxication or Withdrawal
(2) medication use is etiologically related to the disturbance

C. The disturbance is not better accounted for by a Mood Disorder that is not substance induced. Evidence that the symptoms are better accounted for by a Mood Disorder that is not substance induced might include the following: the symptoms precede the onset of the substance use (or medication use); the symptoms persist for a substantial period of time (e.g., about a month) after the cessation of acute withdrawal or severe intoxication or are substantially in excess of what would be expected given the type or amount of the substance used or the duration of use; or there is other evidence that suggests the existence of an independent non-substance-induced Mood Disorder (e.g., a history of recurrent Major Depressive Episodes).
D. The disturbance does not occur exclusively during the course of a delirium.
E. The symptoms cause clinically significant distress or impairment in social, occupational, or other important areas of functioning.

Note: This diagnosis should be made instead of a diagnosis of Substance Intoxication or Substance Withdrawal only when the mood symptoms are in excess of those usually associated with the intoxication or withdrawal syndrome and when the symptoms are sufficiently severe to warrant independent clinical attention.

Code [Specific Substance]–Induced Mood Disorder:
(291.89 Alcohol; 292.84 Amphetamine [or Amphetamine-Like Substance]; 292.84 Cocaine; 292.84 Hallucinogen; 292.84 Inhalant; 292.84 Opioid; 292.84 Phencyclidine [or Phencyclidine-Like Substance]; 292.84 Sedative, Hypnotic, or Anxiolytic; 292.84 Other [or Unknown] Substance)

Specify type:

With Depressive Features: if the predominant mood is depressed

With Manic Features: if the predominant mood is elevated, euphoric, or irritable

With Mixed Features: if symptoms of both mania and depression are present and neither predominates

Specify if (see table for applicability by substance):

With Onset During Intoxication: if the criteria are met for Intoxication with the substance and the symptoms develop during the intoxication syndrome

With Onset During Withdrawal: if criteria are met for Withdrawal from the substance and the symptoms develop during, or shortly after, a withdrawal syndrome

DSM-IV-TR Diagnostic Criteria

Substance-Induced Anxiety Disorder

A. Prominent anxiety, Panic Attacks, or obsessions or compulsions predominate in the clinical picture.
B. There is evidence from the history, physical examination, or laboratory findings of either (1) or (2):

    (1) the symptoms in Criterion A developed during, or within 1 month of, Substance Intoxication or Withdrawal
    (2) medication use is etiologically related to the disturbance

C. The disturbance is not better accounted for by an Anxiety Disorder that is not substance induced. Evidence that the symptoms are better accounted for by an Anxiety Disorder that is not substance induced might include the following: the symptoms precede the onset of the substance use (or medication use); the symptoms persist for a substantial period of time (e.g., about a month) after the cessation of acute withdrawal or severe intoxication or are substantially in excess of what would be expected given the type or amount of the substance used or the duration of use; or there is other evidence suggesting the existence of an independent non-substance-induced Anxiety Disorder (e.g., a history of recurrent non-substance-related episodes).
D. The disturbance does not occur exclusively during the course of a delirium.
E. The disturbance causes clinically significant distress or impairment in social, occupational, or other important areas of functioning.

Note: This diagnosis should be made instead of a diagnosis of Substance Intoxication or Substance Withdrawal only when the anxiety symptoms are in excess of those usually associated with the intoxication or withdrawal syndrome and when the anxiety symptoms are sufficiently severe to warrant independent clinical attention.

Code [Specific Substance]–Induced Anxiety Disorder
(291.89 Alcohol; 292.89 Amphetamine (or Amphetamine-Like Substance); 292.89 Caffeine; 292.89 Cannabis; 292.89 Cocaine; 292.89 Hallucinogen; 292.89 Inhalant; 292.89 Phencyclidine (or Phencyclidine-Like Substance); 292.89 Sedative, Hypnotic, or Anxiolytic; 292.89 Other [or Unknown] Substance)

Specify if:

With Generalized Anxiety: if excessive anxiety or worry about a number of events or activities predominates in the clinical presentation

With Panic Attacks: if Panic Attacks predominate in the clinical presentation

With Obsessive-Compulsive Symptoms: if obsessions or compulsions predominate in the clinical presentation

With Phobic Symptoms: if phobic symptoms predominate in the clinical presentation

Specify if

With Onset During Intoxication: if the criteria are met for Intoxication with the substance and the symptoms develop during the intoxication syndrome

With Onset During Withdrawal: if criteria are met for Withdrawal from the substance and the symptoms develop during, or shortly after, a withdrawal syndrome.

DSM-IV-TR Diagnostic Criteria

Substance-Induced Sexual Dysfunction

A. Clinically significant sexual dysfunction that results in marked distress or interpersonal difficulty predominates in the clinical picture.
B. There is evidence from the history, physical examination, or laboratory findings that the sexual dysfunction is fully explained by substance use as manifested by either (1) or (2):

  (1) the symptoms in Criterion A developed during, or within a month of, Substance Intoxication
  (2) medication use is etiologically related to the disturbance

C. The disturbance is not better accounted for by a Sexual Dysfunction that is not substance induced. Evidence that the symptoms are better accounted for by a Sexual Dysfunction that is not substance induced might include the following: the symptoms precede the onset of the substance use or dependence (or medication use); the symptoms persist for a substantial period of time (e.g., about a month) after the cessation of intoxication, or are substantially in excess of what would be expected given the type or amount of the substance used or the duration of use; or there is other evidence that suggests the existence of an independent non-substance-induced Sexual Dysfunction (e.g., a history of recurrent non-substance-related episodes).

Note: This diagnosis should be made instead of a diagnosis of Substance Intoxication only when the sexual dysfunction is in excess of that usually associated with the intoxication syndrome and when the dysfunction is sufficiently severe to warrant independent clinical attention.

Code [Specific Substance]–Induced Sexual Dysfunction:
(291.89 Alcohol; 292.89 Amphetamine [or Amphetamine-Like Substance]; 292.89 Cocaine; 292.89 Opioid; 292.89 Sedative, Hypnotic, or Anxiolytic; 292.89 Other [or Unknown] Substance)

Specify if:
With Impaired Desire
With Impaired Arousal
With Impaired Orgasm
With Sexual Pain

Specify if:

With Onset During Intoxication: if the criteria are met for Intoxication with the substance and the symptoms develop during the intoxication syndrome.

Diagnostic Criteria

Substance-Induced Sleep Disorder

A. A prominent disturbance in sleep that is sufficiently severe to warrant independent clinical attention.
B. There is evidence from the history, physical examination, or laboratory findings of either (1) or (2):

    (1) the symptoms in Criterion A developed during, or within a month of, Substance Intoxication or Withdrawal
    (2) medication use is etiologically related to the sleep disturbance

C. The disturbance is not better accounted for by a Sleep Disorder that is not substance induced. Evidence that the symptoms are better accounted for by a Sleep Disorder that is not substance induced might include the following: the symptoms precede the onset of the substance use (or medication use); the symptoms persist for a substantial period of time (e.g., about a month) after the cessation of acute withdrawal or severe intoxication or are substantially in excess of what would be expected given the type or amount of the substance used or the duration of use; or there is other evidence that suggests the existence of an independent non-substance-induced Sleep Disorder (e.g., a history of recurrent non-substance-related episodes).
D. The disturbance does not occur exclusively during the course of a delirium.
E. The sleep disturbance causes clinically significant distress or impairment in social, occupational, or other important areas of functioning.

Note: This diagnosis should be made instead of a diagnosis of Substance Intoxication or Substance Withdrawal only when the sleep symptoms are in excess of those usually associated with the intoxication or withdrawal syndrome and when the symptoms are sufficiently severe to warrant independent clinical attention.

Code [Specific Substance]–Induced Sleep Disorder:
(291.89 Alcohol; 292.89 Amphetamine; 292.89 Caffeine; 292.89 Cocaine; 292.89 Opioid; 292.89 Sedative, Hypnotic, or Anxiolytic; 292.89 Other [or Unknown] Substance)

Specify type:
Insomnia Type: if the predominant sleep disturbance is insomnia
Hypersomnia Type: if the predominant sleep disturbance is hypersomnia

Parasomnia Type: if the predominant sleep disturbance is a Parasomnia

Mixed Type: if more than one sleep disturbance is present and none predominates

Specify if

With Onset During Intoxication: if the criteria are met for Intoxication with the substance and the symptoms develop during the intoxication syndrome

With Onset During Withdrawal: if criteria are met for Withdrawal from the substance and the symptoms develop during, or shortly after, a withdrawal syndrome.

Reprinted with permission from the Diagnostic and Statistical Manual of Mental Disorders, Fourth Edition, Text Revision. Copyright 2000 American Psychiatric Association.

The diagnosis of substance abuse and dependence is made by eliciting an appropriate history, performing laboratory tests to confirm drug use, and observing the physiological manifestations of tolerance and withdrawal (see Figure 15-1 for a diagnostic decision tree for SUDs).

The phenomenology and variations in presentation among abused substances are related to the wide range of substance-induced states as well as the conditions under which the

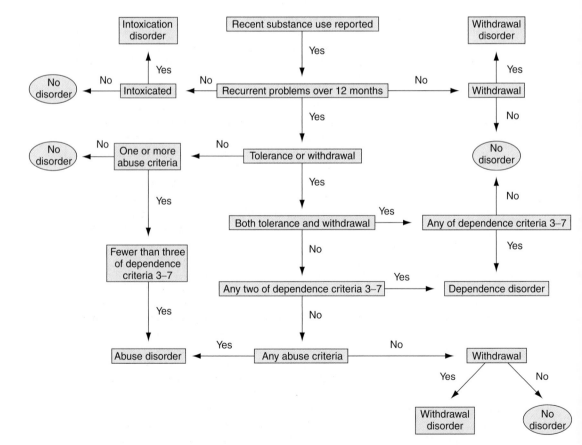

Figure 15-1 *Diagnostic decision tree for substance-use disorders.*

individual using substances is brought to treatment. Many individuals who use illicit *street* drugs may not know precisely what drugs they have ingested and certainly will not have a good idea of the precise amount. In addition, individuals who are dependent on substances producing significant withdrawal syndromes, such as opioids and alcohol, may have a mixed picture of early intoxication and overdose followed by an evolving withdrawal syndrome; alcohol and sedative withdrawal may produce psychiatric complications (e.g., hallucinations) as well as medical complications (e.g., seizures).

The severity of withdrawal symptoms may, in part, be determined by the setting. For example, studies of opioid-dependent individuals have shown that the expression of withdrawal symptoms may be substantially less when no medication treatment is available for symptom relief. As a further example of this phenomenon, individuals with opioid addiction who have been in prison without access to opioids for several years may experience precipitous opiate withdrawal when they return to the neighborhoods where they previously used heroin. This conditioned withdrawal phenomenon further supports the importance of setting in the presentation of withdrawal symptoms.

Finally, the issues of motivation for seeking treatment and a tendency to deny substance abuse can have important influence on the individual's presentation. The individual who presents for treatment because of dysphoric feelings in the context of drug dependence is likely to articulate the severity of his or her problem adequately and even exaggerate some aspects of present discomfort. In contrast, the automobile driver forced to come to a treatment program because of a driving-while-intoxicated offense is likely to minimize her or his alcohol use or any associated complications.

Two special issues in the psychiatric examination of substance dependence include (1) the source of information when obtaining the history of the substance abuse and (2) the management of aberrant behaviors. Information about a individual's substance-abuse history can be provided not only by the individual but also by employers, family members, and school officials. When individuals self-report the amount of substance abused, there is a tendency to underreport the severity and duration of abuse, particularly if the person is being referred to treatment by an outside source such as the family, the employer, or the legal system. Objective verification of the exact amount of substance use is sometimes difficult, but the critical issues in arriving at a diagnosis of substance dependence do not depend on the precise amount of substance abused. Tolerance and withdrawal can be assessed independently by using tests such as the naloxone challenge and the barbiturate tolerance test. In general, significant others' estimates of the amount of drug use by the individual can be a good source of data. Thus, the initial evaluation of substance abuse and dependence may involve a wider range of interviews than would occur with many other types of individuals undergoing psychiatric treatment.

Aberrant behaviors potentially requiring management include intoxication, violence, suicide, impaired cognitive functioning, and uncontrolled affective displays. The evaluation of an intoxicated substance abuser can address only a limited number of issues. These issues are primarily related to the safety of the substance abuser and other individuals who may be affected by his or her actions. Thus, a medical evaluation for signs of overdose or major cognitive impairment is critical, with consideration of detaining the individual for several hours or even days, if severe complications are evident.

Temporary suicidal behavior may be encountered in a variety of substance addictions, particularly those with alcohol and stimulants. Suicidal ideation may be intense but may clear within hours. During the evaluation session, it is important to elicit the precipitants that led the individual to seek treatment at this time and to keep the evaluation focused on specific data needed for the evaluation of substance dependence, its medical complications, and any comorbid mental disorders. Many individuals spend a great deal of time detailing their drug-abusing careers, but, in general, these stories do not provide useful material for the evaluation or for future psychotherapeutic interventions. Similarly, the evaluation should not become focused on the affective aspects of a individual's recent life because affect is frequently used as a defense to avoid discussing issues of more immediate relevance such as precipitants or to act as a pretext for obtaining benzodiazepines or other antianxiety agents from the physician. Abused substances have generally been a way of managing affect and these individuals need to develop alternative coping strategies.

Physical examination is critical for the assessment of substance addiction, particularly before pharmacotherapy is initiated. Many signs of drug withdrawal require a physical examination and cannot rely entirely on history. Because the general medical complications of substance addiction are also substantial, the most clearly ill individuals must have a formal general medical evaluation. Vital signs (blood pressure, pulse, and so on) are an essential beginning but a full examination of heart, lungs, and nervous system is minimally necessary. Transmissible infectious diseases such as AIDS, tuberculosis, and venereal diseases are common among illicit drug users and require screening for adequate detection. This screening for HIV infection also protects health care personnel as well as individuals undergoing treatment. A wide variety of other infectious diseases including hepatitis and endocarditis, are also associated with intravenous drug use and require appropriate blood studies. With alcohol dependence, a wide range of gastrointestinal complications have been described, particularly liver dysfunction.

Urine toxicological screens can be sensitive for detecting drug use within 3 days of use of opiates and cocaine. Urine screens for other abused drugs such as cannabis can remain positive for as long as a month in heavy users. A Breathalyzer can be used for detecting alcohol use within an 8- to 12-hour period after use. Specific biological tests can also aid in the diagnosis of dependence, for example, a naloxone challenge test assesses opioid dependence by precipitating withdrawal symptoms. Associated medical findings on physical examination include *track marks* in intravenous drug users, nasal damage in intranasal drug users, and pulmonary damage in drug smokers.

From a developmental perspective, the most important impact of substance abuse and dependence is in adolescence when substance misuse not only can disrupt schooling but also can have important medical consequences because of its direct hormonal effects. For example, opioids can increase prolactin levels and at the same time decrease corticosteroid and testosterone levels. These hormonal effects can have a direct impact on the expression of secondary sex characteristics as well as sexual behaviors during adolescence. Another critical developmental effect is during the gestational period of unborn children to substance-abusing mothers. These children may be born with a significant neonatal withdrawal syndrome from drugs such as opioids or may have behavioral and congenital abnormalities, secondary to the substance misuse by their mothers—for example, fetal alcohol syndrome in the infants of mothers who are alcohol-dependent during pregnancy and the hyperactivity that has been noted in infants born to cocaine-dependent mothers.

At the other extreme of life, in the geriatric population, substance addiction might have an important iatrogenic contribution. Many chronic debilitating diseases are associated with significant pain and may be treated with opioids. Similarly, sleep disorders in the elderly are often treated with sedatives (such as benzodiazepine and barbiturates) that produce tolerance and dependence. Although most of these individuals will not experience patterns of substance abuse, some individuals may begin to seek out these medications from multiple physicians (so-called doctor shopping), and experience significant psychosocial impairment.

Cultural differences in the presentation of drug addiction can be striking. For example, the use of hallucinogens by Native Americans in religious ceremonies shows none of the abusive characteristics of adolescent hallucinogen addiction in middle-class America. Alcohol abuse can also show widely varying presentations based on the amount of alcohol that is considered culturally acceptable in various geographical settings.

Epidemiology

Wide cultural variations in attitudes toward substance consumption have led to widely varying patterns of substance misuse and prevalence of substance-related disorders. Relatively high prevalence rates for the use of virtually every substance occur between the ages of 18 and 24 years, with intoxication being the initial substance-related disorder, usually beginning in the teens. Tolerance and withdrawal require a sustained period of use and these manifestations of physical dependence for most drugs of abuse typically begin in the twenties and early thirties. Although most substance-related disorders are more common in men than in women, sex ratios can vary considerably with different drugs of abuse.

In both the Epidemiological Catchment Area study and the National Comorbidity Survey, substance abuse and dependence were the most common comorbid disorders, usually appearing in combination with affective and anxiety disorders. In the National Comorbidity Survey (Kessler et al. 1994), the lifetime rate of substance abuse was 27% and the rate of comorbid depression among these substance abusers was 19%. Furthermore, 80% of these depressed substance-abusing subjects had more than one mental disorder; only 20% had only one mental disorder. In the Epidemiological Catchment Area study (Regier et al. 1984), 75% of daily substance users had a comorbid mental disorder. In studies of treatment-seeking substance abusers, the rates of other mental disorders are almost uniformly higher than those in community samples, but the rates of excess comorbidity in these abusers varies with the specific abused drug. For example, in the Epidemiological Catchment Area study, the lifetime rate of major depression in the community was 7%, whereas the major depression rates for substance users seeking treatment were 54% for opioids, 38% for alcohol, and 24% for cocaine. Rates for other disorders are compared in Table 15-2. More recent studies such as the Methods for the Epidemiology of Child and Adolescent Mental Disorders (MECA) Study have focused on adolescents (Kandel et al. 1999). In the MECA study, the rates of mood and disruptive behavior disorders are much higher among adolescents with current SUDs than among adolescents without SUD. Comparison with adult samples suggests that the rates of current comorbidity of SUD with mental disorders are the same among adolescents as in adults, but the comorbidity of lifetime disruptive disorders or antisocial personality disorder with SUD is lower among adolescents than among adults.

Course

The natural history of substance dependence characteristically follows the course of a chronic relapsing disorder, although a large number of individuals who experiment with potentially abusable drugs in adolescence do not go on to acquire dependence. The initial phase of the natural history of experimenting with drugs has been well

Table 15-2	**Lifetime diagnoses in SUD and Community Sample**			
	Patients with Opioid Dependence (N = 533)	**Patients with Alcoholism (N = 321)**	**Cocaine Users (N = 149)**	**New Haven Community (N = 3058)**
Major depression	53.9	38	31.5	6.7
Bipolar disorder I (mania)	0.6	2	3.4	1.1
Schizophrenia	0.8	2	0.7	1.9
Phobia	9.6	27	11.4	7.8
Antisocial personality	25.5	41	34.9	2.1
Alcoholism	34.5	100	63.8	11.5
Drug abuse	100	43	100	5.8

described in studies by Kandel (1975), who has used the concept of gateway drug use and its evolution into more serious drug dependence during adolescence and the early twenties.

The course of substance dependence is variable and may involve full or partial remission with six course specifiers available in the DSM-IV-TR (see below). In order for an individual with dependence to be considered *in remission*, none of the dependence or abuse criteria can be met for at least 1 month. Remission can then be further characterized as either early (less than 12 months) or sustained (lasting 12 months or longer) and partial (one or more criteria for abuse or dependence have been met) or full (no criteria for dependence or abuse). Because the first year of remission carries a particularly high risk for relapse, it has been chosen as the minimum required time for sustained remission. Two additional specifiers apply for special circumstances, such as when the individual is receiving agonist therapy or is in a controlled environment in which access to substances is potentially limited (such as jail or a therapeutic community).

Course Specifiers available for Substance Dependence

The following remission specifiers can be applied only after no criteria for dependence or abuse have been met for at least 1 month. Note that these specifiers do not apply if the individual is on agonist therapy or in a controlled environment (see below).

Early Full Remission. This specifier is used if, for at least 1 month, but for less than 12 months, no criteria for dependence or abuse have been met.

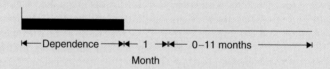

Early Partial Remission. This specifier is used if, for at least 1 month, but less than 12 months, one or more criteria for dependence or abuse have been met (but the full criteria for dependence have not been met).

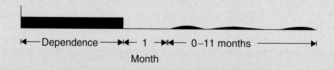

Sustained Full Remission. This specifier is used if none of the criteria for dependence or abuse have been met at any time during a period of 12 months or longer.

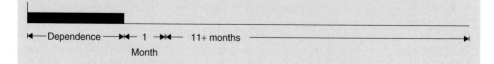

Sustained Partial Remission. This specifier is used if full criteria for dependence have not been met for a period of 12 months or longer; however, one or more criteria for dependence or abuse have been met.

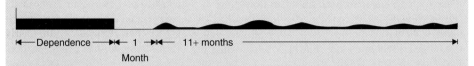

The following specifiers apply if the individual is on agonist therapy or in a controlled environment:

On Agonist Therapy. This specifier is used if the individual is on a prescribed agonist medication such as methadone and no criteria for dependence or abuse have been met for that class of medication for at least the past month (except tolerance to, or withdrawal from, the agonist). This category also applies to those being treated for dependence using a partial agonist or an agonist/antagonist.

In a Controlled Environment. This specifier is used if the individual is in an environment in which access to alcohol and controlled substances is restricted, and no criteria for dependence or abuse have been met for at least the past month. Examples of these environments are closely supervised and substance-free jails, therapeutic communities, or locked hospital units

Reprinted with permission from the Diagnostic and Statistical Manual of Mental Disorders, Fourth Edition, Text Revision. Copyright 2000 American Psychiatric Association.

Population surveys, such as the high school senior surveys and National Institute on Drug Abuse household survey (Wallace et al. 1999), have provided repeated cross-sectional data on changing trends in substance use and its associated problems. These surveys have increasingly recognized cultural differences in the course of drug use. Thus, the natural history of substance abuse and dependence is determined by the type of substance used and, for polysubstance dependence, can be complicated by changing secular trends and epidemics lasting from months to decades.

Differential Diagnosis

The differential diagnosis of substance-induced intoxication and withdrawal can involve a wide range of mental disorders. Distinguishing substance abuse from these disorders is usually facilitated by a structured interview to elicit a wide range of psychiatric symptoms appropriately timed after the most recent substance use. During acute intoxication in polydrug users, the differential diagnosis might include an acute psychotic disorder, mania, delirium, dementia, or several specific anxiety disorders. Among these anxiety disorders are generalized anxiety disorder, panic disorder, and obsessive–compulsive disorder. Distinguishing these disorders from acute intoxication or withdrawal with a mixture of drugs most frequently requires that the clinician wait 24 to 72 hours to determine whether the symptoms persist and, therefore, whether they are independent of the drug use. While the DSM-IV-TR criteria for substance-induced disorders suggest waiting for a "substantial period of time" (e.g., about a month) to distinguish various substance-induced disorders from those not related to substance abuse, the introduction of pharmacological treatments such as antidepressants does not require such a lengthy delay. Thus, diagnostic and therapeutic distinctions may be different when evaluating the individual presenting with substance intoxication or withdrawal.

A previous history of schizophrenia, bipolar disorder, or other major psychiatric disorder that is consistent with the presenting symptoms may also be helpful in arriving at an accurate diagnosis. When individuals present with psychotic or manic behavior during drug intoxication, it may be necessary to use symptomatic treatment such as a benzodiazepine or neuroleptic agent to conduct an examination. A symptomatic response to these medications should not be considered as confirmation of an underlying diagnosis of psychotic disorder, however. Furthermore, some abused drugs such as phencyclidine may produce a sustained psychotic state that lasts longer than the usual 72 hours after acute intoxication.

Antisocial and borderline personality disorders are commonly considered in the differential diagnosis of substance-dependent individuals. Many of the behaviors that characterize these personality disorders are also common to the use of illegal and illicit drugs. In establishing these personality disorders, particularly antisocial personality, it is important to ascertain whether the behaviors are independent of the activities needed to obtain drugs. If many of the antisocial or borderline characteristics are specifically tied to the individual's abuse of drugs, these characteristics should resolve with drug abstinence and should not be considered diagnostic of a personality disorder.

The symptoms of drug withdrawal frequently overlap with those of depressive disorders, and this differential diagnosis can be particularly difficult. Furthermore, the syndrome of protracted withdrawal can include sleep and appetite disturbance as well as dysphoria that mimics dysthymic disorder and other affective disorders. Some drugs, such as opioids, appear to be minimally psychotoxic and are unlikely to produce affective syndromes. Thus, in heroin dependence, a differential diagnosis can be made several days after completing acute detoxification or while the individual is receiving agonist maintenance. With other drugs, such as stimulants, sedatives, and alcohol, depressive symptoms may be more persistent after acute detoxification, which leads to a more difficult differential diagnosis. Thus, conservatively, the clinician should wait 4 to 6 weeks after acute detoxification to determine a diagnosis of affective disorder in these substance-dependent individuals. However, waiting this long is often impractical in the clinical setting in which the maintenance of sustained abstinence may depend on relief of depressive symptoms using either medications or psychotherapy.

Etiology

The cause of substance addiction depends on a variety of biological, psychological, and social factors. Biological factors can include genetic predisposition as well as neurobiological substrates for positive and negative reinforcement by abused substances (Nestler 2000). Family genetic studies have found rates of substance dependence that are three to four times higher in identical twins than in dizygotic twins (Cloninger 1999). Although no single biological marker or specific genetic defect has been confirmed, work has suggested that some alleles associated with variations in the dopamine receptor may be more common in substance-dependent individuals than in those who are not dependent. Similarly, risk factor studies have found that the sons of individuals suffering from alcoholism have a general hyporesponsiveness to alcohol and sedative drugs, when compared with the sons of individuals without alcoholism.

The neurobiological substrates for positive and negative reinforcement by abused substances have been examined in a wide range of animal studies. The neuronal pathways underlying positive reinforcement appear to converge on the dopaminergic pathways leading from the ventral tegmental area in the brain stem to the nucleus accumbens, which is part of the basal ganglia (Spanagel and Weiss 1999). Most drugs of abuse appear to act through this pathway to produce positive reinforcement and reward. Some abused drugs, such as stimulants, affect this pathway directly by increasing the amount of dopamine available to stimulate the cells in the nucleus accumbens. Other drugs, such as opioids, appear to have effects on the dopaminergic cells in the ventral tegmental area through specific opioid receptors and thereby indirectly affect the nucleus accumbens. The reinforcing effects of alcohol and benzodiazepines may be through gamma-aminobutyric acid receptors. These gamma-aminobutyric acid receptors also appear on the dopaminergic cells located in the ventral tegmental area. The positive reinforcing effects of hallucinogenic drugs are less clear. For example, marijuana interacts with a specific cannabinoid receptor that is widely distributed in the brain, and it does not appear to have a direct interaction with the dopaminergic systems in the ventral tegmental area. Other hallucinogenic drugs, such as lysergic acid diethylamide, have critical effects on serotoninergic systems, which may act on the nucleus accumbens to facilitate dopamine neurotransmission indirectly.

The negative reinforcers involved in substance dependence include the relief of withdrawal symptoms (Koob and Le Moa 2001). The neurobiological systems responsible for symptoms of withdrawal are multiply determined. Two brain systems that appear to be particularly important during withdrawal are the noradrenergic system in the locus coeruleus of the brain stem and the dopaminergic system that terminates in the nucleus accumbens. The nucleus accumbens is more broadly a part of the limbic circuit that is generally associated with mood and emotion.

The role of the locus coeruleus in drug withdrawal has been clearly delineated during opiate withdrawal (Kosten and Hollister 2001). The locus coeruleus contains opioid receptors that inhibit locus activity when exposed to morphine. During opiate withdrawal, the locus has high levels of nerve activity, and this nerve activity appears to result from the release of chronic inhibition of the locus by morphine administration.

After chronic administration of cocaine, opioids, or alcohol, there is an increased stimulation threshold in the nucleus accumbens so that the same level of stimulation in the nucleus produces less positive reinforcement. This might be interpreted as a type of negative reinforcement after chronic drug usage. In summary, at least two, and probably more, neural circuits are recruited into the negative reinforcement associated with substance dependence and are thereby important pathophysiological factors.

Psychological factors related to etiology include high rates of depressive disorders and sensation seeking, which are found in substance addiction. The association of sensation seeking with substance addiction suggests not only that drugs enhance pleasant sensations, such as a high, but also that abused drugs may provide potential control of aggressive impulses. Whether abused drugs serve as self-medication for individuals with these psychological disturbances (e.g., depression and impulsivity) has not been resolved clearly because the age at onset for major psychiatric disorders, such as depression, is older than the age at onset for substance abuse and dependence (Khantzian 1985). Childhood precursors of substance abuse and dependence, including shy and aggressive behaviors, can also be precursors of later depressive disorders as well as of antisocial personality disorder—the adult expression of aggressive impulsivity.

Finally, social factors, including peer and family influences, which are not dependent on genetic inheritance, are important in leading to initial drug exposure. Kandel (1975) has conducted longitudinal studies of *gateway drug* usage by adolescents, and these original concepts have been expanded over the last 25 years to recognize their treatment implications. These gateway drugs are tobacco, alcohol, and marijuana. Adolescents who begin using gateway drugs in their early teens are more likely to have substance dependence in their twenties than are adolescents who begin use in their late teens. Delaying the initiation of these gateway drugs and their associated intoxication by 1 to 2 years substantially decreases the later risk of the development of substance dependence.

Treatment

The most important goal of any treatment is abstinence from the abused drug. Issues of *controlled use* are debated by some mental health professionals, but this is usually not a realistic goal for dependent individuals. A critical, first treatment goal with substance addiction is often acute treatment of overdose. A clinician must be aware of specific therapies such as naloxone for opioid overdose and flumazenil for benzodiazepine or other sedative overdose. The polydrug user often has combined toxicity from drug interactions such as alcohol with barbiturates or phencyclidine with cocaine. For dependence on a drug with a significant withdrawal syndrome, such as opioids or alcohol, the initial treatment involves either agonist stabilization, such as methadone maintenance, or medical detoxification when necessary. After detoxification or stabilization, prevention of relapse may occur through a variety of behavioral or other psychotherapeutic approaches. Reduction in drug use without total abstinence using agonist maintenance (e.g., methadone) may be an early priority, together with the provision of essential social services for legal problems, housing, and food. After this stabilization, vocational rehabilitation and various psychotherapeutic issues may be addressed, including the management of affect such as depression. For individuals with psychosis, inpatient treatment or interventions with medication may be required before detoxification can occur.

Other treatment goals in longer-term management include total abstinence and family involvement. A common treatment goal in the longer-term management of individuals who abuse substances is abstinence from all drugs, although the individual often advocates for controlled use of some substances. For example, alcohol use by the individual receiving methadone maintenance or the continued smoking of marijuana or even tobacco by individuals formerly suffering from alcoholism can lead to a serious conflict in treatment goals. Another goal is to change the role of family members from *enablers* or codependents with the substance user to treatment allies. These family members need to be engaged in treatment to work as active collaborators in the therapeutic plan for the individual. Although family treatment is commonly applied to many mental disorders, it can have a particularly powerful impact with adolescent substance users to eliminate family behaviors that reinforce the drug taking.

The first issue in the relationship between the clinician and the individual undergoing treatment is approaching the substance user who denies a problem with abuse. This person must be confronted in such a way that the substance-use problem will become accessible for treatment. This confrontation may involve an *intervention*, in which a variety of the significant others and social supports of the user are brought together to confront the user about his or her substance abuse or dependence problem. Family and employers are important contributors to such an intervention.

Once the abuse is clearly identified as a problem, a series of other issues arise, including confidentiality versus necessary disclosures, comorbid mental disorders, medical evaluations, and potential for relapse. Individuals starting treatment also need to be assured of confidentiality in order to get them to be open with the therapist, since the use of illicit drugs can be associated with a variety of illegal activities. Confidentiality must be balanced against the need to disclose to their family about behaviors that can lead to a relapse of substance use. Psychiatric assessment is critical because of the high rates of depression and risk of suicide in this population. A full medical assessment generally is essential because of the high rates of infectious and gastrointestinal diseases directly related to substance abuse and dependence. Medical assessment is also essential to determine whether active medical detoxification is necessary. Finally, a psychotherapeutic issue early in treatment may be distinguishing between *slips* and a full relapse. Slips are common in substance users, and individuals must be prepared for them and not consider them failures that will inevitably lead to full relapse and dependence.

Somatic Treatments

Pharmacotherapy can have several roles in substance dependence treatment, including treatment of overdose and acute intoxication (naloxone, flumazenil), detoxification or withdrawal symptom relief (benzodiazepines, clonidine), blockage of drug reinforcement (naltrexone), development of responses to the abused substance (disulfiram), treatment of psychiatric comorbidity (antidepressants), and substitution agents to produce cross-tolerance and reduce drug craving (methadone). A key element in the treatment of many dependence-producing drugs is the need for detoxification, which may last from 3 days to as long as 2 weeks. Detoxification is essential if antagonist pharmacotherapies, such as naltrexone for opioid dependence, or aversive agents, such as disulfiram for alcoholism, are to be employed. Conversely, agonist maintenance treatment, such as methadone or buprenorphine for heroin dependence, does not require detoxification before beginning treatment. Using these agonists usually requires regular clinic attendance by the substance user and relatively prolonged treatment of 1 to 2 years, with some individuals continuing agonist therapy for up to 20 years.

Figure 15-2 outlines potential roles for pharmacotherapy and psychotherapy. The general treatment approaches, along with their indications and side effects, are seen in Table 15-3.

Psychosocial Treatments

A wide range of psychosocial treatments are available in SUDs, ranging from long-term residential treatments (6 to 8 months) to relatively low-intervention outpatient medication-free treatments with once-weekly hour-long therapy. In these outpatient treatments, professional interventions may be unavailable, and counseling is provided by nonprofessionals using group therapy. These groups may be based on extensions of self-help groups, such as Alcoholics Anonymous or Narcotics Anonymous, and use a 12-step program and the associated traditions of these fellowships.

Other treatment approaches include inpatient treatment specifically designed for detoxification and day hospital and evening programs focusing on the prevention of relapse. Behavioral treatments that have frequently been used include relapse prevention therapy as developed by Somers and Marlatt (1992) and contingency contracting, in which various

Table 15-3	General Treatment Approaches: Indications and Side Effects	
Treatment	**Indication**	**Side Effects**

Pharmacotherapy
  Detoxifications
	Dependence on
	  Alcohol
	  Opioids
	  Sedatives
		Overmedication, if not carefully monitored

		Undermedication, leading to seizures
Antagonists Aversive agents	Drug-free therapy failed	Precipitated withdrawal
Agonists Continued dependence		Illness from use of abused drugs

Psychotherapy
  Self-help
  Outpatient
  Day hospital
  Residential
	Lower level intervention failed	

Inpatient	Medical detoxification Psychotic behavior Suicidal behavior	Social cost
Urine monitoring Breath alcohol	Outpatient treatment	None

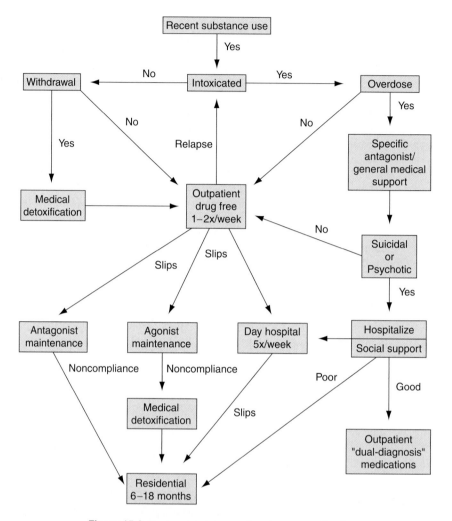

Figure 15-2 *Treatment decision tree for substance use disorders.*

aversive contingencies are put in place for periods of up to 6 months to prevent a relapse to substance abuse and potential dependence.

Special Treatment Factors

Comorbid psychiatric disorders, particularly depressive and anxiety disorders, are extremely common in substance abuse, with lifetime rates approaching 50% in individuals addicted to opioids. Although the rate of major psychotic disorders among SUDs is relatively low, the rate of substance abuse in individuals with schizophrenia or bipolar disorder may be as high as 50%.

Splitting treatment between a mental health clinic and substance-abuse clinic can be a significant problem for the coordinated management of the dual-diagnosis patient. A prominent problem in the management of SUDs with comorbid psychiatric disorders is medication management within a substance-abuse treatment setting, because of limited psychiatric resources. In mental health settings, the need for monitoring, using urine toxicological screens for illicit drugs, and breath testing for alcohol can pose difficult logistic and boundary problems. Integrated dual-diagnosis treatments have been developed using social skills training combined with relapse prevention behavioral therapies as well as pharmacological adjuncts to either typical or atypical neuroleptics for individuals with schizophrenia.

Another special factor in treatment is the relationship between many substance users and the legal system—for example, parole, probation, work release programs, or other alternatives to incarceration—because this requires the clinician to report to these agencies. Contingencies must be developed to clarify the content of this reporting as well as to obtain a specific release of confidentiality so that these reporting requirements can be fulfilled.

Treatment of a comorbid medical condition is essential in SUDs because many substance users do not seek medical care and may be seen only by a mental health professional. The most important current comorbid disorder in SUDs is AIDS that is spread primarily by intravenous drug use but, increasingly, is also spread through sexual activity among drug users. Other areas of medical comorbidity include vitamin deficiencies, infectious diseases, and gastrointestinal disorders such as cirrhosis, gastrointestinal bleeding, and peptic and duodenal ulcers. Stimulant users may experience cerebrovascular accidents. Also, dementing disorders need particular consideration in conjunction with alcoholism, inhalant abuse, and sedative dependence.

Two clinical questions often arise: is use of addictive medication flatly contraindicated in individuals with any kind of substance-abuse history, or is such medication prohibited only in instances of use of drugs of the same class (e.g., alcohol and benzodiazepines, and methylphenidate and cocaine). In general, a physician should never rule out the use of any addictive drug if there are good symptom-based reasons for prescribing it. Nor should the physician assume that an addicting drug of one class (e.g., opiates) will be safe for an individual who abused another class such as stimulants. However, in any situation in which a potentially addicting drug is considered for use in a remitted substance abuser, considerable caution and limit setting is warranted. Finally, inpatient management may become necessary for the evaluation and use of these risky treatment interventions.

Treatment-Refractory Individuals

A variety of escalating treatment interventions can be applied to individuals with substance abuse or dependence who are refractory to treatment. If initial detoxification with outpatient follow-up care is ineffective, several levels of intensified interventions can be applied, such as agonist maintenance with methadone for individuals addicted to opioids, disulfiram treatment for individuals with alcoholism, and perhaps antidepressants for stimulant use disorders. Further interventions can include residential placement for up to 2 years to enable full psychosocial rehabilitation of refractory individuals.

POLYSUBSTANCE DEPENDENCE

This category is often confused with the much more frequently encountered situation in which the individual is dependent on several different substances at the same time. This category does NOT apply in such situations; individuals should instead be given multiple substance-dependence diagnoses, one for each type of substance that the person is dependent on. For example, an individual who smokes crack several times a week, injects heroin daily, and smokes several joints a day would receive three diagnoses: crack dependence, heroin dependence, and marijuana dependence and not a diagnosis of polysubstance dependence.

Polysubstance dependence is intended to be used only in those situations in which there is a pattern of multiple drug use that it fails to meet the criteria for substance dependence on any one class of drug. In such settings, the only viable way to assign a diagnosis of dependence is to consider all the substances that the person uses taken together as if it were one type of drug.

Two typical patterns of drug use fall under the category of polysubstance dependence. In one such pattern, the individual indiscriminantly uses a number of different drugs, so that he or she does not really care what drug is being used, so long as a *high* results. The second pattern is analogous to the old DSM-III concept of *mixed personality disorder* in which an individual would have features from a number of different personality disorders but not one would predominate the picture. In this case, one or two dependence criteria are met for each of several different classes of drug but full criteria for dependence are only met when the drug classes are grouped together as a whole. For example, a diagnosis of polysubstance dependence applies to an individual who, during the same 12-month period, missed work because of his heavy use of alcohol, continued to use marijuana despite the fact that it lead to asthma attacks, and was repeatedly unable to stay within his self-imposed limits regarding his use of cocaine. In this instance, although his problems associated with the use of any one drug were not severe enough to justify a diagnosis of dependence on that drug, his overall use of substances significantly impaired his functioning and thus warrants a diagnosis of polysubstance dependence, that is, on the group of substances taken as a whole.

OTHER SUBSTANCE-USE DISORDERS: ANABOLIC STEROIDS AND NITRITES

This group of substance-induced conditions most notably includes anabolic steroids and nitrite inhalants. Both have psychoactive effects and can have consequences for the individual and broad public health, which suggest that future research may lead to their inclusion in DSM-V as separate disorders.

In 1988, a survey of male high school seniors showed that anabolic steroids had a lifetime use rate of 6.6% (Buckley et al. 1988). Thus, by the late 1980s, widespread abuse of anabolic steroids was occurring among males as well as females. Multiple types of steroid derivatives were being used in order to make the lipid soluble steroids more water soluble and easier to administer than the intramuscular injections that were typically required. Because of this abuse, anabolic steroids were added to Schedule III of the Controlled Substances Act in 1990.

The clinical effects of anabolic steroids are related to a typical *cycle* of 4 to 18 weeks on steroids and 1 month to 1 year off. While taking the steroids, the primary effects sought by abusers are increasing muscle mass and strength, and not euphoria. In the context of an adequate diet and significant physical activity, these individuals appear quite healthy and they are unlikely to appear for treatment of their anabolic steroid abuse. However, some of the adverse cardiovascular, hepatic, and musculoskeletal effects of steroids as well as virilization in women may bring these users to medical attention. Severe cases of acne can also bring some adolescents to medical attention. Abuse of other psychoactive drugs may occur in up to a third of these steroid users, but is generally relatively low compared to other substance abusers.

Heavy use can increase aggression, change libido and sexual functions, and induce mood changes with occasional psychotic features (Brower et al. 1991, Su et al. 1993). In studies comparing doses of 40 to 240 mg/day of methyltestosterone in a double-blind inpatient trial, irritability, mood swings, violent feelings, and hostility were greater during the high-dose period than at baseline. Androgenic steroids' tendency to provoke aggression and irritability has raised concerns about violence toward family members by abusers. Prospective trials have reported mood disturbances in over 50% of body builders using anabolic steroids, as well as cognitive impairment including distractibility, forgetfulness, and confusion.

Dependence symptoms have included a withdrawal syndrome with common symptoms being fatigue, depressed mood, and desire to take more steroids. Other common dependence symptoms are as follows: using the substance more than intended, continuing to use steroids despite problems worsened by its use and the excessive spending of time relating to obtaining steroids. Because few clinical laboratories are equipped to conduct steroid tests and because these tests are quite expensive, these signs of dependence and some common laboratory abnormalities are usually used to make the diagnosis.

Anabolic steroid abuse leads to hypertrophied muscles, acne, oily skin, needle punctures over large muscles, hirsutism in females, and gynecomastia in males. Heavy users can also develop edema and jaundice. Common laboratory abnormalities include elevated hemoglobin and hematocrit, elevated low-density lipoprotein cholesterol, elevated liver function tests, and reduced luteinizing hormone levels.

Mental health professionals may have these individuals come to their attention because of the excessive aggression, loss of sexual ability, or mood disturbances. Treatment approaches are generally symptomatically oriented toward controlling the depressed mood and the psychotic features, but longer-term interventions such as peer counseling by former body builders and group support may be of value for these users.

Nitrite inhalants are sometimes considered within the category of inhalant abuse and produce an intoxication with mild euphoria, muscle relaxation, and a change in time perception. Concern has been raised about their impairing immune functioning, a decrease in oxygen-carrying capacity of the blood and toxicity with severe headache, vomiting, and hypotension. No physical dependence or withdrawal syndrome has been described with these drugs.

Comparison of DSM-IV-TR/ICD-10 Diagnostic Criteria

The ICD-10 Diagnostic Criteria for Research for Substance Dependence are close, but not identical, to the DSM-IV-TR criteria. ICD-10 has included all seven of the DSM-IV-TR items but condenses these into five criteria and adds a sixth item tapping drug-craving behavior. Furthermore, the method for establishing clinical significance differs in the two systems. DSM-IV-TR specifies that there be a maladaptive pattern of substance use leading to clinically significant impairment or distress, whereas the ICD-10 Diagnostic Criteria for Research indicate either a one-month duration or repeated occurrences within a 12-month period.

The ICD-10 Diagnostic Criteria for Research corresponding to Substance Abuse is less specific than the criteria in DSM-IV-TR, requiring that there be "clear evidence that substance use was responsible for (or substantially contributed to) physical or psychological harm, including impaired judgment or dysfunctional behavior, which may lead to disability or have adverse consequences for interpersonal relationships". In ICD-10, this disorder is referred to as *Harmful Use*.

The ICD-10 Diagnostic Criteria for Research for Intoxication are nearly equivalent to the DSM-IV-TR criteria. However, in contrast to the DSM-IV-TR definition of Withdrawal, which specifies that the withdrawal symptoms cause clinically significant distress or impairment, the ICD-10 Diagnostic Criteria for Research for Withdrawal indicates only the presence of characteristic signs and symptoms.

References

Brower KJ, Blow FC, Young JP, et al. (1991) Symptoms and correlates of anabolic-androgenic steroid dependence. *Br J Addict* **86**(6), 759–768.

Buckley WE, Yesalis CE, Freidl KE, et al. (1988) Estimated prevalence of anabolic steroid use among male high school seniors. *J Am Med Assoc* **260**(23), 3441–3445.

Cloninger CR (1999) Genetics of substance abuse. In *Textbook of Substance Abuse Treatment*, 2nd ed., Galanter M and Kleber H (eds). American Psychiatric Press, Washington, DC, pp. 59–66.

Edwards G and Gross MM (1976) Alcohol dependence: provisional description of the clinical syndrome. *Br Med J* **1**, 1058–1061.

Kandel DB (1975) Stages in adolescent involvement in drug use. *Science* **190**, 912–914.

Kandel DB, Johnson JG, Bird HR, et al. (1999) Psychiatric comorbidity among adolescents with substance use disorders: findings from the MECA study. *J Am Acad Child Adolesc Psychiatry* **38**(6), 693–699.

Kessler RC, McGonagle KA, Zhao S, et al. (1994) Lifetime and 12-month prevalence of DSM-III-R psychiatric disorders in the United States: results from the national comorbidity survey. *Arch Gen Psychiatry* **51**, 8–19.

Khantzian EJ (1985) The self-medication hypothesis of addictive disorders: focus on heroin and cocaine dependence. *Am J Psychiatry* **142**, 1259–1264.

Koob GF and Le Moa M (2001) Drug addiction, dysregulation of reward, and allostasis. *Neuropsychopharmacology* **24**, 97–129.

Kosten TR and Hollister L (2001) Drugs of abuse (Chapter 32 Rev.). In *Basic & Clinical Pharmacology*, 8th ed., Katzung GB (ed). Appleton & Lange, Stamford, CT, pp. 532–547.

Nestler EJ (2000) Genes and addiction. *Nat Genet* **26**, 277–281.

Regier DA, Myers JK, Kramer M, et al. (1984) NIMH epidemiologic catchment area program. *Arch Gen Psychiatry* **41**, 934–941.

Somers JM and Marlatt GA (1992) Alcohol problems. In *Principles and Practice of Relapse Prevention*, Wilson PH (ed). Guilford Press, New York, pp. 23–42.

Spanagel R and Weiss F (1999) The dopamine hypothesis of reward: past and current status. *Trends Neurosci* **22**, 521–527.

Su TP, Pagliaro M, Schmidt PJ, et al. (1993) Neuropsychiatric effects of anabolic steroids in male normal volunteers. *J Am Med Assoc* **269**(21), 2760–2764.

Wallace JM Jr., Forman TA, Guthrie BJ, et al. (1999) The epidemiology of alcohol, tobacco and other drug use among black youth. *J Stud Alcohol* **60**(6), 800–809.

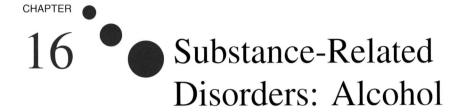

16 Substance-Related Disorders: Alcohol

Alcohol consumption occurs along a continuum, with considerable variability in drinking patterns among individuals. There is no sharp demarcation between "social" or "moderate" drinking and "problem" or "harmful" drinking (Babor et al. 1987a). It is clear, however, that as average alcohol consumption and frequency of intoxication increase, so does the incidence of medical and psychosocial problems (Kranzler et al. 1990). The main focus of this chapter is the alcohol use disorders, which according to the DSM-IV-TR, include alcohol abuse and alcohol dependence. Also included in this chapter are the Alcohol-Induced Disorders, which are those psychiatric disorders caused by the direct effects of alcohol on the central nervous system (CNS) (i.e., Alcohol Intoxication, Alcohol Withdrawal, Alcohol-Induced Persisting Dementia, Alcohol-Induced Persisting Amnestic Disorder, Alcohol-Induced Psychotic Disorder, Alcohol-Induced Mood Disorder, Alcohol-Induced Anxiety Disorder, Alcohol-Induced Sleep Disorder, and Alcohol-Induced Sexual Dysfunction).

The most visible group of people affected by alcohol problems are those who have developed a syndrome of alcohol dependence and who are commonly referred to as alcoholics. In this chapter, the term *alcoholic* is applied specifically to those individuals with alcohol dependence. A less prominent group consists of those persons who experience problems with their drinking but who are not dependent on alcohol. These individuals are variously termed alcohol abusers, problem drinkers, and harmful drinkers. These two "worlds" of alcohol problems may require different approaches to diagnosis and clinical management.

Diagnosis

Diagnostic criteria for alcohol use disorders in DSM-IV-TR are very similar to those employed in the *International Classification of Diseases*, Tenth Edition (ICD-10) (World Health Organization 1992), which in turn were based upon the alcohol dependence syndrome (ADS) concept of Edwards and Gross (1976). ADS is a conception of alcoholism that includes biological, cognitive, and behavioral elements.

Alcohol Dependence and Abuse The DSM-IV-TR diagnosis of *alcohol dependence* is given when three or more of the seven criteria are present (see generic DSM-IV-TR criteria for Substance Dependence, Chapter 15 on page 351). Because physiological dependence is associated with greater potential for acute medical problems (particularly, acute alcohol withdrawal), the first criteria to be considered are tolerance and withdrawal. The remaining criteria reflect the behavioral and cognitive dimensions of ADS: (1) impaired control (i.e., alcohol is consumed in larger amounts or over a longer period of time than was intended; there is a persistent desire or unsuccessful efforts to cut down or control drinking; the individual continues to drink despite knowledge of a persistent or recurrent physical or psychological problem), and (2) increased salience of alcohol (i.e., a great deal of time spent drinking or recovering from its effects; important social, occupational, or recreational activities are given up or reduced because of drinking).

Once a diagnosis of alcohol dependence is given, a specification is made concerning course. *Early remission* is used if no criteria (*full remission*) or fewer than three symptoms (*partial remission*) of alcohol dependence are present for at least 1 month, but less than 12 months. *Sustained remission* is used if no symptoms (*full remission*) or fewer than three symptoms (*partial remission*) of alcohol dependence are present for at least 12 months. Finally, if the individual is in a setting where he or she has no access to alcohol, the course specifier *in a controlled environment* is added (see page 364 for graphical depictions of these patterns of remission).

Alcohol abuse is considered to be present only if the individual's drinking pattern has never met criteria for alcohol dependence and he or she demonstrates a pattern of drinking that leads to clinically significant impairment or distress, as evidenced by one or more of the four criteria in DSM-IV-TR for alcohol abuse (see generic DSM-IV-TR criteria for Substance Abuse, Chapter 15, page 352).

Alcohol Intoxication A DSM-IV-TR diagnosis of alcohol intoxication is given when, shortly after alcohol consumption, there are maladaptive behaviors such as aggression or inappropriate sexual behavior, or there are psychological changes such as labile mood and impaired judgment (see DSM-IV-TR diagnostic criteria below). Clinical signs indicative of alcohol intoxication include slurred speech, lack of coordination, unsteady gait, nystagmus, impairment of attention and memory, and in the most severe cases, stupor and coma. Alcohol intoxication may also present with severe disturbances in consciousness and cognition (alcohol intoxication delirium), especially when large amounts of alcohol have been ingested or after alcoholic intoxication has been sustained for extended periods. Usually, this condition subsides shortly after alcohol intoxication ends. Physical and mental status examinations accompanied by analysis of blood and urine allow the clinician to rule out general medical conditions or mental disorders mimicking this condition. In this regard, urine toxicology is a valuable tool in ruling out intoxication with benzodiazepines, barbiturates, or other sedatives that can present with a similar clinical picture. Collateral information from relatives or friends confirming the ingestion of alcohol is also useful and should be actively pursued by the clinician.

Diagnostic Criteria

303.00 Alcohol Intoxication

A. Recent ingestion of alcohol.
B. Clinically significant maladaptive behavioral or psychological changes (e.g., inappropriate sexual or aggressive behavior, mood lability, impaired judgment, impaired social or occupational functioning) that developed during, or shortly after, alcohol ingestion.
C. One (or more) of the following signs, developing during, or shortly after, alcohol use:

(1) slurred speech
(2) incoordination

(3) unsteady gait

(4) nystagmus

(5) impairment in attention or memory

(6) stupor or coma

D. The symptoms are not due to a general medical condition and are not better accounted for by another mental disorder

The blood alcohol level (BAL) is frequently used as a measure of alcohol intoxication, although this measure is less reliable in persons with a high degree of tolerance to alcohol. Alcohol is metabolized in the average adult at a rate of 1 oz or 7 to 10 g/hour. When this clearance rate is surpassed, signs of alcohol intoxication begin to appear. During the ascending limb of the BAL curve, euphoria, anxiolysis, and mild deficits in coordination, attention, and cognition can be observed at levels between 0.01 and 0.10%. Marked deficits in coordination and psychomotor skills, decreased attention, ataxia, impaired judgment, slurred speech, and mood lability can be observed at a greater BAL. Severe intoxication, characterized by lack of coordination, incoherent thoughts, confusion, nausea, and vomiting can be observed at BALs between 0.20 and 0.30. However, at these levels, some heavy-drinking individuals who have developed tolerance to the effects of alcohol may not appear intoxicated and may perform well on psychomotor or cognitive tasks. Stupor and loss of consciousness often occur when the BAL is between 0.30 and 0.40. Beyond this level, coma, respiratory depression, and death are possible outcomes. It should also be noted that alcohol intoxication is often associated with toxicity and overdose with other drugs, particularly those with depressant effects on the CNS.

Alcohol Withdrawal   Alcohol withdrawal is a condition that follows a reduction in alcohol consumption or an abrupt cessation of drinking in alcohol-dependent individuals (see DSM-IV-TR diagnostic criteria on page 378). In addition to significant distress, alcohol withdrawal is also associated with impairment of social, occupational, and other areas of functioning. Uncomplicated cases of alcohol withdrawal are characterized by signs and symptoms of autonomic hyperactivity, and may include increased heart rate, increased blood pressure, hyperthermia, diaphoresis, tremor, nausea, vomiting, insomnia, and anxiety. Onset of symptoms of uncomplicated alcohol withdrawal usually occurs between 4 and 12 hours following the last drink. Symptom severity tends to peak around the second day, usually subsiding by the fourth or fifth day of abstinence. After this period, less severe anxiety, insomnia, and autonomic symptoms may persist for a few weeks, with some individuals experiencing a protracted alcohol-withdrawal syndrome up to 5 or 6 months after cessation of drinking. A small but significant number of alcohol-dependent individuals (10%) can experience complicated alcohol-withdrawal episodes. Alcohol-withdrawal delirium (also known as delirium tremens) can occur in 5% of the cases, usually between 36 and 72 hours following alcohol cessation. In addition to signs of autonomic hyperactivity, this condition is characterized by illusions, auditory, visual, or tactile hallucinations, psychomotor agitation, fluctuating cloudiness of consciousness, and disorientation. Grand mal seizures associated with alcohol withdrawal occur in 3 to 5% of the cases, typically within the first 48 hours following reduction or cessation of drinking. In both instances of complicated alcohol withdrawal, lack or delay in instituting proper treatment is associated with an increased mortality rate. Prior history of delirium tremens and/or alcohol-withdrawal seizures, older age, poor nutritional status, comorbid medical conditions, and history of high tolerance to alcohol are predictors of increased severity of alcohol withdrawal.

Diagnostic Criteria

291.81 Alcohol Withdrawal

A. Cessation of (or reduction in) alcohol use that has been heavy and prolonged.
B. Two (or more) of the following, developing within several hours to a few days after Criterion A:

  (1) autonomic hyperactivity (e.g., sweating or pulse rate greater than 100)
  (2) increased hand tremor
  (3) insomnia
  (4) nausea or vomiting
  (5) transient visual, tactile, or auditory hallucinations or illusions
  (6) psychomotor agitation
  (7) anxiety
  (8) grand mal seizures

C. The symptoms in Criterion B cause clinically significant distress or impairment in social, occupational, or other important areas of functioning.
D. The symptoms are not due to a general medical condition and are not better accounted for by another mental disorder.

Specify if:

With Perceptual Disturbances.

Reprinted with permission from the Diagnostic and Statistical Manual of Mental Disorders, Fourth Edition, Text Revision. Copyright 2000 American Psychiatric Association.

Alcohol-Induced Persisting Dementia   Continuous heavy drinking is also associated with progressive and gradual development of multiple cognitive deficits characterized by memory impairment, apraxia, agnosia, or disturbances in executive functioning (see generic DSM-IV-TR diagnostic criteria for Substance-Induced Persisting Dementia, Chapter 13, page 299). These deficits cause serious impairment in social and occupational functioning and persist beyond the duration of alcohol intoxication and alcohol withdrawal. History, physical examination, and laboratory tests should be utilized to determine whether these deficits are etiologically related to the toxic effects of alcohol use. Other factors associated with this condition are poor nutritional status and vitamin deficiencies as well as history of head trauma. It is believed that this condition is associated with the repeated occurrence of Wernicke's encephalopathy. Atrophy of frontal lobes and increased ventricular size have been described in this condition. Continuous alcohol consumption exacerbates the dementia, whereas drinking cessation is associated with improvement and even recovery of cognitive deficits.

Alcohol-Induced Persisting Amnestic Disorder   Continuous heavy alcohol consumption can lead to several neurological deficits caused by thiamine deficiency. Among them, alcohol-induced persisting amnestic disorder (AIPAD, also known as a Korsakoff's psychosis due to the fantastic confabulatory stories described by individuals suffering this condition) is prominent (see generic DSM-IV-TR diagnostic criteria for Substance-Induced Persisting Amnestic Disorder, Chapter 13, page 303). Profound deficits in anterograde memory and some deficits in retrograde memory characterize this condition. Individuals cannot retain or learn new information and experience profound disorientation to time and place. The severity of anterograde memory deficits typically leads individuals suffering from Korsakoff's psychosis, who are unaware of their deficit, to reconstruct forgotten events by confabulating. Korsakoff's amnestic disorder is usually preceded by several episodes of Wernicke's encephalopathy, characterized by confusion, ataxia, nystagmus, and gaze palsies. When this condition subsides, the characteristic memory deficits of Korsakoff's psychosis become prominent.

Cessation of drinking can lead to an improvement in memory with approximately 20% of the cases demonstrating complete recovery. However, in most cases, memory deficits remain unchanged, and in some instances, long-term care is needed despite sobriety.

Alcohol-Induced Psychotic Disorder   This disorder is characterized by prominent hallucinations or delusions that are judged by the clinician to be due to the effects of alcohol (see generic DSM-IV-TR diagnostic criteria for Substance-Induced Psychotic Disorder, Chapter 15 on page 355). The psychotic symptoms usually occur within a month of an alcohol intoxication or withdrawal episode, and the individual is characteristically fully alert and oriented, lacking insight that these symptoms are alcohol-induced. Although onset of psychotic symptoms can occur during or shortly after alcohol intoxication, delirium or alcohol-withdrawal delirium, alcohol-induced hallucinations, and/or delusions do not occur exclusively during the course of these conditions. Evidence that hallucinations and delusions are not part of a primary psychotic disorder include: atypical or late age of onset of psychotic symptoms, onset of alcohol drinking preceding the onset of psychiatric symptoms, and remission of psychotic episodes during extended periods of abstinence. Usually, alcohol-induced psychotic symptoms tend to subside within a few weeks of abstinence, although in a subset of individuals, psychotic symptoms can become chronic, requiring long-term treatment with antipsychotic medication. In these cases, clinicians are obligated to consider schizophrenia or delusional disorder as part of the differential diagnosis.

Alcohol-Induced Mood Disorder   Alcohol-induced mood disorder (AIMD), characterized by depressed mood and anhedonia, as well as elevated, expansive, or irritable mood, frequently develops as a consequence of heavy drinking (see generic DSM-IV-TR diagnostic criteria for Substance-Induced Mood Disorder, Chapter 15 on page 356). Onset of symptoms can occur during episodes of alcohol intoxication or withdrawal and may resemble a primary major depressive, manic, hypomanic, or a mixed episode. In contrast to the dysphoria and lack of energy observed during episodes of alcohol withdrawal, the severity and duration of alcohol-induced mood symptoms is greater than what is usually expected, warranting independent attention by the clinician. Although mood disturbances are common among alcoholic individuals entering treatment (occurring in up to 80% of individuals), alcohol-induced mood symptoms tend to subside within 2 to 4 weeks following alcohol cessation. Evidence that the mood disturbances are not better explained by a primary mood disorder should be sought by the clinician. Evidence suggesting a primary mood disorder includes onset of mood symptoms preceding onset of alcohol abuse and persistence of mood symptoms after alcohol cessation or during extended periods of abstinence. Regardless of the primary or secondary nature of mood symptoms, given the high prevalence of suicide among alcoholics, clinicians should closely monitor the individual for emerging suicidal thoughts, implementing more intensive treatment (discussed later) if necessary.

Alcohol-Induced Anxiety Disorder   Although alcohol has anxiolytic properties at low doses, heavy alcohol consumption can induce prominent anxiety symptoms. Alcohol-induced anxiety (AIA) symptoms more commonly include generalized anxiety symptoms, panic attacks, and phobias (see generic DSM-IV-TR diagnostic criteria for Substance-Induced Anxiety Disorder, Chapter 15 on page 357). In order to establish this diagnosis, clinicians must rule out other general medical conditions or mental disorders that can mimic this problem. AIA may develop during alcohol intoxication or withdrawal, but its severity and duration are typically worse than the anxiety normally observed during the course of these conditions. An onset of drinking preceding the anxiety syndrome, and improvement or remission of anxiety during periods of abstinence, suggest alcohol-induced anxiety disorder (AIAD). Monitoring the course of these symptoms for several weeks after alcohol cessation can be useful in determining their nature. Usually, a substantial improvement of anxiety will be observed during this period, suggesting a direct relationship of anxiety to alcohol. In some cases, a full remission of symptoms is not observed until after 3 to 4 weeks of abstinence.

Alcohol-Induced Sleep Disorder

Heavy alcohol consumption can be associated with a prominent disturbance of sleep (see generic DSM-IV-TR diagnostic criteria for Substance-Induced Sleep Disorder, Chapter 15 on page 359). At intoxicating BALs, especially when BALs are declining, sedation and sleepiness can be observed. Alcohol intoxication induces an increase in nonrapid eye movement (NREM) sleep, whereas rapid eye movement (REM) sleep density decreases. Subsequently, there is an increase in wakefulness, restless sleep, and vivid dreams or nightmares related to a reduction in NREM sleep and a rebound in REM sleep density. During alcohol withdrawal, sleep is fragmented and discontinuous with an increase in REM sleep. After withdrawal, individuals frequently complain of sleep difficulties and may experience superficial and fragmented sleep for months or years.

In contrast to the primary sleep disorders (PSD), alcohol-induced sleep disorder (AISD) is characterized by an onset of drinking preceding the sleep disturbance and by remission of symptoms during the course of sustained abstinence. AISD can occur during the course of a typical alcohol intoxication or alcohol-withdrawal episode. However, duration and severity of the sleep disturbances exceed those typically observed during these conditions. Given that protracted alcohol-withdrawal symptoms are frequent among abstinent alcoholics, onset of AISD can occur up to 4 weeks after initiation of alcohol abstinence. History of a previous PSD and/or persistence of sleep disturbances for more than 4 weeks following intoxication or acute withdrawal are highly suggestive of a PSD. Differential diagnosis is complicated by the fact that heavy alcohol consumption can co-occur and exacerbate other mental disorders that present with sleep disturbances (e.g., mood disorders, anxiety). Alcohol consumption can also intensify other sleep problems such as narcolepsy or breathing-related sleep disorders BRSD.

Alcohol-Induced Sexual Dysfunction

Although small doses of alcohol in healthy individuals appear to enhance sexual receptivity in women and facilitate arousal to erotic stimuli in men, continuous and/or heavy drinking may cause significant sexual impairment. Alcohol-induced sexual dysfunction is characterized by impaired desire, impaired arousal, and impaired orgasm, or sexual pain (see generic DSM-IV-TR diagnostic criteria for Substance-Induced Sexual Dysfunction, Chapter 15 on page 358). It is also associated with marked distress or interpersonal conflicts. Onset of these impairments usually occurs during alcohol intoxication but the duration of symptoms exceeds the uncomplicated course of alcohol intoxication. Symptoms usually subside after 3 to 4 weeks of alcohol abstinence. Persistence of symptoms beyond this time may suggest a primary sexual dysfunction (PSD) or a sexual dysfunction due to the medical complications of alcoholism (e.g., neuropathy, alcoholic liver disease). Onset of a recurrent sexual dysfunction preceding the onset of alcohol abuse also suggests a primary disorder. Use of other substances, particularly those prescribed for the treatment of alcohol withdrawal such as benzodiazepines or barbiturates, should be ruled out as a cause of the sexual dysfunction.

Comprehensive assessment provides the basis for an individualized plan of treatment. Depending upon the severity of alcohol dependence, the nature of comorbid medical and psychiatric pathology, the presence of social supports, and evidence of previous response to treatment, decisions can be made concerning the most appropriate intensity, setting, and modality of treatment.

Although denial of alcohol-related problems is legendary among alcoholics, there is substantial evidence that a valid alcohol history can be obtained, given adequate assessment procedures and the right conditions (Babor et al. 1987b). A complete alcohol history should include specific questions concerning average alcohol consumption, maximal consumption per drinking occasion, frequency of heavy-drinking occasions, and drinking-related social problems (e.g., objections raised by family members, friends, or people at work), legal problems (including arrests or near-arrests for driving while intoxicated (DWI)), psychiatric symptoms (e.g., precipitation or exacerbation of mood or anxiety symptoms), and alcohol-related medical problems (e.g., alcoholic gastritis or pancreatitis).

It is crucial that questions concerning alcohol consumption and related problems be asked nonjudgmentally in order to enhance the likelihood of accurate reporting. The optimal approach to history taking in the substance-abuse individual includes reassuring the individual that information provided will be kept confidential. The interview begins with questions that are least likely to make the individual defensive (e.g., a review of systems or psychiatric symptoms, without relating these to alcohol use), and beginning questions with *how*, rather than with *why*, to reduce the appearance of being judgmental (Schottenfeld 1994).

Systematic clinical assessment often begins with routine screening to identify active cases, as well as persons at risk. During the past 25 years, a number of self-report screening tests have been developed to identify alcoholics as well as persons at risk of alcohol problems. The Michigan Alcoholism Screening Test (MAST), developed by Selzer (1971), is one of the most often cited instruments. It contains 25 items that ask about drinking habits, as well as social, occupational, and interpersonal problems associated with excessive drinking. Perhaps the most widely used alcohol-screening test is the CAGE (Ewing 1984), which contains only four questions: (1) Have you ever felt you ought to *cut* (the "C" in CAGE) down on your drinking? (2) Have people *annoyed* (A) you by criticizing your drinking? (3) Have you ever felt bad or *guilty* (G) about your drinking? (4) Have you ever had a drink first thing in the morning to steady your nerves or get rid of a hangover, that is, an *eye* opener (E)? Reliability and validity studies of this test have been conducted in diverse samples (e.g., psychiatric inpatients, ambulatory medical patients, prenatal clinics), with generally acceptable levels of sensitivity (Babor and Kadden 1985).

The Alcohol Use Disorders Identification Test (AUDIT) (Saunders et al. 1993, Babor and Higgins-Biddle 2001a), a 10-item screening instrument, may be used as the first step in a comprehensive and sequential alcohol use history. The AUDIT (Table 16-1) covers the domains of alcohol consumption, symptoms of alcohol dependence, and alcohol-related consequences. It has been shown to be sensitive and specific in discriminating alcoholics from nonalcoholics, and is superior to the MAST in identifying hazardous drinkers, that is, those heavy drinkers who have not yet experienced serious harm from their drinking (Bohn et al. 1995). The AUDIT total score increases with the severity of alcohol dependence and related problems, and can be used as part of a comprehensive approach to early identification and patient placement (Babor and Higgins-Biddle 2001a,b). Because the misuse of both prescribed and illicit drugs is common among alcoholics, screening should include other psychoactive substances, including tobacco products.

Diagnostic assessment in specialized treatment facilities, such as detoxification centers, residential programs, partial hospital programs, and outpatient clinics, should be conducted with a standard interview schedule. If it is not possible to use a complete psychiatric

Table 16-1	Alcohol Use Disorders Identification Test

1. How often do you have a drink containing alcohol?
   (0) Never (1) Monthly or less (2) Two to four times a month (3) Two or three times a week (4) Four or more times a week

2.* How many drinks containing alcohol do you have on a typical day when you are drinking? (Code number of standard drinks)
   (0) 1 or 2 (1) 3 or 4 (2) 5 or 6 (3) 7 or 8 (4) 10 or more

3. How often do you have 6 or more drinks on one occasion?
   (0) Never (1) Less than monthly (2) Monthly (3) Weekly (4) Daily or almost daily

4. How often during the last year have you found that you were not able to stop drinking once you had started?
   (0) Never (1) Less than monthly (2) Monthly (3) Weekly (4) Daily or almost daily

5. How often during the last year have you failed to do what was normally expected from you because of drinking?
   (0) Never (1) Less than monthly (2) Monthly (3) Weekly (4) Daily or almost daily

6. How often during the last year have you needed a first drink in the morning to get yourself going after a heavy-drinking session?
   (0) Never (1) Less than monthly (2) Monthly (3) Weekly (4) Daily or almost daily

7. How often during the last year have you had a feeling of guilt or remorse after drinking?
   (0) Never (1) Less than monthly (2) Monthly (3) Weekly (4) Daily or almost daily

8. How often during the last year have you been unable to remember what happened the night before because you had been drinking?
   (0) Never (1) Less than monthly (2) Monthly (3) Weekly (4) Daily or almost daily

9. Have you or someone else been injured as a result of your drinking?
   (0) No (2) Yes, but not in the last year (4) Yes, during the last year

10. Has a relative or friend or a physician or other health care worker been concerned about your drinking or suggested you cut down?
   (0) No (2) Yes, but not in the last year (4) Yes, during the last year

Record sum of individual item scores here_____.

*In determining the response categories, it has been assumed that one "drink" contains 10 g of alcohol.

interview, such as the Composite International Diagnostic Interview (CIDI) (Robins et al. 1989) or the Structured Clinical Interview for DSM (SCID) (First et al. 1996), then the alcohol sections of these interviews should be used. Given the lack of reliability in unstructured clinical diagnosis, it is imperative that programs specializing in the treatment of alcohol dependence use a structured interview to conduct and report their diagnostic evaluations.

An important purpose of clinical assessment is to obtain an estimate of illness severity. The number of DSM symptoms obtained using a structured interview can serve this purpose or the total score on the AUDIT screening test. The Composite Score from the Drug and Alcohol (CSDA) section of the Addiction Severity Index (ASI) (McLellan et al. 1992) is another useful measure of severity. For lifetime severity, the total score on the MAST is a good measure of severity.

Assessment of psychological function should focus on measures of depression, anxiety, and more global psychological distress. Instruments that are generally reliable, valid, and acceptable in a variety of health care settings include the Beck Depression Inventory (Beck et al. 1961) and the Symptom Checklist 90-Revised (Derogatis 1977). One subscale of the ASI assesses overall psychiatric severity, including number of inpatient and outpatient treatment episodes, medication status, and lifetime and current symptomatology (McLellan et al. 1992).

There has been considerable attention devoted to the role of motivation and readiness of the individual to change, as critical ingredients in treatment planning for alcoholics. The University of Rhode Island Change Assessment Scale (URICA) is a 32-item questionnaire designed to measure the stages of change across diverse problem behaviors (Prochaska and DiClemente 1992). The URICA score profiles have been used to predict treatment response in research on addictive behaviors such as smoking and alcoholism. The readiness to change questionnaire (RCQ) (Rollnick et al. 1992) is a short 12-item instrument developed for the same purpose.

Medical illness is a common consequence of heavy drinking (Babor et al. 1987a, Eckardt et al. 1981) and may be present in the absence of physical dependence. Early in the course, individuals with alcoholism may show no physical or laboratory abnormalities. But as it progresses, it is widely manifested throughout most organ systems. A thorough physical examination is indicated if, in the history, there is evidence of medical problems. The physical examination provides essential information about the presence and extent of end-organ damage, and should be focused on the systems most vulnerable to developing alcohol-related pathology: the cardiovascular system, the gastrointestinal system, and the central and peripheral nervous systems. The physician should also be alert to other acute alcohol-related signs, including alcohol withdrawal or delirium, intoxication or withdrawal from other drugs, and the acute presentation of psychiatric symptomatology. Other systemic or nonspecific health problems associated with alcoholism include malnutrition, muscle wasting, neuritis, specific vitamin deficiencies, infectious diseases (such as tuberculosis, dermatitis, pediculosis, and hepatitis), and trauma secondary to fights and accidents (Arif and Westermeyer 1988) (Table 16-2).

A variety of laboratory tests can be helpful in assessing the effects of alcohol consumption. Individuals experiencing alcohol disorders are typically reluctant to seek help or tend to underreport the frequency and intensity of their drinking. Diagnostic laboratory markers can help detect individuals who deny or minimize their alcohol consumption. Laboratory testing can help resolve diagnostic dilemmas among individuals whose self-report information and physical findings are inconclusive (Allen and Litten 2001).

Laboratory tests can also help detect relapse to the extent they are sensitive to heavy drinking. Early identification of relapse can prevent the reinstatement of alcohol dependence. It can diminish adverse consequences of heavy drinking by promoting modifications to the original treatment plan and by prompting more aggressive therapeutic interventions. Finally, laboratory markers of drinking can be used to evaluate the effectiveness of specific therapeutic interventions and provide funding agencies with objective treatment outcome information (Allen and Litten 2001).

Several laboratory tests, particularly those related to hepatic function (e.g., serum transaminases, bilirubin, prothrombin time, and partial thromboplastin time) have been commonly used by clinicians. Other laboratory tests (e.g., gamma-glutamyl transpeptidase (GGTP), mean corpuscular volume (MCV)) of erythrocytes can be used as objective

Table 16-2	Health Problems Commonly Associated with Alcoholism •
Malnutrition, muscle wasting, neuritis, vitamin deficiencies Infectious diseases (e.g., tuberculosis) Hepatitis, pancreatitis, gastritis Trauma secondary to fights, accidents Cardiovascular disease (e.g., myocardial infarction)	

indicators of heavy drinking (Holt et al. 1981). Elevation in GGTP occurs in approximately three-fourths of alcoholics before there is clinical evidence of liver disease. It is often considered to be the earliest indication of heavy alcohol consumption and is widely available clinically (Holt et al. 1981). GGTP levels usually return to normal limits after 4 to 5 weeks of abstinence (Salaspuro 1986). As with GGTP, elevations of the transaminases serum glutamic oxaloacetic transaminase (SGOT) and serum glutamic pyruvic transaminase (SGPT) are common in other liver diseases. However, elevations in the transaminases are less sensitive indicators of heavy drinking, with SGOT being elevated in 32 to 77% of alcoholics, while elevations in SGPT have been observed in 50% of alcoholics (Holt et al. 1981). In contrast to the use of absolute values of SGPT and SGOT, the ratio of SGPT to SGOT may provide a more accurate indicator of heavy drinking. A ratio greater than 2 is more likely to be related to heavy alcohol consumption, whereas a ratio below 1 would suggest a different etiology (Sharpe et al. 1996). Elevation of MCV, which has also been associated with folate deficiency, is more prominent in alcoholics, especially among those who are smokers. Though MCV can assist clinicians in identifying individuals who drink excessively, particularly when this marker is used in combination with GGTP or carbohydrate-deficient transferrin (CDT), this is not an efficient indicator of relapse because of the 2- to 4-month period of abstinence that is needed for its normalization (Irwin et al. 1988).

CDT is more sensitive than most routine laboratory tests for the identification of heavy alcohol consumption. In one study, CDT was found to have a sensitivity of 91% and a specificity of 100% in distinguishing alcoholics from light drinkers/abstainers (Stibler et al. 1986). In that study, the values of CDT correlated significantly ($r = 0.64$) with the amount of alcohol consumed during the preceding month. A review of subsequent studies (Stibler 1991) showed the test to be somewhat less sensitive (82%) though quite specific (97%). In contrast to GGTP, CDT elevations are associated with few conditions other than heavy drinking (Litten et al. 1995, Murawaki et al. 1997). CDT and GGTP appear to identify two different subsets of alcoholic individuals. Elevations in GGTP values detect alcoholics with hepatic damage secondary to heavy drinking, whereas CDT appears to be more directly related to heavy drinking (Litten et al. 1995, Allen et al. 2001). Whenever possible, CDT and GGTP should be used together by classifying as a case the individuals who have elevated scores in either test. This approach increases the likelihood of identifying individuals experiencing alcohol use disorders (Allen and Litten 2001). CDT appears to detect relapse to heavy drinking among individuals in alcohol treatment more accurately than other laboratory tests (Litten et al. 1995, Allen et al. 2001).

In a clinical setting where laboratory results are generally not immediately available, the alcohol breath test, which measures the amount of alcohol in expired air (providing an estimate of venous ethanol concentration), is valuable. Although its accuracy depends on the individual's cooperation (which in an intoxicated individual is often problematic), the alcohol breath test can be a reliable and inexpensive method for assessing recent alcohol consumption. Venous blood levels should be obtained if dangerously high levels of intoxication are suspected, when an individual is comatose, or for medical–legal purposes. A BAL greater than 150 mg/dL in an individual showing no signs of intoxication (i.e., no dysarthria, motor incoordination, gait ataxia, nystagmus, or impaired attention) can be interpreted to reflect physiological tolerance (Holt et al. 1981). In nontolerant individuals, a BAL in excess of 400 mg/dL can result in death, and 300 mg/dL indicates a need for emergency care.

Another laboratory evaluation that is indicated in alcoholics is a urine toxicology screen. To identify drug use that the individual may not recognize or which he or she denies is a problem, the screen should include opiates, cocaine, cannabis, and benzodiazepines. Routine urinalysis, blood chemistries, hepatitis profile, complete blood count, and serologic test for syphilis and (for women) serum testing for pregnancy should also be obtained.

Gender and Developmental Presentations

There are substantial differences in the prevalence of alcoholism among different gender, age, and racial/cultural groups. Unfortunately, the high prevalence among young adult and middle-aged males often leads to inadequate consideration of the possibility that women and the elderly may drink excessively.

Women Women are more likely to abstain from alcohol, and if they do drink, they are more likely to consume less alcohol than men. Nevertheless, in comparison to men, problem drinking among women is more likely to be associated with negative mood states, particularly depression, anxiety, and somatic symptoms (Lesieur and Blume 1993). Alcoholic women identify negative emotions and interpersonal conflicts as antecedents of a relapse to drinking more frequently than men (Annis and Graham 1995) and substance-dependent women more frequently report depressive and anxiety symptoms as motivators for treatment. These reports are consistent with epidemiological and clinical studies which show that women who are diagnosed with alcohol or drug dependence experience higher rates of mood and anxiety disorders than their male counterparts (Helzer et al. 1987, Hesselbrock et al. 1985). Furthermore, it is more common among women that mood and anxiety disorders precede the onset of substance use and dependence (Kessler et al. 1996, Dunne et al. 1993). Alcoholic women have a *negative profile* of situations surrounding their alcohol use, characterized by solitary drinking and greater severity of alcohol dependence, whereas alcoholic men tend to have a *positive profile*, characterized by social drinking and drinking in the context of positive emotions (Annis and Graham 1995, Skutle 1999). Studies comparing male and female alcoholics (Parrella and Filstead 1988) have found that women are significantly older than men when a variety of alcohol-related milestones occur, including regular drunkenness, loss of control over drinking, first drinking problems, drinking to relieve withdrawal symptoms, first attempt to stop drinking, and realization that alcohol use is a problem. These studies have also found that women exhibit more rapid progression than men between the time of first regular intoxication and first treatment (Randall et al. 1999).

Despite drinking for fewer years at lower levels, women have an increased sensitivity to toxic effects of alcohol on body organs (Nixon 1993). Alcoholic women are more likely to develop liver damage and, in general, alcoholic liver diseases tend to progress faster among women than men (Becker et al. 1996). The five-year mortality rate among alcoholic women is almost twice the mortality rate of alcoholic men. Alcoholic women diagnosed with alcoholic liver disease die almost a decade younger than alcoholic men (Krasner et al. 1977). Alcoholic women appear to be more susceptible to alcohol-induced brain damage, evidenced by greater widening of the cerebral sulci and fissures in CT scans of the brain (Jacobson 1986) as well as poorer performance in cognitive testing (Nixon 1993). The concept of "telescoping" has been used to describe the course of symptom progression observed among women who, despite beginning heavy drinking later than men, experience alcohol-related problems and seek treatment sooner than men (Piazza et al. 1989).

Since alcohol is distributed in the aqueous phase, greater body fat composition among women reduces the volume of distribution. This, combined with smaller average body mass, translates into higher BALs for women in response to a specified level of alcohol consumption (Goldstein 1992). In addition, less first-pass metabolism due to less gastric oxidation of ethanol may also contribute to the higher blood levels obtained by women following an equivalent dose of ethanol (Frezza et al. 1990). Compared with men, women with alcohol problems are also at greater risk of comorbid drug abuse/dependence (Lex

1992). Perhaps as a consequence of these differences, women alcoholics who seek treatment do so earlier in the course of the disorder than do men (Nixon 1993).

Since heavy drinking among women is most prevalent during the child-bearing years, it has important public health implications for prenatal alcohol exposure and possible fetal alcohol effects. A variety of adverse outcomes have been related to heavy drinking in pregnant women, although the minimum amount of alcohol and the pattern of consumption necessary to produce such effects are not known. Heavy drinking in pregnant women may produce malnutrition in both the mother and the fetus, as well as spontaneous abortion, preterm delivery, and intrauterine growth retardation (Hannigan et al. 1992). Alcohol-related birth defects (ARBDs) are estimated to occur in as many as 1 in 100 live births (Finnegan and Kandall 1992). The most severe manifestation of ARBDs is fetal alcohol syndrome (FAS), a constellation of morphological and developmental defects resulting from high-dose prenatal alcohol exposure. FAS is estimated to occur in 1 in 1000 to 1 in 300 live births (Finnegan and Kandall 1992). Prenatal or postnatal growth retardation, CNS involvement, and characteristic facial dysmorphology are necessary for a diagnosis of FAS (Sokol and Clarren 1989).

Since ARBDs can be avoided, the evaluation of alcoholic pregnant women should routinely include questions about alcohol and other substance use. Routine screening with an instrument such as the AUDIT (Saunders et al. 1993), or the T-ACE (Chang 2001), supplemented by questions concerning drug use, may also be useful with pregnant women. Those pregnant women who are identified as heavy drinkers or drug users should be designated as "high risk" and provided with specialized, comprehensive perinatal care, including rehabilitation and appropriate attention to related psychosocial disabilities (Finnegan and Kandall 1992).

Adolescents   There are a number of features that distinguish adolescents with alcohol abuse/dependence from adult alcoholics (Kaminer 1994). As might be expected, adolescents have comparatively short histories of heavy drinking. A corollary to this is the rarity of physiological dependence on alcohol and alcohol-related medical complications among adolescents. Nonetheless, abuse of alcohol and drugs contributes in important ways to morbidity and mortality in adolescents, the leading causes of which are motor vehicle accidents, homicide, and suicide. The values and behavior of the adolescent's peer group are important elements in the evaluation of alcohol use and abuse in the adolescent. The evaluation of adolescents with an alcohol disorder must also take into account other prominent developmental issues that characterize adolescence, including the conflict inherent in asserting one's independence from the family.

A number of instruments have been developed for the assessment of substance use symptoms and disorders in adolescents (Kaminer 1994). As is generally true in dealing with adolescents, given their economic and emotional dependence, whenever possible, a thorough family evaluation is important for understanding the adolescent's substance use and related problems.

The Elderly   Although heavy drinking is less prevalent in the elderly, it is nonetheless an important source of morbidity in this group. Elderly alcoholics suffer from more chronic medical problems and poorer psychosocial functioning than elderly nonalcoholics (Finlayson et al. 1988). The increased use of prescription medications in the elderly increases the potential for adverse pharmacokinetic interactions with alcohol. In addition, decreased cognitive functioning associated with heavy alcohol use can increase medication errors and noncompliance in this group (Ofman 1992).

The manifestations of alcoholism in the elderly are often more subtle and nonspecific than those observed in younger individuals (Ofman 1992; Graham 1986). Because self-reported alcohol consumption may be particularly unreliable in the elderly, other sources of information such as family and neighbors should be used to identify heavy drinkers (Graham 1986). The following areas should be systematically evaluated in the elderly when heavy drinking has been identified: untreated medical illness, prescription drug abuse, psychiatric comorbidity, cognitive impairment, functional assessment, and need for social services (Ofman 1992).

Similar to the approach used with younger adults, alcoholism in the elderly has been classified by age of onset. It has been estimated that about two-thirds of elderly alcoholics began heavy drinking prior to age 60, while the remaining one-third began heavy drinking after the age of 60 (Atkinson and Kofoed 1982). Late-onset alcoholism appears to be more common among women and people of higher socioeconomic status and is less frequently associated with a family history of alcoholism (Ofman 1992). As might be expected, older alcoholics with early onset alcoholism also have more alcohol-related medical and psychosocial problems and are more likely to require alcoholism treatment (Ofman 1992).

Epidemiology

Alcohol in beverage form is among the most widely used psychoactive drugs in the world. Alcohol consumption is highest in the European countries, North America, and Australia. Because of its widespread distribution and the readiness with which it is consumed in a variety of settings, people do not generally conceive of beverage alcohol as a drug. Nonetheless, its complex pharmacologic actions, including a panoply of psychoactive effects, have led societies throughout the world to surround alcoholic beverages with a variety of rules and regulations governing their use (Mäkelä et al. 1981). Despite these efforts at control, excessive drinking with its adverse effects is widespread.

Patterns of drinking and the types of problems associated with alcohol misuse differ markedly throughout the world (Room et al. 2002). In the wine-producing Mediterranean countries (i.e., Spain, Portugal, Italy, France, and Greece), the pattern of drinking and the type of alcoholism have historically been associated with the consumption of wine as a dietary supplement, as well as for its effects as a social lubricant, medicine, and stimulant for manual workers. Drinking tends to be integrated into daily activities and rituals. Wine is typically consumed in moderation by a large segment of the population, and it is used more for its social and presumed nutritional value than for its psychological effects. Drunkenness is uncommon, considering the high level of daily consumption. There are few legal restrictions on the availability of alcoholic beverages. Children are introduced to alcohol gradually and in a culturally appropriate dietary context.

In contrast to the preponderance of wine drinking in the Mediterranean region, the use of distilled spirits predominates in the northern periphery of Europe. In countries such as Norway, Sweden, Finland, Poland, and Russia, there is a separation of drinking from dietary functions and the deliberate use of alcohol to produce intoxication. Heavy drinking is concentrated in a relatively small portion of the male population. As might be expected from this pattern of drinking, problems in spirits-drinking countries consist largely of alcohol-related accidents, public intoxication, and social disruption.

Despite increased availability of alcoholic beverages worldwide, cultural influences continue to exert a strong influence on national patterns of drinking. While the highest alcohol consumption rates are generally found among the industrialized countries of Europe and the North American continent, the lowest consumption rates are found in developing countries that are dominated by Islam, which proscribes the use of alcohol. The percentage of the drinking adult population ranges from a high of 86% in North and Central European countries to less than 10% of adults in Islamic countries such as Pakistan and Iraq (Room et al. 2002).

Recent advances in the assessment of drinking behavior and its consequences have made it possible to estimate the prevalence of alcoholism in different cultural contexts (Helzer and Canino 1992). Cross-national studies employing structured diagnostic interviews have found lifetime prevalence rates of alcohol abuse/dependence that vary from as low as 0.45% (among Chinese in Shanghai) to a high of 23% (among US-born Mexican-Americans) (Helzer and Canino 1992). In addition to the overall differences in lifetime prevalence rates in different countries, the prevalence of alcoholism varies considerably within countries as a function of demographic characteristics, such as sex and age (Helzer and Canino 1992), geographic region (Substance Abuse and Mental Health Services Administration 2000), and population density (Substance Abuse and Mental Health Services Administration 2001).

Table 16-3 shows the prevalence rates of lifetime, past year, and past month drinking, including binge and heavy drinking, for different gender, age and racial/ethnic groups, as determined by the 1999 National Household Survey of Drug Abuse (Substance Abuse and Mental Health Services Administration 2001). As shown in the table, the majority (85.8%) of the US population aged 18 and older has used alcohol in their lifetime, although only half (50.0%) report current drinking. The highest rates of current use are among young adults aged 18 to 25 years, with males predominating. Non-Hispanic whites have the highest prevalence of drinking (89.3% lifetime use and 53.7% past month use), while Asians are least likely to drink (62.7% lifetime and 33.4% current). The prevalence of drinking is positively associated with education level; persons with less than a high school education are almost half as likely to report past-month drinking as college graduates (33.5% compared to 62.6%).

Several large-scale community studies conducted since 1980 have provided estimates of the lifetime and past year prevalence of alcohol use disorders in the general population. For example, the National Comorbidity Study (NCS), a representative household survey of 8098 persons aged 15 to 54 years that was conducted between 1990 and 1992, assessed lifetime and past-year alcohol disorders using DSM-III-R criteria. The NCS estimated that the lifetime prevalence of alcohol abuse and alcohol dependence for adults 18 to 54 years old were 9.4 and 14.1%, respectively, indicating that more than one-in-five young to middle-aged adults in the United States have had a pattern of alcohol use that met criteria for lifetime alcohol disorder (Kessler et al. 1997). The prevalences of alcohol abuse and dependence during the 12 months preceding the interview were 2.5 and 4.4% respectively (Kessler et al. 1997).

Narrow and colleagues (2002) applied "clinically significant" criteria to the NCS data to determine the percentage of the population who were in need of treatment, more in keeping with DSM-IV-TR diagnostic guidelines. The revised estimates of the 12-month prevalence of clinically significant alcohol disorder is 5.2% for adults in the United States (including 6.5% of adults aged 18–54 years and 2% of adults aged 55 years or older).

The 1992 National Longitudinal Alcohol Epidemiologic Survey (NLAES), based on face-to-face interviews with a national probability household sample of 42,862 adults 18 and older, found that the past-year prevalence of DSM-IV alcohol disorder was 7.4%, including 3% with alcohol abuse and 4.4% with alcohol dependence (Grant et al. 1994, Grant 2000). The most recent data on the prevalence of alcohol disorder comes from the 1999 National Household Survey on Drug Abuse (NHSDA), based on interviews with approximately 70,000 persons 12 years of age and older residing in households in the United States (Substance Abuse and Mental Health Services Administration, 2000). The 1999 NHSDA found the one-year prevalence of DSM-IV alcohol dependence among the total population of persons 12 and older to be 3.7%.

able 16-3	**Percentages of Adults Aged 18 or Older Reporting Lifetime Alcohol Use, Past-Month Alcohol Use, Past Month Binge Drinking, Past Month Heavy Alcohol Use, and Past Year Alcohol Dependence, US, 1999**

Demographic Characteristic	Alcohol Use				
	Lifetime	Past Month	Binge Use	Heavy Drinking	Past-Year Dependence
Total	85.8	50	21.4	6.1	3.7
Gender					
Male	90	57.8	30.2	10	5.1
Female	82	42.8	13.4	2.5	2.5
Age					
18–25	83.9	57.2	37.9	13.3	9.2
26+	86.1	48.7	18.6	4.9	2.8
Hispanic origin and race					
Non-Hispanic White	89.3	53.7	22.1	6.5	3.7
Non-Hispanic Black	76.8	37.9	18	4	3.4
American Indian or Alaska native only	79.4	35.7	20.6	6	4.9
Native Hawaiian or other Pacific Islander	*	*	*	*	*
Asian only	62.7	33.4	11.6	2.7	2.3
More than one race	82.5	47.7	23.1	8.9	9
Hispanic	78.9	42.2	23.5	5.9	3.8
<High school	73.9	33.5	19.9	5.9	4.5
High school graduate	85.2	46.2	22.8	6.8	3.3
Some college	90.8	55.9	23.7	7.3	4.4
College graduate	90.9	62.6	18.1	3.8	3

*ow precision; no estimate reported.
e: "Binge" Alcohol Use is defined as drinking five or more drinks on the same occasion on at least 1 day in the past 30 days. By "occasion" meant at the same time or within a couple hours of each other. Heavy Alcohol Use is defined as drinking 5 or more drinks on the same asion on each of 5 or more days in the past 30 days; all Heavy Alcohol Users are also "Binge" Alcohol Users.
*pendence is based on the definition found in the Diagnostic and Statistical Manual of Mental Disorders, 4th ed. (DSM-IV).
rce: Data from Substance Abuse and Mental Health Services Administration (SAMHSA) (2000) Office of Applied Studies, National *usehold Survey on Drug Abuse.

Differences in the rates of disorder across the various studies have been attributed to differences in diagnostic criteria, age ranges of the samples, and sampling approaches (Regier et al. 1998). Regardless of the differences, it should be noted that all of these studies are based on self-reports of drinking behavior and are likely to be conservative estimates of the prevalence of problem drinking due to underreporting.

Adverse consequences of drinking include a variety of social, legal, and medical problems (Babor et al. 1987a). Overall, alcohol-related mortality in 1988 totaled 107,800 deaths, or about 5% of all deaths in the United States, putting it among the top four causes of death (Stinson and DeBakey 1992). Of alcohol-related deaths, approximately 17% were directly attributable to alcohol, 38% resulted from diseases indirectly attributable to alcohol, and 45% were attributable to alcohol-related traumatic injury (US Department of Health and Human Services 1994). Alcohol-related mortality declined during the last few decades of the twentieth century. The age-adjusted mortality rate from liver cirrhosis in 1993 (7.9 deaths/100,000 persons) was almost half the 1970 rate (14.6 deaths/100,000) (Saadatmand et al. 1997), and alcohol-related automobile fatalities fell to a 2-decade low of 33.6% (Lane et al. 1997). Nonetheless, age-adjusted rates of liver cirrhosis in 1988 remained higher for males (43.4 deaths/100,000 population) than females (19.4 deaths/100,000 population) and for nonwhites (57.2 deaths/ 100,000 population) than whites (32 deaths/100,000 population, Stinson and DeBakey 1992).

Alcohol-related morbidity is manifested in virtually all organ systems. The primary chronic health hazard associated with heavy drinking is cirrhosis of the liver, which in 1988 was the ninth leading cause of death in the United States (US Department of Health and Human Services 1994). Although the percentage of drivers in fatal crashes with BALs in excess of the legal limit has declined in recent years, alcohol intoxication remains a major contributor to this and other types of accidental injury, as well as to suicide and homicide (US Department of Health and Human Services 2000). In addition, heavy drinking has been implicated in such health conditions as FAS, esophageal cancer, chronic pancreatitis, nutritional deficiencies, cardiomyopathy, hypertension, and neurological problems (US Department of Health and Human Services 2000). The social consequences of alcohol abuse and dependence are equally serious, with heavy drinking contributing to a variety of family, work, and legal problems. The economic impact of alcoholism is substantial. Alcohol abuse and dependence contribute to unemployment, reduced productivity in the workplace, and crime, as well as increased costs for health care (US Department of Health and Human Services 2000). It has been estimated that the nonhealth related costs associated with alcohol abuse reached approximately \$13 billion in 1992, owing in part to costs associated with crime committed while under the influence of alcohol (Martin 2001). In summary, the annual cost of heavy drinking and alcohol-related disorders in the United States (both in dollars and in suffering) is enormous. Successful efforts to reduce the burden of illness attributable to alcohol could produce substantial reductions in the social, economic, and personal costs of alcohol-related problems.

Comorbidity With Mental Disorders

High rates of comorbid mental disorders have been found in both clinical and community samples of alcohol-dependent individuals (Regier et al. 1990, Kessler et al. 1994, 1997, Ross et al. 1988, Ross 1995, Helzer and Pryzbeck 1988). These studies show a consistent association between alcohol abuse/dependence and a variety of other psychiatric symptoms and disorders. The Epidemiological Catchment Area (ECA) study, for example, revealed that 36.6% of those with a lifetime alcohol use disorder received at least one other psychiatric diagnosis, which is nearly double the rate for community respondents with no lifetime alcohol disorder (Regier et al. 1990). The evidence from the NCS study showed that having a co-occurring disorder is more likely with alcohol dependence than alcohol abuse (Kessler et al. 1997). Among individuals with one or more mental disorders, 22.3% also had a lifetime alcohol disorder, substantially greater than the overall lifetime prevalence of alcohol abuse/dependence (13.5%). Women diagnosed with an alcohol disorder appear to be at greater risk for a comorbid mental disorder. The NCS found that 72% of females with a lifetime alcohol abuse diagnosis had experienced one or more co-occurring mental disorders, compared to 57% of men who had a lifetime history of alcohol abuse. While the prevalence of comorbid disorders was greater with alcohol dependence, the gender differential was smaller: 86% of women and 78% of men with lifetime alcohol dependency had had other lifetime DSM-III-R disorders (Kessler et al. 1997).

The most frequent co-occurring diagnoses are for other drug use disorders, conduct disorder, antisocial personality disorder (ASPD), anxiety disorders, and affective disorders. The relative risks for different types of disorder vary somewhat by gender (Helzer and Pryzbeck 1988, Kessler et al. 1997). Among women, anxiety and affective disorders are the most common co-occurring disorders. Among men with a history of alcohol abuse or dependence, drug disorders and conduct disorder account for the largest proportion of comorbid cases.

Problem drinkers have a significantly increased risk of the ASPD, compared to those in the population with no alcohol-use disorder. Although ASPD was present in only 14.3% of individuals with an alcohol-use disorder in the ECA study, this translated into an odds ratio

(OR) of 21 (Regier et al. 1990). Given that 73.6% of ECA respondents with ASPD also had a drinking pattern that met criteria for alcohol abuse/dependence, there is substantial overlap between the disorders, which is in part attributable to the overlap in diagnostic criteria (e.g., antisocial behavior that is manifest as a consequence of intoxication).

Evidence from multiple studies indicates that individuals with an alcohol-use disorder experience a two- to threefold increased risk of depressive disorders (Swendsen et al. 1998). The ECA study showed mood disorders to be present in 13.4% of those with an alcohol-use disorder (OR = 1.9) (Regier et al. 1990). Conversely, 21.8% of individuals with a mood disorder also had an alcohol-use disorder. Of the mood disorders, bipolar disorder is particularly common among individuals with an alcohol-use disorder, with 5.1% having a form of bipolar disorder. Conversely, among individuals with bipolar disorder, 43.6% have a comorbid alcohol-use disorder (OR = 5.1). Other mood disorders, although generally more common, show substantially lower ORs with alcohol-use disorders. Specifically, major depressive disorder, which is present in 16.5% of individuals with an alcohol-use disorder, has an OR of only 1.3. Similarly, dysthymic disorder, although present in 20.9% of individuals with an alcohol-use disorder, has an OR of only 1.7. Among individuals with an alcohol-use disorder, women were about four times as likely as men to receive a diagnosis of either bipolar disorder or major depressive disorder (Helzer and Pryzbeck 1988). There is also a sex differential with respect to the order of onset of diagnoses. In men, alcoholism is the antecedent diagnosis in 78% of cases of comorbid mood disorder, while for women major depressive disorder is the antecedent diagnosis in 66% of cases of comorbidity (Helzer and Pryzbeck 1988). The NCS study found a similar gender difference in the sequencing of comorbid affective disorders and alcohol use disorders (Kessler et al. 1997).

Anxiety disorders have also been found to be highly prevalent among individuals with an alcohol-use disorder (Regier et al. 1990, Kessler et al. 1997, Swendsen et al. 1998). The ECA study found that 19.4% of those with alcohol abuse/dependence had a comorbid anxiety disorder (Regier et al. 1990). However, because these disorders are also highly prevalent in the general population, they have an OR of only 1.5. Among individuals with an anxiety disorder, 17.9% have a comorbid alcohol-use disorder. Of the anxiety disorders, panic disorder appears to have the strongest association with alcohol-use disorder: 28.7% of individuals with that disorder also have an alcohol use disorder (OR = 2.6). Obsessive–compulsive disorder (OR = 2.1) is intermediate between panic disorder and phobias (OR = 1.4) (Regier et al. 1990). Among individuals with an alcohol-use disorder, women were more than three times as likely as men to have panic disorder and more than twice as likely to have phobia (Helzer and Pryzbeck 1988). Evidence suggests that the onset of social phobia occurs prior to the onset of alcohol use disorder, and that self-medication may play a role in the co-occurrence of the two disorders (Merikangas et al. 1998). A history of posttraumatic stress disorder (PTSD) has been found among 10.3% of men and 26.2% of women with alcohol dependence (Kessler et al. 1997). In the NCS study, the onset of an anxiety disorder appeared to precede the onset of an alcohol-use disorder for women more than men (Kessler et al. 1997).

Among individuals with an alcohol-use disorder, the prevalence of schizophrenia is 3.8%, which is almost three times the rate of that disorder in the general population (Regier et al. 1990). Conversely, among individuals with schizophrenia, the prevalence of a comorbid alcohol use disorder is 33.7% (OR = 3.3). Considerable attention has been focused on the substantial problems encountered in treating individuals with schizophrenia and comorbid alcohol and drug abuse/dependence (National Institute of Mental Health 1990).

Comorbidity influences treatment-seeking behavior. Although the majority of individuals with an alcohol-use disorder do not seek treatment, comorbidity increases the likelihood of using both mental health and substance abuse treatment services (Wu et al. 1999). In the ECA Study, this was evidenced by the fact that 55.0% of individuals with an alcohol-use disorder seeking treatment in a mental health or substance abuse setting had a comorbid nonsubstance use disorder, compared with only 24.4% of individuals with an alcohol-use disorder who had not sought treatment (Regier et al. 1990).

Consistent with the patterns observed in the general population, the most common comorbid disorders are major depressive disorder, ASPD, drug dependence, and anxiety disorders (Hesselbrock et al. 1985, Ross et al. 1988). However, the prevalence of comorbid disorders observed in clinical samples appears to vary as a consequence of a number of factors, including the method of assessment, the sample studied, and the recency of heavy drinking (Grande et al. 1984, Kranzler and Liebowitz 1988). Given the overlap in the diagnostic criteria for alcohol dependence and ASPD, and the effects of chronic heavy drinking on mood and anxiety symptoms, care must be taken to differentiate transient, alcohol-related signs and symptoms from persistent features.

Both community and clinical studies underscore the importance of ASPD and drug abuse/dependence as comorbid diagnoses in individuals with an alcohol disorder. The ORs obtained for these disorders in community studies indicate that these associations are elevated not only as a function of greater treatment-seeking behavior in affected individuals but also because of potential commonalities in the etiology and development of alcohol abuse/dependence. That is, genetic and/or psychosocial risk factors for the development of ASPD are likely to overlap with factors that increase risk for alcohol and drug use disorders. Similarly, the risk factors for alcohol and drug-use disorders may overlap with those for schizophrenia and bipolar disorder. In contrast, although anxiety disorders and depression are highly prevalent in clinical samples of alcohol-dependent individuals, their association with alcohol dependence appears largely due to chance, since these disorders are also highly prevalent in the general population.

Given a high rate of psychiatric comorbidity, it is axiomatic that a careful psychiatric assessment be conducted in individuals being seen for alcohol treatment, and that alcohol use and associated problems be evaluated in individuals being seen primarily for other psychiatric conditions. Because the presence of comorbid disorders may have important implications for the development of alcoholism and its prognosis, the assessment of comorbid psychopathology is an essential element in the clinical evaluation. When comorbid diagnoses are present, an effort should be made to ascertain the order of onset of each disorder since treatment and prognosis may follow from such information (Schuckit 1985).

Course

Schuckit and colleagues (1993) found that the symptoms of alcohol dependence appear in the following sequence in a sample of male veteran alcoholics: heavy drinking during the late twenties; interference with functioning in multiple life areas during their early thirties; loss of control, followed by an intensification of social- and work-related problems, and onset of medical consequences in the mid- to late thirties; and severe long-term consequences by the late thirties and early forties. This relatively predictable order of progression is consistent with previous studies. However, as mentioned above, women appear to experience many of these milestones at a later age than men (Parrella and Filstead 1988, Piazza et al. 1989).

The study by Schuckit and colleagues (1993) showed no effect of onset age, family history of alcoholism, or comorbid psychiatric diagnoses on the order of symptom appearance. However, other features defining the course of alcoholism, particularly the response to treatment, vary as a function of variables related to the individual, including age of onset, severity of alcohol dependence, and comorbid mental disorders. There is consistent evidence that early age of onset is a predictor of greater severity of alcoholism and a poorer response to treatment (Bohn and Meyer 1994, Babor et al. 1992). Greater severity of alcohol dependence has also been shown to predict poorer treatment outcome (Lindstrom 1992).

While considered to be important in the development of alcoholism, comorbid mental disorders also have prognostic significance (Meyer 1986). Rounsaville and colleagues (1987) found that psychiatric diagnosis at the time of treatment intake predicted a variety of 1-year posttreatment outcomes. Among males, the presence of a comorbid lifetime diagnosis of ASPD, major depressive disorder, or drug abuse/dependence was associated with poorer drinking outcomes. Among females, the presence of major depressive disorder predicted a better outcome on drinking-related measures, while those individuals with ASPD or drug abuse/dependence had a poorer prognosis. Three-year posttreatment outcomes in this group of alcoholics also showed comorbid ASPD, major depressive disorder, and drug abuse/dependence to be associated with poorer outcomes, irrespective of gender. It is notable, however, that at the 3-year follow-up, major depressive disorder was not associated with a protective effect for women alcoholics (Kranzler et al. 1996b).

Other investigators have found no difference in drinking outcomes when comparing primary alcoholics (i.e., those for whom alcohol dependence is the first and predominant disorder) and alcoholics with a comorbid mood disorder (Schuckit 1985, O'Sullivan et al. 1988, Powell et al. 1992). However, as might be expected, alcoholics with comorbid depression have greater psychiatric severity at follow-up than primary alcoholics (O'Sullivan et al. 1988, Powell et al. 1992). Variable findings have also been reported concerning the prognostic significance of ASPD and drug abuse among alcoholics. Both Powell and colleagues (1992) and Schuckit (1985) found that, compared with primary alcoholics, alcoholics with either primary ASPD or a primary drug abuse diagnosis (i.e., individuals in whom these disorders preceded the onset of alcohol dependence) did not differ on alcohol-related outcomes. However, in one study (Schuckit 1985), alcoholics with these primary diagnoses reported more illicit drug use and poorer social functioning during the posttreatment period. Furthermore, Liskow and colleagues (1990) found that alcoholics with a lifetime drug diagnosis in combination with ASPD had poorer alcohol-related outcomes.

Etiology

Alcoholism is a complex, multifaceted disorder that has long been recognized to run in families. There is substantial evidence from twin research and adoption studies that a major genetic component is operative in the development of alcoholism. Nonetheless, the disorder is etiologically complex, with a variety of other vulnerability factors (Goldman 1993, Gelernter 1995). It has been estimated that there is a sevenfold risk of alcoholism in first-degree relatives of alcohol-dependent individuals, with male relatives of male alcohol-dependent individuals having the greatest risk for the disorder (Merikangas 1990). However, the majority of alcohol-dependent individuals do not have a first-degree relative who is alcohol dependent. This underscores the fact that the risk for alcohol dependence is also determined by environmental factors, which may interact in complex ways with genetics.

Genetic/Environmental Factors

In a review of population-based twin studies of alcoholism published since 1992, heritability estimates (i.e., the proportion of risk attributable to genetic factors) ranged between 0.52 and 0.64, with no substantial sex difference (Kendler 2001). One study conducted in Sweden using data from temperance board registration showed that the estimate of the genetic contribution to risk of the disorder was stable across four birth cohorts over a 50-year period, despite a rapidly changing social environment (Kendler et al. 1997).

The majority of adoption studies has shown an excess of alcoholism in adopted-away offspring of biological parents (McGue 1994). Among studies conducted in the past 30 years, the risk ratio has varied between 1.6 and 3.6 in males and between 0.5 (an effect statistically indistinguishable from 1 or no effect) and 6.3 in females (McGue 1994).

Despite evidence that a genetic factor is influential in the transmission of alcohol dependence, exactly how risk of the disorder is transmitted remains unknown. Alcohol dependence appears to be a polygenic disorder with multiple genes acting either in additive or interactive ways.

Candidate Gene Studies   The best-known example of genetic variation affecting risk for alcohol dependence involves candidate genes that are not directly relevant to alcohol's neuropharmacologic effects, including variant forms of the alcohol-metabolizing enzymes alcohol dehydrogenase (ADH) and aldehyde dehydrogenase (ALDH) (Goldman 1988, Gelernter 1995). The mechanism of this effect depends upon the metabolism of alcohol, first to acetaldehyde by ADH and then to acetate by acetaldehyde dehydrogenase. Acetaldehyde is toxic and produces a flushing reaction characterized by a set of uncomfortable symptoms including facial flushing, lightheadedness, palpitations, and nausea. Thus, increased metabolism of ethanol or decreased metabolism of acetaldehyde, either of which can result in increased acetaldehyde concentrations, produces an aversive effect that could decrease the risk of alcohol dependence (Goedde et al. 1979). There is, in fact, evidence that a variant that greatly reduces or eliminates ALDH function (occurring mostly in Asian populations) is protective against alcohol dependence, and ADH variants that increase function may also be protective (Thomasson et al. 1991).

No replicated positive findings have been shown for several other candidate genes relating to the D_2 dopamine receptor protein, serotonergic and opioidergic neurotransmitters, or the μ-opioid receptor.

Genes encoding proteins in the serotonergic and opioidergic neurotransmitter systems have also been targeted as candidate genes for alcohol dependence. A polymorphism consisting of a repetitive sequence of base pairs in the promoter region of the serotonin transporter protein (genetic locus SLC6A4) is of particular interest. The allele with the smallest number of repeats, commonly called the "short" (S) allele, has lower transcriptional activity, leading to marked reductions in messenger ribonucleic acid (mRNA) levels, serotonin binding, and serotonin uptake in both platelets and lymphoblasts, compared with the "long" (L) allele (Lesch et al. 1996, Greenberg et al. 1999). Findings from studies examining whether 5′-HTTLPR alleles are associated with alcoholism in humans are not consistent: five studies report no association to alcoholism (Ishiguro et al. 1999, Gorwood et al. 2000, Edenberg et al. 1998b, Gelernter et al. 1997) and three studies report an association (Hallikainen et al. 1999, Hammoumi et al. 1999, Lichtermann et al. 2000).

Similarly, studies focusing on the gene encoding the μ-opioid receptor (genetic locus OPRM1) have failed to provide convincing evidence of association to alcohol dependence. The polymorphism receiving the most attention in this regard is a nonsynonymous substitution (Asn40Asp), which has been shown to affect the affinity for beta-endorphin (Bond et al. 1998). Studies of this polymorphism in Southwest American Indians, Finns, and European Americans have found no association to alcohol dependence (Bergen et al. 1997, Gelernter et al. 1999).

Linkage Studies   Two large linkage studies have been conducted in an effort to identify chromosomal regions that contain genes that modify risk for alcohol dependence. The larger of these two projects, the Collaborative Study on the Genetics of Alcoholism (COGA), includes more than 9,000 adults and nearly 1500 children and adolescents (Hesselbrock et al. 2001). A genomic scan of the COGA samples showed that chromosomes 1 and 7 each have a region containing one or more genes that increase risk of alcohol dependence (Hesselbrock et al. 2001). In addition, COGA found evidence for a "protective factor" on chromosome 4 (Reich et al. 1998).

A linkage study has also been reported from a sample of 152 subjects belonging to extended pedigrees in a southwestern American-Indian tribe (Long et al. 1998). A genome-wide scan was performed on 172 sibling pairs from this sample. Evidence for linkage to alcohol dependence was obtained for regions on chromosomes 4 and 11. Three closely linked loci on chromosome 4 map onto the Type I ADH gene cluster in proximity to the region on this chromosome that was identified as linked to a "protective factor" by COGA.

These linkage studies, in parallel with candidate gene studies, may help explain the specific mechanisms involved in the increased risk for alcohol dependence that are attributable to genetic factors. As we learn more about the genetic basis for alcoholism risk, a clearer understanding will emerge concerning the interaction of genetic and environmental factors in the etiology of alcohol dependence.

Etiological Subtypes of Alcoholics   Another approach to understanding the etiology of alcoholism is to identify distinct subtypes of alcoholics. A variety of typologic approaches have been proposed to simplify the diverse phenomena associated with alcoholism (Nixon 1993, Bohn and Meyer 1994, Babor and Lauerman 1986). The best known of these typologies is the Type 1/Type 2 distinction developed by Cloninger and colleagues (1981) from studies of adopted sons of Swedish alcoholics (see Table 16-4).

Type 1 alcoholics are characterized by the late onset of problem drinking, rapid development of behavioral tolerance to alcohol, prominent guilt and anxiety related to drinking, and infrequent fighting and arrests when drinking. Cloninger also termed this subtype *milieu-limited*, which emphasizes the etiologic role of environmental factors. In contrast, Type 2 alcoholics are characterized by early onset of an inability to abstain from alcohol, frequent fighting and arrests when drinking, and the absence of guilt and fear concerning drinking. Cloninger postulated that transmission of alcoholism in Type 2 alcoholics was from fathers to sons, hence the term *male-limited* alcoholism. Differences in the two subtypes are thought to result from differences in three basic personality (i.e., temperament) traits, each of which has a unique neurochemical and genetic substrate (Cloninger 1987). Type 1 alcoholics are characterized by high reward dependence, high harm avoidance, and low novelty seeking. In contrast, Type 2 alcoholics are characterized by high novelty seeking, low harm avoidance, and low reward dependence.

More recently, Babor and colleagues (1992) used statistical clustering techniques to derive a dichotomous typology similar to that proposed earlier by Cloninger. The analysis identified two homogeneous subtypes that may have important implications for the etiology of alcoholism, as well as for treatment outcome. Cloninger's Type 1 alcoholic shares with the Type A alcoholic a later onset of alcohol-related problems and the absence of antisocial characteristics. Cloninger's Type 2 alcoholic shares with the Type B alcoholic an early onset of alcohol-related problems and the presence of antisocial characteristics, particularly when intoxicated.

able 16-4	Cloninger's Alcoholism Typology	
	Type 1	**Type 2**
nset of problem drinking	Late onset	Early onset
olerance	Rapid development of behavioral tolerance	Not specified
lood issues	Prominent guilt and anxiety about drinking	Absence of guilt and anxiety about drinking
ersonality traits	High reward dependence	Low reward dependence
	High harm avoidance	Low harm avoidance
	Low novelty seeking	High novelty seeking

rce: Adapted from Cloninger CR, Bohman M, and Sigvardsson S (1981) Inheritance of alcohol abuse: Cross-fostering analysis of adopted . *Arch Gen Psychiatr* **38**, 861–868. Copyright 1981 American Medical Association.

The Type A/Type B classification (Babor et al. 1992) has been successful in predicting outcome following alcoholism treatment (Litt et al. 1992). However, its relevance to the matching of alcoholics to different psychotherapies has been supported by some studies (Litt et al. 1992) but not by others (Project MATCH Research Group 1997a,b).

Implicit in the subtyping theories that have been developed to explain different clinical varieties of alcoholism is the notion that there are a variety of plausible etiological factors in addition to or mediated by genetic predisposition. Three such factors are pharmacological vulnerability, affective dysregulation, and personality disorder. The evidence for pharmacological vulnerability as an etiological factor is based on studies showing reduced sensitivity to the effects of alcohol in adult children of alcoholics (Schuckit and Smith 1996, Pollock 1992). Other evidence comes from research on the effects of $ALDH_2$, ADH_2, and ADH_3 polymorphisms in individuals of Asian ancestry where aversive reactions to the effects of alcohol are associated with reduced risk of alcohol dependence (Thomasson et al. 1993). A second etiological factor is affect dysregulation, which proposes that alcoholism is caused by repeated use of alcohol to "self-medicate" negative affective states such as anxiety and depression. This theory is supported by research indicating strong associations between alcohol problems, mood disorders, and life stress (Schuckit 1985, Kessler et al. 1997, Helzer and Pryzbeck 1988). The third etiological factor that has received considerable research support is deviance proneness or behavioral undercontrol, as indicated by hyperactivity, distractibility, sensation seeking, impulsivity, difficult temperament, and conduct disorder. These conditions are hypothesized to contribute to school failure and association with deviant peers, which then provide a context for heavy drinking and drug use (Sher and Trull 1994, Sher 1991).

In summary, despite considerable progress in the identification of risk factors for alcoholism, the interactions among genetic, familial, psychological, interpersonal, and environmental influences remain so complex that there is little consensus about etiology at this time.

Biological Factors

Taken in large doses, alcohol is considered to have anesthetic or depressive properties. It also has the ability to elicit euphoria when administered in small doses to susceptible persons (Begleiter and Porjesz 1999). This phenomenon appears to be mediated by direct activation by alcohol of the mesolimbic dopaminergic circuit, particularly the ventral tegmental area (VTA) and the nucleus accumbens (NAc) (Brodie et al. 1999). Anxiolysis and relaxation also appear to be part of the spectrum of the rewarding effects of alcohol, though these effects appear to be mediated by activation of GABAergic neurotransmitter system.

In contrast to other addictive substances (e.g., nicotine, cocaine, and opioids) and despite its significant effect on dopaminergic neurotransmission, the existence of specific alcohol-binding sites on neuronal membranes has not been conclusively established. The lack of an alcohol receptor has led to the hypothesis that some alcohol effects, particularly those observed when it is administered at large doses, may be explained by disturbances in fluidity of the bilayer lipid neuronal membrane. Changes in fluidity of neuronal membranes may affect the structure and function of neurotransmitter receptors and ion channels. However, this hypothesis has failed to explain alcohol-rewarding effects that occur at lower doses.

On the other hand, alcohol administration appears to have effects across the major neurotransmitter systems (i.e., opioidergic, serotonergic, GABAergic, and glutamatergic). These systems are affected by both acute and chronic alcohol administration. They appear to play a major role in mediating the rewarding effects of alcohol by modulating the firing of dopaminergic neurons in the VTA and the release of dopamine in the NAc.

Opioidergic Neurotransmission   Findings derived from animal models of alcoholism support a relationship between alcohol administration and opioidergic neurotransmission. Hypothalamic synthesis, release, and binding of endogenous opioids such as beta-endorphin and enkephalin to μ-opiate receptors have been shown to be stimulated by alcohol administration (Eskelson et al. 1980). Disturbances in opioidergic neurotransmission have been reported among alcoholic individuals and their unaffected adult children (i.e., paternal history–positive or PHP, Topel 1988, Trachtenberg and Blum 1987). Both groups show lower plasma and cerebrospinal fluid (CSF) concentrations of beta-endorphin than adult children of nonalcoholic subjects (i.e., paternal history–negative or PHN; Gianoulakis et al. 1989), and after alcohol administration, PHP individuals show a greater increase or normalization of their beta-endorphin levels (Gianoulakis et al. 1989, 1996). These findings suggest that an inherited or acquired deficiency in endogenous opioid activity may be present among the offspring of alcoholics. This deficiency might lead them to drink to remediate this deficiency (opioid deficiency hypothesis; Reid 1990, Gianoulakis et al. 1996). Further support for the opioidergic hypothesis of alcoholism derives from the study of opioid antagonism on alcohol consumption. Opioid antagonists reliably decrease alcohol preference across a range of experimental conditions and across different animal species. Several placebo-controlled clinical trials in humans show efficacy of the opioid antagonists naltrexone (Volpicelli et al. 1992, O'Malley et al. 1992, Anton et al. 1999, Kranzler et al. 1998) and nalmefene (Mason et al. 1999) as adjuncts to the psychosocial treatment of alcoholism (discussed later).

Serotonergic Neurotransmission   Serotonin (5-HT) also appears to play a role in modulating alcohol consumption (LeMarquand et al. 1994a, Soubrie 1986). In rodents, acute administration of alcohol is associated with an increment in the brain concentration of 5-HT, and central infusion of 5-HT enhances dopaminergic tone in the VTA (Brodie and Bunney 1996). In contrast, chronic administration of alcohol is associated with low CNS concentrations of 5-HT. This reduction in serotonergic tone after chronic ethanol administration appears to be associated with behavioral disinhibition and impulsive aggression (Higley et al. 1992, 1996). Administration of serotonin reuptake inhibitors decreases alcohol consumption in rodents that show preference for alcohol (Gill and Amit 1989). Whether this phenomenon is due to a dampening of the reinforcing effects of alcohol or to a generalized reduction of consummatory behaviors is unclear (Gill and Amit 1989).

  Data derived from humans has also suggested that disturbances in central serotonergic functioning may be involved in alcohol and drug dependence, particularly among substance-dependent individuals diagnosed with a comorbid ASPD. For example, in comparison to controls, antisocial alcoholics have lower basal CSF levels of 5-HIAA (Limson et al. 1991, Virkkunen et al. 1994). Substance-dependent individuals and antisocial men also have blunted cortisol and prolactin responses to a challenge with the 5-HT agonists fenfluramine and D-fenfluramine (O'Keane et al. 1992, Moss et al. 1990). Additionally, children with a positive parental history of substance abuse or criminal behavior have a decreased number of 5-HT_{2A} receptors on platelets (Pine et al. 1996). Consistent with preclinical findings, treatment with ondansetron, a 5-HT_3 antagonist, attenuates the subjective effects of low alcohol doses and reduces relapse rates among early-onset alcoholic individuals (Johnson et al. 2000).

GABAergic Neurotransmission   Behavioral responses to alcohol resemble the effects of pharmacological agents that predominantly affect GABAergic neurotransmission (i.e., benzodiazepines, barbiturates, and neurosteroids), suggesting a significant involvement of this system in the pharmacological effects of alcohol. Cross-tolerance with alcohol and the effectiveness of benzodiazepines and barbiturates in treating alcohol-withdrawal symptoms also support this notion. Neurons that express $GABA_A$ receptors containing the alpha-1 subunit, such as cerebellar Purkinje neurons, appear to be sensitive to the effects of alcohol (Criswell et al. 1993). However, electro-physiologic responses to alcohol in neurons expressing $GABA_A$ receptors appear to be inconsistent (Harris 1999). It has been suggested that such inconsistencies may be due to the existence of alcohol-sensitive receptors and alcohol resistant receptors, determined by subunit composition and posttranslational processes (Mihic and Harris 1995). Strains of mice that differ in sleep sensitivity to alcohol (i.e., short sleep/long sleep ((SS/LS)) mice) show differential alcohol sensitivity of $GABA_A$ receptors. $GABA_A$ receptors in SS mice are resistant to alcohol, whereas $GABA_A$ receptors in LS mice are alcohol-sensitive (Allan and Harris 1986). Interestingly, individuals who are children of alcoholic fathers show increased resistance to induction of body sway and incoordination by alcohol administration. This finding suggests that people at risk for alcoholism experience decreased sensitivity to the effects of alcohol on the GABAergic system, and that this abnormality may be under genetic control (Schuckit 1994).

Glutamatergic Neurotransmission   Alcohol also affects the glutamatergic neurotransmitter system. Acute administration of alcohol antagonizes N-methyl-D-aspartate (NMDA) receptors (where glutamate acts as an agonist), whereas chronic administration increases these receptor sites (Snell et al. 1993, Hoffman et al. 1994, Chu et al. 1995). This latter finding reflects the fact that alcohol-withdrawal symptoms and other neurotoxic effects of alcohol are mediated by glutamate. Furthermore, alcohol withdrawal appears to be associated with increased glutamate concentrations and decreased dopamine levels in the NAc (Rossetti and Carboni 1995, Dahchour et al. 1998). Findings concerning the efficacy of acamprosate (which exerts effects on the NMDA receptor) in the treatment of alcohol dependence suggest that this neurotransmitter system may have a major role in the disorder (Kranzler et al. 2000).

Cholinergic Neurotransmission   Studies in rodents have shown that the alcohol-induced dopamine release in the NAc can be antagonized by the central nicotinic receptor antagonist mecamylamine (Söderpalm et al. 2000, Blomqvist et al. 1993, 1996, 1997, Ericson et al. 1998, Nadal et al. 1998). These findings suggest that the mesolimbic dopamine-activating and reinforcing effects of alcohol are both mediated in part by central nicotinic acetylcholine receptor activation. In healthy humans (Blomqvist et al. 2002), pharmacological manipulation of the nicotinic cholinergic receptor with mecamylamine reduces the stimulant effects of acute alcohol administration during the ascending limb of the blood alcohol curve. This finding suggests that blockade of nicotinic receptors may be a useful strategy in reducing alcohol consumption in alcoholics.

Treatment

When a determination has been made that an individual is drinking excessively, the nature, setting, and intensity of the intervention must be determined in order to address the specific treatment needs of the individual. Among heavy drinkers without evidence of alcohol dependence, a brief intervention aimed at the reduction of drinking may suffice. In contrast, among alcoholics, there are typically a variety of associated disabilities, so it is necessary to address both the excessive drinking *and* problems related to it. Consequently, alcoholism treatment is best conceived of as multimodal. Table 16-5 provides an overview of the goals of alcoholism treatment, many of which have been discussed by Schuckit (1994). It should be noted that while total abstinence is a primary goal of treatment for persons with alcohol dependence, moderate drinking can be considered as a goal for persons with alcohol abuse.

Figure 16-1 describes a process for the management of individuals with alcohol abuse and dependence. The algorithm is written from the perspective of a community-based

Table 16-5	Goals of Alcoholism Treatment

Promote complete abstinence from alcohol.
Stabilize acute medical (including alcohol withdrawal) and psychiatric conditions, as needed.
Increase motivation for recovery.
Initiate treatment for chronic medical and psychiatric conditions, as needed.
Assist the patient in locating suitable housing (e.g., moving from a setting where drinking is widespread), as needed.
Enlist social support for recovery (e.g., introduce to 12-step programs and, when possible, help the patient to repair damaged marital and other family relationships).
Enhance coping and relapse prevention skills (including social skills, identification and avoidance of high-risk situations).
Improve occupational functioning.
Promote maintenance of recovery through ongoing participation in structured treatment or self-help groups.

or consultation/liaison clinician who does not necessarily have specialized training in addiction medicine. Following the initial assessment, using a screening test such as the CAGE or AUDIT, the individual is referred to either a diagnostic evaluation with a likely treatment recommendation or a brief intervention with further monitoring. Brief interventions are characterized by their low intensity and short duration. They typically consist of one to three sessions of counseling and education. They are intended to provide early intervention, before or soon after the onset of alcohol-related problems. Brief interventions seek to motivate high-risk drinkers to moderate their alcohol consumption, rather than promote total abstinence with specialized treatment techniques. They are simple enough to be delivered by primary care practitioners and are especially appropriate for individuals whose at-risk drinking meets criteria for alcohol abuse rather than dependence.

During the past 2 decades, more than 40 randomized controlled trials have been conducted to evaluate the efficacy of brief interventions. The results of these trials have been summarized in several integrative literature reviews and meta-analyses (Bien et al. 1993, Babor 1994, Kahan et al. 1995, Wilk et al. 1997, Poikolainen 1999). The cumulative evidence shows that clinically significant effects on drinking behavior and related problems can follow from brief interventions. Nevertheless, the results have not always been consistent across studies (Poikolainen 1999). Furthermore, there is little evidence that these interventions are beneficial for alcohol-dependent individuals (Mattick and Jarvis 1994).

If the individual's screening results and diagnostic evaluation provide evidence of alcohol dependence, the next step is to differentiate between mild and more severe levels of physical dependence to determine the need for detoxification. If withdrawal risk is low, the individual may be referred directly to outpatient therapy. If the withdrawal risk is moderate or high, outpatient or inpatient detoxification is indicated.

There are a number of potentially life-threatening conditions for which alcoholics are at increased risk. The presence of any of the following requires immediate attention: acute alcohol withdrawal (with the potential for seizures and delirium tremens), serious medical or surgical disease (e.g., acute pancreatitis, bleeding esophageal varices), and serious psychiatric illness (e.g., psychosis, suicidal intent). In the presence of any of these emergent conditions, acute stabilization should be the first priority of treatment.

The presence of complicating medical or psychiatric conditions is an important determinant of whether detoxification and rehabilitation are initiated in an inpatient or an outpatient setting. Other considerations are the alcoholic's current living circumstances and social support network. Women with children are sometimes unwilling to enter residential treatment unless their family needs are taken care of. Homeless people may be eager to enter residential treatment even when their medical or psychiatric condition does not warrant it.

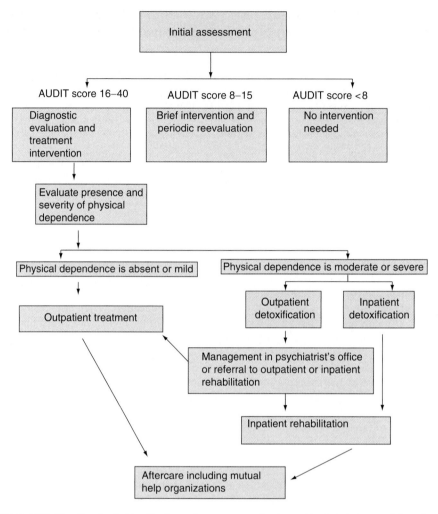

Figure 16-1 *Algorithm for the identification and management of patients with alcohol abuse and dependence.*

In the alcoholic individual whose condition is stabilized or in the individual without these complicating features, the major focus should be on the establishment of a therapeutic alliance, which provides the context within which rehabilitation can occur. The presence of a trusting relationship facilitates the individual's acknowledgement of alcohol-related problems and encourages open consideration of different treatment options. In addition to participation in structured rehabilitation treatment, the individual should be made aware of the widespread availability of Alcoholics Anonymous (AA) and the wide diversity of its membership.

Another approach to individual placement and treatment matching is based on the notion that individuals should initially be matched to the least intensive level of care that is appropriate, and then stepped up to more intensive treatment settings if they do not respond (Institute of Medicine 1990). This approach is consistent with the American Society of Addiction Medicine (ASAM) criteria, which specify that inpatient treatment should not be recommended unless the individual has failed at outpatient treatment. Matching can also be guided by theoretically derived hypotheses. This strategy relies on the cumulative evidence of research to suggest the kinds of treatments most likely to produce favorable outcomes with different types of individuals. An example is the assignment of individuals with ASPD to cognitive behavioral treatment, based on evidence (Kadden et al. 1989) that these individuals have better outcomes with structured therapy.

The possibility of rational treatment/patient matching continues to attract interest, and there is some evidence to suggest that individuals with certain characteristics (e.g., severe dependence, high levels of anger, social networks that support drinking) respond marginally better to certain types of therapy (e.g., Twelve Step Facilitation, motivational enhancement, cognitive behavioral; Project MATCH Research Group 1997a,b, 1998, Ouimette et al. 1999). In one study, McLellan and colleagues (1993) compared the range and intensity of service delivery and associated outcomes in two inpatient and two outpatient substance abuse treatment programs for alcohol- or cocaine-dependent employed individuals. In areas of functioning of the individual other than substance use (i.e., health, employment, family, and psychiatric), those who were treated in programs with services that met their particular areas of need showed the greatest improvement in those areas after discharge. These findings suggest the importance of incorporating a range of services within specialized treatment facilities to meet the diverse psychosocial needs of alcoholic individuals.

Despite treatment, some alcoholics relapse repeatedly. For many emergency department personnel, the multiple recidivist alcoholic has come to personify the disorder. For clinicians involved in the delivery of alcoholism rehabilitation services, these individuals' apparent unresponsiveness to treatment may contribute to frustration and a sense of futility. Presently, long-term residential treatment appears to be the only option for alcoholics who do not respond to more limited efforts at rehabilitation. Unfortunately, the availability of such care in many states is limited as a consequence of the effort to deinstitutionalize psychiatric patients.

Finally, the importance of continuing care by means of aftercare groups, and other mutual help organizations cannot be overestimated. The value of these resources as well as the newer pharmacological and nonpharmacological interventions developed in the past 2 decades are discussed in subsequent sections of this chapter.

Management of Alcohol Withdrawal

An important initial intervention for a substantial number of alcohol-dependent individuals is the management of alcohol withdrawal through detoxification. The objectives in treating alcohol withdrawal are the relief of discomfort, prevention or treatment of complications, and preparation for rehabilitation. Successful management of the alcohol-withdrawal syndrome provides a basis for subsequent efforts at rehabilitation.

Careful screening for concurrent medical problems is an important element in detoxification (Naranjo and Sellers 1986). Administration of thiamine (50–100 mg by mouth or IM) and multivitamins is a low-cost, low-risk intervention for the prophylaxis and treatment of alcohol-related neurological disturbances. Good supportive care and treatment of concurrent illness, including fluid and electrolyte repletion, are essential (Naranjo and Sellers 1986).

Social detoxification, which involves the nonpharmacological treatment of alcohol withdrawal has been shown to be effective (Naranjo et al. 1983, Sellers et al. 1983). It consists of frequent reassurance, reality orientation, monitoring of vital signs, personal attention, and general nursing care (Naranjo and Sellers 1986). Social detoxification is most appropriate for individuals in mild-to-moderate withdrawal. The medical problems commonly associated with alcoholism (Eckardt et al. 1981) may substantially complicate therapy, so care must be taken to refer those individuals whose condition requires medical management.

Increasingly, detoxification is being done on an ambulatory basis, which is much less costly than inpatient detoxification (Hayashida et al. 1989). Inpatient detoxification is indicated for serious medical or surgical illness, and for those individuals with a past history of adverse withdrawal reactions or with current evidence of more serious withdrawal (e.g., delirium tremens) (Feldman et al. 1975).

A variety of medications have been used for the treatment of alcohol withdrawal. However, owing to their favorable side effect profile, the benzodiazepines have largely supplanted all other medications (Naranjo and Sellers 1986). Although any benzodiazepine will suppress alcohol-withdrawal symptoms, diazepam and chlordiazepoxide are often used, since they are metabolized to long-acting compounds, which in effect are self-tapering. Because metabolism of these drugs is hepatic, impaired liver function may complicate their use. Oxazepam and lorazepam are not oxidized to long-acting metabolites and thus carry less risk of accumulation.

Although carbamazepine appears useful as a primary treatment of withdrawal (Malcolm et al. 1989), the liver dysfunction that is common in alcoholics may affect its metabolism, which makes careful blood level monitoring necessary. Antipsychotics are not indicated for the treatment of withdrawal except in those instances where hallucinations or severe agitation are present (Naranjo and Sellers 1986), in which case they should be added to a benzodiazepine. In addition to their potential to produce extrapyramidal side effects, antipsychotics lower seizure threshold, which may be particularly problematic during alcohol withdrawal.

Psychosocial Treatments

A variety of treatment components are delivered within the context of rehabilitation services. In many programs, a combination of therapeutic interventions is provided to all individuals, based on the assumption that multiple components have a greater chance of meeting at least some of each individual's needs. Therapeutic approaches most often employed in both residential and outpatient programs include behavior therapy, group therapy, family treatment, and pharmacotherapy. Regarding specific treatment modalities, the weight of evidence suggests that behavioral treatments are likely to be more effective than insight-oriented or family therapies (Miller and Hester 1986). Nevertheless, recent research (Project MATCH Research Group 1997a,b, 1998, Ouimette et al. 1999) also indicates that the Twelve Step Facilitation, which is based on the principles of AA, is as effective as more theory-based therapies. Controlled studies provide little support for the effectiveness of psychodynamic psychotherapy, although such treatment has been shown to be helpful in the treatment of drug abuse (Institute of Medicine 1989, Miller and Hester 1980).

Cognitive and behavior therapies are among the most investigated theory-based treatments. Behavioral elements most frequently employed in treatment programs are relapse prevention, social skills and assertiveness training, contingency management, deep muscle relaxation, self-control training, and cognitive restructuring (Miller and Mastria 1977). Aversion therapy, based on Pavlovian conditioning theory, has been virtually abandoned in this country. Although it has been shown that the sight, smell, and taste of alcohol will acquire aversive properties if repeatedly paired with noxious stimuli (e.g., chemically induced nausea and vomiting), the procedure is expensive and has not been shown to be superior to less heroic methods.

Behavior therapists stress the importance of teaching new, adaptive skills designed to alter the conditions that precipitate and reinforce drinking, as well as developing alternative ways of coping with persons, events, and feelings that serve to maintain drinking (Miller and Mastria 1977). A number of studies have demonstrated the benefits of teaching social and other coping skills (Institute of Medicine 1990, Oei and Jackson 1982). Chaney and colleagues (1978) tested a model of treatment characterized as "relapse prevention" because of its focus on identifying and coping with situations that represent high risk for heavy drinking. Individuals who received skills training attended aftercare more regularly and they had less severe (though no less frequent) relapses than individuals in control groups.

These and other trials of cognitive–behavioral treatments (Institute of Medicine 1989) have provided the empirical basis for elaboration of a generalized relapse prevention strategy (Marlatt 1985).

The deleterious effects of alcoholism on marriages and families have been a source of concern to both clinicians and researchers. Alcoholism creates major stress on the family system by threatening health, interpersonal relations, and the economic functioning of family members. Although research has shown a strong association between healthy family functioning and positive outcome following alcoholism treatment (Moos and Moos 1984), little systematic evaluation has been undertaken to assess the efficacy of family approaches, either to reduce alcohol problems or to improve family functioning.

The majority of studies have involved marital rather than family treatment. A trial of behavioral marital therapy was conducted by O'Farrell and colleagues (1985). Alcoholics and their spouses were treated in aftercare for 10 weeks. At follow-up, behavioral marital therapy was found to have enhanced marital well-being more than interactional couples therapy, while a no-marital-therapy control group showed no significant change. There was no differential improvement in drinking behavior among the three groups. Subsequently, McCrady and colleagues (1986) showed behavioral marital therapy to be superior to control treatments in both the reduction of drinking and maintenance of sobriety.

In addition to specific treatment for alcoholic couples or families, self-help groups for family members of alcoholics have grown substantially. Al-Anon, although not formally affiliated with AA, shares the structure and many of the tenets of the 12 steps of AA. Al-Anon and AA meetings are often held jointly. Alateen groups, sponsored by Al-Anon for children of alcoholics, are available as well.

Somatic Treatments

Although the benzodiazepines have played a key role in the treatment of alcohol withdrawal, pharmacotherapy has not yet had a demonstrable effect on other aspects of alcoholism treatment. Disulfiram, an alcohol-sensitizing drug, has been approved for clinical use in the United States since the 1940s, but it has not been widely prescribed. During the past decade, however, medications have begun to play a more important role both in the treatment of comorbid mental disorders in alcoholics and in the rehabilitation of alcohol dependence. In dually diagnosed individuals, medications that reduce psychiatric symptomatology may also reduce the risk of drinking. Independent of their effects on comorbid psychopathology, medications that reduce drinking may enhance the alcoholic's participation in psychosocial treatment. This rationale is similar to that underlying the combination of medications with psychotherapy in the treatment of depressive or anxiety disorders.

In the following sections, we discuss two types of pharmacotherapy for alcoholics: alcohol-sensitizing drugs and medications to directly reduce drinking. The reader is referred to detailed reviews of these topics for additional information (Swift 1999, Garbutt et al. 1999, Kranzler 2000).

Alcohol-Sensitizing Drugs Medications such as disulfiram or calcium carbimide cause an unpleasant reaction when combined with alcohol. The efficacy of such drugs in the prevention or limitation of relapse in alcoholics has not been demonstrated. However, these drugs may be of utility in selected samples of alcoholics with whom special efforts are made to ensure compliance.

Disulfiram (Antabuse) is the most commonly used alcohol-sensitizing medication and the only one approved for use in the United States. When given in a single daily dose of 125 to 500 mg, disulfiram binds irreversibly to ALDH, permanently inactivating this enzyme. When alcohol is consumed, it is metabolized to acetaldehyde, which accumulates because of inhibition of the enzyme that metabolizes it. Elevated levels of acetaldehyde are responsible for the aversive effects associated with the disulfiram-ethanol reaction (DER).

Although disulfiram has been used in the treatment of alcoholism for more than 50 years, the few placebo-controlled studies that have been conducted have not shown the drug to have substantial efficacy. In a multicenter trial conducted by the US Department of Veterans Affairs (VA), more than 600 male alcoholics were assigned randomly to groups receiving either 1 mg of disulfiram per day or 250 mg/day, or to a control group that was told that they were not receiving disulfiram (Fuller et al. 1986). Results revealed a direct relationship between compliance with any of the three treatment regimens and complete abstinence. Among individuals who resumed drinking, those taking the 250-mg dosage of disulfiram had significantly fewer drinking days than did individuals in the other two groups. However, there was no significant difference among the three groups with respect to a variety of outcome measures, including length of time to first drink, unemployment, social stability, or number of men totally abstinent.

Disulfiram is usually given orally. Although the daily dosage prescribed in the United States has been limited to 250–500 mg/day, some individuals require in excess of 1 g/day of disulfiram to reach blood levels sufficient to produce the DER (Brewer 1984). The requirement that disulfiram undergo bioactivation before it can inhibit ALDH (Yourick and Faiman 1991) may explain the need for a higher dosage in some individuals. At the dosage that is used clinically, faulty bioactivation in some individuals may yield too low a concentration of the active metabolite to inhibit ALDH.

Given the limited efficacy of disulfiram for the prevention of relapse, it should not be used as a first-line treatment for alcohol dependence. However, if an individual has not responded to other pharmacological treatments and is motivated to take disulfiram, it may be beneficial. Whenever disulfiram is prescribed, individuals should be warned about its hazards, including the need to avoid over-the-counter (OTC) preparations with alcohol and drugs that interact adversely with disulfiram, as well as the potential for a DER to result from alcohol used in food preparations.

Drugs That May Directly Reduce Alcohol Consumption   A number of specific neurotransmitter systems have been implicated in the control of alcohol consumption, including endogenous opioids, catecholamines, especially dopamine, and serotonin. Although these systems appear to function interactively in their effects on drinking behavior, efforts to use medications to treat excessive drinking have increasingly focused on agents that have selective effects on specific neurotransmitter systems.

An extensive literature supports the role of opioidergic neurotransmission in the pathophysiology of alcohol consumption and related phenomena. For example, small doses of morphine increase alcohol intake in experimental animals (Hubbell et al. 1986). In contrast, opioid antagonists, such as naltrexone, decrease ethanol consumption and self-administration (Altschuler et al. 1980, Siviy et al. 1982).

Effects similar to those in animals have been reported in some, but not all, studies of naltrexone for the treatment of alcohol dependence (Kranzler and Van Kirk 2001). The considerable variability in findings concerning the efficacy of naltrexone underscores the need to identify the circumstances under which the medication exerts its therapeutic effects.

Naltrexone appears to produce a modest effect on drinking behavior among alcoholics (Kranzler and Van Kirk 2001). However, given the comparatively small overall effect of the medication, a variety of other factors, including medication compliance, the severity and chronicity of alcohol dependence, and the choice of concomitant psychotherapy, may determine whether an effect of the medication is observed.

Another major focus of research on medications to treat alcoholism has been the role of the indoleamine neurotransmitter, serotonin (5-HT). 5-HT has been shown consistently to exert an influence over alcohol consumption in preclinical models of drinking behavior (McBride et al. 1990, LeMarquand et al. 1994a). In contrast to this preclinical literature, data on the effects of serotonergic medications on human drinking behavior are more limited, and the results are less consistent (LeMarquand et al. 1994b, Kranzler 2000).

Naranjo and colleagues (1990) found that fluoxetine 60 mg/day reduced average daily alcohol consumption by approximately 17% from baseline levels, while treatment with fluoxetine 40 mg/day or placebo had no effect. When alcoholics on an inpatient unit were given the opportunity to drink alcohol, fluoxetine pretreatment (80 mg/day) initially reduced alcohol consumption, but the effect did not persist (Gorelick and Paredes 1992). In a crossover comparison of fluoxetine 40 mg/day, acamprosate, and placebo in family history–positive (FHP) and family history–negative (FHN) alcoholics (Gerra et al. 1992), both active medications were superior to placebo in reducing the number of drinks consumed. Fluoxetine was effective only in the FHP individuals, while acamprosate produced a significant reduction only in the FHN individuals. A placebo-controlled trial of fluoxetine 60 mg/day in combination with coping skills psychotherapy in outpatient alcoholics showed no overall advantage to the active drug on drinking outcomes (Kranzler et al. 1995). However, among the subgroup of individuals with high levels of both premorbid vulnerability and alcohol-related problems, fluoxetine appeared to reduce the beneficial effects of coping skills training (Kranzler et al. 1996a). Kabel and Petty (1996) showed no effect of fluoxetine 60 mg/day, compared with placebo, among veterans with severe alcoholic problems.

Another selective serotonin reuptake inhibitor (SSRI) whose effects on alcohol consumption have been extensively examined is citalopram. At a dosage of 40 mg/day, citalopram was initially reported to reduce the number of drinks consumed per day and increase the number of abstinent days in a sample of nondepressed, early stage problem drinkers (Naranjo et al. 1987). Using a similar design, these findings were replicated (Naranjo et al. 1992). However, when citalopram 40 mg/day was combined with a brief psychosocial intervention, there was a drug effect only during the first week of treatment; the overall reduction in drinking during the 12-week treatment trial was comparable for the citalopram and placebo groups (Naranjo et al. 1995). Balldin and colleagues (1994) found no effect of citalopram 40 mg/day on alcohol intake among heavy drinkers. However, in a *post hoc* analysis based on pretreatment drinking level, citalopram-treated subjects in the lighter drinking subgroup showed lower daily alcohol intake. Tiihonen and colleagues (1996) compared citalopram 40 mg with placebo in a 3-month study. Study retention was significantly better in the active medication group, with individuals' condition being rated by collateral informants as more improved. There was also a trend for decreased alcohol consumption and GGTP levels in the citalopram group.

One explanation for the variable findings in studies of whether SSRIs reduce drinking is the diversity of study samples. The initial studies were conducted in nontreatment-seeking heavy drinkers. Subsequent studies, which have shown differential effects based on severity, suggest that SSRIs are efficacious only in subgroups of alcoholics. For example, Gerra and colleagues (1992) found an effect of fluoxetine only in alcoholics with a positive family history of alcoholism. In contrast, Kranzler and colleagues (1996a) found that high risk/severity alcoholics (i.e., Type B, who have an earlier age of alcoholism onset, more sociopathic features, greater concomitant drug use) had poorer drinking outcomes when treated with fluoxetine, compared with placebo, and that low risk/severity alcoholics (Type A) had somewhat better outcomes on the active medication. Balldin and colleagues (1994) found an effect of citalopram only among drinkers in the lower range of alcohol consumption in their sample. Pettinati and colleagues (2000) found that later-onset alcoholics drank on fewer days and were more likely to be abstinent in a 12-week treatment trial if they received sertraline than if they were treated with placebo.

In a similar vein, although not an SSRI, ondansetron (a 5-HT$_3$ antagonist) was shown to produce a selective beneficial effect in alcoholics with onset of problem drinking before age 25 (Johnson et al. 2000). At a dosage substantially lower than that used to exert the antiemetic effects for which the medication is FDA approved, ondansetron was superior to placebo in terms of days abstinent and the intensity of alcohol intake on days when individuals did drink. Among alcoholics with onset of problem drinking at age 25 years or later, the effects of ondansetron on drinking behavior were, in nearly all respects, comparable to those of placebo. These findings suggest that prospective studies that aim to match alcoholic subtypes with serotonergic medications may reveal a useful role for such medications in the treatment of alcohol dependence.

Acamprosate, an amino acid derivative, affects both gamma-aminobutyric acid (GABA) and excitatory amino acid (i.e., glutamate) neurotransmission (the latter effect most likely being the one that is important for its therapeutic effects in alcoholism). The medication is approved for use throughout Europe, and is likely to be approved soon for use in the United States.

Together, studies involving more than 4000 individuals provide consistent evidence of the efficacy of acamprosate in alcoholism rehabilitation (Kranzler and Van Kirk 2001). On the basis of these findings, and the benign side effect profile of the medication, it appears to hold considerable value for the treatment of alcohol dependence.

Considerable additional research is required before medications are likely to play a meaningful role in the postwithdrawal treatment of alcohol dependence. One currently useful strategy is the identification of comorbid psychopathology in alcoholics, with pharmacotherapy directed toward reducing both psychiatric symptoms and alcohol consumption. In addition, the opioid antagonist naltrexone, which is capable of yielding a modest effect overall in reducing drinking behavior, appears to be of considerable value in some individuals. Further research is required with naltrexone to determine the optimal dosage, duration of treatment, and psychosocial treatment strategies with which to use the medication. The question of whether the medication is most efficacious for alcoholics with high levels of craving for alcohol remains an important one. The SSRIs fluoxetine, citalopram, and sertraline may be of value in subgroups of heavy drinkers, particularly those with a later onset of problem drinking. In contrast, ondansetron may be useful in alcoholics with an early onset of problem drinking. Prospective replication of this serotonergic matching strategy is required, however, before it can be recommended for general clinical use. Finally, acamprosate, once it is approved by the FDA, could assume a prominent role in the pharmacological management of alcohol dependence in the United States.

Alcoholics Anonymous (AA) and Mutual Help Organizations

Although mutual help societies composed of recovering alcoholics are not considered a formal treatment, they are often used as a substitute, an alternative, and an adjunct to treatment (McCrady and Miller 1993). Mutual help groups based on the Twelve Steps of AA have proliferated throughout the world (Mäkelä 1993). To the extent that AA and other mutual help groups are more numerous than outpatient treatment, they may constitute a significant resource for problem drinkers who are attempting to reduce or stop drinking.

With an estimated 87,000 groups in 150 countries, AA is by far the most widely utilized source of help for drinking problems in the United States and throughout the world. In addition, a number of self-help organizations have modeled themselves after AA, basing recovery from drug abuse, overeating, and other behavioral disorders on the 12 Steps of AA (see Table 16-6). Unfortunately, clinicians often refer individuals to self-help groups such as AA without consideration of the individual's needs and without adequate monitoring of the individual's response (Emrick 1994). Not all people are willing to endorse the AA emphasis on spirituality and its disease concept of alcoholism, which requires lifelong abstinence as the only means to recovery. Greater familiarity with AA may help clinicians to identify those individuals who might benefit from this approach.

Although it is regarded as one of the most useful resources for recovering alcoholics, the research literature supporting the efficacy of AA is limited (Miller and McCrady 1993). Attendance at AA tends to be correlated with long-term abstinence (Vaillant 1983, Polich et al. 1980, Hoffman et al. 1983) but this may reflect motivation for recovery. The type of motivated alcoholic that persists with AA might do just as well with other forms of supportive therapy. In fact, the few random assignment studies that have been conducted (Walsh et al. 1991, Brandsma et al. 1980) do not indicate that AA (or similar programs) is more effective than other types of treatment.

Personality variables do not appear to differentiate between alcoholics who affiliate with AA and those who do not (Ogborne and Glaser 1981), although there is some evidence that AA is less successful among persons with major psychiatric disorders and those of low socioeconomic status (Ogborne and Glaser 1981).

Infrequent attempts have been made to assess the efficacy of AA using controlled research designs because of methodological challenges, such as self-selection and ethical concerns about random assignment to treatment conditions. Nevertheless, several large-scale, well-designed studies (Project MATCH Research Group 1997a, 1998, Ouimette et al. 1999, Walsh et al. 1991) suggest that AA can have an incremental effect when combined with formal treatment, and AA attendance alone may be better than no intervention.

Walsh and colleagues (1991) showed that workers who were randomly assigned to a 3-week inpatient alcoholism rehabilitation program had significantly better alcohol-related outcomes than workers who were assigned to mandatory AA attendance only. Workers assigned to a third group were allowed to choose their treatment. This group had outcomes that were intermediate between the other two groups. Outcomes were worse among individuals abusing both alcohol and cocaine. A study of long-term outcomes of treated and untreated alcoholics (Timko et al. 2000) indicates that individuals who obtain help for a drinking problem, especially in a timely manner, have better outcomes over 8 years than those who do not receive help, but the type of help they receive (e.g., self-help or formal treatment) makes little difference in long-term outcomes.

Table 16-6	The 12 Steps of Alcoholics Anonymous

1. We admitted we were powerless over alcohol—that our lives had become unmanageable.
2. Came to believe that a Power greater than ourselves could restore us to sanity.
3. Made a decision to turn our will and our lives over to the care of God *as we understood Him.*
4. Made a searching and fearless moral inventory of ourselves.
5. Admitted to God, to ourselves, and to another human being the exact nature of our wrongs.
6. Were entirely ready to have God remove all these defects of character.
7. Humbly asked Him to remove our shortcomings.
8. Made a list of all persons we had harmed, and became willing to make amends to them all.
9. Made direct amends to such people wherever possible, except when to do so would injure them or others.
10. Continued to take personal inventory and when we were wrong, promptly admitted it.
11. Sought through prayer and meditation to improve our conscious contact with God *as we understood Him*, praying only for knowledge of His will for us and the power to carry that out.
12. Having had a spiritual awakening as the result of these steps, we tried to carry this message to alcoholics, and to practice these principles in all our affairs.

Source: The 12 Steps are reprinted with permission of Alcoholics Anonymous World Services, Inc. Permission to reprint this material does not mean that AA has reviewed or approved the contents of this publication, nor that AA agrees with the views expressed herein. AA is a program of recovery from alcoholism. Use of the 12 Steps in connection with programs and activities that are patterned after AA but address other problems does not imply otherwise

Treatment of Psychiatric Comorbidity

Comorbid psychiatric disorders may contribute to the development or maintenance of heavy drinking (Meyer 1986). Efforts to treat the comorbidity may have beneficial effects on drinking outcomes. Following detoxification, many alcoholics complain of persistent anxiety, insomnia, and general distress. These symptoms may last for weeks or months and may be difficult to differentiate from the emergence of diagnosable mental disorders. Irrespective of their etiology, negative emotional states, including frustration, anger, anxiety, depression, and boredom, have been shown to contribute to relapse in a substantial proportion of alcoholics (Marlatt 1985).

A variety of medications have been employed to treat comorbid psychiatric symptoms and disorders in alcoholics. Indications for the use of these medications in alcoholics are similar to those for nonalcoholic populations, but there is added potential for adverse effects due to comorbid medical disorders and the pharmacokinetic effects of acute and chronic alcohol consumption. The use of these medications in alcoholics therefore entails additional considerations that can only be arrived at through careful psychiatric diagnosis.

Treatment of Depressive Symptoms/Disorders

Depressive symptoms are common early in alcohol withdrawal, but they often remit spontaneously with time (Dorus et al. 1987). For depression that persists beyond the period of acute withdrawal, an antidepressant is probably warranted.

Although it has been argued that most instances of postwithdrawal depression will spontaneously remit within a few days to several weeks (Schuckit 1983, Brown and Schuckit 1988), there are still a substantial number of individuals whose severe and persistent depression requires treatment. Given the superior safety profile of SSRIs, particularly in relation to risk of suicide by medication overdose, use of these drugs is preferable to the use of TCAs.

Treatment of Anxiety Symptoms/Disorders

A number of studies have shown chlordiazepoxide to be effective in the maintenance of alcoholics in long-term outpatient treatment (Kissin 1975, Rosenberg 1974). However, the potential for additive CNS depression produced by the concurrent use of alcohol and benzodiazepines is well recognized. Furthermore, the use of benzodiazepines may itself result in tolerance and dependence and may increase depressive symptoms (Schuckit 1983). Although this concern may be exaggerated (Ciraulo et al. 1988) and all benzodiazepines may not be equal in their capacity to produce dependence in alcoholics (Jaffe et al. 1983), generally speaking, the use of benzodiazepines in alcoholics is probably best limited to detoxification.

Buspirone (Taylor et al. 1985) is a non-benzodiazepine anxiolytic that is less sedating than diazepam or clorazepate, does not interact with alcohol to impair psychomotor skills, and has a low potential for abuse. When combined with appropriate psychosocial treatment, buspirone appears useful in the treatment of alcoholics with persistent anxiety.

Currently, antipsychotics are indicated only in alcoholics with a coexistent psychotic disorder or for the treatment of alcoholic hallucinosis (Naranjo and Sellers 1986). Several placebo-controlled studies have found no advantage in the use of phenothiazines for treatment of anxiety, tension, and depression following detoxification (Jaffe et al. 1992). Because of their capacity to lower seizure threshold, antipsychotics should be used with caution in this population.

Comparison of DSM-IV-TR/ICD-10 Diagnostic Criteria

The ICD-10 and DSM-IV-TR criteria sets are nearly identical except for the following: The ICD-10 Diagnostic Criteria for Research for Alcohol Intoxication also lists flushed face and conjunctival injection as symptoms but does not include the DSM-IV-TR item for impairment in attention; the ICD-10 Diagnostic Criteria for Research for Alcohol Withdrawal require three symptoms from a list of 10 which includes headache and splits tachycardia and sweating into two separate items.

References

Allan AM and Harris RA (1986) Gamma-aminobutyric acid and alcohol actions: neurochemical studies of long sleep and short sleep mice. *Life Sci* **39**, 2005–2015.

Allen JP and Litten RZ (2001) The role of laboratory tests in alcoholism treatment. *J Subst Abuse Treat* **20**, 81–85.

Allen JP, Litten RZ, Fertig JB, et al. (2001) Carbohydrate-deficient transferrin: an aid to early recognition of alcohol relapse. *Am J Addict* **10**(Suppl.), 24–28.

Altschuler HL, Phillips PE, and Feinhandler DA (1980) Alterations of ethanol self-administration by naltrexone. *Life Sci* **26**, 679–688.

Annis HM and Graham GM (1995) Profile types of the inventory of drinking situations: implications for relapse prevention counseling. *Psychol Addict Behav* **9**, 176–182.

Anton RF, Moak DH, Waid R, et al. (1999) Naltrexone and cognitive behavioral therapy for the treatment of outpatient alcoholics: results of a placebo-controlled trial. *Am J Psychiatry* **156**, 1758–1764.

Arif A and Westermeyer J (eds). (1988) *Manual of Drug and Alcohol Abuse: Guidelines for Teaching in Medical and Health Institutions.* Plenum Press, New York, pp. 167–191.

Atkinson RM and Kofoed LL (1982) Alcohol and drug abuse in old age: a clinical perspective. *Subst Alcohol Actions/Misuse* **3**, 353–368.

Babor TF (1994) Avoiding the horrid and beastly sin of drunkenness: does dissuasion make a difference? *J Consult Clin Psychol* **62**, 1127–1140.

Babor TF and Higgins-Biddle JC (2001a) *AUDIT The Alcohol Use Disorders Identification Test: Guidelines for use in Primary Care*, 2nd ed. World Health Organization, Geneva, Switzerland.

Babor TF and Kadden R (1985) Screening for alcohol problems: conceptual issues and practical considerations. In *Early Identification of alcohol abuse, NIAAA National Institute on Alcohol Abuse and Alcoholism Research Monograph 17*, DHHS Pub. No. (ADM) 85–1258, Chang N and Chao HM (eds). US Government Printing Office, Washington, DC, pp. 1–30.

Babor TF and Lauerman RJ (1986) Classification and forms of inebriety: historical antecedents of alcoholic typologies. In *Recent Developments in Alcoholism*, Vol. IV, Galanter M (ed). Plenum Press, New York, pp. 113–144.

Babor TF, Hofmann M, DelBoca FK, et al. (1992) Types of alcoholics: evidence for an empirically-derived typology based on indicators of vulnerability and severity. *Arch Gen Psychiatry* **8**, 599–608.

Babor TF, Kranzler HR, and Lauerman RL (1987a) Social drinking as a health and psychosocial risk factor: Anstie's limit revisited. In *Recent Developments in Alcoholism*, Vol. 5, Galanter M (ed). Plenum Press, New York, pp. 373–402.

Babor TF, Stephens RS, and Marlatt GA (1987b) Verbal report methods in clinical research on alcoholism: response bias and its minimization. *J Stud Alcohol* **48**, 410–424.

Balldin J, Berggren U, Engel J, et al. (1994) Effect of citalopram on alcohol intake in heavy drinkers. *Alcohol Clin Exp Res* **18**, 1133–1136.

Beck AT, Ward CH, Mendelson M, et al. (1961) An inventory for measuring depression. *Arch Gen Psychiatry* **4**, 561–571.

Becker U, Deis A, Sorensen TI, et al. (1996) Prediction of risk of liver disease by alcohol intake, sex, and age: a prospective population study. *Hepatology* **23**, 1025–1029.

Begleiter H and Porjesz B (1999) What is inherited in the predisposition toward alcoholism? A proposed model. *Alcohol Clin Exp Res* **23**, 1125–1135.

Bergen AW, Kokoszka J, Peterson R, et al. (1997) Mu opioid receptor gene variants: lack of association with alcohol dependence. *Mol Psychiatry* **2**, 490–494.

Bien TH, William R, and Tonigan S (1993) Brief interventions for alcohol problems: a review. *Addiction* **88**, 315–336.

Blomqvist O, Engel JA, Nissbrandt H, et al. (1993) The mesolimbic dopamine-activating properties of ethanol are antagonized by mecamylamine. *Eur J Pharmacol* **249**, 207–213.

Blomqvist O, Ericson M, Engel JA, et al. (1997) Accumbal dopamine overflow after ethanol: localization of the antagonizing effect of mecamylamine. *Eur J Pharmacol* **334**, 149–156.

Blomqvist O, Ericson M, Johnson DH, et al. (1996) Voluntary ethanol intake in the rat: effects of nicotinic acetylcholine receptor blockage or subchronic nicotine treatment. *Eur J Pharmacol* **314**, 257–267.

Blomqvist O, Hernandez-Avila CA, Van Kirk J, et al. (2002) Mecamylamine modifies the pharmacokinetics and reinforcing effects of alcohol. *Alcohol Clin Exp Res* **26**, 326–331.

Bohn MJ and Meyer RE (1994) Typologies of addiction. In *Textbook of Substance Abuse Treatment*, Galanter M and Kleber HD (eds). American Psychiatric Press, Washington, DC, pp. 11–24.

Bohn MJ, Babor TF, and Kranzler HR (1995) The Alcohol Use Disorders Identification Test (AUDIT): validation of a screening instrument for use in medical settings. *J Stud Alcohol* **56**, 423–432.

Bond C, LaForge KS, Tian M, et al. (1998) Single-nucleotide polymorphism in the human mu opioid receptor gene alters b-endorphin binding and activity: possible implications for opiate addiction. *Proc Natl Acad Sci U S A* **95**, 9608–9613.

Brandsma JM, Maultsby MC, and Welsh RJ (1980) *The Outpatient Treatment of Alcoholism: A Review and Comparative Study*. University Park Press, Baltimore, MD.

Brewer C (1984) How effective is the standard dose of disulfiram? A review of the alcohol-disulfiram reaction in practice. *Br J Psychiatry* **144**, 200–202.

Brodie MS and Bunney EB (1996) Serotonin potentiates dopamine inhibition of ventral tegmental area neurons in vitro. *J Neurophysiol* **76**, 2077–2082.

Brodie MS, Pesold C, and Appel SB (1999) Ethanol directly excites dopaminergic ventral tegmental area reward neurons. *Alcohol Clin Exp Res* **23**, 1848–1852.

Brown SA and Schuckit MA (1988) Changes in depression among abstinent alcoholics. *J Stud Alcohol* **49**, 412–417.

Chaney E, O'Leary M, and Marlatt GA (1978) Skill training with alcoholics. *J Consult Clin Psychol* **46**, 1092–1104.

Chang G (2001) Alcohol-screening instruments for pregnant women. *Alcohol Res Health* **25**, 204–209.

Chu B, Anantharam V, and Treistman SN (1995) Ethanol inhibition of recombinant heteromeric NMDA channels in the presence and absence of modulators. *J Neurochem* **65**, 140–148.

Ciraulo DA, Sands BF, and Shader RI (1988) Critical review of liability for benzodiazepine abuse among alcoholics. *Am J Psychiatry* **145**, 1501–1506.

Cloninger CR (1987) Neurogenetic adaptive mechanisms in alcoholism. *Science* **236**, 410–416.

Cloninger CR, Bohman M, and Sigvardsson S (1981) Inheritance of alcohol abuse: cross-fostering analysis of adopted men. *Arch Gen Psychiatry* **38**, 861–868.

Criswell HE, Simson PE, Duncan GE, et al. (1993) Molecular basis for regional specification of ethanol on gamma-aminobutyric acid A receptors: generalization to other ligand-gated ion channels. *J Pharmacol Exp Ther* **267**, 522–537.

Dahchour A, De Witte P, Bolo N, et al. (1998) Central effects of acamprosate: Part 1. Acamprosate blocks the glutamate increase in the nucleus accumbens microdialysate in ethanol withdrawn rats. *Psychiatr Res* **82**, 107–114.

Derogatis LR (1977) *SCL-90 Manual-I*. John Hopkins, Baltimore, MD.

Dorus W, Kennedy J, Gibbons RD, et al. (1987) Symptoms and diagnosis of depression in alcoholics. *Alcohol Clin Exp Res* **11**, 150–154.

Dunne FJ, Galatopoulos C, and Schipperheijn JM (1993) Gender differences in psychiatric morbidity among alcohol misusers. *Compr Psychiatry* **34**, 95–101.

Eckardt MJ, Harford TC, Kaelber CT, et al. (1981) Health hazards associated with alcohol consumption. *J Am Med Assoc* **246**, 648–666.

Edenberg HJ, Reynolds J, Koller DL, et al. (1998b) A family-based analysis of whether the functional promoter alleles of the serotonin transporter gene HTT affect the risk for alcohol dependence. *Alcohol Clin Exp Res* **22**, 1080–1085.

Edwards G and Gross MM (1976) Alcohol dependence: provisional description of a clinical syndrome. *Br Med J* **1**, 1058–1061.

Emrick CD (1994) Alcoholics Anonymous and other 12-step groups. In *Textbook of Substance Abuse Treatment*, Galanter M and Kleber HD (eds). American Psychiatric Press, Washington, DC, pp. 351–358.

Ericson M, Blomqvist O, Engel JA, et al. (1998) Voluntary ethanol intake in the rat and the associated accumbal dopamine overflow is blocked by ventral tegmental mecamylamine. *Eur J Pharmacol* **358**, 189–196.

Eskelson CD, Hameroff SR, and Kanel JS (1980) Ethanol increases serum beta-endorphin levels in rats. *Anesth Analg* **59**, 537–538.

Ewing JA (1984) Detecting alcoholism: the CAGE questionnaire. *J Am Med Assoc* **252**, 1905–1907.

Feldman DJ, Pattison EM, Sobell LC, et al. (1975) Outpatient alcohol detoxification: initial findings on 564 patients. *Am J Psychiatry* **132**, 407–412.

Finlayson RE, Hurt RD, Davis LJ, et al. (1988) Alcoholism in elderly persons: a study of the psychiatric and psychosocial features of 216 inpatients. *Mayo Clin Proc* **63**, 753–760.

Finnegan LP and Kandall SR (1992) Maternal and neonatal effects of alcohol and drugs. In *Substance Abuse: A Comprehensive Textbook*, 2nd ed., Lowinson JH, Ruiz P, and Millman RB (eds). Williams & Wilkins, Philadelphia, pp. 628–656.

First MB, Spitzer RL, Gibbon M, et al. (1996) *Structured Clinical Interview for DSM-IV Axis I Disorders, Clinician Version (SCID-CV)*. American Psychiatric Press, Washington, DC.

Frezza M, DiPadova C, Pozzato G, et al. (1990) High blood alcohol levels in women: the role of decreased gastric alcohol dehydrogenase activity and first-pass metabolism. *N Engl J Med* **322**, 95–99.

Fuller RK, Branchey L, Brightwell DR, et al. (1986) Disulfiram treatment of alcoholism: A Veteran's Administration Cooperative Study. *J Am Med Assoc* **256**, 1449–1455.

Garbutt JC, West SL, Carey TS, et al. (1999) Pharmacological treatment of alcohol dependence: a review of the evidence. *J Am Med Assoc* **281**, 1318–1325.

Gelernter J (1995) Genetic factors in alcoholism: evidence and implications. In *The Pharmacology of Alcohol Abuse*, Kranzler HR (ed). Springer-Verlag, New York, pp. 297–313.

Gelernter J, Kranzler H, and Cubells J (1999) Genetics of two μ receptor gene (OPRM1) exon I polymorphisms: population studies, and allele frequencies in alcohol and drug dependent subjects. *Mol Psychiatry* **4**, 476–483.

Gelernter J, Kranzler H, and Cubells JF (1997) Serotonin transporter protein (SLC6A4) allele and haplotype frequencies and linkage disequilibria in African- and European-American and Japanese populations and in alcohol-dependent subjects. *Hum Genet* **101**, 243–246.

Gerra G, Caccavari R, Delsignore R, et al. (1992) Effects of fluoxetine and Ca-acetyl-homotaurinate on alcohol intake in familial and nonfamilial alcohol patients. *Curr Ther Res* **52**, 291–295.

Gianoulakis C, Beliveau D, Angelogianni P, et al. (1989) Different pituitary beta-endorphin and adrenal cortisol response to ethanol in individuals with high and low risk for future development of alcoholism. *Life Sci* **45**, 1097–1109.

Gianoulakis C, Krishnan B, and Thavundayil J (1996) Enhanced sensitivity of pituitary beta-endorphin to ethanol in subjects at high risk of alcoholism. *Arch Gen Psychiatry* **53**, 250–257.

Gill K and Amit Z (1989) Serotonin uptake blockers and voluntary alcohol consumption: a review of recent studies. *Recent Dev Alcohol* **7**, 225–248.

Goedde HW, Harada S, and Agarwal DP (1979) Racial differences in alcohol sensitivity: a new hypothesis. *Hum Genet* **51**, 331–334.

Goldman D (1988) Molecular markers for linkage of genetic loci contributing to alcoholism. In *Recent Developments in Alcoholism*, Vol. 6, Galanter M (ed). Plenum Press, New York, pp. 333–349.

Goldman D (1993) Genetic transmission. In *Recent Developments in Alcoholism*, Vol. 11, Galanter M (ed). Plenum Press, New York, pp. 231–248.

Goldstein DB (1992) Pharmacokinetics of alcohol. In *Medical Diagnosis and Treatment of Alcoholism*, Mendelson JH and Mello NK (eds). McGraw-Hill, New York, pp. 25–54.

Gorelick DA and Paredes A (1992) Effect of fluoxetine on alcohol consumption in male alcoholics. *Alcohol Clin Exp Res* **16**, 261–265.

Gorwood P, Batel P, Ades J, et al. (2000) Serotonin transporter gene polymorphisms, alcoholism, and suicidal behavior. *Biol Psychiatry* **48**, 259–264.

Graham K (1986) Identifying and measuring alcohol abuse among the elderly: serious problems with existing instrumentation. *J Stud Alcohol* **47**, 322–326.

Grande TP, Wolf AW, Schubert DSP, et al. (1984) Associations among alcoholism, drug abuse, and antisocial personality disorder: a review of literature. *Psychol Rep* **55**, 455–474.

Grant BF (2000) Theoretical and observed subtypes of DSM-IV alcohol abuse and dependence in a general population sample. *Drug Alcohol Depend* **60**, 287–293.

Grant BF, Harford TC, Dawson DA, et al. (1994) Prevalence of DSM-IV alcohol abuse and dependence: United States, 1992. *Alcohol Health Res World* **18**, 243–248.

Greenberg BD, Tolliver TJ, Huang SJ, et al. (1999) Genetic variation in the serotonin transporter promoter region affects serotonin uptake in human blood platelets *Am J Med Genet (Neuropsychiatr Genet)* **88**, 83–87.

Hallikainen T, Saito T, Lachman HM, et al. (1999) Association between low activity serotonin transporter promoter genotype and early onset alcoholism with habitual impulsive violent behavior. *Mol Psychiatry* **4**, 385–388.

Hammoumi S, Payen A, Favre JD, et al. (1999) Does the short variant of the serotonin transporter linked polymorphic region constitute a marker of alcohol dependence? *Alcohol* **17**, 107–112.

Hannigan JH, Welch RA, and Sokol RJ (1992) Recognition of fetal alcohol syndrome and alcohol-related birth defects. In *Medical Diagnosis and Treatment of Alcoholism*, Mendelson JH and Mello NK (eds). McGraw-Hill, New York, pp. 639–667.

Harris RA (1999) Ethanol actions on multiple ion channels: Which are important? *Alcohol Clin Exp Res* **23**, 1563–1570.

Hayashida M, Alterman AI, McLellan T, et al. (1989) Comparative effectiveness and costs of inpatient and outpatient detoxification of patients with mild-to-moderate alcohol withdrawal syndrome. *N Engl J Med* **320**, 358–365.

Helzer JE and Canino GJ (1992) Comparative analysis of alcoholism in ten cultural regions. In *Alcoholism in North America, Europe, and Asia*, Helzer JE and Canino GJ (eds). Oxford University Press, New York, pp. 289–308.

Helzer J and Pryzbeck T (1988) The co-occurrence of alcoholism with other psychiatric disorders in the general population and its impact on treatment. *J Stud Alcohol* **49**, 210–224.

Helzer JE, Robins LN, and McEvoy L (1987) Post-traumatic stress disorder in the general population. Findings of the epidemiologic catchment area survey. *N Engl J Med* **317**, 1630–1634.

Hesselbrock MN, Meyer RE, and Keener JJ (1985) Psychopathology in hospitalized alcoholics. *Arch Gen Psychiatry* **42**, 1050–1055.

Hesselbrock VM, Foroud T, Edenberg H, et al. (2001) Genetics and alcoholism: the COGA Project. In *Alcohol in Health and Disease*, Agarwal DP and Seitz HK (eds). Marcel-Dekker, New York, pp. 103–124.

Higley JD, Mehlman PT, Taub DM, et al. (1992) Cerebrospinal fluid monoamine and adrenal correlates of aggression in free-ranging rhesus monkeys. *Arch Gen Psychiatry* **49**, 436–441.

Higley JD, Suomi SJ, and Linnoila M (1996) A nonhuman primate model of type II excessive alcohol consumption? Part 2. Diminished social competence and excessive aggression correlates with low cerebrospinal fluid 5-hydroxyindoleacetic acid concentrations. *Alcohol Clin Exp Res* **20**, 643–650.

Hoffman NB, Harrison PA, and Belille CA (1983) Alcoholics Anonymous after treatment: attendance and abstinence. *Int J Addict* **18**, 311–318.

Hoffman PL, Snell LD, Bhave SV, et al. (1994) Ethanol inhibition of NMDA receptor function in primary cultures of rat cerebellar granule cells and cerebral cortical cells. *Alcohol Alcohol*, 2(Suppl.), 199–204.

Holt S, Skinner HA, and Israel Y (1981) Early identification of alcohol abuse. II. Clinical and laboratory indicators. *Can Med Assoc J* **124**, 1279–1295.

Hubbell C, Czirr S, Hunter G, et al. (1986) Consumption of ethanol solution is potentiated by morphine and attenuated by naloxone persistently across repeated daily administrations. *Alcohol* **3**, 39–54.

Institute of Medicine (1989) Treatment modalities: process and outcome. In *Prevention and Treatment of Alcohol Problems: Research Opportunities*. National Academy Press, Washington, DC, pp. 169–213.

Institute of Medicine (1990) *Broadening the Base of Treatment for Alcohol Problems*. National Academy Press, Washington, DC.

Irwin M, Baird S, Smith TL, et al. (1988) Use of laboratory tests to monitor heavy drinking by alcoholic men discharged from a treatment program. *Am J Psychiatry* **145**, 595–599.

Ishiguro H, Saito T, Akazawa S, et al. (1999) Association between drinking-related antisocial behavior and a polymorphism in the serotonin transporter gene in a Japanese population. *Alcohol Clin Exp Res* **23**, 1281–1284.

Jacobson R (1986) The contributions of sex and drinking history to the CT brain scan changes in alcoholics. *Psychol Med* **16**, 547–559.

Jaffe JH, Ciraulo DA, Nies A, et al. (1983) Abuse potential of halazepam and diazepam in patients recently treated for acute alcohol withdrawal. *Clin Pharmacol Ther* **34**, 623–630.

Jaffe JH, Kranzler HR, and Ciraulo D (1992) Drugs used in the treatment of alcoholism. In *Medical Diagnosis and Treatment of Alcoholism*, 3rd ed., Mendelson JH and Mello NK (eds). McGraw-Hill, New York, pp. 421–461.

Johnson BA, Roache JD, Javors MA, et al. (2000) Ondansetron for reduction of drinking among biologically predisposed alcoholic patients: a randomized controlled trial. *J Am Med Assoc* **284**, 963–971.

Kabel DI and Petty F (1996) A double blind study of fluoxetine in severe alcohol dependence: adjunctive therapy during and after inpatient treatment. *Alcohol Clin Exp Res* **20**, 780–784.

Kadden RM, Cooney NL, Getter H, et al. (1989) Matching alcoholics to coping skills or interactional therapies: posttreatment results. *J Consult Clin Psychol* **57**, 698–704.

Kahan M, Wilson L, and Becker L (1995) Effectiveness of physician-based interventions with problem drinkers: a review. *Can Med Assoc J* **152**, 851–859.

Kaminer Y (1994) *Adolescent Substance Abuse: A Comprehensive Guide to Theory and Practice*. Plenum Press, New York.

Kendler KS (2001) Twin studies of psychiatric illness. *Arch Gen Psychiatry* **58**, 1005–1014.

Kendler KS, Prescott CA, Neale MC, et al. (1997) Temperance board registration for alcohol abuse in a national sample of male twins born 1902–1949. *Arch Gen Psychiatry* **54**, 178–184.

Kessler RC, McGonagle KA, Zhao S, et al. (1994) Lifetime and 12-month prevalence of DSM-III-R psychiatric disorders in the United States. *Arch Gen Psychiatry* **51**, 8–19.

Kessler RC, Crum RM, Warner LA, et al. (1997) Lifetime co-occurrence of DSM-III-R alcohol abuse and dependence with other psychiatric disorders in the National Comorbidity Survey. *Arch Gen Psychiatry* **54**, 313–321.

Kessler RC, Nelson CB, McGonagle KA, et al. (1996) The epidemiology of co-occurring addictive and mental disorders: implications for prevention and service utilization. *Am J Orthopsychiatry* **66**, 17–31.

Kissin B (1975) The use of psychoactive drugs in the long-term treatment of chronic alcoholics. *Ann N Y Acad Sci* **52**, 385–395.

Kranzler HR (2000) Pharmacotherapy of alcoholism: gaps in knowledge and opportunities for research. *Alcohol Alcohol* **35**, 537–547.

Kranzler HR and Liebowitz N (1988) Depression and anxiety in substance abuse: clinical implications. In *Anxiety and Depression, Medical Clinics of North America*, Vol. 72, Frazier S (ed). Williams & Wilkins, Philadelphia, pp. 867–885.

Kranzler HR and Van Kirk J (2001) Naltrexone and acamprosate in the treatment of alcoholism: a meta-analysis. *Alcohol Clin Exp Res* **25**, 1335–1341.

Kranzler HR, Babor TF, and Lauerman R (1990) Problems associated with average alcohol consumption and frequency of intoxication in a medical population. *Alcohol Clin Exp Res* **14**, 119–126.

Kranzler HR, Burleson JA, Brown J, et al. (1996a) Fluoxetine treatment seems to reduce the beneficial effects of cognitive–behavioral therapy in Type B alcoholics. *Alcohol Clin Exp Res* **20**, 1534–1541.

Kranzler HR, Burleson JA, Korner P, et al. (1995) Placebo-controlled trial of fluoxetine as an adjunct to relapse prevention in alcoholics. *Am J Psychiatry* **152**, 391–397.

Kranzler HR, Del Boca FK, and Rounsaville BJ (1996b) Comorbid psychiatric diagnosis predicts three-year outcomes in alcoholics: a post-treatment natural history study. *J Stud Alcohol* **57**, 619–626.

Kranzler HR, Modesto-Lowe V, and Nuwayser ES (1998) A sustained-release naltrexone preparation for treatment of alcohol dependence, *Alcoholism: Clin Exp Res* **22**, 1074–1079.

Kranzler HR, Modesto-Lowe V, and Van Kirk J (2000) Naltrexone vs. nefazodone for treatment of alcohol dependence: a placebo-controlled trial. *Neuropsychopharmacology* **22**, 493–503.

Krasner N, Davis M, Portmann B, et al. (1977) Changing pattern of alcoholic liver disease in Great Britain: relation to sex and signs of autoimmunity. *Br Med J* **1**, 1497–1500.

Lane JD, Stinson FS, and Bertolucci D (1997) *Trends in Alcohol-Related Fatal Traffic Crashes, United States, 1977–95*, Surveillance Report No. 42. National Institute on Alcohol Abuse and Alcoholism, Rockville, MD.

LeMarquand D, Pihl RO, and Benkelfat C (1994a) Serotonin and alcohol intake, abuse, and dependence: findings of animal studies. *Biol Psychiatry* **36**, 395–421.

LeMarquand D, Pihl RO, and Benkelfat C (1994b) Serotonin and alcohol intake, abuse, and dependence: clinical evidence. *Biol Psychiatry* **36**, 326–337.

Lesch PK, Bengel D, Heils A, et al. (1996) Association of anxiety-related traits with a polymorphism in the serotonin transporter gene regulatory region. *Science* **274**, 1527–1531.

Lesieur HR and Blume SB (1993) Pathological gambling, eating disorders, and the psychoactive substance use disorders. *J Addict Dis* **12**, 89–102.

Lex BW (1992) Alcohol problems in special populations. In *Medical Diagnosis and Treatment of Alcoholism*, Mendelson JH and Mello NK (eds). McGraw-Hill, New York, pp. 71–154.

Lichtermann D, Hranilovic D, Trixler M, et al. (2000) Support for allelic association of a polymorphic site in the promoter region of the serotonin transporter gene with risk for alcohol dependence. *Am J Psychiatry* **157**, 2045–2047.

Limson R, Goldman D, Roy A, et al. (1991) Personality and cerebrospinal fluid monoamine metabolites in alcoholics and controls. *Arch Gen Psychiatry* **48**, 437–444.

Lindstrom L (1992) *Managing Alcoholism: Matching Clients to Treatments*. Oxford University Press, New York.

Liskow BI, Powell BJ, Nickel EJ, et al. (1990) Diagnostic subgroups of antisocial alcoholics: outcome at 1 year. *Compr Psychiatry* **31**, 549–556.

Litt MD, Babor TF, Del Boca FK, et al. (1992) Types of Alcoholics: II. Application of an empirically-derived typology to treatment matching. *Arch Gen Psychiatry* **8**, 609–614.

Litten RZ, Allen JP, and Fertig JB (1995) Gamma-glutamyltranspeptidase and carbohydrate deficient transferrin: alternative measures of excessive alcohol consumption. *Alcohol Clin Exp Res* **19**, 1541–1546.

Long JC, Knowler WC, Hanson RL, et al. (1998) Evidence for genetic linkage to alcohol dependence on chromosomes 4 and 11 from an autosome-wide scan in an American Indian population. *Am J Med Genet* **81**, 216–221.

Mäkelä K (1993) International comparisons of Alcoholics Anonymous. *Alcohol Health Res World* **17**, 228–234.

Mäkelä K, Room R, Single E, et al. (1981) *Alcohol, Society, and the State: 1. A Comparative Study of Alcohol Control*. Addiction Research Foundation, Toronto.

Malcolm R, Ballenger JC, Sturgis ET, et al. (1989) Double-blind controlled trial comparing carbamazepine to oxazepam treatment of alcohol withdrawal. *Am J Psychiatry* **146**, 617–621.

Marlatt GA (1985) Relapse prevention: theoretical rationale and overview of the model. In *Relapse Prevention: Maintenance Strategies in the Treatment of Addictive Behaviors*, Marlatt GA and Gordon JR (eds). Guilford Press, New York, pp. 3–70.

Martin SE (2001) The links between alcohol, crime and the criminal justice system: explanations, evidence and interventions. *Am J Addict* **10**, 136–158.

Mason BJ, Salvato FR, Williams LD, et al. (1999) A double-blind, placebo-controlled study of oral nalmefene for alcohol dependence. *Arch Gen Psychiatry* **56**, 719–724.

Mattick RP and Jarvis T (1994) Brief or minimal intervention for "alcoholics"? The evidence suggests otherwise. *Drug Alcohol Rev* **13**, 137–144.

McBride WJ, Murphy JM, Lumeng L, et al. (1990) Serotonin, dopamine and GABA involvement in alcohol drinking of selectively bred rats. *Alcohol* **7**, 199–205.

McCrady BS and Miller WR (eds) (1993) *Research on Alcoholics Anonymous: Opportunities and Alternatives*. Rutgers Center of Alcohol Studies, New Brunswick, NJ, pp. 41–78.

McCrady BS, Noel NE, Abrams DB, et al. (1986) Comparative effectiveness of three types of spouse involvement in outpatient behavioral alcoholism treatment. *J Stud Alcohol* **47**, 459–467.

McGue M (1994) Genes, environment, and the etiology of alcoholism. In *The Development of Alcohol Problems: Exploring the Biopsychosocial Matrix of Risk*, NIAAA Research Monograph No. 26, Zucker R, Boyd G, Howard J (eds). US Department of Health and Human Services, Rockville, MD, pp. 1–40.

McLellan AT, Grissom GR, Brill P, et al. (1993) Private substance abuse treatments: are some programs more effective than others? *J Subst Abuse Treat* **10**, 243–254.

McLellan AT, Kushner H, Metzger D, et al. (1992) The fifth edition of the addiction severity index. *J Subst Abuse Treat* **9**, 199–213.

Merikangas KR (1990) The genetic epidemiology of alcoholism. *Psychol Med* **20**, 11–22.

Merikangas KR, Stevens DE, Fenton B, et al. (1998) Comorbidity and familial aggregations of alcoholism and anxiety disorders. *Psychol Med* **28**, 773–788.

Meyer RE (1986) How to understand the relationship between psychopathology and addictive disorders: another example of the chicken and the egg. In *Psychopathology and Addictive Disorder*, Meyer RE (ed). Guilford Press, New York, pp. 3–16.

Mihic SJ and Harris RA (1995) Alcohol actions at the GABA$_A$ receptor/chloride channel complex. In *Pharmacological Effects of Ethanol on the Nervous System*, Dietrich RA and Erwin VG (eds). CRC Press, Boca Raton, Florida, pp. 51–72.

Miller WR and Hester RK (1980) Treating the problem drinker: modern approaches. In *The Addictive Behaviors*, Vol. 11, Miller WR (ed). Pergamon Press, New York, pp. 11–141.

Miller WR and Hester RK (1986) Inpatient alcoholism treatment: Who benefits? *Am Psychol* **41**, 794–805.

Miller PM and Mastria MA (1977) *Alternatives to Alcohol Abuse: A Social Learning Model*. Research Press, IL.

Miller WR and McCrady BS (1993) The importance of research on Alcoholics Anonymous. In *Research on Alcoholics Anonymous: Opportunities and Alternatives*, McCrady BS and Miller WR (eds). Rutgers Center of Alcohol Studies, New Brunswick, pp. 3–11.

Moos RH and Moos BS (1984) The process of recovery from alcoholism. III. Comparing functioning in families of alcoholics and matched control families. *J Stud Alcohol* **45**, 111–118.

Moos RH and Moos BS (2003) Long-term influence of duration and intensity of treatment on previously untreated individuals with alcohol use disorders. *Addiction* **98**, 325–337.

Moss HB, Yao JK, and Panzak GL (1990) Serotoninergic responsivity and behavioral dimensions in antisocial personality disorder with substance abuse. *Biol Psychiatry* **28**, 325–338.

Murawaki Y, Sugisaki H, Yuasa I, et al. (1997) Serum carbohydrate-deficient transferrin in patients with nonalcoholic liver disease and with hepatocellular carcinoma. *Clin Chim Acta* **259**, 97–108.

Nadal R, Chappell AM, and Samson HH (1998) Effects of nicotine and mecamylamine microinjections into the nucleus accumbens on ethanol and sucrose self-administration. *Alcohol Clin Exp Res* **22**, 1190–1198.

Naranjo CA and Sellers EM (1986) Clinical assessment and pharmacotherapy of the alcohol withdrawal syndrome. In *Recent Developments in Alcoholism*, Vol. 4, Galanter M (ed). Plenum Press, New York, pp. 265–281.

Naranjo CA, Bremner KE, and Lanctot KL (1995) Effects of citalopram and a brief psycho-social intervention on alcohol intake, dependence, and problems. *Addiction* **90**, 87–99.

Naranjo CA, Kadlec KE, Sanhueza P, et al. (1990) Fluoxetine differentially alters alcohol intake and other consummatory behaviors in problem drinkers. *Clin Pharmacol Ther* **47**, 490–498.

Naranjo CA, Poulos CX, Bremner KE, et al. (1992) Citalopram decreases desirability, liking, and consumption of alcohol in alcohol-dependent drinkers. *Clin Pharmacol Ther* **51**, 729–739.

Naranjo CA, Sellers EM, Chater K, et al. (1983) Nonpharmacologic interventions in acute alcohol withdrawal. *Clin Pharmacol Ther* **34**, 214–219.

Naranjo CA, Sellers EM, Sullivan JT, et al. (1987) The serotonin uptake inhibitor citalopram attenuates ethanol intake. *Clin Pharmacol Ther* **41**, 266–274.

Narrow WE, Rae DS, Robins LN, et al. (2002) Revised prevalence estimates of mental disorders in the United States: using a clinical significance criterion to reconcile 2 surveys' estimates. *Arch Gen Psychiatry* **59**, 115–123.

National Institute of Mental Health (NIMH) (1990) Substance abuse comorbidity in schizophrenia. *Schizophr Bull* **16**.

Nixon SJ (1993) Typologies in women. In *Recent Developments in Alcoholism*, Vol. 11, Galanter M (ed). Plenum Press, New York, pp. 305–323.

Oei TPS and Jackson PR (1982) Social skills and cognitive–behavioral approaches to the treatment of problem drinking. *J Stud Alcohol* **43**, 532–547.

O'Farrell T, Cutter HSG, and Floyd FJ (1985) Evaluating behavioral marital therapy for male alcoholics: effects on marital adjustment and communication before and after treatment. *Behav Ther* **16**, 147–167.

Ofman D (1992) Alcoholism and geriatric practice. In *Medical Diagnosis and Treatment of Alcoholism*, Mendelson JH and Mello NK (eds). McGraw-Hill, New York, pp. 501–573.

Ogborne AC and Glaser FB (1981) Characteristics of affiliates of Alcoholics Anonymous: a review of the literature. *J Stud Alcohol* **42**, 661–675.

O'Keane V, Moloney E, O'Neill H, et al. (1992) Blunted prolactin responses to D-fenfluramine in sociopathy: evidence for subsensitivity of central serotoninergic function. *Br J Psychiatry* **160**, 643–646.

O'Malley SS, Jaffe AJ, Chang G, et al. (1992) Naltrexone and coping skills therapy for alcohol dependence: a controlled study. *Arch Gen Psychiatry* **49**, 894–898.

O'Sullivan K, Rynne C, Miller J, et al. (1988) A follow-up study on alcoholics with and without co-existing affective disorder. *Br J Psychiatry* **152**, 813–819.

Ouimette PC, Finney JW, Gima K, et al. (1999) A comparative evaluation of substance abuse treatment: examining mechanisms underlying patient-treatment matching hypotheses for 12-step and cognitive–behavioral treatments for substance abuse, *Alcohol Clin Exp Res* **23**, 545–551.

Parrella DP and Filstead WJ (1988) Definition of onset in the development of onset-based alcoholism typologies. *J Stud Alcohol* **49**, 85–92.

Pettinati HM, Volpicelli JR, Kranzler HR, et al. (2000) Sertraline treatment for alcohol dependence: interactive effects of medication and subtype. *Alcohol Clin Exp Res* **24**, 1041–1049.

Piazza NJ, Vrbka JL, and Yeager RD (1989) Telescoping of alcoholism in women alcoholics. *Int J Addict* **24**, 19–28.

Pine DS, Wasserman GA, Coplan J, et al. (1996) Platelet serotonin 2A (5HT$_{2A}$) receptor characteristics and parenting factors for boys at risk for delinquency: a preliminary report. *Am J Psychiatry* **153**, 538–544.

Poikolainen K (1999) Effectiveness of brief interventions to reduce alcohol intake in primary health care populations: a meta-analysis. *Prev Med* **28**, 503–509.

Polich JM, Armor DJ, and Braiker HB (1980) Patterns of alcoholism over four years. *J Stud Alcohol* **41**, 397–416.

Pollock VE (1992) Meta-analysis of subjective sensitivity to alcohol in sons of alcoholics. *Am J Psychiatry* **149**, 1534–1538.

Powell BJ, Penick EC, Nickel EJ, et al. (1992) Outcomes of comorbid alcoholic men: a 1-year follow-up. *Alcohol Clin Exp Res* **16**, 131–138.

Prochaska J and DiClemente C (1992) Stages of change in the modification of problem behavior. In *Progress in Behavior Modification* Vol. 28, Hersen J, Eisler R, and Miller PM (eds). Sycamore Publishing, Sycamore, IL.

Project MATCH Research Group (1997a) Matching alcoholism treatments to client heterogeneity: project MATCH posttreatment drinking outcomes. *J Stud Alcohol* **58**, 7–29.

Project MATCH Research Group (1997b) Project MATCH secondary a priori hypotheses. *Addiction* **92**, 1671–1698.

Project MATCH Research Group (1998) Matching alcoholism treatments to client heterogeneity: project MATCH three-year drinking outcomes. *Alcohol Clin Exp Res* **22**, 1300–1311.

Randall CL, Roberts JS, Del Boca FK, et al. (1999) Telescoping of landmark events associated with drinking: a gender comparison. *J Stud Alcohol* **60**, 252–260.

Reid LD (1990) Summary. In *Opioids, Bulimia, and Alcohol Abuse and Alcoholism*, Reid LD (ed). Springer-Verlag, New York, pp. 289–304.

Regier DA, Farmer ME, Rae DS, et al. (1990) Comorbidity of mental disorders with alcohol and other drug abuse: results from the Epidemiologic Catchment Area (ECA) study. *J Am Med Assoc* **264**, 2511–2518.

Regier DA, Kaelber CT, Rae DS, et al. (1998) Limitations of diagnostic criteria and assessment instruments for mental disorders. Implications for research and policy. *Arch Gen Psychiatry* **55**, 109–115.

Reich T, Edenberg HJ, Goate A, et al. (1998) Genome-wide search for genes affecting the risk for alcohol dependence. *Am J Med Genet* **81**, 207–215.

Robins LN, Wing J, Wittchen HU, et al. (1989) The Composite International Diagnostic Interview: an epidemiological instrument suitable for use in conjunction with different diagnostic systems and in different cultures. *Arch Gen Psychiatry* **45**, 1069–1077.

Rollnick S, Heather N, Gold R, et al. (1992) Development of a short "Readiness to Change" questionnaire for use in brief, opportunistic interventions among excessive drinkers. *Br J Addict* **87**, 743–754.

Room R, Jernigen D, and Carlini-Marlatt (2002) *Alcohol in Developing Societies*. Finnish Foundation for Alcohol Studies, Helsinki, Finland.

Rosenberg CM (1974) Drug maintenance in the outpatient treatment of chronic alcoholism. *Arch Gen Psychiatry* **30**, 373–377.

Ross HE (1995) DSM-III-R alcohol abuse and dependence and psychiatric comorbidity in Ontario: results from the Mental Health Supplement to the Ontario Health Survey. *Drug Alcohol Depend* **39**, 111–128.

Ross HE, Glaser FB, and Germanson T (1988) The prevalence of psychiatric disorders in patients with alcohol and other drug problems. *Arch Gen Psychiatry* **45**, 1023–1031.

Rossetti ZL and Carboni S (1995) Ethanol withdrawal is associated with increased extracellular glutamate in the rat striatum. *Eur J Pharmacol* **283**, 177–183.

Rounsaville BJ, Dolinsky ZS, Babor TF, et al. (1987) Psychopathology as a predictor of treatment outcome in alcoholics. *Arch Gen Psychiatry* **44**, 505–513.

Saadatmand F, Stinson FS, Grant FB, et al. (1997) *Liver Cirrhosis Mortality in the United States, 1970–94*, Surveillance Report No. 45. National Institute on Alcohol Abuse and Alcoholism, Rockville, MD.

Salaspuro M (1986) Conventional and coming laboratory markers of alcoholism and heavy drinking. *Alcohol Clin Exp Res* **10**(Suppl.), 5–12.

Saunders JB, Aasland OG, Babor TF, et al. (1993) Development of the Alcohol Use Disorders Identification Test (AUDIT): WHO collaborative project on early detection of persons with harmful alcohol consumption—II. *Addiction* **88**, 791–804.

Schottenfeld RS (1994) Assessment of the patient. In *Textbook of Substance Abuse Treatment*, Galanter M and Kleber HD (eds). Am Psychiatric Press, Washington, DC, pp. 25–33.

Schuckit MA (1983) Alcoholic patients with secondary depression. *Am J Psychiatry* **140**, 711–714.

Schuckit MA (1985) The clinical implications of primary diagnostic groups among alcoholics. *Arch Gen Psychiatry* **42**, 1043–1049.

Schuckit MA (1994) Goals of treatment. In *Textbook of Substance Abuse Treatment*, Galanter M and Kleber HD (eds). American Psychiatric Press, Washington, DC, pp. 3–10.

Schuckit MA and Smith T (1996) An 8-year follow-up of 450 sons of alcoholic and control subjects. *Arch Gen Psychiatry* **53**, 202–210.

Schuckit MA, Smith TL, Anthenelli R, et al. (1993) Clinical course of alcoholism in 636 male inpatients. *Am J Psychiatry* **150**, 786–792.

Sellers EM, Naranjo CA, Harrison M, et al. (1983) Diazepam loading: simplified treatment of alcohol withdrawal. *Clin Pharmacol Ther* **34**, 822–826.

Selzer ML (1971) The Michigan Alcoholism Screening Test: the quest for a new diagnostic instrument. *Am J Psychiatry* **127**, 1653–1658.

Sharpe PC, McBride R, and Archbold GP (1996) Biochemical markers of alcohol abuse. *QJM* **89**, 137–144.

Siviy S, Calcagnetti D, and Reid L (1982) A temporal analysis of naloxone's suppressant effect on drinking. *Pharmacol Biochem Behav* **16**, 173–175.

Sher KJ (1991) *Children of Alcoholics: A Critical Appraisal of Theory and Research*. University of Chicago Press, Chicago.

Sher KJ and Trull T (1994) Personality and disinhibitory psychopathology: alcoholism and antisocial personality disorder. *J Abnormal Psychol* **203**, 92–102.

Skutle A (1999) Association between gender and marital status and confidence in remaining abstinent among alcohol abusers in treatment. *Addiction* **94**, 1219–1225.

Snell LD, Tabakoff B, and Hoffman PL (1993) Radioligand binding to the N-methyl-d-aspartate receptor/ionophore complex: alterations by ethanol *in vitro* and by chronic *in vivo* ethanol ingestion. *Brain Res* **602**, 91–98.

Söderpalm B, Ericson M, Olausson P, et al. (2000) Nicotinic mechanisms involved in the dopamine activating and reinforcing properties of ethanol. *Behav Brain Res* **113**, 85–96.

Sokol RJ and Clarren SK (1989) Guidelines for use of terminology describing the impact of prenatal alcohol on the offspring. *Alcohol Clin Exp Res* **13**, 597–598.

Soubrie P (1986) Reconciling the role of central serotonin neurons in human and animal behavior. *Behav Brain Sci* **9**, 319–364.

Stibler H (1991) Carbohydrate deficient transferrin in serum: a new marker of potentially harmful alcohol consumption reviewed. *Clin Chem* **37**, 2029–2037.

Stibler H, Borg S, and Jousta M (1986) Microanion exchange chromatography of carbohydrate deficient transferrin in serum in relation to alcohol consumption (Swedish patient 8400587–5) *Alcohol Clin Exp Res* **10**, 535–544.

Stinson FS and DeBakey SF (1992) Alcohol-related mortality in the United States, 1979–1988. *Br J Addict* **87**, 777–783.

Substance Abuse and Mental Health Services Administration (SAMHSA) (2000) Office of Applied Studies, National Household Survey on Drug Abuse.

Substance Abuse and Mental Health Services Administration (SAMHSA) (2001) *Summary of Findings from the 2000 National Household Survey on Drug Abuse*, NHSDA Series: H-13, DHHS Publication No. SMA 01–3549. Rockville, MD.

Swendsen JD, Merikangas KR, Canino GJ, et al. (1998) The comorbidity of alcoholism with anxiety and depressive disorders in four geographic communities. *Compr Psychiatry* **39**, 176–184.

Swift RM (1999) Drug therapy for alcohol dependence. *N Engl J Med* **340**, 1482–1490.

Taylor DP, Eison M, Riblet LA, et al. (1985) Pharmacological and clinical effects of buspirone. *Pharmacol Biochem Behav* **23**, 687–694.

Thomasson HR, Crabb DW, Edenberg HJ, et al. (1993) Alcohol and aldehyde dehydrogenase polymorphins and alcoholism. *Behav Gen* **23**, 131–136.

Thomasson HR, Edenberg HJ, Crabb DW, et al. (1991) Alcohol and aldehyde dehydrogenase genotypes and alcoholism in Chinese men. *Am J Hum Gen* **48**, 677–681.

Tiihonen J, Ryynanen OP, Kauhanen J, et al. (1996) Citalopram in the treatment of alcoholism: a double-blind placebo-controlled study. *Pharmacopsychiatry* **29**, 27–29.

Timko C, Moos RH, Finney JW, et al. (2000) Long-term outcomes of alcohol use disorders: comparing untreated individuals with those in Alcoholics Anonymous and formal treatment. *J Stud Alcohol* **61**, 529–538.

Topel H (1988) Beta-endorphin genetics in the etiology of alcoholism. *Alcohol* **5**, 159–165.

Trachtenberg M and Blum K (1987) Alcohol and opioid peptides: neuropharmacological rationale for physical craving of alcohol. *Am J Drug Alcohol Abuse* **13**, 365–372.

US Department of Health and Human Services (DHHS) (1994) *Eighth Special Report to the US Congress on Alcohol and Health*. NIH Publication No. 94–3699.

US Department of Health and Human Services (DHHS) (2000) *Tenth Special Report to the US Congress on Alcohol and Health*. NIH Publication No. 00–1583.

Vaillant GE (1983) *The Natural History of Alcoholism*. Harvard University Press, Cambridge, MA.

Virkkunen M, Rawlings R, Tokola R, et al. (1994) CSF biochemistries, glucose metabolism, and diurnal activity rhythms in alcoholic violent offenders, fire setters, and healthy volunteers. *Arch Gen Psychiatry* **51**, 20–27.

Volpicelli JR, Alterman AI, Hayashida M, et al. (1992) Naltrexone in the treatment of alcohol dependence. *Arch Gen Psychiatry* **49**, 876–880.

Walsh DC, Hingson RW, Merrigan DM, et al. (1991) A randomized trial of treatment options for alcohol-abusing workers. *N Engl J Med* **325**, 775–782.

Wilk AI, Jensen NM, and Havighurst TC (1997) Meta-analysis of randomized control trials addressing brief interventions in heavy alcohol drinkers. *J Gen Intern Med* **12**, 274–283.

World Health Organization (1992) *The ICD-10 Classification of Mental and Behavioural Disorders: Clinical Descriptions and Diagnostic Guidelines*. World Health Organization, Geneva, Switzerland.

Wu LT, Kouzis AC, and Leaf PJ (1999) Influence of comorbid alcohol and psychiatric disorders on utilization of mental health services in the National Comorbidity Survey. *Am J Psychiatry* **156**, 1230–1236.

Yourick JJ and Faiman MD (1991) Disulfiram metabolism as a requirement for the inhibition of rat liver mitochondrial low Km aldehyde dehydrogenase. *Biochem Pharmacol* **42**, 1361–1366.

17 Substance-Related Disorders: Amphetamine

Kevin A. Sevarino

Most mental health and medical professionals in the United States consider the psychostimulant cocaine as representative of the entire class of psychostimulant drugs. While far less literature exists regarding other psychostimulants, illicit abuse of substances such as methamphetamine and illicit use of prescribed substances such as methylphenidate (Ritalin) represent a growing health concern (Anglin et al. 2002). While the major abused psychostimulant in the United States is cocaine, this is not the case in several Western US cities, nor in the state of Hawaii (Rawson et al. 2002a). Worldwide abuse or regular use of amphetamines is more than double that of cocaine.

Consistent with the schema put forward by the DSM-IV-TR, this chapter defines the amphetamine-like substances to include the phenylisopropylamines amphetamine (AMPH), methamphetamine (METH), and phenylpropanolamine (PPA), the natural substances ephedrine and pseudoephedrine, and phenylethylamines including methylphenidate and pemoline. While METH and AMPH cause the vast majority of abuse and dependence, use of any of these substances has been associated with abuse and dependence, so as a class these will be referred to as amphetamine-type stimulants, or ATS, in this chapter.

By far, the most widely abused ATS is METH, which is commonly known as meth, speed, crank, CR, wire, and jib, and in its recrystallized smoked form, ice, crystal, or glass. Legitimate forms of METH prescribed for attention-deficit/hyperactivity disorder (ADHD) and weight control (Methedrine, Desoxyn, and Adipex) undoubtedly represent a miniscule source of the total amount abused each year. AMPH, most prevalent in Western Europe, is commonly known as amp, bennies, dex, or black beauties, and is prescribed as Adderall, Dexedrine, and Dextrostat in the treatment of ADHD, narcolepsy, weight control, and depression. Other agents that have been designated as Schedule II controlled substances by the Drug Enforcement Administration are methylphenidate (Ritalin, Concerta) and phenmetrazine (Preludin). Given the widespread prescription of Ritalin in the United States for ADHD and narcolepsy, its diversion to abuse appears rare (Kollins et al. 2002). On the street, Ritalin is known as Rits or Vitamin R. Pemoline (Cylert) is a Schedule IV agent, also used to treat ADHD and narcolepsy. A large number of Schedule III and IV phenylethylamines (benzphetamine, diethylproprion, mazindol, phendimetrazine, phenmetrazine, and phentermine) are used for weight control. There is no specific evidence that these substances represent a significant source of illicit diversion, and they are not further discussed in this chapter. ATS agents are also widely available in over-the-counter (OTC) preparations. As discussed below, PPA has been removed from the market, but ephedrine and pseudoephedrine are still very widely used as decongestants, and less so, phenylephrine and propylhexidrine (Gorelick and Cornish 2003). An excellent tabulation of currently available formulations of prescribed ATS agents is found in Greenhill et al. 2003.

Diversion of prescription medications for illicit use is not a major source of illicit precursor synthesis of METH or AMPH. Unfortunately, a large amount of stimulant abuse that is not easily quantified occurs at rave parties and other venues for experimentation (Poulin 2001). Drug use among such individuals probably represents substance misuse and is less likely to meet formal criteria for abuse. However, it is uncommon that those that go on to amphetamine dependence continue to supply their habit through licit sources. Further, medically appropriate use of synthetic stimulants does not appear to pose a significant risk for the induction of substance-use disorders. This has been most closely examined for the widely prescribed methylphenidate (Ritalin) for ADHD; in this case, treatment may actually reduce the risk of developing substance abuse by controlling ADHD, itself a risk factor for substance abuse (Biederman et al. 1999). Further, methylphenidate poses a low risk for medical complications (Rappley 1997). With increasing distribution in the adult population, there may be concern that this picture may change (Levin et al. 1999). It has been postulated that the persistence of peripheral autonomic effects, as well as much longer half-life in the striatum, accounts for its low abuse potential relative to cocaine (Volkow et al. 1995, Volkow et al. 1999).

The socially acceptable and very desirable effects of prescribed ATS, weight loss and productivity enhancement, make widespread use, and thus abuse, unavoidable. Students and athletes appear particularly at risk for development of stimulant abuse, given that both exposure to licit and illicit sources and the pressures to use are high (Murray 1998, Teter et al. 2003). Of course, those whose jobs require sleep cycle reversal, long hours and so on, such as truck drivers, also appear at high risk (Akerstedt and Ficca 1997).

AMPH-like substances, especially METH, are most commonly injected or smoked by heavy users (Murray 1998). Its low melting point, similar to crack cocaine, makes it well suited as a smokable agent (Cho 1990). These routes provide the most rapid onset of action, though peak blood levels and half-lives are approximately the same as for the oral route (Cook et al. 1993, Lebish et al. 1970). Most likely, abuse by those experimenting with the agent is oral. Through the mid 1990s, the oral and intravenous routes were still the most popular (Hall and Hando 1993). Methylphenidate displays a significantly shorter half-life (2–4 hours) than AMPH and METH, reaching peak levels in 1 to 3 hours (Volkow et al. 1995). Methylphenidate abuse, however, is mainly through the intravenous route with crushed tablets (Parran and Jasinski 1991) though it may also be snorted (Garland 1998).

Diagnosis

Consistent with the DSM-IV-TR perspective functionally equating amphetamines with cocaine, those diagnostic categories that are included are identical to those for Cocaine-Related Disorders, with the sole exception of omitting the specifier "With Onset During Withdrawal" from the diagnostic category Amphetamine-Induced Anxiety Disorder. For the substance use disorders, amphetamine (ATS) abuse and dependence will be discussed below. Of the substance-induced disorders, the critical diagnoses of ATS intoxication and withdrawal are described. The specific complications of delirium, psychotic disorders, mood disorders, anxiety disorders, sexual dysfunctions, and sleep disorders all are described under intoxication. Amphetamine-induced mood and sleep disorders also allow for specifiers of onset during withdrawal.

Amphetamine Dependence   ATS dependence is diagnosed when a maladaptive pattern of use leads to clinically significant impairment or distress, as defined by three or more of the following that occur during the same 12-month period: (1) evidence of tolerance, (2) occurrence of withdrawal, or the reuse of the substance to alleviate withdrawal, and (3) compulsive use of amphetamines as defined by three or more of the following: using more than intended, (4) desire or efforts to reduce use, (5) occupying significant time in drug-related activities, (6) loss of social, occupational, or recreational pursuits, or (7) continued use despite known adverse, physical, or psychological consequences (see DSM-IV-TR diagnostic criteria for Substance Dependence in Chapter 15 on page 351).

Amphetamine Abuse   The diagnosis of ATS abuse requires a maladaptive pattern of use that does not meet the criteria for dependence, and that results in clinically significant impairment or distress. In the preceding 12 months, recurrent substance use must result in one or more of the following: failure to meet major role obligations, placement of the user in physical danger, legal entanglements, or social/interpersonal problems (see DSM-IV-TR diagnostic criteria for Substance Abuse in Chapter 15 on page 352).

Amphetamine Intoxication   Specific diagnostic criteria are provided for ATS intoxication (see DSM-IV-TR diagnostic criteria below). These include recent use of an ATS (criterion A), clinically significant maladaptive behavioral or psychological changes occurring after the use of the ATS (criterion B), two or more specified physiological changes after the use of the ATS (criterion C), and the requirement that the condition is not accounted for by another mental or medical condition (criterion D). A specifier "with perceptual disturbances" is included.

DSM-IV-TR Diagnostic Criteria

292.89 Amphetamine Intoxication

A. Recent use of amphetamine or a related substance (e.g., methylphenidate).
B. Clinically significant maladaptive behavioral or psychological changes (e.g., euphoria or affective blunting; changes in sociability; hypervigilance; interpersonal sensitivity; anxiety, tension, or anger; stereotyped behaviors; impaired judgment; or impaired social or occupational functioning) that developed during, or shortly after, use of amphetamine or a related substance.
C. Two (or more) of the following, developing during, or shortly after, use of amphetamine or a related substance:

1. tachycardia or bradycardia
2. pupillary dilation
3. elevated or lowered blood pressure
4. perspiration or chills
5. nausea or vomiting
6. evidence of weight loss
7. psychomotor agitation or retardation
8. muscular weakness, respiratory depression, chest pain, or cardiac arrhythmias
9. confusion, seizures, dyskinesias, dystonias, or coma

D. The symptoms are not due to a general medical condition and are not better accounted for by another mental disorder.

Specify if:

With Perceptual Disturbances.

The specifics of criteria B and C provide a useful clinical consensus of the syndrome of ATS intoxication (see Table 17-1 for a list of the maladaptive behaviors of Criterion B, with comments by the author in parentheses). Importantly, psychosis and paranoia are experienced by approximately one-third of ATS-dependent subjects (Williamson et al. 1997, Harris and Batki 2000) and occur at a significantly greater rate than for cocaine or Ecstasy. With chronic use, the incidence of psychosis increases (Hall et al. 1996). Furthermore, the occurrence of psychotic symptoms correlates with heavier use, co-use of benzodiazepines, and preexisting mental illness (Vincent 1998). Cognitive disturbances include visual, tactile, and auditory hallucinations. Visual hallucinations often suggest an underlying "organic" cause to psychosis, and formication, the feeling of "bugs crawling under the skin" is highly suggestive of ATS or cocaine intoxication. Psychosis in the presence of an intact sensorium, where the subject is aware that the hallucinations are not real, may differentiate ATS-induced psychosis from psychotic states such as schizophrenia. Nonetheless, ATS-induced psychosis shares many features with other acute psychotic states (Griffith et al. 1969, Snyder 1973, Flaum and Schulz 1996). A wide range of ATS dosages can induce psychosis, likely because individuals vary in tolerance (Bell 1973). Of concern, ATS-induced psychosis can sometimes persist for months following cessation of drug use (Buffenstein et al. 1999). Recently, an intriguing finding is that such prolonged METH-induced psychosis is associated with the presence of nine or fewer repeat alleles in the VNTR polymorphism of the human *DAT1* gene (Ujike et al. 2003). This 3′ untranslated (i.e., the region of RNA not coding for proteins) region polymorphism could affect mRNA half-life, and relate to the prolonged depression of DAT levels following chronic METH exposure. Interestingly, while psychosis would appear to be a fairly drastic symptom during intoxication, it appears to be a relatively common drug reaction among nonabusing methylphenidate users. Cherland and Fitzpatrick (1999) found 6 of 98 children with signs of psychosis. Appropriate use of PPA also is associated with psychosis (Goodhue et al. 2000, Norvenius et al. 1979). Women appear to be at greater risk, as do those with preexisting mood or psychotic disorders (Marshall and Douglas 1994).

Table 17-1	Maladaptive Behaviors Listed in Criterion B of Amphetamine Intoxication, with Comments and Explications in Parentheses
Euphoria or affective blunting (felt to occur in longer-term users)	
Changes in sociability (e.g., being hypertalkative, more interactive or more withdrawn, increased libido)	
Hypervigilance (with ideas of reference that can proceed to frank paranoia)	
Interpersonal sensitivity	
Anxiety, tension, or anger (agitated behavior and altercations are common)	
Stereotyped behavior (picking at skin, grooming, pacing, disassembly/reassembly of objects)	
Impaired judgment (often seen as sexual promiscuity)	
Impaired social or occupational functioning	

Table 17-2	Physiological Disturbances Listed in Criterion C of Amphetamine Intoxication, with Comments and Explications in Parentheses

Tachycardia or reflex bradycardia
Papillary dilatation
Elevated or lowered blood pressure
Perspiration or chills
Nausea or vomiting
Evidence of weight loss
Psychomotor agitation or retardation (an excited delirium is described as for cocaine, along with tremor)
Muscle weakness, respiratory depression, chest pain, or cardiac arrhythmia
Confusion, seizures, dyskinesias, dystonias or coma (Headaches and tinnitus are additional neurological symptoms that have also been described as occurring)

The physiological disturbances in criterion C are listed in Table 17-2, again with author's comments in parentheses.

Amphetamine Withdrawal While the intoxicated state is characterized as euphoric, expansive, and activated, and often presents with agitation, violence, and/or psychosis, ATS withdrawal is characterized by decreased energy and mood. The clinician often evaluates such individuals who become suicidal during the "crash." The period of most intense withdrawal may last days, though a protracted state of depression and low energy often persists for weeks (Kramer et al. 1967, Murray 1998). Resurgence of craving when exposed to drug-associated environmental cues probably persists for years, as is the case with other substance-dependence disorders. The occurrence of ATS withdrawal usually occurs in those that have progressed from the diagnosis of abuse to dependence.

The ATS withdrawal diagnosis requires cessation or reduction of ATS use that has been heavy or prolonged (criterion A), dysphoric mood and at least two physiologic changes that occur from a few hours to days after cessation of use (i.e., fatigue; vivid, unpleasant dreams; insomnia and hypersomnia; increased appetite; psychomotor retardation or agitation) which cause clinically significant distress or impairment in social, occupational, or other important areas of functioning (criteria B and C); and the requirement that the condition is not accounted for by another mental or medical condition (criterion D) (see DSM-IV-TR diagnostic criteria below).

DSM-IV-TR Diagnostic Criteria

292.0 Amphetamine Withdrawal

A. Cessation of (or reduction in) amphetamine (or a related substance) use that has been heavy and prolonged.
B. Dysphoric mood and two (or more) of the following physiological changes, developing within a few hours to several days after Criterion A:

1. fatigue
2. vivid, unpleasant dreams
3. insomnia or hypersomnia
4. increased appetite
5. psychomotor retardation or agitation

C. The symptoms in Criterion B cause clinically significant distress or impairment in social, occupational, or other important areas of functioning.
D. The symptoms are not due to a general medical condition and are not better accounted for by another mental disorder

Both the longer half-lives of ATS relative to other psychostimulants, as well as the broader-spectrum effects on nerve terminal catecholamine levels, result in prolonged withdrawal and abstinence states. ATS withdrawal states occur in some 87% of users (Cantwell and McBride 1998, Schuckit et al. 1999). The acute phase appears to last up to 5 days, with some symptoms persisting for weeks, possibly months, following the acute phase (Srisurapanont 2001a, Watson et al. 1972).

Since neurocognitive impairment occurs early in withdrawal, clinicians should be cognizant that instructions to individuals in withdrawal be kept simple and written out (Kalechstein et al. 2003). Decision making, as has been known anecdotally for years, appears affected (Paulus et al. 2003). If individuals with amphetamine dependence fail to appear in follow-up, outreach attempts are necessary to keep the individuals engaged. EEG data support alterations during early withdrawal (Newton et al. 2003). Over months, these cognitive deficits may partially remit to a greater extent than in opiate abusers (Rogers et al. 1999, Ornstein et al. 2000). Severe craving marks the early withdrawal phase, leading to high recidivism. Sleep disturbance is accompanied by increase in REM sleep (Watson et al. 1972).

Epidemiology

After cannabis, worldwide ATS (principally METH and AMPH) are regularly used or abused by some 35 million individuals (United Nations Drug Control Program 2003). In contrast, cocaine is used by 15 million worldwide, and heroin by 10 million. The United Nations Office of Drug Control Report (2003) showed that, except for cannabis, more new countries reported use of ATS than any other illicit substance. Interestingly, while cocaine is the most widely used psychostimulant in the Americas, outside of these areas, especially in the Far East and Southeast Asia, Oceana, and Western Europe, ATS abuse is far more prevalent (United Nations Drug Control Program 2003). It is estimated that two-thirds of the world's ATS abusers live in Asia, with Thailand experiencing perhaps the most severe epidemic (Ahmad 2003). The long half-life and relatively inexpensive nature (approximately 25% the cost of use of cocaine) make it possible to continue use for years without adverse sequelae necessitating treatment or incarceration. (Simon et al. 2002b). However, it seems likely that users in the workplace may suffer increased use of other health care services, loss of workplace attendance and so on.

It is estimated that 5 to 10% of adults have a lifetime prevalence of nonprescription ATS use, 0.5% in the last year, and 0.2% in the prior month (SAMHSA 2003). Roughly, 5% of adults in the United States have had a history of nonprescribed use of ATS drugs, 1% in the prior year, and 0.4% in the prior month. ATS dependence and abuse combined have approximately a 1.5% lifetime prevalence according to DSM-IV-TR. The performance-enhancing effects of ATS place students faced with competitive stress such as high-achievers and athletes at high risk (Bailey 1987, Conrad et al. 1988). Since performance enhancement is much more pronounced under conditions of sleep deprivation, abuse by those in repetitive, sleep-shifted occupations, such as truck drivers, is also high (Heishman 1998).

The prevalence of ATS use appears particularly related to supply routes, perhaps because its sole source of production is synthetic, and not grown. While originally diverted from pharmaceutical supplies (such as via the US armed forces into Japan in the 1950s), and synthesized by biker gangs, it is now produced by a more wide variety of small producers, as well as "superlabs" producing 10–100 lb batches in Mexico where precursor supplies are not legislatively limited (Karch 2002). Small production sites are likely to remain because its synthesis is relatively easy, and provides for personal use as well as excellent profit margins. Further, precursor supply interdiction appears to affect large producers to a far greater extent than the small backyard labs (Cunningham and Liu 2003).

METH is the predominant form of ATS used in the world today. This is especially true in the United States west of the Mississippi, in Hawaii, Taiwan, Japan, and Southeast Asia (Rawson et al. 2002a). METH-related emergency room admissions represent a small but rapidly growing problem in these regions (Karch 2002). The demographics of METH use are also unusual for the United States. METH use, as well as deaths related to METH use, is predominantly male (86%) and Caucasian (75%), as well as surprisingly old (mean 36.8 years of age). (Karch 2002). Use in the last several years appears to be spreading beyond the typical unemployed, single Caucasian males that originally characterized users during past epidemics (Baberg et al. 1996).

The clandestine nature of production in small "mom and pop" labs, and the release of easily detected noxious fumes, makes rural production, and thus rural use, a particular problem. These demographics present problems for smaller health-treatment resources ill equipped to handle mental health issues integrally linked to antisocial and violent behavior.

Patterns and Routes of Use

ATS is regarded as highly addictive, with some 50% who initially experiment illicitly with ATSs progressing to dependence (Woody et al. 1993). Heavy users, especially of METH, most commonly inject or smoke. These routes appear to have the highest potential to result in dependence (Gorelick and Cornish 2003). Its low melting point, similar to crack cocaine, makes it well suited as a smokable substance. Most likely, abuse by those experimenting with the agent is oral. Indeed, even OTC preparations containing ephedrine and pseudoephedrine are commonly abused (Tinsley and Watkins 1998). Through the mid 1990s the oral route, and intravenous, were still the most popular (Hall and Hando 1993). Methylphenidate abuse, however, is mainly through IV route with crushed tablets (Parran and Jasinski 1991), though it may also be snorted (Garland 1998).

It is believed that ATS smoking and IV abuse lead to more rapid dependence than oral and snorted abuse. By the smoking route METH reach the brain in seconds, and the initial "rush" occurs soon thereafter, with peak effects at 2 to 4 minutes. Intravenously, ATS probably peak slightly later, though this conclusion is based on the extension of studies with cocaine (Telang et al. 1999).

There are two main patterns of heavy use—binge use and chronic use. In binge use ("speed runs"), increasing amounts are used over a few days, usually ended by exhaustion of resources, the user, or the onset of adverse events, such as intense agitation or psychosis. The second pattern of use in dependent individuals is chronic, repeated use over long periods. This pattern is sustained both by IV and smoking routes, as well as oral use.

Methylphenidate is believed to be less addictive than other ATS for several reasons. It appears to be cleared from human brain sites far more slowly than cocaine (Volkow et al. 1995) and so should show a reduced addictive potential. Further, it appears to cause less euphoria than AMPH (Klein and Wender 1995). In the main, ATS taken by the oral route reach maximum plasma level in 1 to 3 hours, but half-life of effect is more varied.

Methylphenidate, PPA, and phenylephrine have half-lives of 2 to 2.5 hours, significantly shorter than those for AMPH (7–34 hours) and METH (6–15 hours) (Baselt 1999).

As with other stimulants, adverse subjective effects experienced by users may be tempered by co-use of depressants, including alcohol and benzodiazepines, but there are no large studies of such comorbidity.

METH is cleared from the body by several routes. Approximately 45% is excreted unchanged in the urine, though this can be increased by acidification of the urine (Cook et al. 1993, Wan et al. 1978); conversely, ingestion of sodium bicarbonate can reduce elimination and concentrations in the urine (to hinder detection) (Braithwaite et al. 1995). Approximately 20% is N-demethylated to form AMPH (Caldwell et al. 1972). This fact is used to advantage in distinguishing METH positive urines that result artifactually from current analytic processes with ephedrine testing (where no AMPH is found) to positives where both METH and AMPH are present (supporting actual METH use). These compounds undergo further metabolism via oxidation (forming norephedrine and other active metabolites), parahydroxylation (also to active compounds), and deamination (to inactive products). All phenylisopropylamines competitively inhibit CYP2D6 (Wu et al. 1997).

Medical Complications

For heavy users, a number of general consequences of ATS dependence will be obvious; malnutrition and cachexia from sleep deprivation, exposure to the elements and so on. Skin disorders, including infections and lesions from "picking" are common. More serious are ATS-related deaths due to cardiac arrhythmias, stroke, and rhabdomyolysis that have been documented since the 1950s. These problems were similar to those reported for the more widely abused cocaine. Concern over unique toxicity further increased when "ice," the smokable form of METH, began to be seen in Japan in the late 1970s (Cho and Wright 1978). Still there is only approximately 1 METH-related death for every 10 related to cocaine, and the reasons that may be are described below. Also as described below, a number of factors place ATS users at high risk for contraction of HIV, and likely Hepatitis B and C, infection.

Some of the medical complications result from exposure to contaminants during ATS use. The production methods for ATS determine what contaminants are present in illicit manufacture. Contaminants are both toxic, as well as stimulants in their own right (Soine 1986). In the United States, the "red phosphorous" route of conversion of (−) ephedrine (to METH) and (+) pseudoephedrine (to DEX) is nearly exclusive today. Contaminants such as 2-phenylmethyl-phenylethylamine are common to both processes. Now that it is recognized that ephedrine is being illicitly diverted in the United States, its importation is also being regulated. METH cooks occasionally resort to other cold remedies and stimulants, but these appear to represent minor supply sources, for example, substitution of phenylpropylamine (PPA) leads to production of DEX.

For methylphenidate, the principal complications occur only when the drug is diverted to illicit intravenous use. Its formulation makes talcosis resulting from IV use prominent, where the lungs (Schmidt et al. 1991) and eyes (Lederer and Sabates 1982) are most affected. There are case reports of catecholamine toxicity with intentional overdose, and the complication pattern is not unique compared to METH.

Many of the cardiovascular complications for ATS described below result from peripheral catecholamine toxicity. This explains why the principal drug interactions of concern involve the psychotropics that are meant to augment catecholamine function. Of most concern are the monoamine oxidase inhibitors, whose action can potentiate ATS toxicity for 2 to 3 weeks following cessation of use. Similarly, tricyclic antidepressants can potentiate effects of ATS, as well as increase absorption and slow hepatic metabolism (Gorelick and Cornish

2003). However, off-label use of ATS to augment tricyclics is not uncommon, and at least one study has found that desipramine and stimulants (i.e., methylphenidate and dexadrine) have no clinically significant interaction in children (Cohen et al. 1999).

HIV and Immunomodulatory Effects

It is now appreciated that intravenous drug use is the fastest growing route for transmission of HIV infection (NIDA Research Report, 2002). In addition, ATS use is associated with unsafe sexual behaviors, including participation in unprotected sex and involvement with multiple sexual partners (Molitor et al. 1998, Chesney et al. 1998, Zule and Desmond 1999). This results from the drug's acute effect of enhancing libido and impairing judgment, and from the association of ATS use with sexual behavior among gays (Shoptaw et al. 2002). In the Shoptaw study, two-thirds of treatment-seeking ATS users were HIV positive. Once HIV has been contracted, ATS abuse leads to accelerated CNS and cardiovascular toxicity (Nath et al. 2001, Yu et al. 2003). METH and AMPH are immunomodulators, and in fact, may be immunotoxic to peripheral T cells, mitogen-stimulated lymphocytes, and spleen cells (Yu et al. 2003). METH use and HIV infection may synergistically interact to accelerate the course of the HIV infection (Phillips et al. 2000).

Pulmonary

In the Karch autopsy series (1999) of individuals who died from ATS use, pulmonary edema was present in 70% of cases, as well as pneumonia (8.2%), and emphysema (5.1%). Birefringent crystals at bifurcation of pulmonary vessels is associated with intravenous abuse of crushed pills that contain insoluble fillers such as talc, microcrystalline cellulose, corn starch, or cotton fibers. With sufficient deposition, small vessel thrombosis and granuloma formation ensues (Tomashefski and Hirsch 1980). The changes ultimately reduce pulmonary perfusion, and increase pulmonary vascular resistance (Kringsholm and Christoffersen 1987). Possibly because of an increased ratio of intravenous drug abuse to other routes, heroin abusers are more prone to progress to pulmonary thromboembolic complications than are stimulant abusers. Less commonly, oral tablet consumption by the IV route results in pulmonary amyloid formation (Shah et al. 1998).

Gastrointestinal

In METH-related deaths, the sum of liver-related complications was second highest among organ systems. Fatty liver (16.2%), cirrhosis (9.0%), portal triaditis (6.1%), and hepatitis (4.1%) were detected (Karch et al. 1999b). This may relate to the high comorbidity with alcohol dependence, though the exact contribution is unknown. One pathophysiological connection may be hepatotoxicity secondary to excessive alpha2-adrenergic stimulation (Roberts et al. 1997). ATS, including pemoline (Cylert) and methylphenidate (Ritalin) have been specifically implicated as hepatotoxins, though this appears to be rare, idiosyncratic hepatocellular damage (Nehra et al. 1990, Mehta et al. 1984).

Cardiovascular

Both cocaine and ATS cause similar vascular toxicity, largely related to catecholamine excess (Todd et al. 1985a,b). Hearts of stimulant abusers develop areas of fibrosis and contraction band necrosis, and usually are increased in weight. Typically, interstitial fibrosis with myocyte hypertrophy is found at autopsy (Karch 2002). As well, coronary artery disease is accelerated. At autopsy, 16.4% of METH-related deaths showed moderate to severe coronary artery disease (Karch et al. 1999b). Aortic dissection is a less well known but catastrophic complication of METH use (Swalwell and Davis 1999). Yu et al. (2003) also argue that immunosuppressive effects of ATS lead to enhanced cardiotoxicity. Cardiotoxic effects are partly reversible (Islam et al. 1995).

Case reports of myocardial infarction that occurs following ATS are known for use by any route (Furst et al. 1990 Packe et al. 1990, Derreza et al. 1997). Limited data indicate that infarctions result from coronary spasm rather than the results of fixed lesions. Why are myocardial infarction rates with METH so much less than those with cocaine? Karch hypothesizes that the prolonged nature of insult required to damage the fairly hardy cardiovascular system is more the exception than the rule in human users; many more people experiment with ATS than become regular users. Further, hyperthermia, more common with METH than cocaine results in the production of heat shock proteins that may be protective of ischemic damage (Maulik et al. 1995). Cardiomyopathy also appears more rarely in METH use than for cocaine (Smith et al. 1976, Call et al. 1982, Jacobs 1989). The phenomenon clearly occurs at increased rates relative to controls with METH (Matoba et al. 1986, Hong et al. 1991). While most ATS seem similar, methylphenidate may produce a unique pattern of lamellated ultrastructural lesions in the heart (Henderson and Fischer 1995). Of note, heart failure in children treated with Ritalin is so rare as to be at the case report level.

Central Nervous System   As opposed to the medical complications described above, which often are discerned at autopsy, CNS effects including psychosis and stroke are common presenting symptoms in emergency departments.

Seizures are one of the most common presentations of ATS intoxication to emergency rooms (Alldredge et al. 1989). In association with an uncontrollable delirium, they can quickly lead to death if not controlled. Following decreases in ATS blood levels, individuals who abuse ATS are not left at increased risk for reoccurrence of seizures unless CNS lesions from prior stroke have developed.

Strokes associated with ATS can be ischemic or hemorrhagic in nature. These are seen with METH that is taken IV (Imanse and Vanneste 1990, Yen et al. 1994, O'Brien 1998, Pettiti et al. 1998), smoked (Rothrock et al. 1988, Yen et al. 1994), or taken orally (Delaney and Estes 1980). Intracerebral hemorrhage, or a combination of intracerebral and subarachnoid hemorrhage, appear to be the most common stroke type (Harrington et al. 1983). Similar to cocaine, the frontal lobes are most commonly involved, followed by the basal ganglia. These are the same areas where dopamine depletion appears to be the most prominent, and differs from the areas of highest involvement with hyptertensive hemorrhagic stroke, where the basal ganglia and hypothalamus are most commonly involved.

The alleged connection between hemorrhagic stroke and phenylpropylamine (PPA; ±norephedrine) prompted its withdrawal from the market in 2000 (Kernan et al. 2000). Widely used in cold and cough remedies, it was also popular as an appetite suppressant. Compared to METH and AMPH, it has much higher affinity for alpha-adrenergic receptors than beta. Thus, the agent has greater affects on peripheral blood pressure. However, its overall pattern of toxicity is again consistent with catecholamine excess, though cerebral vasculature seems more affected than coronary or pulmonary vessels (Karch 2002).

Ischemic stroke most commonly follows embolism (Pettiti et al. 1998). In some cases, this appears related to an intimal fibrinoid necrosis and mixed cellular infiltrates that results in luminal compromise (Citron et al. 1970, Stafford et al. 1975, Bostwick 1981). A number of oral agents, including methylphenidate and ephedrine, have been implicated in vasculitis (Trugman 1988, Schteinschnaider et al. 2000).

Hyperthermia is related to a number of causes in those presenting with METH intoxication. Increased motor activity, with reduced heat dissipation from peripheral vasoconstriction is the proximate cause. It is also likely that direct affects on hypothalamic thermal regulation exist.

In humans, METH use is correlated over time with declines in N-acetylaspartate levels in basal ganglia and frontal white matter (Ernst et al. 2000, Nordahl et al. 2001). These changes, however, are not correlated with gross histopathologic changes in METH-related deaths. A clue that dopamine declines might be related to functional incapacities, however, is the fact that hyperthermic crises during METH use appear to be related to basal ganglia depletion of dopamine (DA) (Bowyer et al. 1994).

Renal Rhabdomyolysis is clearly the major concern for renal impairment; there does not appear to be independent toxicity to the kidney (Karch 2002). However, METH is an increasingly common cause of rhabdomyolysis (Richards et al. 1999), and is often associated with hyperthermia. Myoglobin and myoglobin breakdown products cause tubular obstruction. Renal damage results from hypotension and renal ischemia secondary to metabolic derangements secondary to rhabdomyolysis, including phosphorus and potassium imbalance, and tubular obstruction due to catabolic product accumulation.

Effects on the Fetus Fetal loss, developmental delay, and subsequent learning disabilities are potential complications of ATS use during pregnancy. While widely quoted, it appears that perinatal complications may be more rare than expected (Catanzarite and Stein 1995, also see Plessinger and Woods 1998). This is despite the fact that fetal exposure is widespread (Oro and Dixon 1987). Karch puts forward the argument that the about-to-be-born fetus is protected from AMPH-related toxicity because it has already been prepared for the catecholamine surge that occurs during childbirth by downregulation of catecholinergic receptors. Preclinical studies indicate METH also concentrates in the fetus (Stek et al. 1993), supported by a limited number of human autopsy cases (Stewart and Meeker 1997). In reported cases, fetal death was not attributable to drug presence; conversely pregnancy may increase the risk of METH use (more common than cocaine) (Vega et al. 1993). METH also concentrates in breast milk (Steiner et al. 1984), but ill effects on children remain controversial (Briggs et al. 1975, Eriksson et al. 1978, Little et al. 1988 a,b, Joffe and Kasnic 1994). Most recent studies support a small effect of newborn birthweight, and a low incidence (4%) of overt ATS withdrawal in newborns of METH-dependent mothers (Smith et al. 2003).

Etiology

ATS operate as indirect sympathomimetics to enhance catecholamine release, and at higher doses, serotonin release. Practically speaking, these agents increase peripheral norepinephrine (NE) levels in the sympathetic nervous system, and centrally, dopamine, norepinephrine, and serotonin levels. Release of central dopamine appears to be the primary action mediating the addictive potential of ATS, but release of NE mediates many of the toxic and peripheral effects (Wilens and Spencer 1998, Sevarino et al. 2000). Postsynaptically, the principal peripheral effects are to stimulate alpha and beta adrenergic receptors. In virtually all actions, the D-stereoenantiomer of the compounds at their alpha-carbon center is 3 to 5 times more active than the L-enantiomer (Gorelick and Cornish 2003). The precise mechanisms by which these agents affect synaptic levels of neurotransmitters is best understood for AMPH, METH, and methylphenidate.

Acutely there are four identified molecular targets of AMPH. In the dopamine system, AMPH acts as a false substrate for the dopamine transporter (DAT) (Amara and Sonders 1998). This transporter is the principal exchange mechanism by which released dopamine (DA) is cleared from the synapse and recycled into the synaptic nerve terminals. Elegant studies have now determined that AMPH results in elevation of intracellular sodium, causing the kinetics of DA exchange through the DAT to favor outward movement of DA (Khoshbouei et al. 2003, Jones et al. 1999). AMPH is internalized where it enhances release of vesicular stores of DA (and NE) into the cytoplasm where exchange via the DAT occurs. This appears to be through inhibition of vesicular monoamine transporter (VMAT) (Boja and Meil 1998), an action shared by cocaine (Brown et al. 2001). VMAT partial knockout mice show enhanced locomotor stimulation by AMPH, reduced reward, and absent sensitization (Uhl et al. 2000). AMPH is selective for releasing newly synthesized cytoplasmic catecholamine stores before enhancing vesicular release; methylphenidate acts more on vesicular pools (Greenhill et al. 2003). A key difference appears to be METH's selectivity for action at the DAT, and not on vesicular transport or cytoplasmic DA release (Seiden et al. 1993, Volkow et al. 1995). Third, AMPH inhibits the DA degradative enzyme catechol-o-methyltransferase (COMT), which would sustain extracellular levels of dopamine. Finally, intracellular monoamine oxidase A is inhibited, an action not found for cocaine. This last action would raise levels of both DA and NE, but it is unclear if levels reached *in vivo* would achieve this effect (Rothman et al. 2001). A prominent difference between cocaine and ATS agents is the lack of sodium transporter inhibition by the latter (Hoffman and Lefkowitz 1990).

ATS has similar effects on the NE system. In fact, ATS may be more potent at releasing NE centrally than DA (Rothman et al. 2001). Both AMPH and METH appear to affect both the DAT and NET, while methylphenidate is more selective for the DAT (Giros et al. 1996). Whether this relates to the abuse-liability hierarchy, where both METH and AMPH appear more addictive than methylphenidate, is unknown (Langer et al. 1986). Norepinephrine transporter (NET) knockout mice are hypersensitive to the locomotor stimulating effects of AMPH (Xu et al. 2000). Serotonin system effects of ATS are even less well understood, though the serotonin transporter (5HTT) is also antagonized by ATS.

The neuroanatomical substrates of ATS agents are also being characterized. By virtue of their lipophilicity, these agents easily cross the blood–brain barrier and show selective accumulation in various brain loci. In particular, the striatum is an area of accumulation for methylphenidate (Volkow et al. 1995). The neostriatum (caudatoputamen and nucleus accumbens) is particularly activated by ATS agents, as well as projections to the orbitofrontal regions and other limbic areas. The neocortex appears inhibited. In more primitive areas of the brain, the ascending reticular activating system and medullary respiratory centers are activated.

A rich literature exists in animal studies supporting the development of neurobiological adaptations to chronic ATS exposure. In humans, the development of tolerance to acute effects such as euphoria and anorexia, the persistent potential for relapse once one has become addicted, and the ability to reexperience psychotic symptoms with low doses of ATS exposure long after chronic use, support long-term changes in humans as well (Sato et al. 1983, 1992, Wilens and Spencer 1998). Sensitization to amphetamines can be demonstrated with eye blink in humans (Strakowski et al. 2001) but only if subjects have not had prior exposure to amphetamines (Comer et al. 2001). This would argue that at least to this marker, sensitization is achieved quickly. Tolerance to ATS also can develop after only several exposures (Gorelick and Cornish 2003).

The DA depletion hypothesis has long been used to explain the long-term effects of psychostimulant abuse (Dackis and Gold 1985). In animals, METH and AMPH dose-dependently reduce the activity of tyrosine hydroxylase, the rate-limiting enzyme in catecholamine synthesis, and DA levels in the nerve terminals decline (Koda and Gibb 1973). AMPH seems to be less neurotoxic than METH in these models (Ellison and Switzer 1993). Nonetheless, DA recovery in rat striatum is remarkably slow, taking months, more consistent with neuroadaptations such as neuronal sprouting rather than resynthesis of depleted stores (Cass and Manning 1999).

The issue of whether DA is depleted in chronic users is critical to understanding imaging findings in chronic METH-dependent individuals that support long-term changes in the DAT. Reductions in DAT can be demonstrated in the caudate and putamen (Wilson et al. 1996, McCann et al. 1998, Volkow et al. 2001a). These reductions correlated with motor and cognitive impairments, and were present in users abstinent for over 11 months. While animal studies support nerve terminal degeneration with high-dose METH administration, in humans it appears other neuronal markers, for example VAMT, are still present, and recovery may be possible over a period of years (Wilson et al. 1996, Volkow et al. 2001b). Sekine and colleagues have demonstrated that DAT reductions are also prominent after chronic METH use in the orbitofrontal and dorsolateral prefrontal cortices, the amygdala, and the nucleus accumbens (Sekine et al. 2001, 2003). Except for the amygdala, these reductions correlated with length of use, and the positive subscale of the Brief Psychiatric Rating Scale. The fact that dopamine D2 receptor function is reduced in the striatum may explain orbitofrontal dysfunction (Volkow et al. 2001c). These findings clearly support long-term alterations caused by METH, but it is unclear why DAT levels would be reduced in the presence of depleted DA levels. There are limited data that oxidative products of DA might specifically inactivate the DAT (Cho and Melega 2002, Hastings et al. 1996, Bindoli et al. 1992).

METH also is neurotoxic to striatal serotonin nerve terminals, again inducing long-term changes in animals (Cass 2000). At high doses, METH appears to permanently destroy serotonin nerve terminals (Woolverton et al. 1989). Surprisingly, little is known about the effects of acute or chronic ATS exposure on the NET.

Preclinical studies also support the importance of glutamatergic transmission in modu-lating dopaminergic areas, and in turn affecting the development of sensitization to psychostimulants (Vanderschuren and Kalivas 2000). Animal studies (Zhang et al. 2001) show METH and cocaine do not acutely elevate the glutamate in the striatum or nucleus accumbens. After chronic exposure, rechallenge with METH increased caudate glutamate and decreased nucleus accumbens glutamate, while cocaine increased gluta-mate in both regions. Acute METH decreased glutamate in substantia nigra and ventral tegmentum, while cocaine increased glutamate in the same regions. Thus, glutamate effects remain to be discerned, but support important differences between cocaine and ATS. Kalivas and colleagues (Pierce and Kalivas 1997) hypothesize that chronic AMPH exposure will recruit glutamatergic cortical inputs to the nucleus accumbens, mirroring environment cue association with drug reward. Further, glutamate antago-nists block the development of locomotor sensitization to stimulants (Vanderschuren and Kalivas 2000).

While the long-term adaptations to ATS and cocaine are usually held to be similar, the bulk of studies have been with cocaine only (White and Kalivas 1998, Robinson and Berridge 2000). Cross sensitization between cocaine and AMPH can be demonstrated (Bonate et al. 1997). However, given the differing pharmacology of cocaine and ATS, it is not surprising that evidence does exist that long-term processes such as sensitization can vary between cocaine, AMPH, and methylphenidate (Vanderschuren and Kalivas 2000).

Treatment

There are few studies that specifically address the treatment of ATS use disorders. This reflects the traditional focus on cocaine use disorders. Even for cocaine, effective pharma-cotherapies are lacking compared to treatment of alcohol- and opiate-dependent individuals. Behavioral treatment approaches remain the mainstay of treatment of psychostimulant use disorders, and those whose efficacy is supported in the cocaine use disorders are assumed will be effective for ATS use disorders. Outcomes in psychosocial treatment cohorts do appear to be similar (Huber et al. 1997, Rawson et al. 2000).

Several unique aspects of ATS addiction must be addressed for treatment to be effective. Because ATS users begin to experience adverse consequences of their use later than com-parable cocaine addicts, they appear to be more ambivalent to enter treatment, probably because they reason that since they have gotten along fairly well up to that point, why should they begin the difficult process of treatment? Thus, treatment entry and retention rates are lower than those for individuals with cocaine dependence, and necessitates outreach programs to enhance treatment engagement (Huber et al. 1997). A number of co-occurring problems, such as high HIV and hepatitis infection rates, homelessness, and child-rearing difficulties must be integrated into the treatment approach. Further, the continued neurocognitive deficits in METH-dependent individuals increase the need to apply outreach attempts to noncompliant individuals (Simon et al. 2000a).

Association with difficult-to-alter behaviors (sexual/social and weight loss) means those "rewards" must be coopted by substitution of other options, such as referral to self-help groups for weight loss. As for any addiction, the need to separate reinforcing social contacts from the addict's lifestyle is a difficult process. Abuse by those seeking performance enhancement may be targeted through education programs and drug screening programs, such as those that have been so successful in the military (Rawson et al. 2002a).

Treatment of ATS Intoxication

Management of acute intoxication is guided by the presenting medical and psychiatric symptoms. In ATS intoxication, there are no direct receptor targets to achieve blockade; though dopamine receptor blockade theoretically should be useful in blocking acute and or chronic affects of ATS, this has not proven to be the case (Sevarino et al. 2000). Anxiety and agitation are first treated by an environment that reduces stimulation and provides orientation, with staff providing reassurance and talk downs (Khantzian and McKenna 1979). Physical restraints should be avoided, as these may worsen rhabdomyolysis or hyperthermia. When nonpharmacological means are insufficient, benzodiazepines, typically lorazepam or diazepam, are first-line treatments since they protect against imminent seizures. Antipsychotics for agitation should be avoided because of the risk of worsening hyperthermia or rhabdomyolysis if neuroleptic malignant syndrome were to occur, and their ability to lower seizure threshold. However, since benzodiazepines run the risk of disinhibiting some individuals, typical antipsychotics are often the preferred choice. Indeed, in one controlled trial, intravenous droperidol was significantly faster than intravenous lorazepam in sedating ATS-intoxicated psychotic individuals (Richards 1997, 1998).

For psychosis and paranoia, high potency antipsychotics, typically haloperidol, are used. This avoids the anticholinergic effects that may worsen delirium and hyperthermia. There is no reason to assume that atypical antipsychotics, such as intramuscular ziprasidone, might not be effective in this population, though there are no trials examining this. While there are no controlled trials on the treatment of ATS-induced psychosis (Srisurapanant et al. 2001c), it appears the psychotic symptoms do not differ from those in schizophrenia in their response to acute intramuscular injection of typical neuroleptics (Angrist 1974). While preclinical literature would argue that DA or serotonin blockade should block the acute subjective effects of ATS use, clinical evidence has not supported this (Wachtel et al. 2002).

The management of medical sequelae of ATS intoxication, most commonly nontraumatic chest pain, is well described in Wilkins et al. (2003). If oral use of the ATS is suspected or confirmed, charcoal gastric lavage is indicated. Acidification of the urine with ammonium chloride solution or cranberry juice may be used to enhance ATS excretion, though should be avoided if rhabdomyolysis is a concern, since this would worsen dissociation and precipitation of myoglobin (Karch 2002), or where renal or hepatic dysfunction are an issue (Hurlbut 1991). Basic life support and initial management are needed for critical conditions such as myocardial ischemia or arrythmia, stroke or seizures, hyperthermia and rhabdomyolysis. Hypertension and tachycardia, if not responsive to benzodiazepine sedation, may require treatment with an alpha-adrenergic blocker, typically phentolamine.

Agents with beta blockade activity, such as propanolol and labetolol, must be avoided as alpha-adrenergic tone can increase, leading to a worsening of the clinical condition (Ramoska and Sacchetti 1985).

Treatment of ATS Withdrawal

Emergency considerations in the withdrawal phase of ATS intoxication are principally psychiatric. The week following cocaine withdrawal is associated with increased risk of silent myocardial ischemia (Nademanee et al. 1989). Because this is hypothesized to result from coronary vasospasm, this may not generalize to ATS withdrawal. Otherwise, medical complications of ATS withdrawal, such as myalgias, involuntary motor movements and so on can be treated symptomatically and should spontaneously remit.

The use of antidepressants for 3 to 4 weeks following cessation of ATS use is suggested, because depression is a hallmark of ATS withdrawal (Watson et al. 1972, Ellinwood 1975). Often, allowing the individual increased time to sleep and reestablishment of normal nutrition is quite helpful. Where needed, the use of trazodone for sleep or short-term benzodiazepines for anxiety is needed along with antidepressant therapy.

Psychosocial Treatments for ATS Dependence

Cognitive behavioral therapy forms the basis of many treatments for psychostimulant dependence (NIDA Research Report 2002). NIDA-sponsored treatment efforts mainly have focused on those with cocaine dependence, but there is no reason to assume that these approaches cannot form the basis of treatment for ATS use disorders. Contingency incentives, skills training, and family member participation are helpful for maintaining cocaine abstinence (Higgins et al. 1993). An extension of such a combined approach, termed the community-reinforcement-plus-vouchers approach, is described in the Treatment Improvement Protocol Series (TIPS) 33: Treatment for Stimulant Use Disorders (CSAT 1999). This approach combines couples counseling, vocational training and skills training (community reinforcement, see Meyers and Smith 1995), and contingency management through rewards for negative urine testing. This combined approach for treatment of cocaine dependence is shown to improve treatment retention and decrease drug use (Higgins et al. 1993, 1994). Further, the approach has been manualized to improve consistency among clinicians (Budney and Higgins 1998).

Contingency management by itself is likely to improve outcomes in ATS use disorders (Stitzer and Higgins 1995, Petry and Martin 2002). Besides rewards for negative urines, more general targets such as improved compliance with treatment, improved employment efforts, and decreased legal involvement can be utilized to more broadly impact the consequences of ATS use. In fact, the drug court approach (i.e., an alternative corrections system that routes addicts to the "drug court" rather than the traditional court system) may be particularly applicable to stimulant dependence because it is so concretely consequence based (Rawson et al. 2002a). Coordination between mental health services, social services resources, and the criminal justice system will be critical in reducing overall ATS use (Rawson et al. 2002a).

The manualized Matrix Model is a second integrated treatment approach utilized in southern California for ATS-dependent individuals (Rawson et al. 1990). This combined approach of group and individual counseling, along with encouragement to participate in 12-step programs, incorporates elements of drug counseling, psychoeducation, motivational enhancement, relapse prevention (see below), family involvement, and case management. The Matrix approach is associated with large reductions in METH use, a decrease in high-risk sexual behavior, improved employment status, and reduced paranoia, though problems with depression persist (Shoptaw et al. 1994, Huber et al. 1997, Rawson et al. 2002b). More focused application of motivational interviewing and motivational enhancement therapy to stimulant use disorders, developed to improve treatment engagement and achievement of abstinence, is in its infancy (Carroll et al. 2002).

Several other psychosocial treatments might be applied to individuals with ATS use disorders (Marlatt and Gordon 1985). Relapse prevention is also recommended in the TIPS protocol. This approach, easily combined with widely used drug counseling, systematically teaches individuals the skills needed to avoid drug use through training in assertiveness and refusal skills, how to cope with craving, how to deal with relapses, and how to recognize patterns of behavior or thinking that lead to relapse. Again, controlled trials support the efficacy of this approach for individuals with cocaine dependence (Carroll 1994).

Network therapy, meant to engage family and community in supporting drug-free functioning, appears well suited to ATS abuse and dependence, where acquisition appears more linked to community networks than stressful street "buys."

There is some controversy as to whether these various treatment modalities, applied under real-world conditions, are superior to the widely applied "drug counseling," whether or not through certified addiction counselors, which loosely applies group counseling, supportive expression session, and case management (Wells et al. 1994, Woody 2003). The NIDA Cocaine Psychotherapy Study examined the effects of psychotherapy (cognitive behavioral therapy or supportive-expressive psychotherapy), individual drug counseling, or no additional treatment, on cocaine-dependent subjects participating in group-drug counseling. Though all groups displayed reductions in cocaine use and risky sexual behaviors, the combined group–individual drug counseling cohort had superior outcomes to the other three groups, which did not differ significantly from each other (Crits-Christoph et al. 1999).

Residential treatment for pregnant women and the homeless is likely to be of benefit for stabilization of ATS-dependent subjects, though there is no specific indication for stimulants (Hughes et al. 1995). The prolonged nature of ATS-induced withdrawal, and the association with aggressivity and violence, will often make inpatient psychiatric stabilization necessary. It is unknown whether transition to therapeutic communities or half-way houses will be of greater benefit to ATS-dependent subjects that those with other substance use disorders, or be superior in outcome to outpatient-based programs (Mueller and Wyman 1997).

Pharmacotherapy for ATS Dependence

As is the case with cocaine use disorders, effective pharmacotherapies for amphetamine use disorders are not available (Sevarino et al. 2000). Pharmacotherapy trials for ATS agents have not focused on dopaminergic mechanisms, but on serotonergic/noradrenergic mechanisms (Srisurapanont et al. 2001b). Galloway et al. (1996) reported that the tricyclic antidepressant imipramine, improved treatment retention (33.0 median days versus 10.5 days) in 32 METH-dependent subjects. However, craving, use, and depression scores were not significantly affected. While open-label trials indicated that fluoxetine might be effective in reducing AMPH use in dependent outpatients, Batki et al. (2000), in a randomized, double-blind study failed to confirm this using fluoxetine at 40 mg/day in METH-dependent subjects.

It had long been known that depletion of DA and NE with alpha-methyltyrosine would antagonize the acute euphoric affects of AMPH in humans, though tolerance to the effect developed within a week (Jonsson et al. 1971). In a very small study involving four subjects, desipramine, a tricyclic antidepressant with prominent norepinephrine effects, reduced amphetamine use and craving, but did not improve treatment retention (Tennant et al. 1986).

In parallel to the successful use of opiate agonist maintenance therapy for heroin dependence, there are open trials of dexamphetamine elixir, at 10 to 90 mg per day being used for controlled maintenance of ATS-dependent subjects (Charnaud and Griffiths 1998,

White 2000). While randomized, prospective studies are not yet reported, a reduction of intravenous use of one-half to two-thirds was seen in these prior studies.

In conclusion, the main role of pharmacotherapy is acute symptomatic relief, and treatment of comorbid conditions. Behavioral treatments and self-help groups remain the mainstay of treatment for the many individuals suffering from ATS dependence.

Comparison of DSM-IV-TR/ICD-10 Diagnostic Criteria

The ICD-10 criteria sets for other stimulant intoxication and withdrawal are almost the same as the DSM-IV-IR criteria sets for amphetamine intoxication and withdrawal except that the ICD-10 diagnostic criteria for research include drug craving as an additional item. ICD-10 combines amphetamines and caffeine into a single substance class, referred to as "other stimulants, including caffeine".

References

Ahmad K (2003) Asia grapples with spreading amphetamine abuse. *Lancet* **361**, 1878–1879.

Akerstedt T and Ficca G (1997) Alertness-enhancing drugs as a counter-measure to fatigue in irregular work hours. *Chronobiol Int* **14**(2), 145–158.

Alldredge BK, Lowenstein DH, and Simon RP (1989) Seizures associated with recreational drug use. *Neurology* **39**, 1037–1039.

Amara SG and Sonders MS (1998) Neurotransmitter transporters as molecular targets for addictive drugs. *Drug Alcohol Depend* **51**, 87–96.

Anglin MD, Rawson RA, and Ling W (2002) Will the methamphetamine problem go away: special issue. *J Addict Dis* **21**(1), 5–19.

Angrist B, Lee HK, and Gershon S (1974) The antagonism of amphetamine-induced symptomatology by a neuroleptic. *Am J Psychiatry* **131**, 817–819.

Baberg HT, Nelesen RA, and Dimsdale JE (1996) Amphetamine use: return of an old scourge in a consultation psychiatry setting. *Am J Psychiatry* **153**, 789–793.

Bailey DN (1987) Amphetamine detection during toxicology screening of a university medical center patient population. *J Toxicol-Clin Toxicol* **25**, 399–409.

Baselt RC (1999) *Disposition of Toxic Drugs and Chemicals in Man*, 5th ed., Chemical Toxicology Institute, Foster City, CA.

Batki SL, Moon J, Bradley M, et al. (2000) *Problems of Drug Dependence 1999: Proceedings of the 61st annual scientific meeting of the College on Problems on Drug Dependence, Inc.* NIDA Research Monograph, 180, NIH Pub. No. 00–4737. Government Printing Office, Washington, DC 235, Harris LS.

Bell DS (1973) The experimental reproduction of amphetamine psychosis. *Arch Gen Psychiatry* **29**, 35–40.

Biederman J, Wilens T, Mick E, et al. (1999) Pharmacotherapy of attention-deficit/hyperactivity disorder reduces risk for substance abuse disorder. *Pediatrics* **104**(2), e20.

Bindoli A, Rigobello MP, and Deeble DJ (1992) Biochemical and toxicological properties of the oxidation products of catecholamines. *Free Radic Biol Med* **13**(4), 391–405.

Boja JW and Meil WM (1998) The dopamine transporter and addiction. In *Drug Abuse Handbook*, Karch SB (ed). CRC Press, Boca Raton, FL, pp. 397–412.

Bonate PL, Swann A, and Silverman PB (1997) Context-dependent cross-sensitization between cocaine and amphetamine. *Life Sci* **60**(1), PL1–PL7.

Bostwick DG (1981) Amphetamine induced cerebral vasculitis. *Hum Pathol* **12**(11), 1031–1033.

Bowyer JF, Davies DL, Schmued L, et al. (1994) Further studies of the role of hyper thermia in methamphetamine neurotoxicity. *J Pharmacol Exp Ther* **268**(3), 1571–1580.

Braithwaite RA, Jarvie DR, Minty PS, et al. (1995) Screening for drugs of abuse. I: Opiates, amphetamines and cocaine. *Ann Clin Biochem* **32**(Pt 2), 123–153.

Briggs GC, Samson JH, and Crawford DJ (1975) Lack of abnormalities in a newborn exposed to amphetamine during gestation. *Am J Dis Child* **129**(2), 249–250.

Brown JM, Hanson GR, and Fleckenstein AE (2001) Regulation of the vesicular monoamine transporter-2: a novel mechanism for cocaine and other psychostimulants. *J Pharmacol Exp Ther* **296**, 762–767.

Budney AJ and Higgins ST (1998) A community reinforcement plus vouchers approach: treating cocaine addiction. *Therapy Manuals for Drug Addiction, Manual 2*, DHHS Pub. No. (ADM) 98–4309, National Institute on Drug Abuse, Rockville, MD. See http://165.112.78.61/TXManuals/CRA/CRA1.html

Buffenstein A, Heaster J, and Ko P (1999) Chronic psychotic illness from methamphetamine. *Am J Psychiatry* **156**(4), 662.

Caldwell J, Dring JG, and Williams RT (1972) Metabolism of (C-14) methamphetamine in man, the guinea pig and the rat. *Biochem J* **129**(1), 11–22.

Call TD, Hartneck J, Dickinson WA, et al. (1982) Acute Cardiomyopathy secondary to intravenous amphetamine abuse. *Ann Intern Med* **97**(4), 59–60.

Cantwell B and McBride AJ (1998) Self detoxification by amphetamine dependent patients: a pilot study. *Drug Alcohol Depend* **49**, 157–163.

Carroll KM, Farentinos C, Ball SA, et al. (2002) MET meets the real world: design issues and clinical strategies in the clinical trials network. *J Subst Abuse Treat* **23**(2), 73–80.

Carroll KM, Rounsaville BJ, Gordon LT, et al. (1994) Psychotherapy and pharmacotherapy for ambulatory cocaine users. *Arch Gen Psychiatry* **51**, 177–187.

Cass WA (2000) Attenuation and recovery of evoked overflow of striatal serotonin in rats treated with neurotoxic doses of methamphetamine. *J Neurochem* **74**, 1079–1085.

Cass WA and Manning MW (1999) Recovery of presynaptic dopaminergic functioning in rats treated with neurotoxic doses of methamphetamine. *J Neurosci* **19**(17), 7653–7660.

Catanzarite VA and Stein DA (1995) 'Crystal' and pregnancy- methamphetamine-associated maternal deaths. *West J Med* **165**(5), 454–457.

Charnaud B and Griffiths V (1998) Levels of intravenous drug misuse among clients prescribed oral dexamphetamine or oral methadone: a comparison. *Drug Alcohol Depend* **52**, 79–84.

Chesney MA, Barrett DC, and Stall R (1998) Histories of substance use and risk behavior: precursors to HIV seroconversion in homosexual men. *Am J Public Health* **88**(1), 113–116.

Cherland E and Fitzpatrick R (1999) Psychotic side effects of psychostimulants: a 5-year Review. *Can J Psychiatry* **44**(8), 811–813.

Cho A and Wright J (1978) Minireview: pathways of metabolism of amphetamine. *Life Sci* **22**, 363–372.

Cho AK (1990) Ice: a new dosage form of an old drug. *Science* **249**, 631–634.

Cho AK and Melega WP (2002) Patterns of methamphetamine abuse and their consequences. *J Addict Dis* **21**, 21–34.

Citron BP, Halpern M, McCarron MJ, et al. (1970) Necrotizing angiitis associated with drug abuse. *N Engl J Med* **283**(19), 1003–1011.

Cohen LG, Prince J, Biederman J, et al. (1999) Absence of effect of stimulants on the phamacokinetics of desipramine in children. *Pharmacotherapy* **19**, 746–752.

Comer SD, Hart CL, Ward AS, et al. (2001) Effects of repeated oral methamphetamine administration in humans. *Psychopharmacology* **155**(4), 397–404.

Conrad S, Hughes P, Baldwin DC Jr., et al. (1988) Substance use by fourth-year students at 13 U.S. medical schools. *J Med Educ* **63**, 747–758.

Cook CE, Jeffcoat AR, Hill JM, et al. (1993) Pharmacokinetics of methamphetamine self-administered to human subjects by smoking S- (+)-methamphetamine hydrochloride. *Drug Metab Dispos* **21**(4), 717–723.

Crits-Christoph P, Siqueland L, Blaine J, et al. (1999) Psychosocial treatments for cocaine dependence: results of the national institute on drug abuse collaborative cocaine treatment study. *Arch Gen Psychiatry* **56**(6), 493–502.

CSAT (Center for Substance Abuse Treatment) (1999) Treatment Improvement Protocol 33: Treatment for Stimulant Use Disorders: Methamphetamine and Cocaine, DHHS Publication No. (SMA) 99–3296.

Cunningham JK and Liu LM (2003) Impacts of federal ephedrine and pseudoephedrine regulations on methamphetamine-related hospital admissions. *Addiction* **98**(9), 1229–1237.

Dackis CA and Gold MS (1985) New concepts in cocaine addiction: the dopamine depletion hypothesis. *Neurosci Biobehav Rev* **9**, 469–477.

Delaney P and Estes M (1980) Intracranial hemorrhage with amphetamine abuse. *Neurology* **30**(10), 1125–1128.

Derreza H, Fine MD, and Sadaniantz A (1997) Acute myocardial infarction after use of pseudoephedrine for sinus congestion. *J Am Board Fam Pract* **10**(6), 436–438.

Ellinwood EH (1975) Treatment of reactions to amphetamine-type stimulant. *Curr Psychiatr Rev* **15**, 163–169.

Ellison G and Switzer RCD (1993) Dissimilar patterns of degeneration in brain following four different addictive stimulants. *Neuroreport* **5**(1), 17–20.

Eriksson M, Larsson G, Winbladh B, et al. (1978) The influence of amphetamine addiction on pregnancy and the newborn infant. *Acta Paedriatica Scandinavica* **67**, 95–99.

Ernst T, Chang L, Leonido-Yee M, et al. (2000) Evidence for long-term neurotoxicity associated with methamphetamine abuse: a 1H MRS study. *Neurology* **54**(6), 1344–1349.

Flaum M and Schulz SK (1996) When does amphetamine-induced psychosis become schizophrenia? *Am J Psychiatry* **153**, 812–815.

Furst SR, Fallon SP, Reznik GN, et al. (1990) Myocardial infarction after inhalation of methamphetamine. *N Engl J Med* **323**(16), 1147–1148.

Galloway GP, Newmeyer J, Knapp T, et al. (1996) A controlled trial of imipramine for the treatment of methamphetamine dependence. *J Subst Abuse Treat* **13**(6), 493–497.

Garland EJ (1998) Intranasal abuse of prescribed methylphenidate. *J Am Acad Child Adolesc Psychiatry* **37**(12), 1242–1243.

Giros B, Jaber M, Jones SR, et al. (1996) Hyperlocomotion and indifference to cocaine and amphetamine in mice lacking the dopamine transporter. *Nature* **379**(6566), 606–612.

Goodhue A, Bartel RL, and Smith NB (2000) Exacerbation of psychosis by phenylpropanolamine. *Am J Psychiatry* **157**(6), 1021–1022.

Gorelick DA and Cornish JL (2003) The pharmacology of cocaine, amphetamines, and other stimulants. In *Principals of Addiction Medicine*, 3rd ed., Graham AW (ed). American Society of Addiction Medicine, Chevy Chase, MD, pp. 157–190.

Greenhill LL, Shockey E, Halperin J, et al. (2003) Stimulants. In *Psychiatry Therapeutics*, Tasman A, Kay J, and Lieberman JA (eds). John Wiley & Sons, INC, Hoboken, NJ, pp. 364–397.

Griffith JD, Cavanaugh J, and Oates J (1969) Schizophreniform psychosis induced by large-dose administration of D-amphetamine. *J Psychedelic Drugs* **2**, 42–48.

Hall W and Hando J (1993) Illicit amphetamine use as a public health problem in Australia. *Med J Aust* **159**(10), 643–644.

Hall W, Hando J, Darke S, et al. (1996) Psychological morbidity and route of administration among amphetamine users in Sydney, Australia. *Addiction* **91**(1), 81–87.

Harrington H, Heller HA, Dawson D, et al. (1983) Intracerebral hemorrhage and oral amphetamine. *Arch Neurol* **40**, 503–507.

Harris D and Batki SL (2000) Stimulant psychosis: symptom profile and acute clinical Course. *Am J Addict* **9**(1), 28–37.

Hastings TG, Lewis DA, and Zigmond MJ (1996) Role of oxidation in the neurotoxic effects of intrastriatal dopamine injections. *Proc Natl Acad Sci U S A* **93**, 1956–1961.

Heishman SJ (1998) Effects of abused drugs on human performance: laboratory assessment. In *Drug Abuse Handbook*, Karch SB (ed). CRC Press, Boca Raton, FL, pp. 206–235.

Henderson TA and Fischer VW (1995) Effects of methylphenidate (Ritalin) on mammalian myocardial ultrastructure. *Am J Cardiovasc Pathol* **5**(1), 68–78.

Higgins ST, Budney AJ, Bickel WK, et al. (1993) Achieving cocaine abstinence with a behavioral approach. *Am J Psychiatry* **150**(5), 763–769.

Higgins ST, Budney AJ, Bickel WK, et al. (1994) Incentives improve outcome in outpatient behavioral treatment of cocaine dependence. *Arch Gen Psychiatry* **51**, 568–576.

Hoffman BB and Lefkowitz RJ (1990) Catecholamines and sympathomimetic drugs. In *The pharmacological Basis of Therapeutics*, Gilman AG, Rall TW, Nies AS, et al. (eds). New York, Pergamon, pp. 187–220.

Hong R, Matsuyama E, and Nur K (1991) Cardiomyopathy associated with the smoking of crystal methamphetamine. *J Am Med Assoc* **265**, 1152–1154.

Huber A, Ling W, Shoptaw S, et al. (1997) Integrating treatments for methamphetamine abuse: a psychosocial perspective. *J Addict Dis* **16**(4), 41–50.

Hughes PH, Coletti SD, Neri RL, et al. (1995) Retaining cocaine-abusing women in a therapeutic community: the effect of a child live-in program. *Am J Public Health* **85**, 1149–1152.

Hurlbut KM (1991) Drug-induced psychoses. *Emerg Med Clin North Am* **9**(1), 31–52.

Imanse J and Vanneste J (1990) Intracentricular hemorrhage following amphetamine abuse. *Neurology* **40**, 1318–1319.

Islam MN, Kuroki H, Hongcheng B, et al. (1995) Cardiac lesions, and their reversibility after long term administration of methamphetamine. *Forensic Sci Int* **75**(1), 29–43.

Jacobs LJ (1989) Reversible dilated cardiomyopathy induced by methamphetamine. *Clin Cardiol* **12**(12), 725–727.

Joffe GM and Kasnic T (1994) Medical prescription of dextroamphetamine during pregnancy. *J Perinatol* **14**(4), 301–303.

Jones SR, Joseph JD, Barak LS, et al. (1999) Dopamine neuronal transport kinetics and effects of amphetamine. *J Neurochem* **73**(6), 2406–2414.

Jonsson LE, Anggard E, and Gunne L (1971) Blockade of intravenous amphetamine euphoria in man. *Clin Pharmacol Ther* **12**(6), 889–896.

Kalechstein AD, Newton TF, and Green M (2003) Methamphetamine dependence is associated with neurocognitive impairment in the initial phases of abstinence. *J Neuropsychiatr Clin Neurosci* **15**, 215–220.

Karch SB (2002) Synthetic stimulants, Chapter 3. In *Karch's Pathology of Drug Abuse*, CRC Press, New York, pp. 233–280.

Karch SB, Stephens BG, and Ho CH (1999b) Methamphetamine-related deaths in San Francisco: demographic, pathologic, and toxicologic profiles. *J Forensic Sci* **44**(2), 359–368.

Kernan WN, Viscoli CM, Brass LM, et al. (2000) Phenylpropanolamine and the risk of hemorrhagic stroke. *N Engl J Med* **343**(25), 1826–1832.

Khantzian EJ and McKenna GJ (1979) Acute toxic and withdrawal reactions associated with drug use and abuse. *Ann Intern Med* **90**, 361–372.

Khoshbouei H, Wang H, Lechleiter JD, et al. (2003) Amphetamine-induced dopamine efflux. *J Biol Chem* **278**(14), 12070–12077.

Klein R and Wender P (1995) The role of methylphenidate in psychiatry. *Arch Gen Psychiatry* **52**, 429–433.

Koda LY and Gibb JW (1973) Adrenal and striatal tyrosine hydroxylase activity after methamphetamine. *J Pharmacol Exp Ther* **185**(1), 42–48.

Kollins SH, MacDonald EK, and Rush CR (2002) Assessing the abuse potential of methylphenidate in nonhuman and human subjects: a review. *Pharmacol Biochem Behav* **68**, 611–627.

Kramer JC, Fischman VS, and Littlefield DC (1967) Amphetamine abuse: pattern and effects of high doses taken intravenously. *J Am Med Assoc* **201**, 305–309.

Kringsholm B and Christoffersen P (1987) Lung and heart pathology in fatal drug addiction. A consecutive autopsy study. *Forensic Sci Int* **34**(1–2), 39–51.

Langer DH, Sweeney KP, Bartenbach DE, et al. (1986) Evidence of lack of abuse or dependence following pemoline treatment: results of a retrospective survey. *Drug Alcohol Depend* **17**, 213–227.

Lebish P, Finkle BS, and Brackett JW Jr. (1970) Determination of amphetamine, methamphetamine, and related amines in blood and urine by gas chromatography with hydrogen-flame ionization detector. *Clin Chem* **16**(3), 195–200.

Lederer CM Jr. and Sabates FN (1982) Ocular findings in the intravenous drug abuser. *Ann Ophthalmol* **14**(5), 436–438.

Levin FR, Evans SM, and Kleber HD (1999) Practical guidelines for the treatment of substance abusers with adult attention-deficit hyperactivity disorder. *Psychiatr Serv* **50**(8), 1001–1003.

Marlatt GA and Gordon JR (1985) *Relapse Prevention*. Guilford Press, New York, NY.

Marshall RD and Douglas CJ (1994) Phenylpropanolamine-induced psychosis. Potential predisposing factors. *Gen Hosp Psychiatry* **16**(5), 358–360.

Matoba R, Shikata I, and Fujitani N (1986) Cardiac lesions in methamphetamine abusers. *Acta Medicinae Legalis et Socialis (liege)* **36**(1), 51–55.

Maulik N, Engelman RM, Wei Z, et al. (1995) Drug-induced heat-shock preconditioning improves post-ischemic ventricular recovery after cardiopulmonary bypass. *Circulation* **92**(9 suppl. II), 381–388.

McCann UD, Wong DF, Yokoi F, et al. (1998) Reduced striatal dopamine transporter density in abstinent methamphetamine and methcathinone users: evidence from positron emission tomography studies with [11C]WIN-35, 428. *J Neurosci* **18**(20), 8417–8422.

Mehta H, Murray B, and Loludice TA (1984) Hepatic dysfunction due to intravenous abuse of methylphenidate hydrochloride. *J Clin Gastroenterol* **6**(2), 149–151.

Meyers RJ and Smith JE (1995) *Clinical Guide to Alcohol Treatment: The Community Reinforcement Approach*. New York, New York.

Molitor F, Traux SR, Ruiz JD, et al. (1998) Association of methamphetamine use during sex with risky sexual behaviors and HIV infection among non-injection drug users. *West J Med* **168**(2), 93–97.

Mueller MD and Wyman JR (1997) Study sheds new light on the state of drug abuse treatment nationwide. *NIDA Notes* **12**(5), 1–7.

Murray JB (1998) Psychophysiological aspects of amphetamine-methamphetamine abuse. *J Psychol* **132**(2), 227–237.

Nademanee K, Gorelick DA, Josephson MA, et al. (1989) Myocardial ischemia during cocaine withdrawal. *Ann Intern Med* **111**, 876–880.

Nath A, Maragos WF, Avison MJ, et al. (2001) Acceleration of HIV dementia with methamphetamine and cocaine. *J Neurovirol* **7**, 66–71.

Nehra A, Mullick F, Ishak KG, et al. (1990) Pemoline-associated Hepatic injury. *Gastroenterology* **99**(5), 1517–1519.

Newton TF, Cook IA, Kalechstein AD, et al. (2003) Quantitative EEG abnormalities in recently abstinent methamphetamine dependent individuals. *Clin Neurophysiol* **114**(3), 410–415.

NIDA Research Report (2002) Methamphetamine Abuse and Addiction, *NIH Publication* No. 02–4210, Printed April 1998, Reprinted January 2002.

Nordahl TE, Salo RE, and Poissin K (2001) Low N-acetyl-aspartate and high choline in the Anterior cingulum of recently abstinent methamphetamine dependent subjects: a Proton MRS study. *Presented at the Annual Meeting of Social Neuroscience*.

Norvenius G, Widerlov E, and Lonnerholm G (1979) Phenylpropanolamine and mental disturbances. *Lancet* **2**(8156–8157), 1367–1368.

O'Brien CP (1998) Stroke in young women who use cocaine or amphetamines. *Epidemiology* **9**(6), 587–588.

Ornstein TJ, Iddon JL, Baldaccino AM, et al. (2000) Profiles of cognitive dysfunction in chronic amphetamine and heroin abusers. *Neuropsychopharmacology* **23**(2), 113–126.

Oro AS and Dixon SD (1987) Perinatal cocaine and methamphetamine exposure: maternal and neonatal correlates. *J Pediatr* **111**(4), 571–578.

Packe GE, Garton MJ, and Jennings K (1990) Acute myocardial infarction caused by Intravenous amphetamine abuse. *Br Heart J* **64**(1), 23–24.

Parran TV Jr. and Jasinski DR (1991) Intravenous methylphenidate abuse. Prototype for prescription drug abuse. *Arch Intern Med* **151**(4), 781–783.

Paulus MP, Hozack N, Frank L, et al. (2003) Decision making by methamphetamine-dependent subjects is associated with error-rate-independent decrease in prefrontal and parietal activation. *Biol Psychiatry* **53**(1), 65–74.

Pettiti DB, Sidney S, Quesenberry C, et al. (1998) Stroke and cocaine or amphetamine use. *Epidemiology* **9**(6), 596–600.

Petry NM and Martin B (2002) Low-cost contingency management for treating cocaine- and opioid-abusing methadone patients. *J Consult Clin Psychol* **70**(2), 398–405.

Phillips TR, Billaud JN, and Henriksen SJ (2000) Methamphetamine and HIV-1: potential interactions and the use of the FIV/cat model. *J Psychopharmacol* **14**(3), 244–250.

Pierce RC and Kalivas PW (1997) A circuitry model of the expression of behavioral sensitization to amphetamine-like psychostimulants. *Brain Res Rev* **25**(2), 192–216.

Plessinger MA and Woods JR Jr. (1998) Cocaine in pregnancy on maternal and fetal risks. *Obstet Gynecol Clin North Am* **25**(1), 99–118.

Poulin C (2001) Medical and nonmedical stimulant use among adolescents: from sanctioned to unsanctioned use. *Can Med Assoc J* **165**, 1039–1044.

Rappley MD (1997) Safety issues in the use of methylphenidate. An American perspective. *Drug Saf* **17**(3), 143–148.

Rawson R, Anglin MD, and Ling W (2002a) Will the methamphetamine problem go Away? *J Addict Dis* **21**(1), 5–19.

Rawson RA, Huber A, Brethen P, et al. (2002b) Status of Methamphetamine users 2–5 years after outpatient treatment. *J Addict Dis* **21**(1), 107–119.

Rawson R, Huber A, Brethen P, et al. (2000) Methamphetamine and cocaine users: differences in characteristics and treatment retention. *J Psychoactive Drugs* **32**(2), 233–238.

Rawson RA, Obert JL, McCann MJ, et al. (1990) Neurobehavioral treatment for cocaine dependency. *J Psychoactive Drugs* **22**, 159–171.

Richards JR, Johnson EB, Stark RW, et al. (1999) Methamphetamine abuse and rhabdomyolysis in The ED: a 5-year study. *Am J Emerg Med* **17**(7), 681–685.

Richards JR, Derlet RW, and Duncan DR (1998) Chemical restraint for the agitated patient in the emergency department: Lorazepam versus droperidol. *J Emerg Med* **16**(4), 567–573.

Richards JR, Derlet RW, and Duncan DR (1997) Methamphetamine toxicity: treatment with a benzodiazepine versus a butyrophenone. *Eur J Emerg Med* **4**, 130–135.

Roberts SM, DeMott RP, and James RC (1997) Adrenergic modulation of hepatotoxicity. *Drug Metab Rev* **29**(1–2), 329–353.

Robinson TE and Berridge KC (2000) The psychology and neurobiology of addiction: an incentive-sensitization view. *Addiction* **95**, S91–S117.

Rogers RD, Everitt BJ, Baldacchino A, et al. (1999) Dissociable deficits in the decision-making cognition of chronic amphetamine abusers, opiate abusers, patients with focal damage to prefrontal cortex, and tryptophan-depleted normal volunteers: evidence for monoaminergic mechanisms. *Neuropsychopharmacology* **20**, 322–339.

Rothman RB, Baumann MH, Dersch CM, et al. (2001) Amphetamine-type central nervous system stimulants release norepinephrine more potently than they release dopamine and serotonin. *Synapse* **39**(1), 32–41.

Rothrock JF, Rubenstein R, and Lyden PD (1988) Ischemic stroke associated with methamphetamine inhalation. *Neurology* **38**(4), 589–592.

SAMHSA (2003) *Results from the 2002 National Survey on Drug Use and Health: National Findings* NHSDA Series H-22, DHHS Publication No. SMA 03–3836, Office of Applied Studies, Rockville, MD.

Sato M, Chen C, Akiyama K, et al. (1983) Acute exacerbation of paranoid psychotic state after long-term abstinence in patients with previous methamphetamine psychosis. *Biol Psychiatry* **18**, 429–440.

Sato M, Numachi Y, and Hamamura T (1992) Relapse of paranoid psychotic state in methamphetamine model of schizophrenia. *Schizophr Bull* **18**, 115–122.

Schmidt RA, Glenny RW, Godwin JD, et al. (1991) Panlobular emphysema in young intravenous Ritalin abusers. *Am Rev Respir Dis* **143**(3), 649–656.

Schuckit MA, Daeppen J-B, and Danko GP (1999) Clinical implications for four drugs of the DSM-IV distinction between substance dependence with and without a physiological component. *Am J Psychiatry* **156**, 41–49.

Schteinschnaider A, Plaghos LL, Garbugino S, et al. (2000) Cerebral arteritis following methylphenidate use. *J Child Neurol* **15**(4), 265–267.

Seiden LS, Sabol KE, and Ricaurte GA (1993) Amphetamine: effects on catecholamine systems and behavior. *Annu Rev Pharmacol Toxicol* **32**, 639–677.

Sekine Y, Iyo M, Ouchi Y, et al. (2001) Methamphetamine-related psychiatric symptoms and reduced brain dopamine transporters studied with PET. *Am J Psychiatry* **158**(8), 1206–1214.

Sekine Y, Minabe Y, Ouchi Y, et al. (2003) Association of dopamine transporter loss in the orbitofrontal and dorsolateral prefrontal cortices with methamphetamine-related psychiatric symptoms. *Am J Psychiatry* **160**, 1699–1701.

Sevarino KA, Oliveto A, and Kosten TR (2000) Neurobiological adaptations to psychostimulants and opiates as a basis of treatment development. *Ann N Y Acad Sci* **909**, 51–87.

Shah SP, Khine M, Anigbogu J, et al. (1998) Nodular amyloidosis of the lung from intravenous drug abuse: an uncommon cause of multiple pulmonary nodules. *South Med J* **91**(4), 402–404.

Shoptaw S, Reback CJ, and Freese TE (2002) Patient characteristics, HIV serostatus, and risk behaviors among gay and bisexual males seeking treatment for methamphetamine abuse and dependence in Los Angeles. *J Addict Dis* **21**(1), 91–105.

Shoptaw S, Rawson RA, McCann MJ, et al. (1994) The Matrix Model of outpatient stimulant abuse treatment: Evidence of efficacy. *J Addict Dis* **13**(4), 23–35.

Simon SL, Domier CP, Sim T, Richardson K, Rawson RA, and Ling W (2002a) Cognitive performance of current methamphetamine and cocaine abusers. *J Addic Dis* **21**(1), 61–74.

Simon SL, Richardson K, Dacey J, et al. (2002b) A comparison of patterns of methamphetamine and cocaine use. *J Addict Dis* **21**(1), 35–44.

Smith H, Roche AH, Jausch MF, et al. (1976) Cardiomyopathy associated with amphetamine administration. *Am Heart J* **91**, 792–797.

Smith L, Yonekura ML, Wallace T, et al. (2003) Effects of prenatal methamphetamine exposure on fetal growth and drug withdrawal symptoms in infants born at term. *J Dev Behav Pediatr* **24**(1), 17–23.

Snyder SH (1973) Amphetamine psychosis: A "model" schizophrenia mediated by catecholamines. *Am J Psychiatry* **130**, 61–67.

Stitzer ML and Higgins ST (1995) Behavioral treatment of drug and alcohol abuse. In *Psychopharmacology: The Fourth Generation of Progress*, Bloom FE and Kupfer DJ (eds). Raven Press, New York, pp. 1807–1819.

Soine WH (1986) Clandestine drug synthesis. *Med Res Rev* **6**, 41–74.

Srisurapanont M, Jarusuraisin N, and Kittiratanapaiboon P (2001a) Treatment of amphetamine withdrawal. *Cochrane Database Syst Rev* 2001(4):CD003021. Review.

Srisurapanont M, Jarusuraisin N, and Kittiratanapaiboon P (2001b) Treatment of amphetamine dependence and abuse. *The Cochrane Database Syst Rev* **2001**(4), CD003022. Review.

Srisurapanont M, Kittiratanapaiboon P, and Jarusuraisin N (2001c) Treatment of amphetamine psychosis. *Cochrane Database Syst Rev* **2001**(4), CD003026. Review.

Stafford CR, Bogdanoff BM, Green L, et al. (1975) Mononeuropathy multiplex as a complication of amphetamine angiitis. *Neurology* **25**(6), 570–572.

Steiner E, Villen T, Hallberg M, et al. (1984) Amphetamine secretion in breast milk. *Eur J Clin Pharmacol* **27**, 123–124.

Stek AM, Fisher BK, Baker RS, et al. (1993) Maternal and fetal cardiovascular responses to methamphetamine in the pregnant sheep. *Am J Obstet Gynecol* **169**(4), 888–897.

Stewart JL and Meeker JE (1997) Fetal and infant deaths associated with maternal methamphetamine abuse. *J Anal Toxicol* **21**(6), 515–517.

Strakowski SM, Sax KW, Rosenberg HL, et al. (2001) Human response to repeated low-dose d-amphetamine: evidence for behavioral enhancement and tolerance. *Neuropsychopharmacology* **25**(4), 548–554.

Swalwell CI and Davis GG (1999) Methamphetamine as a risk factor for acute aortic dissection. *J Forensic Sci* **44**(1), 23–26.

Telang FW, Volkow ND, Levy A, et al. (1999) Distribution of tracer levels of cocaine in human brain as assessed with averaged (^{11}C) cocaine images. *Synapse* **31**, 290–296.

Tennant FS Jr., Tarver A, Pumphrey E, et al. (1986) Double-blind comparison of desipramine and placebo for treatment of phencyclidine or amphetamine dependence. *NIDA Res Monogr* **67**, 310–317.

Teter CJ, McCabe SE, Boyd CJ, et al. (2003) 2003 Illicit methylphenidate use in an undergraduate student sample: prevalence and risk factors. *Pharmacotherapy* **23**(5), 609–617.

Tinsley JA and Watkins DD (1998) Over-the-counter stimulants: abuse and addiction. *Mayo Clin Proc* **73**, 977–982.

Todd GL, Baroldi G, Pieper GM, Clayton FC, and Eliot RS (1985a) Experimental catecholamine-induced myocardial necrosis. I. Morphology, quantification and regional distribution of acute contraction band lesions. *J Mol Cell Cardiol* **17**(4), 317–338.

Todd GL, Baroldi G, Pieper GM, Clayton FC, and Eliot RS (1985b) Experimental catecholamine-induced myocardial necrosis. II. Temporal development of isoproterenol-induced contraction band lesions correlated with ECG, hemodynamic and biochemical changes. *J Mol Cell Cardiol* **17**(7), 647–656.

Tomashefski JF Jr. and Hirsch C (1980) The pulmonary vascular lesions of intravenous drug abuse. *Hum Pathol* **11**, 133–145.

Trugman JM (1988) Cerebral arteritis and oral methylphenidate. *Lancet* **1**(8585), 584–585.

Uhl GR, Li S, Takahashi N, et al. (2000) The VMAT2 gene in mice and humans: amphetamine responses, locomotion, cardiac arrhythmias, aging, and vulnerability to dopaminergic toxins. *FASEB J* **14**, 2459–2465.

Ujike H, Harano M, Inada T, et al. (2003) Nine- or fewer repeat alleles in VNTR polymorphism of the dopamine transporter gene is a strong risk factor for prolonged methamphetamine psychosis. *Pharmacogenomics J* **3**(4), 242–247.

United Nations Office on Drugs and Crime (2003) *Global Illicit Drug Trends*. See www.unodc.org/unodc/en/global_illicit_drug_trends.html.

United Nations Drug Control Program (2003) *Global Illicit Drug Trends*. United Nations Office on Drugs and Crime, Vienna, Austria, pp. 1–351.

Vanderschuren LJ and Kalivas PW (2000) Alterations in dopaminergic and glutamatergic transmission in the induction and expression of behavioral sensitization: a critical review of preclinical studies. *J Neurosci* **151**(2–3), 99–120.

Vega WA, Kolody B, Hwang J, et al. (1993) Prevalence and magnitude of perinatal substance exposure in California. *N Engl J Med* **329**(12), 850–854.

Vincent N, Shoobridge J, Ask A, et al. (1998) Physical and mental health Problems in amphetamine users from metropolitan Adelaide, Australia. *Drug Alcohol Rev* **17**, 187–195.

Volkow ND, Chang L, Wang G, et al. (2001a) Association of dopamine transporter reduction with psychomotor impairment in methamphetamine abusers. *Am J Psychiatry* **158**(3), 377–382.

Volkow ND, Chang L, Wang GJ, et al. (2001b) Loss of dopamine transporters in methamphetamine abusers recovers with protracted abstinence. *J Neurosci* **21**(23), 9414–9418.

Volkow ND, Chang L, Wang GJ, et al. (2001c) Low level of brain dopamine D2 receptors in methamphetamine abusers: association with metabolism in the orbitoprefrontal cortex. *Am J Psychiatry* **158**, 2015–2021.

Volkow ND, Wang GJ, Fowler JS, et al. (1999) Methylphenidate and cocaine have a similar in vivo potency to block dopamine transporters in the human brain. *Life Sci* **65**(1), L7–L12.

Volkow ND, Ding Y, Fowler JS, et al. (1995) Is methylphenidate like cocaine? *Arch Gen Psychiatry* **52**, 456–463.

Wachtel SR, Ortengren A, and de Wit H (2002) The effects of acute haloperidol or risperidone on subjective responses to methamphetamine in healthy volunteers. *Drug Alcohol Depend* **68**, 23–33.

Wan SH, Matin SB, and Azarnoff DL (1978) Kinetics: salivary excretion of amphetamine isomers and effects of urinary pH. *Clin Pharmacol Ther* **23**(5), 585–590.

Watson R, Hartmann E, and Schildkraut JJ (1972) Amphetamine withdrawal: affective state, sleep patterns, and MHPG excretion. *Am J Psychiatry* **129**, 263–269.

Wells EA, Petersen PL, Gainey RR, et al. (1994) Outpatient treatment for cocaine abuse: a controlled comparison of relapse prevention and twelve-step approaches. *Am J Drug Alcohol Abuse* **20**, 1–17.

White R (2000) Dexamphetamine substitution in the treatment of amphetamine abuse: an initial Investigation. *Addiction* **95**, 229–238.

White FJ and Kalivas PW (1998) Neuroadaptations involved in amphetamine and cocaine addiction. *Drug Alcohol Depend* **51**(1–2), 141–153.

Wilens TE and Spencer TJ (1998) Pharmacology of Amphetamines. *Handbook Subst Abuse: Neurobehav Pharmacol* **30**, 501–513.

Wilkins JN, Mellott KG, Markvista R, et al. (2003) Management of stimulant, hallucinogen, marijuana, phencyclidine and club drug intoxication and withdrawal. In *Principals of Addiction Medicine*, 3rd ed., Graham AW (ed). American Society of Addiction Medicine, Chevy Chase, MD, pp. 671–695.

Williamson S, Gossop M, Powis B, et al. (1997) Adverse effects of stimulant drugs in a community sample of drug users. *Drug Alcohol Depend* **44**, 87–94.

Wilson JM, Kalasinsky KS, Levey AI, et al. (1996) Striatal dopamine nerve terminal markers in human, chronic methamphetamine users. *Nat Med* **2**(6), 699–703.

Woody GE, Cottler LB, and Cacciola J (1993) Severity of dependence: data from DSM-IV field trials. *Addiction* **88**, 1573–1579.

Woody GE (2003) Research findings on psychotherapy of addictive disorders. *Am J Addict* **12**(Suppl. 2), S19–S26.

Woolverton WL, Ricaurte GA, Forno LS, et al. (1989) Long-term effects of chronic methamphetamine administration in rhesus monkeys. *Brain Res* **486**, 73–78.

Wu D, Otton SV, Inaba T, et al. (1997) Interactions of amphetamine analogs with human liver CYP2D6. *Biochem Pharmacol* **53**(11), 1605–1612.

Xu F, Gainetdinov RR, Wetsel WC, et al. (2000) Mice lacking the norepinephrine transporter are supersensitive to psychostimulants. *Nat Neurosci* **3**(5), 465–471.

Yen DJ, Wang SJ, Ju TH, et al. (1994) Stroke associated with methamphetamine inhalation. *Eur Neurol* **34**(1), 16–22.

Yu Q, Larson DF, and Watson RR (2003) Minireview: heart disease, methamphetamine and AIDS. *Life Sci* **73**, 129–140.

Zhang Y, Loonam TM, Noailles PA, et al. (2001) Comparison of cocaine- and methamphetamine-evoked dopamine and glutamate overflow in somatodendritic and terminal field regions of the rat brain during acute, chronic, and early withdrawal conditions. *Ann N Y Acad Sci* **937**, 93–120.

Zule WA and Desmond DP (1999) An ethnographic comparison of HIV risk behaviors among heroin and methamphetamine injectors. *Am J Drug Alcohol Abuse* **25**, 1–23.

Substance-Related Disorders: Caffeine

Caffeine is the most widely consumed psychoactive substance in the world (Gilbert 1984). In North America, it is estimated that more than 80% of adults and children consume caffeine regularly (Graham 1978, Hughes and Oliveto 1997). Throughout the world caffeine use occurs in a variety of different but culturally well-integrated social contexts, such as the coffee break in the United States, teatime in the United Kingdom, and kola nut chewing in Nigeria. In the United States, for example, habitual consumption of coffee or caffeinated soda drinks with meals is extremely common and may not be readily recognized as caffeine consumption. This cultural integration of caffeine use can make the recognition of mental disorders associated with caffeine use particularly difficult. However, it is important for the clinician to recognize the role of caffeine as a psychoactive substance capable of producing a variety of psychiatric syndromes, despite the pervasive and well-accepted use of caffeine. In this chapter, five disorders associated with caffeine use are reviewed: caffeine intoxication, caffeine withdrawal, caffeine dependence, caffeine-induced anxiety disorder, and caffeine-induced sleep disorder.

CAFFEINE INTOXICATION

Diagnosis

DSM-IV-TR defines caffeine intoxication as a set of symptoms that develop during or shortly after caffeine use. There may be two kinds of presentation associated with caffeine intoxication. The first presentation is associated with the *acute* ingestion of a large amount of caffeine and represents an acute drug overdose condition. The second presentation is associated with the *chronic* consumption of large amounts of caffeine and results in a more complicated presentation.

Caffeine intoxication has long been recognized as a syndrome produced by the ingestion of an excessive amount of caffeine. For example, Rugh (1896) reported the case of a traveling salesman who had nervousness, involuntary contractions in the arms and legs, a sense of impending danger, and sleep disturbance in the context of excessive coffee consumption used to maintain a highly active pace of work. Similar reports of caffeine intoxication can be found throughout the medical literature of the 1800s and early 1900s with observations of motor unrest, insomnia, tachycardia, irritability, headache, emotional lability, anxiety, and gastrointestinal disturbances associated with excessive use of caffeine (Bullard 1889, Cole 1833, Bram 1913, King 1903, Powers 1925, Love 1891, Orendorff 1914). Thus, caffeine intoxication represents a mental disorder that has been well described for at least 100 years.

The primary features of caffeine intoxication can be found in the diagnostic criteria from DSM-IV-TR (see DSM-IV-TR diagnostic criteria below). The diagnostic decision tree for caffeine intoxication, caffeine-induced anxiety disorder, and caffeine-induced sleep disorder is shown in Figure 18-1. One study that utilized a random-digit–dial telephone interview survey of 162 users of caffeine, examined the types of symptoms reported by persons who had experienced some features of caffeine intoxication (Hughes et al. 1998b). Results from that study showed that two-thirds of participants had experienced at least one of the DSM-IV-TR symptoms related to caffeine intoxication in the previous year. The most common symptoms reported in decreasing order of frequency were frequent urination, restlessness, insomnia, nervousness, and excitement (all which were at rates greater than 20%). In addition, 24% reported heart pounding in response to high caffeine use (although this is not one of the DSM-IV-TR criteria).

DSM-IV-TR Diagnostic Criteria

305.90 Caffeine Intoxication

A. Recent consumption of caffeine, usually in excess of 250 mg (e.g., more than 2–3 cups of brewed coffee).

B. Five (or more) of the following signs, developing during, or shortly after, caffeine use:

(1) restlessness
(2) nervousness
(3) excitement

(4) insomnia
(5) flushed face
(6) diuresis
(7) gastrointestinal disturbance
(8) muscle twitching
(9) rambling flow of thought and speech
(10) tachycardia or cardiac arrhythmia
(11) periods of inexhaustibility
(12) psychomotor agitation

C. The symptoms in Criterion B cause clinically significant distress or impairment in social, occupational, or other important areas of functioning.
D. The symptoms are not due to a general medical condition and are not better accounted for by another mental disorder (e.g., an anxiety disorder).

Reprinted with permission from the Diagnostic and Statistical Manual of Mental Disorders, Fourth Edition, Text Revision. Copyright 2000 American Psychiatric Association.

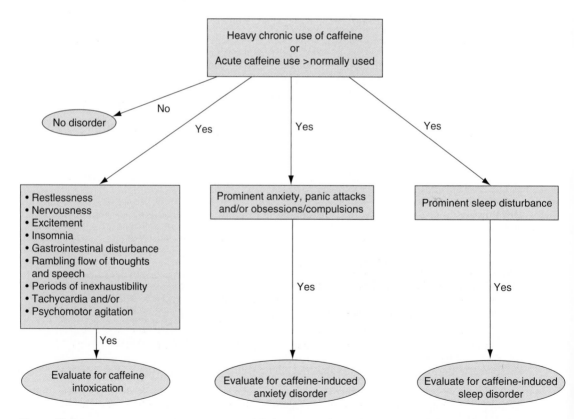

Figure 18-1 *Diagnostic decision tree for caffeine intoxication disorder, caffeine-induced anxiety disorder, and caffeine-induced sleep disorder.*

In a study of 124 general hospital patients, the most common somatic symptoms that individuals reported as associated with caffeine intake (i.e., symptoms not specified as associated with either caffeine intoxication or caffeine withdrawal) were in descending order of frequency: diuresis, insomnia, withdrawal headaches, diarrhea, anxiety, tachycardia, and tremulousness (Victor et al. 1981).

In addition to the characteristics of caffeine intoxication noted in DSM-IV-TR, there have been reports of fever (Reimann 1967), irritability, tremors, sensory disturbances, tachypnea (Greden 1974), and headaches (Shirlow and Mathers 1985, Stoffer 1979) associated with cases of caffeine intoxication. Although a wide variety of symptoms of caffeine intoxication have been reported, the most common signs and symptoms appear to be anxiety and nervousness, diuresis, insomnia, gastrointestinal disturbances, tremors, tachycardia, and psychomotor agitation.

Epidemiology

Despite the long history of recognition of caffeine intoxication, there is little information available about the prevalence or incidence of caffeine intoxication either in the general community or in selected populations. There is one study that has examined caffeine intoxication in the community, and four that have examined rates of caffeine intoxication in special populations.

The study that addresses the prevalence of caffeine intoxication in the community was a telephone survey conducted in Vermont (Hughes et al. 1998b)., and 162 caffeine users provided self-report information on caffeine intoxication (as well as dependence). In this study, 7% of the subjects had symptoms that met DSM-IV-TR criteria for caffeine intoxication. However, it is also worth noting that two-thirds of the subjects reported at least one caffeine intoxication symptom (DSM-IV-TR criterion) in the previous year. These results suggest caffeine intoxication and symptoms related to excessive caffeine use may be quite common in the general community.

Four studies have examined the rate of caffeine intoxication in special populations. In a 1975 survey of 220 psychiatric patients and control subjects, none of the participants had symptoms of caffeine intoxication (Furlong 1975). A 1976 survey of 135 inpatients in a psychiatric unit found two cases (1.5%) of caffeine intoxication (Winstead 1976). A 1981 survey of college students found 1.3% with high caffeine consumption, and these high caffeine consumers had higher levels of symptoms associated with caffeine intoxication (Gilliland and Andress 1981). Finally, a 1990 survey of college students found that 19% reported a history of caffeine intoxication (Bradley and Petree 1990).

Course

In an individual who is not tolerant to caffeine, acute caffeine ingestion producing caffeine intoxication is a time-limited condition that will rapidly resolve with cessation of caffeine use, consistent with the relatively short half-life of caffeine (3–6 hours) (Balogh et al. 1992). In an individual who has caffeine intoxication superimposed on chronic caffeine use, abrupt termination of all caffeine use may lead to caffeine-withdrawal symptoms (described in detail in the section on caffeine withdrawal). Because symptoms of caffeine withdrawal can partially overlap with symptoms of caffeine intoxication (e.g., nervousness and anxiety), the time course of symptom resolution can be expected to be protracted, lasting several days to a week or more.

While many people may experience some of the symptoms of caffeine intoxication at some point in their lives, caffeine users do not generally seek out the experience of caffeine intoxication (unlike many other drugs of abuse). The symptoms of caffeine intoxication tend to be perceived as unpleasant, and caffeine users tend to titrate their dose of caffeine to avoid intoxication.

Table 18-1	Differential Diagnosis of Caffeine Intoxication
Manic episode	Panic disorder
Amphetamine/cocaine intoxication	Generalized anxiety disorder
Sedative, hypnotic or anxiolytic withdrawal	Medication-induced side effects (e.g., akathisia)
Nicotine withdrawal	Sleep disorders

Differential Diagnosis

The diagnosis of caffeine intoxication is based on the history and clinical presentation of the individual. Ideally, the extent of caffeine exposure can also be assessed by a serum or saliva assay of the caffeine level. In the past, caffeine use has often been overlooked in individuals presenting with symptoms consistent with a caffeine use disorder (Doucette and Willoughby 1980). However, it may be that there is presently a greater awareness of the deleterious effects of caffeine, making clinicians more sensitive to the inclusion of caffeine in a differential diagnosis, and individuals that ingest caffeine more aware of the possible role of excessive caffeine in somatic and psychological symptoms.

Several conditions should be included in the differential diagnosis of caffeine intoxication (Table 18-1). These include other substance-abuse-related disorders (amphetamine or cocaine intoxication; withdrawal from sedatives, hypnotics, anxiolytics, or nicotine), other psychiatric disorders (panic disorder, generalized anxiety disorder, mania, and sleep disorders), medication-induced side effects (e.g., akathisia), and somatic disorders (e.g., pheochromocytoma, hyperthyroidism, gastroesophageal reflux, and arrhythmia). Caffeine intoxication may present with a wide variety of clinical features, and the possibility of caffeine intoxication should be included in the differential diagnosis for individuals with nonspecific complaints, or presentations that do not readily fit into a known diagnostic pattern.

Etiology

Although caffeine intoxication is clearly related to caffeine ingestion, it is not simply the result of a person consuming a high dose of caffeine. Rather, caffeine intoxication represents the relationship between the dose of caffeine consumed, the degree of acquired tolerance to caffeine in that person, and the individual's sensitivity to caffeine.

Tolerance represents an acquired change in responsiveness by an individual as a result of exposure to a drug, such that an increased amount of the drug is required to produce the same effect, or a lesser effect is produced by the same dose of the drug. In a person who regularly consumes caffeine, tolerance may occur to the acute effects of caffeine. Thus, a sensitive person with no tolerance to caffeine might have signs and symptoms of caffeine intoxication in response to a relatively low dose of caffeine (such as 100 mg, the amount found in a typical cup of brewed coffee) (Table 18-2), whereas another person with a high daily consumption of caffeine would show no evidence of intoxication with a similar dose.

In addition to individual differences due to acquired tolerance, substantial differences in sensitivity to caffeine effects have been documented. For instance, drug discrimination studies have shown that the threshold for caffeine discrimination can vary over a tenfold range of doses (Griffiths et al. 1990a, Mumford et al. 1994). There may also be a genetic basis to individual differences to caffeine intoxication. While this evidence is limited, one study used a twin registry to examine genetic influences on caffeine toxicity (Kendler and Prescott 1999). Interestingly, monozygotic versus dizygotic twins had significantly higher concordance rates of caffeine toxicity, suggesting genetic vulnerabilities may contribute to experiencing this disorder. (For a more complete review of genetic vulnerabilities to caffeine use, see also the section on caffeine dependence later.)

Table 18-2	Typical Caffeine Content of Foods and Medications
Substance	**Caffeine content (mg)**
Brewed coffee	100 mg/6 oz
Instant coffee	70 mg/6 oz
Espresso	40 mg/1 oz
Decaffeinated coffee	4 mg/6 oz
Brewed tea	40 mg/6 oz
Instant tea	30 mg/6 oz
Canned or bottled tea	20 mg/12 oz
Caffeinated soda	40 mg/12 oz
Cocoa beverage	7 mg/6 oz
Chocolate milk	4 mg/6 oz
Dark chocolate	20 mg/1 oz
Milk chocolate	6 mg/1 oz
Caffeinated water	100 mg/16.9 oz
Coffee ice cream or yogurt	50 mg/8 oz
Caffeinated gum	50 mg/stick
Caffeine-containing analgesics	32–65 mg/tablet
Stimulants	100–200 mg/tablet
Weight-loss aids	40–100 mg/tablet
Sports nutrition	100 mg/tablet

Source: Griffiths RR, Juliano LM, and Chausmer AL (in press) Caffeine pharmacology and clinical effects. In *Principles of Addiction Medicine*, Graham AN, Schultz TK, Mayo-Smith M, et al. (eds). Chevy Chase, Maryland.

Although caffeine intoxication can occur in the context of habitual chronic consumption of high doses, probably most often it occurs after inadvertent overdosing. Examples include overdosing of intravenous caffeine to children in medical settings (e.g., for respiratory stimulating effects), excessive caffeine consumption in tablet form by students who fail to appreciate the dose being ingested (e.g., to study through the night), and the person who unknowingly consumes a highly concentrated form of caffeine (e.g., caffeinated coffee brewed with caffeine-containing water to create an especially high dose of caffeine in the coffee).

Biological Factors

The principal cellular site of action of caffeine is the adenosine receptor, where caffeine functions as an antagonist (Snyder et al. 1981, Daly 1993, Fredholm et al. 1999). Adenosine produces a wide variety of physiological effects, including decreasing spontaneous electrical activity in brain, inhibiting neurotransmitter release in brain, decreasing spontaneous and operant motor activity, dilating central vasculature, producing antidiuresis, inhibiting renin release, and inhibiting gastric secretion and lipolysis (Daly 1993). As an antagonist of adenosine, many of caffeine's actions are opposite to those produced by adenosine (e.g., central nervous system stimulation, decreased cerebral blood flow, increased renin release and diuresis, increased gastric secretions, and stimulation of respiration).

Caffeine's effects may be related to the direct effects on adenosine as well as indirect effects that are mediated by adenosine. In the latter case, the relationship between adenosine and dopamine functioning has become a particular area of interest and study. Caffeine enhances dopaminergic activity by competitive antagonism of A_{2A} and possibly A_1 receptors that are colocalized and functionally interact with dopamine receptors (Fredholm et al. 1999). Basal adenosine functioning is thought to exert a negative modulation of dopaminergic functioning. Thus, by antagonizing adenosine, caffeine increases dopaminergic activity. Consistent with this mechanism, preclinical behavioral studies show that caffeine produces behavioral effects similar to classic dopaminergically mediated stimulants, such as cocaine and amphetamine, including increased locomotor activity and stimulant-like discriminative stimulus effects. Furthermore, a number of these effects are blocked by dopamine antagonists (Fredholm et al. 1999, Powell et al. 1999, Garrett and Griffiths 1997), or abolished in adenosine receptor knockout mice (El Yacoubi et al. 2000). Although dopaminergically mediated effects may be important to understanding the amphetamine-like stimulant effects of low and moderate doses of caffeine, dopaminergic mechanisms may not be as relevant in understanding the clinical manifestation of caffeine intoxication that emerge at high toxic doses of caffeine.

Caffeine's direct effects on adenosine and indirect effects on dopamine occur at concentrations similar to those attained after typical dietary doses of caffeine. Caffeine can also exert effects on phosphodiesterase and intracellular calcium, although with typical dietary doses of caffeine, blood levels of caffeine are believed to be too low to appreciably affect these nonadenosine mechanisms of actions. Thus, adenosine antagonism appears to be the primary mechanism for caffeine's effects. It is not known whether these other mechanisms may mediate some of the clinical effects produced when caffeine concentrations are elevated (e.g., as may occur with caffeine intoxication).

Treatment

The first step in evaluating an individual with a possible diagnosis of caffeine intoxication is to obtain a careful history about all recent caffeine consumption. The possible use of beverages and medications—both prescription and over-the-counter (OTC) diet aids and energy pills—should be reviewed. Some beverages (e.g., caffeine-containing soft drinks) and medications (e.g., energy pills, aids to combat sleep, or diet pills) may not be recognized by the individual as containing caffeine. The amount of caffeine acutely consumed should help clarify the diagnosis of caffeine intoxication, although it is important to determine whether the individual has been chronically consuming high doses of caffeine. If this is the case, the individual may be tolerant and therefore less likely to be experiencing caffeine intoxication. However, some clinicians have reported that caffeine intoxication can occur even in the context of chronic caffeine use.

If the individual is unable to provide an accurate history of recent caffeine consumption (e.g., because of delirium after a caffeine overdose), the individual should be evaluated on an emergency basis and medically monitored.

The primary approach to the treatment of caffeine intoxication is to teach the individual about the effects of excessive caffeine consumption. In individuals who are resistant to accepting the role of caffeine in their presenting symptoms, it may be useful to suggest a trial-off of caffeine as both a diagnostic and a potentially therapeutic probe.

CAFFEINE WITHDRAWAL

Diagnosis

Like caffeine intoxication, there is a long history of recognition that some people also can experience symptoms of caffeine withdrawal. For example, Bridge (1893) reported on a series of individuals who had various conditions he thought were associated with the use of coffee or tea. He concluded that the cessation of coffee could be beneficial, although individuals were at risk for developing a severe headache acutely with abrupt termination, and he recommended "reducing the rations of coffee gradually through a week or more of time." This observation of headaches associated with the cessation of caffeine use has been repeatedly observed and is now a well-established characteristic of caffeine

Table 18-3	Signs and Symptoms Associated with Caffeine Withdrawal

Headache
Fatigue, lethargy, sluggishness
Sleepiness, drowsiness
Dysphoric mood
Difficulty concentrating
Work difficulty, unmotivated
Depression
Anxiety
Irritability
Nausea or vomiting
Muscle aches or stiffness

withdrawal. Other symptoms, in roughly decreasing order of frequency, are fatigue, sleepiness/drowsiness, dysphoric mood (e.g., miserable, decreased well-being/contentedness), difficulty concentrating, work difficulty, depression, anxiety, irritability, and influenza-like symptoms (e.g., nausea/vomiting, muscle aches/stiffness, hot and cold spells, heavy feelings in arms or legs) (Table 18-3). In addition to these symptoms, caffeine withdrawal may produce impairment in psychomotor, vigilance and cognitive performances, increases in cerebral blood flow, and changes in quantitative electroencephalography (EEG) activity (Jones et al. 2000, Phillips-Bute and Lane 1997, Garrett and Griffiths 1998, Streufert et al. 1995, Griffiths et al. 1990b, Griffiths and Woodson 1988a).

In 1994, the Substance Use Disorders Work Group for DSM-IV had several concerns about the inclusion of a diagnosis of caffeine withdrawal in DSM-IV: only headache, fatigue, and drowsiness were well-validated symptoms, the symptoms of fatigue and drowsiness appeared to overlap, and the three caffeine abstinence symptoms had a high prevalence in the general population and also had several other etiologies (Hughes 1994). The research literature on caffeine withdrawal has almost doubled since 1994 (Griffiths and Chausmer 2000), now providing much better validation of a wider range of symptoms (Table 18-3). The proposed criteria for a DSM-IV-TR research diagnosis of caffeine withdrawal require the presence of headache and one or more of the following: marked fatigue or drowsiness, marked anxiety or depression, and nausea or vomiting. Problems with this approach are that it does not reflect the independence of headache and nonheadache withdrawal symptoms and it excludes several withdrawal symptoms that have been repeatedly documented: difficulty concentrating, work difficulty or feeling unmotivated, and irritable or dysphoric mood (see DSM-IV-TR research criteria below).

DSM-IV-TR Research Criteria

Caffeine Withdrawal

A. Prolonged daily use of caffeine.
B. Abrupt cessation of caffeine use, or reduction in the amount of caffeine used, closely followed by headache and one (or more) of the following symptoms:

   (1) marked fatigue or drowsiness
   (2) marked anxiety or depression
   (3) nausea or vomiting

C. The symptoms in Criterion B cause clinically significant distress or impairment in social, occupational, or other important areas of functioning.

D. The symptoms are not due to the direct physiologic effects of a general medical condition (e.g., migraine, viral illness) and are not better accounted for by another mental disorder.

Reprinted with permission from the Diagnostic and Statistical Manual of Mental Disorders, Fourth Edition, Text Revision. Copyright 2000 American Psychiatric Association.

On the basis of the expanded research literature, we now propose that the diagnosis of caffeine withdrawal requires the presence of three or more of the following five symptom clusters: (1) headache, (2) fatigue or drowsiness, (3) dysphoric mood (including irritability, depression, or anxiety), (4) difficulty concentrating or work difficulty, and (5) nausea or vomiting. The new criteria address the 1994 DSM-IV Work Group concerns that there were too few validated symptoms and there may be an overlap between fatigue and drowsiness. Although it remains true that some of the proposed symptoms have high prevalence and may have other etiologies, this is also true of other withdrawal diagnoses recognized by DSM (e.g., cocaine withdrawal, nicotine withdrawal, and opioid withdrawal). The only study to evaluate the incidence of caffeine withdrawal using the criteria for the DSM-IV-TR research diagnosis was a random-digit telephone survey of the general population (Hughes et al. 1998). Among individuals who reported trying to stop caffeine use permanently, 24% had symptoms that met criteria for the diagnosis of caffeine withdrawal.

The key steps in establishing a diagnosis of caffeine withdrawal are to determine the history of the person's caffeine consumption from all dietary sources, and then establish whether there has been a significant decrease in caffeine intake. The diagnostic decision tree for caffeine-dependence and caffeine-withdrawal is shown in Figure 18-2. Caffeine withdrawal is probably more common than is generally recognized, and it seems there is a tendency for people to attribute the symptoms of caffeine withdrawal to other etiologies besides caffeine (e.g., having the flu, or a bad day). Caffeine withdrawal may be particularly common in medical settings where individuals are required to abstain from food and fluids, such as before surgical procedures and certain diagnostic tests. In addition, caffeine withdrawal may occur in settings where the use of caffeine-containing products is restricted or banned, such as inpatient psychiatric wards.

The most common feature of caffeine withdrawal is headache (Table 18-4) (Griffiths and Woodson 1988a, Griffiths et al. in press, Lader et al. 1996, Griffiths and Mumford 1995). Caffeine-withdrawal headache is typically described as gradual in development, diffuse, throbbing, and sometimes accompanied by nausea and vomiting (Griffiths and Woodson 1988a, Lader et al. 1996, Griffiths and Mumford 1995). It is relieved with caffeine consumption and it may be worsened with physical exercise and Valsalva maneuver (Dreisbach and Pfeiffer 1943). Careful double-blind studies of caffeine withdrawal have shown that headache generally occurs 12 to 24 hours after the last dose of caffeine (Griffiths et al. 1986, 1990b) (mean 19 hours), although headache onset as late as about 40 hours has been documented (Griffiths et al. 1990b). Caffeine-withdrawal headache usually resolves

Table 18-4	Features of Caffeine-Withdrawal — Headache

Gradual onset between 12 and 40 hours
Worse with exercise, Valsalva maneuver
Can be accompanied by flu-like symptoms (including nausea, vomiting)
Diffuse, throbbing, severe

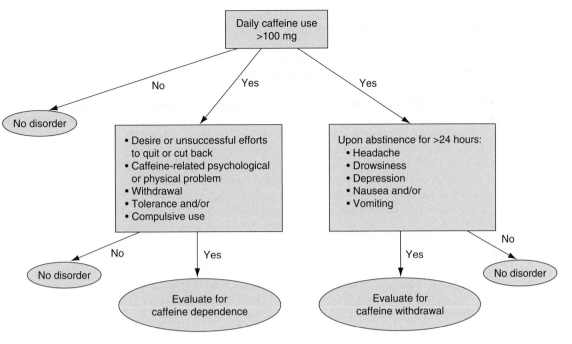

Figure 18-2 *Diagnostic decision tree for caffeine-dependence disorder and caffeine-withdrawal disorder.*

within 2 to 4 days, although some subjects continue to report sporadic headaches for as long as 11 days after cessation of caffeine use (Griffiths et al. 1986, 1990b).

Clinical reports, correlation analyses, and cluster analysis of withdrawal symptoms indicate that nonheadache signs and symptoms of caffeine withdrawal do not always covary with the presence of headache, and can occur in the absence of headache (Garrett and Griffiths 1998, Griffiths et al. 1990b, Griffiths and Woodson 1988a, Evans and Griffiths 1999, Lader et al. 1996). This indicates that nonheadache symptoms represent distinct features of the caffeine-withdrawal syndrome that can occur independently of headache.

When symptoms of caffeine withdrawal occur, the severity can vary from mild to extreme. At its worst, caffeine withdrawal has been repeatedly documented to produce clinically significant distress or impairment in daily functioning and, on rare occasions, to be totally incapacitating (Bridge 1893, Griffiths et al. 1990b, Lader et al. 1996, Strain et al. 1994, Dreisbach and Pfeiffer 1943, Kingdon 1833, Silverman et al. 1992, Greden et al. 1980, Cobbs 1982, Goldstein and Kaizer 1969, Rainey 1985). For example, in a double-blind caffeine-withdrawal evaluation, 73% of individuals whose pattern of caffeine use met criteria for DSM-IV-TR substance dependence on caffeine reported functional impairment in normal activities during an experimental withdrawal phase (Strain et al. 1994).

The proportion of regular caffeine consumers who are at risk for experiencing such functional impairment during caffeine withdrawal is difficult to estimate. Several rigorous blind studies indicate that the incidence of moderate to severe headache is about 50% in healthy normal subjects abstaining from caffeine (Lader et al. 1996, Dreisbach and Pfeiffer 1943, Silverman et al. 1992). One of these studies reported that 28% of those reporting headache also reported nausea and sickness (Lader et al. 1996). Dews and colleagues (1999) reported that 22% of 18 subjects who previously reported experiencing withdrawal symptoms showed substantial decreases in their ratings of daily functioning (e.g., work and leisure activities) during caffeine abstinence. The relatively lower rate of severe withdrawal symptoms in this study may be due to methodological shortcomings (Griffiths et al. in press).

Although most research on caffeine withdrawal has been conducted in adults, several studies document that children also experience withdrawal effects during caffeine abstinence (Goldstein and Wallace 1997, Bernstein et al. 1998, 2002, Hale et al. 1995). There is also one report of eight infants with suspected caffeine withdrawal born to mothers who had heavy caffeine consumption during their pregnancies (range: 200–1800 mg/day) (McGowan et al. 1988). Symptoms that began on an average of 19 hours after birth were primarily irritability, jitteriness, and vomiting, and resolved spontaneously.

Individuals with high daily caffeine consumption (Evans and Griffiths 1999, Weber et al. 1997), or individuals with a history of frequent headaches (Weber et al. 1997) may be at increased risk for developing caffeine withdrawal or caffeine-withdrawal headaches.

Caffeine abstinence has been shown to contribute to the incidence and severity of postoperative headache after general anesthesia. Studies in individuals required to abstain from caffeine in preparation for an operative procedure have shown that a history of preoperative caffeine is associated with an increased risk for postoperative headache (Nikolajsen et al. 1994) and that this risk may be dose-related (Fennelly et al. 1991, Galletly et al. 1989). In individuals with a history of caffeine consumption who received caffeine on the day of a surgical procedure, the rate of postoperative headaches was lower than in those who received placebo (Weber et al. 1997, Hampl et al. 1995).

Epidemiology

There are two types of studies that have examined the prevalence/incidence of caffeine withdrawal. In the first, caffeine withdrawal is experimentally induced, and in the second, there is an epidemiologic assessment of the prevalence/incidence of caffeine withdrawal, usually through the use of some form of a retrospective questionnaire. The results of eight blind experimental studies in healthy normal caffeine users who abstained for ≥ 24 hours indicated that the incidence of headache is about 50% (ranging from 30 to 86%) (Griffiths et al. in press). A similar incidence of headache has been reported in studies of subjects specifically selected for reporting problems with caffeine use or withdrawal (Strain et al. 1994, Dews et al. 1999). Not surprisingly, the incidence is higher (ranging from 39 to 100%) when withdrawal symptoms in addition to headache are considered (Griffiths et al. 1990b, Hughes et al. 1993, Lader et al. 1996, Strain et al. 1994, Dews et al. 1999).

Survey studies have also been conducted to determine the prevalence/incidence of caffeine withdrawal. In a population-based random digit-dial telephone survey study (Hughes et al. 1998b), 44% of caffeine users reported having stopped or reduced caffeine use for at least 24 hours in the past year. Of those, 41% reported that they experienced one or more DSM-IV-TR-defined caffeine-withdrawal symptoms. Among individuals who stopped caffeine use in an attempt to abstain permanently, 71% reported experiencing one or more DSM-IV-TR-defined symptoms, and 24% reported having headache plus other symptoms that interfered with performance. In another study, which surveyed individuals who called about possible participation in a clinical research trial, only 11% of caffeine users indicated that they had problems or symptoms on stopping caffeine in the past (Dews et al. 1999). However, the number of individuals who actually abstained from caffeine was not determined, nor was there an assessment of whether symptoms may have been underreported because of the desire to participate in a research trial.

It seems likely that survey studies may underestimate the rate of caffeine withdrawal. Many caffeine consumers may be unaware of their vulnerability to caffeine-withdrawal symptoms, because their routine habitual consumption never involves a period of sustained abstinence, and they may misattribute withdrawal symptoms such as headache, nausea, and muscle aches to other ailments such as viral infection. Furthermore, since as little as 25 mg/day of caffeine is sufficient to suppress withdrawal (Evans and Griffiths 1999), even small amounts of caffeine that are unknowingly consumed during presumed caffeine abstinence may result in underestimates of the frequency of withdrawal.

Course

Caffeine withdrawal generally begins within 12 to 24 hours after discontinuing caffeine use. The peak of caffeine withdrawal generally occurs within 24 to 48 hours, and the duration of caffeine withdrawal is generally 2 days to about 1 week. In this study, four volunteers, who initially received 100 mg/day of caffeine in capsules, were switched under double-blind conditions to placebo for a period of 12 days (Griffiths et al. 1990b). Symptoms of headache, lethargy/fatigue/tired/sluggish, and impaired concentration peaked on days 1 or 2 after placebo substitution and progressively returned toward prewithdrawal levels over about a week.

There is considerable variability, both between people and within the same person across episodes, in the manifestations, time course and severity of caffeine withdrawal. No studies have examined the possibility of a protracted caffeine-withdrawal syndrome. See Griffiths and Woodson (1988a), Griffiths and Mumford (1995), Griffiths and colleagues (in press) for a review of human and laboratory animal studies of caffeine withdrawal.

Differential Diagnosis

Caffeine withdrawal should be considered when evaluating individuals presenting with headaches, fatigue, sleepiness, mood disturbances, or impaired concentration. The differential diagnosis of caffeine withdrawal includes: viral illnesses; sinus conditions; other types of headaches such as migraine, tension, postanesthetic; other drug withdrawal states such as amphetamine or cocaine withdrawal; and idiopathic drug reactions.

Etiology

Caffeine withdrawal is the result of a decrease in the amount of caffeine consumed by an individual who has been using it regularly (daily or almost daily). Studies of caffeine withdrawal have generally focused upon the complete cessation of caffeine use, although one study has also shown that a partial decrease (i.e., changing intake from 300 to 100 mg/day) can also produce withdrawal symptoms (Evans and Griffiths 1999).

Several studies have found either the presence of caffeine withdrawal, or its severity are more likely as the daily maintenance dose of caffeine is increased (Evans and Griffiths 1999, Nikolajsen et al. 1994, Fennelly et al. 1991, Galletly et al. 1989), although this relationship is relatively weak because it has not been observed in some studies (Hofer and Battig 1994, Hughes et al. 1993, Lader et al. 1996), and some studies have shown no or only very mild symptoms after stopping high doses of caffeine in some individuals (Griffiths et al. 1986, Strain et al. 1994). It has been shown that caffeine withdrawal can occur with surprisingly low doses of caffeine—as low as 100 mg/day (Griffiths et al. 1990b, Evans and Griffiths 1999), which is the equivalent of about one cup of brewed coffee or two to three caffeinated sodas per day (Table 18-2).

Caffeine withdrawal has been shown to occur after relatively short-term exposure to daily caffeine (Evans and Griffiths 1999, Dreisbach and Pfeiffer 1943). One study showed that significant withdrawal occurred after only three consecutive days of 300 mg/day caffeine, with somewhat greater severity shown after 7 and 14 consecutive days of exposure (Evans and Griffiths 1999). Another study showed that caffeine-withdrawal headache occurred in three individuals who normally abstained from caffeinated beverages but were given 600 to 750 mg/day caffeine for 6 or 7 days (Dreisbach and Pfeiffer 1943).

Low doses of caffeine are capable of suppressing caffeine withdrawal (Watson et al. 2000). One study showed that a small dose of only 25 mg/day was sufficient to suppress caffeine-withdrawal headache in people maintained on 300 mg/day (Evans and Griffiths 1999). This finding suggests that a substantial percentage reduction in caffeine consumption is necessary to manifest the full caffeine-withdrawal syndrome.

Biological Factors

Antagonism of adenosine at adenosine receptors is the primary molecular mechanism underlying most of the central and peripheral physiological effects of caffeine after acute administration (Daly 1993, Fredholm et al. 1999). Chronic caffeine consumption has been shown to produce compensatory upregulation of the adenosine system, resulting in an increase in functional sensitivity to adenosine during caffeine withdrawal (Paul et al. 1993, Kaplan et al. 1993, Varani et al. 1999) (see section on "caffeine intoxication"). Because adenosine produces sedation and cerebral vasodilation (Daly 1993) has been implicated in headache (Guieu et al. 1998), increased sensitivity to endogenous adenosine, particularly in vascular and neural tissue in brain, may be a mechanism underlying the common caffeine-withdrawal symptoms of fatigue and headache. Studies have shown that caffeine abstinence produces increase in cerebral blood flow and cerebral blood flow velocities (Jones et al. 2000, Couturier et al. 1997, Mathew and Wilson 1985). These findings are consistent with a vascular explanation of caffeine-withdrawal symptoms since blood flow has been implicated in headache (Moskowitz et al. 1989, Olesen 1991). Another physiological effect documented during caffeine abstinence is a change in quantitative EEG. Two studies (Jones et al. 2000, Reeves et al. 1995) showed increases in theta activity, an effect generally correlated with drowsiness which is a common caffeine-withdrawal symptom.

Treatment

There have been few studies attempting to address the treatment of caffeine withdrawal, although it has frequently been observed that the symptoms of caffeine withdrawal can be alleviated with the consumption of caffeine (Evans and Griffiths 1999, Dreisbach and Pfeiffer 1943), and this approach is probably best. There has been one report that experimentally induced caffeine-withdrawal headaches responded to aspirin (Dreisbach and Pfeiffer 1943). If the medical recommendation is made to eliminate or substantially reduce caffeine consumption, then it may be useful to recommend a tapering dose schedule rather than abrupt discontinuation. Caffeine tapering (or "fading") is described in more detail in the section on "caffeine dependence".

CAFFEINE DEPENDENCE

Diagnosis

Caffeine dependence, a diagnosis not officially included in DSM-IV-TR, may be an unrecognized condition with a higher prevalence than is generally appreciated (see Figure 18-2). Clinicians do not typically think to inquire about caffeine use and about problematic use consistent with a diagnosis of caffeine dependence. However, probing for evidence of caffeine dependence may be useful, and it would be reasonable to focus upon the DSM-IV-TR criteria for dependence that are more appropriate for a substance that is widely available and generally culturally accepted. Thus, the clinician should probe for evidence of tolerance, withdrawal, and continued use despite a doctor's recommendation that the person cut down or stop using caffeine, use despite other problems associated with caffeine, often using larger amounts or over a longer period than intended, or persistent desires and/or difficulties in decreasing or discontinuing use. For research purposes, a section for the diagnosis of caffeine dependence according to DSM-IV-TR or ICD-10 criteria is now available on the Composite International Diagnostic Interview-Substance Abuse Module (CIDI-SAM), which is a reliable and valid structured interview focused on substance use disorders (Cottler et al. 1989, Compton et al. 1996).

In a study by Strain and colleagues (1994), which characterized DSM-IV-diagnosed caffeine dependence in 16 adults, it was found that two subjects (13%) had an additional current psychiatric diagnosis (both being anxiety disorders), and 69% had other mental disorders in remission. Most commonly, these other disorders were other psychoactive substance use disorders (63%) followed by mood disorders (44%), anxiety disorders (25%), or eating disorders (19%). Among the psychoactive substance use disorders, the most commonly abused substance was alcohol; 57% of the participants in the study had a past diagnosis of alcohol abuse or dependence. Five of the subjects in the study (32%) were nicotine cigarette smokers and, notably, four of these five had a history of an alcohol disorder (suggesting a clustering of caffeine dependence, smoking and alcohol abuse/dependence). One study showed that the severity of caffeine dependence is significantly correlated with the severity of the alcohol dependence, however, dependence on caffeine and nicotine were not correlated (Hughes et al. 2000).

Epidemiology

Caffeine is the most widely used mood-altering drug in the world. In North America, dietary surveys indicate that weekly or more frequent consumption of caffeine-containing foods occurs in 80 to 90% of children and adults (Gilbert 1984, Hughes and Oliveto 1997). In the United States, average daily caffeine consumption among caffeine consumers is 280 mg (Barone and Roberts 1996).

Course

While there are no studies that have specifically examined the course and natural history of caffeine dependence like other drug-dependence syndromes, caffeine dependence appears to be a chronic relapsing disorder. In the study described above by Strain and colleagues (1994), caffeine-dependence participants reported recurrent efforts to discontinue caffeine use, with failures to discontinue use or frequent relapses.

Differential Diagnosis

The diagnosis of caffeine dependence includes symptoms that can also contribute to a diagnosis of caffeine intoxication and caffeine withdrawal, and both of these conditions should be included in the differential diagnosis of an individual with possible caffeine dependence. Since intoxication and withdrawal symptoms can contribute to the diagnosis of dependence, conditions that overlap with these caffeine-related disorders should also be considered (and are reviewed above in their respective sections). When considering an individual for a possible diagnosis of caffeine dependence, the clinician should also consider other substance-dependence syndromes—especially those related to stimulants—in the differential diagnosis. Finally, the possible presence of other psychiatric conditions, such as depressive and anxiety disorders, should be assessed. These disorders may be more commonly found among individuals with caffeine dependence, and some of their presenting features (e.g., low mood, anxiety, and disturbed sleep) can overlap with the symptoms of caffeine intoxication and withdrawal, which commonly occur in caffeine dependence.

Etiology

Factors Influencing Caffeine Consumption

Many studies have shown that caffeine in low to moderate doses (20–200 mg) produces mild positive subjective effects of increased feelings of well-being, alertness, energy, concentration, self-confidence, motivation for work, and a desire to talk to people (Griffiths et al. 1990a, Robelin and Rogers 1998, Griffiths and Woodson 1988b). The profile of positive effects with caffeine is qualitatively similar to that produced by *D*-amphetamine and cocaine, which may reflect a common dopaminergic mechanism of action (Fredholm et al. 1999, Garrett and Griffiths 1997). High doses of caffeine (e.g., 800 mg) produce negative subjective effects such as anxiety and nervousness, especially in people who are not tolerant to caffeine (Griffiths and Woodson 1988b, Chait 1992, Evans and Griffiths 1991).

Consistent with its ability to produce mild positive subjective effects, low to moderate doses of caffeine have also been shown to function as a reinforcer in humans—that is, when given the choice under experimental conditions, some people will consistently choose to consume caffeine rather than placebo (Hughes et al. 1992, 1993, Griffiths and Woodson 1988b, Silverman et al. 1994, Griffiths et al. 1989, Evans et al. 1994). The profile of positive, subjective, and reinforcing effects may help explain the wide and regular consumption of caffeine-containing substances. However, not everyone uses caffeine, and it appears that some people tend to prefer caffeine and others do not.

Studies have shown that repeated pairing of a novel flavored drink with caffeine results in increased ratings of flavor preference, while pairing of a novel flavored drink with placebo results in decreased ratings of pleasantness (Rogers et al. 1995, Richardson et al. 1996, Yeomans et al. 1998, 2000). In caffeine dependence, it seems likely that the development of such conditioned flavor preferences over many days of self-administration plays a role in the development of strong preferences for specific types or even brands of caffeine-containing beverages.

Tolerance refers to a decrease in responsiveness to a drug because of drug exposure. Complete tolerance to caffeine's subjective, pressor, and neuroendocrine (e.g., increases in plasma epinephrine, norepinephrine and renin) effects have been demonstrated when very high doses of caffeine (750–1200 mg/day spread throughout the day) are administered daily (Evans and Griffiths 1992, Robertson et al. 1981). Partial tolerance to the sleep-disruptive effects of caffeine has also been demonstrated (Bonnet and Arand 1992). At lower doses similar to those usually consumed, complete caffeine tolerance does not occur. Survey data indicate 17% of current caffeine users reported tolerance (Hughes et al. 1998b), whereas 75% of a group of caffeine-dependent individuals reported tolerance (Strain et al. 1994). Although tolerance is one of the criteria for making a diagnosis of caffeine dependence (see DSM-IV-TR criteria for substance dependence on page 351), it is not clear what role the development of tolerance may have in the development of clinical dependence upon caffeine.

Caffeine withdrawal, described in detail above, is a distinct clinical syndrome characterized by symptoms including headache, fatigue, sleepiness, dysphoric mood, difficulty concentrating, work difficulty, depression, anxiety, irritability, nausea/vomiting, and muscle aches/stiffness (Table 18-3). Caffeine consumption alleviates caffeine-withdrawal symptoms (Dreisbach and Pfeiffer 1943), and avoidance of withdrawal symptoms associated with caffeine abstinence has been shown to be an important mechanism of the reinforcing effects of caffeine among regular consumers (Garrett and Griffiths 1998, Hughes et al. 1993, Schuh and Griffiths 1997). It is likely that caffeine consumption in people with caffeine dependence may be related in part to the avoidance of caffeine-withdrawal symptoms.

Genetic studies suggest that caffeine use problems have an underlying biological basis, part of which may be shared with other commonly abused substances. Twin studies comparing monozygotic and dizygotic twins showed heritabilities of heavy caffeine use, caffeine tolerance, and caffeine withdrawal which ranged between 35 and 77% (Kendler and Prescott 1999, Swan et al. 1997, Pedersen 1981, Partanen et al. 1966). Other twin studies examining caffeine use, alcohol use, and cigarette smoking concluded that a common genetic factor (polysubstance use) underlies the use of these three substances, with 28 to 41% of the heritable effects of caffeine use (or heavy use) shared with alcohol and smoking (Swan et al. 1997, Hettema et al. 1999).

The conclusion suggested by the genetic studies described above is that a common genetic factor underlies joint use of caffeine, alcohol, and cigarettes. This is consistent with findings of studies on the co-occurrence of use of these three substances (Kozlowski et al. 1993, Talcott et al. 1998). Kozlowski and colleagues (1993) found that severity of alcoholism was directly related to use of caffeine and cigarettes, and they conclude that dependence on caffeine, nicotine and alcohol may be governed by the same factors. Other studies indicate that heavy use of caffeine is related to heavy use of alcohol (Istvan and Matarazzo 1984) and that the severity of caffeine dependence increases as the severity of alcohol dependence increases (Hughes et al. 2000). A study of individuals whose pattern of caffeine use fulfilled DSM-IV-TR diagnostic criteria for substance dependence on caffeine found that almost 60% had a past diagnosis of alcohol abuse or dependence (Strain et al. 1994).

Epidemiological studies have shown that cigarette smokers consume more caffeine than nonsmokers (Istvan and Matarazzo 1984, Swanson et al. 1994), and experimental studies have shown that cigarette smoking and coffee drinking tend to covary temporally within individuals (Emurian et al. 1982, Lane 1996). As described above, twin studies and a study by Kozlowski and colleagues (1993) also indicate the co-occurrence of caffeine use and cigarette smoking, however, dependence on caffeine and nicotine were not correlated in one study (Hughes et al. 2000). Preclinical research indicates that caffeine can enhance the reinforcing effects of nicotine (Shoaib et al. 1999, Tanda and Goldberg 2000).

Surveys of psychiatric patients (typically inpatients) have found high rates of caffeine consumption, particularly among individuals with schizophrenia (Hughes et al. 1998a, Mayo et al. 1993, Greden et al. 1978, Rihs et al. 1996). Other groups at risk may include substance abusers (Russ et al. 1988, Hays et al. 1998) and individuals with anorexia nervosa (Sours 1983). Interestingly, daily coffee consumption shows a J-shaped relation with the risk of suicide, with very high rates of coffee consumption (>7 cups/day) showing the greatest suicide risk, and joint heavy use of coffee, alcohol and cigarettes showing a fourfold increase in risk (Tanskanen et al. 2000a,b, Kawachi et al. 1996).

While preliminary work suggests there may be some factors (such as heritability) that contribute to the predisposition to use caffeine, there are no studies that have examined the possible etiologic role of such factors in the development of caffeine dependence as a specific diagnosis. Caffeine dependence, like other drug-dependence syndromes, in all likelihood represents the interaction of social and cultural forces, and individual histories and predispositions, operating in the context of a psychoactive substance that produces pleasant subjective effects and is reinforcing. A particular value to understanding the etiology to caffeine dependence may be the light it sheds upon the understanding of drug-dependence syndromes generally.

Biological Factors

As has been discussed in the sections on caffeine intoxication and caffeine withdrawal, antagonism of the endogenous neuromodulator adenosine at adenosine receptors is the primary cellular mechanism underlying most of the effects of caffeine, including the mood and performance stimulant effects (Daly 1993, Fredholm et al. 1999) as well as the physiological effects and symptoms accompanying caffeine abstinence.

Table 18-5	A Method for Eliminating or Reducing Caffeine Use

Step 1: Use a daily diary to have the person identify all sources of caffeine in their diet, including different forms (i.e., brewed vs. instant coffee) and doses, for 1 week.

Step 2: Educate the patient about sources of caffeine. For example, some individuals might not be aware that caffeine is present in noncola soft drinks or analgesics. Calculate the total milligrams of caffeine consumed on a daily basis.

Step 3: With the collaboration of the patient, generate a graded dose reduction (i.e., fading schedule) of caffeine use. Reasonable decreases would be 10% of the initial dose every few days. Allow for individualization of the caffeine fading. Rather than attempting to progressively eliminate consumption of the preferred caffeine beverage, it may be useful to suggest that the patient substitute decaffeinated for caffeinated beverages. In the case of coffee or tea, caffeine fading can be accomplished by mixing caffeinated and decaffeinated beverages together and progressively increasing the proportion of decaffeinated beverage. It may be useful to have the patient maintain a diary throughout the time they are progressively decreasing their caffeine use, in order to monitor their progress.

Step 4: Discuss the possibility of relapse with the patient. Discuss triggers (i.e., antecedent conditions) for caffeine use and offer coping suggestions for high risk relapse situations. Suggest that the patient continue to self-monitor caffeine consumption.

Treatment

In a survey of physicians' practices, it was found that over 75% of medical specialists recommend that patients reduce or eliminate caffeine for certain conditions including anxiety, insomnia, arrhythmias, palpitations, and tachycardia, esophagitis/hiatal hernia, and fibrocystic disease (Hughes et al. 1988). However, stopping caffeine use can be difficult for some people. For example, in the diagnostic study of caffeine dependence (Strain et al. 1994), subjects reported physical conditions such as acne rosacea, pregnancy, palpitations, and gastrointestinal problems that led physicians to recommend that they reduce or eliminate caffeine; all reported that they were unable to follow their doctors' recommendations.

While there have been no systematic studies which have examined the treatment of people with a clearly established diagnosis of caffeine dependence, several studies with heavy caffeine consumers demonstrated efficacy of a structured caffeine reduction treatment program (i.e., caffeine fading) in achieving substantial reductions in caffeine consumption (James et al. 1985, 1988, Bernard et al. 1981, Foxx and Rubinoff 1979). These reports have generally noted success with a combination of gradual tapering of caffeine, self-monitoring of daily caffeine use, and reinforcement for decreased use. When attempting to reduce or eliminate caffeine use, several steps may be useful (Table 18-5). Since many individuals are not knowledgeable about sources of caffeine in their diets, education and history taking are likely to be important components of treatment. During caffeine tapering it may be useful for the individual to consume extra noncaffeinated fluids, to avoid herbal preparations which contain caffeine or other psychoactive drugs, to avoid the use of anxiolytics, and to maintain a diary throughout the time they are progressively decreasing their caffeine use in order to monitor their progress. Abrupt cessation of caffeine should be avoided in order to minimize withdrawal symptoms and increase the likelihood of long-term compliance with the dietary change. No data about the probability of relapse is currently available, although relapse after caffeine reduction has been reported (James et al. 1988).

CAFFEINE-INDUCED ANXIETY DISORDER

Diagnosis

In addition to the symptom of anxiety that can be a component of caffeine intoxication and caffeine withdrawal, caffeine can also produce an anxiety disorder, caffeine-induced anxiety disorder (see generic DSM-IV-TR criteria in Chapter 15 on page 357). Although there has been no research using this specific set of diagnostic criteria, there have been several studies examining the relationship between caffeine and anxiety in general, and this work is reviewed here.

Substance-induced anxiety disorders in general are distinguished by prominent anxiety symptoms that are directly related to a psychoactive substance. Whereas the form of the disorder can resemble panic disorder, generalized anxiety disorder, social phobia, or obsessive–compulsive disorder, an individual with a substance-induced anxiety disorder does not need to manifest all the diagnostic criteria of one of these conditions to justify making the diagnosis of a substance-induced anxiety disorder.

The diagnosis of caffeine-induced anxiety disorder is based on evidence of an anxiety disorder etiologically related to caffeine (see previous diagnostic decision tree for caffeine intoxication, caffeine-induced anxiety disorder, and caffeine-induced sleep disorder). Other diagnostic considerations besides caffeine-induced anxiety disorder include caffeine intoxication and caffeine withdrawal, a primary anxiety disorder, and an anxiety disorder due to a general medical condition. Caffeine-induced anxiety disorder can occur in the context of caffeine intoxication or caffeine withdrawal, but the anxiety symptoms associated with the caffeine-induced anxiety disorder should be excessive relative to the anxiety seen in caffeine intoxication or caffeine withdrawal. In addition to these conditions, substance-induced anxiety disorder can be produced by a variety of other psychoactive substances (e.g., cocaine).

Etiology

Caffeine-induced anxiety disorder by definition is etiologically related to caffeine. Caffeine's primary cellular site of action appears to be the adenosine receptor, where it functions as an antagonist (Snyder et al. 1981, Daly 1993, Fredholm et al. 1999, Nehlig et al. 1992), as reviewed in more detail in the caffeine intoxication section above.

Caffeine's ability to produce anxiety has been studied in two populations: persons without an anxiety disorder, and those with an anxiety disorder. While these studies do not directly assess for a caffeine-induced anxiety disorder, they provide evidence that caffeine can be etiologically related to anxiety.

Finally, it has also been shown that individuals with high caffeine consumption have higher rates of minor tranquilizer use (benzodiazepine or meprobamate) than individuals with moderate or low caffeine use (Greden et al. 1981). It is not known whether some individuals consume higher levels of caffeine to antagonize the sedative effects of minor tranquilizers, whether minor tranquilizers are prescribed in response to the anxiogenic effects produced by higher doses of caffeine (Roache and Griffiths 1987), or whether some underlying factors (e.g., personality) may account for the increased use of caffeine and minor tranquilizers together.

Treatment

Although there are no studies on the treatment of caffeine-induced anxiety disorder, guidelines for treatment should generally follow those recommended for the treatment of caffeine dependence (see Caffeine Dependence). Thus, an initial, careful assessment of caffeine consumption should be conducted, and a program of gradual decreasing caffeine use should be instituted (see Table 18-5). Abrupt cessation of caffeine use should be avoided to minimize withdrawal symptoms and to increase the likelihood of long-term compliance with the dietary change. Given the etiological role of caffeine in caffeine-induced anxiety disorder, the prudent course of treatment would avoid the use of pharmacological agents such as benzodiazepines for the treatment of the anxiety disorder until caffeine use has been eliminated. A temporary caffeine-free trial may be useful in persuading skeptical individuals about the role of caffeine in their anxiety symptoms.

CAFFEINE-INDUCED SLEEP DISORDER

Diagnosis

Psychoactive substances can produce sleep disorders distinct from the sleep disturbances associated with intoxication or withdrawal produced by that substance. It has long been recognized that caffeine-containing products can produce sleep disturbances, primarily in the form of insomnia. For example, Chavanne (1911) wrote that "black coffee will make some people lie awake and try to stare through the ceiling . . .." Although caffeine primarily produces insomnia, there are case reports of hypersomnia associated with acute use of caffeine (Regestein 1989).

The primary feature of a substance-induced sleep disorder is a sleep disturbance directly related to a psychoactive substance (see generic DSM-IV-TR diagnostic criteria for Substance-Induced Sleep Disorder, Chapter 15 on page 359). The form of the disorder can be insomnia, hypersomnia, parasomnia, or mixed, although caffeine typically produces insomnia. In general, sleep disturbance can often be a feature of substance intoxication or withdrawal (although sleep disturbance does not typically occur with caffeine withdrawal), and caffeine-induced sleep disorder should be diagnosed in individuals who are having caffeine intoxication only if the symptoms of the sleep disturbance are excessive relative to what would typically be expected.

In addition to caffeine-induced sleep disorder, it is worth noting that complaints of poor sleep that are not severe enough to qualify as a "disorder" may also be related to caffeine use. It is not uncommon for individuals to complain of sleep difficulties while failing to recognize the possible role of caffeine ingestion in their complaints (Brown et al. 1995). A careful assessment of caffeine use, including time of use and quantity, should be included in the evaluation of an individual with sleep difficulties, even if these sleep problems do not constitute a sleep disorder.

The diagnosis of a caffeine-induced sleep disorder is based on evidence of a sleep disorder etiologically related to caffeine (see previous diagnostic decision tree for caffeine intoxication, caffeine-induced anxiety disorder, and caffeine-induced sleep disorder). Other diagnostic considerations include caffeine intoxication and caffeine withdrawal, a primary sleep disorder, insomnia or hypersomnia related to another mental disorder, and a sleep disorder due to a general medical condition. A caffeine-induced sleep disorder can occur in the context of caffeine intoxication or caffeine withdrawal, but the sleep symptoms associated with the caffeine-induced sleep disorder should be excessive relative to the sleep disturbance seen in caffeine intoxication or caffeine withdrawal.

Although caffeine consumption may decrease with age, the elderly commonly report increased sleeping problems, which may be exacerbated by caffeine (Curless et al. 1993). Occult caffeine consumption in the form of analgesic medication may produce sleep problems in the elderly (Brown et al. 1995).

As with caffeine-induced anxiety disorder, a trial of caffeine abstinence may be useful in confirming the diagnosis and helping to convince a skeptical individual about the etiological significance of caffeine in their sleep disorder.

Course

There is little information available on the course or natural history of caffeine-induced sleep disorder. Sleep disturbances due to caffeine are more likely to occur in people who are not regular caffeine consumers (Colton et al. 1968). In a study of caffeine use as a model of acute and chronic insomnia, subjects maintained on a high dose of caffeine (1200 mg/day) for 1 week demonstrated some adaptation to the sleep-altering effects of caffeine (Bonnet and Arand 1992). Thus, caffeine-induced sleep disorder may be a time-limited condition that reflects relatively acute responses to the effects of caffeine.

Etiology

Caffeine-induced sleep disorder by definition is etiologically related to caffeine. Caffeine's effects on sleep can depend on a variety of factors, such as the dose of caffeine ingested, the individual's tolerance to caffeine, the time between caffeine ingestion and attempted sleep onset, and the ingestion of other psychoactive substances. The effects of caffeine on various measures of sleep quality are an increasing function of dose (Karacan et al. 1976, Hindmarch et al. 2000, Alford et al. 1996). Caffeine administered immediately prior to bedtime or throughout the day has been shown to delay onset of sleep and rapid eye-movement sleep, reduce total sleep time, alter the normal stages of sleep, and decrease the reported quality of sleep (Hindmarch et al. 2000, Alford et al. 1996, Goldstein 1964, Snel 1993).

Caffeine–induced sleep disturbance is greatest among individuals who are not regular caffeine users (Snel 1993, Colton et al. 1968). It is not known if this difference is due to acquired caffeine tolerance or to preexisting population differences in sensitivity to caffeine (Goldstein 1964, Snel 1993, Goldstein et al. 1965). Although some acquired tolerance to the sleep disrupting effects of caffeine has been demonstrated (Bonnet and Arand 1992, Zwyghuizen-Doorenbos et al. 1990), complete tolerance may not occur. Therefore, regular consumers of caffeine may still experience caffeine-induced sleep problems (Goldstein 1964, Goldstein et al. 1965). In addition to caffeine's well-documented ability to disrupt sleep, a few studies have shown that caffeine withdrawal after acute abstinence from chronic caffeine can increase sleep duration and quality (Goldstein et al. 1965, James 1998).

The mechanism for caffeine-induced sleep disorder is not known, although caffeine's primary action appears to be that of an adenosine antagonist (as described in the section on "caffeine intoxication").

Although caffeine can produce a sleep disorder, it should be noted that caffeine's effects on sleep may also serve beneficial effects under certain circumstances. Studies have examined the use of caffeine to counteract the effects of sleep deprivation. In general, it appears that caffeine dose-dependently reverses the effects of 1 to 2 days of sleep deprivation (Wesensten et al. 2002, Penetar et al. 1993, Borland et al. 1986). Compared to lower acute doses, 600 mg of caffeine shows greater efficacy in attenuating the effects of sleep deprivation over a several hour period of time, although lower doses of caffeine are not necessarily ineffective and may exert beneficial effects that are primarily shorter in duration (Reyner and Horne 2000). However, naps can also improve performance in sleep-deprived individuals, and combining caffeine with naps may be particularly effective in counteracting the effects of sleep deprivation (Reyner and Horne 1998, Bonnet et al. 1995).

Treatment

There are no studies on the treatment of caffeine-induced sleep disorder. As for other conditions associated with caffeine use, such as caffeine dependence, caffeine intoxication, and caffeine-induced anxiety disorder, general guidelines for caffeine reduction can be recommended. These include an initial assessment of total caffeine consumption followed by a program of gradually decreasing caffeine use (see Table 18-5). Abrupt cessation of caffeine use should be avoided to minimize withdrawal symptoms and to increase the likelihood of long-term compliance with the dietary change. Given the etiological role of caffeine in caffeine-induced sleep disorder, the use of pharmacological agents or other interventions to improve sleep should be avoided until an adequate trial-off caffeine establishes the presence of a noncaffeine-related sleep disorder.

Comparison of DSM-IV-TR/ICD-10 Diagnostic Criteria
ICD-10 includes caffeine-related disorders in its "Other Stimulant" class which also includes amphetamines. This results in the ICD-10 Diagnostic Criteria for Research for Caffeine Intoxication being the same as those for amphetamine intoxication.

References

Alford C, Bhatti J, Leigh T, et al. (1996) Caffeine-induced sleep disruption: effects on waking the following day and its reversal with an hypnotic. *Hum Psychopharmacol* **11**, 185–198.

Balogh A, Harder S, Vollandt R, et al. (1992) Intra-individual variability of caffeine elimination in healthy subjects. *Int J Clin Pharmacol Ther Toxicol* **30**(10), 383–387.

Barone JJ and Roberts HR (1996) Caffeine consumption. *Food Chem Toxicol* **34**(1), 119–129.

Bernard ME, Dennehy S, and Keefauver LW (1981) Behavioral treatment of excessive coffee and tea drinking: a case study and partial replication. *Behav Ther* **12**, 543–548.

Bernstein GA, Carroll ME, Dean NW, et al. (1998) Caffeine withdrawal in normal school-age children. *J Am Acad Child Adolesc Psychiatry* **37**(8), 858–865.

Bernstein GA, Carroll ME, Thuras PD, et al. (2002) Caffeine dependence in teenagers. *Drug Alcohol Depend* **66**(1), 1–6.

Bonnet MH and Arand DL (1992) Caffeine use as a model of acute and chronic insomnia. *Sleep* **15**(6), 526–536.

Bonnet MH, Gomez S, Wirth O, et al. (1995) The use of caffeine versus prophylactic naps in sustained performance. *Sleep* **18**(2), 97–104.

Borland RG, Rogers AS, Nicholson AN, et al. (1986) Performance overnight in shiftworkers operating a day–night schedule. *Aviat Space Environ Med* **57**(3), 241–249.

Bradley JR and Petree A (1990) Caffeine consumption, expectancies of caffeine-enhanced performance, and caffeinism symptoms among university students. *J Drug Educ* **20**(4), 319–328.

Bram I (1913) The truth about coffee drinking. *Med Summary* **35**, 168–173.

Bridge N (1893) Coffee-drinking as a frequent cause of disease. *Trans Assoc Am Phys* **8**, 281–288.

Brown SL, Salive ME, Pahor M, et al. (1995) Occult caffeine as a source of sleep problems in an older population. *J Am Geriatr Soc* **43**(8), 860–864.

Bullard WN (1889) The relation of tea drinking to disorders of the nervous system. *Med Commun Mass Med Soc* **14**, 71–87.

Chait LD (1992) Factors influencing the subjective response to caffeine. *Behav Pharmacol* **3**(3), 219–228.

Chavanne H (1911) Coffee. *J Med Soc N J* **8**, 19–22.

Cobbs LW (1982) Lethargy, anxiety, and impotence in a diabetic. *Hosp Pract* **17**(8), 67, 70, 73.

Cole J (1833) On the deleterious effects produced by drinking tea and coffee in excessive quantities. *Lancet* **2**, 274–278.

Colton T, Gosselin RE, and Smith RP (1968) The tolerance of coffee drinkers to caffeine. *Clin Pharmacol Ther* **9**(1), 31–39.

Compton WM, Cottler LB, Dorsey KB, et al. (1996) Comparing assessments of DSM-IV substance dependence disorders using CIDI-SAM and SCAN. *Drug Alcohol Depend* **41**(3), 179–187.

Cottler LB, Robins LN, and Helzer JE (1989) The reliability of the CIDI-SAM: a comprehensive substance abuse interview. *Br J Addict* **84**(7), 801–814.

Couturier EG, Laman DM, van Duijn MA, et al. (1997) Influence of caffeine and caffeine withdrawal on headache and cerebral blood flow velocities. *Cephalalgia* **17**(3), 188–190.

Curless R, French JM, James OF, et al. (1993) Is caffeine a factor in subjective insomnia of elderly people? *Age Ageing* **22**(1), 41–45.

Daly JW (1993) Mechanism of action of caffeine. In *Caffeine, Coffee and Health*, Garattini S (ed). Raven Press, New York, pp. 97–150.

Dews PB, Curtis GL, Hanford KJ, et al. (1999) The frequency of caffeine withdrawal in a population-based survey and in a controlled, blinded pilot experiment. *J Clin Pharmacol* **39**(12), 1221–1232.

Doucette SR and Willoughby A (1980) Relevance of caffeine symptomatology to alcohol rehabilitation efforts. *US Navy Med* **71**(10), 6–13.

Dreisbach RH and Pfeiffer C (1943) Caffeine-withdrawal headache. *J Lab Clin Med* **28**, 1212–1219.

El Yacoubi M, Ledent C, Parmentier M, et al. (2000) The anxiogenic-like effect of caffeine in two experimental procedures measuring anxiety in the mouse is not shared by selective A(2A) adenosine receptor antagonists. *Psychopharmacology (Berl)* **148**(2), 153–163.

Emurian HH, Nellis MJ, Brady JV, et al. (1982) Event time-series relationship between cigarette smoking and coffee drinking. *Addict Behav* **7**(4), 441–444.

Evans SM and Griffiths RR (1991) Dose-related caffeine discrimination in normal volunteers: individual differences in subjective effects and self-reported cues. *Behav Pharmacol* **2**,(4–5), 345–356.

Evans SM and Griffiths RR (1992) Caffeine tolerance and choice in humans. *Psychopharmacology* **108**,(1–2), 51–59.

Evans SM and Griffiths RR (1999) Caffeine withdrawal: a parametric analysis of caffeine dosing conditions. *J Pharmacol Exp Ther* **289**(1), 285–294.

Evans SM, Critchfield TS, and Griffiths RR (1994) Caffeine reinforcement demonstrated in a majority of moderate caffeine users. *Behav Pharmacol* **5**(3), 231–238.

Fennelly M, Galletly DC, and Purdie GI (1991) Is caffeine withdrawal the mechanism of postoperative headache? *Anesth Analg* **72**(4), 449–453.

Foxx RM and Rubinoff A (1979) Behavioral treatment of caffeinism: reducing excessive coffee drinking. *J Appl Behav Anal* **12**(3), 335–344.

Fredholm BB, Battig K, Holmen J, et al. (1999) Actions of caffeine in the brain with special reference to factors that contribute to its widespread use. *Pharmacol Rev* **51**(1), 83–133.

Furlong FW (1975) Possible psychiatric significance of excessive coffee consumption. *Can Psychiatr Assoc J* **20**(8), 577–583.

Galletly DC, Fennelly M, and Whitwam JG (1989) Does caffeine withdrawal contribute to postanaesthetic morbidity? *Lancet* **1**(8650), 1335.

Garrett BE and Griffiths RR (1997) The role of dopamine in the behavioral effects of caffeine in animals and humans. *Pharmacol Biochem Behav* **57**(3), 533–541.

Garrett BE and Griffiths RR (1998) Physical dependence increases the relative reinforcing effects of caffeine versus placebo. *Psychopharmacology (Berl)* **139**(3), 195–202.

Gilbert RM (1984) Caffeine consumption. In *The Methylxanthine Beverages and Foods: Chemistry, Consumption, and Health Effects*, Spiller GA (ed). Alan R. Liss, New York, pp. 185–213.

Gilliland K and Andress D (1981) Ad lib caffeine consumption, symptoms of caffeinism, and academic performance. *Am J Psychiatry* **138**(4), 512–514.

Goldstein A (1964) Wakefulness caused by caffeine. *Naunyn Schmiedebergs Arch Pharmacol* **248**, 269–278.

Goldstein A and Kaizer S (1969) Psychotropic effects of caffeine in man. 3. A questionnaire survey of coffee drinking and its effects in a group of housewives. *Clin Pharmacol Ther* **10**(4), 477–488.

Goldstein A, Warren R, and Kaizer S (1965) Psychotropic effects of caffeine in man. I. Individual differences in sensitivity to caffeine-induced wakefulness. *J Pharmacol Exp Ther* **149**(1), 156–159.

Goldstein A and Wallace ME (1997) Caffeine dependence in schoolchildren? *Exp Clin Psychopharmacol* **5**(4), 388–392.

Graham DM (1978) Caffeine—its identity, dietary sources, intake and biological effects. *Nutr Rev* **36**(4), 97–102.

Greden JF (1974) Anxiety or caffeinism: a diagnostic dilemma. *Am J Psychiatry* **131**(10), 1089–1092.

Greden JF, Fontaine P, Lubetsky M, et al. (1978) Anxiety and depression associated with caffeinism among psychiatric inpatients. *Am J Psychiatry* **135**(8), 963–966.

Greden JF, Procter A, and Victor B (1981) Caffeinism associated with greater use of other psychotropic agents. *Compr Psychiatry* **22**(6), 565–571.

Greden JF, Victor BS, Fontaine P, et al. (1980) Caffeine-withdrawal headache: a clinical profile. *Psychosomatics* **21**(5), 411–413, 417–418.

Griffiths RR, Bigelow GE, and Liebson IA (1986) Human coffee drinking: reinforcing and physical dependence producing effects of caffeine. *J Pharmacol Exp Ther* **239**(2), 416–425.

Griffiths RR, Bigelow GE, and Liebson IA (1989) Reinforcing effects of caffeine in coffee and capsules. *J Exp Anal Behav* **52**(2), 127–140.

Griffiths RR and Chausmer AL (2000) Caffeine as a model drug of dependence: recent developments in understanding caffeine withdrawal, the caffeine dependence syndrome, and caffeine negative reinforcement. *Nihon Shinkei Seishin Yakurigaku Zasshi* **20**(5), 223–231.

Griffiths RR, Evans SM, Heishman SJ, et al. (1990a) Low-dose caffeine discrimination in humans. *J Pharmacol Exp Ther* **252**(3), 970–978.

Griffiths RR, Evans SM, Heishman SJ, et al. (1990b) Low-dose caffeine physical dependence in humans. *J Pharmacol Exp Ther* **255**(3), 1123–1132.

Griffiths RR, Juliano LM, and Chausmer AL (in press) Caffeine pharmacology and clinical effects. In *Principles of Addiction Medicine*, Graham AN, Schultz TK, Mayo-Smith M, et al. (eds). Chevy Chase, MD.

Griffiths RR and Mumford GK (1995) Caffeine—a drug of abuse? In *Psychopharmacology: The Fourth Generation of Progress*, Bloom FE and Kupfer DJ (eds). Raven Press, New York, pp. 1699–1713.

Griffiths RR and Woodson PP (1988a) Caffeine physical dependence: a review of human and laboratory animal studies. *Psychopharmacology* **94**(4), 437–451.

Griffiths RR and Woodson PP (1988b) Reinforcing effects of caffeine in humans. *J Pharmacol Exp Ther* **246**(1), 21–29.

Guieu R, Devaux C, Henry H, et al. (1998) Adenosine and migraine. *Can J Neurol Sci* **25**(1), 55–58.

Hale KL, Hughes JR, Oliveto AH, et al. (1995) Caffeine self-administration and subjective effects in adolescents. *Exp Clin Psychopharmacol* **3**(4), 364–370.

Hampl KF, Schneider MC, Ruttimann U, et al. (1995) Perioperative administration of caffeine tablets for prevention of postoperative headaches. *Can J Anaesth* **42**(9), 789–792.

Hays LR, Farabee D, and Miller W (1998) Caffeine and nicotine use in an addicted population. *J Addict Dis* **17**(1), 47–54.

Hettema JM, Corey LA, and Kendler KS (1999) A multivariate genetic analysis of the use of tobacco, alcohol, and caffeine in a population based sample of male and female twins. *Drug Alcohol Depend* **57**(1), 69–78.

Hindmarch I, Rigney U, Stanley N, et al. (2000) A naturalistic investigation of the effects of day-long consumption of tea, coffee and water on alertness, sleep onset and sleep quality. *Psychopharmacology (Berl)* **149**(3), 203–216.

Hofer I and Battig K (1994) Cardiovascular, behavioral, and subjective effects of caffeine under field conditions. *Pharmacol Biochem Behav* **48**(4), 899–908.

Holle C, Heimberg RG, Sweet RA, et al. (1995) Alcohol and caffeine use by social phobics: an initial inquiry into drinking patterns and behavior. *Behav Res Ther* **33**(5), 561–566.

Hughes JR (1994) Caffeine withdrawal, dependence, and abuse. In *DSM-IV Sourcebook*, Widiger TA, Frances AJ, and Pincus HA (eds). American Psychiatric Association, Washington, DC, pp. 129–134.

Hughes JR, Amori G, and Hatsukami DK (1988) A survey of physician advice about caffeine. *J Subst Abuse* **1**(1), 67–70.

Hughes JR, Hunt WK, Higgins ST, et al. (1992) Effect of dose on the ability of caffeine to serve as a reinforcer in humans. *Behav Pharmacol* **3**(3), 211–218.

Hughes JR, McHugh P, and Holtzman S (1998a) Caffeine and schizophrenia. *Psychiatr Serv* **49**(11), 1415–1417.

Hughes JR and Oliveto AH (1997) A systematic survey of caffeine intake in Vermont. *Exp Clin Psychopharmacol* **5**(4), 393–398.

Hughes JR, Oliveto AH, Bickel WK, et al. (1993) Caffeine self-administration and withdrawal: incidence, individual differences and interrelationships. *Drug Alcohol Depend* **32**(3), 239–246.

Hughes JR, Oliveto AH, Liguori A, et al. (1998b) Endorsement of DSM-IV dependence criteria among caffeine users. *Drug Alcohol Depend* **52**(2), 99–107.

Hughes JR, Oliveto AH, and MacLaughlin M (2000) Is dependence on one drug associated with dependence on other drugs? The cases of alcohol, caffeine and nicotine. *Am J Addict* **9**(3), 196–201.

Istvan J and Matarazzo JD (1984) Tobacco, alcohol, and caffeine use: a review of their interrelationships. *Psychol Bull* **95**(2), 301–326.

James JE (1998) Acute and chronic effects of caffeine on performance, mood, headache, and sleep. *Neuropsychobiology* **38**(1), 32–41.

James JE, Paull I, Cameron-Traub E, et al. (1988) Biochemical validation of self-reported caffeine consumption during caffeine fading. *J Behav Med* **11**(1), 15–30.

James JE, Stirling KP, and Hampton BAM (1985) Caffeine fading: behavioral treatment of caffeine abuse. *Behav Ther* **16**, 15–27.

Jones HE, Herning RI, Cadet JL, et al. (2000) Caffeine withdrawal increases cerebral blood flow velocity and alters quantitative electroencephalography (EEG) activity. *Psychopharmacology (Berl)* **147**(4), 371–377.

Kaplan GB, Greenblatt DJ, Kent MA, et al. (1993) Caffeine treatment and withdrawal in mice: relationships between dosage, concentrations, locomotor activity and A1 adenosine receptor binding. *J Pharmacol Exp Ther* **266**(3), 1563–1572.

Karacan I, Thornby JI, Anch M, et al. (1976) Dose-related sleep disturbances induced by coffee and caffeine. *Clin Pharmacol Ther* **20**(6), 682–689.

Kawachi I, Willett WC, Colditz GA, et al. (1996) A prospective study of coffee drinking and suicide in women. *Arch Intern Med* **156**(5), 521–525.

Kendler KS and Prescott CA (1999) Caffeine intake, tolerance, and withdrawal in women: a population-based twin study. *Am J Psychiatry* **156**(2), 223–228.

King E (1903) Tea and coffee intoxication. *Am Med* **5**, 182–183.

Kingdon (1833) Effects of tea and coffee drinking. *Lancet* **II**, 47–48.

Kozlowski LT, Henningfield JE, Keenan RM, et al. (1993) Patterns of alcohol, cigarette, and caffeine and other drug use in two drug abusing populations. *J Subst Abuse Treat* **10**(2), 171–179.

Lader M, Cardwell C, Shine P, et al. (1996) Caffeine withdrawal symptoms and rate of metabolism. *J Psychopharmacol* **10**(2), 110–118.

Lane JD (1996) Association of coffee drinking with cigarette smoking in the natural environment. *Exp Clin Psychopharmacol* **4**(4), 409–412.

Love IN (1891) Coffee, its use and abuse. *JAMA* **16**, 219–221.

Mathew RJ and Wilson WH (1985) Caffeine consumption, withdrawal and cerebral blood flow. *Headache* **25**(6), 305–309.

Mayo KM, Falkowski W, and Jones CA (1993) Caffeine: use and effects in long-stay psychiatric patients. *Br J Psychiatry* **162**, 543–545.

McGowan JD, Altman RE, and Kanto WP Jr. (1988) Neonatal withdrawal symptoms after chronic maternal ingestion of caffeine. *S Med J* **81**(9), 1092–1094.

Moskowitz MA, Buzzi MG, Sakas DE, et al. (1989) Pain mechanisms underlying vascular headaches. Progress report 1989. *Rev Neurol* **145**(3), 181–193.

Mumford GK, Evans SM, Kaminski BJ, et al. (1994) Discriminative stimulus and subjective effects of theobromine and caffeine in humans. *Psychopharmacology (Berl)* **115**,(1–2), 1–8.

Nehlig A, Daval JL, and Debry G (1992) Caffeine and the central nervous system: mechanisms of action, biochemical, metabolic and psychostimulant effects. *Brain Res Rev* **17**(2), 139–170.

Nikolajsen L, Larsen KM, and Kierkegaard O (1994) Effect of previous frequency of headache, duration of fasting and caffeine abstinence on perioperative headache. *Br J Anaesth* **72**(3), 295–297.

Olesen J (1991) Cerebral and extracranial circulatory disturbances in migraine: pathophysiological implications. *Cerebrovasc Brain Metab Rev* **3**(1), 1–28.

Orendorff O (1914) A caffeine addict with asthenopic symptoms. *JAMA* **62**, 1828–1829.

Partanen J, Bruun K, and Markkenen T (1966) *Inheritance of Drinking Behavior: A Study of Intelligence, Personality, and Use of Alcohol in Adult Twins*. The Finnish Foundation for Alcohol Studies, Helsinki.

Paul S, Kurunwune B, and Biaggioni I (1993) Caffeine withdrawal: apparent heterologous sensitization to adenosine and prostacyclin actions in human platelets. *J Pharmacol Exp Ther* **267**(2), 838–843.

Pedersen N (1981) Twin similarity for usage of common drugs. In *Twin Research 3. Part C: Epidemiological and Clinical Studies*, Gedda L, Parisi P, and Nance W (eds). Alan R. Liss, New York, pp. 53–59.

Penetar D, McCann U, Thorne D, et al. (1993) Caffeine reversal of sleep deprivation effects on alertness and mood. *Psychopharmacology* **112**,(2–3), 359–365.

Phillips-Bute BG and Lane JD (1997) Caffeine withdrawal symptoms following brief caffeine deprivation. *Physiol Behav* **63**(1), 35–39.

Powell KR, Koppelman LF, and Holtzman SG (1999) Differential involvement of dopamine in mediating the discriminative stimulus effects of low and high doses of caffeine in rats. *Behav Pharmacol* **10**(8), 707–716.

Powers H (1925) The syndrome of coffee. *Med J Rec* **121**, 745–747.

Rainey JT (1985) Headache related to chronic caffeine addiction. *Texas Dent J* **102**(7), 29–30.

Reeves RR, Struve FA, Patrick G, et al. (1995) Topographic quantitative EEG measures of alpha and theta power changes during caffeine withdrawal: preliminary findings from normal subjects. *Clin Electroencephalogr* **26**(3), 154–162.

Regestein QR (1989) Pathologic sleepiness induced by caffeine. *Am J Med* **87**(5), 586–588.

Reimann HA (1967) Caffeinism: a cause of long-continued, low-grade fever. *JAMA* **202**(12), 1105–1106.

Reyner LA and Horne JA (1998) Evaluation "in-car" countermeasures to sleepiness: cold air and radio. *Sleep* **21**(1), 46–50.

Reyner LA and Horne JA (2000) Early-morning driver sleepiness: effectiveness of 200 mg caffeine. *Psychophysiology* **37**(2), 251–256.

Richardson NJ, Rogers PJ, and Elliman NA (1996) Conditioned flavour preferences reinforced by caffeine consumed after lunch. *Physiol Behav* **60**(1), 257–263.

Rihs M, Muller C, and Baumann P (1996) Caffeine consumption in hospitalized psychiatric patients. *Eur Arch Psychiatr Clin Neurosci* **246**(2), 83–92.

Roache JD and Griffiths RR (1987) Interactions of diazepam and caffeine: behavioral and subjective dose effects in humans. *Pharmacol Biochem Behav* **26**(4), 801–812.

Robelin M and Rogers PJ (1998) Mood and psychomotor performance effects of the first, but not of subsequent, cup-of-coffee equivalent doses of caffeine consumed after overnight caffeine abstinence. *Behav Pharmacol* **9**(7), 611–618.

Robertson D, Wade D, Workman R, et al. (1981) Tolerance to the humoral and hemodynamic effects of caffeine in man. *J Clin Invest* **67**(4), 1111–1117.

Rogers PJ, Richardson NJ, and Elliman NA (1995) Overnight caffeine abstinence and negative reinforcement of preference for caffeine-containing drinks. *Psychopharmacology (Berl)* **120**(4), 457–462.

Rugh JT (1896) Profound toxic effects from the drinking of large amounts of strong coffee. *Med Surg Rep* **75**, 549–550.

Russ NW, Sturgis ET, Malcolm RJ, et al. (1988) Abuse of caffeine in substance abusers. *J Clin Psychiatry* **49**(11), 457.

Schuh KJ and Griffiths RR (1997) Caffeine reinforcement: the role of withdrawal. *Psychopharmacology (Berl)* **130**(4), 320–326.

Shirlow MJ and Mathers CD (1985) A study of caffeine consumption and symptoms: indigestion, palpitations, tremor, headache and insomnia. *Int J Epidemiol* **14**(2), 239–248.

Shoaib M, Swanner LS, Yasar S, et al. (1999) Chronic caffeine exposure potentiates nicotine self-administration in rats. *Psychopharmacology (Berl)* **142**(4), 327–333.

Silverman K, Evans SM, Strain EC, et al. (1992) Withdrawal syndrome after the double-blind cessation of caffeine consumption. *N Engl J Med* **327**(16), 1109–1114.

Silverman K, Mumford GK, and Griffiths RR (1994) Enhancing caffeine reinforcement by behavioral requirements following drug ingestion. *Psychopharmacology (Berl)* **114**(3), 424–432.

Snel J (1993) Coffee and caffeine sleep and wakefulness. In *Caffeine, Coffee, and Health*, Garattini S (ed). Raven Press, New York, pp. 255–290.

Snyder SH, Katims JJ, Annau Z, et al. (1981) Adenosine receptors and behavioral actions of methylxanthines. *Proc Natl Acad Sci U S A* **78**(5), 3260–3264.

Sours JA (1983) Case reports of anorexia nervosa and caffeinism. *Am J Psychiatry* **140**(2), 235–236.

Stoffer SS (1979) Coffee consumption. *Arch Intern Med* **139**(10), 1194–1195.

Strain EC, Mumford GK, Silverman K, et al. (1994) Caffeine dependence syndrome. Evidence from case histories and experimental evaluations. *JAMA* **272**(13), 1043–1048.

Streufert S, Pogash R, Miller J, et al. (1995) Effects of caffeine deprivation on complex human functioning. *Psychopharmacology (Berl)* **118**(4), 377–384.

Swan GE, Carmelli D, and Cardon LR (1997) Heavy consumption of cigarettes, alcohol and coffee in male twins. *J Stud Alcohol* **58**(2), 182–190.

Swanson JA, Lee JW, and Hopp JW (1994) Caffeine and nicotine: a review of their joint use and possible interactive effects in tobacco withdrawal. *Addict Behav* **19**(3), 229–256.

Talcott GW, Poston WS II, and Haddock CK (1998) Co-occurrent use of cigarettes, alcohol, and caffeine in a retired military population. *Mil Med* **163**(3), 133–138.

Tanda G and Goldberg SR (2000) Alteration of the behavioral effects of nicotine by chronic caffeine exposure. *Pharmacol Biochem Behav* **66**(1), 47–64.

Tanskanen A, Tuomilehto J, Viinamaki H, et al. (2000a) Joint heavy use of alcohol, cigarettes and coffee and the risk of suicide. *Addiction* **95**(11), 1699–1704.

USDA (2001) Food consumption, prices, and expenditures, 1970–1999.

Varani K, Portaluppi F, Merighi S, et al. (1999) Caffeine alters A2A adenosine receptors and their function in human platelets. *Circulation* **99**(19), 2499–2502.

Victor BS, Lubetsky M, and Greden JF (1981) Somatic manifestations of caffeinism. *J Clin Psychiatry* **42**(5), 185–188.

Watson JM, Lunt MJ, Morris S, et al. (2000) Reversal of caffeine withdrawal by ingestion of a soft beverage. *Pharmacol Biochem Behav* **66**(1), 15–18.

Weber JG, Klindworth JT, Arnold JJ, et al. (1997) Prophylactic intravenous administration of caffeine and recovery after ambulatory surgical procedures. *Mayo Clin Proc* **72**(7), 621–626.

Wesensten NJ, Belenky G, Kautz MA, et al. (2002) Maintaining alertness and performance during sleep deprivation: Modafinil versus caffeine. *Psychopharmacology (Berl)* **159**(3), 238–247.

Winstead DK (1976) Coffee consumption among psychiatric inpatients. *Am J Psychiatry* **133**(12), 1447–1450.

Yeomans MR, Jackson A, Lee MD, et al. (2000) Expression of flavour preferences conditioned by caffeine is dependent on caffeine deprivation state. *Psychopharmacology (Berl)* **150**(2), 208–215.

Yeomans MR, Spetch H, and Rogers PJ (1998) Conditioned flavour preference negatively reinforced by caffeine in human volunteers. *Psychopharmacology (Berl)* **137**(4), 401–409.

Zwyghuizen-Doorenbos A, Roehrs TA, Lipschutz L, et al. (2002) Effects of caffeine on alertness. *Psychopharmacology* **100**(1), 36–39.

Substance-Related Disorders: Cannabis

Cannabis preparations, derived from the female *Cannabis sativa* plant, have been widely used for their psychotropic effects since the beginning of history. The drug is prepared in different ways in different parts of the world. The flowering tops and resin secreted by the female plant contain the highest concentrations of Δ-9-tetrahydrocannabinol (Δ-9-THC), the primary psychoactive component. Marijuana, the most common preparation, is made by drying and shredding the upper leaves, tops, stems, flowers, and seeds of the plant. Hashish is a more potent preparation made by extracting and drying the resin and sometimes also the compressed flowers. Hashish oil, which is even more potent, is distilled from hashish. Marijuana and hashish can be smoked either in the form of cigarettes or by using a pipe. Hashish, hashish oil, and less commonly marijuana, can be mixed with tea or food and taken orally (Ashton 2001, Hall and Solowij 1998). For the remainder of this chapter, we will refer to these preparations collectively as *cannabis*.

Selective breeding and improved growing methods have produced cannabis plants that contain significantly higher Δ-9-THC concentrations than naturally occurring plants. Thus, although there is a great deal of variation, the potency of illicit cannabis available in the United States has increased substantially, on average, over the last 30 years (Ashton 2001, Hall and Solowij 1998).

Intoxication occurs within minutes after smoking cannabis and typically persists for several hours. After eating foods containing cannabis, intoxication occurs after approximately an hour and can persist for 8 to 24 hours. The onset of intoxication after drinking cannabis steeped in tea is shorter, but not as rapid as after smoking, and has an intermediate duration of intoxication. Smoking cannabis induces intoxication more quickly than ingesting cannabis because first-pass metabolism in the liver is avoided and the combustion causes enhanced release of Δ-9-THC from pyrolysis of acids in cannabis preparations. Smoking is the predominant method of taking cannabis in most parts of the world including the United States, probably because of the more rapid onset of action and because the potency of the drug when it is smoked is about three times that experienced when an equivalent amount is eaten (Ashton 2001, Hall and Solowij 1998).

Δ-9-THC and other cannabinoids are highly lipophilic and are quickly and widely distributed throughout the body. Δ-9-THC can cross the placenta and enter breast milk; it may interact with other drugs by inducing liver enzymes and competing for plasma binding sites. Δ-9-THC is metabolized in the liver by hydroxylation to at least 20 different metabolites. Some, such as 11-hydroxy-THC, are psychoactive and have half-lives exceeding 2 days. Δ-9-THC may also be conjugated to more water-soluble metabolites that are excreted predominantly into the gut where they may be reabsorbed, and also into the bile, urine, sweat, and hair. Δ-9-THC is stored in the adipose tissue from which it is released slowly; in regular users, it can often be detected more than 30 days after the individual's last exposure to cannabis (Johnson 1990). If an individual uses cannabis regularly, the stores of Δ-9-THC in the adipose tissue result in a constant supply of cannabinoids to the body including the brain (Ashton 2001).

There are two types of G-protein-coupled cannabinoid receptors. CB_1 receptors are found in the lipid membranes of neurons in the central nervous system, including the cerebral cortex, basal ganglia, thalamus, and brain stem, with high densities in the hippocampus, cerebellum, and striatum. CB_2 receptors are found in the lipid membranes of various types of cells in the immune system. Δ-9-THC is a partial agonist, activating both CB_1 and CB_2 receptors (Hall and Solowij 1998). Activation of cannabinoid receptors mediates the inhibitory effect of adenylate cyclase, decreasing cyclic adenosine monophosphate, and also inhibits calcium and potassium transport. Receptor activation also mediates the excitatory effect of mitogen-activated protein kinase (Ameri 1999). The cannabinoid system plays a modulatory role in regulating many different functions including mood, motor control, perception (including pain perception), appetite, sleep, memory and cognition, reproductive function, and immune response (Hall and Solowij 1998). Δ-9-THC can potentiate the effects of alcohol, barbiturates, caffeine, and amphetamines (Solomons and Neppe 1989).

As with other substances of abuse, DSM-IV-TR distinguishes a number of different cannabis-related diagnoses. These fall into two basic groups. The first group is defined by adverse effects resulting from cannabis use; these include cannabis abuse and cannabis dependence. The category of cannabis dependence includes a number of specifiers that indicate the presence or absence of physiological dependence, type of remission, and whether or not the individual has been in a controlled environment. The second set of cannabis-related disorders in DSM-IV-TR includes psychiatric syndromes presumed to be induced by cannabis. This group includes the following: cannabis intoxication, which is almost certainly induced by cannabis and consists of the common signs and symptoms that normally follow cannabis use; cannabis intoxication delirium, a degree of disturbance beyond that normally expected with ordinary intoxication; cannabis-induced psychotic disorder which is subdivided into categories of psychosis with delusions and psychosis with hallucinations; and cannabis-induced anxiety disorder, which is also subdivided into several types as shown in Table 19-1.

To diagnose any of the cannabis-related disorders, it is important to obtain a detailed history of the individual's pattern of substance abuse (including abuse not only of cannabis but also of other substances) and to attempt to substantiate this report with toxicology screening for drugs of abuse. Individuals who smoke cannabis regularly can have substantial accumulations of THC in their fat stores. Thus, for weeks after cessation of smoking, detectable levels of cannabinoids may be found in the urine (Johnson 1990). However, a positive response on toxicology screening for cannabinoids cannot establish any of the cannabis-related diagnoses; it is useful only as an indicator that these diagnoses should be considered. A diagnostic decision tree for cannabis-related disorders is presented in Figure 19-1.

Table 19-1	Cannabis-Related Disorders

Cannabis-Use Disorders
304.3   Cannabis dependence
                With physiological dependence
                Without physiological dependence
                Early full remission
                Early partial remission
                Sustained full remission
                Sustained total remission
                In a controlled environment
305.20   Cannabis abuse

Cannabis-Induced Disorders
292.89   Cannabis intoxication
                With perceptual disturbances
292.81   Cannabis intoxication delirium
292.11   Cannabis-induced psychotic disorder, with delusions
                With onset during intoxication
292.12   Cannabis-induced psychotic disorder, with hallucinations
                With onset during intoxication
292.89   Cannabis-induced anxiety disorder
                With onset during intoxication
                With generalized anxiety
                With panic attacks
                With obsessive-compulsive symptoms
                With phobic symptoms
292.9   Cannabis-related disorder not otherwise specified

CANNABIS-USE DISORDERS

Diagnosis

Cannabis Dependence It is uncommon to see individuals who exhibit cannabis dependence as their only diagnosis because such individuals rarely seek treatment, as they generally do not acknowledge that they have a problem and are unaware that treatment is available. However, some individuals with this disorder will respond to offers for treatment because they realize that they are unable to stop use on their own and because they notice the deleterious effect of compulsive use (Roffman and Barnhart 1987). Therefore, the diagnosis of cannabis dependence will most often be made in individuals who present with other psychiatric problems, such as mood and anxiety disorders, and other substance-use disorders (see generic DSM-IV-TR diagnostic criteria for Substance dependency, Chapter 15, page 351). Another manner in which individuals with cannabis dependence may come to the attention of clinicians is when they are arrested for possession of the substance or some crime related to cannabis abuse, such as driving under the influence of the drug. Nevertheless, cannabis dependence is probably underdiagnosed in both psychiatric and general medical populations because it is not considered.

The diagnosis of cannabis dependence cannot be made without obtaining a history indicating that the cannabis use is impairing the individual's ability to function either physically or psychologically. Areas to inquire about include the individual's performance at work, ability to carry out social and family obligations, and physical health. It is also important to find out how much of the individual's time is spent on cannabis-related activities and whether the individual has tried unsuccessfully to stop or cut down on use in the past. Although it has been our experience that people who have used cannabis daily over a period of years almost invariably report tolerance to many of the effects of cannabis

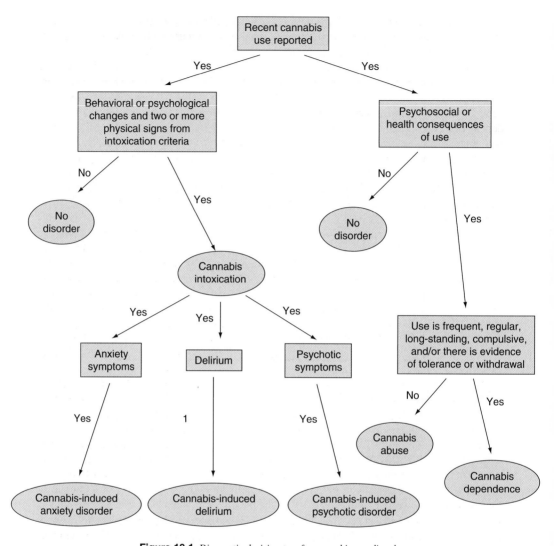

Figure 19-1 *Diagnostic decision tree for cannabis-use disorders.*

and experience an unpleasant withdrawal state if use is discontinued, neither tolerance nor withdrawal is necessary for the diagnosis of cannabis dependence. When this diagnosis is made, it can be described further by the following specifiers: with or without physiological dependence, early full or partial remission, sustained full or partial remission, or in a controlled environment. These diagnostic distinctions must be based on the pattern of use reported by the individual.

Cannabis Abuse   Most individuals who are diagnosed with cannabis abuse have only recently started using cannabis (see DSM-IV-TR diagnostic criteria for substance abuse in Chapter 15 on page 352). As with cannabis dependence, cannabis abuse is unlikely to be diagnosed unless some additional condition or circumstance brings the individual to medical attention. Teenagers often fall into this category because they spend time in supervised environments like school and home where responsible adults may intervene.

Also, teenagers are more likely to have motor vehicle accidents while intoxicated because they are inexperienced drivers, and are more likely to be arrested for possession because they have a greater tendency to participate in risky behaviors of all types.

Although virtually all individuals with cannabis dependence meet the inclusion criteria for cannabis abuse, they cannot be given this diagnosis because the presence of cannabis dependence is an exclusion criterion. Undoubtedly, the vast majority of people with cannabis dependence would have been given the diagnosis of cannabis abuse until they developed dependence. It is probable that individuals qualifying for a diagnosis of cannabis abuse will either cease use (see Course section) or develop cannabis dependence. The criteria for cannabis abuse focus on adverse consequences of cannabis use that could potentially result from just a single use such as failure to fulfill obligations at work, school, or home, participating in potentially dangerous activities like driving while intoxicated with cannabis, having cannabis-related legal problems, or social or interpersonal difficulties. Even though these adverse consequences can occur following a single episode of cannabis use, the consequences must be recurrent, requiring multiple episodes of use. Since the number of episodes necessary for "recurrent" is not defined, and the pattern of use is often dependent on individual self-report, it is often difficult to distinguish between abuse and dependence. This difficulty is easier to recognize if one looks at the extremes. On one end of the continuum, a high school student who actually has only used cannabis twice, but who was unfortunate enough to be caught and suspended from school on both occasions, would appropriately be diagnosed with cannabis abuse. At the other end of the continuum, a high school student who had actually been using cannabis every day for 3 years and met the criteria for dependence, who was also caught and suspended from school twice but denied symptoms of dependence, would incorrectly be diagnosed with cannabis abuse.

The difference between people with cannabis abuse and those with cannabis dependence is that the people with dependence have been using more regularly (one or more times per day) and for a longer duration (one or more years), and the acute problems associated with abuse have turned into the chronic problems associated with dependence. For example, what started as failure to fulfill obligations at work or school has resulted in dropping out of school or working at jobs with extremely low expectations. Multiple car accidents or arrests have led to chronic injuries (often associated with obtaining SSDI), loss of licenses, probation, and even periods of time in prison. Social or interpersonal problems have resulted in isolation or at least separation from people who are not regular cannabis users. If there is a committed relationship where the partner is typically cannabis-dependent, and if children are involved, chronic neglect is present if caring for children while intoxicated with cannabis represents neglect.

Epidemiology

Cannabis is probably the most commonly used illicit substance in the world, with an estimated 200 to 300 million regular users (Johnson 1990). In the United States, cannabis is generally thought to be the most widely used illicit drug, with more than 50% of Americans reporting at least one episode of use (Johnson 1990, Mueser et al. 1992, Chen and Kandel 1998, Hubbard et al. 1999). As with most other illicit drugs, cannabis use occurs more often in men though the difference between the sexes is decreasing (Greenfield and O'Leary 1999). Also, like other illicit drugs, cannabis use typically begins in adolescence and is most prevalent in people between the ages of 18 and 30 years (Chen and Kandel 1995, 1998, Johnston et al. 2001, Kandel and Chen 2000). The age of first cannabis use in America has been decreasing; in 1997 the average age of first use was reported to be 14 by the National Household Survey on Drug Abuse (NHSDA) (SAMHSA 1997). The annual, Monitoring the Future Study of high school students, reported that in 2000, 15.6% of 8th graders,

32.2% of 10th graders, and 36.5% of 12th graders reported using cannabis in the past year. Approximately 20% of 12th grade cannabis users reported daily use (Johnston et al. 2001).

Adolescents appear more vulnerable to developing cannabis dependence than adults, becoming dependent after using cannabis at a lower dose and frequency of use (Chen et al. 1997). Although earlier onset of use during adolescence is a predictor for continued use and the development of dependency, frequency of use is a stronger predictor (Chen and Kandel 1998, Kandel and Chen 2000, DeWit et al. 2000, SAMHSA 2000). Of those adolescents who use cannabis more than once, about a third will subsequently use cannabis regularly for some period of time, with 20% using daily, and an additional 10 to 20% using nearly daily (Hall and Solowij 1998, Johnston et al. 2001, Zoccollilo et al. 1999). It is estimated that a third of those who use cannabis daily meet the criteria for cannabis dependence, and that of all adolescents who use cannabis at least once, approximately 9%, will develop dependence (Anthony et al. 1994, Chen et al. 1997). However, most adolescents who use cannabis regularly will have stopped use by the time they are 30 (Chen and Kandel 1995, 1998).

Studies have reported that individuals with cannabis-use disorders have high rates of other substance abuse disorders (Miller et al. 1990) as well as other types of Axis I disorders (Regier et al. 1990, Troisi et al. 1998). It is possible, however, that these findings reflect "spurious comorbidity" (Smoller et al. 2000) because individuals with cannabis dependence and other Axis I disorders are probably more likely to present for treatment or research studies than those with cannabis dependence alone.

Conversely, studies of several psychiatric populations (Brady et al. 1991, Alterman et al. 1982, Miller et al. 1989, Cantwell et al. 1999, Menezes et al. 1996, Johns 2001) with a number of different Axis I diagnoses other than panic disorder (Szuster et al. 1988) have found high rates of cannabis use. The course of the Axis I illnesses is often adversely affected by cannabis use; cannabis may exacerbate psychotic symptoms in individuals with schizophrenia, possibly precipitate schizophrenia in predisposed individuals (Andreasson et al. 1987, 1989), precipitate hypomanic or manic episodes in bipolar individuals (Gruber and Pope 1994), and trigger panic reactions in individuals with panic disorder (Szuster et al. 1988). Cannabis use, abuse, and dependence are also commonly comorbid, with conduct disorder in children and adolescents and with antisocial personality disorder in adults (Weller and Halikas 1985, Henry et al. 1993, True et al. 1999, Crowley et al. 1998). Despite these findings of comorbidity, cannabis use has not been shown to induce any mental disorders *de novo* in nonpredisposed individuals (Hall and Degenhardt 2000, Johns 2001).

Course

As discussed in the Epidemiology section, about a third of those adolescents who try cannabis will use it regularly for some period of time, whereas only about 10% will go on to develop long-term dependence lasting into adulthood (Hall and Solowij 1998). Even among these persistent users, the majority will stop use by age 30 years. Thus, it is possible to extrapolate from these figures that less than 2% of adults will exhibit cannabis dependence during their 20s and that probably less than 1% of adults will continue use into their 30s, suggesting a good prognosis for the majority of cannabis-dependent individuals under age 30 years. However, for the small minority who continue to suffer from cannabis dependence into their 30s, most follow a chronic or relapsing course similar to those who suffer from dependence on other substances (Miller et al. 1989, Hall and Solowij 1998, Johnston et al. 2001, Zoccollilo et al. 1999, Anthony et al. 1994, Chen and Kandel 1995, 1998, Chen et al. 1997, Kandel and Chen 2000, Stephens et al. 1993a,b, 1994, 2000, Baer et al. 1998, Hser et al. 2001, Hubbard et al. 1985).

Cannabis abuse and dependence appear to pursue a benign course in many individuals; many studies have suggested that individuals suffering from these disorders do not differ in ability to function in society from matched control subjects who are not users (Kouri et al.

1995, Simon et al. 1974, Pope et al. 1990, 2001b, Zinberg and Weil 1970, Comitas 1976, Hochman and Brill 1973, Boulougouris et al. 1976, Robins et al. 1970, Mendelson et al. 1976, Brill and Christie 1974, Pope and Yurgelun-Todd 1996). However, a few studies have described an "amotivational syndrome" associated with chronic cannabis use, characterized by subjective reports of lack of direction, motivation, and ambition (Mellinger et al. 1976, Lessin and Thomas 1976, Kupfer et al. 1973, Burdsal et al. 1973, Campbell 1976, Hendin and Haas 1985, Musty and Kaback 1995, Gruber et al. in press). This "amotivational syndrome" appears to result from the effects of continuous intoxication and resolves when cannabis is discontinued (Johns 2001).

Etiology

Cannabis dependence develops as a result of repeated use of the drug, and frequency of use is one of the most important predictors of developing dependence (Chen and Kandel 1998, Kandel and Chen 2000). Like most other dependence-producing drugs, cannabis produces its reinforcing effects by activating the mesolimbic dopaminergic "reward" pathway, which consists of dopaminergic neurons in the ventral tegmental area (VTA) that project to the nucleus accumbens, increasing dopamine levels in the shell of the nucleus accumbens (Diana et al. 1998a, Gardner 1999, Tanda et al. 1997). Naloxone, an opiate antagonist at the μ_1 opioid receptor in the VTA, blocks this increase in dopamine, which suggests that Δ-9-THC and opiates share the same mechanism of activating this pathway (Tanda et al. 1997). Studies have shown that people choose higher-potency cannabis preparations over lower-potency preparations, a finding which suggests that increased potency may result in an increased risk of progression to addiction and dependence (Chait and Burke 1994, Harder and Reitbrock 1997).

Regular use of cannabis for periods as short as 1 to 3 weeks can produce tolerance to many of its acute physiological and psychological effects (Jones et al. 1976, 1981, Jones 1983). Such tolerance may cause some individuals to increase their use in order to continue to experience desired effects. As with other addictive drugs, discontinuation of cannabis use increases corticotropin-releasing factor (CRF) in the central amygdala and decreases dopaminergic transmission in the limbic system, resulting in withdrawal symptoms (Diana et al. 1998b, Rodriguez de Fonseca et al. 1997).

The core symptoms of cannabis withdrawal are irritability, anxiety, physical tension, and decreases in mood and appetite. Restlessness, tremors, sweating, insomnia, increased aggressiveness, and very vivid dreams have also been reported (Budney et al. 1999, Haney et al. 1999, Kouri et al. 1999, Kouri and Pope 2000, Kaymakcalan 1973, 1981, Tennant 1986, Compton et al. 1990, Jones et al. 1976, 1981, Jones 1983, Wiesbeck et al. 1996). The symptoms of cannabis withdrawal are similar to those of opiate withdrawal, except that their intensity is milder and their course is delayed and prolonged because cannabis is cleared from the body gradually as it is released slowly from storage in the adipose tissue. Symptoms typically begin the day after the last use, do not reach maximal intensity until the third day, and then resolve over the following week. The severity of the withdrawal syndrome varies considerably among individuals. In a recent study of 108 chronic, long-term cannabis users, the authors observed a number of individuals who experienced severe withdrawal symptoms that precluded their completion of the month-long abstinence period required by the study protocol, suggesting that, for at least some individuals, the withdrawal syndrome is an important factor in the development and persistence of dependence (Pope et al. 2001a, Gruber et al. in press).

Environment appears to play a major role in determining whether an individual will initiate cannabis use, but only a minor role in determining whether an individual will go on to develop cannabis dependence. Genetic factors, on the other hand, appear to play only a moderate role in determining whether an individual will initiate cannabis use, but a major role in determining whether an individual who initiates use will subsequently develop cannabis dependence.

In addition to the addictive properties of cannabis and the genetic predisposition of individuals, another possible etiology for cannabis dependence is that some individuals may be "self-medicating" themselves for underlying psychiatric symptoms. Some individuals with depression, anxiety, or negative symptoms of schizophrenia report that marijuana use alleviates their symptoms (Peralta and Cuesta 1992, Disxon et al. 1991, Estroff and Gold 1986, Warner et al. 1994, Gruber et al. 1996). In addition, a large portion of adolescents and young adults with cannabis dependence have reported using marijuana to self-treat anger, boredom, or lack of direction (Chen and Kandel 1998, Gruber et al. in press, Johnston et al. 2001, Newcombe and Bentler 1988).

However, contrary to the beliefs of the users, cannabis may also contribute to the symptoms enumerated above (Miller et al. 1989, Lex et al. 1989, Mirin et al. 1971, Chen and Kandel 1998, Baigent et al. 1995, Green and Ritter 2000).

Treatment

Up until the last few years, the prevailing opinion was that cannabis use did not produce addiction and dependence and that cannabis users could discontinue use without the help of treatment programs. In fact, this was the prevailing attitude even amongst users, many of whom had tried unsuccessfully to discontinue use (Weiner et al. 1999). Although it is undeniably true that the majority of cannabis users are able to stop without assistance, it is also becoming apparent that many cannabis-dependent individuals cannot stop without help. The generally held opinion among cannabis users is that there are few substance-abuse programs that will accept them if their primary substance is cannabis and that those programs that do exist are not effective for cannabis users (Weiner et al. 1999).

However, mounting evidence documents the existence of a population of cannabis-dependent individuals who desire treatment (Roffman and Barnhart 1987, Budney et al. 1999, Stephens et al. 1993a,b, 1994, 2000, Weiner et al. 1999). For example, a survey of 335 adolescent cannabis users reported that 80% had considered quitting, 52% had tried unsuccessfully to quit, and only 24% believed that they would never quit (Weiner et al. 1999). In one investigation, a public-service announcement directed at chronic marijuana users resulted in interviews of 225 people who responded. It was found that 74% reported negative consequences of their marijuana use and 92% wanted to be treated (Roffman and Barnhart 1987). In 1998, 48% of adolescent admissions to state-funded substance abuse programs were for primary cannabis dependence, indicating a significant need for treatment programs for cannabis dependence (SAMHSA 1999).

With the recognition that cannabis use produces dependence and withdrawal, and that cannabis-dependent individuals may benefit from treatment, many substance abuse programs have started offering treatment to people whose primary drug of abuse or dependence is marijuana. Unfortunately, these programs are not generally designed specifically for cannabis dependence and they have not achieved high success rates (Baer et al. 1998, Hser et al. 2001, Hubbard et al. 1985, SAMHSA 2000). Similarly, many nonprofessional organizations that offer support groups, such as Alcoholics Anonymous (AA), Narcotics Anonymous (NA), and Self-Management and Recovery Training (SMART) have also begun to welcome people whose primary drug is cannabis. In addition, there is now a nonprofessional support organization, Marijuana Anonymous (MA), started by and run for cannabis-dependent individuals.

We are aware of only four controlled studies of treatment of cannabis-dependent individuals. In three of the studies, the subjects were seeking treatment specifically for cannabis dependence, whereas the fourth study involved schizophrenic individuals undergoing treatment for marijuana dependence. The first study found no difference in the outcome between a cognitive–behavioral relapse-prevention group and a support group—overall, 16% of subjects had decreased use and 15% were abstinent when assessed 12 months after treatment (Stephens et al. 1994). Higher quantity and frequency of marijuana use prior to treatment were strongly correlated with poorer outcome (Stephens et al. 1993b). A second study compared a motivational enhancement group, a motivational enhancement plus cognitive–behavioral therapy group, and a motivational enhancement plus cognitive–behavioral therapy group combined with a voucher-based incentive program that rewarded biweekly urine screens that were negative with vouchers for retail items. The group that received the voucher-based incentive program achieved a higher rate of abstinence during the study period and at the end of the study than either of the other two treatment groups (Budney et al. 2000). Similar success using monetary rewards for negative urines was also reported in a small trial of schizophrenic individuals undergoing treatment for marijuana dependence (Sigmon et al. 2000). The last study compared brief motivational therapy with a cognitive–behavioral relapse-prevention support group and a control group consisting of subjects put on a waiting list. Although no difference was found between the two active-treatment groups, subjects in both treatment groups were using significantly less marijuana and reported significantly fewer symptoms of dependence and fewer marijuana-related problems than subjects in the control group. Nevertheless, only 22% of the subjects in the active-treatment groups remained abstinent throughout a 16-month follow-up period (Stephens et al. 2000).

The strongest predictor of successful outcome is longer retention in treatment programs (Simpson 1981). Predictors of dropping out of an outpatient treatment program and presumably continuing use were found to be young age, financial difficulties, and psychological stress (Crits-Christoph and Siqueland 1996, Grella et al. 1999, Hser et al. 2001, Simpson et al. 1997, Roffman et al. 1993). More research is clearly required to discover effective ways to retain cannabis-dependent individuals in treatment.

Currently, there are few substance abuse programs specifically designed to treat cannabis dependence. Most programs are designed to treat all types of substance abuse, so that cannabis-dependent individuals typically receive the same treatment as individuals with other types of substance abuse. Since many cannabis-dependent individuals are also dependent on other substances, this is often a satisfactory treatment strategy. Also, a number of basic principles of treatment of substance-use disorders are equally applicable to cannabis dependence and other types of substance dependence.

One of these principles, critical for selecting the most appropriate intervention, is the importance of assessing an individual's stage in the recovery process (Prochaska and Velicer 1997). Individuals in early stages, such as "precontemplation" and "contemplation," benefit most from strategies aimed at using reliable sources to convey accurate information about cannabis that will help individuals identify personal reasons for discontinuing use. Individuals in later stages, such as "action" and "maintenance," benefit most from cognitive–behavioral relapse-prevention strategies (Botvin 2000, Prochaska and Velicer 1997).

As with all other drugs of abuse, the ultimate goal in the treatment of cannabis dependence is abstinence. In a phenomenon similar to that seen in alcohol-dependent people, many cannabis-dependent people have exposure to others who are able to use cannabis in a nonproblematic manner, and will often insist that their goal is to moderate their use, rather than cease use altogether. Unfortunately, if a person is susceptible to cannabis dependence, the most frequent outcome of trying to use moderately after a period of abstinence is that within a few weeks or months they have returned to their preabstinence pattern of use. Although physicians can tell cannabis-dependent people that this is the likely outcome, only after going through this process one or more times do people whose goal is moderation rather than abstinence recognize that like alcoholics, moderation is not an option for them.

The process of treatment begins with detoxification followed by maintenance. As discussed in the section on Etiology, chronic users usually experience a withdrawal syndrome during detoxification. Since the cannabis withdrawal syndrome is not life-threatening, detoxification generally does not require hospitalization unless it is complicated by detoxification from other drugs or by comorbid Axis I disorders that do require hospitalization for safe treatment. The intensity of the cannabis withdrawal syndrome varies widely, with some individuals reporting very mild symptoms and others reporting more severe symptoms (Budney et al. 1999, Haney et al. 1999, Kouri and Pope 2000, Kaymakcalan 1973, 1981, Tennant 1986, Compton et al. 1990, Jones et al. 1976, 1981, Jones 1983, Wiesbeck et al. 1996).

To help an individual tolerate the 7- to 10-day withdrawal period, practitioners should provide psychological support (e.g., reassurance that the symptoms will resolve in a little over a week) and in some cases, provide pharmacological support (Miller et al. 1989, Haney et al. 2001a, 2001b). Research into possible pharmacological interventions is just getting under way. One author suggested the use of long-acting benzodiazepines if the level of discomfort is high or there are abnormal vital signs (Miller et al. 1989). A small placebo-controlled, crossover study of 10 subjects showed that the antidepressant bupropion (Wellbutrin, Zyban) worsened irritability, restlessness, depression, and insomnia associated with marijuana withdrawal (Haney et al. 2001a). A second small placebo-controlled, crossover study of seven subjects showed that the antidepressant nefazodone (Serzone) decreased anxiety, muscleaches, and restlessness associated with marijuana withdrawal, but not irritability or insomnia (Haney et al. 2001b).

The foundation of maintenance treatment, as with other types of substance- use disorders, is regular attendance at groups that provide education and support. It is hypothesized that such groups are effective because fellow group members are best able to confront each other's denial and minimization of the substance abuse problem and the rationalizations put forth by the substance abuser for continued use despite negative consequences. Also, substance users typically report that they are most likely to believe information if it is provided by former users (Weiner et al. 1999). Since cannabis dependence, like other types of substance abuse, is characterized by a chronic, relapsing course, these groups provide an important function by addressing issues around relapse prevention and provide support for dealing with relapses when they do occur.

Several approaches that are more important to the treatment of cannabis dependence should be employed in addition to the basic, general substance abuse program. Recent studies examining reasons for cannabis use have provided information to guide treatment strategies. For example, both adolescent and adult cannabis users frequently report that they use cannabis to relax, or as a stress reduction or coping mechanism. This observation suggests that treatment programs should teach healthier and more effective coping mechanisms and cognitive–behavioral strategies for relaxation and stress reduction (Botvin 2000, Hendin and Haas 1985, Weiner et al. 1999).

The most salient feature of cannabis abuse or dependence is that it is often comorbid with other Axis I disorders as discussed earlier. Toxicology screening for other drugs of abuse is imperative because the most common comorbid Axis I disorders are other types of substance abuse. Even in the absence of an obvious Axis I diagnosis, psychological reasons for cannabis use should be investigated. For example, use of cannabis for relaxation or improving mood may be indicative of efforts to "self-medicate" underlying anxiety or mood disorders (Chen and Kandel 1998, Latimer et al. 2000). Thus, treatment programs for cannabis dependence should include a dual-diagnosis component. Because of the high frequency of comorbidity among cannabis-dependent individuals, diagnosing and treating the underlying disorder or symptomatology may be a necessary condition for the individual to stop using marijuana (Brady et al. 1991, Cantwell et al. 1999, Crits-Christoph and

Siqueland 1996, Johns 2001, Menezes et al. 1996, Regier et al. 1990, Rounds-Bryant et al. 1999, Simpson 1981, Simpson et al. 1997, Troisi et al. 1998).

Another treatment situation frequently encountered is that of an individual with a known Axis I disorder that is being exacerbated by cannabis use. Some studies, performed in populations of individuals with schizophrenia, have found that cannabis use worsens the course of the illness, whereas others have found that it does not affect the course (Negrete et al. 1986, Treffert 1978, Cuffel et al. 1993, Linszen et al. 1994). It is a reasonable assumption that at least some individuals with Axis I disorders are adversely affected by cannabis use even if they use the drug only occasionally. In such cases, the role of cannabis as an exacerbating factor must be assessed and discussed with the individual. These patients may or may not be suitable for support groups directed primarily at substance abuse because cannabis may represent a relatively minor portion of the individual's overall clinical picture.

Refractory Individuals

Like alcohol, the most common problem in managing cannabis-use disorders is the high rate of relapse due to the wide availability of the drug and the large number of people who are users. Users are therefore tempted to resume use soon after a period of treatment when they find themselves in situations where they are surrounded by people using the substance. It is often useful for families and other people important in the individual's life to get involved in the treatment to understand the role that they play in the individual's substance abuse. Some treaters advocate periodic random urine testing, which is an inexpensive and reliable method of monitoring abstinence, because THC remains present for a long time and can be detected with infrequent testing (Miller et al. 1989).

A difficult treatment situation arises when it is hypothesized that the individual is using cannabis to self-medicate a primary Axis I disorder such as depression or an anxiety disorder. In these individuals, abstinence is difficult to achieve because the individual believes that cannabis will alleviate his or her symptoms. Relapse may occur repeatedly until the underlying Axis I disorder is effectively treated (Peralta and Cuesta 1992, Dixon et al. 1991, Estroff and Gold 1986, Warner et al. 1994).

In the given treatment decision tree, a diagnosis of cannabis-use disorders is presented Figure 19-2.

CANNABIS-INDUCED DISORDERS

Diagnosis

Cannabis Intoxication   There are four criteria necessary to make this diagnosis (see DSM-IV-TR criteria for intoxication on page 476). The first is that recent use of cannabis must be established. This cannot be done with toxicology screening because the result may be negative after a single episode of smoking or, alternatively, may be positive even if the individual has not used the drug for a time much longer than the period of intoxication. Thus, the recent use of cannabis must be reported by the individual or another person who witnessed the individual's use. In addition, the symptoms resulting from cannabis use must produce "clinically significant maladaptive behavioral or psychological changes." Third, the individual must exhibit some physical signs of cannabis use. DSM-IV-TR requires the individual to have at least two of four signs—conjunctival injection, increased appetite, dry mouth, and tachycardia—within 2 hours of cannabis use. Fourth, symptoms cannot be accounted for by a general medical condition or another mental disorder. There is a specifier, "with perceptual disturbances," that can be used if the individual

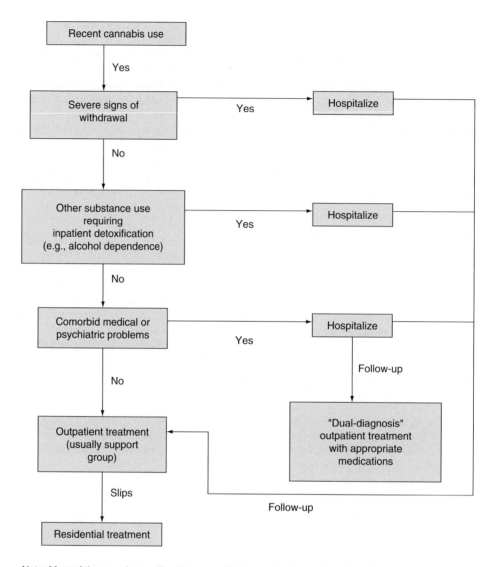

Note: Most of these patients will not be committable and will have to voluntarily seek treatment.

Figure 19-2 *Treatment decision tree for cannabis-use disorders.*

is experiencing illusions or hallucinations while not delirious and while maintaining intact reality testing.

DSM-IV-TR Diagnostic Criteria

292.89 Cannabis Intoxication

A. Recent use of cannabis.

B. Clinically significant maladaptive behavioral or psychological changes (e.g., impaired motor coordination, euphoria, anxiety, sensation of slowed time, impaired judgment, social withdrawal) that developed during or shortly after cannabis use.

C. Two (or more) of the following signs, developing with 2 hours of cannabis use:

(1) conjunctival injection
(2) increased appetite
(3) dry mouth
(4) tachycardia

D. The symptoms are not due to a general medical condition and are not better accounted for by another mental disorder.

Reprinted with permission from the Diagnostic and Statistical Manual of Mental Disorders, Fourth Edition, Text Revision. Copyright 2000 American Psychiatric Association.

There has been extensive research on the effects of acute cannabis intoxication. In addition to the symptoms and signs required for a DSM-IV-TR diagnosis, many psychological and physiological effects have been reported. Awareness of these may enhance the clinician's ability to recognize cannabis intoxication. Physiological effects are listed in Table 19-2, and are divided into commonly observed effects and rare effects that have been described only after the use of very high doses of cannabis (Hall and Solowij 1998, Ameri 1999, Perez-Reyes 1999). Cannabis has low toxicity, and to our knowledge, no deaths from cannabis overdose have been reported (Hall and Solowij 1998). Similarly, psychological effects are listed in Table 19-3, divided into commonly observed effects and uncommon effects. Most

Table 19-2	Physiological Effects of Cannabis Intoxication

Common and Transient
Tachycardia
Hypertension
Thirst
Increased appetite
Constipation
Decreased intraocular pressure
Mydriasis
Mild bronchoconstriction followed by bronchodilation
Increased reaction time
Impaired coordination
Distorted time perception
Decreased libido
Mild analgesia
Mild anti-emetic effects

Uncommon and Transient
Ataxia
Ptosis
Miosis
Drowsiness
Bradycardia
Hypotension
Peripheral vasoconstriction
Hypothermia

Table 19-3	Psychological Effects of Cannabis Intoxication

Common and Transient
Euphoria
Distortions in perception, including time perception
Enhancement of sensations

Uncommon and Transient
Dysphoria
Anxiety, and less commonly panic reactions
Restlessness
Depersonalization
Derealization
Paranoid ideation

people find the commonly experienced psychological effects enjoyable. However, some individuals, especially women (Thomas 1996) and inexperienced users in an unfamiliar environment, find them frightening and experience anxiety and even have panic reactions (Hall and Solowij 1998, Johns 2001, Thomas 1996). Although all of these effects typically persist only for the period of acute intoxication, some reports have described individuals who report "flashbacks" of cannabis intoxication long after use, and depersonalization persisting long after acute intoxication (Keeler et al. 1968, 1971, Levi and Miller 1990, Annis and Smart 1973, Stanton and Bardoni 1972). At this time, there is insufficient evidence to ascertain whether these reports are attributable to cannabis itself, to confounding factors such as the concomitant use of other drugs, or the presence of other Axis I disorders (Johns 2001).

In addition, cannabis use produces deficits in a number of neuropsychological functions, both during acute intoxication and after up to a week or more of abstinence in chronic, long-term users. These tasks include short-term memory, sustained or divided attention, and complex decision making (Ehrenreich et al. 1999, Pope et al. 1995, 1997, 2001a, Pope and Yurgelun-Todd 1996, Schwartz et al. 1989, Solowij et al. 1991, 1995, Solowij 1995, 1998). A study of chronic, long-term users found that these deficits were reversible after 28 days of abstinence (Pope et al. 2001a). However, a few studies have found that subtle electrophysiologic changes, of uncertain clinical significance, may persist even after years of abstinence (Solowij 1995, 1998, Struve et al. 1998).

Cannabis Intoxication Delirium   We have not located any original reports of this entity, although it is mentioned in various reviews and is included in DSM-IV-TR (see generic DSM-IV-TR diagnostic criteria for Substance Intoxication Delirium in Chapter 13, page 271). Thus, if cannabis intoxication delirium does occur in neurologically intact individuals, it is probably a rare complication. If the delirium does not resolve within 24 to 48 hours, it is almost certainly a result of an underlying neurological or medical condition. Therefore, in an individual with delirium, even if recent cannabis use has been reported, a full diagnostic workup should be performed to rule out a concomitant, treatable neurological condition (Halikas 1974, Johns 2001).

The following two substance-induced conditions are not generally diagnosed unless the symptoms are in excess of those usually associated with the intoxication or withdrawal state and are sufficiently severe to warrant independent clinical attention.

Cannabis-Induced Psychotic Disorder   There are two subtypes of cannabis-induced psychotic disorder: one featuring delusions, the other hallucinations (see generic DSM-IV-TR diagnostic criteria for Substance-Induced Psychotic Disorder in Chapter 15, page 355). The diagnosis of this disorder is readily made in individuals who have psychotic symptoms that appear immediately after ingestion of cannabis. However, a careful history is required to establish whether the individual has a preexisting psychotic disorder (as is often the case in such situations) or whether the symptoms arose *de novo* after cannabis consumption. There is little evidence that cannabis-induced psychotic disorders can arise in previously asymptomatic individuals (Gruber and Pope 1994). Therefore, if psychotic symptoms persist for 24 to 48 hours after the period of acute intoxication, they are likely due to an underlying mental disorder, which must be diagnosed and treated (Hall and Degenhardt 2000, Johns 2001, Gruber and Pope 1994).

Cannabis-Induced Anxiety Disorder This disorder may be further described by the following specifiers: with generalized anxiety, with panic attacks, with obsessive–compulsive symptoms, and with phobic symptoms (see generic DSM-IV-TR diagnostic criteria Substance-Induced Anxiety Disorder in Chapter 15, page 357). The literature contains papers that report individuals who have anxiety, panic reactions, and paranoid ideation during the period of acute intoxication, but we are unaware of any papers that report obsessive–compulsive or phobic symptoms. People who experience anxiety after using cannabis are typically inexperienced users who react to the novel experiences of perceptual distortions and intensified sensations with anxiety and even panic reactions, rather than enjoyment (Thomas 1996, Johns 2001, Szuster et al. 1988). Women are more likely than men to experience cannabis-induced anxiety (Thomas 1996). As with cannabis-induced psychotic disorders, we have been unable to find clear cases of cannabis-induced anxiety disorders in individuals without a preexisting Axis I disorder. Again, if symptoms of severe anxiety or panic persist for 24 to 48 hours after the period of acute intoxication, they are likely due to an underlying mental disorder that must be diagnosed and treated (Johns 2001).

Epidemiology

The prevalence of cannabis intoxication should be approximately the same as the prevalence of cannabis use described at the beginning of this section. No formal epidemiological data exist regarding the prevalence of cannabis intoxication delirium, cannabis-induced psychotic disorder, or cannabis-induced anxiety disorder. In fact, it is not entirely certain that any of these three entities actually occurs in individuals free of preexisting DSM-IV-TR Axis I disorders (Hall and Degenhardt 2000, Johns 2001).

For example, no original reports of cannabis-induced delirium in the literature were found except for comments about it in review articles. Whereas cannabis use occasionally causes anxiety, or even panic reactions, especially among inexperienced users, there is again no known published study exhibiting a cohort of previously asymptomatic subjects who developed clinically significant cannabis-induced anxiety disorder. One investigator (Pillard 1970) observed that there were five to seven cases of cannabis-associated anxiety reactions reported to a university health service per year; he hypothesized that more cases occurred but were not reported. However, he noted that reassurance was all the treatment necessary, suggesting that these individuals had not developed clinically significant anxiety disorders. Finally, although anecdotal reports and even case series of cannabis-induced psychotic disorder have appeared, many of these have been collected outside the United States and most provide insufficient evidence to assess whether the subjects studied were suffering from preexisting psychotic disorders before their ingestion of cannabis (Gruber and Pope 1994). In one US study, the investigators reviewed approximately 10,000 discharges from two psychiatric units. All cases of possible cannabis-induced mental disorders were investigated by chart review. No cases of clear-cut cannabis-induced psychotic disorder or cannabis-induced anxiety disorder were found. Thus, it appears that these disorders, at least of sufficient magnitude to prompt a psychiatric admission, are rare or do not exist at all (Gruber and Pope 1994, Hall and Degenhardt 2000, Johns 2001).

Course

Cannabis intoxication is a self-limiting state that remits as cannabis is metabolized and eliminated from the body. If symptoms suggestive of cannabis intoxication persist, other diagnoses should be considered. Similarly, although there are few data regarding the course of the other cannabis-induced disorders, it appears that cannabis-induced psychotic and anxiety disorders as well as cannabis intoxication delirium rarely persist beyond the period of acute intoxication with the drug. For example, although there have been reports of cannabis-induced psychoses persisting for days or even weeks beyond the time of acute intoxication, a review of the literature (as discussed earlier) was unable to exhibit a series of unequivocal cases in which such symptoms persisted in the absence of an underlying Axis I disorder. Therefore, symptoms of delirium, psychosis, or anxiety persisting more than 24 to 48 hours after acute cannabis intoxication suggest that another Axis I disorder, rather than cannabis itself, is responsible for the symptoms (Gruber and Pope 1994, Hall and Degenhardt 2000, Johns 2001).

Etiology

The mechanism causing the euphoria experienced during cannabis intoxication is activation of the mesolimbic dopaminergic "reward" pathway, and is described earlier (Diana et al. 1998a, Gardner 1999, Tanda et al. 1997). The mechanisms causing the physiological signs and symptoms associated with cannabis intoxication are thought to result from the action of the cannabinoid system on other major neurotransmitter systems including the noradrenergic, cholinergic, serotonin, and opioid systems (Ameri 1999).

There are no adequate data regarding the mechanism by which cannabis intoxication delirium, cannabis-induced psychotic disorder, or cannabis-induced anxiety disorder can occur *de novo* in individuals without preexisting medical or psychiatric disorders. In a review of studies of individuals with cannabis-induced psychotic disorder, it was found that most of the studies had not excluded individuals with a preexisting Axis I disorder, such as schizophrenia or a major mood disorder, which would render the individual vulnerable to psychotic symptoms even in the absence of cannabis use. At present, therefore, it seems possible that the majority of cannabis-induced psychotic or anxiety disorders represent exacerbations of preexisting DSM-IV-TR Axis I psychiatric disorders in individuals who become intoxicated with the drug (Gruber and Pope 1994).

Treatment

Uncomplicated cannabis intoxication rarely comes to clinical attention, and if it does, it does not require treatment other than reassurance, as it is a self-limiting condition. Similarly, as suggested in the previous sections, symptoms of delirium, psychosis, or anxiety associated with cannabis use typically resolve promptly after the period of acute intoxication is past. Again, no treatment is necessary other than keeping the individual safe and providing reassurance that symptoms caused by the drug will stop, as these are also self-limiting conditions. If the symptoms continue after more than 24 to 48 hours of abstinence from the drug, the possibility of another Axis I diagnosis must be considered. In such cases, treatment should then be directed at the primary Axis I disorder.

References

Alterman AI, Erdlen DL, LaPorte DJ, et al. (1982) Effects of illicit drug use in an inpatient psychiatric population. *Addict Behav* **7**, 231–242.

Ameri A (1999) The effects of cannabinoids on the brain. *Prog Neurobiol* **58**(4), 315–348.

Andreasson S, Allebeck P, Engstrom A, et al. (1987) Cannabis and schizophrenia: a longitudinal study of Swedish conscripts. *Lancet* **2**(8574), 1483–1486.

Andreasson S, Allebeck P, and Rydberg U (1989) Schizophrenia in users and nonusers of cannabis. A longitudinal study in Stockholm County. *Acta Psychiatr Scand* **79**(5), 505–510.

Annis HM and Smart RG (1973) Adverse reactions and recurrences from marijuana use. *Br J Addict* **68**, 315–319.

Anthony JC, Warner LA, and Kessler RC (1994) Comparative epidemiology of dependence on tobacco, alcohol, controlled substances and inhalants: basic findings from the National comorbidity study. *Clin Exp Psychopharmacol* **2**, 244–268.

Ashton CH (2001) Pharmacology and effects of cannabis: a brief review. *Br J Psychiatr* **178**, 101–106.

Baer JS, MacLean MG, and Marlatt GA (1998) Linking etiology and treatment for adolescent substance abuse: toward a better match. In *New Perspectives on Adolescent Risk Behavior*, Jessor R (ed). Cambridge University Press, New York, pp. 182–220.

Baigent M, Holme G, and Hafner RJ (1995) Self reports of the interaction between substance abuse and schizophrenia. *Aust NZ J Psychiatr* **29**, 69–74.

Botvin GJ (2000) Preventing drug abuse in schools: social and competence enhancement approaches targeting individual-level etiologic factors. *Addict Behav* **25**(6), 887–897.

Boulougouris JC, Liakos A, and Stefanis C (1976) Social traits of heavy hashish users and matched controls. *Ann NY Acad Sci* **282**, 17–23.

Brady K, Casto S, Lydiard RB, et al. (1991) Substance abuse in an inpatient psychiatric sample. *Am J Drug Alcohol Abuse* **17**, 389–397.

Brill NQ and Christie RL (1974) Marijuana use and psychosocial adaptation. *Arch Gen Psychiatr* **31**, 713–719.

Budney AJ, Higgins ST, Radonovich KJ, et al. (2000) Voucher-based incentives to coping skills and motivational enhancement improves outcomes during treatment for marijuana dependence. *J Consult Clin Psychol* **68**(6), 1051–1061.

Budney AJ, Novy PL, and Hughes JR (1999) Marijuana withdrawal among adults seeking treatment for marijuana dependence. *Addiction* **94**(9), 1311–1322.

Burdsal C, Greenberg G, and Timpe R (1973) The relationship of marijuana usage to personality and motivational factors. *J Psychol* **85**, 45–51.

Campbell I (1976) The amotivational syndrome and cannabis use with emphasis on the Canadian scene. *Ann NY Acad Sci* **282**, 33–36.

Cantwell R, Brewin J, Glazebrook C, et al. (1999) Prevalence of substance misuse in first-episode psychosis. *Br J Psychiatr* **174**, 150–153.

Chait LD and Burke KA (1994) Preference for high-versus low-potency marijuana. *Pharmacol Biochem Behav* **49**(3), 643–647.

Chen K and Kandel DB (1995) The natural history of drug use from adolescence to the mid-thirties in a general population sample. *Am J Pub Health* **85**(1), 41–47.

Chen K and Kandel DB (1998) Predictors of cessation of marijuana use: an event history analysis. *Drug Alcohol Depend* **50**, 109–121.

Chen K, Kandel DB, and Davies M (1997) Relationships between frequency and quantity of marijuana use and last year proxy dependence among adolescents and adults in the United States. *Drug Alcohol Depend* **46**(1–2), 53–67.

Comitas L (1976) Cannabis and work in Jamaica: a refutation of the amotivational syndrome. *Ann NY Acad Sci* **282**, 24–35.

Compton DR, Dewey WL, and Martin BR (1990) Cannabis dependence and tolerance production. *Adv Alcohol Subst Abuse* **9**, 129–147.

Crits-Christoph P and Siqueland L (1996) Psychosocial treatment for drug abuse. Selected review and recommendations for national health care. *Arch Gen Psychiatr* **53**(8), 749–756.

Crowley TJ, Macdonald MJ, Whitmore EA, et al. (1998) Cannabis dependence, withdrawal, and reinforcing effects among adolescents with conduct symptoms and substance use disorders. *Drug Alcohol Depend* **50**(1), 27–37.

Cuffel BJ, Heithoff KA, and Lawson W (1993) Correlates of patterns of substance abuse among patients with schizophrenia. *Hosp Comm Psychiatr* **44**, 247–251.

DeWit DJ, Hance J, Offord DR, et al. (2000) The influence of early and frequent use of marijuana on the risk of desistance and of progression to marijuana-related harm. *Prev Med* **31**(5), 455–464.

Diana M, Melis M, and Gessa GL (1998a) Increase in meso-prefrontal dopaminergic activity after stimulation of CB1 receptors by cannabinoids. *Eur J Neurosci* **10**(9), 2825–2830.

Diana M, Melis M, Muntoni AL, et al. (1998b) Mesolimbic dopaminergic decline after cannabinoid withdrawal. *Proc Natl Acad Sci U S A* **95**(17), 10269–10273.

Dixon L, Haas G, Weiden PJ, et al. (1991) Drug abuse in schizophrenic patients: clinical correlates and reasons for use. *Am J Psychiatry* **148**, 224–230.

Ehrenreich H, Rinn T, Kunert HJ, et al. (1999) Specific attentional dysfunction in adults following early start of cannabis use. *Psychopharmacology* **142**(3), 295–301.

Estroff TW and Gold MS (1986) Psychiatric presentations for marijuana abuse. *Psychiatr Ann* **16**, 221–224.

Gardner EL (1999) Cannabinoid interaction with brain reward systems. In *Marijuana and Medicine*, Nahas GG, Sutin KM, Harvey DJ, et al. (eds). Humana Press, Totowa, NJ, pp. 187–205.

Green BE and Ritter C (2000) Marijuana use and depression. *J Health Soc Behav* **41**(1), 40–49.

Greenfield SF and O'Leary G (1999) Sex differences in marijuana use in the United States. *Harv Rev Psychiatry* **6**(6), 297–303.

Grella CE, Hser YI, Joshi V, et al. (1999) Patient histories, retention, and outcome models for younger and older adults in DATOS. *Drug Alcohol Depend* **57**(2), 151–166.

Gruber AJ and Pope HG Jr (1994) Cannabis psychotic disorder: Does it exist? *Am J Addict* **3**, 72–83.

Gruber AJ, Pope HG Jr., and Brown ME (1996) Do patients use marijuana as an antidepressant? *Depression* **4**(2), 77–80.

Gruber AJ, Pope HG Jr., Hudson JI, et al. (in press) Attributes of long-term heavy cannabis users: a case–control study.

Halikas JA (1974) Marijuana use and psychiatric illness. In *Marijuana: Effects on Human Behavior*, Miller LL (ed). Academic Press, New York, pp. 265–302.

Hall W and Degenhardt L (2000) Cannabis use and psychosis: a review of clinical and epidemiological evidence. *Aust N Z J Psychiatry* **34**(1), 26–34.

Hall W and Solowij N (1998) Adverse effects of cannabis. *Lancet* **352**(9140), 1611–1616.

Haney M, Ward AS, Comer SD, et al. (1999) Abstinence symptoms following smoked marijuana in humans. *Psychopharmacologia* **141**(4), 395–404.

Haney M, Ward AS, Comer SD, et al. (2001a) Bupropion SR worsens mood during marijuana withdrawal in humans. *Psychopharmacologia* **155**, 171–179.

Haney M, Ward AS, Hart CL, et al. (2001b) Effects of nefazodone on marijuana withdrawal in humans. College on problems of drug dependence. *63rd Annual Scientific Meeting*, Scottsdale, AZ, June 16–21, appears as abstract #241. *Drug Alcohol Depend* **63**(Suppl. 1), S62.

Harder S and Reitbrock S (1997) Concentration–effect relationship of delta-9-tetrahydrocannabinol and prediction of psychotropic effects after smoking marijuana. *Int J Clin Pharmacol Ther* **35**(4), 155–159.

Hendin H and Haas AP (1985) The adaptive significance of chronic marijuana use for adolescents and adults. *Adv Alcohol Subst Abuse* **4**(3–4), 99–115.

Henry B, Feehan M, McGee R, et al. (1993) The importance of conduct problems and depressive symptoms in predicting adolescent substance use. *J Abnorm Child Psychol* **21**, 469–480.

Hochman JS and Brill NQ (1973) Chronic marijuana use and psychosocial adaptation. *Am J Psychiatry* **130**, 132–140.

Hser Y-I, Grella CE, Hubbard RL, et al. (2001) An evaluation of drug treatments for adolescents in 4 US cities. *Arch Gen Psychiatry* **58**, 689–695.

Hubbard RL, Cavanaugh ER, and Craddock SG (1985) Characteristics, behaviors, and outcomes for youth in the TOPS. In *Treatment Services for Adolescent Substance Abusers*, Friedman AS and Beschner G (eds). National Institute on Drug Abuse, Rockville, MD, pp. 49–65.

Hubbard JR, Franco SE, and Onaivi ES (1999) Marijuana: medical implications. *Am Fam Physician* **60**(9), 2583–2588, 2593.

Johns A (2001) Psychiatric effects of cannabis. *Br J Psychiatry* **178**, 116–122.

Johnson BA (1990) Psychopharmacological effects of cannabis. *Br J Hosp Med* **43**, 114–122.

Johnston LD, O'Malley PM, and Bachman JG (2001) *Monitoring the Future National Results on Adolescent Drug Use: Overview of Key Findings, 2000*, NIH Publication No. 01-4923. National Institute on Drug Abuse, Bethesda, MD.

Jones RT (1983) Cannabis tolerance and dependence. In *Cannabis and Health Hazards*, Fehr KO and Kalant H (eds). Addiction Research Foundation, Toronto, pp. 617–689.

Jones RT, Benowitz N, and Bachman J (1976) Clinical studies of cannabis tolerance and dependence. *Ann N Y Acad Sci* **282**, 221–239.

Jones RT, Benowitz NL, and Herning RI (1981) Clinical relevance of cannabis tolerance and dependence. *J Clin Pharmacol* **21**, 143S–152S.

Kandel DB and Chen K (2000) Types of marijuana users by longitudinal course. *J Stud Alcohol* **61**(3), 367–378.

Kaymakcalan S (1973) Tolerance to and dependence on cannabis. *Bull Narc* **25**, 39–47.

Kaymakcalan S (1981) The addictive potential of cannabis. *Bull Narc* **33**, 21–31.

Keeler MH, Ewing JA, and Rouse BA (1971) Hallucinogenic effects of marijuana as currently used. *Am J Psychiatry* **128**, 213–216.

Keeler MH, Reifler CB, and Liptzin MB (1968) Spontaneous recurrence of marijuana effect. *Am J Psychiatry* **125**, 384–386.

Kouri EM and Pope HG Jr. (2000) Abstinence symptoms during withdrawal from chronic marijuana use. *Exp Clin Psychopharmacol* **8**(4), 483–492.

Kouri EM, Pope HG Jr., and Lukas SE (1999) Changes in aggressive behavior during withdrawal from long-term cannabis use. *Psychopharmacology* **143**, 302–308.

Kouri E, Pope HG Jr., Todd E, et al. (1995) Attributes of heavy versus occasional marijuana smokers in a college population. *Biol Psychiatry* **38**, 475–481.

Kupfer DJ, Detre T, Koral J, et al. (1973) A comment on the "amotivational syndrome" in marijuana smokers. *Am J Psychiatry* **130**, 1319–1321.

Latimer WW, Winters KC, Stinchfield R, et al. (2000) Demographic, individual, and interpersonal predictors of adolescent alcohol and marijuana use following treatment. *Psychol Addict Behav* **14**(2), 162–173.

Lessin PJ and Thomas SA (1976) Assessment of the chronic effect of marijuana on motivation and achievement: a preliminary report. In *The Pharmacology of Marijuana*, Braude MC and Szara S (eds). Raven Press, New York, pp. 681–690.

Levi L and Miller NR (1990) Visual illusions associated with previous drug abuse. *J Clin Neuroophthalmol* **10**, 103–110.

Lex BW, Griffin ML, Mello NK, et al. (1989) Alcohol, marijuana, and mood states in young women. *Int J Addict* **24**, 405–424.

Linszen DH, Dingemans PM, and Lenior ME (1994) Cannabis abuse and the course of recent-onset schizophrenic disorder. *Arch Gen Psychiatry* **51**, 273–279.

Mellinger GD, Somers RH, Davidson ST, et al. (1976) The amotivational syndrome and the college student. *Ann N Y Acad Sci* **282**, 37–55.

Mendelson JH, Kuehnle JC, Greenberg I, et al. (1976) The effects of marijuana use on human operant behavior: individual data. In *The Pharmacology of Marijuana*, Braude MC and Szara S (eds). Raven Press, New York, pp. 643–653.

Menezes PR, Johnson S, Thornicroft G, et al. (1996) Drug and alcohol problems among individuals with severe mental illness in south London. *Br J Psychiatry* **168**, 612–619.

Miller FT, Busch F, and Tanenbaum JG (1989) Drug abuse in schizophrenia and bipolar disorder. *Am J Drug Alcohol Abuse* **15**, 291–295.

Miller NS, Klahr AL, Gold MS, et al. (1990) Cannabis diagnosis of patients receiving treatment for cocaine dependence. *J Subst Abuse* **2**(1), 107–111.

Mirin SM, Shapiro LM, Meyer RE, et al. (1971) Casual versus heavy use of marijuana: a redefinition of the marijuana problem. *Am J Psychiatry* **127**(9), 1134–1140.

Mueser KT, Yarnold PR, and Bellak AS (1992) Diagnostic and demographic correlates of substance abuse in schizophrenia and major affective disorder. *Acta Psychiatr Scand* **85**, 48–55.

Musty RE and Kaback L (1995) Relationships between motivation and depression in chronic marijuana users. *Life Sci* **56**(23–24), 2151–2158.

Negrete JC, Knapp WP, Douglas DE, et al. (1986) Cannabis affects the severity of schizophrenic symptoms: results of a clinical survey. *Psychol Med* **16**, 515–520.

Newcombe MD and Bentler P (1988) *Consequences of Adolescent Drug Use: Impact on the Lives of Young Adults*. Sage Publications, Newbury Park, CA.

Peralta V and Cuesta MJ (1992) Influence of cannabis abuse on schizophrenic psychopathology. *Acta Psychiatr Scand* **85**, 127–130.

Perez-Reyes M (1999) The psychologic and physiologic effects of active cannabinoids. In *Marijuana and Medicine*, Nahas GG, Sutin KM, Harvey DJ, et al. (eds). Humana Press, Totowa, NJ, pp. 245–252.

Pillard RC (1970) Marijuana. *N Engl J Med* **283**, 294–303.

Pope HG Jr., Gruber AJ, Hudson JI, et al. (2001a) Neuropsychological performance in long-term cannabis users. *Arch Gen Psychiatry* **58**, 909–915.

Pope HG Jr., Gruber AJ, and Yurgelun-Todd D (1995) The residual neuropsychological effects of cannabis: the current status of research. *Drug Alcohol Depend* **38**(1), 25–34.

Pope HG Jr., Ionescu-Pioggia M, Aizley HG, et al. (1990) Drug use and lifestyle among college undergraduates in 1989: a comparison with 1969 and 1978. *Am J Psychiatry* **147**, 998–1001.

Pope HG Jr., Ionescu-Pioggia M, and Pope KW (2001b) Drug use and life style among college undergraduates: a 30-year longitudinal study. *Am J Psychiatry* **158**(9), 1519–1521.

Pope HG, Jacobs A, Mialet JP, et al. (1997) Evidence for a sex-specific residual effect of cannabis on visuospatial memory. *Psychother Psychosom* **66**(4), 179–184.

Pope HG and Yurgelun-Todd D (1996) The residual cognitive effects of heavy marijuana use. *JAMA* **275**, 521–527.

Prochaska JO and Velicer WF (1997) The transtheoretical model of health behavior change. *Am J Health Promot* **12**(1), 38–48.

Regier DA, Farmer ME, Rae DS, et al. (1990) Comorbidity of mental disorders with alcohol and other drug abuse. Results from the epidemiologic catchment area (ECA) study. *JAMA* **264**(19), 2511–2518.

Robins LN, Darvish HS, and Murphy GE (1970) The long-term outcome for adolescent drug users: a follow-up study of 76 users and 146 non-users. In *The Psychopathology of Adolescence*, Zubin J and Freedman AM (eds). Grune & Stratton, New York, pp. 159–180.

Roffman RA and Barnhart R (1987) Assessing need for marijuana dependence treatment through an anonymous telephone interview. *Int J Addict* **22**(7), 639–651.

Roffman RA, Klepsch R, Wertz JS, et al. (1993) Predictors of attrition from an outpatient marijuana-dependence counseling program. *Addict Behav* **18**, 553–566.

Rounds-Bryant JL, Kristiansen PL, and Hubbard RL (1999) Drug abuse treatment outcome study of adolescents: a comparison of client characteristics and pretreatment behaviors in three treatment modalities. *Am J Drug Alcohol Abuse* **25**(4), 573–591.

Schwartz RH, Gruenewald PJ, Klitzner M, et al. (1989) Short-term memory impairment in cannabis-dependent adolescents. *Am J Dis Child* **143**(10), 1214–1219.

Sigmon SC, Steingard S, Badger GJ, et al. (2000) Contingent reinforcement of marijuana abstinence among individuals with serious mental illness: a feasibility study. *Exp Clin Psychopharmacol* **8**(4), 509–517.

Simon WE, Primavera LH, Simon MG, et al. (1974) A comparison of marijuana users and nonusers on a number of personality variables. *J Consult Clin Psychol* **42**, 917–918.

Simpson DD (1981) The relation of time spent in drug abuse treatment to posttreatment outcome. *Am J Psychiatry* **136**, 1449–1453.

Simpson DD, Joe GW, and Brown BS (1997) Treatment retention and follow-up outcomes in the drug abuse treatment outcome study (DATOS). *Psychol Addict Behav* **11**(4), 294–307.

Smoller JW, Lunetta KL, and Robins J (2000) Implications of comorbidity and ascertainment bias for identifying disease genes. *Am J Med Genet* **96**, 817–822.

Solomons K and Neppe VM (1989) Cannabis—its clinical effects. *S Afr Med J* **76**, 102–104.

Solowij N (1995) Do cognitive impairments recover following cessation of cannabis use? *Life Sci* **56**(23–24), 2119–2126.

Solowij N (1998) *Cannabis and Cognitive Functioning*. Cambridge University Press, Cambridge, UK.

Solowij N, Michie PT, and Fox AM (1991) Effects of long-term cannabis use on selective attention: an event-related potential study. *Pharmacol Biochem Behav* **40**(3), 683–688.

Solowij N, Michie PT, and Fox AM (1995) Differential impairments of selective attention due to frequency and duration of cannabis use. *Biol Psychiatry* **37**(10), 731–739.

Stanton MD and Bardoni A (1972) Drug flashbacks: reported frequency in a military population. *Am J Psychiatry* **129**, 751–755.

Stephens RS, Roffman RA, and Curtin L (2000) Comparison of extended versus brief treatments for marijuana use. *J Consult Clin Psychol* **68**(5), 898–908.

Stephens RS, Roffman RA, and Simpson EE (1993a) Adult marijuana users seeking treatment. *J Consult Clin Psychol* **61**(6), 1100–1104.

Stephens RS, Roffman RA, and Simpson EE (1994) Treating adult marijuana dependence: a test of the relapse prevention model. *J Consult Clin Psychol* **62**(1), 92–99.

Stephens RS, Wertz JS, and Roffman RA (1993b) Predictors of marijuana treatment outcomes: the role of self-efficacy. *J Subst Abuse* **5**(4), 341–353.

Struve FA, Patrick G, Straumanis JJ, et al. (1998) Possible EEG sequelae of very long duration marijuana use: pilot findings from topographic quantitative EEG analysis of subjects with 15 to 24 years of cumulative daily exposure to THC. *Clin Electroencephalogr* **29**, 31–36.

Substance Abuse and Mental Health Services Administration, Office of Applied Studies (1997) *Preliminary Results from the 1996 National Household Survey on Drug Abuse*. SAMHSA, Rockville, MD.

Substance Abuse and Mental Health Services Association, Office of Applied Studies (1999) *National Admissions to Substance Abuse Treatment Services: The Treatment Episode Data Set (TEDS) 1992–1997*. US Government Printing Office, Washington, DC.

Substance Abuse and Mental Health Services Administration, Office of Applied Studies (2000) *Summary of Findings from the 1999 National Household Survey on Drug Abuse*. SAMHSA, Rockville, MD.

Szuster RR, Pontuis EB, and Campos PE (1988) Marijuana sensitivity and panic anxiety. *J Clin Psychiatry* **49**, 427–429.

Tanda G, Pontieri FE, and Di Chiara G (1997) Cannabinoid and heroin activation of mesolimbic dopamine transmission by a common micro1 opioid receptor mechanism. *Science* **276**(5321), 2048–2050.

Tennant FS (1986) The clinical syndrome of marijuana dependence. *Psychiatr Ann* **16**, 225–234.

Thomas H (1996) A community survey of adverse effects of cannabis use. *Drug Alcohol Depend* **42**, 201–207.

Treffert DA (1978) Marijuana use in schizophrenia: a clear hazard. *Am J Psychiatry* **135**, 1213–1215.

Troisi A, Pasini A, Saracco M, et al. (1998) Psychiatric symptoms in male cannabis users not using other illicit drugs. *Addiction* **93**(4), 487–492.

True WR, Heath AC, Scherrer JF, et al. (1999) Interrelationship of genetic and environmental influences on conduct disorder and alcohol and marijuana dependence symptoms. *Am J Med Genet* **88**(4), 391–397.

Warner R, Taylor D, Wright J, et al. (1994) Substance use among the mentally ill: prevalence, reasons for use, and effects on illness. *Am J Orthopsychiatry* **64**, 30–39.

Weiner MD, Sussman S, McCuller WJ, et al. (1999) Factors in marijuana cessation among high-risk youth. *J Drug Educ* **29**(4), 337–357.

Weller RA and Halikas JA (1985) Marijuana use and psychiatric illness: a follow-up study. *Am J Psychiatry* **142**, 848–850.

Wiesbeck GA, Schuckit MA, Kalmijn JA, et al. (1996) An evaluation of the history of a marijuana withdrawal syndrome in a large population. *Addiction* **91**(10), 1469–1478.

Zinberg NE and Weil AT (1970) A comparison of marijuana users and non-users. *Nature* **226**, 119–123.

Zoccollilo M, Vitaro F, and Tremblay RE (1999) Problem drug and alcohol use in a community sample of adolescents. *J Am Acad Child Adolesc Psychiatry* **38**(7), 900–907.

20 Substance-Related Disorders: Cocaine

Cocaine, a central nervous system stimulant produced by the coca plant, is consumed in several preparations. Cocaine hydrochloride powder is usually snorted through the nostrils, or it may be mixed in water and injected intravenously. Cocaine hydrochloride powder is also commonly heated ("cooked up") with ammonia or baking soda and water to remove the hydrochloride, thus forming a gel-like substance that can be smoked ("freebasing"). "Crack" cocaine is a precooked form of cocaine alkaloid that is sold on the street as small "rocks." Abundant supplies and falling prices for cocaine (the equivalent of 1 gram of cocaine can be purchased for as little as $25 to $50 and a vial of crack (two or three small "rocks") can be had for about $10) have contributed greatly to the prevalence of cocaine abuse and dependence as well as other related cocaine-use disorders.

Diagnosis

The state of intense euphoria produced by cocaine intoxication is a powerful reinforcer and can lead to the development of cocaine-use disorders in many individuals, although only 10 to 16% of those who try the drug go on to develop these disorders (Gawin 1991, Warner et al. 1995, Ensminger et al. 1997, Van Etten and Anthony 1999). Some experience the stimulant effects of cocaine as anxiogenic; others discontinue use because of lack of easy drug availability, fear of loss of control over use, or apprehension regarding possible legal consequences of cocaine abuse. The route of administration is strongly correlated with the development of cocaine-use disorders, in that the intravenous and smoked routes of administration allow rapid transport of the drug to the brain, producing intense effects that are short-lived. Rapid tolerance to euphoria occurs and plasma concentrations are not correlated with peak euphoria, producing a need for frequent dosing to regain euphoric effects (binge use) that can place the cocaine abuser at a risk for medical and psychiatric complications of cocaine abuse.

While the question of whether cocaine is physiologically addictive is not completely clear, the psychological addiction alone is powerful and can completely dominate the life of the cocaine abuser. Binge use of cocaine may be followed by what has been described as a mild withdrawal syndrome characterized by dysphoria and anhedonia. Cocaine withdrawal may resemble a depressive disorder, in some cases requiring emergent treatment. Some combinations of these consequences of cocaine abuse are usually responsible for the identification and diagnosis of individuals with cocaine-use disorders and referral to substance-abuse treatment.

When evaluating an individual regarding the possible presence of a cocaine-related disorder, the initial evaluation period should include the collection of a complete history of all substance abuse, which is essential to accurate diagnosis and appropriate treatment. Figure 20-1 shows a diagnostic decision tree for cocaine-related disorders. The history includes the circumstances under which each drug was used, the psychoactive effects sought and obtained, the route of administration, and the frequency and amount of each drug used. Cocaine abusers frequently abuse other drugs and alcohol to enhance euphoria or to alleviate dysphoric effects associated with cocaine abuse (agitation, paranoia). A thorough history with diagnosis of other substance-use disorders is important to treatment planning. Individuals may need detoxification from other substances prior to initiation of cocaine abuse treatment. It is also important to monitor clinically for relapses to any substance abuse during treatment for cocaine-use disorders because the use of other drugs and alcohol often leads to resumption of cocaine abuse. In addition, a thorough history of current and previous substance abuse is important so that treatment can be individualized and individuals can be helped in developing coping skills that will assist them in specific situations that they identify as placing them at high risk for relapse.

A careful psychiatric history with particular attention to onset of psychiatric symptoms in relation to drug use is essential. The determination of a premorbid psychiatric illness is critical to providing appropriate treatment. For persons in whom substance abuse is an attempt to self-medicate an underlying mental illness, the introduction of psychotropic medication in conjunction with ongoing treatment for the substance abuse will improve both the mental disorder as well as the substance-use disorder(s). Conversely, the evaluation of temporal onset of psychiatric symptoms may preclude erroneous use of psychotropic medication in cases in which the psychiatric symptoms are in fact cocaine-induced and spare the individual exposure to the potential side effects of these medications.

Cocaine Dependence   The DSM-IV-TR defines the essential features of substance dependence as a cluster of cognitive, behavioral, and physiological symptoms indicating continued use of the substance despite significant consequences of use (see Chapter 15, page 351 for the DSM-IV-TR diagnostic criteria for Substance Dependence). There is a pattern of administration that usually results in tolerance to and compulsive self-administration of the drug and may produce a withdrawal syndrome on cessation of drug use. Cocaine dependence can develop quickly after initiation of use because of the potent euphoria produced by the drug. The route of administration is related to the development of cocaine dependence; smoked and intravenous routes are more highly correlated with dependence than the intranasal route of administration.

Cocaine has a short half-life requiring frequent dosing to maintain the "high" (binge use). Persons with cocaine dependence often spend large amounts of money for the drug and may be involved in illegal activities to obtain cocaine. Binges may be separated by several days while the individual recovers or attempts to obtain more money for drug purchase. Illegal activities such as theft and prostitution are often engaged in to obtain cash for cocaine. Obligations such as employment and childcare are often neglected. Tolerance to cocaine effects develops quickly, resulting in larger amounts of drug use with time. This is often associated with mental or physical complications of use including paranoia, aggressive behavior, anxiety and agitation, depression, and weight loss. Withdrawal symptoms, most prominently dysphoric mood, may be seen, but are usually short-lived and clear within several days of abstinence.

Cocaine Abuse   Substance abuse is described by DSM-IV-TR as a maladaptive pattern of substance use demonstrated by recurrent and significant adverse consequences related to repeated use (see Chapter 15, page 352 for the DSM-IV-TR diagnostic criteria for Substance

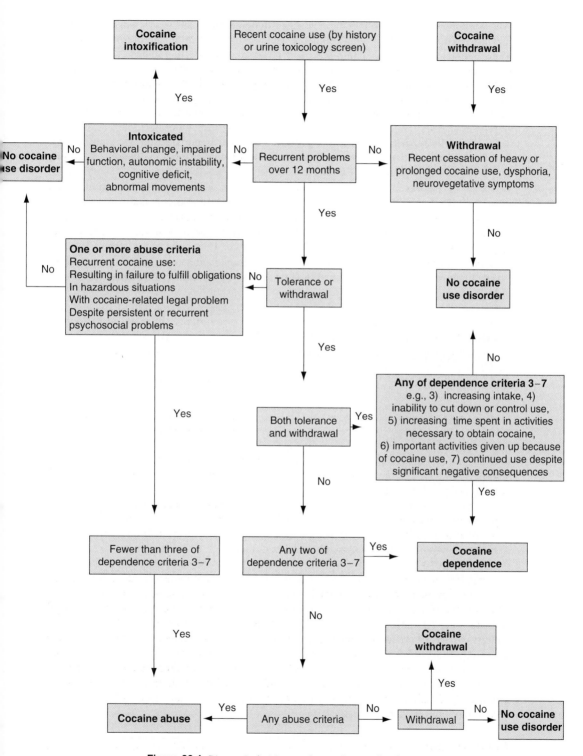

Figure 20-1 *Diagnostic decision tree for cocaine-use disorders.*

Abuse). For example, there may be neglect of obligations to family or employer, repeated use in hazardous situations, legal problems, and recurrent social or interpersonal problems. These problems must recur within the same 12-month period. The intensity and frequency of use are less in cocaine abuse than in cocaine dependence. Episodes of abuse may occur around paydays or special occasions and may be characterized by brief periods (hours to days) of high-dose binge use followed by longer periods of abstinence or nonproblem use.

Cocaine Intoxication The clinical effects of cocaine intoxication are characterized initially by euphoria (referred to as "high") and also include agitation, anxiety, irritability or affective lability, grandiosity, impaired judgment, increased psychomotor activity, hyper-vigilance or paranoia, and sometimes hallucinations (visual, auditory, or tactile) may occur (see DSM-IV-TR diagnostic criteria below). Physical symptoms that can accompany cocaine intoxication include hypertension, tachycardia, hyperthermia, pupillary dilation, nausea, vomiting, tremor, diaphoresis, chest pain, arrhythmia, confusion, seizures, dysk-inetic movements, dystonia, and, in severe cases, coma. These effects are more frequently seen in high-dose binge users of cocaine. Cardiovascular effects are probably a result of sympathomimetic properties of cocaine (i.e., release of norepinephrine and blockade of norepinephrine reuptake.)

DSM-IV-TR Diagnostic Criteria

292.89 Cocaine Intoxication

A. Recent use of cocaine.
B. Clinically significant maladaptive behavioral or psychological changes (e.g., euphoria or affective blunting; changes in sociability; hypervigilance; interpersonal sensitivity; anxiety, tension, or anger; stereotyped behaviors; impaired judgment; or impaired social or occupational functioning) that developed during, or shortly after, use of cocaine.
C. Two (or more) of the following developing during or shortly after cocaine use:

  (1) tachycardia or bradycardia
  (2) pupillary dilation
  (3) elevated or lowered blood pressure
  (4) perspiration or chills
  (5) nausea or vomiting
  (6) evidence of weight loss
  (7) psychomotor agitation or retardation
  (8) muscular weakness, respiratory depression, chest pain, or cardiac arrhythmias
  (9) confusion, seizures, dyskinesias, dystonias, or coma.

D. The symptoms are not due to a general medical condition and are not better accounted for by another mental disorder.

Specify if:

With perceptual disturbances

Cocaine Withdrawal The principal feature of substance withdrawal is development of a substance-specific maladaptive behavioral change, which may have associated physiological and cognitive components, resulting from the cessation of or reduction in heavy and prolonged substance use. The syndrome is characterized by significant distress or impairment in function. Symptoms must not be better explained by a mental or physical disorder. Cocaine withdrawal develops within a few hours to a few days after stopping or reducing cocaine use that has been heavy and prolonged (see DSM-IV-TR diagnostic criteria below). The syndrome is characterized by dysphoria and two or more physiological changes including fatigue, vivid and unpleasant dreams, insomnia or hypersomnia, increased appetite, and psychomotor agitation or retardation. Anhedonia and craving for cocaine can be part of the withdrawal syndrome. Depression and suicidal ideation are the most serious complications and require individualized assessment and treatment. The syndrome may last up to several days but generally resolves without treatment.

DSM-IV-TR Diagnostic Criteria

292.0 Cocaine Withdrawal

A. Cessation of (or reduction in) cocaine use that has been heavy and prolonged.
B. Dysphoric mood and two (or more) of the following physiological changes, developing within a few hours to several days after Criterion A:

  (1) fatigue
  (2) vivid, unpleasant dreams
  (3) insomnia or hypersomnia
  (4) increased appetite
  (5) psychomotor retardation or agitation.

C. The symptoms in Criterion B cause clinically significant distress or impairment in social, occupational, or other important areas of functioning.
D. The symptoms are not due to a general medical condition and are not better accounted for by another mental disorder.

Other Cocaine-Induced Disorders DSM-IV-TR also specifies additional cocaine-induced disorders described in other diagnostic groupings with which they share phenomenology (Table 20-1). These include cocaine intoxication delirium, cocaine-induced psychotic disorder, cocaine-induced mood disorder, cocaine-induced anxiety disorder, cocaine-induced sleep disorder, and cocaine-induced sexual dysfunction. These disorders are diagnosed instead of intoxication or withdrawal only if symptoms are in excess of those usually associated with cocaine intoxication or cocaine withdrawal and warrant independent clinical attention. In addition, the clinician should pay careful attention to the temporal relationship of the psychiatric symptoms and cocaine abuse. Symptoms that are severe enough to warrant consideration of one of these diagnoses should also dissipate with continued abstinence from cocaine. Symptoms that worsen after cessation of cocaine use

Table 20-1	Other DSM-IV-TR Cocaine-Induced Disorders
292.89	Cocaine intoxication
	Specify if: with perceptual disturbances
292.0	Cocaine withdrawal
292.81	Cocaine intoxication delirium
292.11	Cocaine-induced psychotic disorder, with delusions
	Specify if: with onset during intoxication
292.12	Cocaine-induced psychotic disorder, with hallucinations
	Specify if: with onset during intoxication
292.84	Cocaine-induced mood disorder
	Specify if: with onset during intoxication/with onset during withdrawal
292.89	Cocaine-induced anxiety disorder
	Specify if: with onset during intoxication/with onset during withdrawal
292.89	Cocaine-induced sexual dysfunction
	Specify if: with onset during intoxication
292.89	Cocaine-induced sleep disorder
	Specify if: with onset during intoxication/with onset during withdrawal
292.9	Cocaine-related disorder not otherwise specified

Source: Data Reprinted with permission from the Diagnostic and Statistical Manual of Mental Disorders, Fourth Edition, Text Revision. Copyright 2000 American Psychiatric Association.

in a period of 1 to 4 weeks should be reevaluated and other Axis I or Axis III disorders considered with modification of the treatment plan as clinically indicated.

Epidemiology

The National Household Survey on Drug Abuse (NHSDA) reported that in 2000, 1.2 million Americans were current cocaine users representing 0.5% of the population over the age of 12 (SAMHSA 2000a). Since 1975, the Monitoring The Future (MTF) study has annually examined the extent of drug abuse among 8th to 12th graders. Use of cocaine decreased significantly among 12th graders, from 6.2% in 1999 to 5.0% in 2000; crack cocaine use in the year 2000 decreased from 2.7 to 2.2% for 12th graders. This was the first decrease in cocaine and crack cocaine use among 12th graders since the early 1990s. Crack use by 8th graders also decreased from a 10-year high of 2.1% in 1998 to 1.8% in 1999, which remained constant in 2000 (Johnson et al. 2001). While cocaine use has shown a downward trend, several statistics indicate that cocaine abuse is still a serious threat to the public. For example, cocaine-related emergency department visits constituted 29% of all drug-related visits in 2000, more than for any other illicit substance (SAMHSA 2001b). The National Drug Threat Assessment 2001 (National Drug Threat Assessment 2001—The Domestic Perspective, by the National Drug Intelligence Center, NDIC) reported that availability and demand for cocaine continues to be high. The assessment also indicated that the transportation, distribution, abuse, and criminal activity related to powder and crack cocaine continue to constitute the greatest drug threat to the United States. Of the 412 state and local agencies responding to the survey, 109 rated cocaine as one of the greatest drug threats in their areas (Johnston PA 2000).

Earlier epidemiological surveys had failed to identify demographic characteristics, personality traits, or features of early cocaine use that differentiate noncompulsive and heavy use (Schnoll et al. 1985). However, recent studies suggest that a particular personality trait known as novelty or sensation seeking may play an important role in the initiation of cocaine use (Laviola et al. 1999).

Course

Cocaine produces a sense of intensified pleasure in most activities and a heightened sense of alertness and well-being. Anxiety and social inhibition are decreased. Energy, self-esteem, and self-perception of ability are increased. There is enhancement of emotion and sexual feeling (Bolla et al. 1998, Leshner and Koob 1999). Pleasurable experiences, although heightened, are not distorted and hallucinations are usually absent. The person engaging in low-dose cocaine use often receives positive feedback from others responding to the user's increased energy and enthusiasm. This, in combination with the euphoria experienced by the user, can be reinforcing, and cocaine use is perceived as free of any adverse consequences. The duration of cocaine's euphoric effects depends on the route of administration. The faster the drug is absorbed and occupies receptors of the "brain rewarding region," the more intense the euphoric effects (Ward et al. 1997a, Leshner and Koob 1999, Koob 1999).

Cocaine and alcohol are often consumed together. In addition to the synergistic effects of cocaine and alcohol in humans, an active metabolite, cocaethylene, with cocaine-like pharmacological properties is formed and users of both drugs simultaneously report enhanced euphoria (McCance-Katz et al. 1993, Andrews 1997, McCance-Katz et al. 1998a, Hart et al. 2000).

Cocaine users quickly learn that higher doses are associated with intensified and prolonged euphoria, resulting in increasing use of the drug and progression to cocaine dependence. The abuser is focused on the cocaine-induced euphoria and begins to compulsively pursue this effect. These behaviors become pivotal in the lives of cocaine abusers who continue drug abuse despite the presence of increasing personal and social consequences (Ward et al. 1997a, Bolla et al. 1998).

The psychoactive effects of cocaine are similar to those of amphetamine; the main difference in terms of abuse liability is in cocaine's much shorter duration of action. Whereas the plasma elimination half-life for cocaine is approximately 90 minutes, this drug produces pharmacodynamic tachyphylaxis, resulting in rapidly diminishing psychoactive effects in the presence of continued cocaine in the plasma. This phenomenon explains the "half-life" of cocaine-induced euphoria, (which is approximately 45 minutes after intranasal use and 5 minutes after intravenous and smoking administration) as well as characteristic binge use in which cocaine is repetitively administered over short intervals (Mendelson et al. 1999, Jufer et al. 2000, Moolchan et al. 2000). During binge use, the drug may be administered as frequently as every 10 minutes, resulting in rapid mood changes. Cocaine binges reportedly can last as long as 7 days, although the average length is 12 hours (Pottieger et al. 1995, Foltin and Fischman 1997, Ward et al. 1997b, Foltin and Fischman 1998, Evans et al. 1999).

Uncontrolled use of cocaine often begins with either increased access and resultant escalating dosages and frequency of administration or a change from intranasal use to a route of administration with more rapid onset of effects (i.e., intravenous or smoked) (Ward et al. 1997a, Foltin and Fischman 1998). These characteristics are integral to the development of high-dose binging with cocaine. Such binges produce extreme euphoria and vivid memories. These memories are later contrasted with current dysphoria to produce intense craving, which perpetuates the binge-use pattern (Margolin et al. 1996, Uslaner et al. 1999). Addicts report that during binge use, thoughts are focused exclusively on the cocaine-induced effects. Normal daily needs, including sleep and nourishment, are neglected. Responsibilities to family and employer and social obligations are given up. This continues until the supply of cocaine is exhausted.

Binges are often separated by several days of abstinence; cocaine-dependent individuals average one to three binges per week. This is in contrast to use patterns for opiate and alcohol dependence, which often produce physiological dependence necessitating daily consumption to prevent withdrawal symptoms. This differentiation is crucial to an understanding of the syndrome of cocaine dependence (Pottieger et al. 1995, Evans et al. 1999). Although the prediction of development of cocaine-use disorders is not possible on an individual basis, it is clear that those who progress to binge use of the drug will be significantly affected and constitute the treatment-seeking population. The cocaine abuser is likely to be ambivalent about the need for treatment, and the treatment dropout rate is high (ranging from 38 to 73%). Dropout usually occurs early in treatment (during the initial evaluation process) (Siqueland et al. 1998, Simpson et al. 1997, Chou et al. 1998, Fiocchi and Kingree 2001).

Newly abstinent cocaine abusers may experience a triphasic abstinence pattern, although this varies by individual, that includes a period of acute abstinence, sometimes referred to as the "crash," lasting several hours to several days consisting of dysphoria, fatigue, insomnia or hypersomnia, increased appetite, and either psychomotor agitation or retardation, subsequent to the more intensive "crash" phase. A more chronic withdrawal period sometimes occurs characterized by minor depressive symptoms and cocaine craving lasting 2 to 10 weeks. This may then be followed by an extinction phase characterized by intermittent drug craving that becomes increasingly manageable with continued abstinence.

Like other drug and alcohol use disorders, cocaine-use disorders are chronic relapsing illnesses that present substantial challenges in the treatment process. Cocaine abusers are at high risk for relapse, particularly in the first few months of treatment related to acute craving often in the context of ongoing psychosocial stressors that result from or have been exacerbated by cocaine abuse. Newly abstinent cocaine abusers often lack adequate coping skills necessary to avoid cocaine use, which take time to acquire in the treatment process. Although the ability to cope with cocaine craving improves with continued abstinence, relapse to cocaine abuse or other drug and alcohol abuse will continue to be a risk for those with a history of a cocaine-use disorder who relapse to cocaine abuse. Repeated treatments may be required for those with cocaine-use disorders. Treatment modalities include inpatient hospitalization for medical or psychiatric complications of cocaine abuse, partial hospital programs, self-help groups, psychotherapy (usually group or family therapy for individuals with primary cocaine-use disorders), or some combination of these treatments according to the clinical presentation of the individual (see later in the chapter).

Comorbidity with Other Mental Disorders

Comorbid conditions related to cocaine abuse are abuse of other substances (Withers et al. 1995, Birnbach et al. 2001, Usdan et al. 2001) and comorbid mental disorder (Volkow 2001). Several studies have documented the high rate of comorbid mental disorders in cocaine abusers entering treatment. These disorders include mood disorders (major depressive disorder, bipolar disorders), schizophrenia, posttraumatic stress disorder, attention-deficit/hyperactivity disorder, anxiety disorders, and antisocial personality disorder (Marlowe et al. 1997, Najavits et al. 1997, Westermeyer et al. 1997, Brady et al. 1998, Eames et al. 1998, Brown et al. 1998, Thomas et al. 1999, Dixon 1999, Clure et al. 1999, Schmitz et al. 2000, Sherwood Brown et al. 2001, Skinstad and Swain 2001, Cassidy et al. 2001). Mood disorders often temporally follow the onset of cocaine abuse in individuals presenting for treatment, while attention-deficit/hyperactivity disorder and antisocial personality disorder precede the onset of cocaine abuse (McMahon et al. 1999, Clure et al. 1999). However, while high levels of depressive symptoms during treatment were associated with greater craving for cocaine, alcohol, and other substances, only limited evidence exists regarding the influence of depression on treatment course and outcome (Carroll et al. 1995a, Brown et al. 1998, Simpson et al. 1999).

It is important to note that comorbid psychiatric illnesses are common among cocaine users. Furthermore, the diagnosis of a comorbid primary mental disorder can be challenging to make in cocaine abusers because psychiatric symptoms may be the result of cocaine abuse or acute abstinence. When mental disorders co-occur with cocaine-use disorders, it is important to provide treatment for both disorders. Cocaine-use disorders will not generally resolve with treatment of the mental disorder alone, nor will substance-abuse treatment resolve a comorbid mental disorder.

Medical Complications of Cocaine Abuse

Cardiac toxicity is one of the leading causes of morbidity and mortality associated with cocaine use. The risk of myocardial infarct is well established in cocaine use (Pitts et al. 1997, 1998) and is not related to dose, route, or frequency of administration (Lange and Hillis 2001). The risk of acute myocardial infarction is increased 24-fold in 1 hour immediately following cocaine use in persons who are otherwise at a relatively low risk for such events (Mittleman et al. 1999). Detection of recent cocaine use by urine toxicology screen has been observed in 25% of those reporting to urban emergency departments and 7% of those evaluated at suburban hospitals and found to have evidence of myocardial infarct (Hollander et al. 1995). About half of the individuals with cocaine-related myocardial infarction have no evidence of atherosclerotic coronary artery disease (Hollander et al. 1997a,b). Identifying and diagnosing cocaine-related myocardial infarction can be difficult. The hallmarks of myocardial infarct are a constellation of physical symptoms including chest pain, electrocardiogram (ECG) abnormalities, and elevated creatine kinase. Cocaine abusers with chest pain may have ECG abnormalities that are not specific for myocardial infarct (Hollander et al. 1994, 1998a, Hamad and Khan 2000, Weber et al. 2000). Cocaine abusers also are often found to have nonspecific elevations in creatine kinase without myocardial infarction (Hollander et al. 1998b). Therefore, the diagnosis of cocaine-related myocardial infarction is often based on the physician's clinical judgment. Evaluation of serum troponin I, a cardiac marker that is not affected by recent cocaine use, can be helpful in the determination of whether a myocardial infarct has occurred (Hollander et al. 1998b, Lange and Hillis 2001).

According to new treatment guidelines for emergency cardiovascular care, nitroglycerine and benzodiazepines are first-line agents and phentolamine is a second-line agent for individuals with cocaine-related myocardial ischemia or infarction. Propranolol is contraindicated as it exacerbates cocaine-induced vasoconstriction of coronary arteries (American Psychiatric Association 2000a,b). Thrombolysis is not recommended unless evidence of evolving myocardial infarction persists despite medical therapy and an occluded coronary artery is shown to be present on angiography (American Psychiatric Association 2000a,b Lange and Hillis 2001).

Cocaine use is associated with a wide range of cardiac dysrhythmias including sinus tachycardia, sinus bradycardia, supraventricular and ventricular tachycardia, ventricular premature contractions, ventricular tachycardia and fibrillation, torsades de pointes and asystole (Kerns et al. 1997, Perera et al. 1997, Castro and Nacht 2000, Gamouras et al. 2000, Singh et al. 2001). While the precise arrhythmogenic mechanism of cocaine is unclear, limited evidence suggests that it may be owing to cocaine's sodium-channel-blocking property similar to class I antidysrhythmic drugs that prolong the QRS and QT intervals on ECG (Kerns et al. 1997, Brady and Chan 1999). Life-threatening dysrhythmia caused by cocaine in the absence of myocardial ischemia is rare. In many instances, cardiac dysrhythmias have occurred in the context of profound hemodynamic or metabolic disturbances (Wang 1999). Individuals with cocaine-induced ventricular dysrhythmias and heart block should receive standard therapy including the treatment of ischemia if present, the correction of metabolic disturbances, and the administration of appropriate antiarrhythmic agents (Lange and Hillis 2001). Class IA antiarrhythmic drugs, such as quinidine, procainamide, and di-isopyramide, should be avoided since they may exacerbate prolongation of the QRS and QT intervals and slow the metabolism of cocaine.

Several cases of cardiomyopathy and left ventricular hypertrophy attributed to cocaine use have been reported (Fineschi et al. 1997, Missouris et al. 2001). The condition is often associated with chronic cocaine use and cocaine-related myocardial ischemia and infarction. While the exact underlying mechanisms of cocaine-induced cardiomyopathy and hypertrophy are still unclear, the process may involve repetitive sympathetic stimulation of cocaine with altered myocardial collagen and myosin composition in endothelial cells (Mao et al. 1997, Besse et al. 1997, Woolf et al. 1997, Huang et al. 1997, He et al. 2000, 2001, Xiao et al. 2000). A few cases of aortic dissection have also been reported in association with cocaine abuse (Baumgartner and Omari 1997, Perron and Gibbs 1997, Madu et al. 1999). This adverse event might be associated with sudden increase in blood pressure after cocaine use.

Intranasal abuse of cocaine has been associated with a number of medical complications including chronic sinusitis, septal perforation, subperiosteal abscess, pneumomediastinum, pneumothorax, and pulmonary edema (Gendeh et al. 1998). The presence of pulmonary edema in a young, otherwise healthy individual, without predisposing risk factors, should alert the physician to the possibility of cocaine abuse (Albertson et al. 1995, Boghdadi and Henning 1997, Bird and Markey 1997, Cuenca Carvajal et al. 1998).

Cerebrovascular accidents related to cocaine use have been well documented in the medical literature (Petitti et al. 1998, Kaufman et al. 1998, Blanco et al. 1999, Tolat et al. 2000, Alves and Gomes 2000, Neiman et al. 2000, Nwosu et al. 2001, Kaufman et al. 2001, Daras et al. 2001, Qureshi et al. 2001). Cerebral infarct, subarachnoid hemorrhage, intraparenchymal hemorrhage, and intraventricular hemorrhage have been observed as acute complications of cocaine use. The physiological etiology of these events appears to be related to adrenergic stimulation resulting in a sudden surge in blood pressure. Abrupt increases in blood pressure in otherwise normotensive individuals may precipitate spontaneous bleeding (Strickland et al. 1998, Neiman et al. 2000). Additional risk would be encountered by a cocaine user with an arteriovenous malformation or cerebral artery aneurysm.

Seizures were one of the earliest-known complications of cocaine abuse (Koppel et al. 1996, Winbery et al. 1998, Chiarotti and Fucci 1999, O'Connell and Heffron 2000, Steele et al. 2000). Cocaine produces hyperpyrexia, which in combination with its effects on neurotransmitters may contribute to the development of seizures (Boghdadi and Henning 1997, Winbery et al. 1998). Seizures may occur as a primary effect of cocaine owing to its ability to lower the seizure threshold or may be secondary to other central nervous system or cardiac events precipitated by cocaine use (Koppel et al. 1996). One study retrospectively analyzed 474 cases of cocaine-related seizures. Of these, 403 had no history of seizures. It was found that the majority of seizures were single, generalized, and induced by intravenous or "crack" cocaine abuse not associated with any lasting neurological deficits. Seizures that were focal, multiple, or occurred with nasal cocaine use were more frequently associated with an acute intracerebral complication or concurrent use of other drugs (Pascual-Leone et al. 1990, Koppel et al. 1996, Chiarotti and Fucci 1999). While anticonvulsants have not been helpful in preventing cocaine-related seizures, intravenous diazepam has been effective in acute management (Koppel et al. 1996). These findings imply that there is no clinical benefit to the institution of anticonvulsant therapy in cocaine-related seizure, rather substance-abuse treatment for the cocaine-use disorder is indicated.

Recently, acute renal failure as a result of rhabdomyolysis has been recognized as an important complication of cocaine abuse (Lampley et al. 1996, Horowitz et al. 1997, Ruttenber et al. 1999, Richards 2000, van der Woude 2000). Pregnancy may increase the risk of rhabdomyolysis and renal failure (Lampley et al. 1996). Renal failure may progress

Table 20-2	Major Medical Complications Associated with Cocaine Abuse

Cardiovascular
Myocardial infarct
Arrhythmias
Aortic dissection
Cardiomyopathy

Respiratory
Pneumonitis (associated with smoked cocaine)
Pulmonary edema
Nasal septal perforation, chronic sinusitis (associated with intranasal inhalation)

Central Nervous System
Hyperpyrexia
Seizure
Cerebral infarct
Subarachnoid hemorrhage
Intraparenchymal hemorrhage
Intraventricular hemorrhage

Renal
Renal failure secondary to rhabdomyolysis
Obstetrical
Premature labor
Placental abruption

Complications of Intravenous Use
Infectious diseases (HIV, hepatitis)
Endocarditis
Cellulitis Abscesses

Psychiatric
Depression
Suicidality
Psychosis

rapidly in the context of cocaine-induced rhabdomyolysis and dialysis may be necessary for some individuals. The mechanism for this complication is unclear. Some possibilities include increased muscle activity, muscle compression, hyperthermia, and vasospasm with muscle ischemia (Ruttenber et al. 1999, van der Woude 2000, Richards 2000).

The major medical complications of cocaine abuse are summarized in Table 20-2.

Etiology

Genetic Vulnerability

Heritability or genetic vulnerability may play an important role in the development of cocaine addiction. Epidemiological studies of twins suggest that while both genetic and environmental factors play a role in twin concordance of cocaine use, concordance of abuse and dependence appear to be more influenced by genetic factors (Kendler and Prescott 1998). While no single gene has been linked to cocaine-use disorders, certain alleles may play a role in the development of cocaine-use disorders and/or clinical manifestations of these disorders. Population-based genetic association studies have yielded some interesting preliminary results. For example, an association between cocaine-induced paranoia and an allelic polymorphism in the dopamine transporter protein (DAT) (allele 9) has been described (Gelernter et al. 1994). A second study reported on a haplotype at the dopamine beta-hydroxylase (DBH) locus associated with low plasma DBH activity that appears to be associated with cocaine-associated paranoia (Gelernter et al. 1994). These results together with candidate gene studies using genetic engineering techniques and genome mapping may contribute to important advances in our understanding of genetic vulnerability to cocaine abuse and dependence (Kuhar et al. 2001).

Neurobiological Changes

Cocaine has effects on multiple neurotransmitters, including release and reuptake blockade of dopamine, serotonin (5-hydroxytryptamine [5-HT]), and norepinephrine (Hemby 1999, Koob 1999). The most widely accepted explanation of cocaine-induced euphoria is that dopamine reuptake inhibition results in increased extracellular dopamine concentration in the mesolimbic and mesocortical reward pathways in the brain. Numerous studies have provided evidence for the importance of dopamine in the reinforcing properties of cocaine. For example, 6-hydroxydopamine lesions of dopaminergic terminals in the nucleus accumbens produce extinction-like responding and a reduction in cocaine self-administration. Similar lesions in other areas of the brain (frontal cortex and caudate nucleus) do not alter cocaine self-administration (Schenk et al. 1991, Brown and Fibiger 1993, Reavill et al. 1998).

In vivo brain microdialysis and neuroimaging studies using functional magnetic resonance imaging (fMRI), PET, and SPECT, have provided additional direct evidence that the limbic region and other dopamine rich structures in the brain are associated with cocaine reward (Gatley and Volkow 1998, London et al. 1999, Hommer 1999). Cocaine-induced euphoria has been associated with activity in many areas of the brain, but primarily in the prefrontal cortex as evidenced by reduced cerebral glucose metabolism (London et al. 1996, Bolla et al. 1998, London et al. 1999) and reduced cerebral blood flow (rCBF) (Pearlson et al. 1993, Breiter et al. 1997, Gollub et al. 1998). Moreover, SPECT neuroimaging has shown that the euphoric effects of cocaine are associated with blockade of the dopamine transporter (Malison et al. 1995, 1998a, Volkow et al. 1999). Cue-induced craving increases activation in the limbic regions including dorsolateral prefrontal cortex, cerebellum, anterior cingulate, and amygdala (London et al. 1990, Childress et al. 1999, Garavan et al. 2000). These structures have been linked to memory and learning. The amygdala, in particular, is linked to the emotional aspect of memory (Rolls 2000, Cahill 2000, LeDoux 2000). Studies using fMRI technology showed that cocaine-specific cues activated the same limbic regions activated by other pleasurable stimuli (such as sex in cocaine users) but had almost no effect on nonusers (Childress et al. 1999, Garavan et al. 2000, Stein 2001).

Another important phenomenon related to acute cocaine administration is that of "acute tolerance." A single dose of cocaine has been shown experimentally to reduce the response to a second identical dose given 100 minutes later as measured by extracellular dopamine levels and motor activity (Bradberry 2000). The finding of "acute tolerance" is consistent with the binge pattern of cocaine use in which abusers consume escalating doses of cocaine in an attempt to recapture the intense euphoria of the initial cocaine dose (Bradberry 2000).

A growing body of evidence indicates that chronic cocaine administration can result in sustained neurophysiological changes in brain systems that regulate psychological processes, specifically pleasure and hedonic responsivity (Bolla et al. 1998). This has been postulated to underlie a physiological addiction to cocaine with associated withdrawal phenomena that are manifested clinically as a psychological syndrome (Koob and Nestler 1997). Long-term cocaine administration in animals is associated with an increase in dopamine transporter–binding sites, a decrease in intracranial electrical self-stimulation in dopaminergic brain-reward areas, such as the nucleus accumbens, and an increase in the voltage required to elicit intracranial electrical self-stimulation (Richter et al. 1995, Weiss et al. 2001b). These findings imply that an alteration in brain-reward regions affected by cocaine occurs with chronic use and is also associated with blunted responses to usual reward stimuli such as sex and food.

Treatment

Treatments for cocaine-use disorders continue to evolve and have been shown to be effective. In a large-outcome study, a comparison of short-term inpatient treatment programs, outpatient drug-free programs, and long-term residential programs specifically for those with cocaine-use disorders was undertaken. Of those who received any treatment, 24% relapsed to weekly cocaine use, a large decrease over the 73% relapse rate in the year prior to treatment. Some required an additional treatment program (18%) in the year following treatment, which is not an uncommon scenario for this chronic, relapsing disorder. Those with high levels of psychosocial, medical, or psychiatric problems at intake or less than 90 days of treatment had higher cocaine use in the follow-up period. Treatment periods of 90 days or more were associated with better substance-abuse outcomes (Crits-Christoph et al. 1999).

The two primary goals of cocaine treatment are (1) the initiation of abstinence through disruption of binge cycles and (2) the prevention of relapse. Treatment planning to achieve these goals must be considered in the context of the individual clinical presentation of the patient. Initial assessment to determine immediate needs is necessary to determine the most appropriate level of care (inpatient or outpatient treatment) as well as other psychiatric and medical considerations important to the development of the treatment plan.

The majority of those with cocaine-use disorders are most appropriately treated in an outpatient setting. Outpatient treatment may vary with provider but generally includes multiple weekly contacts for the initial months of treatment because less-frequent contact is not effective in the initiation or maintenance of abstinence (Weinstein et al. 1997, Gottheil et al. 1998, Katz et al. 2001, Coviello et al. 2001). These sessions consist of some combination of individual drug counseling, peer support groups, family or couples therapy, urine toxicology monitoring, education sessions, psychotherapy, and psychiatric treatment that may include pharmacotherapy for cocaine addiction or comorbid mental disorders. Inpatient treatment is reserved for those who have been refractory to outpatient treatment, whose compulsive use of cocaine represents an imminent danger (e.g., suicidality associated with cocaine toxicity or acute abstinence), who have other comorbid mental disorder or general medical conditions, or who are dependent on more than one substance and require monitored detoxification.

Cocaine abusers may present to urgent care settings in the context of cocaine toxicity or severe psychiatric symptoms associated with acute abstinence including anxiety, depression, or psychosis. Symptoms may be of a severity that requires emergent use of benzodiazepines or antipsychotics. Lorazepam is a good choice for the treatment of anxiety, agitation, or psychosis because it can be administered orally; it is also well absorbed by the intramuscular route. The use of benzodiazepines in the severely agitated cocaine user may decrease the need to employ the use of restraints. Antipsychotics should be used sparingly because, like cocaine, these drugs may lower the seizure threshold. In considering the choice of an antipsychotic, low-potency antipsychotics (e.g. chlorpromazine) may be more likely than high-potency neuroleptics (e.g. haloperidol) to lower seizure threshold and therefore should be avoided. Psychiatric management must also include clinical observation because suicidal ideation is not uncommon. Symptoms resembling those of a major depressive episode occur frequently in newly abstinent cocaine abusers. The occurrence of major depressive disorder must be excluded by observation over several days following the initiation of abstinence.

The treatment of cocaine-use disorders should be undertaken in the context of a thorough understanding of the disease (Table 20-3). One of the greatest challenges in the early stages of cocaine treatment is to prevent an early drop out. It has been estimated that up to 80% of individuals drop out of treatment programs (Higgins et al. 1994). Frequent clinical contacts especially in the early weeks of treatment can help establish a therapeutic alliance that will assist in engaging the cocaine user in the treatment process. Many programs offer 3 to 6 days per week of substance-abuse treatment sessions within outpatient partial hospital programs or intensive outpatient chemical dependency programs. Assessments by the program physician and counseling staff can identify other areas requiring specific interventions (comorbid general medical condition or mental disorders) and can expedite the initiation of appropriate pharmacotherapies. These interventions will increase treatment retention. Often, cocaine users must be helped to realize that their drug use is having a significant and adverse impact on their lives. Many individuals come to treatment because of family, legal, or social pressures. They can be ambivalent about the need for treatment and require education about their addiction and assistance in reviewing the consequences of cocaine use in their lives. This inventory should occur in the initial visits to the substance-abuse treatment program.

Initial treatment should include the encouragement of abstinence from all drug and alcohol use. Individuals who abuse alcohol and marijuana often do not perceive these drugs as problems. Education regarding the use of such drugs as conditioned stimuli to the use of cocaine should be emphasized. The "disease model" of chemical dependency may be used to assist in the initiation of abstinence. Emphasis is placed on the individuals recognizing chemical dependency as a disease needing treatment to control, but one for which there is no cure. Comprehensive drug education should also be provided in the initial treatment phase. Frequent contact with a drug counselor is an important part of treatment. Individual, group, and (where clinically indicated) family or marital therapy should be available. Attendance at 12-step or other self-help groups is often a useful adjunct to treatment and can be particularly helpful during the early stages of treatment when support for sobriety is essential.

The early recovery phase of treatment varies in duration from 3 to 12 months and is characterized by multiple weekly contacts and participation in therapeutic modalities with the goal of initiation and maintenance of abstinence. The focus during early recovery should be on relapse prevention and development of new and adaptive coping skills, healthy relationships, and lifestyle changes that will facilitate abstinence.

Relapses are common during early recovery. Individuals often feel pleased about their progress in treatment, become overly confident about their ability to control use, and test themselves by deliberately encountering what they know to be a high-risk situation for their drug use. Experimentation with cocaine to prove that drug use can be controlled often results in relapse and is associated with guilt. Individuals should be informed about the potential for relapse from the start of the treatment process. Relapse should be reviewed

Table 20-3	Cocaine-use Disorders: Recovery and Treatment		
Parameter	**Acute Abstinence**	**Withdrawal Phase**	**Extinction Phase**
Duration	Several hours to four days	2 to 10 weeks	3 to 12 months
Treatment	Symptomatic	Initiate psychotherapy	Continue psychotherapy,
	May need hospitalization for medical or psychiatric care and assessment	Individual/group therapy Self-help groups, other therapies, e.g., family, marital, individual, as needed	decrease intensity with continued abstinence; self-help groups and additional interventions developed for patients as needed
Pharmacotherapy	Benzodiazepines for anxiety, agitation, paranoia	None approved specific for cocaine-use disorders	Unusual to initiate in this phase
	Antipsychotics (sparingly) for severe psychosis or agitation	Consider disulfiram for cocaine–alcohol abuse previously refractory to treatment; psychotropics for comorbid psychiatric disorders or cocaine-related disorders; pharmacotherapies for other substance use disorders	Taper and discontinue pharmacotherapy for cocaine abuse and monitor clinically

with the individual in a supportive way with an emphasis on helping the individual to gain an understanding of the events leading to relapse. Relapse should, however, also trigger a review of the treatment plan and consideration of the need for additional interventions or whether a higher level of care is needed to assist the individual in the recovery process.

Success with initiating and maintaining abstinence over several months is followed by a reduced frequency of contact (e.g., a decrease to weekly group or individual therapy sessions). The focus should be on maintaining a commitment to abstinence, addressing renewed denial, and continued improvement of interpersonal skills. Participation in self-help groups should continue to be encouraged. Self-help groups based on 12-step principles encourage individuals to continue to view themselves as addicts in recovery—a cognitive structuring that many recovering drug abusers find helpful in maintaining sobriety.

Psychosocial Treatments

A variety of psychotherapeutic strategies for the treatment of cocaine-use disorders have been described (Higgins et al. 1993, Carroll et al. 1994a, 1995b, Crits-Christoph and Siqueland 1996, Barber et al. 1997, Crits-Christoph et al. 1998, 1999, Barber et al. 2001) (Table 20-4). In contrast to opiate addiction, for which psychotherapies alone are insufficient (Woody et al. 1995, Woody and Munoz 2000), there appear to be at least some subpopulations of cocaine abusers for whom psychotherapy alone may be adequate (Crits-Christoph et al. 1997, 1998, 1999). Behavioral therapies, in particular cognitive–behavioral therapy (Carroll 1998) and contingency management approaches have been demonstrated to be effective treatments for some cocaine-dependent individuals (Higgins et al. 1991, Elk et al. 1998, Milby et al. 2000, Jones et al. 2001).

The lack of a medically dangerous withdrawal syndrome from cocaine also suggests that some cocaine abusers may respond to psychotherapy alone in an outpatient treatment setting, compared with opiate- or alcohol-dependent persons for whom hospitalization may be required for detoxification. Another important reason for the development of psychotherapies for the treatment of cocaine-use disorders is that no medication is currently approved for the treatment of these disorders. Psychotherapies are also important platforms on which any pharmacological treatment may be supported. Furthermore, individuals not eligible for pharmacological treatment or who do not respond to pharmacological treatment require treatment alternatives such as psychotherapeutic interventions.

Interpersonal or psychodynamically oriented treatment approaches such as interpersonal psychotherapy (IPT) are based on the concept that many mental disorders, including cocaine dependence, are integrally related to disorders in interpersonal functioning that may be associated with the genesis or perpetuation of the disorder. IPT, as adapted for cocaine-use disorders treatment, includes four characteristics: (1) adherence to a medical model of mental disorders, which views these illnesses as chronic relapsing disorders, (2) focus on individuals' difficulties in current interpersonal functioning, (3) brevity and

Table 20-4	Psychotherapies: the Mainstay of Treatment for Cocaine-use Disorders
Interpersonal therapy	
Supportive expressive therapy	
Cognitive–behavioral therapy/Relapse-prevention therapy	
Voucher-based treatment	
Individual and group drug counseling	
Systematic cue exposure	
Self-help groups (e.g., Cocaine Anonymous)	

consistency of focus, and (4) use of an exploratory stance by the therapist (Carroll and Rounsaville 1993).

Supportive–expressive therapy is a time-limited, focused psychotherapy. The therapy has two main components: supportive techniques to help individuals feel comfortable in discussing their personal experiences related to drug abuse and expressive techniques to help individuals identify and work through difficulties in interpersonal relationships. Special attention is paid to the role of drugs in relation to problem feelings and behaviors, and how problems may be solved without recourse to drugs (NIDA 1999b). The efficacy of individual supportive–expressive psychotherapy has been studied with cocaine-abusing opiate-dependent individuals in methadone maintenance treatment who had comorbid psychiatric diagnoses (Woody et al. 1995). It was found that supportive–expressive psychotherapy, when added to drug counseling, improved substance-abuse treatment outcomes. Those receiving supportive–expressive therapy had fewer cocaine-positive urine toxicologies and required lower doses of methadone.

Cognitive–behavioral coping skills treatment (CBT) is a short-term, focused approach to help cocaine users become abstinent from cocaine and other substances. The underlying assumption is that learning processes play an important role in the development and continuation of maladaptive behaviors such as cocaine abuse. CBT techniques can be used to help cocaine abusers identify and correct behaviors associated with cocaine use (Carroll 1998). Relapse-prevention therapy (RPT) is based on cognitive–behavioral principles and attempts to address the serious problem of relapse in substance use disorders through the development of self-control strategies (Carroll et al. 1994a, 1994b). RPT may be especially well suited as a psychotherapeutic intervention for cocaine abusers because it encompasses several distinctive features important to treating this population. Relapse prevention is oriented toward symptom control. Although the name implies focus on the prevention of relapse, in fact this method employs several strategies intended to facilitate abstinence. Specific techniques in cocaine-addiction treatment include exploring the positive and negative consequences of continued use, self-monitoring to recognize drug cravings early on and to identify high-risk situations for use, and developing strategies for coping with and avoiding high-risk situations and the desire to use. Research indicates that the skills individuals learn through relapse-prevention therapy remain after the completion of treatment. In two long-term outcome studies, most people receiving this cognitive–behavioral approach maintained the gains they made in treatment throughout the year following treatment and a proportion of study participants continued to make gains following the termination of the 12-week CBT treatment period (Carroll et al. 1994a, 2000).

Relapse-prevention techniques are easily integrated into other treatment modalities. These techniques have been employed in the context of pharmacotherapy, group therapy, and brief psychoeducational groups for individuals entering drug-free treatment programs, and intervention for persons at risk for HIV infection (1999b). RPT is effective given either in a group format or individually (Schmitz et al. 1997). Other studies have shown that CBT/RPT is an effective platform on which cocaine pharmacotherapy can be based. In a double-blind, placebo-controlled, clinical trial examining the joint action of naltrexone (NTX) in combination with RPT, individuals receiving the combination treatment had less cocaine use over time than those receiving pharmacotherapy or RPT alone (Schmitz et al. 2001b). In a study of the effectiveness of disulfiram alone, CBT or 12-Step Facilitation therapies alone, or disulfiram in combination with either psychotherapy, those assigned to medication plus a psychotherapy had better outcomes in terms of reduced cocaine use and longer periods of abstinence than those receiving either medication or psychotherapy alone (Carroll et al. 1998).

Developed from the theory of alternative reinforcement, the voucher-based treatment approach is another example of behavioral therapy. A model that has been effective for the treatment of cocaine-use disorders is that of community reinforcement plus vouchers. Using this model delivered over a 24-week outpatient period, two specific treatment goals are addressed. One goal is the achievement of cocaine abstinence for a period long enough to help individuals learn new skills that will help sustain abstinence, and the second is the reduction of alcohol consumption in those who consume cocaine and alcohol together. In one to two individual counseling sessions weekly, individuals focus on improving family relations, learning skills to minimize drug abuse, receiving vocational counseling, and developing new sober social contacts and new recreational activities. Those who abuse alcohol also receive treatment with disulfiram (Antabuse). Urine samples for toxicology screen are submitted two to three times weekly and vouchers are received for cocaine-free urines. Vouchers can be exchanged for retail goods that would support a drug-free lifestyle (e.g., gift certificates to local stores). This approach has been shown to facilitate patient engagement in treatment and support abstinence both in urban and rural settings in which it has been used (Higgins et al. 1994, Bickel et al. 1995, Silverman et al. 1996).

Psychotherapeutic approaches are often delivered in the context of multimodal treatment programs and nearly all substance-abuse clinicians emphasize the importance of self-help groups such as Cocaine Anonymous. The efficacy of psychotherapy for drug abuse was initially established in several studies conducted in opiate-dependent individuals receiving methadone maintenance treatment (Rounsaville et al. 1983, Kleinman et al. 1990, Woody et al. 1995, Woody and Munoz 2000). It was found that the individuals receiving psychotherapies in addition to routine drug counseling had better outcomes than those receiving drug counseling alone.

Individual and group drug counseling focuses directly on reducing or stopping the use of drugs. It also addresses related areas of impaired social and occupational function as well as the content and structure of the patient's individualized recovery program. Through its emphasis on short-term behavioral goals, drug counseling helps the patient develop coping strategies and tools for abstaining from drug use and then maintaining abstinence (McLellan et al. 1993).

This premise of increased efficacy of psychotherapy in drug abuse treatment was examined in a multicenter clinical trial, the Drug Abuse Collaborative Cocaine Treatment Study (CCTS), which compared the efficacy of four common psychosocial treatments for cocaine-dependent individuals. Participants ($N = 487$) were randomly assigned to one of four manual-guided treatments: individual drug counseling + group drug counseling, cognitive–behavioral therapy + group drug counseling, supportive–expressive therapy + group drug counseling, or group drug counseling alone. In this study, those receiving individual drug counseling + group drug counseling showed the greatest improvement in substance-use outcomes (Crits-Christoph et al. 1999). This study shows that comprehensive drug counseling treatments that provide both individual and group counseling can be effective for the treatment of cocaine-use disorders.

One factor that may be an important precipitant to relapse to drug use is that of conditioned responses produced by repeated drug administration in the presence of specific stimuli. First described by Pavlov in 1927, this phenomenon has been reported for cocaine and other psychoactive drugs in animals and humans (Ehrman et al. 1992, O'Brien et al. 1993, Robbins et al. 1997, 1999). Neuroimaging studies have linked cue-induced craving to the limbic region involved in memory, learning, and pleasurable activities such as sex (Childress et al. 1999, Garavan et al. 2000). Research has shown that cocaine abusers exhibit increased limbic activation when watching videos containing cocaine-related scenes. Control subjects with no history of cocaine use show no limbic activation in response to these cues (Childress et al. 1999). Furthermore, while sexually explicit scenes activate the same brain structures in cocaine users and nonusers, the level of activation is less for the cocaine users (Garavan et al. 2000).

Cocaine abusers often report intense craving, arousal, and palpitations when they encounter objects, persons, or situations that remind them of cocaine use. Such cues often result in relapse. Systematic cue exposure and extinction has been studied as a treatment for cocaine addiction (Ehrman et al. 1992, Monti et al. 1997, Rohsenow et al. 2000). To reduce cue-triggered relapse, a treatment technique has been developed that links cue exposure in a clinical setting and teaches cocaine users to control drug use by recognizing these cues (also called *triggers*) and their responses. Cue exposure is combined with the teaching of coping skills to address high-risk situations. Individuals develop skills for how to avoid or modify the trigger situation when possible. For unavoidable triggers, individuals are helped to establish a repertoire of cognitive and behavioral skills to disrupt the behavioral chain leading to cocaine abuse. A controlled trial showed that individuals in cue-exposure therapy who relapsed had significantly fewer cocaine-using days than did a control group (Monti et al. 1997).

Somatic Therapies

The development of pharmacological treatments for cocaine abuse has been based on the premise that an altered neurochemical substrate underlies the chronic, high-intensity (binge) use and acute abstinence/withdrawal that follows binge use. This neuroadaptation model has also served as a basis for a number of studies that have evaluated the clinical utility of psychotropic agents that, based on their pharmacological profile, might possess anticraving properties, block euphoria, or decrease cocaine abstinence symptoms. To date, no medication has emerged as an accepted effective pharmacotherapy.

Dopaminergic agents have been evaluated to ameliorate early withdrawal symptoms associated with cocaine abstinence. The theoretical basis of this treatment is that habitual use of cocaine results in central dopamine depletion and dopamine receptor supersensitivity. This altered state of dopaminergic function (or hypofunction) could be related to drug craving and other withdrawal symptoms that lead to repeated drug use, but might be corrected by use of a medication that enhances dopaminergic function. Dopaminergic medications that have been evaluated in clinical trials and found not to be effective for the treatment of cocaine-use disorders include amantadine (Gawin et al. 1989b, Handelsman et al. 1995, Kampman et al. 1996, Perez de los Cobos et al. 2001), bromocriptine, (Preston et al. 1992, Eiler et al. 1995, Handelsman et al. 1997, McCance-Katz and Kosten 1998, Boyarsky and McCance-Katz 2000) methylphenidate (Roache et al. 2000), mazindol (Stine et al. 1995, Margolin et al. 1995a, Malison et al. 1998b), bupropion (Margolin et al. 1995b, Oliveto et al. 2001), flupenthixol (Gawin et al. 1996, Evans et al. 2001), haloperidol (Ohuoha et al. 1997, Kosten 1997), risperidone (Grabowski et al. 2000), and the D1 antagonist ecopipam (Nann-Vernotica et al. 2001, Haney et al. 2001, McCance-Katz et al. 2001). Although preclinical studies implicate dopamine in the reinforcing effects of cocaine, the lack of efficacy in the many clinical trials conducted with dopaminergic agents provides indirect evidence that reinforcing effects are likely to be mediated by multiple neurotransmitters and/or intracellular processes.

Desipramine was one of the earliest drugs explored as a potential cocaine pharma-cotherapy. The rationale of using this tricyclic antidepressant as a treatment for cocaine-use disorders was that desipramine treatment might reverse cocaine-induced postsynaptic dopaminergic receptor supersensitivity (McCance-Katz and Kosten 1998). Rather than acting as a general antidepressant in cocaine abusers who do not have major affective disor-ders, desipramine could act as a specific antianhedonic agent in this population. Whereas the positive aspects of antidepressants such as desipramine for treatment of cocaine abuse include a relatively benign side effect profile, lack of abuse liability, and acceptance by individuals, a significant disadvantage lies in the delayed onset of effect (approximately 2 weeks). Findings from controlled clinical trials with desipramine in cocaine abusers have been mixed. An early study of 72 cocaine-abusing participants yielded encouraging results (Gawin et al. 1989a). Desipramine at dosages of 200 to 250 mg/day significantly decreased cocaine use. However, other clinical trials reported mixed results that were overall negative in terms of desipramine's effectiveness for the treatment of cocaine dependence (Levin and Lehman 1991, Arndt et al. 1992).

Treatment Refractoriness

The term "treatment refractoriness" sometimes implies a lack of response to a therapeutic trial of a pharmacotherapy. In the case of cocaine dependence, however, there is no effective pharmacotherapy with which to treat the disorder; therefore, the term relates to a different set of occurrences in the treatment setting. Recidivism to cocaine use, treatment dropout, and multiple treatment experiences are common. Such problems are a reflection of the severity of illness and parameters of relative treatment refractoriness. Comorbid substance use and mental disorders contribute to treatment refractoriness. Lack of accurate diagnosis and treatment contributes to relapse potential in the form of continued exposure to high-risk situations and lifestyle instability that are associated with ongoing substance abuse. Continued psychiatric symptoms that individuals attempt to relieve through cocaine use contribute to poor treatment outcome.

The psychological addiction associated with cocaine abuse can be disabling. Because physiological dependence, if it does occur, generally does not require pharmacotherapy, treatment referrals for individuals with primary cocaine dependence but no other acute mental disorder or general condition, are generally to an outpatient drug abuse treatment clinic. Those unable to initiate and maintain sobriety in an outpatient drug treatment program should be evaluated for more intensive forms of treatment. Management of these individuals should include consideration of a variety of options including pharmacotherapy (see the earlier section on pharmacotherapy for cocaine abuse) and programs that offer a graded increase in structure. Such individuals may need initial detoxification from another drug or alcohol that could require several days of inpatient treatment. Those who are determined to need intensive outpatient treatment often attend these programs 5 days a week initially, and sessions last an average of about 4 hours. There is a gradual reduction in the number of sessions per week as the period of sobriety lengthens. Such programs are of flexible duration, but a full program usually requires at least 12 weeks. This program can be followed with resumption of the outpatient treatment clinic level of care, which takes place fewer days per week and with shorter sessions. Those with comorbid psychiatric disorders should be referred to dual diagnosis specialty treatment programs when available. Dual diagnosis speciality programs differ from traditional substance-abuse treatment programs in that they have a dual diagnosis treatment orientation, with an increased use of psychotropic medication, longer lengths of stay, and greater tolerance for relapse and medication nonadherence. As compared to standard abuse treatment programs, they tend to have a more severe case mix, a higher 180-day readmission rate, and a higher rate of psychiatric aftercare in the 30 days after discharge (Swindle et al. 1995).

Individuals who have failed other forms of treatment may be referred to residential programs, although the number of these programs is shrinking, given the constraints on treatment that have occurred as a result of managed care and erosion of benefits provided by health insurers for treating substance-use disorders. Residential programs vary in length and must be tailored to the needs of the patient. Such programs can be important to the initiation of abstinence. These programs allow sufficient time in a drug-free and supportive environment so that the recovery process can begin, as well as provide adequate time for reduction of drug craving and acquisition of effective relapse-prevention skills.

Comparison of DSM-IV-TR/ICD-10 Diagnostic Criteria

The ICD-10 and DSM-IV-TR criteria sets for cocaine intoxication and withdrawal are almost the same except that ICD-10 criteria set for withdrawal includes drug craving as an additional item.

References

Albertson TE, Walby WF, and Derlet RW (1995) Stimulant-induced pulmonary toxicity. *Chest* **108**, 1140–1149.

Alves LG (2000) Cocaine-related acute subdural hematoma: an emergent cause of cerebrovascular accident. *Acta Neurochir (Wien)* **142**, 819–821.

American Heart Association (2000a) Guidelines 2000 for Cardiopulmonary Resuscitation and Emergency Cardiovascular Care. Part 6: Advanced cardiovascular life support. Section 1: Introduction to ACLS 2000: Overview of recommended changes in ACLS from the guidelines 2000 conference. The American Heart Association in collaboration with the International Liaison Committee on Resuscitation. *Circulation* **102**(Suppl. 8), 186–189.

American Heart Association (2000b) Guidelines 2000 for Cardiopulmonary Resuscitation and Emergency Cardiovascular Care. Part 8: Advanced challenges in resuscitation. Section 3: Special challenges in ECC. The American Heart Association in collaboration with the International Liaison Committee on Resuscitation. *Circulation* **102**(Suppl. 8), 1229–1252.

American Psychiatric Association (2000) *Diagnostic and Statistical Manual of Mental Disorders*, 4th ed., Text Rev. APA, Washington, DC.

Andrews P (1997) Cocaethylene toxicity. *J Addict Dis* **16**, 75–84.

Arndt IO, Dorozynsky L, Woody GE, et al. (1992) Desipramine treatment of cocaine dependence in methadone-maintained patients. *Arch Gen Psychiatry* **49**, 888–893.

Avants SK, Margolin A, Holford TR, et al. (2000) A randomized controlled trial of auricular acupuncture for cocaine dependence. *Arch Intern Med* **160**, 2305–2312.

Barber JP, Krakauer I, Calvo N, et al. (1997) Measuring adherence and competence of dynamic therapists in the treatment of cocaine dependence. *J Psychother Pract Res* **6**, 12–24.

Barber JP, Luborsky L, Gallop R, et al. (2001) Therapeutic alliance as a predictor of outcome and retention in the National Institute on Drug Abuse Collaborative Cocaine Treatment Study. *J Consult Clin Psychol* **69**, 119–124.

Baumann BM, Perrone J, Hornig SE, et al. (2000) Cardiac and hemodynamic assessment of patients with cocaine-associated chest pain syndromes. *J Toxicol Clin Toxicol* **38**, 283–290.

Baumgartner FJ and Omari BO (1997) Method of repair of cocaine-induced chronic type A aortic dissection. *Ann Thorac Surg* **64**, 1518–1519.

Bennett ME, Bellack AS, and Gearon JS (2001) Treating substance abuse in schizophrenia. An initial report. *J Subst Abuse Treat* **20**, 163–175.

Besse S, Assayag P, Latour C, et al. (1997) Molecular characteristics of cocaine-induced cardiomyopathy in rats. *Eur J Pharmacol* **338**, 123–129.

Bickel WK, DeGrandpre RJ, and Higgins ST (1995) The behavioral economics of concurrent drug reinforcers: a review and reanalysis of drug self-administration research. *Psychopharmacology (Berl)* **118**, 250–259.

Biederman J, Wilens T, Mick E, et al. (1999) Pharmacotherapy of attention-deficit/hyperactivity disorder reduces risk for substance use disorder. *Pediatrics* **104**, E20.

Biegon A, Dillon K, Volkow ND, et al. (1992) Quantitative autoradiography of cocaine binding sites in human brain postmortem. *Synapse* **10**, 126–130.

Bird DJ and Markey JR (1997) Massive pulmonary edema in a habitual crack cocaine smoker not chemically positive for cocaine at the time of surgery. *Anesth Analg* **84**, 1157–1159.

Birnbach DJ, Browne IM, Kim A, et al. (2001) Identification of polysubstance abuse in the parturient. *Br J Anaesth* **87**, 488–490.

Blanco M, Diez-Tejedor E, Vivancos F, et al. (1999) Cocaine and cerebrovascular disease in young adults. *Rev Neurol* **29**, 796–800.

Boghdadi MS and Henning RJ (1997) Cocaine: Pathophysiology and clinical toxicology. *Heart Lung* **26**, 466–483.

Bolla KI, Cadet JL, and London ED (1998) The neuropsychiatry of chronic cocaine abuse. *J Neuropsychiatr Clin Neurosci* **10**, 280–289.

Boyarsky BK and McCance-Katz EF (2000) Improving the quality of substance dependency treatment with pharmacotherapy. *Subst Use Misuse* **35**, 2095–2125.

Bradberry CW (2000) Acute and chronic dopamine dynamics in a nonhuman primate model of recreational cocaine use. *J Neurosci* **20**, 7109–7115.

Bradberry CW, Nobiletti JB, Elsworth JD, et al. (1993) Cocaine and cocaethylene: microdialysis comparison of brain drug levels and effects on dopamine and serotonin. *J Neurochem* **60**, 1429–1435.

Brady KT and Randall CL (1999) Gender differences in substance use disorders. *Psychiatr Clin North Am* **22**, 241–252.

Brady KT, Dansky BS, Sonne SC, et al. (1998) Posttraumatic stress disorder and cocaine dependence. Order of onset. *Am J Addict* **7**, 128–135.

Brady WJ and Chan TC (1999) Electrocardiographic manifestations: benign early repolarization. *J Emerg Med* **17**, 473–478.

Breiter HC, Gollub RL, Weisskoff RM, et al. (1997) Acute effects of cocaine on human brain activity and emotion. *Neuron* **19**, 591–611.

Brookoff D, Rotondo MF, Shaw LM, et al. (1996) Coacaethylene levels in patients who test positive for cocaine. *Ann Emerg Med* **27**, 316–320.

Brown EE and Fibiger HC (1993) Differential effects of excitotoxic lesions of the amygdala on cocaine-induced conditioned locomotion and conditioned place preference. *Psychopharmacology (Berl)* **113**, 123–130.

Brown RA, Monti PM, Myers MG, et al. (1998) Depression among cocaine abusers in treatment: relation to cocaine and alcohol use and treatment outcome. *Am J Psychiatry* **155**, 220–225.

Buckley PF (1998) Substance abuse in schizophrenia: a review. *J Clin Psychiatry* **59**, 26–30.

Buehler BA (1995) Cocaine: How dangerous is it during pregnancy? *Nebr Med J* **80**, 116–117.

Buehler BA, Conover B, and Andres RL (1996) Teratogenic potential of cocaine. *Semin Perinatol* **20**, 93–98.

Cahill L (2000) Neurobiological mechanisms of emotionally influenced, long-term memory. *Prog Brain Res* **126**, 29–37.

Carlezon WA Jr., Thome J, Olson VG, et al. (1998) Regulation of cocaine reward by CREB. *Science* **282**, 2272–2275.

Carmona GN, Jufer RA, Goldberg SR, et al. (2000) Butyrylcholinesterase accelerates cocaine metabolism: in vitro and in vivo effects in nonhuman primates and humans. *Drug Metab Dispos* **28**, 367–371.

Carmona GN, Schindler CW, Shoaib M, et al. (1998) Attenuation of cocaine-induced locomotion activity by butyrylcholinesterase. *Exp Clin Psychopharmacol* **6**, 274–279.

Carrera MR, Ashley JA, Wirsching P, et al. (2001) A second-generation vaccine protects against the psychoactive effects of cocaine. *Proc Natl Acad Sci U S A* **98**, 1988–1992.

Carrera MR, Ashley JA, Zhou B, et al. (2000) Cocaine vaccines: antibody protection against relapse in a rat model. *Proc Natl Acad Sci U S A* **97**, 6202–6206.

Carroll K (1998) *A Cognitive–Behavioral Approach: treating Cocaine Addiction*. National Institute on Drug Abuse, Rockville, MD.

Carroll KM and Rounsaville BJ (1993) History and significance of childhood attention deficit disorder in treatment-seeking cocaine abusers. *Compr Psychiatry* **34**, 75–82.

Carroll KM, Nich C, Ball SA, et al. (1998) Treatment of cocaine and alcohol dependence with psychotherapy and disulfiram. *Addiction* **93**, 713–727.

Carroll KM, Nich C, Ball SA, et al. (2000) One-year follow-up of disulfiram and psychotherapy for cocaine-alcohol users: sustained effects of treatment. *Addiction* **95**, 1335–1349.

Carroll KM, Nich C, and Rounsaville BJ (1995a) Differential symptom reduction in depressed cocaine abusers treated with psychotherapy and pharmacotherapy. *J Nerv Ment Dis* **183**, 251–259.

Carroll KM, Nich C, and Rounsaville BJ (1997) Variability in treatment-seeking cocaine abusers: implications for clinical pharmacotherapy trials. *NIDA Res Monogr* **175**, 137–157.

Carroll KM, Rounsaville BJ, Gordon LT, et al. (1994a) Psychotherapy and pharmacotherapy for ambulatory cocaine abusers. *Arch Gen Psychiatry* **51**, 177–187.

Carroll KM, Rounsaville BJ, Nich C, et al. (1994b) One-year follow-up of psychotherapy and pharmacotherapy for cocaine dependence. Delayed emergence of psychotherapy effects. *Arch Gen Psychiatry* **51**, 989–997.

Carroll KM, Rounsaville BJ, Nich C, et al. (1995b) Integrating psychotherapy and pharmacotherapy for cocaine dependence: results from a randomized clinical trial. *NIDA Res Monogr* **150**, 19–35.

Carroll KM, Ziedonis D, O'Malley SS, et al. (1993) Pharmacologic interventions for abusers of alcohol and cocaine: disulfiram versus naltrexone. *Am J Addict* **2**, 77–79.

Cashman JR, Berkman CE, and Underiner GE (2000) Catalytic antibodies that hydrolyze (−)-cocaine obtained by a high-throughput procedure. *J Pharmacol Exp Ther* **293**, 952–961.

Cassidy F, Ahearn EP, and Carroll BJ (2001) Substance abuse in bipolar disorder. *Bipolar Disord* **3**, 181–188.

Castro VJ and Nacht R (2000) Cocaine-induced bradyarrhythmia: an unsuspected cause of syncope. *Chest* **117**, 275–277.

Chang L, Ernst T, Strickland T, et al. (1999) Gender effects on persistent cerebral metabolite changes in the frontal lobes of abstinent cocaine users. *Am J Psychiatry* **156**, 716–722.

Chiarotti M and Fucci N (1999) Comparative analysis of heroin and cocaine seizures. *J Chromatogr, B: Biomed Sci Appl* **733**, 127–136.

Childress AR, Hole AV, Ehrman RN, et al. (1993) Cue reactivity and cue reactivity interventions in drug dependence. *NIDA Res Monogr* **137**, 73–95.

Childress AR, Mozley PD, McElgin W, et al. (1999) Limbic activation during cue-induced cocaine craving. *Am J Psychiatry* **156**, 11–18.

Chou CP, Hser YI, and Anglin MD (1998) Interaction effects of client and treatment program characteristics on retention: an exploratory analysis using hierarchical linear models. *Subst Use Misuse* **33**, 2281–2301.

Ciccocioppo R, Sanna PP, and Weiss F (2001) Cocaine-predictive stimulus induces drug-seeking behavior and neural activation in limbic brain regions after multiple months of abstinence: reversal by D(1) antagonists. *Proc Natl Acad Sci U S A* **98**, 1976–1981.

Clay LH, Mazzio EA, Kolta MG, et al. (1998) Repeated administration of cocaine alters dopamine uptake and release in the striatum nucleus accumbens. *Ann N Y Acad Sci* **844**, 346–355.

Clure C, Brady KT, Saladin ME, et al. (1999) Attention-deficit/hyperactivity disorder and substance use: symptom pattern and drug choice. *Am J Drug Alcohol Abuse* **25**, 441–448.

Compton WM, Cottler LB, Ben Abdallah A, et al. (2000) Substance dependence and other psychiatric disorders among drug dependent subjects: race and gender correlates. *Am J Addict* **9**, 113–125.

Coviello DM, Alterman AI, Rutherford MJ, et al. (2001) The effectiveness of two intensities of psychosocial treatment for cocaine dependence. *Drug Alcohol Depend* **61**, 145–154.

Crits-Christoph P and Siqueland L (1996) Psychosocial treatment for drug abuse. Selected review and recommendations for national health care. *Arch Gen Psychiatry* **53**, 749–756.

Crits-Christoph P, Siqueland L, Blaine J, et al. (1997) The National Institute on Drug Abuse Collaborative Cocaine Treatment Study. Rationale and methods. *Arch Gen Psychiatry* **54**, 721–726.

Crits-Christoph P, Siqueland L, Blaine J, et al. (1999) Psychosocial treatments for cocaine dependence: National Institute on Drug Abuse Collaborative Cocaine Treatment Study. *Arch Gen Psychiatry* **56**, 493–502.

Crits-Christoph P, Siqueland L, Chittams J, et al. (1998) Training in cognitive, supportive-expressive, and drug counseling therapies for cocaine dependence. *J Consult Clin Psychol* **66**, 484–492.

Cuenca Carvajal C, Gomez Antunez M, Ortiz Vega M, et al. (1998) Cocaine intoxication and acute pulmonary edema. *Ann Med Intern* **15**, 232.

Daras M, Kakkouras L, Tuchman AJ, et al. (1995) Rhabdomyolysis and hyperthermia after cocaine abuse: a variant of the neuroleptic malignant syndrome? *Acta Neurol Scand* **92**, 161–165.

Daras MD, Orrego JJ, Akfirat GL, et al. (2001) Bilateral symmetrical basal ganglia infarction after intravenous use of cocaine and heroin. *Clin Imag* **25**, 12–14.

Dixon L (1999) Dual diagnosis of substance abuse in schizophrenia: prevalence and impact on outcomes. *Schizophr Res* **35**, S93–S100.

Eames SL, Westermeyer J, and Crosby RD (1998) Substance use and abuse among patients with comorbid dysthymia and substance disorder. *Am J Drug Alcohol Abuse* **24**, 541–550.

Ehrman RN, Robbins SJ, Childress AR, et al. (1992) Conditioned responses to cocaine-related stimuli in cocaine abuse patients. *Psychopharmacology (Berl)* **107**, 523–529.

Eiler K, Schaefer MR, Salstrom D, et al. (1995) Double-blind comparison of bromocriptine and placebo in cocaine withdrawal. *Am J Drug Alcohol Abuse* **21**, 65–79.

Elk R, Mangus L, Rhoades H, et al. (1998) Cessation of cocaine use during pregnancy: effects of contingency management interventions on maintaining abstinence and complying with prenatal care. *Addict Behav* **23**, 57–64.

Ensminger ME, Anthony JC, and McCord J (1997) The inner city and drug use: initial findings from an epidemiological study. *Drug Alcohol Depend* **48**, 175–184.

Evans SM, Haney M, Fischman MW, et al. (1999) Limited sex differences in response to "binge" smoked cocaine use in humans. *Neuropsychopharmacology* **21**, 445–454.

Evans SM, Walsh SL, Levin FR, et al. (2001) Effect of flupenthixol on subjective and cardiovascular responses to intravenous cocaine in humans. *Drug Alcohol Depend* **64**, 271–283.

Farren CK, Hameedi FA, Rosen MA, et al. (2000) Significant interaction between clozapine and cocaine in cocaine addicts. *Drug Alcohol Depend* **59**, 153–163.

Fineschi V, Wetli CV, Di Paolo M, et al. (1997) Myocardial necrosis and cocaine. A quantitative morphologic study in 26 cocaine-associated deaths. *Int J Legal Med* **110**, 193–198.

Fiocchi FF and Kingree JB (2001) Treatment retention and birth outcomes of crack users enrolled in a substance abuse treatment program for pregnant women. *J Subst Abuse Treat* **20**, 137–142.

Foltin RW and Fischman MW (1997) Residual effects of repeated cocaine smoking in humans. *Drug Alcohol Depend* **47**, 117–124.

Foltin RW and Fischman MW (1998) Effects of "binge" use of intravenous cocaine in methadone-maintained individuals. *Addiction* **93**, 825–836.

Fox BS (1997) Development of a therapeutic vaccine for the treatment of cocaine addiction. *Drug Alcohol Depend* **48**, 153–158.

Fox BS, Kantak KM, Edwards MA, et al. (1996) Efficacy of a therapeutic cocaine vaccine in rodent models. *Nat Med* **2**, 1129–1132.

Frank DA, Augustyn M, Knight WG, et al. (2001) Growth, development, and behavior in early childhood following prenatal cocaine exposure: a systematic review. *JAMA* **285**, 1613–1625.

Frank DA, McCarten KM, Robson CD, et al. (1999) Level of in utero cocaine exposure and neonatal ultrasound findings. *Pediatrics* **104**, 1101–1105.

Gamouras GA, Monir G, Plunkitt K, et al. (2000) Cocaine abuse: repolarization abnormalities and ventricular arrhythmias. *Am J Med Sci* **320**, 9–12.

Gan X, Zhang L, Berger O, et al. (1999) Cocaine enhances brain endothelial adhesion molecules and leukocyte migration. *Clin Immunol* **91**, 68–76.

Garavan H, Pankiewicz J, Bloom A, et al. (2000) Cue-induced cocaine craving: neuroanatomical specificity for drug users and drug stimuli. *Am J Psychiatry* **157**, 1789–1798.

Gatley SJ and Volkow ND (1998) Addiction and imaging of the living human brain. *Drug Alcohol Depend* **51**, 97–108.

Gawin FH (1991) Cocaine addiction: psychology and neurophysiology. *Science* **251**, 1580–1586.

Gawin FH, Khalsa-Denison ME, and Jatlow P (1996) Flupentixol-induced aversion to crack cocaine. *N Engl J Med* **334**, 1340–1341.

Gawin FH, Kleber HD, Byck R, et al. (1989a) Desipramine facilitation of initial cocaine abstinence. *Arch Gen Psychiatry* **46**, 117–121.

Gawin FH, Morgan C, Kosten TR, et al. (1989b) Double-blind evaluation of the effect of acute amantadine on cocaine craving. *Psychopharmacology (Berl)* **97**, 402–403.

Gelernter J, Kranzler HR, Satel SL, et al. (1994) Genetic association between dopamine transporter protein alleles and cocaine-induced paranoia. *Neuropsychopharmacology* **11**, 195–200.

Gendeh BS, Ferguson BJ, Johnson JT, et al. (1998) Progressive septal and palatal perforation secondary to intranasal cocaine abuse. *Med J Malaysia* **53**, 435–438.

Giannini AJ, Folts DJ, Feather JN, et al. (1989) Bromocriptine and amantadine in cocaine detoxification. *Psychiatr Res* **29**, 11–16.

Gollub RL, Breiter HC, Kantor H, et al. (1998) Cocaine decreases cortical cerebral blood flow but does not obscure regional activation in functional magnetic resonance imaging in human subjects. *J Cereb Blood Flow Metab* **18**, 724–734.

Gorelick DA (1997) Enhancing cocaine metabolism with butyrylcholinesterase as a treatment strategy. *Drug Alcohol Depend* **48**, 159–165.

Gottheil E, Weinstein SP, Sterling RC, et al. (1998) A randomized controlled study of the effectiveness of intensive outpatient treatment for cocaine dependence. *Psychiatr Serv* **49**, 782–787.

Gottschalk C, Beauvais J, Hart R, et al. (2001) Cognitive function and cerebral perfusion during cocaine abstinence. *Am J Psychiatry* **158**, 540–545.

Grabowski J, Rhoades H, Elk R, et al. (1995) Fluoxetine is ineffective for treatment of cocaine dependence or concurrent opiate and cocaine dependence: two placebo-controlled double-blind trials. *J Clin Psychopharmacol* **15**, 163–174.

Grabowski J, Rhoades H, Silverman P, et al. (2000) Risperidone for the treatment of cocaine dependence: randomized, double-blind trial. *J Clin Psychopharmacol* **20**, 305–310.

Grant BF and Harford TC (1990) Concurrent and simultaneous use of alcohol with cocaine: results of national survey. *Drug Alcohol Depend* **25**, 97–104.

Grella CE, Anglin MD, and Wugalter SE (1997) Patterns and predictors of cocaine and crack use by clients in standard and enhanced methadone maintenance treatment. *Am J Drug Alcohol Abuse* **23**, 15–42.

Hamad A and Khan M (2000) ST-segment elevation in patients with cocaine abuse and chest pain: Is there a pattern? *Am J Cardiol* **86**, 1054.

Hameedi FA, Rosen MI, McCance-Katz EF, et al. (1995) Behavioral, physiological, and pharmacological interaction of cocaine and disulfiram in humans. *Biol Psychiatry* **37**, 560–563.

Handelsman L, Limpitlaw L, Williams D, et al. (1995) Amantadine does not reduce cocaine use or craving in cocaine-dependent methadone maintenance patients. *Drug Alcohol Depend* **39**, 173–180.

Handelsman L, Rosenblum A, Palij M, et al. (1997) Bromocriptine for cocaine dependence. A controlled clinical trial. *Am J Addict* **6**, 54–64.

Haney M, Ward AS, Foltin RW, et al. (2001) Effects of ecopipam, a selective dopamine D1 antagonist, on smoked cocaine self-administration by humans. *Psychopharmacology (Berl)* **155**, 330–337.

Hart CL, Jatlow P, Sevarino KA, et al. (2000) Comparison of intravenous cocaethylene and cocaine in humans. *Psychopharmacology (Berl)* **149**, 153–162.

He J, Xiao Y, and Zhang L (2000) Cocaine induces apoptosis in human coronary artery endothelial cells. *J Cardiovasc Pharmacol* **35**, 572–580.

He J, Xiao Y, and Zhang L (2001) Cocaine-mediated apoptosis in bovine coronary artery endothelial cells: role of nitric oxide. *J Pharmacol Exp Ther* **298**, 180–187.

Hemby SE (1999) Recent advances in the biology of addiction. *Curr Psychiatr Rep* **1**, 159–165.

Henning RJ and Wilson LD (1996) Cocaethylene is as cardiotoxic as cocaine but is less toxic than cocaine plus ethanol. *Life Sci* **59**, 615–627.

Hersh D, Van Kirk JR, and Kranzler HR (1998) Naltrexone treatment of comorbid alcohol and cocaine use disorders. *Psychopharmacology (Berl)* **139**, 44–52.

Higgins ST and Budney AJ (1993) Treatment of cocaine dependence through the principles of behavior analysis and behavioral pharmacology. *NIDA Res Monogr* **137**, 97–121.

Higgins ST, Budney AJ, Bickel WK, et al. (1993) Disulfiram therapy in patients abusing cocaine and alcohol. *Am J Psychiatry* **150**, 675–676.

Higgins ST, Budney AJ, Bickel WK, et al. (1994) Incentives improve outcome in outpatient behavioral treatment of cocaine dependence. *Arch Gen Psychiatry* **51**, 568–576.

Higgins ST, Delaney DD, Budney AJ, et al. (1991) A behavioral approach to achieving initial cocaine abstinence. *Am J Psychiatry* **148**, 1218–1224.

Hollander JE (2001) Cocaine-associated acute coronary syndromes. *Ann Emerg Med* **38**, 95–96; discussion 97–98.

Hollander JE, Brooks DE, and Valentine SM (1998a) Assessment of cocaine use in patients with chest pain syndromes. *Arch Intern Med* **158**, 62–66.

Hollander JE, Hoffman RS, Gennis P, et al. Cocaine Associated Chest Pain (COCHPA) Study Group (1994) Prospective multicenter evaluation of cocaine-associated chest pain. *Acad Emerg Med* **1**, 330–339.

Hollander JE, Levitt MA, Young GP, et al. (1998b) Effect of recent cocaine use on the specificity of cardiac markers for diagnosis of acute myocardial infarction. *Am Heart J* **135**, 245–252.

Hollander JE, Shih RD, Hoffman RS, et al. Cocaine-Associated Myocardial Infarction (CAMI) Study Group (1997a) Predictors of coronary artery disease in patients with cocaine-associated myocardial infarction. *Am J Med* **102**, 158–163.

Hollander JE, Todd KH, Green G, et al. (1995) Chest pain associated with cocaine: an assessment of prevalence in suburban and urban emergency departments. *Ann Emerg Med* **26**, 671–676.

Hollander JE, Vignona L, and Burstein J (1997b) Predictors of underlying coronary artery disease in cocaine associated myocardial infarction: a meta-analysis of case reports. *Vet Hum Toxicol* **39**, 276–280.

Hommer DW (1999) Functional imaging of craving. *Alcohol Res Health* **23**, 187–196.

Horowitz BZ, Panacek EA, and Jouriles NJ (1997) Severe rhabdomyolysis with renal failure after intranasal cocaine use. *J Emerg Med* **15**, 833–837.

Huang L, Woolf JH, Ishiguro Y, et al. (1997) Effect of cocaine and methylecgonidine on intracellular Ca2+ and myocardial contraction in cardiac myocytes. *Am J Physiol* **273**, H893–H901.

Hwang CK, D'Souza UM, Eisch AJ, et al. (2001) Dopamine receptor regulating factor, DRRF: a zinc finger transcription factor. *Proc Natl Acad Sci U S A* **98**, 7558–7563.

Jacobsen LK, Staley JK, Malison RT, et al. (2000) Elevated central serotonin transporter binding availability in acutely abstinent cocaine-dependent patients. *Am J Psychiatry* **157**, 1134–1140.

Jatlow P, Elsworth JD, Bradberry CW, et al. (1991) Cocaethylene: a neuropharmacologically active metabolite associated with concurrent cocaine-ethanol ingestion. *Life Sci* **48**, 1787–1794.

Jensen PS (2000) Current concepts and controversies in the diagnosis and treatment of attention-deficit/hyperactivity disorder. *Curr Psychiatr Rep* **2**, 102–109.

Johnson LD, O'Malley PM, and Bachman JC (2001) *Monitoring the Future National Survey Results on Drug Use, 1975–2000*. National Institute on Drug Abuse, Bethesda, MD.

Johnston PA (2000) *The National Drug Threat Assessment 2001—The Domestic Perspective*. National Drug Intelligence Center, US Department of Justice.

Jones HE, Haug N, Silverman K, et al. (2001) The effectiveness of incentives in enhancing treatment attendance and drug abstinence in methadone-maintained pregnant women. *Drug Alcohol Depend* **61**, 297–306.

Jufer RA, Wstadik A, Walsh SL, et al. (2000) Elimination of cocaine and metabolites in plasma, saliva, and urine following repeated oral administration to human volunteers. *J Anal Toxicol* **24**, 467–477.

Kampman K, Volpicelli JR, Alterman A, et al. (1996) Amantadine in the early treatment of cocaine dependence: a double-blind, placebo-controlled trial. *Drug Alcohol Depend* **41**, 25–33.

Kampman KM, Volpicelli JR, Alterman AI, et al. (2000) Amantadine in the treatment of cocaine-dependent patients with severe withdrawal symptoms. *Am J Psychiatry* **157**, 2052–2054.

Kantak KM, Collins SL, Bond J, et al. (2001) Time course of changes in cocaine self-administration behavior in rats during immunization with the cocaine vaccine IPC-1010. *Psychopharmacology (Berl)* **153**, 334–340.

Kantak KM, Collins SL, Lipman EG, et al. (2000) Evaluation of anti-cocaine antibodies and a cocaine vaccine in a rat self-administration model. *Psychopharmacology (Berl)* **148**, 251–262.

Katz EC, Gruber K, Chutuape MA, et al. (2001) Reinforcement-based outpatient treatment for opiate and cocaine abusers. *J Subst Abuse Treat* **20**, 93–98.

Kaufman MJ, Levin JM, Maas LC, et al. (2001) Cocaine-induced cerebral vasoconstriction differs as a function of sex and menstrual cycle phase. *Biol Psychiatry* **49**, 774–781.

Kaufman MJ, Levin JM, Ross MH, et al. (1998) Cocaine-induced cerebral vasoconstriction detected in humans with magnetic resonance angiography. *JAMA* **279**, 376–380.

Kelz MB, Chen J, Carlezon WA Jr., et al. (1999) Expression of the transcription factor deltaFosB in the brain controls sensitivity to cocaine. *Nature* **401**, 272–276.

Kendler KS and Prescott CA (1998) Cocaine use, abuse and dependence in a population-based sample of female twins. *Br J Psychiatry* **173**, 345–350.

Kerns W, Garvey L, and Owens J (1997) Cocaine-induced wide complex dysrhythmia. *J Emerg Med* **15**, 321–329.

King DE, Herning RI, Gorelick DA, et al. (2000) Gender differences in the EEG of abstinent cocaine abusers. *Neuropsychobiology* **42**, 93–98.

Kissin WB, Svikis DS, Morgan GD, et al. (2001) Characterizing pregnant drug-dependent women in treatment and their children. *J Subst Abuse Treat* **21**, 27–34.

Kleinman PH, Woody GE, Todd TC, et al. (1990) Crack and cocaine abusers in outpatient psychotherapy. *NIDA Res Monogr* **104**, 24–35.

Kolodgie FD, Farb A, and Virmani R (1995) Pathobiological determinants of cocaine-associated cardiovascular syndromes. *Hum Pathol* **26**, 583–586.

Kolodgie FD, Wilson PS, Mergner WJ, et al. (1999) Cocaine-induced increase in the permeability function of human vascular endothelial cell monolayers. *Exp Mol Pathol* **66**, 109–122.

Koob GF (1999) Cocaine reward and dopamine receptors: Love at first site. *Arch Gen Psychiatry* **56**, 1107–1108.

Koob GF and Nestler EJ (1997) The neurobiology of drug addiction. *J Neuropsychiatr Clin Neurosci* **9**, 482–497.

Koppel BS, Samkoff L, and Daras M (1996) Relation of cocaine use to seizures and epilepsy. *Epilepsia* **37**, 875–878.

Kosten TA (1997) Enhanced neurobehavioral effects of cocaine with chronic neuroleptic exposure in rats. *Schizophr Bull* **23**, 203–213.

Kosten TR (1998) The pharmacotherapy of relapse prevention using anticonvulsants. *Am J Addict* **7**, 205–209.

Kosten TR and Kleber HD (1988) Rapid death during cocaine abuse: a variant of the neuroleptic malignant syndrome? *Am J Drug Alcohol Abuse* **14**, 335–346.

Kosten TA, Gawin FH, Kosten TR, et al. (1993) Gender differences in cocaine use and treatment response. *J Subst Abuse Treat* **10**, 63–66.

Kosten TR, Kosten TA, McDougle CJ, et al. (1996) Gender differences in response to intranasal cocaine administration to humans. *Biol Psychiatry* **39**, 147–148.

Kosten TR, Morgan CM, Falcione J, et al. (1992) Pharmacotherapy for cocaine-abusing methadone-maintained patients using amantadine or desipramine. *Arch Gen Psychiatry* **49**, 894–898.

Krystal JH, D'Souza DC, Madonick S, et al. (1999) Toward a rational pharmacotherapy of comorbid substance abuse in schizophrenic patients. *Schizophr Res* **35**, S35–S49.

Kugelmass AD, Oda A, Monahan K, et al. (1993) Activation of human platelets by cocaine. *Circulation* **88**, 876–883.

Kuhar MJ and Pilotte NS (1996) Neurochemical changes in cocaine withdrawal. *Trends Pharmacol Sci* **17**, 260–264.

Kuhar MJ, Joyce A, and Dominguez G (2001) Genes in drug abuse. *Drug Alcohol Depend* **62**, 157–162.

Lampley EC, Williams S, and Myers SA (1996) Cocaine-associated rhabdomyolysis causing renal failure in pregnancy. *Obstet Gynecol* **87**, 804–806.

Lange RA and Hillis LD (2001) Cardiovascular complications of cocaine use. *N Engl J Med* **345**, 351–358.

Laviola G, Adriani W, Terranova ML, et al. (1999) Psychobiological risk factors for vulnerability to psychostimulants in human adolescents and animal models. *Neurosci Biobehav Rev* **23**, 993–1010.

LeDoux JE (2000) Emotion circuits in the brain. *Annu Rev Neurosci* **23**, 155–184.

Lee HO, Eisenberg MJ, Drew D, et al. (1995) Intraventricular thrombus after cocaine-induced myocardial infarction. *Am Heart J* **129**, 403–405.

Leshner AI and Koob GF (1999) Drugs of abuse and the brain. *Proc Assoc Am Phys* **111**, 99–108.

Levin FR and Lehman AF (1991) Meta-analysis of desipramine as an adjunct in the treatment of cocaine addiction. *J Clin Psychopharmacol* **11**, 374–378.

Levin FR, Evans SM, and Kleber HD (1998a) Prevalence of adult attention-deficit/hyperactivity disorder among cocaine abusers seeking treatment. *Drug Alcohol Depend* **52**, 15–25.

Levin FR, Evans SM, McDowell DM, et al. (1998b) Methylphenidate treatment for cocaine abusers with adult attention-deficit/hyperactivity disorder: a pilot study. *J Clin Psychiatry* **59**, 300–305.

Levin JM, Holman BL, Mendelson JH, et al. (1994) Gender differences in cerebral perfusion in cocaine abuse: Technetium-99m-HMPAO SPECT study of drug-abusing women. *J Nucl Med* **35**, 1902–1909.

Lima AR, Lima MS, Soares BG, et al. (2001) Carbamazepine for cocaine dependence (Cochrane Review). *Cochrane Database Syst Rev* **4**, CD002023.

London ED, Bonson KR, Ernst M, et al. (1999) Brain imaging studies of cocaine abuse: implications for medication development. *Crit Rev Neurobiol* **13**, 227–242.

London ED, Cascella NG, Wong DF, et al. (1990) Cocaine-induced reduction of glucose utilization in human brain. A study using positron emission tomography and [fluorine 18]-fluorodeoxyglucose. *Arch Gen Psychiatry* **47**, 567–574.

London ED, Stapleton JM, Phillips RL, et al. (1996) PET studies of cerebral glucose metabolism: acute effects of cocaine and long-term deficits in brains of drug abusers. *NIDA Res Monogr* **163**, 146–158.

Lukas SE, Sholar M, Lundahl LH, et al. (1996) Sex differences in plasma cocaine levels and subjective effects after acute cocaine administration in human volunteers. *Psychopharmacology (Berl)* **125**, 346–354.

Luthar SS, Cushing G, Merikangas KR, et al. (1998) Multiple jeopardy: risk and protective factors among addicted mothers' offspring. *Dev Psychopathol* **10**, 117–136.

Madu EC, Shala B, and Baugh D (1999) Crack-cocaine-associated aortic dissection in early pregnancy—a case report. *Angiology* **50**, 163–168.

Magura S, Kang SY, Rosenblum A, et al. (1998) Gender differences in psychiatric comorbidity among cocaine-using opiate addicts. *J Addict Dis* **17**, 49–61.

Malison RT, Best SE, van Dyck CH, et al. (1998a) Elevated striatal dopamine transporters during acute cocaine abstinence as measured by [123I] beta-CIT SPECT. *Am J Psychiatry* **155**, 832–834.

Malison RT, Best SE, Wallace EA, et al. (1995) Euphorigenic doses of cocaine reduce [123I]beta-CIT SPECT measures of dopamine transporter availability in human cocaine addicts. *Psychopharmacology (Berl)* **122**, 358–362.

Malison RT, McCance E, Carpenter LL, et al. (1998b) [123I]beta-CIT SPECT imaging of dopamine transporter availability after mazindol administration in human cocaine addicts. *Psychopharmacology (Berl)* **137**, 321–325.

Mao JT, Zhu LX, Sharma S, et al. (1997) Cocaine inhibits human endothelial cell IL-8 production: the role of transforming growth factor-beta. *Cell Immunol* **181**, 38–43.

Margolin A, Avants SK, and Kosten TR (1995a) Mazindol for relapse prevention to cocaine abuse in methadone-maintained patients. *Am J Drug Alcohol Abuse* **21**, 469–481.

Margolin A, Avants SK, and Kosten TR (1996) Abstinence symptomatology associated with cessation of chronic cocaine abuse among methadone-maintained patients. *Am J Drug Alcohol Abuse* **22**, 377–388.

Margolin A, Kosten TR, Avants SK, et al. (1995b) A multicenter trial of bupropion for cocaine dependence in methadone-maintained patients. *Drug Alcohol Depend* **40**, 125–131.

Markou A and Koob GF (1992) Bromocriptine reverses the elevation in intracranial self-stimulation thresholds observed in a rat model of cocaine withdrawal. *Neuropsychopharmacology* **7**, 213–224.

Marlowe DB, Kirby KC, Festinger DS, et al. (1997) Impact of comorbid personality disorders and personality disorder symptoms on outcomes of behavioral treatment for cocaine dependence. *J Nerv Ment Dis* **185**, 483–490.

Martino S, McCance-Katz E, and Workman OJ (1995) The development of a dual diagnosis partial hospital program. *Dev Ambul Ment Health Care* **2**, 145–165.

Mash DC, Staley JK, Izenwasser S, et al. (2000) Serotonin transporters upregulate with chronic cocaine use. *J Chem Neuroanat* **20**, 271–280.

McCance EF, Price LH, Kosten TR, et al. (1995) Cocaethylene: Pharmacology, physiology, and behavioral effects in humans. *J Pharmacol Exp Ther* **274**, 215–223.

McCance-Katz E and Kosten T (1998) Psychopharmacological treatment. In *Clinical Textbook of Addictive Disorders*, Miller S and Frances R (eds). Guilford Press, New York, pp. 596–624.

McCance-Katz E and Schottenfeld R (1995) Attention-deficient/hyperactivity disorder and cocaine abuse. *Am J Addict* **4**, 88–99.

McCance-Katz EF, Boyarsky BK, Hart C, et al. (2001) Repeated administration of cocaine and alcohol to humans: gender effects. *Sixty-Third Annual Scientific Meeting of the College on Problem of Drug and Alcohol Dependence*, Vol. 63, Drug and Alcohol Dependence. Scottsdale, AZ, p. 101.

McCance-Katz EF, Carroll KM, and Rounsaville BJ (1999) Gender differences in treatment-seeking cocaine abusers—implications for treatment and prognosis. *Am J Addict* **8**, 300–311.

McCance-Katz EF, Kosten TR, and Jatlow P (1998a) Concurrent use of cocaine and alcohol is more potent and potentially more toxic than use of either alone—a multiple-dose study. *Biol Psychiatry* **44**, 250–259.

McCance-Katz EF, Kosten TR, and Jatlow P (1998b) Disulfiram effects on acute cocaine administration. *Drug Alcohol Depend* **52**, 27–39.

McCance-Katz EF, Price LH, McDougle CJ, et al. (1993) Concurrent cocaine-ethanol ingestion in humans: pharmacology, physiology, behavior, and the role of cocaethylene. *Psychopharmacology (Berl)* **111**, 39–46.

McLellan AT, Arndt IO, Metzger DS, et al. (1993) The effects of psychosocial services in substance abuse treatment. *JAMA* **269**, 1953–1959.

McMahon RC, Malow R, and Loewinger L (1999) Substance abuse history predicts depression and relapse status among cocaine abusers. *Am J Addict* **8**, 1–8.

Mello NK and Negus SS (2001) Effects of indatraline and buprenorphine on self-administration of speedball combinations of cocaine and heroin by rhesus monkeys. *Neuropsychopharmacology* **25**, 104–117.

Mendelson JH, Mello NK, Sholar MB, et al. (1999) Cocaine pharmacokinetics in men and in women during the follicular and luteal phases of the menstrual cycle. *Neuropsychopharmacology* **21**, 294–303.

Mets B, Winger G, Cabrera C, et al. (1998) A catalytic antibody against cocaine prevents cocaine's reinforcing and toxic effects in rats. *Proc Natl Acad Sci U S A* **95**, 10176–10181.

Milby JB, Schumacher JE, McNamara C, et al. (2000) Initiating abstinence in cocaine abusing dually diagnosed homeless persons. *Drug Alcohol Depend* **60**, 55–67.

Miner LL, Drago J, Chamberlain PM, et al. (1995) Retained cocaine conditioned place preference in D1 receptor deficient mice. *NeuroReport* **6**, 2314–2316.

Missouris CG, Swift PA, and Singer DR (2001) Cocaine use and acute left ventricular dysfunction. *Lancet* **357**, 1586.

Mittleman MA, Mintzer D, Maclure M, et al. (1999) Triggering of myocardial infarction by cocaine. *Circulation* **99**, 2737–2741.

Modesto-Lowe V, Burleson JA, Hersh D, et al. (1997) Effects of naltrexone on cue-elicited craving for alcohol and cocaine. *Drug Alcohol Depend* **49**, 9–16.

Moliterno DJ, Lange RA, Gerard RD, et al. (1994) Influence of intranasal cocaine on plasma constituents associated with endogenous thrombosis and thrombolysis. *Am J Med* **96**, 492–496.

Monti PM, Rohsenow DJ, Michalec E, et al. (1997) Brief coping skills treatment for cocaine abuse: substance use outcomes at three months. *Addiction* **92**, 1717–1728.

Moolchan ET, Cone EJ, Wstadik A, et al. (2000) Cocaine and metabolite elimination patterns in chronic cocaine users during cessation: plasma and saliva analysis. *J Anal Toxicol* **24**, 458–466.

Najavits LM, Weiss RD, and Shaw SR (1997) The link between substance abuse and posttraumatic stress disorder in women. *Am J Addict* **6**, 273–283.

Nann-Vernotica E, Donny EC, Bigelow GE, et al. (2001) Repeated administration of the D1/5 antagonist ecopipam fails to attenuate the subjective effects of cocaine. *Psychopharmacology (Berl)* **155**, 338–347.

National Institute on Drug Abuse (1999b) *Principles of Drug Addiction Treatment: a Research-Based Guide*. Rockville, MD.

Negus SS, Gatch MB, and Mello NK (1998) Discriminative stimulus effects of a cocaine/heroin "speedball" combination in rhesus monkeys. *J Pharmacol Exp Ther* **285**, 1123–1136.

Neiman J, Haapaniemi HM, and Hillbom M (2000) Neurological complications of drug abuse: pathophysiological mechanisms. *Eur J Neurol* **7**, 595–606.

Nestler EJ (1997) Molecular mechanisms of opiate and cocaine addiction. *Curr Opin Neurobiol* **7**, 713–719.

Nestler EJ (2001) Neurobiology. Total recall—the memory of addiction. *Science* **292**, 2266–2267.

Nolla-Salas J, Felez MA, Iglesias MI, et al. (1996) Fatal neuroleptic malignant syndrome caused by cocaine and amphetamine overdose. *Med Clin (Barc)* **106**, 717–718.

Nwosu MC, Nwosu MN, Nwabueze AC, et al. (2001) Brain cardiac events in Nigerian patients with cocaine abuse. *W Afr J Med* **20**, 65–72.

O'Brien CP, Childress AR, McLellan AT, et al. (1993) Developing treatments that address classical conditioning. *NIDA Res Monogr* **135**, 71–91.

O'Connell D and Heffron JJ (2000) Rapid analysis of illicit drugs by mass spectrometry: results from seizures in Ireland. *Analyst* **125**, 119–121.

Ohuoha DC, Maxwell JA, Thomson LE, et al. (1997) Effect of dopamine receptor antagonists on cocaine subjective effects: a naturalistic case study. *J Subst Abuse Treat* **14**, 249–258.

Oliveto A, McCance-Katz FE, Singha A, et al. (2001) Effects of cocaine prior to and during bupropion maintenance in cocaine-abusing volunteers. *Drug Alcohol Depend* **63**, 155–167.

Oslin DW, Pettinati HM, Volpicelli JR, et al. (1999) The effects of naltrexone on alcohol and cocaine use in dually addicted patients. *J Subst Abuse Treat* **16**, 163–167.

Parsons LH, Koob GF, and Weiss F (1995) Serotonin dysfunction in the nucleus accumbens of rats during withdrawal after unlimited access to intravenous cocaine. *J Pharmacol Exp Ther* **274**, 1182–1191.

Pascual-Leone A, Dhuna A, Altafullah I, et al. (1990) Cocaine-induced seizures. *Neurology* **40**, 404–407.

Pearlson GD, Jeffery PJ, Harris GJ, et al. (1993) Correlation of acute cocaine-induced changes in local cerebral blood flow with subjective effects. *Am J Psychiatry* **150**, 495–497.

Perera R, Kraebber A, and Schwartz MJ (1997) Prolonged QT interval and cocaine use. *J Electrocardiol* **30**, 337–339.

Perez de los Cobos J, Duro P, Trujols J, et al. (2001) Methadone tapering plus amantadine to detoxify heroin-dependent inpatients with or without an active cocaine use disorder: two randomised controlled trials. *Drug Alcohol Depend* **63**, 187–195.

Perron AD and Gibbs M (1997) Thoracic aortic dissection secondary to crack cocaine ingestion. *Am J Emerg Med* **15**, 507–509.

Petitti DB, Sidney S, Quesenberry C, et al. (1998) Stroke and cocaine or amphetamine use. *Epidemiology* **9**, 596–600.

Pilotte NS, Sharpe LG, Rountree SD, et al. (1996) Cocaine withdrawal reduces dopamine transporter binding in the shell of the nucleus accumbens. *Synapse* **22**, 87–92.

Pitts WR, Lange RA, Cigarroa JE, et al. (1997) Cocaine-induced myocardial ischemia and infarction: pathophysiology, recognition, and management. *Prog Cardiovasc Dis* **40**, 65–76.

Pitts WR, Vongpatanasin W, Cigarroa JE, et al. (1998) Effects of the intracoronary infusion of cocaine on left ventricular systolic and diastolic function in humans. *Circulation* **97**, 1270–1273.

Pottieger AE, Tressell PA, Surratt HL, et al. (1995) Drug use patterns of adult crack users in street versus residential treatment samples. *J Psychoact Drugs* **27**, 27–38.

Preston KL, Sullivan JT, Strain EC, et al. (1992) Effects of cocaine alone and in combination with bromocriptine in human cocaine abusers. *J Pharmacol Exp Ther* **262**, 279–291.

Qureshi AI, Suri MF, Guterman LR, et al. (2001) Cocaine use and the likelihood of nonfatal myocardial infarction and stroke: data from the third national health and nutrition examination survey. *Circulation* **103**, 502–506.

Reavill C, Hatcher JP, Lewis VA, et al. (1998) 5-HT4 receptor antagonism does not affect motor and reward mechanisms in the rat. *Eur J Pharmacol* **357**, 115–120.

Rezkalla SH, Mazza JJ, Kloner RA, et al. (1993) Effects of cocaine on human platelets in healthy subjects. *Am J Cardiol* **72**, 243–246.

Richards JR (2000) Rhabdomyolysis and drugs of abuse. *J Emerg Med* **19**, 51–56.

Richardson GA (1998) Prenatal cocaine exposure. A longitudinal study of development. *Ann N Y Acad Sci* **846**, 144–152.

Richardson GA, Hamel SC, Goldschmidt L, et al. (1999) Growth of infants prenatally exposed to cocaine/crack: comparison of a prenatal care and a no prenatal care sample. *Pediatrics* **104**, E18.

Richter RM, Pich EM, Koob GF, et al. (1995) Sensitization of cocaine-stimulated increase in extracellular levels of corticotropin-releasing factor from the rat amygdala after repeated administration as determined by intracranial microdialysis. *Neurosci Lett* **187**, 169–172.

Rinder HM, Ault KA, Jatlow PI, et al. (1994) Platelet alpha-granule release in cocaine users. *Circulation* **90**, 1162–1167.

Ritz MC, Boja JW, George FR, et al. (1989) Cocaine binding sites related to drug self-administration. *NIDA Res Monogr* **95**, 239–246.

Roache JD, Grabowski J, Schmitz JM, et al. (2000) Laboratory measures of methylphenidate effects in cocaine-dependent patients receiving treatment. *J Clin Psychopharmacol* **20**, 61–68.

Robbins SJ, Ehrman RN, Childress AR, et al. (1997) Relationships among physiological and self-report responses produced by cocaine-related cues. *Addict Behav* **22**, 157–167.

Robbins SJ, Ehrman RN, Childress AR, et al. (1999) Comparing levels of cocaine cue reactivity in male and female outpatients. *Drug Alcohol Depend* **53**, 223–230.

Rohsenow DJ, Monti PM, Martin RA, et al. (2000) Brief coping skills treatment for cocaine abuse: 12-month substance use outcomes. *J Consult Clin Psychol* **68**, 515–520.

Rolls ET (2000) Memory systems in the brain. *Annu Rev Psychol* **51**, 599–630.

Rosenblum A, Fallon B, Magura S, et al. (1999) The autonomy of mood disorders among cocaine-using methadone patients. *Am J Drug Alcohol Abuse* **25**, 67–80.

Ross DL (1998) Factors associated with excited delirium deaths in police custody. *Mod Pathol* **11**, 1127–1137.

Rounsaville BJ, Glazer W, Wilber CH, et al. (1983) Short-term interpersonal psychotherapy in methadone-maintained opiate addicts. *Arch Gen Psychiatry* **40**, 629–636.

Roy A (2001) Characteristics of cocaine-dependent patients who attempt suicide. *Am J Psychiatry* **158**, 1215–1219.

Ruttenber AJ, McAnally HB, and Wetli CV (1999) Cocaine-associated rhabdomyolysis and excited delirium: different stages of the same syndrome. *Am J Forens Med Pathol* **20**, 120–127.

Schenk S, Horger BA, Peltier R, et al. (1991) Supersensitivity to the reinforcing effects of cocaine following 6-hydroxydopamine lesions to the medial prefrontal cortex in rats. *Brain Res* **543**, 227–235.

Schmitz JM, Averill P, Stotts AL, et al. (2001a) Fluoxetine treatment of cocaine-dependent patients with major depressive disorder. *Drug Alcohol Depend* **63**, 207–214.

Schmitz JM, Oswald LM, Jacks SD, et al. (1997) Relapse prevention treatment for cocaine dependence: group vs. individual format. *Addict Behav* **22**, 405–418.

Schmitz JM, Stotts AL, Averill PM, et al. (2000) Cocaine dependence with and without comorbid depression: a comparison of patient characteristics. *Drug Alcohol Depend* **60**, 189–198.

Schmitz JM, Stotts AL, Rhoades HM, et al. (2001b) Naltrexone and relapse prevention treatment for cocaine-dependent patients. *Addict Behav* **26**, 167–180.

Schnoll SH, Karrigan J, Kitchen SB, et al. (1985) Characteristics of cocaine abusers presenting for treatment. *NIDA Res Monogr* **61**, 171–181.

Schubiner H, Tzelepis A, Milberger S, et al. (2000) Prevalence of attention-deficit/hyperactivity disorder and conduct disorder among substance abusers. *J Clin Psychiatry* **61**, 244–251.

Serper MR, Chou JC, Allen MH, et al. (1999) Symptomatic overlap of cocaine intoxication and acute schizophrenia at emergency presentation. *Schizophr Bull* **25**, 387–394.

Sherwood Brown E, Suppes T, Adinoff B, et al. (2001) Drug abuse and bipolar disorder: comorbidity or misdiagnosis? *J Affect Disord* **65**, 105–115.

Siegel AJ, Sholar MB, Mendelson JH, et al. (1999) Cocaine-induced erythrocytosis and increase in von Willebrand factor: evidence for drug-related blood doping and prothrombotic effects. *Arch Intern Med* **159**, 1925–1929.

Silverman K, Higgins ST, Brooner RK, et al. (1996) Sustained cocaine abstinence in methadone maintenance patients through voucher-based reinforcement therapy. *Arch Gen Psychiatry* **53**, 409–415.

Simpson DD, Joe GW, Fletcher BW, et al. (1999) A national evaluation of treatment outcomes for cocaine dependence. *Arch Gen Psychiatry* **56**, 507–514.

Simpson DD, Joe GW, and Rowan-Szal GA (1997) Drug abuse treatment retention and process effects on follow-up outcomes. *Drug Alcohol Depend* **47**, 227–235.

Singer AJ, McCance-Katz E, Petrakis I, et al. (1999) The effects of naltrexone and isradipine on the behavioral response to cocaine in human subjects. *NIDA Res Monogr* **180**,.

Singh N, Singh HK, Singh PP, et al. (2001) Cocaine-induced torsades de pointes in idiopathic long Q-T syndrome. *Am J Ther* **8**, 299–302.

Siqueland L, Crits-Christoph P, Frank A, et al. (1998) Predictors of dropout from psychosocial treatment of cocaine dependence. *Drug Alcohol Depend* **52**, 1–13.

Skinstad AH and Swain A (2001) Comorbidity in a clinical sample of substance abusers. *Am J Drug Alcohol Abuse* **27**, 45–64.

Smeriglio VL and Wilcox HC (1999) Prenatal drug exposure and child outcome: past, present, future. *Clin Perinatol* **26**, 1–16.

Smith BH, Waschbusch DA, Willoughby MT, et al. (2000) The efficacy, safety, and practicality of treatments for adolescents with attention-deficit/hyperactivity disorder (ADHD). *Clin Child Fam Psychol Rev* **3**, 243–267.

Sofuoglu M, Brown S, Babb DA, et al. (2001) Depressive symptoms modulate the subjective and physiological response to cocaine in humans. *Drug Alcohol Depend* **63**, 131–137.

Sora I, Hall FS, Andrews AM, et al. (2001) Molecular mechanisms of cocaine reward: combined dopamine and serotonin transporter knockouts eliminate cocaine place preference. *Proc Natl Acad Sci U S A* **98**, 5300–5305.

Sora I, Wichems C, Takahashi N, et al. (1998) Cocaine reward models: conditioned place preference can be established in dopamine- and in serotonin-transporter knockout mice. *Proc Natl Acad Sci U S A* **95**, 7699–7704.

Steele MT, Westdorp EJ, Garza AG, et al. (2000) Screening for stimulant use in adult emergency department seizure patients. *J Toxicol Clin Toxicol* **38**, 609–613.

Stein EA (2001) fMRI: A new tool for the in vivo localization of drug actions in the brain. *J Anal Toxicol* **25**, 419–424.

Stine SM, Krystal JH, Kosten TR, et al. (1995) Mazindol treatment for cocaine dependence. *Drug Alcohol Depend* **39**, 245–252.

Strickland TL, Miller BL, Kowell A, et al. (1998) Neurobiology of cocaine-induced organic brain impairment: contributions from functional neuroimaging. *Neuropsychol Rev* **8**, 1–9.

Substance Abuse and Mental Health Services Administration (1996) *Trends in the Incidence of Drug Use in the United States*. Rockville, MD.

Substance Abuse and Mental Health Service Administration (1999) *The 1999 National Household Survey on Drug Abuse*. Rockville, MD.

Substance Abuse and Mental Health Service Administration (2000) *The 2000 National Household Survey on Drug Abuse*. Rockville, MD.

Substance Abuse and Mental Health Administration (2001a) *DASIS Report: Women in Treatment for Smoked Cocaine*. The Office of Applied Studies, Arlington, VA.

Substance Abuse and Mental Health Service Administration (2001b) *Mid-Year 2000 Preliminary Emergency*. Department Data from the Drug Abuse Warning Network. Rockville, MD.

Suchman NE and Luthar SS (2000) Maternal addiction, child maladjustment and socio-demographic risks: implications for parenting behaviors. *Addiction* **95**, 1417–1428.

Swindle RW, Phibbs CS, Paradise MJ, et al. (1995) Impatient treatment for substance abuse patients with psychiatric disorders: a national study of determinants of readmission. *J Subst Abuse* **7**, 79–97.

Thomas VH, Melchert TP, and Banken JA (1999) Substance dependence and personality disorders: comorbidity and treatment outcome in an inpatient treatment population. *J Stud Alcohol* **60**, 271–277.

Tolat RD, O'Dell MW, Golamco-Estrella SP, et al. (2000) Cocaine-associated stroke: three cases and rehabilitation considerations. *Brain Inj* **14**, 383–391.

Uhl GR, Vandenbergh DJ, and Miner LL (1996) Knockout mice and dirty drugs. Durg addiction. *Curr Biol* **6**, 935–936.

Usdan SL, Schumacher JE, Milby JB, et al. (2001) Crack cocaine, alcohol, and other drug use patterns among homeless persons with other mental disorders. *Am J Drug Alcohol Abuse* **27**, 107–120.

Uslaner J, Kalechstein A, Richter T, et al. (1999) Association of depressive symptoms during abstinence with the subjective high produced by cocaine. *Am J Psychiatry* **156**, 1444–1446.

van der Woude FJ (2000) Cocaine use and kidney damage. *Nephrol Dial Transplant* **15**, 299–301.

Van Etten ML and Anthony JC (1999) Comparative epidemiology of initial drug opportunities and transitions to first use: Marijuana, cocaine, hallucinogens and heroin. *Drug Alcohol Depend* **54**, 117–125.

Volkow ND (2001) Drug abuse and mental illness: progress in understanding comorbidity. *Am J Psychiatry* **158**, 1181–1183.

Volkow ND, Fowler JS, and Wang GJ (1999) Imaging studies on the role of dopamine in cocaine reinforcement and addiction in humans. *J Psychopharmacol* **13**, 337–345.

Wang RY (1999) pH-dependent cocaine-induced cardiotoxicity. *Am J Emerg Med* **17**, 364–369.

Ward AS, Haney M, Fischman MW, et al. (1997a) Binge cocaine self-administration by humans: smoked cocaine. *Behav Pharmacol* **8**, 736–744.

Ward AS, Haney M, Fischman MW, et al. (1997b) Binge cocaine self-administration in humans: intravenous cocaine. *Psychopharmacology (Berl)* **132**, 375–381.

Warner LA, Kessler RC, Hughes M, et al. (1995) Prevalence and correlates of drug use and dependence in the United States. Results from the National Comorbidity Survey. *Arch Gen Psychiatry* **52**, 219–229.

Weber JE, Chudnofsky CR, Boczar M, et al. (2000) Cocaine-associated chest pain: How common is myocardial infarction? *Acad Emerg Med* **7**, 873–877.

Weinstein SP, Gottheil E, and Sterling RC (1997) Randomized comparison of intensive outpatient vs. individual therapy for cocaine abusers. *J Addict Dis* **16**, 41–56.

Weiss F, Ciccocioppo R, Parsons LH, et al. (2001a) Compulsive drug-seeking behavior and relapse. Neuroadaptation, stress, and conditioning factors. *Ann N Y Acad Sci* **937**, 1–26.

Weiss F, Maldonado-Vlaar CS, Parsons LH, et al. (2000) Control of cocaine-seeking behavior by drug-associated stimuli in rats: effects on recovery of extinguished operant-responding and extracellular dopamine levels in amygdala and nucleus accumbens. *Proc Natl Acad Sci U S A* **97**, 4321–4326.

Weiss F, Martin-Fardon R, Ciccocioppo R, et al. (2001b) Enduring resistance to extinction of cocaine-seeking behavior induced by drug-related cues. *Neuropsychopharmacology* **25**, 361–372.

Weiss RD, Martinez-Raga J, Griffin ML, et al. (1997) Gender differences in cocacine dependent patients: a 6 month follow-up study. *Drug Alcohol Depend* **44**, 35–40.

Westermeyer J, Kopka S, and Nugent S (1997) Course and severity of substance abuse among patients with comorbid major depression. *Am J Addict* **6**, 284–292.

Wetli CV, Mash D, and Karch SB (1996) Cocaine-associated agitated delirium and the neuroleptic malignant syndrome. *Am J Emerg Med* **14**, 425–428.

Winbery S, Blaho K, Logan B, et al. (1998) Multiple cocaine-induced seizures and corresponding cocaine and metabolite concentrations. *Am J Emerg Med* **16**, 529–533.

Withers NW, Pulvirenti L, Koob GF, et al. (1995) Cocaine abuse and dependence. *J Clin Psychopharmacol* **15**, 63–78.

Woody GE and Munoz A (2000) Efficacy, individual effectiveness, and population effectiveness in substance abuse treatment. *Curr Psychiatr Rep* **2**, 505–507.

Woody GE, McLellan AT, Luborsky L, et al. (1995) Psychotherapy in community methadone programs: a validation study. *Am J Psychiatry* **152**, 1302–1308.

Woolf JH, Huang L, Ishiguro Y, et al. (1997) Negative inotropic effect of methylecgonidine, a major product of cocaine base pyrolysis, on ferret and human myocardium. *J Cardiovasc Pharmacol* **30**, 352–359.

Xiao Y, He J, Gilbert RD, et al. (2000) Cocaine induces apoptosis in fetal myocardial cells through a mitochondria-dependent pathway. *J Pharmacol Exp Ther* **292**, 8–14.

Yui K, Goto K, Ikemoto S, et al. (1999) Neurobiological basis of relapse prediction in stimulant-induced psychosis and schizophrenia: the role of sensitization. *Mol Psychiatry* **4**, 512–523.

Zimmet SV, Strous RD, Burgess ES, et al. (2000) Effects of clozapine on substance use in patients with schizophrenia and schizoaffective disorder: a retrospective survey. *J Clin Psychopharmacol* **20**, 94–98.

Human ingestion of hallucinogens can be traced back thousands of years. In the Americas, Europe, and Africa, hallucinogens were used for consecration during religious ceremonies, for divination, and as tools for rites of passage and shamanic healing. It is possible that the soma of the 3500-year-old Hindu–Aryan Rig Veda (Smith 2000), the kykeon of the ancient Greek rites of the Eleusinian Mysteries (Wasson 1961), and the manna of the Judeo–Christian Old Testament (Merkur 2000) may all have been hallucinogen-containing substances.

The majority of these botanicals grow in the Americas. In South and North America, cacti containing the hallucinogen mescaline are still widely used by a number of Native American tribes. In South America, boiled potions are made from *Trichocereus* species, a cactus containing about 1% mescaline. A much more potent mescaline-containing cactus, peyote (*Lophophora williamsii*), grows naturally in northern Mexico and along a long strip of the Texas–Mexico border. The Huichol of Mexico have used peyote as a religious sacrament continuously for 3000 years (Schaefer and Furst 1998), as have the Native American Church (NAC) of the United States and Canada. In the NAC, peyote is treasured as the holy sacrament from God to be ingested in all-night prayer vigils. Currently, the NAC has as many as 300,000 members and is federally protected by the Act of Congress. Several reports in the medical literature allude to participation in NAC meetings as a successful, culturally sensitive therapy for alcoholism and other drug addictions among Native Americans (Bergman 1971, Albaugh and Anderson 1974).

Hallucinogenic mushrooms containing psilocybin (4-phosphoryloxy-N,N-dimethyltryptamine) and psilocin (4-hydroxy-N,N-dimethyltryptamine), especially from the genus *Psilocybe*, are found throughout the Americas, Europe, and Asia. *Psilocybe cubensis* typically contains 1.6-mg psilocybin per gram of dried mushroom; a dose of 40 μg/kg induces a 3- to 4-hour intoxication. The ancient cultures of Mesoamerica almost certainly venerated the *Psilocybe* experience (Wasson 1961), and some Native Americans of Oaxaca, Mexico continue to use these mushrooms in religious ceremonies to this day. Easily grown and indigenous to many parts of the United States, *Psilocybe* mushrooms are commonly trafficked as hallucinogens in the illicit market. Dimethyltryptamine (DMT), a short-acting hallucinogen, is also present in a wide variety of botanicals. Many tribes of the Amazon and elsewhere ingest potent DMT snuffs prepared from seeds of *Anadenanthera peregrina*, *Anadenanthera columbrina*, and other botanicals (Schultes and Hofmann 1992).

The dawn of modernity for hallucinogenic drugs can be placed to the moment in 1943 when Albert Hofmann, a Swiss chemist, discovered the potent psychological effects of LSD. Within a decade the drug was being tested as an agent of chemical warfare in the United States and Europe. Within two decades it assumed cult status among the ministry, academics, and students, culminating in an epidemic of abuse in its third decade starting in the late 1960s. Congressional reaction came in the form of the Drug Abuse Control Amendments of 1965 and 1968, which choked off drug supplies to researchers, and criminalized drug sale and use. The scientific impact of these laws was to retard the advance of knowledge in this field for a generation.

The development and chemical identification of additional agents causing LSD-like mental symptoms, however, proceeded apace. This work has both clarified aspects of their mechanisms of action, and created a challenge to defining hallucinogens. Two classes of drugs appear to have more in common with LSD than not. These include other substituted indolealkylamines (psilocybin, psilocin, ibogaine, dimethyltryptamine, and bufotenine, *inter alia*) and phenethylamines (mescaline, MDMA, MDA, 2CB [4-bromo-2,5-dimethoxyphenethylamine], and DOM [2,5-dimethoxy-4-methylamphetamine] *inter alia*). Shulgin has synthesized and tested nearly 200 compounds, largely of the phenethylamine class, for hallucinogenic properties (Shulgin 1991).

The definition of a hallucinogenic drug has been a matter of controversy (Hollister 1968, Jarvik 1970, Brawley and Duffield 1972, LaBarre 1975, Martin and Sloan 1977, Grinspoon and Bakalar 1979, Schultes and Hofmann 1980). More than 90 species of hallucinogenic plants afford an anthropological definition. Hundreds of substituted phenylethylamines and tryptamines lend themselves to chemical characterization. Because few have been systematically studied in humans, hallucinogens have been defined by their botanical or chemical rubrics rather than their psychophysiological affects. To address the problem of classification, one may define as hallucinogenic "any agent which has alterations in perception, cognition, or mood as its primary psychobiological actions in the presence of an otherwise clear sensorium. Most commonly this includes indolealkylamines and phenethylamines, and excludes, *inter alia*, the anticholinergics, the arylcyclohexylamine dissociative anesthetics such as phencyclidine, stimulants such as amphetamine and cocaine, bromism and heavy metal intoxication" (Abraham et al. 1996) (either because changes in perception, mood, or cognition are not the primary effect or because they cloud the sensorium). Instruments are now available that objectify the human factor in hallucinogenic responses (Hermle et al. 1994, Strassman et al. 1994). Future definitions may likely be refined on the basis of neuroreceptor and second-messenger drug effects.

HALLUCINOGEN INTOXICATION

Diagnosis

Criteria for the diagnosis of acute hallucinogen intoxication are shown below.

DSM-IV-TR Diagnostic Criteria

292.89 Hallucinogen Intoxication

A. Recent use of a hallucinogen.
B. Clinically significant maladaptive behavioral or psychological changes (e.g., marked anxiety or depression, ideas of reference, fear of losing one's mind, paranoid ideation, impaired judgment, or impaired social or occupational function) that developed during, or shortly after, hallucinogen use.
C. Perceptual changes occurring in a state of full wakefulness and alertness (e.g., subjective intensification of perceptions, depersonalization, derealization, illusions, hallucinations, synesthesias) that developed during, or shortly after, hallucinogen use.
D. Two (or more) of the following signs, developing during, or shortly after, hallucinogen use:

(1) pupillary dilation
(2) tachycardia
(3) sweating
(4) palpitations
(5) blurring of vision
(6) tremors
(7) incoordination

E. The symptoms are not due to a general medical condition and are not better accounted for by another mental disorder.

Reprinted with permission from the Diagnostic and Statistical Manual of Mental Disorders, Fourth Edition, Text Revision. Copyright 2000 American Psychiatric Association.

Chemical identification of hallucinogens in emergency specimens with methods such as gas chromatography–mass spectrometry remain costly and time consuming. Thus, clinicians in emergency settings must rely on a careful drug history, the information from the less drug-affected friends of the individual, the mental status examination, and signs apparent from the physical examination. The high potency of this class of drugs permits their distribution in venues of single drops of solution. Thus, blotter paper (often marked with stamps of cartoon characters or New Age symbols) or a single sugar cube can easily carry more than the 50 to 100 µg of LSD necessary for the user to trip 6 to 12 hours. Routes of administration other than by ingestion are rare. Autonomic arousal is the rule, with tachycardia, increased deep tendon reflexes, and dilated pupils present regardless of whether euphoria or panic is present. Hypersensitivity to visual and auditory stimuli is common, with atypical affective responses as the result.

Motor function is reduced, so that such individuals are not likely to act out aggressively. Emergency presentations of the proverbial "bad trip" have apparently declined in recent years despite continued use by a significant percentage of American youth. "Bad trips" are drug-induced panic attacks in the context of a hallucinogenic experience, associated with prepossessing feelings of unreality, confusion, and the flooding of the senses with unbidden imagery.

Epidemiology

Among hallucinogens, LSD remains the most popular in its class among American high school students. An annual drug survey of 45,000 students by the Monitoring the Future Program of the University of Michigan has been performed since 1975. There is a stable long-term trend of LSD lifetime use among 1 in 10 seniors. In the year 2001, 10.9% of the seniors had used LSD at least once. Attitudes among seniors have relaxed regarding their perception of dangers from LSD use. In 1990, 44.7% of the students believed users were risking harming themselves from the drug if taken once or twice. A decade later, 34.3% of the students felt the same way. Nearly half the seniors in 2001 (44.7%) reported that LSD is "fairly easy" or "very easy" to get (Johnston et al. 2002). A single dose of LSD is available now to any adolescent for less than $5. Despite apparently easy availability and easing apprehensions about its effects, the prevalence of lifetime LSD use among students has remained steady.

Differential Diagnosis

The differential diagnosis of an acute hallucinogenic intoxication includes intoxication by other agents (such as phencyclidine (PCP), cocaine, amphetamines, anticholinergics, and inhalants, among others). It also includes acute schizophrenia or affective disorder, panic disorder, head injury, sedative, hypnotic, anxiolytic, or alcohol withdrawal (including gamma-hydroxybutyrate [GHB]), metabolic disorders such as hypoglycemia and hyperthyroidism, epilepsy, acute vascular events, release hallucinations of ophthalmologic disease, and the complications of central nervous system (CNS) tumors. Age, along with prior clinical history, the history of the current event, physical examination, and toxicology screen for suspected nonhallucinogenic agents usually reveal the diagnosis.

An individual presenting with a history of taking LSD is only correct approximately 50% of the time, judging from analysis of street samples analyzed by the Massachusetts Department of Public Health in the last decade. The street practice of adulteration or mislabeling of the drug is common. Psychosis following a smoked agent suggests phencyclidine. Differentiating between PCP and LSD is clinically important, since LSD-induced panic responds well to oral benzodiazepines, while PCP delirium requires high potency antipsychotic medications such as haloperidol. A "palm test" can be employed to differentiate PCP from LSD toxicity (Abraham and Aldridge 1993). This is performed by the examiner holding an open palm in front of the individual and asking "the names of all the colors you see in my palm." The LSD individual often ticks off a series of vivid colors and occasional images. The dissociated, aggressive PCP individual attempts to attack the hand.

Etiology

The acute effects of "tripping" on LSD-like (i.e., with similar psychic effects, e.g., psilocybin or mescaline) hallucinogens are variable and profound. Classic descriptions are to be found by Albert Hofmann (1980) and Aldous Huxley (1954). Subjects given LSD without their knowledge suffer more anxiety, hypomotility, and speech disruption than those who take it knowingly. LSD is active within 30 minutes of the ingestion of a dose of 50 to 100 μg. Physically the drug stimulates the autonomic nervous system rapidly, resulting in tachycardia, hypertension, and dilated pupils, the last being present for much of the trip. The flood of rapidly changing perceptual, affective, and cognitive effects are by alternate turns exhilarating, nerve wracking, and incapacitating. Table 21-1 illustrates a typical time course for the psychiatric effects of LSD.

The effective hallucinogenic doses vary widely between drugs in this class, and between individuals. Thus, a dose of 1 μg/kg of LSD is approximately equivalent to 150 to 200 μg/kg of psilocybin and 5 to 6 mg/kg of mescaline (Hollister 1984). Adverse reactions have been observed following 40 μg of LSD in some individuals, but absent in others taking as much as 2000 μg. The conventional explanation of this variability of response is instructional set, anticipation of drug effects due to previous experience, and environmental setting–affect outcome. Additionally, personality, preexisting mental illness, and genetic vulnerability are also likely to be important.

Unlike the chronic use of stimulants like amphetamine and cocaine, chronic use of hallucinogens does not lead to physiological dependence. On the other hand, tolerance to LSD rapidly builds in 4 to 7 days, and lasts 3 days (Abramson et al. 1956). LSD shows cross-tolerance with psilocybin and mescaline, but not with amphetamines, dimethyltryptamine, or cannabis. There is no withdrawal or documented fatalities from overdose. Homicide and suicide in the acute drug state have been reported (Cohen 1960, Reich and Hepps 1972) but are rare, ostensibly because of drug-induced hypomotility. The mechanism of action of hallucinogens is complex. Titeler and colleagues (1988) have shown that hallucinogenic potency of LSD and selected phenylisopropylamines correlates with the drug's ability to bind at the postsynaptic 5-HT_2 receptor.

Neurophysiologic studies in animals support the involvement of postsynaptic 5-HT_2 and 5-HT_{1C} receptors for hallucinogenic activity (Abraham et al. 2002). Hallucinogens simultaneously decrease spontaneous activity in the locus coeruleus, considered a novelty detector in the midbrain, while enhancing sensory responses of the locus coeruleus by activating N-methyl-D-aspartate receptors. In the cerebral cortex, the drugs both inhibit and induce activity by exciting GABAergic and glutamatergic neurons respectively.

The presence of selective serotonin reuptake inhibitors blunts hallucinogenic effects, possibly through the activation of 5-HT_1 receptors (Aghajanian and Marek 1999). GABA-_A antianxiety agents (e.g., benzodiazepines) promptly bring a bad trip to an end, presumably by inhibition of the locus coeruleus. Opiates are likely to have a similar outcome by reducing glutamatergic excitation of cortical systems. This may explain why hallucinogen abuse appears to be so uncommon among active opioid abusers.

Table 21-1	Time Course for the Psychiatric Effects of LSD-like Hallucinogens
Time	**Psychiatric Effects**
0–30 minutes	Dizziness, nausea, weakness, anxiety
30–60 minutes	Blurred vision, visual pseudohallucinations and hallucinations, afteримagery, geometric and imagistic imagery with eyes closed, decreased concentration, dissociation, depersonalization, out of body sensations, reduced coordination
60–240 minutes	Intensified afterimagery, false perceptions of movement (walls appearing to breathe or melt), loss of rectilinearity of perceptions, a rapid flood of emotions including anxiety, euphoria, and oceanic unity, loss of the sense of time
4–12 hours	Gradual return to previous mental state, but with continued arousal, headache, fatigue, contemplative frame of reference, sense of profundity

Source: Modified from Hollister L (1984) Effects of hallucinogens in humans. In *Hallucinogens: Neurochemical, Behavioral, and Clinical Perspectives*, Jacobs B (ed). Raven Press, New York.

Several European groups have published neuroimaging studies of the acute effects of hallucinogens (Hermle et al. 1994, Vollenweider et al. 1997). Hermle and colleagues using single photon emission computed tomography (SPECT) in healthy volunteers found that mescaline resulted in increased metabolic activity in the temporofrontal cortex, in distinction to individuals with schizophrenia, who show hypofrontality. Vollenweider and colleagues administered psilocybin to healthy volunteers who were then studied with ^{18}F-fluorodeoxyglucose positron-emission tomography (PET). The hallucinogen globally increased brain metabolic activity, with special activation of the anterior cingulate, frontal, and medial temporal cortex. Metabolic activation correlated with the intensity of subjective symptoms.

Treatment

Treatment of hallucinogen intoxication with panic is easily managed with oral benzodiazepines (diazepam 20 mg or lorazepam 2 mg), which bring the terror, as well as the trip, to an end within 30 minutes. This knowledge, along with the availability of benzodiazepines in the environment, has reduced the need of psychiatric emergency interventions.

HALLUCINOGEN-INDUCED PSYCHOTIC DISORDERS

Criteria for substance-induced psychotic disorder are shown in Chapter 15 on page 355.

Among the hallucinogens, LSD has been associated with the majority of, but not all, prolonged psychotic reactions following acute drug use. These have been reviewed extensively (Abraham et al. 1996, Abraham and Aldridge 1993, Strassman 1984). Psychoses are apparently rare with the abuse of botanical preparations, in all likelihood because such agents are of low potency, not widely abused, and often controlled by religious sanctions. By comparison, psychoses have been seen following the administration of LSD to patients and experimental subjects (Opitz 1963, Fink et al. 1966, Leuner 1967, Baker 1967, McFarling 1980). Rates for the development of psychosis following experimentally administered LSD range from 0.08 (Malleson 1971, Titeler et al. 1988) to 4.6% (Fink 1966, Hollister 1984), with patients being at higher risk. Psychosis is associated with LSD use in two longitudinal studies (McLellan et al. 1979, Bowers 1977), six cross-sectional studies (Abraham 1980, Smart and Jones 1970, Breakey et al. 1974, Bowers 1972, Safer 1987, Vardy and Kay 1983), 13 case series (Cohen 1960, Anonymous 1966, Ungerleider et al. 1966, Smart and Bateman 1967, Tietz 1967, Blumenfield and Glickman 1967, Hekimian and Gershon 1968, Frosch 1969, Malleson 1971, Sanborn and Daniels 1971, Abruzzi 1977, McLellan and Druley 1977, Kornblith 1981), and 75 case reports (Riech and Hepps 1972, Cooper 1955, Cohen and Ditman 1963, Frosch et al. 1965, Metzner 1969, Hatrick and Dewhurst 1970, Muller 1971, Dewhurst and Hatrick 1972, Fookes 1972, Horowitz 1975, Lake et al. 1981, Bowers 1987, Schwartz et al. 1987, Abraham 1983). The potency of LSD in this respect cannot be generalized to other agents in this class.

In addition to exhibiting positive signs of schizophrenia, individuals with post-LSD psychoses show affective lability and the novel addition of visual hallucinations uncommon in non-drug-related psychoses (Abraham 1980). Individuals with post-LSD psychosis in one study had healthier premorbid personalities and an earlier age of onset than non-drug-using schizophrenics (Bowers 1972), a finding confirmed by Breakey and colleagues (1974). The uniqueness of post-LSD psychosis remains controversial. One comparison of post-LSD psychosis and non-drug-related schizophrenia found no essential clinical differences between the two (Vardy and Kay 1983). Bowers (1972) found that LSD psychosis is associated with a reduced serotonin metabolite in cerebrospinal fluid (CSF), while Tsuang and colleagues (1982) found more visual hallucinations, depression, and families with affective disorder in drug-abusing psychotics than a drug-abstinent schizophrenia comparison group.

Differential Diagnosis

The differential diagnosis of posthallucinogen psychosis is the same as that for any acute psychotic disorder. This includes protracted psychoses following the use of the dissociative anesthetics phencyclidine and ketamine, amphetamines, and cocaine; schizophrenia and affective disorders, migraine, deliria from CNS infections, closed head injuries, tumors, vascular events, and the toxic effects of bromine, heavy metals, and anticholinergic drugs. Central to diagnosis is a careful premorbid history, complemented by data from friends and family on the individual's recent medical history and behavior. Neurological examination, urine for toxicological screening, and computed tomography or magnetic resonance imaging of the brain are helpful in ruling out treatable non-LSD-related psychotic disorders.

Etiology

Sandison and colleagues (1954) first described LSD-like experiences recurring days to weeks following the ingestion of LSD in 1954. Subsequent clinical reports of this phenomenon adopted the street label of "flashbacks" to describe persisting imagery and LSD-associated affect (Rosenthal 1964, Robbins et al. 1967, Holsten 1976, Horowitz 1969, Shick and Smith 1970). Anderson and O'Malley (1972) first suggested that the term "flashback" was a misnomer, since many individuals described not simply flashes of imagery but also continuous visual disturbances. A description of the visual phenomenology subsequently confirmed this impression.

This study found that in 123 LSD users visual symptoms predominated, and lasted for at least 5 years in half of the samples. Clinical follow-ups of individuals with hallucinogen persisting perception disorder (HPPD) find that these symptoms have been stable for the last three decades, suggesting that in at least some individuals HPPD appears to be permanent. Controlled studies of individuals with HPPD suggest that the disorder is the product of chronic visual disinhibition of information processing in which ordinarily filtered visual noise is perceived. This hypothesis is supported by psychophysical (Abraham 1982, Abraham and Wolf 1988) and electrophysiological data (Abraham and Duffy 1991). In the eyes-closed state, when visual disturbances are heightened, EEG coherence, a measure of cortical synchrony, and ostensible disinhibition between cortical regions, increases in the primary visual cortex (Abraham and Duffy 2001).

Further support for hallucinogen-mediated disinhibition of neurobehavioral systems comes from animal data in which the hallucinogenic 5-HT$_{2A}$ agonist 2,5-dimethoxy-4-iodoamphetamine (DOI) has been shown to disrupt sensory gating (Sipes et al. 1995).

Treatment

Treatment for post-LSD psychoses has been described in 15 case series. Four studies reported success with neuroleptics (Cohen 1960, Reich and Hepps 1972, Hatrick and Dewhurst 1970, Dewhurst and Hatrick 1972), four with electroconvulsive therapy (ECT) (Metzner 1969, Hatrick and Dewhurst 1970, Muller 1971, Fookes 1972), two with lithium (Horowitz 1975, Lake et al. 1981), and one a controlled clinical trial of the serotonin precursor 5-hydroxytryptophan (Abraham 1983).

HALLUCINOGEN PERSISTING PERCEPTION DISORDER (HPPD)

Diagnosis

The DSM-IV-TR diagnostic criteria for hallucinogen persisting perception disorder is shown below.

DSM-IV-TR Diagnostic Criteria

292.89 Hallucinogen Persisting Perception Disorder (Flashbacks)

A. The reexperiencing, following cessation of use of a hallucinogen, of one or more of the perceptual symptoms that were experienced while intoxicated with the hallucinogen (e.g., geometric hallucinations, false perception of movement in the peripheral visual fields, flashes of color, intensified colors, trails of images of moving objects, positive afterimages, halos around objects, macropsia, and micropsia).

B. The symptoms in Criterion A cause clinically significant distress or impairment in social, occupational, or other important areas of functioning.

C. The symptoms are not due to a general medical condition (e.g., anatomical lesions and infections of the brain, visual epilepsies) and are not better accounted for by another mental disorder (e.g., delirium, dementia, schizophrenia) or hypnopompic hallucinations.

Reprinted with permission from the Diagnostic and Statistical Manual of Mental Disorders, Fourth Edition, Text Revision. Copyright 2000 American Psychiatric Association.

It is not uncommon for an individual suffering from HPPD to consult multiple clinicians before a diagnosis is made. Because the symptoms are primarily perceptual, an HPPD subject may consult an ophthalmologist, neurologist, or psychologist before seeing a mental health professional. Often individuals come for help having made their own diagnoses using the DSM-IV-TR or internet chat groups devoted to HPPD. Despite an individual's certainty about their diagnosis, the clinician is obligated to rule out other sources of chronic organic hallucinosis, including other drug toxicities, strokes, CNS tumors, infections, and head trauma. Magnetic resonance images of the brain are usually negative. Quantitative electroencephalography shows accelerated alpha and visual evoked potentials, especially in the posterior cerebrum.

Treatment

Treatment at the present time is palliative. Benzodiazepines, olanzapine, sertraline, naltrexone, and clonidine have anecdotally been reported to help in selected cases (Lerner et al. 1997, 1998, 2000, 2001, Aldurra and Crayton 2001, Alcantara 1998, Young 1997). Risperidone has been reported to exacerbate HPPD symptoms (Abraham and Mamen 1996). Marijuana can chronically induce an exacerbation of HPPD. Because HPPD is also exacerbated by CNS arousal, affect, stress, and stimulants, these are to be reduced or avoided. HPPD is worse with one's eyes closed, or when entering a dark environment. Thus, sunglasses, which serve to reduce the difference between outdoor and indoor luminance, may reduce HPPD symptoms when the individual enters an interior space.

MDMA ("ECSTASY")-RELATED DISORDERS

3,4-methylenedioxymethamphetamine (MDMA, commonly known as "ecstasy," and chemically N-methyl-1-[3,4-methylene-dioxyphenyl]-2-aminopropane) is a synthetic amphetamine analogue that is also similar to mescaline. It was originally synthesized by Dr E. Merck and patented in Germany as an appetite suppressant in 1914 (Merck 1914). It was never marketed and did not attract attention until the 1970s when it was studied as a hallucinogen analogue (Hardman et al. 1973). During the "psychedelic" 1970s, recreational use of MDMA took root because of its psychological effects and the fact that it was available legally. Recreational use was partially fueled by reports of the use of MDMA as a psychotherapeutic adjunct (Shulgin and Nichols 1978). In 1985, guided by reports that a structurally related congener, 3,4-methylenedioxyamphetamine (MDA), damages serotonergic neurons in rodents (Ricaurte et al. 1985), the Drug Enforcement Administration (DEA) placed MDMA on Schedule 1 of controlled substances (Lawn 1986). The actions of the DEA were validated when subsequent reports found that MDMA is toxic to the animal (Stone et al. 1986, O'Hearn et al. 1988, Fischer et al. 1995, Hatzidimitriou et al. 1999) and the human (Reneman et al. 2002, McCann et al. 1998, Semple et al. 1999) brain. This is not surprising since MDA is the major metabolite of MDMA (Helmlin et al. 1996, de la Torre et al. 2000).

The publicity that followed the scheduling of MDMA only served to increase its popularity, particularly in college campuses (Peroutka 1987). Recognition of this trend led the National Institute of Drug Abuse (NIDA) to begin formal collection of epidemiologic data in the 1989 Monitoring the Future Study. Recently, the use of MDMA has increased and its pattern of use has changed. These factors have heightened public awareness of the drug and paradoxically led to an increase in use and adverse consequences. Emerging evidence supports the hypothesis that MDMA is a neurotoxin in humans with long-lived sequelae on cognition, memory, and emotions.

Diagnosis

A typical MDMA user is a college student (Pope et al. 2001, Peroutka et al. 1988). In a survey of 14,000 college students in 119 American colleges, MDMA users were more likely to use marijuana, smoke cigarettes, and engage in binge alcohol consumption (Strote et al. 2002). They were also more likely to have multiple sex partners (Strote et al. 2002). They considered art and parties important, but they were not academic underachievers (Strote et al. 2002). In a study of 132 pregnant MDMA users compared with 122 nonusers, several characteristics stood out (Ho et al. 2001). The MDMA-using women were younger (23.2 versus 31.2 years old, $P < 0.0001$), experienced more unplanned pregnancies (84.2% versus 54.3%, $P < 0.05$), and were more likely to be single parents (57% versus 18.3%, $P < 0.001$) (Ho et al. 2001). Over half abused alcohol (66.4% versus 37.3%, $P < 0.001$), and a greater fraction abused other drugs (not significant) (Ho et al. 2001). Over a third reported some psychiatric problem, but only 6.5% had a psychiatric diagnosis (Ho et al. 2001). While other drug use appears more common in subjects using MDMA, it is of interest to note that in over a third, their first exposure to illicit drugs is in the setting of MDMA use (Gervin et al. 2001).

Unlike many drugs of abuse that are frequently used alone, MDMA is almost always used in the company of others. Most MDMA users report positive mood and emotional effects as they relate to others. In a survey of 44 experienced MDMA users, subjects report a greater capacity for empathy, communication, and understanding (Table 21-2). Subjects also reported increased self-esteem, high energy, relaxation, and dissociation. In a similar study of 21 subjects with previous MDMA experience, using doses in the range of 1.75 to 4.18 mg/kg, most subjects reported a euphoria, increased physical and

Table 21-2	A Survey of 44 Experienced MDMA Users Regarding Reported Effects of Ecstasy Use	
Reported Effect of MDMA in the		**% Reporting**
Range of 50 to 700 mg		80
Increase in communication and empathy		68
Changes in cognition or mental associations		68
Increase in euphoria or ecstasy		63
Changes in perception*		44

*Illusions or hallucinations are usually associated with higher doses.
Source: Cohen S (1960) Lysergic acid diethylamide: Side effects and complications. *J Nerv Ment Disord* **130**, 20–40.

emotional energy, and a heightened sensual awareness (Downing 1986). In a double-blind, placebo-controlled study of 13 MDMA-naïve subjects given 1.7 mg/kg (about 119 mg to a 70-kg person), MDMA-induced enhanced mood, a sense of improved well-being, increased emotional sensitivity, increased energy, and a heightened sensory awareness (Vollenweider et al. 1998). Similar findings were reported in another double-blind study (Grab et al. 1996). In a double-blind, placebo-controlled comparison study of MDMA 75 mg, MDMA 125 mg, and amphetamine 40 mg, all subjects reported a euphoria, but this feeling was greatest in the MDMA 125-mg group (Mas et al. 1999). In another blinded comparison of escalating MDMA doses and *meta*-chlorophenylpeperazine (mCPP), a serotonin releasing agent, both agents produced euphorogenic and hallucinogenic effects to a similar degree (Tancer and Johanson 2001). One of the most common reasons for using ecstasy is its effect on sexual drive. More than 90% of users report a moderate-to-profound increase in sexual desire and satisfaction (Tancer and Johanson et al. 2001). Orgasm is reported as delayed but more intense (Zemishlany et al. 2001). However in males, erection can be impaired in as many as 40% of subjects (Zemishlany et al. 2001). As stated earlier, individuals in couples treatment who were given MDMA as part of a therapeutic trial reported a sense of increased closeness to their significant-other (Greer and Tolbert 1986).

Altered perceptions (Siegel 1986, Mas et al. 1999, Vollenweider et al. 1998) may be experienced by some MDMA users as a negative consequence of the drug. In the above-mentioned double-blind, placebo-controlled study of 13 MDMA-naïve subjects, most reported anxiety, a mild depersonalization or derealization, a moderate thought disorder, and poor coordination (Vollenweider et al. 1998). In a study of 21 previous MDMA users given doses ranging from 1.75 to 4.18 mg/kg (an average of 175 mg for a 70-kg person), 40% reported impaired decision-making ability and 30% reported decreased mathematics performance (Downing 1986). When given as an adjunct for psychotherapy, all 29 subjects reported some adverse event (Greer and Tolbert 1986). Fatigue was the most common psychosomatic complaint (Greer and Tolbert 1986). Worsening or precipitation of panic attacks has been reported by several authors in different settings (Greer and Tolbert 1986). At least 12 cases of acute psychosis associated with MDMA use have been reported (Vaiva et al. 2001, Creighton et al. 1991, Cox 1993). In most of these cases, there is use of concomitant substances (Vaiva et al. 2001, Creighton et al. 1991, Cox 1993). In at least one case with long-term follow-up, psychotic symptoms were evident 6 months later (Vaiva et al. 2001). A wide range of impulsive or irrational behaviors have been associated with MDMA use (Dowling et al. 1987, Cadier and Clarke 1993, Hooft et al. 1994, Cifasi and Long 1996). Most of these reports were published because they resulted in a major medical problem or death. There is no *a priori* reason to expect that MDMA use would produce impulsivity, but many "ecstasy" users have an increase in impulsive behaviors (Strote et al. 2002, Ho et al. 2001).

MDMA users generally limit the frequency of use of the drug. Most report limiting use of MDMA to twice per month or less. Fridays and Saturdays are the most common days of use because users say they need 1 day to recover after use (Peroutka et al. 1988, Liester et al. 1992). More frequent use is associated with a loss of the desired effect of the drug (Gerhard et al. 2001).

Prior to its placement on Schedule 1 by the DEA, MDMA was considered as an adjunct to psychotherapy (Shulgin and Nichols 1978, Greer and Tolbert 1986, 1998). In this setting, a dosage of 50 to 200 mg (with modal doses ranging from 100 to 150 mg), with a booster of 50 to 75 mg several hours later, was used. There are no controlled studies of the use of MDMA in psychotherapy. However, there is one open study of 29 subjects in which the dosage used was 75 to 150 mg after a 6-hour fast with an offered second dose of 50 to 75 mg. All subjects reported positive attitudinal and emotional changes. Twenty-two felt that their insight into their own psychopathology was enhanced. Twenty-one subjects in couples treatment reported increased closeness and communication with their partner (Greer and Tolbert 1986). All subjects reported adverse consequences similar to those reported by recreational drug users. While the use of MDMA as a psychotherapeutic adjunct appears to have advocates (Greer and Tolbert 1998), the documentation of neurotoxicity in humans (Reneman et al. 2002, McCann et al. 1998, Semple et al. 1999) makes such use dubious.

Physical Consequences of MDMA Use

Animals receiving MDMA will exhibit signs that are consistent with sympathomimetic activation. These include increased heart rate, locomotion, and body temperature in rats, and mydriasis, salivation, and piloerection in dogs and monkeys (Hardman et al. 1973). Humans exhibit complications that are related to both the sympathomimetic and serotonergic properties of MDMA. These include nausea, vomiting, anorexia, hypertension, palpitations, diaphoresis, headaches, difficulty walking, muscle aches and tension, hot and cold flashes, urinary urgency, nystagmus, blurred vision, insomnia, and dry mouth (Peroutka et al. 1988, Topp et al. 1999, Downing 1986, Liester et al. 1992, Greer and Tolbert 1986, Solowij et al. 1992). The common complaints of trismus and bruxism may reflect MDMA enhancement of serotonin activation of the $5HT_{1B}$ receptors of the trigeminal motor nuclei (Tancer and Johanson 2001).

In a survey study of 44 experienced MDMA users at an average dose of 120 mg (range 50–700 mg), all reported muscle tension, 91% reported diaphoresis, and 77% reported blurred vision or ataxia (Siegel 1986). Muscle tension in the form of trismus is a commonly reported adverse event (Downing 1986, Vollenweider et al. 1998). A transient gait disturbance was also common in a group of subjects who received MDMA as a psychotherapeutic adjunct, 21 MDMA users who received doses averaging 175 mg for a 70-kg subject (Downing 1986), and 13 MDMA-naïve healthy controls (Vollenweider et al. 1998). Other frequently reported acute physical consequences of MDMA use are hyperreflexia (Downing 1986), tachycardia, and hypertension (Grab et al. 1996).

Twenty-four hours after a single dose of MDMA averaging 119 mg in a 70-kg MDMA-naïve subject, a detailed evaluation revealed the presence of decreased energy, decreased appetite, restlessness, insomnia, and trismus (Vollenweider et al. 1998).

The acute motoric abnormalities have been related to driving impairment. A review of the literature noted at least 18 reports of driving impairment in people using MDMA (usually along with other drugs) (Logan and Couper 2001). These reports include six users stopped for speeding, eight for erratic driving, and five involved in collisions (Logan and Cooper 2001). At least two MDMA-related deaths have been associated with automobiles (Hooft et al. 1994, Cifasi and Long 1996).

MDMA has been associated with a wide range of somatic toxic events. These include thrombotic or hemorrhagic strokes (Harries and DeSilva 1992, Gledhill et al. 1993, Hughes et al. 1993, Manchanda and Connolly 1993, Rothwell and Grant 1993), leukoencephalopathy (Bertram et al. 1999), myocardial infarction (Qasim et al. 2001), arrhythmias (Dowling et al. 1987, Henry et al. 1992), and pneumothorax (Mazur and Hitchcock 2001). The wide range of manifestations suggests that most of these cases are either idiosyncratic or related to impurities remaining from the synthetic process. Since much of the MDMA supply is synthesized in small "basement" laboratories, the quality control of the manufacturing process may not be adequate. The results of weekly drug sampling in the Netherlands found that most (75% in 1996) "ecstasy" pills contained MDMA (Spruit 2001). The percentage dropped in 1997 and increased again in 1998 (Spruit 2001). About one-third of the pills contained amphetamine or other derivatives (Spruit 2001). These non-MDMA drugs might explain some of the heterogeneity of medical complications of "ecstasy" use. Certainly, the cases of hepatotoxicity (Henry et al. 1992, Shearman et al. 1992, Ijzermans et al. 1993, Khakoo et al. 1995, Ellis et al. 1996, Andreu et al. 1998, DeCarlis et al. 2001, Lawler et al. 2001) and aplastic anemia (Marsh et al. 1994, Clark and Butt 1997) most likely are idiosyncratic or secondary to contaminants.

Cases of severe medical illness or death due to electrolyte and fluid abnormalities (Maxwell et al. 1993, Kessel 1994, Matthai et al. 1996, Hall 1997, Ajaelo et al. 1998, Magee et al. 1998, Holmes et al. 1999, O'Connor et al. 1999) and cases of multiple organ system failure (Henry et al. 1992, Brown and Osterloh 1987, Chadwick et al. 1991, Campkin and Davies 1992, Roberts and Wright 1993, Lehmann et al. 1995, Coore 1996, Demirkiran et al. 1996) are more likely due to MDMA use. These complications may be related to the specific environment in raves. In raves, people are exposed to hot, crowded environments. In association with the increased body temperature caused by MDMA (Liechti and Vollenweider 2000), dehydration and its consequences are likely. Crowding has been shown to increase amphetamine toxicity in animals, a phenomenon labeled *aggregation toxicity* (Chance 1946, Hohn and Lasagna 1960). A similar phenomenon may occur in crowded raves in humans.

MDMA may also cause serotonergic hyperstimulation and produce a fatal serotonin–syndrome-like (Sternback 1991) illness (Demirkiran et al. 1996, Mueller and Korey 1998).

Clinical Manifestations of Long-Term MDMA Neurotoxicity

Former chronic "ecstasy" users (an average of 527 tablets) have higher self-reported depression as measured by the Beck's Depression Scale than non-drug-using controls (MacInnes et al. 2001). The predictors of developing this depressive syndrome are maximum quantity of pills consumed over a 12-hour period, and mild, frequent life stress (MacInnes et al. 2001). Heavy MDMA use has also been associated with higher rates of psychopathology including obsessive and compulsive behaviors, anxiety, somatization, and loss of libido (Parrott et al. 2001). The cause-and-effect relationship between MDMA use and these psychiatric syndromes is unclear, but since these syndromes involve serotonergic mechanisms, additional investigation into these potential long-term sequelae is warranted.

MDMA users have been noted to have problems with memory, attention, reasoning, impulse control, and sleep abnormalities (Reneman et al. 2001b, Verkes et al. 2001, Krystal and Price 1992, Allen et al. 1993, McGuire 2000, Reneman et al. 2000, Parrott and Lasky 1998, McCann et al. 1999, Gouzoulis-Mayfrank et al. 2000, Bhattachary and Powell 2001, Croft et al. 2001, Zakzanis and Young 2001). In a study of 22 recent MDMA users, 16 ex-users (abstinent for over 1 year), and 13 normal controls who underwent the Rey Auditory Verbal Learning Test, the immediate recall score (47, 48, and 60, respectively, $P = 0.001$) and the delayed recall score (9.8, 10.1, and 13.1, respectively, $P = 0.003$) were significantly less in recent and remote MDMA users than in normal controls, suggesting that the memory dysfunction persists for more than 1 year (Reneman et al. 2001b). The memory difficulties persisted despite recovery of serotonergic abnormalities on SPECT (Reneman et al. 2001b). Similarly, 15 MDMA users were tested initially after a 2-week abstinence, and again a year later (Zakzanis and Young 2001). The subjects who continued to use MDMA experienced a progressive decline of both immediate and delayed recall (Zakzanis and Young 2001). In 21 heavy users, 21 moderate users, and 20 nonusers, there was a "statistically significant but clinically small" decline in memory and prolongation of reaction time (Verkes et al. 2001). Heavy users were more affected than moderate users (Verkes et al. 2001).

In 80 subjects, which included novice users, regular users, ex-users, compared with nonusers, all subjects exposed to MDMA had decreased verbal fluency, decreased immediate prose recall, and decreased delayed prose recall, but no change in visual recall (Bhattachary and Powell 2001). The number of days since last MDMA use and total lifetime dose accounted for over 50% of variance suggesting both a dose-response effect and a possible recovery process (Bhattachary and Powell 2001). The relative sparing of visual recall is of interest since decline in 5-HT_{2A} receptor density after MDMA use is a characteristic of all brain regions except the occipital cortex in rats and humans, where MDMA upregulates the receptor density (Reneman et al. 2002a). Similarly, a study of NAA, a marker of cellular health on magnetic resonance spectroscopy, found that the NAA signal was decreased in the frontal cortex, but not in the occipital or parietal cortices (Reneman et al. 2002b).

Since many MDMA users also use other drugs, Croft and colleagues (2001) studied 18 pure cannabis abusers, 11 that use both cannabis and MDMA, and 31 subjects who use neither cannabis nor MDMA. They report that both cannabis and MDMA/cannabis users showed equal impairment in memory, learning, work fluency, speed of processing, and manual dexterity compared to normal controls (Croft et al. 2001). This suggests that most of the reported cognitive decline attributed to MDMA use may be due to concomitant use of cannabis. This view is not shared by many other researchers based on both clinical studies (Krystal and Price 1992, Allen et al. 1993, McGuire 2000, Reneman et al. 2000, Parrott and Lasky 1998, McCann et al. 1999, Gouzoulis-Mayfrank et al. 2000, Battachary and Powell 2001, Zakzanis and Young 2001) and animal and basic studies of the toxicity of MDMA (Stone et al. 1986, Hatzidimitriou et al. 1999, Simantov and Tauber 1997, Taffe et al. 2001).

Epidemiology

Despite its existence for nearly 90 years, the recreational use of MDMA appears to have had its origins in the 1960s (Pope et al. 2001). Initial drug use centered around college campuses (Pope et al. 2001, Peroutka et al. 1988). At that time, use of MDMA was generally in small groups in private places (Peroutka et al. 1988). Accurate epidemiologic data are not available for the 1960s. However, by 1977 about 2.8% of US college students used MDMA (Strote et al. 2002). College is the first time that people are likely to begin use of MDMA (Cuomo et al. 1994, Randell 1992). Nonetheless, use in high school students has also increased, so that in 1998, 4.4% of 10th graders and 5.6% of high school seniors had tried MDMA (Johnston et al. 1999). In a survey of 14,000 college students at 119 American colleges by the Harvard School of Public Health College Alcohol Study, there was a 69% increase in use between 1997 and 1999 (from 2.8 to 4.7%) (Strote et al. 2002). At 10 high-use schools with a 1997 rate of 4.7%, the rate increased to 10.6% by the year 2000 (Strote et al. 2002). Over the same time, the use of marijuana did not significantly change (38.5% in 1997 and 37.6% in 2000) (Strote et al. 2002). MDMA is the only illicit drug to see continued increase in use. In surveys of a large New England college performed in 1969, 1978, 1989, and 1999, all drug use peaked in 1978 and dropped thereafter, but MDMA use has continued to increase. The increasing popularity of MDMA is not just an American phenomenon, but is also seen in both Europe (Cregg and Traqcey 1993, Christophersen 2000) and Australia (Topp et al. 1999).

In addition to increased popularity of MDMA, the pattern of use appears to have changed. Initial use was in small groups at doses ranging from 75 to 150 mg with an occasional booster of 50 to 100 mg (Peroutka et al. 1988, Downing 1986, Siegel 1986, Liester 1992). The 1990s saw the onset of the rave phenomenon. These are generally large gatherings in warehouses or dance clubs. Dosages utilized in raves are much more variable ranging from 100 to 750 mg and as high as 1250 mg/night (Brown et al. 1995, Forsyth 1996). Concomitant drug use is also more common in raves (Strote et al. 2002, Gervin et al. 2001, Gerhard 2001). These include alcohol, marijuana, and opiates. Furthermore, the term "ecstasy", which was originally used to refer specifically to MDMA, has grown to refer to other related compounds such as 3,4-methylenedioxyamphetamine (MDA) and 3,4-methylenedioxyethylamphetamine (MDE or Eve) (Gerhard 2001). The combination of these variables increases the risks of adverse consequences associated with MDMA use (see later).

Etiology

MDMA is usually present in two optical isomers. The dextrorotary form, S-(+)-MDMA, is more potent in the CNS than the levorotary form, R-(−)-MDMA (Anderson et al. 1978). MDMA is broken down by N-demethylation, O-dealkylation, deamination, and conjugation. MDMA is broken down into MDA (which is sometimes used recreationally), 4-hydroxy-3-methoxymethamphetamine (HMMA), and 3,4-dihydroxymethamphetamine (HHMA) (Helmlin et al. 1996, Fallon et al. 1999, Maurer et al. 2000). MDA can also be metabolized to HHMA and HMMA, which are either excreted unchanged in the urine or are glucuronidated prior to urinary excretion (Helmlin et al. 1996, Fallon et al. 1999, Maurer et al. 2000). HHMA plasma levels will peak at approximately the same concentration as the parent drug but ultimately accounts for only 17.7% of total drug recovered in a 24-hour urine collection (Segura et al. 2001). The combination of MDMA and HHMA accounts for 58% of total drug in the urine over 24 hours (McFarling 1980). The MDA metabolite peaks at around 2 to 6 hours after an oral MDMA dose of 50 to 150 mg (Helmlin et al. 1996, de la Torre et al. 2000, Verebey et al. 1988). MDA accounts for less than 5% to 28% of MDMA (Helmlin et al. 1996, de la Torre et al. 2000, Verebey et al. 1988).

Maximum plasma MDMA concentrations are achieved 2 to 4 hours after ingestion. (Extensive metabolizers possess enzymes that metabolize the drug at a faster rate than the general population.)

The peak MDMA concentration increases disproportionately in a nonlinear fashion compared to the metabolites. This suggests that the demethylating enzyme step is saturable with increasing MDMA dose (de la Torre et al. 2000).

The more active S-(+)-MDMA isomer is metabolized faster (Fallon et al. 1999, Cho et al. 1990) and more extensively (Fallon et al. 1999, Fitzgerald et al. 1989) than the levorotary form so that the half-life of S-(+)-MDMA is 73.8 to 210 minutes while the half-life of R-(−)-MDMA is 100.7 to 350 minutes (Fallon et al. 1999, Verebey et al. 1988, Pacifici et al. 2001). The mean plasma concentration of the levorotatory form is 2.4 times higher than the S-(+) isomer and a significantly greater amount is excreted unchanged in the urine (Fallon et al. 1999). MDMA in brain microsomes is metabolized primarily through O-dealkylation (Lin et al. 1992). Isomer-specific brain metabolism has not been studied.

MDMA causes a calcium-independent release of serotonin from nerve endings (Johnson et al. 1986, McKenna and Peroutka 1990) with concomitant inhibition of serotonin reuptake (Steele et al. 1987). MDMA has a very low affinity for postsynaptic serotonin receptors (Lyon et al. 1986, Bettaglia et al. 1988). It also increases dopamine release (Yamamoto and Spanos 1988, Hiramatsu and Cho 1990, Nash et al. 1990) but this effect is less than the effect on serotonin (Johnson et al. 1986, McKenna and Peroutka 1990, Steele et

1987). There is also a dose-related increase in cortical acetylcholine (ACh) release (Acquas et al. 2001). The cortex is more sensitive to MDMA than the striatum: 3.2 mg/kg MDMA increases ACh release in the cortex some 141%, but only 32% in the striatum (Acquas et al. 2001). It is believed that the effects on serotonin mediate most of the psychological effects of MDMA.

MDMA is toxic to serotonergic neurons. This has been documented in several species including rats (Stone et al. 1986, Schmidt et al. 1986, Schmidt 1987, Commins et al. 1987, O'Hearn et al. 1988, Slikker et al. 1988, 1989), mice (Stone et al. 1986), guinea pigs (Schmidt et al. 1986), and monkeys (Slikker et al. 1988, 1989, Ricaurte et al. 1988, 1992, Insel et al. 1989, Wilson et al. 1989, Fischer et al. 1995, Hatzidimitriou et al. 1999). Serotonergic loss is evident through several markers that include reduced brain serotonin, 5-hydroxyindoleacetic acid (5-HIAA), and the serotonin transporter (Acquas et al. 2001, Schmidt et al. 1986, Schmidt 1987, Commins et al. 1987, O'Hearn et al. 1988, Slikker et al. 1988, 1989, Battaglia et al. 1987). Immunocytochemical studies suggest that serotonergic neurons are damaged, but the cell bodies are preserved (O'Hearn et al. 1988, Wilson et al. 1989, Molliver et al. 1990). Recovery from MDMA-induced serotonergic damage can occur. While rodents appear to recover (Scanzello et al. 1993), in monkeys the damage persists for at least 7 years (Ricaurte et al. 1992, Fischer et al. 1995, Hatzidimitriou et al. 1999).

In humans, serotonergic damage after repeated MDMA use is evident through several different types of studies. CSF 5-HIAA levels are reduced in MDMA users (McCann et al. 1994). For unclear reasons, this effect is more pronounced in women than in men (McCann et al. 1994). N-acetyl aspartate (NAA, a marker of cellular health) was quantified with magnetic resonance spectroscopy in 15 MDMA users and 12 age-matched controls. NAA was significantly reduced in the frontal cortex, but not in the parietal or occipital cortex (Reneman et al. 2001c, 2002b). The extent of previous MDMA use and frontal cortical neuronal loss were significantly associated indicating that cortical damage is directly related to the extent of MDMA use. McCann and colleagues (1998) used PET and a radioligand, (^{11}C)-McN5652, that binds to serotonin transporter to quantify serotonergic damage after MDMA use. They found that MDMA use is associated with a reduction in (^{11}C)-McN5652 binding, and that the extent of MDMA use correlated with the severity of serotonin transporter loss (McCann et al. 1998). Semple and colleagues (1999) found similar results with SPECT in MDMA users compared to controls. Reneman and colleagues (2001b, 2001a) also used SPECT and (^{123}I)-2beta-carbomethoxy-3beta-(4-iodophenyl) tropane, which binds to both the serotonin and dopamine transporters with high affinity (Laruelle et al. 1994, Lew et al. 1996), and found that serotonin transporter binding was reduced in female heavy users but not male users (Reneman et al. 2001b, 2001a). This provides independent support to the finding that women are more susceptible to damage by MDMA. In subjects abstinent from MDMA for over 1 year, recovery to normal levels was evident (Reneman et al. 2001a).

Indirect evidence of serotonergic involvement is found in neuroendocrine studies. In animals, MDMA treatment produces a profound increase in serum corticosterone and prolactin (Nash et al. 1988, Poland et al. 1997). This effect is attenuated or blocked by pretreatment with the serotonin neurotoxin, p-chlorophenylalanine (Nash et al. 1988), suggesting that the process is mediated by serotonin. MDMA at doses of 75 mg are associated with an increase in serum cortisol, while doses greater than 75 mg increase both cortisol and prolactin (Grob et al. 1996, Mas et al. 1999). The prolactin response to serotonin agonists, such as fenfluramine, is generally blunted in MDMA users compared to controls (Price et al. 1989, Verkes et al. 2001, Gerra et al. 1998, 2000, Gouzoulis-Mayfrank et al. 2002). However, since concomitant drug use, particularly marijuana, is so common in ecstasy users, all these studies are confounded by potential cannabis effects (Gouzoulis-Mayfrank et al. 2002). Consequently, this may be one of the reasons that studies using L-tryptophan as a neuroendocrine challenge have been negative (L-tryptophan is a serotonin precursor and increases brain serotonin levels) (Price et al. 1990, McCann et al. 1994). Alternatively, L-tryptophan challenge may be insufficiently sensitive.

Treatment

There have been no studies examining the treatment of MDMA use. The issue of how a practitioner may help the individual seeking treatment discontinue MDMA use is never addressed in the literature. This may be due to the rarity of presentation of subjects seeking treatment for MDMA addiction. Nonetheless, MDMA has abuse potential. Baboons will self-administer MDMA (Lamb and Griffiths 1987). Rhesus monkeys trained to self-administer cocaine prefer MDMA over vehicle (Beardsley et al. 1986). Also, 50% of these animals will administer MDMA at a rate higher than they had administered cocaine. In several animal species that are trained to discriminate amphetamine from saline, MDMA easily substitutes for amphetamine (Glennon and Young 1984, Kamien et al. 1986). Animals treated with high-dose MDMA (40 mg/kg for 4 days) exhibit increased cocaine self-administration with rates twice those of saline-treated controls (Fletcher et al. 2001). Intracranial self-administration of MDMA lowers the threshold to a rewarding electrical stimulus to the medial forebrain bundle (Hubner et al. 1988). These data suggest that if MDMA itself is not abused (users tend to limit their use to twice monthly) (Peroutka et al. 1988, Liester et al. 1992), it may facilitate the abuse of other substances.

Serotonin reuptake inhibiting antidepressants may offer a possible treatment for individuals who present with an MDMA addiction. In rats, preadministration of fluoxetine 10 mg/kg given prior to or concurrent with MDMA 15 mg/kg protects against MDMA-induced serotonergic toxicity (Sanchez et al. 2001). Similarly, citalopram preadministration to healthy volunteers (40 mg intravenously) prior to MDMA 1.5 mg/kg orally blocks the increased pulse and blood pressure induced by MDMA, but does not block the hyperthermia (Liechti and Vollenweider 2000).

Comparison of DSM-IV-TR/ICD-10 Diagnostic Criteria
The ICD-10 and DSM-IV-TR diagnostic criteria are nearly identical.

References

Abraham HD (1980) Psychiatric illness in drug abusers. *N Engl J Med* **302**, 868–869.

Abraham HD (1982) A chronic impairment of colour vision in users of LSD. *Br J Psychiatry* **140**, 518–520.

Abraham HD (1983) L-5-hydroxytryptophan for LSD-induced psychosis. *Am J Psychiatry* **140**, 456–458.

Abraham HD and Aldridge A (1993) Adverse consequences of lysergic acid diethylamide. *Addiction* **88**, 1327–1334.

Abraham HD, Aldridge AM, and Gogia P (1996) The psychopharmacology of hallucinogens. *Neuropsychopharmacology* **14**, 285–298.

Abraham HD and Duffy FH (1991) Computed EEG abnormalities in panic disorder with and without premorbid drug abuse. *Biol Psychiatry* **29**, 687–690.

Abraham HD and Duffy FH (2001) EEG coherence in post-LSD visual hallucinations. *Psychiatr Res* **107**, 151–163.

Abraham HD and Mamen A (1996) LSD-like panic from risperidone in post-LSD visual disorder. *J Clin Psychopharmacol* **16**, 238–241.

Abraham HD, McCann UD, and Ricaurte GA (2002) Psychedelic drugs. In *Neuropsychopharmacology: The Fifth Generation of Progress*, Davis KL, et al. (eds). Lippincott, Williams & Wilkins, Philadelphia, pp. 1545–1556.

Abraham HD and Wolf E (1988) Visual function in past users of LSD: psychophysical findings. *J Abnorm Psychol* **97**, 443–447.

Abramson HA, Jarvik ME, Gorin MH, et al. (1956) Tolerance development and its relation to a theory of psychosis. *J Psychol* **41**, 81.

Abruzzi W (1977) Drug-induced psychosis. *Int J Addict* **12**, 183–193.

Acquas E, Marrocu P, Pisanu A, et al. (2001) Intravenous administration of ecstasy (3,4-methylenedioxymethamphetamine) enhances cortical and striatal acetylcholine release *in vivo*. *Eur J Pharmacol* **418**, 207–211.

Aghajanian GK and Marek GJ (1999) Serotonin and hallucinogens. *Neuropsychopharmacology* **21**, 18S–23S.

Ajaelo I, Koenig K, and Snoey E (1998) Severe hyponatremia and inappropriate antidiuretic hormone secretion following ecstasy use. *Acad Emerg Med* **5**, 839–840.

Albaugh BJ and Anderson PO (1974) Peyote in the treatment of alcoholism among American Indians. *Am J Psychiatry* **131**, 1247–1250.

Alcantara AG (1998) Is there a role for the alpha-2 antagonism in the exacerbation of hallucinogen-persisting perception disorder with risperidone? *J Clin Psychopharmacol* **18**, 487–488.

Aldurra G and Crayton JW (2001) Improvement of hallucinogen persisting perception disorder by treatment with a combination of fluoxetine and olanzapine: case report. *J Clin Psychopharmacol* **21**, 343–344.

Allen RP, McCann UD, and Ricaurte GA (1993) Persistent effects of +/− 3,4-methylenedioxymethamphetamine (MDMA, "Ecstasy") on human sleep. *Sleep* **16**, 560–564.

Anderson GM, Braun G, Braun U, et al. (1978) Absolute configuration and psychomimetic phenylalkylamines. NIDA Res Monogr 22. Rockville, MD.

Anderson WH and O'Malley JE (1972) Trifluoperazine for the "trailing" phenomenon. *JAMA* **220**, 1244–1245.

Andreu V, Mas A, Bruguera M, et al. (1998) Ecstasy: a common cause of severe acute hepatotoxicity. *J Hepatol* **29**, 394–397.

Anonymous (1966) Public Health Committee, Subcommittee on Narcotics Addiction, County of New York. *N Y Med* **22**, 241.

Baker E (1967) Second international conference on the use of LSD in psychotherapy and alcoholism. In *LSD Psychotherapy*, Abramson H (ed). Bobbs-Merrill, Indianapolis.

Battaglia G, Yeh SY, O'Hearn E, et al. (1987) 3,4-Methylenedioxymethamphetamine and 3,4-methylenedioxyamphetamine destroy serotonin terminals in rat brain: qualification of neurodegeneration by measurement of [^{3}H]paroxetine-labeled serotonin uptake sites. *J Pharmacol Exp Ther* **242**, 911–916.

Beardsley PM, Balster RL, and Harris LS (1986) Self-administration of methylenedioxymethamphetamine (MDMA) by rhesus monkey. *Drug Alcohol Depend* **18**, 149–157.

Bergman RL (1971) Navajo peyote use: its apparent safety. *Am J Psychiatry* **128**, 695–699.

Bertram M, Egelhoff T, Schwarz S, et al. (1999) Toxic leukoencephalopathy following "ecstasy" ingestion. *J Neurol* **146**, 617–618.

Bettaglia G, Brooks BP, Kulsakdinum C, et al. (1988) Pharmacologic profile of MDMA (3,4-methylenedioxyamphetamine) at various brain recognition sites. *Eur J Pharmacol* **149**, 159–163.

Bhattachary S and Powell JH (2001) Recreational use of 3,4-methylenedioxymethamphetamine (MDMA) or 'ecstasy': evidence for cognitive impairment. *Psychol Med* **31**, 647–658.

Blumenfield M and Glickman L (1967) Ten months experience with LSD users admitted to county psychiatric receiving hospital. *N Y State J Med* **67**, 1849–1853.

Bowers MB (1972) Acute psychosis induced by psychotomimetic drug abuse, II: neurochemical findings. *Arch Gen Psychiatry* **27**, 440–442.

Bowers MB (1977) Psychoses precipitated by psychotomimetic drugs: a follow-up study. *Arch Gen Psychiatry* **34**, 832–835.

Bowers M (1987) The role of drugs in the production of schizophreniform psychoses and related disorders. In *Psychopharmacology: The Third Generation of Progress*, Meltzer HY (ed). Raven Press, New York, pp. 819–823.

Brawley P and Duffield JC (1972) The pharmacology of hallucinogens. *Pharmacol Rev* **24**, 31–66.

Breakey WR, Goodell H, Lorenz PC, et al. (1974) Hallucinogenic drugs as precipitants of schizophrenia. *Psychol Med* **4**, 225–261.

Brown ER, Jarvie DR, and Simpson D (1995) Use of drugs at 'raves'. *Scot Med J* **40**, 168–171.

Brown C and Osterloh J (1987) Multiple complications from recreational ingestion of MDMA ("Ecstasy"). *J Am Med Assoc* **258**, 780–781.

Cadier MA and Clarke JA (1993) Ecstasy and Whizz at a rave resulting in a major burn plus complications. *Burns* **19**, 239–240.

Campkin NTA and Davies UM (1992) Another death from ecstasy. *J R Soc Med* **85**, 61.

Chadwick IS, Linsley A, Freemont AJ, et al. (1991) Ecstasy, 3,4-methylenedioxymethamphetamine (MDMA), a fatality associated with coagulopathy and hyperthermia. *J R Soc Med* **84**, 371.

Chance M (1946) Aggregation as a factor influencing the toxicity of sympathomimetic amines in mice. *J Pharmacol Exp Ther* **198**, 214–219.

Cho AK, Hiramatsu M, DiStefano EW, et al. (1990) Stereochemical differences in the metabolism of 3,4-methylenedioxymethamphetamine *in vivo* and *in vitro*: a pharmacokinetic analysis. *Drug Metab Dispos* **18**, 686–691.

Christophersen AS (2000) Amphetamine designer drugs—an overview and epidemiology. *Toxicol Lett* **112–113**, 127–131.

Cifasi J and Long C (1996) Traffic fatality related to the use of methylenedioxymethamphetamine. *J Forens Sci* **41**, 1082–1084.

Clark AD and Butt N (1997) Ecstasy-induced very severe aplastic anaemia complicated by invasive pulmonary mucormycosis treated with allogeneic peripheral blood progenitor cell transplant. *Clin Lab Haematol* **19**, 279–281.

Cohen S (1960) Lysergic acid diethylamide: side effects and complications. *J Nerv Ment Disord* **130**, 20–40.

Cohen S and Ditman K (1963) Prolonged adverse reactions to lysergic acid diethylamide. *Arch Gen Psychiatry* **8**, 475–480.

Commins DL, Vosmer G, Virus RM, et al. (1987) Biochemical and histological evidence that methylene-dioxymethamphetamine (MDMA) is toxic to neurons in the rat brain. *J Pharmacol Exp Ther* **241**, 338–345.

Cooper H (1955) Hallucinogenic drugs. *Lancet* **268**, 1078–1079.

Coore JR (1996) A fatal trip with ecstasy: a case of 3,4-methylenedioxy-methamphetamine/3,4-methylenedioxy-ampthetamine toxicity. *J R Soc Med* **89**, 51P–52P.

Cox DE (1993) "Rave" to the grave. *Forens Sci Int* **60**, 5–6.

Cregg MT and Traqcey JA (1993) Ecstasy abuse in Ireland. *Ir Med J* **86**, 118–120.

Creighton FJ, Black DL and Hyde CE (1991) 'Ecstasy' psychosis and flashbacks. *Br J Psychiatry* **159**, 713–715.

Croft RJ, Mackay AJ, Mills AT, et al. (2001) The relative contributions of ecstasy and cannabis to cognitive impairment. *Psychopharmacology* **153**, 373–379.

Cuomo MJ, Dyment PG and Gammino VM (1994) Increasing use of "ecstasy" (MDMA) and other hallucinogens on a college campus. *J Am Coll Health* **42**, 272–274.

DeCarlis L, DeGasperi A, Slim AO, et al. (2001) Liver transplantation of ecstasy-induced fulminant hepatic failure. *Transplant Proc* **33**, 2743–2744.

de la Torre R, Farre M, Ortuno J, et al. (2000) Nonlinear pharmacokinetics of MDMA ("ecstasy") in humans. *Br J Clin Pharmacol* **49**, 104–109.

Demirkiran M, Jankovic J, and Dean JM (1996) Ecstasy intoxication: an overlap between serotonin syndrome and neuroleptic malignant syndrome. *Clin Neuropsychopharmacol* **19**, 157–164.

Dewhurst K and Hatrick JA (1972) Differential diagnosis and treatment of lysergic acid diethylamide induced psychosis. *Practitioner* **209**, 327–332.

Dowling GP, McDonough ET, and Bost RD (1987) 'Eve' and 'Ecstasy'. A report of five deaths associated with the use of MDEA and MDMA. *J Am Med Assoc* **257**, 1615–1617.

Downing J (1986) The psychological and physiological effects of MDMA on normal volunteers. *J Psychoact Drugs* **18**, 335–340.

Ellis AJ, Wendon JA, Portmann B, et al. (1996) Acute liver damage and ecstasy ingestion. *Gut* **38**, 454–458.

Fallon JK, Kicman AT, Henry JA, et al. (1999) Stereospecific analysis and enantiomeric disposition of 3,4-methylenedioxymethamphetamine (ecstasy) in humans. *Clin Chem* **45**, 1058–1069.

Fischer CA, Hatzidimitriou G, Katz JL, et al. (1995) Reorganization of ascending serotonin axon projections in animals previously exposed to the recreational drug 3,4-methylenedioxymethamphetamine. *J Neurosci* **15**, 5476–5485.

Fitzgerald RL, Blanke RV, Rosecrans JA, et al. (1989) Stereochemistry of the metabolism of MDMA to MDA. *Life Sci* **45**, 295–301.

Fletcher PJ, Robinson SR, and Slippoy DL (2001) Pre-exposure to (+/−) 3,4-methylenedioxymethamphetamine (MDMA) facilitates acquisition of intravenous cocaine self-administration in rats. *Neuropsychopharmacology* **25**, 195–203.

Fookes BH (1972) Psychosis after L.S.D. *Lancet* **1**, 1074–1075.

Forsyth AJ (1996) Places and patterns of drug use in the Scottish dance scene. *Addiction* **91**, 511–521.

Frosch W (1969) *Adverse Reactions to Hallucinogenic Drugs*. US Government NIMH PHS Pub. 1910.

Frosch W, Robbins E, and Stern M (1965) Untoward reactions to lysergic acid diethylamide (LSD) resulting in hospitalization. *N Engl J Med* **273**, 1235–1239.

Gerhard H (2001) Party-drugs: sociocultural and individual background and risks. *Int J Clin Pharmacol Ther* **39**, 362–366.

Gerra G, Zaimovic A, Ferri M, et al. (2000) Long-lasting effects of (+/−)3,4-methylenedioxymethamphetamine (ecstasy) on serotonin system function in humans. *Biol Psychiatry* **47**, 127–136.

Gerra G, Zaimovic A, Giucastro G, et al. (1998) Serotonergic function after (+/−)3,4-methylenedioxymetham-phetamine ('Ecstasy') in humans. *Int Clin Psychopharmacol* **13**, 1–9.

Gervin M, Hughes R, Bamford L, et al. (2001) Heroin smoking by "chasing the dragon" in young opiate users in Ireland: stability and associations with use to "come down" of "Ecstasy." *J Subst Abuse Treat* **20**, 297–300.

Gledhill JA, Moore DF, Bell D, et al. (1993) Subarachnoid hemorrhage associated with MDMA abuse. *J Neurol Neurosurg Psychiatry* **56**, 1036–1037.

Glennon RA and Young RY (1984) Further investigations of the discriminative stimulus properties of MDA. *Pharmacol Biochem Behav* **20**, 501–505.

Gouzoulis-Mayfrank E, Becker S, Pelz S, et al. (2002) Neuroendocrine abnormalities in recreational ecstasy (MDMA) users: Is it ecstasy or cannabis? *Biol Psychiatry* **51**, 766–769.

Gouzoulis-Mayfrank E, Daumann J, Tuchtenhagen F, et al. (2000) Impaired cognitive performance in drug free users of recreational ecstasy (MDMA). *J Neurol Neurosurg Psychiatry* **68**, 719–725.

Grab CS, Poland RE, Chang L, et al. (1996) Psychobiologic effects of 3,4-methylenedioxymethamphetamine in humans: methodological considerations and preliminary observations. *Behav Brain Res* **73**, 103–107.

Greer G and Tolbert P (1986) Subjective reports of the effects of MDMA in a clinical setting. *J Psychoact Drugs* **18**, 319–327.

Greer GR and Tolbert P (1998) A method of conducting therapeutic sessions with MDMA. *J Psychoact Drugs* **30**, 371–379.

Grinspoon L and Bakalar JB (1979) *Psychedelic Drugs Reconsidered*. Basic Books, New York.

Grob CS, Poland RE, Chang L, et al. (1996) Psychobiologic effects of 3,4-methylenedioxymethamphetamine in humans: methodological considerations and preliminary observations. *Behav Brain Res* **73**, 103–107.

Hall AP (1997) Hyponatremia, water intoxication and 'ecstasy.' *Intens Care Med* **23**, 1289.

Hardman HF, Haavik CO, and Seevers MH (1973) Relationship of the structure of mescaline and seven analogs to toxicity and behavior in five species of laboratory animals. *Toxicol Appl Pharmacol* **25**, 299–309.

Harries DP and DeSilva R (1992) 'Ecstacy' and intracerebral haemorrhage. *Scot Med* **37**, 476.

Hatrick JA and Dewhurst K (1970) Delayed psychosis due to L.S.D. *Lancet* **2**, 742–744.

Hatzidimitriou G, McCann UD, and Ricaurte GA (1999) Aberrant serotonin innervation in the forebrain of monkeys exposed to MDMA seven years previously: factors influencing abnormal recovery. *J Neurosci* **19**, 5096–5107.

Hekimian LJ and Gershon S (1968) Characteristics of drug abusers admitted to a psychiatric hospital. *JAMA* **205**, 125–130.

Helmlin H-J, Bracher K, Bourquin D, et al. (1996) Analysis of 3,4-methylenedioxymethamphetamine (MDMA) and its metabolites in plasma and urine by HPLC-DAD and GC-MS. *J Anal Toxicol* **20**, 432–440.

Henry JA, Jeffreys KJ, and Dowling S (1992) Toxicity and deaths from 3,4-methylenedioxymethamphetamine ("ecstasy"). *Lancet* **340**, 384–387.

Hermle L, Spitzer M, and Gouzoulis E (1994) Arylalkanamine-induced effects in normal volunteers: on the significance of research in hallucinogenic agents for psychiatry. In *Fifty Years of LSD: Current Status and Perspectives of Hallucinogens*, Pletscher A and Ladewig D (eds). Parthenon, New York.

Hiramatsu M and Cho AK (1990) Enantiomeric differences in the effects of 3,4-methylenedioxymethamphetamine on extracellular monoamines and metabolites in the striatum of freely-moving rats. *Neuropharmacology* **29**, 269–275.

Ho E, Karimi-Tabesh L, and Koren G (2001) Characteristics of pregnant women who use ecstasy (3,4-methylenedioxymethamphetamine). *Neurotoxicol Teratol* **23**, 561–567.

Hofmann A (1980) *LSD: My Problem Child*. McGraw Hill, New York.

Hohn R and Lasagna L (1960) Effects of aggregation and temperature on amphetamine toxicity in mice. *Psychopharmacologia* **1**, 2210–2220.

Hollister L (1968) *Chemical Psychoses: LSD and Related Drugs*. Thomas, Springfield, IL.

Hollister L (1984) Effects of hallucinogens in humans. In *Hallucinogens: Neurochemical, Behavioral, and Clinical Perspectives*, Jacobs B (ed). Raven Press, New York.

Holmes SB, Banerjee AK, and Alexander WD (1999) Hyponatremia and seizures after ecstasy use. *Postgrad Med J* **75**, 32–33.

Holsten F (1976) Flashbacks. Clinical and social significance 1 1/2–4 years after the 1st admission. [Norwegian]. *Tidsskrift for Den Norske Laegeforening* **96**, 875–878.

Hooft PJ and Van der Voorde HP (1994) Reckless behavior related to the use of 3,4-methylenedioxymethamphetamine (ecstasy): apropos of fatal accident during car surfing. *Int J Legal Med* **106**, 328–329.

Horowitz MJ (1969) Flashbacks: Recurrent intrusive images after the use of LSD. *Am J Psychiatry* **126**, 565–569.

Horowitz HA (1975) The use of lithium in the treatment of the drug-induced psychotic reaction. *Dis Nerv Syst* **36**, 159–163.

Hubner CB, Bird M, Ressnick S, et al. (1988) The threshold lowering effects of MDMA (ecstasy) on brain-stimulation reward. *Psychopharmacology* **95**, 49–51.

Hughes JC, McCube M, and Evans RJ (1993) Intracranial haemorrhage associated with ingestion of "Ecstasy." *Arch Emerg Med* **10**, 372–374.

Huxley A (1954) *The Doors of Perception*. Chatto and Windus, London.

Ijzermans JNM, Tilanus HW, DeMan RA, et al. (1993) Ecstasy and liver transplantation. *Ann Med Int* **144**, 568.

Insel TR, Battaglia G, Johannessen JN, et al. (1989) 3,4-methylenedioxymethamphetamine ("ecstasy") selectively destroys brain serotonin terminals in rhesus monkeys. *J Pharmacol Exp Ther* **249**, 713–720.

Jarvik M (1970) *Drugs, Hallucinations, and Memory: Origin and Mechanisms of Hallucinations*. Plenum Press, New York.

Johnson MP, Hoffman AH, and Nichols DE (1986) Effects of the enantiomers of MDA, MDMA and related analogues on [³H]-serotonin and [³H]-dopamine release from superfused rat brain slices. *Eur J Pharmacol* **132**, 269–276.

Johnston L, Bachman J, and O'Malley P (2002) *Monitoring the Future—National Results on Adolescent Drug Use*. National Institute on Drug Abuse, Bethesda, MD.

Johnston LD, O'Malley PM, and Bachman JG (1999) *National Survey Results on Drug Use from the Monitoring the Future Study, 1975–1998*, Vol. I, *Secondary School Students*. NIH Publication No. 99–4660, US Department of Health and Human Services, Washington, DC.

Kamien JB, Johanson CE, Schuster CR, et al. (1986) The effects of (+)-methylenedioxymethamphetamine and (+)-methylenedioxyamphetamine in monkeys trained to discriminate (+)-amphetamine from saline. *Drug Alcohol Depend* **18**, 139–147.

Kessel B (1994) Hyponatremia after ingestion of "ecstasy." *Br Med J* **308**, 414.

Khakoo SI, Coles CJ, Armstrong JS, et al. (1995) Hepatotoxicity and accelerated fibrosis following 3,4-methylenedioxymethamphetamine ("Ecstasy") usage. *J Clin Gastroenterol* **20**, 244–247.

Kornblith AB (1981) Multiple drug abuse involving nonopiate, nonalcoholic substances. II. Physical damage, long-term psychological effects and treatment approaches and success. *Int J Addict* **16**, 527–540.

Krystal JH and Price LH (1992) Chronic 3,4-methylenedimethoxymethamphetamine (MDMA) use: effects on mood and neuropsychological function? *Am J Drug Alcohol Abuse* **18**, 331–341.

LaBarre W (1975) *Anthropological Perspectives on Hallucination and Hallucinogens: Hallucinations*. John Wiley, New York.

Lake CR, Stirba AL, Kinneman R Jr., et al. (1981) Mania associated with LSD ingestion. *Am J Psychiatry* **138**, 1508–1509.

Lamb RJ and Griffiths RR (1987) Self-injection of 3,4-methylenedioxy methamphetamine (MDMA) in the baboon. *Psychopharmacology* **91**, 268–272.

Laruelle M, Wallace E, Seibyl JP, et al. (1994) Graphical, kinetic, and equilibrium analyses of *in vivo* [123I] β-CIT binding to dopamine transporters in healthy human subjects. *J Cereb Blood Flow Metab* **14**, 982–994.

Lawler LP, Abraham S, and Fishman EK (2001) 3,4-methylenedioxymethamphetamine (ecstasy)-induced hepatotoxicity: Multidetector CT and pathology findings. *J Comput Assist Tomgr* **25**, 649–652.

Lawn JC (1986) Schedules of controlled substances: scheduling of 3,4-methylenedioxymethamphetamine (MDMA) into schedule I of the controlled substances act. *Fed Reg* **51**, 36552–36560.

Lehmann ED, Thom CH, and Croft DN (1995) Delayed severe rhabdomyolysis after taking ecstasy. *Postgrad Med J* **71**, 186–187.

Lerner AG, Finkel B, Oyffe I, et al. (1998) Clonidine treatment for hallucinogen persisting perception disorder. *Am J Psychiatry* **155**, 1460.

Lerner AG, Gelkopf M, Oyffe I, et al. (2000) LSD-induced hallucinogen persisting perception disorder treatment with clonidine: an open pilot study. *Int Clin Psychopharmacol* **15**, 35–37.

Lerner AG, Oyefe I, Isaacs G, et al. (1997) Naltrexone treatment of hallucinogen persisting perception disorder. *Am J Psychiatry* **154**, 437.

Lerner AG, Skladman I, Kodesh A, et al. (2001) LSD-induced hallucinogen persisting perception disorder treated with clonazepam: two case reports. *Isr J Psychiatr Rel Sci* **38**, 133–136.

Leuner H (1967) Present state of psycholytic therapy and its possibilities. In *Second International Conference on the Use of LSD in Psycho therapy and Alcoholism*, Abramson HA (ed). Bobbs-Merrill, Indianapolis.

Lew R, Sabol KE, Chou C, et al. (1996) Methylenedioxymethamphetamine-induced serotonin deficits are followed by partial recovery over a 52-week period, part II: Radioligand binding and autoradioligand binding and autoradiography studies. *J Pharmacol Exp Ther* **276**, 855–865.

Liechti ME and Vollenweider FX (2000) The serotonin uptake inhibitor citalopram reduces acute cardiovascular and vegetative effects of 3,4-methylenedioxymethamphetamine ("Ecstasy") in healthy volunteers. *J Psychopharmacol* **14**, 269–274.

Liester MB, Grob CS, Bravo GL, et al. (1992) Phenomenology and sequelae of 3,4-methylenedioxymethamphetamine use. *J Nerv Ment Dis* **180**, 345–352.

Lin LY, Kamagai Y, and Cho AK (1992) Enzymatic and chemical demethylation of (methylenedioxy) amphetamine and (methylenedioxy) methamphetamine by rat brain microsomes. *Chem Res Toxicol* **5**, 401–406.

Logan BK and Couper FJ (2001) 3,4-methylenedioxymethamphetamine (MDMA, ecstasy) and driving impairment. *J Forens Sci* **46**, 1426–1433.

Lyon RA, Glennon RA, and Titeler M (1986) 3,4-methylenedioxymethamphetamine (MDMA): stereoselective interactions at brain 5-HT$_1$ and 5-HT$_2$ receptors. *Psychopharmacology* **88**, 525–526.

MacInnes N, Handley SL, and Harding GF (2001) Former chronic methylenedioxymethamphetamine (MDMA or ecstasy) users report mild depressive symptoms. *J Psychopharmacol* **15**, 181–186.

Magee C, Staunton H, Tormey W, et al. (1998) Hyponatremia, seizures and stupor associated with ecstasy ingestion in a female. *Ir Med J* **91**, 178.

Malleson N (1971) Acute adverse reactions to LSD in clinical and experimental use in the United Kingdom. *Br J Psychiatry* **118**, 229–230.

Manchanda S and Connolly MJ (1993) Cerebral infarction in association with ecstasy abuse. *Postgrad Med J* **69**, 874–875.

Marsh JC, Abboudi ZH, Gibson FM, et al. (1994) Aplastic anemia following exposure to 3,4-methylenedioxy-methamphetamine ("Ecstasy"). *Br J Haematol* **88**, 281–285.

Martin W and Sloan J (1977) Pharmacology and classification of LSD-like hallucinogens. In *Drug Addiction II*, Martin W (ed). Springer-Verlag, Berlin.

Mas M, Farre M, de la Torre R, et al. (1999) Cardiovascular and neuroendocrine effects and pharmacokinetics of 3,4-methylenedioxymethamphetamine in humans. *J Pharmacol Exp Ther* **290**, 136–145.

Matthai SM, Davidson DC, Sills JA, et al. (1996) Cerebral oedema after ingestion of MDMA ("Ecstasy") and unrestricted intake of water. *Br Med J* **312**, 1359.

Maurer HH, Bickeboeller-Friedrich J, Kraemer T, et al. (2000) Toxicokinetics and analytical toxicology of amphetamine-derived designer drugs ("Ecstasy"). *Toxicol Lett* **112–113**, 133–142.

Maxwell DL, Polkey MI, and Henry JA (1993) Hyponatremia and catatonia stupor after taking 'ecstasy.' *Br Med J* **27**, 1399.

Mazur S and Hitchcock T (2001) Spontaneous pneumomediastinum, pneumothorax and ecstasy abuse. *Emerg Med (Fremantle, West Austral)* **13**, 121–123.

McCann UD, Mertl M, Eligulashvili V, et al. (1999) Cognitive performance in (+/−) 3,4-methylenedioxymethamphetamine (MDMA, "Ecstasy") users: a controlled study. *Psychopharmacology* **143**, 417–425.

McCann UD, Ridenour A, Shaham Y, et al. (1994) Brain serotonergic neurotoxicity after MDMA ("Ecstasy"): a controlled study in humans. *Neuropsychopharmacology* **10**, 129–138.

McCann UD, Szabo Z, Scheffel U, et al. (1998) Positron emission tomographic evidence of toxic effect of MDMA ("Ecstasy") on brain serotonin neurons in human beings. *Lancet* **352**, 1433–1437.

McFarling D (1980) *LSD Follow-up Study Report*. United States Army Medical Department, United States Army Health Services Command.

McGuire P (2000) Long-term psychiatric and cognitive effects of MDMA use. *Toxicol Lett* **112–113**, 153–156.

McKenna DJ and Peroutka SJ (1990) Neurochemistry and neurotoxicity of 3,4-methylenedioxymethamphetamine (MDMA, "Ecstasy"). *J Neurochem* **54**, 14–22.

McLellan AT and Druley KA (1977) Non-random relation between drugs of abuse and psychiatric diagnosis. *J Psychiatr Res* **13**, 179–184.

McLellan AT, Woody GE, and O'Brien CP (1979) Development of psychiatric illness in drug abusers. *N Engl J Med* **301**, 1310–1314.

Merck E (1914) Verfahren zur darstellung von alkyloxyaryl-dialyloxyaryl und alkylenedioxy-arylaminopropanen bzw deren am stickstoffmonalkylieten derivaten. German Patent #273,350. Berlin, Germany.

Merkur D (2000) *The Mystery of Manna: The Psychedelic Sacrament of the Bible*. Park Street Press, Vermont.

Metzner R (1969) A note on the treatment of LSD psychosis. *Behav Neuropsychiatry* **1**, 29–32.

Molliver ME, Berger UV, Mamounas LA, et al. (1990) Neurotoxicity of MDMA and related compounds: anatomic studies. *Ann N Y Acad Sci* **600**, 640–664.

Mueller PD and Korey WS (1998) Death by "Ecstasy": the serotonin syndrome? *Ann Emerg Med* **32**, 377–380.

Muller DJ (1971) ECT in LSD psychosis. A report of three cases. *Am J Psychiatry* **128**, 351–352.

Nash JF Jr., Meltzer HY, and Gudelsky GA (1988) Elevation of serum prolactin and corticosterone concentrations in the rat after the administration of 3,4-methylenedioxymethamphetamine. *J Pharmacol Exp Ther* **245**, 873–879.

Nash JF, Meltzer HY, and Gudelsky GA (1990) Effect of 3,4-methylenedioxymethamphetamine accumulation in the striatum and nucleus accumbens. *J Neurochem* **54**, 1062–1067.

O'Connor A, Cluroe A, Couch R, et al. (1999) Death from hyponatremia-induced cerebral oedema associated with MDMA ("Ecstasy") use. *N Z Med J* **112**, 255–256.

O'Hearn EG, Battaglia G, DeSouza EB, et al. (1988) Methylenedioxyamphetamine (MDA) and methylenedioxymethamphetamine (MDMA) cause selective ablation of serotonergic axon terminals in forebrain: immunocytochemical evidence for neurotoxicity. *J Neurosci* **8**, 2788–2803.

Opitz E (1963) Die klinische therapie seelischer Strungen mit lysergsaure. *Psychiatr Neurol Med Psychol* **15**, 366–372.

Pacifici R, Farre M, Pichini S, et al. (2001) Sweat testing of MDMA with the Drugwipe analytical device: a controlled study with two volunteers. *J Anal Toxicol* **25**, 144–146.

Parrott AC and Lasky J (1998) Ecstasy (MDMA) effects upon mood and cognition: before, during, and after a saturday night dance. *Psychopharmacology* **139**, 261–268.

Parrott AC, Milani RM, Parmar R, et al. (2001) Recreational ecstasy/MDMA and other drug users from the UK and Italy: psychiatric symptoms and psychobiological problems. *Psychopharmacology* **159**, 77–82.

Peroutka SJ (1987) Incidence of recreational use of 3,4-methylenedi oxymethamphetamine (MDMA, "Ecstasy") on an undergraduate campus. *N Engl J Med* **317**, 1542–1543.

Peroutka SJ, Newman H, and Harris H (1988) Subjective effects of 3,4-methylenedioxymethamphetamine in recreational users. *Neuropsychopharmacology* **1**, 273–277.

Poland RE, Lutchmansingh P, McCracken JT, et al. (1997) Abnormal ACTH and prolactin responses to fenfluramine in rats exposed to single and multiple doses of MDMA. *Psychopharmacologia (Berl)* **131**, 411–419.

Pope HG Jr., Ionescu-Pioggia M, and Pope KW (2001) Drug use and life style among college undergraduates: a 30-year longitudinal study. *Am J Psychiatry* **158**, 1519–1521.

Price LH, Charney DS, Delgado PL, et al. (1990) Clinical studies of 5-HT function using I.V. L-tryptophan. *Prog Neuro-psychopharmacol Biol Psychiatry* **14**, 459–472.

Price LH, Ricaurte GA, Krystal JH, et al. (1989) Neuroendocrine and mood responses to intravenous L-tryptophan in MDMA users. *Arch Gen Psychiatry* **46**, 20–22.

Qasim A, Townend J, and Davies MK (2001) Ecstasy induced acute myocardial infarction. *Heart Br Cardiac Soc* **85**, E10.

Randell T (1992) Rave scene, ecstasy use, leap Atlantic. *J Am Med Assoc* **268**, 1506.

Reich P and Hepps RB (1972) Homicide during a psychosis induced by LSD. *JAMA* **219**, 869–871.

Reneman L, Booij J, de Bruin K, et al. (2001a) Effects of dose, sex, and long-term abstention from use on toxic effects of MDMA (ecstasy) on brain serotonin neurons. *Lancet* **358**, 1864–1869.

Reneman L, Booij J, Schmand B, et al. (2000) Memory disturbances in "Ecstasy" users are correlated with altered brain serotonin neurotransmission. *Psychopharmacology* **148**, 322–324.

Reneman L, Endert E, de Bruin K, et al. (2002a) The acute and chronic effects of MDMA ("Ecstasy") on cortical 5-HT$_{2A}$ receptors in rat and human brain. *Neuropsychopharmacology* **26**, 387–396.

Reneman L, Lavalaye J, Schmand B, et al. (2001a) Cortical serotonin transporter density and verbal memory in individuals who stopped using 3,4-methylenedioxymethamphetamine (MDMA or "Ecstasy"): preliminary findings. *Arch Gen Psychiatry* **58**, 907–908.

Reneman L, Majoie CB, Flick H, et al. (2002b) Reduced N-acetylaspartate levels in the frontal cortex of 3,4-methylenedioxymethamphetamine (Ecstasy) users: preliminary results. *Am J Neuroradiol* **23**, 231–237.

Reneman L, Majoie CB, Schmand B, et al. (2001c) Prefrontal N-acetylaspartate is strongly associated with memory performance in (abstinent) ecstasy users: Preliminary report. *Biol Psychiatry* **50**, 550–554.

Ricaurte G, Bryan G, Strauss L, et al. (1985) Hallucinogenic amphetamine selectively destroys brain serotonin nerve terminals. *Science* **229**, 986–988.

Ricaurte GA, DeLanney LE, Irwin I, et al. (1988) Toxic effects of MDMA on central serotonergic neurons in the primate: importance of route and frequency of drug administration. *Brain Res* **446**, 165–168.

Ricaurte GA, Katz JL, and Martello MB (1992) Lasting effects of (+/−)-3,4-methylenedioxymethamphetamine (MDMA) on central serotonergic neurons in nonhuman primates: neurochemical observations. *J Pharmacol Exp Ther* **261**, 616–622.

Robbins E, Frosch WA, and Stern M (1967) Further observations on untoward reactions to LSD. *Am J Psychiatry* **124**, 393–395.

Roberts L and Wright H (1993) Survival following intentional massive overdose of 'Ecstasy.' *J Accid Emerg Med* **11**, 53–54.

Rosenthal S (1964) Persistent hallucinosis following repeated administration of hallucinogenic drugs. *Am J Psychiatry* **124**, 238–244.

Rothwell PM and Grant R (1993) Cerebral venous thrombosis induced by "Ecstasy." *J Neurol Neurosurg Psychiatry* **56**, 1035–1039.

Safer DJ (1987) Substance abuse by young adult chronic patients. *Hosp Comm Psychiatry* **38**, 511–514.

Sanborn B and Daniels J (1971) LSD reaction: a family research approach. *Int J Addict* **6**, 497–507.

Sanchez V, Camarero J, Esteban B, et al. (2001) The mechanisms involved in the long-lasting neuroprotective effect of fluoxetine against MDMA ('ecstasy')-induced degeneration of 5-HT nerve endings in rat blind. *Br J Pharmacol* **134**, 46–57.

Sandison RA, Spencer AM, and Whitelaw JDA (1954) The therapeutic value of lysergic acid diethylamide in mental illness. *J Ment Sci* **100**, 491.

Scanzello CR, Hatzidimitriou G, Martello AL, et al. (1993) Serotonergic recovery after (+) 3,4-(methylenedioxy) methamphetamine injury: observations in rodents. *J Pharmacol Exp Ther* **264**, 1484–1491.

Schaefer SB and Furst PT (eds). (1998) *People of the Peyote: Huichol Indian History, Religion and Survival.* University of New Mexico Press, Albuquerque, NM.

Schmidt CJ (1987) Neurotoxicity of the psychedelic amphetamine, methylenedioxymethamphetamine. *J Pharmacol Exp Ther* **240**, 1–7.

Schmidt CJ, Wu L, and Lovenberg W (1986) Methylenedioxymethamphetamine: a potentially neurotoxic amphetamine analog. *Eur J Pharmacol* **124**, 175–178.

Schultes R and Hofmann A (1980) *The Botany and Chemistry of Hallucinogens.* Thomas, Springfield, IL.

Schultes RE and Hofmann A (1992) *Plants of the Gods: their Sacred, Healing, and Hallucinogenic Powers.* Healing Arts Press, Rochester, VT, p. 192.

Schwartz RH, Comerci GD, and Meeks JE (1987) LSD: patterns of use by chemically dependent adolescents. *J Pediatr* **111**, 936–938.

Segura M, Ortuno J, Farre M, et al. (2001) 3,4-Dihydroxymethamphetamine (HHMA): a major *in vivo* 3,4-methylenedioxymethamphetamine (MDMA) metabolite in humans. *Chem Res Toxicol* **14**, 1203–1208.

Semple DM, Ebmeier KP, Glabus MF, et al. (1999) Reduced *in vivo* binding to the serotonin transporter in the cerebral cortex of MDMA ("Ecstasy") users. *Br J Psychiatry* **175**, 63–69.

Shearman JD, Satsangi J, Chapman RWG, et al. (1992) Misuse of Ecstasy. *Br Med J* **305**, 309.

Shick J and Smith D (1970) Analysis of the LSD flashback. *J Psychedel Drugs* **3**, 13–19.

Shulgin A (1991) *Pihkal, A Chemical Love Story.* Transform Press, Berkeley.

Shulgin AT and Nichols DE (1978) Characterization of three new psychomimetics. In *The Psychopharmacology of Hallucinogens*, Stillman R and Willette R (eds). Pergamon Press, New York, pp. 74–83.

Siegel RK (1986) MDMA: nonmedical use and intoxication. *J Psychoact Drugs* **18**, 349–354.

Simantov R and Tauber M (1997) The abused drug MDMA (ecstasy) induces programmed death of human serotonergic cells. *FASEB J* **11**, 141–146.

Sipes TE and Geyer MA (1995) DOI disruption of prepulse inhibition of startle in the rat is mediated by 5-HT(2A) and not by 5-HT(2C) receptors. *Behav Pharmacol* **6**, 839–842.

Slikker W, Ali SF, Scallet C, et al. (1988) Neurochemical and neurohistological alterations in the rat and monkey produced by orally administered methylenedioxymethamphetamine (MDMA). *Toxicol Appl Pharmacol* **94**, 448–457.

Slikker W Jr., Holson RR, Ali SF, et al. (1989) Behavioral and neurochemical effects of orally administered MDMA in the rodent and nonhuman primate. *Neurotoxicology* **10**, 529–549.

Smart RG and Bateman K (1967) Unfavourable reactions to LSD: a review and analysis of the available case reports. *Can Med Assoc J* **97**, 1214–1221.

Smart RG and Jones D (1970) Illicit LSD users: their personality characteristics and psychopathology. *J Abnorm Psychol* **75**, 286–292.

Solowij N, Hall W, and Lee N (1992) Recreational MDMA use in Sydney: a profile of "Ecstacy" users and their experiences with the drug. *Br J Addict* **87**, 1161–1172.

Smith H (2000) *Cleansing the Doors of Perception: The Religious Significance of Entheogenic Plants and Chemicals*. Penguin Putnam, New York.

Spruit IP (2001) Monitoring synthetic drug markets, trends, and public health. *Subst Use Misuse* **36**, 23–47.

Steele TD, Nichols DE, and Yim GKW (1987) Stereochemical effects of 3,4-methylenedioxymethamphetamine (MDMA) and related amphetamine derivatives on inhibition of uptake of [^{3}H]-monoamines into synaptosomes from different regions of rat brain. *Biochem Pharmacol* **36**, 2297–2303.

Sternback H (1991) The serotonin syndrome. *Am J Psychiatry* **148**, 705–713.

Stone DM, Stahl DC, Hanson GR, et al. (1986) The effects of 3,4-methylenedioxymethamphetamine (MDMA) and 3,4-methylendioxyamphetamine (MDA) on monoaminergic systems in the rat brain. *Eur J Pharmacol* **128**, 41–48.

Strassman RJ (1984) Adverse reactions to psychedelic drugs. A review of the literature. *J Nerv Ment Dis* **172**, 577–595.

Strassman RJ, Qualls CR, Uhlenhuth EH, et al. (1994) Dose–response study of N,N-dimethyltryptamine in humans II. Subjective effects and preliminary results of a new rating scale. *Arch Gen Psychiatry* **51**, 98–108.

Strote J, Lee JE, and Wechsler H (2002) Increasing MDMA use among college students: results of a national survey. *J Adolesc Health* **30**, 64–72.

Taffe MA, Weed MR, Davis S, et al. (2001) Functional consequences of repeated (+/−)3,4-methylenedioxymethamphetamine (MDMA) treatment in rhesus monkeys. *Neuropsychopharmacology* **24**, 230–239.

Tancer ME and Johanson CE (2001) The subjective effects of MDMA and mCPP in moderate MDMA users. *Drug Alcohol Depend* **65**, 97–101.

Tietz W (1967) Complications following ingestion of LSD in a lower class population. *Calif Med* **107**, 396–398.

Titeler M, Lyon RA, and Glennon RA (1988) Radioligand binding evidence implicates the brain 5-HT$_2$ receptor as a site of action for LSD and phenylisopropylamine hallucinogens. *Psychopharmacology* **94**, 213–216.

Topp L, Hando J, Dillon P, et al. (1999) Ecstasy use in Australia: patterns of use and associated harm. *Drug Alcohol Depend* **55**, 105–115.

Tsuang MT, Simpson JC, and Kronfol Z (1982) Subtypes of drug abuse with psychosis. Demographic characteristics, clinical features, and family history. *Arch Gen Psychiatry* **39**, 141–147.

Ungerleider JT, Fisher DD, and Fuller M (1966) The dangers of LSD. Analysis of seven months' experience in a university hospital's psychiatric service. *JAMA* **197**, 389–392.

Vaiva G, Boss V, Bailly D, et al. (2001) An "accidental" acute psychosis with ecstasy use. *J Psychoact Drugs* **33**, 95–98.

Vardy MM and Kay SR (1983) LSD psychosis or LSD-induced schizophrenia? A multimethod inquiry. *Arch Gen Psychiatry* **40**, 877–883.

Verebey K, Alrazi J, and Jaffe JU (1988) The complications of "ecstasy" (MDMA). *J Am Med Assoc* **259**, 1649–1650.

Verkes RJ, Gijsman HJ, Pieters RC, et al. (2001) Cognitive performance and serotonergic function in users of ecstasy. *Psychopharmacology* **153**, 186–202.

Vollenweider FX, Gamma A, Liechti M, et al. (1998) Psychological and cardiovascular effects and short-term sequelae of MDMA ("Ecstasy") in MDMA-naïve healthy volunteers. *Neuropsychopharmacology* **19**, 241–251.

Vollenweider FX, Leenders KL, Scharfetter C, et al. (1997) Positron emission tomography and fluorodeoxyglucose studies of metabolic hyperfrontality and psychopathology in the psilocybin model of psychosis. *Neuropsychopharmacology* **16**, 257–272.

Wasson RG (1961) The hallucinogenic fungi of Mexico: an inquiry into the origins of the religious idea among primitive peoples. *Bot Mus Leaflets Harv Univ* **19**, 137–162.

Wilson MA, Ricaurte GA, and Molliver ME (1989) Distinct morphological classes of serotonergic axons in primates exhibit differential vulnerability to the psychotropic drug 3,4-methylenedioxymethamphetamine. *Neuroscience* **28**, 121–137.

Yamamoto BK and Spanos LJ (1988) The acute effects of methylenedioxymethamphetamine on dopamine release in the awake-behaving rat. *Eur J Pharmacol* **148**, 195–203.

Young CR (1997) Sertraline treatment of hallucinogen persisting perception disorder. *J Clin Psychiatry* **58**, 85.

Zakzanis KK and Young DA (2001) Memory impairment in abstinent MDMA ("Ecstasy") users: a longitudinal investigation. *Neurology* **56**, 966–969.

Zemishlany Z, Aizenberg D, and Weizman A (2001) Subjective effects of MDMA ("Ecstasy") on human sexual function. *Eur Psychiatr. J Assoc Eur Psychiatry* **16**, 127–130.

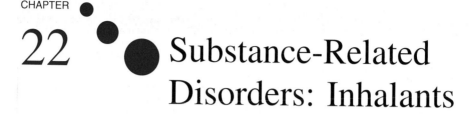

Substance-Related Disorders: Inhalants

The term *inhalant abuse* is used to describe a variety of drug-using behaviors that cannot be classified by their pharmacology or toxicology but are grouped on the basis of their primary mode of administration. Although other substances can be inhaled (e.g., tobacco, marijuana with or without phencyclidine, and even heroin or crack), this is not the primary route of administration; therefore, they do not fall into this classification. Several subcategories of inhalants can be established on the basis of chemical classes of products and primary abuse groups as follows: (1) industrial or household cleaning and paint-type solvents including paint thinners or solvents, degreasers or dry cleaning solvents, solvents in glues, art or office supply solvents such as correction fluids, and solvents in magic markers (gasoline is similar to these products); (2) propellant gases used in household or commercial products, such as butane in lighters, or fluorocarbons in electronic (personal computer, office equipment) cleaners or refrigerant gases; (3) household aerosol sprays such as paint, hair, and fabric protector sprays; (4) medical anesthetic gases such as ether, chloroform, halothane, and nitrous oxide; and (5) aliphatic nitrites. Nitrous oxide is also available in whipped cream dispensers (e.g., whippets) and for octane boosters in car racing, and is used outside the medical theater by nonprofessionals. Most of the foregoing compounds affect the central nervous system (CNS) directly, whereas nitrites act on cardiovascular smooth muscle rather than as an anesthetic in the CNS. The nitrites are also used primarily as sexual enhancers rather than as mood alterants. Therefore, when discussing "inhalant abuse," we will be referring primarily to substances other than nitrites. One item worthy of note: the exclusion of anesthetics from the inhalant-related disorders section in the DSM-IV-TR is not medically correct, as almost all of the inhalants act physiologically as would any anesthetic and some, particularly the anesthetics nitrous oxide and trichloroethylene (TCE), are abused by the primary inhalant abuser discussed herein. Thus, the following discussion includes the abuse of selected anesthetics but does not discuss the problems of the anesthetic state.

Table 22-1 enumerates the solvents (frequently noted on the labels) contained in corresponding popular products currently used for recreational purposes. Despite the widespread availability and inhalation of these substances, it was not until the 1950s that reporters (Kerner 1988) and judicial action focused nationwide attention on "glue sniffing." The term "glue sniffing" is still widely used today to describe the abuse of most of these substances. It is important to keep in mind that there are many different chemicals in these different products, all of which have different physiological effects and toxicities as well as different chemical properties. Sometimes the substances are listed on the product label; however, many times the container lacks sufficient detail to identify the potential toxin(s).

Table 22-1	Chemicals Commonly Found in Inhalants
Inhalant	**Chemicals**
Adhesives	
Airplane glue	Toluene, ethyl acetate
Other glues	Hexane, toluene, methyl chloride, acetone, methyl ethyl ketone, methyl butyl ketone
Special cements	Trichloroethylene, tetrachloroethylene
Aerosols	
Paint sprays	Butane, propane, fluorocarbons, toluene, hydrocarbons
Hair sprays	Butane, propane
Deodorants, air fresheners	Butane, propane
Analgesic spray	Fluorocarbons
Asthma spray	Fluorocarbons
Fabric spray	Butane, trichloroethane
Personal computer cleaners	Dimethyl ether, hydrofluorocarbons
Anesthetics	
Gaseous	Nitrous oxide
Liquid	Halothane, enflurane
Local	Ethyl chloride
Cleaning Agents	
Dry cleaners	Tetrachloroethylene, trichloroethane
Spot removers	Xylene, petroleum distillates, chlorohydrocarbons
Degreasers	Tetrachloroethylene, trichloroethane, trichloroethylene
Solvents and Gases	
Nail polish remover	Acetone, ethyl acetate, toluene
Paint remover	Toluene, methylene chloride, methanol, acetone, ethyl acetate
Paint thinners	Petroleum distillates, esters, acetone
Correction fluids and thinners	Trichloroethylene, trichloroethane
Fuel gas	Butane, isopropane
Cigar or cigarette lighter fluid	Butane, isopropane
Fire extinguisher propellant	Bromochlorodifluoromethane
Food Products	
Whipped cream aerosols	Nitrous oxide
Whippets	Nitrous oxide
Room Odorizers	
Poppers, fluids (Rush, Locker Room)	Isoamyl, isobutyl, isopropyl, or butyl nitrite (now illegal) or cyclohexyl

The disorders described in this chapter are classified under the inhalant-related disorders section in DSM-IV-TR and are subdivided into two groups: inhalant use disorders and inhalant-induced disorders.

Diagnosis

The practice of "sniffing," "snorting," "huffing," "bagging," or inhaling to get high describes various methods of inhalation (Sharp et al. 1992). These terms refer to the inhalation of volatile substances from (1) filled balloons, (2) bags, and (3) soaked rags and/or sprayed directly into oral orifices. Abusers can be identified by various telltale clues such as organic odors in the breath or clothes, stains on the clothes or around the mouth, empty spray paint or solvent containers, and other unusual paraphernalia. These clues may enable one to identify a serious problem of solvent abuse before it causes serious health problems or death.

Most volatile substances are widely available and are inhaled to provide a quick high, often to make users forget their problems and relieve boredom. Solvent abusers, more than other drug users, are poor, come from broken homes, and do poorly in school (Korman et al. 1981, Oetting and Webb 1992). There are also many other types of inhalant abusers, for example, medical personnel (Spencer et al. 1976, Jastak 1991, England and Jones 1992), college students, who inhale one or another of these solvents to get high or feel good.

There is an interesting observation that includes alcohol and solvents. Some time ago, "degreaser's flush" (so described because of a flushing of the face) was observed when occupational workers left their degreasing vats and drank alcohol after leaving work (Pardys and Brotman 1974, Stewart et al. 1974). Also, heavy drinking has been associated with occupational toluene exposure (Antti-Poika et al. 1985). Both humans and rats have been noted to be thirsty when exposed to toluene and alcohol (Pryor et al. 1985, Kira et al. 1988). Whether either substance may accentuate the use of the other is unknown; an attempt to study the acute effects of low levels of alcohol and toluene in human volunteers failed to produce any identifiable interaction.

The following Inhalant-Related Disorders are included in DSM-IV-TR:

Inhalant Dependence   Dependence on inhalants is primarily psychological, with a less dramatic associated physical dependence occurring in some heavy users (see generic DSM-IV-TR diagnostic criteria Chapter 15, page 351). Physical tolerance of some solvents has been documented by animal studies only under unusual conditions (Evans and Balster 1993). The urgent need to continue use of inhalants has been reported among individuals with heavy use, although the nature of this phenomenon is unknown. There is at least a psychological dependence and often a weak physical dependence on these substances. A mild withdrawal syndrome occurs in 10 to 24 hours after cessation of use (only in those who have excessively abused inhalants) and lasts for several days. Symptoms include general disorientation, sleep disturbances, headaches, muscle spasms, irritability, nausea, and fleeting illusions. However, this is not an easily identified or a characteristic withdrawal syndrome that is useful for many practitioners in a clinical setting. The need to continue use is undeniably strong in many individuals; specific treatments for inhalant dependence, other than the drug therapy and/or psychotherapy used for other drug dependence, need to be developed.

Inhalant Abuse   Abuse of inhalants may lead to harm to individuals (e.g., accidents involving automobiles, falling from buildings when in an impaired or intoxicated state (illusionary feelings), or self-inflicted harm such as attempted or successful suicide) (see generic DSM-IV-TR diagnostic criteria Chapter 15, page 352). Frozen lips caused by rapidly expanding gases (Wheeler et al. 1992) or serious burns (Scerri et al. 1992) may also occur. Chronic inhalant use is often associated with familial conflict and school problems.

Inhalant-Induced Disorders   The primary disorder is inhalant intoxication, which is characterized by the presence of clinically significant maladaptive behavioral or psychological changes (e.g., belligerence, assaultiveness, apathy, impaired judgment, impaired social or occupational functioning) that develop during the intentional short-term, high-dose exposure to volatile inhalants (see DSM-IV-TR diagnostic criteria on page 541). The maladaptive changes occurring after intentional and nonintentional exposure include disinhibition, excitedness, light-headedness, visual disturbances (blurred vision, nystagmus), incoordination, dysarthria, an unsteady gait, and euphoria. Higher doses of inhalants may lead to depressed reflexes, stupor, coma, and death, sometimes caused by cardiac arrhythmia. Lethargy, generalized muscle weakness, and headaches may occur some hours later depending on the dose.

DSM-IV-TR Diagnostic Criteria

292.89 Inhalant Intoxication

A. Recent intentional use or short-term, high-dose exposure to volatile inhalants (excluding anesthetic gases and short-acting vasodilators).

B. Clinically significant maladaptive behavioral or psychological changes (e.g., belligerence, assaultiveness, apathy, impaired judgment, impaired social or occupational functioning) that developed during, or shortly after, use of or exposure to volatile inhalants.

C. Two (or more) of the following signs developing during, or shortly after, inhalant use or exposure:

   (1) dizziness
   (2) nystagmus
   (3) incoordination
   (4) slurred speech
   (5) unsteady gait
   (6) lethargy
   (7) depressed reflexes
   (8) psychomotor retardation
   (9) tremor
   (10) generalized muscle weakness
   (11) blurred vision or diplopia
   (12) stupor or coma
   (13) euphoria

D. The symptoms are not due to a general medical condition and are not better accounted for by another mental disorder.

Reprinted with permission from the Diagnostic and Statistical Manual of Mental Disorders, Fourth Edition, Text Revision. Copyright 2000 American Psychiatric Association.

There is little evidence that inhalant abuse either coexists with other mental disorders or leads to any such altered state. Mental disorders related to solvent abuse were reviewed (Ron 1986); it was concluded that psychiatric morbidity is "highest in those referred to psychiatric hospitals and lowest in clinics dealing exclusively with VS (volatile substance (solvent) abuse." There have been few studies of comorbidity in psychiatric hospital populations and almost no studies in other populations. In an analysis of dual diagnoses, drug abuse was stated to coexist with depression and anxiety disorders (Anthenelli and Schuckit 1993); however, neither this study nor another on dual diagnoses of drug abuse disorders and mental disorders (Ries 1993) identified an inhalant abuse disorder in its subjects. The reason may be that the latter populations are seldom identified or characterized because of lack of recognition of this area of drug abuse and are thus not available in treatment for study.

On the other hand, there is little doubt that personality disorders of an antisocial type are common in solvent abusers. A study of older drug users (Dinwiddie et al. 1987) observed that most of the subjects had antisocial personality disorders. Most were admitted for their drug dependence, with a prominent use of solvents (for 5–13 years); they also used marijuana, alcohol, stimulants, and other drugs. The interpretation was that an age-dependent progression of antisocial behavior occurred for those previously self-selecting solvent use.

In another study of psychiatric emergency room admittants (Korman et al. 1980), "inhalant users differed significantly from matched other drug users in that they displayed significantly more self-directed destructive behavior, as well as some degree of recent suicidal and homicidal behavior." Cognitive measures of these groups supported the antisocial and self-destructive nature of inhalant abusers (Oetting and Webb 1992). Overall, there is accepted knowledge that long-term solvent abusers are among the most difficult to work with based on antisocial traits; also, it is likely that inhalants prevent their continued growth and development (Oetting et al. 1988, Oetting and Webb 1992).

Reports of suicides in the inhalant abusing population (Garriott 1992) raise the question of an association of mental disorders with inhalant exposure, which bears further investigation. This situation may be related to the earlier studies (Korman et al. 1981) identifying self-aggressive tendencies in inhalant abusers.

Epidemiology

An analysis of questionnaire responses of lifetime use in surveys regarding the inhalation of various products (Table 22-2) indicated that gasoline and glue were most popular (Substance Abuse and Mental Health Services Administration 2001). Also frequently mentioned are spray paints, nitrous oxide, correction fluids, and butane-type gases. A Texas high-school survey (Liu and Maxwell 2001) of lifetime use ranked correction fluids at the top with spray paint; gasoline and nitrous oxide (the rate of use of these latter substances were much lower in earlier Texas surveys) were also frequently mentioned. Glue and paint thinner are half as frequently mentioned compared to spray paint; the use of fluorocarbons even less frequently. Although fluorocarbons may be less readily available, the outbreaks of theft of air conditioner fluids (by breaking the conduit lines) and numerous deaths attributed to the inhalation abuse of these fluorocarbons indicate the use to still be a major problem (Litovitz et al. 2001). Many aerosols now use low-molecular-weight hydrocarbons (e.g., butane and propane) as the propellant instead of fluorocarbons. The fad of inhaling butane lighter and other cooking gases, as well as isobutane–propane propellants of aerosol products, in the United States and in England (Evans and Raistrick 1987a, b, Mathew et al. 1989a, Ramsey et al. 1989, Siegel and Wason 1990, Field-Smith et al. 2001) is an example that demonstrates that the replacement of one toxin with something else is not a solution for diminishing the problems of inhalation abuse. The availability of the pure gas in pressurized containers (lighter replenishers) makes it even easier to attain a desired gas without other solvents, and especially without undesired particulates in aerosols. Even medications are susceptible to misuse, as some individuals have overdosed on their asthma inhalers in order to get "high" on the fluorocarbons that are used to deliver the medication in them (Thompson et al. 1983, O'Callaghan and Milner 1988). This is one of the few marketable uses of fluorocarbons in products available for public use.

Inhalant abuse is a worldwide problem. Countries are increasingly evaluating the abuse of solvents (Smart 1988, Ramsey et al. 1989, Kozel et al. 1995). The pattern of inhalant abuse is exemplified by two national studies in the United States, the annual Monitoring the Future (Johnston et al. 2001) and National Household surveys (Substance Abuse and Mental Health Services Administration 2001), and also by state surveys such as the New York (Johnson et al. 1998) and Texas (Liu and Maxwell 2001) surveys. Also, a survey of the drug abuse problem in institutional populations (e.g., those in group homes, halfway houses, psychiatric and correctional institutions) was published as the Washington DC Metropolitan Area Drug Study: 1991 (National Institutes of Health 1994).

Current estimates of sniffing volatile substances to "get high" rank inhalants high in the "ever use" category of substance abuse, especially for the younger population. Some

Table 22-2	Inhalant Use (Percent), 2000 Data					
Solvent or Gas	Age 12–17 Yr ($n = 23,360$)		Age 18–25 Yr ($n = 28,914$)		Age 26–36 Yr ($n = 170,656$)	
	Life-1999	Life-2000	Life-1999	Life-2000	Life-1999	Life-2000
Gasoline	3.4	3.3	2.7	2.5	0.9	0.9
Spray paint	1.0	2.2	1.3	1.1	0.3	0.4
Glue or Toluene	3.8	3.9	2.4	1.9	1	1
Correction fluids	2.1	2.0	1.9	1.4	0.6	0.4
Degreaser						
Nitrous oxide	2.0	2.0	9.5	9.2	2.8	3.0
Aerosol sprays	1.8	1.7	1.4	1.3	0.4	0.5
Thinners	1.7	1.6	1.5	1.2	0.5	0.4
Butane, Propane	1.1	1.0	1.1	0.8	0.2	0.2
Organic nitrites	1.8	1.7	3.3	2.7	3.6	3.2

Source: Data from Substance Abuse and Mental Health Services Administration (2001) *National Household Survey on Drug Abuse: Population Estimates 2000*. US Government Printing Office, Washington, DC. http://www.samhsa.gov/oas/2k2/inhalNS/inhalNS.cfm.

surveys of teenage use showed that one in six had tried an inhalant and that over 2,20,000 persons of the US population had done so in the past month during the year 2000 (Substance Abuse and Mental Health Services Administration 2001, Johnston et al. 2001). As many as 20,000 to 40,000 youth got high on inhalants several times a month. Some of the highest rates were noted for 8th graders (Edwards 1993) (Table 22-3). Although the "ever use" rate for 8th graders exceeded that for marijuana in 1993, the reverse is now reported. Adults also use inhalants at a lower rate than observed for the youthful population and they seem more selective in the products they use. Nitrous oxide and organic nitrites are two types of substances abused more by adult populations; the reason for inhaling appears to be for different purposes. Thus, the rate of "ever use" of nitrous oxide by the 18 to 25 age group is twice that noted in the last review in 1993.

Toxicology of Inhalant Abuse

The majority of inhalant abusers are never seen in a hospital or outpatient facility. Although many do not need medical attention for their inhalant habit, of those who do, many often die before reaching the hospital as a result of asphyxia, cardiac arrhythmia, or related overdose effects after inhaling fluorocarbons, low-molecular-weight hydrocarbon gases (butane, propane), nitrous oxide, or other solvents including toluene during either the first or a subsequent episode (Bass 1970, Wason et al. 1986, Ramsey et al. 1989,

Table 22-3	Inhalant Use (Percent), Data					
	High School* Year 2001			Household[†] Year 2000		
	8th Grade	10th Grade	12th Grade	Age 12–17 Yr ($n = 23,360$)	Age 18–25 Yr ($n = 28,914$)	Age 26–36 Yr ($n = 170,656$)
Lifetime	17.1	15.2	13.0	8.9	12.8	6.4
Annual	9.1	6.6	4.5	3.5	2.4	0.2
30-day	4.0	2.4	1.7	1.0	0.6	0.1

Source: *Johnston LD, O'Malley PM, and Bachman JG (2001) *Monitoring the future national survey results on drug use, 1994–2001*. National Institute on Drug Abuse. US Government Printing Office, Washington, DC. http://monitoringthefuture.org/; [†]Substance Abuse and Mental Health Services Administration (2001) *National Household Survey on Drug Abuse: Population Estimates 2000*. US Government Printing Office, Washington, DC. http://www.samhsa.gov/oas/nhsda/2kdetailedtabs/Vol_1_Part_1/sect1v1.htm#1.2a, http://www.samhsa.gov/centers/clearinghouse/clearinghouses.html.

Al-Alousi 1989, Siegel and Wason 1990, Garriott 1992, Fitzgerald et al. 1993, Groppi et al. 1994, Broussard et al. 1997, Rohrig 1997, Bowen et al. 1999, Hobara et al. 2000, Field-Smith et al. 2001, Beauvais et al. 2002). Death may also occur after inhalation of toluene-containing substances as a result of metabolic acidosis or related kidney failure if left untreated (Garriott 1992). Although it is not common, anesthetics abused by medical personnel or others have also been a cause of death; death related to nitrous oxide use is often due to asphyxia (Clark et al. 1985, Suruda and McGlothlin 1990, Wagner et al. 1992). Some of the more common acute syndromes of the intoxicated state are listed in Table 22-4.

Neurotoxic Manifestations

Chronic high-level exposure to organic solvents occurs in the inhalant abuse setting at levels several thousand times higher than in the occupational setting and results in numerous irreversible disease states. Some toxicities have been validated through animal studies; others have been only tentatively correlated with certain substances. Table 22-5 describes several well-characterized disorders and identifies the solvent when corroborated by animal studies. Some substances have been strongly correlated with the development of a disorder through numerous case studies. The following discussion briefly describes these conditions and the important associated symptoms.

The nervous system may be affected at many levels by organic solvents as well as other neurotoxic substances. Because of their nonfocal presentation, neurotoxic disorders may be confused with metabolic, degenerative, nutritional, or demyelinating diseases (Schaumburg and Spencer 1987). This is illustrated in the setting of chronic toluene abuse, which clinically may resemble the multifocal demyelinating disease, multiple sclerosis, in the findings on neurological examination (Lazar et al. 1983, Fornazzari et al. 1983, Hormes et al. 1986). In addition, neurotoxic syndromes rarely have specific identifying features on diagnostic tests such as computed tomography, magnetic resonance imaging (MRI), or nerve conduction studies (Schaumburg and Spencer 1987). As a result, subjects who only inhale for a limited time or to a limited extent may be difficult to diagnose. High-level chronic inhalant abuse, on the other hand, produces a specific MRI picture with a combination of diffuse white matter changes and low signal intensity in the basal ganglia and thalamus (Rosenberg et al.

Table 22-4	Symptoms Related to Solvent Abuse (Not All for Gases and Nitrites)

Moderate Intoxication
Dizziness
Headache
Lethargy
Disorientation, incoherence
Ataxia, gait (uncoordinated movement)
Odoriferous, foul breath (solvent vapors)

Strong Intoxication
Blurred vision
Belligerence
Nausea, vomiting
Irritability
Delirium
Slurred speech

Severe (Rare)
Seizures
Violent actions

able 22-5	**Diseases Observed in Humans After Chronic Inhalant Abuse**		
ondition	Syndrome	Substance	Animal Studies*
Slowly Reversible and/or Irreversible Syndromes			
ncephalopathy	Cognitive dysfunction	"Toluene,"[†] other solvents	—
erebellar syndrome	Limb dysmetria	"Toluene"	Rat
	Dysarthria		—
ensorineural optic ensorineural	High-frequency hearing loss	TCE, toluene	Rat, mouse
ptic nerve	Visual loss	"Toluene"	—
culomotor	Oculomotor disturbances (nystagmus)	Xylene, TCE	Rabbits
Iyeloneuropathy	Sensory loss Spasticity	Nitrous oxide	Rat, mouse
xonal neuropathy	Distal sensory loss, limb weakness	Hexane, methyl butyl ketone	Rat, monkey
ardiotoxicity	Arrhythmia	Chlorofluorocarbons, butanes, propanes	Mouse, rat, dog
eukemia	Myelocytic	Benzene	Rat, mouse
Mostly Reversible Syndromes			
rigeminal neuropathy	Numbness, paresthesia	TCE and/or dichloroacetylene	Rat
.enal acidosis	Metabolic acidosis Hypokalemia	"Toluene"	Rat —
arboxyhemoglobin	Hypoxia	Methylene chloride, tobacco	Human, rat
Iethemoglobinemia	Syncope, blue	Nitrites, organic	Rat
leonatal syndrome	Retarded growth, development	"Toluene"	Rat
lepatotoxicity	Fatty vacuoles, plasma liver enzymes	Chlorohydrocarbons	Rat
mmunomodulatory	Loss of immune cell function	Nitrites, organic	Rat

mptoms observed in animal studies with these solvents.
.1otation marks around substance indicates uncertainty about this solvent (alone) producing these symptoms.

1988a, Caldmeyer et al. 1993, Unger et al. 1994, Yamanouchi et al. 1995, 1997, Kamran and Bakshi 1998, Rosenberg et al. 2002).

Many organic solvents produce nonspecific effects (e.g., encephalopathy) after exposure to extremely high concentrations; a few produce relatively specific neurological syndromes with chronic administration. Two specific neurotoxic syndromes, a peripheral neuropathy and an ototoxicity, are well correlated with organic solvents. Most common, however, is a clinical syndrome consisting of cognitive impairment, cerebellar ataxia, and spasticity syndrome (Lazar et al. 1983, Fornazzari et al. 1983, Hormes et al. 1986). In addition, a myopathy may occur alone or in combination with any of these clinical syndromes.

Encephalopathy Grabski (1961) first reported a case of persistent neurological consequences of chronic inhalation of toluene-containing solvents; this was further described by Knox and Nelson (1966). Other types of severe neurotoxicity were subsequently described, including cognitive dysfunction (Lazar et al. 1983, Fornazzari et al. 1983, Hormes et al. 1986, Kamran and Bakshi 1998) and cerebellar ataxia (Boor and Hurtig 1977, Malm and Lying-Tunell 1980, Streicher et al. 1981, Takeuchi et al. 1981, Lazar et al. 1983, Fornazzari et al. 1983). This encephalopathy was characterized using computed tomography (Schikler et al. 1982, Fornazzari et al. 1983) and, more extensively, MRI (Rosenberg et al. 1988b,

Filley et al. 1990, Ikeda and Tsukagoshi 1990, Poungvarin 1991, Xiong et al. 1993, Cald-meyer et al. 1993, Kornfeld et al. 1994, Yamanouchi et al. 1995, 1997, Kamran and Bakshi 1998, Rosenberg et al. 2002). The most common syndrome is that of multifocal CNS involvement (Streicher et al. 1981, Metrick and Brenner 1982, Schikler et al. 1982, Fornaz-zari et al. 1983, Hormes et al. 1986, Rosenberg et al. 1988b, Poungvarin 1991, Xiong et al. 1993, Caldmeyer et al. 1993); in only one study was abstinence documented before clin-ical evaluation (Hormes et al. 1986). Abstinence from solvent use is necessary to not have intoxication symptoms interfering with neurologic measures. Microencephalopathy is now emerging as a possible embryopathic syndrome in infants of women exposed during preg-nancy to solvents containing toluene (Arnold et al. 1994, Pearson et al. 1994).

Most reports emphasized the cerebellar and cognitive dysfunction, with most cases showing combined impairment of cerebral and cerebellar functions as well as pyramidal changes. Neurological abnormalities varied from mild cognitive impairment to severe dementia, associated with elemental neurological signs such as cerebellar ataxia, corti-cospinal tract dysfunction, oculomotor abnormalities, tremor, deafness, and hyposmia. Cognitive dysfunction was the most disabling and frequent feature of chronic toluene toxi-city and may be the earliest sign of permanent damage. Dementia, when present, was typically associated with cerebellar ataxia and other signs (Hormes et al. 1986).

Rosenberg and colleagues (1988b, 2002) utilized MRI to study the brains of chronic abusers of toluene-containing substances and interpreted the encephalopathy as a diffuse CNS white matter change with the following abnormalities: (1) diffuse cerebral, cerebellar, and brain stem atrophy; (2) loss of differentiation of the gray and white matter throughout the CNS; and (3) increased periventricular white matter signal intensity on T2-weighted images (Filley et al. 1990). These MRI measures seemed to correlate with the extent of exposure and the impairment of the individual's capabilities as measured on several neuropsychological tests (Filley et al. 1990). Others (Xiong et al. 1993, Caldmeyer et al. 1993, Yamanouchi et al. 1995, 1997, Kamran and Bakshi 1998) corroborated these findings.

MRI results (Unger et al. 1994) may suggest a possible mechanism for the abnormalities in the basal ganglia and thalamus. The MRI analyses of eight chronic toluene abusers revealed diffuse white matter changes and marked hypointensity in the basal ganglia and thalamus, all seen on T2-weighted images. Thus, the hypointensity of the basal ganglia and thalamus on T2-weighted magnetic resonance images of brains of chronic toluene abusers may be related to partitioning of toluene into the lipid membranes in these areas. An interaction of toluene with GABAergic systems has also been studied.

Few detailed pathological studies have been done (Escobar and Aruffo 1980, Rosenberg et al. 1988a, Kornfeld et al. 1994). The predominant feature in these studies is that of a leukoencephalopathy. A study of three cases (Kornfeld et al. 1994)—one of which was previously reported by Rosenberg and colleagues (1988)—found pathological changes similar to those in adrenoleukodystrophy, a rare hereditary disorder affecting the white matter. Gross pathological study revealed a patchy loss of myelin. The overall pathological study revealed a demyelinating process grossly manifest as brain atrophy, including macrophages containing unusual cytoplasmic bodies with an increase of long-chain fatty acids similar to that seen in adrenoleukodystrophy (Kornfeld et al. 1994). These findings suggest that toluene is a white matter toxin.

Toxicities similar to those already noted may be caused by tetraethyllead (or its metabolite triethyllead) after prolonged or extensive inhalation of gasoline (Robinson 1978, Seshia et al. 1978, Valpey et al. 1978, Coodin et al. 1980, Prockop and Karampelas 1981, Goldings and Stewart 1982, Remington and Hoffman 1984, Eastwell 1985, Reese and Kimbrough 1993, Goodheart and Dunne 1994, Maruff et al. 1998). It is less clear whether unleaded gasoline, which contains some of the previously described solvents, produces similar encephalopathies. In cases in which high lead levels are observed, hallucinations

Table 22-6	Mostly Irreversible Syndromes Caused by Chronic Inhalant Use Observed in Humans	
Condition	Syndrome	Substance
Encephalopathy	Cognitive dysfunction, possible delirium, possible seizures	Lead (gasoline)
Cerebellar syndrome	Limb dysmetria, dysarthria, truncal ataxia, tremors	Lead (gasoline)
Sensorineural (optic)	Nystagmus	Lead (gasoline)
Peripheral nerves	Possible slower nerve conduction	

and disorientation, dysarthria, chorea, and convulsions have been reported (Table 22-6). The symptoms have also included moderate to severe ataxia, insomnia, anorexia, slowed peripheral nerve conduction, limb tremors, dysmetria, and sometimes limb paralysis. In most cases, the electroencephalogram is normal, but in severe states, an abnormal to severely depressed cortical electroencephalogram is observed. Because many of these symptoms in the early stages of the disease can be reversed by chelation therapy with ethylenediaminetetraacetic acid, dimercaprol, or penicillamine, it is important to check the serum lead levels in any chronic inhalant abuser.

Ototoxicity   Sensorineural hearing loss (Rybak 1992) is one of the more commonly occurring clinical neurotoxic syndromes related to inhalant abuse, along with a related equilibrium disorder (Sasa et al. 1978). Neural conduction, most readily diagnosed by brain stem auditory evoked responses, was abnormal in several case studies (Biscaldi et al. 1981, Metrick and Brenner 1982, Lazar et al. 1983, Ehyai and Freemon 1983, Rosenberg et al. 1988b, Morrow et al. 1992). These studies suggest that brain stem auditory evoked responses would detect early CNS injury related to toluene or other solvent inhalation at a time when the neurological examination and MRI scans are normal. Brain stem auditory evoked responses may be a sensitive screening test for monitoring individuals at risk from toluene exposure and for early detection of CNS injury. However, although specific in revealing abnormalities characteristic of CNS involvement in chronic inhalant abuse, brain stem auditory evoked responses revealed abnormalities in less than 10 individuals of a chronic inhalant abuse population (Levisohn et al. 1992).

The hearing loss was originally classified as one of high frequency (it probably still is for humans). It is now more clearly delineated as a midfrequency hearing loss when measured in rats exposed to solvents (Crofton and Zhao 1993, Jaspers et al. 1993). A recent study of rats observed no change in the outer hair cells after exposure to TCE but revealed a loss of spiral ganglion cells in the middle turn of hair cells (Fechter et al. 1998). As hearing loss has been identified in humans, more careful studies of those affected might clarify the nature of the problem.

This neuropathy can be produced in days after high exposures of animals to specific solvents and is considered to originate with the destruction of cochlear cells, which contributes to a central conduction pathology as observed in the human studies noted earlier (Pryor et al. 1983, Rebert et al. 1983, 1991). Because of the quantitative animal model available, Pryor's group (Pryor 1995) has conducted a structure–activity study of many solvents in an effort to define the basic moiety responsible. Table 22-7 lists the different compounds and their activities. Niklasson and colleagues (1993) also analyzed the effects of some of these compounds on the vestibular function and correlated the changes with nystagmus in humans.

Table 22-7	Auditory Response After Exposure to Different Solvents
Solvent	**Hearing Loss**
Benzene	No
Toluene	Yes
Ethylbenzene	Yes
n-Propylbenzene	Yes
Isopropylbenzene (cumene)	No
Methoxybenzene	Yes
1,4-Dimethylbenzene (*p*-xylene)	Yes
1,2-Dimethylbenzene (*o*-xylene)	No
1,3-Dimethylbenzene (*m*-xylene)	No
Styrene	Yes
Monochlorobenzene	Yes
Carbon disulfide	Yes
Dichloromethane	No
Trichloroethane	No
TCE	Yes
Tetrachloroethylene	No
Acetone	No
Methyl ethyl ketone	No
Ethyl alcohol	No
n-Hexane	No

Other Cranial Nerve Involvement A study of four subjects (Maas et al. 1991) supported earlier observations of pendular nystagmus and related eye movement disorders in sniffers of various solvents. Oculomotor dysfunction and tremor were seen only in severely affected individuals (Hormes et al. 1986). Optical neuropathy (Keane 1978, Takeuchi et al. 1981, Ehyai and Freemon 1983, Channer and Stanley 1983, Rosenberg et al. 1988a, Takeuchi 1988, Kiyokawa et al. 1999) and oculomotor dysfunction (Lazar et al. 1983, Maas et al. 1991, Poblano et al. 2000) have been observed after exposure to toluene-containing substances, pupillary damage after exposure to TCE (Feldman et al. 1985), and optical neuritis after methyl ethyl ketone (MEK) exposure (Berg 1971). Hollo and Varga (1992) suggested that visual function measures may be useful in detecting early toxic effects in solvent abusers. All of these neuropathies can be identified with specific cranial nerves (Table 22-8).

These changes have yet to be specifically correlated with TCE or other chemicals (Odkvist et al. 1980). Optic damage needs to be corroborated through animal studies. A study of the effects of TCE exposure in rabbits for 12 weeks measured a decreased amplitude of visual evoked responses; the responses slowly returned to normal 6 weeks after exposure (Blain et al. 1992).

Hexane is not usually considered a CNS toxin; however, some clinical studies have indicated that *n*-hexane affects the CNS. Also, experimental animal studies have shown

Table 22-8	Cranial Nerve Abnormalities Noted in Inhalant Abuse
Cranial Nerve	**Dysfunction**
I	Hyposmia, anosmia
II	Optic neuropathy
III, IV, VI	Oculomotor disorders: nystagmus, opsoclonus, ocular dysmetria
VIII	Sensorineural hearing loss

that *n*-hexane causes axonal degeneration in the CNS (Schaumburg and Spencer 1976, Bruhn et al. 1981, Frontali et al. 1981). Clinically, cranial neuropathy, spasticity, and autonomic dysfunction occasionally occur (Altenkirch et al. 1982). Of all these possible actions, animal studies have demonstrated only the optical-toxic effects of 2,5-hexanedione, a toxic metabolite of hexane, in rats (Backstrom and Collins 1992). Until these issues are further clarified through human and animal studies, *n*-hexane should be primarily considered a peripheral nervous system toxin.

Anosmia is an often described syndrome of inhalant abuse. It would be expected that solvents would diminish the olfactory responses; however, it has seldom been studied. Mergler and Beauvais (1992) found that olfactory perception was reduced after 7 hours of exposure to toluene and returned to normal a couple of hours after cessation of exposure. Anosmia or hyposmia was detected on clinical examination utilizing simple bedside measures in chronic inhalant abusers (Hormes et al. 1986).

Trigeminal Neuropathy One neurological manifestation associated with TCE intoxication is a slowly reversible trigeminal neuropathy (Ruijten et al. 1991, Feldman et al. 1992). Cranial neuropathies were noted after general anesthesia with TCE more than 40 years ago. Individuals developed paresthesia around the lips, which then spread to involve the entire trigeminal distribution bilaterally. Motor weakness also occasionally occurred. Resolution of the trigeminal neuropathy occurs slowly, which is thought to indicate segmental or nuclear trigeminal involvement.

There has been a long-term controversy about whether or not unmetabolized TCE causes trigeminal neuralgia or if the neurotoxicity is due to dichloroacetylene, an environmental breakdown product of TCE (Laureno 1993, Lash and green 1993). The incidence of trigeminal neuralgia in humans can be disputed; however, animal studies do demonstrate the production of trigeminal neuralgia by TCE, as well as dichloroacetylene (Barret et al. 1992). There are no reports of trigeminal neuropathy noted for solvent abusers despite common inhalation of TCE from different products (Levy 1986).

Myeloneuropathy Nitrous oxide is not an organic solvent; however, it is widely abused by adolescents (Schwartz and Calihan 1984, Wagner et al. 1992), adults (Wagner et al. 1992, Brett 1997, Butzkueven and King 2000), and professional personnel (Jastak 1991, Vishnubhakat and Beresford 1991, Gillman 1992). Nitrous oxide is a common anesthetic widely used in dentistry; it is also used as a propellant for whipped cream. High levels of nitrous oxide exposure produce a myeloneuropathy with both central and peripheral components, even in the presence of adequate oxygen (Layzer 1978, Pema et al. 1998, Maze and Fujinaga 2000). The symptoms include numbness and weakness in the limbs, loss of dexterity, sensory loss, and loss of balance. The early neurological features indicate sensorimotor polyneuropathy; however, with persistent abuse, a myelopathy with severe spasticity may develop. There is also a combined degeneration of the posterior and lateral columns of the spinal cord resembling that in vitamin B_{12} deficiency (Layzer 1978). Studies focusing on the mechanism of this action indicate that cobalamins (vitamin B_{12}) are inactivated by nitrous oxide, primarily at the level of the enzyme methionine synthase, which needs vitamin B_{12} to function (Nunn 1987). This enzyme is important in the maintenance of the myelin sheath (Flippo and Holder 1993). Flippo and Holder (1993) noted that paresthesia and other neuropathic symptoms resulting from spinal cord degeneration were produced after prolonged anesthesia in vitamin B_{12}-deficient individuals. Administration of vitamin B_{12} (or folinic acid) dramatically aids recovery of these surgical patients and may assist recovery in solvent abusers (Vishnubhakat and Beresford 1991), especially once the myelopathy appears. The use of methionine should also be considered (Fujinaga and Baden 1994). Recent studies have identified the role of GABA receptors in mediating these neurologic actions; thus, use of GABA agonists may be useful in some treatment regimens (Maze and Fujinaga 2000, Jevtovic-Todorovic et al. 2000).

In regard to dependence on nitrous oxide, studies of mice selectively bred for alcohol dependence showed a cross-dependence on nitrous oxide (Belknap et al. 1987). These studies also observed handling-induced convulsions shortly after cessation of nitrous oxide, which could be prevented by either alcohol or nitrous oxide. This might indicate a physical dependence on nitrous oxide that needs to be dealt with in treatment of this drug abuse state.

Peripheral Neuropathy Two organic solvents were identified as neurotoxins after an investigation of peripheral neuropathies in an industrial setting when the solvent methyl isobutyl ketone was replaced by methyl butyl ketone (MBK) (Allen et al. 1975). Cases of *n*-hexane polyneuropathy have been reported both after occupational exposure (Herskowitz et al. 1971, Mendell et al. 1974, Mallov 1976) and after deliberate inhalation of vapors from products containing *n*-hexane such as glues (Gonzalez and Downey 1972, Goto et al. 1974, Korobkin et al. 1975, Means et al. 1976, Oh and Kim 1976, Towfighi et al. 1976, King et al. 1985b, Dittmer et al. 1993, Takeuchi 1993), gasoline (Gallassi et al. 1980, Hall et al. 1986), and naphtha (Tenenbein et al. 1984). Both *n*-hexane and MBK (Menkes 1976) are metabolized to the same neurotoxin, 2,5-hexanedione, and produce a peripheral neuropathy. 2,5-Hexanedione is responsible for most, if not all, of the neurotoxic effects of exposure to *n*-hexane or MBK (Spencer et al. 1980, Graham et al. 1982). MEK alone produces neither clinical nor pathological evidence of a peripheral neuropathy in experimental animals (Spencer et al. 1980); however, it acts synergistically with MBK or *n*-hexane in experimental animals and probably in humans (Saida et al. 1976, Altenkirch et al. 1978, 1982, Ichihara et al. 1998). This potentiation of toxicity of one compound (MBK or *n*-hexane) by an otherwise nontoxic compound (MEK) underscores the difficulty in sorting out toxic effects of individual solvents contained in a mixture.

Clinically and pathologically, the neuropathy occurring with *n*-hexane or MBK is that of a distal axonopathy (Schaumburg and Spencer 1976). The clinical syndrome is an initially painless sensorimotor polyneuropathy, which begins after chronic exposure; weight loss may be an early symptom. Sensory and motor disturbances are noted initially in the hands and feet, and sensory loss involves primarily small fiber sensation (i.e., light touch, pin prick, temperature) with relative sparing of large fiber sensation (i.e., position and vibration). Electrophysiological studies reveal an axonal polyneuropathy and pathologically multifocal axonal degeneration, multiple axonal swellings, and neurofilamentous accumulation at paranodal areas (Spencer et al. 1975). Overlying the axonal swellings, thinning of the myelin sheath occurs. These findings are typical of a distal axonopathy or dying-back neuropathy described in relation to other toxic and metabolic causes of peripheral neuropathy.

Prognosis for recovery correlates directly with the intensity and duration of the toxic exposure and the severity of the neuropathy. Residual neuropathy is seen only in the most severely affected individuals with motor as well as sensory involvement, some of whom still continue to inhale despite warnings of further debilitation.

Nonnervous System Toxicity

Most of the known adverse clinical effects of inhalant abuse relate to its effects on the nervous system. There are, however, other significant adverse effects on other organ systems including the kidney, liver, lung, heart, and hemopoietic systems.

Renal Toxicity Some time ago, Gabow (Streicher et al. 1981) and others (Bennett and Forman 1980, Will and McLaren 1981) described the effects of toluene-containing substances on the kidneys, which often result in hospitalization of inhalant abusers. Young people present with renal disease most often; however, adults do so also after sniffing glue, spray paint, and other solvent products (Miller et al. 1985, Patel and Benjamin 1986, Batlle et al. 1988, Davidman and Schmitz 1988, Jone and Wu 1988, Marjot and McLeod 1989, Mizutani et al. 1989, Nelson et al. 1990, Carlisle et al. 1991, Gupta et al. 1991, Wilkins-Haug and Gabow 1991, Kaneko et al. 1992, Caravati 1997).

This dysfunction, which may rapidly reappear in individuals who return to their habit after release from the hospital, is characterized by hyperchloremic metabolic acidosis, hypokalemia, hypocalcemia, and other electrolyte imbalances. Solvents usually cause a unique distal-type tubular acidosis, but proximal tubules are also affected (the distal tubule is responsible for the known electrolyte and metabolic imbalance; the proximal type is responsible for the wasting of amino acids and other proteins). These subjects often have associated gastrointestinal involvement, including nausea, vomiting, and severe abdominal cramps. Severe rhabdomyolysis may render some subjects nearly paralyzed. Other renal disorders related to solvents were reviewed by Lauwerys and colleagues (1985), and cases of glomerulonephritis in commercial settings (painters, degreasers) were described by Daniell and coworkers (1988). An unusual, possibly high-risk category of individuals with diabetes who might present with both acetone (not from a solvent) and other solvents in their breaths in an unconscious state at the emergency department are of concern (Brown et al. 1991). This may cover up the diabetic coma. In addition to the other disease states, an interstitial nephritis leading to renal failure has been reported by Taverner and associates (1988).

On the basis of these reports, renal dysfunction appears to be one of the most common toxic effects noted for solvent abusers. Although this renal damage is usually reversible, other organs, particularly brain, are the target of repetitive acidosis and any depletion of important amino acids. This may be the basis for some of the observed neurological deficits (Yamamoto et al. 1992).

Of all the solvents, toluene is most often correlated with this disease; however, other solvents, including chlorinated hydrocarbons, are frequently the basis for renal disease in these populations. Further animal studies are necessary to clarify specific solvent toxicities similar to those associated with nephrotic changes after exposure to halogenated hydrocarbons (Kimbrough et al. 1985, Lock 1989) and petroleum hydrocarbons (Short et al. 1987).

Clinicians especially need to be alert for pregnant women who abuse these solvents. Not only do they present to the clinic with renal tubular acidosis but the fetuses are also affected (Goodwin 1988, Lindemann 1991, Wilkins-Haug 1997). This condition places the mother at risk for hypokalemia and associated cardiac dysrhythmias and rhabdomyolysis (Wilkins-Haug 1997). Preterm labor therapy (β-mimetics and intravenous fluids) exacerbated the maternal and fetal problems. Fatty livers may also be observed in these pregnant subjects (Paraf et al. 1993). Treatment for their metabolic imbalance needs immediate attention.

For pregnant women as well as other individuals, electrolyte repletion usually restores the kidney function and eliminates the muscle spasms even in the more severely affected individuals in a few days. Correction of salt and electrolyte imbalance, including potassium, calcium, magnesium, phosphate, and bicarbonate (Davidman and Schmitz 1988, Wilkins-Haug and Gabow 1991), is important and may be considered in the treatment of solvent abusers for muscle fatigue even in the absence of more severe kidney disorders. Caution about the use of bicarbonate early in the treatment of these subjects has been discussed by Lavoie and coworkers (1987).

Hepatotoxicity Chlorohydrocarbons (e.g., TCE, chloroform, carbon tetrachloride, halo-thane, methylene chloride) have been noted to be hepatotoxic (Litt and Cohen 1969, Clearfield 1970, Baerg and Kimberg 1970, Benjamin et al. 1985, Farrell et al. 1985, Hutchens and Kung 1985, Mizutani et al. 1988, Hodgson et al. 1989, Hakim et al. 1992, Stewart and Witts 1993, Koporec et al. 1995, Yamanouchi et al. 1997, Soni et al. 1998,

Chang et al. 1999, Omae et al. 2000). In animals, acetone and more complex ketones potentiate this halocarbon hepatotoxicity (Plaa 1988).

Inhalation of correction fluids (Greer 1984), which contain TCE and trichloroethanes and tetrachloroethanes (Ong et al. 1993), increases the likelihood of these toxicities in inhalant abusers. Methylene chloride may be hepatotoxic (Cordes et al. 1988, Chang et al. 1999) as reported after ingestion or abuse and is a solvent in thinners and other inhalants. Also, a user of butanes, who also added carburetor cleaner to his repertoire, presented with "fatal fulminant hepatic failure" (McIntyre and Long 1992); this raises the possibility that there are other hepatotoxicities that go undetected in inhalant users.

Pulmonary Toxicity   Solvents do irritate the lungs; however, few pulmonary problems have been reported (Devathasan et al. 1984). In two studies, mild pulmonary hypertension, acute respiratory distress, increased airway resistance and residual volume, and restricted ventilation were noted. Increased airway resistance or residual volume may be more clearly noted after an exercise challenge (Schikler et al. 1984, Reyes de la Rocha et al. 1987). An increase in the frequency of respiratory (viral) illnesses, often noted in clinical reports, may be related to solvent exposure. In Australia (Currie et al. 1994), aspiration pneumonia was noted as a major cause of death in aboriginal sniffers. In sniffers in the United States, aspiration pneumonia has not been a major cause of death. How to generalize the impact of dual exposure to solvent and infection is uncertain, but animal studies have measured decreased pulmonary bactericidal activity after exposure to solvents (e.g., dichloroethylene) (Sherwood et al. 1987). Animal studies have also measured pulmonary fibrosis in mice after solvent (TCE) (Forkert and Forkert 1994) exposure. Also, a recent outbreak of respiratory illnesses has been associated with the leather treatment process using specific fluorocarbon aerosolized sprays (Hubbs et al. 1997).

Any pulmonary change may not be readily detected early on; it also may be enhanced by the other substances volatilized along with the solvent (e.g., polystyrenes, tars), utilized by the individual (e.g., tobacco and marijuana), or related to other conditions (Cartwright et al. 1983). Because of the potential for cause and augmentation by other substances, the amount of smoking should always be considered in any treatment of these individuals.

Cardiotoxicity   One of the most common causes of solvent-induced deaths is cardiac arrhythmia, especially ventricular fibrillation and cardiac arrest (Wright and Strobl 1984, King et al. 1985a, Boon 1987, Cunningham et al. 1987, McLeod et al. 1987, Zakhari and Salem 1991, Ong et al. 1988, Bowen et al. 1999). Bass (1970) reported deaths related to fluorocarbons; subsequently, fluorocarbons were demonstrated to cause arrhythmias in animals (Taylor and Harris 1970). Since then, most fluorocarbon propellants have been replaced by butanes and propane. However, similar arrhythmias were observed after the abuse of these newly designed aerosols (with butanes etc.), lighter (gas) fluids, and cooking gases (Bass 1984, Siegel and Wason 1990, Roberts et al. 1990). Chenoweth (1977) has shown that butane, hexane, heptanes, gasoline, some anesthetics, and toluene also produce these arrhythmias. Although less common, glue sniffing exposure (Cunningham et al. 1987, Knight et al. 1991, Wernisch et al. 1991) and TCE-containing stain removers (Wright and Strobl 1984, Hantson et al. 1990) have been linked to arrhythmias, myocarditis, and cardiac arrest. Organic nitrites have also been reported to produce bradycardia (Rosoff and Cohen 1986).

When arrhythmias are observed, antiarrhythmic therapy should be used (McLeod et al. 1987). Recovery from cardiopulmonary arrest is not common; however, a successful resuscitation from fluorocarbon overexposure has been reported (Brilliant and Grillo 1993). Cardiopulmonary resuscitation (mouth to mouth) followed by electrodefibrillation within

7 minutes was the primary aspect of the emergency treatment. Exercise and epinephrine exacerbate these cardiotoxicities.

Hematopoietic Toxicity

Of great concern are the incidences of neoplasm in solvent abusers. A common solvent, benzene, has long been identified as causing aplastic anemia and acute myelocytic leukemia (Austin et al. 1988, Yardley-Jones et al. 1991). Benzene is present in thinners, varnish removers and other solvents, and gasoline, which may lead to various neoplasms (Lauwerys et al. 1985, Knight et al. 1991). On the basis of the release of the nitrite ion in blood after the administration of organic nitrites, the ability to produce nitrosamines has fueled the speculation that nitrites are carcinogenic (Osterloh and Goldfield 1984, Mirvish and Haverkos 1987, Yamamoto et al. 1987, Dunkel et al. 1989).

Also of concern are the hematological changes caused by various solvents, most of which are reversible because of the regenerative nature of red blood cells. Carbon monoxide, at high levels, produces cerebral hypoxia, which may subsequently have permanent neurological sequelae; it also produces carboxyhemoglobin. This occurs with exposure to a common solvent, methylene chloride (Horowitz 1986, Chang et al. 1999), as well as to cigarette smoke. The acute elevation of carboxyhemoglobin after exposure to methylene chloride has been studied in controlled experiments in humans (Stewart et al. 1972, Gamberale et al. 1975, Winneke 1981). The elevation is a result of the metabolism of the solvent methylene chloride to carbon monoxide (Stewart and Fisher 1972, Kubic et al. 1974, Ratney et al. 1974, Astrand et al. 1975), and therefore the hypoxic effect of carbon monoxide as well as its narcotic actions must be taken into account in considering the actions of methylene chloride. The levels of carboxyhemoglobin may become sufficiently high to cause brain damage (Barrowcliff and Knell 1979) or death (Manno et al. 1989).

One group of substances—the organic nitrites—produces a different hematological change, the formation of methemoglobin and hemolytic anemia (Wason et al. 1980, Brandes et al. 1989). This group of substances includes the volatile liquids amyl, butyl, isopropyl, and cyclohexyl organic nitrites. These drugs are not the typical solvents of most solvent abusers. A study could not correlate changes in regional blood flow with any psychological measures or somatic changes (Mathew et al. 1989b); also, isoamyl nitrite did not substitute for barbiturates as a reinforcing agent as do toluene and other solvents (Rees et al. 1987). These studies do not offer any explanation for why individuals become dependent on nitrites. However, the finding by Mathew and colleagues (1989b) that nitrites reduce anger, fatigue, and depression may offer a clue.

The nitrites are not usually considered toxic during inhalation because of syncope (fainting), and overdose is unlikely. However, Guss and coworkers (1985) noted a dangerously high methemoglobin level in a normal subject who had used isobutyl nitrite. Methemoglobinemia is the major identified toxicity of organic nitrites and is the cause of several deaths (Wood and Cox 1981). However, there is a specific treatment for nitrite overdose. The high and slowly reversible reduction of methemoglobin can be aided by the use of methylene blue (Smith et al. 1980).

Organic nitrites have also been reported to alter immune function as measured by direct lymphocytic actions (Soderberg and Barnett 1995) or in whole-animal studies (Gaworski et al. 1992). These effects are of special concern in the development of acquired immunodeficiency syndrome (AIDS). Haverkos and associates (1994) reviewed the possible link between the development of Kaposi's sarcoma and high amyl or butyl nitrite use. Seage and colleagues (1992), however, proposed that the link is related to enhancement of the accessibility of the human immunodeficiency virus.

Early studies did not show major effects of organic nitrites on isolated immune or bacterial cells (Lewis and Lynch 1988, Jacobs et al. 1983); however, studies by Soderberg's group (Soderberg and Barnett 1995) showed that isobutyl nitrite inhalation resulted in disruption of T-dependent immune mechanisms, including the induction of antibodies and cytotoxic T-cells and of macrophage tumoricidal activity. This loss of immunity depended on habitual exposure and lasted for up to 5 to 7 days after exposures were terminated. The inhalant apparently produces this immunotoxicity by altering accessory cell functions, probably macrophage functions.

Neonatal Syndrome   Newborns of mothers who chronically abuse solvents (Hersh 1989, Hersh et al. 1985, Goodwin 1988, Donald et al. 1991, Wilkins-Haug 1997) present with abnormal growth similar to that in the fetal alcohol syndrome. The mothers inhaled paint thinner and paint sprays and some also drank various quantities of alcohol. Thus, toluene may augment the fetal alcohol syndrome when alcohol is also consumed. It is also worth noting that the mothers of the infants in one (Hersh 1989) study showed ataxia, mild tremors, and slurred speech, and the mothers in the other studies presented with severe renal tubular acidosis. Newborns of these women showed growth retardation and some dysmorphic features including microcephaly and also distal acidosis and aminoaciduria (Wilkins-Haug 1997, Lindemann 1991). Some of these abnormalities were also observed in rodents exposed to toluene (Donald et al. 1991); however, the extent and severity of the effects are unclear. Embryonic death may result from high doses of these solvents.

Nitrous oxide has been shown to produce some "major visceral and minor skeletal (fetal) abnormalities" (Mazze et al. 1988). Also, animal studies demonstrated fetal toxicities of the liver caused by carbon tetrachloride (Cagen and Klaassen 1979) and malformations by chloroform (Murray et al. 1979). It is thus important that pregnant women not be exposed to high concentrations of solvents. It is encouraging to know that a critical prospective study of female workers exposed to low levels of solvent showed no more fetal abnormalities than in the carefully matched control subjects (Eskenazi et al. 1988). This does not, however, diminish the need for pregnant women to avoid exposure to most solvents, especially at the high levels incurred through deliberate abuse.

Treatment

Individuals need different treatments based on the severity of the dependence and any medical complications. Primary care physicians should address the medical issues identified earlier as well as other medical concerns before dealing with the dependence on solvents and other drugs. During this period, sedatives, neuroleptics, and other forms of pharmacotherapy are not useful in the treatment of inhalant abusers and should be avoided in most cases as they are likely to exacerbate the depressed state. Once it is determined that the individual is detoxified, that is, has low levels of solvent or other depressant drug, then therapy with other drugs, such as antianxiety drugs, may be useful. The determination of detoxification, even in the absence of drug (solvent) administration, is not well defined or systematic. It may take several days for the major "reversible" intoxication state to be reduced to a level at which coherent cognition can occur. The use of various psychological assessment tools can assist not only in evaluating the intoxication but also in following the progress of the treatment. Little can be done during this period other than to facilitate improvement of the basic health of these individuals, provide supportive care, and build the individual's self-esteem.

There is no accepted treatment approach for inhalant abuse. It should also be emphasized that there are various categories of solvent abusers, from those who may use only one substance (e.g., only nitrous oxide or butanes) to heavy users of a variety of solvents and gases. Many drug treatment facilities refuse treatment of the inhalant abuser because many feel that inhalant abusers are resistant to treatment (Jumper-Thurman and Beauvais 1992) or that there is no standard or accepted treatment. One facility that focuses solely on the comprehensive treatment of inhalant abusers, the International Institute on Inhalant

Abuse based in Colorado (www.allaboutinhalants.com), uses a three-phase model that allows longer periods of treatment. Longer periods of treatment are needed to be able to address the complex psychosocial, economic, and biophysical issues of the inhalant abuser. When brain injury, primarily in the form of cognitive dysfunction, is present, the rate of progression in the treatment process is even slower and assumes a comprehensive neurological rehabilitation approach similar to that in individuals with traumatic brain injury. As few treatment approaches with solvent abusers have been evaluated, none on a broad scale, all treatments should consider several important parameters including the following:

- Culture
- Family structure
- Living environment
- Peer interactions
- Individual's ability to learn and adapt
- Establishment of self-image
- Individual attitudes and behavioral characteristics
- Building basic life skills
- Social bonding

Some of these issues may be dealt with only through treating these individuals separately, especially in the early periods of treatment.

The inhalant abuser typically does not respond to usual drug rehabilitation treatment modalities. Several factors may be involved, particularly for the chronic abuser who may have significant psychosocial problems as well as irreversible brain injury. Treatment becomes slower and progressively more difficult when the severity of brain injury worsens as abuse progresses through transient social use (experimenting in groups) to chronic use in isolation. For these and other reasons, longer therapies are necessary than are utilized in most drug treatment facilities. Also, neurological impairment, the breadth of which still needs to be established, may be a major complication slowing the progress of rehabilitation. This is not as significant a problem with other forms of drug abuse.

Drug screening would be useful in monitoring inhalant abusers. Routine urine screening for hippuric acid (the major metabolite of toluene metabolism) performed two or three times weekly can detect the high level of exposure to toluene commonly seen in inhalant abusers. More frequently performed expired breath analysis for toluene or other abused compounds is also available. As alcohol is a common secondary drug of abuse among inhalant abusers, alcohol abuse should be monitored and considered in the approach to treatment.

Comparison of DSM-IV-TR/ICD-10 Diagnostic Criteria
The DSM and ICD-10 criteria are nearly identical.

References

Al-Alousi LM (1989) Pathology of volatile substance abuse: a case report and a literature review. *Med Sci Law* **29**, 189–208.

Allen N, Mendell JR, Billmaier DJ, et al. (1975) Toxic polyneuropathy due to methyl *n*-butyl ketone: an industrial outbreak. *Arch Neurol* **32**, 209–218.

Altenkirch H, Stoltenburg G, and Wagner HM (1978) Experimental studies on hydrocarbon neuropathies induced by methyl-ethyl-ketone. *J Neurol* **219**, 159–170.

Altenkirch H, Wagner HM, Stoltenburg-Didinger G, et al. (1982) Potentiation of hexacarbon-neurotoxicity by methyl-ethyl-ketone (MEK) and other substances: clinical and experimental aspects. *Neurobehav Toxicol Teratol* **4**, 623–627.

Anthenelli RM and Schuckit MA (1993) Affective and anxiety disorders and alcohol and drug dependence: diagnosis and treatment. *J Addict Dis* **12**, 73–87.

Antti-Poika M, Juntunen J, Matikainen E, et al. (1985) Occupational exposure to toluene: neurotoxic effects with special emphasis on drinking habits. *Int Arch Occup Environ Health* **56**, 31–40.

Arnold GL, Kirby RS, Langendoerfer S, et al. (1994) Toluene embryopathy: clinical delineation and developmental follow-up. *Pediatrics* **93**, 216–220.

Astrand I, Ovrum P, and Carlsson A (1975) Exposure to methylene chloride. I. Its concentration in alveolar air and blood during rest and exercise and its metabolism. *Scand J Work Environ Health* **1**, 78–94.

Austin H, Delzell E, and Cole P (1988) Benzene and leukemia. a review of the literature and a risk assessment. *Am J Epidemiol* **127**, 419–439.

Backstrom B and Collins VP (1992) The effects of 2,5-hexanedione on rods and cones of the retina of albino rats. *Neurotoxicology* **13**, 199–202.

Baerg RD and Kimberg DV (1970) Centrilobular hepatic necrosis and acute renal failure in "solvent sniffers". *Ann Intern Med* **73**, 713–720.

Barret L, Torch S, Leray CL, et al. (1992) Morphometric and biochemical studies in trigeminal nerve of rat after trichloroethylene or dichloroacetylene oral administration. *Neurotoxicology* **13**, 601–614.

Barrowcliff DF and Knell AJ (1979) Cerebral damage due to endogenous chronic carbon monoxide poisoning caused by exposure to methylene chloride. *J Soc Occup Med* **29**, 12–14.

Bass M (1970) Sudden sniffing death. *JAMA* **212**, 2075–2079.

Bass M (1984) Abuse of inhalation anesthetics (letter). *JAMA* **251**, 604.

Batlle DC, Sabatini S, and Kurtzman NA (1988) On the mechanism of toluene-induced renal tubular acidosis. *Nephron* **49**, 210–218.

Beauvais F, Wayman JC, Thurman PJ, et al. (2002) Inhalant abuse among American Indian, Mexican American, and non-Latino white adolescents. *Am J Drug Alcohol* **28**, 171–187.

Belknap JK, Laursen SE, and Crabbe JC (1987) Ethanol and nitrous oxide produce withdrawal-induced convulsions by similar mechanisms in mice. *Life Sci* **41**, 2033–2040.

Benjamin SB, Goodman ZD, Ishak KG, et al. (1985) The morphologic spectrum of halothane-induced hepatic injury: analysis of 77 cases. *Hepatology* **5**, 1163–1171.

Bennett RH and Forman HR (1980) Hypokalemic periodic paralysis in chronic toluene exposure. *Arch Neurol* **37**, 673.

Berg EF (1971) Retrobulbar neuritis. *Ann Ophthalmol* **3**, 1351–1353.

Biscaldi GP, Mingardi M, Pollini G, et al. (1981) Acute toluene poisoning. Electroneurophysiological and vestibular investigations. *Toxicol Eur Res* **3**, 271–273.

Blain L, Lachapelle P, and Molotchnikoff S (1992) Evoked potentials are modified by long-term exposure to trichloroethylene. *Neurotoxicology* **13**, 203–206.

Boon NA (1987) Solvent abuse and the heart (editorial). *Br Med J (Clin Res)* **294**, 722.

Boor JW and Hurtig HI (1977) Persistent cerebellar ataxia after exposure to toluene. *Ann Neurol* **2**, 440–442.

Bowen SE, Daniel J, and Balster RL (1999) Deaths associated with inhalant abuse in Virginia from 1987–1996. *Drug Alcohol Depend* **53**, 239–245.

Brandes JC, Bufill JA, and Pisciotta AV (1989) Amyl nitrite–induced hemolytic anemia. *Am J Med* **86**, 252–254.

Brett A (1997) Myeloneuropathy from whipped cream bulbs presenting as conversion disorder. *Aust N Z J Psychiatry* **31**, 131–132.

Brilliant LC and Grillo A (1993) Successful resuscitation from cardiopulmonary arrest following deliberate inhalation of Freon refrigerant gas. *Del Med J* **65**, 375–378.

Broussard LA, Brustowicz T, Pittman T, et al. (1997) Two traffic fatalities related to the use of dichloroethane. *J Forensic Sci* **42**, 1186–1187.

Brown JH, Hadden DR, and Hadden DS (1991) Solvent abuse, toluene acidosis and diabetic ketoacidosis. *Arch Emerg Med* **8**, 65–67.

Bruhn P, Arlien-Soborg P, Gyldensted C, et al. (1981) Prognosis in chronic toxic encephalopathy. *Acta Neurol Scand* **64**, 259–272.

Butzkueven H and King JO (2000) Nitrous oxide myelopathy in an abuser of whipped cream bulbs. *J Clin Neurosci* **7**, 73–75.

Cagen SZ and Klaassen CD (1979) Hepatotoxicity of carbon tetrachloride in developing rats. *Toxicol Appl Pharmacol* **50**, 347–354.

Caldmeyer KS, Pascuzzi RM, Moran CC, et al. (1993) Tolune abuse causing reduced MR signal intensity in the brain. *AJR* **161**, 1259–1261.

Caravati EM (1997) Acute toluene ingestion toxicity. *Ann Emerg Med* **30**, 838–839.

Carlisle EJ, Donnelly SM, Vasuvattakul S, et al. (1991) Glue-sniffing and distal renal tubular acidosis: Sticking to the facts. *J Am Soc Nephrol* **1**, 1019–1027.

Cartwright TR, Brown ED, and Brashear RE (1983) Pulmonary infiltrates following butane "fire-breathing". *Arch Intern Med* **143**, 2007–2008.

Chang YL, Yang CC, Deng JF, et al. (1999) Diverse manifestations of oral methylene chloride poisoning: report of 6 cases. *J Toxicol-Clin Toxic* **37**, 497–504.

Channer KS and Stanley S (1983) Persistent visual hallucination secondary to chronic solvent encephalopathy: case report and review of the literature. *J Neurol Neurosurg Psychiatry* **46**, 83–86.

Chenoweth MB (1977) Abuse of inhalation anesthetic drugs. *NIDA Res Monogr* **15**, 102–111.

Clark MA, Jones JW, Robinson JJ, et al. (1985) Multiple deaths resulting from shipboard exposure to trichlorotrifluoroethane. *J Forensic Sci* **30**, 1256–1259.

Clearfield HR (1970) Hepatorenal toxicity from sniffing spot-remover (trichloroethylene). *Digest Dis* **15**, 851–856.

Coodin FJ, Dawes C, Dean GW, et al. (1980) Riposte to "Environmental lead and young children". *Can Med Assoc J* **123**, 469–471.

Cordes DH, Brown WD, and Quinn KM (1988) Chemically induced hepatitis after inhaling organic solvents. *West J Med* **148**, 458–460.

Crofton KM and Zhao X (1993) Mid-frequency hearing loss in rats following inhalation exposure to trichloroethylene: evidence from reflex modification audiometry. *Neurotoxicol Teratol* **15**, 413–423.

Cunningham SR, Dalzell GWN, McGirr P, et al. (1987) Myocardial infarction and primary ventricular fibrillation after glue sniffing. *Br Med J (Clin Res)* **294**, 739–740.

Currie B, Burrow J, Fisher D, et al. (1994) Petrol sniffer's encephalopathy. *Med J Aust* **160**, 800–801.

Daniell WE, Couser WG, and Rosenstock L (1988) Occupational solvent exposure and glomerulonephritis. *JAMA* **259**, 2280–2283.

Davidman M and Schmitz P (1988) Renal tubular acidosis. A pathophysiologic approach. *Hosp Pract (Off ed)* **23**, 77–81, 84–88, 93–96.

Devathasan G, Low D, and Teoh PC (1984) Complications of chronic glue (toluene) abuse in adolescents. *Aust N Z J Med* **14**, 39–43.

Dinwiddie SH, Zorumski CF, and Rubin EH (1987) Psychiatric correlates of chronic solvent abuse. *J Clin Psychiatry* **48**, 334–337.

Dittmer DK, Jhamandas JH, and Johnson ES (1993) Glue-sniffing neuropathies. *Can Fam Phys* **39**, 1965–1971.

Donald JM, Hooper K, and Hopenhayn-Rich C (1991) Reproductive and developmental toxicity of toluene: a review. *Environ Health Perspect* **94**, 237–244.

Dunkel VC, Rogers-Back AM, Lawlor TE, et al. (1989) Mutagenicity of some alkyl nitrites used as recreational drugs. *Environ Mol Mutagen* **14**, 115–122.

Eastwell HD (1985) Elevated lead levels in petrol "sniffers". *Med J Aust* **143**, 563–564.

Edwards RW (1993) Drug use among 8th grade students is increasing. *Int J Drug Addict* **28**, 1621–1623.

Ehyai A and Freemon FR (1983) Progressive optic neuropathy and sensorineural hearing loss due to chronic glue sniffing. *J Neurol Neurosurg Psychiatry* **46**, 349–351.

England A and Jones RM (1992) Inhaled anaesthetic agents: from halothane to the present day. *Br J Hosp Med* **48**, 254–257.

Escobar A and Aruffo C (1980) Chronic thinner intoxication: clinicopathologic report of a human case. *J Neurol Neurosurg Psychiatry* **43**, 986–994.

Eskenazi B, Gaylord L, Bracken MB, et al. (1988) In utero exposure to organic solvents and human neurodevelopment. *Dev Med Child Neurol* **30**, 492–501.

Evans AC and Raistrick D (1987a) Patterns of use and related harm with toluene-based adhesives and butane gas. *Br J Psychiatry* **150**, 773–776.

Evans EB and Balster RL (1993) Inhaled 1,1,1-trichloroethane–produced physical dependence in mice: effects of drugs and vapors on withdrawal. *J Pharmacol Exp Ther* **264**, 726–733.

Farrell G, Prendergast D, and Murray M (1985) Halothane hepatitis. Detection of a constitutional susceptibility factor. *N Engl J Med* **313**, 1310–1314.

Fechter LD, Liu Y, Herr DW, et al. (1998) Trichloroethylene ototoxicity: evidence for a cochlear origin. *Toxicol Sci* **42**, 28–35.

Feldman RG, Niles C, Proctor SP, et al. (1992) Blink reflex measurement of effects of trichloroethylene exposure on the trigeminal nerve. *Muscle Nerve* **15**, 490–495.

Feldman RG, White RF, Currie JN, et al. (1985) Long-term follow-up after single toxic exposure to trichloroethylene. *Am J Ind Med* **8**, 119–126.

Field-Smith ME, Taylor JC, Norman CL, et al. (2001) Trends in Deaths Associated with Abuse of Volatile Substances, 1971–1999. Report 14. St. George's Hospital Medical School, London.

Filley CM, Heaton RK, and Rosenberg NL (1990) White matter dementia in chronic toluene abuse. *Neurology* **40**, 532–534.

Fitzgerald RL, Fishel CE, and Bush LL (1993) Fatality due to recreational use of chlorodifluoromethane and chloropentafluoroethane. *J Forensic Sci* **38**, 477–483.

Flippo TS and Holder WD Jr. (1993) Neurologic degeneration associated with nitrous oxide anesthesia in patients with vitamin B_{12} deficiency. *Arch Surg* **128**, 1391–1395.

Forkert PG and Forkert L (1994) Trichloroethylene induces pulmonary fibrosis in mice. *Can J Physiol Pharmacol* **72**, 205–210.

Fornazzari L, Wilkinson DA, Kapur BM, et al. (1983) Cerebellar, cortical and functional impairment in toluene abusers. *Acta Neurol Scand* **67**, 319–329.

Frontali N, Amantini MC, Spagnolo A, et al. (1981) Experimental neurotoxicity and urinary metabolites of the C5–C7 aliphatic hydrocarbons used as glue solvents in shoe manufacture. *Clin Toxicol* **18**, 1357–1367.

Fujinaga M and Baden JM (1994) Methionine prevents nitrous oxide–induced teratogenicity in rat embryos grown in culture. *Anesthesiology* **81**, 184–189.

Gallassi R, Montagna P, Pazzaglia P, et al. (1980) Peripheral neuropathy due to gasoline sniffing—a case report. *Eur Neurol* **19**, 419–421.

Gamberale F, Annwall G, and Hultengren M (1975) Exposure to methylene chloride. II. Psychological functions. *Scand J Work Environ Health* **1**, 95–103.

Garriott J (1992) Death among inhalant abusers. In *A Volatile Research Agenda on Inhalant Abuse*, Sharp CW, Spence R, and Beauvais F (eds). A NIDA Res Monogr. US Government Printing Office, Department of Health and Human Services publication (ADM) 93–3480, Washington, DC, pp. 181–192.

Gaworski CL, Aranyi C, Hall A, III, et al. (1992) Prechronic inhalation toxicity studies of isobutyl nitrite. *Fund Appl Toxicol* **19**, 169–175.

Gillman MA (1992) Nitrous oxide abuse in perspective. *Clin Neuropharmacol* **15**, 297–306.

Goldings AS and Stewart RM (1982) Organic lead encephalopathy: behavioral change and movement disorder following gasoline inhalation. *J Clin Psychiatry* **43**, 70–72.

Gonzalez EG and Downey JA (1972) Polyneuropathy in a glue sniffer. *Arch Phys Med Rehab* **53**, 333–337.

Goodheart RS and Dunne JW (1994) Petrol sniffer's encephalopathy. A study of 25 patients. *Med J Aust* **160**, 178–181.

Goodwin TM (1988) Toluene abuse and renal tubular acidosis in pregnancy. *Obstet Gynecol* **71**, 715–718.

Goto I, Matsumura M, Inove N, et al. (1974) Toxic polyneuropathy due to glue sniffing. *J Neurol Neurosurg Psychiatry* **37**, 848–853.

Grabski DA (1961) Toluene sniffing producing cerebellar degeneration. *Am J Psychiatry* **118**, 461–462.

Graham DG, Anthony DC, and Boekelheide K (1982) *In vitro* and *in vivo* studies of the molecular pathogenesis of *n*-hexane neuropathy. *Neurobehav Toxicol Teratol* **4**, 629–634.

Greer JE (1984) Adolescent abuse of typewriter correction fluid. *South Med J* **77**, 297–298.

Groppi A, Polettini A, Lunetta P, et al. (1994) A fatal case of trichlorofluoromethane (Freon 11) poisoning. Tissue distribution study by gas chromatography–mass spectrometry. *J Forensic Sci* **39**, 871–876.

Gupta RK, van der Meulen J, and Johny DV (1991) Oliguric acute renal failure due to glue-sniffing. Case report. *Scand J Urol Nephrol* **25**, 247–250.

Hakim A, Jain AK, and Jain R (1992) Chloroform ingestion causing toxic hepatitis. *J Assoc Phys Ind* **40**, 477.

Hall DMB, Ramsey J, Schwartz MS, et al. (1986) Neuropathy in a petrol sniffer. *Arch Dis Child* **61**, 900–901.

Hantson P, Vandenplas O, Dive A, et al. (1990) Trichloroethylene and cardiac toxicity: Report of two consecutive cases. *Acta Clin Belg* **45**, 34–37.

Hersh JH (1989) Toluene embryopathy: two new cases. *J Med Genet* **26**, 333–337.

Hersh JH, Podruch PE, Rogers G, et al. (1985) Toluene embryopathy. *J Pediatry* **106**, 922–927.

Herskowitz A, Ishii N, and Schaumburg H (1971) *n*-hexane neuropathy: a syndrome occurring as a result of industrial exposure. *N Engl J Med* **285**, 82–85.

Hobara T, Okuda M, Gotoh M, et al. (2000) Estimation of the lethal toluene concentration from the accidental death of painting workers. *Ind Health* **38**, 228–231.

Hodgson MJ, Heyl AT, and Van Thiel DH (1989) Liver disease associated with exposure to 1,1,1-trichloroethane. *Arch Intern Med* **149**, 1793–1798.

Hollo G and Varga M (1992) Toluene and visual loss (letter; comment). Comment on: Neurology 42, 266. *Neurology 1991* **41**, 282–285.

Hormes JT, Filley CM, and Rosenberg NL (1986) Neurologic sequelae of chronic solvent vapor abuse. *Neurology* **36**, 698–702.

Horowitz BZ (1986) Carboxyhemoglobinemia caused by inhalation of methylene chloride. *Am J Emerg Med* **4**, 48–51.

Hubbs AF, Castranova V, Ma JYC, et al. (1997) Acute lung injury induced by a commercial leather conditioner. *Toxicol Appl Pharmacol* **143**, 37–46.

Hutchens KS and Kung M (1985) "Experimentation" with chloroform. *Am J Med* **78**, 715–718.

Ichihara G, Saito I, Kamijima M, et al. (1998) Urinary 2,5-hexanedione increases with potentiation of neurotoxicity in chronic coexposure to n-hexane and methyl ethyl ketone. *Int Arch Occup Environ Health* **71**, 100–104.

Ikeda M and Tsukagoshi H (1990) Encephalopathy due to toluene sniffing. Report of a case with magnetic resonance imaging. *Eur Neurol* **30**, 347–349.

Jacobs RF, Marmer DJ, Steele RW, et al. (1983) Cellular immunotoxicity of amyl nitrite. *J Toxicol-Clin Toxicol* **20**, 421–449.

Jaspers RM, Muijser H, Lammers JH, et al. (1993) Mid-frequency hearing loss and reduction of acoustic startle responding in rats following trichloroethylene exposure. *Neurotoxicol Teratol* **15**, 407–412.

Jastak JT (1991) Nitrous oxide and its abuse. *J Am Dent Assoc* **122**, 48–52.

Jevtovic-Todorovic V, Benshoff N, and Olney JW (2000) Ketamine potentiates cerebral cortical damage induced by the common anaesthetic agent nitrous oxide in adult rats. *Br J Pharmacol* **130**, 1692–1698.

Johnson BD, Marel R, and Raimone G (1998) Statewide Household Survey of Substance Abuse, 1998: Illicit Substance Use Among Adults in New York State's Transient Population, New York.

Johnston LD, O'Malley PM, and Bachman JG (2001) *Monitoring the Future National Survey Results on Drug Use, 1994–2001*. National Institute on Drug Abuse. US Government Printing Office, Washington, DC. http://monitoringthefuture.org/

Jone CM and Wu AH (1988) An unusual case of toluene-induced metabolic acidosis. *Clin Chem* **34**, 2596–2599.

Jumper-Thurman P and Beauvais F (1992) Treatment of volatile solvent abusers. In *A Volatile Research Agenda on Inhalant Abuse*, Sharp CW, Spence R, and Beauvais F (eds). NIDA Res Monogr. US Government Printing Office, DHHS publication (ADM) 93–3480, Washington, DC, pp. 203–213.

Kamran S and Bakshi R (1998) MRI in chronic toluene abuse: low signal in the cerebral cortex on T2-weighted images. *Neuroradiology* **40**, 519–521.

Kaneko T, Koizumi T, Takezaki T, et al. (1992) Urinary calculi associated with solvent abuse. *J Urol* **147**, 1365–1366.

Keane JR (1978) Toluene optic neuropathy. *Ann Neurol* **4**, 390.

Kerner K (1988) Current topics in inhalant abuse. *NIDA Res Monogr* **85**, 8–29.

Kimbrough RD, Mitchell FL, and Houk VN (1985) Trichloroethylene: an update. *J Toxicol Environ Health* **15**, 369–383.

King GS, Smialek JE, and Troutman WG (1985a) Sudden death in adolescents resulting from the inhalation of typewriter correction fluid. *JAMA* **253**, 1604–1606.

King PJL, Morris JGL, and Pollard JD (1985b) Glue sniffing neuropathy. *Aust N Z J Med* **15**, 293–299.

Kira S, Ogata M, Ebara Y, et al. (1988) A case of thinner sniffing: Relationship between neuropsychological symptoms and urinary findings after inhalation of toluene and methanol. *Ind Health* **26**, 81–85.

Kiyokawa M, Mizota A, Takasoh M, et al. (1999) Pattern visual evoked cortical potentials in patients with toxic optic neuropathy caused by toluene abuse. *Jpn J Ophthalmol* **43**, 438–442.

Knight AT, Pawsey CG, Aroney RS, et al. (1991) Upholsterers' glue associated with myocarditis, hepatitis, acute renal failure, and lymphoma. *Med J Aust* **154**, 360–362.

Knox JW and Nelson JR (1966) Permanent encephalopathy from toluene inhalation. *N Engl J Med* **275**, 1494–1496.

Koporec KP, Kim HJ, Mackenzie WF, et al. (1995) Effect of oral dosing vehicles on the subchronic hepatotoxicity of carbon-tetrachloride in the rat. *J Toxicol Environ Health* **44**, 13–27.

Korman M, Matthews RW, and Lovitt R (1981) Neuropsychological effects of abuse of inhalants. *Percept Mot Skills* **53**, 547–553.

Korman M, Semler I, and Trimboli F (1980) A psychiatric emergency room study of 162 inhalant users. *Addict Behav* **5**, 143–147.

Kornfeld M, Moser AB, Moser HW, et al. (1994) Solvent vapor abuse leukoencephalopathy. Comparison to adrenoleukodystrophy. *J Neuropathol Exp Neurol* **53**, 389–398.

Korobkin R, Asbury AK, Sumner AJ, et al. (1975) Glue-sniffing neuropathy. *Arch Neurol* **32**, 158–162.

Kozel N, Sloboda Z, and de la Rosa M (1995) *Epidemiology of Inhalant Abuse: An International Perspective. NIDA Res Monogr*. US Government Printing Office, NIH publication 95–3831, Washington, DC, p. 148.

Kubic VL, Andres MW, Engel RR, et al. (1974) Metabolism of dihalomethanes to carbon monoxide. I. *In vivo* studies. *Drug Metab Dispos* **2**, 53–57.

Laureno R (1993) Trichloroethylene does not cause trigeminal neuropathy (letter). *Muscle Nerve* **16**, 217.

Lauwerys R, Bernard A, Viau C, et al. (1985) Kidney disorders and hematotoxicity from organic solvent exposure. *Scand J Work Environ Health* **11**(Suppl. 1), 83–90.

Lavoie FW, Dolan MC, Danzl DF, et al. (1987) Recurrent resuscitation and "no code" orders in a 27-year-old spray paint abuser (clinical conference). *Ann Emerg Med* **16**, 1266–1273.

Layzer RB (1978) Myeloneuropathy after prolonged exposure to nitrous oxide. *Lancet* **2**, 1227–1230.

Lazar RB, Ho SU, Melen O, et al. (1983) Multifocal central nervous system damage caused by toluene abuse. *Neurology* **33**, 1337–1340.

Levisohn PM, Kramer RE, and Rosenberg NL (1992) Neurophysiology of chronic cocaine and toluene abuse. *Neurology* **42**(Suppl. 3), 434.

Levy AB (1986) Delirium induced by inhalation of typewriter correction fluid. *Psychosomatics* **27**, 665–666.

Lewis DM and Lynch DW (1988) Toxicity of inhaled isobutyl nitrite in BALB/c mice: systemic and immunotoxic studies. *NIDA Res Monogr* **83**, 50–58.

Lindemann R (1991) Congenital renal tubular dysfunction associated with maternal sniffing of organic solvents. *Acta Paediatr Scand* **80**, 882–884.

Litovitz TL, Klein-Schwartz W, White S, et al. (2001) 2000 annual report of the american association of poison control centers toxic exposure surveillance system. *Am J Emerg Med* **19**, 337–395.

Litt IF and Cohen MI (1969) Danger... vapor harmful: spot-remover sniffing. *N Engl J Med* **281**, 543–544.

Liu LY and Maxwell JC (2001) Texas School Survey of Substance Use Among Students: Grades 7–12, 2000 Texas Commission on Alcohol and Drug Abuse. http://www.tcada.state.tx.us/research/.

Lock EA (1989) Mechanism of nephrotoxic action due to organohalogenated compounds. *Toxicol Lett* **46**, 93–106.

Maas EF, Ashe J, Spiegel P, et al. (1991) Acquired pendular nystagmus in toluene addiction. *Neurology* **41**, 282–285.

Mallov JS (1976) MBK neuropathy among spray painters. *JAMA* **235**, 1455–1457.

Malm G and Lying-Tunell U (1980) Cerebellar dysfunction related to toluene sniffing. *Acta Neurol Scand* **62**, 188–190.

Manno M, Chirillo R, Daniotti G, et al. (1989) Carboxyhaemoglobin and fatal methylene chloride poisoning (letter). *Lancet* **2**, 274.

Marjot R and McLeod AA (1989) Chronic nonneurological toxicity from volatile substance abuse. *Hum Toxicol* **8**, 301–306.

Maruff P, Burns CB, Tyler P, et al. (1998) Neurological and cognitive abnormalities associated with chronic petrol sniffing. *Brain* **121**, 1903–1917.

Mathew RJ, Wilson WH, and Tant SR (1989b) Regional cerebral blood flow changes associated with amyl nitrite inhalation. *Br J Addict* **84**, 293–299.

Maze M and Fujinaga M (2000) Recent advances in understanding the actions and toxicity of nitrous oxide. *Anaesthesia* **55**, 311–314.

Mazze RI, Fujinaga M, and Baden JM (1988) Halothane prevents nitrous oxide teratogenicity in Sprague-Dawley rats; folinic acid does not. *Teratology* **38**, 121–127.

McIntyre AS and Long RG (1992) Fatal fulminant hepatic failure in a "solvent abuser". *Postgrad Med J* **68**, 29–30.

McLeod AA, Marjot R, Monaghan MJ, et al. (1987) Chronic cardiac toxicity after inhalation of 1,1,1-trichloroethane. *Br Med J (Clin Res)* **294**, 727–729.

Means ED, Prockop LD, and Hooper GS (1976) Pathology of lacquer thinner induced neuropathy. *Ann Clin Lab Sci* **6**, 240–250.

Mendell JR, Saida K, Ganansia MF, et al. (1974) Toxic polyneuropathy produced by methyl *n*-butyl ketone. *Science* **185**, 787–789.

Menkes JH (1976) Toxic polyneuropathy due to methyl *n*-butyl ketone (letter). *Arch Neurol* **33**, 309.

Mergler D and Beauvais B (1992) Olfactory threshold shift following controlled 7-hour exposure to toluene and/or xylene. *Neurotoxicology* **13**, 211–215.

Metrick SA and Brenner RP (1982) Abnormal brain stem auditory evoked potentials in chronic paint sniffers. *Ann Neurol* **12**, 553–556.

Miller L, Pateras V, Friederici H, et al. (1985) Acute tubular necrosis after inhalation exposure to methylene chloride. Report of a case. *Arch Intern Med* **145**, 145–146.

Mirvish SS and Haverkos HW (1987) Butyl nitrite in the induction of Kaposi's sarcoma in AIDS (letter). *N Engl J Med* **317**, 1603.

Mizutani K, Shinomiya K, and Shinomiya T (1988) Hepatotoxicity of dichloromethane. *Forensic Sci Int* **38**, 113–128.

Mizutani T, Oohashi N, and Naito H (1989) Myoglobinemia and renal failure in toluene poisoning: a case report. *Vet Hum Toxicol* **31**, 448–450.

Morrow LA, Steinhauer SR, and Hodgson MJ (1992) Delay in P300 latency in patients with organic solvent exposure. *Arch Neurol* **49**, 315–320.

Murray FJ, Schwetz BA, McBride JG, et al. (1979) Toxicity of inhaled chloroform in pregnant mice and their offspring. *Toxicol Appl Pharmacol* **50**, 515–522.

National Institutes of Health Technical Report 8 (1994) *Prevalence of Drug Use in the DC Metropolitan Area Household and Nonhousehold Populations: 1991.* National Institute on Drug Abuse, Washington, DC.

Nelson NA, Robins TG, and Port FK (1990) Solvent nephrotoxicity in humans and experimental animals. *Am J Nephrol* **10**, 10–20.

Nunn JF (1987) Clinical aspects of the interaction between nitrous oxide and vitamin B$_{12}$. *Br J Anaes* **59**, 3–13.

O'Callaghan C and Milner AD (1988) Aerosol treatment abuse. *Arch Dis Child* **63**, 70.

Odkvist LM, Larsby B, Fredrickson JMF, et al. (1980) Vestibular and oculomotor disturbances caused by industrial solvents. *J Otolaryngol* **9**, 57–58.

Oetting ER and Webb J (1992) Psychosocial characteristics and their links with inhalants, a research agenda. In *A Volatile Research Agenda on Inhalant Abuse,* Sharp CW, Spence R, and Beauvais F (eds). NIDA Res Monogr. US Government Printing Office, DHHS publication 129 (ADM) 93–3475, Washington, DC, pp. 59–98.

Oetting ER, Edwards RW, and Beauvais F (1988) Social and psychological factors underlying inhalant abuse. *NIDA Res Monogr* **85**, 172–203.

Oh SJ and Kim JM (1976) Giant axonal swelling in "huffer's" neuropathy. *Arch Neurol* **33**, 583–586.

Omae K, Takabayashi T, Tanaka S, et al. (2000) Acute and recurrent hepatitis induced by 2,2-dichloro-1,1,1-trifluoroethane (HCFC-123). *J Occup Health* **42**, 235–238.

Ong CN, Koh D, Foo SC, et al. (1993) Volatile organic solvents in correction fluids: Identification and potential hazards. *Bull Environ Contam Toxicol* **50**, 787–793.

Ong TK, Rustage KJ, Harrison KM, et al. (1988) Solvent abuse. An anaesthetic management problem. *Br Dent J* **164**, 150–151.

Osterloh J and Goldfield D (1984) Butyl nitrite transformation in vitro, chemical nitrosation reactions, and mutagenesis. *J Anal Toxicol* **8**, 164–169.

Paraf F, Lewis J, and Jothy S (1993) Acute fatty liver of pregnancy after exposure to toluene. A case report. *J Clin Gastroenterol* **17**, 163–165.

Pardys S and Brotman M (1974) Trichloroethylene and alcohol: a straight flush (letter). *JAMA* **229**, 521–522.

Patel R and Benjamin J Jr. (1986) Renal disease associated with toluene inhalation. *Clin Toxicol* **24**, 213–223.

Pearson MA, Hoyme HE, Seaver LH, et al. (1994) Toluene embryopathy: delineation of the phenotype and comparison with fetal alcohol syndrome. *Pediatrics* **93**, 211–215.

Pema PJ, Horak HA, and Wyatt RH (1998) Myelopathy caused by nitrous oxide toxicity. *Am J Neuroradiol* **19**, 894–896.

Plaa GL (1988) Experimental evaluation of haloalkanes and liver injury. *Fund Appl Toxicol* **10**, 563–570.

Poblano A, Ishiwara K, Ortega P, et al. (2000) Thinner abuse alters optokinetic nystagmus parameters. *Arch Med Res* **31**, 182–185.

Poungvarin N (1991) Multifocal brain damage due to lacquer sniffing: the first case report of Thailand. *J Med Assoc Thai* **74**, 296–300.

Prockop LD and Karampelas D (1981) Encephalopathy secondary to abusive gasoline inhalation. *J Fla Med Assoc* **68**, 823–824.

Pryor GT (1995) Solvent-induced neurotoxicity: effects and mechanisms. In *Handbook of Toxicology*, Chang LW and Dyer RS (eds). Marcel Dekker, New York.

Pryor GT, Dickinson J, Howd RA, et al. (1983) Transient cognitive deficits and high-frequency hearing loss in weanling rats exposed to toluene. *Neurobehav Toxicol Teratol* **5**, 53–57.

Pryor GT, Howd RA, Uyeno ET, et al. (1985) Interactions between toluene and alcohol. *Pharmacol Biochem Behav* **23**, 401–410.

Ramsey J, Anderson HR, Bloor K, et al. (1989) An introduction to the practice, prevalence, and chemical toxicology of volatile substance abuse. *Hum Toxicol* **8**, 261–269.

Ratney RS, Wegman DH, and Elkins HB (1974) In vivo conversion of methylene chloride to carbon monoxide. *Arch Environ Health* **28**, 223–226.

Rebert CS, Day VL, Matteucci MJ, et al. (1991) Sensory-evoked potentials in rats chronically exposed to trichloroethylene: predominant auditory dysfunction. *Neurotoxicol Teratol* **13**, 83–90.

Rebert CS, Sorenson SS, Howd RA, et al. (1983) Toluene-induced hearing loss in rats evidenced by the brain stem auditory-evoked response. *Neurobehav Toxicol Teratol* **5**, 59–62.

Rees DC, Knisely JS, Balster RL, et al. (1987) Pentobarbital-like discriminative stimulus properties of halothane, 1,1,1-trichloroethane, isoamyl nitrite, flurothyl and oxazepam in mice. *J Pharmacol Exp Ther* **241**, 507–515.

Reese E and Kimbrough RD (1993) Acute toxicity of gasoline and some additives. *Environ Health Perspect* **101**(Suppl. 6), 115–131.

Remington G and Hoffman BF (1984) Gas sniffing as a form of substance abuse. *Can J Psychiatry* **29**, 31–35.

Reyes de la Rocha S, Brown MA, and Fortenberry JD (1987) Pulmonary function abnormalities in intentional spray paint inhalation. *Chest* **92**, 100–104.

Ries RK (1993) The dually diagnosed patient with psychotic symptoms. *J Addict Dis* **12**, 103–122.

Roberts MJD, McIvor RA, and Adgey AAJ (1990) Asystole following butane gas inhalation. *Br J Hosp Med* **44**, 294.

Robinson RO (1978) Tetraethyl lead poisoning from gasoline sniffing. *JAMA* **240**, 1373–1374.

Rohrig TP (1997) Sudden death due to butane inhalation. *Am J For Med Pathol* **18**, 299–302.

Ron MA (1986) Volatile substance abuse: a review of possible long-term neurological, intellectual, and psychiatric sequelae. *Br J Psychiatry* **148**, 235–246.

Rosenberg NL, Grigsby J, Dreisbach J, et al. (2002) Neuropsychologic impairment and MRI abnormalities associated with chronic solvent abuse. *J Toxicol-Clin Toxicol* **40**(1), 1–14.

Rosenberg NL, Kleinschmidt-DeMasters BK, Davis KA, et al. (1988a) Toluene abuse causes diffuse central nervous system white matter changes. *Ann Neurol* **23**, 611–614.

Rosenberg NL, Spitz MC, Filley CM, et al. (1988b) Central nervous system effects of chronic toluene abuse—clinical, brain stem evoked response and magnetic resonance imaging studies. *Neurotoxicol Teratol* **10**, 489–495.

Rosoff MH and Cohen MV (1986) Profound bradycardia after amyl nitrite in patients with a tendency to vasovagal episodes. *Br Heart J* **55**, 97–100.

Ruijten MW, Verberk MM, and Salle HJ (1991) Nerve function in workers with long-term exposure to trichloroethene. *Br J Ind Med* **48**, 87–92.

Rybak LP (1992) Hearing: the effects of chemicals. *Otolaryngol Head Neck Surg* **106**, 677–686.

Saida K, Mendell JR, and Weiss HS (1976) Peripheral nerve changes induced by methyl n-butyl ketone and potentiated by methyl ethyl ketone. *J Neuropathol Exp Neurol* **35**, 207–225.

Sasa M, Igarashi S, Miyazaki T, et al. (1978) Equilibrium disorders with diffuse brain atrophy in long-term toluene sniffing. *Arch Otorhinolaryngol* **221**, 163–169.

Scerri GV, Regan PJ, Ratcliffe RJ, et al. (1992) Burns following cigarette lighter fluid abuse. *Burns* **18**, 329–331.

Schaumburg HH and Spencer PS (1976) Degeneration in central and peripheral nervous systems produced by pure n-hexane: an experimental study. *Brain* **99**, 183–192.

Schaumburg HH and Spencer PS (1987) Recognizing neurotoxic disease. *Neurology* **37**, 276–278.

Schikler KN, Lane EE, Seitz K, et al. (1984) Solvent abuse associated pulmonary abnormalities. *Adv Alcohol Subs Abuse* **3**, 75–81.

Schikler KN, Seitz K, Rice JF, et al. (1982) Solvent abuse associated cortical atrophy. *J Adolesc Health Care* **3**, 37–39.

Schwartz RH and Calihan M (1984) Nitrous oxide: a potentially lethal euphoriant inhalant. *Am Fam Pract* **30**, 171–172.

Seshia SS, Rajani KR, Boeckx RL, et al. (1978) The neurological manifestations of chronic inhalation of leaded gasoline. *Dev Med Child Neurol* **20**, 323–334.

Sharp CW, Spence R, and Beauvais F (eds) (1992) *A Volatile Research Agenda on Inhalant Abuse*. NIDA Res Monogr. US Government Printing Office, DHHS publication 129 (ADM) 93–3475, Washington, DC, pp. 1–10.

Sherwood RL, O'Shea W, Thomas PT, et al. (1987) Effects of inhalation of ethylene dichloride on pulmonary defenses of mice and rats. *Toxicol Appl Pharmacol* **91**, 491–496.

Short BG, Burnett VL, Cox MG, et al. (1987) Site-specific renal cytotoxicity and cell proliferation in male rats exposed to petroleum hydrocarbons. *Lab Invest* **57**, 564–577.

Siegel E and Wason S (1990) Sudden death caused by inhalation of butane and propane (letter). *N Engl J Med* **323**, 1638.

Smart RG (1988) Inhalant use and abuse in Canada. *NIDA Res Monogr* **85**, 121–139.

Smith M, Stair T, and Rolnick MA (1980) Butyl nitrite and a suicide attempt. *Ann Intern Med* **5**, 719–720.

Soderberg LSF and Barnett JB (1995) Inhalation exposure to isobutyl nitrite inhibits macrophage tumoricidal activity and modulates inducible nitric oxide. *J Leukocyte Biol* **57**, 135–140.

Soni MG, Mangipudy RS, Mumtaz MM, et al. (1998) Tissue repair response as a function of dose during trichloroethylene hepatotoxicity. *Toxicol Sci* **42**, 158–165.

Spencer JD, Raasch FO, and Trefny FA (1976) Halothane abuse in hospital personnel. *JAMA* **235**, 1034–1035.

Spencer PS, Schaumburg HH, Raleigh RL, et al. (1975) Nervous system degeneration produced by the industrial solvent methyl *n*-butyl ketone. *Arch Neurol* **32**, 219–222.

Spencer PS, Schaumburg HH, Sabri MI, et al. (1980) The enlarging view of hexacarbon neurotoxicity. *Crit Rev Toxicol* **7**, 279–357.

Stewart A and Witts LJN (1993) Chronic carbon tetrachloride intoxication (1944 classical article). *Br J Ind Med* **50**, 8–18.

Stewart RD and Fisher TN (1972) Carboxyhemoglobin elevation after exposure to dichloromethane. *Science* **176**, 295–296.

Stewart RD, Fisher TN, Hosko MJ, et al. (1972) Experimental human exposure to methylene chloride. *Arch Environ Health* **25**, 342–348.

Stewart RD, Hake CL, and Peterson JE (1974) "Degreasers' flush," dermal response to trichloroethylene and ethanol. *Arch Environ Health* **29**, 1–5.

Streicher HZ, Gabow PA, Moss AH, et al. (1981) Syndromes of toluene sniffing in adults. *Ann Int Med* **94**, 758–762.

Substance Abuse and Mental Health Services Administration (2001) *National Household Survey on Drug Abuse: Population Estimates 2000*. US Government Printing Office, Washington, DC.

Suruda AJ and McGlothlin JD (1990) Fatal abuse of nitrous oxide in the workplace. *J Occup Med* **32**, 682–684.

Takeuchi Y (1988) Visual disorders due to organic solvent poisoning. *Jpn J Ind Health* **30**, 236–247.

Takeuchi Y (1993) *n*-Hexane polyneuropathy in Japan: a review of n-hexane poisoning and its preventive measures. *Environ Res* **62**, 76–80.

Takeuchi Y, Hisanaga N, Ono Y, et al. (1981) Cerebellar dysfunction caused by sniffing of toluene-containing thinner. *Ind Health* **19**, 163–169.

Taverner D, Harrison DJ, and Bell GM (1988) Acute renal failure due to interstitial nephritis induced by "glue-sniffing" with subsequent recovery. *Scott Med J* **33**, 246–247.

Taylor GJ and Harris W (1970) Cardiac toxicity of aerosol propellants. *JAMA* **214**, 81–85.

Tenenbein M, deGroot W, and Rajani KR (1984) Peripheral neuropathy following intentional inhalation of naphtha fumes. *Can Med Assoc J* **131**, 1077–1079.

Thompson PJ, Dhillon P, and Cole P (1983) Addiction to aerosol treatment: the asthmatic alternative to glue sniffing. *Br Med J (Clin Res)* **287**, 1515–1516.

Towfighi J, Gonatas NK, Pleasure D, et al. (1976) Glue sniffer's neuropathy. *Neurology* **26**, 238–243.

Unger E, Alexander A, Fritz T, et al. (1994) Toluene abuse: physical basis for hypointensity of the basal ganglia on T2-weighted MR images. *Radiology* **193**, 473–476.

Valpey R, Sumi SM, Copass MK, et al. (1978) Acute and chronic progressive encephalopathy due to gasoline sniffing. *Neurology* **28**, 507–510.

Vishnubhakat SM and Beresford HR (1991) Reversible myeloneuropathy of nitrous oxide abuse: serial electrophysiological studies. *Muscle Nerve* **14**, 22–26.

Wagner SA, Clark MA, Wesche DL, et al. (1992) Asphyxial deaths from the recreational use of nitrous oxide. *J Forensic Sci* **37**, 1008–1015.

Wason S, Detsky AS, Platt OS, et al. (1980) Isobutyl nitrite toxicity by ingestion. *Ann Intern Med* **92**, 637–638.

Wason S, Gibler WB, and Hassan M (1986) Ventricular tachycardia associated with non-Freon aerosol propellants. *JAMA* **256**, 78–80.

Wernisch M, Paya K, and Palasser A (1991) Cardiovascular arrest after inhalation of leather glue. *Wien Med Wochenschr* **141**, 71–74.

Wheeler MG, Rozycki AA, and Smith RP (1992) Recreational propane inhalation in an adolescent male. *J Toxicol Clin Toxicol* **30**, 135–139.

Wilkins-Haug L (1997) Teratogen update: Toluene. *Teratol* **55**, 145–51.

Wilkins-Haug L and Gabow PA (1991) Toluene abuse during pregnancy: Obstetric complications and perinatal outcomes. *Obstet Gynecol* **77**, 504–509.

Will AM and McLaren EH (1981) Reversible renal damage due to glue sniffing. *Br Med J* **283**, 525–526.

Winneke G (1981) The neurotoxicity of dichloromethane. *Neurobehav Toxicol Teratol* **3**, 391–395.

Wood RW and Cox C (1981) Acute oral toxicity of butyl nitrite. *J Appl Toxicol* **1**, 30–31.

Wright MF and Strobl DJ (1984) 1,1,1-Trichloroethane cardiac toxicity: report of a case. *J Am Osteopath Assoc* **84**, 285–288.

Xiong L, Matthes JD, Li J, et al. (1993) MR imaging of spray heads: Toluene abuse via aerosol paint inhalation. *AJNR* **14**, 1195–1199.

Yamamoto M, Ishiwata H, Yamada T, et al. (1987) Studies in the guinea-pig stomach on the formation of N-nitrosomethylurea, from methylurea and sodium nitrite, and its disappearance. *Food Chem Toxicol* **25**, 663–668.

Yamamoto S, Mori NYH, Miyata M, et al. (1992) Neurogenic bladder caused by toluene abuse. *Acta Urol Jpn* **38**, 459–462.

Yamanouchi N, Okada S, Kodama K, et al. (1995) White matter changes caused by chronic solvent abuse. *Am J Neuroradiol* **16**, 1643–1649.

Yamanouchi N, Okada S, Kodama K, et al. (1997) Effects of MRI abnormalities on WAIS-R performance in solvent abusers. *Acta Neurol Scand* **96**, 34–39.

Yardley-Jones A, Anderson D, and Parke DV (1991) The toxicity of benzene and its metabolism and molecular pathology in human risk assessment. *Br J Ind Med* **48**, 437–444.

Zakhari S and Salem H (1991) Cardiac toxicology of solvents. In *Principles of Cardiac Toxicology*, Baskin SI (ed). CRC Press, Boca Raton, FL, pp. 465–501.

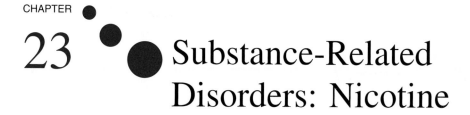

23 Substance-Related Disorders: Nicotine

Nicotine dependence is the most common substance use disorder in the United States with about 25% of the population addicted to tobacco. Tobacco addiction has serious health consequences for the user, family members, and others who breathe second hand environmental tobacco smoke or are exposed during pregnancy. Tobacco addiction increases morbidity and mortality. Most individuals with mental illness or other addictions are nicotine dependent, and about 44% of all the cigarettes consumed in the United States are by these individuals (Lasser et al. 2000).

Diagnosis

Nicotine dependence was first included as a substance use disorder in the DSM-III in 1980. In the DSM-IV-TR, a specifier is used to designate the presence or absence of physiological dependence, depending on whether tolerance or withdrawal is present or whether both are absent (see generic DSM-IV-TR diagnostic criteria for Substance Dependence in Chapter 15, page 351). Further specifiers can be used to denote course (e.g., early full remission or sustained partial remission). Of note, the DSM distinguishes nicotine from other substances by not including a diagnosis of nicotine abuse because most individuals transit quickly and directly from use to dependence (meeting criteria of tolerance and withdrawal).

The nicotine withdrawal syndrome occurring after abstinence was also first classified as a disorder in DSM-III (American Psychiatric Association 1980). The DSM-IV-TR nicotine withdrawal syndrome describes a characteristic set of symptoms that develops after abrupt cessation or a reduction in the use of nicotine products after at least several weeks of daily use (see DSM-IV-TR diagnostic criteria on page 565). Other symptoms that may be associated with nicotine withdrawal include craving for nicotine, a factor thought to be significant in relapse; a desire for sweets; and impaired performance on tasks requiring vigilance. To some extent, the degree of physiological dependence predicts severity of the withdrawal syndrome and difficulty stopping smoking. The Fagerstrom Tolerance Questionnaire (FTQ) is an instrument that was developed to assess the degree of physical dependence on nicotine (Fagerstrom 1978). Its two primary measures are number of cigarettes smoked per day and time in the morning until the first cigarette (see section on evaluation and assessment). A score of five or higher on the FTQ is indicative of higher severity of nicotine dependence, but does not constitute a definitive diagnosis. In addition to frank symptoms, other objective biological and physiological changes are associated with nicotine withdrawal, such as generalized slowing of electroencephalographic activity, decreases in catecholamine and cortisol levels, changes in rapid eye movement, impairment on neuropsychological testing, and decreased metabolic rate.

Diagnostic Criteria for

292.0 Nicotine Withdrawal

A. Daily use of nicotine for at least several weeks.

B. Abrupt cessation of nicotine use, or reduction in the amount of nicotine used, followed within 24 hours by four (or more) of the following signs:

    (1) dysphoric or depressed mood
    (2) insomnia
    (3) irritability, frustration, or anger
    (4) anxiety
    (5) difficulty concentrating
    (6) restlessness
    (7) decreased heart rate
    (8) increased appetite or weight gain

C. The symptoms in Criterion B cause clinically significant distress or impairment in social, occupational, or other important areas of functioning.

D. The symptoms are not due to a general medical condition and are not better accounted for by another mental disorder.

Reprinted with permission from the Diagnostic and Statistical Manual of Mental Disorders, Fourth Edition, Text Revision. Copyright 2000 American Psychiatric Association.

Epidemiology

Nicotine dependence is the most prevalent substance use disorder in the United States (Fagerstrom 1978). Cigarette smoking is the primary preventable cause of morbidity and mortality in the United States, with an estimated 434,000 premature deaths occurring each year from tobacco-caused illnesses and 50,000 additional deaths occurring in nonsmokers from exposure to environmental tobacco smoke (Office on Smoking and Health 1988, Centers for Disease Control 1991). Smoking is the cause of 90% of all lung cancers and nearly all cases of chronic obstructive pulmonary disease and is associated with two times greater risk of death from stroke and coronary heart disease (Office on Smoking and Health 1988). It is also associated with an increased incidence of cancer at a number of other sites, including the larynx, oral cavity, esophagus, cervix, bladder, pancreas, and kidney, and is associated with complications of pregnancy and negative effects on the fetus, including low birth weight (Office on Smoking and Health 1988). Detrimental effects on nonsmokers exposed to tobacco smoke have been demonstrated, particularly in children (Office on Smoking and Health 1988). Smoking causes 10 times the morbidity and mortality of all other substances of abuse combined and results in a total of $22 billion in direct medical costs for treating smoking-related illness and $43 billion in lost productivity per year (US Department of Health and Human Services 1989). The Morbidity and Mortality Weekly Report stated that every pack of cigarettes smoked costs the US about $7.18 in medical costs and lost productivity. The prevalence of smoking is increasing in most developing countries, whereas it is decreasing in most industrialized countries. In the United States, there has been increasing societal pressures for individuals to stop smoking; however, despite an increase in the proportion of smokers quitting, about 25% of the US population continues to smoke, with a lifetime prevalence of nicotine dependence of 20% (Office on Smoking and Health 1988). Only 45% of the population has never smoked.

The prevalence of cigarette smoking is higher at lower socioeconomic levels. Slightly more males than females smoke, although more males than females are successful in stopping smoking. There is evidence that the number of cigarettes per smoker is increasing, leaving a more hard-core and potentially more dependent group of smokers. There has also been a recent increase in the rate of smoking among adolescents, particularly in the number of teenage girls smoking. This increased smoking rate among adolescents is particularly alarming, as smokers typically start smoking at an early age, with more than 60% of smokers beginning by age 14 years and nearly all by age 18 years.

Comorbidity with Psychiatric Disorders

Nicotine dependence and smoking are two to three times more common in individuals with mental and other substance use disorders than in the general population (Hughes et al. 1986, Glassman 1993, Dierker et al. 2002). Smoking-related illnesses are the primary cause of death among those in recovery from other substances. It is estimated that 55 to 90% of individuals with mental disorders smoke versus the 23% of the general population. The prevalence of smoking is especially high in individuals with schizophrenia (70–90%), affective disorders (42–70%), and alcohol dependence (60–90%) or other substance use disorders (70–95%). The odds ratio for "ever smoked" is 4.7 in persons suffering from alcohol dependence, 2.4 for individuals with major depressive disorder (MDD), 1.8 for persons with agoraphobia, 1.6 for individuals with dysthymia, and 1.6 for individuals with panic disorder (PD) (Glassman 1993). Conversely, there is also evidence that affective, anxiety, and substance use disorders may be more common in individuals who smoke than in those who do not or in those who have never smoked (Glassman 1993). Finally, there is evidence to suggest that in one study up to 75% of smokers with a history of MDD developed depressed mood during the first week of withdrawal versus only 30% of those with no depressive history, and that the withdrawal syndrome may be more severe in smokers with a history of depression (Covey et al. 1990). The presence of depressive symptoms during withdrawal is also associated with failed cessation attempts (West et al. 1989, Hughes 1992). Self-reported depressive symptoms during adolescence also predict later frequency and duration of smoking (Kandel and Davies 1986). Several studies suggest a genetic predisposition to both nicotine dependence and co-occurring depression (Carmelli et al. 1990, Kendler et al. 1993, Dierker et al. 2002, Glassman et al. 1990).

There is no simple reason why so many individuals with a mental disorder smoke. As with other addictive disorders, a combination of complex biological and psychosocial factors is likely. Potential biological factors in this group include a greater likelihood of susceptibility to nicotine dependence, with persons experiencing a greater sense of reward from nicotine. Other possibilities include using nicotine to reduce the side effects of psychiatric medications, both as a stimulant to counter sedation as well as a dopamine modulator that can diminish neuroleptic-induced parkinsonism. Subjectively, individuals report that using nicotine improves their cognitive functioning and reduces stress, although research data is mixed in this regard (West and Hack 1991). In individuals with schizophrenia, an abnormality in P50 gating, which is believed to relate clinically to the ability to filter out distracting auditory stimuli, is reversed with nicotine. Social and behavioral factors are also important in understanding nicotine dependence, and psychiatric and addictive comorbidity. Smoking has been ignored and is a part of the pervasive culture in most mental health and substance abuse treatment centers and residential facilities. This is beginning to change. Historically, smoking was often used as a behavioral reward in psychiatric inpatient units and continues to serve as a social connector for many individuals with a mental disorder. Additionally, individuals coping with persistent psychiatric symptoms and reduced social and occupational functioning report smoking to fill the voids of boredom and disappointment (Ziedonis et al. 1994, Hall et al. 1991, Anda et al. 1990).

Course

The National Health Interview Survey found that 70% of smokers interviewed reported they wanted to quit smoking at some point in their lifetime, and about 33% of smokers try to quit each year. Only about 3% of quit attempts without formal treatment are successful, and in recent years, about 30% of smokers who want to quit are seeking treatment. Outcomes for nicotine dependence treatment vary by the type of treatment and the intensity of treatment with specific reports ranging from about 15 to 45% 1-year abstinence rates following treatment. Cessation attempts result in high relapse rates, with the relapse curve for smoking cessation paralleling that for opiates. Most individuals relapse during the first 3 days of withdrawal and most others will relapse within the first 3 months. Withdrawal symptoms are most severe within the first 1 to 3 days of abstinence, often continue for 3 to 4 weeks, and in some persons last for up to 6 months or longer (Hughes 1992). Current depressive symptoms and a history of depression are predictors of relapse. Weight gain may also contribute to relapse, particularly in women. In contrast, several factors have been found to predict worse outcomes at smoking cessation (Kabat and Wynder 1987) (Table 23-1). Predictors include individual factors, manifestations of the addiction such as severity of withdrawal, and social and environmental circumstances.

Nicotine dependence, like other substance use disorders, can be thought of as a chronic relapsing illness with a course of intermittent episodes alternating with periods of remission for most smokers. About 65% of those who stop smoking relapse in 3 months and another 10% relapse in 3 to 6 months (Hunt et al. 1971), and with treatment the overall relapse rate is still about 75 to 80% by 1 year. However, these reported lower outcome rates do not consider the additive effects over time related to multiple quit attempts, since about 40 to 50% of smokers in the United States have been able to quit smoking in their lifetime. Less than 25% of the individuals who have quit smoking are successful in their first attempt. Repeated failures are common before successful abstinence, with the average smoker attempting to quit five or six times before success. Recent prior attempts at quitting do increase the odds that individuals will be able to quit smoking on a future attempt. Relapse can occur even after a long time of abstinence, with about 33% of former smokers who are abstinent for 1 year eventually relapsing 5 to 10 years after cessation.

Treatment of nicotine dependence with resultant abstinence can result in highly beneficial health effects (US Department of Health and Human Services 1990). Educating individuals and families about these benefits of abstinence from smoking can be helpful. Short-term effects (within 1 month) include a significant reduction in respiratory symptoms and respiratory infections such as influenza, pneumonia, and bronchitis. Excess risk of death from coronary heart disease is reduced after 1 year and continues to decline over time. In individuals with coronary heart disease, smoking cessation decreases the risk of recurrent

Table 23-1	Factors Predicting Worse Outcomes in Nicotine Dependence Treatment
Physical reactivity (pulse, blood pressure, etc.) to smoking-related cues Family and friends who are current smokers Lack of social support from spouses, partners, family members, friends Deficits in social skills and assertiveness Higher severity of withdrawal symptoms Limited ability to cope with effects occurring in response to cues or triggers Depressed mood	

myocardial infarction and cardiovascular death by 50%. By 10 to 15 years of abstinence, the mortality rate from all causes returns to that of a person who has never smoked. Pulmonary function can also return to normal if chronic obstructive changes have not already occurred at the time of cessation, and even with obstructive changes pulmonary function can improve with abstinence.

Etiology

Nicotine dependence has been called a "pediatric disease" since most smokers started during adolescence. By the age of 18, 90% of those who will ever try a cigarette have done so, and age 18 years is the average age at which individuals become daily smokers. As with other substance use disorders, the etiology of nicotine dependence is multifactorial and includes biological, psychological, and social factors, including genetic factors.

Nicotine is the primary psychoactive agent in tobacco smoke and smokeless tobacco and has powerful addictive properties (Benowitz 1988). As an indication of the addictive potential of this substance, one-third to one half of all children and adolescents who smoke one cigarette progress to become habitual users. Nicotine is considered to be the "gateway drug" to the use of other substances (Henningfield et al. 1990). Nicotine is readily absorbed in the lung from tobacco smoke or through the mucous membranes with smokeless tobacco. When smoking tobacco, nicotine enters the blood stream and is available to the brain within 7 to 9 seconds (even more quickly than with intravenous administration). Its peak effect occurs within 1 minute, and effects are present after a single puff of smoke. With a half-life of approximately 2 hours, the level of nicotine in the blood stream gradually accumulates during the day, dropping but persisting overnight. Smokers, especially those with severe dependence, awaken in the morning with nicotine withdrawal and rapidly dose themselves.

Nicotine has a multitude of effects. Some are acute, while others appear only after chronic usage. It acts in two primary areas of the brain—the mesolimbic dopaminergic system (the brain reward pathway), which is related to the euphoriant effects of the drug, and the locus coeruleus, which mediates stress reactions and vigilance and relates to the higher mental and cognitive functions. There are specific nicotine receptor sites (the nicotinic cholinergic receptors) throughout the central nervous system in the hypothalamus, hippocampus, thalamus, midbrain, brain stem, and cerebral cortex. In addition, nicotine affects nearly all aspects of the endocrine–neuroendocrine system, including the catecholamine, serotonin, corticosteroid, and pituitary hormones. Its endocrine effects are mediated via the hypothalamic–pituitary axis and the adrenal medullary cortex. Centrally, it causes release of acetylcholine, norepinephrine, serotonin, dopamine, vasopressin, growth hormone, corticotropin, cortisol, prolactin, and endorphins.

Nicotine has stimulant and depressive effects on both the central and the peripheral nervous systems. It also affects the cardiovascular system, the gastrointestinal system, and the skeletal motor system. Nicotine stimulates the cholinergic nervous system (sympathetic and parasympathetic). Through this variety of central and peripheral actions, nicotine improves mood and decreases anxiety; decreases distress in response to stressful stimuli and decreases aggression; improves overall cognitive function and performance (improves reaction time, concentration, vigilance, and stimulus-processing capacity, increases attention, memory and learning, improves the ability to disregard irrelevant stimuli); and decreases the appetite for simple carbohydrates, decreases stress-induced eating, and increases resting metabolic rate. Many individuals soon become tolerant to these effects so that they smoke not to achieve them, but rather to avoid withdrawal symptoms.

Nicotine is a highly addictive substance that causes physical and psychological dependence that is similar to that of opiates and other substances of abuse (Office on Smoking and Health 1988, Henningfield 1984, Jarvik and Henningfield 1988). It is highly reinforcing, leading to compulsive use (Henningfield and Goldberg 1983). From a neurobiological perspective, there is strong evidence that the rewarding effects of smoking are mediated through the dopamine reward pathway, the mesolimbic dopamine (Balfour and Fagerstrom 1996). Nicotinic acetylcholine receptors, the site of action of nicotine, have been found on mesolimbic dopamine neurons (Clark and Pert 1985). Effects are related to dose, and tolerance to its actions develops rapidly, resulting in increased intake. Smokers adjust smoking behavior to regulate and maintain the level of nicotine in the blood stream. A withdrawal syndrome develops in response to reduced intake or total abstinence and involves both physiological and psychological symptoms (Benowitz 1988). Withdrawal symptoms overlap with those of alcohol and other substances of abuse (Hughes et al. 1994). The literature on the biology of the nicotine withdrawal state points to reduced dopaminergic, adrenergic, and norepinephrine function (Fung et al. 1996, Ward et al. 1991). In addition to the physiologically addictive aspects of nicotine, smoking is highly conditioned to cues in the environment.

In addition to nicotine being in tobacco, unprocessed tobacco smoke includes more than 2500 compounds, and when manufactured additives and other compounds are taken into account, about 4000 compounds are present (US Department of Health and Human Services 1988). Research has demonstrated that the vast majority of harm associated with cigarettes is attributable to the by-products of smoking rather than to the effects of nicotine (Slade 1999). Tobacco (not nicotine) is metabolized by the P450/1a2 isoenzyme and enhances the metabolism of psychiatric medications that are also similarly metabolized by this isoenzyme (Lee and D'Alonzo 1993, Goldstein et al. 1991). Quitting smoking will eliminate tobacco's effects on the P450/1a2 isoenzyme, which will typically cause an increase in the blood levels of those medications also metabolized by that isoenzyme, potentially resulting in increased side effects or other adverse events, including increased noncompliance due to the side effects (Lee and D'Alonzo 1993).

Treatment

Nicotine dependence treatment targets severity of the problem, co-occurring disorders, and the different motivational levels to change. Treatment is provided in a range of levels of intensity of care (self-help, brief treatment, and once or twice per week outpatient treatment) and may include different modalities (self-help guides, internet resources, medications, and individual or group therapy). Formal treatment options have expanded rapidly in the past 25 years to include six FDA-approved medications, a range of effective psychosocial interventions including internet and phone-line services. Unfortunately, most insurance plans do not cover nicotine dependence treatment, and only some prescription plans will cover the medications. Few individuals receive combined medications and therapy treatment. Most receiving treatment get medication treatments, and only about 3% of the individuals receiving medication treatments will also receive psychosocial treatment despite the fact that this combination improves outcomes by 50%. Primary care treatment providers tend to offer brief counseling treatment services with follow-up visits. In addition, many individuals receive minimal formal treatment and either purchase over-the-counter nicotine replacement patch or gum, or go to Nicotine Anonymous or other self-help groups in attempting to quit on their own.

Before formal intervention is undertaken, it is beneficial and important to perform a comprehensive evaluation to determine the biological, psychological, and social factors that are most significant in the initiation and maintenance of nicotine use and dependence. Comprehensive evaluation of the individual is outlined in Table 23-2 (American Psychiatric Association 1996, Ziedonis et al. 1998). The assessment often begins with an assessment of the patterns of tobacco usage (number of cigarettes smoked per day, times during the day, location, and circumstances). The severity of nicotine dependence can be assessed with the Fagerstrom Tolerance Questionnaire (Fagerstrom 1978). It assesses factors such as the

Table 23-2	Assessing Nicotine Use and Nicotine Dependence

Current and past patterns of tobacco use
(include multiple sources of nicotine)
Current motivation to quit
Objective measures: breath CO level or cotinine level (saliva, blood, urine)
Assess prior quit attempts (number and what happened in each attempt)
  Why quit? How long abstinent? Why relapsed?
  What treatment was used (how used and for how long)
Assess withdrawal symptoms and dependence criteria
Psychiatric and other substance use history
Medical conditions
Their common triggers (car, people, moods, home, phone calls, meals, etc.)
Perceived barriers against and supports for treatment success
Preference for treatment strategy

amount of time until the first cigarette in the morning, the number of cigarettes smoked in one day, smoking when ill, difficulty refraining from smoking, the degree to which the first cigarette of the day is the most difficult to give up, and smoking more in the morning than in the afternoon. In addition, the amount of tobacco usage can be assessed through cotinine levels or carbon monoxide (CO) levels. Cotinine levels can be obtained from the urine, blood, or saliva to assess the amount of nicotine ingested. Cotinine is a primary metabolite of nicotine and remains in the body for several weeks. Despite the advantage of this longer opportunity for detecting nicotine usage, the cotinine tests are costly and may require several days for a lab to report the results. In contrast, the expired-air test for a CO level is less costly and can be obtained within a minute by any clinician with a CO meter. The CO meter is useful at intake and to monitor for relapse. Higher cotinine and CO levels are associated with a higher number of cigarettes per day and also with the severity of nicotine withdrawal. For the 20-cigarette per day smoker, expired-air CO levels are typically in the 10 to 30 parts per million (ppm) range and cotinine levels 250 to 300 ng/mL range.

A history of prior cessation attempts should include the nature of prior treatments, length of abstinence, timing of relapse, and factors specifically related to relapse (e.g., environmental or interpersonal triggers). Assessing prior treatments includes assessing medications and psychosocial treatments. The five Food and Drug Administration (FDA)-approved medications for nicotine dependence treatment are the four nicotine replacement therapies (NRT) of the patch, gum, spray, and inhaler; and the nonnicotine pill bupropion (Zyban). Sometimes, other medications have been prescribed for nicotine dependence treatment. Assessment about medications includes asking about what dose of medications and how long it was taken, any side effects that developed, and how the individual actually took the medication (especially relevant for NRT). For example, the individual may report taking off the NRT patch prior to a shower and then replacing the same patch, rendering it ineffective. Psychosocial treatments might include group or individual treatment, American Lung Association and other community support groups, hypnosis, acupuncture, or Nicotine Anonymous. A history of specific withdrawal symptoms and their severity and duration is critical, as is an assessment of the smoker's social and environmental contexts, for example, whether other household members smoke, and available family and social supports.

An assessment should be made of the person's reasons for quitting, his or her motivation and commitment and self-efficacy (perceived ability to quit). The individual's stage of readiness for stopping smoking is also important, that is, whether the person is not yet seriously considering stopping smoking (precontemplation), is considering attempting to quit but not for several months (contemplation), is seriously considering quitting in the next month and has begun to think about the necessary steps to stop smoking (preparation), or is actually attempting to stop smoking (action) (Prochaska 1983). It is also important to access the smoker's knowledge about smoking and nicotine dependence because deficits in knowledge and information can have a deleterious effect on smoking cessation attempts.

Assessment of the psychiatric history is also important. Numerous studies have shown the significance of current and past depression in relation to smoking, as well as the increased prevalence rates of cigarette smoking in individuals with a variety of mental disorders, such as MDD, schizophrenia, and alcohol and substance abuse. The presence of these comorbid disorders may also make successful smoking cessation less likely, especially if undiagnosed and untreated.

Assessing the individual for a history of current alcohol or other substance abuse is also important, as the prevalence of smoking in persons with alcohol dependence as well as in other substance abusers is much higher than in the general population. It may also be more difficult for individuals with current or prior substance abuse or dependence to stop smoking, as there is evidence that persons with alcohol dependence and other substance abusers start smoking earlier and are more physiologically dependent on nicotine (Hughes 1993b). In addition, the use of alcohol or other substances may be intimately linked to smoking cigarettes and can serve as a strong trigger for craving and ultimate relapse.

A careful medical history should also be obtained. The presence of significant tobacco-related medical illness can sometimes serve as crucial leverage to help motivate the individual to attempt cessation. Current medications and medical conditions may also be important considerations in determining the approach to cessation, especially with regard to pharmacotherapy. For example, a history of seizures or an eating disorder is usually a contraindication to the use of bupropion/Zyban (nonnicotine pill medication). The individual should be assessed for pulmonary symptoms and signs (cough), and if there is a long history of significant nicotine use, pulmonary function tests should be considered. The presence of significant cardiovascular disease, especially a history of recent myocardial infarction, is especially relevant to planning psychopharmacological interventions. If the individual is already taking a psychiatric medication, consider it important to realize that quitting smoking may result in an increase in medication blood levels and side effects.

Phases of Treatment

The general approach to the treatment of nicotine dependence considers three phases of treatment (engagement, quitting, and relapse prevention) (Table 23-3). Each phase of treatment includes consideration of three primary biological, psychological, and social factors affecting nicotine dependence outcomes. The biological or physiological dependence has already been described and parallels the characteristics of other physiologically addicting substances (dose-related effects, rapid tolerance leading to increased intake and the presence of a withdrawal syndrome, compulsive use). Psychological dependence involves the perceived benefits/reasons a person smokes, such as a perception that they are able to improve mood and sense of well-being, to satisfy craving, and to provide stimulation and relaxation (Goldstein et al. 1991). The social component involves environmental and social cues that become associated with the behavior of smoking cigarettes, such as the association with drinking coffee or alcohol, talking on the telephone, taking a work break, or smoking at parties or social functions. The direct beneficial effects of nicotine on mood and concentration become highly positive reinforcements, as do associated social context and behaviors linked with smoking, which then can act as powerful triggers for relapse during attempts at cessation.

The importance of each of the biopsychosocial factors in initiating and maintaining smoking can vary considerably in different individuals. As a result, smoking cessation interventions should be tailored to the individual and his or her particular circumstances.

Table 23-3	Three Phases of Nicotine Dependence Treatment

Engagement Phase
- Do a comprehensive evaluation of nicotine use and dependence
- Provide MET personalized feedback from the assessment
- Assess motivational level to quit and attempt to set a target quit date
- Explore previous quit attempts—what worked? What did not work? What triggered the return to tobacco use?
- Assess patient preference for treatment (medications, psychosocial treatments, group vs. individual, self-help, etc.) and provide education on treatment
- Create a treatment plan
- Strengthen and renew patient's motivation to quit smoking (MET orientation)
- Identify cues and triggers for usage
- Self-monitoring of smoking behavior (write down when use)
- Help patients gain understanding of their own tobacco use patterns
- Help increase knowledge about triggers and cues
- Help patients understand environmental influences on their smoking
- Begin education about nicotine, tobacco addiction, withdrawal symptoms, etc.
- Begin disconnecting smoking behavior and linked behaviors (no smoking while driving car, talking on phone, during meal time, etc.)
- Help them get medication evaluation and medications for the quitting phase.

Quitting Phase
- Start medications on quit date (NRT) or before quit date (bupropion), sometimes begin NRT (gum, spray, inhaler, not patch) in small amounts and reduce tobacco usage in an equivalent or greater amount
- Teach specific coping techniques for handling withdrawal symptoms, cues/triggers, and how to enhance social support
- Help patient prepare emotionally, behaviorally, and physically for the quit date and the early abstinence period
- Help identify support systems, anticipate challenges, and address ways to handle people, places, things, and mood challenges
- Address nutrition and exercise components
- Address role of family/friends in supporting or sabotaging treatment
- Continue to strengthen client's resolve to quit
- Continue relapse prevention therapy approaches
- Assess triggers to craving and use and high-risk situations
- Coping with cravings, thoughts, and urges
- Problem solving
- Smoke refusal skills
- Planning for emergencies
- Seemingly irrelevant decisions
- Relapse analysis for slips.

Relapse Prevention Phase
- Continue relapse prevention strategies for long-term abstinence
- Reinforce specific coping skills, including mood management and patient specific triggers
- Teach positive coping skills for dealing with frustration and anxiety
- Compliment success and provide encouragement
- Continue focus on maintaining motivation and commitment for abstinence
- Monitor progress
- Provide treatment within your discipline and make referrals when appropriate
- Encourage the use of peer support such as Nicotine Anonymous, help the client gain personal insight, and keep growing in their recovery
- Manage any relapses/slips to continue the course
- Continue medications as needed.

This may be one reason why "one size fits all" generic treatment interventions have had such a low success rate. It must also be kept in mind that nicotine dependence is as complex in its components and determinants as other addictions and that more comprehensive multicomponent treatments may be required.

Algorithms and primers for nicotine dependence treatment have been developed, including those from the American Psychiatric Association (1996) and the US Public Health Service (Fiore et al. 2000). For smokers not yet ready to quit, use of interventions to increase motivation and presentation of information about treatment options are appropriate. Discussing reasons for the person to consider quitting—for example, health consequences specific to the individual—and the factors that may have prevented an attempt is important. Written materials and brief advice from the physician are methods of providing such information and increasing motivation. Preparation for quitting may include self-monitoring or keeping a diary of smoking, planning rewards for successful abstinence, and making a list of reasons for and potential benefits of quitting. Sources of social support should also be identified.

When a smoker is ready for a cessation attempt, a "quit date" should be selected. After cessation, close monitoring should occur during the early period of abstinence. Before the quit date, the person should be encouraged to explore and organize social support for the self-attempt. Plans to minimize cues associated with smoking (e.g., avoiding circumstances likely to contribute to relapse) are important, as is considering alternative coping behaviors for situations with a higher potential for relapse. A telephone or face-to-face follow-up during the first few days after cessation is critical because this is the time that withdrawal symptoms are most severe, with 65% of individuals relapsing by 1 week. A follow-up face-to-face meeting within 1 to 2 weeks allows a discussion of problems that have occurred (e.g., difficulties managing craving) and serves as an opportunity to provide reinforcement for ongoing abstinence. Even after the early period of abstinence, periodic telephone or face-to-face contacts can provide continued encouragement to maintain abstinence, allow problems with maintaining abstinence to be addressed, and provide feedback regarding the health benefits of abstinence.

If an initial attempt at cessation using only information and brief advice from the physician has been unsuccessful, pharmacotherapy may be used unless contraindications are present or unless the person has had few or no significant withdrawal symptoms. The most common pharmacotherapy approaches are nicotine replacement therapies (NRTs—patch, gum, spray, or inhaler) or bupropion (Zyban for nicotine dependence = Wellbutrin for depression). Combining different types of NRT and bupropion is becoming more common in clinical practice, including using these medications for at least several months and in some cases 1 year or longer. Maintenance medications are being considered in an effort of harm reduction in a more select group of individuals. If a detoxification/quit attempt with pharmacotherapy alone fails, psychosocial treatments and the use of higher NRT dosages/multiple medications are the next possible clinical steps. Psychosocial treatments are often available through organizations such as the American Cancer Society, American Lung Association, the American Heart Association, or through local hospitals that provide health prevention and public education programs (American Cancer Society/National Cancer Institute 1989). If pharmacotherapy is unacceptable or contraindicated, behavioral therapy (BT) alone should be provided. Failure with pharmacotherapy or BT alone suggests the need for more detailed in-depth assessment and more intensive and multimodal interventions.

Self-Help

Many smokers have successfully quit smoking without participating in formal treatment (Fiore et al. 1990). Although only about 3 to 4% are successful during the past year, this success rate improves with multiple attempts and probable self-learning through trial and error and learning from others. Eventually, about 50% of smokers are able to quit and more than 90% of successful quitters have been able to do so without the assistance of professionals or formal programs. These numbers reflect multiple factors including the limitations on access to treatment (nonexistent health insurance coverage and limited number of providers with expertise to help), the cumulative process of multiple attempts, learning from others and from self-help materials, and the severity of the nicotine dependence. The advantage of quitting without professional intervention is the decreased expense and time commitment; however, professional treatment may be necessary for higher severity cases that are often complicated by other behavioral health problems. The primary unassisted method of detoxification from nicotine dependence is precipitous cessation (cold turkey), which is used by more than 80% of smokers. This is followed by spontaneous strategies to handle cravings and triggers. Some smokers attempt to limit intake, taper the number of cigarettes smoked, or switch to a reduced tar or nicotine brand. Special filters and holders are also available to decrease the amount of smoke that is available from a cigarette. These methods are usually less successful because smokers have been shown to alter smoking behavior by increasing the frequency, volume, or duration of the inhalation to ensure maintenance of blood levels of nicotine adequate to prevent withdrawal symptoms (Moss and Prue 1982, Russell 1987). Some smokers use nonprescription pills that are analogs of nicotine, such as lobeline, to help manage or prevent withdrawal symptoms. These agents have not been shown to be effective in controlled studies (Hughes 1994a).

Some geographical areas have Nicotine Anonymous groups that are structured similar to Alcoholics Anonymous or Narcotics Anonymous groups. These groups are based on the 12-Step approach to recovery from addictions. Nicotine Anonymous is a relatively new organization (founded in 1985) and does not have the extensive network that other 12-Step programs like Alcoholics Anonymous or Narcotics Anonymous have developed. No formal controlled studies of the benefits of this intervention have been carried out. In addition, self-help written materials can play an important role in educating individuals about the negative health effects of nicotine, the benefits of quitting, and the nature of the addiction. Self-help literature, internet resources, and Nicotine Anonymous can be effectively integrated into formal treatments of brief interventions and individual and group treatments. Even smokers with major health conditions, such as chronic obstructive pulmonary disease or cardiovascular disease, often have a difficult time attaining and maintaining abstinence. Numerous psychological and pharmacological treatments have been developed to assist in smoking cessation.

Brief or Minimal Medical Professional-Delivered Interventions/Advice

Even a brief face-to-face intervention by a physician or other medical staff can increase the likelihood of cessation two- to tenfold (Klesges et al. 1990). The impact of physicians' brief advice to quit has received the most study relative to other disciplines such as nursing; however, clearly all disciplines have opportunity to make an impact. Physicians can inquire about an individual's smoking status, urge the individual to stop smoking, and spend a brief time counseling the individual about cessation strategies. Multiple follow-up interventions, even telephone contacts by other medical staff, can further improve the cessation rate. Resources are available to assist physicians in providing effective antismoking interventions, which can even be used by those not highly skilled in counseling. Physicians' advice appears to be most successful with individuals with a serious medical problem or specific medical reason for quitting (e.g., pregnancy or congestive heart disease). In addition, because an estimated 70% of smokers in the United States visit their physicians at least once a year, an important opportunity exists for providing this type of smoking cessation intervention.

Formal Treatment Options

There are now numerous effective psychosocial and pharmacological approaches that can be used in nicotine dependence treatment. Psychosocial intervention alone, pharmacotherapy alone, or combined approaches may be used. Given individuals' preferences and current concerns with cost-effectiveness, less costly single-modality interventions are often used initially, whereas more costly multimodal interventions are often reserved for persons for whom cessation attempts have failed. This may not be the wisest strategy, but it is the most common. Whether failure with unaided or minimal intervention attempts may have a negative effect on future cessation attempts is not known; however, some research suggests that with each repeated cessation attempt, the person gains additional knowledge and experience that may contribute to success in future cessation attempts.

Somatic Treatments

Pharmacological interventions have become an important component of treating nicotine dependence. Approaches used parallel other addictions in treating acute withdrawal (detoxification), protracted withdrawal, and even maintenance for harm reduction. The primary medications are NRT and bupropion. All six of these modalities are FDA approved and have demonstrated efficacy. Other medications may have some potential; however, they are not FDA approved and have limited empirical foundation to support their use (Table 23-4).

Nicotine replacement therapy (NRT) is the most widely used medication option and is available over the counter (patch and gum) or by prescription (patch, gum, spray, and inhaler). The principle behind nicotine replacement is that nicotine is the dependence producing constituent of cigarette smoking, and that smoking cessation and abstinence can be achieved by replacing nicotine without the harmful impurities in cigarette smoke. The abuse liability of nicotine replacement appears to be minimal. The intent is to substitute a safer, medically prescribed substance for nicotine and then to taper the substance in a manner that prevents or minimizes withdrawal. This agonist approach is similar to the use of benzodiazepines to treat acute alcohol withdrawal or methadone substitution and taper in the treatment of heroin addiction. The substituted nicotine initially prevents significant withdrawal symptoms that may lead to relapse during the early period of smoking cessation. The substituted nicotine is then gradually tapered and discontinued. Replacement produces a lower overall plasma level of nicotine than that experienced with smoking. Replacement not only avoids the strongly reinforcing peaks in plasma level but also prevents the emergence of withdrawal symptoms by maintaining the nicotine plasma level above a threshold. Typically, each cigarette contains about 13 mg of nicotine and about 2 mg is absorbed into the body.

Nicotine gum, approved in 1984, was the first NRT approved. It slowly releases nicotine from an ion exchange resin when chewed. The nicotine released is absorbed through the buccal mucous membranes. The NRT gum is available in doses of 2 and 4 mg, and the recommended dosing is in the range of 9 to 16 pieces per day. Peak blood nicotine levels achieved are low (approximately 10–15 ng/mL) compared to those in dependent smokers (15–100 ng/mL). Placebo-controlled studies of nicotine gum treatment in smoking cessation clinics show a doubling of abstinence rates (Lam et al. 1987) with the 4-mg dose possibly providing a better outcome than the 2-mg dose for persons who are highly nicotine dependent (Tonnesen et al. 1988). Nicotine gum is more effective when used in conjunction with some type of psychosocial intervention, particularly BT (Lam et al. 1987). Outcome is more positive when a definite schedule for gum use is prescribed—for example, one piece of gum per hour while awake—than when used on an as-needed basis (Fagerstrom and Melen 1985, Goldstein et al. 1989). Some studies suggest that it is also more effective when used for longer than 3 months (Fagerstrom and Melen 1985). Tapering may be necessary after 4

Table 23-4	Approaches to the Pharmacological Treatment of Nicotine Dependence

Nicotine replacement or substitution (agonist administration)—FDA-approved nicotine patch, gum, spray, lozenge, and inhaler
Nonnicotine pill—bupropion/Zyban—FDA approved
Combinations of nicotine replacement types and/or bupropion
Non-FDA-approved experimental options:
  Blockade therapy (antagonist administration)
  Nonspecific attenuation therapy
  Deterrent therapy

to 6 months of use, especially for individuals using higher total daily doses of gum. Nicotine gum is often not effectively utilized in individuals with temporomandibular joint problems, dental problems, and dentures. Nicotine gum requires a highly motivated individual and a good deal of time in instructing the individual in proper use of the gum. Many individuals find the gum difficult to learn to use properly. Individuals must be instructed that nicotine gum is not like bubble gum and that the gum is crunched a few times and "parked" between the gum and cheek. It should not be used soon after drinking acidic substances such as coffee, soda, or orange juice because the acidic environment in the mouth interferes with its release and absorption. Specifics of the proper use of nicotine gum are provided by Schneider (1988). Side effects and adverse effects include local irritation in the mouth, tongue, and throat, mouth ulcers, hiccups, jaw ache, gastrointestinal symptoms (flatulence, indigestion, nausea), anorexia, and palpitations. About 6 to 9% continue to use nicotine gum for 1 year—this may reflect some risk for dependence. However, most individuals report that they still prefer the tobacco product and are using the nicotine gum only to avoid the tobacco usage (Hajek et al. 1988). The nicotine lozenge was FDA approved in 2002, and is similar in dosing to the nicotine gum and less complicated to use.

The *nicotine patch* transdermal delivery system provides continual sustained release of nicotine, which is absorbed through the skin. This form of nicotine replacement more than doubles the 1-year cessation rate (Hughes 1994b). There is a dose–response relationship, with individuals receiving higher doses attaining higher cessation rates. The nicotine patch eliminates the conditioning of repeated nicotine use, which remains present with the use of other NRT products. Compliance rates are higher because it involves once-daily dosing and its administration is simple and discreet. The typical starting dose of NRT patch is 21 or 15 mg patch; however, in some cases multiple patches are used. Lower dose patches available at 7 and 14 mg are used to taper after smoking cessation. The patch delivers approximately 0.9 mg of nicotine/hour. Steady-state nicotine levels are 13 to 25 ng/mL and the highest levels are seen soon after patch application. The nicotine patch is often used for a total of 6 to 12 weeks but can be used for much longer (American Psychiatric Association 1996). The transdermal patch does not allow for self-titrated dosing, craving, and nicotine withdrawal symptoms like the other NRT routes (gum, spray, inhaler); however, the nicotine blood levels are significantly less than with smoking. The patch can be used more discreetly and can be used despite dental or temporomandibular joint problems. Specifics on the proper use of transdermal nicotine are provided by Gourley (1994).

Although the nicotine patch is well tolerated, about 25% of individuals have significant local skin irritation or erythema and 10% discontinue the patch because of intolerable side effects. Other side effects include sleep problems with the 24-hour patches. In a few cases, nicotine toxicity developed when smokers continued their usual heavy cigarette smoking while using the transdermal nicotine patch. However, transdermal nicotine may cause less activation of blood coagulation and have less impact on the sympathetic nervous system than nicotine polacrilex gum; therefore, it may be preferable in the presence of cardiac disease (Rennard et al. 1991, Benowitz et al. 1993). One study found that it could be safely used in individuals with stable coronary artery disease (Anonymous 1994, Gross et al. 1989, Hughes 1995).

Some experts suggest using nicotine gum concurrently with transdermal nicotine on an as-needed basis to cover emergent withdrawal symptoms or craving not controlled by replacement from the transdermal patch, whereas others suggest simply increasing the dose of the transdermal patch or using gum initially and then switching to the patch (Gourley 1994, Fagerstrom et al. 1993). Combining transdermal nicotine and nicotine gum increases the potential for significant side effects.

The *nicotine nasal spray* is rapidly absorbed and produces a higher nicotine blood level than does transdermal nicotine or gum. A single dose of the spray delivers 0.5 mg to each nostril and it can be used one to three times/hour. It has been suggested that the effective daily dose in nicotine dependent smokers is 15 to 20 sprays (8–10 mg) per day (Balfour and Fagerstrom 1996). Onset of action of the spray is the most rapid of all nicotine replacements; nicotine levels in plasma reach 10 to 20 ng/mL (Balfour and Fagerstrom 1996). An initial concern about the nasal spray had been the potential for abuse because it has the most rapid absorption rate of the NRTs. It replicates repeated administration of nicotine in smoking, resulting in reinforcing peaks in the plasma level of the drug. Side effects of the spray include local airway irritation (i.e., coughing, rhinorrhea, lacrimation, nasal irritation), but tolerance to these local effects appears to develop. Systemic effects include nausea, headache, dizziness, tachycardia, and sweating (Balfour and Fagerstrom 1996, Sutherland et al. 1992).

The *nicotine inhaler* provides nicotine through a cartridge that must be "puffed." It mimics the upper airway stimulation experienced with smoking; however, absorption is primarily through the oropharyngeal mucosa. Although the blood level of nicotine is lower than with other forms of nicotine replacement (8–10 ng/mL), the inhaler has been shown to be effective (Tonneson et al. 1993). Controlled trials (Schneider 1996) indicate 1-year abstinence rates of 17% for the nicotine inhaler and 8% for placebo. Side effects of the inhaler and spray include local irritation, cough, headache, nausea, dyspepsia, the need for multiple dosing, and the impossibility of discreet use.

Bupropion, the nonnicotine pill FDA-approved medication option, is a heterocyclic, atypical antidepressant that blocks the re-uptake of both dopamine and norepinephrine. Its efficacy as an aid to smoking cessation was first demonstrated in three double-blind placebo-controlled trials in nondepressed chronic cigarette smokers (Hurt 1997) (28% versus 4% abstinence at 12 weeks) (Ferry et al. 1992). It was well tolerated and did not produce weight gain. The effects in smoking cessation appear to be unrelated to its antidepressant properties (Hurt 1997). Smoking cessation rates appear to improve further when bupropion is combined with the nicotine patch (Nides 1997). In all studies, adverse events had a low incidence and included dry mouth, insomnia, nausea, and skin rash. There have been no reports of seizures in any smoking cessation studies to date; however, this agent should not be used in individuals with a history of seizure disorders.

Antidepressants have been used in an attempt to attenuate withdrawal symptoms, to treat or prevent emergent depressive symptoms or episodes in the early phase of cessation, and to prevent relapse of depressive episodes in individuals with a history of depression. Antidepressants may provide significant benefits in special populations of individuals with current or prior major depressive disorder (MDD), dysthymic disorder, or current depressive symptoms when these factors predict a poor outcome. Given that negative affect has been shown to be the most common antecedent of a smoking relapse, this approach appears promising (Shiffman 1982). If antidepressants are used, pretreatment is necessary because the benefit of the medication may not be apparent for 1 to 3 weeks.

Combined NRTs/bupropion or serial pharmacotherapeutic approaches may also be beneficial, especially in more difficult to treat cases of nicotine dependence. For example, combining the patch with other nicotine replacement medications like nicotine gum or the spray allows for both more rapid onset of action and reduction of withdrawal symptoms through steady levels of nicotine released by the patch. Combining nicotine replacement with nonnicotine replacement strategies (e.g., bupropion and nicotine patch) has been beneficial in further improving outcomes in some studies and is common in clinical practice. The combination approach offers the advantage of multiple neurobiological mechanisms of actions. In addition, many researchers increasingly believe that periods of pharmacotherapy should be extended, although the issue of whether longer-term pharmacotherapy is beneficial in improving cessation rates remains unresolved. There may be some smokers who are unable to stop smoking without ongoing nicotine replacement, similar to individuals dependent on heroin who must be maintained on methadone. Although long-term/maintenance use of NRT requires further study, successful maintenance in smokers who have chronic relapses would potentially reduce a number of the serious health risks associated with smoking, inspite of individuals still being exposed to the effects of nicotine. Ongoing maintenance antidepressant treatment may also be necessary for a time for some individuals with a history of serious depressive illness or for those who have had significant depressive symptoms emerge on cessation that do not improve with time.

Non-FDA-approved pharmacotherapy approaches are being evaluated or have limited empirical support. Given the FDA-approved options availability, these approaches have less clinical relevance at this time. This includes the use of mecamylamine, clonidine, and silver acetate.

Psychosocial Treatments

In contrast with the treatment of other substance use disorders, psychosocial treatment is underutilized and has not evolved to be the cornerstone of treatment. This limited utilization of psychosocial treatments does not match the very positive outcomes from either psychosocial treatments alone (25% 1-year abstinence with BT) or when combined with NRT or bupropion (50% improvement compared to NRT or bupropion alone); however, it does match the lack of health care coverage for this service. The underutilization of psychosocial treatment has become the cultural norm in nicotine dependence treatment. This may be due to several important considerations. These include the following: (1) Primary care practitioners most frequently attempt to address nicotine dependence and do not traditionally integrate BTs. (2) Nicotine dependence treatment is often not paid for by health care insurance companies (3) Few behavioral health specialists have been formally trained in nicotine dependence treatments. (4) Mental health and addiction treatment programs have ignored addressing tobacco in those treatment settings, although this appears to be changing. (5) Individuals are unaware of this treatment modality and its success rates, and believe that medications or quitting cold turkey is all that is needed.

A great variety of psychosocial interventions have been developed to help in the treatment of nicotine dependence (Table 23-5). As in treating other substance use disorders, the core psychotherapy approaches are motivational enhancement therapy (MET), cognitive–behavioral therapy (CBT) (relapse prevention), and 12-Step facilitation. Psychosocial interventions, particularly BT, have been shown to increase abstinence rates significantly (Ferry et al. 1992). However, only 7% of smokers attempting to quit smoking are willing to participate in BT (Ferry et al. 1992). In addition, it is more expensive than pharmacotherapy and more labor-intensive.

Motivational enhancement therapy (MET) is especially helpful for the smoker who continues to be ambivalent about quitting. MET aims to enhance the smoker's commitment

Table 23-5	Psychosocial Interventions for the Treatment of Nicotine Dependence

Self-help materials
Brief advice from the physician
Multiple component therapies
Motivational enhancement therapy
Cognitive–behavioral therapies/relapse prevention
Nicotine fading
Nicotine anonymous
Others used, but with limited empirical support: hypnosis and acupuncture

and motivation to quit smoking. The therapist maintains an approach that is tailored to the individual and is empathic and optimistic. The therapist adopts a focused but nonconfrontational style while examining the effect of tobacco use on the smoker's life and collaborating with the smoker to develop and implement a treatment plan. MET is compatible with Prochaska and DiClemente's stages of change model, in which individuals are assessed as being in either the precontemplation, contemplation, preparation, action, or maintenance stage of change. This model also emphasizes the importance of tailoring interventions to the individual's motivational level (Prochaska et al. 1992). Interventions aimed at immediate cessation of tobacco are often ineffective for individuals in the contemplation and precontemplation stages especially since there is usually not a powerful external motivator to maintain compliance. Without an external motivator, a confrontational approach is likely to provoke resistance and treatment dropout. Realistic goals for the poorly motivated individual are to simply increase awareness of the impact of tobacco and the possibility of change. Later interventions may involve creating a change of plan and discussing feelings of ambivalence, including the individuals' perceived benefits of using tobacco and reasons to stop using tobacco (Miller et al. 1995). An important initial component of MET is to provide personalized feedback on how tobacco may be affecting their lives and others. Feedback that has impact might include the cost of tobacco products during a year, negative health consequences, likelihood for health improvement in case of abstinence, social stigma towards smoking, CO levels, interaction of tobacco metabolism and specific medications, and other health consequences (wrinkles, impotence, etc.).

Behavioral and cognitive–behavioral therapy (CBT) approaches have been developed to be effective treatments for nicotine dependence, and as for any other addiction CBTs are one of the core therapy approaches. BTs often include a self-monitoring assessment phase that is linked with specific treatment interventions. The self-monitoring involves the identification of affective, cognitive, and environmental cues that trigger smoking behavior. Understanding the cues and triggers for usage are helpful in guiding the CBT approach of relapse prevention.

Relapse prevention training helps clients develop problem-solving skills for coping with situations or emotions that might be likely to precipitate relapse, as well as alternative behaviors appropriate for high-risk situations. Individuals learn to manage an abstinence violation ("slip" or "lapse") in a way that prevents a relapse to smoking. Discussing ways of managing withdrawal symptoms, such as sleep disturbance and irritability, can also be useful and, if performed in a group setting, can allow individuals to learn from others struggling with cessation. Stress management and relaxation training are often also used as adjunctive interventions, individually or in a group setting. Problems with the group format include a generally low compliance rate, lack of availability of groups in all geographical areas or at a given point in time, and individuals' reluctance to participate. Problems with the individual format include higher cost and the need for a larger number of counselors per population (Hajek et al. 1985).

In relapse prevention coping skills training, individuals are taught skills to manage situations without resorting to smoking. Cognitive approaches involve specific techniques such as reframing or restricting thoughts related to smoking or replacing thoughts about smoking with thoughts intended to enhance motivation or self-efficacy. Assertiveness training can contribute to improved coping by helping individuals to ask for assistance from significant others and to request that others refrain from smoking in their presence. One controlled trial found that a cognitive intervention focused on enhancing the regulation of affect produced a better outcome in smokers with a history of MDD, suggesting some potential benefit of providing more expensive, time-intensive interventions to specific populations of individuals (Hall et al. 1992). *Stimulus control strategies* involve removing or altering cues that have been strongly associated with smoking, for example, avoiding certain situations that are likely to increase craving or trigger smoking. Cue extinction involves repeated exposure of the individual to cues or triggers associated with smoking. Through repeated episodes of exposure that are not followed by smoking, these cues and triggers gradually lose their power to provoke craving. *Nicotine fading* contrasts with an abrupt discontinuation of tobacco. In some cases, this includes switching to a different brand of cigarettes with lower nicotine, and it usually also focuses on gradually reducing the number of cigarettes smoked on a schedule over time, usually several weeks. Nicotine fading sometimes helps to make the transition from several packs of cigarettes per day to the reduced amount of nicotine during NRT and other treatments. Nicotine fading may help any smoker try to quit; however, the research results are mixed and more research must be done in this area. Another nicotine fading strategy focuses on disconnecting specific triggers and tobacco usage, for example, helping individuals not to smoke while in the car, on the phone, or during mealtime. Sometimes this reduces the overall nicotine consumption in the day, and it has the effect of increasing the individual's self-efficacy that they can begin to shape their behaviors and develop coping strategies to handle specific situations (American Psychiatric Association 1996). *Aversive techniques* include the use of rapid smoking and smoke holding. Rapid smoking involves inhaling cigarette smoke every 6 seconds until the smoker becomes ill. Several repetitions over several sessions are usually planned. Smoke holding involves holding smoke in the mouth and continuing to breathe. Both techniques have been found effective and safe even in individuals with medical complications from smoking. A limiting factor in the use of these techniques is acceptability by the individual. In *contingency contracting*, the individual participates in developing rewards for not smoking or punishment for smoking. As an example, an individual might give money to a friend or person overseeing the treatment. The money would be returned only if the individual successfully stopped smoking for a prescribed period.

Despite the fact that there has been little controlled research examining whether psychosocial intervention with spouses and significant others or families can increase abstinence rates, overall social support for individuals who are attempting to stop smoking appears to improve the outcome. Others in the smoker's immediate family or social circle can be involved in their treatment through education about appropriate supportive behaviors. Concerned others can also be engaged in treatment to provide assessment information or to help enhance the individual's motivation.

Hypnosis and acupuncture are two approaches that some individuals believe have helped them in their efforts to quit smoking; however, there is limited research support for these approaches and treatment guidelines still list them as potentially promising approaches. Studies suggest that hypnosis has little more than a weak positive effect on outcome in smoking cessation (Schwartz 1987, 1991). In addition, not all people are hypnotically suggestive; therefore, the technique may have limited applicability, availability, and acceptability. Meta-analysis of studies on the effect of acupuncture shows no evidence of efficacy on the outcome of smoking cessation (Ter Riet et al. 1990). Positive effects likely represent a placebo effect related to the individual's expectations. Controlled trials have not consistently shown the efficacy of acupuncture and hypnosis and the American Psychiatric Association (APA) guidelines determined that these treatments lacked sufficient evidence to be recommended (American Psychiatric Association 1996).

Combined Psychosocial and Psychopharmacological Therapies

All nicotine dependence treatment practice guidelines recommend the integration of nicotine dependence treatment medications (NRT and bupropion) with behavioral and supportive psychosocial treatment approaches. Empirical evidence supports the finding that medications double the quit rate compared to placebo, and face-to-face BT can double the quit rate compared to minimal psychosocial intervention. BT also can increase medication compliance. Integrated treatment further increases the quit rate by another 50% and triples the outcome rate compared to a control group (Fiore et al. 1990). Nicotine dependence treatment guidelines by the American Psychiatric Association (1996), Agency for Health Care Policy Research (1996), and the US Public Health Service (Fiore et al. 2000) support integrated treatment, and are excellent sources of clinical and research information. Recent reviews and meta-analyses by Hughes (1995), Fiore and colleagues (1990), Baille and colleagues (1994), and Ziedonis and colleagues (2001) also support integrated treatment.

Compared with treating other addictions, there is philosophical support among clinicians for integrated treatment for nicotine dependence. This support is probably due to the fact that there are effective medications for nicotine dependence and the absence of controversies that have plagued other fields of addiction, particularly with regard to abstinence versus controlled use and medical versus behavioral approaches. Unfortunately, few smokers use BT because of the added cost, lack of local expertise, waiting time for treatment, and preference against group therapy. Efforts are being made to make BT more acceptable to smokers and to triage smokers to more intensive therapies as needed.

Hughes (1995) performed a meta-analysis of existing studies of combined psychosocial and pharmacological treatments for smoking cessation and found that the addition of nicotine gum to psychosocial therapies resulted in a 60 to 80% increase in abstinence, whereas addition of transdermal nicotine produced a 40 to 80% increase in abstinence. Addition of psychosocial therapies to nicotine replacement (gum or transdermal) resulted in a 60 to 80% increase in abstinence with nicotine gum and an odds ratio of 3 : 1 for transdermal nicotine. Studies of combined nicotine gum and psychosocial treatment showed additive, possibly synergistic positive effects.

Managing Repeated Relapses

Although generally effective treatments have been developed for nicotine dependence, research is limited on treatment matching and determining the timing and duration of interventions. Questions regarding treatment specificity become even more complicated when treating smokers who have experienced repeated relapses, those who have been totally unable to stop smoking, or those who are able to maintain abstinence for only brief periods (Table 23-6). Treatment algorithms applied to the general population of smokers may have little relevance to the smoker who suffers chronic relapses. Given the lack of data regarding treatment specificity, the key to planning interventions with smokers who have had repeated relapses is a comprehensive reevaluation to determine the unique set of factors related to repeated relapse in a given individual. This analysis can serve as the basis for developing an individualized comprehensive treatment program.

In approaching evaluation and treatment planning, it is important not to view the smoker as a "failure" but rather to understand how neglecting to adequately understand the illness of nicotine dependence as it presents in the particular individual has resulted in ineffective treatment with a poor outcome. It is also important to realize that even our

Table 23-6	Effectiveness of Nicotine Dependence Treatment Interventions
No professional or formal intervention	5%
Physicians' advice	10%
Nicotine polacrilex	15–20%
Nicotine patch, gum, inhaler	20–25%
Bupropion	25%
Behavioral therapy	25–30%
Medication and behavioral therapy	40%

"intensive" nicotine dependence treatments pale compared to the intensity of addiction treatment for other substances (residential treatment, intensive outpatient programs, partial hospitalizations, etc.). In some cases, the repeat relapsing smoker would appear to benefit from more intensive interventions, multiple-component interventions, or both. However, in some cases, these smokers did not receive an adequate single intervention and did not ever receive an adequate "dose" of treatment. In the latter case, treating with a previously used single therapy and ensuring the adequacy of all aspects of the treatment may be appropriate. For example, an individual may have relapsed despite being treated with NRT gum because an intermittent dosing schedule was prescribed or because of improper use of the gum, both of which resulted in an inadequate overall dose of nicotine replacement followed by withdrawal symptoms and relapse. Such an individual might be treated with NRT transdermal patch to improve compliance and ensure a stable plasma level of nicotine to prevent withdrawal symptoms. Alternatively, the dose of nicotine the individual was prescribed may have been too low and the withdrawal symptoms too substantial to refrain from relapsing. In some rarer cases, the dose may have been too high, leading to adverse effects, discontinuation of the transdermal patch, and subsequent relapse. Providing a lower dose that is tolerated may lead to successful cessation with a single previously used treatment. An inappropriate single treatment may also have been provided, as in the case of a male treated with one of the non-FDA-approved medications of clonidine for the management of nicotine withdrawal symptoms when research data show that clonidine is effective primarily in women. A single treatment may have been inappropriate in that it was focused on an area that is not critical, whereas an area critical to the maintenance of abstinence has been overlooked. An individual without a high degree of physiological dependence on nicotine may have been treated with nicotine replacement while the fact that her husband is a heavy smoker was not addressed. A future cessation attempt might be preceded by conjoint sessions with the spouse to motivate him also to stop smoking, to educate him about the psychological effects of smoking and the behavioral changes that may accompany cessation, and to enlist his aid in providing a more supportive environment for nicotine dependence treatment (e.g., not smoking at home or in her presence).

Even with multiple interventions, an important aspect of relapse may have been overlooked. For example, both nicotine replacement and group therapy may have been provided to a woman who then made a conscious decision to start smoking again to lose the weight gained during the cessation attempt. In this case, educating the woman about the effects of nicotine on metabolism, helping her develop a healthy diet and exercise plan, and providing her with a cognitive intervention to assist her in reframing and accepting the weight gain as a return to a normal weight that was abnormally lowered by nicotine might make a critical difference in the success of the cessation attempt. Planning to address weight loss at a future time after abstinence has been solidly established is an example of how serial treatment interventions might be used successfully. Alternative modalities might also be appropriate. For example, a group BT might have been prescribed for a person who was so anxious and uncomfortable in the presence of others that he or she avoided attending many of the sessions and was unable to participate even when present. Providing individual sessions in which key elements of the BT are presented and discussed might lead to more successful cessation.

The degree of aggressiveness in treating smokers who have repeated relapses will depend in part on the immediacy and seriousness of the consequences of continued smoking. For example, a pregnant woman endangering the health of a developing fetus is a situation that requires immediate intervention. Likewise, a man with severe cardiac or vascular disease in whom continued smoking poses a serious threat to health or life may require immediate aggressive multimodal interventions.

The skills, knowledge, and experience of a nicotine dependence treatment specialist may be required in complex cases in which more intensive or aggressive individualized treatment is indicated or when more complex psychosocial interventions such as relapse prevention are tailored to the individual. Smokers who suffer repeated relapses may require more frequent monitoring as well as coordination of multiple services or interventions that can involve considerable expenditure of clinical time. This is especially true for persons with serious medical or psychiatric problems, or for pregnant women who require careful coordination of treatment through active collaboration with medical caretakers. The person providing or overseeing treatment for smokers who have chronic relapses must accept the reality of an ongoing long-term relationship that may be demanding of her or his time and attention as well as clinical acumen if appropriate support and monitoring are to be available.

With regard to reassessing specifics of treatment, it is important to determine if prior pharmacotherapy has been used. If nicotine replacement has not been used previously, if there are no contraindications to its use, and if it is acceptable to the smoker, it should be included as an element of a future treatment plan. As noted previously, assessing whether prior pharmacotherapy has been adequate in its focus, dose and duration is also important. Some smokers who have had repeated relapses may require multiple pharmacological agents, a longer duration of treatment, long-term maintenance with nicotine replacement, or a combination of these modalities.

When pharmacotherapy has been assessed as adequate, the addition of BT should be considered, as data show a significant benefit in improving cessation rates when BT is added to pharmacotherapy (Hughes 1995). A history of depressive episodes or current depressive symptoms may have been overlooked. In such a case, or when significant depressive symptoms have emerged during the acute withdrawal period, pretreatment with antidepressant medication added to the prior treatment regimen may result in successful cessation.

It is important to determine if prior psychosocial interventions (e.g., group BT) have been provided. Group BT most often includes components with several foci: providing information and education about nicotine dependence; developing and improving coping skills, especially those related to situations in which relapse is likely; and providing emotional support during withdrawal and early abstinence. If prior group therapy has not been used or does not appear to have been adequate, referral to an appropriate group may be indicated. Whether more dynamically oriented group therapy is beneficial has not been investigated in a controlled fashion.

If adequate group BT has previously been provided, and there does not appear to be a deficit in knowledge, an individual behavioral approach focusing on specific aspects of relapse may be useful. Some individuals may have idiosyncratic factors related to relapse that can be adequately addressed only in individual psychotherapy. The person may also have more of an opportunity in individual psychotherapy to discuss the difficulties of cessation, grieve the loss of smoking and its role in his or her life, express anger, and discuss stresses in life that may have contributed to relapse. Finally, individuals who find participation in a group therapy format unacceptable may be candidates for individual psychotherapy.

The family and home environment should also be reassessed to determine if the smoker is receiving adequate support from the spouse, significant other, family, and general social circle. Conjoint marital or family sessions may be beneficial to educate family members about smoking cessation and the psychological, physiological, and behavioral changes that can occur with cessation. The family can also be counseled about what types of behaviors can undermine rather than support the nicotine dependence treatment effort. Family members can also assist and support the smoker in complying with treatment, for example, attending group meetings or encouraging the smoker to call the physician, rather than discontinuing treatment, if adverse effects result from pharmacotherapy. The presence of one or more active smokers in the household may also need to be addressed, as this factor predicts relapse.

Alterations in various aspects of the smoker's lifestyle also may be required. The person may need to change deeply ingrained behavioral patterns such as socializing and smoking during the morning work break with coworkers. Alterations in diet and the addition of an exercise regimen may also be helpful, although there are no controlled studies to support this.

Finally, ongoing monitoring and feedback regarding improvement in medical conditions related to cigarette smoking and nicotine use may be helpful in maintaining a high level of motivation for continued abstinence, particularly in smokers with more serious medical conditions.

Some smokers may not be able to achieve successful abstinence with outpatient treatment despite intensive multiple interventions. Inpatient treatment represents a drastic intervention that should be reserved for the most treatment-resistant individual who have been completely unsuccessful despite repeated attempts and treatment with a variety of interventions. Inpatient treatment can provide the most intensive and aggressive program of treatment interventions coupled with close monitoring and prevention of access to nicotine. It requires a commitment of both time and money, however, as almost no insurance policies reimburse for such treatment. Inpatient nicotine dependence treatment is usually 1 week in duration. Follow-up data from the few programs in existence suggest that it may be effective for some highly treatment-resistant smokers (Hurt et al. 1992, Docherty 1991).

Treatment with Co-Occurring Mental Illness or Other Addictions

Individuals with nicotine dependence and either a co-occurring mental illness, another addiction, or all three are more likely to be seeking treatment and require some modifications in the traditional nicotine treatment approach. A critical issue in the treatment planning is the timing of the nicotine dependence treatment. There is literature supporting treating all together and also in delaying the nicotine dependence treatment until the other problems are stabilized. Successful nicotine dependence treatment in persons with active alcohol dependence is less likely than in individuals recovering from alcohol dependence; however, a few addiction treatment programs have addressed both problems simultaneously with success. Nicotine replacement appears to be especially beneficial in helping smokers with co-occurring mental illness and addiction. Appropriate treatment of the mental illness or other addiction is also important, including appropriate medications and therapy approaches. These individuals often benefit from clinicians beginning with a motivational enhancement approach that enhances the smoker's readiness to change and self-efficacy. Adding BT may address the social and other skills deficits that are often present in persons suffering from these co-occurring problems (Hughes 1993b). Successful nicotine dependence treatment has been shown in several studies to be associated with successful recovery from alcohol dependence (Hughes 1993a, b, Burling and Ziff 1988, Budney et al. 1993, Sellers et al. 1987).

There is a growing literature supporting that treatment can be effective with these harder to treat smokers when motivational enhancement, NRT medications, psychiatric medications, and BTs are integrated (Ziedonis et al. 1994, American Psychiatric Association 1996). Several authors summarize ways to modify and integrate medication and BT approaches for use among smokers with schizophrenia (Ziedonis and George 1997, Hughes and McHugh 1995), with depression (Hall et al. 1998), and with substance use disorders (Bobo 1989, Clemmey et al. 1997, Istvan and Matarazzo 1984).

Comparison of DSM-IV-TR/ICD-10 Diagnostic Criteria

The DSM-IV-TR and ICD-10 symptom lists for nicotine withdrawal include some different items: the ICD-10 list has craving, malaise, increased cough, and mouth ulceration and does not include the DSM-IV-TR decreased heart rate item.

References

Agency for Health Care Policy and Research (1996) Smoking cessation clinical practice guidelines. *JAMA* **275**, 1270–1280.

American Cancer Society/National Cancer Institute (1989) *Quit for Good: A Practitioners' Stop-Smoking Guide*, Publication 89–1825. National Institutes of Health, Bethesda, MD.

American Psychiatric Association (1980) *Diagnostic and Statistical Manual of Mental Disorders*, 3rd ed. APA, Washington, DC.

American Psychiatric Association (1996) *Practice Guideline for the Treatment of Patients with Nicotine Dependence*. APA, Washington, DC.

Anda RF, Williamson DF, Escobedo LG, et al. (1990) Depression and the dynamics of smoking: a national perspective. *JAMA* **264**, 1541–1545.

Anonymous (1994) Nicotine replacement therapy for patients with coronary artery disease. Working group for the study of transdermal nicotine in patients with coronary artery disease. *Arch Intern Med* **154**, 989–995.

Baille A, Mattick R, Hall W, et al. (1994) Meta-analytic review of the efficacy of smoking cessation interventions. *Drug Alcohol Rev* **13**, 179–192.

Balfour DKJ and Fagerstrom KO (1996) Pharmacology of nicotine and its therapeutic use in smoking cessation and neurodegenerative disorders. *Pharmacol Ther* **72**, 51–81.

Benowitz NL (1988) Pharmacological aspects of cigarette smoking and nicotine addiction. *N Engl J Med* **319**, 1318–1330.

Benowitz NL, Fitzgerald GA, Wilson M, et al. (1993) Nicotine effects on eicosanoid formation and hemostatic function: comparison of transdermal nicotine and cigarette smoking. *J Am Coll Cardiol* **22**, 1159–1167.

Bobo JK (1989) Nicotine dependence and alcoholism epidemiology and treatment. *J Psychoact Drugs* **21**, 323–329.

Budney AJ, Higgins ST, Hughes JR, et al. (1993) Nicotine and caffeine use in cocaine-dependent individuals. *J Subst Abuse* **5**, 117–130.

Burling TA and Ziff DC (1988) Tobacco smoking: a comparison between alcohol and drug abuse inpatients. *Addict Behav* **13**, 185–190.

Carmelli D, Swan GE, Robinette D, et al. (1990) Heritability of substance use in the NAS-NRC twin registry. *Acta Genet Med Gemel (Roma)* **39**, 91–98.

Centers for Disease Control (1991) *Smoking-Attributable Mortality and Years of Potential Life Lost—United States, 1988*, DHHS Publication CDC 91–8017. Centers for Disease Control, Atlanta.

Clark PBS and Pert A (1985) Autoradiographic evidence of nicotine receptors on nigrostriatal and mesolimbic dopamine neurons. *Brain Res* **348**, 355–359.

Clemmey P, Brooner R, Chutuage MA, et al. (1997) Smoking habits and attitudes in a methadone maintenance treatment population. *Drug Alcohol Depend* **44**, 123–132.

Covey LS, Glassman AH, and Stetner F (1990) Depression and depressive symptoms in smoking cessation. *Compr Psychiatry* **31**, 350–354.

Dierker L, Avenevoli S, Stolar M, et al. (2002) Smoking and depression: an examination of mechanisms of comorbidity. *Am J Psychiatry* **159**, 947–953.

Docherty JP (1991) Residential treatment. In *The Clinical Management of Nicotine Dependence*, Cocores JA (ed). Springer-Verlag, New York, pp. 266–279.

Fagerstrom K-O (1978) Measuring the degree of physical dependence to tobacco smoking with reference to individualization of treatment. *Addict Behav* **3**, 235–241.

Fagerstrom KO and Melen B (1985) Nicotine chewing gum in smoking cessation: efficacy, nicotine dependence, therapy duration, clinical recommendations. In *Pharmacological Adjuncts in Smoking Cessation*, Grabowski J and Hall SM (eds). National Institute on Drug Abuse, Bethesda, MD, pp. 102–109.

Fagerstrom KO, Schneider NG, and Lunell E (1993) Effectiveness of nicotine patch and nicotine gum in individual versus combined treatments for tobacco withdrawal symptoms. *Psychopharmacology (Berl)* **11**, 271–277.

Ferry LH, Robbins AS, Scariati AM, et al. (1992) Enhancement of smoking cessation using the antidepressant bupropion (abstract). *Circulation* **86**(Suppl.), 1–167.

Fiore MC, Bailey WC, Cohen SJ, et al. (2000) *Treating Tobacco Use and Dependence. Quick Reference Guide for Clinicians*. Public Health Service, US Department of Health and Human Services, Rockville, MD.

Fiore MC, Novonty TE, Pierce JP, et al. (1990) Methods used to quit smoking in the United States. Do cessation programs help? *JAMA* **263**, 2760–2765.

Fung YK, Schmid MJ, Andreson TM, et al. (1996) Effects on nicotine withdrawal on central dopaminergic systems. *Pharmacol Biochem Behav* **53**, 633–640.

Glassman AH (1993) Cigarette smoking: implications for psychiatric illness. *Am J Psychiatry* **150**, 546–553.

Glassman AH, Helzer JE, Covey LS, et al. (1990) Smoking, smoking cessation and major depression. *JAMA* **264**, 1546–1549.

Goldstein MG, Niaura R, and Abrams DB (1991) Pharmacological and behavioral treatment of nicotine dependence: nicotine as a drug of abuse. In *Medical Psychiatric Practice*, Stoudemire A and Fogel BS (eds). American Psychiatric Press, Washington, DC.

Goldstein MG, Niaura R, Follick MJ, et al. (1989) Effects of behavioral skills training and schedule of nicotine gum administration on smoking cessation. *Am J Psychiatry* **146**, 56–60.

Gourley S (1994) The pros and cons of transdermal nicotine therapy. *Med J Aust* **160**, 152–159.

Gross J, Stitzer ML, and Maldonado J (1989) Nicotine replacement: effects of post-cessation weight gain. *J Consult Clin Psychol* **57**, 87–92.

Hajek P, Belcher M, and Stapleton J (1985) Enhancing the impact of groups: an evaluation of two group formats for smokers. *Br J Clin Psychol* **24**, 289–294.

Hajek P, Jackson P, and Belcher M (1988) Long-term use of nicotine chewing gum. *JAMA* **260**, 1593–1596.

Hall SM, Munoz R, and Reus V (1991) Smoking cessation, depression and dysphoria. *NIDA Res Monogr* **105**, 312–313.

Hall SM, Munoz R, and Reus V (1992) Depression and smoking treatment: a clinical trial of an affect regulation treatment. *NIDA Res Monogr* **119**, 326.

Hall SM, Reus VI, Munoz RF, et al. (1998) Nortryptyline and cognitive behavior therapy in treatment of cigarette smoking. *Arch Gen Psychiatry* **55**, 683–690.

Henningfield JE (1984) Pharmacologic basis and treatment of cigarette smoking. *J Clin Psychiatry* **45**, 24–34.

Henningfield JE, Clayton R, and Pollin W (1990) Involvement of tobacco in alcoholism and illicit drug use. *Br J Addict* **85**, 279–292.

Henningfield JE and Goldberg SR (1983) Control of behavior by intravenous nicotine injections in human subjects. *Pharmacol Biochem Behav* **19**, 989–992.

Hughes JR (1992) Tobacco withdrawal in self-quitters. *J Consult Clin Psychol* **60**, 689–697.

Hughes JR (1993a) Possible effects of smoke-free inpatient units on psychiatric diagnosis and treatment. *J Clin Psychiatry* **54**, 109–114.

Hughes JR (1993b) Treatment of smoking cessation in smokers with past alcohol/drug problems. *J Subst Abuse Treat* **10**, 181–187.

Hughes JR (1994a) Non-nicotine pharmacotherapies for smoking cessation. *J Drug Dev* **6**, 197–203.

Hughes JR (1994b) Pharmacotherapy of nicotine dependence. In *Pharmacological Aspects of Drug Dependence: Towards an Integrative Neurobehavioral Approach. Handbook of Experimental Pharmacology*, Schuster CR, Gust SW, and Kuhar MJ (eds). Springer-Verlag, Forchheim, Germany.

Hughes JR (1995) Combining behavioral therapy and pharmacotherapy for smoking cessation: an update. In *Integrating Behavior Therapies with Medication in the Treatment of Drug Dependence*, NIDA Res Monogr. Oken LS, Blaine JD, and Boren JJ (eds). US Government Printing Office, Washington, DC, pp. 92–109.

Hughes JR, Hatkusami DK, Mitchell JE, et al. (1986) Prevalence of smoking among psychiatric outpatients. *Am J Psychiatry* **143**, 993–997.

Hughes JR, Higgins ST, and Bickel WK (1994) Nicotine withdrawal versus other drug withdrawal syndromes: similarities and dissimilarities. *Addiction* **89**, 1461–1470.

Hughes JR and McHugh P (1995) Nicotine and neuropsychiatric disorders: schizophrenia. In *Effects of Nicotine on Biological Systems II. Advances in Pharmacological Sciences*, Clarke P, Quik M, Thureau K, et al. (eds). Birkhauser Verlag, Basel, pp. 301–305.

Hunt WA, Barnett LW, and Branch LG (1971) Relapse rates in addiction process. *J Clin Psychol* **27**, 455–461.

Hurt RD (1997) A comparison of sustained-release bupropion and placebo for smoking cessation. *N Engl J Med* **337**, 1195–1202.

Hurt RD, Lowell CD, Offord KP, et al. (1992) Inpatient treatment of severe nicotine dependence. *Mayo Clin Proc* **67**, 823–828.

Istvan J and Matarazzo JD (1984) Tobacco, alcohol and caffeine use: a review of their interrelationships. *Psychol Bull* **95**, 301–326.

Jarvik ME and Henningfield JE (1988) Pharmacologic treatment of tobacco dependence. *Pharmacol Biochem Behav* **30**, 279–294.

Kabat GC and Wynder EL (1987) Determinants of quitting smoking. *Am J Pub Health* **77**, 1301–1305.

Kandel DB and Davies M (1986) Adult sequelae of adolescent depressive symptoms. *Arch Gen Psychiatry* **43**, 255–262.

Kendler KS, Neale MC, MacClean CJ, et al. (1993) Smoking and major depression. *Arch Gen Psychiatry* **50**, 36–43.

Klesges RC, Klesges LM, Myers AW, et al. (1990) The effects of phenylpropanolamine on dietary intake, physical activity, and body weight after smoking cessation. *Clin Pharmacol Ther* **47**, 747–754.

Lam WL, Sze PC, Sacks HS, et al. (1987) Meta-analysis of randomized controlled trials of nicotine chewing gum. *Lancet* **2**, 27–29.

Lasser K, Boyd JW, Woolhandler S, et al. (2000) Smoking and mental illness: a population-based prevalence study. *JAMA* **284**, 2606–2610.

Lee EW and D'Alonzo GE (1993) Cigarette smoking, nicotine addiction, and its pharmacologic treatment. *Arch Intern Med* **153**, 34–48.

Miller WR, Zweben A, DiClemente CC, et al. (1995) *Motivational Enhancement Therapy Manual*, Publication No. 94–3723. US Department of Health and Human Services, National Institute of Health, Rockville, MD.

Moss RA and Prue DM (1982) Research on nicotine regulation. *Behav Ther* **13**, 31–46.

Nides M (1997) *Oral Presentation to the Society for Research on Nicotine and Tobacco (SRNT) (June 13)*. Nashville, TN.

Office on Smoking and Health, Public Health Service (1988) *The Health Consequences of Smoking: Nicotine Addiction: A Report of the US Surgeon General*, Office on Smoking and Health, DHHS Publication CDC 88–8406. Public Health Service, Rockville, MD.

Prochaska JO (1983) Stages and process of self-change of smoking: toward an integrative model of change. *J Consult Clin Psychol* **51**, 390–395.

Prochaska JO, Di Clemente CC, and Norcross J (1992) In *search of how people change: applications to addictive behavior*. *Am Psychol* **47**, 1102–1114.

Rennard S, Daughton D, Fortmann S, et al. (1991) Transdermal nicotine enhances smoking cessation in coronary artery disease patients (abstract). *Chest* **100**, 55.

Russell MAH (1987) Nicotine intake and its regulation by smokers. In *Tobacco, Smoking and Nicotine: A Neurobiological Approach*, Martin WR, VanLoon GR, Iwamoto ET, et al. (eds). Plenum Press, New York, p. 25.

Schneider N (1988) *How to Use Nicotine Gum and Other Strategies to Quit Smoking*. Pocket Books, New York.

Schneider NG (1996) Efficacy of a nicotine inhaler in smoking cessation: a double-blind, placebo-controlled trial. *Addiction* **91**, 1293–1306.

Schwartz JL (1987) *Review and Evaluation of Smoking Cessation Methods: The US and Canada, 1978–1985*, NCI Publication 87–2940. National Institutes of Health, Bethesda, MD.

Schwartz J (1991) Methods for smoking cessation. *Clin Chest Med* **12**, 737–753.

Sellers EM, Naranjo CA, and Kadlec K (1987) Do serotonin uptake inhibitors decrease smoking? observations in a group of heavy drinkers. *J Clin Psychopharmacol* **7**, 417–420.

Shiffman S (1982) Relapse following smoking cessation: a situational analysis. *J Consult Clin Psychol* **50**, 71–86.

Slade J (1999) Nicotine. In *Addictions: A Comprehensive Guidebook*, McCrady BS and Epstein EE (eds). Oxford University Press, New York.

Sutherland G, Stapleton JA, Russell MAH, et al. (1992) Randomised controlled trial of nasal nicotine spray in smoking cessation. *Lancet* **340**, 324–329.

Ter Riet G, Kleijnen J, and Knipschild P (1990) A meta-analysis of studies into the effects of acupuncture on addiction. *Br J Gen Pract* **40**, 379–382.

Tonnesen P, Fryd V, Hansen M, et al. (1988) Two and four mg nicotine chewing gum and group counseling in smoking cessation: an open, randomized controlled trial with a 22 month follow-up. *Addict Behav* **13**, 17–27.

Tonnesen P, Norregaard J, Mikkelsen K, et al. (1993) A double-blind trial of a nicotine inhaler for smoking cessation. *JAMA* **269**, 1268–1271.

US Department of Health and Human Services (1988) *The Health Consequences of Smoking: Nicotine Addiction*, DHHS Publication CDC-88-8406, A Report of the Surgeon General. Office on Smoking and Health, Rockville, MD.

US Department of Health and Human Services (1989) *Smoking Tobacco and Health. A Fact Book*, Rev. ed. (Oct). DHHS Publication CDC 87–8397. US Department of Health and Human Services, Washington, DC.

US Department of Health and Human Services (1990) *The Health Benefits of Smoking Cessation: A Report of the Surgeon General*. US Department of Health and Human Services, Washington, DC.

Ward KD, Garvey AJ, Bliss Re, et al. (1991) Changes in urinary catecholamine excretion after smoking cessation. *Pharmacol Biochem Behav* **40**, 937–940.

West RJ and Hack S (1991) Effect of cigarettes on memory search and subjective ratings. *Pharmacol Biochem Behav* **38**, 281–286.

West RJ, Hajek P, and Belcher M (1989) Severity of withdrawal symptoms as a predictor of outcome of an attempt to quit smoking. *Psychol Med* **19**, 981–985.

Ziedonis DM and George TP (1997) Schizophrenia and nicotine use: report of a pilot smoking cessation program and review of neurobiological and clinical issues. *Schizophr Bull* **23**(2), 247–254.

Ziedonis DM, Kosten TR, Glazer WM, et al. (1994) Nicotine dependence and schizophrenia. *Hosp Comm Psychiatry* **45**, 204–206.

Ziedonis DM, Krejci J, and Atdjian S (2001) Integrating medications and Psychotherapy in the treatment of alcohol, tobacco, and other drug addictions. In *Integrated Treatment*, Kay J (ed). American Psychiatric Press, Washington, DC, pp. 79–111.

Ziedonis DM, Wyatt SA, and George TP (1998) Current issues in nicotine dependence and treatment. In *New Treatments for Chemical Addictions*, McCance-Katz E and Kosten TR (eds). American Psychiatric Press, Washington, DC, pp. 1–34.

The term *opioids* describes a class of substances that acts on opioid receptors. Numerous opioid receptors have been identified, but the physiologic and pharmacologic responses in man are best understood for the mu (μ) and kappa (κ) receptors. The μ receptor, for which morphine is a prototypical agonist, appears to be the one most closely related to opioid analgesic and euphorigenic effects. Opioids can be naturally occurring substances such as morphine, semisynthetics such as heroin, and synthetics with morphine-like effects such as meperidine. These drugs are prescribed as analgesics, anesthetics, antidiarrheal agents, or cough suppressants. In addition to morphine and heroin, the opioids include codeine, hydromorphone, methadone, oxycodone, and fentanyl among others. Drugs such as buprenorphine, a partial agonist at the μ receptor, and pentazocine, an agonist–antagonist, are also included in this class because their physiologic and behavioral effects are mediated through opioid receptors (Table 24-1).

Opioids are the most effective medications for relief of severe pain and are widely used for that purpose. Their euphoric properties can also result in inappropriate use, abuse, and dependence (i.e., "addiction"), which is why they have been placed under the Controlled Substances Act. The more potent opioids approved for medical use are under schedule II—examples are fentanyl, hydromorphone, methadone, and morphine; others are under schedules III and IV.

Diagnosis

As with other substances, there are two general categories of opioid-related disorders: opioid use disorders and opioid-induced disorders. Opioid use disorders include opioid dependence and opioid abuse. Opioid dependence has two sets of specifiers, the first set being with physiologic features (i.e., tolerance and/or withdrawal), or without physiologic features. The second set consists of course specifiers: early full remission, early partial remission, sustained full remission, sustained partial remission, on agonist therapy, and in a controlled environment. The agonist therapy specifier is used only to note the status of opioid dependence, and not for other opioid-related disorders or substance dependencies.

Opioid-induced disorders include opioid intoxication, opioid withdrawal, opioid intoxication delirium (see generic DSM-IV-TR diagnostic criteria for Substance Intoxication Delirium in Chapter 13, page 271), opioid-induced psychotic disorders (see generic DSM-IV-TR diagnostic criteria for Substance-Induced Psychotic Disorder, Chapter 15, page 355), opioid-induced mood disorders (see generic DSM-IV-TR diagnostic criteria for

le 24-1	Opioids*						
g	**Active Metabolite**	**Route of Administration**	**Relative Potency**	**Medical Use**	**Plasma Half-Life (Hours)**	**Duration of Action (Hours)**	
phine		IM	1	Analgesia	2	4–6	
oin	Morphine	IM	1–2	None	0.5	3–5	
eine		PO	0.05	Analgesia, antitussive	2–4	4–6	
tanyl		IM	40–100	Analgesia	3–4	1–2	
dromorphone		IM	13	Analgesia	2–3	4–6	
codone		PO	0.5–1	Analgesia		4–6	
hadone		PO	0.50	Analgesia, opioid substitution	15–40	18–30	
acetylmethadol (_AAM)		PO	0.40	Opioid substitution	14–104†	48–80	
	Nor-LAAM				13–130†		
	Dinor-LAAM				97–430†		
renorphine		SL	N/A (partial agonist)	Analgesia (opioid substitution, investigational)	6–12	4–6 (for analgesia) 12–48‡	

ntramuscular; PO, by mouth; SL, sublingual; N/A, not applicable.
eady state.
ars to be dose dependent.

Substance-Induced Mood Disorder in Chapter 15, page 356), opioid-induced sexual dysfunctions (see generic DSM-IV-TR diagnostic criteria for Substance-Induced Sexual Dysfunction in Chapter 15, page 358), opioid-induced sleep disorder (see generic DSM-IV-TR diagnostic criteria for Substance-Induced Sleep Disorder in Chapter 15, page 359).

The defining features, according to DSM-IV-TR, for opioid dependence, and abuse are similar to those for other substance use disorders. Essentially, opioid dependence is a cluster of cognitive, behavioral, and physiological symptoms indicating that the affected person is using high doses of opioids in a compulsive manner, for no legitimate medical reason, with loss of control over use and adverse medical or psychiatric consequences. Unlike cocaine, hallucinogens, solvents, and other substances that do not always produce withdrawal symptoms, opioid dependence is almost always accompanied by significant physiological tolerance and a defined withdrawal–abstinence syndrome. Opioid abuse is a less severe disorder that consists of intermittent use of one or more opioids, in the absence of compulsive use and significant tolerance and/or withdrawal, but resulting in recurrent social, legal, or personal problems, or in use that is physically hazardous. Opioid intoxication consists of clinically significant maladaptive behaviors or psychological changes that are associated with acute opioid effects. Opioid withdrawal is a syndrome associated with abrupt cessation or reduction of opioid use in persons who have been taking opioids regularly and have developed neuroadaptation to their agonist effects. Opioid withdrawal symptoms are generally opposite to those of intoxication.

Opioid Dependence Opioid dependence is diagnosed by the signs and symptoms associated with compulsive, prolonged self-administration of opioids that are used for no legitimate medical purpose, or if a medical condition exists that requires opioid treatment, are used in doses that greatly exceed the amount needed for pain relief (see generic DSM-IV-TR diagnostic criteria for Substance Dependence in Chapter 15, page 351). Persons with opioid dependence typically demonstrate continued use in spite of adverse physical, behavioral, and psychological consequences. Almost all persons meeting criteria for opioid dependence have significant levels of tolerance and will experience withdrawal upon abrupt discontinuation of opioid drugs. Persons with opioid dependence tend to develop such regular patterns of compulsive use that daily activities are typically planned around obtaining and administering drugs.

Opioids are usually purchased on the illicit market, but they can also be obtained by forging prescriptions, faking or exaggerating medical problems, or by receiving simultaneous prescriptions from several physicians. Physicians and other health care professionals who are dependent will often obtain opioids by writing prescriptions or by diverting opioids that have been prescribed for their own patients.

Opioid Abuse   Opioid abuse is a maladaptive pattern of intermittent use in hazardous situations (driving under the influence, being intoxicated while using heavy machinery, working in dangerous places, etc.), or periodic use resulting in adverse social, legal, or interpersonal problems (see generic DSM-IV-TR diagnostic criteria for Substance Abuse in Chapter 15, page 351). All of these signs and symptoms can also be seen in persons who are dependent; abuse is characterized by less regular use than dependence (i.e., compulsive use not present) and by the absence of significant tolerance or withdrawal. As with other substance use disorders, opioid abuse and dependence are hierarchical and thus, persons diagnosed as having opioid abuse must never have met criteria for opioid dependence.

Opioid Intoxication   Opioid intoxication is characterized by maladaptive and clinically significant behavioral changes developing within minutes to a few hours after opioid use (see DSM-IV-TR diagnostic criteria on page 591). Symptoms include an initial euphoria sometimes followed by dysphoria or apathy. Psychomotor retardation or agitation, impaired judgment, and impaired social or occupational functioning are commonly seen. Intoxication is accompanied by pupillary constriction unless there has been a severe overdose with consequent anoxia and pupillary dilatation. Persons with intoxication are often drowsy (described as being "on the nod") or even obtunded, have slurred speech, impaired memory, and demonstrate inattention to the environment to the point of ignoring potentially harmful events. Dryness of secretions in the mouth and nose, slowing of gastrointestinal activity, and constipation are associated with both acute and chronic opioid use. Visual acuity may be impaired as a result of pupillary constriction. The magnitude of the behavioral and physiologic changes depends on the dose as well as individual characteristics of the user such as rate of absorption, chronicity of use, and tolerance. Symptoms of opioid intoxication usually last for several hours, but are dependent on the half-life of the particular opioid that has been used. Severe intoxication following an opioid overdose can lead to coma, respiratory depression, pupillary dilatation, unconsciousness, and death (Table 24-2).

Table 24-2	Signs and Symptoms of Opioid Intoxication
Symptoms Euphoria, dysphoria, or apathy Psychomotor retardation or agitation Impaired judgment, social, or occupational functioning **Signs** Pupillary constriction Drowsy or obtunded Slurred speech, impaired memory, and inattention to environment Dryness in mouth or nose Slowed gastrointestinal activity and constipation Severe intoxication can lead to coma, respiration depression, pupillary dilation, unconsciousness, and death.	

Diagnostic Criteria

292.89 Opioid Intoxication

A. Recent use of an opioid.
B. Clinically significant maladaptive behavioral or psychological changes (e.g., initial euphoria followed by apathy, dysphoria, psychomotor agitation or retardation, impaired judgment, or impaired social or occupational functioning) that developed during, or shortly after, opioid use.
C. Pupillary constriction (or pupillary dilation due to anoxia from severe overdose) and one (or more) of the following signs, developing during, or shortly after, opioid use:

1. drowsiness or coma
2. slurred speech
3. impairment in attention or memory

D. The symptoms are not due to a general medical condition and are not better accounted for by another mental disorder.

Specify if:

With perceptual disturbances

Reprinted with permission from the Diagnostic and Statistical Manual of Mental Disorders, Fourth Edition, Text Revision. Copyright 2000 American Psychiatric Association.

Opioid Withdrawal   Opioid withdrawal is a clinically significant, maladaptive behavioral and physiological syndrome associated with cessation or reduction of opioid use that has been heavy and prolonged (see DSM-IV-TR criteria for Opioid Withdrawal on page 592). It can also be precipitated by administration of an opioid antagonist such as naloxone or

Table 24-3	Signs and Symptoms of Opioid Withdrawal
Symptoms	
Anxiety, irritability, restlessness	
Muscle aching	
Craving for opioids	
Increased pain sensitivity	
Signs	
Dysphoric or depressed mood	
Nausea/vomiting/diarrhea	
Lacrimation/rhinorrhea	
Sweating	
Yawning	
Insomnia	
Pupillary dilatation	
Piloerection	
Fever	

naltrexone. Individuals in opioid withdrawal typically demonstrate a pattern of signs and symptoms that are opposite the acute agonist effects. The first of these are subjective and consist of complaints of anxiety, restlessness, and an "achy feeling" that is often located in the back and legs. These symptoms are accompanied by a wish to obtain opioids (sometimes called "craving") and drug-seeking behavior, along with irritability and increased sensitivity to pain. Additionally, individuals typically demonstrate three or more of the following: dysphoric or depressed mood, nausea or vomiting, diarrhea, muscle aches, lacrimation or rhinorrhea, increased sweating, yawning, fever, insomnia, pupillary dilatation, fever, and piloerection. Piloerection and withdrawal-related fever are rarely seen in clinical settings (other than prison) as they are signs of advanced withdrawal in persons with a very significant degree of physiologic dependence; opioid-dependent persons with "habits" of that magnitude usually manage to obtain drugs before withdrawal becomes so far-advanced (Table 24-3).

Diagnostic Criteria

292.0 Opioid Withdrawal

A. Either of the following:

    (1) cessation of (or reduction in) opioid use that has been heavy and prolonged (several weeks or longer)

    (2) administration of an opioid antagonist after a period of opioid use

B. Three (or more) of the following, developing within minutes to several days after Criterion A:

    (1) dysphoric mood
    (2) nausea or vomiting
    (3) muscle aches
    (4) lacrimation or rhinorrhea
    (5) papillary dilation, piloerection, or sweating
    (6) diarrhea
    (7) yawning
    (8) fever
    (9) insomnia

C. The symptoms in Criterion B cause clinically significant distress or impairment in social, occupational, or other important areas of functioning.

D. The symptoms are not due to a general medical condition and are not better accounted for by another mental disorder

For short-acting drugs such as heroin, withdrawal symptoms occur within 6 to 24 hours after the last dose in most dependent persons, peak within 1 to 3 days, and gradually subside over a period of 5 to 7 days. Symptoms may take 2 to 4 days to emerge in the case of longer-acting drugs such as methadone or levo-alpha-acetylmethadol (LAAM). Less acute withdrawal symptoms are sometimes present and can last for weeks to months. These more persistent symptoms can include anxiety, dysphoria, anhedonia, insomnia, and drug craving.

Opioid use disorders can occur at any age, including adolescence and the geriatric years, but most affected persons are between 20 and 45 years. There have recently been increasing numbers of reports of adolescents presenting for treatment with opioid problems, but good data are hard to find. Neonates whose mothers are addicted can also experience opioid withdrawal. Rarely, young children are affected with some cases of dependence having been reported in persons who are 8 to 10 years of age. Males are more commonly affected, with the male–female ratio typically being 3 or 4 to 1.

A nonjudgmental and supportive yet firm approach to these individuals is especially important. They typically have engaged in antisocial or other forms of problematic behavior. They are often embarrassed or afraid to describe the extent of their behavior, and have extremely low self-esteem. At the same time, they are prone to be impulsive, manipulative, and to act-out when frustrated. Communicating a feeling of nonjudgmental support in the context of setting limits, along with a clear and informed effort to provide appropriate help will encourage optimum therapeutic opportunities.

On physical examination, sclerosed veins ("tracks") and puncture marks on the lower portions of the upper extremities are common in intravenous users. When these veins become unusable or otherwise unavailable, persons will usually switch to veins in the legs, neck, or groin. Veins sometimes become so badly sclerosed that peripheral edema develops. When intravenous access is no longer possible, persons will often inject directly into their subcutaneous tissue ("skin-popping") resulting in cellulitis, abscesses, and circular-appearing scars from healed skin lesions. Tetanus is a relatively rare but extremely serious consequence of injecting into the subcutaneous tissues. Infections also occur in other organ systems, including bacterial endocarditis, hepatitis B and C, and HIV infection.

Persons who "snort" heroin or other opioids often develop irritation of the nasal mucosa. Difficulties in sexual function are common, as are a variety of sexually transmitted diseases. Males often experience premature ejaculation associated with opioid withdrawal, and impotence during intoxication or chronic use. Females commonly have disturbances of reproductive function and irregular menses.

During dependence, routine urine toxicology tests are often positive for opioid drugs and remain positive for most opioids for 12 to 36 hours. Methadone and LAAM, because they are longer acting, can be identified for several days. Fentanyl is not detected by standard urine tests but can be identified by more specialized procedures. Oxycodone, hydrocodone, and hydromorphone are often not routinely included on urine toxicology tests though they can be identified by gas chromatography/mass spectrometry. Testing for fentanyl is not necessary in most programs, but needs to be performed in assessing and treating health care professionals such as anesthesiologists who have access to this drug. Concomitant laboratory evidence of other abusable substances such as cocaine, marijuana, alcohol, amphetamines, and benzodiazepines is common.

Hepatitis screening tests are often positive, either for hepatitis B antigen (signifying active infection) or hepatitis B and/or C antibody (signifying past infection). Mild to moderate elevations of liver function tests are common, usually as a result of chronic infection with hepatitis C but also from toxic injury to the liver due to contaminants that have been mixed with injected opioids, or from heavy use of other hepatotoxic drugs such as alcohol. Low platelet count, anemia, or neutropenia, as well as positive HIV tests or low CD-4 cell counts are often signs of HIV infection. HIV is commonly acquired via the practice of sharing injection equipment, or by unprotected sexual activity that may be related to the substance use disorder, for example, exchanging sex for drugs or money to buy drugs.

Epidemiology

Heroin is the most commonly abused drug of this class. The 2000 National Household Survey obtained information on nonmedical use of analgesics and heroin separately. For heroin, the survey showed that 1.3% of the population had used it in their lifetime; in the adolescent groups, 0.6% of 16- to 17-year olds had used it in their lifetime, but by age 18 to 20 the percentage was the same as in the adult population, 1.3%. When the data for nonmedical use of opioid pain relievers are examined, particularly in adolescent populations, the numbers are more alarming, with 12.4% of 16- to 17-year olds having used these agents and 15.8% of 18- to 20-year olds. It is unclear what proportion of the users met criteria for dependence or abuse since diagnoses were not part of the Household Survey (National Household Survey on Drug Abuse 2000). The Epidemiologic Catchment Area Study, completed in 1985 and using DSM-III criteria, found that 0.7% of the target population had ever met criteria for opioid dependence or abuse. Among those who had ever met criteria, 18% reported use in the last month, and 42% reported having had a problem with opioids in the last year (Robins and Regier 1991). This study, and other similar epidemiological surveys, may underestimate the true prevalence of opioid use disorders since they do not often include persons in prisons or who are homeless. More recent estimates indicate that there may be as many as 2 million persons with opioid dependence in the United States, though exact figures are difficult to obtain.

Heroin addiction has traditionally been associated with large urban areas in the United Stated, especially those in the northeast and mid-Atlantic states. There also appears to have been an increase in the abuse of prescription opioids, mainly in nonurban areas. Oxycodone and hydrocodone-containing products have traditionally been the main prescription opioids of abuse. Attention has recently focused on oxycontin, a long-acting formulation of oxycodone that contains doses up to 80 mg/tablet. Though the slow absorption of this medication is unlikely to result in abuse when taken as prescribed, addicts have discovered that the tablets can be crushed, freeing much of the oxycodone that can then be inhaled or injected to produce a potent euphoria

Heroin is usually taken by injection, though it can be smoked, inhaled ("snorted"), or taken orally. Smoking and inhalation are commonly seen only when very pure heroin is available and is currently on the rise in the northeastern United States; tar heroin is also commonly smoked in the Pacific Northwest. Hydromorphone (Dilaudid), morphine, and meperidine (Demerol) are also usually injected though they can be taken orally; fentanyl is always injected. Codeine and other analgesics made for oral ingestion (such as Percodan or Percocet) are usually taken orally. All of these drugs can cause intoxication, withdrawal, dependence, and abuse.

Course

Opioid dependence can begin at any age, but problems associated with opioid use are most commonly first observed in the late teens or early twenties. Once dependence occurs, it is usually continuous over a period of many years even though periods of abstinence are frequent. Reoccurrence is common even after many years of forced abstinence, such as occurs during incarceration. Increasing age appears to be associated with a decrease in prevalence. This tendency for dependence to remit generally begins after age 40 and has been called "maturing out." However, many persons have remained opioid dependent for 50 years or longer. Thus, though spontaneous remission can and does occur, most cases of untreated opioid dependence follow a chronic, relapsing course for many years.

Differential Diagnosis

Individuals who are dependent on "street" opioids are usually easy to diagnose because of the physical signs of intravenous use, drug-seeking behavior, reports from independent observers, the lack of medical justification for opioid use, urine test results, and the signs and symptoms of intoxication or withdrawal.

The signs and symptoms of opioid withdrawal are fairly specific, especially lacrimation and rhinorrhea, which are not associated with withdrawal from any other abusable substances. Other psychoactive substances with sedative properties such as alcohol, hypnotics, or anxiolytics can cause a clinical picture that resembles opioid intoxication. A diagnosis can usually be made by the absence of pupillary constriction, or by the lack of response to a naloxone challenge. In some cases, intoxication is due to opioids along with alcohol or other sedatives. In these cases, the naloxone challenge will not reverse all of the sedative drug effects.

Difficult diagnostic situations are seen among persons who fabricate or exaggerate the signs and symptoms of a painful illness (such as kidney stones, migraine headache, back pain, etc.). Because pain is subjective and difficult to measure, and because some of these individuals can be very skillful and deceptive, diagnosis can be difficult and time-consuming. Drugs that are obtained in such deceptions may be used by the individual in the service of his/her dependence or abuse, or may be sold on the illicit drug market for profit. These individuals cause problems not only for physicians but also for individuals with disorders that need opioids for pain relief. Individuals who have pain that should be treated promptly with opioids are sometimes denied treatment or given inadequate amounts of opioids because of uncertainty or disbelief about the legitimacy of their complaints. Individuals with cancer, kidney stones, or other painful conditions have sometimes suffered considerably from this type of "reverse discrimination."

Persons with opioid dependence will often present with psychiatric signs and symptoms such as depression or anxiety. Such subjective distress often serves to motivate the individual to seek treatment, and thus can be therapeutically useful. These symptoms can be the result of opioid intoxication or withdrawal, or they might result from the pharmacological effects of other substances that are also being abused such as cocaine, alcohol, or benzodiazepines. They may also represent independent, non-substance-induced psychiatric disorders that require long-term treatment. The correct attribution of psychiatric symptoms that are seen in the context of opioid dependence and abuse follows the principles that are outlined in the substance-related section and other relevant parts of DSM-IV-TR.

Opioids are much less likely to produce psychopathology than most other drugs of abuse, and in some instances, they reduce psychiatric symptoms. In these cases, symptoms will emerge not during opioid use, but after it is discontinued. Examples have been observed by clinicians in methadone maintenance programs, who occasionally see an exacerbation of symptoms of schizophrenia, posttraumatic stress disorder (PTSD), or other problems in individuals who discontinue chronic opioid use.

Etiology

Opioid-related disorders, as in the case of other substance-related disorders, are felt to arise from a variety of social, psychological, and biological factors that interact to produce a "case." Among those identified as especially important are opioid use within the individual's immediate social environment and peer group; availability of opioids; a history of childhood conduct disorder or adult antisocial personality disorder; and a family history of one or more substance use disorders. The families of persons with opioid dependence are likely to have higher levels of psychopathology, especially an increased incidence of alcohol and drug use disorders, and antisocial personality disorder (Rounsaville et al. 1982). These findings suggest that there is a genetic susceptibility to substance use disorders. However, more exact information regarding the nature or location of potential genetic factors is not available at this time nor is information on the influence of psychological and environmental factors on the expression of a presumed genetic predisposition.

The exact mechanism or mix of factors that produce opioid dependence or abuse are unknown, as are the factors that contribute to the chronic relapsing pattern that is typically seen in many of these individuals. Studies by Dole and others suggest that persons who have used opioids regularly over extended periods of time experience physiological alterations as a consequence of chronic use, which are permanent and which contribute to an inability to achieve periods of sustained remission (Dole and Nyswander 1965, Kreek 1986). The exact nature of these physiological alterations has not yet been identified. Studies by Wikler and others have demonstrated the existence of conditioned drug responses that can persist for years and that may contribute to relapse in formerly dependent individuals (Wikler, 1980, O'Brien et al. 1997).

Treatment

There are currently a number of effective pharmacological and behavioral therapies for the treatment of opioid dependence, with these two approaches often combined to optimize outcome. There are also some newer treatment options, which may take various forms. For example, methadone maintenance is an established treatment, while the use of buprenorphine/naloxone in an office-based setting represents a new variation on that theme. Clonidine has been used extensively to treat opioid withdrawal while lofexidine is a structural analog that appears to have less hypotensive and sedating effects. The depot dosage form of naltrexone may increase compliance with a medication that has been an effective opioid antagonist, but which has been underutilized because of poor acceptance by individuals. In almost every treatment episode using pharmacotherapy, it is combined with some type of psychosocial or behavioral treatment. Recent research has documented the value of these additional treatments and provided insight into the ones that are the most effective.

Detoxification: Long-Term, Short-Term, Rapid, and Ultrarapid

Detoxification from opioids, for most individuals, is only the first phase of a longer treatment process. Pharmacological detoxification is generally ineffective in achieving sustained remission unless combined with long-term pharmacologic, psychosocial, or behavioral therapies. Most individuals seeking treatment have been addicted to heroin or other opioids for 2 to 3 years, and some for 30 years or more. Thus, treatment usually involves changes in individuals' lifestyles. Though generally ineffective in achieving sustained remission unless combined with long-term pharmacological, psychosocial, or behavioral therapies, detoxification alone continues to be widely used. It is sometimes the only option available for individuals who do not meet the Food and Drug Administration (FDA) criteria for, do not desire, or do not have access to agonist medications such as methadone or methadyl acetate (LAAM).

The detoxification process may include use of opioid agonists (e.g., methadone), partial agonists (e.g., buprenorphine), antagonists (e.g., naloxone, naltrexone), or nonopioid alternatives such as clonidine, benzodiazepines, or nonsteroidal anti-inflammatory agents. In many cases, one or more medications are combined, such as naloxone with clonidine and a benzodiazepine (Table 24-4). The choice of detoxification medication and the duration of the process depend on numerous factors including individual preference, clinician expertise and experience, type of treatment facility, licensing, and available resources. Ultimately, however, the goal of detoxification is the achievement (and maintenance) of a drug-free state while minimizing withdrawal.

Opioid detoxification paradigms are frequently categorized according to their duration: long-term (typically 180 days), short-term (up to 30 days), rapid (typically 3–10 days), and

Table 24-4	Pharmacologic Agents in Opioid Detoxification

Opioid agonists (methadone)
Partial agonists (buprenorphine)
Antagonists (naloxone, naltrexone)
Nonopioid alternatives (clonidine, benzodiazepines,
    nonsteroidal anti-inflammatory agents)
Combinations of above medications

ultrarapid (1–2 days). These temporal modifiers provide only a coarse description of the paradigm; they do not provide other important information such as the medications used or whether postdetoxification pharmacological, psychosocial, or behavioral therapy is provided. However, some general guidelines typically apply.

The most common detoxification protocols, and those for which the most data are available, are the long-term (typically 180 days) and short-term (up to 30 days) paradigms involving the use of methadone. Unfortunately, these strategies have not generally been associated with acceptable treatment response using relapse to opioid use as an outcome criterion. For example, one study (Banys et al. 1994) reported that more than half of the individuals participating in a 180-day detoxification program were using opioids illicitly during the medication taper phase. Six-month follow-up indicated that 38.5% of the urine samples ($n = 26$) tested negative for illicit opioids, only 3 of 31 individuals reported remaining free of illicit opioids for the entire 6 months prior to follow-up, and 22 participated in some other form of treatment (Reilly et al. 1995). Results from more rapid detoxification evaluations using short- or even intermediate-term (up to 70 days) medication-tapering protocols are even less encouraging and have an unfortunately low success rate. It should be noted, however, that provision of additional services such as counseling, behavioral therapy, treatment of underlying psychopathologies, job skills training, and family therapy to address concomitant treatment needs can improve outcome though success rates remain low, even with these services (Kleber 1999).

Rapid detoxification involves the use of an opioid antagonist, typically naltrexone or naloxone, in combination with other medications (such as clonidine and benzodiazepines) to mitigate the precipitated withdrawal syndrome. The procedure is intended to expedite and compress withdrawal in order to minimize discomfort and decrease treatment time. Ultrarapid detoxification also utilizes other medications, along with an opioid antagonist, to moderate withdrawal effects. However, rather than individuals being awake as they are during the rapid detoxification process, they are placed under general anesthesia or alternatively, deeply sedated. A comprehensive review of the rapid and ultrarapid detoxification literature was recently published (O'Connor and Kosten 1998).

A major concern regarding ultrarapid detoxification is the occurrence of potentially serious adverse effects, such as respiratory distress (San et al. 1995), or other pulmonary and renal complications (Pfab et al. 1999) during or immediately following the procedure. A high frequency of vomiting has also been reported (Cucchia et al. 1998). The degree to which serious adverse events occur has not yet been determined; however, there have been reports of sudden death occurring shortly after the procedure, which was not caused by relapse to opioid use and overdose (O'Brien et al. personal communication 2001).

In spite of the emerging evidence about serious adverse events, ultrarapid detoxification may be appropriate for highly selected individuals based on considerations of previous treatment history, economic factors, and individual choice. However, individuals seeking this treatment must be thoroughly informed that serious adverse events, including sudden unexpected deaths, have occurred in association with this procedure and its use should probably be limited to inpatient settings where monitoring by anesthesiologists and other highly trained staff is available.

Buprenorphine, a µ-opioid partial agonist, has also been used as a detoxification agent. Results from inpatient (Cheskin et al. 1994, Parran et al. 1994, Vignau 1998) and outpatient (O'Connor et al. 1997, Diamant et al. 1998) studies have shown that it is safe, well tolerated, and mitigates opioid withdrawal signs and symptoms over a range of doses and detoxification schedules. Clonidine, an alpha-2-adrenergic agonist, has been shown to suppress many of the autonomic signs and symptoms of opioid withdrawal. It can cause sedation and hypotension but has been used with few problems when appropriate monitoring is available. It does not suppress the subjective discomfort of withdrawal, and probably for that reason, is not well accepted by most individuals.

Other alpha-2-adrenergic agonists have also been evaluated in order to find agents that are as or more effective, but less sedating and hypotensive than clonidine. Lofexidine, a medication that was originally promoted as an antihypertensive but was shown to lack clinically significant hypotensive effects, has been the most studied. When compared to clonidine, it has been found to equally suppress autonomic signs and symptoms of opioid withdrawal but with less sedation and hypotension (Kahn et al. 1997, Lin et al. 1997, Carnwath and Hardman 1998). When compared to methadone dose tapering, lofexidine detoxification was associated with opioid withdrawal effects that peaked sooner, but resolved to negligible levels more rapidly (Bearn et al. 1996). In another study (Bearn et al. 1998), an accelerated 5-day lofexidine treatment regimen attenuated opioid withdrawal symptoms more rapidly than 10 days of either lofexidine or methadone, with similar blood pressure responses observed for the lofexidine groups. Data regarding the potential effectiveness of guanabenz and guanfacine have also been reported, but further studies are required to assess the potential utility of these medications. In summary, recent studies have shown that lofexidine is likely to be a useful opioid detoxification agent whose efficacy approximates that of clonidine but with fewer side effects.

Opioid Agonist Pharmacotherapy

Methadone maintenance was developed by Dole and Nyswander (1968) and has become the most commonly used pharmacotherapy for opioid dependence. Methadone acts at the µ-opioid receptor and its ability to suppress opioid withdrawal for 24 to 36 hours following a single oral dose makes it an ideal medication for this purpose. Another µ-opioid agonist, LAAM, received FDA approval for maintenance treatment in 1993. LAAM is a long-acting congener of methadone, which suppresses withdrawal for 48 to 72 hours, and thus has the advantage of requiring less frequent clinic visits than methadone, which must be taken daily. A third medication, buprenorphine, has unique properties that are likely to result in it being used with fewer regulatory controls than methadone and LAAM.

Both methadone and LAAM are Schedule II controlled substances and can only be used for maintenance and detoxification in programs that are licensed and regulated by the FDA and the Drug Enforcement Administration (DEA). The regulations specify who is eligible for treatment, procedures that are required for its administration, the number of take-home doses permitted, and the type of medication storage security needed. Treatment programs have been inspected approximately every 3 years for the past 30 years and violations have resulted in sanctions ranging from administrative citations to criminal prosecution.

This combination of FDA and DEA regulations has resulted in a treatment system that is separated from the mainstream of other medical care and that consists almost entirely of specially licensed and inspected clinics. Clinics are often located in old buildings that have been converted to comply with regulations but that were never intended for medical use. At the present time, it is estimated that approximately 179,000 individuals are being maintained on methadone or LAAM at 940 or more sites, and that this number represents only about 20% of all persons with opioid dependence in the United States (Addiction Treatment Forum 2000). This situation is very unlike that of some other western countries such as Spain and Switzerland where 50% or more of persons with opioid dependence are reported to be on agonist therapy, with substantial numbers of others in residential treatment (Suarez, personal communication, 1998, Unchtenhagen, personal communication, 2002).

The appropriate dose of agonist medication has been a subject of both federal and state regulations, although there has been a gradual shift toward allowing more clinical judgment in its determination. A number of studies have been done during the last 25 years to determine the optimal dose and, although it is clear that some individuals do well on low doses of methadone or LAAM (about 20–50 mg), studies have consistently shown that most individuals need higher doses if they are to achieve maximum benefit from agonist treatment (Ball and Ross 1991). The results of these comparison studies are generally supportive of the guidelines originally proposed by Dole and Nyswander, who recommended doses in the 80 to 120 mg/day range (Dole and Nyswander 1968). Clear relationships between methadone blood levels and clinical response have not been observed consistently. One recent study found significant correlations between oral dose and methadone concentration, but only among individuals who complained of low dosing (Hiltunen et al. 1999). These findings suggest that some individuals may be more sensitive to dose changes and that clinical response, including subjective complaints, is a more important guide to adequate dosing than blood levels. No controlled studies have been done examining doses above 120 mg; thus, the upper limits of dosing effectiveness are not well understood.

Perhaps the most important pending regulatory change is to amend the Controlled Substances Act with respect to registration requirements for practitioners using drugs approved for detoxification and/or maintenance that are in Schedules III, IV, and V (Drug Addiction Treatment Act 2000). Physicians who choose to treat persons with opioid dependence under the new regulations will need to notify the Secretary of Health and Human Services in writing of their intent and show that they are qualified to provide addiction treatment by virtue of certification or experience. No physician will be allowed to treat more than 30 individuals at one time without special approval according to the proposed legislation.

This change in the regulations will be especially important for buprenorphine and the buprenorphine/naloxone combination, as it will provide better access to treatment for persons who are unwilling or unable to be treated in the current methadone or LAAM system. The overall intent of the proposed regulatory reform is to better integrate maintenance treatment into the mainstream of medical care, and to make it more available and improve its quality.

As mentioned above, these changes are likely to influence the ways that buprenorphine is used in opioid addiction treatment. Buprenorphine is marketed internationally as an analgesic (both without naloxone, and with naloxone to deter abuse) and as a treatment for opioid addiction. The most widespread use of buprenorphine is in France where it was approved for addiction treatment in 1996. Buprenorphine has been used almost exclusively sublingually in addiction treatment due to its poor oral bioavailability. Most of the early clinical trials used a sublingual solution of buprenorphine, although a more commercially suitable sublingual tablet formulation is now being used.

The greatest advantage of buprenorphine compared to full agonists such as methadone and LAAM is the plateau effect of μ-agonist activity. Parenteral doses as high as 12 mg intravenously (Umbricht-Schneiter et al. 1998) have been given to individuals who are not tolerant to opioids with only limited adverse effects (e.g., sedation, irritability, nausea, itching). A number of large trials have confirmed the utility of buprenorphine for agonist maintenance therapy. These studies include comparisons of buprenorphine to placebo (Johnson et al. 1995, Fudala et al. 1998a), a buprenorphine/naloxone combination and placebo (Fudala et al. 1998a), and a multiple-dose comparison study (Ling et al. 1998). In one of the most recent trials (Johnson et al. 2000), buprenorphine (given three times weekly) was compared with LAAM (given three times weekly) and methadone (given daily) in a 17-week study. Mean retention in treatment was higher for buprenorphine, LAAM, and high-dose methadone compared to low-dose methadone, and for high-dose methadone compared to LAAM. Opioid-positive urine samples decreased most for the LAAM-treated group and least for low-dose methadone. Self-reports of individuals for opioid use did not differ between the groups, but showed decreases of about 90% over the course of the study.

Buprenorphine has the potential to be abused and can produce addiction; however, most persons who abuse buprenorphine initiated opioid use with other drugs. Abuse may take the form of using greater than prescribed dosages for analgesia, using buprenorphine in place of a more desired but less available opioid, or using buprenorphine for its positive reinforcing effects (Baumevieille et al. 1997, Dore et al. 1997). Only one study has characterized the behavioral and physiologic effects of a wide range of buprenorphine analgesic doses in nonusers of opioids (Zacny et al. 1997) and the results indicated that buprenorphine given intravenously has a low abuse liability in this population.

Buprenorphine, in combination with naloxone, has less potential for abuse than buprenorphine alone (Fudala et al. 1998b, Mendelson et al. 1999). The therapeutic utility of combining naloxone with buprenorphine derives from the low sublingual bioavailability of naloxone as compared to buprenorphine. Parenteral misuse of the combination by persons addicted to opioids would be expected to produce antagonist-like effects; thus, most persons with opioid dependence would be unlikely to inject the combination more than once. The use of the buprenorphine/naloxone combination in an office-based setting represents an innovative alternative to the restrictive methadone or LAAM maintenance paradigm described previously and should expand the availability of agonist maintenance treatment with a relatively low risk for abuse or diversion. In addition, the partial agonist activity of buprenorphine results in a much lower risk for overdose death than is the case with methadone or LAAM.

Antagonist Maintenance

Naltrexone is the prototypical opioid antagonist used in abstinence therapy, blocking the effects of heroin and other opioids through competitive receptor inhibition. Naltrexone has no opioid agonist effects and is a competitive opioid antagonist. It is orally effective and can block opioid effects for 24 hours when administered as a single daily dose of 50 mg; doses of 100 to 150 mg can block opioid effects for 48 to 72 hours (Lee et al. 1998). Despite a favorable adverse event profile (nausea is typically the most common side effect), naltrexone is generally not favored by opioid addicts because, unlike opioid agonists and partial agonists, it produces no positive, reinforcing effects. Furthermore, it may be associated with the precipitation of an opioid withdrawal syndrome if used too soon after opioid use stops, an effect that can be minimized by administering a naloxone challenge prior to giving the first dose of naltrexone.

While there is a literature spanning more than 25 years on naltrexone treatment, work continues on increasing compliance and improving outcomes. Some of these more recent efforts include work to develop a depot form that will block opioid effects for 14 to 28 days. This dosage form is currently in Phase II clinical trials. Presently, an individual treated with naltrexone has only to stop the medication for 1 to 3 days in order to experience the full effects of subsequent opioid use. A depot dosage form of naltrexone would provide more time for individuals to overcome ambivalence about stopping opioid use and could result in more long-term success than has currently been the case. Another variant on antagonist treatment is nalmefene, an orally effective but somewhat longer-acting (about 48 hours at dosages of 50–100 mg/day) opioid antagonist that has been effective for alcohol treatment (Mason et al. 1994) and shows promise as an alternative to naltrexone for opioid dependence (Jones et al. 2000).

Psychosocial Treatments

Recent research has called attention to the fact that, as in other substance use disorders, most individuals with opioid dependence and abuse are ambivalent about stopping use (Miller and Rollnick 1991, Rollnick et al. 1999). This ambivalence presents a challenge as it contributes to varying levels of motivation to enter and remain in treatment, to early dropout, and to partial or (in some cases) nontreatment response. Studies have emphasized that clinicians must be aware of this "normal" ambivalence, and make reasonable efforts to resolve it in favor of treatment participation and cessation of use (Rollnick et al. 1999). Suggestions that have been made regarding initial steps to maximize the chances for engagement in treatment and cessation of drug use include avoiding unnecessary delays in entering treatment, expressing a hopeful and nonjudgmental attitude, performing a comprehensive evaluation, and developing a treatment plan that is responsive to the individual's self-identified goals (Miller and Rollnick 1991).

In addition to challenges related to ambivalence, individuals often have serious problems with nonopioid substance abuse and/or with medical, psychiatric, legal, employment, and family/social issues that preexist or result from the addiction. Research has found that addressing these additional problems can be helpful, but is complex and requires coordination between agonist pharmacotherapy staff, and other medical and psychosocial services (McLellan et al. 1993, Umbricht-Schneiter et al. 1994).

The most common type of psychosocial treatment in opioid agonist maintenance is individual drug counseling. Counselors are typically persons at the masters level or below who deliver a behaviorally focused treatment aimed to identify specific problems, help the individual access services that may not be provided in the clinic (e.g., medical, psychiatric, legal, family/social), stop substance use, and improve overall adjustment. Functions that counselors perform include monitoring methadone and LAAM doses and requesting changes when needed, reviewing urine test results, responding to requests for take-home doses, assisting with family problems, responding to crises, writing letters for court or social welfare agencies, recommending inpatient treatment when necessary, and providing support and encouragement for a drug-free lifestyle.

Counseling usually addresses both opioid and nonopioid use. Although nicotine (tobacco) use is not always included, the increased emphasis on adverse health effects of smoking has resulted in more attention to stop smoking at all levels, including drug counseling. Counselors and substance-dependent individuals typically have weekly, 30- to 60-minute sessions during the first weeks or months of treatment with reductions in frequency to biweekly or monthly depending on progress. The frequency of counseling can vary widely depending on the severity of the individual's problems, clinic requirements, and counselor workload.

The importance of regular counseling was clearly demonstrated in a study by McLellan and coworkers (1993) in which individuals were randomly assigned to minimal counseling (one 5- to 10-minute session per month), standard counseling (one 45-minute session per week), or enhanced counseling (standard plus on-site referral to psychiatric, medical, and family/social services). Results showed a dose–response relationship with the minimal condition doing significantly worse than standard, and enhanced counseling doing the best overall; however, about 30% of individuals did well in the minimal counseling condition. This study clearly demonstrated the positive benefits achieved by drug counseling and showed that, for most individuals, counseling is necessary to bring out the maximum benefits from agonist maintenance.

Though most counseling is individual, some programs use group therapy exclusively and others do not use it at all. Most agonist programs that use groups have them only for individuals with focal problems such as HIV disease, PTSD, homelessness, or loss of close personal relationships. Many programs encourage individuals to participate in self-help groups, but ask them to select a group that accepts persons who are on agonist maintenance treatment. Some programs have self-help groups that meet on site. Counselors, like psychotherapists, can vary widely in the results they achieve (McLellan et al. 1988). This variability seems more related to the ability to form a positive, helping relationship than to specific techniques (Luborsky et al. 1985).

Contingency management techniques are always included in drug counseling, if for nothing else but to fulfill regulations about requiring progress in treatment as a condition of providing take-home doses; studies have shown that such contingencies can be helpful. For example, an opportunity to receive take-home medications in return for drug-free urine tests is a powerful and practical motivator for many individuals (Iguchi et al. 1996). More flexibility in dispensing take-home doses as contingencies for positive behaviors could be an additionally useful result of the regulatory reforms that were described earlier. Another contingency that is easily applicable, and that some programs have used with positive results, is requiring a negative alcohol breath test prior to dispensing the daily dose of methadone or LAAM.

Though counseling and other services are effective enhancements of agonist treatment, compliance is often an issue and clinics vary in the way they respond to this problem. Some remind individuals of appointments, others do not permit individuals to be medicated unless they keep appointments, and others suspend individuals who miss appointments. For noncompliant individuals, a powerful contingency is requiring certain behaviors for individuals to remain on the program, a procedure that is often formalized in a "treatment contract." Here, the individual is given the option of stopping heroin and other drug use, keeping regular counseling appointments, looking for work, or correcting other behaviors that need improvement as a condition for remaining in treatment. Individuals who fail are administratively detoxified, suspended for months to years, and referred to another program, although the referrals are not always successful.

The long-term effects of this form of contingency management have not been well studied. For example, relatively little is known about negative effects on individuals who might have improved with methadone and counseling, but not to the degree required by the contingency, and are subsequently discharged for failing a contract. A recent study done in Philadelphia (Zanis and Woody 1998) found that among 110 individuals who were administratively discharged or dropped out of a Veterans Affairs (VA) maintenance program, 8.2% (9/110) died within the following year as compared to only 1% (4/397) who remained in treatment. Among the 43 individuals (from the 110) who were discharged for failing a treatment contract, 5 (11.6%) died within a year. None of these five were in treatment at the time of death and all died as a result of overdoses. No overdose deaths occurred among individuals remaining in treatment and, interestingly, there were no deaths in those who were suspended for violating program rules (mainly drug dealing or giving a false urine specimen). These results are consistent with recent data from New South Wales (NSW), Australia, where there has been a sharp rise in heroin-related deaths. Though it is estimated that 20 to 30% of the heroin addicts in NSW are receiving methadone maintenance, only 3% of the 953 heroin-related fatalities occurred among individuals receiving methadone maintenance

(Darke et al. 1996). These data emphasize the fine line between use of suspension as a contingency and the dangers associated with program dismissal.

The above data, when considered along with studies showing a protective effect of maintenance on acquiring HIV infection (Metzger et al. 1998), have made some clinicians increasingly hesitant to suspend individuals from maintenance treatment for positive urine test results alone. This caution may be especially relevant in environments where the potency of heroin is high, such as Philadelphia, where the average "bag" of heroin is now 71% pure (Community Epidemiology Work Group 1999). The concept of a "risk/benefit" ratio seems appropriate—the risk of serious adverse events among those who are suspended for failing to meet the contingency, without making provision for them to enter another form of treatment, appears to be substantial.

Therapeutic community (TC) programs are another approach that has been shown useful for treating opioid dependence, especially individuals with a long history of addiction and a strong motivation to become drug-free, either as a result of internal processes or from external pressures such as being given the choice of entering prison for a drug-related crime, or getting treatment in a TC. These programs are very selective, self-governing, and long-term (6–18 months). They occur in residential settings where individuals share responsibilities for maintaining the treatment milieu (cleaning, cooking, and leading group therapy). Confrontation of denial and behaviors such as lying and "conning," combined with group support for healthy, positive change are used to restructure character and the addictive lifestyle. Medications such as methadone, LAAM, or naltrexone are rarely used; however, medications for specific psychiatric or medical conditions are usually available after careful screening and evaluation. Many TCs have large numbers of individuals who have been referred by the criminal justice system including some who have tried but not responded to agonist maintenance on repeated occasions. Though dropout rates are high, studies have shown that over 80% of individuals who complete TCs have a sustained remission and demonstrate significant improvement in psychiatric symptoms, employment, and criminal behavior (Inciardi et al. 1997, DeLeon 1999).

Addressing Comorbidity

Individuals seeking treatment for opioid dependence are typically using one or more other substances (cocaine, alcohol, benzodiazepines, amphetamines, marijuana, nicotine), and have additional problems in the psychiatric, medical, family/social, employment, or legal areas. In fact, it is rare to find a person with only opioid dependence and no other substance use, or without a psychiatric, medical, or family/social problem. The presence of these problems, perhaps with the exception of nicotine dependence, tends to magnify the severity of the opioid dependence and makes the individual even more difficult to treat.

Among the mental disorders seen in persons with opioid dependence, antisocial personality disorder is one of the most common. Diagnostic studies of persons with opioid dependence have typically found rates of antisocial personality disorder ranging from 20 to 50%, as compared to less than 5% in the general population. PTSD is also seen with increased frequency.

Opioid-dependent persons are especially at risk for the development of brief depressive symptoms, and for episodes of mild to moderate depression that meet symptomatic and duration criteria for major depressive disorder or dysthymia. These syndromes represent both substance-induced mood disorders as well as independent depressive illnesses. Brief periods of depression are especially common during chronic intoxication or withdrawal, or in association with psychosocial stressors that are related to the dependence. Insomnia is common, especially during withdrawal; sexual dysfunction, especially impotence, is common during intoxication. Delirium or brief, psychotic-like symptoms are occasionally seen during opioid intoxication.

The data on psychiatric comorbidity among opioid addicts and its negative effect on outcome (McLellan et al. 1983) have stimulated research on the effect of combining psychiatric and substance abuse treatment. Studies have shown that tricyclic antidepressants can be useful for chronically depressed opioid-dependent persons who are treated with methadone maintenance (Nunes et al. 1998). Two other studies have shown that professional psychotherapy can be useful for psychiatrically impaired, methadone-maintained opioid addicts (Woody et al. 1984, 1999), although another found no psychotherapy effect (Rounsaville et al. 1983). The main result in most pharmacotherapy and psychotherapy studies with methadone-maintained addicts has usually been a reduction in psychiatric symptoms such as depression, although some have shown reductions in substance use as well (Nunes et al. 1998, Woody et al. 1985, 1995).

Less than 5% of persons with opioid dependence have psychotic disorders such as bipolar illness or schizophrenia; however, these individuals can present special problems since programs typically have few psychiatric staff. As a result, these individuals are sometimes excluded from methadone treatment because they cannot be effectively managed within the constraints of the available resources. Others are treated with methadone, counseling, and the same medications used for nonaddicted individuals with similar disorders. Though studies evaluating the outcome of combining opioid agonist treatment with antipsychotic or antimanic medications have not been done, there is little controversy that these medications are useful for persons with opioid dependence and psychotic disorders.

Women with opioid dependence can present special challenges because many have been sexually abused as children, have other mental disorders, and are involved in difficult family/social situations (Blume 1999). Abusive relationships with addicted males are common, sometimes characterized by situations in which the male exerts control by providing drugs. These complex psychiatric and relationship issues have emphasized the need for comprehensive psychosocial services that include psychiatric assessment and treatment, and access to other medical, family, and social services.

Medical comorbidity is a major problem among persons with opioid dependence; HIV infection, AIDS, and hepatitis B and C have become some of the most common problems. Sharing injection equipment including "cookers" and rinse water, or engaging in high-risk sexual behaviors are the main routes of infection. Sexual transmission appears to be a more common route of HIV transmission among females than males because the HIV virus is spread more readily from males to females than from females to males. Females who are intravenous drug users and also engage in prostitution or other forms of high-risk sex are at extremely high risk for HIV infection (Blume 1999). Cocaine use has been found to be a significant risk factor as a single drug of abuse or when used in combination with heroin or other opioids (Booth et al. 2000).

After rising rapidly in the late 1970s and early 1980s, the incidence of new HIV infections among intravenous drug users, of whom opioid-dependent individuals constitute a large proportion, has decreased (Seage et al. 2001). However, as a result of high levels of needle sharing and other risky behavior in the early phases of the epidemic, HIV infection rates are as high as 60% in some areas of the United States. Owing to the long incubation period prior to the development of AIDS, it is expected that future years will continue to see high levels of morbidity and mortality associated with HIV, although the advent of new pharmacotherapies for HIV has extended many lives.

Recent studies have identified several important interactions between methadone and drugs to treat HIV. Information is not complete, however, and more studies are needed to map out the full extent of these interactions. One important interaction is that methadone increases plasma levels of zidovudine; the associated symptoms resemble methadone withdrawal. There have been instances in which methadone doses have been increased in response to complaints of withdrawal with increasing doses compounding the problem.

Another important interaction involves decreased methadone blood levels secondary to nevirapine that may result in mild to moderate withdrawal. This interaction can be important if the individual is taken off either of these two drugs while on methadone, since the result may be a sudden rise in methadone blood levels with signs and symptoms of over medication (Altice et al. 1999, Otero et al. 1999).

As mentioned earlier, mortality is high and studies have found annual death rates of approximately 10 per 1000 or greater, which is substantially higher than demographically matched samples in the general population (Gronbladh et al. 1990). Common causes of death are overdose, accidents, injuries, and medical complications such as cellulitis, hepatitis, AIDS, tuberculosis, and endocarditis. The cocaine and alcohol dependence that is often seen among opioid-dependent persons contributes to cirrhosis, cardiomyopathy, myocardial infarction and cardiac arrhythmias.

Tuberculosis has become a particularly serious problem among intravenous drug users, especially heroin addicts. In most cases, infection is asymptomatic and evident only by the presence of a positive tuberculin skin test. However, many cases of active tuberculosis have been found, especially among those who are infected with HIV.

Other medical complications of heroin dependence are seen in children born to opioid-dependent women. Perhaps the most serious is premature delivery and low birth weight, a problem that can be reduced if the mother is on methadone maintenance and receiving prenatal care (Finnegan 1991). Another is physiological dependence on opioids, seen in about half the infants born to women maintained on methadone or dependent on heroin or other opioids. Effective treatments for neonatal withdrawal are available and long-term adverse effects of opioid withdrawal have not been demonstrated. Adverse neonatal effects associated with LAAM or buprenorphine have not been observed, but few studies have been done since neither medication is approved for use in pregnancy.

A recent study found that methadone is present in the breast milk of women maintained on doses as high as 180 mg but that the concentration is very low and no adverse effects were observed in the infants (McCarthy and Posey 2000). HIV infection is seen in about one-third of infants born to HIV-positive mothers, but can be reduced to about 10% if HIV-positive pregnant women are given zidovudine prior to delivery (Connor et al. 1994). HIV can also be transmitted by breast-feeding, and thus formula is recommended for HIV-positive mothers with the exception of countries where it is unavailable or unaffordable. Thorough washing of infants born to HIV-infected mothers immediately after delivery also appears to reduce the incidence of HIV infection.

The comorbidity data have led to research that has demonstrated the positive effects of integrating psychiatric and medical care within agonist and other substance abuse treatment programs (Kessler et al. 1996). Clinical experience and National Institute on Drug-Abuse demonstration projects have shown that integration of these services can be done, and with very positive results since individuals are seen frequently and treatment retention is high (Umbricht-Schneiter et al. 1994). Related to this line of research are studies that have shown improved compliance with directly observed antituberculosis pharmacotherapy (Chaulk et al. 1995). These findings have important implications for tuberculosis control policies in methadone programs since intravenous drug users are at very high risk for tuberculosis infection and because maintenance programs provide settings in which directly observed therapy can be easily applied. Similar principles apply to administration of psychotropic medication in noncompliant individuals with schizophrenia or other major Axis I disorders.

Harm Reduction

Harm reduction is concerned with minimizing various negative consequences of addiction. As such, the focus is shifted away from drug use to the consequences of use and its attendant behaviors (Marlatt 1996). Examples of harm reduction include needle exchange programs, efforts directed at reducing drug use–associated behaviors that may result in the transmission of HIV, and making changes in policies (including increasing treatment availability) that reduce heroin use and the criminal behavior associated with drug procurement. Harm reduction refers not only to reducing harm to the individual addict, but also to family, friends, and to society generally. Other terms sometimes used synonymously with harm reduction include harm minimization, risk reduction, and risk minimization (Riley et al. 1999).

A number of authors have identified the limitations of harm reduction when it is used as a sole strategy to combat the adverse effects of addiction. For example, Reuter and Caulkins (1995) point out the benefit of balancing drug use reduction and harm-reduction components into a single framework, since the chances for harm may be lowered by reducing either component. Roche and colleagues (1997) have proposed a model for an integrated addiction treatment strategy that incorporates harm reduction and use reduction with abstinence and nonuse, in addition to other critical elements such as factors related to culture and gender. Additionally, MacCoun (1998) has provided a template for integrating harm reduction with prevalence reduction (discouraging the engagement in drug use) and quantity reduction (encouraging the reduction in frequency or extent of drug use).

With regard to opioids, much of the health-related harm from their improper or illicit use is secondary to elements other than the substances themselves (Kalant 1999). Sequelae from unhygienic methods of administration and poor injection technique are typically more serious than the constipation or other side effects of the drugs themselves, acute overdoses notwithstanding. At current levels of use, greater harm is expected to result from the use of alcohol and tobacco than from opioids. With regard to opioid addiction treatment, medications such as methadone, LAAM, and buprenorphine, among others (including supervised heroin substitution) used for maintenance agonist treatment, may be considered harm-reduction measures. All have the potential to reduce morbidity, mortality, and crime associated with the addict lifestyle and in this sense, their outcomes on the target symptoms bear some resemblance to the results of other medical therapies that control but do not cure, such as those used for the treatment of hypertension, diabetes, or asthma.

Needle/syringe exchange has been one of the most controversial strategies for harm reduction. Recent research indicates that these programs may have beneficial effects in a number of areas, including a reduction in the spread of blood-borne infections such as hepatitis and HIV, and acting as a conduit to more comprehensive drug-abuse treatment services (Normand et al. 1995). In one study (Bluthenthal et al. 2000), the initiation and continuation of participation in a syringe exchange program by high-risk injection drug users was independently associated with a cessation of syringe sharing. In another (Strathdee et al. 1999), participation in a needle exchange program was associated with individuals entering detoxification treatment for both HIV-infected and noninfected groups. Not all findings have been positive, however. In a study designed to assess the association between risk behaviors and HIV infection among injection drug users, risk elevations for HIV associated with needle exchange programs were substantial and consistent despite adjustment for confounding factors (Bruneau et al. 1997). However, an examination of potential bias in nonrandomized comparisons (Hagan et al. 2000) suggested that injection drug users participating in needle exchange programs at a given point in time may include a high proportion of individuals whose pattern of drug use puts them at greater risk for blood-borne viral infections. Further, a prospective cohort study (Schechter et al. 1999) found no evidence of a causal association between needle exchange program participation and transmission of HIV.

Harm reduction related to psychoactive substance abuse has gone through a number of stages. The current phase has been described as the development of an integrated public health perspective for all drugs in which a multifaceted, strategic approach is taken (Erickson 1999). The direction of this approach will be guided, in part, by whether biases against a harm-reduction philosophy can be overcome by those who see it as synonymous with acceptance of drug abuse or legalization, and how harm-reduction objectives relate to an overall strategy to improve public health.

Comparison of DSM-IV-TR/ICD-10 Diagnostic Criteria

The DSM-IV-TR and ICD-10 criteria sets for opioid intoxication are almost the same. The DSM-IV-TR and ICD-10 symptom lists for opioid withdrawal include some different items: the ICD-10 list has craving, abdominal cramps, and tachycardia and does not include the fever and dysphoric mood items from the DSM-IV-TR criteria set.

References

Addiction Treatment Forum (2000) The Quarterly Newsletter Of Addiction Treatment for Clinical Health Care Professionals IX (2), 2.

Altice FL, Friedland GH, and Cooney EL (1999) Nevirapine induced opiate withdrawal among injection drug users with HIV infection receiving methadone. *AIDS* **13**, 957–962.

Ball JC and Ross A (1991) *The Effectiveness of Methadone Maintenance Treatment*. Springer-Verlag, New York.

Banys P, Tusel DJ, Sees KL, et al. (1994) Low (40 mg) versus high (80 mg) dose methadone in a 180-day heroin detoxification program. *J Subst Abuse Treat* **11**, 225–232.

Baumevieille M, Haramburu F, and Bégaud B (1997) Abuse of prescription medicines in southwestern France. *Ann Pharmacother* **31**, 847–850.

Bearn J, Gossop M, and Strang J (1996) Randomized double-blind comparison of lofexidine and methadone in the inpatient treatment of opiate withdrawal. *Drug Alcohol Depend* **43**, 87–89.

Bearn J, Gossop M, and Strang J (1998) Accelerated lofexidine treatment regimen compared with conventional lofexidine and methadone treatment for inpatient opiate detoxification. *Drug Alcohol Depend* **50**, 227–232.

Blume SB (1999) Addiction in women. In *Textbook of Substance Abuse Treatment*, Galanter M and Kleber HD (eds). American Psychiatric Association Press, Washington, DC, pp. 485–494.

Bluthenthal RN, Kral AH, Gee L, et al. (2000) The effect of syringe exchange use on high-risk injection drug users: a cohort study. *AIDS* **14**, 605–611.

Booth RE, Kwiatkowski CF, and Chitwood DD (2000) Sex related HIV risk behaviors: differential risks among injection drug users, crack smokers, and injection drug users who smoke crack. *Drug Alcohol Depend* **58**, 219–226.

Bruneau J, Lamothe F, Franco E, et al. (1997) High rates of HIV infection among injection drug users participating in needle exchange programs in Montreal: results of a cohort study. *Am J Epidemiol* **146**, 994–1002.

Carnwath T and Hardman J (1998) Randomized double-blind comparison of lofexidine and clonidine in the outpatient treatment of opiate withdrawal. *Drug Alcohol Depend* **50**, 251–254.

Chaulk CP, Moore-Rice K, Rizzo R, et al. (1995) Eleven years of community-based directly observed therapy for tuberculosis. *J Am Med Assoc* **274**, 945–951.

Cheskin LJ, Fudala PJ, and Johnson RE (1994) A controlled comparison of buprenorphine and clonidine for acute detoxification from opioids. *Drug Alcohol Depend* **36**, 115–121.

Community Epidemiology Work Group (1999) Epidemiologic Trends in Drug Abuse: Advance Report (Dec).

Connor EM, Sperling RS, Gelber R, et al. (1994) Reduction of maternal-infant transmission of human immuno-deficiency virus type 1 with zidovudine treatment. *N Engl J Med* **331**, 1173–1180.

Cucchia AT, Monnat M, Spagnoli J, et al. (1998) Ultra-rapid opiate detoxification using deep sedation with or midazolam: short and long-term results. *Drug Alcohol Depend* **52**, 243–250.

Darke S, Ross J, Zador D, et al. (1996) Heroin-related deaths in New South Wales, Australia. *Drug Alcohol Depend* **60**, 141–150.

DeLeon G (1999) Therapeutic communities. In *Textbook of Substance Abuse Treatment*, Galanter M and Kleber HD (eds). American Psychiatric Association Press, Washington, DC, pp. 447–462.

Diamant K, Fischer G, Schneider C, et al. (1998) Outpatient opiate detoxification treatment with buprenorphine: preliminary investigation. *Eur Addict Res* **4**, 198–202.

Dole VP and Nyswander ME (1965) A medical treatment for diacetylmorphine (heroin) addiction. *JAMA* **193**, 646–650.

Dole VP and Nyswander M (1968) Successful treatment of 750 criminal addicts. *J Am Med Assoc* **26**, 2708–2710.

Dore GM, Hargreaves G, and Niven BE (1997) Dependent opioid users assessed for methadone treatment in Otago: patterns of drug use. *N Z Med J* **110**, 162–165.

Drug Addiction Treatment Act of 2000. Public Law 106–310. 106th Congress.

Erickson PG (1999) Introduction: the three phases of harm reduction. An examination of emerging concepts, methodologies, and critiques. *Subst Use Misuse* **34**, 1–7.

Finnegan LP (1991) Treatment issues for opioid-dependent women during the perinatal period. *J Psychoact Drugs* **23**, 191–201.

Fudala PJ, Bridge TP, Herbert S, et al. (1998a) *A Multisite Efficacy Evaluation of a Buprenorphine/Naloxone Product for Opiate Dependence Treatment*, NIDA Res Monogr 179. Government Printing Office, Rockville, USA, p. 105.

Fudala PJ, Yu E, Macfadden W, et al. (1998b) Effects of buprenorphine and naloxone in morphine-stabilized opioid addicts. *Drug Alcohol Depend* **50**, 1–8.

Gronbladh L, Ohlund LS, and Gunne LM (1990) Mortality in heroin addiction: impact of methadone treatment. *Acta Psychiatr Scand* **82**, 223–227.

Hagan H, McGough JP, Thiede H, et al. (2000) Volunteer bias in nonrandomized evaluations of the efficacy of needle-exchange programs. *J Urb Health* **77**, 103–112.

Hiltunen AJ, Beck O, Hjemdahl P, et al. (1999) Rated well-being in relation to plasma concentrations of l- and d-methadone in satisfied and dissatisfied patients on methadone maintenance treatment. *Psychopharmacology* **143**, 385–393.

Iguchi MY, Lamb RJ, Belding MA, et al. (1996) Contingent reinforcement of group participation versus abstinence in a methadone maintenance program. *Exp Clin Psychopharmacol* **4**, 315–321.

Inciardi JA, Martin SS, Butzin CA, et al. (1997) An effective model of prison-based treatment for drug-involved offenders. *J Drug Issues* **27**, 261–278.

Johnson RE, Chutuape MA, Strain EC, et al. (2000) A comparison of levomethadyl acetate, buprenorphine, and methadone as treatments for opioid dependence. *N Engl J Med* **343**, 1290–1297.

Johnson RE, Eissenberg T, Stitzer ML, et al. (1995) A placebo-controlled trial of buprenorphine as a treatment for opioid dependence. *Drug Alcohol Depend* **40**, 17–25.

Jones HE, Johnson RE, Fudala PJ, et al. (2000) Nalmefene: Blockade of intravenous morphine challenge effects in opioid abusing humans. *Drug Alcohol Depend* **60**, 29–37.

Kahn A, Mumford JP, Rogers GA, et al. (1997) Double-blind study of lofexidine and clonidine in the detoxification of opiate addicts in hospital. *Drug Alcohol Depend* **44**, 57–61.

Kalant H (1999) Differentiating drugs by harm potential: the rational versus the feasible. *Subst Use Misuse* **34**, 25–34.

Kessler RC, Nelson CB, McGonagle KA, et al. (1996) The epidemiology of co-occurring addictive and mental disorders: implications for prevention and service utilization. *Am J Orthopsychiatry* **66**, 17–31.

Kleber HD (1999) Opioids: Detoxification. In *Textbook of Substance Abuse Treatment*, 2nd ed., Galanter M and Kleber HD (eds). American Psychiatric Association, Washington, DC, pp. 251–269.

Kreek MJ (1986) Tolerance and dependence: implications for the pharmacological treatment of addiction. In *Problems of Drug Dependence*, Harris LS (ed). *Proceedings of the 48th Annual Scientific Meeting of the Committee on Problems of Drug Dependence*. DHHS Publication No (ADM) 87–1508, Rockville, MD, pp. 77–86.

Lee MC, Wagner HN, Tanada S, et al. (1998) Duration of occupancy of opiate receptors by naltrexone. *J Nucl Med* **29**, 1207–1211.

Lin SK, Strang J, Su LW, et al. (1997) Double blind randomized controlled trial of lofexidine versus clonidine in the treatment of heroin withdrawal. *Drug Alcohol Depend* **48**, 127–133.

Luborsky L, McLellan AT, Woody GE, et al. (1985) Therapist success and its determinants. *Arch Gen Psychiatry* **42**, 602–611.

MacCoun RJ (1998) Toward a psychology of harm reduction. *Am Psychol* **53**, 1199–1208.

Marlatt GA (1996) Harm reduction: come as you are. *Addict Behav* **21**, 779–788.

Mason BJ, Ritvo EC, Morgan RO, et al. (1994) A double-blind, placebo-controlled pilot study to evaluate the efficacy and safety of oral nalmefene HCl for alcohol dependence. *Alcohol Clin Exp Res* **18**, 1162–1167.

McCarthy JJ and Posey BL (2000) Methadone levels in human milk. *J Hum Lac* **16**, 115–120.

McLellan AT, Arndt IO, Metzger DS, et al. (1993) The effects of psychosocial services on substance abuse treatment. *J Am Med Assoc* **269**, 1953–1959.

McLellan AT, Luborsky L, Woody GE, et al. (1983) Predicting response to alcohol and drug abuse treatments: role of psychiatric severity. *Arch Gen Psychiatry* **40**, 620–625.

McLellan AT, Woody GE, Luborsky L, et al. (1988) Is the counselor an "active ingredient" in substance abuse treatment? *J Nerv Ment Dis* **176**, 423–430.

Mendelson J, Jones RT, Welm S, et al. (1999) Buprenorphine and naloxone combinations: the effects of three dose ratios in morphine-stabilized, opiate-dependent volunteers. *Psychopharmacology* **141**, 37–46.

Metzger DS, Navaline H, and Woody GE (1998) *Drug Abuse Treatment as AIDS Prevention*, Pub Health Rep 113S. pp. 97–106.

Miller WR and Rollnick S (1991) *Motivational Interviewing: Preparing People to Change Addictive Behavior*. Guilford Press, New York.

National Household Survey on Drug Abuse (2000) *Population Estimates*, 2nd Rev., DHHS Publication No. (ADM) 92–1887. US Department of Health and Human Services, Public Health Service, Alcohol, Drug Abuse and Mental Health Administration.

Normand J, Vlahov D, and Moses L (eds) (1995) *Preventing HIV Transmission: The Role of Sterile Needles and Bleach*. National Research Council, Institute of Medicine. National Academy Press, Washington, DC.

Nunes EV, Quitkin FM, Donovan S, et al. (1998) Imipramine treatment of opiate dependent patients with depressive disorders: a placebo-controlled trial. *Arch Gen Psychiatry* **55**, 153–160.

O'Brien CP, Testa T, O'Brien TJ, et al. (1997) Conditioned narcotic withdrawal in humans. *Science* **195**, 1000–1002.

O'Connor PG, Carroll KM, Shi JM, et al. (1997) Three methods of opioid detoxification in a primary care setting: a randomized trial. *Ann Intern Med* **127**, 526–530.

O'Connor PG and Kosten TR (1998) Rapid and ultrarapid opioid detoxification techniques. *J Am Med Assoc* **279**, 229–234.

Otero MJ, Fuentes A, Sanchezn R, et al. (1999) Nevirapine-induced withdrawal symptoms in HIV patients on methadone maintenance programme: an alert. *AIDS* **13**, 1004–1005.

Parran TV Jr., Adelman CL, and Jasinski DR (1994) A buprenorphine stabilization and rapid-taper protocol for the detoxification of opioid dependent patients. *Am J Addict* **3**, 306–313.

Pfab R, Hirtl C, and Zilker T (1999) Opiate detoxification under anesthesia: no apparent benefit but suppression of thyroid hormones and risk of pulmonary and renal failure. *J Toxicol Clin Toxicol* **37**, 43–50.

Reilly PM, Banys P, Tusel DJ, et al. (1995) Methadone transition treatment: a treatment model for 180-day methadone detoxification. *Int J Addict* **30**, 387–402.

Reuter P and Caulkins JP (1995) Redefining the goals of national drug policy: recommendations from a working group. *Am J Pub Health* **85**, 1059–1063.

Riley D, Sawka E, Conley P, et al. (1999) Harm reduction: concepts and practice. A policy discussion paper. *Subst Use Misuse* **34**, 9–24.

Robins LN and Regier DA (1991) *Psychiatric Disorders in America: The Epidemiologic Catchment Area Study.* Free Press, New York, pp. 116–154.

Roche AM, Evans KR, and Stanton WR (1997) Harm reduction: roads less travelled to the Holy Grail. *Addiction* **92**, 1207–1212.

Rollnick S, Mason P, and Butler C (1999) *Health Behavior Change: A Guide for Practitioners.* Churchill Livingstone, New York.

Rounsaville BJ, Glazer W, Wilber CH, et al. (1983) Short-term interpersonal psychotherapy in methadone maintained opiate addicts. *Arch Gen Psychiatry* **39**, 161–166.

Rounsaville BJ, Weissman MM, and Wilber CH (1982) The heterogeneity of psychiatric diagnosis in treated opiate addicts. *Arch Gen Psychiatry* **39**, 161–166.

San L, Puig M, Bulbena A, et al. (1995) High risk of ultrashort noninvasive opiate detoxification. *Am J Psychiatry* **152**, 956.

Schechter MT, Strathdee SA, Cornelisse PG, et al. (1999) Do needle exchange programmes increase the spread of HIV among injection drug users? An investigation of the Vancouver outbreak. *AIDS* **13**, F45–F51.

Seage GR, Holte SE, Metzger D, et al. (2001) Are US populations appropriate for trials of human immunodeficiency virus vaccine?. *Am J Epidemiol* **153**, 619–627.

Strathdee SA, Celentano DD, Shah N, et al. (1999) Needle-exchange attendance and health care utilization promote entry into detoxification. *J Urb Health* **76**, 448–460.

Umbricht-Schneiter A, Ginn DH, Pabst KM, et al. (1994) Providing medical care to methadone clinic patients: referral vs. on-site care. *Am J Pub Health* **84**, 207–210.

Umbricht-Schneiter A, Huestis MA, Cone EJ, et al. (1998) *Safety of Buprenorphine: Ceiling for Cardio-Respiratory Effects at High IV Doses.* NIDA Res Monogr 179. Government Printing Office, Rockville, USA, p. 225.

Vignau J (1998) Preliminary assessment of a 10-day rapid detoxification programme using high dosage buprenorphine. *Eur Addict Res* **4**, 29–31.

Wikler A (1980) *Opioid Dependence: Mechanisms and Treatment.* Plenum Press, New York.

Woody GE, McLellan AT, Luborsky L, et al. (1984) Psychiatric severity as a predictor of benefits from psychotherapy the Penn-VA study. *Am J Psychiatry* **141**, 1172–1177.

Woody GE, McLellan AT, Luborsky L, et al. (1985) Sociopathy and psychotherapy outcome. *Arch Gen Psychiatry* **42**, 1081–1086.

Woody GE, McLellan AT, Luborsky L, et al. (1995) Psychotherapy in community methadone programs: a validation study. *Am J Psychiatry* **152**(9), 1302–1308.

Woody GE, Mercer DS, and Luborsky L (1999) Individual psychotherapy for substance use disorders. In *Textbook of Substance Abuse Treatment*, 3rd ed., Kleber HD and Galanter M (eds). American Psychiatric Association, Washington DC, pp. 343–352.

Zacny JP, Conley K, and Galinkin J (1997) Comparing the subjective, psychomotor and physiological effects of intravenous buprenorphine and morphine in healthy volunteers. *J Pharmacol Exp Ther* **282**, 1187–1197.

Zanis DA and Woody GE (1998) One-year mortality rates following methadone treatment discharge. *Drug Alcohol Depend* **52**, 257–260.

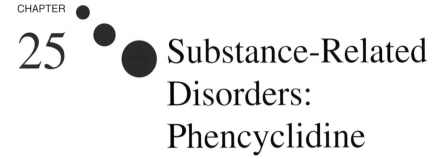

25 Substance-Related Disorders: Phencyclidine

Phencyclidine (1-(1-phenylcyclohexyl)piperidine, PCP) was developed as a general anesthetic agent in the 1950s under the brand name Sernyl (Collins et al. 1960, Greifenstein et al. 1958, Johnstone et al. 1958). The drug was considered physiologically promising because of its lack of respiratory and cardiovascular depressant effects. In fact, individuals under PCP anesthesia rather than manifesting a state of relaxed sleep such as that induced by typical anesthetic agents appeared semiconscious with open eyes, fixed staring, flat facies, open mouth, rigid posturing, and waxy flexibility. Because of this apparent sharp dissociation from the environment without true unconsciousness, PCP and the related drug ketamine were classified as dissociative anesthetics (Corssen and Domino 1966).

Approximately 50% of individuals anesthetized with PCP developed behavioral syndromes including agitation and hallucinations during emergence from anesthesia (Collins et al. 1960, Greifenstein et al. 1958, Johnstone et al. 1958). A substantial number of individuals developed postoperative psychotic reactions, which in some cases persisted up to 10 days (Greifenstein et al. 1958, Johnstone et al. 1958, Corssen and Domino 1966, Meyer et al. 1959). Trials of subanesthetic doses of PCP for treatment of chronic pain led to similar although less severe adverse reactions (Meyer et al. 1959). As a result, after 1965, PCP was limited to veterinary applications. Ketamine remains available for human anesthesia; side effects are less frequent and less severe owing to the lower potency and shorter duration of ketamine action compared to PCP.

Despite its well-documented aversive and disruptive behavioral effects, PCP emerged during the 1970s as a popular drug of abuse, increasing in popularity to the point that in 1979, 13% of high school seniors had tried it (Johnston et al. 1994). Although PCP has never regained that remarkable level of popularity, it has remained a significant public health problem among certain populations and in certain geographical areas. Compared to most other drugs of abuse, PCP has more complex and potentially more harmful effects.

Diagnosis

Physicians must be alert to the wide spectrum of PCP effects on multiple-organ systems. Because fluctuations in serum levels may occur unpredictably, an individual being treated for apparently selective psychiatric or behavioral complications of PCP abuse may suddenly undergo radical alterations in medical status; emergency medical intervention may become necessary to avoid permanent organ damage or death. Any individual manifesting significant cardiovascular, respiratory, neurological, or metabolic derangement subsequent to PCP use should be evaluated and treated in a medical service; the mental health professional plays a secondary role in diagnosis and treatment until physiological stability has been reached and sustained.

PCP-intoxicated individuals may come to medical attention on the basis of alterations in mental status, bizarre or violent behavior, injuries sustained while intoxicated, or medical complications, such as rhabdomyolysis, hyperthermia, or seizures (Baldridge and Bessen 1990). As illicit ketamine use has increased significantly as part of the "club drug" phenomenon, it is important to remember that ketamine can induce the same spectrum of effects and complications, the chief difference from PCP being the much shorter duration of action of ketamine. In a series of 20 ketamine users presenting in Connecticut, the most frequent complications of ketamine abuse were severe agitation and rhabdomyolysis (Weiner et al. 2000).

The presenting symptoms may be predominantly or exclusively psychiatric, without significant alterations in the level of consciousness, and may closely resemble an acute schizophrenic decompensation (Luisada 1978) with concrete or illogical thinking, bizarre behavior, negativism, catatonic posturing, and echolalia (see DSM-IV-TR diagnostic criteria below). Subjective feelings and objective signs of "drunkenness" may or may not be present. Retrospective studies conducted during the period of widespread PCP abuse demonstrated that PCP psychosis could not reliably be distinguished from schizophrenia on the basis of presenting symptoms (Erard et al. 1980, Yesavage and Freeman 1978).

DSM-IV-TR Diagnostic Criteria

292.89 Phencyclidine Intoxication

A. Recent use of phencyclidine (or a related substance).
B. Clinically significant maladaptive behavioral changes (e.g., belligerence, assaultiveness, impulsiveness, unpredictability, psychomotor agitation, impaired judgment, or impaired social or occupational functioning) that developed during, or shortly after, phencyclidine use.
C. Within an hour (less when smoked, "snorted," or used intravenously), two (or more) of the following signs:

   (1) Vertical or horizontal nystagmus
   (2) Hypertension or tachycardia
   (3) Numbness or diminished responsiveness to pain
   (4) Ataxia
   (5) Dysarthria
   (6) Muscle rigidity
   (7) Seizures or coma
   (8) Hyperacusis

D. The symptoms are not due to a general medical condition and are not better accounted for by another mental disorder.

Specify if:

With perceptual disturbances

Studies of normal volunteers suggested that the acute psychosis induced by a single low dose of PCP usually lasts for 4 to 6 hours (Javitt and Zukin 1991). However, in some PCP users, psychotic symptoms including hallucinations, delusions, paranoia, thought disorder, and catatonia, with intact consciousness, have been reported to persist from days to weeks after single doses (Burns and Lerner 1976, Allen and Young 1978, Rainey and Crowder 1975, McCarron et al. 1981). The frequency of such prolonged psychotic states after single doses has not been determined systematically. However, one study indicated that 25% of PCP-intoxicated individuals required inpatient psychiatric admission (Allen and Young 1978). PCP psychosis can occur at undetectably low serum or urinary levels of the drug (Walberg et al. 1983, Pearce 1976). Sudden and impulsive violent and assaultive behaviors have been reported in PCP-intoxicated individuals without previous histories of such conduct.

In PCP intoxication, the central nervous, cardiovascular, respiratory, and peripheral autonomic systems are affected to degrees ranging from mild to catastrophic (Table 25-1).

The level of consciousness may vary from full alertness to coma. Coma of variable duration may occur spontaneously or after an episode of bizarre or violent behavior (McCarron et al. 1981). Prolonged coma due to continued drug absorption from ruptured ingested packages of PCP has been described (Jackson 1989).

Nystagmus (which may be horizontal, vertical, or rotatory) has been described in 57% of a series of 1000 individuals with PCP intoxication (McCarron et al. 1981). Consequences of PCP-induced central nervous system hyperexcitability may range from mildly increased deep tendon reflexes to grand malseizures (observed in 31 of a series of 1000 PCP-intoxicated individuals) or status epilepticus (McCarron et al. 1981, Kessler et al. 1974). Seizures are usually generalized, but focal seizures or neurological deficits have been reported, probably on the basis of focal cerebral vasoconstriction (Crosley and Binet 1979). Other motor signs have been observed, such as generalized rigidity, localized dystonias, facial grimacing, and athetosis (McCarron et al. 1981).

Hypertension, one of the most frequent physical findings, was described in 57% of 1000 PCP-intoxicated individuals evaluated, and it was found to be usually mild and selflimiting, but 4% had severe hypertension, and some remained hypertensive for days (McCarron et al. 1981). One fatal case of hypertensive crisis late in the course of PCP intoxication has been described (Eastman and Cohen 1975). Tachycardia occurs in 30% of individuals with PCP intoxication. PCP-induced tachypnea can progress to periodic breathing and respiratory

Table 25-1	**Nonpsychiatric Findings in Phencyclidine Intoxication**
Altered level of consciousness	
Central nervous system changes including nystagmus, hyperreflexia, and motor abnormalities	
Hypertension	
Cholinergic or anticholinergic signs	
Hypothermia or hyperthermia	
Myoglobinuria	

arrest (Hurlbut 1991). Autonomic signs seen in PCP intoxication may be cholinergic (diaphoresis, bronchospasm, miosis, salivation, bronchorrhea) or anticholinergic (mydriasis, urinary retention) (McCarron et al. 1981).

Hypothermia and hyperthermia have been observed (McCarron et al. 1981). Hyperthermia may reach malignant proportions (Thompson 1979).

Rhabdomyolysis frequently results from a combination of PCP-induced muscle contractions and trauma occurring in relation to injuries sustained as a result of behavioral effects. Acute renal failure can result from myoglobinuria (Patel and Connor 1986).

In children, PCP intoxication may result from ingestion of remnants of used PCP-impregnated cigarettes or from inhalation of sidestream smoke (Karp et al. 1980, Schwartz and Einhorn 1986, Welch and Correa 1980). Young children often present with impaired consciousness, ataxia, nystagmus, staring (Karp et al. 1980, Schwartz and Einhorn 1986, Welch and Correa 1980), or apnea (Burns et al. 1975). Aggressive or violent behavior is unusual in this population (Baldridge and Bessen 1990).

The disruption of normal cognitive and memory function by PCP frequently renders individuals incapable of giving an accurate history, including a history of having used PCP. Therefore, assay of urine or blood for drugs may be the only way to establish the diagnosis. PCP is frequently taken in forms in which it has been used to adulterate other drugs, such as marijuana and cocaine, often without the user's knowledge. One of the most recent and alarming manifestations of this phenomenon is a preparation known variously as *illy*, *hydro*, *wet*, or *fry*, consisting of a marijuana cigarette or blunt containing formaldehyde/formalin (which is advertised) and PCP (which often is not); PCP precursors and synthesis by-products as well as PCP have been detected in toxicological screens of users who have consumed these preparations (Nelson et al. 1999).

By disrupting sensory pathways, PCP frequently renders users hypersensitive to environmental stimuli to the extent that physical examination or psychiatric interview may cause severe agitation. If PCP intoxication is suspected, measures should be taken from the outset to minimize sensory input. The individual should be evaluated in a quiet, darkened room with the minimal necessary number of medical staff present. Assessments may need to be interrupted periodically.

Vital signs should be obtained immediately on presentation. Temperature, blood pressure, and respiratory rate are dose-dependently increased by PCP and may be of a magnitude requiring emergency medical treatment to avoid the potentially fatal complications of malignant hyperthermia, hypertensive crisis, and respiratory arrest. In all cases, monitoring of vital signs should continue at 2- to 4-hour intervals throughout treatment, because serum PCP levels may increase spontaneously as a result of mobilization of drug from lipid stores or enterohepatic recirculation.

Analgesic and behavioral changes induced by PCP not only predispose individuals to physical injury but also mask these injuries, which may be found only with careful physical examination (Baldridge and Bessen 1990).

On neurological examination, nystagmus and ataxia, although not conclusive, are strongly suggestive of PCP intoxication. Examination of deep tendon reflexes helps establish the degree of nervous system hyperexcitability. Crossed or clonic deep tendon reflexes alert the physician to the possibility of subsequent seizures.

Because PCP is usually supplied in combination with other drugs and is often misrepresented, toxicological analysis of urine or blood is essential. However, there may be circumstances in which PCP may not be detected in urine even if it is present in the body, for example, when the urine is alkaline. On the other hand, in chronic PCP users, drug may be detected in urine up to 30 days after the last use (Simpson et al. 1982–1983). It must be kept in mind that false-positive PCP results can be caused by the presence of venlafaxine and *O*-desmethylvenlafaxine (Sena et al. 2002), or dextromethorphan (Shier 2000). Urine should be tested for heme because of the possible complication of myoglobinuria.

Blood and urine samples should be sent for toxicological analysis. In addition, serum uric acid, creatine kinase, aspartate transaminase, and alanine transaminase elevations, common findings in PCP intoxication, were found to be associated with rhabdomyolysis in 22 of 1000 cases (McCarron et al. 1981).

Epidemiology

Illicit use of phencyclidine was first noted in 1965 in Los Angeles (Lerner and Burns 1978). The spread of the drug from California throughout the country was facilitated by its ease of synthesis compared to other drugs. At least six synthetic methods, some simple, are published in scientific journals (Allen et al. 1993). Surveys of street drug samples indicated that PCP was sold under many street names (Table 25-2) and frequently combined with or misrepresented as other substances (Lerner and Burns 1978, Siegel 1978). During the late 1970s and early 1980s, PCP gained considerable notoriety in the popular press not only as a leading drug of abuse but also as one with particularly novel and devastating effects.

In more recent years, indicators of PCP use have remained generally low; however, localized increases have been observed in some cases associated with the use of new dosage forms, in particular, the use of "blunts" (cigars filled with PCP-impregnated marijuana) (Community Epidemiology Work Group 1994).

As of 2000, the highest rates of PCP use during the previous year were observed among 18- to 20-year olds, followed by 12- to 17-, 21- to 25-, and 26- to 34-year olds. In 2000, among Americans aged 12 or older, it was estimated that 54,000 had used PCP within the previous month, 264,000 within the previous year, and 5,693,000 (2% of the population) within their lifetimes (Substance Abuse and Mental Health Services Administration 2001). In the same year, PCP ranked 31st among the top 50 drugs mentioned most frequently in drug-related emergency department episodes nationwide showing a 48% increase in emergency room mentions compared to 1999 (Substance Abuse and Mental Health Services Administration 2002).

Course

As drug levels decline, the clinical picture recedes in 5 to 21 days through periods of moderating neurological, autonomic, and metabolic impairments to a stage at which only psychiatric impairments are apparent. Once the physical symptoms and signs have cleared,

Table 25-2	Street Names for Phencyclidine and Mixtures
Phencyclidine	**Phencyclidine Mixtures and Analog**
Angel dust Animal trank	Beam me up Scottie (crack dipped in PCP)
Baby doll Black whack	Blunt (marijuana and PCP in cigar wrapper)
Butt naked	Love boat (marijuana dipped in PCP)
Devil's dust Elephant tranquilizer	Peanut butter (PCP mixed in peanut butter)
Embalming fluid	Special K (ketamine)
Gorilla biscuits	Tragic magic (crack dipped in PCP)
Heaven	Wet
HogJet fuel	Illy (marijuana treated with formaldehyde/formalin and PCP)
Mad dog	Hydro
Peace pill	Fry
Rocket fuel	
Talk to the angels	
Yellow fever	
Zombie weed	

the period of simple PCP psychosis may last from 1 day to 6 weeks, whether or not neuroleptics are administered, during which the psychiatric symptoms and signs abate gradually and progressively. Even after complete recovery, flashbacks may occur if PCP sequestered in lipid stores is mobilized. Any underlying mental disorders can be detected and evaluated only after complete resolution of the drug-induced psychosis. Although systematic studies in humans have not been carried out, clinical experience predicts a high likelihood of resumption of PCP use after recovery from PCP psychosis.

Differential Diagnosis

The presence of nystagmus and hypertension with mental status changes should raise the possibility of PCP intoxication. Because of the close resemblance of both the acute and the prolonged forms of PCP psychosis to schizophrenia, and the increased sensitivity of individuals with schizophrenia to the psychotomimetic effects of the drug, an underlying schizophrenia spectrum disorder should be considered, particularly if paranoia or thought disorder persists beyond 4 to 6 weeks after the last use of PCP. PCP psychosis may also resemble mania or other mood disorders. Therefore in all cases, a detailed psychiatric history should be obtained. Robust response of psychotic symptoms to treatment with neuroleptics would favor a diagnosis other than simple PCP psychosis.

PCP psychosis is readily distinguishable from lysergic acid diethylamide (LSD) psychosis in normal as well as in individuals with schizophrenia by the lack of typical LSD effects, such as synesthesia. The cluster of psychotic symptoms, hypertension, and stereotypy may be seen in both PCP psychosis and chronic amphetamine psychosis; in such cases, accurate histories and toxicological analysis are particularly important.

In cases involving prominent PCP-induced neurological, cardiovascular, or metabolic derangement, encephalitis, head injury, postictal state, and primary metabolic disorders must be ruled out (Lerner and Burns 1978). Either intoxication with or withdrawal from sedative–hypnotics may be associated with nystagmus (Baldridge and Bessen 1990). Neuroleptic malignant syndrome should be ruled out in the differential diagnosis of PCP-induced hyperthermia and muscle rigidity (Baldridge and Bessen 1990).

Etiology

The psychotomimetic effects of PCP result from its interaction with a unique high-affinity PCP receptor, demonstrated in 1979 (Zukin and Zukin 1979, Sircar et al. 1987), that selectively binds PCP-like drugs in rank order proportional to their behavioral potencies. In contrast, a wide variety of other drugs of abuse and neurotransmitters fail to bind to the PCP receptor at physiologically relevant concentrations (Zukin and Zukin 1979, Vincent et al. 1979, Sircar et al. 1987, Wong et al. 1988, Zukin et al. 1983). The PCP receptor is located within the ion channel gated by the N-methyl-D-aspartate (NMDA) receptor complex (Figure 25-1). When activated by binding of the major excitatory amino acid neurotransmitter of brain, L-glutamate, in the presence of the coagonist glycine, the cation channel gated by the NMDA receptor is activated, permitting influx of calcium ions. Binding of PCP-like drugs uncompetitively inhibits NMDA receptor activation by L-glutamate, thus disrupting NMDA receptor-mediated glutamatergic neurotransmission in a fashion that cannot be surmounted by increasing L-glutamate concentration. Such disruption of NMDA receptor function results in impairment of a number of mental functions including learning and memory (Handelman et al. 1987, Balster and Chait 1976, Thompson et al. 1987, Butelman 1989, Moerschbaecher and Thompson 1983). In animals, exposure to PCP-type drugs has been shown to result in reversible microscopic changes, including vacuolization, in specific populations of brain neurons (Olney et al. 1989). The applicability of these findings to humans remains to be established.

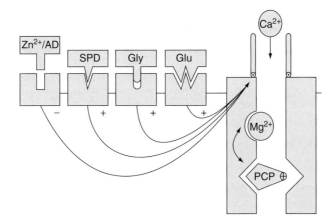

Figure 25-1 *Schematic model of N-methyl-D-aspartate (NMDA) receptor functioning. After magnesium blockade is relieved by membrane depolarization, the cation channel gated by the NMDA receptor can be activated by binding of L-glutamate and glycine. Binding of PCP within the channel blocks ion flux. There are a number of other regulatory sites external to the channel, of which two are illustrated: a site at which polyamines such as spermidine (SPD) positively modulate activation induced by L-glutamate (Glu) and glycine (Gly); and a site at which zinc and tricyclic antidepressants (AD) negatively modulate activation.*

Table 25-3	Single-Dose Effects of Intravenous Phencyclidine
Withdrawal	
Negativism	
Catatonic posturing in some cases	
Concrete, idiosyncratic, and bizarre thinking	
Absence of significant physical or neurological findings	

The effects of low-dose PCP administration have been extensively studied in volunteers. In normal subjects (Table 25-3), single intravenous doses of 0.05 to 0.1 mg/kg induced withdrawal, negativism, and in some cases catatonic posturing; thinking processes became concrete, idiosyncratic, and bizarre in the absence of significant physical or neurological findings; and drug effects persisted for 4 to 6 hours (Bakker and Amini 1961, Luby et al. 1959, Ban et al. 1961, Davies and Beech 1960, Domino and Luby 1981, Rodin et al. 1959). In contrast to lysergic acid diethylamide (LSD) or amphetamine (Domino and Luby 1981, Cohen et al. 1961), PCP was noted to induce disturbances in symbolic thinking (Davies and Beech 1960, Cohen et al. 1961), perception (Luby et al. 1959, Rosenbaum et al. 1959), and attention (Domino and Luby 1981), strikingly similar to those observed in schizophrenia. Administration of PCP to schizophrenic subjects caused exacerbation of illness-specific symptoms persisting up to several weeks (Luby et al. 1959, Domino and Luby 1981), suggesting that schizophrenic or preschizophrenic individuals may be at significantly increased risk of behavioral effects from PCP abuse. At the doses used in these studies, which were equivalent to the typical 5-mg street dose (Burns and Lerner 1976), serum PCP concentrations of 0.01 to 0.1 μM are attained. At such levels, the PCP receptor is the only target site that would be significantly occupied by the drug (Figure 25-2).

Abusers often use PCP in higher or repeated doses leading to significantly higher serum concentrations than those associated selectively with psychotomimetic effects. In general, concentrations greater than 0.4 μM are associated with impairment of consciousness; at concentrations greater than 1 μM, coma, seizures, and respiratory arrest are common

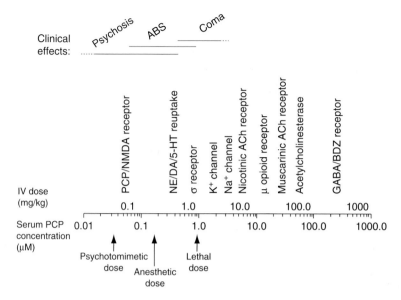

Figure 25-2 *Dose range of PCP effects. Relationship of dose of PCP and PCP affinities for brain target sites to clinical effects is illustrated. Low psychotomimetic doses of PCP act selectively at the PCP site of the NMDA receptor–channel complex. (ABS, acute brain syndrome; ACh, acetylcholine; BDZ, benzodiazepine; DA, dopamine; GABA, γ-aminobutyric acid; 5-HT, 5-hydroxytryptamine; NE, norepinephrine).*

(Walberg et al. 1983, Pearce 1976). These neurological and metabolic effects result in part from interaction of PCP with sites other than the PCP–NMDA receptor, including catecholamine and indoleamine reuptake sites (see Figure 25-2).

PCP is extremely lipid soluble. As a result, it can reach its brain target sites after oral, parenteral, smoked, inhaled (McCarron et al. 1981), or topical administration. Another consequence of its lipophilicity is its tendency to accumulate in lipid tissues throughout the body, including the brain (James and Schnoll 1976, Misra et al. 1979). Flashbacks may result from mobilization of adipose stores, for example, by exercise (James and Schnoll 1976, Misra et al. 1979).

Because of its pK_a of 8.5, PCP is largely ionized in the stomach or urinary tract. However, in the nonacidic environment of the small intestine, PCP becomes nonionized and is readily reabsorbed across the intestinal mucosa; subsequent enterohepatic recirculation may account for the fluctuating clinical course that is often observed.

Metabolism of PCP occurs primarily in the liver. Both PCP (Cook et al. 1982) and hydroxylated metabolites (Wong and Biemann 1976) are excreted in the urine. The serum half-life of PCP has been reported to vary from 4 to 72 hours (Cook et al. 1982, Done et al. 1977). Its volume of distribution is 6.2 L/kg (Cook et al. 1982).

Tolerance to and dependence on PCP have not been formally investigated in humans. Clinical observations suggest that chronic PCP users are significantly less sensitive to a given dose than are casual users. In the case of ketamine, which shares the same fundamental mechanism of action as PCP, tolerance has been more formally observed in burn patients who require increased doses after a time to maintain the same level of analgesia (Carroll 1985). In laboratory animals, a twofold to fourfold shift to the right in the behavioral dose-response curve for PCP is observed in most studies, with indications that tolerance develops to a much greater extent with continuous administration (Balster 1986).

Signs of severe physical withdrawal have been noted in experimental animals when PCP is withdrawn after long-term administration (Balster 1986). In monkeys, even under

·circumstances in which physical withdrawal symptoms are minimal, normal behaviors are disrupted for a week or more after cessation of long-term PCP administration (Slifer et al. 1984). In humans, a single study indicated that one-third of 68 chronic PCP users had sought treatment to help them withdraw from PCP in the face of depressed mood, craving for the drug, and alterations in sleep and appetite that occurred when they attempted to cease drug use on their own (Tennant et al. 1981).

Treatment

The hierarchy of treatment goals begins with detection and treatment of physical manifestations of PCP intoxication. Equally important are measures to anticipate PCP-induced impulsive, violent behaviors and provide appropriate protection for the PCP user and others. The individual must then be closely observed during the period of PCP-induced psychosis, which may persist for weeks after resolution of physical symptoms and signs. Finally, the possibly dramatic medical and psychiatric presentation and its resolution must not divert the attention of the clinician from full assessment and treatment of the individual's drug-seeking behavior.

In contrast to psychotic states induced by drugs such as LSD, in which "talking the individual down" (by actively distracting the individual from his LSD-induced sensory distortions and convincing the individual that his or her distress stems from nothing more than the temporary effects of a drug that soon will wear off) may be highly effective, no such effort should be made in the case of PCP psychosis, particularly during the period of acute intoxication, because of the risk of sensory overload that can lead to dramatically increased agitation. The risk of sudden and unpredictable impulsive, violent behavior can also be increased by sensory stimulation.

Somatic Treatments

There is no pharmacological competitive antagonist for PCP, in contrast to opiates and benzodiazepines. Any compound competing with PCP for binding to its recognition site within the NMDA receptor–gated ion channel would also block the channel and prevent ion flux, thus exerting PCP-like effects. Oral or intramuscular benzodiazepines are recommended for agitation. Neuroleptics usually have little or no effect on acute or chronic PCP-induced psychosis or thought disorder. Because they lower the seizure threshold, neuroleptics should be used with caution. Physical restraint may be lifesaving if the individual's behavior poses an imminent threat to his or her safety or that of others; however, such restraint risks triggering or worsening rhabdomyolysis.

Because of the large volume of distribution of PCP, dialysis is ineffective as a means of clearing the drug from circulation. The "trapping" of PCP in acidic body compartments suggests either gastric gavage or urinary acidification as a measure to reduce levels of PCP in the body. However, these should be considered measures of last resort because of the possibility of electrolyte imbalance and additional nephrotoxic effects. Administration of activated charcoal has been shown to bind PCP and to diminish toxic effects of PCP in animals (Picchioni and Consroe 1979).

Special Features Influencing Treatment

PCP psychosis may be clinically indistinguishable from schizophrenia (Luby et al. 1959, Luisada 1978) or mania (Slavney et al. 1977). It has been suggested that some individuals who remain psychotic for weeks after PCP ingestion may have an underlying predisposition to schizophrenia or mania. In some series, significant percentages of individuals suffering prolonged PCP-induced psychosis are subsequently hospitalized with nondrug-induced schizophrenic disorders (Luisada 1978). In the case of an individual with schizophrenia, responsiveness to neuroleptic treatment may resume after recovery from prolonged PCP psychosis.

Individuals with preexisting neurological, cardiovascular, respiratory, or renal disorders are at increased risk for complications of PCP intoxication, such as seizures, stroke, hypertensive crisis, respiratory arrest, or renal failure. Abusers of more than one drug may be at increased risk from the presence of other drugs exerting toxic effects on the same organ systems (e.g., cardiovascular effects of cocaine and amphetamine) or because of damage to specific organs secondary to infectious complications of parenteral drug use.

Comparison of DSM-IV-TR/ICD-10 Diagnostic Criteria
ICD-10 does not have a separate class for PCP-related disorder and instead includes PCP in the hallucinogen class.

References

Allen AD, Robles J, Dovenski W, et al. (1993) PCP: a review of synthetic methods for forensic clandestine investigation. *Forensic Sci Int* **61**, 85–100.

Allen RM and Young SJ (1978) Phencyclidine-induced psychosis. *Am J Psychiatry* **135**, 1081–1084.

Bakker CB and Amini FB (1961) Observations on the psychotomimetic effects of Sernyl. *Compr Psychiatry* **2**, 269–280.

Baldridge BE and Bessen HA (1990) Phencyclidine. *Emerg Med Clin North Am* **8**, 541–550.

Balster RL (1986) Clinical implications of behavioral pharmacology research on phencyclidine. *NIDA Res Monogr* **64**, 148–162.

Balster RL and Chait LD (1976) The behavioral pharmacology of phencyclidine. *Clin Toxicol* **9**, 513–528.

Ban AT, Lohrenz JJ, and Lehmann HE (1961) Observations on the action of Sernyl—a new psychotropic drug. *Can Psychiatr Assoc J* **6**, 150–156.

Burns RS and Lerner SE (1976) Perspectives: acute phencyclidine intoxication. *Clin Toxicol* **9**, 477–501.

Burns RS, Lerner SE, and Corrado R (1975) Phencyclidine—states of acute intoxication and fatalities. *West J Med* **123**, 345–349.

Butelman ER (1989) A novel NMDA antagonist, MK-801, impairs performance in a hippocampal-dependent spatial learning task. *Pharmacol Biochem Behav* **34**, 13–16.

Carroll ME (1985) PCP: the dangerous angel. In *The Encyclopedia of Psychoactive Drugs*, Snyder SH (ed). Chelsea House, New York, p. 41. (Updated 1992).

Cohen BD, Rosenbaum G, Luby ED, et al. (1961) Comparison of phencyclidine hydrochloride (Sernyl) with other drugs. *Arch Gen Psychiatry* **6**, 79–85.

Collins VJ, Gorospe CA, and Rovenstine EA (1960) Intravenous nonbarbiturate, nonnarcotic analgesics: preliminary studies. Cyclohexylamines. *Anesth Analg* **39**, 303–306.

Community Epidemiology Work Group (1994) *Epidemiologic Trends in Drug Abuse*, Vol. 1. National Institute on Drug Abuse, NIH publication 94–3853, Rockville, MD.

Cook CD, Brine DR, and Jeffcoat AR (1982) Phencyclidine disposition after intravenous and oral doses. *Clin Pharmacol Ther* **31**, 625–634.

Corssen G and Domino EF (1966) Dissociative anesthesia: further pharmacologic studies and first clinical experience with the phencyclidine derivative CI-581. *Anesth Analg* **45**, 29–40.

Crosley CJ and Binet EF (1979) Cerebrovascular complications in phencyclidine intoxication. *J Pediatry* **94**, 316–318.

Davies BM and Beech HR (1960) The effect of 1-arylcyclohexylamine (Sernyl) on 12 normal volunteers. *J Ment Sci* **106**, 912–924.

Domino EF and Luby E (1981) Abnormal mental states induced by phencyclidine as a model of schizophrenia. In *PCP (Phencyclidine): Historical and Current Perspectives*, Domino EF (ed). NPP Books, Ann Arbor, MI.

Done AK, Aronow R, and Miceli JN (1977) Pharmacokinetic observations in the treatment of phencyclidine poisoning: a preliminary report. In *Management of the Poisoned Patient*, Rumack BH and Temple AR (eds). Science Press, Princeton, NJ, pp. 79–95.

Eastman JW and Cohen SN (1975) Hypertensive crisis and death associated with phencyclidine poisoning. *N Engl J Med* **231**, 1270–1271.

Erard R, Luisada PV, and Peele R (1980) The PCP psychosis: prolonged intoxication or drug-precipitated functional illness? *J Psychedel Drugs* **12**, 235–245.

Greifenstein FE, Yoskitake J, DeVault M, et al. (1958) A study of 1-aryl-cyclohexylamine for anesthesia. *Anesth Analg* **37**, 283–294.

Handelman GE, Contreras PC, and O'Donohue TL (1987) Selective memory impairment by phencyclidine in rats. *Eur J Pharmacol* **140**, 69–73.

Hurlbut KM (1991) Drug-induced psychosis. *Emerg Med Clin North Am* **9**, 31–53.

Jackson JE (1989) Phencyclidine pharmacokinetics after a massive overdose. *Ann Int Med* **111**, 613–615.

James SH and Schnoll SH (1976) Phencyclidine: Tissue distribution in the rat. *Clin Toxicol* **9**, 573–582.

Javitt DC and Zukin SR (1991) Recent advances in the phencyclidine model of schizophrenia. *Am J Psychiatry* **148**, 1301–1308.

Johnston LD, O'Malley PM, and Bachman JG (1994) National survey results on drug use from the monitoring the future study, 1975–1993, Vol. I, Secondary School Students. National Institute on Drug Abuse, NIH publication 94–3809, Rockville, MD.

Johnstone M, Evans V, and Baigel S (1958) Sernyl (CI-395) in clinical anesthesia. *Br J Anaesth* **31**, 433–439.

Karp HN, Kaufman ND, and Anand SK (1980) Phencyclidine poisoning in young children. *J Pediatry* **97**, 1006–1009.

Kessler GF, Demers LM, and Berlin C (1974) Phencyclidine and fatal status epilepticus (letter). *N Engl J Med* **291**, 979.

Lerner SE and Burns RS (1978) Phencyclidine use among youth: history, epidemiology, and chronic intoxication. *NIDA Res Monogr* **21**, 66–118.

Luby ED, Cohen BD, Rosenbaum F, et al. (1959) Study of a new schizophrenomimetic drug, Sernyl. *Arch Neurol Psychiatry* **81**, 363–369.

Luisada PV (1978) The phencyclidine psychosis: phenomenology and treatment. *NIDA Res Monogr* **21**, 241–253.

McCarron MM, Schulze BW, Thompson GA, et al. (1981) Acute phencyclidine intoxication: incidence of clinical findings in 1,000 cases. *Ann Emerg Med* **10**, 237–242.

McCarron MM, Schulze BW, Thompson GA, et al. (1981) Acute phencyclidine intoxication: clinical patterns, complications, and treatment. *Ann Emerg Med* **10**, 290–297.

Meyer JS, Greifenstein F, and DeVault M (1959) A new drug causing symptoms of sensory deprivation. *J Nerv Ment Dis* **129**, 54–61.

Misra AL, Pontani RB, and Bartolemeo J (1979) Persistence of phencyclidine (PCP) and metabolites in brain and adipose tissue and implications for long-lasting behavioral effects. *Res Commun Chem Pathol Pharmacol* **24**, 3431–3445.

Moerschbaecher JM and Thompson DM (1983) Differential effects of prototype opioid agonists on the acquisition of conditional discriminations in monkeys. *J Pharmacol Exp Ther* **226**, 738–748.

Nelson LS, Holland JA, and Ravikumar PR (1999) Dangerous form of marijuana. *Ann Emer Med* **34**(1), 115–116.

Olney JW, Labruyere J, and Price MT (1989) Pathological changes induced in cerebrocortical neurons by phencyclidine and related drugs. *Science* **244**, 1360–1362.

Patel R and Connor G (1986) A review of 30 cases of rhabdomyolysis-associated acute renal failure among phencyclidine users. *Clin Toxicol* **23**, 547–556.

Pearce DS (1976) Detection and quantitation of phencyclidine in blood by use of [2H5]phencyclidine and select ion monitoring applied to nonfatal cases of phencyclidine intoxication. *Clin Chem* **22**, 1623–1626.

Picchioni AL and Consroe PF (1979) Activated charcoal—a phencyclidine antidote, or hog in dogs (letter). *N Engl J Med* **300**, 202.

Rainey JM and Crowder MK (1975) Prolonged psychosis attributed to phencyclidine: report of three cases. *Am J Psychiatry* **132**, 1076–1078.

Rodin EA, Luby ED, and Meyer JS (1959) Electroencephalographic findings associated with Sernyl infusion. *Electroencephalogr Clin Neurophysiol* **11**, 796–798.

Rosenbaum G, Cohen BD, Luby ED, et al. (1959) Comparisons of Sernyl with other drugs. *Arch Gen Psychiatry* **1**, 651–656.

Schwartz RH and Einhorn A (1986) PCP intoxication in seven young children. *Pediatr Emerg Care* **2**, 238–241.

Sena SF, Kazimi S, and Wu AH (2002) False-positive phencyclidine immunoassay results caused by venlafaxine and O-desmethylvenlafaxine. *Clin Chem* **48**(4), 676–677.

Shier J (2000) Avoid unfavorable consequences: dextromethorphan can bring about a false-positive phencyclidine urine drug screen. *J Emerg Med* **18**(3), 379–381.

Siegel RK (1978) Phencyclidine and ketamine intoxication: a study of four populations of recreational users. *NIDA Res Monogr* **21**, 119–147.

Simpson JM, Khajawallam AM, and Alatorre E (1982–1983) Urinary phencyclidine excretion in chronic abusers. *J Toxicol Clin Toxicol* **19**, 1051–1059.

Sircar R, Rappaport M, Nichtenhauser R, et al. (1987) The novel anticonvulsant MK-801: a potent and specific ligand of the brain phencyclidine/receptor. *Brain Res* **435**, 235–240.

Slavney PR, Rich GB, Pearlson GD, et al. (1977) Phencyclidine abuse and symptomatic mania. *Biol Psychiatry* **12**, 697–700.

Slifer BL, Balster RL, and Woolverton WL (1984) Behavioral dependence produced by continuous phencyclidine infusion in rhesus monkeys. *J Pharmacol Exp Ther* **230**, 339–406.

Substance Abuse and Mental Health Services Administration (2001) *Summary of Findings from the 2000 National Household Survey on Drug Abuse*. Office of Applied Studies, NHSDA Series H-13, DHHS Publication No. (SMA) 01–3549, Rockville, MD.

Substance Abuse and Mental Health Services Administration (2002) Office of Applied Studies. Emergency Department Trends from the Drug Abuse Warning Network, Preliminary Estimates January–June 2001 with Revised Estimates 1994–2000, DAWN Series D-20, DHHS Publication No. (SMA) 02–3634, Rockville, MD.

Tennant FS Jr. Rawson RA, and McCann M (1981) Withdrawal from chronic phencyclidine dependence with desipramine. *Am J Psychiatry* **138**, 845–847.

Thompson TN (1979) Malignant hyperthermia from PCP (letter). *J Clin Psychiatry* **40**, 327.

Thompson DM, Winsauer PJ, and Mastropaolo J (1987) Effects of phencyclidine, ketamine, and MDMA on complex operant behavior in monkeys. *Pharmacol Biochem Behav* **26**, 401–405.

Vincent JP, Kartalovski B, Geneste P, et al. (1979) Interaction of phencyclidine ("angel dust") with a specific receptor in rat brain membranes. *Proc Natl Acad Sci U S A* **76**, 4678–4682.

Walberg CB, McCarron MM, and Schulze BW (1983) Quantitation of phencyclidine in serum by enzyme immunoassay: results in 405 patients. *J Anal Toxicol* **7**, 106–110.

Weiner AL, Vieira L, McKay CA, et al. (2000) Ketamine abusers presenting to the emergency department: a case series. *J Emerg Med* **18**(4), 447–451.

Welch MJ and Correa GA (1980) PCP intoxication in young children and infants. *Clin Pediatry* **19**, 510–514.

Wong LK and Biemann K (1976) Metabolites of phencyclidine. *Clin Toxicol* **9**, 583–591.

Wong EHF, Knight AR, and Woodruff GN (1988) [^{3}H]MK-801 labels a site on the N-methyl-d-aspartate receptor channel complex in rat brain membranes. *J Neurochem* **50**, 274–281.

Yesavage JA and Freeman AM (1978) Acute phencyclidine (PCP) intoxication: psychopathology and prognosis. *J Clin Psychiatry* **44**, 664–665.

Zukin SR and Zukin RS (1979) Specific [^{3}H]phencyclidine binding in rat central nervous system. *Proc Natl Acad Sci U S A* **76**, 5372–5376.

Zukin SR, Fitz-Syage L, Nichtenhauser R, et al. (1983) Specific binding of [^{3}H]phencyclidine in rat central nervous tissue: Further characterization and technical considerations. *Brain Res* **258**, 277–284.

26 Substance-Related Disorders: Sedative, Hypnotic, and Anxiolytics

Sedative–hypnotics and anxiolytics include prescription sleeping medications and most medications used for the treatment of anxiety. Pharmacologically alcohol is appropriately included among sedative–hypnotics; however, it is generally considered separately as it is in DSM-IV-TR and in this book.

The medications usually included in the category of sedative–hypnotics are listed in Table 26-1. The sedative–hypnotics include a chemically diverse group of medications. Although buspirone is marketed for the treatment of anxiety, its pharmacological profile is sufficiently different that it is not usually included among the sedative–hypnotics. Antidepressant medications may also have antianxiety properties, and their sedative effects are often of clinical utility in sleep induction; however, they too are usually excluded from the sedative–hypnotic classification.

For treatment of anxiety and insomnia, the benzodiazepines have largely supplanted the older sedative–hypnotics. The benzodiazepines have a major advantage over the older compounds. In an overdose, the older sedative–hypnotics are lethal at 10 to 15 times the usual therapeutic doses. Benzodiazepines, if taken alone, have a therapeutic ratio exceeding 100. In combination with alcohol or other drugs, the benzodiazepines may contribute to the lethality, but death from a benzodiazepine overdose is rare. Some atavistic uses of the older compounds remain driven primarily by economic considerations and misguided attempts to reduce abuse of benzodiazepines by addicts and perceived overprescription of benzodiazepines by physicians.

Most people do not like the subjective effects of benzodiazepines, especially in high doses. Even among drug addicts, the benzodiazepines alone are not common intoxicants. They are, however, widely used by drug addicts to self-medicate opiate withdrawal and to alleviate the side effects of cocaine and amphetamines. Individuals receiving methadone maintenance use benzodiazepines to boost (enhance) the effects of methadone. Some alcoholic individuals use benzodiazepines either in combination with alcohol or as a second-choice intoxicant, if alcohol is unavailable. Fat-soluble benzodiazepines that enter the central nervous system (CNS) quickly are usually the benzodiazepines preferred by addicts.

Table 26-1	Medications Usually Included in the Category of Sedative–Hypnotics		
Generic Name	**Trade Names**	**Common Therapeutic Use**	**Therapeutic-Dose Range (mg/d)**
Barbiturates			
Amobarbital	Amytal	Sedative	50–150
Butabarbital	Butisol	Sedative	45–120
Butalbital	Fiorinal, Sedapap	Sedative/analgesic	100–300
Pentobarbital	Nembutal	Hypnotic	50–100
Secobarbital	Seconal	Hypnotic	50–100
Benzodiazepines			
Alprazolam	Xanax	Antianxiety	0.75–6
Chlordiazepoxide	Librium	Antianxiety	15–100
Clonazepam	Klonopin	Anticonvulsant	0.5–4
Clorazepate	Tranxene	Antianxiety	15–60
Diazepam	Valium	Antianxiety	5–40
Estazolam	ProSom	Hypnotic	1–2
Flunitrazepam	Rohypnol*	Hypnotic	1–2
Flurazepam	Dalmane	Hypnotic	15–30
Halazepam	Paxipam	Antianxiety	60–160
Lorazepam	Ativan	Antianxiety	1–16
Midazolam	Versed	Anesthesia	–
Oxazepam	Serax	Antianxiety	10–120
Prazepam	Centrax	Antianxiety	20–60
Quazepam	Doral	Hypnotic	15
Temazepam	Restoril	Hypnotic	7.5–30
Triazolam	Halcion	Hypnotic	0.125–0.5
Others			
Chloral hydrate	Noctec, Somnos	Hypnotic	250–1000
Ethchlorvynol	Placidyl	Hypnotic	200–1000
Glutethimide	Doriden	Hypnotic	250–500
Meprobamate	Miltown, Equanil, Equagesic	Antianxiety	1200–1600
Methyprylon	Noludar	Hypnotic	200–400
Zaleplon	Sonata, (Stilnox, other countries)	Hypnotic	5–20
Zolpidem	Ambien	Hypnotic	5–10

*Rohypnol is not marketed in the United States.

Addicts whose urine is being monitored for benzodiazepines prefer benzodiazepines with high milligram potency, such as alprazolam or clonazepam. These benzodiazepines are excreted in urine in such small amounts that they are often not detected in drug screens, particularly with thin-layer chromatography.

Diagnosis

Sedative–hypnotics are among the most commonly prescribed medications. They are also often misused and abused and can produce severe, life-threatening dependence. With the exception of the benzodiazepines and newer hypnotics (e.g., zaleplon, zopiclone and zolpidem), overdose with sedative–hypnotics can be lethal. Benzodiazepines and the newer hypnotics are rarely lethal if taken alone; in combination with alcohol or other drugs, however, they can be lethal.

In common use, ideas about drug abuse, misuse, and addiction are deeply rooted in social values and attitudes. These social values in mainstream culture are reflected in drug abuse policy and drug control laws. For example, moderate use of alcohol is widely sanctioned for adults, but public intoxication or driving with an alcohol blood level above 0.8 to 1 mg/dL is generally considered alcohol abuse and criminal behavior. Prescription medications are not sanctioned as intoxicants.

The term *misuse* is commonly applied to prescription sedative–hypnotics, but the DSM-IV-TR does not provide explicit criteria for misuse as it does for abuse and dependence. When medications are taken in higher doses or more frequently than prescribed, or by someone other than the person for whom the medication was prescribed, or for reasons other than what would normally be considered medical use, the behavior is generally considered misuse of the medication.

DSM-IV-TR defines abuse and dependence in terms of behavioral and physiological consequences to the person taking the medication. The criteria for abuse and dependence are intended to apply as uniformly as possible across classes of drugs, and the criteria do not distinguish the source of the medication or the intended purpose for which it was taken. Further, when most people, including physicians, speak of drug dependence, they are referring to physical dependence. DSM-IV-TR uses the term *dependence* to denote a more severe form of substance use disorder than abuse, and it uses the specifier "with or without physiological dependence" to indicate whether the individual has significant physical dependence. Physiological dependence is not necessarily required for a diagnosis of drug dependence. A diagnosis of substance dependence is made only when an individual has dysfunctional behaviors that are a result of the drug use.

The qualification that the dysfunctional behavior is the "result" of drug use is extremely important, and observation of the individual over time in a medication-free state may be necessary to determine which is driving which. The drug user, the drug user's family members, and the treating clinician may disagree about what is causing symptoms or behavioral dysfunction. Likewise, the underlying motivation for "drug-seeking" behavior may vary. For example, an individual whose panic attacks are ameliorated by a medication may exhibit what may be interpreted as drug-seeking behavior if access to the medication is threatened. The terms *anxiolytic* and *minor tranquilizer* are also frequently sources of confusion. In classic pharmacology, sedative–hypnotics are drugs or medications that produce a dose-related depression of consciousness. Drug classes are formed by combining drugs or medications that have similar pharmacological profiles.

Sedative-Hypnotic-Anxiolytic Dependence   Sedative–hypnotics can produce tolerance and physiological dependence (see generic DSM-IV-TR diagnostic criteria for Substance Dependence in Chapter 15, page 351). Physiological dependence can be induced within several days with continuous infusion of anesthetic doses. Individuals who are taking barbiturates daily, for example, for a month or more above the upper therapeutic range listed in Table 26-1 should be presumed to be physically dependent and in need of medically managed detoxification.

Sedative-Hypnotic-Anxiolytic Abuse   Abuse may occur on its own or in conjunction with use of other substances (e.g., while using high doses of sedatives in order to "come down" from a cocaine or amphetamine high). Abuse of sedatives in hazardous situations (e.g., getting "high" and then driving while intoxicated) is among the more common reasons for a diagnosis of Sedative-Hypnotic-Anxiolytic Abuse (see generic DSM-IV-TR diagnostic criteria for Substance Abuse in Chapter 15, page 352).

Sedative-Hypnotic-Anxiolytic Intoxication   The acute toxicity of sedative–hypnotics consists of slurred speech, incoordination, ataxia, sustained nystagmus, impaired judgment, and mood lability. When taken in large amounts, sedative–hypnotics produce progressive respiratory depression and coma. The amount of respiratory depression produced by the benzodiazepines is much less than that produced by the barbiturates and other sedative–hypnotics. Consistent with its general approach, the DSM-IV-TR diagnosis of intoxication requires "clinically significant maladaptive behavioral or psychological changes" developing after drug use in addition to the signs and symptoms of acute toxicity. The DSM-IV-TR criteria for intoxication are shown below.

DSM-IV-TR Criteria

292.89 Sedative, Hypnotic, or Anxiolytic Intoxication

A. Recent use of a sedative, hypnotic, or anxiolytic.
B. Clinically significant maladaptive behavioral or psychological changes (e.g., inappropriate sexual or aggressive behavior, mood lability, impaired judgment, impaired social or occupational functioning) that developed during, or shortly after, sedative, hypnotic, or anxiolytic use.
C. One (or more) of the following signs, developing during, or shortly after, sedative, hypnotic, or anxiolytic use:

    (1) slurred speech
    (2) incoordination
    (3) unsteady gait
    (4) nystagmus
    (5) impairment in attention or memory
    (6) stupor or coma.

D. The symptoms are not due to a general medical condition and are not better accounted for by another mental disorder.

Reprinted with permission from the Diagnostic and Statistical Manual of Mental Disorders, Fourth Edition, Text Revision. Copyright 2000 American Psychiatric Association.

Sedative-Hypnotic-Anxiolytic Withdrawal The withdrawal syndrome arising from the discontinuation of short-acting sedative–hypnotics is similar to that from stopping or cutting down on the use of alcohol (see DSM-IV-TR diagnostic criteria given below). Signs and symptoms of sedative–hypnotic withdrawal include anxiety, tremors, nightmares, insomnia, anorexia, nausea, vomiting, postural hypotension, seizures, delirium, and hyperpyrexia. The syndrome is qualitatively similar for all sedative–hypnotics; however, the time course of symptoms depends on the particular drug. With short-acting sedative–hypnotics (e.g., pentobarbital, secobarbital, meprobamate, oxazepam, alprazolam, and triazolam), withdrawal symptoms typically begin 12 to 24 hours after the last dose and peak in intensity between 24 and 72 hours (symptoms may develop more slowly in individuals with liver disease or in the elderly because of decreased drug metabolism). With long-acting drugs (e.g., phenobarbital, diazepam, and chlordiazepoxide), withdrawal symptoms peak on the fifth to eighth day.

Diagnostic Criteria

292.0 Sedative, Hypnotic, or Anxiolytic Withdrawal

A. Cessation of (or reduction in) sedative, hypnotic, or anxiolytic use that has been heavy and prolonged.

B. Two (or more) of the following, developing within several hours to a few days after Criterion A:

    (1) autonomic hyperactivity (e.g., sweating or pulse rate greater than 100)

    (2) increased hand tremor

    (3) insomnia

    (4) nausea or vomiting

    (5) transient visual, tactile, or auditory hallucinations or illusions

    (6) psychomotor agitation

    (7) anxiety

    (8) grand mal seizures.

C. The symptoms in Criterion B cause clinically significant distress or impairment in social, occupational, or other important areas of functioning.

D. The symptoms are not due to a general medical condition and are not better accounted for by another mental disorder.

Specify if:

With Perceptual Disturbances.

Reprinted with permission from the Diagnostic and Statistical Manual of Mental Disorders, Fourth Edition, Text Revision. Copyright 2000 American Psychiatric Association.

During untreated sedative–hypnotic withdrawal, the electroencephalogram (EEG) may show paroxysmal bursts of high-voltage, low-frequency activity that precedes the development of seizures. The withdrawal delirium may include confusion, and visual and auditory hallucinations. The delirium generally follows a period of insomnia. Some individuals may have only delirium; others only seizures; and some may have both delirium and convulsions.

Studies of humans have established that large doses of chlordiazepoxide (Hollister et al. 1961) and diazepam (Hollister et al. 1963) taken for 1 month or more produce a withdrawal syndrome that is clinically similar to the withdrawal syndrome produced by high doses of barbiturates that had been previously described (Isbell 1950). Other benzodiazepines have not been studied under such precise conditions, but numerous case reports leave no doubt that they also produce a similar withdrawal syndrome when taken in excess of the upper therapeutic range.

Many people who have taken benzodiazepines in therapeutic doses for months to years can abruptly discontinue the drug without developing withdrawal symptoms. But other individuals, taking similar amounts of a benzodiazepine develop symptoms ranging from mild to severe when the benzodiapine is stopped or when the dosage is substantially reduced. Characteristically, individuals tolerate a gradual tapering of the benzodiazepine until they are at 10 to 20% of their peak dose. Further reductions in benzodiazepine dose then cause individuals to become increasingly symptomatic. In addition, in medicine literature, the low-dose withdrawal may be called therapeutic-dose withdrawal, normal-dose withdrawal, or benzodiazepine discontinuation syndrome. The symptoms can ultimately be categorized as symptom reemergence, symptom rebound, or a prolonged withdrawal syndrome.

Many individuals experience a transient increase in symptoms for 1 to 2 weeks after benzodiazepine withdrawal. The symptoms are an intensified return of the symptoms for which the benzodiazepine was prescribed. This transient form of symptoms intensification is called *symptom rebound*. The term comes from sleep research where rebound insomnia is commonly observed after sedative–hypnotic use. Symptom rebound lasts a few days to weeks after discontinuation (American Psychiatric Association Task Force on Benzodiazepine Dependency 1990). Symptom rebound is the most common withdrawal consequence of prolonged benzodiazepine use.

The symptoms for which the benzodiazepine has been taken may return to the same level as before the benzodiazepine therapy. This is called symptom reemergence (or recrudescence). In other words, the individual's symptoms, such as anxiety, insomnia, or muscle tension, that had abated during benzodiazepine treatment return.

The reason for making a distinction between symptom rebound and symptom reemergence is that symptom reemergence suggests that the original symptoms are still present and must be treated. Symptom rebound is a transient withdrawal syndrome that will disappear over time.

Some drugs or medications may facilitate neuroadaptation by increasing the affinity of benzodiazepines for their receptors. Phenobarbital, for example, increases the affinity of diazepam to benzodiazepine receptors (Skolnick et al. 1981, Olsen and Loeb-Lundberg 1981) and prior treatment with phenobarbital has been found to increase the intensity of chlordiazepoxide (45 mg/day) withdrawal symptoms (Covi et al. 1973). Individuals at increased risk for development of the low-dose withdrawal syndrome are those with a family or personal history of alcoholism, those who use alcohol daily, and those who concomitantly use other sedatives. Case-control studies suggest that individuals with a history of addiction, particularly to other sedative–hypnotics, are at high risk for low-dose benzodiazepine dependence. The short-acting, high-milligram-potency benzodiazepines appear to produce a more intense low-dose withdrawal syndrome (Rickels et al. 1990).

A few individuals experience a severe, protracted withdrawal syndrome that includes symptoms (e.g., paresthesia and psychosis) that were not present before. This withdrawal syndrome has generated much of the concern about the long-term safety of the benzodiazepines. Protracted benzodiazepine withdrawal may consist of relatively mild withdrawal symptoms such as anxiety, mood instability, and sleep disturbance similar to the protracted withdrawal syndrome described for alcohol and other drugs. In some individuals, the protracted withdrawal syndrome from benzodiazepines can be severe and disabling and lasts many months.

There is considerable controversy surrounding even the existence of this syndrome, which evolves primarily from the addiction medicine literature. Many symptoms are nonspecific and often mimic an obsessive–compulsive disorder (OCD) with psychotic features. As a practical matter, it is often difficult in the clinical setting to separate symptom reemergence from protracted withdrawal. New symptoms, such as increased sensitivity to sound, light, and touch and paresthesia, are particularly suggestive of low-dose withdrawal.

The protracted benzodiazepine withdrawal has no pathognomonic signs or symptoms, and the broad range of nonspecific symptoms produced by the protracted benzodiazepine withdrawal syndrome could also be the result of agitated depression, GAD, panic disorder, partial complex seizures, and schizophrenia. The time course of symptom resolution is the primary differentiating feature between symptoms generated by withdrawal and symptom reemergence. Symptoms from withdrawal gradually subside with continued abstinence, whereas symptom reemergence and symptom sensitization do not.

The waxing and waning of symptom intensity are characteristic of the low-dose protracted benzodiazepine withdrawal syndrome. Individuals are sometimes asymptomatic for several days, and then, without apparent reason they become acutely anxious. Often there are concomitant physiological signs (e.g., dilated pupils, increased resting heart rate, and increased blood pressure). The intense waxing and waning of symptoms are important in distinguishing low-dose withdrawal symptoms from symptom reemergence.

Assessment Issues

The individual's drug use history is usually the first source of information that is used in assessing sedative–hypnotic abuse or dependence. If the sedative–hypnotics were being used for treatment of insomnia or anxiety, the history is often best obtained as part of the history of the primary disorder and its response to treatment. A detailed history of use of all sedative–hypnotics, including alcohol, should be elicited from the individual. When framed in terms of the presenting disorder, individuals are generally more candid about their drug use and their relationship with past treating physicians.

For many reasons, individuals may minimize or exaggerate their drug use and not accurately report the behavioral consequences of their use. High doses of benzodiazepines or therapeutic doses of benzodiazepines in combination with alcohol may disrupt memory. Individuals are likely to attribute impairment of function to the underlying disorder rather than to the medication use. Observations of the individual's behavior by family members can be a source of valuable information. Whenever possible, the individual's history should be supplemented by medical records to help piece together as accurate a picture of drug use as possible. Pharmacy records may be helpful in establishing and verifying the individual's drug use history, and urine testing can be useful in verifying recent drug use history.

Individuals who obtain some or all of their medication from street sources may not know what they have been taking, as deception in the street-drug marketplace is common. For example, tablets sold as methaqualone have been found to contain phenobarbital or diazepam.

Sustained horizontal nystagmus is a reliable indicator of sedative–hypnotic intoxication. Onset of tremor, abnormal sweating, and blood pressure or pulse increase may be produced by sedative–hypnotic withdrawal.

Urine toxicology can be useful in monitoring the individual's use of drugs and in confirming a history of drug or medication use. The detection time varies widely for benzodiazepines. Diazepam or chlordiazepoxide may be detected for weeks following chronic or high-dose use, whereas others, such as alprazolam or clonazepam, may not be detectable in routine toxicology urinalysis. Because of the variability in laboratory cut-offs and detection time, and different drugs included in the screening panel, the analytical laboratory should be asked about what they routinely screen for as well as the detection limits.

Epidemiology

The prevalence of sedative–hypnotic disorders is not known with precision. Unlike most drugs of abuse (e.g., cocaine or heroin) that are manufactured in clandestine laboratories and distributed through the street-drug black markets, sedative–hypnotics are exclusively manufactured by pharmaceutical companies. Sedative–hypnotics that are used and abused by addicts are obtained either from the black market, where they have been diverted from medical channels, or from physicians and pharmacies under treatment subterfuge. Drug dependence may arise as an inadvertent consequence of medical treatment or through an individual's self-administration of sedative–hypnotics obtained from illicit sources or sequential visits to different physicians. The prevalence of abuse of a particular sedative–hypnotic is to some extent a reflection of its availability through medical channels.

The usual data sources for monitoring the prevalence of drug use in the United States, for example, the National Household Survey and the Drug Abuse Warning Network (DAWN), do not directly measure dependence on sedative–hypnotics. Furthermore, the interpretations that can be made of abuse and dependence are limited because the data are confounded by appropriate medical use.

By some indicators, tranquilizer and sedative–hypnotic use is increasing. Estimates from the 1999 National Household Survey on drug abuse show that between 1990 and 1998, the number of individuals who initiated tranquilizer use increased by 132% and the number of new sedative users increased by 90%. An estimated 1.3 million people in the United States use sedatives and tranquilizers. DAWN, which collects data on drug-related visits in hospital emergency departments, noted a 102% increase in mentions of clonazepam compared to 1992 (National Institute on Drug Abuse 2002).

Insomnia and anxiety disorders are common, and sedative–hypnotics are among the most commonly prescribed medications worldwide. Sedative–hypnotic abuse and dependence disorders are common, but involve only a small percentage of the people who use these medications. Most people do not find the subjective effects of sedative–hypnotics pleasant or appealing beyond their therapeutic effects (e.g., relief of anxiety or facilitation of sleep). Many addicts, on the other hand, have a subjectively different response to sedative–hypnotics and like the subjective effects of sedative–hypnotics (Griffiths and Roache 1985). The qualitative difference in subjective response to medications by addicts is one extremely important factor in understanding why medications that are safe and efficacious for nonaddicts cannot be safely prescribed for addicts. In addition, addicts may take doses of medications far in excess of recommended dosage, take them by injection or means other than prescribed (e.g., dissolving tablets and injecting them, crushing tablets and snorting them), or take them in combination with other prescription medications or street drugs such as heroin or cocaine that are extremely likely to produce adverse consequences.

Most individuals with sedative–hypnotic dependence are either patients whose dependence evolved during a course of medical treatment (generally with dosage escalation), or drug abusers (including alcohol) who also use sedative–hypnotics in addition to other drugs as primary intoxicants or to self-medicate adverse effects of other drugs of abuse.

Patterns of Use/Abuse

Some sedative–hypnotics, such as the short-acting barbiturates, are primary drugs of abuse—that is, they are injected for the "rush" or are taken orally to produce a state of disinhibition similar to that achieved with alcohol. Sedative hypnotics may also be taken in combination with other primary intoxicants, such as alcohol or heroin, to intensify the desired subjective effects.

Drug addicts may also use sedative–hypnotics to self-medicate withdrawal of drugs such as heroin. When the avowed intent is to stop the use of drugs such as heroin, physicians may be lured into thinking that addicts' self-administration of sedative–hypnotics is not an "abuse" but rather a reasonable approximation of medical use. While on occasion this may be the case, often it is not. Addicts' episodic attempts to stop using heroin by self-medicating opiate-withdrawal symptoms with sedative–hypnotics without entering drug abuse treatment is rarely successful, and may result in the secondary development of sedative–hypnotic dependence.

Addicts may also use sedative–hypnotics to reduce unpleasant side effects of stimulants, particularly cocaine or methamphetamine. Impairment of judgment and memory produced by the sedative–hypnotic in combination with wakefulness of a stimulant may result in unpredictable behavior.

Barbiturates
During the late 1960s and early 1970s, the short-acting barbiturates, secobarbital and pentobarbital, were common drugs of abuse. Addicts dissolved the tablets or the contents of capsules in water and injected the solution. The desired effect was the "rush," a dreamy, floaty feeling lasting a few minutes after the injection. After the rush, the addict was intoxicated, but the primary appeal to injection was the rush. The intoxication is not qualitatively different from that produced by oral ingestion of a short-acting barbiturate.

Injection of a barbiturate is associated with the usual infectious risk of injecting street drugs, but the barbiturates are particularly pernicious if inadvertently injected into an artery or if the solution is injected or leaked from a vein or artery into tissue surrounding the vessel. Barbiturates are irritating to the tissue, and the affected tissue becomes indurated and may abscess. In addition, barbiturate solution injected into an artery produces intense vasoconstriction and blockage of the arterioles, resulting in gangrene of areas supplied by the artery.

Methaqualone   Methaqualone (Quaalude) was removed from the US market in 1984 because of its abuse. Subsequently, it has continued to be sold on the street-drug black market. Some tablets sold on the black market as Quaalude contain methaqualone, apparently diverted from countries where methaqualone is still available; others contain diazepam, phenobarbital, or another sedative–hypnotic.

Benzodiazepines   Benzodiazepines are often used or misused by addicts to self-medicate opiate withdrawal, to intensify the CNS effects of methadone, or to ameliorate the adverse effects of cocaine or methamphetamine.

The benzodiazepine, flunitrazepam (Rohypnol, Narcozep), is singled out for additional discussion in this chapter on benzodiazepine abuse because of the media and legislative attention it received during the 1990s, and because it is still widely abused in Europe and other areas of the world. Flunitrazepam, a potent benzodiazepine hypnotic, was never marketed in the United States but is widely available by prescription in many other countries in 1- or 2-mg oral dosage forms and for injection.

Flunitrazepam has many street names, including rophies, ropies, roopies, roofies, ruffes, rofinol, loops, and wheels (Calhoun et al. 1996). Tablets of Rohypnol have the name of the manufacturer Roche engraved on them and a number indicating the milligram strength (either 1 or 2). Drug abusers usually prefer the 2-mg tablets, which are often called "Roche dos" or just "Roche" (usually pronounced "row-shay"). Although flunitrazepam is similar in many respects to other benzodiazepines in abuse potential (Woods and Winger 1997), flunitrazepam is among the benzodiazepines with the highest abuse potential (Farre et al. 1996, Bond et al. 1994) and has considerable appeal among heroin addicts (Thirion et al. 2002, Salvaggio et al. 2000).

In the mid-1990s, Rohypnol achieved notoriety as the "date-rape drug. Subsequently, GHB (gamma-hydroxybutyric acid), which has some properties of a sedative–hypnotic, was also called a *date-rape drug.*" Because of the media attention, considerable public debate ensued and the US Congress was prompted to pass legislation increasing penalties for rape when Rohypnol or other drugs were used to facilitate it.

Flunitrazepam and other benzodiazepines have also been associated with deaths among opiate addicts taking buprenorphine in France (Reynaud et al. 1998, Tracqui et al. 1998). Although buprenorphine alone or benzodiazepines alone are rarely fatal, the combination appears to increase the risk of overdose. Benzodiazepines and buprenorphine may have synergistic action in suppressing respiration (Gueye et al. 2002).

Zolpidem   Zolpidem (Ambien) is an imidazopyridine hypnotic, chemically unrelated to the benzodiazepines. However, it binds to a subunit of the same gamma-aminobutyric acid (GABA)–benzodiazepine complex as the benzodiazepines (Byrnes et al. 1992), and its sedative effects are reversed by the benzodiazepine antagonist flumazenil (Wesensten et al. 1995). Zolpidem has been available for prescription since 1993 in the United States and in Europe for several years before.

A few case reports of abuse suggest that some individuals increase the dosage many times above what is prescribed and that zolpidem produces a withdrawal syndrome similar to that of other sedative–hypnotics (Aragona 2000). The case histories also describe significant tolerance to the sedative effects of zolpidem.

Zolpidem is rapidly absorbed and has a short half-life (2.2 hours). Its sedative effects are additive with alcohol. Like triazolam, zolpidem decreases brain metabolism of glucose (Piercey et al. 1991).

The data concerning zolpidem's ability to produce tolerance and physical dependence have shown conflicting results. In some animal models, zolpidem does not produce tolerance or physical dependence (Perrault et al. 1992). Mice were administered zolpidem or midazolam (both 30 mg/kg) by gastric intubation for 10 days. Those treated with midazolam, but not zolpidem, showed tolerance to the drug's sedative effects and a lowered seizure threshold after the drug was stopped. Further, the benzodiazepine antagonist flumazenil precipitated withdrawal in the midazolam-treated animals but not in those treated with zolpidem.

Studies of baboons suggested that zolpidem is reinforcing and that it produces tolerance and physical dependence (Griffiths et al. 1992). In a free-choice paradigm, baboons consistently self-administered zolpidem intravenously at higher rates than either the vehicle solution alone or the triazolam. After 2 weeks of zolpidem self-administration, substitution of the vehicle solution alone resulted in suppression of food-pellet intake, which the investigators interpreted as zolpidem withdrawal. Baboons trained to discriminate oral doses of either phenobarbital (10 mg/kg) or lorazepam (1.8 mg/kg) from placebo responded to zolpidem as though it were an active drug more than 80% of the time. In another experiment, animals developed tolerance to zolpidem-induced ataxia and sedation during 7 days of drug administration. The investigators concluded that the rates of self-administration of zolpidem were similar to those of pentobarbital and higher than those maintained by 11 benzodiazepines that they had studied.

In addition to dependence, zolpidem has produced idiosyncratic psychotic reactions. A report from Belgium described two cases of transient psychosis after the first dose of 10 mg of zolpidem (Ansseau et al. 1992). Neither individual had a history of drug abuse or misuse nor were they using alcohol at the time. Both individuals experienced a transient psychosis with visual hallucinations beginning 20 to 30 minutes after 10 mg of zolpidem. Both individuals previously used benzodiazepines without difficulty and both were amnestic for the psychotic episode.

A report from Spain described a 20-year-old woman with severe anorexia who became terrified by visual hallucinations and illusions 20 minutes after taking a 10-mg dose of zolpidem (Iruela et al. 1993). She had full recall of the psychotic episode. A week later she took a 5-mg dose of zolpidem and experienced a similar episode of reduced intensity. A week later, she took 2.5 mg and again experienced visual distortions. Additional case reports of psychosis have been reported in the United States (Markowitz and Brewerton 1996, Pitner et al. 1997).

Zaleplon Zaleplon (Sonata) is a pyrazolopyrimidine approved by the Food and Drug Administration (FDA) for marketing in the United States in 1999. Like zolpidem, it is chemically unrelated to the benzodiazepines and binds to the omega-1 receptor, which is a subunit of the GABA-benzodiazepine receptor. Studies in baboons (Ator et al. 2000) and healthy volunteers with a history of drug abuse (Rush et al. 1999) suggest abuse potential similar to triazolam. Peak plasma concentration occurs about 1 hour following oral ingestion. It is rapidly metabolized with a half-life of about 1 hour. Impairment of short-term memory may occur at dosages of 10 to 20 mg.

Course

Once a diagnosis of sedative–hypnotic dependence is manifested, it is unlikely that an individual will be able to return to controlled, therapeutic use of sedative–hypnotics. All sedative–hypnotics, including alcohol, are cross-tolerant, and physical dependence and tolerance are quickly reestablished if an individual resumes use of sedative–hypnotics.

If after sedative–hypnotic withdrawal the individual has another mental disorder, such as generalized anxiety disorder (GAD), panic attacks, or insomnia, alternate treatment strategies other than sedative–hypnotics should be used if possible. Definitive diagnosis of a mental disorder during early abstinence is often not possible because protracted withdrawal symptoms may mimic anxiety disorders, and disruption of sleep architecture for days to months after drug withdrawal is extremely common.

If the sedative–hypnotic dependence has developed secondary to stimulant or alcohol use, primary treatment of the chemical dependence should be a priority. Often the symptom that was driving the sedative–hypnotic use disappears after the individual is drug-abstinent.

Differential Diagnosis

The diagnosis of sedative–hypnotic abuse and dependence is based primarily on drug use history and the DSM-IV-TR criteria of continuing behavior dysfunction caused by the drug. With dependence developing from prescribed use, the practical difficulty is determining when the dysfunction is a result of the drug use rather than the disorder for which the medication was prescribed.

Long-term use of benzodiazepines can result in physical dependence in nondrug-dependent medical patients. Withdrawal symptoms or return of symptoms suppressed by the benzodiazepines may make discontinuation difficult.

Some individuals who are physically dependent on or unable to discontinue a medication do not necessarily have a substance use disorder. Physical dependence results from neuroadaptive changes resulting from long-term exposure to a medication. Inability to discontinue the medication may simply mean that individuals are unwilling to tolerate the severity of postwithdrawal symptoms that develop. In the absence of medication-produced dysfunction, the continuation of the medication may be an appropriate choice. Individuals who do not have a substance use disorder take medications in the quantity prescribed. They follow their physicians' recommendations, and they do not mix them with drugs of abuse.

Abusers of alcohol and other drugs rarely present for primary treatment of sedative–hypnotic dependency. From the drug-abusing individual's point of view, sedative–hypnotic use is an effort to self-medicate anxiety or insomnia, which is often the result of alcohol or stimulant abuse. Despite their assertion that the medication is being taken for symptom relief, they often take the medication in larger than physician-prescribed doses, combine the medication with intoxicating amounts of alcohol or other drugs, and purchase medications from street sources. They may also use the sedative–hypnotic as an intoxicant when other drugs are not available.

There are marked class and ethnic differences in beliefs and values about the use of intoxicants and medications. The dominant culture in the United States prohibits the use of any intoxicant other than alcohol and places limits on tolerated behaviors while intoxicated (e.g., public intoxication, driving an automobile while intoxicated).

Many individuals view the distinction between medication and recreational drugs as arbitrary and pharmacologically irrational. For some, medications such as methaqualone simply extend the number of available intoxicants. A strength of the drug abuse and dependence criteria of DSM-IV-TR is that the diagnostic criteria for abuse and dependence are dysfunctional behaviors that most people would agree are pathological.

Etiology

Biological Factors

Many neurons in the CNS have receptors for the neurotransmitter gamma-aminobutyric acid (GABA). There are two main subtypes of GABA receptors: $GABA_A$, which is a ligand-gated chloride ion channel (ionophore) and $GABA_B$, which is a member of the G protein-coupled receptor family. $GABA_A$ receptors are made up of subunits. Benzodiazepines attach to receptors that are allosteric to the $GABA_A$ receptor, that is, occupancy of the benzodiazepine receptor potentiates GABA at the GABA$_A$ receptor. The molecular pharmacology of the receptor is exceedingly complex. Chronic exposure to benzodiazepines may uncouple the benzodiazepine receptor from the GABA$_A$ receptor (Wong et al. 1994, Klein et al. 1994). The uncoupling may explain in part why over time benzodiazepines appear to become less effective in controlling symptoms in some individuals, which give them an impetus to increase dosage (Lader 1994).

There is also evidence in animals that benzodiazepine receptor density is increased by stress and corticosterone and that the effects are affected by sex hormones (Wilson and Biscardi 1994).

Genetic Factors

There is considerable evidence that the propensity to develop alcohol dependence has a genetic component. In sons of alcoholics, diazepam produces significantly less effects on eye movement tasks but produces significantly greater pleasurable effects (Cowley et al. 1994). The differential response of sons of alcoholics may reflect altered functional sensitivity of the central GABA–benzodiazepine receptor system.

Treatment

Treatment of sedative–hypnotic dependence that has developed as a result of treatment of an underlying mental disorder is almost always a lengthy undertaking. The goals of the first phase of treatment are to establish the diagnosis and, to the extent possible, to delineate the comorbid psychiatric diagnoses and to establish a therapeutic relationship with the individual. The art of treatment is to know when the therapeutic alliance is sufficiently established to institute drug withdrawal, and knowing when outpatient treatment is not progressing adequately.

Somatic Treatments

Detoxification Three general strategies are used for withdrawing individuals from sedative–hypnotics, including benzodiazepines. The first is to use decreasing doses of the agent of dependence. The second is to substitute phenobarbital or some other long-acting barbiturate for the addicting agent, and gradually withdraw the substitute medication (Smith and Wesson 1970, 1971). The third, used for individuals with a dependence on both alcohol and a benzodiazepine, is to substitute a long-acting benzodiazepine, such as chlordiazepoxide, and taper it during 1 to 2 weeks.

The pharmacological rationale for phenobarbital substitution is that phenobarbital is long-acting and little change in blood levels of phenobarbital occurs between doses. This allows the safe use of a progressively smaller daily dose. Phenobarbital is safer than the shorter-acting barbiturates; lethal doses of phenobarbital are many times higher than toxic doses, and the signs of toxicity (e.g., sustained nystagmus, slurred speech, and ataxia) are easy to observe. Finally, phenobarbital intoxication usually does not produce euphoria or behavioral disinhibition, so most individuals view it as a medication, not as a drug of abuse.

The withdrawal strategy selected depends on the particular benzodiazepine, the involvement of other drugs of dependence, and the clinical setting in which the detoxification program takes place. The gradual reduction of the benzodiazepine of dependence is used primarily in medical settings for dependence arising from treatment of an underlying condition. The individual must be cooperative, must be able to adhere to dosing regimens, and must not be abusing alcohol or other drugs.

Substitution of phenobarbital can also be used to withdraw individuals who have lost control of their benzodiazepine use or who are polydrug-dependent. Phenobarbital substitution has the broadest use for all sedative–hypnotic drug dependencies and is widely used in drug treatment programs.

For high-dose benzodiazepine dependence, the pharmacological treatment strategy is the same as that for barbiturates. The phenobarbital conversion equivalents are shown in Table 26-2. The dose conversions computed using Table 26-2 prevent the emergence of severe withdrawal of the classic sedative–hypnotic type.

For treatment of protracted benzodiazepine withdrawal, the phenobarbital conversions based on Table 26-2 are not adequate to suppress symptoms. For example, someone discontinuing 20 mg of diazepam would have a computed phenobarbital conversion of 60 mg. In managing low-dose withdrawal, an approach is to begin with about 200 mg/day of phenobarbital and then taper the phenobarbital, slowly as tolerated. If palpitations or other symptoms of autonomic hyperactivity are bothersome, beta-adrenergic blockers, such as propranolol or alpha-2-adrenergic agonists, such as clonidine, may be useful adjuncts. Reports on the use of clonidine to reduce benzodiazepine withdrawal severity have yielded mixed results.

Stabilization Phase   The individual's history of drug use during the month before treatment is used to compute the stabilization dose of phenobarbital. Although many addicts exaggerate the number of pills they are taking, the individual's history is the best guide to initiating pharmacotherapy for withdrawal. Individuals who have overstated the amount of drug that they have taken will become intoxicated during the first day or two of treatment. Intoxication is easily managed by omitting one or more doses of phenobarbital and reducing the daily dose.

To compute the initial daily starting dose of phenobarbital, the individual's average daily use of each sedative–hypnotic is estimated. Next, the individual's average daily sedative–hypnotic dose for each drug is converted to its phenobarbital withdrawal equivalent by multiplying the average daily dose by the drug's phenobarbital conversion constant shown in both Tables 26-2 and 26-3. Finally, the phenobarbital withdrawal equivalences for each drug are added together. In any case, the maximum daily phenobarbital dose is limited to 500 mg/day. The total daily amount of phenobarbital is divided into three doses per day.

Table 26-2	Phenobarbital Withdrawal Equivalents of Benzodiazepines		
Generic Name	**Trade Name**	**Dose Equal to 30 mg of Phenobarbital for Withdrawal*(mg)**	**Phenobarbital Conversion Constant**
Alprazolam	Xanax	1	30
Chlordiazepoxide	Librium	25	1.2
Clonazepam	Klonopin	2	15
Clorazepate	Tranxene	7.5	4
Diazepam	Valium	10	3
Estazolam	ProSom	1	30
Flurazepam	Dalmane	15	2
Halazepam	Paxipam	40	0.75
Lorazepam	Ativan	2	15
Oxazepam	Serax	10	3
Prazepam	Centrax	10	3
Quazepam	Doral	15	2
Temazepam	Restoril	15	2
Triazolam	Halcion	0.25	120

*Phenobarbital withdrawal conversion equivalence is not the same as therapeutic-dose equivalence.

Table 26-3	Phenobarbital Withdrawal Equivalents of Nonbenzodiazepines		
Generic Name	Trade Name	Dose Equal to 30 mg of Phenobarbital for Withdrawal*(mg)	Phenobarbital Conversion Constant
Barbiturates			
Amobarbital	Amytal	100	0.33
Butabarbital	Butisol	100	0.33
Butalbital†	Fiorinal	100	0.33
Pentobarbital	Nembutal	100	0.33
Secobarbital	Seconal	100	0.33
Others			
Chloral hydrate	Noctec, Somnos	500	0.06
Ethchlorvynol	Placidyl	500	0.06
Glutethimide	Doriden	250	0.12
Meprobamate	Miltown	1200	0.025
Methyprylon	Noludar	200	0.15
Zaleplon	Sonata	10	3
Zolpidem	Ambien	5	6

*Phenobarbital withdrawal conversion equivalence is not the same as therapeutic-dose equivalence.
†Butalbital is in combination with opiate or nonopiate analgesics.

Before receiving each dose of phenobarbital, the individual is checked for signs of phenobarbital toxicity: sustained nystagmus, slurred speech, or ataxia. Of these, sustained nystagmus is the most reliable. If nystagmus is present, the scheduled dose of phenobarbital is withheld. If all three signs are present the next two doses of phenobarbital are withheld, and the daily dosage of phenobarbital for the next day is halved.

If the individual is in acute withdrawal and has had, or is in danger of having withdrawal seizures, the initial dose of phenobarbital is administered by intramuscular injection. If nystagmus and other signs of intoxication develop 1 to 2 hours after the intramuscular dose, the individual is in no immediate danger from barbiturate withdrawal. Individuals are maintained with the initial dosing schedule of phenobarbital for 2 days. If the individual has neither signs of withdrawal nor phenobarbital toxicity (slurred speech, nystagmus, unsteady gait), phenobarbital withdrawal is begun.

Withdrawal Phase Unless the individual develops signs and symptoms of phenobarbital toxicity or sedative–hypnotic withdrawal, phenobarbital is decreased by 30 mg/day. Should signs of phenobarbital toxicity develop during withdrawal, the daily phenobarbital dose is decreased by 50% and the 30-mg/day withdrawal is continued from the reduced phenobarbital dose. Should the individual have objective signs of sedative–hypnotic withdrawal, the daily dose is increased by 50% and the individual is restabilized before continuing the withdrawal.

Psychosocial Treatments

Psychotherapy in treatment of drug dependence has been much maligned; two reasons for this deserve consideration: first, some psychotherapists treat drug dependence as a symptom of an underlying disorder and use a self-medication model of drug abuse that assumes that the drug abuse will cease if the underlying causes are understood. Second, during the early recovery of individuals from drug dependence, some therapists mobilize strong affect, memories, or emotions that the individuals they are treating are unable to tolerate, and consequently, they relapse to drug abuse.

The self-medication model, even if accurate in a particular case, is not a good one because once drug abuse or dependence becomes established, the drug use takes on a life of its own regardless of the underlying reason for initiation. Rarely is treatment with insight-oriented psychotherapy successful in stopping the drug use. During early recovery, most individuals are coping with subtle withdrawal symptoms, repairing relationships, and learning to function without reliance on psychoactive drugs. Individuals with underlying mental disorders may have the additional burden of emergence of symptoms that had been ameliorated by their drug use. Psychotherapy during early recovery should be supportive and focused on coping with current life difficulties. Psychotherapists should remain vigilant for symptoms of panic attacks, generalized anxiety, depression, or sleep disturbances that interfere with current function and should initiate appropriate psychopharmacological or somatic treatments when appropriate.

Psychotherapy can, however, have an important role in motivating an individual for primary treatment of drug dependency. Therapists can help break down the individual's denial of their drug dependence by helping them see how drug use is interfering with relationships and undermining their ability to function. In some instances, it is desirable to continue the psychotherapeutic relationship while the individual is undergoing treatment for chemical dependence. With drug abusers, it is often desirable to separate the medication management from psychotherapy to prevent the psychotherapy from becoming bogged down in discussions of medications and medication side effects.

Alcoholics Anonymous, Narcotics Anonymous, and Cocaine Anonymous groups are important treatment adjuncts for many people recovering from alcohol and other forms of drug dependence. Although many groups are becoming more tolerant of appropriate use of pharmacotherapies, many individuals who attend 12-step recovery meetings are adamantly opposed to any form of psychotropic medication use and counsel fellow members to stop their use. Strong opposition to medications is usually based on their own or friends' bad experience with medications. Some individuals recover without medications and believe that recovery is of better quality if not supported by a pharmacological crutch.

Individuals with underlying mental disorders and the need for treatment with psychopharmacotherapeutic medications often require ongoing support from their psychotherapist if they must have medication.

Treatment of Individuals With Comorbid Disorders

Most individuals who are being prescribed long-term benzodiazepine therapy have underlying major depressive disorder, panic disorder, or GAD. The clinical dilemma is deciding which individuals are receiving appropriate maintenance therapy for a chronic mental disorder. Physical dependence on benzodiazepines may be acceptable if the individual's disabling anxiety symptoms are ameliorated. The reason for the individual's request for benzodiazepine withdrawal from long-term, stable dosing should be carefully explored. Valid reasons to discontinue benzodiazepine treatment include: (1) breakthrough of symptoms that were previously well controlled; (2) impairment of memory or other neurocognitive functions; and (3) abuse of alcohol, cocaine, or other medications.

Individuals with severe underlying mental disorders may have unrealistic hopes of becoming medication-free. Often the origin of request for benzodiazepine withdrawal comes from concerned friends or relatives. The individual's "problems" may be reframed as the use of "addictive medications" or "dependence" rather than the underlying psychopathology. As a practical matter, a trial of medication discontinuation may be undertaken with the understanding that return to a benzodiazepine or use of an antidepressant or other medications may be appropriate.

Many abusers of alcohol or other drugs have symptoms that would reasonably indicate treatment with benzodiazepines or other sedatives if they were not drug abusers. Treating drug abusers with benzodiazepines or other sedatives, while they are still abusing drugs, is, however, generally not helpful. Such individuals are at high risk of misusing or abusing the medications, and the medication may enable them to continue abuse of their primary drug. Drug abusers who are symptomatic because of drug toxicity need hospitalization and detoxification. In individuals with drug dependence disorders, abstinence from all abusable medications is the preferred treatment goal, particularly during the first 6 months of abstinence. In individuals who do not have a drug dependence disorder, return to benzodiazepine use after detoxification may have a different implication than among individuals with a drug dependence disorder. The term *relapse*, which is clearly pejorative, could reasonably be applied to individuals who self-administer a benzodiazepine when benzodiazepine abstinence is the agreed goal of treatment. However, the term relapse should not be applied to individuals without a substance abuse disorder who return to prescribed benzodiazepine use because emerging symptoms are not otherwise manageable.

Numerous studies have documented a high prevalence of psychopathological conditions among alcohol and drug abusers. Although the abuse of drugs can induce a psychopathological condition, and there is considerable uncertainty as to the extent to which drug abuse itself contributes to estimates of psychopathology, it is clinically apparent that some drug abusers have severe underlying psychopathological conditions that must be treated if they are to remain abstinent and functional.

Comparison of DSM-IV-TR/ICD-10 Diagnostic Criteria

The DSM-IV-TR and ICD-10 Criteria sets for Sedative, Hypnotic, or Anxiolytic Intoxication are almost equivalent (except that ICD-10 also includes "erythematous skin lesions or blisters.") The DSM-IV-TR and ICD-10 symptom lists for Sedative, Hypnotic, or Anxiolytic Withdrawal include some different items: the ICD-10 list has craving, postural hypotension, headache, malaise or weakness, and paranoid ideation and do not include the DSM-IV-TR anxiety item.

References

American Psychiatric Association Task Force on Benzodiazepine Dependency (1990) *Benzodiazepine Dependency, Toxicity, and Abuse*. American Psychiatric Press, Washington, DC.

Ansseau M, Pitchot W, Hansenne M, et al. (1992) Psychotic reactions to zolpidem (letter). *Lancet* **339**(8796), 809.

Aragona M (2000) Abuse, dependence, and epileptic seizures after zolpidem withdrawal: review and case report. *Clin Neuropharmacol* **23**(5), 281–283.

Ator NA, Weerts EM, Kaminski BJ, et al. (2000) Zaleplon and triazolam physical dependence assessed across increasing doses under a once-daily dosing regimen in baboons. *Drug Alcohol Depend* **61**(1), 69–84.

Bond A, Seijas D, Dawling S, et al. (1994) Systemic absorption and abuse liability of snorted flunitrazepam. *Addiction* **89**(7), 821–830.

Byrnes JJ, Greenblatt DJ, and Miller LG (1992) Benzodiazepine receptor binding of nonbenzodiazepines *in vivo*: Alpidem, zolpidem and zopiclone. *Brain Res Bull* **29**(6), 905–908.

Calhoun SR, Wesson DR, Galloway GP, et al. (1996) Abuse of flunitrazepam (rohypnol) and other benzodiazepines in Austin and south Texas. *J Psychoact Drugs* **28**(2), 183–189.

Covi L, Lipman RS, Pattison JH, et al. (1973) Length of treatment with anxiolytic sedatives and response to their sudden withdrawal. *Acta Psychiatr Scand* **49**, 51–64.

Cowley DS, Roy-Byrne PP, Radant A, et al. (1994) Eye movement effects of diazepam in sons of alcoholic fathers and male control subjects. *Alcohol Clin Exp Res* **18**(2), 324–332.

Farre M, Teran MT, and Cami J (1996) A comparison of the acute behavioral effects of flunitrazepam and triazolam in healthy volunteers. *Psychopharmacology (Berl)* **125**(1), 1–12.

Griffiths R and Roache J (1985) Abuse liability of benzodiazepines. A review of human studies evaluating subjective and/or reinforcing effects. In *The Benzodiazepines: Current Standards for Medical Practice*, Smith D and Wesson D (eds). MTP Press, Hingham, MA, pp. 209–225.

Griffiths RR, Sannerud CA, Ator NA, et al. (1992) Zolpidem behavioral pharmacology in baboons: self-injection, discrimination, tolerance and withdrawal. *J Pharmacol Exp Ther* **260**(3), 1199–1208.

Gueye PN, Borron SW, Risede P, et al. (2002) Buprenorphine and midazolam act in combination to depress respiration in rats. *Toxicol Sci* **65**(1), 107–114.

Hollister LE, Bennett LL, Kimbell I, et al. (1963) Diazepam in newly admitted schizophrenics. *Dis Nerv Syst* **24**(12), 746–750.

Hollister L, Motzenbecker E, and Degan R (1961) Withdrawal reactions from chlordiazepoxide (librium). *Psychopharmacologia* **2**, 63–68.

Iruela L, Ibanez-Rojo V, and Baca E (1993) Zolpidem-induced macropsia in anorexic woman (letter). *Lancet* **342**(8868), 443–444.

Isbell H (1950) Addiction to barbiturates and the barbiturate abstinence syndrome. *Ann Intern Med* **33**, 108–120.

Klein RL, Whiting PJ, and Harris RA (1994) Benzodiazepine treatment causes uncoupling of recombinant GABA$_A$ receptors expressed in stably transfected cells. *J Neurochem* **63**(6), 2349–2352.

Lader M (1994) Biological processes in benzodiazepine dependence. *Addiction* **89**(11), 1413–1418.

Markowitz JS and Brewerton TD (1996) Zolpidem-induced psychosis. *Ann Clin Psychiatry* **8**(2), 89–91.

National Institute on Drug Abuse (2002) National Institute on Drug Abuse Research Report Series (Feb 21). www.drugabuse.gov/ResearchReports/Prescription/html.

Olsen R and Loeb-Lundberg F (1981) Convulsant and anti-convulsant drug binding sites related to GABA-regulated chloride ion channels. In *GABA and Benzodiazepine Receptors*, Costa E, DiChiari G, and Gessa G (eds). The Raven Press, New York.

Perrault G, Morel E, Sanger DJ, et al. (1992) Lack of tolerance and physical dependence upon repeated treatment with the novel hypnotic zolpidem. *J Pharmacol Exp Ther* **263**(1), 298–303.

Piercey MF, Hoffmann WE, and Cooper M (1991) The hypnotics triazolam and zolpidem have identical metabolic effects throughout the brain: implications for benzodiazepine receptor subtypes. *Brain Res* **554**(1–2), 244–252.

Pitner JK, Gardner M, Neville M, et al. (1997) Zolpidem-induced psychosis in an older woman. *J Am Geriatr Soc* **45**(4), 533–534.

Reynaud M, Tracqui A, Petit G, et al. (1998) Six deaths linked to misuse of buprenorphine–benzodiazepine combinations (letter). *Am J Psychiatry* **155**(3), 448–449.

Rickels K, Schweizer E, Case WG, et al. (1990) Long-term therapeutic use of benzodiazepines. I. Effects of abrupt discontinuation. *Arch Gen Psychiatry* **47**(10), 899–907.

Rush CR, Frey JM, and Griffiths RR (1999) Zaleplon and triazolam in humans: acute behavioral effects and abuse potential. *Psychopharmacology (Berl)* **145**(1), 39–51.

Salvaggio J, Jacob C, Schmitt C, et al. (2000) Abuse of flunitrazepam in opioid addicts. *Ann Med Interne (Paris)* **151**(Suppl. A),, A6–A9.

Skolnick P, Concada V, Barker J, et al. (1981) Pentobarbital: dual action to increase brain benzodiazepine receptor affinity. *Science* **211**, 1448–1450.

Smith DE and Wesson DR (1970) A new method for treatment of barbiturate dependence. *JAMA* **213**(2), 294–295.

Smith DE and Wesson DR (1971) Phenobarbital technique for treatment of barbiturate dependence. *Arch Gen Psychiatry* **24**(1), 56–60.

Thirion X, Lapierre V, Micallef J, et al. (2002) Buprenorphine prescription by general practitioners in a French region. *Drug Alcohol Depend* **65**(2), 197–204.

Tracqui A, Kintz P, and Ludes B (1998) Buprenorphine-related deaths among drug addicts in France: a report on 20 fatalities. *J Anal Toxicol* **22**(6), 430–434.

Wesensten NJ, Balkin TJ, Davis HQ, et al. (1995) Reversal of triazolam- and zolpidem-induced memory impairment by flumazenil. *Psychopharmacology (Berl)* **121**(2), 242–249.

Wilson MA and Biscardi R (1994) Sex differences in GABA/benzodiazepine receptor changes and corticosterone release after acute stress in rats. *Exp Brain Res* **101**(2), 297–306.

Wong G, Lyon T, and Skolnick P (1994) Chronic exposure to benzodiazepine receptor ligands uncouples the gamma-aminobutyric acid type A receptor in WSS-1 cells. *Mol Pharmacol* **46**(6), 1056–1062.

Woods JH and Winger G (1997) Abuse liability of flunitrazepam. *J Clin Psychopharmacol* **17**(3 Suppl. 2),, 1S–57S.

Schizophrenia and Other Psychotic Disorders

SCHIZOPHRENIA

Diagnosis

Schizophrenia is the most severe and debilitating mental illness, and it has long been the focus of medical, scientific, and societal attention. The term schizophrenia is relatively new to our vocabulary, yet chronic psychotic illnesses have most likely been in existence throughout civilized times. The words used historically to describe psychotic symptoms included madness, folie, insanity, and dementia. They depict a constellation of symptoms that have been poorly understood and shrouded in mystery and fear. Even in the twenty-first century, the layperson's conception of schizophrenia is influenced by these early beliefs. It is only with our modern understanding of the pathophysiology and manifestations of this debilitating illness that the stigmata associated with schizophrenia can be overcome.

In DSM-IV-TR, criterion A of schizophrenia includes delusions, hallucinations, disorganized speech, disorganized or catatonic behavior, and negative symptoms (see DSM-IV-TR diagnostic criteria below). Two or more of these symptoms are required during the active phase of the illness. However, if the individual describes bizarre delusions or auditory hallucinations consisting of a voice commenting on the individual's behavior or voices conversing, only one of these symptoms is required to reach the diagnosis. It is important to distinguish negative symptoms, which are often difficult to appreciate, from the myriad factors that may contribute to the severity and serious morbidity associated with schizophrenia. Individuals who are not motivated to attend to their personal hygiene or suffer from alogia and a flattened affect are sadly at a disadvantage in society. The addition of negative symptoms as a separate criterion in DSM-IV recognizes the prominence of these symptoms in individuals with schizophrenia.

DSM-IV-TR Diagnostic Criteria

295.xx Schizophrenia

A. *Characteristic symptoms*: Two (or more) of the following, each present for a significant portion of time during a 1-month period (or less if successfully treated):

(1) delusions
(2) hallucinations
(3) disorganized speech (e.g., frequent derailment or incoherence)
(4) grossly disorganized or catatonic behavior
(5) negative symptoms, i.e., affective flattening, alogia, or avolition

Note: Only one criterion A symptom is required if delusions are bizarre or hallucinations consist of a voice keeping up a running commentary on the person's behavior or thoughts, or two or more voices conversing with each other.

B. *Social/occupational dysfunction*: For a significant portion of the time since the onset of the disturbance, one or more major areas of functioning such as work, interpersonal relations, or self-care are markedly below the level achieved prior to the onset (or when the onset is in childhood or adolescence, failure to achieve expected level of interpersonal, academic, or occupational achievement).

C. *Duration*: Continuous signs of the disturbance persist for at least 6 months. This 6-month period must include at least 1 month of symptoms (or less if successfully treated) that meet criterion A (i.e., active-phase symptoms) and may include periods of prodromal or residual symptoms. During these prodromal or residual periods, the signs of the disturbance may be manifested by only negative symptoms or two or more symptoms listed in criterion A present in an attenuated form (e.g., odd beliefs, unusual perceptual experiences).

D. *Schizoaffective and mood disorder exclusion*: Schizoaffective disorder and mood disorder with psychotic features have been ruled out because either (1) no major depressive, manic, or mixed episodes have occurred concurrently with the active-phase symptoms; or (2) if mood episodes have occurred during active-phase symptoms, their total duration has been brief relative to the duration of the active and residual periods.

E. *Substance/general medical condition exclusion*: The disturbance is not due to the direct physiological effects of a substance (e.g., a drug of abuse, a medication) or a general medical condition.

F. *Relationship to a pervasive developmental disorder*: If there is a history of autistic disorder or another pervasive developmental disorder, the additional diagnosis of schizophrenia is made only if prominent delusions or hallucinations are also present for at least a month (or less if successfully treated).

Reprinted with permission from the Diagnostic and Statistical Manual of Mental Disorders, Fourth Edition, Text Revision. Copyright 2000 American Psychiatric Association.

Criterion B addresses loss of social and occupational functioning, not exclusively because of any one of the items in criterion A. Individuals may have difficulties maintaining employment, relationships, or academic achievements. If the illness presents at an early age, rather than as a degeneration or reversal of function, there may be a break from continued academic and social gains that are developmentally appropriate so that the person never achieves what had been expected.

Criterion C eliminates individuals with less than 6 months of continued disturbance and again requires at least 1 month of the symptoms from criterion A. Criterion C allows prodromal and residual periods to include only negative symptoms or a less severely manifested version of the other symptoms of the A criteria.

Criterion D excludes individuals who have a more compelling mood aspect of their illness and therefore their symptoms might instead meet criteria for schizoaffective disorder or a mood disorder. Both of these restrictions force a narrower view of the diagnosis of schizophrenia, which lessens the tendency of clinicians to overdiagnose schizophrenia.

Criterion E clarifies the fact that individuals with schizophrenia are not suffering from other medical illnesses or the physiological effects of substances that might mimic the symptoms of schizophrenia. Finally, criterion F acknowledges that schizophrenia can be diagnosed in individuals with autistic disorder or developmental disorder, as long as there have been prominent delusions or hallucinations that have lasted at least 1 month.

In an attempt to describe schizophrenia in a way that was different from prevailing psychodynamic principles of the day, McGhie and Chapman (1961) reported that individuals with schizophrenia demonstrated profound deficits in selective attention. This idea had also been described earlier by both Kraepelin (1919) and Bleuler (1950). At present, there is a growing body of literature supporting this observation. By now, it is widely accepted that individuals with schizophrenia experience neuropsychological deficits that can be characterized by difficulties with attention, information processing, executive function, learning, and memory, which leads to a generalized performance deficit. Typically, there is a wide variance with some aspects of performance being more impaired then others. Interestingly, a small subgroup of individuals with schizophrenia have cognitive functioning within the normal range (Palmer et al. 1997). Most individuals with schizophrenia have only modest reductions in their IQs with an average of 90 (Frith et al. 1991), and about 0.67 standard deviation below that of the general population. In contrast, their performance is usually worse (Heaton et al. 1994) even in first-episode individuals (Gold et al. 1999, Riley et al. 2000). Usually, individuals with schizophrenia underperform relative to estimates of their premorbid functioning (Harvey 2001). Cognitive impairments involving verbal learning, verbal delayed recall, working memory, vigilance, and executive functioning have a significant negative impact on social and occupational functioning (Green 1996, Harvey et al. 1998). Two meta-analyses of 24 and 9 studies respectively suggest that treatment with novel antipsychotic agents improve cognitive function compared to typical antipsychotic agents (Keefe et al. 1999, Harvey 2001).

The degree of cognitive deficit appears to be more strongly associated with severity of negative symptoms, symptoms of disorganization, and adaptive dysfunction (Tollefson et al. 1997, Beasley et al. 1996) than with positive symptoms (Blin et al. 1996). Verbal fluency is severely impaired in individuals with psychotic disorders and the use of atypical antipsychotic medications results in significant improvement (Keefe et al. 1999, Velligan and Miller 1999). Motor functions (e.g., reaction time, motor and graphomotor speed) improve with clozapine, olanzapine, and risperidone (Myer-Lindenberg et al. 1997, Gallhoffer et al. 1996, Purdon et al. 2000). Olanzapine improves motor functions more than either haloperidol or risperidone (Purdon et al. 2000). Furthermore, motor functions are related to outcome, underscoring the importance of this domain. The digit symbol test has been among the most responsive tests to atypical antipsychotic treatment (Keefe et al. 1999).

In general, individuals with schizophrenia have impairments in information processing, especially when they are exposed to increasing demands on their attentional capabilities, such as under timed conditions or in stressful situations. Therefore, these deficits are not only viewed as trait linked (i.e., a manifestation of the illness itself) but may also be compounded when state linked (i.e., when there are increases in symptoms) (Sacuzzo and Braff 1981). The trait-linked disturbances in neuropsychological parameters are seen in those at high risk for developing schizophrenia, those who have schizophrenia, and relatives who appear clinically unaffected, which may indicate a genetic vulnerability (Braff 1993, Cannon et al. 1994).

Although there are generally no consistent gross deficits of memory in individuals with schizophrenia, close examination of certain aspects of learning and memory has revealed striking abnormalities. Individuals with schizophrenia have been shown to be poorer in recall of word lists if the words are not grouped into categories (Koh 1978). Furthermore, unlike normal control subjects, schizophrenic individuals do not seem to show an improvement in memory when asked to recall words with latent positive emotional meaning (Koh 1978). These findings have been attributed to poor cognitive organization in individuals with schizophrenia (Harvey et al. 1986).

Mental Status Examination in Schizophrenia

There is no specific laboratory test, neuroimaging study, or clinical presentation of an individual that yields a definitive diagnosis of schizophrenia. Schizophrenia can present with a wide variety of symptoms, and a longitudinal history of symptoms and comorbid clinical variables such as medical illness and a history of substance abuse must necessarily be reviewed before a diagnosis can be considered. The Mental Status Examination, much like the physical examination, is an additional clinical tool that aids the clinician in generating a differential diagnosis and appropriate treatment recommendations.

Appearance   Although a disheveled look is not pathognomonic for schizophrenia, individuals with this disorder often present, especially acutely, with a disordered appearance.

The description of an individual's appearance is an objective verbal sketch, much like the description of a heart murmur, that can uniquely identify a particular individual.

A person with schizophrenia often has difficulty attending to activities of daily living, either because of negative symptoms (apathy, social withdrawal, or motor retardation) or because of the presence of positive symptoms, such as psychosis, disorganization, or catatonia, that interfere with the ability to maintain personal hygiene. Also, schizophrenic individuals often present with odd or inappropriate attire, such as a coat and hat worn during the summer or dark sunglasses worn during an interview. It is generally thought that the inappropriate dress is a manifestation of symptoms such as disorganization or paranoid ideation. It should be noted that some individuals are quite neatly groomed. Thus, appearance is noted but is not diagnostic.

Attitude   Individuals with schizophrenia may be friendly and cooperative, or they may be hostile, annoyed, and defensive during an interview. The latter may be secondary to paranoid symptoms, which can make individuals quite cautious and guarded in their responses to questions.

Behavior   Schizophrenic individuals can have bizarre mannerisms or stereotyped movements that can make them look unusual. Individuals with catatonia can stay in one position for weeks, even to the point of causing serious physical damage to their body; for example, an individual who stands in one place for days may develop stress fractures, peripheral edema, and even pulmonary emboli. Individuals with catatonia may have waxy flexibility, maintaining a position after someone else has moved them into it. Individuals with catatonic excitement exhibit odd posturing or purposeless, repetitive, and often strange movements.

Behaviors seen in schizophrenic individuals include choreoathetoid movements, which may be related to neuroleptic exposure but have been reported in individuals even before neuroleptic use. Other behaviors or movement disorders may be seen as parkinsonian features, such as a shuffling gait or a pill-rolling tremor.

Psychomotor retardation may be present and may be a manifestation of catatonia or negative symptoms. On close observation, it is usually characterized, in this group of individuals, as a lack of motor movements rather than slowed movements.

Individuals may present with agitation, ranging from minimal to extreme. This agitation is often seen in the acute state and may require immediate pharmacotherapy. However, agitation may be secondary to neuroleptic medications, as in akathisia, which is felt as an internal restlessness making it difficult for the person to sit still. Akathisia can manifest itself in limb shaking, pacing, or frequent shifting of position. Severely agitated individuals may be unresponsive to verbal limits and may require measures to ensure their safety and the safety of others around them.

Eye Contact   Paranoid individuals may look hypervigilant, scanning a room or glancing suspiciously at an interviewer. Psychotic individuals may make poor eye contact, looking away, or appear to stare vacuously at the interviewer, making a conversational connection seem distant. Characteristic responding to internal stimuli is seen when a individual appears to look toward a voice or an auditory hallucination, which the individual may hear. A nystagmus may also be observed. This clinical finding has a large differential diagnosis, including Wernicke–Korsakoff syndrome; alcohol, barbiturate, or phenytoin intoxication; viral labyrinthitis; or brain stem syndromes including infarctions or multiple sclerosis (Adams and Victor 1989).

Speech   In a mental status examination, one usually comments on the rate, tone, and volume of an individual's speech, as well as any distinct dysarthrias that may be present. Pressured speech is usually thought of in conjunction with mania; however, it can be seen in schizophrenic individuals, particularly on acute presentation. This is often difficult to assess, as it may be a normal variant or a cultural phenomenon, because some languages are spoken faster than others.

Tone refers to prosody, or the natural singsong quality of speech. Negative symptoms may include a lack of prosody, resulting in monotonous speech. Furthermore, odd tones may be consistent with neurological disorders or bizarre behavior.

Speech volume is important for a number of reasons. Loud speech can be a measure of agitation, it can occur in conjunction with psychosis, or it could even be an indication of hearing loss. Speech that is soft may be an indication of guardedness or anxiety.

Dysarthrias are notable because they can be idiopathic and long-standing, or they can be an indication of neurological disturbance. In individuals who have been exposed to neuroleptics, orobuccal tardive dyskinesia should be considered when there is evidence of slurred speech.

Mood and Affect   Affect, which is the observer's objective view of the individual's emotional state, is often constricted or flat in individuals with schizophrenia. In fact, this is one of the hallmark negative symptoms. Flattened affect may also be a manifestation of pseudoparkinsonism, an extrapyramidal side effect of typical neuroleptics.

Inappropriate affect is commonly seen in individuals with more predominant positive symptoms. A smile or a laugh while relating a sad tale is an example. Individuals with catatonic excitement or hebephrenia may have bizarre presentations or affective lability, laughing and crying out of context with the situation. Emotional reactivity must alert the clinician to the possibility of neurological impairment as well, as in the case of pseudobulbar palsy (Adams and Victor 1989).

Mood is based on an individual's subjective report of how he or she feels, emotionally, at the time of the interview. It is not uncommon for individuals with schizophrenia to be depressed (especially individuals with history of higher premorbid functioning who may have some insight into the losses they are facing) or to be indifferent, with seemingly no emotional awareness of their situation.

Thought Process   Because actual thoughts cannot be measured, thought processes are assessed by extrapolation from the organization of speech. Thought disorders can be more or less obvious, and a trained listener, much like a cardiologist who listens for heart murmurs or a neurologist who detects aphasias, is one who appreciates the normal logical pattern of flow of words and ideas in speech and can thus sense abnormalities.

There are many different versions of thought disorders: lack of logical connections of ideas (looseness of associations); shift of the original theme because of weak connections of ideas (tangentiality); overinclusiveness to the point of loss of the theme (circumstantiality); use of words and phrases with no relation to grammatical rules (word salad); repetition of words spoken by others (echolalia); use of sounds of other words, such as "yellow bellow, who is this fellow?" (clang associations); use of made-up words (neologisms); and repetition of a particular word or phrase, such as "this and that, this and that" (perseveration).

Other thought disorders are part of a constellation of negative symptoms. Examples would be thoughts that appear to stop abruptly, either because of interruption by an auditory hallucination or because the thought is lost (thought blocking); absence of thoughts (paucity of thought content); and a delayed response to questions (increased latency of response).

Thought Content   Although not necessarily present in every individual, characteristic symptoms of schizophrenia include the belief that outside forces control a person's thought or actions. An individual might report that others can insert thoughts into her or his head (thought insertion), broadcast them to others (thought broadcasting), or take thoughts away (thought withdrawal). Other delusions, or fixed false beliefs, may also be prominent. Individuals may describe ideas of reference, which is the phenomenon of feeling that some external event or report relates to oneself specifically; for example, an individual may infer special meaning from an image seen on television or a broadcast heard on the radio.

Paranoid ideation may be manifested as general suspiciousness or frank, well-systematized delusions. The themes may be considered bizarre, such as feeling convinced that aliens are sending signals through wires in the individual's ear, or nonbizarre, such as being watched by the Central Intelligence Agency or believing that one's spouse is having an affair. These symptoms can be quite debilitating and lead to a great deal of personal loss, which individuals may not understand because the ideas are so real to them.

Individuals with schizophrenia commonly express an abundance of vague somatic concerns, and a particular individual might develop a delusion around a real physiological abnormality. Therefore, somatic symptoms should be evaluated appropriately in their clinical context without automatically dismissing them as psychotic. Preoccupations and obsessions are also seen commonly in this population, and certain individuals have comorbid obsessive–compulsive disorder.

The mortality rate for suicide in schizophrenia is approximately 10% (Hare 1987, Drake et al. 1985). It is therefore imperative to evaluate an individual for both suicidal and homicidal ideation. Individuals with mental disorders, and particularly those with schizophrenia, may not spontaneously articulate suicidal or homicidal ideation and must therefore be asked directly about such feelings. Moreover, psychotic individuals may feel compelled by an auditory hallucination telling them to hurt themselves.

Perceptions   Perceptual disturbances involve illusions and hallucinations. Hallucinations may be olfactory, tactile, gustatory, visual, or auditory, although hallucinations of the auditory type are more typical of schizophrenia. Hallucinations in the other sensory modalities are more commonly seen in other medical or substance-induced conditions. Auditory hallucinations can resemble sounds, background noise, or human voices. Auditory hallucinations that consist of a running dialogue between two or more voices or a commentary on the individual's behavior are typical of schizophrenia. These hallucinations are distinct from verbalized thoughts that most humans experience. They are often described as originating from outside the individual's head, as if they were emanating from the walls or the radiators in the room. Less commonly, an individual with schizophrenia describes illusions or misperceptions of a real stimulus, such as seeing demons in a shadow.

Consciousness and Orientation   One of the observations that struck Kraepelin in his first descriptions of dementia praecox was that individuals did not have clouding of consciousness. Individuals with schizophrenia most likely have a clear sensorium unless there is some comorbid medical illness or substance-related phenomenon. A schizophrenic individual may be disoriented, but this could be a result of inattentiveness to details or distraction secondary to psychotic preoccupation. In fact, there is some literature suggesting that a subgroup of individuals may present as disoriented to temporal relations such as the date or their own age (Crow 1986).

Attention and Concentration   Studies utilizing continuous performance task paradigms have demonstrated repeatedly that individuals with schizophrenia have pervasive deficits in attention in both acute and residual phases (Walker 1981, Straube and Oades 1992). On a mental status examination, these deficits may present themselves as the inability to perform mental exercises, such as spelling the word "earth" backward or serial subtractions.

Memory Careful assessment of memory in individuals with schizophrenia may yield some deficits. Acquisition of new information, immediate recall, and recent and remote memory may be impaired in some individuals. Furthermore, answers to questions regarding memory may lead to idiosyncratic responses related to delusions, thought disorder, or other overriding symptoms of the illness. In general, individuals with schizophrenia do not show gross deficits of memory such as may be seen in individuals with dementia or head trauma (Adams and Victor 1989, Straube and Oades 1992).

Fund of Knowledge Schizophrenia is not the equivalent of mental retardation, although these syndromes can coexist in some individuals. Individuals with schizophrenia generally experience a slight shift in intellectual functioning after the onset of their illness, yet they typically demonstrate a fund of knowledge consistent with their premorbid level. Schizophrenic individuals manifest a characteristic discrepancy on standardized tests of intelligence, with the nonverbal scores being lower than the verbal scores (Straube and Oades 1992). Furthermore, some reports suggest that individuals who have been chronically hospitalized or those with some cerebral atrophy may evidence diminished intellectual function (Johnstone et al. 1978).

Abstraction A classical aberration of mental function in an individual with schizophrenia involves the inability to utilize abstract reasoning, which is similar to metaphorical thinking, or the ability to conceptualize ideas beyond their literal meaning. For example, when the individual is asked what brought him or her to the hospital, a typical answer might be "an ambulance." On a mental status examination, this concrete thinking is best elicited by asking an individual to interpret a proverb or state the similarities between two objects. For example, "a rolling stone gathers no moss" may mean, to the individual with schizophrenia, that "if a stone just stays in one place, the moss won't be able to collect." More profound difficulties in abstraction and executive function, often seen in schizophrenia, such as inability to shift cognitive focus or set, may be assessed by neuropsychological tests.

Judgment and Insight Individuals suffering from schizophrenia often display a lack of insight regarding their illness. Whether it is a reflection of a negative symptom, such as apathy, or a constricted display of emotion, individuals often appear to be emotionally disconnected from their illness and may even deny that anything is wrong. Poor judgment, which is also characteristic and may be related to lack of insight, may lead to potentially dangerous behavior. For example, an individual walking barefoot in the snow because of the feeling that her or his shoes could be traced by surveillance cameras would be displaying both poor judgment and poor insight. On a formal mental status examination, judgment is commonly assessed by asking individuals what they would do if they saw a fire in a movie theater or if they saw a stamped, addressed envelope on the street. Insight can be ascertained by asking individuals about their understanding of why they are being evaluated by a mental health professional or why they are receiving a certain medication.

Physical Examination

Although there are no pathognomonic physical signs of schizophrenia, some individuals have neurological "soft" signs on physical examination. The neurological deficits include nonspecific abnormalities in reflexes, coordination (as seen in gait and finger-to-nose tests), graphesthesia (recognition of patterns marked out on the palm), and stereognosis (recognition of three-dimensional pictures). Other neurological findings include odd or awkward movements (possibly correlated with thought disorder), alterations in muscle tone, an increased blink rate, a slower habituation of the blink response to repetitive glabellar tap, and an abnormal pupillary response (Straube and Oades 1992).

The exact etiology of these abnormalities is unknown, but they have historically been associated with minimal brain dysfunction and may be more likely in individuals with poor premorbid functioning and a chronic course (Straube and Oades 1992). These neurological abnormalities have been seen in neuroleptic-naive individuals as well as those with exposure to traditional antipsychotic medication. Overall, the literature suggests that these findings may be associated with the disease itself, although further research is needed to determine the role of neuroleptic exposure in the manifestation of neurological signs and the extent to which schizophrenia is itself associated with neurological abnormalities (Johnstone and Owens 1981).

Neuroophthalmological investigations have shown that individuals with schizophrenia have abnormalities in voluntary saccadic eye movements (rapid eye movement toward a stationary object) as well as in smooth pursuit eye movements. The influence of attention and distraction, neuroleptic exposure, and the specificity of smooth pursuit eye movements for schizophrenia have raised criticisms of this area of study, and further investigation is necessary to determine its potential as a putative genetic marker for schizophrenia.

Clinical Subtypes of Schizophrenia

In DSM-IV-TR, schizophrenia has been divided into clinical subtypes on the basis of field trials of the reliability of symptom clusters. The subtypes are divided by the most prominent symptoms, although it is acknowledged that the specific subtype may exist simultaneously with or change over the course of the illness. DSM-IV-TR also includes an optional dimensional descriptor (included in the appendix for criteria sets and axes provided for further study), which allows the condition to be characterized by the presence or absence of a psychotic, disorganized, or negative symptom dimension over the entire course of the illness.

Paranoid Type In DSM-IV-TR, paranoid-type schizophrenia is marked by hallucinations or delusions in the presence of a clear sensorium and unchanged cognition (see DSM-IV-TR diagnostic criteria below). Disorganized speech, disorganized behavior, and flat or inappropriate affect are not present to any significant degree. The delusions (usually of a persecutory or grandiose nature) and the hallucinations most often revolve around a particular theme or themes. Because of their delusions, these individuals may attempt to keep the interviewer at bay, and thus they may appear hostile or angry during an interview. This type of schizophrenia may have a later age of onset and a better prognosis than the other subtypes.

DSM-IV-TR Diagnostic Criteria

295.30 Paranoid Type

A type of schizophrenia in which the following criteria are met:

A. Preoccupation with one or more delusions or frequent auditory hallucinations.

> B. None of the following is prominent: disorganized speech, disorganized or catatonic behavior, or flat or inappropriate affect.

Disorganized Type   Disorganized schizophrenia, historically referred to as hebephrenic schizophrenia, presents with the hallmark symptoms of disorganized speech and/or behavior, along with flat or inappropriate (incongruent) affect (see DSM-IV-TR diagnostic criteria below). Any delusions or hallucinations, if present, also tend to be disorganized and are not related to a single theme. Furthermore, these individuals would not be classified as having catatonic schizophrenia. These individuals in general have more severe deficits on neuropsychological tests. According to DSM-IV-TR, these individuals tend to have an earlier age at onset, an unremitting course, and a poor prognosis.

DSM-IV-TR Diagnostic Criteria

295.10 Disorganized Type

A type of schizophrenia in which the following criteria are met:

A. All of the following are prominent:

   (1) disorganized speech
   (2) disorganized behavior
   (3) flat or inappropriate affect

B. The criteria are not met for catatonic type.

Catatonic Type   Catatonic schizophrenia has unique features that distinguish it from the other subtypes of schizophrenia (see DSM-IV-TR diagnostic criteria on page 649). During the acute phase of this illness, individuals may demonstrate marked negativism or mutism, profound psychomotor retardation or severe psychomotor agitation, echolalia (repetition of words or phrases in a nonsensical manner), echopraxia (mimicking the behaviors of others), or bizarreness of voluntary movements and mannerisms. Some individuals demonstrate a waxy flexibility, which is seen when a limb is repositioned on examination and remains in that position as if the individual were made of wax. Individuals with catatonic stupor must be protected against bodily harm resulting from the profound psychomotor retardation. They may remain in the same position for weeks at a time. Because of extreme mutism or agitation, individuals may not be able to report any difficulties. Some individuals may experience extreme psychomotor agitation, with grimacing and bizarre postures. These individuals may require careful monitoring to safeguard them from injury or deterioration in nutritional status or fluid balance.

▬ DSM-IV-TR Diagnostic Criteria

295.20 Catatonic Type

A type of schizophrenia in which the clinical picture is dominated by at least two of the following:

A. motoric immobility as evidenced by catalepsy (including waxy flexibility) or stupor
B. excessive motor activity (that is apparently purposeless and not influenced by external stimuli)
C. extreme negativism (an apparently motiveless resistance to all instructions or maintenance of a rigid posture against attempts to be moved) or mutism
D. peculiarities of voluntary movement as evidenced by posturing (voluntary assumption of inappropriate or bizarre postures), stereotyped movements, prominent mannerisms, or prominent grimacing
E. echolalia or echopraxia

Reprinted with permission from the Diagnostic and Statistical Manual of Mental Disorders, Fourth Edition, Text Revision. Copyright 2000 American Psychiatric Association.

Undifferentiated Type   There is no hallmark symptom of undifferentiated schizophrenia; thus, it is the subtype that meets the criterion A for schizophrenia but does not fit the profile for paranoid, disorganized, or catatonic schizophrenia (see DSM-IV-TR diagnostic criteria below).

▬ DSM-IV-TR Diagnostic Criteria

295.90 Undifferentiated Type

A type of schizophrenia in which symptoms that meet criterion A are present, but the criteria are not met for the paranoid, disorganized, or catatonic type.

Reprinted with permission from the Diagnostic and Statistical Manual of Mental Disorders, Fourth Edition, Text Revision. Copyright 2000 American Psychiatric Association.

Residual Type   The diagnosis of residual schizophrenia, according to DSM-IV-TR, is appropriately used when there is a past history of an acute episode of schizophrenia but at the time of presentation, the individual does not manifest any of the associated psychotic or positive symptoms (see DSM-IV-TR diagnostic criteria on page 650). However, there is continued evidence of schizophrenia manifested in either negative symptoms or low-grade symptoms of criterion A. These may include odd behavior, some abnormalities of thought processes, or delusions or hallucinations that exist in a minimal form. This type of schizophrenia has an unpredictable, variable course.

DSM-IV-TR Diagnostic Criteria

295.60 Residual Type

A type of schizophrenia in which the following criteria are met:

A. Absence of prominent delusions, hallucinations, disorganized speech, and grossly disorganized or catatonic behavior.
B. There is continuing evidence of the disturbance, as indicated by the presence of negative symptoms or two or more symptoms listed in criterion A for schizophrenia, present in an attenuated form (e.g., odd beliefs, unusual perceptual experiences).

Reprinted with permission from the Diagnostic and Statistical Manual of Mental Disorders, Fourth Edition, Text Revision. Copyright 2000 American Psychiatric Association.

Other Subgroupings of Schizophrenia

The idea that schizophrenia can be divided into subgroups has been explored since the illness was first described. Attempts to subdivide schizophrenia have been based on multiple factors including symptom patterns, as in paranoid versus nonparanoid or reactive versus process schizophrenia, or outcome, such as the good versus poor prognosis subtypes. Biological and clinical factors, including platelet monoamine oxidase activity, amphetamine induction of psychosis, neurological soft signs, and perinatal complications, have also been considered in subgrouping this complex illness, although these classifications have generally not withstood the test of time as valid means of subdividing schizophrenia.

Positive and Negative Symptoms   There has been an emphasis on positive and negative symptom clusters in some individuals with schizophrenia. Positive and negative symptoms were first described by Sir John Russell Reynolds, a British neurologist who had worked with epileptic individuals. In 1857, in a presentation to a division of the London Medical Society, he proposed that physical signs could manifest themselves in positive and negative forms (Berrios 1985). The prominent neurologist Hughlings-Jackson (Jackson 1987) expanded on Reynolds' statement by positing that negative symptoms could be thought of in terms of an upper motor neuron deficit that leads to the lower motor neuron hyperactivity, which he identified as a positive symptom. By definition, then, both negative and positive symptoms would be found in the same individual and there would be a causative relationship between them. In the psychiatric literature, positive symptoms have come to mean those that are actively expressed, such as hallucinations, thought disorder, delusions, and bizarre behavior, whereas negative symptoms reflect deficit states such as avolition, flattened affect, and alogia.

How these distinct symptom patterns are related in schizophrenia remains unresolved. Bleuler had conceptualized fundamental and accessory symptoms, and Schneider had divided symptoms into those of first and second rank, but neither specifically addressed positive and negative symptom subdivisions. Strauss and colleagues (1974) considered positive and negative symptoms as distinct symptom patterns associated with clinical course over time, with negative symptoms being more associated with poor long-term outcome. Subsequent hypotheses considered positive and negative symptoms to be either two end points of a spectrum of symptoms or a single disease process in which either the positive or negative symptoms are primary and the other symptoms become a secondary response.

That schizophrenia could be divided into a two-syndrome concept was put forth by Crow (1980) of the Clinical Research Center at Northwick Park Hospital in England. According to his theory, individuals with type I schizophrenia are those who present, often more acutely, with a predominantly positive symptom profile and who have a good response to neuroleptics. In contrast, individuals with type II schizophrenia are those who have a more chronic illness, more frequent evidence of intellectual impairment, enlarged ventricular size, and cortical atrophy as seen on CT or MRI scans, a poorer response to neuroleptics, and predominantly negative symptoms. Crow further postulated that type I schizophrenia may be secondary to a hyperdopaminergic state, whereas type II disease may be due to structural abnormality of the brain.

The idea that positive and negative symptoms may be overlapping end points along a single continuum of biological and clinical manifestations has been described by Andreasen and colleagues (1982). In their study of 52 schizophrenic individuals, they found that negative symptoms correlated with the presence of ventricular enlargement and that individuals with small ventricles were more likely to manifest positive symptoms. In a separate report, Andreasen and Olsen (1982) posited that negative and positive symptoms reflect opposite extremes of a spectrum and that a mixed symptom pattern can exist and may be present 30% of the time. Others have suggested that although the positive and negative characteristics may be part of a continuum, they may not be related to the presence or absence of structural brain abnormalities; rather, there may be a relationship between the symptom pattern and outcome, depending on the clinical course.

A categorical scheme for differentiation of so-called primary and secondary negative symptoms was developed by Carpenter and colleagues (1985). This distinction is based in part on the fact that negative symptoms are not pathognomonic of schizophrenia. The negative symptoms that can be seen in a number of other illnesses, including depression and medical illness, and as a result of positive symptoms themselves or the side effects of medication, particularly extrapyramidal symptoms (EPS), are considered "secondary." The negative symptoms that are a core element of schizophrenia are deemed "primary" or "deficit" symptoms. This distinction enables further exploration of outcome variables and the heterogeneity of this illness and in many ways aids treatment decisions.

Because positive and negative symptoms may be seen differently by individual clinicians, valid psychometric scales have become important clinical and research tools. The Brief Psychiatric Rating Scale (BPRS) (Overall and Gorham 1961), for example, includes subscales for positive and negative symptoms, as does the Positive and Negative Syndrome Scale (PANSS) for schizophrenia (Kay et al. 1988). Others have more broadly defined negative symptoms. Crow (1985) proposed the use of a narrow definition, that is, flattened affect and poverty of speech, for negative symptoms, and Andreasen (1981) supported a broader definition in the widely used Scale for the Assessment of Negative Symptoms (SANS). This psychometric scale includes categories of alogia and flattened affect as well as items such as anhedonia, asociality, avolition, apathy, and deficits in attention.

Subgroupings Based on Symptom Cluster Analysis

Although the dichotomous positive–negative distinction has gained clinical and research recognition, several reports suggest that this division is incomplete. Much of the current interest in understanding the heterogeneity of schizophrenia has involved a more detailed look at the symptoms of schizophrenia. Sophisticated statistical techniques utilize factor analysis to reduce data to elucidate clusters of symptoms that are most likely to group together or be found independently.

An application of this approach found that there are three, rather than two, symptom dimensions that better subdivide schizophrenia. Correlational relationships between symptoms reveal that positive symptoms can be divided into two distinct groups. The first includes psychotic symptoms such as hallucinations and delusions, and the second includes symptoms of disorganization, consisting of thought disorder, bizarre behavior, and inappropriate affect. A third group is that of negative symptoms. Although these patterns of symptoms may be seen in different proportions in individuals and may change over time, they can be shown to have distinct clinical courses and may be related to independent neuropsychological deficits in a given individual (Andreasen et al. 1995).

In a 2-year follow-up study of these different symptom patterns, negative symptoms were found to remain stable and the other two dimensions were found to have a more fluctuating pattern (Arndt et al. 1995). This study found that the three symptom dimensions changed independently.

An earlier report supporting three distinct symptom dimensions came from a study of neuropsychological and neurological findings in relation to schizophrenic symptoms (Liddle 1987). In this study, individuals with a predominantly negative symptom dimension were shown to have cognitive deficits related to the frontal lobe, as were individuals with thought disorder and inappropriate affect, but the specific deficits appeared to be related to different regions of the frontal lobe. Furthermore, individuals who presented primarily with delusions and hallucinations appeared to have neuropsychological deficits associated with the temporal lobe.

Further investigation is warranted to understand the role of these three symptom dimensions in the onset, course, and treatment of schizophrenia. In addition, this factor analytical division of schizophrenic symptoms must be evaluated to understand their relationship to genetic and neurochemical mechanisms.

Late-Onset Schizophrenia   The phenomenology of late-onset compared with early-onset schizophrenia may be distinct, with later-onset cases having a higher level of premorbid social functioning and exhibiting paranoid delusions and hallucinations more often than formal thought disorder, disorganization, and negative symptoms (Howard et al. 1994, Almeida et al. 1995, Jeste et al. 1995). Studies have also shown a high comorbid risk of sensory deficits, such as loss of hearing or vision, in individuals with late-onset schizophrenia (Pearlson et al. 1989). Specifically, late-onset individuals are more likely to report visual, tactile, and olfactory hallucinations and are less likely to display affective flattening or blunting (Jeste et al. 1995, Howard et al. 2000). For individuals over the age of 65, community prevalence estimates range from 0.1 to 0.5% (Copeland et al. 1998, Castle and Murray 1993). One of the most robust finding among the late-onset cases is the higher prevalence seen in women (Howard et al. 1994, Almeida et al. 1995, Castle and Murray 1993, Howard et al. 2000). This does not appear to be due to sex differences in seeking care, societal role expectations (Hambrecht et al. 1992), or delay between emergence of symptoms and service contact (Riecher et al. 1989). The International Late-onset Schizophrenia group has suggested a new classification system of *late-onset schizophrenia* (onset after the age of 40 years) and a *very late-onset schizophrenia-like psychosis* (onset after age 60) (Howard et al. 2000). Future studies will clarify how meaningful these categories are.

Epidemiology

Three major studies conducted by the World Health Organization (WHO) have provided clinicians and researchers with invaluable information regarding the epidemiology of schizophrenia. By utilizing consistent diagnostic criteria, having large sample sizes across several countries of diverse cultures and development, and including follow-up data, the WHO has collected a significant data set from which we can derive epidemiological information.

The first of these studies is known as the International Pilot Study of Schizophrenia and was conducted from 1969 to 1977. This study assessed 1202 individuals across nine countries (Taiwan, Colombia, Czechoslovakia, Denmark, India, Nigeria, UK, US, and former USSR) utilizing Wing's Present State Examination, which was translated and back-translated to ensure consistency in diagnostic assessment across languages. A second major study, the Assessment and Reduction of Psychiatric Disability, examined social adjustment in 520 individuals with schizophrenia in seven countries: Bulgaria, Federal Republic of Germany, Netherlands, Sudan, Switzerland, Turkey, and Yugoslavia. From 1978 to 1986, the Determinants of Outcome of Severe Mental Disorders studied 1379 individuals in 10 countries who had sought help for mental illness and were diagnosed with probable schizophrenia (Jablensky et al. 1988). All 3 of these studies included long-term follow-up with assessments of the initial cohort for a period of up to 10 years. Although these studies were conducted with large sample sizes in different cultural settings, the methodology was consistent, with diagnostic assessments made by trained professionals, enhancing the reliability and validity of the conclusions.

One of the most comprehensive epidemiological undertaking in the United States to date, the Epidemiological Catchment Area (ECA) program, was planned as a result of a need for comprehensive data that would answer questions regarding the prevalence of mental disorders that could be utilized to implement services for those in need. Funded by the National Institute of Mental Health, the ECA program began in 1978 as a multisite program designed primarily to determine accurate prevalence rates of specific mental illnesses (Robins et al. 1984). Structured diagnostic interviews were administered to a population of almost 20,000 people residing in designated areas, and the corresponding DSM-III diagnoses were registered in a central data set.

Incidence   The incidence of schizophrenia is defined as the number of new cases in a given population, usually per 1000 persons, during a specific period of time (1 year by convention). In an illness with an insidious onset, such as schizophrenia, accurate incidence rates can be difficult to determine. Incidence rates are often calculated from first hospital admission data, which may not correspond to the time when the illness first presented. Incidence rates can also be calculated from retrospective interviews or chart reviews, which may misrepresent accurate incidence rates because of imperfect charting, unreliable historical information given by individuals and their families, and nonvalidated retrospective diagnoses. In any case, the incidence varies depending on the methods and the diagnostic criteria used. For example, the US–UK study is often cited as an example of epidemiological variation based on different diagnostic criteria (Kramer 1969). This study, conducted in the 1960s, found a lower incidence of schizophrenia in the United Kingdom than in the United States. It is now widely accepted that this difference was found because a broader definition of schizophrenia was being used in the United States, and it did not reflect true differences in the incidence of schizophrenia in each country.

The data obtained from the WHO studies are important in part because the same diagnostic criteria were used in all countries studied. According to the results of the International Pilot Study of Schizophrenia, schizophrenia is found in all cultures and the incidence rates per 1000 people annually ranged from 0.15 in Denmark to 0.42 in India (World Health Organization 1973). This finding is corroborated by a review of the literature, in which the incidence of schizophrenia across 13 studies representing seven countries is found to range between 0.11 (UK) and 0.54 (US) per 1000 people per year (Eaton 1985). Small variations in these incidence rates, because they are so low, have little meaning epidemiologically. Furthermore, the range of incidence rates for schizophrenia decreases significantly when consistent, tightly defined diagnostic criteria are employed. It is reassuring that when investigators replicated studies using the design of the WHO 10-country study, results similar to the original study were reported from India (Rajkumar et al. 1993), the United Kingdom (McNaught et al. 1997, Brewin et al. 1997), and Barbados (Hickling and Rodgers-Johnson 1995, Mahy et al. 1999).

Because schizophrenia is a chronic illness, the incidence rates must, by definition, be much lower than the prevalence rates. Prevalence is defined as the number of cases present in a specified population at a given time or time interval (e.g., at a specific point in time, during a time period, or over a lifetime). Lifetime prevalence represents the proportion of persons who have ever had the illness at a given time.

Prevalence Lifetime prevalence rates of schizophrenia, based on the ECA data, were approximately 1% (range across three sites, 1–1.9%) (Robins et al. 1984). Point prevalence rates based on International Pilot Study of Schizophrenia data showed no significant differences across study centers: schizophrenia was found universally with relatively equal frequencies in a wide variety of cultures. Eaton's review of the literature showed a range of point prevalence between 0.6 and 8.3 cases of schizophrenia per 1000 persons in the population. The rate of schizophrenia per 1000 persons fell within a similar range when looking at lifetime prevalence, point prevalence and period prevalence, which Eaton hypothesized was related to the fact that schizophrenia is a chronic but not fatal illness (Eaton 1985). In an update of Eaton's review, it was noted that methodological differences may have partly accounted for statistical outliers in studies examining the incidence and prevalence of schizophrenia in different countries regardless of the type of prevalence (Eaton 1991). Specific studies of smaller populations, such as Helgason's study of Iceland, found a 0.9% morbidity risk (which approximates point prevalence rates) of schizophrenia (Helgason 1964). This study has been highlighted because it examined 99% of individuals in a closed population and supports the findings of the larger studies such as the ECA study.

Interestingly, smaller studies have found specific populations with either a higher or a lower prevalence of schizophrenia (Jablensky 1986, Hare 1987, Hovatta 1997). For example, a higher rate of schizophrenia has been found in a specific community in the north of Sweden, in northeastern Finland (Lehtinen 1996), in northwestern Croatia, and in western Ireland. Lower rates of schizophrenia have been found in, for example, parts of Tonga, Papua New Guinea, Taiwan, and Micronesia. In the United States, schizophrenia was almost nonexistent in the Hutterite community, a Protestant sect living in South Dakota. Epidemiologists generally agree that these communities may represent aberrant findings. However, if these differences in prevalence rates are accurate, several theories have been offered as explanations, including genetic preloading, differences in diet, or even differences in factors such as maternal age (Hare 1987). A suggestion has been raised that there might a decline in the incidence of schizophrenia (Bojholm and Stromgren 1989) but the evidence so far is inconsistent and conflicting (Jeffreys et al. 1997, Brewin et al. 1997). This issue awaits further clarification.

Age at onset An investigation of late-onset schizophrenia found that 28% of individuals had the onset of illness after age 44 years and 12% after age 63 years, based on 470 chart reviews of individuals who had sought psychiatric help during a period of 20 years (Castle and Murray 1993). Other studies have demonstrated that 23% of schizophrenic individuals had an onset after their forties (Lacro et al. 1993). The 1-year prevalence rate for schizophrenia in individuals between 45 and 64 years of age was found to be 0.6% according to the ECA study (Keith et al. 1991). Furthermore, in a study of individuals with onset after the age of 44 years, the majority of individuals had symptoms that met all the criteria for schizophrenia found in DSM-III except for the age requirement, lending support to the need to discard the maximal age at onset limitation of DSM-III (Rabins et al. 1984). Thus, although the majority of individuals have an early age at onset, a certain subgroup of individuals may have a disturbance that meets all the criteria of schizophrenia with onset in their forties or later.

Sex Differences   A large body of data suggests that although men and women have an equivalent lifetime risk, the age at onset varies with sex. Although some sites showed different prevalence rates of schizophrenia in men and women, the overall prevalence rates, as reported in the ECA survey, did not differ significantly between sexes (Bourdon et al. 1992). However, there is strong evidence that onset of schizophrenia is on average 3.5 to 6 years earlier in men than in women (Flor-Henry 1985, Hafner 2000, Riecher-Rossler and Hafner 2000). The WHO 10-country study observed this phenomenon in most cultures studied (Jablensky et al. 1992). Therefore, incidence and prevalence rates of schizophrenia across sexes may vary according to age. Interestingly, in some cultural populations (e.g., West Ireland, Micronesia), the ratio of prevalence of schizophrenia for men could be as high as 2 : 1 (Kendler and Walsh 1995, Myles-Worsley et al. 1999).

Many studies have used criteria for schizophrenia that require onset before the age of 45 years, which also has accounted for some of the discrepancy in findings. There is undoubtedly a subgroup of individuals who have a later onset of illness (after age 45 years), and this subgroup is made up predominantly of women (Flor-Henry 1985, Loranger 1984, Howard 2000, Almeida et al. 1995). Among these female schizophrenic individuals, there is a higher incidence of comorbid affective symptoms (Flor-Henry 1985, Loranger 1984). When the effects of gender, premorbid personality, marital status, and family history of psychosis on the age at onset were removed in a reanalysis of WHO 10-country study data, there was a significant attenuation of the sex differences (Jablensky and Cole 1997).

Race and Ethnicity   The ECA data have shown that there is no significant difference in the prevalence of schizophrenia between black and white persons when corrected for age, sex, socioeconomic status, and marital status (Robins and Regier 1991). This finding is significant because it refutes prior studies that have shown the prevalence of schizophrenia to be much greater in the black population than in the white population. Adebimpe (1994) proposed several factors, including racial differences in help-seeking behavior, research populations, commitment status, and treatment, as explanations for some of these discrepancies. Efforts are being made to correct for some of these issues so that the epidemiological variables and heterogeneity of schizophrenia can be better understood in terms of race, whether black, white, Asian, or any other.

Marriage and Fertility Rates   A study of marriage and fertility rates of individuals with schizophrenia compared with the general population showed that on average, by the age of 45 years, three times as many of those with schizophrenia as of the general population are still unmarried (40% of men and 30% of women with schizophrenia are still single by age 45) (Slater et al. 1971). Studies have also shown that fertility rates are lower in individuals with schizophrenia compared with the general population (Vogel 1979). These observations may be related, and further investigation of the role of premorbid function, negative symptoms, and fertility rates, including rates among unmarried individuals, is warranted. With the advent of the newer and more effective antipsychotic medications, and their increased use in first-episode individuals, it is possible that we may witness improved fertility and marriage rates in individuals with schizophrenia.

Socioeconomic Status   For many years, epidemiological studies revealed a higher incidence and prevalence of schizophrenia in groups with lower socioeconomic status (Mishler and Scotch 1963). With these findings came the hypothesis that lower social class could be considered a plausible risk factor for schizophrenia, possibly because of a higher risk of obstetrical complications, poorer nutrition, increased exposure to environmental toxins or infectious disease, or exposure to greater life stressors. In the past half century, studies have found that the actual incidence of schizophrenia does not vary with social class, based on first admission rates, adoption studies, and a series of studies examining the social class of the fathers of people with schizophrenia (Goldberg and Morrison 1963, Noreik and Odegard 1967).

When these findings did not validate the original theory, it became clear that lower socioeconomic status was more a result than a cause of schizophrenia. This led to the acceptance of the downward drift hypothesis, which stated that because of the nature of schizophrenic symptoms, people who develop schizophrenia are unable to attain employment and positions in society that would allow them to achieve a higher social status (Myerson 1940). Thus, these individuals drift down the socioeconomic ladder, and because of the illness itself they may become dependent on society for their well-being.

Immigration   Epidemiological studies of immigrant populations in the early part of the twentieth century led to the supposition that the stress of immigration increased the risk for psychosis (Odegard 1932). However, further investigations of acculturation as a risk factor for schizophrenia have yielded mixed results (Eaton 1985). The opposite idea, that having a mental illness increased the likelihood of emigrating, has also been reviewed (Hare 1987, Eaton 1985). At this time, there is no conclusive evidence that emigration increases the risk of schizophrenia. Furthermore, immigration screening has become more rigorous since the earlier studies, and legal immigrants may therefore be less likely to have an increased risk for developing schizophrenia (Rosenthal et al. 1974).

The remarkably high incidence and prevalence rates of schizophrenia observed in second-generation Afro-Caribbean, and Suriname and Dutch Antilles migrants to the United Kingdom and Netherlands respectively are baffling. These findings have been replicated and data from 17 studies show a wide range of relative risk from 1.7 to 13.2 (Eaton and Harrison 2000). Diagnostic bias, misclassification (Sharpley et al. 2001), or biological risk factors (Hutchinson 1997, Selten et al. 1998) do not account for these findings. Thus, environmental risk factor(s), currently unknown, have been proposed to underlie this phenomenon. The relationship between migration and schizophrenia is complex and needs further clarification (Bhugra 2000).

Industrialization   With the increasing presence of the mentally ill on the streets of modern urban locations, the question has often been raised of whether urban life, or industrialized society, is a risk factor for the development of schizophrenia. In fact, there seems to be data suggesting that people in urban areas have a higher relative risk for schizophrenia than those in rural areas (Torrey 1980, Eaton 1974, Mortensen et al. 1999, Allardyce et al. 2001). Torrey and colleagues (1997) reanalyzed the US 1880 census data and found that urban residence was associated with a higher risk for psychosis. Marcelis and colleagues (1998) analyzed all first admissions for schizophrenia and other psychosis in Holland between 1942 and 1978 by place of birth and found a statistically significant relationship between size of urban areas and incidence of schizophrenia, affective, and other psychosis. Furthermore, in the WHO follow-up studies of the International Pilot Study of Schizophrenia, there was a significant difference in the course of schizophrenia between industrialized and developing nations, with individuals with schizophrenia in developing countries having a less severe and less chronic course of the illness (World Health Organization 1979, Waxler 1979).

Various explanations for these discrepancies have been postulated (Cooper and Sartorius 1977). For example, in industrialized areas the family structure may impose more social stresses on the ill relative, who is often unable to work and perform by society's standards, whereas in developing countries the family structure may be protective, with other relatives supporting the ill relative. Another possible explanation is a selection factor in developing countries resulting from the higher infant mortality in nonindustrialized societies. According to this hypothesis, children in less-developed countries who would be at risk for schizophrenia would not be as likely to survive, thus skewing the prevalence rates of schizophrenia in these areas (Cooper and Sartorius 1977). However, some suggest that this risk factor of increased incidence of psychosis in urban areas is more ecological then genetic (Jablensky 2000). Further investigation is needed to provide definitive answers as to why schizophrenia may have a higher prevalence and more severe course in industrialized nations.

Season of Birth and Onset
That season of birth differs between individuals with schizophrenia and the general population has by now gained wide acceptance. This factor has been studied in the twentieth century, with the predominant view that the birth rate of people with schizophrenia is highest in late winter (Jablensky 1986, Hare 1987, Eaton 1985). Torrey and colleagues (1997) confirmed this, reviewing approximately 250 studies and concluding that there is an excess of schizophrenia births during winter. In fact, there is approximately a 5 to 8% greater likelihood for individuals with schizophrenia to be born during winter months compared with the general population. This higher incidence of winter births has been found in both hemispheres, offering further evidence that this phenomenon is related to the colder months rather than specific calendar months.

It is clear that even though only a small proportion of all those with schizophrenia are born during winter months, the deviation from the seasonality of birth of the general population (the number of general births peaks in the spring) is a striking phenomenon. This finding is not unique to schizophrenia, and differences in seasonality of birth have been described for mania (Hare 1983), diabetes mellitus (Christy et al. 1982), Down syndrome, congenital hip dislocation, and certain cardiovascular malformations (Jongbloet et al. 1982). It is therefore debatable whether this observation has etiological significance unique to schizophrenia.

Season of onset has also been considered in epidemiological investigations of schizophrenia. A preponderance of data dating back to the early 1800s indicates that the summer season is associated with a higher incidence of the onset of symptoms. Suicide rates also vary according to season, with a spring peak, indicating that the interaction of environment and psychopathology may be of some significance (Silverman 1968).

Course
The most influential model for the long-term course of schizophrenia was proposed by Kraepelin. Inherent in the term *dementia praecox* was the view that the course of this illness was similar to that of the dementias in that they were progressive with worsening over time. This downhill trajectory had profound clinical and research implications throughout the century. For example, if individuals with schizophrenia recovered or even had a prolonged remission, it was generally considered that they had been erroneously diagnosed. Indeed, even in DSM-III, individuals with schizophrenia were described as rarely recovering. Moreover, pathophysiological theories were influenced by this model in that disease processes that were progressive were given strong consideration.

The Kraepelinian model for this illness went essentially unchallenged for more than 50 years until well-designed epidemiological studies of schizophrenia were conducted. In long-term follow-up studies of 20 years or more, surprisingly favorable outcomes were observed: between 40 and 66% of individuals had either recovered or were only mildly impaired at follow-up (Table 27-1). In the Vermont Longitudinal Study of Schizophrenia (Harding et al. 1987a,b), 269 backward individuals who were chronically institutionalized

Table 27-1	Long-Term Follow-up Studies of Schizophrenia			
Study	Location	Length of Follow-up (mean, year)	Sample Size (*N*)	Recovered or Significantly Improved (%)
DeSisto et al. (1992)	Maine	36	117	45
Harding et al. (1987a)	Vermont	32	82	67
Tsuang et al. (1979)	Iowa	35	186	46
Huber et al. (1982)	Bonn	22	502	57
Ciompi et al. (1982)	Lausanne	37	289	53
Bleuler (1987)	Zurich	23	208	53

in the 1950s were followed up an average of 32 years later. The individuals who met rigorously applied retrospective DSM-III diagnostic criteria for schizophrenia ($N = 118$) during their index admission in the 1950s were found on follow-up to have outcomes that varied widely; 82% were not hospitalized in the year of the follow-up, 68% displayed slight or no symptoms, 81% were able to meet their own basic needs, and more than 60% had good social functioning. Thus, these data indicate that the long-term outcome of schizophrenia is heterogeneous, with substantially larger numbers of individuals having better outcomes than would have been predicted by the Kraepelinian model.

On the basis of current epidemiological data, a new model of the natural course of schizophrenia has been proposed (Breier et al. 1991). This model has three phases: an early phase marked by deterioration from premorbid levels of functioning; a middle phase characterized by a prolonged period of little change termed the stabilization phase; and the last period, which incorporates the long-term outcome data just cited, which is called the improving phase.

An enormous clinical and research effort is directed internationally toward individuals in very early stages of their illness and especially during their first psychotic break with a focus on early and effective intervention. First episode provides a unique opportunity to intervene early and effectively and possibly change the course of illness. It is well known that there is a delay of 1 to 2 years on an average between onset of psychosis and starting of treatment (Lieberman and Fenton 2000). This duration of untreated psychosis (DUP) is recognized by many, though not all, as an important indicator of subsequent clinical outcome (Norman 2001, Larsen et al. 2000). Larsen and colleagues (2000) examined 1-year outcome in 43 first-episode individuals and at 1-year follow-up, 56% were in remission, 26% were still psychotic, and 18% suffered multiple relapses. Both longer DUP and poor premorbid functioning predicted more negative symptoms and poor global functioning. DUP remained a strong predictor of outcome even after controlling for premorbid functioning. Clinical deterioration appears to be correlated with the duration of psychosis and number of episodes of psychosis (Wyatt 1991). The deterioration usually occurs during the first 5 years after onset and then stabilizes at a level where the individual has persistent symptoms and is impaired in social and vocational function. After that point, additional exacerbation may occur, but they are not usually associated with further deterioration (Lieberman 1999a).

Long-term studies of schizophrenia suggest that negative symptoms tend to be less common and less severe in the early stages of the illness but increase in prevalence and severity in the later stages. Positive symptoms such as delusions and hallucinations are more common earlier on while thought disorganization, inappropriate affect, and motor symptoms occur more commonly in the later stages of illness (McGlashan and Fenton 1993, Fenton and McGlashan 1994). A possible decline in the prevalence of the hebephrenic and catatonic subtypes of schizophrenia may be attributed to effective treatment and possible arrest of the progression of illness (Wyatt 1991). Thus with effective treatment, and with long-term compliance, it is possible to produce favorable outcomes.

Following onset of the illness, individuals experience substantial decline in cognitive functions from their premorbid levels (Saykin et al. 1994). However, it is unclear whether, after the first episode, there is further cognitive decline due to the illness. Some studies even suggest a slight and gradual improvement (Gur et al. 1998). Increased number of episodes and the longer DUP are associated with greater cognitive dysfunction (Waddington 1995, 1997).

Individuals with first-episode psychosis usually have excellent clinical response to antipsychotic treatment early in their course of illness when compared to individuals with chronic multiple episodes. *Effective and early intervention does help achieve clinical remission and good outcome* (Lieberman et al. 1993, Robinson et al. 1999). Some suggest that atypical antipsychotic medication should be used preferentially in the treatment of individuals with first-episode psychosis (Lieberman 1996) as they are a highly treatment-responsive group, and may be best able to optimize the outcome. In addition, individuals with first-episode psychosis are sensitive to side effects, especially extrapyramidal and weight gain side effects. They require lower doses of medication to achieve therapeutic responses. The issue of treatment adherence is of critical importance in individuals in their first-episode of psychosis. Although these individuals respond very well with 1-year remission rates of greater than 80%, the 1-year attrition rates are as high as 60%. This important issue undermines management of individuals with first-episode psychosis during this critical period of their illness.

Morbidity and Mortality

The economic costs of schizophrenia have been estimated to be six times the costs of myocardial infarction (Andrews 1985). The WHO has estimated that mental illness accounts for as much as two-fifths of all disability funding in the US (Jablensky et al. 1980). Amongst the homeless in New York City, a significant percentage of cost of hospital admissions were associated with individuals with schizophrenia (Salit et al. 1998). In the United States, the cost of schizophrenia in 1994 was $44.9 billion and rising (Rice 1999). In the United Kingdom, 5.4% of total national health service in patient costs was attributed to schizophrenia. When all services were combined together, approximately £2.6 billion was spent annually taking care of individuals with schizophrenia (Knapp 1997). In Australia, it is estimated that schizophrenia costs approximately $3 billion for treatment and due to lost productivity (Mowry and Nancarrow 2001). Much of the cost of schizophrenia is due to the high morbidity of this chronic illness. Premorbid deficits, cognitive deficits, and negative symptoms account for much of the disability (Johnstone et al. 1979). Also, schizophrenic individuals with more severe courses may require repeated hospitalizations and may not be capable of maintaining independent living or stable employment.

The mortality rate of schizophrenia is estimated to be twice that of the general population. Approximately 10% of the mortality is secondary to suicide (Hare 1987). Young men with schizophrenia are most likely to complete suicide attempts, especially early in their illness (Drake et al. 1985, Breier and Astrachan 1984). Degree of social isolation, agitation, depression, a sense of hopelessness, a history of prior suicide attempts, and recent loss may be associated with increased risk of suicide among schizophrenic individuals (Breier and Astrachan 1984). There is also some evidence that an increased number of relapses, rehospitalizations, and discharges lead to an increased risk of suicide. There have been observations that suicide rates of individuals with schizophrenia may be increasing in the era of shorter hospital stays and community treatment (Drake et al. 1985). However, with the advent of the novel antipsychotic medications and especially with clozapine use, it is possible that this risk of suicide may even out or decrease owing to their possible protective effects against suicide (Meltzer and Okayli 1995). Other factors leading to increased mortality rates in schizophrenic individuals include an increased incidence of accidents as well as a more frequent association with other medical illnesses (including cardiovascular disease), comorbid substance abuse, a general neglect of health, an increased rate of damaging behaviors such as smoking and poor diet, decreased access to health services and depression (Vieweg et al. 1995, Ruschena et al. 1998, Harris and Barraclough 1998, Ameddeo et al. 1995, Musselman et al. 1998, Schulz et al. 2000, Allebech et al. 1986, Zarate and Patel 2001).

Differential Diagnosis

Making an accurate diagnosis of schizophrenia requires high levels of clinical acumen, extensive knowledge of schizophrenia, and sophisticated application of the principles of differential diagnosis. It is unfortunately common for individuals with psychotic disorders to be misdiagnosed and consequently treated inappropriately. The importance of accurate diagnosis is underlined by an emerging database indicating that early detection and prompt pharmacological intervention may improve the long-term prognosis of the illness.

Possibly the most difficult diagnostic dilemma in cases in which an individual has both psychotic symptoms and affective symptoms is in the differentiation between schizophrenia and schizoaffective disorder. The term *schizoaffective disorder* was first coined by Kasanin (1933). Since then, there has been some controversy regarding this diagnostic entity. It has been included in studies of both affective disorder and schizophrenia and has at times been considered part of a continuum between the two, which has contributed to some of the diagnostic confusion.

In DSM-IV-TR, schizoaffective disorder is treated as a unique clinical syndrome. A individual with schizoaffective disorder must have an uninterrupted period of illness during which, at some time, they have symptoms that meet the diagnostic criteria for a major depressive episode, manic episode, or a mixed episode concurrently with the diagnostic criteria for the active phase of schizophrenia (criterion A for schizophrenia). Additionally, *the individual must have had delusions or hallucinations for at least 2 weeks in the absence of prominent mood disorder symptoms* during the same period of illness. The mood disorder symptoms must be present for a substantial part of the active and residual psychotic period. The essential features of schizoaffective disorder must occur within a single uninterrupted period of illness where the "period of illness" refers to the period of active or residual symptoms of psychotic illness and this can last for years and decades. The total duration of psychotic symptoms must be at least 1 month to meet the criterion A for schizophrenia and thus, the minimum duration of a schizoaffective episode is also 1 month.

The criteria for major depressive episode requires a minimum duration of 2 weeks of either depressed mood or markedly diminished interest or pleasure. As the symptoms of loss of pleasure or interest commonly occur in nonaffective psychotic disorders, to meet the criteria for schizoaffective disorder criterion A, the major depressive episode must include pervasive depressed mood. Presence of markedly diminished interest or pleasure is not sufficient to make a diagnosis as it is possible that these symptoms may occur with other conditions too.

The distinctions among brief psychotic disorder, schizophreniform disorder, and schizophrenia are based on duration of active symptoms. As discussed earlier, DSM-III adopted a 6-month rule from the St. Louis group criteria. DSM-IV-TR has maintained the requirement of 6 months of active, prodromal, and/or residual symptoms for a diagnosis of schizophrenia. Brief psychotic disorder is a transient psychotic state, not caused by medical conditions or substance use, which lasts for at least 1 day and up to 1 month. Schizophreniform disorder falls in between and requires symptoms for at least 1 month and not exceeding 6 months, with no requirement for loss of functioning.

If the delusions that an individual describes are not bizarre (e.g., examples of bizarre delusions include the belief that an outside force or person has taken over one's body or that radio signals are being sent through the caps in one's teeth), it is wise to consider delusional disorder in the differential diagnosis. Delusional disorder is usually characterized by specific types of false fixed beliefs such as erotomanic, grandiose, jealous, persecutory, or somatic types. Delusional disorder, unlike schizophrenia, is not associated with a marked social impairment or odd behavior. Moreover, individuals with delusional disorder do not experience hallucinations or typically have negative symptoms.

If the individual experiences psychotic symptoms solely during times when affective symptoms are present, the diagnosis is more likely to be mood disorder with psychotic features. If the mood disturbance involves both manic and depressive episodes, the diagnosis is bipolar disorder. According to DSM-IV-TR, affective disorders that are seen in individuals with schizophrenia may fall in the category of depressive disorder not otherwise specified or bipolar disorder not otherwise specified.

Psychotic disorders, delirium, and dementia that are caused by substance use, in DSM-IV-TR, are distinguished from schizophrenia by virtue of the fact that there is clear-cut evidence of substance use leading to symptoms. Examples of psychotomimetic properties of substances include a phencyclidine psychosis (PCP) that can resemble schizophrenia clinically, chronic alcohol intoxication (Korsakoff's psychosis), and chronic amphetamine administration, which can lead to paranoid states. Therefore, individuals who have symptoms that meet criterion A of schizophrenia in the presence of substance use must be reevaluated after a significant period away from the suspected substance, and proper toxicology screens must be performed to rule out recent substance abuse.

General medical conditions ranging from vitamin B_{12} deficiency to Cushing's syndrome have been associated with a clinical presentation resembling that of schizophrenia. The most common neurological disorder appearing clinically similar to schizophrenia is epilepsy (Flor-Henry 1983), particularly of the temporal lobe. Other medical illnesses with symptoms similar to those of schizophrenia include basal ganglia calcifications and acute intermittent porphyria (Propping 1983). Imbalances of endocrine function as well as certain infectious diseases can present with symptoms that mimic schizophrenic psychosis. Because the prognosis for the associated medical condition is better than that for schizophrenia and the stigma attached to schizophrenia is significant, it is imperative to provide individuals with a thorough medical workup before giving a diagnosis of schizophrenia. This includes a physical examination; laboratory analyses including thyroid function tests, syphilis screening, and folate and vitamin B_{12} levels; a CT or MRI scan; and a lumbar puncture when indicated in new-onset cases.

Etiology

The cause of schizophrenia is currently not known. However, fast-paced developments in neuroscience combined with advances in psychiatric research have resulted in increased optimism about discovering the cause(s) and delineating the pathophysiology of this mysterious illness. A leading view is that schizophrenia may be heterogeneous with respect to etiology. Thus, multiple causative mechanisms may give rise to distinct disease subtypes. If this is true, it is important for psychiatric researchers to differentiate the homogeneous subtypes of this illness. Moreover, it has been proposed that more than one causative mechanism might interact (the so-called double-hit hypothesis) to cause the illness in some individuals. In this section, the main etiological theories of schizophrenia are examined.

Genetics

Schizophrenia represents a daunting challenge for genetic researchers for several reasons: the paucity of extended multigenerational family histories containing large numbers of affected individuals; the possibility of genetic heterogeneity, such as more than one phenotype or more than one genetic variant; and a lack of agreement on the mode of transmission. Following genetic modeling of epidemiological data and the results of several genome screens for susceptibility genes, it appears that the probability of schizophrenia being a single-gene disorder is unlikely. The probability that several genes of large effects may confer vulnerability to schizophrenia is diminishing too. Thus, the focus has shifted to multiple genes of small to moderate effects which may compound their effects through interactions with each other and with other nongenetic risk factors. (See Mowry and Nancarrow 2001 for more discussion). Despite these formidable obstacles, enormous progress has been made in the search of a genetic basis for schizophrenia. Moreover, the proteins expressed by the genes (proteome) are equally important in understanding the working of the cells being studied. Thus, genomics or the study of how genes control normal neuronal function is now moving on to proteomics or the study of different proteins expressed by the genome (Stahl 2000).

Wide agreement now exists that the rate of schizophrenia among first-degree family members of persons with schizophrenia is higher than in control families. The chance of occurrence is approximately 10 times greater among these individuals than among individuals with no first-degree relatives with schizophrenia (Kendler and Diehl 1993). There is approximately 6 times and 2 times greater chance of developing schizophrenia in second- and third-degree relatives of individuals with schizophrenia (Tsuang et al. 2001). In addition, the higher prevalence of schizophrenia spectrum disorders among family members of individuals with schizophrenia, such as schizoaffective disorder and schizoid and schizotypal personality disorders, provides support for a common genetic basis for this family of schizophrenia-like illnesses. Different studies have provided evidence for and against an increased prevalence of other psychotic disorders and nonpsychotic affective illnesses among relatives of persons with schizophrenia.

Adoption studies constitute a powerful experimental strategy for examining the role of genetic versus environmental factors. In these studies, the rates of schizophrenia are compared in relatives of adoptees with and without schizophrenia. Danish adoption studies conducted in the 1960s and 1970s provided compelling evidence that adoptees with schizophrenia had higher rates of schizophrenia in their first-degree relatives than control adoptees (Kety et al. 1968, Kety 1987). A reanalysis of these data in the late 1980s confirmed the original finding that biological relatives of schizophrenia adoptees had significantly higher rates of schizophrenia (4.1%) than biological relatives of nonschizophrenia (control) adoptees (0.5%).

In Finland, a large study of adopted-away offspring of mothers with schizophrenia found that significantly more offspring of mothers with schizophrenia themselves developed schizophrenia (9.1%) than did control offspring (1.1%) (Tienari 1991). An interesting aspect of the Finnish study was the examination of family environment in the adoptive families. A relationship was found between a disruptive family environment and occurrence of schizophrenia in adoptees. This suggests that environmental factors might play a role in the manifestation of the illness in genetically susceptible individuals. However, the study did not make clear whether the schizophrenia adoptee caused the disruptive home environment or the disruptive environment contributed to the manifestation of the illness. Longitudinal assessment of environmental conditions throughout childhood before the onset of illness will be important in resolving this issue.

Another approach to examining genetic contributions to schizophrenia involves concordance studies of dizygotic (nonidentical) and monozygotic (identical) twin pairs. Available data indicate that the concordance of schizophrenia among dizygotic twins is approximately 8 to 12%. This is much greater than the 1% rate found in the general population and comparable to the rate of concordance of schizophrenia among first-degree siblings. The concordance of schizophrenia among monozygotic twins is approximately 50% (Kendler and Diehl 1993). Even though the high rate of concordance among monozygotic twin pairs is compelling evidence for genetic contributions, the fact that it is not higher than 50% suggests a role for additional, perhaps nongenetic, factors in the etiology of schizophrenia. Moreover, although monozygotic twins share the same genetic information, it is possible for a mutation to occur in one member of the twin pair and not the other. Birth order of twin pairs and different intrauterine effects are other factors to consider. An attractive and robust experimental design is provided by adoption away of monozygotic twin pairs, which effectively combines the strengths of both adoption and twin methodologies. The number of sets of adopted-away, monozygotic twin pairs affected with schizophrenia is relatively small. However, data available on the limited number of pairs meeting these criteria support the strong concordance of schizophrenia in monozygotic twins.

There was tremendous enthusiasm and hope riding on the two promising approaches to identify the faulty gene(s) responsible for schizophrenia: *linkage studies* and *association studies*. Linkage studies use polymorphic genetic markers to attempt to identify statistical agreement (known as a logarithm of the odds score) between the presence of the marker and illness in families under investigation. The human genome project has established a set of markers for the entire human genome that will make it possible to scan the entire genome for schizophrenia linkage. It should be noted that genetic markers mark a segment of DNA presumably where the gene of interest resides; they do not necessarily identify mutant genes themselves. Once linkage is established, the second stage of work begins, which entails searching the identified segment of DNA for the faulty gene. However, the linkage studies have a limited power to detect susceptibility genes of small effect, a most likely scenario in complex disease genetics such as schizophrenia. This can be overcome by association studies (Lichtermann et al. 2000).

Association studies actually use the candidate genes themselves and test the highly specific hypothesis that a mutation in the candidate gene occurs at a greater rate in the population of interest (in this case, schizophrenic individuals) than in nonaffected control populations. More recently, family-based samples such as *trios* (consisting of the affected person and both parents, if available), are collected to avoid population stratification. The results have so far been equivocal. Serotonin 5-HT$_{2A}$ receptor gene and dopamine D$_3$ receptor gene are weakly associated with schizophrenia susceptibility (O'Donnell et al. 1999). The NMDA receptor holds promise based on animal models (Mohn et al. 1999). One limitation of this approach is that it is all or none; that is, the candidate gene either is or is not associated with the illness.

The Human Genome Project with its 3 billion base pairs and approximately 35,000 genes has ushered us into the "Genomic Era." However, systematic genome scans done recently have not resulted in strong evidence for linkage to any chromosomal region. Regions currently attracting most support are 6p (Schizophrenia Collaborative Linkage Group 1996), 6q (Cao et al. 1997, Levinson et al. 1998), 8p (Pulver et al. 1995, Schizophrenia Collaborative Linkage Group 1996), 13q (Blouin et al. 1998, Levinson et al. 2000), 3p (Schizophrenia Collaborative Linkage Group 1996), 22q (Gill et al. 1996, Moises et al. 1995), 5q (Levinson 1991), and 10p (Levinson et al. 2000, Faraone et al. 1998, Straub et al. 1998).

Velocardiofacial syndrome (VCFS) is associated with small interstitial deletions of chromosome 22q11 and a high rate of psychiatric comorbidity, specifically schizophrenia. This has generated enormous interest in this disorder especially because of evidence suggesting that the migration of mesencephalic and cardiac neural crest cells may be associated with pathogenesis of midfacial and cardiac abnormalities; similarities of this process to the neurodevelopment theory of schizophrenia has raised interesting speculations (Murphy et al. 1999, Chow et al. 1994).

Studies focused on 15q14 (Freedman et al. 1997, 2001) have shown some interesting findings especially considering its location close to the gene for nicotinic receptors, a system possibly involved with aspects of cognition. Ongoing and future studies will clarify the relevance of these findings.

At the time of this writing, no genetic linkage or association related to schizophrenia has been discovered. There have been reports of suggestive linkages but there has been a failure to replicate these findings. It has become painfully clear that the replication studies are, in many ways, more important to establishing linkage than the initial report. Genes that have been found not to be associated with schizophrenia include the dopamine D_2 and D_4 genes.

The initial enthusiasm for these strategies has waned to some extent as no gene has yet been isolated for schizophrenia or bipolar disorder. According to Merikangas (2002), the impediments that limited the success of linkage and association studies are etiologic and phenotypic heterogeneity of schizophrenia, lack of power, and high false-positive rates. Thus, newer approaches such as multi-investigator collaborative studies to increase the power have already been implemented.

Meanwhile, modern functional genomic approaches such as DNA microarrays, based on the principles of nucleic acid hybridization, can check a tissue sample for presence of thousands of genes simultaneously. For example, Mirnics and colleagues (2000) employed cDNA microarrays and compared transcriptomes in schizophrenia and matched control subjects and found that only a few gene groups consistently differed between subjects and controls. In all subjects with schizophrenia, the most changed gene group was related to *presynaptic group secretory function* (PSYN) gene group and in particular, the "mechanics" of neurotransmitter release. Thus, Mirnics and colleagues (2000) postulate that as the most affected genes in the PSYN group varied across study subjects (suggesting that the illness has "distinct molecular signatures"), schizophrenia therefore may involve a combination of different sequence-related polygenic susceptibility factors and physiological adaptations that lead to impairment of the signaling between neurons. They find additional support for their hypothesis from reports of reduced expression of regulator of G-protein signaling 4 (RGS4) in individuals with schizophrenia. In the brain, RGS4 is one of the 20 or more RGS family members that serve as GTPase-activating proteins (GAPs), which reduce response duration of postsynaptic neurons after the release of presynaptic neurotransmitters that bind to G-protein coupled receptors. Thus, Mirnics and colleagues (2001) suggest that the deficits in PSYN and RGS4 expression may produce synaptic changes with pathophysiologic consequences relevant to schizophrenia.

Weinberger and colleagues (2001) suggest that the gene that encodes the postsynaptic enzyme catechol-*o*-methyl transferase (COMT) is preferentially involved in the metabolism of dopamine in the frontal lobe. Dopamine is hypothesized to underlie aspects of cognition in the frontal lobe such as information processing. On the basis of animal studies, family-based association studies, and fMRI studies in individuals with schizophrenia and the general population, Weinberger and colleagues propose an interesting hypothesis that the COMT genotype with valenine allele (val/val type) may increase the risk of developing schizophrenia due to its effect on dopamine-mediated prefrontal information processing. Clearly, faster, innovative, and sophisticated techniques have ushered genetic research into a new era with a renewed promise to explore the genetic basis of mental illnesses.

Researchers are urgently searching for schizophrenia phenotypes for subgroups or dimensions that may define etiologically or genetically distinct subtypes. Similarly, the field is yearning for *endophenotypes* with simpler architecture than schizophrenia to possibly guide to newer leads in research (Mowry and Nancarrow 2001). Latent genetically influenced traits, which may be related only indirectly to the classic disease symptoms defined in major classification systems are known as *endophenotypes* (Gottesman 1997). They reflect an underlying susceptibility to the disease phenotype (or some form of it). In schizophrenia, we are interested in endophenotypes that are measurable by neurophysiological or neuropsychological means. Crucial characteristics of any endophenotype include the fact that it can be measured before the explicit onset of the illness, and that it represents the genetic liability of nonaffected relatives of probands with the disorder. For example, in genetically complex disorders such as schizophrenia, separate genetic loci could contribute to distinct aspects of the illness phenotype (e.g., evoked potentials, aspects of cognition, etc.).

Multinational studies are underway using *simple tandem-repeat polymorphic* (STRP) markers genome screen technology to detect genes of small to moderate effect. Also, large-scale *single-nucleotide polymorphism* (SNP) analysis will allow genome screen of extremely small densities. Thus, advances in proteomics and genomics provide more powerful approaches in identifying gene products involved in schizophrenia pathogenesis.

Viral Hypotheses

The suggestion that psychotic illnesses may be related to an infectious process has a long history. Jean Etienne Esquirol, in 1845, noted that some forms of psychotic illness followed "epidemic" illness patterns. In the early part of this century, Karl Menninger observed an association between the onset of schizophrenia and influenza epidemics. In addition, it has long been known that clinical features of viral encephalitis may include psychosis and other features resembling those of schizophrenia.

Two lines of evidence that have provoked the most interest in the possibility that viral infections are causative of schizophrenia are an increase, during influenza epidemics, in birth of individuals who subsequently develop schizophrenia and an increase in winter births among individuals with schizophrenia because of the higher rate of viral infections in winter months. Mednick and colleagues (1988) reported a strong association between pregnancies during the 1957 influenza epidemic in Helsinki, Finland, and subsequent development of schizophrenia. Moreover, it was learned that the relationship between viral exposure and schizophrenia appears strongest when exposure occurred during the second trimester of pregnancy. This is of interest because the second trimester is a critical period for cortical and limbic development. It was therefore reasoned that second-trimester viral exposure might disrupt neuronal development in key areas of the brain, such as the hippocampus and prefrontal cortex, which have been implicated in this illness. In fact, there is some experimental evidence from animal models that viral exposure to these regions in the developing brain produces neuropathological changes resembling those observed in some postmortem studies of schizophrenia. However, reanalysis of previous data failed to detect significant association between *in utero* exposure to influenza epidemics and schizophrenia (Grech et al. 1997, Selten et al. 1998). Similarly, data from Australia failed to find an association between six influenza epidemics and schizophrenia (Morgan et al. 1997). These and other negative results (Crow and Done 1992) have raised serious questions about this theory. Interestingly, in the North Finland birth cohort, a significant association was found with laboratory confirmed diagnosis of viral infection, especially Coxsackie B5 meningitis in the neonatal period and risk of schizophrenia later on (Rantakallio et al. 1997).

Several studies have demonstrated an excess of winter births among individuals with schizophrenia. Although statistically significant, the association between winter births and schizophrenia appears relatively small, occurring in less than 10% of cases. Thus, season of birth remains an interesting (and unresolved) research issue but has little use as a risk factor for the illness from a clinical perspective.

Exposure to influenza *in utero* and excess winter births are interesting although indirect lines of evidence for a viral cause of schizophrenia. To date, there has been no direct confirmation for any viral agent causing this illness, such as viral isolates or consistent findings of specific viral antibodies. Advances in neurovirology, however, are providing new insights into the role of viruses in brain diseases, leading to new hypotheses about schizophrenia. One area involves the search for neurotropic retroviruses. For example, Borna virus is a naturally occurring neurotropic agent in horses and sheep. The development of a serological assay method to detect antibodies for Borna virus led to the discovery that its hosts also include humans and that it has relative tropism for the hippocampus. Moreover, its clinical manifestations range from asymptomatic infection to profound behavioral abnormalities that resemble some aspects of schizophrenia. An association between deficit symptoms, Borna virus antibodies, and summer birth excess has been reported (Waltrip et al. 1997). There is now an active research effort to determine whether Borna and other neurotropic viruses are more common in schizophrenia.

Immune Dysfunction

Several research groups are exploring the possibility that schizophrenia may be associated with impaired immune function including alterations in autoimmunity (Muller and Ackenheil 1998). Anticardiolipin antibody and antinuclear antibody, two autoantibodies that are used as markers of autoimmune vulnerability, have been shown to be increased in individuals with schizophrenia in some but not all studies of this illness. Specific histocompatibility antigens (human leukocyte antigens (HLA)) have also been linked to several autoimmune diseases and have been investigated in schizophrenia with conflicting results (Miyanaga et al. 1984). Two other markers relevant to autoimmune function, impaired T-lymphocyte proliferative response to the mitogen phytohemagglutinin and impaired interleukin-2 production, have shown more consistent alterations in individuals with schizophrenia than in control populations (Coffey et al. 1983). Some of the most intriguing work in this area is focused on finding autoantibodies to brain tissue. Recent reports of atypical antipsychotic medications having immunomodulatory effects (Muller et al. 1997, Lin et al. 1998) and selective COX-2 inhibitor (a new type of nonsteroidal anti-inflammatory drug used as a pain killer) having positive effects on schizophrenia symptoms are interesting and provide yet another avenue of research in understanding the complexity of schizophrenia (Muller et al. 2002).

Birth Complications

Numerous studies have reported a higher rate of pregnancy and birth complications in individuals with schizophrenia than in control populations (Jones et al. 1998, Dalman et al. 1999, PretI et al. 2000, McNeil et al. 1994, Cannon et al. 2002). The complication rates vary widely among studies, probably because of the inherent difficulties in obtaining reliable and valid retrospective data in this area. In one study, two-thirds of individuals with schizophrenia and less than one-third of control subjects had histories of obstetrical complications. Hypoxia is one possible result of pregnancy and birth complications that has been shown to disrupt brain development. The hippocampus and some neocortical regions are particularly sensitive to shortfalls in oxygen. Thus, one proposed mechanism for a role of pregnancy and birth complications in the cause of schizophrenia involves hypoxia-mediated damage to these areas. While some investigators agree with this theory (Geddes et al. 1999, Rosso et al. 2000, Zornberg 2000), others do not (McCreadie et al. 1994, Byrne et al. 2000, Kendell et al. 2000). Interestingly, some studies suggest that the rate of obstetric complications are higher in early-onset schizophrenia (Verdoux et al. 1997, Smith et al. 1998, Rosso et al. 2000), occur more often in males, in people with prominent negative symptoms, and no family history of schizophrenia (McNeil 1995, Verdoux et al. 1997, Smith et al. 1998, Rosso et al. 2000).

A meta-analysis of data involving 854 individuals from 11 research groups (Verdoux et al. 1997) suggests that the relationship between birth complications and age at onset tends to be linear and may indicate a causal effect. Jones and colleagues (1998), using North Finland birth cohort involving 11,017 individuals reported a sevenfold excess among schizophrenic individuals of perinatal brain injury. In a recent historical and meta-analytic review by Cannon and colleagues (2002), complications of pregnancy, abnormal fetal growth and development, and complications of delivery were significantly associated with developing schizophrenia but the effect sizes were generally small with odds ratios of less than 2. They elaborate current methodological shortcomings and suggest need for newer and better approaches to inform our understanding of these important associations.

Association with General Medical Conditions

Schizophrenia is associated with an increased frequency of tuberculosis (not accounted for by institutionalization), celiac disease, myxedema, and arteriosclerotic heart disease (Baldwin 1979, Hare 1987, Eaton 1985, Jablensky 1986, Harris and Barraclough 1998, Musselman et al. 1998, Schulz et al. 2000). Individuals who present with atypical psychoses have been noted to have an increased risk of ankylosing spondylitis and uroarthritis, which may indicate a relationship between the histocompatibility complex and schizophrenia (Jablensky 1986, Osterberg 1978).

Along these lines, there is a strikingly decreased risk for rheumatoid arthritis among individuals with schizophrenia (Jablensky 1986, Eaton 1985). Many of the studies supporting this observation were conducted before the use of phenothiazines, which eliminates any potential protective role of neuroleptics (Eaton 1985). It has been postulated that further investigation of this link may yield significant genetic or biological markers for both diseases.

Such studies of potential biological markers have yielded some interesting findings. Illnesses such as rheumatoid arthritis and ankylosing spondylitis are autoimmune disorders that are associated with HLA. The associated risks for these disorders and schizophrenia have led to speculation that some subgroup of individuals with schizophrenia may be manifesting symptoms related to an autoimmune process. For example, studies have shown that there may be an association between HLA and types of schizophrenia (Ganguli et al. 1993, Zamani et al. 1994). In one recent study, the HLA frequency was increased for HLA A10, A11, and A29 and decreased for HLA A2 in individuals with schizophrenia (Ozcan et al. 1996). Thus, although the presence of HLA is not universal among persons with schizophrenia, further investigation into this area may point to an alternative hypothesis regarding etiology and treatment of a certain population of individuals with schizophrenia.

Neuroanatomical Theories

The brains of individuals with psychotic illnesses have been examined for hundreds of years. At the end of the nineteenth century, Alzheimer described loss of cortical neurons in individuals with dementia precox. In 1915, Southard noted cerebral atrophy in individuals. Although these early reports were suggestive of a brain lesion in schizophrenia, only recently have the investigative tools become available to probe the human brain in enough detail to confirm cerebral abnormalities in this illness.

Advances in *in vivo* brain imaging and postmortem methodology have provided powerful new tools for neuroanatomical investigations of this illness. *In vivo* structural brain analysis began in earnest with computed tomography (CT), which provided the most compelling evidence for morphological abnormalities in this illness. CT has been replaced by magnetic resonance imaging (MRI) for morphological studies because of its superior anatomical resolution (1 mm or less in-plane resolution), ability to provide true volumetric and three-dimensional analysis of even minute brain regions, tissue segmentation capability, and because it involves no radiation exposure. Positron emission tomography (PET), single-photon emission computed tomography (SPECT), functional MRI (fMRI), and MR spectroscopy (MRS) are imaging tools used to assess the functional and neurochemical activity of specific brain regions. Diffusion Tensor Imaging (DTI) and Line Scan Diffusion Imaging (LSDI) are newer MRI approaches that can provide sophisticated information on the orientation and integrity of neuron fibers *in vivo*. Advances in postmortem methodology include rapid access to brains after death, well-matched control groups, controls for neuroleptic exposure including studies of neuroleptic-naive populations, and application of new molecular biological techniques. The following is an examination of the brain structures most often implicated in the pathophysiology of schizophrenia.

Enlarged Ventricles   Ventricles are fluid-filled spaces in the center of the brain. The most consistent morphological finding in the literature of schizophrenia is enlarged ventricles, which has been confirmed by a large number of CT and MRI studies (Pahl et al. 1990, Wolkin et al. 1998, McCarley et al. 1999, Henn and Braus 1999). The effective size of ventriculomegaly has been reported to be 0.7 (Raz and Raz 1990). Seventy-nine percent of the well-designed studies report enlargement of lateral ventricles (Henn and Braus 1999). CT studies have tended to use ventricle–brain ratios to assess lateral ventricular size, and MRI studies have used more sophisticated quantifications. Lawrie and Abukmeil (1998), in a review report approximately 40% difference in volume between individuals with schizophrenia and controls across all volumetric MRI studies. It should be noted that although the ventricular increases are statistically significant, the ventricles are not grossly enlarged in most cases. In fact, radiologists most often read CT and MRI scans of individuals with schizophrenia as normal. In addition, most studies of ventricular size demonstrate overlap between individuals with schizophrenia and normal control subjects, indicating that many individuals with schizophrenia have ventricles in the normal range. Nonetheless, enlargement of the ventricles is the first consistently reported finding confirming a brain abnormality in schizophrenia.

The pathophysiological significance of larger than normal ventricles is unclear (Lawrie and Abukmeil 1998). There have been reports that enlarged ventricles may be more prominent in more severely ill individuals, and related to poor response to neuroleptic medication, although these findings have not been consistently replicated. Ventricular enlargement, particularly third-ventricle and temporal horn enlargement, has been found in first-episode individuals with schizophrenia, which suggests that it is not secondary to chronic neuroleptic exposure or a progressive disease process. However, frontal horn enlargement is usually seen in chronic cases, suggesting possible progressive changes following onset of the illness (Bilder et al. 1994). Enlarged ventricles are most likely a secondary manifestation of brain atrophy or some other process resulting in either focal or generalized reductions in brain mass. Indeed, there have been many reports of brain atrophy and reduced mass in the illness. Enlarged ventricles have also been reported in first-degree relatives of subjects with schizophrenia (Cannon et al. 1998, Seidman et al. 1997) and in persons suffering from schizotypal personality disorder (Buchsbaum et al. 1997), raising interesting speculations of whether ventriculomegaly may be an indicator of neurodevelopmental risk for schizophrenia (Lencz et al. 2001).

Limbic System   The limbic structures that have been implicated in schizophrenia are the hippocampus, entorhinal cortex, anterior cingulate, and amygdala. These structures have important functions for memory (hippocampus), attention (anterior cingulate), and emotional expression and social affiliation (amygdala). The entorhinal cortex serves as a "way station" between hippocampus and neocortex in that neurotransmissions between these regions synapse in the entorhinal cortex. The entorhinal cortex, hippocampus, and other components of the parahippocampal gyrus are often considered *mesiotemporal* structures because of their close anatomical and functional relationship.

There are more reports of abnormalities in hippocampal and related mesiotemporal structures than other limbic structures in schizophrenia. In fact, mesiotemporal pathology is consistently found in studies of schizophrenia and mesiotemporal structures are leading candidates for the neuroanatomical site of this illness (Goldstein et al. 1999, Wright et al. 1999). This region has been implicated by converging brain imaging and postmortem lines of evidence. One of the most consistent MRI morphological findings is reduction in size of the hippocampus (Breier et al. 1992). In addition, more than 25 postmortem studies have reported morphological and cytoarchitectural abnormalities in this structure. The findings have included reduced size and cellular number (Benes et al. 1998), white matter reductions, and abnormal cell arrangement. Nelson and colleagues (1998) conclude from a meta-analysis of 18 studies that there is a bilateral reduction of approximately 4% hippocampal volume in schizophrenia. However, reduced hippocampal volume is not reported by all studies (Harrison 1999, Maier et al. 2000). In another review, Lawrie and Abukmeil (1998) reported approximately 6% reduction in amygdala hippocampal complex. Reduction in the volume of amygdala is reported by some but not all (Altshuler et al. 1998). In a very interesting preliminary report from Australia, subjects who went on to develop schizophrenia had larger left hippocampal volumes compared to controls at baseline (during the prodrome) with subsequent reduction in volume after the onset of schizophrenia (Pantelis et al. 1999).

The anterior cingulate has been implicated in schizophrenia largely because of post-mortem findings of reduced gamma-aminobutyric acid (GABA) interneurons (Benes et al. 1991). In addition, functional imaging studies have demonstrated altered metabolic activity both at rest and during selective attention tasks in the anterior cingulate in individuals with schizophrenia (Baker 1997, Carter et al. 1997, Erkwoh et al. 1997, Fletcher 1999, Haznedar et al. 1997). Data from many studies suggest possible neurodevelopmental abnormalities in anterior cingulate in individuals with schizophrenia (Benes 2000, Harrison 1999, Honer et al. 1997, Kalus et al. 1999). Bouras and colleagues (2001) reported that mean total and laminar cortical thickness as well as mean pyramidal neuron size were significantly decreased in the dorsal and subgenual parts of anterior cingulate in individuals with schizophrenia. Thirty-one studies evaluated one or more of the medial temporal lobe structures—hippocampus, amygdala, parahippocampal gyrus, entorhinal cortex—with 77% reporting positive findings; this is one of the higher percentages of abnormalities reported in all regions of interest throughout the brain.

Prefrontal Cortex   The prefrontal cortex is the most anterior portion of the neocortex, sitting behind the forehead. It has evolved through lower species to become one of the largest regions of the human brain, constituting approximately one-third of the cortex. It is responsible for some of the most sophisticated human functions. It contains a heteromodal association area that is responsible for integrating information from all other cortical areas as well as from several subcortical regions for the execution of purposeful behavior. Among its specific functions are working memory, which involves the temporary storage (seconds to minutes) of information, attention, and suppression of interference from internal and external sources. The most inferior portion of the prefrontal cortex, termed the *orbital frontal cortex*, is involved in emotional expression. Given its unique role, it is not surprising that the prefrontal cortex has been considered in the etiology of schizophrenia.

Indeed, several lines of evidence have implicated the prefrontal cortex in schizophrenia. CT studies have provided evidence for prefrontal atrophy, and some, although not all, MRI studies have found evidence for decreased volume of this structure (Breier et al. 1992, Andreasen et al. 1986, McCarley et al. 1999). One of the earliest observations from functional imaging studies of schizophrenia was reduced perfusion of the frontal lobes (Ingvar and Franzen 1974). This finding was subsequently replicated by several PET studies suggesting decreased frontal glucose utilization and blood flow, which came to be known as *hypofrontality*. Subsequent functional imaging studies provided further support for hypofrontality by demonstrating that individuals with schizophrenia failed to activate their frontal lobes to the same degree as normal control subjects when performing frontal cognitive tasks (Weinberger and Berman 1988, 1996, Kindermann et al. 1997). This finding has been questioned because individuals with schizophrenia typically perform poorly in many cognitive paradigms, so it is unclear whether their lack of frontal activation is a primary frontal deficit or secondary to poor cognitive task performance related to factors such as lack of motivation, inattention, or cognitive impairment stemming from nonfrontal regions. Auditory hallucinations were found to be associated with increases in Broca's area, a portion of the frontal cortex responsible for language production (McGuire et al. 1993). This finding was of interest because it supported a hypothesis that auditory hallucinations were a form of abnormal "inner speech."

MRI studies employing diffusion tensor imaging have reported changes suggestive of an abnormality in white matter connectivity possibly due to reduced myelination of fiber tracts in individuals with schizophrenia (Lim et al. 1999, Buchsbaum et al. 1998). Magnetic resonance spectroscopy (MRS) studies have reported reduced levels of neuronal membrane constituents (phosphomonoesters) and/or increased levels of their breakdown products (phosphodiesters) in individuals with schizophrenia, primarily in the frontal cortex (Keshavan et al. 2000). Such abnormalities have been observed in treatment-naive individuals during their first-episode (Stanley et al. 1995) and have been correlated with traitlike negative symptoms and neurocognitive performance (Shioiri et al. 1994, Deicken et al. 1995).

Though sometimes contradictory, the neuroimaging studies consistently report abnormalities in orbitofrontal region; often, these abnormalities tend to correlate with severity of schizophrenia symptomatology, show gender differences in relation to spatial localization, and the gray matter deficits may be more widespread in chronic as compared to medication-naive individuals having their first-episode (Lencz et al. 2001, Szeszko et al. 1999). Additional support for prefrontal cortical involvement in schizophrenia comes from postmortem studies with a range of findings. There have been reports of reduced cortical thickness, loss of pyramidal cells, malformed cellular architecture, loss of GABA interneurons, and evidence of failed neuronal migration. The Stanley Foundation Neuropathology Consortium is reported to be "the most extensively characterized collection of pathological specimens from individuals with major mental illnesses" (Knable et al. 2001). Their exploratory analyses of prefrontal cortex from individuals suffering from schizophrenia, bipolar disorder, and depression compared with samples from normal controls found the largest number of abnormalities in schizophrenia with an overlap with bipolar disorder. A majority of the abnormalities represented a decline in function suggesting a widespread failure of gene expression. Specifically, abnormalities involving the glycoprotein Reelin were observed in schizophrenia, a finding reported previously by other postmortem studies also (Impagnatiello et al. 1998, Guidotti 2000). Reelin, an extracellular matrix glycoprotein secreted from different GABAergic interneurons during development and adult life, may be important for the transcription of specific genes necessary for synaptic plasticity and morphological changes associated with learning. Future studies will clarify the role of Reelin in the pathology of schizophrenia.

Thus, a substantial body of evidence is converging on the prefrontal cortex as a site of pathophysiology in schizophrenia (Bunney and Bunney 2000, Weinberger et al. 2001). The genetics of the prefrontal neurons, the cortical circuits, and its underlying neurochemistry in the brains of individuals with schizophrenia is one of the most intensely investigated areas.

Temporal Lobe   The superior temporal gyrus is involved in auditory processing and, with parts of the inferior parietal cortex, is a heteromodal association area that includes Wernicke's area, a language center. Because of the important role it plays in audition, it was hypothesized to be involved in auditory hallucinations. Indeed, MRI studies have found the superior temporal gyrus to be reduced in size in schizophrenia and have found a significant relationship between these reductions and the presence of auditory hallucinations (Barta et al. 1990). Similarly, Wernicke's area, which is involved in the conception and organization of speech, has been hypothesized to mediate the thought disorder of schizophrenia, particularly conceptual disorganization. Support for this hypothesis comes from a report of an individual with vascular and other lesions of this region that produce Wernicke's aphasia, a disruption in the organization of speech that resembles the thought disorder of schizophrenia. MRI studies have found a relationship between morphological abnormalities in this region and conceptual disorganization in schizophrenia (Shenton et al. 1992). McCarley and colleagues (1999) reviewed 118 MRI studies published from 1988 to 1998; 62% of the 37 studies of the whole temporal lobe showed volume reduction and/or abnormal asymmetry. Of the 15 studies surveyed, 80% showed abnormalities in the superior temporal gyrus, the *highest* percentage of any cortical region of interest. This difference appears to be largely due to gray matter. Most studies, including those involving individuals in their first-episode of schizophrenia (Hirayasu et al. 1998), report abnormalities in *planum temporale* (area related to language) with specific reductions of left posterior superior temporal gyrus gray matter. According to the authors, the higher percentage of abnormalities in specifically defined regions of interest of medial temporal lobe and superior temporal gyrus suggests a nondiffuse distribution of temporal lobe structural changes.

Striatum   The striatum, consisting of the caudate, putamen, globus pallidus, substantia nigra, and accumbens, is an output center for the cortex and has been traditionally thought to have a primary role in the execution of motor programs. Subsequent studies have demonstrated an important cognitive role for this structure as well. Moreover, in primary diseases of the striatum, such as Parkinson's and Huntington's diseases, clinical manifestations include psychosis and other schizophrenia-type behavior, which has contributed to interest in this region in the pathophysiology of schizophrenia.

Two related bodies of data are most frequently cited regarding the role of the striatum in schizophrenia; these concern the mechanism of antipsychotic drugs and postmortem studies of altered dopamine D_2 receptor numbers. The dorsal striatum (caudate and putamen) is the site of the vast majority of D_2 receptors in brain. All effective antipsychotic drugs antagonize this receptor and thus, by extrapolation, it was reasoned that this region might be central to the pathophysiology of schizophrenia (Creese et al. 1975). Moreover, the most consistent postmortem finding in the schizophrenia literature is an increased density of striatal D_2 receptors. However, neuroleptic exposure causes upregulation of D_2 receptors, which may account for this postmortem finding. A current view of the antipsychotic mechanism is that the dorsal striatum is involved in mediating the extrapyramidal side effects of antipsychotic medications and, based on rodent studies of antipsychotic drug mechanisms, the ventral striatum (nucleus accumbens) may be involved in antipsychotic efficacy. Thus, attention has shifted toward the possible role of the accumbens in mediating the psychosis of schizophrenia.

Several MRI studies have found an increased volume of the caudate, putamen, and globus pallidus in schizophrenia (Breier et al. 1992, Elkashef et al. 1994). In all cases, the individuals included in these studies had exposure to typical neuroleptic treatment, which raised the possibility that striatal enlargement may be secondary to neuroleptic exposure. In a longitudinal study of neuroleptic-naive individuals who were subsequently treated with typical neuroleptics, it was found that striatal size was not enlarged before antipsychotic drug treatment but increased after neuroleptic exposure, which supports the notion that (typical) neuroleptics may account for this consistent morphological finding (Chakos et al. 1994). This was further confirmed when increased size of caudate nucleus following long-term antipsychotic exposure normalized after switching to clozapine, an atypical antipsychotic drug that has significantly less activity in the striatal region (Chakos et al. 1995).

Thalamus   The thalamus is a nucleus that receives subcortical input and outputs it to the cortex. One theory posits that the thalamus provides a filtering function for sensory input to the cortex. A deficit in thalamic filtering was proposed to account in part for the experiential phenomena of being overwhelmed by sensory stimuli reported by many individuals with schizophrenia. Preclinical studies have demonstrated that antipsychotic drugs modulate thalamic input to the cortex, which has been offered as a model for antipsychotic drug action. Several MRI studies have reported reduced volume (Andreasen et al. 1994, Gur et al. 1998, Dasari et al. 1999, Hazlett et al. 1999) and functional abnormalities (Buchsbaum and Hazlett 1998, Hazlett et al. 1999) of the thalamus in individuals with schizophrenia. Postmortem studies have also found cell loss and reductions in tissue volume in thalamic nuclei. This thalamic tissue reduction is considered as a possible evidence of abnormal circuitry linking the cortex, thalamus, and cerebellum (Andreasen 1997).

Neural Circuits

Because of the large number of different neuroanatomical findings in studies of schizophrenia and the appreciation that brain function involves integration of several brain regions, current thinking about the neuroanatomy of this illness is centered on neural circuits. Thus, investigators are attempting to examine the integrity of a variety of cortical–cortical and cortical–subcortical neural networks that function together to execute behavioral programs. It is conceivable that an isolated lesion anywhere in a neural circuit could result in dysfunction of the entire network, and therefore spurious conclusions could be drawn by investigating only one component of a neural network. Evidence suggests that schizophrenia may be associated with a decrease in synaptic connectivity of the dorsal prefrontal cortex though this is not reported by all studies. McGlashan and Hoffman (2000) have proposed the Developmentally Reduced Synaptic Connectivity (DRSC) model which proposes that cortical gray matter deficits may arise from either reduced baseline synaptic density due to genetic and/or perinatal factors, or excessive pruning of synapses during adolescence and early adulthood or both. Margolis and colleagues (1994) propose that there could be graded apoptosis rather than a necrotic fulminant process. Apoptosis is a form of cell death that occurs in many neurodegenerative disorders in which intra- or extracellular physiologic events trigger a programmed sequence of cellular actions resulting in cell destruction and evacuation (Bredesen 1995). According to Goldman-Rakic and Selemon (1997), there is regionally specific decreased neuronal size in cortical layer III with cytoplasmic atrophy and generally reduced neuropil. The reduced size and increased density of neurons or glia and decreased cortical thickness suggest that cell processes and synaptic connections are reduced in schizophrenia. This is consistent with reports of decreased concentrations of synaptic proteins (e.g., synaptophysin). These cell processes and synapses could be lost as a consequence of a neurochemically mediated (through dopamine and or glutamate) synaptic apoptosis that would compromise cell function and alter brain morphology without, however, producing serious cell injury (and thus inducing glial reactions). However, McCarley and colleagues (1999) suggest that the main neural abnormality in schizophrenia involves neural connectivity (dendrite/neuropil/gray matter changes) rather than the number of neurons or network size. They suggest that a "failure of inhibition" on the cellular level is present in schizophrenia and may be linked to a "failure of inhibition" at the cognitive level. According to Lafargue and Brasic (2000), abnormalities involving the temporolimbic–prefrontal cerebral circuitry is postulated to underlie the organizational and memory deficits commonly observed in schizophrenic individuals. Furthermore, as reviewed by these authors, a possible insult or injury to the mechanism of GABAergic and glutamatergic influence during early corticogenesis may largely contribute to the later manifestation of clinical schizophrenia. Malfunction of the cooperating sensory systems of excitation and inhibition during the early stages of development of the brain could result in the failure of "pioneer neurons" to properly differentiate and migrate to their appropriate cerebral locations. Consequently, the later migrating projection neurons may fail to reach or invade their preselected area-specific brain sites. A disturbance of the proper GABAergic and glutamatergic influences would upset NMDA mechanisms and normal cortical development. If such a disturbance is actively occurring from the onset of cerebral ontogeny, the affected individual may suffer from the signs and symptoms observed in schizophrenia. A challenge for the future is developing new approaches to examining the brain as an integrated and highly interactive system. An unanswered question is whether the morphological differences reflect hypoplasia (failure to develop) or atrophy (shrinkage).

Electrophysiology

An electroencephalogram (EEG) records the electrical activity of the brain, which may reflect the mental functions carried out by the neurons possibly in "real time." However, the precise localization of this event in the specific brain region is poor. When EEG activity from repeated presentations of a specific stimulus is summed across trials, some potentials related to the specific processing of the target stimulus can be extracted from the EEG and are referred to as *event-related potentials* (ERPs).

The P300 ERP, a positive deflection occurring approximately 300 ms after the introduction of a stimulus, is regarded as a putative biological marker of risk for schizophrenia (Bharath et al. 2000, Blackwood 2000). The P300 amplitudes are smaller in individuals with schizophrenia and are among the most replicated electrophysiological findings (Bruder 1999, Ford et al. 1999, McCarley et al. 1997). The P300 ERP is often elicited with an oddball paradigm, wherein two stimuli are presented in a random series such that one of them occurs relatively infrequently and subjects are instructed to respond to the infrequent target stimulus (Polich and Herbst 2000). Though the exact neural location of the normal P300 generation is uncertain (Halgren et al. 1995, McCarthy et al. 1997), it is thought that discriminating the target from a standard stimulus should involve frontal lobe. If the neuroelectric events that underlie P300 generation are related to an interaction between frontal lobe and hippocampal/temporal–parietal function (Knight 1996, 1997, Kirino et al. 2000, Demiralp et al. 2001), disease states that affect frontal and temporal/parietal lobe function should also affect P300 measures. This hypothesis has been supported by findings of smaller P300 amplitudes over left temporal scalp locations relative to the homologous right temporal locations for individuals with schizophrenia compared to controls (O'Donnell et al. 1999, McCarley et al. 1993). Remarkably, reductions in the left posterior superior temporal gyrus gray matter volume (using MRI) correlated with the reduction in the temporal P300 amplitude in chronic and first-episode schizophrenia (McCarley et al. 1993, 2002). Even though the magnitude of P300 component differences between individuals with schizophrenia and control subjects is highly reliable across individual studies (Jeon and Polich 2001), variation for the group effect size is systematically associated with disease definition, stimulus parameters, task conditions, and recording methods (Polich 1998).

N400 is a negative deflection in the ERP occurring approximately 400 ms after introduction of a stimulus, whose latency is thought to reflect the speed of linguistic operations related to semantic search (Van Petten and Kutas 1990). Abnormalities in the N400 amplitude in schizophrenia have been reported (Niznikiewicz et al. 1997, Nestor et al. 1997, Mathalon et al. 2002). Investigators suggest that individuals with schizophrenia do not use the context of the preceding portion of the sentence and fill-in responses to phrases on the basis of the immediately preceding word rather than the whole sentence or passage.

Investigations using newer probes such as atypical antipsychotic agents and their effects on ERPs are interesting; clozapine, in a small sample using a double-blind paradigm, improved the amplitude of the P300 but chlorpromazine did not (Patel et al. 2001). Thus, future studies promise interesting information in this area.

Neurochemical Theories

Dopamine   Dopamine is the most extensively investigated neurotransmitter system in schizophrenia. In 1973, it was proposed that schizophrenia is related to hyperactivity of dopamine (Matthysee 1973). This proposition became the dominant pathophysiological hypothesis for the next 15 years. Its strongest support came from the fact that all commercially available antipsychotic agents have antagonistic effects on the dopamine D_2 receptor in relation to their clinical potencies (Creese et al. 1975). In addition, dopamine agonists, such as amphetamine and methylphenidate, exacerbate psychotic symptoms in a subgroup of individuals with schizophrenia. Moreover, as noted earlier, the most consistently reported postmortem finding in the literature of schizophrenia is elevated D_2 receptors in the striatum.

The dopamine hyperactivity hypothesis and the primacy of D_2 antagonism for antipsychotic drug action were seriously questioned largely because of the advent of clozapine, an atypical antipsychotic drug. Clozapine has proved to be the most efficacious treatment for chronic schizophrenia and yet it has one of the lowest levels of D_2 occupancy of all antipsychotic drugs. *In vivo* brain-imaging studies demonstrated that clozapine D_2 occupancy levels were as low as 20% more than 12 hours after the last dose of medication in individuals deriving excellent antipsychotic efficacy (compared with more than 80% D_2 occupancy for haloperidol) (Farde et al. 1988, 1989, 1990, 1992). This started an extensive search for explanations underlying the extraordinary efficacy of clozapine. However, new information from PET studies has once again highlighted the central role that the dopaminergic system plays in the treatment of psychosis. The typical and atypical antipsychotics are effective only when their D_2 receptor occupancy exceeds 65%, reinforcing the importance of D_2 antagonism in producing antipsychotic effects. However, an important difference between typical and atypical antipsychotics is in their affinity for the D_2 receptors. Medications like clozapine attach loosely to and dissociate rapidly from the dopamine D_2 receptors compared to typical antipsychotic agents (like haloperidol) that have strong affinity for and bind tightly to these receptors. Thus, Kapur and Seeman propose that this fast dissociation from the D_2 receptors and the low receptor affinity may explain the atypicality of clozapine.

Five subtypes of dopamine receptor have now been discovered, D_1, D_2, D_3, D_4, and D_5, and interest in dopamine receptors other than the D_2 receptor has arisen. Reduced levels of D_1-like dopamine receptors in the prefrontal cortex of individuals with schizophrenia including in those never exposed to antipsychotic agents have been reported. The D_1 receptors are expressed predominantly by pyramidal neurons on their dendritic spines, where they possibly modulate glutamate-mediated inputs to these neurons—inputs that mainly come from other pyramidal and thalamic neurons. Thus the reduced D_1-like receptors seen in the prefrontal cortex of schizophrenic individuals may underlie aspects of cognitive dysfunction and severity of negative symptoms (Nestler 1997).

There was hope that D_4 receptor could be a possible pathophysiological candidate for schizophrenia as clozapine was initially reported to have differential affinity for this receptor (van Tol et al. 1991). Contrary to initial expectations, D_4 receptors do not uniquely distinguish atypical antipsychotic medications from typical ones (Seeman et al. 1997, Tarazi 2000). Short-term clinical trials involving a limited range of doses of at least two drugs with high D_4 potency failed to show antipsychotic effects (Kramer et al. 1997, Truffinet et al. 1999).

Clinical trials of dopamine agonists have resulted in improvements in the negative symptoms of schizophrenia. A new model of dopamine dysfunction was proposed which stated that deficits in dopamine, perhaps in the prefrontal cortex, may result in negative symptoms and that concomitant dopamine dysregulation in the striatum, perhaps related to faulty presynaptic control of dopamine release, may be involved in positive symptoms. This bidirectional model is under investigation.

The dopamine (DA) hypothesis of schizophrenia has been critical in guiding schizophrenia research for several decades. Until recently, a main shortcoming of this hypothesis was absence of direct evidence linking DA dysfunction to schizophrenia. Sophisticated *in vivo* techniques have provided fascinating data directly implicating dopamine in developing psychosis. When the synthesis of dopamine in the brain was measured using PET scan following administration of radiolabeled fluro-L-DOPA, a dopamine precursor, an increase in dopamine was observed in drug-naïve schizophrenic individuals compared to age-matched controls (Hietala et al. 1994, Dao-Costellano et al. 1997, Lindstrom et al. 1999). Similarly, dopamine release in the basal ganglia was elevated in drug-naïve schizophrenic individuals compared to age-matched controls when measured by PET and SPECT scans following an amphetamine challenge. This dopamine elevation correlated to the induction of positive symptoms of schizophrenia (Laruelle et al. 1996, Breier et al. 1997, Abi-Dargham et al. 1998). Furthermore, SPECT studies using alpha-methyltyrosine showed that unchallenged release of dopamine was elevated in individuals with schizophrenia compared to controls (Laruelle et al. 1996). Arvid Carlsson, the Nobel laureate, and his colleagues (2001), whose work led to the original dopamine hypothesis, appreciate the significance of this data but observe that a wide scatter exists with some values of dopamine release being within normal range in individuals with schizophrenia. They suggest that these findings may reflect heterogeneity where dopamine dysfunction may be limited to a subgroup of individuals with schizophrenia. Furthermore, the observation that the elevated dopamine release correlates with a good clinical response to antipsychotic medications leads Carlsson and colleagues to suggest that DA release may be state dependent such that studies done in acute conditions may yield different results than in a chronic remitted individual. However, it is also becoming clear that dopamine works closely with serotonin, glutamate, and other systems such that changes in one system affects the balance of the other systems too (see later).

Serotonin   Interest in serotonin as a pathophysiological candidate in schizophrenia arose in the 1950s with the discovery that the hallucinogen lysergic acid diethylamide (LSD) had primary effects on serotonin neurotransmission. Several studies were conducted to characterize its behavioral profile to determine whether LSD psychosis was a suitable model of schizophrenia. Indeed, LSD produces some features of schizophrenia, including a profound psychotic state, distractibility, social withdrawal, referential thinking, and delusions. However, the most prominent feature of LSD psychosis is visual hallucinations, and auditory hallucinations are exceedingly rare. Visual hallucinations are quite rare among individuals with schizophrenia and auditory hallucinations are among the most common symptoms of the illness. Thus, because of the failure to mimic key features of schizophrenia and the growing interest in dopamine at that time, enthusiasm for serotonin's involvement in the pathophysiology of schizophrenia waned for some time (Breier 1995).

Clozapine has a relatively high affinity for specific serotonin (5-hydroxytryptamine (5-HT)) receptors (5-HT$_{2A}$ and 5-HT$_{2C}$) and risperidone has even greater serotonin antagonistic properties (Schotte et al. 1996). Clozapine, risperidone, olanzapine, quetiapine, and ziprasidone, the novel antipsychotic agents, have a greater ratio of serotonin 5-HT$_{2A}$ to dopamine D$_2$ binding affinity. This has led to the hypothesis that the balance between serotonin and dopamine may be altered in schizophrenia (Meltzer et al. 1989c). Serotonin 5-HT$_{2A}$ (and other serotonin) receptor occupancy by the antipsychotic drugs, depending on the areas of the brain involved, could be associated with improvement in cognition, depression, and D$_2$ receptor-mediated EPS (Kasper et al. 1999).

In addition to the renewed interest in serotonin because of the action of new antipsychotic drugs, several postmortem studies have found elevations of serotonin and its metabolites in the striatum of individuals with schizophrenia. Again, as was the case with striatal D$_2$ receptors, previous neuroleptic exposure may have contributed to this finding. Another common finding is decreased 5-HT$_{2A}$ receptor densities in prefrontal cortex. Several postmortem studies (Gurevich and Joyce 1997, Burnet et al. 1997) and a recent *in vivo* PET study (Tauscher et al. 2002) have shown elevation of 5-HT$_{1A}$ receptor density in the cortex of individuals with schizophrenia. The relevance of these findings is not clear. Some, but not all, investigators have reported that the partial serotoninergic agonist *m*-chlorophenylpiperazine causes psychotic exacerbations in individuals with schizophrenia but has no psychosis-inducing properties in normal control subjects.

There has been an explosion of new information about the structure and function of 5-HT receptors (Breier 1995). To date, 15 serotonin receptor subtypes have been identified. Two receptors, 5-HT$_6$ and 5-HT$_7$, have been proposed as candidates for atypical drug action and are therefore reasonable targets for pathophysiological studies of schizophrenia. It is clear that the field is in the early stages of understanding the possible involvement of serotonin in schizophrenia.

Glutamate and N-Methyl-D-Aspartate Receptor

Glutamate is a major brain excitatory amino acid neurotransmitter and is critically involved in learning, memory, and brain development. There are five excitatory amino acid receptors in brain: *N*-methyl-D-aspartate (NMDA), AMPA, kainate, metabotropic, and L-AP-4. Interest in glutamate and the NMDA receptor in schizophrenia arose because of the similarity between PCP-induced psychosis and the psychosis of schizophrenia. PCP is a noncompetitive antagonist of the NMDA receptor and produces a psychotic state that includes conceptual disorganization, auditory hallucinations, delusions, and negative symptoms. PCP produces more symptoms that are similar to those of schizophrenia than most other pharmacological agents. It should be noted that PCP produces behaviors that are not commonly seen in schizophrenia as well, including spatial and temporal distortion, dreamlike states, and violence. Other findings that support a hypoglutamatergic function in schizophrenia are decreased glutamate levels in cerebrospinal fluid and increased NMDA receptor number and decreased glutamate binding in neocortex in postmortem studies.

PCP and other highly potent NMDA receptor antagonists, such as MK-801, cause neuronal damage and therefore are not used as research tools in clinical populations. However, ketamine, a widely used dissociative anesthetic, is another noncompetitive NMDA antagonist, and at subanesthetic doses, produces a PCP-like psychosis resembling schizophrenia (Krystal et al. 1994, Tamminga 1999). In a PET study of healthy volunteers, subanesthetic ketamine administration produced a robust psychotic state and focal activation of the prefrontal cortex, suggesting that prefrontal NMDA receptors may mediate this schizophrenia-like behavioral syndrome. The Glutamate hypothesis of schizophrenia is one of the most active areas of research currently. Postmortem studies have reported alterations in NMDA receptors or expression in certain brain areas of individuals with schizophrenia (Gao et al. 2000). NMDA receptor is reported to play a critical role in guiding axons to their final destination during neurodevelopment. Also, abnormalities with glutamate transmission are reported in many areas of the brain such as frontal cortex, hippocampus, limbic cortex, striatum, and thalamus. Moreover, there are changes reported in the gene expression also in these areas. In animal models of NMDA receptor antagonists, atypical antipsychotic agents are more effective in ameliorating symptoms (Gainetdinov et al. 2001). Thus, hypoglutamatergia in schizophrenia may have very important downstream modulatory effects on catecholaminergic neurotransmission and play a critical role during neurodevelopment. It also plays an important role in synaptic pruning and underlies important aspects of neurocognition.

GABA

GABA is the major inhibitory neurotransmitter in the brain. Support for GABA's involvement in schizophrenia comes from two lines of investigation. First, clinical trials have demonstrated that benzodiazepines, administered both in conjunction with antipsychotic drugs and as the sole treatment, are effective at reducing symptoms in subgroups of individuals with schizophrenia (Wolkowitz and Pickar 1991). Benzodiazepines are agonists at $GABA_A$ receptors. Second, postmortem studies have found a deficit in GABA interneurons in the anterior cingulum and prefrontal cortex and decreased GABA uptake sites in hippocampus (Benes et al. 1991). GABAergic neurons are especially vulnerable to glucocorticoid hormones and also to glutamatergic excitotoxicity.

Peptides   Several peptides have been hypothesized to play a pathophysiological role in schizophrenia. Interest in neurotensin arose because of the discovery that it is colocalized in some dopaminergic neurons and acts as a neuromodulator of this and other neurotransmitters. In preclinical studies, neurotensin was found to have effects that resembled those of antipsychotic drugs (Kasckow and Nemeroff 1991, Binder et al. 2001) and antipsychotic drugs cause increases in neurotensin levels in rat brain (Bisette et al. 1988). In addition, individuals with schizophrenia were found to have lower cerebrospinal fluid neurotensin levels than healthy control subjects and other individuals with neuropsychiatric disorders. Another peptide with neuromodulatory actions that was found to be colocalized with dopamine and was therefore of interest in relation to schizophrenia is cholecystokinin. Unlike the case of neurotensin, however, there has been a lack of consistent data from postmortem and cerebrospinal fluid studies of individuals with schizophrenia. Moreover, a clinical trial of CCK-8, a cholecystokinin analog, has failed to demonstrate antipsychotic efficacy (Montgomery and Green 1988). Other peptides that are under consideration for a pathophysiological role in schizophrenia are somatostatin, dynorphin, substance P, and neuropeptide Y.

Norepinephrine   Heightened noradrenergic function has been implicated in psychotic relapse in subgroups of individuals with schizophrenia (van Kammen et al. 1990). In addition, clozapine, but not other neuroleptic drugs, consistently produces increases in central and peripheral indices of noradrenergic function, and one study found a significant relationship between increases in plasma norepinephrine and improvement in positive symptoms (Breier et al. 1994).

Carlsson and colleagues (2001) provide a multineurotransmitter theory of schizophrenia which improves upon previous biochemical theories of schizophrenia. Accumulating evidence suggests that hyperdopaminergia in schizophrenia is probably secondary to some other phenomena. The data involving glutamatergic system suggests that NMDA receptor antagonism enhances the spontaneous and amphetamine-induced release of dopamine and thus raises the possibility that *hypoglutamatergia* could be related to the *hyperdopaminergia*. Carlsson and colleagues (2001) propose that psychotogenesis depends on an interaction between dopamine and glutamate pathways projecting to the striatum from the lower brain stem and cortex respectively. These neurotransmitters are predominantly antagonistic to each other, the former being inhibitory and the latter stimulatory when acting on striatal GABAergic projection neurons. These GABAergic neurons belong to striatothalamic pathways, which exert an inhibitory action on thalamocortical glutamatergic neurons, thereby filtering off part of the sensory input to the thalamus to protect the cortex from a sensory overload and hyperarousal. Hyperactivity of dopamine or hypofunction of the corticostriatal glutamate pathway should reduce this protective influence and could thus lead to confusion or psychosis. As a result, the indirect striatothalamic pathways have an inhibitory influence on the thalamus with the corresponding direct pathways exerting an opposite and excitatory influence. Both pathways are controlled by glutamatergic corticostriatal pathways enabling the cortex to regulate the thalamic gating in opposite directions. Thus, according to Carlsson and colleagues (2001), they appear to serve as *brakes* and *accelerators*.

It has been suggested that the activity of the direct pathways is predominantly phasic and of the indirect pathways is mainly tonic. This difference could have important consequences for a different responsiveness of the direct and indirect pathways to drugs. Thus the NMDA receptor antagonists are behavioral stimulants. AMPA receptor antagonists act in the same direction as NMDA antagonists in some and the opposite direction in other experiments. Thus, the two most important animal models of psychosis are those induced by hyperfunction of dopamine and hypofunction of glutamate. The relationship between glutamate and serotonin is very important and interesting. Serotonin appears to play a more important role than dopamine in the behavioral stimulation induced by hypoglutamatergia. In two models of psychosis, haloperidol is quite powerful in alleviating the hyperdopaminergic stimulation induced by amphetamine but is least efficacious in the hypoglutamatergic behavioral stimulation induced by MK-801. However, M100907, a selective serotonin 5-HT$_{2A}$ antagonist, is clearly more powerful in counteracting MK-801 than amphetamine-induced stimulation. These observations indicate that serotonin may play a more prominent role than dopamine in the behavioral stimulation induced by hypoglutamatergia. Schizophrenia is a syndrome of heterogeneous etiology and pathology. If one neurotransmitter is disturbed, it will inevitably have an impact on other neurotransmitters (Carlsson et al. 2001).

Neurodevelopmental versus Neurodegenerative Disease Processes

Neurodevelopmental hypotheses of schizophrenia posit that a disruption in normal development causes the illness (Weinberger 1987, Cannon et al. 2000). Thus, the "lesion" occurs well before the onset of the illness and interacts with maturation events such as neuronal precursor, glial proliferation and migration; axonal and dendritic proliferation; myelination of axons; programmed cell death and synaptic pruning (Lieberman 1999a); and is in all likelihood a nonprogressive disease process (Lewis 1997). Support for the neurodevelopment hypothesis includes the fact that the majority of individuals with schizophrenia do not have a course of illness marked by progressive deterioration such as found in dementias. In addition, brain morphological abnormalities commonly found in this illness, such as enlarged ventricles and reduced mesolimbic structures, do not appear to be progressive and, in fact, are present at the onset of the illness. Moreover, gliosis, which occurs during active pathological processes as part of the cellular reparative process in mature brains, is not commonly found in postmortem studies of schizophrenia.

That illness onset typically occurs in the teenage years and early twenties, as opposed to earlier in life when the proposed pathogenic insult occurs, has been explained by the fact that brain regions implicated in this illness, such as prefrontal cortex, are still undergoing myelination during the adolescent years and are therefore not fully functional until that time. Thus, an early lesion involving this region could remain silent until adolescence, when its normal functional capacity is expected to be realized. However, these assumptions have been questioned on the basis of the MRI findings of changes in the volume of brain areas in individuals with schizophrenia over a period of time (Woods 1998, Lieberman 1999b). As reviewed by Weinberger and McClure (2002), this has generated interest in the "neurodegenerative hypothesis" of schizophrenia as originally proposed by Kraepelin and others. However, based on the evidence available thus far, they suggest that it is unlikely that the MRI changes imply neurodegeneration. The argument is supported by the contradictory findings of clinical improvement in individuals in the face of progressive changes in MRI. Furthermore, the magnitude of the changes suggested by some of the MRI studies are large enough to be observed in neurodegenerative diseases like Alzheimer's without the postmortem evidence of neurodegeneration. Thus, Weinberger and McClure caution against overinterpretation of the MRI data without converging information from other areas. They suggest that there may be other possible explanations for these findings including physiological variations, neuroadaptation, and so on. Newer and more sophisticated techniques will help interpret MRI data more coherently.

Treatment

It could be argued that the successful treatment of schizophrenia requires a greater level of clinical knowledge and sophistication than the treatment of most other mental disorders and medical illnesses. It begins with the formation of a therapeutic relationship between the clinician and the individual with schizophrenia and must combine the latest developments in pharmacological and psychosocial therapeutics and interventions.

The relationship between the clinician and the patient is the foundation for treating individuals with schizophrenia. Because of the clinical manifestations of the illness, the formation of this relationship is often difficult. Paranoid delusions may lead to mistrust of the clinician. Conceptual disorganization and cognitive impairment make it difficult for individuals with schizophrenia to attend to what the clinician is saying and to follow even the simplest directions. Negative symptoms result in lack of emotional expression and social withdrawal, which can be demoralizing for the clinician who is attempting to "connect" with the individual.

It is important for the clinician to understand the ways in which the psychopathology of the illness affects the therapeutic relationship. The clinician should provide constancy to the individual with schizophrenia, which helps "anchor" individuals in their turbulent world. The qualities of the relationship should include consistency, acceptance, appropriate levels of warmth that respect the individual's needs for titrating emotional intensity, nonintrusiveness, and, most important, caring. "Old-fashioned" family doctors who know their patients well, are easily approachable, have a matter-of-fact style, attend to a broad range of needs, and are available and willing to reach out during crises provide a useful model for the relationship between the clinician and the patient in the treatment of schizophrenia.

Psychopharmacological Treatment

One hundred years ago, Philippe Pinel changed the philosophy of treating the mentally ill when he unchained patients and provided them with well-balanced diets in the hope that these interventions would ameliorate their symptoms (Weiner 1992). Attempts to treat these individuals medically included interventions such as insulin shock, dialysis, and frontal lobotomies. These methods appeared effective at times, yet it was clear that something else was needed to help the poorly understood symptoms of schizophrenia.

Although chlorpromazine had been around since the late 1800s, it was not until 1952 that it was first used to treat psychosis. The seminal work of Delay and Deniker (1952) provided a pharmacological strategy that would forever change the face of schizophrenia. The implementation of chlorpromazine became the turning point for psychopharmacology. Individuals who had been institutionalized for years were able to receive treatment as outpatients and live in community settings. The road was paved for the deinstitutionalization movement, and scientific understanding of the pathophysiology of schizophrenia burgeoned.

The discovery of chlorpromazine led to the development of other phenothiazines and new classes of antipsychotic medications, now totaling 11 different classes available in the US today. The word *neuroleptic*, literally "nerve cutting," was used to describe the tranquilizing effects of these medications. The enormous efforts to understand the mechanism of action of typical antipsychotics uncovered the intimate association of dopamine D_2 receptor blockade to the antipsychotic effects. This formed the basis of the hypothesis suggesting that symptoms of schizophrenia were possibly related to the hyperactivity of the (mesolimbic and mesocortical) dopaminergic systems in the brain. Antipsychotics developed subsequent to chlorpromazine such as haloperidol, thiothixene, and so on, were modeled on the (misguided) belief that induction of EPS was an integral part of having an antipsychotic efficacy. Over the years, another belief developed that all antipsychotics were similar in their efficacy and varied only in their side effects. However, clozapine challenged these beliefs by being significantly superior in efficacy than the existing antipsychotics and having minimal to no EPS! This started the era of antipsychotic agents being referred to as either *typical* (*conventional or traditional*) or *atypical* (*or novel*) antipsychotic drugs. If chlorpromazine started the first revolution in the psychopharmacological treatment of schizophrenia, then clozapine ushered in the second and more profound revolution whose impact is felt beyond schizophrenia and its full extent is yet to be realized. Moreover, clozapine has invigorated the psychopharmacology of schizophrenia and rekindled one of the most ambitious searches for new antipsychotic compounds by the pharmaceutical industry. Following approval of clozapine in 1990, FDA has already approved five novel antipsychotics—risperidone, olanzapine, quetiapine, ziprasidone, and aripiprazole.

Though clozapine, a dibenzodiazepine compound, was approved for use in the US in 1990, it had been available in European markets during the 1970s but had been found to be associated with agranulocytosis, a potentially fatal side effect, which led to its removal from clinical trials. The need for improved treatment of schizophrenia, particularly for individuals who do not respond to traditional neuroleptics, generated interest in resuming investigations of clozapine's clinical efficacy.

Double-blind, controlled studies demonstrated the superior clinical efficacy of clozapine compared to standard neuroleptics, without the associated EPS (Kane et al. 1988, Breier et al. 1994). It is clearly superior to traditional neuroleptics for psychosis. A summary of the US studies of individuals with chronic and treatment-resistant schizophrenia suggests that approximately 50% of individuals derive a better response from clozapine than from traditional neuroleptics (Table 27-2). Its effect on negative symptoms is somewhat controversial and has started an intense and a passionate debate as to whether the efficacy of the medication is with primary or secondary negative symptoms or both (Meltzer 1995, Carpenter et al. 1995). There is substantial evidence that clozapine decreases relapses, improves stability in the community, and diminishes suicidal behavior. There have also been reports that clozapine may cause a gradual reduction in preexisting tardive dyskinesia (Tamminga et al. 1994).

Unfortunately, clozapine is associated with agranulocytosis, and because of this risk, it requires weekly white blood cell testing. Approximately 0.8% of individuals taking clozapine and receiving weekly white blood cell monitoring develop agranulocytosis. Women and the elderly are at higher risk than other groups (Alvir et al. 1993). The period of highest risk is the first 6 months of treatment. These data have led to monitoring of white cell counts less frequently after first 6 months to every other week if a person has a history of white cell counts within normal range in the preceding 6 months. Current guidelines

Table 27-2	Clozapine Responder Rates in Chronic Schizophrenia: US Studies			
Study	**Number of Inpatients**	**Illness Severity**	**Trial Duration**	**Responders (%)**
Kane (1988)	126	++++	6 weeks	30
Meltzer (1990)	51	+++	6 months	61
Conley (1992)	25	++++	1 year	60
Wilson (1992)	37	++++	6 months	62
Breier (1993)	30	++	1 year	60
Zito (1993)	152	++++	1 year	43
Pickar (1994)	40	+++	4 months	50

state that the medication must be held back if the total white blood cell count is 3000/mm³ or less or if the absolute polymorphonuclear cell count is 1500/mm³ or less. Individuals who stop clozapine treatment continue to require blood monitoring for at least 4 weeks after the last dose according to current guidelines. Other side effects of clozapine include orthostatic hypotension, tachycardia, sialorrhea, sedation, elevated temperature, and weight gain (Baldessarini and Frankenburg 1991). Furthermore, clozapine can lower the seizure threshold in a dose-dependent fashion, with a higher risk of seizures seen particularly at doses greater than 600 mg/day.

Clozapine has an affinity for dopamine receptors (D_1, D_2, D_3, D_4, and D_5), serotonin receptors (5-HT_{2A}, 5-HT_{2C}, 5-HT_6, and 5-HT_7), alpha-1- and alpha-2-adrenergic receptors, nicotinic and muscarinic cholinergic receptors, and H_1 histaminergic receptors. As clozapine has a relatively shorter half-life, it is usually administered twice a day.

The superior antipsychotic efficacy of clozapine has inspired an abundance of research in the field of modern psychopharmacology for the treatment of schizophrenia. Clozapine and the other novel compounds have an array of biochemical profiles, with affinities to dopaminergic, serotoninergic, and noradrenergic receptors. Research on the atypical antipsychotic compounds has led to a greater understanding of the biochemical effects of antipsychotic agents, leaving the basic dopamine hypothesis of schizophrenia insufficient to explain schizophrenic symptoms. Clozapine shows selectivity for mesolimbic neurons and does not increase the prolactin level. Binding studies have shown it to be a relatively weak D_1 and D_2 antagonist, compared to traditional neuroleptics (Farde et al. 1989). Clozapine shares the property of higher serotonin 5-HT_{2A} to dopamine D_2 blockade ratio reported to impart atypicality. The noradrenergic system may also have a role in the mechanism of action of clozapine (Breier 1994). Clozapine, but not traditional neuroleptics, causes up to fivefold increases in plasma norepinephrine. Moreover, these increases in norepinephrine correlated with clinical response.

Following clozapine, risperidone was the first novel antipsychotic medication approved by FDA in 1994. Risperidone is a benzisoxazol compound with a high affinity for 5-HT_{2A} and D_2 receptors and has a high serotonin–dopamine receptor antagonism ratio. It has high affinity for alpha-1-adrenergic and H_1 histaminergic receptors and moderate affinity for alpha-2-adrenergic receptors. Risperidone is devoid of significant activity against the cholinergic system and the D_1 receptors. The efficacy of this medication is equal to that of other first-line atypical antipsychotic agents (Marder and Meibach 1994, Peuskens 1995) and is well tolerated and can be given once or twice a day. It is available in a liquid form as well. The most common side effects reported are drowsiness, orthostatic hypotension, lightheadedness, anxiety, akathisia, constipation, nausea, nasal congestion, prolactin elevation, and weight gain. At doses above 6 mg/day, EPS can become a significant issue. The risk of tardive dyskinesia at the regular therapeutic doses is low.

Olanzapine is a thienobenzodiazepine compound approved in 1996. It has antagonistic effects at dopamine D_1 through D_5 receptors and serotonin 5-HT_{2A}, 5-HT_{2C}, and 5-HT_6 receptors. The antiserotonergic activity is more potent than the antidopaminergic one. It also has affinity for alpha-1-adrenergic, M_1 muscarinic acetylcholinergic and H_1 histaminergic receptors. It differs from clozapine by not having high affinity for the 5-HT_7, alpha-2-adrenergic, and other cholinergic receptors (Bymaster et al. 1999). It has significant efficacy against positive and negative symptoms and also improves cognitive functions (Beasley et al. 1997). EPS is minimal when used in the therapeutic range with the exception of mild akathisia. As the compound has a long half-life, it is used once a day and as it is well tolerated, it can be started at a higher dose or rapidly titrated to the most effective dose. It is available as a rapidly disintegrating wafer form (Zyprexa Zydis), which dissolves immediately in the mouth. An intramuscular form has also been approved by FDA for agitation. The major side effects of olanzapine include weight gain, sedation, dry mouth, nausea, lightheadedness, orthostatic hypotension, dizziness, constipation, headache, akathisia, and transient elevation of hepatic transaminases. The risk of tardive dyskinesia and neuroleptic malignant syndrome (NMS) is low (Tollefson et al. 1997, Tran et al. 1997). Though used as a once-a-day medication, it is often administered twice a day with an average dose of 15 to 20 mg/day. However, doses higher than 20 mg/day are often used clinically and are thus being evaluated in clinical trials (Volavka et al. 2002, Lindenmayer et al. 2001, CATIE 1999).

Quetiapine, a dibenzothiazepine compound approved in 1997, has a greater affinity for serotonin 5-HT$_2$ receptors than for dopamine D$_2$ receptors; it has considerable activity at dopamine D$_1$, D$_5$, D$_3$, D$_4$, serotonin 5-HT$_{1A}$, and alpha-1-, alpha-2-adrenergic receptors. Unlike clozapine, it lacks affinity for the muscarinic cholinergic receptors. It is usually administered twice a day due to a short half-life. Quetiapine is as effective as typical agents and also appears to improve cognitive function. Among 2035 individuals enrolled in seven controlled studies, quetiapine at all doses used did not have an EPS rate greater than a placebo. This is in contrast to olanzapine, risperidone, and ziprasidone, where there were dose-related effects on EPS levels. The rate of treatment-emergent EPS was very low even in high at-risk populations such as adolescents, parkinsonian individuals with psychosis, and geriatric individuals. There was no elevation of prolactin (Kasper and Muller-Spahn 2001). Major side effects include somnolence, postural hypotension, dizziness, agitation, dry mouth, and weight gain (Small et al. 1997). Akathisia occurs on rare occasions. The package insert warns about developing lenticular opacity or cataracts and advises periodic eye examination based on data from animal studies. However, recent data suggest that this risk may be minimal.

Ziprasidone, approved by FDA in 2001, has the strongest 5-HT$_{2A}$ receptor binding relative to D$_2$ binding amongst the atypical agents currently in use. Interestingly, ziprasidone has 5-HT$_{1A}$ agonist and 5-HT$_{1D}$ antagonist properties with a high affinity for 5-HT$_{1A}$, 5-HT$_{2C}$, and 5-HT$_{1D}$ receptors. As it does not interact with many other neurotransmitter systems, it does not cause anticholinergic side effects and produces little orthostatic hypotension and relatively little sedation. Just like some antidepressants, ziprasidone blocks presynaptic reuptake of serotonin and norepinephrine. Ziprasidone has a relatively short half-life and thus it should be administered twice a day and along with food for best absorption. Ziprasidone is not completely dependent on CYP3A4 system for metabolism, thus inhibitors of the cytochrome system do not significantly change the blood levels. Data for efficacy, side effects, and dosing come from a number of studies (Keck et al. 1998, Daniel et al. 1999, Goff et al. 1998, Arato et al. 1998). Ziprasidone at doses between 80 and 160 mg/day is probably the most effective for treating symptoms of schizophrenia. To assess the cardiac risk of ziprasidone and other antipsychotic agents, Pfizer and FDA designed a landmark study to evaluate the cardiac safety of the antipsychotic agents, given at high doses alone and with a known metabolic inhibitor in a randomized study involving individuals with schizophrenia. This was done to replicate the possible worst-case scenario (overdose or dangerous combination treatment) in the real world. All antipsychotic agents studied caused some degree of QTc prolongation. Oral form of haloperidol was associated with the least and thioridazine with the greatest change (Figure 27-1). Major side effects reported with the use of ziprasidone are somnolence, nausea, insomnia, dyspepsia, and prolongation of QTc interval. Dizziness, weakness, nasal discharge, orthostatic hypotension, and tachycardia occur less commonly.

Ziprasidone should not be used in combination with other drugs that cause *significant* prolongation of the QTc interval. It is also contraindicated for individuals with a known history of significant QTc prolongation, recent myocardial infarction, or symptomatic heart failure. Ziprasidone has low EPS potential, does not elevate prolactin levels, and causes approximately 1-lb weight gain in short-term studies (Allison et al. 1999).

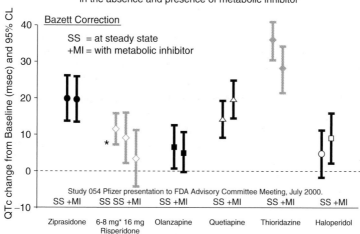

Figure 27-1 *Study 054 was an open label, parallel-group study in patients with schizophrenia to assess the effect of oral doses of ziprasidone, risperidone, olanzapine, quetiapine, thioridazine and haloperidol on the QT interval of the EKG. EKGs were measured to correspond to T_{max} of the given drug. There were 25 patients per group. The highest dose for each drug was reached on the basis of US package insert. For Risperidone, two different doses were used on the basis of common practice of using lower than approved doses. Later in the study, a CYP 450 metabolism inhibitor was coadministered and EKGs were obtained. QTc was calculated using Bazett's correction. Data from this study resulted in "black box" warning from FDA for mesoridazine and thioridazine. (FDA Psychopharmacological Drugs Advisory Committee: Briefing documents for ziprasidone, July 2000.) (Source: Pfizer Pharmaceuticals and www.fda.gov/ohrms/dockets/ac/00&col;/backgrd/361961a.pdf).*

Aripiprazole was approved by the FDA for the treatment of schizophrenia in 2003. It has a unique pharmacodynamic profile compared to the other atypical neuroleptics—partial agonist activity (rather than full antagonist activity) at both dopaminergic (D_2) (Burris et al. 2002) and serotonergic (5-HT_{1A}) (Jordan et al. 2002) receptors and full antagonist activity at (5-HT_{2A}) receptions (McQuade et al. 2002). The efficacy of aripiperazole as a treatment for the acute relapse of schizophrenia was demonstrated in four short-term, double-blind, placebo-controlled trials; among them was a pivotal multicenter study comparing aripiprazole (15 or 30 mg) with placebo (Kane et al. 2002). The recommended starting and target dose is 10–15 mg a day. The most commonly reported adverse events from a pooled analysis of safety and tolerability data (Marder et al. 2003) were headache, insomnia, agitation, and anxiety, but these were also the most frequently reported events in the placebo, haloperidol, and risperidone comparison groups. The incidence of adverse events was similar in the aripiperazole and placebo groups. There was also a similar incidence of EPS-related adverse events in the aripiperazole and placebo groups. There were also only minimal changes in mean body weight and no increases in prolactin level.

At present, with respect to efficacy, it does not appear that any one of the novel antipsychotic agents (except clozapine) is better than another one in treating schizophrenia. The randomized controlled trials suggest that, on average, these antipsychotic agents are each associated with 20% improvement in symptoms. However, clozapine is the only new antipsychotic agent that is more effective than haloperidol in managing treatment-resistant schizophrenia (Kane et al. 1988, 2001). Unfortunately, its potential for treatment-emergent agranulocytosis, seizures, and the new warning of myocarditis precludes its use as a first-line agent for schizophrenia. A major difference amongst the newer antipsychotic agents is the side effect profile and its effect on the overall quality of life of the individual.

Acute Treatment   Until recently, the typical antipsychotics were the mainstay of the treatment for acute episodes of psychosis. In the last few years, the use of novel antipsychotics has surpassed the use of typical ones in the management of acute phase symptoms of schizophrenia, except for the use of parenteral and liquid forms of antipsychotics where typical antipsychotic agents still hold an upper hand. However, this trend will most likely change once the injectable preparations of the novel antipsychotics enter the market starting with olanzapine (already approved by FDA) (Breier et al. 2002) and followed by ziprasidone and aripiprazole. The primary goal of acute treatment is the amelioration of any behavioral disturbances that would put the individual or others at risk of harm. Acute symptom presentation or relapses are heralded by the recurrence of positive symptoms, including delusions, hallucinations, disorganized speech or behavior, severe negative symptoms, or catatonia. Quite frequently, a relapse is a result of antipsychotic discontinuation, and resumption of antipsychotic treatment aids in the resolution of symptoms. There is a high degree of variability in response rates among individuals. When treatment is initiated, improvement in clinical symptoms can be seen over hours, days, or weeks of treatment.

Studies have shown that although typical neuroleptics are undoubtedly effective, a significant percentage (between 20 and 40%) of individuals show only a poor or partial response to traditional agents (Cole et al. 1964, Kane 1987). Furthermore, there is no convincing evidence that one typical antipsychotic is more efficacious as an antipsychotic than any other, although a given individual may respond better to a specific drug. Once an informed choice has been made between using a novel or a typical antipsychotic medication by the patient and the clinician, selection of a specific antipsychotic agent should be based on efficacy, side effect profile, history of prior response (or nonresponse) to a specific agent, or history of response of a family member to a certain antipsychotic agent. (For a pharmacotherapy decision tree based on Texas Medication Algorithm Project, see Figure 27-2.) Amongst the typical antipsychotic medications, low-potency, more sedating agents, such as chlorpromazine, were long thought to be more effective for agitated individuals, yet there are no consistent data proving that high-potency agents are not equally useful in this context. The low-potency antipsychotics, however, are more associated with orthostatic hypotension and lowered seizure threshold and are often not as well tolerated at higher doses. Higher potency neuroleptics, such as haloperidol and fluphenazine, are safely used at higher doses and are effective in reducing psychotic agitation and psychosis itself. However, they are more likely to cause EPS than the low-potency agents.

The efficacy of novel antipsychotic drugs on positive and negative symptoms is comparable to or even better than the typical antipsychotic drugs (Robinson et al. 1999, Aravantis and Miller 1997, Beasley et al. 1997, Peuskens and Link 1997, Small et al. 1997, Tollefson et al. 1997, Borison et al. 1996, Fabre et al. 1995, Marder and Meibach 1994, Ceskova and Svestka 1993, Chouinard et al. 1993, Hoyberg et al. 1993, Lieberman et al. 1993, Chakos et al. 2001, Geddes et al. 2000). The significantly low potential to cause EPS or dystonic reaction and thus the decreased long-term consequences of TD has made the novel agents more tolerable and acceptable in acute treatment of schizophrenia. Other significant advantages adding to the popularity of novel antipsychotics include their beneficial impact on mood symptoms, suicidal risk, and cognition. The selection of the first-line treatment with novel antipsychotic (and occasionally typical antipsychotic agent) also depends on the circumstances under which the medications are started, for example, extremely agitated or catatonic individuals would require intramuscular preparation of the antipsychotic agents, which would limit the choice. Except for clozapine, which is not considered first-line treatment because of substantial and potentially life-threatening side effects, there is no convincing data supporting the preference of one atypical antipsychotic over the other. However, if the individual does not respond to one, a trial with another atypical antipsychotic is reasonable and may produce response.

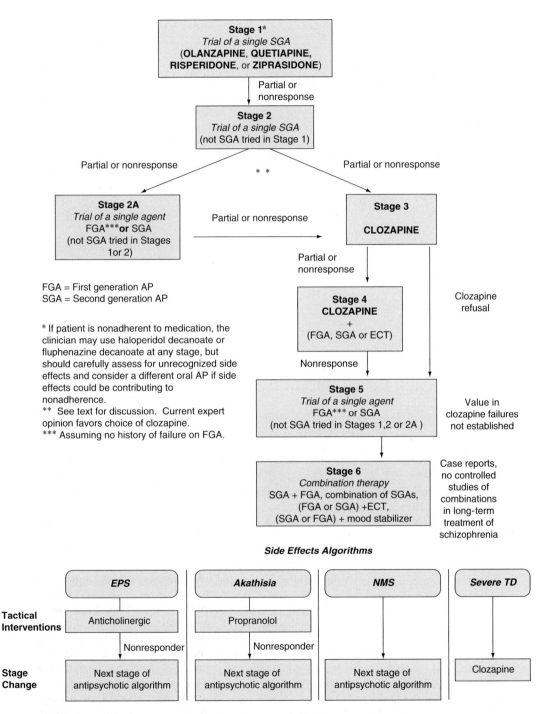

Figure 27-2 *Selecting antipsychotic treatment using Texas medication algorithm for schizophrenia. Choice of antipsychotic (AP) should be guided by considering the clinical characteristics of the patient and the efficacy and side effect profiles of the medication. Any stage(s) can be skipped depending on the clinical picture or history of antipsychotic failures. Texas medication algorithm project for choosing antipsychotic treatment, managing side effects, and coexisting symptoms. This project is a public–academic collaborative effort to develop, implement, and evaluate medication treatment algorithms for public sector patients. For more information or to view the most current version of the algorithm, visit www.mhmr.state.tx.us/centraloffice/medicaldirector/tmaptoc.html).*

Coexisting Symptoms Algorithms

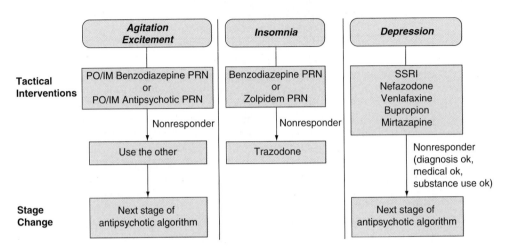

Figure 27-2 *(Continued).*

Once the decision is made to use an antipsychotic agent, an appropriate dose must be selected. Initially, higher doses or repeated dosing may be helpful in preventing grossly psychotic and agitated individuals from doing harm. In general, there is no clear evidence that higher doses of neuroleptics (more than 2000 mg chlorpromazine equivalents per day) have any advantage over standard doses (400–600 chlorpromazine equivalents per day) (Kane 1987).

In an open trial, 80 schizophrenia inpatients were assigned to receive haloperidol at a dose of 5, 10, or 20 mg/day for 4 weeks (Van Putten et al. 1990). In this study, the individuals receiving the highest dose of haloperidol initially demonstrated the most effective treatment of psychotic symptoms, but they were later found to have a higher incidence of EPS and emotional withdrawal. In a 6-week double-blind randomized study of 31 nonchronic treatment-refractory individuals with schizophrenia standard doses of fluphenazine (20 mg/day) led to greater clinical improvement than very high doses (up to 120 mg/day) (Quitkin et al. 1975). EPS seemed to account in part for the poorer response rate in the group treated with the higher doses. In general, the studies indicated that doses of high-potency neuroleptics such as haloperidol can be maintained at a total of 10 mg/day in an acute setting, and that there is no generalizable benefit of using higher doses. Early adjuvant treatment with anticholinergic medication may facilitate compliance with medication by decreasing intolerable side effects.

Some individuals who are extremely agitated or aggressive may benefit from concomitant administration of high-potency benzodiazepines such as lorazepam, at 1 to 2 mg, until they are stable. Benzodiazepines rapidly decrease anxiety, calm the person, and help with sedation to break the cycle of agitation. They also help decrease agitation due to akathisia. The use of these medications should be limited to the acute stages of the illness to prevent tachyphylaxis and dependency. Benzodiazepines are quite beneficial in the treatment of catatonic or mute individuals but the results are only temporary though of enough duration to help with body functions and nutrition.

Maintenance Treatment   There is by now a great deal of evidence from long-term follow-up studies that individuals with schizophrenia have a higher risk of relapse and exacerbations if not maintained with adequate antipsychotic regimens (Hogarty et al. 1974,

Davis 1975). Noncompliance with medication, possibly because of intolerable neuroleptic side effects, may contribute to increased relapse rates. In a double-blind placebo-controlled study of relapse rates, 50% of patients in a research ward demonstrated clinically significant exacerbation of their symptoms within 3 weeks of stopping neuroleptic treatment (Pickar and Pinals 1995). Furthermore, in a comprehensive review of the literature on neuroleptic withdrawal examining 4365 subjects, 53.2% of individuals withdrawn from neuroleptics relapsed, compared with 15.6% of control subjects who were maintained with neuroleptic treatment (Gilbert et al. 1995). The length of follow-up was related to the risk of relapse. Unfortunately, in this review there were no clear demographical or clinical characteristics that consistently predicted relapse. Others have estimated that two-thirds of individuals relapse after 9 to 12 months without neuroleptic medication, compared with 10 to 30% who relapse when *typical* neuroleptics are maintained (Straube and Oades 1992). Long-term outcome studies showed that persistent symptoms that do not respond to standard neuroleptic therapy are associated with a greater risk of rehospitalization (Breier et al. 1991). Nonpharmacological interventions may help decrease relapse rates.

Long-term treatment of schizophrenia is a complex issue. It is clear that the majority of individuals require maintenance medication. Some individuals do well with stable doses of neuroleptics for years without any exacerbations. However, many individuals who are maintained with a stable neuroleptic dose have episodic breakthroughs of their psychotic symptoms. In a study by Hogarty and associates (1974), 374 schizophrenic individuals were followed up for 2 years after hospitalization and randomized to receive placebo alone, placebo and sociotherapy, chlorpromazine alone, or chlorpromazine and sociotherapy. In this study, the placebo-only group had a relapse rate that was almost twice that of the chlorpromazine-treated group. Unfortunately, the difficulty in tolerating neuroleptic side effects often results in noncompliance with medication. Furthermore, intensive case management and rehabilitation counseling did prevent relapse but only after a delayed period. Sociotherapy and drug treatment were found to have additive effects in preventing relapse.

Given the findings of Hogarty and colleagues, it would be prudent to assess individuals for medication compliance when signs of relapse are suspected. Prodromal cues may be present before an exacerbation of psychotic symptoms. For example, any recent change in sleep, attention to activities of daily living, or disorganization may be a warning sign of an impending increase in psychosis.

With the increased use of novel antipsychotics, it is widely anticipated that compliance will improve proportionately due to significantly less neurological side effects and possible beneficial effects on negative symptoms and neurocognition. In a landmark study comparing risperidone to haloperidol for effects on maintenance treatment, at the end of 1 year, individuals taking risperidone were significantly better clinically, more individuals were compliant with it and fewer individuals had relapses. In this double-blind prospective study, 397 stable outpatients were randomized to receive either risperidone or haloperidol for a minimum of 1 year. The Kaplan–Meier estimate of the risk of relapse at the end of study was 34% for the risperidone group and 60% for the haloperidol group. Early discontinuation of treatment for any reason was more frequent among haloperidol-treated individuals. The risperidone group had greater reductions in the mean severity of both psychotic symptoms and extrapyramidal side effects than those in the haloperidol group (Csernansky et al. 2002). This led to an FDA indication for its use in maintenance treatment. Olanzapine, at 5 to 15 mg/day has been reported to be superior to placebo and olanzapine 1 mg/day in preventing relapses in a 1-year double-blind study (Dellva et al. 1997). Long-term use of quetiapine and ziprasidone are also reported to have significant beneficial effects. The data from treatment with clozapine suggest its significant superiority compared to other treatments. In treatment-refractory individuals, long-term randomized trials found significant reduction in rehospitalization (Essock et al. 1996, Rosenheck et al. 1997) and suicide rates (Meltzer and Okayli 1995).

For individuals for whom compliance is a problem, long-acting, depot neuroleptics are available in the US for both fluphenazine and haloperidol. The antipsychotic drug is esterified in an oily solution, which is injected every 1 to 6 weeks to circumvent the need for daily oral antipsychotic medications in most cases (although some individuals benefit from adjuvant oral medication). This form of medication delivery guarantees that the medication is in the system of the person taking it and eliminates the need to monitor daily compliance. This alternative should be considered if noncompliance with oral agents has led to relapses and rehospitalization. With these individuals, maintenance treatment using long-acting preparations should begin as early as possible (Barnes and Curson 1994). In a meta-analysis done by Adams and colleagues (2001), 3348 individuals were randomized in trials of fluphenazine decanoate. The study attrition rates were remarkably low at only 14% of those randomized compared to 40 to 60% in trials of oral atypical antipsychotic agents (Thornley and Adams 1998). Depot antipsychotic drugs are effective maintenance therapy for individuals with schizophrenia. However, currently we only have esters of typical antipsychotic agents and thus the significantly elevated risk of bothersome neurological side effects is an unfortunate limitation to their use. Fortunately, novel antipsychotic depot preparations are currently being investigated.

Many studies have investigated appropriate maintenance doses of standard antipsychotics. Effective maintenance treatment is defined as that which prevents or minimizes the risks of symptom exacerbation and subsequent morbidity. A series of interesting dose-finding studies were performed by Kane and colleagues (1983, 1985) to determine the minimal dosage required to prevent relapse and to reduce the risk of EPS and tardive dyskinesia. This group found that the relapse rate (56%) of individuals treated with lower doses of fluphenazine decanoate (1.25–5 mg every 2 weeks) was significantly greater than the relapse rate (14%) of individuals receiving standard doses (12.5–50 mg every 2 weeks). Other investigators have found that this low dosage range may appear to prevent relapse for a certain period (Marder et al. 1984) but fails to do so if individuals are followed up for more than 1 year (Marder et al. 1987). Unfortunately, no specific dosage reliably prevents relapse, and there is no way to predict future relapse. This is true for the novel antipsychotic agents as well.

Plasma drug levels and their correlation with clinical response have also been considered in determining dosage requirements. However, the results remain controversial. Some studies have found that levels that were in excess of a certain therapeutic window led to an exacerbation of symptoms (Kane 1987). There is no strong evidence with which to sort out whether this finding was indeed a result of higher plasma levels, secondary to higher dosing for treatment-resistant individuals, or due to the fact that the side effects associated with higher doses of neuroleptics may mimic exacerbations of the primary illness (Kane 1987). At this time, plasma drug levels are not recommended for dosage determination. They are clinically useful, however, for confirming compliance with medication and may provide information regarding toxicity or altered metabolism.

Depression and Schizophrenia Symptoms of depression occur in a substantial percentage of individuals with schizophrenia with a wide range of 7 to 75% and a modal rate of 25% and is associated with poor outcome, impaired functioning, suffering, higher rates of relapse or rehospitalization, and suicide (Heila et al. 1997, Siris 2000, Addington et al. 2002). It is important to distinguish depression as a symptom or as a syndrome when it occurs. There is an important overlap of symptoms of depression with the negative symptoms. Differentiating these states can sometimes be difficult, especially in individuals who lack the interpersonal communication skills to articulate their internal subjective states well. A link between typical antipsychotic use and depression has been suggested with some considering depression to be a form of medication-induced akinesia. Many individuals have a reaction of disappointment, a sense of loss or powerlessness, or awareness of psychotic symptoms or psychological deficits that contributes to depression

(Lysaker et al. 1995). Depression in schizophrenia is heterogeneous and requires careful diagnostic clarification. DSM-IV-TR suggests that the term *postpsychotic depression* be used to describe depression that occurs at any time after a psychotic episode of schizophrenia, even after a prolonged interval. The atypical antipsychotic medications, with less potential to cause motor side effects and different mechanisms of action at receptor levels, themselves may contribute substantially towards a decrease in the rate of depression. Moreover, the atypical antipsychotic medications appear to be superior to standard neuroleptics in treatment of negative symptoms (Tandon et al. 1997, Borison et al. 1996, Beasley et al. 1996, Buchanan 1995, Franz et al. 1997). The clear advantage of atypical antipsychotic medications over the typical ones in treatment of psychosis itself can possibly further decrease the rate of depression. The impact of clozapine on the rate of suicide is significantly superior compared to the conventional agents (Meltzer and Okayli 1995). However, a large number of individuals still end up with a depression that will require treatment with an antidepressant.

Risks and Side Effects of Typical Neuroleptics   Extrapyramidal symptoms (EPS) are side effects of typical antipsychotic medications that include dystonias, oculogyric crisis, pseudoparkinsonism, akinesia, and akathisia. They are referred to collectively as EPS because they are mediated at least in part by dopaminergic transmission in the extrapyramidal system. Prevalence rates vary among the different types of EPS. When present, they can be uncomfortable for the individual and a reason for noncompliance.

Dystonias are involuntary muscular spasms that can be brief or sustained, involving any muscle group. They can occur with even a single dose of medication (Ayd 1961). When they develop suddenly, these spasms can be quite frightening to the individual and potentially dangerous, as in the case of laryngeal dystonias. They are more likely to be seen in young individuals. Studies differ as to whether the prevalence is higher in males (Boyer et al. 1987) or females (Chakos et al. 1992). Prevalence rates for dystonias secondary to typical neuroleptic exposure range from 2 to 20% (Marsden et al. 1986).

Pseudoparkinsonism and akinesia are characterized by muscular rigidity, tremor, and bradykinesia, much as in Parkinson's disease. On examination, individuals typically have masked facies, cogwheel rigidity, slowing, and decreased arm swing with a shuffling gait. This condition is reported to be more prevalent than the dystonias, presenting with a frequency ranging from 15% (Ayd 1961, Marsden et al. 1986) to 35% (Chakos et al. 1992).

Akathisia is more common, affecting more than 20% of individuals taking neuroleptic medications (Ayd 1961, Marsden et al. 1986). This clinical entity presents as motor restlessness or an internal sense of restlessness. Often, individuals experiencing akathisia are unable to sit still during an interview. Akathisia is difficult to differentiate from agitation. The tendency to treat agitation with neuroleptics may exacerbate akathisia, making treatment decisions challenging.

Treatment of EPS can be difficult but usually involves administration of anticholinergic medications. Some advocate the use of prophylactic anticholinergic agents when beginning typical neuroleptic treatment to decrease the incidence of EPS. This option may be appropriate, but it should be used with caution, considering the side effects associated with anticholinergic agents (Levinson 1991) and their potential for abuse (Land et al. 1991).

Treatment of acute dystonic reactions usually involves acute intramuscular administration of either an anticholinergic or diphenhydramine. Akathisia may not respond to anticholinergic medications. Both neuroleptic dosage reduction and the use of beta-blocking agents such as propranolol have been found to be efficacious in the treatment of akathisia.

Nonextrapyramidal side effects of the typical antipsychotic agents include those that are secondary to blockade of muscarinic, histaminic, and alpha-adrenergic receptors. These side effects, which are more commonly seen with the low-potency neuroleptics, include sedation, tachycardia, and anticholinergic side effects such as urinary hesitancy or retention, blurred vision, or constipation. Other nonextrapyramidal side effects include some cardiac conduction disturbances, retinal changes, sexual dysfunction, weight gain, lowered seizure threshold, and a risk of agranulocytosis.

Neuroleptic malignant syndrome (NMS) is a relatively rare but serious phenomenon seen in approximately 1% of individuals taking neuroleptics (Dickey 1991). It can be fatal in 15% of cases if not properly recognized and treated (Levinson 1991, Dickey 1991). Because the symptoms of NMS may reflect multiple etiologies, making diagnosis difficult, Levenson (Levenson 1985) has proposed clinical guidelines. According to Levenson, three or two major and four minor manifestations are indicative of a high probability of NMS. Major manifestations of NMS comprise fever, rigidity, and increased creatine kinase levels, and minor manifestations include tachycardia, abnormal blood pressure, tachypnea, altered consciousness, diaphoresis, and leukocytosis. Others do not subscribe to the major–minor manifestation distinctions. In general, NMS is considered to be a constellation of symptoms that usually develops during 1 to 3 days. Although its pathogenesis is poorly understood, it has been associated with all antidopaminergic neuroleptic agents and presents at any time during treatment. It must be distinguished from other clinical entities, including lethal catatonia and malignant hyperthermia (Dickey 1991).

The mainstay of treatment is cessation of neuroleptic treatment and supportive care, including intravenous hydration, reversal of fever with antipyretics and cooling blankets, and careful monitoring of vital signs because of the risk of cardiac and respiratory disturbance. Rhabdomyolysis is one of the most serious sequelae of NMS; it can lead to renal failure unless individuals are well hydrated (Levenson 1985). In some cases, dantrolene and bromocriptine have been reported to be effective pharmacological treatments (Granato et al. 1983). Though quite rare, NMS has been reported even with the use of novel antipsychotic agents. The decision to rechallenge the individual with neuroleptics after an episode of NMS must be made with caution.

One of the major risks of neuroleptic treatment with the traditional antipsychotic agents is that of tardive dyskinesia, a potentially irreversible syndrome of involuntary choreoathetoid movements and chronic dystonias associated with long-term neuroleptic exposure. These buccal, orofacial, truncal, or limb movements can be exacerbated by anxiety and disappear during sleep. They can present with a range of severity, from subtle tongue movements to truncal twisting and pelvic thrusting movements and even possible respiratory dyskinesias. The prevalence rates for this syndrome range from less than 10% to more than 50% (American Psychiatric Association Task Force 1980), but it is generally accepted that the risk increases 3 to 5% per year for each year the individual is treated with typical neuroleptics (Kane et al. 1988). Older age is a considerable risk factor for tardive dyskinesia, and there is some evidence that women are at increased risk for the development of this condition (American Psychiatric Association Task Force 1980). Of note, a withdrawal dyskinesia that resembles tardive dyskinesia may appear on cessation of the neuroleptic. The specific mechanism involved in tardive dyskinesia remains unclear, although supersensitivity of dopaminergic receptors has been implicated.

All individuals receiving traditional neuroleptic treatment should be monitored regularly for any signs of a movement disorder. DSM-IV-TR includes a diagnosis of neuroleptic-induced tardive dyskinesia. If tardive dyskinesia is suspected, the benefits of antipsychotic treatment must be carefully weighed against the risk of tardive dyskinesia. This should be discussed with the individual, and the antipsychotic should be removed if clinically feasible or at least maintained at the lowest possible dose that provides antipsychotic effect. This would also be an indication to switch to the novel antipsychotic agents with significantly reduced risk of TD or in the case of clozapine no risk of TD. In many instances, clozapine (and possibly quetiapine or olanzapine) may be the best treatment that can be offered for the TD itself (Tamminga et al. 1994). Unfortunately, there is no specific treatment of tardive dyskinesia, although some investigators have proposed the use of adrenergic agents such as clonidine, calcium channel blockers, vitamin E, benzodiazepines, valproic acid, or reserpine to reduce the spontaneous movements (American Psychiatric Association Task Force 1980).

Sudden death in psychiatric patients treated with typical antipsychotic drugs has been reported for a long time (Hollister and Kosek 1965). Sudden cardiac deaths probably occur from prolongation of the ventricular action potential duration represented as the QT interval (or QTc when corrected for heart rate) on the electrocardiogram resulting in a polymorphic ventricular tachycardia termed *torsades de pointes* that can degenerate into ventricular fibrillation (Tamargo 2000). The incidence of *torsades de pointes* is unknown and the specific duration of the QTc interval at which the risk of an adverse cardiac event is greatest has not been established. QTc prolongation alone does not appear to explain *torsades de pointes*; several other risk factors must be present simultaneously with QT prolongation before *torsades de pointes* occurs. These risk factors may include hypokalemia, hypomagnesemia, hypocalcemia, bradycardia, preexisting cardiac diseases (life-threatening arrhythmias, cardiac hypertrophy, heart failure, and congenital QT syndrome), female gender, advancing age, baseline QTc interval of more than 460 m/s and a long list of medications (Tamargo 2000). In some instances, *torsades de pointes* may be associated with an increase in drug plasma concentrations (e.g., combination with drugs that inhibit the cytochrome P450 systems) (Tamargo 2000, Yap and Camm 2000). Thus, the increase in polypharmacy in psychiatry is especially of concern (Frye et al. 2000). The frequency of ECG abnormalities in individuals treated with antipsychotic drugs is unclear (Warner et al. 1996, Mehtonen et al. 1991). QTc prolongation has been reported with virtually all antipsychotic drugs (Thomas 1994, Cohen et al. 2000, Czekalla et al. 2001). QTc prolongation by more than 2 standard deviations was reported in 8% of individuals treated with antipsychotics and especially in those receiving thioridazine (Ray et al. 2001). Of the typical antipsychotic drugs, haloperidol, chlorpromazine, trifluoperazine, mesoridazine, prochlorperazine, droperidol, and fluphenazine have all been reported to cause QTc prolongation and *torsades de pointes*, but thioridazine may be the worst offender (Buckley et al. 1995, Haverkamp et al. 2000, Ray et al. 2001). Pimozide, another typical antipsychotic, has also been associated with QTc prolongation, *torsades de pointes*, and deaths (Committee on Safety of Medicines and Medicines Control Agency 1995). A reevaluation by the FDA of the cardiac safety parameters of thioridazine, mesoridazine, and droperidol resulted in a black box warning due to significant QTc prolongation. Thus, it is important to monitor QTc interval in the high-risk population to prevent this rare, but potentially fatal side effect.

Side Effects of Atypical Antipsychotic Agents

One of the most significant advantages of the newer antipsychotic agent is the relatively less risk of developing EPS and TD. However, treatment-emergent substantial weight gain is a harbinger for long-term health consequences and frequently an important reason for noncompliance with medication. According to a meta-analysis done by Allison and colleagues (1999), clozapine and olanzapine are associated with a weight gain of about 10 lb over 10 weeks and ziprasidone was among the agents with the lowest weight gain at an average of 1 lb over the same period. Risperidone and quetiapine are intermediate with approximately 5 lb. Individuals with schizophrenia, independent of the use of antipsychotic agents are at higher risk of developing diabetes mellitus relative to the general population (Fucetola et al. 1999, Dixon et al. 2000, Thakore et al. 2002). The data from Patient Outcome Research Team (PORT) suggest that the rate of diabetes mellitus and obesity amongst individuals with major mental illness was substantially higher even before the advent of the novel antipsychotic drugs. This was more so in women and nonwhite population (Dixon et al. 2000). Thakore and colleagues (2002) investigated visceral fat distribution in drug-naïve and drug-free individuals with schizophrenia. Compared to controls, individuals with schizophrenia had central obesity and significantly higher levels of plasma cortisol. Thus individuals with schizophrenia are at a higher risk to develop major medical problems even before they are exposed to antipsychotic medications. However, this risk has been exacerbated with the introduction of the novel antipsychotic agents as seen by the dramatic rise in the number of published cases and reports of significant hyperglycemia associated with the use of these medications, particularly olanzapine and clozapine (Masand 2000, Wirshing et al. 1998, Henderson et al. 2000, Hagg et al. 1998, Newcomer et al. 2002) and a few reports with quetiapine (Procyshyn et al. 2000) and risperidone (Haupt and Newcomer 2001). The risk of antipsychotic-induced weight gain and secondary diabetes with clozapine and olanzapine may result from changes in glucose metabolism and insulin resistance induced by these agents. In approximately 40% of the cases of hyperglycemia, insulin resistance appears to occur even in the absence of significant weight gain, raising some interesting questions about how these medications may interact with the insulin-glycemic control (e.g. Wirshing et al. 1998, Hagg et al. 1998, Newcomer et al. 2002). Unfortunately, in the case of clozapine, the risk of developing abnormal glucose and diabetes mellitus appears to be cumulative over the years as reported by Henderson and colleagues (2000). There are no effective countermeasures available to help with weight gain and hyperglycemia. The substantial increased risk to the health of individuals with schizophrenia due to these effects is worrisome and an important shortcoming of these efficacious and important medications.

Amongst the novel agents, risperidone, due to its potent dopamine D_2 blockade, removes the inhibitory dopaminergic tone in the tuberoinfundibular neurons resulting in significant increase in prolactin levels. This increase in prolactin is significantly more than usually seen with the typical antipsychotic agents. It is likely that the serotonin system is also involved along with dopamine in raising the prolactin levels. Clozapine and quetiapine, on the other hand, are less potent at the D_2 receptors and thus are unlikely to cause prolactin elevations. In some individuals, these elevations of prolactin lead to amenorrhea, galactorrhea, gynecomastia, and may possibly decrease bone mineral density. Ziprasidone and olanzapine, within the therapeutic dose range do not cause significant increases in prolactin levels.

Cases of sudden death while receiving clozapine therapy (in physically healthy young adults with schizophrenia) from myocarditis and cardiomyopathy (Kilian et al. 1999, Modai et al. 2000, Grenade et al. 2001) led to a black box warning from FDA.

Treatment Resistance and Negative Symptoms   The concept of treatment resistance has entered into common clinical judgment with the burgeoning interest in atypical antipsychotics, particularly clozapine. Treatment resistance was originally defined for research purposes (Kane et al. 1988). Individuals who had failed to respond to or could not tolerate adequate trials of standard neuroleptics from three different biochemical classes and who had a clinically significant psychopathology rating based on the Brief Psychiatric Rating Scale qualified as treatment resistant. However, this research definition did not necessarily encompass individuals who, by clinical standards, would meet the definition of treatment resistance. Marder and Van Putten (1988) suggested that backward schizophrenic individuals, who are severely symptomatic or with severe tardive dyskinesia or EPS, especially those with suboptimal responses to traditional agents, should be eligible for a trial of the atypical antipsychotic agent clozapine. One might also think of clinical treatment resistance as seen in individuals who had an early age of illness onset with subsequent repeated hospitalizations and neuroleptic trials and who cannot achieve a level of social and occupational function commensurate with their age and level of education.

The concept of treatment resistance has undergone significant modification in recent years and is reviewed by Conley and Kelly (2001). The original concept of treatment refractory applied to the use of typical antipsychotic agents. With the advent of the novel agents, which are generally more effective than the traditional ones, the individual should fail at least one novel antipsychotic agent before initiating a trial of clozapine mainly to avoid its side effects. The definition of the duration of a drug trial has also evolved over the years. It is increasingly appreciated that a 4- to 6-week duration of treatment with an antipsychotic agent at therapeutic doses can be considered an adequate trial. The recommended dosing has also undergone changes. The original recommendation considered a trial of 1000 mg equivalent of chlorpromazine as a necessary minimum requirement, but this threshold has now been reduced to 400 to 600 mg/day equivalent on the basis of the knowledge that these doses block enough dopamine D_2 receptors with higher doses providing no additional benefit. Thus, a 4- to 6-week trial of 400 to 600 mg of chlorpromazine equivalent is accepted as an adequate antipsychotic trial.

In treatment-refractory individuals, typical antipsychotic use results in less than 5% response rate (Kane et al. 1988). Clozapine is the only antipsychotic drug proven more efficacious in rigorously defined treatment-refractory groups. Chakos and colleagues (2001) did a meta-analysis of 12 controlled studies involving 1916 individuals. Seven studies involved clozapine. The data showed that treatment-resistant schizophrenia individuals had more favorable outcomes when treated with clozapine rather than a typical antipsychotic agent. However, monitoring of blood counts and fear of its side effects makes it one of most underused effective treatment for schizophrenia.

There is a dearth of good clinical data that indicates how effective risperidone is in this group. In one well-controlled double-blind study, risperidone was more effective and better tolerated than haloperidol though the efficacy was not comparable to clozapine (Wirshing et al. 1999). Two other studies have compared risperidone to clozapine in refractory individuals and showed the efficacy of risperidone to be similar to clozapine, but the definition used of "treatment refractory" status and the study design are either not comparable or have limitations (Klieser et al. 1995, Bondolfi et al. 1998). From these and other open label–studies, risperidone clearly appears to be superior to typical antipsychotics in treatment-refractory individuals but does not appear to be as efficacious as clozapine.

Olanzapine has been reported to have better outcome than haloperidol in the treatment-resistant schizophrenia group from a double-blind study (Breier and Hamilton 1999). However, when olanzapine was compared to chlorpromazine in a treatment-refractory group using a double-blind study design, the outcome with olanzapine was not comparable to what is typically seen with the use of clozapine (Conley et al. 1998). When individuals refractory to olanzapine in this trial were subsequently treated with clozapine, the response rate was similar to what is seen with the use of clozapine in the treatment-refractory group. Similar findings were reported from an open label–study of olanzapine in a treatment-refractory group (Sanders and Mossman 1999). Thus, it appears that though olanzapine was better than standard treatment, it was not as efficacious as clozapine for treatment-refractory individuals. However, these studies were conducted using the standard doses of olanzapine. Recent studies using higher doses of olanzapine, up to 50 mg/day, appear to be better and comparable to clozapine in efficacy (Volavka et al. 2002, Lindenmayer et al. 2001, Tollefson et al. 2001), suggesting that the treatment-refractory group may need higher doses of olanzapine to have a meaningful outcome.

Negative symptoms, such as apathy, amotivational syndrome, flattened affect, and alogia, are often the most problematic for individuals with schizophrenia, accounting for much of the morbidity associated with this illness. In addition, these symptoms are often the most difficult to treat and do not respond well to traditional neuroleptics. The atypical antipsychotic agents are more effective against the negative symptoms than the typical agents (Kane et al. 1988, Chouinard et al. 1993, Tollefson et al. 1997). However, the magnitude of the effect of these compounds on primary negative symptoms is not clear. Clearly, one of the goals of psychopharmacological research is to develop new antipsychotic agents with low associated risk, a more effective treatment for negative and cognitive symptoms, a further reduction in positive symptoms, and an improvement in long-term relapse rate for individuals with chronic schizophrenia.

Augmentation of Typical Neuroleptics   When an individual has shown an inadequate response to traditional neuroleptic agents from different classes and there is a good reason for not switching to a novel antipsychotic drug, other strategies may be necessary to ameliorate residual symptoms. Adding a different type of psychotropic medication may augment the neuroleptic response in some individuals. Several neuroleptic augmentation strategies have been studied, including the addition of beta-blockers, thyrotropin-releasing hormone, clonidine, and valproic acid, with mixed results (Meltzer 1992). Carbamazepine was initially shown to be effective when added to neuroleptic treatment for schizophrenic individuals with electroencephalographic abnormalities and violent outbursts (Hakola and Laulumaa 1982). Later investigation showed that carbamazepine provided adjunctive amelioration of psychotic and affective symptoms when combined with neuroleptics (Klein et al. 1984). Another study reported a significant antipsychotic effect of the addition of carbamazepine to neuroleptics in only one of six treatment-resistant individuals (Herrera et al. 1987). However, the group as a whole improved significantly in terms of anxiety, withdrawal, and depression.

Lithium has been evaluated extensively for its efficacy as an additional treatment of schizophrenia (Meltzer 1992, Delva and Letemendia 1982). In one study, lithium seemed to improve psychotic symptoms of individuals who had not adequately responded to neuroleptics alone (Small et al. 1975). Although lithium does not seem to affect positive or negative symptoms specifically, it may be beneficial for individuals who present at the depressed end of the spectrum (Meltzer 1992).

The use of benzodiazepines as augmenting agents in the treatment of schizophrenia has also been extensively studied (Meltzer 1992, Wolkowitz et al. 1990). There may be some individuals who show improvement in psychotic symptoms, and others who show improvement in negative symptoms. Interestingly, there has been a suggestion that the triazolobenzodiazepines may be more effective than other types of benzodiazepines in augmenting the neuroleptic response (Wolkowitz et al. 1990).

Antidepressant medications have also been considered in the treatment of depression associated with schizophrenia. Although there is some evidence that typical neuroleptics themselves cause depression (Galdi 1983), there undoubtedly are schizophrenic individuals who have primary depressive symptoms. Negative symptoms are often difficult to distinguish from depression (both have features of amotivation, apathy, and social withdrawal), but those that are secondary to depression may respond to the addition of an antidepressant to the individual's medication regimen (Carpenter et al. 1985). One study reported that fluoxetine as an adjuvant agent was effective in treating both positive and negative symptoms in individuals (Goff et al. 1990), although other reports of selective serotonin reuptake inhibitors have been less encouraging. In a separate study, tranylcypromine combined with a typical neuroleptic agent was shown to be helpful in treating negative symptoms (Bucci 1987).

Others have hypothesized a more specific role of the noradrenergic system in the treatment of schizophrenia. For example, Litman and colleagues (1993) noted the improvement of individuals with chronic schizophrenia given idazoxan, a highly selective alpha-2-antagonist, in combination with fluphenazine. Levodopa and d-amphetamine have also been used to enhance treatment of negative symptoms (Meltzer 1992). Although this may be promising, these treatments are associated with the risk of exacerbation of positive symptoms and must therefore be used with caution.

The use of electroconvulsive therapy with concomitant neuroleptic treatment has also been evaluated (Salzman 1980). With electroconvulsive therapy as an adjuvant treatment, it appears that the individual may improve initially, but relapse is likely. However, individuals with comorbid affective symptoms may have some increased benefit (Meltzer 1992). In general, however, this option should be considered only if the individual is not a candidate for a trial with an atypical antipsychotic agent and only if the individual has severe persistent symptoms.

When agonists of the glycine site of the NMDA receptor were added to typical antipsychotic agents in a placebo-controlled study, a significant improvement was reported in negative symptoms and aspects of cognitive functioning (Heresco-Levy et al. 1999). D-cycloserine, a partial agonist at the glycine site, produced a selective improvement of negative symptoms at 6 weeks (Goff et al. 1999). Augmentation with another endogenous full agonist, D-serine, was associated with significant improvement in negative, positive, and cognitive symptoms when added to conventional agents in an 8-week trial (Tsai et al. 1998).

Nonpharmacological Treatment of Schizophrenia

Although psychopharmacological intervention has proved to be the foundation on which the treatment of schizophrenia depends, other approaches to the management of these individuals serve a critical function. Studies have shown repeatedly that symptoms of schizophrenia have not only a genetic component but also an environmental aspect, and interactions with family and within the community can alter the course of the illness.

For many years, a dichotomous view of treatment options was tenaciously debated as dynamic psychiatry was challenged by developments in the neurosciences. A more unified view is now accepted as it has become clear that psychopharmacological treatment strategies are most efficacious if combined with some type of psychosocial intervention and vice versa. It can be said that because of the chronic nature of schizophrenia, one or more treatments may be required throughout the illness and they are likely to have to be modified as symptoms change over time.

Psychosocial Rehabilitation   Bachrach has defined psychosocial rehabilitation as "a therapeutic approach that encourages a mentally ill person to develop his or her fullest capacities through learning and environmental supports" (Bachrach 2000). According to the author, the rehabilitation process should appreciate the unique life circumstances of each person and respond to the individual's special needs while promoting both the treatment of the illness and the reduction of its attendant disabilities. The treatment should be provided in the context of the individual's unique environment taking into account social support network, access to transportation, housing, work opportunities, and so on. Rehabilitation should exploit the individual's strengths and improve his/her competencies. Ultimately, rehabilitation should focus on the positive concept of restoring hope to those who have suffered major setbacks in functional capacity and their self-esteem due to major mental illness. To have this hope grounded in reality, it requires promoting acceptance of one's illness and the limitations that come with it. While work offers the ultimate in sense of achievement and mastery, it must be defined more broadly for the mentally ill and should include prevocational and nonvocational activities along with independent employment. It is extremely important that work is individualized to the talents, skills, and abilities of the individual concerned. However, psychosocial rehabilitation has to transcend work to encompass medical, social, and recreational themes. Psychosocial treatment's basic principle is to provide comprehensive care through active involvement of the individual in his or her own treatment. Thus, it is important that a holding environment be created where individuals can safely express their wishes, aspirations, frustrations, and reservations such that they ultimately mold the rehabilitation plan. Clearly, to achieve these goals, the intervention has to be ongoing.

Given the chronicity of the illness, the process of rehabilitation must be enduring to encounter future stresses and challenges. These goals cannot be achieved without a stable relationship between the individual and the rehabilitation counselor, which is central to an effective treatment and positive outcome. Thus, psychosocial rehabilitation is intimately connected to the biological intervention and forms a core component of the biopsychosocial approach to the treatment of schizophrenia. In the real world, programs often deviate from the aforementioned principles and end up putting excessive and unrealistic expectations on individuals, thus achieving exactly the opposite of the intended values of the program (see Bachrach 2000 for more details).

Psychodynamic Approach   Many attempts have been made to understand the psycho-dynamic implications and meaning of schizophrenic symptoms. To mention all of the contributors who laid the foundations of psychodynamic theory is beyond the scope of this chapter. However, several names are important to put this vast field into historical perspective. Adolph Meyer (1866–1950), for example, contributed to our appreciation of a longitudinal, rather than a cross-sectional, perspective of the individual. He was one of the first to consider that maladjustment early on may have some influence on later psychotic development (Arieti 1955). In his work with schizophrenic individuals, Sigmund Freud (1855–1939) thought that schizophrenia was an illness that represented a regression and a subsequent turning away from social supports because of unresolved conflicts. He observed that these individuals had difficulties in developing transference, which was a necessary step to effective analysis. Freud concluded that schizophrenic individuals could not benefit from this treatment (Gabbard 1990). Carl Jung (1875–1960) concentrated specifically on the psychotic content, looking for symbolic meaning through word association tests while working with individuals with schizophrenia at the Bergozoli Hospital in Switzerland. He believed that humans shared images and mythological symbols or archetypes through a collective unconscious, which was reflected in the psychotic processes of the schizophrenic (Arieti 1955). Harry Stack Sullivan (1892–1949) focused his life's work on interpersonal therapy with schizophrenic individuals. He thought that even the most severe schizophrenic individual was capable of a relational attachment (Arieti 1955, Gabbard 1990).

The psychotherapeutic technique held promise for many years as a potential for unraveling the mystery of individuals' symptoms, with the hope of improvement in course and symptoms and even cure. On the basis of derivations of the classical analytical school, symptoms of schizophrenia were thought of in terms of conflict and defense mechanisms. For example, when paranoid individuals believe that they are being preyed on, they are projecting onto others their own internal, unconscious wish to kill. Thus, unconscious conflicts became manifest as psychotic symptoms. To the psychodynamic therapist then, affectively laden material elicits an increase in thought disorder or psychotic responses, as it touches on the individual's unconscious feelings. These conceptualizations of schizophrenia influenced early work with these individuals.

Although the psychodynamic understanding of intrapsychic events has been of historical interest, the application of traditional psychodynamic principles as primary treatment modalities is not recommended. One of the first studies that compared outcomes between medication-treated individuals and psychotherapy-treated individuals was conducted at the Camarillo State Hospital in 1968. This study found that the group of individuals who received neuroleptic medication showed greater improvement than those who received psychotherapy alone (May 1968). Subsequent studies have replicated these findings even when different types of therapy are examined. Evidence suggests that insight-oriented individual psychotherapy may not be as helpful for individuals with schizophrenia as supportive, goal-directed individual therapy combined with medication treatment and social skills training.

Individual Psychotherapy   Individual therapy in a nontraditional sense can begin on meeting the individual with schizophrenia. Even the briefest of normalizing contacts with an agitated, acutely psychotic individual can have therapeutic value. Psychodynamic interpretations are not helpful during the acute stages of the illness and may actually agitate the individual further. The clinician using individual psychotherapy should focus on forming and maintaining a therapeutic alliance (which is also a necessary part of psychopharmacological treatment) (Frank and Gunderson 1990) and providing a safe environment in which the individual is able to discuss symptoms openly. A sound psychotherapist provides clear structure about the therapeutic relationship and helps the individual to focus on personal goals.

Often, an individual is not aware of or does not have insight into the fact that some beliefs are part of a specific symptom. A psychotherapist helps an individual to check whether his or her reality coincides with that of the therapist. The therapeutic intervention then becomes a frank discussion of what schizophrenia is and how symptoms may feel to the individual. This objectifying of psychotic or negative symptoms can prove of enormous value in allowing the individual to feel more in control of the illness. A good analogy is to diabetic individuals, who know they have a medical illness and are educated about the symptoms associated with exacerbation. Just as these individuals can check blood glucose levels, schizophrenic individuals can discuss with a therapist their sleep patterns, their interpersonal relationships, and their internal thoughts, which may lead to earlier detection of relapses.

Schizophrenia often strikes just as a person is leaving adolescence and entering young adulthood. The higher the premorbid level of social adjustment and functioning, the more devastating and confusing the onset of symptoms becomes. Young males with a high level of premorbid function are at increased risk of suicide, presumably in part because of the tremendous loss they face (Drake et al. 1985). These feelings can continue for years, with schizophrenic individuals feeling isolated and robbed of a normal life. Therefore, a component of individual work (which can also be achieved to some degree in a group setting) with these individuals is a focus on the impact schizophrenia has had on their lives. Helping individuals to grieve for these losses is an important process that may ultimately help them achieve a better quality of life.

Group Psychotherapy   Acutely psychotic individuals do not benefit from group interaction. In fact, a quiet place with decreased social contact is most useful until medications have controlled acute symptoms (Kanas et al. 1980). It is common in inpatient settings to slowly integrate individuals into the ward community only as they appear less agitated and are able to remain in good behavioral control with improvement in psychotic symptoms. As their condition improves, inpatient group therapy prepares individuals for interpersonal interactions in a controlled setting. After discharge, individuals may benefit from day treatment programs and outpatient groups, which provide ongoing care for individuals with schizophrenia living in the community.

Because one of the most difficult challenges of schizophrenia is the inherent deficits in relatedness, group therapy is an important means of gathering individuals with schizophrenia together and providing them with a forum for mutual support. Insight-oriented groups may be disorganizing for individuals with schizophrenia, but task-oriented, supportive groups provide structure and a decreased sense of isolation for this population of individuals. Keeping group focus on structured topics, such as daily needs or getting the most out of community services, is useful for these individuals (Gabbard 1990). In the era of community treatment and brief hospitalizations, many individuals are being seen in medication groups, which they attend regularly to discuss any side effects or problems and to get prescriptions.

Psychoeducational Treatment   One of the inherent deficits from which schizophrenic individuals suffer is an inability to engage appropriately in social or occupational activities. This debilitating effect is often a lasting feature of the illness, despite adequate psychopharmacological intervention. This disability often isolates individuals and makes it difficult for them to advocate appropriate social support or community services. Furthermore, studies have found that there is a correlation between poor social functioning and incidence of relapse (Linn et al. 1980). One of the challenges of this area of study is the great deal of variability in each individual. However, standardized measures have been developed to ascertain objective ratings of social deficits. These assessments have become important tools in the determination of effective nonpharmacological treatment strategies.

The literature suggests that schizophrenic individuals can benefit from social skills training (Wallace et al. 1980, Brady 1984). This model is based on the idea that the course of schizophrenia is, in part, a product of the environment, which is inherently stressful because of the social deficits from which these individuals suffer. The hypothesis is that if individuals are able to monitor and reduce their stress, they could potentially decrease their risk of relapse.

For this intervention to be successful, individuals must be aware of and set their own goals. Goals such as medication management, activities of daily living, and dealing with a roommate are achievable examples. Social skills and deficits can be assessed by individuals' self-report, observation of behavioral patterns by trained professionals, or a measurement of physiological responses to specific situations (e.g., increased pulse when asking someone to dinner). Individuals can then begin behavioral training in which appropriate social responses are shaped with the help of instructors.

One example of such a program, discussed by Liberman and colleagues (1985), is a highly structured curriculum that includes a training manual, audiovisual aids, and role-playing exercises. Behaviors are broken down into small bits, such as learning how to maintain eye contact, monitor vocal volume, or ameliorate body language. The modules are learned one at a time, with role-playing, homework, and feedback provided to the participants. In several studies, Liberman and coworkers (1986) have shown that individuals who were treated with social skills training and medication spent less time hospitalized, with fewer relapses than those treated with holistic health measures (e.g., yoga, stress management) on a 2-year follow-up. Research such as this in the field of social skills training is growing as the inherent deficits in information processing, executive function, and interpersonal skills are further elucidated.

Earlier studies have suggested that educational interventions influence both knowledge and drug use errors. Similarly, educating the individual improves compliance. Merinder (2000) reviewed patient education in seven randomized trials, four naturalistic studies, and eight studies with mixed samples. The author concludes that knowledge and compliance can be improved by the interventions used, and in some circumstances, relapse and symptomatology can be partly influenced. The didactic format influences knowledge more readily while interventions with behavioral contents influence compliance. Education programs for the individual tend to use more didactic interactive format, enabling a more thorough negotiation of illness attitudes.

In a large number of individuals, deficits in social competence persist despite antipsychotic treatment. These deficits can lead to social distress, whereas social competence can alleviate distress related to social discomfort. The "token economy" programs with operant conditioning paradigms were used in the past to discourage undesirable behavior. However, nowadays there are better ways to deal with these behaviors. Paradigms using instruction, modeling, role-playing, and positive reinforcement are helpful. Controlled studies suggest that individuals with schizophrenia are able to acquire lasting social skills after attending such programs and apply these skills to everyday life. Besides reducing anxiety, social skills training also improve the level of social activity and foster new social contacts. This in turn improves the quality of life and significantly shortens the duration of inpatient care. However, their impact on symptom resolution and relapse rates is unclear.

Individuals with schizophrenia generally demonstrate poor performance in various aspects of information processing. Cognitive dysfunction can be a rate-limiting factor in learning and social functioning. Additionally, impaired information processing can lead to increased susceptibility to stress and thus to an increased risk of relapse. Practice appears to improve some of the cognitive dysfunction. Remediation of cognitive dysfunctions with social skills training has been reported to have positive impact. Mojtabai and colleagues (1998) performed a comprehensive meta-analysis of 106 controlled studies that were published between 1966 and 1994. They found that various types of cognitive behavioral therapies were particularly effective. Social skills training program, cognitive training program to improve neurocognitive functioning, and cognitive behavioral therapy approaches are oriented toward coping with symptoms, the disorder, and everyday problems.

Cognitive adaptation training (CAT) is a novel approach to improve adaptive functioning and compensate for the cognitive impairments associated with schizophrenia. A thorough functional needs assessment is done to measure current adaptive functioning. Besides measuring adaptive functioning and quantifying apathy and disinhibition, a neurocognitive assessment using tests to measure executive function, attention, verbal and visual memory, and visual organization is also completed. Treatment plans are adapted to the individual's level of functioning, which includes the individual's level of apathy. Interventions include removal of distracting stimuli, and use of reminders such as checklists, signs, and labels. In a randomized trial, 45 individuals with schizophrenia were randomized to a standard medication plus CAT group, standard medication follow-up group, and a control group that included standard medication plus a condition designed to control for therapist time. At 9 months, there was a significant improvement in positive and negative symptoms in the CAT group compared with the two other groups, namely, the follow-up group and the control group of standard medication plus controlled therapist time. The most consistent improvement was in favor of CAT group and involved motivation as measured by rating instruments. The Global Assessment of Functioning (GAF) scores also differed significantly between the groups. The relapse rates for CAT, control, and follow-up groups were significantly different (13.33, 67.67, and 33.33%, respectively) (Velligan et al. 2000).

Family Therapy

A large body of the literature explores the role of familial interactions and the clinical course of schizophrenia. Many of these studies have examined the outcome of schizophrenia in relation to the degree of expressed emotion (EE) in family members. EE is generally defined as excessive criticism and overinvolvement of relatives. Schizophrenic individuals have been found to have a higher risk of relapse if their relatives have high EE levels. Clearly, an individual's disturbing symptoms at the time of relapse may affect the level of criticism and overinvolvement of family members, but evidence suggests that preexisting increased EE levels in relatives predict increased risk of schizophrenic relapse and that interventions that decrease EE levels can decrease relapse rates.

Specifically, studies have demonstrated that effective strategies lower the risk of relapse with the use of family intervention and measurements of EE levels (Leff et al. 1982, Falloon et al. 1982, 1985, Hogarty et al. 1986). For example, in a study by Falloon and colleagues (1982, 1985), 37 individuals were randomly assigned to one of two treatment groups. One group received family therapy, the other received individual therapy. In both groups, the individuals were maintained with appropriate neuroleptic doses. Family therapy was done in the home, with a focus on education about schizophrenia and ways in which families could achieve lowered stress levels and improved problem-solving skills. Specific problem-solving mechanisms were rehearsed and modeled by trained therapists. The individual treatment was supportive psychotherapy, which was conducted at the clinic. At the end of 9 months, family therapy was found to be a more effective means of preventing relapse (one relapsed out of 18) than individual therapy (eight relapsed out of 19). Moreover, the advantages of the family therapy persisted after a second year of less intensive follow-up (Falloon et al. 1985).

Barbato and D'Avanzo (2000) critically reviewed family interventions in 25 randomized studies involving 1744 individuals. Though the studies suffer from methodological limitations, the efficacy of family intervention on relapse rate is fairly well supported. This efficacy was particularly evident when contrasted with low quality or uncontrolled individual treatments. The addition of family intervention to standard treatment of schizophrenia has a positive impact on outcome to a moderate extent. Family intervention effectively reduces the short-term risk of clinical relapse after remission from an acute episode. There is evidence of effect on the individual's mental state and social functioning, or on any family-related variables. The elements common to most effective interventions are inclusion of the individual in at least some phases of the treatment, long duration, and information and education about the illness provided within a supportive framework. There is sufficient data only for males with chronic schizophrenia living with high EE parents. Evidence is limited for recent onset individuals, women, and people in different family arrangements and families with low EE. Research in family intervention is still a growing field. Thus, at present it is unclear if the effect seen with family therapy is due to family treatment or more intensive care.

Leff (2000) concluded from his review that family interventions reduced relapse rates by one half over the first year of combined treatment with medications and family therapy. Medications and family therapy augment each other. Psychoeducation by itself is not enough. It also seems that multiple family groups are more efficacious than single family sessions. Attempts are being made to generalize training of mental health workers in effectively implementing these strategies.

On the basis of these findings, it is clear that there is a significant interaction between the level of emotional involvement and criticism of relatives of probands with schizophrenia and the outcome of their illness. Identifying the causative factors in familial stressors and educating involved family members about schizophrenia lead to long-term benefits for individuals. Future work in this field must examine these interactions with an understanding of modern sociological and biological advances in genetics, looking at trait carriers, social skills assessments, positive and negative symptoms, and medication management with the novel antipsychotic agents.

Case Management   Assertive Community Treatment (ACT) is a community care model with a caseload per worker of 15 individuals or less in contrast to standard case management (SCM) with a caseload of 30 to 35 individuals. Intensive clinical case management (ICCM) differs from ACT by the case manager not sharing the caseload. In the ACT model, most services are provided in the community rather than in the office; the caseloads are shared across clinicians rather than individual caseloads. These are time unlimited services provided directly by the ACT team and not brokered out, and 24-hour coverage is provided. Research on the ACT model confirms that it is successful in making individuals comply with treatment and leads to less inpatient admissions. ACT also improves housing conditions (fewer homeless individuals, more individuals in stable housing), employment, quality of life, and patient satisfaction. No clear differences between ACT and standard or intensive clinical case management are reported with mental condition, social functioning, self-esteem, or number of deaths.

Combining Pharmacological and Psychosocial Treatments

The combination of pharmacological and psychosocial interventions in schizophrenia can have complex interactions. For example, psychotherapies improve medication compliance on the one hand and are more effective in the presence of antipsychotic treatment on the other. Family psychoeducation has been reported to decrease the level of EE in the family, resulting in better social adjustment and a need for lower dose of antipsychotic medications. Marder and colleagues (1996) found in their study that pharmacological and psychosocial treatments affect different outcome dimensions. Medications affect relapse risk whereas skills training affect social adjustment. The VA cooperative study by Rosenheck and colleagues (1998) found that individuals who received clozapine were more likely to participate in these treatments that led to an improved quality of life. The qualitative differences in the interactions between the newer antipsychotic agents and psychotherapy suggest a hopeful trend of better utilization of psychosocial treatments (Marder 2000).

Self-Directed Treatment

Groups such as the National Alliance for Mentally Ill (NAMI) and the Manic–Depressive Association offer tremendous resources to individuals with psychiatric problems and their relatives. They provide newsletters, neighborhood meetings, and support groups to interested persons. These nonprofessional self-help measures may feel less threatening to individuals and their families and provide an important adjunct to professional settings.

Structured self-help clubs have also been effective means of bolstering individuals' social, occupational, and living skills. The Fountain House was the first such club aimed at social rehabilitation (Beard 1982). Individuals who are involved are called members of the club, giving them a sense of belonging to a group. They are always made to feel welcome, useful, and productive members of the club community.

The clubhouse model has expanded to provide services such as transitional employment programs, apartment programs, outreach programs, and medication management and consultation services, to name a few. A self-supportive rehabilitation program for mentally ill individuals is an important option for many schizophrenic individuals who might otherwise feel isolated and out of reach.

SCHIZOAFFECTIVE DISORDER

Kraepelin's landmark classification at the dawn of the twentieth century could not accurately classify those individuals who manifested both psychotic (schizophrenia-like) and affective symptoms and had a better course of illness then schizophrenia (Kraepelin 1919). It was Kasanin (1933), who coined the term *schizoaffective disorder* to describe some of these individuals. However, over the decades, these individuals were often classified as having atypical schizophrenia, good prognosis schizophrenia, remitting schizophrenia, or cycloid psychosis. Inherent within these diagnoses was the implication that they shared similarities to schizophrenia and also appeared to have a relatively better course of illness. With the advent of effective treatment of bipolar disorder with lithium salts, some of these individuals started responding to lithium, and the term *schizoaffective disorder* gained further momentum and evolved in the direction of bipolar disorder. Unfortunately, this lack of diagnostic clarity has plagued the diagnosis of schizoaffective disorder such that there is much that is unknown about the illness.

Diagnosis

Schizoaffective disorder criteria have evolved over the years and undergone major changes (see DSM-IV-TR diagnostic criteria on page 702). According to the DSM-IV-TR, an individual with schizoaffective disorder must have an uninterrupted period of illness during which, at some time, they meet the diagnostic criteria for a major depressive episode, manic episode, or a mixed episode concurrently with the diagnostic criteria for the active phase of schizophrenia (criterion A for schizophrenia). Additionally, "the individual must have had delusions or hallucinations for at least 2 weeks in the absence of prominent mood disorder symptoms" during the same period of illness. The mood disorder symptoms must be present for a substantial part of the active and residual psychotic period. The essential features of schizoaffective disorder must occur within a single uninterrupted period of illness where the "period of illness" refers to the period of active or residual symptoms of psychotic illness and this can last for years and decades. The total duration of psychotic symptoms must be at least 1 month to meet the criterion A for schizophrenia and thus, the minimum duration of a schizoaffective episode is also 1 month.

DSM-IV-TR Diagnostic Criteria

295.70 Schizoaffective Disorder

A. An uninterrupted period of illness during which, at some time, there is either a major depressive episode, a manic episode, or a mixed episode concurrent with symptoms that meet criterion A for schizophrenia.

Note: The major depressive episode must include criterion A1: depressed mood.

B. During the same period of illness, there have been delusions or hallucinations for at least 2 weeks in the absence of prominent mood symptoms.
C. Symptoms that meet criteria for a mood episode are present for a substantial portion of the total duration of the active and residual periods of the illness.
D. The disturbance is not due to the direct physiological effects of a substance (e.g., a drug of abuse, a medication) or a general medical condition.

Specify type:

Bipolar type: if the disturbance includes a manic or a mixed episode (or a manic or a mixed episode and major depressive episodes)
Depressive type: if the disturbance only includes major depressive episodes

---

The criteria for major depressive episode requires a minimum duration of 2 weeks of either depressed mood or markedly diminished interest or pleasure. As the symptoms of loss of pleasure or interest commonly occur in nonaffective psychotic disorders, to meet the criterion A for schizoaffective disorder the major depressive episode must include pervasive depressed mood. Presence of markedly diminished interest or pleasure is not sufficient to make a diagnosis as it is possible that these symptoms may occur with other conditions too.

The clinical signs and symptoms of schizoaffective disorder include all the signs and symptoms of schizophrenia, and a manic episode and/or a major depressive episode. The schizophrenia and mood symptoms may occur together or in an alternate sequence. The clinical course can vary from one of exacerbations and remissions to that of a long-term deterioration. Presence of mood-incongruent psychotic features—where the psychotic content of hallucinations or delusions is not consistent with the prevailing mood—more likely indicate a poor prognosis.

The DSM-IV-TR diagnosis of schizoaffective disorder can be further classified as schizoaffective disorder *bipolar type* or schizoaffective disorder *depressive type*. For a person to be classified as having the bipolar subtype, he/she must have a disorder that includes a manic or mixed episode with or without a history of major depressive episodes. Otherwise, the person is classified as having depressive subtype having had symptoms that meet the criteria for a major depressive episode with no history of having had mania or mixed state.

Epidemiology

As discussed earlier, the diagnosis of schizoaffective disorder has undergone numerous changes through the decades making it difficult to get reliable epidemiology information. When data was pooled together from various clinical studies, approximately 2 to 29% of those individuals diagnosed as having mental illness at the time of the study were suffering from schizoaffective disorder with women having a higher prevalence (Keck et al. 2001). This could possibly be explained by a higher rate of depression in women. Relatives of women suffering from schizoaffective disorder have a higher rate of schizophrenia and depressive disorders compared to relatives of male schizoaffective subjects. The estimated lifetime prevalence of schizoaffective disorder is possibly in the range of 0.5 to 0.8%. In the inpatient settings of New York State psychiatric hospitals, approximately 19% of 6000 individuals had a diagnosis of schizoaffective disorder (Levinson et al. 1999).

The depressive type of schizoaffective disorder appears to be more common in older people while the bipolar type probably occurs more commonly in younger adults. The higher prevalence of the disorder in women appears to occur particularly amongst those who are married. As in schizophrenia, the age of onset for women is later than that for men. Depression tends to occur more commonly in women.

Course

Owing to the evolving nature of the diagnosis and limited studies done thus far, much remains unknown. However, to the extent that this illness has symptoms from both a major mood disorder and schizophrenia, theoretically one can confer a relatively better prognosis than schizophrenia and a relatively poorer prognosis than bipolar disorder. In one study in which individuals with DSM-III and DSM-IV schizoaffective disorder were followed for 8 years, the outcome of these individuals more closely resembled schizophrenia than mood disorder with psychosis. Some data indicate that individuals with a diagnosis of schizoaffective disorder bipolar type have a 2- to 5-year course similar to that of bipolar disorder, while individuals diagnosed as having schizoaffective disorder depressive type have a course similar to schizophrenia on outcome measures such as occupational and social functioning after the index episode (Grossman et al. 1991). Regardless of the subtype, the following variables are harbingers of a poor prognosis:

(a) a poor premorbid history
(b) an insidious onset
(c) absence of precipitating factors
(d) a predominance of psychotic symptoms, especially deficit or negative ones
(e) an early age of onset
(f) an unremitting course, and
(g) a family history of schizophrenia.

The corollary would be that the opposite of each of these characteristics would suggest a better prognosis. Interestingly, the presence or the absence of Schneiderian first-rank symptoms does not seem to predict the course of illness. The incidence of suicide in individuals with schizoaffective disorder is at least 10%. Some data indicate that the suicidal behavior may be more common in women then men.

In a small sample comparing 27 schizoaffective disorder with 27 bipolar disorder individuals, first-rank symptoms and mood-incongruent psychosis did not differ between the two groups (Strakowski et al. 1999). Over 70% of the sample included unemployed or unskilled laborers. A few studies have reported that low socioeconomic status is a strong predictor of poor outcome (Strakowski et al. 1998, 1999).

In one study, 82% of those individuals who were suffering from a first episode of schizoaffective disorder and had recovered, experienced psychotic relapse within 5 years. These individuals had high rates of second and third relapses despite careful monitoring. Medication discontinuations in first-episode individuals who are stable for 1 year substantially increase relapse risks. Aside from medication status, premorbid social adjustment was the only predictor of relapse in their study. Poor adaptation to school and premorbid social isolation predicted initial relapse independent of medication status. Thus, like schizophrenia, the risk of relapse is diminished by antipsychotic maintenance treatment (Robinson et al. 1999).

Differential Diagnosis

The possible differential diagnosis consists of bipolar disorder with psychotic features, major depressive disorder with psychotic features, and schizophrenia. Clearly, substance-induced states and symptoms caused by coexisting medical conditions should be carefully ruled out. All conditions listed in differential diagnosis of schizophrenia, bipolar disorder, and major depressive disorder should be considered including but not limited to those individuals undergoing treatment with steroids, those abusing substances such as PCP, and medical conditions such as temporal lobe epilepsy. In circumstances where there is ambiguity, it may be prudent to delay making a final diagnosis until the most acute symptoms of psychosis have subsided and time is allowed to establish a course of illness and collect collateral information.

Etiology

The etiology of schizoaffective disorder is unknown. There is a dearth of data relating to this illness. Studies involving families of schizoaffective probands suggest that they have significantly higher rates of relatives with mood disorder than families of schizophrenia probands. It is possible that some of the same environmental theories that apply to schizophrenia and bipolar disorder may also apply to schizoaffective disorder.

Over the years, the concept of schizoaffective disorder has evolved such that many view it as either a type of schizophrenia or a type of mood disorder. Evans and colleagues (1999) suggest that schizoaffective disorder represents a variant of schizophrenia in terms of clinical symptoms, family history and treatment. Moreover, in their study and others', schizophrenia individuals did not differ from schizoaffective ones on cognitive impairment (Bornstein et al. 1990, Beatty et al. 1993). Williams and associates (1987) suggest that the disorder represents a variant of either schizophrenia or mood disorder while others consider it to be on a continuum of illness intermediate between schizophrenia or mood disorder (Taylor 1992, Kendler et al. 1995a). Lapierre's (1994) opinion is that schizoaffective disorder represents a phenotypic variation of either schizophrenia or mood disorder and over a long term becomes a subtype of either one. Alternatively, some view schizoaffective disorder as the simultaneous expression of schizophrenia and a mood disorder. However, Kendler and colleagues (1995b) observe that schizoaffective individuals differ significantly from both schizophrenic and mood disorder individuals. Specifically, schizoaffective individuals have more affective symptoms, fewer negative symptoms, and a better course and outcome than schizophrenia. Bertelsen and Gottesman (1995) reviewed the literature relevant to genetic predisposition to schizoaffective disorder. Though variable, the results generally suggest that schizoaffective disorder is either a phenotypic variation or an expression of a genetic interform between schizophrenia and mood disorder, a position similar to Kendler. However, the possibility that schizoaffective disorder is distinct from schizophrenia and mood disorders is not supported by the observations that only a small percentage of the relatives of schizoaffective disorder probands have schizoaffective disorder.

It is most likely that schizoaffective disorder is a heterogeneous condition that includes all of the possibilities mentioned above. Thus, depending on the type of schizoaffective disorder studied, an increased prevalence of either schizophrenia or mood disorders may be found in their relatives. As a group, individuals with schizoaffective disorder have a prognosis intermediate between mood disorders and schizophrenia. Thus, on an average, they have a better course than those suffering from schizophrenia, respond to mood stabilizers more often, and tend to have a relatively nondeteriorating course.

Treatment

With the shifting definitions of schizoaffective disorder, evaluating the treatment of schizoaffective disorder is not easy. Mood stabilizers, antidepressants, and antipsychotic medications clearly have a role in the management of these individuals. The presenting symptoms, their duration and intensity, and the choices of the individual need to be incorporated into deciding what treatment(s) to choose.

Atypical antipsychotic medications are reported to be more effective than the typical ones in the treatment of schizoaffective disorder (Levinson et al. 1999, Keck et al. 1999). They appear to have a more broad-spectrum effect than the typical agents. Optimizing antipsychotic treatment, especially with the novel agents is more likely to be effective than the routine use of adjunctive antidepressants or mood stabilizers. However, when indicated, the use of antidepressants is well supported in schizoaffective individuals who present with a full depressive syndrome after stabilization of psychosis.

Olanzapine is effective against symptoms of psychosis, mania, and depression. Tollefson and colleagues (1997) studied 300 individuals with schizoaffective disorder bipolar type, one of the largest studies of its kind in schizoaffective disorder, and reported that olanzapine was significantly superior to haloperidol in treating affective and psychotic symptoms.

Ziprasidone was studied in 115 hospitalized individuals with acute episode of schizoaffective disorder using a double-blind randomized design. Ziprasidone was significantly superior to placebo and was well tolerated (Keck et al. 2001). Ziprasidone also has significant antidepressant effects at doses of 120 to 160 mg/day.

Vieta and colleagues (2001) studied 102 schizoaffective disorder bipolar type individuals where risperidone was added to their existing regimen of mood stabilizers in the absence of an antipsychotic agent. Risperidone had significant clinical efficacy and a favorable safety profile when combined with mood stabilizers in individuals with schizoaffective disorders. The response rate was comparatively better than what is typically observed in schizophrenia studies (Keck et al. 1999). Hillert and associates (1992) also reported that treatment with risperidone reduced both psychotic and mood symptoms in individuals with schizoaffective disorder depressed type. However, Janicak and colleagues (2001), in a small sample, did not find significant differences between haloperidol and risperidone in a short-term 6-week double-blind randomized study. However, risperidone produced significantly greater responders in the individuals with severe depression and also improved the sleep factor. Moreover, risperidone did not exacerbate manic symptoms, a prevailing concern at the time when this study was conducted. Furthermore, the risperidone group had less EPS compared to haloperidol. Efficacy of clozapine in schizoaffective disorder has been reported in several short-term studies or chart reviews (Naber et al. 1989, Banov et al. 1994). Clozapine monotherapy has been reported to be effective in treatment up to 16 months in a small sample (Zarate et al. 1995). Presence of affective symptoms predicted good response to clozapine. When clozapine use was compared in treatment-refractory schizophrenia, bipolar disorder, and schizoaffective disorder, the outcomes were significantly better in bipolar disorder and schizoaffective disorder (Banov et al. 1994, Zarate et al. 1995, Green et al. 2000, CiapparellI et al. 2000). Persistent and enduring improvement with clozapine lasting 1 to 2 years have been reported (CiapparellI et al. 2000). Clozapine also helps decrease suicidality (CiapparellI et al. 2000, Meltzer 1998). Thus, clozapine use may be beneficial in treatment-refractory schizoaffective disorder as it has both mood stabilizing and antipsychotic properties, a substantial advantage.

Two small open label–studies suggest that valproic acid is effective in treating the manic symptoms associated with schizoaffective disorder bipolar type (Puzynski and Klosiewicz 1984, Emrich et al. 1985) with 65.2% reduction in manic episodes in 5 individuals after 29 to 51 months. Similar results were reported by Hayes (1989) where 79% of the individuals reported improvement after a 1-year treatment with valproic acid. Bogan and associates (2000) also reported 75% improvement in Clinical Global Impression scale in a small sample.

Three double-blind, parallel-group studies examined the efficacy of lithium carbonate in schizoaffective mania. One study found that chlorpromazine alone was as effective as the combination of chlorpromazine and lithium. Another study with a small sample found that the combination of lithium and haloperidol was more effective than haloperidol itself in individuals with predominantly affective symptoms compared to those with predominantly psychotic symptoms. Reports of carbamazepine use is sparse and difficult to draw conclusions from. Lamotrigine was also reported to be useful in three cases of schizoaffective disorder (Erfurth et al. 1998).

The novel antipsychotic agents are often efficacious against depression in individuals who suffer from both depression and psychosis negating the need for routine use of antidepressants. However, there are individuals who remain depressed even with optimal antipsychotic and mood stabilizer treatment. SSRIs are widely used in individuals who present with schizoaffective disorder with depression. If the SSRIs and newer antidepressants do not show efficacy, tricyclic antidepressants do have a role. Interestingly, chlorpromazine in combination with amitriptyline was reported to be as effective as chlorpromazine alone. Many studies suggest that addition of antidepressants helps in effective treatment of depression in schizoaffective disorder. Occasionally, antidepressants may worsen the course. For individuals suffering from depression where they are not responding adequately and are at risk for suicide, ECT is an effective alternative.

To the extent that schizoaffective disorder shares symptoms with schizophrenia, most of the psychosocial treatments used in the treatment of schizophrenia are likely to be useful in the treatment of schizoaffective disorder. Specifically, individuals benefit from individual supportive therapy, family therapy, group therapy, cognitive–behavioral therapy, and social skills training. Many individuals would be suitable candidates for assertive community therapy (ACT). Depending on the level of recovery, some of the individuals may need rehabilitation services to assist them with either developing skills for some form of employment or assistance to maintain a job. Family members benefit from support groups such as NAMI or MDA groups.

BRIEF PSYCHOTIC DISORDER

Diagnosis

Brief psychotic disorder is defined by DSM-IV-TR as a psychotic disorder that lasts more than 1 day and less than a month (see DSM-IV-TR diagnostic criteria on page 707). Moreover, the disorder may develop in response to severe psychosocial stressors or group of stressors.

DSM-IV-TR Diagnostic Criteria

298.8 Brief Psychotic Disorder

A. Presence of one (or more) of the following symptoms:

 (1) delusions
 (2) hallucinations
 (3) disorganized speech (e.g., frequent derailment or incoherence)
 (4) grossly disorganized or catatonic behavior

Note: Do not include a symptom if it is a culturally sanctioned response pattern.

B. Duration of an episode of the disturbance is at least 1 day but less than 1 month, with eventual full return to premorbid level of functioning.
C. The disturbance is not better accounted for by a mood disorder with psychotic features, schizoaffective disorder, or schizophrenia and is not due to the direct physiological effects of a substance (e.g., a drug of abuse, a medication) or a general medical condition.

Specify if:

With marked stressor(s) (brief reactive psychosis): if symptoms occur shortly after and apparently in response to events that, singly or together, would be markedly stressful to almost anyone in similar circumstances in the person's culture

Without marked stressor(s): if psychotic symptoms do not occur shortly after, or are not apparently in response to events that, singly or together, would be markedly stressful to almost anyone in similar circumstances in the person's culture

With postpartum onset: if onset within 4 weeks postpartum

Reprinted with permission from the Diagnostic and Statistical Manual of Mental Disorders, Fourth Edition, Text Revision. Copyright 2000 American Psychiatric Association.

European and Scandinavian countries have traditionally diagnosed this type of psychosis as *psychogenic psychoses*, *reactive psychosis*, or *brief reactive psychosis*. Some have also referred to this condition as *hysterical psychosis*. These terms are probably more commonly used in Scandinavian countries due to Langfeldt and Leonhard's contributions to the classification of psychosis that does not have a course like schizophrenia. In the United States, brief reactive psychosis was formally included as a diagnostic category in DSM-III. Subsequently, it has undergone a change in its name to *brief psychotic disorder*.

The DSM-IV-TR diagnostic criteria specify the presence of at least one clear psychotic symptom lasting a minimum of 1 day to a maximum of 1 month. Furthermore, DSM-IV-TR allows the specification of two additional features: the presence or the absence of one or more marked stressors and a postpartum onset. DSM-IV-TR describes a continuum of diagnosis for psychotic disorder based primarily on the duration of the symptoms. Once the duration criteria are met, other conditions such as etiological medical illnesses and substance- induced psychosis need to be excluded. In those cases where the duration of psychosis lasts more than 1 month, appropriate diagnoses to be considered are other psychotic conditions based on reevaluation of the clinical features, duration of psychosis, and presence of mood symptoms.

People suffering from this disorder usually present with an acute onset, manifest at least one major symptom of psychosis, and do not always include the entire symptom constellation seen in schizophrenia. Affective symptoms, confusion, and impaired attention may be more common in brief psychotic disorders than in chronic psychotic conditions. Some of the characteristic symptoms include emotional lability, outlandish behavior, screaming or muteness, and impaired memory for recent events. Some of the symptoms suggest a diagnosis of *delirium* and may warrant a more complete medical workup. The symptom patterns include acute paranoid reactions, reactive confusions, excitations, and depressions. In French psychiatry, *Bouffee delirante* is similar to brief psychotic disorder.

The precipitating stressors most commonly encountered are major life events that would cause any person significant emotional turmoil. Such events include the death of a close family member or severe accidents. Rarely, it could be accumulation of many smaller stresses.

Epidemiology

This illness is not uncommon, but, unfortunately, reliable estimates of the incidence, prevalence, sex ratio, and average age of onset are not available. It is believed that this disorder is more common among young people with occasional cases involving older people. This disorder may be seen more commonly in individuals from low socioeconomic classes and in those with personality disorders such as histrionic, paranoid, schizotypal, narcissistic, and borderline. Though immigrants and people who have experienced major disasters are reported to be at a higher risk, well-controlled studies have failed to show this.

Course

As defined by DSM-IV-TR, the duration of the disorder is less than 1 month. Nonetheless, the development of such a significant mental disorder may indicate an individual's mental vulnerability. An unknown percentage of individuals who are first classified as having brief psychotic disorder later display chronic mental disorder such as schizophrenia and bipolar disorder. Individuals with brief psychotic disorders generally have good prognosis, and European studies indicate that 50 to 80% of all individuals have no further major psychiatric problems.

The length of the acute and residual symptoms is often just a few days. Occasionally, depressive symptoms follow the resolution of the psychosis. Suicide is a concern during both the psychotic phase and the postpsychotic depressive phase. Indicators of good prognosis are good premorbid adjustment, few premorbid schizoid traits, severe precipitating stressors, sudden onset of symptoms, confusion and perplexity during psychosis, little affective blunting, short duration of symptoms, and absence of family history of schizophrenia.

Differential Diagnosis

Although the classical presentation may be short in duration and associated with stressors, a thorough and careful evaluation is necessary. Additional information is critical to rule out other major psychotic conditions as temporal association of stressors to the acute manifestation of symptoms may be coincidental and thus misleading. Other conditions to be ruled out include psychotic disorder due to a general medical condition, substance-induced psychosis, factitious disorder with predominantly psychological signs and symptoms, and malingering. Individuals with epilepsy and delirium may also present with similar symptoms. Additional conditions to be considered are dissociative identity disorder and psychotic episodes associated with borderline and schizotypal personality disorder that may last for less than a day.

Etiology

As with other psychotic illnesses, this condition appears to be heterogeneous; clearly, more research is necessary. The development of psychosis is an important indication of severity of this illness and may suggest either a breakdown of or inadequate coping mechanisms.

Treatment

These individuals may require short-term hospitalizations for a comprehensive evaluation and safety. Antipsychotic drugs are often most useful along with benzodiazepines. Long-term use of medication is often not necessary and should be avoided. If maintenance medications are necessary, the diagnoses may need to be revised. Clearly, the newer antipsychotic agents have a better neurological side effect profile and would be preferred over the typical agents.

Psychotherapy is necessary to help the person reintegrate the experience of psychosis and possibly the precipitating trauma. Individual, family, and group therapies may be necessary in some individuals. Many individuals need help to cope with the loss of self-esteem and confidence.

SCHIZOPHRENIFORM DISORDER

Diagnosis

Gabriel Langfeldt (1939) suggested the term *Schizophreniform Disorder* in 1937 for a heterogeneous group of individuals characterized by the similarity of their symptoms to those of schizophrenia, albeit with a good clinical outcome. Langfeldt observed that those individuals whose diagnosis was questionable as schizophrenia had a much better outcome than those whose diagnosis was confirmed as schizophrenia; these individuals were thus classified as having schizophreniform psychosis. Langfeldt also noted that these individuals often had good premorbid adjustment, an abrupt onset of symptoms, frequent presence of psychosocial stressor(s), and a good prognosis.

Schizophreniform disorder shares a majority of the DSM-IV-TR diagnostic features with schizophrenia (see DSM-IV-TR diagnostic criteria on page 710) except the following two criteria: (1) the total duration of the illness which includes the prodrome, active, and residual phases is at least 1 month but less than 6 months in duration; (2) though impairment in social and occupational functioning may occur during the illness, it is not required or necessary. Thus, the duration of more than 1 month eliminates brief psychotic disorder as a possible diagnosis; if the illness lasts or has lasted for more than 6 months, the diagnosis has to be reevaluated for other possible conditions including schizophrenia. Therefore, the diagnosis of schizophreniform disorder is intermediate between brief psychotic disorder and schizophrenia. Hence, those individuals whose duration of episode lasted more than a month and less than 6 months, and have recovered would be diagnosed as having schizophreniform disorder. On the other hand, those individuals who have not recovered from an episode, which is less than 6 months but more than one month in duration, and are likely to have schizophrenia would be diagnosed to have schizophreniform disorder until the 6 months criteria is met for schizophrenia. The diagnosis of 'provisional' schizophreniform disorder is made while the clinician monitors the evolving course of the illness, waits for the symptoms to resolve, or when the clinician cannot obtain a reliable history from an individual about the duration of the symptoms.

DSM-IV-TR Diagnostic Criteria

295.40 Schizophreniform Disorder

A. Criteria A, D, and E of schizophrenia are met.
B. An episode of the disorder (including prodromal, active, and residual phases) lasts at least 1 month but less than 6 months. (When the diagnosis must be made without waiting for recovery, it should be qualified as "provisional.")

Specify if:

Without good prognostic features

With good prognostic features: as evidenced by two (or more) of the following:

   (1) onset of prominent psychotic symptoms within 4 weeks of the first noticeable change in usual behavior or functioning
   (2) confusion or perplexity at the height of the psychotic episode
   (3) good premorbid social and occupational functioning
   (4) absence of blunted or flat affect

Reprinted with permission from the Diagnostic and Statistical Manual of Mental Disorders, Fourth Edition, Text Revision. Copyright 2000 American Psychiatric Association.

DSM-IV-TR has specifiers for the presence or absence of good prognostic features. These features include a rapid onset (within 4 weeks) of prominent psychotic symptoms, presence of (psychogenic) confusion or perplexity at the height of the psychotic episode, good premorbid adjustment as evidenced by social and occupational functioning, and the absence of deficit symptoms such as blunted or flat affect.

Epidemiology

Little is known about the incidence, prevalence, and sex ratio of schizophreniform disorder (Poulton et al. 2000). A strong linear relationship has been reported between self-reported psychotic symptoms in childhood at age 11 years and subsequent development of adult schizophreniform disorder. Those children with strong symptoms were 16 times more likely to have a schizophreniform diagnosis by age 26 years compared to a control group. Forty-two percent of those who developed schizophreniform psychosis by age 26 years in the cohort had reported one or more psychotic symptoms at age 11 years. Interestingly, these psychotic symptoms that appeared at age 11 years did not predict mania or depression at age 26 years (Poulton 2000). Over the years, schizophreniform psychosis has moved much closer to the diagnosis of schizophrenia. ECA studies indicate prevalence of 0.2% lifetime prevalence and 1-year prevalence of 0.1%.

Course

The course is, as anticipated, variable. The DSM-IV-TR specifiers "with good prognostic features" and "without good prognostic features" though helpful in guiding the clinician, require further validation. However, confusion or perplexity at the height of the psychotic episode is the feature best correlated with good outcome. Also, the shorter the period of illness, the better the prognosis is likely to be. There is a significant risk of suicide in these individuals. Postpsychotic depression is quite likely and should be addressed in psychotherapy. Psychotherapy may help speed up the recovery and improve the prognosis. By definition, schizophreniform disorder resolves within 6 months with a return to baseline mental functioning.

Differential Diagnosis

This is similar to schizophrenia. Psychotic disorder caused by a general medical condition and substance-induced psychotic disorder must be ruled out. General medical conditions to be considered are HIV infection, temporal lobe epilepsy, CNS tumors, and cerebrovascular disease, all of which can also be associated with relatively short-lived psychotic episodes. The increasing number of reports of psychosis associated with the use of anabolic steroids by young men who are attempting to build up their muscles to perform better in athletic activities require careful history. Factitious disorder with predominantly psychological signs and symptoms and malingering may need to be ruled out in some instances.

Etiology

Schizophreniform psychosis, similar to other psychoses, is probably heterogeneous and due to an unknown cause. In general, some individuals have a disorder similar to schizophrenia, whereas others have a disorder similar to mood disorders. Some data, however, indicate a close relation to schizophrenia. Several studies have shown that individuals with schizophreniform disorder, as a group, have more affective symptoms (especially mania) and a better outcome than do individuals with schizophrenia. In addition, the increased presence of mood disorders in the relatives of individuals with schizophreniform disorder indicates a relation to mood disorders. Thus, the biological and epidemiological data are most consistent with the hypothesis that the current diagnostic category defines a group of individuals, some of whom have a disorder similar to schizophrenia and others similar to a mood disorder.

As in schizophrenia, a relative activation deficit in the inferior prefrontal region of the brain while the individual is performing the Wisconsin Card Sorting Test is reported. One study showed that the deficit was limited to the left hemisphere indicating a similarity to schizophrenia. More studies are needed to determine the long-term course, which is often variable and sometimes similar to schizophrenia but more often a shortened course quite different from schizophrenia. Some data indicate that individuals with schizophreniform disorder may have enlarged ventricles, as seen on CT scans and MRI, while other data indicate that unlike the enlargement seen in schizophrenia, the ventricular enlargement in schizophreniform disorder is not correlated with outcome measures or other biological measures.

Although brain-imaging studies suggest a similarity between schizophreniform disorder and schizophrenia, one study of electrodermal activity has indicated a difference. Individuals with schizophrenia born during the winter and spring months had hyporesponsive skin conductances, but this association was absent in individuals with schizophreniform disorder. Though the significance of this one study would be difficult to interpret, the results do suggest caution in assuming similarity between individuals with schizophrenia and those with schizophreniform disorder. Data from a study of eye tracking in the two groups also indicate that there are differences on some biological measures between schizophrenia and schizophreniform psychosis.

Treatment

Hospitalization is often necessary and allows for effective assessment, treatment, and supervision of an individual's behavior. The psychotic symptoms, usually treated with a 3- to 6-month course of antipsychotic drugs, respond more rapidly than in individuals with schizophrenia. One study found that 75% of the individuals with schizophreniform psychosis compared to 20% of those with schizophrenia responded to antipsychotic agents within 8 days. ECT may be indicated for some individuals, especially those with marked catatonic features or depression. If an individual has recurrent episodes, trials of lithium carbonate, valproic acid, or carbamazepine may be warranted for prophylaxis. Psychotherapy is usually necessary to help individuals integrate the psychotic experience into their understanding of their minds, brains, and lives.

DELUSIONAL DISORDER

Diagnosis

Delusional disorder refers to a group of disorders, the chief feature of which is the presence of *nonbizarre* delusions (see DSM-IV-TR diagnostic criteria below). People suffering from this illness generally do not regard themselves as mentally ill and actively oppose psychiatric referral. Because they may experience little impairment, they generally remain outside hospital settings, appearing reclusive, eccentric, or odd, rather than ill. They are more likely to have contacts with professionals such as lawyers and other medical specialists for health concerns. The current shift in diagnosis from *paranoid* to *delusional* helps avoid the ambiguity around the term "paranoid." This also emphasizes that other delusions besides the paranoid ones are included in this diagnosis. It is important to understand the definition of nonbizarre delusion so as to reach an unambiguous diagnosis. Nonbizarre delusions typically involve situations or circumstances that can occur in real life (e.g., being followed, infected, or deceived by a lover) and are believable.

DSM-IV-TR Diagnostic Criteria

297.10 Delusional Disorder

A. Nonbizarre delusions (i.e., involving situations that occur in real life, such as being followed, poisoned, infected, loved at a distance, or deceived by spouse or lover, or having a disease) of at least 1 month's duration.
B. Criterion A for schizophrenia has never been met.

Note: Tactile and olfactory hallucinations may be present in delusional disorder if they are related to the delusional theme.

C. Apart from the impact of the delusion(s) or its ramifications, functioning is not markedly impaired and behavior is not obviously odd or bizarre.
D. If mood episodes have occurred concurrently with delusions, their total duration has been brief relative to the duration of the delusional periods.
E. The disturbance is not due to the direct physiological effects of a substance (e.g., a drug of abuse, a medication) or a general medical condition.

Specify type (the following types are assigned based on the predominant delusional theme):

Erotomanic type: delusions that another person, usually of higher status, is in love with the individual

Grandiose type: delusions of inflated worth, power, knowledge, identity, or special relationship to a deity or famous person

Jealous type: delusions that the individual's sexual partner is unfaithful

> **Persecutory type:** delusions that the person (or someone to whom the person is close) is being malevolently treated in some way
>
> **Somatic type:** delusions that the person has some physical defect or general medical condition
>
> **Mixed type:** delusions characteristic of more than one of the above types but no one theme predominates
>
> **Unspecified type**

Reprinted with permission from the Diagnostic and Statistical Manual of Mental Disorders, Fourth Edition, Text Revision. Copyright 2000 American Psychiatric Association.

According to DSM-IV-TR, the diagnosis of delusional disorder can be made when a person exhibits nonbizarre delusions of at least 1 month's duration that cannot be attributed to other mental disorders. Nonbizarre delusions must be about phenomena that, although not real, are within the realm of being possible. In general, the individual's delusions are well systematized and have been logically developed. If the person experiences auditory or visual hallucinations, they are not prominent except for tactile or olfactory hallucinations where they are tied in to the delusion (e.g., a person who believes that he emits a foul odor might experience an olfactory hallucination of that odor). The person's behavioral and emotional responses to the delusions appear to be appropriate. Usually, the person's functioning and personality are well preserved and show minimal deterioration if at all.

Subtypes

Persecutory Type   This is the most common form of delusional disorder (Yamada et al. 1998). Here, the person affected believes that he or she is being followed, spied on, poisoned or drugged, harassed, or conspired against. The person affected may get preoccupied by small slights that can become incorporated into the delusional system. These individuals may resort to legal actions to remedy perceived injustice. Individuals suffering from these delusions often become resentful and angry with a potential to get violent against those believed to be against them.

Jealous Type   Individuals with this subtype have the delusional belief that their spouses/lovers are unfaithful. This is often wrongly inferred from small bits of benign evidence, which is used to justify the delusion. Delusions of infidelity have also been called *conjugal paranoia*. The term *Othello syndrome* has been used to describe morbid jealousy. This delusion usually affects men, with no history of prior psychiatric problems. The condition is difficult to treat and may diminish only on separation, divorce, or death of the spouse. Marked jealousy (pathological jealousy or morbid jealousy) is a symptom of many disorders including schizophrenia and is not unique to delusional disorder. Jealousy is a powerful emotion and when it occurs in delusional disorder or as part of another condition, it can be potentially dangerous and has been associated with violence including suicidal and homicidal behavior.

Erotomanic Type   These individuals have delusions of secret lovers. Most frequently, the individual is a woman, though men are also susceptible to these delusions. The individual believes that a suitor, usually more socially prominent than herself, is in love with her. This can become the central focus of the individual's existence and the onset can be sudden.

Erotomania is also referred to as *de Clerambault's syndrome*. Again, these delusions can occur as part of other disorders too. Generally women (but not exclusively so), unattractive in appearance, working at a lower-level jobs, who lead withdrawn, lonely single lives with few sexual contacts are reported to be more prone to develop this condition. They select lovers who are substantially different from them. They exhibit what has been called paradoxical conduct, the delusional phenomenon of interpreting all denials of love no matter how clear as secret affirmations of love. Separation from the love object may be the only satisfactory means of intervention. When it affects men, it can manifest with more aggressive and possibly violent pursuit of love. Thus, such people are often in the forensic system. The object of aggression is often companions or protectors of the love object who are viewed as trying to come between the lovers. However, resentment and rage in response to an absence of reaction from all forms of love communication may escalate to a point that the love object may be in danger too.

Approximately 10% of stalkers have a primary diagnosis of erotomania (Meloy 1996). Menzies and colleagues (1995) conducted the first predictive study of violence among erotomanic males and found that serious antisocial behavior (a criminal history) unrelated to the delusion and concurrent multiple objects of fixations discriminated between the dangerous and the nondangerous men. In a review by Meloy (1996), if violence occurred, the object of love was the target at least 80% of the time. The next most likely target was a third party perceived as impeding access to the object. He referred to this latter behavior as *triangulation*. Triangulation when present in jealousy, whether delusional or not, is motivated by a perceived competition for the love object (Meloy 1999).

Somatic Type   Delusional disorder with somatic delusions has been called *monosymptomatic hypochondriacal psychosis*. This disorder differs from other conditions with hypochondriacal symptoms in degree of reality impairment. Munro (1988, 1991) has described the largest series of cases and has used content of delusions to define three main types:

Delusional parasitosis is one of the most common presentations of monohypochondriacal psychosis, which occurs in absence of other psychiatric illness (Munro 1982). In one study involving 52 individuals, 88% of the cases were above 45 years of age (Bhatia et al. 2000). The prevalence of this condition is unknown (Berrios 1985). There appears to be a higher incidence of illness among middle-aged and elderly individuals. In the study mentioned above, 65% of the individuals were females (Bhatia et al. 2000). This is similar to some reports but not all. The onset is insidious and chronic (Lyell 1983).

Matchbox sign describes the common phenomenon that occurred not so long ago in individuals suffering from this condition. During their clinic visit, the individual would present with peeled skin, and other substances connected to delusional thinking in an empty old-fashioned matchbox as evidence that they were infested with insects (Lancet 1983, Morris 1991). Delusional parasitosis has been described in association with many physical illnesses such as vitamin B_{12} deficiency, pellagra, neurosyphilis, multiple sclerosis, thalamic dysfunction, hypophyseal tumors, diabetes mellitus, severe renal disease, hepatitis, hypothyroidism, mediastinal lymphoma, and leprosy. Use of cocaine and presence of dementia has also been reported.

Psychogenic parasitosis was also known as *Ekbom's syndrome* before being referred to as *delusional parasitosis*. Females experienced this disorder twice as often as males. Entomologists, pest control specialists, and dermatologists had often seen the individual before seen by a mental health professional. All investigators have been impressed by the concurrent medical illnesses associated with this condition. Others have attempted to distinguish between delusional and nondelusional aspects of presentation to establish clearer diagnosis and thus management.

Other delusions that are included in the Somatic Type include delusions of Dymorphophobia (e.g., delusions of misshapenness, personal ugliness, or exaggerated size of body parts) and delusions of foul body odors or halitosis (also called *olfactory reference syndrome*).

The frequency of these conditions is low, but they may be underdiagnosed because individuals present to dermatologists, plastic surgeons, and infectious disease specialists more often than to psychiatrists. Individuals with these conditions do respond to pimozide, a typical antipsychotic medication and also to SSRIs. Usually prognosis is poor without treatment. It affects both sexes equally. Suicide apparently motivated by anguish is not uncommon.

Grandiose Type   This is also referred to as *megalomania*. In this subtype, the central theme of the delusion is the grandiosity of having made some important discovery or having great talent. Sometimes there may be a religious theme to the delusional thinking such that the person believes that he or she has a special message from God.

Mixed Type   This subtype is reserved for those with two or more delusional themes. However, it should be used only where it is difficult to clearly discern one theme of delusion.

Unspecified Type   This subtype is used for cases in which the predominant delusion cannot be subtyped within the above-mentioned categories. A possible example is certain delusions of misidentification, for example, *Capgras's syndrome*, named after the French psychiatrist who described the "illusions of doubles." The delusion here is the belief that a familiar person has been replaced by an imposter. A variant of this is *Fregoli's syndrome* where the delusion is that the persecutors or familiar persons can assume the guise of strangers and the very rare delusion that familiar persons could change themselves into other persons at will (intermetamorphosis). Each disorder is not only a rare delusion but is highly associated with other conditions such as schizophrenia and dementia.

Epidemiology

Though the existence of delusional disorder has been known for a long time, relatively little is known about the demographics, incidence, and prevalence. Unfortunately, people suffering from this illness function reasonably well in the community and lack insight resulting in minimal or no contact with the mental health system. However, the crude incidence is roughly 0.7 to 3.0 per 100,000 with a more frequent occurrence in females. Some have associated this condition with widowhood, celibacy, and history of substance abuse. In one study, 1.2% of 4144 consecutively attending subjects in an outpatient clinic were diagnosed to have delusional disorder. Half of the subjects were diagnosed to have *persecutory* type of delusional disorder. Females suffering from this disorder were significantly older than males. In a retrospective study from China, 0.83% of 10,418 outpatients met DSM-IV criteria of delusional disorder with equal gender distribution. The age range was 17 to 86 years with an average age of 42 ± 15 years. Women were significantly older than men at age of onset (46 versus 38.7). The mean duration of symptom onset to first psychiatry visit was 2.4 years and did not differ significantly between the sexes. Auditory hallucinations were reported in 11.6%, tactile hallucinations in 5.8%, visual hallucinations in 2.3%, and olfactory hallucinations in 2.3%. The delusional disorder subtypes were persecutory type 70.9%, mixed 14%, jealous 8.1%, somatic 2.3%, unspecified 2.1%, erotomanic 1.2%, and grandiose 1.2% (Hsiao 1999). Kendler (1982) reported a prevalence of 0.24 to 0.3% with a sex ratio of female to male of 1.18 : 1. Yamada and associates (1998) reported a 3 : 1 female to male ratio among the individuals treated from

Japan. Hwu and colleagues (1989) reported the lifetime prevalence of 0.48% in cities, 0.67% in townships, and 0.33% in rural villages. The gender ratios were not significantly different in their studies. Someya and colleagues (1987) reported that persecutory type of delusional disorder was more common (64%) followed by jealous type (19%) in their cohort. Yamada and associates (1998) reported that persecutory type was most common at 51% followed by somatic type at 27.5% and jealous type at 13.7%. Both Yamada's and Hsiao's group did not find significant differences in the frequency of subtypes of delusional disorder between the sexes. Depressive symptomatology was present in 43% of the individuals at their first visit (Hsiao et al. 1999). Higher frequency of depression has been reported by others (Marino et al. 1993) at 50.7%. Both depression before the onset of delusions and after the onset of delusions have been reported (Marino et al. 1993, Chiu et al. 1990). The subgroup of individuals who have hallucinations may have a poorer outcome depending on the intensity of the hallucinations (SerrettI et al. 1999).

Course

Though the onset can occur in adolescence, generally it begins from middle to late adulthood with variable patterns of course, including lifelong disorder in some cases. Delusional disorder does not lead to severe impairment or change in personality, but rather to a gradual, progressive involvement with the delusional concern. Suicide has often been associated with this disorder. The base rate of spontaneous recovery may not be as low as previously thought, especially because only the more severely afflicted are referred for psychiatric treatment. Retterstol (Retterstol and Opjordsmoen 1991, Retterstol 1970) has provided much information on this. The more chronic forms of the illness tend to have their onset early in the fifth decade. Onset is acute in nearly two-thirds of the cases and gradual in the remainder. In almost half of the cases, the delusion disappears at follow-up, improves in 10%, and is unchanged in 31%. In the more acute forms of the illness, the age of onset is in the fourth decade, a lasting remission occurs in over half of the individuals, and a pattern of chronicity develops in only 10%; a relapsing course has been observed in 37%. Thus, the more acute and earlier the onset of the illness, the more favorable the prognosis. The presence of precipitating factors, married status, and female gender are associated with better outcome. The persistence of delusional thinking is most favorable for cases with persecutory delusions and somewhat less favorable for delusions of grandeur and jealousy. However, the outcome in terms of overall functioning appears somewhat more favorable for the jealous subtype.

Etiology

Etiology of the delusional disorder is unknown. Risk factors associated with the disorder include advanced age, sensory impairment/isolation, family history, social isolation, personality features (e.g., unusual interpersonal sensitivity), and recent immigration. Some have reported higher association of delusional disorder with widowhood, celibacy, and history of substance abuse. Age of onset is later than schizophrenia and earlier in men compared to women.

Treatment

Though generally considered resistant to treatment and interventions, the management is focused on managing the morbidity of the disorder by reducing the impact of the delusion on the individual's (and family's) life. However, in recent years, the outlook has become less pessimistic or restricted in planning effective treatment for these conditions. An effective and therapeutic clinician–patient relationship is important but difficult to establish.

Overall, treatment results suggest that 80.8% of cases recover either fully or partially. Pimozide, the most frequently reported treatment, produced full remission in 68.5% and partial recovery in 22.4% ($N = 143$). There are reports of treatment with other typical antipsychotic agents with variable success in a small number of subjects. SSRIs have been used and reported to be helpful. The newer atypical antipsychotic agents have been used in a small number of cases with success but the data is anecdotal. Bhatia and colleagues (2000) report that pimozide, fluoxetine, and amitriptyline were used in their study with pimozide showing good response.

As mentioned earlier, developing a therapeutic relationship is very important and yet significantly difficult, and requires a frank and supportive attitude. Supportive therapy is very helpful in dealing with emotions of anxiety and dysphoria generated because of delusional thinking. Cognitive therapy, when accepted and implemented, is helpful. Confrontation of the delusional thinking usually does not work and can further alienate the individual.

SHARED PSYCHOTIC DISORDER

Diagnosis

Shared psychotic disorder is a rare disorder, which is also referred to as *shared paranoid disorder, induced psychotic disorder, folie a deux,* and *double insanity* (see DSM-IV-TR diagnostic criteria below). Jules Baillarger, in 1860, first described the syndrome and called it *folie a communiquee,* while Lasegue and Falret, in 1877, first described *folie a deux.* In this disorder, the transfer of delusions takes place from one person to another. Both persons are closely associated for a long time and typically live together in relative social isolation. In its more common form, *folie imposee,* the individual who first has the delusion is often chronically ill and typically is the influential member of the close relationship with another individual, who is more suggestible and who develops the delusion too. The second individual is frequently less intelligent, more gullible, more passive, or more lacking in self-esteem than the primary case. If the two people involved are separated, the second individual may abandon the delusion. However, this is not seen consistently. Other forms of shared psychotic disorder reported are *folie simultanee,* where similar delusional systems develop independently in two closely associated people. Occasionally, more than two individuals are involved (e.g. *folie a trois, quatre, cinq;* also *folie a famille*) but such cases are very rare. The most common dyadic relationships who develop this disorder are sister–sister, husband–wife, and mother–child. Almost all cases involve members of a single family.

DSM-IV-TR Diagnostic Criteria

297.3 Shared Psychotic Disorder

A. A delusion develops in an individual in the context of a close relationship with another person(s), who has an already-established delusion.

B. The delusion is similar in content to that of the person who already has the established delusion.

C. The disturbance is not better accounted for by another Psychotic Disorder (e.g., Schizoprenia) or a Mood Disorder with Psychotic Features and is not due to the direct physiological effects of a substance (e.g., a drug of abuse, a medication) or a general condition.

An important feature in the diagnosis is that the person with shared psychotic disorder does not have a preexisting psychotic disorder. The delusions arise in the context of a close relationship with a person who suffers from delusional thinking and resolve on separation from that person. The key symptom of shared psychosis is the unquestioning acceptance of another person's delusions. The delusions themselves are often in the realm of possibility and usually not as bizarre as those seen in individuals with schizophrenia. The content of the delusion is often persecutory or hypochondriacal. Symptoms of a coexisting personality disorder may be present, but signs and symptoms that meet criteria for schizophrenia, mood disorders, and delusional disorder are absent. The individual may have ideation about suicide or pacts about homicide; clinicians must elicit this information during the interview.

Epidemiology
More than 95% of all cases of shared psychotic disorder involve two members of the same family. About a third of the cases involve two sisters, another one-third involve husband and wife or a mother and her child. The dominant person is usually affected by schizophrenia or a similar psychotic disorder. In 25% of all cases, the submissive person is usually affected with physical disabilities such as deafness, cerebrovascular diseases, or other disability that increases the submissive person's dependence on the dominant person. This condition is more common in people from low socioeconomic groups and in women.

Course
Though separation of the submissive person from the dominant person should resolve the psychosis, this probably occurs only in 10 to 40 % of the cases. Unfortunately, when these individuals are discharged from hospital, they usually move back together.

Differential Diagnosis
Malingering, factitious disorder with predominantly psychological sign and symptoms, psychotic disorder due to a general medical condition, and substance-induced psychotic disorder must be considered.

Etiology
There is some data that suggest that people suffering from shared psychotic disorder may have a family history of schizophrenia. The dominant person suffering from this illness often has schizophrenia or a related psychotic illness. The dominant person is usually older, more intelligent, better educated, and has stronger personality traits than the submissive person, who is usually dependent on the dominant person. The affected individuals usually live together or have an extremely close personal relationship, associated with shared life experiences, common needs and hopes, and often, a deep emotional rapport with each other. The relationship between the people involved is usually somewhat or completely isolated from external societal cultural inputs. The submissive person may be predisposed to a mental disorder and may have a history of a personality disorder with dependent or suggestible qualities as well as a history of depression, suspiciousness, and social isolation.

The dominant person's psychotic symptoms may develop in the submissive person through the process of identification. By adopting the psychotic symptoms of the dominant person, the submissive person gains acceptance by the other.

Treatment

The initial step in treatment is to separate the affected person from the source of the delusions, the dominant individual. Antipsychotic agents may be used if the symptoms have not abated in a week after separation. Psychotherapy with the nondelusional members of the individual's family should be undertaken, and psychotherapy with both the individual and the person sharing the delusion may be indicated later in the course of treatment. To prevent redevelopment of the syndrome, the family may need family therapy and social support to modify the family dynamics and to prevent redevelopment of the syndrome. Steps to decrease the social isolation may also help prevent the syndrome from reemerging.

Comparison of DSM-IV-TR/ICD-10 Diagnostic Criteria

The ICD-10 and DSM-IV-TR criteria sets for schizophrenia are similar in many important ways although not identical. The ICD-10 Diagnostic Criteria for Research provide two ways to satisfy the criteria for schizophrenia: having one Schneiderian first-rank symptom or having at least two of the other characteristic symptoms (hallucinations accompanied by delusions, thought disorder, catatonic symptoms, and negative symptoms). In contrast to DSM-IV-TR which requires 6 months of symptoms (including prodromal, active, and residual phases), the ICD-10 definition of schizophrenia requires only a 1-month duration, thereby encompassing the DSM-IV-TR diagnostic categories of both schizophrenia and schizophreniform disorder. Thus, cases of DSM-IV-TR schizophreniform disorder are diagnosed in ICD-10 as schizophrenia.

The DSM-IV-TR and ICD-10 definitions of schizoaffective disorder differ with regard to the relationship of the schizoaffective disorder category with the category mood disorder with psychotic features. In DSM-IV-TR, the differentiation depends on the temporal relationship between the mood and psychotic symptoms (i.e., mood disorder with psychotic features is diagnosed whenever the psychotic symptoms occur only in the presence of a mood episode, regardless of the characteristics of the psychotic symptoms). In contrast, the ICD-10 definition of schizoaffective disorder is much broader. It includes situations in which certain specified psychotic symptoms (i.e., thought echo, insertion, withdrawal, or broadcasting; delusions of control or passivity; voices giving a running commentary; disorganized speech, catatonic behavior) occur even if they are confined to a mood episode. Therefore, many cases of DSM-IV-TR mood disorder with mood-incongruent psychotic features would be considered to be schizoaffective disorder in ICD-10. Furthermore, the ICD-10 definition suggests that there should be an "approximate balance between the number, severity, and duration of the schizophrenic and affective symptoms." For delusional disorder, the ICD-10 Diagnostic Criteria for Research specify a minimum 3-month duration in contrast to the 1-month minimum duration in DSM-IV-TR.

In contrast to the single DSM-IV-TR category brief psychotic disorder, ICD-10 has a much more complex way of handling brief psychotic disorders. It includes criteria sets for four specific brief psychotic disorders that differ on the basis of types of symptoms (i.e., with or without symptoms of schizophrenia) and course (i.e., whether they change rapidly or not). Furthermore, the maximum duration of these brief psychotic episodes varies depending on the type of symptoms (i.e., 1 month for schizophrenia-like symptoms and 3 months for predominantly delusional). In contrast, DSM-IV-TR has a single criteria set and a maximum 1-month duration.

Finally, the ICD-10 and DSM-IV-TR definitions of shared psychotic disorder are almost identical.

References

Adams CE, Fenton MK, Quraishi S, et al. (2001) Systematic meta-review of depot antipsychotic drugs for people with schizophrenia. *Br J Psychiatry* **179**, 290–299.

Adams RD and Victor M (1989) *Principles of Neurology*, 4th ed., McGraw-Hill, New York.

Adebimpe VR (1994) Race, racism and epidemiological surveys. *Hosp Comm Psychiatry* **45**, 27–31.

Addington DD, Azorin JM, Falloon IRH, et al. (2002) Clinical issues related to depression in schizophrenia: an international survey of psychiatrists. *Acta Psychiatr Scand* **105**, 189–195.

Allardyce J, Boydell J, Van Os J, et al. (2001) Comparison of the incidence of schizophrenia in rural Dumfries and Galloway and urban Camberwell. *Br J Psychiatry* **179**, 335–339.

Allebech P, Varia A, and Wistedt B (1986) Suicide and violent death among patients with schizophrenia. *Acta Psychiatr Scand* **74**, 43–49.

Allison DB, Mentore JL, Heo M, et al. (1999) Antipsychotic-induced weight gain: a comprehensive research synthesis. *Am J Psychiatry* **156**, 1686–1696.

Almeida O, Howards R, Levy R, et al. (1995) Psychotic states rising in late life (late paraphrenia): psychopathology and nosology. *Br J Psychiatry* **166**, 205–214.

Altshuler LL, Bartzokis G, Grieder T, et al. (1998) Amygdala enlargement in bipolar disorder and hippocampal reduction in schizophrenia: an MRI study demonstrating neuroanatomic specificity. *Arch Gen Psychiatry* **55**, 663–664.

Alvir JM, Lieberman JA, Safferman AZ, et al. (1993) Clozapine-induced agranulocytosis: incidence and risk factors in the United States. *N Engl J Med* **329**, 162–167.

Ameddeo F, Bisoffi G, Bonizzato P, et al. (1995) Mortality among patients with psychiatric illness: a ten-year case register study in an area with community-based system of care. *Br J Psychiatry* **166**, 783–788.

American Psychiatric Association (1994) *Diagnostic and Statistical Manual of Mental Disorders*, 4th ed., APA, Washington, DC.

American Psychiatric Association (APA) Task Force (1980) Task force on late neurological effects of antipsychotic drugs: Tardive dyskinesia. *Am J Psychiatry* **137**, 1163–1172.

Andreasen NC (1981) *Scale for the Assessment of Negative Symptoms (SANS)*. University of Iowa, Iowa City, IA.

Andreasen NC (1997) The role of the thalamus in schizophrenia. *Can J Psychiatry* **42**, 27–33.

Andreasen NC and Olsen SA (1982) Negative vs. positive schizophrenia: definition and validation. *Arch Gen Psychiatry* **39**, 789–794.

Andreasen NC, Arndt S, Alliger R, et al. (1995) Symptoms of schizophrenia: methods, meanings and mechanisms. *Arch Gen Psychiatry* **52**, 341–351.

Andreasen NC, Arndt S, Swayze V, et al. (1994) Thalamic abnormalities in schizophrenia visualized through magnetic resonance image averaging. *Science* **266**, 294–298.

Andreasen NC, Nasrallah HA, Dunn VD, et al. (1986) Structural abnormalities in the frontal system in schizophrenia: a magnetic resonance imaging study. *Arch Gen Psychiatry* **43**, 135–144.

Andreasen NC, Olsen SA, Dennert JW, et al. (1982) Ventricular enlargement in schizophrenia: relationship to positive and negative symptoms. *Am J Psychiatry* **139**, 297–302.

Andrews G, Hall W, Goldstein G, et al. (1985) The economic costs of schizophrenia: implications for public policy. *Arch Gen Psychiatry* **42**, 537–543.

Arato M, O'Conner R, Bradbury JE, et al. (1998) Ziprasidone in the long-term treatment of negative symptoms and prevention of exacerbation of schizophrenia. *Eur Psychiatry* **13**(Supp. 4), 303.

Aravantis LA and Miller BG (1997) Multiple fixed doses of "Seroquel" (quetiapine) in patients with acute exacerbation of schizophrenia: a comparison with haloperidol and placebo, The Seroquel Trial 13 Study Group. *Biol Psychiatry* **42**, 233–246.

Arieti S (1955) *Interpretation of Schizophrenia*. Robert Brunner, New York.

Arndt S, Andreasen NC, Flaum M, et al. (1995) A longitudinal study of symptom dimensions in schizophrenia. Prediction and patterns of change. *Arch Gen Psychiatry* **52**, 341–351.

Ayd FJ (1961) A survey of drug induced extrapyramidal reactions. *JAMA* **175**, 1054–1061.

Bachrach LL (2000) Psychosocial rehabilitation and psychiatry in the treatment of schizophrenia: what are the boundaries? *Acta psychiatr Scand* **102**(Suppl. 407), 6–10.

Baker SC, Frith CD, and Dolan RJ (1997) The interaction between mood and cognitive function studied with PET. *Psychol Med* **27**, 565–578.

Baldessarini RJ and Frankenburg FR (1991) Clozapine: a novel antipsychotic agent. *N Engl J Med* **324**, 746–754.

Baldwin JA (1979) Schizophrenia and physical disease. *Psychol Med* **9**, 611–618.

Barbato A and D'Avanzo B (2000) Family interventions in schizophrenia and related disorders: a critical review of clinical trials. *Acta Psychiatr Scand* **102**, 81–97.

Barta PE, Pearlson GD, Powers RE, et al. (1990) Auditory hallucinations and smaller superior temporal gyral volume in schizophrenia. *Am J Psychiatry* **147**, 1457–1462.

Banov MD, Zarate CA Jr., Tohen M, et al. (1994) Clozapine therapy in refractory affective disorders: polarity predicts response in long-term follow-up. *J Clin Psychiatry* **55**, 411–414.

Barnes TR and Curson DA (1994) Long-term depot antipsychotics. A risk-benefit assessment. *Drug Safety* **10**, 464–479.

Beard JH, Propst RN, and Malamud TJ (1982) The Fountain House model of psychiatric rehabilitation. *Psychosoc Rehabil J* **5**, 47–53.

Beasley CM Jr., Hamilton SH, Crawford AM, et al. (1997) Olanzapine versus haloperidol: acute phase results of the international double-blind olanzapine trial. *Eur Neuropsychopharmacol* **7**, 125–137.

Beasley CM Jr., Tollefson G, Tran P, et al. (1996) Olanzapine versus placebo and haloperidol: acute phase results of the North American double-blind olanzapine trial. *Neuropsychopharmacology* **14**, 111–123.

Beatty WW, Jocic Z, Monson N, et al. (1993) Memory and frontal lobe dysfunction in schizophrenia and schizoaffective disorder. *J Nerv Ment Dis* **181**, 448–453.

Benes FM (2000) Emerging principles of altered neural circuitry in schizophrenia. *Brain Res Brain Res Rev* **31**, 251–269.

Benes FM, Kwok EW, Vincent MS, et al. (1998) A reduction of nonpyramidal cells in sector CA2 of schizophrenics and manic depressives. *Biol Psychiatry* **44**, 88–97.

Benes FM, McSparren J, Bird ED, et al. (1991) Deficits in small interneurons in prefrontal and cingulate cortices of schizophrenic and schizoaffective patients. *Arch Gen Psychiatry* **48**, 996–1001.

Berrios GE (1985) Positive and negative symptoms and Jackson. A conceptual history. *Arch Gen Psychiatry* **42**, 95–97.

Bertelsen A and Gottesman II (1995) Schizoaffective psychoses: genetical clues to classification. *Am J Med Genet* **60**, 7–11.

Bharath S, Gangadhar BN, and Janakiramaiah N (2000) P300 in family studies of schizophrenia: review and critique. *Int J Psychophysiol* **38**, 43–54.

Bhatia MS, Jagawat T, and Choudhary S (2000) Delusional Parasitosis: a clinical profile. *Int J Psychiatr Med* **30**, 83–91.

Bhugra D (2000) Migration and schizophrenia. *Acta Psychiatr Scand* **102**(Suppl. 407), 68–73.

Bilder RM, Bogerts B, Wu H, et al. (1994) Independence of morphological markers in schizophrenia. *Biol Psychiatry* **35**, 730.

Binder EB, Kinkead B, Owens MJ, et al. (2001) The role of neurotensin in the pathophysiology of schizophrenia and the mechanism of action of antipsychotic drugs. *Biol Psychiatry* **50**, 856–872.

Bisette G, Dole K, Johnson M, et al. (1988) Antipsychotic drugs increase neurotensin concentrations after destruction of dopamine neurons by 6–OHDA. *Soc Neurosci Abstr* **14**, 1211.

Blackwood D (2000) P300, a state and a trait marker in schizophrenia. *Lancet* **355**, 771–772.

Bleuler E and Zinkin J (trans) (1950) *Dementia Praecox or the Group of Schizophrenics*. International Universities Press, New York.

Blin O, Azorin JM, and Bouhours P (1996) Antipsychotic and anxiolytic properties of risperidone, haloperidol, and methotrimeprazine in schizophrenic patients. *J Clin Psychopharmacol* **16**, 38–44.

Blouin JL, Dombroski BA, Nath SK, et al. (1998) Schizophrenia susceptibility loci on chromosomes 13q32 and 8p21. *Nat Genet* **20**, 70–73.

Bogan AM, Brown ES, and Suppes T (2000) Efficacy of divalproex therapy for schizoaffective disorder. *J Clin Psychopharmacol* **20**, 520–522.

Bojholm S and Stromgren E (1989) Prevalence of schizophrenia on the island of Bornholm in 1935 and in 1983. *Acta Psychiatr Scand* **79**(Suppl. 348), 157–166.

Bondolfi G, Dufour H, Patris M, et al. (1998) Risperidone versus clozapine in treatment-resistant chronic schizophrenia: a randomized double-blind study. *Am J Psychiatry* **155**, 499–504.

Borison RL, Aravantis LA, and Miller BG, US Seroquel Study Group (1996) ICI 204,636, an atypical antipsychotic: efficacy and safety in a multicenter, placebo-controlled trial in patients with schizophrenia. *J Clin Psychopharm* **16**, 158–169.

Bornstein RA, Nasrallah HA, Olson SC, et al. (1990) Neuropsychological deficit in schizophrenic subtypes: paranoid, nonparanoid, and schizoaffective subgroups. *Psychiatr Res* **31**, 15–24.

Bouras C, Kovari E, Hof PR, et al. (2001) Anterior cingulate cortex pathology in schizophrenia and bipolar disorder. *Acta Neuropathol* **102**, 373–379.

Bourdon KH, Rae DS, Lacke BZ, et al. (1992) Estimating the prevalence of mental disorders in US adults from the epidemiological catchment area survey. *Pub Health Rep* **107**, 663–668.

Boyer WF, Bakalar NH, and Lake CR (1987) Anticholinergic prophylaxis of acute haloperidol-induced acute dystonic reactions. *J Clin Psychopharmacol* **7**, 164–166.

Brady JP (1984) Social skills training for psychiatric patients. I: Concepts, methods, and clinical results. *Am J Psychiatry* **141**, 333–340.

Braff DL (1993) Information processing and attention dysfunctions in schizophrenia. *Schizophr Bull* **19**, 233–259.

Bredesen DE (1995) Neural apoptosis. *Ann Neurol* **38**, 839–851.

Breier A (1994) Clozapine and noradrenergic function: support for a novel hypothesis for superior efficacy. *J Clin Psychiatry* **55**, 122–125.

Breier A (1995) Serotonin, schizophrenia and antipsychotic drug action. *Schizophr Res* **14**, 187–202.

Breier A and Astrachan BM (1984) Characterization of schizophrenic patients who commit suicide. *Am J Psychiatry* **141**, 610–611.

Breier A and Hamilton SH (1999) Comparative efficacy of olanzapine and haloperidol for patients with treatment-resistant schizophrenia. *Biol Psychiatry* **45**(4), 403–411.

Breier A, Buchanan RW, Elkashef A, et al. (1992) Brain morphology and schizophrenia: an MRI study of limbic, prefrontal cortex and caudate structures. *Arch Gen Psychiatry* **49**, 921–926.

Breier A, Buchanan RW, Waltrip RW, et al. (1994) The effect of clozapine on plasma norepinephrine: relationship to clinical efficacy. *Neuropsychopharmacology* **10**, 1–7.

Breier A, Meehan K, Birkett M, et al. (2002) A double-blind, placebo-controlled dose-response comparison of intramuscular olanzapine and haloperidol in the treatment of acute agitation in schizophrenia. *Arch Gen Psychiatry* **59**, 441–448.

Breier A, Schreiber JL, Dyer J, et al. (1991) National Institute of Mental Health longitudinal study of chronic schizophrenia: prognosis and prediction of outcome. *Arch Gen Psychiatry* **48**, 239–246.

Breier A, Su T-P, Saunders R, et al. (1997) Schizophrenia is associated with elevated amphetamine-induced synaptic dopamine concentrations: evidence from a novel positron emission tomography method. *Proc Natl Acad Sci U S A* **94**, 2569–2574.

Brewin J, Cantwell R, Dalkin T, et al. (1997) Incidence of schizophrenia in Nottingham. *Br J Psychiatry* **171**, 140–144.

Bruder G, Kayser J, Tenke C, et al. (1999) Left temporal lobe dysfunction in schizophrenia: Event-related potential and behavioral evidence from phonetic and tonal dichotic listening tasks. *Arch Gen Psychiatry* **56**, 267–276.

Bucci L (1987) The negative symptoms of schizophrenia and the monoamine oxidase inhibitors. *Psychopharmacology* **91**, 104–108.

Buchanan RW (1995) Clozapine: efficacy and safety. *Schizophr Bull* **21**, 579–591.

Buchsbaum MS and Hazlett E (1998) Positron emission tomography studies of abnormal glucose metabolism in schizophrenia. *Schizophr Bull* **24**, 343–364.

Buchsbaum MS, Tang CY, Peled S, et al. (1998) MRI white matter diffusion anisotropy and PET metabolic rate in schizophrenia. *Neuroreport* **9**, 425–430.

Buchsbaum MS, Yang S, Hazlett E, et al. (1997) Ventricular volume and asymmetry in schizotypal personality disorder and schizophrenia assessed with magnetic resonance imaging. *Schizophr Res* **27**, 45–53.

Buckley NA, Whyte IM, and Dawson AH (1995) Cardiotoxicity more common in thioridazine overdose than with other neuroleptics. *J Toxicol Clin Toxicol* **33**, 199–204.

Bunney WE and Bunney BG (2000) Evidence for a compromised dorsolateral prefrontal cortical parallel circuit in schizophrenia. *Brain Res Brain Res Rev* **31**, 138–146.

Burnet PW, Eastwood SL, and Harrison PJ (1997) [3H]WAY-100635 for 5-HT$_{1A}$ receptor autoradiography in human brain: a comparison with [3H]8-OH-DPAT and demonstration of increased binding in the frontal cortex in schizophrenia. *Neurochem Int* **30**, 565–574.

Burris KD, Molski TF, Xu C, et al. (2002) Aripiprazole, a novel antipsychotic, is a high affinity partial agonist at human dopamine D$_2$ receptors. *J Pharmacol Exp Ther* **203**, 318–389.

Bymaster F, Perry KW, Nelson DL, et al. (1999) Olanzapine: a basic science update. *Br J Psychiatry* **174**(Suppl. 37), 36–40.

Byrne M, Browne R, Mulryan N, et al. (2000) Labor and delivery complications and schizophrenia: case control study using contemporaneous labour ward records. *Br J Psychiatry* **176**, 531–536.

Cannon M, Jones PB, and Murray RM (2002) Obstetric complications and schizophrenia: historical and meta-analytic review. *Am J Psychiatry* **159**, 1080–1092.

Cannon TD, Rosso IM, Hollister JM, et al. (2000) A prospective cohort study of genetic and perinatal influences in the etiology of schizophrenia. *Schizophr Bull* **26**, 249–256.

Cannon TD, van Erp TG, Huttunen M, et al. (1998) Regional gray matter, white matter, and cerebrospinal fluid distributions in schizophrenic patients, their siblings, and controls. *Arch Gen Psychiatry* **55**, 1084–1091.

Cannon TD, Zorilla LE, and Shtasel D (1994) Neuropsychological function in siblings discordant for schizophrenia and healthy volunteers. *Arch Gen Psychiatry* **51**, 651–661.

Cao Q, Martinez M, Zhang J, et al. (1997) Suggestive evidence for a schizophrenia susceptibility locus on chromosome 6q and a confirmation in an independent series of pedigrees. *Genomics* **43**, 1–8.

Carlsson A, Waters N, Holm-Waters S, et al. (2001) Interactions between monoamines glutamate, and GABA in schizophrenia: new evidence. *Annu Rev Pharmacol Toxicol* **41**, 237–260.

Castle DJ and Murray RM (1993) The epidemiology of late-onset schizophrenia. *Schizophr Bull* **19**, 691–700.

Carpenter WT, Heinrichs DS, and Alphs LD (1985) Treatment of negative symptoms. *Schizophr Bull* **11**, 440–452.

Carpenter WT Jr., Conley RR, Buchanan RW, et al. (1995) Patient response and resource management: another view of clozapine treatment of schizophrenia. *Am J Psychiatry* **152**, 827–832.

Carter CS, Mintun M, Nichols T, et al. (1997) Anterior cingulate gyrus dysfunction and selective attention deficits in schizophrenia: [^{15}O]H$_2$0 PET study during single-trial Stroop task performance. *Am J Psychiatry* **154**, 1670–1675.

CATIE (1999) (Clinical Antipsychotic Trials of Intervention Effectiveness) funded by National Institute of Mental Health and coordinated by University of North Carolina at Chapel Hill (www.nih.nimh.gov; www.catie.unc.edu).

Ceskova E and Svestka J (1993) Double-blind comparison of risperidone and haloperidol in schizophrenic and schizoaffective psychoses. *Pharmacopsychiatry* **26**, 121–124.

Chakos MH, Lieberman JA, Alvir J, et al. (1995) Caudate nuclei volumes in schizophrenic patients treated with typical antipsychotics or clozapine. *Lancet* **345**, 456–457.

Chakos MH, Lieberman JA, Bilder RM, et al. (1994) Increase in caudate nuclei volumes of first-episode schizophrenic patients taking antipsychotic drugs. *Am J Psychiatry* **151**, 1430–1436.

Chakos MH, Lieberman JA, Hoffman E, et al. (2001) Effectiveness of second-generation antipsychotics in patients with treatment-resistant schizophrenia: a review and meta-analysis of randomized trials. *Am J Psychiatry* **158**, 518–526.

Chakos MH, Mayerhoff DI, Loebel AD, et al. (1992) Incidence and correlates of acute extrapyramidal symptoms in first episode of schizophrenia. *Psychopharmacol Bull* **28**, 81–86.

Chiu S, McFarlane AH, and Dobson N (1990) The treatment of nondelusional psychosis associated with depression. *Br J Psychiatry* **156**, 112–115.

Chouinard G, Jones B, Remington G, et al. (1993) A Canadian multicenter placebo-controlled study of fixed doses of risperidone and haloperidol in the treatment of chronic schizophrenic patients. *J Clin Psychopharmacol* **13**, 25–40.

Chow EWC, Bassett AS, and Weksberg R (1994) Velo-cardio-facial syndrome and psychotic disorders: implications for psychiatric genetics. *Am J Med Genet* **54**, 107–112.

Christy M, Christau B, Molbak AG, et al. (1982) Diabetes and month of birth (Letter). *Lancet* **2**, 216.

Ciapparelli A, Dell'Osso L, Pini S, et al. (2000) Clozapine for treatment-refractory schizophrenia, schizoaffective disorder, and psychotic bipolar disorder: A 24-month naturalistic study. *J Clin Psychiatry* **61**, 329–334.

Coffey CE, Sullivan JL, and Rice JR (1983) T lymphocytes in schizophrenia. *Biol Psychiatry* **18**, 113–119.

Cohen HW, Gibson G, and Alderman MH (2000) Excess risk of myocardial infarction in patients treated with antidepressant medications: association with use of tricyclic agents. *Am J Med* **108**, 2–8.

Cole JO, Klerman GL, and Goldberg SC (1964) Phenothiazine treatment in acute schizophrenia. *Arch Gen Psychiatry* **10**, 246–261.

Conley RR and Kelly DL (2001) Management of treatment resistance in schizophrenia. *Biol Psychiatry* **50**, 898–911.

Conley RR, Tamminga CA, Bartko JJ, et al. (1998) Olanzapine compared with chlorpromazine in treatment-resistant schizophrenia. *Am J Psychiatry* **155**(7), 914–920.

Committee on Safety of Medicines and Medicines Control Agency (1995) Cardiac arrhythmias with pimozide (Orap). *Curr Prob Pharmacovigil* **21**, 1.

Cooper JE and Sartorius N (1977) Cultural and temporal variations in schizophrenia: a speculation on the importance of industrialization. *Br J Psychiatry* **130**, 50–55.

Copeland JRM, Dewey ME, Scott A, et al. (1998) Schizophrenia and delusional disorder in older age: community prevalence, incidence, comorbidity, and outcome. *Schizophr Bull* **24**, 153–161.

Creese I, Burt DR, and Snyder SH (1975) Dopamine receptor binding predicts clinical and pharmacological potencies of antischizophrenic drugs. *Science* **192**, 481–483.

Crow TJ (1980) Molecular pathology of schizophrenia: more than one disease process? *Br Med J* **280**, 66–68.

Crow TJ (1985) The two-syndrome concept: origins and current status. *Schizophr Bull* **11**, 471–486.

Crow TJ (1986) Temporal disorientation in chronic schizophrenia. The implications of an "organic" psychological impairment for the concept of functional psychosis. In *Contemporary Issues in Schizophrenia*, Kerr TA and Snaith RP (eds). Gaskall, Royal College of Psychiatrists, London, pp. 168–174.

Crow TJ and Done DJ (1992) Prenatal influenza does not cause schizophrenia. *Br J Psychiatry* **161**, 390–393.

Csernansky JG, Mahmoud R, Brenner R, et al. (2002) A comparison of risperidone and haloperidol for the prevention of relapse in patients with schizophrenia. *N Engl J Med* **346**, 16–22.

Czekalla J, Beasley CM Jr., Dellva MA, et al. (2001) Analysis of the QTc interval during olanzapine treatment of patients with schizophrenia and related psychosis. *J Clin Psychiatry* **62**, 191–198.

Dalman C, Allebech P, Cullberg J, et al. (1999) Obstetric complications and the risk of schizophrenia: a longitudinal study of a national birth cohort. *Arch Gen Psychiatry* **56**, 234–240.

Daniel DG, Zimbaroff DL, Potkin SG, et al. (1999) Ziprasidone 80 mg/day and 160 mg/day in acute exacerbation of schizophrenia and schizoaffective disorder: a 6-week placebo-controlled trial. *Neuropsychopharmacology* **20**, 491–505.

Dasari M, Friedman L, Jesberger J, et al. (1999) A magnetic resonance imaging study of thalamic area in adolescent patients with either schizophrenia or bipolar disorder as compared to healthy controls. *Psychiatr Res* **91**, 155–162.

Davis JM (1975) Overview: maintenance therapy in psychiatry-I. Schizophrenia. *Am J Psychiatry* **132**, 1237–1245.

Deicken RF, Merrin EL, Floyd TC, et al. (1995) Correlation between left frontal phospholipids and Wisconsin card sort test performance in schizophrenia. *Schizophr Res* **14**, 177–181.

Delay J and Deniker P (1952) Trente-huit cas de psychoses traités par la cure prolongée et continué de 4560 RP. LeCongres des Al et Neurol. de Langue Fr. *Comptes Rendu du Congrès*. Masson et Cie, Paris.

Dellva MA, Tran P, Tollefson GD, et al. (1997) Standard olanzapine versus placebo and ineffective-dose olanzapine in the maintenance treatment of schizophrenia. *Psychiatr Serv* **48**, 1571–1577.

Delva NJ and Letemendia FJJ (1982) Lithium treatment in schizophrenia and schizoaffective disorders. *Br J Psychiatry* **141**, 387–400.

Demiralp T, Ademoglu A, Comerchero M, et al. (2001) Wavelet analysis of P3a and P3b. *Brain Topogr* **13**, 251–267.

Dickey W (1991) The neuroleptic malignant syndrome. *Prog Neurobiol* **36**, 425–436.

Dixon L, Weiden P, Delahanty J, et al. (2000) Prevalence and correlates of diabetes in national schizophrenia samples. *Schizophr Bull* **26**, 903–912.

Drake RE, Gates C, Whitaker A, et al. (1985) Suicide among schizophrenics: a review. *Compr Psychiatry* **26**, 90–100.

Eaton WW (1974) Residence, social class and schizophrenia. *J Health Soc Behav* **15**, 289–299.

Eaton WW (1985) Epidemiology of schizophrenia. *Epidemiol Rev* **7**, 105–126.

Eaton WW (1991) Update on the epidemiology of schizophrenia. *Epidemiol Rev* **13**, 320–328.

Eaton WW and Harrison G (2000) Ethnic disadvantage and schizophrenia. *Acta Psychiatr Scand* **1102**(Suppl. 407), 38–43.

Elkashef AM, Buchannan RW, Gellad F, et al. (1994) Basal ganglia pathology in schizophrenia and tardive dyskinesia: an MRI quantitative study. *Am J Psychiatry* **151**, 752–755.

Emrich HM, Dose M, and von Zerssen D (1985) The use of sodium divalproex, carbamazepine and oxycarbazepine in patients with affective disorders. *J Affect Disord* **8**, 243–250.

Erfurth A, Walden J, and Grunze H (1998) Lamotrigine in the treatment of schizoaffective disorder. *Neuropsychobiology* **38**, 204–205.

Erkwoh R, Sabri O, Steinmeyer EM, et al. (1997) Psychopathological and SPECT findings in never-treated schizophrenia. *Acta Psychiatr Scand* **96**, 51–57.

Essock SM, Hargreaves WA, Covell NH, et al. (1996) Clozapine's effectiveness for patients in state hospitals: results from a randomized trial. *Psychopharmacol Bull* **32**, 683–697.

Evans JD, Heaton RK, Paulsen JS, et al. (1999) Schizoaffective disorder: a form of schizophrenia or affective disorder? *J Clin Psychiatry* **60**, 874–882.

Fabre LFJ, Aravantis L, Pultz J, et al. (1995) ICI 204,636, a novel atypical antipsychotic: Early indication of safety and efficacy in patients with chronic and subchronic schizophrenia. *Clin Ther* **17**, 366–378.

Falloon IRH, Boyd JL, McGill CW, et al. (1982) Family management in the prevention of exacerbations of schizophrenia: a controlled study. *N Engl J Med* **306**, 1437–1440.

Falloon IRH, Boyd JL, McGill CW, et al. (1985) Family management in the prevention of morbidity of schizophrenia: clinical outcome of a two-year longitudinal study. *Arch Gen Psychiatry* **42**, 887–896.

Faraone SV, Matise T, Svrakic D, et al. (1998) Genome scan of European-American schizophrenia pedigrees: results of the NIMH genetics initiative and millennium consortium. *Am J Med Genet* **81**, 290–295.

Farde L, Nordstrom AL, Wiesel FA, et al. (1992) PET-analysis of central D_1 and D_2 dopamine receptor occupancy in patients treated with classical neuroleptics and clozapine-relation to extrapyramidal side effects. *Arch Gen Psychiatry* **49**, 538–544.

Farde L, Wiesel FA, Halldin C, et al. (1988) Central D_2-dopamine receptor occupancy in schizophrenic patients treated with antipsychotic drugs. *Arch Gen Psychiatry* **45**, 71–76.

Farde L, Wiesel FA, Nordstrom AL, et al. (1989) D_1 and D_2 dopamine receptor occupancy during treatment with conventional and atypical neuroleptics. *Psychopharmacology* **99**, S28–S29.

Farde L, Wiesel FA, Stone-Elander S, et al. (1990) D_2 dopamine receptors in neuroleptic-naive schizophrenic patients: a positron emission tomography study with [^{11}C] raclopride. *Arch Gen Psychiatry* **47**, 213–219.

Fenton WS and McGlashan TM (1994) Antecedents, symptom progression, and long-term outcome of the deficit syndrome in schizophrenia. *Am J Psychiatry* **151**, 351–356.

Fletcher P, McKenna PJ, Friston KJ, et al. (1999) Abnormal cingulate modulation of fronto-temporal connectivity in schizophrenia. *Neuroimage* **9**(3), 337–342.

Flor-Henry P (1983) *Cerebral Basis of Psychopathology*. John Wright, Boston.

Flor-Henry P (1985) Schizophrenia: sex differences. *Can J Psychiatry* **30**, 319–322.

Ford JM, Mathalon DH, Marsh L, et al. (1999) P300 amplitude is related to clinical state in severely and moderately ill patients with schizophrenia. *Biol Psychiatry* **46**, 94–101.

Frank AF and Gunderson JG (1990) The role of the therapeutic alliance in the treatment of schizophrenia: relationship to course and outcome. *Arch Gen Psychiatry* **47**, 228–236.

Franz M, Lis S, Pluddemann K, et al. (1997) Conventional versus atypical neuroleptics: Subjective quality of life in schizophrenic patients. *Br J Psychiatry* **170**, 422–425.

Freedman R, Coon H, Myles-Worsley M, et al. (1997) Linkage of a neurophysiological deficit in schizophrenia to a chromosome 15 locus. *Proc Natl Acad Sci U S A* **94**, 587–592.

Freedman R, Leonard S, Gault J, et al. (2001) Linkage disequilibrium for schizophrenia at the chromosome 15q13–14 locus of the alpha-7-nicotinic acetylcholine receptor subunit gene (CHRNA7). *Am J Med Genet* **105**, 20–22.

Frith CD, Leary J, Cahill C, et al. (1991) Performance on psychological tests. Demographic and clinical correlates of the results of these tests. *Br J Psychiatry* **13**(Suppl.), 26–29.

Frye MA, Ketter TA, Leverich GS, et al. (2000) The increasing use of polypharmacotherapy for refractory mood disorder: 22 years of study. *J Clin Psychiatry* **61**, 9–15.

Fucetola R, Newcomer JW, Craft S, et al. (1999) Age- and dose-dependent glucose-induced increases in memory and attention in schizophrenia. *Psychiatr Res* **88**, 1–13.

Gabbard GO (1990) *Psychodynamic Psychiatry in Clinical Practice*. American Psychiatric Press, Washington, DC.

Gainetdinov RR, Mohn AR, and Caron MG (2001) Genetic animal models: focus on schizophrenia. *Trends Neurosci* **24**, 527–533.

Galdi J (1983) The causality of depression in schizophrenia. *Br J Psychiatry* **142**, 621–625.

Gallhoffer B, Bauer U, Lis S, et al. (1996) Cognitive dysfunction in schizophrenia: Comparison of treatment with atypical antipsychotic agents and conventional neuroleptic drugs. *Eur Neuropsychopharmacol* **6**, 13–20.

Ganguli R, Brar JS, Roy Chengappa KN, et al. (1993) Autoimmunity in schizophrenia: a review of recent findings. *Ann Med* **25**, 489–496.

Gao XM, Sakai K, Roberts RC, et al. (2000) Ionotropic glutamate receptors and expression of N-methyl-d-aspartate receptor subunits in subregions of human hippocampus: Effects of schizophrenia. *Am J Psychiatry* **157**, 1141–1149.

Geddes J, Freemantle N, Harrison P, et al. (2000) Atypical antipsychotics in the treatment of schizophrenia: systematic overview and meta-regression analysis. *Br Med J* **321**, 1371–1376.

Geddes JR, Verdoux H, Takei N, et al. (1999) Schizophrenia and complications of pregnancy and labor: an individual-patient data meta-analysis. *Schizophr Bull* **25**, 413–423.

Gilbert PL, Harris MJ, McAdams LA, et al. (1995) Neuroleptic withdrawal in schizophrenic patients: a review of the literature. *Arch Gen Psychiatry* **52**, 173–188.

Gill M, Vallada H, Collier D, et al. (1996) A combined analysis of $D_2 2S278$ marker alleles in affected sib-pairs: support for a susceptibility locus for schizophrenia at chromosome 22q12. Schizophrenia Collaborative Linkage Group (Chromosome 22). *Am J Med Genet* **67**, 40–45.

Goff DC, Brotman AW, Waites M, et al. (1990) Trial of fluoxetine added to neuroleptics for treatment-resistant schizophrenic patients. *Am J Psychiatry* **147**, 492–494.

Goff DC, Posever T, Herz L, et al. (1998) An exploratory haloperidol-controlled dose-finding study of ziprasidone in hospitalized patients with schizophrenia or schizoaffective disorder. *J Clin Psychopharmacol* **18**, 296–304.

Goff DC, Tsai G, Levitt J, et al. (1999) A placebo-controlled crossover trial of d-cycloserine added to conventional neuroleptics in patients with schizophrenia. *Arch Gen Psychiatry* **56**, 21–27.

Gold S, Arndt S, Nopoulos P, et al. (1999) Longitudinal study of cognitive function in first-episode and recent-onset schizophrenia. *Am J Psychiatry* **156**, 1342–1348.

Goldberg EM and Morrison SL (1963) Schizophrenia and social class. *Br J Psychiatry* **109**, 785–802.

Goldman-Rakic PS and Selemon LD (1997) Functional and anatomical aspects of prefrontal pathology in schizophrenia. *Schizophr Bull* **23**, 437–458.

Goldstein JM, Goodman JM, Seidman LJ, et al. (1999) Cortical abnormalities in schizophrenia identified by structural magnetic resonance imaging. *Arch Gen Psychiatry* **56**, 537–547.

Gottesman II (1997) Twins: En route to QTLs for cognition. *Science* **276**, 1522–1523.

Granato JE, Stern BJ, Ringel A, et al. (1983) Neuroleptic malignant syndrome: successful treatment with dantrolene and bromocriptine. *Ann Neurol* **14**, 89–90.

Grech A, Takei N, and Murray RM (1997) Maternal exposure to influenza and paranoid schizophrenia. *Schizophr Res* **26**(2–3), 121–125.

Green AI, Tohen M, Patel JK, et al. (2000) Clozapine in treatment refractory psychotic mania. *Am J Psychiatry* **157**, 982–986.

Green MF (1996) What are the functional consequences of neurocognitive deficits in schizophrenia? *Am J Psychiatry* **153**, 321–330.

Grenade LL, Graham D, and Trontell A (2001) Myocarditis and cardiomyopathy associated with clozapine use in the United States. *N Engl J Med* **345**, 224.

Grossman LS, Harrow M, Goldberg JF, et al. (1991) Outcome of schizoaffective disorder at two long-term follow-ups: comparisons with outcome of schizophrenia and affective disorders. *Am J Psychiatry* **148**, 1359.

Guidotti A, Auta J, Davis JM, et al. (2000) Decrease in reelin and glutamic acid decarboxylase 67 ($GAD_6 7$) expression in schizophrenia and bipolar disorder: a postmortem brain study. *Arch Gen Psychiatry* **57**, 1061–1069.

Gur RE, Cowell P, Turetsky BI, et al. (1998) A follow-up MRI study of schizophrenia: relationship of neuroanatomic changes with clinical and neurobehavioral measures. *Arch gen Psychiatry* **55**, 145–152.

Gurevich EV and Joyce JN (1997) Alterations in the cortical serotonergic system in schizophrenia: a postmortem study. *Biol Psychiatry* **42**, 529–545.

Hafner H (2000) Onset and early course as determinants of the further course of schizophrenia. *Acta Psychiatr Scand* **102**(Suppl. 407), 44–48.

Hagg S, Joelsson L, Mjorndal T, et al. (1998) Prevalence of diabetes and impaired glucose tolerance in patients treated with clozapine compared with patients treated with conventional depot neuroleptic medications. *J Clin Psychiatry* **59**, 294–299.

Hakola HPA and Laulumaa VA (1982) Carbamazepine in treatment of violent schizophrenics (Letter). *Lancet* **1**, 1358.

Halgren E, Baudena P, Clarke J, et al. (1995) Intracerebral potentials to rare target and distractor auditory and visual stimuli II. Medial, lateral, and posterior temporal lobe. *Electroencephalogr Clin Neurophysiol* **94**, 229–250.

Hambrecht M, Maurer K, Hafner H, et al. (1992) Transnational stability of gender differences in schizophrenia? An analysis based on the WHO study on determinants of outcome of severe mental disorders. *Eur Arch Psychiatr Clin Neurosci* **242**, 6–12.

Harding CM, Brooks GW, Ashikaga T, et al. (1987a) The Vermont longitudinal study of persons with severe mental illness. I. Methodology, study sample, and overall status 32 years later. *Am J Psychiatry* **144**, 718–726.

Harding CM, Brooks GW, Ashikaga T, et al. (1987b) The Vermont longitudinal study of persons with severe mental illness II. Long-term outcome of subjects who retrospectively met DSM-III criteria for schizophrenia. *Am J Psychiatry* **144**, 727–735.

Hare EH (1983) Epidemiological evidence for a viral factor in the aetiology of the functional psychoses. *Adv Biol Psychiatry* **12**, 52.

Hare EH (1987) Epidemiology of schizophrenia and affective psychoses. *Br Med Bull* **43**, 514–530.

Harris EC and Barraclough B (1998) Excess mortality of mental disorder. *Br J Psychiatry* **173**, 11–33.

Harrison PJ (1999) The neuropathology of schizophrenia: a critical review of the data and their interpretation. *Brain* **122**, 593–624.

Harvey PD (2001) Abbreviated cognitive assessment in schizophrenia: recent data on feasibility. *J Adv Schizophr Brain Res* **3**, 73–78.

Harvey PD, Earle-Boyer EA, Wielgus MS, et al. (1986) Encoding memory and thought disorder in schizophrenia and mania. *Schizophr Bull* **12**, 252–261.

Harvey PD, Howanitz E, Parrella M, et al. (1998) Symptoms, cognitive functioning, and adaptive skills in geriatric patients with lifelong schizophrenia: a comparison across treatment sites. *Am J Psychiatry* **155**, 1080–1086.

Haupt DW and Newcomer JW (2001) Risperidone-associated diabetic ketoacidosis. *Psychosomatics* **42**, 279–280.

Haverkamp W, Breithardt G, Camm AJ, et al. (2000) The potential for QT prolongation and proarrhythmia by non-antiarrhythmic drugs: clinical and regulatory implications, Report on a Policy Conference of the European Society of Cardiology. *Cardiovasc Res* **47**, 219–233.

Hayes SG (1989) Long-term use of valproate in primary psychiatric disorders. *J Clin Psychiatry* **5**(Suppl. 3), 35–39.

Hazlett EA, Buchsbaum MS, Byne W, et al. (1999) Three-dimensional analysis with MRI and PET of the size, shape and function of the thalamus in the schizophrenia spectrum. *Am J Psychiatry* **156**, 1190–1199.

Haznedar MM, Buchsbaum MS, Luu C, et al. (1997) Decreased anterior cingulate gyrus metabolic rate in schizophrenia. *Am J Psychiatry* **154**, 682–684.

Heaton RK, Paulsen JS, McAdams LA, et al. (1994) Neuropsychological deficits in schizophrenics relationship to age, chronicity and dementia. *Arch Gen Psychiatry* **51**, 469–476.

Heila H, Isometsa ET, Henriksson MM, et al. (1997) Suicide and schizophrenia: a nationwide psychological autopsy study on age- and sex-specific clinical characteristics of 92 suicide victims with schizophrenia. *Am J Psychiatry* **154**, 1235–1242.

Helgason T (1964) Epidemiology of mental disorders in Iceland. *Acta Psychiatr Scand* **40**(Suppl.), 173.

Henderson DC, Cagliero E, Gray C, et al. (2000) Clozapine, diabetes mellitus, weight gain and lipid abnormalities: a five-year naturalistic study. *Am J Psychiatry* **157**, 975–981.

Henn FA and Braus DF (1999) Structural neuroimaging in schizophrenia: an integrative view of neuromorphology. *Eur Arch Psychiatr Clin Neurosci* **249**(Suppl. 4), IV/48–IV/56.

Herrera JM, Sramek JJ, and Costa JF (1987) Efficacy of adjunctive carbamazepine in the treatment of chronic schizophrenia. *Drug Intel Clin Pharm* **21**, 355–358.

Hickling F and Rodgers-Johnson P (1995) The incidence of first contact schizophrenia in Jamaica. *Br J Psychiatry* **167**, 474–481.

Hietala E, Syvalaht K, Vuorio K, et al. (1994) Striatal dopamine receptor characteristics in neuroleptic-naïve schizophrenic patients studied with positron emission tomography. *Arch Gen Psychiatry* **51**, 116–123.

Hillert A, Maier W, Wetzel H, et al. (1992) Risperidone in the treatment of disorders with a combined psychotic and depressive syndrome: a functional approach. *Pharmacopsychiatry* **25**, 213–217.

Hirayasu Y, Shenton ME, Salisbury DF, et al. (1998) Lower left temporal lobe MRI volumes in patients with first-episode schizophrenia compared with psychotic patients with first-episode affective disorder and normal subjects. *Am J Psychiatry* **155**, 1384–1391.

Hogarty GE, Anderson CM, Reiss DJ, et al. (1986) Family psychoeducation, social skills training, and maintenance chemotherapy in the aftercare treatment of schizophrenia. I. One-year effects of a controlled study on relapse and expressed emotion. *Arch Gen Psychiatry* **43**, 633–642.

Hogarty GE, Goldberg SC, Scholler NR, et al. (1974) Drugs and sociotherapy in the aftercare of schizophrenia patients. *Arch Gen Psychiatry* **31**, 603–608.

Hollister LE and Kosek JC (1965) Sudden death during treatment with phenothiazine derivatives. *JAMA* **192**, 1035–1038.

Honer WG, Falkai P, Young C, et al. (1997) Cingulate cortex synaptic terminal proteins and neural cell adhesion molecule in schizophrenia. *Neuroscience* **78**, 99–110.

Hovatta I, Terwilliger JD, Lichtermann D, et al. (1997) Schizophrenia in the genetic isolate of Finland. *Am J Med Genet Neuropsychiatr Genet* **74**, 353–360.

Howard R, Almeida OP, and Levy R (1994) Phenomenology, demography and diagnosis in late paraphrenia. *Psychol Med* **24**, 397–410.

Howard R, Rabins PV, Seeman MV, et al. (2000) Late-onset schizophrenia and very-late-onset schizophrenia-like psychosis: an international consensus. *Am J Psychiatry* **157**, 172–178.

Hoyberg OJ, Fensbo C, Remvig J, et al. (1993) Risperidone versus pepehnazine in the treatment of chronic schizophrenic patients with acute exacerbations. *Acta Psychiatr Scand* **88**, 395–402.

Hsiao MC, Liu CY, Yang YY, et al. (1999) Delusional disorder: retrospective analysis of 86 Chinese outpatients. *Psychiatr Clin Neurosci* **53**, 673–676.

Hutchinson G, Takei N, Bhugra D, et al. (1997) Increased rate of psychosis among African-Caribbeans in Britain is not due to an excess of pregnancy and birth complications. *Br J Psychiatry* **171**, 145–147.

Hwu HG, Yeh EK, and Chang LY (1989) Prevalence of psychiatric disorders in Taiwan defined by the Chinese diagnostic interview schedule. *Acta Psychiatr Scand* **79**, 136–147.

Impagnatiello F, Guidotti A, Pesold C, et al. (1998) A decrease of reelin expression as a putative vulnerability factor in schizophrenia. *Proc Natl Acad Sci U S A* **95**, 15718–15723.

Ingvar DH and Franzen G (1974) Abnormalities of cerebral blood flow distribution in patients with chronic schizophrenia. *Acta Psychiatr Scand* **50**, 425–462.

Jablensky A (1986) Epidemiology of schizophrenia: a European perspective. *Schizophr Bull* **12**, 52–73.

Jablensky A (2000) Epidemiology of schizophrenia: the global burden of disease and disability. *Eur Arch Psychiatr Clin Neurosci* **250**, 274–285.

Jablensky A and Cole SW (1997) Is the earlier age at onset of schizophrenia in males a confounded finding? Results from a cross-cultural investigation. *Br J Psychiatry* **170**, 234–240.

Jablensky A, Sartorius N, Ernberg G, et al. (1988) *Schizophrenia: Manifestation, Incidence and Course in Different Cultures*. World Health Organization, Geneva.

Jablensky A, Sartorius N, Ernberg G, et al. (1992) Schizophrenia: manifestations, incidence and course in different cultures. A world health organization ten-country study. *Psychological Medicine Monograph*, (Suppl 20). Cambridge University Press, Cambridge.

Jablensky A, Schwarz R, and Tomov T (1980) WHO collaborative study on impairments and disabilities associated with schizophrenic disorders. *Acta Psychiatr Scand* **62**(Suppl. 285), 152–163.

Jackson JH (1987) Remarks on evolution and dissolution of the nervous system. *J Ment Sci* **33**, 25–48.

Janicak PG, Keck PE Jr., Davis JM, et al. (2001) A double-blind, randomized, prospective evaluation of the efficacy and safety of risperidone versus haloperidol in the treatment of schizoaffective disorder. *J Clin Psychopharm* **21**, 360–368.

Jeffreys SE, Harvey CA, McNaught AS, et al. (1997) The Hampstead Schizophrenia Survey 1991. I: Prevalence and service use comparisons in an inner London health authority, 1986–1991. *Br J Psychiatry* **170**, 301–306.

Jeon YW and Polich J (2001) P300 asymmetry in schizophrenia: a meta-analysis. *Psychiatr Res* **104**, 61–74.

Jeste DV, Harris MJ, Krull A, et al. (1995) Clinical and neuropsychological characteristics of patients with late-onset schizophrenia. *Am J Psychiatry* **152**, 722–730.

Johnstone EC and Owens DGC (1981) Neurological changes in a population of patients with chronic schizophrenia and their relationship to physical treatment. *Acta Psychiatr Scand* **63**(Suppl. 291), 103–110.

Johnstone EC, Crow TJ, Frith CD, et al. (1978) The dementia of dementia praecox. *Acta Psychiatr Scand* **57**, 305–324.

Johnstone EC, Frith CD, Gold A, et al. (1979) The outcome of severe acute schizophrenic illnesses after one year. *Br J Psychiatry* **134**, 28–33.

Jones PB, Rantakallio P, Hartikainen AL, et al. (1998) Schizophrenia as a long-term outcome of pregnancy, delivery, and perinatal complications: a 28-year follow-up of the 1966 North Finland general population birth cohort. *Am J Psychiatry* **155**, 355–364.

Jongbloet PH, Mulder A, and Hamers AJ (1982) Seasonality of preovulatory nondisjunction and the etiology of down syndrome. A European collaborative study. *Hum Genet* **62**, 134–138.

Jordan S, Koprivica V, Chen R, et al. (2002) The antipsychotic aripiprazole is a potent, partial agonist at the human 5-HT$_{1A}$ receptor. *Eur J Pharmacol* **441**, 137–140.

Kalus P, Senitz D, Lauer M, et al. (1999) Inhibitory catridge synapses in the anterior cingulate cortex of schizophrenics. *J Neural Transm* **106**, 763–771.

Kanas N, Rogers M, Dreth E, et al. (1980) The effectiveness of group psychotherapy during the first three weeks of hospitalization: a controlled study. *J Nerv Ment Dis* **168**, 487–492.

Kane JM (1987) Treatment of schizophrenia. *Schizophr Bull* **13**, 133–156.

Kane JM, Carson WH, Saha AR et al. (2002) Efficacy and safety of aripiprazole and haloperidol vs placebo in patients with schizophrenia and schizoaffective disorder. *J Clin Psychiatry* **53**, 763–771.

Kane JM, Marder SR, Schooler NR, et al. (2001) Clozapine and haloperidol in moderately refractory schizophrenia: a 6-month randomized and double-blind comparison. *Arch Gen Psychiatry* **58**, 965–972.

Kane JM, Rifkin A, Woerner MG, et al. (1983) Low-dose neuroleptic treatment of outpatient schizophrenics. *Arch Gen Psychiatry* **40**, 893–896.

Kane JM, Rifkin A, Woerner MG, et al. (1985) High-dose versus low-dose strategies in the treatment of schizophrenia. *Psychopharmacol Bull* **21**, 533–537.

Kane JM, Woerner M, and Lieberman J (1988) Tardive dyskinesia: prevalence, incidence and risk factors. *J Clin Psychopharmacol* **8**, 525–565.

Kasanin J (1933) The acute schizoaffective psychoses. *Am J Psychiatry* **13**, 97–126.

Kasckow J and Nemeroff C (1991) The neurobiology of neurotensin: focus on neurotensin-dopamine interactions. *Regul Peptides* **36**, 153–164.

Kasper S and Muller-Spahn F (2001) Review of quetiapine and its clinical applications in schizophrenia. *Expert Opin Pharmacother* **1**, 783–801.

Kasper S, Tauscher J, Kufferle B, et al. (1999) Dopamine- and serotonin-receptors in schizophrenia: results of imaging-studies and implications for pharmacotherapy in schizophrenia. *Eur Arch Psychiatr Clin Neurosci* **249**(Suppl. 4), IV/83–IV/89.

Kay SR, Opler LA, and Lindemayer JP (1988) Reliability and validity of the positive and negative syndrome scale for schizophrenics. *Psychiatr Res* **23**, 99–110.

Keck P Jr., Buffenstein A, Ferguson J, et al. (1998) Ziprasidone 40 and 120 mg/day in the acute exacerbation of schizophrenia and schizoaffective disorder: a 4-week placebo-controlled trial. *Psychopharmacology* **140**, 173–184.

Keck PE, McElroy SL, and Strakowski SM (1999) Schizoaffective disorder: role of atypical antipsychotic. *Schizophr Res* **35**(Suppl.), 121–125.

Keefe RS, Perkins D, Silva SG, et al. (1999) The effects of atypical antipsychotic drugs on neurocognitive impairment in schizophrenia. *Schizophr Bull* **25**, 201–222.

Keith SJ, Regier DA, and Rae DS (1991) Schizophrenic disorders. In *Psychiatric Disorders in America*, Robins LN and Regier DA (eds). Free Press, New York, pp. 33–52.

Kendell RE, McInneny K, Jusczak E, et al. (2000) Obstetric complications and schizophrenia: two case-control studies based on structured obstetric records. *Br J Psychiatry* **174**, 516–522.

Kendler KS (1982) Demography of paranoid psychosis (delusional disorder): a review and comparison with schizophrenia and affective illness. *Arch Gen Psychiatry* **39**, 890–902.

Kendler KS and Diehl SR (1993) The genetics of schizophrenia: a current, genetic-epidemiologic perspective. *Schizophr Bull* **19**, 261–285.

Kendler KS and Walsh D (1995) Gender and schizophrenia. Results of an epidemiologically-based family study. *Br J Psychiatry* **167**, 184–192.

Kendler KS, McGuire M, Gruenberg AM, et al. (1995b) Examining the validity of DSM-III-R schizoaffective disorder and its putative subtypes in the Roscommon family study. *Am J Psychiatry* **152**, 755–764.

Keshavan MS, Stanley JA, and Pettegrew JW (2000) Magnetic resonance spectroscopy in schizophrenia: methodological issues and findings. Part II. *Biol Psychiatry* **48**, 369–380.

Kety SS (1987) The significance of genetic factors in the etiology of schizophrenia: results from the national study of adoptees in Denmark. *J Psychiatr Res* **21**, 423–429.

Kety SS, Rosenthal D, Wender PH, et al. (1968) The types and prevalence of mental illness in the biological and adoptive families of adopted schizophrenics. *J Psychiatr Res* **6**, 345–362.

Kilian JG, Kerr K, Lawrence C, et al. (1999) Myocarditis and cardiomyopathy associated with clozapine. *Lancet* **354**, 1841–1845.

Kindermann SS, Karimi A, Symonds L, et al. (1997) Review of functional magnetic resonance imaging in schizophrenia. *Schizophr Res* **27**, 143–156.

Kirino E, Belger A, Goldman-Rakic P, et al. (2000) Prefrontal activation evoked by infrequent target and novel stimuli in a visual target detection task: an event-related functional magnetic resonance study. *J Neurosci* **20**, 6612–6618.

Klein E, Beutal E, Lerer B, et al. (1984) Carbamazepine and haloperidol versus placebo and haloperidol in excited psychosis: a controlled study. *Arch Gen Psychiatry* **41**, 165–170.

Klieser E, Lehmann E, Kinzler E, et al. (1995) Randomized, double-blind, controlled trial of risperidone versus clozapine in patients with chronic schizophrenia. *J Clin Psychopharmacol* **1**(Suppl. 1), 45S–51S.

Knable MB, Torrey EF, Webster MJ, et al. (2001) Multivariate analysis of prefrontal cortical data from the stanley foundation neuropathology consortium. *Brain Res Bull* **55**, 651–659.

Knapp M (1997) Costs of schizophrenia. *Br J Psychiatry* **171**, 509–518.

Knight RT (1996) Contribution of human hippocampal region to novelty detection. *Nature* **383**, 256–259.

Knight RT (1997) Distributed cortical network for visual attention. *J Cogn Neurosci* **9**, 75–91.

Koh SD (1978) Remembering of verbal materials by schizophrenic young adults. In *Language and Cognition in Schizophrenia*, Schwartz S (ed.). Lawrence Erlbaum, Hillsdale, NJ.

Kraepelin E and Barclay RM (trans) (1919) *Dementia Praecox and Paraphrenia*, Robertson GM (ed.). E & S Livingstone, Edinburgh.

Kramer M (1969) Cross-national study of diagnosis of the mental disorders: origin of the problem. *Am J Psychiatry* **10**(Suppl.), 1–11.

Kramer MS, Last B, Getson A, et al. (1997) The effects of a selective D_4 dopamine receptor antagonist (L-745,870) in acutely psychotic inpatients with schizophrenia. D_4 Dopamine Antagonist Group. *Arch Gen Psychiatry* **54**, 567–572.

Krystal JH, Karper LP, Siebyl JP, et al. (1994) Subanesthetic effects of the noncompetitive NMDA antagonist, ketamine, in humans, psychotomimetic, perceptual, cognitive, and neuroendocrine responses. *Arch Gen Psychiatry* **51**, 199–214.

Lacro JP, Harris MJ, and Jeste DV (1993) Late life psychosis. *Int J Geriatr Psychiatry* **8**, 49–57.

Lafargue T and Brasic J (2000) Neurodevelopmental hypothesis of schizophrenia: a central sensory disturbance. *Med Hypotheses* **55**, 314–318.

Lancet (1983) The matchbox sign. *Lancet* **1**, 26.

Land W, Pinsky D, and Salzman C (1991) Psychopharmacology: abuse and misuse of anticholinergic medications. *Hosp Comm Psychiatry* **42**, 580–581.

Langfeldt G (1939) *The Schizophreniform States*. Oxford University Press, London.

Lapierre YD (1994) Schizophrenia and manic depression: separate illnesses or a continuum? *Can J Psychiatry* **39**, S59–S64.

Larsen TR, Moe LC, Vibe-Hansen L, et al. (2000) Premorbid functioning versus duration of untreated psychosis in 1-year outcome in first-episode psychosis. *Schizophr Res* **45**, 1–9.

Laruelle M, Abi-Dargham A, van Dyck CH, et al. (1996) Single photon emission computerized tomography imaging of amphetamine-induced dopamine release in drug-free schizophrenic subjects. *Proc Natl Acad Sci U S A* **20**, 9235–9240.

Lawrie SM and Abukmeil SS (1998) Brain abnormality in schizophrenia: a systematic and quantitative review of volumetric magnetic resonance imaging studies. *Br J Psychiatry* **172**, 110–120.

Leff J (2000) Family work for schizophrenia: practical application. *Acta Psychiatr Scand* **102**(Suppl. 407), 78–82.

Leff J, Kuipers L, Berkowitz R, et al. (1982) A controlled trial of social intervention in the families of schizophrenic patients. *Br J Psychiatry* **141**, 121–134.

Lehtinen V (1996) The epidemiology of mental disorders in Finland. *Nord J Psychiatry* **50**(Suppl. 36), 25–30.

Lencz T, Bilder RM, and Cornblatt B (2001) The timing of neurodevelopmental abnormality in schizophrenia: an integrative review of the neuroimaging literature. *CNS Spectrums* **6**, 233–255.

Levenson JL (1985) Neuroleptic malignant syndrome. *Am J Psychiatry* **142**, 1137–1145.

Levinson DF (1991) Pharmacologic treatment of schizophrenia. *Clin Ther* **13**, 326–352.

Levinson DF, Holmans P, Straub RE, et al. (2000) Multicenter linkage of schizophrenia candidate region of chromosomes 5q, 6q, 10p, and 13q: Schizophrenia linkage collaborative group III. *Am J Hum Genet* **67**, 652–663.

Levinson DF, Mahtani MM, Nancarrow DJ, et al. (1998) Genome scan of schizophrenia. *Am J Psychiatry* **155**, 741–750.

Levinson DF, Umapathy C, and Musthaq M (1999) Treatment of schizoaffective disorder and schizophrenia with mood symptoms. *Am J Psychiatry* **156**, 1138–1148.

Lewis DA (1997) Development of the prefrontal cortex during adolescence: Insights into vulnerable neural circuits in schizophrenia. *Neuropsychopharamacology* **16**, 358–398.

Lieberman JA (1996) Atypical antipsychotic drugs as a first-line treatment of schizophrenia: a rationale and hypothesis. *J Clin Psychiatr* **57**(Suppl. 11), 68–71.

Lieberman JA (1999a) Is schizophrenia a neurodegenerative disorder? A clinical and neurobiological perspective. *Biol Psychiatry* **46**, 729–739.

Lieberman JA (1999b) Searching for the neuropathology of schizophrenia: neuroimaging strategies and findings. *Am J Psychiatry* **156**, 1133–1136.

Lieberman JA and Fenton W (2000) Delayed detection of psychosis: causes, consequences, and effect on public health. *Am J Psychiatry* **157**, 1727–1730.

Liberman RP, Massel HK, Mosk MD, et al. (1985) Social skills training for chronic mental patients. *Hosp Comm Psychiatry* **36**, 396–403.

Liberman RP, Mueser KT, and Wallace CJ (1986) Social skills training for schizophrenic individuals at risk for relapse. *Am J Psychiatry* **143**, 523–526.

Lichtermann D, Karbe E, and Maier W (2000) The genetic epidemiology of schizophrenia and of schizophrenia spectrum disorders. *Eur Arch Psychiatr Clin Neurosci* **250**, 304–310.

Liddle PF (1987) Schizophrenic syndromes, cognitive performance and neurological dysfunction. *Psychol Med* **17**, 49–57.

Lim KO, Hedehus M, Moseley M, et al. (1999) Compromised white matter tract integrity in schizophrenia inferred from diffusion tensor imaging. *Arch Gen Psychiatry* **56**, 367–374.

Lin A, Kenis G, Bignotti S, et al. (1998) The inflammatory response system in treatment-resistant schizophrenia: increased serum interleukin-6. *Schizophr Res* **32**, 9–15.

Lindenmayer JP, Volavka J, Lieberman J, et al. (2001) Olanzapine for schizophrenia refractory to typical and atypical antipsychotics: an open-label prospective trial. *J Clin Psychopharm* **21**, 448–453.

Lindstrom L, Gefvert O, Hogberg G, et al. (1999) Increased dopamine synthesis rate in medial prefrontal cortex and striatum in schizophrenia indicated by L(-beta-11C) DOPA and PET. *Biol Psychiatry* **46**, 681–688.

Linn MW, Klett J, and Caffey FM (1980) Foster home characteristics and psychiatric patient outcome. *Arch Gen Psychiatry* **37**, 129–132.

Litman RE, Hong WW, Weissman EM, et al. (1993) Idazoxan, an a_2 antagonist, augments fluphenazine in schizophrenic patients: a pilot study. *J Clin Psychopharmacol* **13**, 264–267.

Loranger AW (1984) Sex difference in age at onset of schizophrenia. *Arch Gen Psychiatry* **41**, 157–161.

Lyell A (1983) Delusions of parasitosis. *Br J Psychiatry* **108**, 485–499.

Lysaker PH, Bell MD, Bioty SM, et al. (1995) The frequency of associations between positive and negative symptoms and dysphoria in schizophrenia. *Compr Psychiatry* **36**, 113–117.

Mahy C, Mallet R, Leff J, et al. (1999) First contact incidence rate of schizophrenia in Barbados. *Br J Psychiatry* **175**, 28–33.

Maier M, Mellers J, Toone B, et al. (2000) Schizophrenia, temporal lobe epilepsy and psychosis: an *in vivo* magnetic resonance spectroscopy and imaging study of the hippocampus/amygdala complex. *Psychol Med* **30**(3), 571–581.

Marcelis M, Navarro-Mateu F, Murray R, et al. (1998) Urbanization and psychosis: study of 1942–1978 birth cohorts in the Netherlands. *Psychol Med* **28**, 871–879.

Marder SR (2000) Integrating pharmacological and psychosocial treatments for schizophrenia. *Acta Psychiatr Scand* **102**(Suppl. 407), 87–90.

Marder SR and Meibach RC (1994) Risperidone in the treatment of schizophrenia. *Am J Psychiatry* **151**, 825–835.

Marder SR and Van Putten T (1988) Who should receive clozapine? *Arch Gen Psychiatry* **45**, 865–867.

Marder SR, Van Putten T, Mintz J, et al. (1984) Costs and benefits of two doses of fluphenazine. *Arch Gen Psychiatry* **41**, 1025–1029.

Marder SR, Van Patten T, Mintz J, et al. (1987) Low- and conventional-dose maintenance therapy with fluphenazine decanoate: two-year outcome. *Arch Gen Psychiatry* **44**, 518–521.

Marder SR, Wirshing W, Mintz J, et al. (1996) Two-year outcome of social skills training and group psychotherapy for outpatients with schizophrenia. *Am J Psychiatry* **153**, 1585–1592.

Margolis RL, Chuang DM, and Post RM (1994) Programmed cell death: implications for neuropsychiatric disorders. *Biol Psychiatry* **35**, 946–956.

Marino C, Nobile M, Bellodi L, et al. (1993) Delusional disorder and mood disorder: can they coexist? *Psychopathology* **26**, 53–61.

Marder SR, McQuade RD, Stock E, et al. (2003) Aripiprazole in the treatment of schizophrenia: safety and tolerability in short-term placebo-controlled trials. *Schizphr Res* **61**, 123–136.

Marsden CD, Mindham RHS, and Mackay AVP (1986) Extrapyramidal movement disorders produced by antipsychotic drugs. In *The Psychopharmacology and Treatment of Schizophrenia*, Bradley PB and Hirsch SR (eds). Oxford University Press, Oxford.

Masand PS (2000) Weight gain associated with psychotropics. *Expert Opin Psychopharmacol* **1** 377–389.

Mathalon DH, Faustman WO, and Ford JM (2002) N400 and automatic semanting processing abnormalities in patients with schizophrenia. *Arch Gen Psychiatry* **59**, 641–648.

Matthysee S (1973) Antipsychotic drug actins: a clue to a neuropathology of schizophrenia? *Fed Proc* **32**, 200–205.

May PRA (1968) *Treatment of Schizophrenia a Comparative Study of Five Treatment Methods*. Science House, New York.

McCarley RW, O'Donnell BF, Niznikiewicz MA, et al. (1997) Update on electrophysiology in schizophrenia. *Int Rev Psychiatry* **9**, 373–386.

McCarley RW, Salisbury DF, Hirayasu Y, et al. (2002) Association between smaller left posterior superior temporal gyrus volume on magnetic resonance imaging and smaller left temporal P300 amplitude in first-episode schizophrenia. *Arch Gen Psychiatry* **59**, 321–331.

McCarley RW, Shenton ME, O'Donnell BF, et al. (1993) Auditory P300 abnormalities and left posterior temporal gyrus reduction in schizophrenia. *Arch Gen Psychiatry* **50**, 190–197.

McCarley RW, Wible CG, Frumin M, et al. (1999) MRI anatomy of schizophrenia. *Biol Psychiatry* **45**, 1099–1119.

McCarthy G, Luby M, Gore J, et al. (1997) Infrequent events transiently activate human prefrontal and parietal cortex as measured by functional MRI. *J Neurophysiol* **77**, 1630–1634.

McCreadie RG, Connolly MA, Williamson DJ, et al. (1994) The Nithsdale Schizophrenia Surveys. XII: "Neurodevelopmental" schizophrenia: a search for clinical correlates and putative aetiological factors. *Br J Psychiatry* **165**, 340–346.

McGhie A and Chapman J (1961) Disorders of attention and perception in early schizophrenia. *Br J Med Psychol* **34**, 103–116.

McGlashan TH and Fenton WS (1993) Subtype progression and pathophysiologic deterioration in early schizophrenia. *Schizophr Bull* **19**, 71–84.

McGlashan TH and Hoffman RE (2000) Schizophrenia as a disorder of developmentally reduced synaptic connectivity. *Arch Gen Psychiatry* **57**, 637–648.

McGuire PK, Shah GMS, and Murray RM (1993) Increased blood flow in Broca's area during auditory hallucinations in schizophrenia. *Lancet* **324**, 703–706.

McNeil TF (1995) Perinatal risk factors and schizophrenia: selective review and methodological concerns. *Epidemiol Rev* **17**, 107–112.

McQuade RD, Burns KD, Jordan S, et al. (2002) Aripiprazole: a dopamine-serotonin system stabilizer (abstract). *Int J Neuropsychopharmacol* **5**(Suppl 1), S176.

Mednick SA, Machon RA, Huttunen MO, et al. (1988) Adult schizophrenia following prenatal exposure to an influenza epidemic. *Arch Gen Psychiatry* **45**, 189–192.

Mehtonen O-P, Aranko K, Malkonen L, et al. (1991) A survey of sudden death associated with the use of antipsychotic or antidepressant drugs: 49 cases in Finland. *Acta Psychiatr Scand* **84**, 58–64.

Meloy JR (1996) Stalking (obsessional following): a review of some preliminary studies. *Aggr Viol Behav* **1**, 147–162.

Meloy JR (1999) Case report: erotomania, triangulation, and homicide. *J Forensic Sci* **44**, 421–424.

Meltzer HY (1992) Treatment of the neuroleptic–nonresponsive schizophrenic patient. *Schizophr Bull* **18**, 515–542.

Meltzer HY (1995) Clozapine: is another view valid? *Am J Psychiatry* **152**, 821–825.

Meltzer HY (1998) Suicide in schizophrenia: risk factors and clozapine treatment. *J Clin Psychiatry* **59**(Suppl. 3), 15–20.

Meltzer HY and Okayli G (1995) The reduction of suicidality during clozapine treatment in neuroleptic-resistant schizophrenia: impact on risk-benefit assessment. *Am J Psychiatry* **152**, 183–190.

Menzies R, Federoff JP, Green CM, et al. (1995) Prediction of dangerous behaviour in male erotomania. *Br J Psychiatry* **166**, 529–536.

Merikangas K (2002) Genetic epidemiology: bringing genetics to the population—the NAPE Lecture 2001. *Acta Psychiatr Scand* **105**, 3–13.

Merinder LB (2000) Patient education in schizophrenia: a review. *Acta Psychiatr Scand* **102**, 98–106.

Mirnics K, Middleton FA, Lewis DA, et al. (2001) Analysis of complex brain disorders with gene expression microarrays: schizophrenia as a disease of the synapse. *Trends Neurosci* **24**, 479–486.

Mirnics K, Middleton FA, Marquez A, et al. (2000) Molecular characterization of schizophrenia viewed by microarray analysis of gene expression in prefrontal cortex. *Neuron* **28**, 53–67.

Mishler EG and Scotch NA (1963) Sociocultural factors in the epidemiology of schizophrenia: a review. *Psychiatry* **26**, 315–351.

Miyanaga K, Machiyama T, and Juji T (1984) Schizophrenic disorders and HLA-DR antigens. *Biol Psychiatry* **19**, 121–129.

Modai I, Hirschmann S, Rava A, et al. (2000) Sudden death in patients receiving clozapine treatment: a preliminary investigation. *J Clin Psychopharmacol* **20**, 325–327.

Mohn AR, Gainetdinov RR, Caron MG, et al. (1999) Mice with reduced NMDA receptor expression display behaviors related to schizophrenia. *Cell* **98**, 427–436.

Moises HW, Yang L, Kristbjarnarson H, et al. (1995) An international two-stage genome-wide search for schizophrenia. *Am J Hum Genet* **34**, 630–649.

Mojtabai R, Nicholson RA, and Carpenter PN (1998) Role of psychosocial treatments in management of schizophrenia: a meta-analytic review of controlled outcome studies. *Schizophr Bull* **24**, 569–587.

Montgomery SA and Green M (1988) The use of cholecystokinin in schizophrenia: a review. *Psychol Med* **18**, 593–603.

Morgan V, Castle D, Page A, et al. (1997) Influenza epidemics and incidence of schizophrenia, affective disorders and mental retardation in Western Australia: no evidence of major effect. *Schizophr Res* **26**, 25–39.

Morris M (1991) Delusional parasitosis. *Br J Psychiatry* **159**, 83–87.

Mortensen PB, Pederson CB, Westergaard T, et al. (1999) Effects of family history and place and season of birth on the risk factors for schizophrenia. *N Engl J Med* **340**, 603–608.

Mowry BJ and Nancarrow DJ (2001) Molecular genetics of schizophrenia: proceedings of the Australian neuroscience society symposium. *Clin Exp Pharmacol Physiol* **28**, 66–69.

Muller N and Ackenheil M (1998) Psychoneuroimmunology and the cytokine action in the CNS: implications for psychiatric disorders. *Prog Neuropsychopharmacol Biol Psychiatry* **22**, 1–33.

Muller N, Empel M, Riedel M, et al. (1997) Neuroleptic treatment increases soluble IL-2 receptors and decreases soluble IL-6 receptors in schizophrenia. *Eur Arch Psychiatr Clin Neurosci* **247**, 308–313.

Muller N, Riedel M, Scheppach C, et al. (2002) Beneficial antipsychotic effects of celecoxib add-on therapy compared to risperidone alone in schizophrenia. *Am J Psychiatry* **159**, 1029–1034.

Munro A (1982) Paranoia revisited. *Br J Psychiatry* **141**, 344–349.

Munro A (1988) Monosymptomatic hypochondriacal psychosis. *Br J Psychiatry* **153**(Suppl. 2), 37–40.

Munro A (1991) Phenomenologic aspects of monodelusional disorders. *Br J Psychiatry* **159**(Suppl. 14), 62–64.

Murphy KC, Jones LA, and Owen MJ (1999) High rates of schizophrenia in adults with velocardio-facial syndrome. *Arch Gen Psychiatry* **56**, 940–945.

Musselman DL, Evans DL, and Nemeroff CB (1998) The relationship of depression to cardiovascular disease: epidemiology, biology, and treatment. *Arch Gen Psychiatry* **55**, 580–592.

Myerson A (1940) Review: mental disorders in urban areas. *Am J Psychiatry* **96**, 995–997.

Naber D, Leppig M, Grohmann R, et al. (1989) Efficacy and adverse effects of clozapine in the treatment of schizophrenia and tardive dyskinesia: a retrospective study of 387 patients. *Psychopharmacology (Berl)* **99**, 73–76.

Nelson MD, Saykin AJ, Flashman LA, et al. (1998) Hippocampal volume reduction in schizophrenia as assessed by magnetic resonance imaging: a meta-analytic study. *Arch Gen Psychiatry* **55**, 433–440.

Nestler EJ (1997) Schizophrenia: an emerging pathophysiology. *Nature* **385**, 578–579.

Nestor PG, Kimble MO, O'Donnell BF, et al. (1997) Aberrant semantic activation in schizophrenia: a neurophysiological study. *Am J Psychiatry* **157**, 640–646.

Newcomer JW, Haupt DW, Fucetola R, et al. (2002) Abnormalities in glucose regulation during antipsychotic treatment of schizophrenia. *Arch Gen Psychiatry* **59**, 337–345.

Niznikiewicz MA, O'Donnell BF, Nestor PG, et al. (1997) ERP assessment of visual and auditory language processing in schizophrenia. *J Abnorm Psychol* **106**, 85–94.

Noreik K and Odegard O (1967) Age at onset of schizophrenia in relation to socio-economic factors. *Br J Soc Psychiatry* **1**, 243–249.

Norman RM and Malla AK (2001) Duration of untreated psychosis: a critical examination of the concept and its importance. *Psychol Med* **31**, 381–400.

Odegard O (1932) Emigration and insanity: a study of mental disease among the Norwegian-born population of Minnesota. *Acta Psychiatr Neurol Scand* **7**(Suppl. 4), 1–206.

O'Donnell BF, McCarley RW, Potts GF, et al. (1999) Identification of neural circuits underlying P300 abnormalities in schizophrenia. *Psychophysiology* **36**(3), 253–257.

Osterberg E (1978) Schizophrenia and rheumatic disease. *Acta Psychiatr Scand* **58**, 339–359.

Overall JE and Gorham DE (1961) The Brief Psychiatric Rating Scale. *Psychol Rep* **10**, 799–812.

Ozcan ME, Taskin R, Banoglu R, et al. (1996) HLA antigens in schizophrenia and mood disorders. *Biol Psychiatry* **39**, 891–895.

Pahl JJ, Swayze VW, and Andreasen NC (1990) Diagnostic advances in anatomical and functional brain imaging in schizophrenia. In *Recent Advances in Schizophrenia*, Kales A, Stefanis CN, and Talbott J (eds). Springer-Verlag, New York, pp. 163–189.

Palmer BW, Heaton RK, Paulsen JS, et al. (1997) Is it possible to be schizophrenic yet neuropsychologically normal? *Neuropsychology* **11**, 437–446.

Pantelis C, Barber FZ, Barbes TR, et al. (1999) Comparison of set-shifting ability in patients with chronic schizophrenia and frontal lobe damage. *Schizophr Res* **37**, 251–270.

Patel JK, Niznikiewicz MA, Shafa R, et al. (2001) Clozapine enhances P300 amplitude in patients with schizophrenia (Abstract). *Schizophr Res* **49**(Suppl.), 255.

Pearlson GP, Kreger L, Rabins PW, et al. (1989) A chart review study of late-onset and early-onset schizophrenia. *Am J Psychiatry* **146**, 1568–1574.

Peuskens J (1995) Risperidone in the treatment of patients with chronic schizophrenia: a multinational, multicentre, double-blind, parallel-group study versus haloperidol. *Br J Psychiatry* **166**, 712–726.

Peuskens J and Link CG (1997) A comparison of quetiapine and chlorpromazine in the treatment of schizophrenia. *Acta Psychiatr Scand* **96**, 265–273.

Pickar D and Pinals D (1995) Drug-free symptoms in schizophrenia. Presented at the 34th Annual Meeting of the American College of Neuropsychopharmacology, San Juan, PR.

Polich J (1998) P300 clinical utility and control of variability. *J Clin Neurophysiol* **15**, 14–33.

Polich J and Herbst KL (2000) P300 as a clinical assay: rationale, evaluation, and findings. *Int J Psychophysiol* **38**, 3–19.

Poulton R, Caspi A, Moffitt TE, et al. (2000) Children's self-reported psychotic symptoms and adult schizophreniform disorder: 15-year longitudinal study. *Arch Gen Psychiatry* **57**, 1053–1058.

Preti A, Cardascia L, Zen T, et al. (2000) Risk for obstetric complications and schizophrenia. *Psychiatr Res* **96**, 127–139.

Procyshyn RM, Pande S, and Tse G (2000) New-onset diabetes mellitus associated with quetiapine. *Can J Psychiatry* **45**, 668–669.

Propping P (1983) Genetic disorders presenting as "schizophrenia": Karl Bonhoeffer's early view of the psychoses in the light of medical genetics. *Hum Genet* **65**, 1–10.

Pulver AE, Lasseter VK, Kasch L, et al. (1995) Schizophrenia: a genome scan targets chromosomes 3p and 8p as potential sites of susceptibility genes. *Am J Med Genet* **60**, 252–260.

Purdon SE, Jones BDW, Stip E, et al. (2000) Neuropsychological change in early phase schizophrenia during 12 months of treatment with olanzapine, risperidone, or haloperidol. *Arch Gen Psychiatry* **57**, 249–258.

Puzynski S and Klosiewicz L (1984) Divalproex amide in the treatment of affective and schizoaffective disorders. *J Affect Disord* **6**, 115–121.

Quitkin AF, Rifkin A, and Klein DF (1975) Very high doses vs. standard dosage fluphenazine in schizophrenia. *Arch Gen Psychiatry* **32**, 1276–1281.

Rabins P, Pauker S, and Thomas J (1984) Can schizophrenia begin after age 44? *Compr Psychiatry* **25**, 290–293.

Rajkumar S, Padmavati R, Thara R, et al. (1993) Incidence of schizophrenia in an urban community in Madras. *Indian J Psychiatry* **35**, 18–21.

Rantakallio P, Jones P, Moring J, et al. (1997) Association between central nervous system infections during childhood and adult onset schizophrenia and other psychoses: a 28-year follow-up. *Int J Epidemiol* **26**, 837–843.

Ray WA, Meredith S, Thapa PB, et al. (2001) Antipsychotics and the risk of sudden cardiac death. *Arch Gen Psychiatry* **58**, 1161–1167.

Raz S and Raz N (1990) Structural brain abnormalities in the major psychoses: a quantitative review of the evidence from computerized imaging. *Psychol Bull* **108**, 93–108.

Rice DP (1999) The economic impact of schizophrenia. *J Clin Psychiatry* **60**(Suppl. 1), 4–6.

Riecher A, Maurer K, Loffler W, et al. (1989) Schizophrenia: a disease of single young males? Preliminary results from an investigation on a representative cohort admitted to hospital for the first time. *Eur Arch Psychiatr Neurosci* **239**, 210–212.

Riecher-Rossler A and Hafner H (2000) Gender aspects in schizophrenia: bridging the border between social and biological psychiatry. *Acta Psychiatr Scand* **102**(Suppl. 407), 58–62.

Riley JG, Ayis SA, Ferrier IN, et al. (2000) QTc-interval abnormalities and psychotropic drug therapy in psychiatric patients. *Lancet* **355**, 1048–1052.

Retterstol N (1970) *Prognosis in Paranoid Psychoses*. Charles Thomas, Springfield, IL.

Retterstol N and Opjordsmoen S (1991) Fatherhood, impending or newly established, precipitating delusional disorders: long-term course and outcome. *Psychopathology* **24**, 232.

Robins LN and Regier DA (eds) (1991) *Psychiatric Disorders in America: The Epidemiologic Catchment Area Study*. Free Press, New York.

Robins LN, Helzer JE, Weissman MM, et al. (1984) Lifetime prevalence of specific psychiatric disorders in 3 sites. *Arch Gen Psychiatry* **41**, 949–958.

Robinson D, Woerner MG, Alvir JMJ, et al. (1999) Predictors of relapse following response from a first episode of schizophrenia or schizoaffective disorder. *Arch Gen Psychiatry* **56**, 241–247.

Rosenheck R, Cramer J, Xu W, et al. (1997) A comparison of clozapine and haloperidol in hospitalized patients with refractory schizophrenia: department of veterans affairs cooperative study group on clozapine in refractory schizophrenia. *N Engl J Med* **337**, 809–815.

Rosenheck R, Teckett J, Peters J, et al. (1998) Does participation in psychosocial treatment augment the benefit of clozapine? *Arch Gen Psychiatry* **55**, 618–625.

Rosenthal D, Goldberg I, Jacobsen B, et al. (1974) Migration, heredity, and schizophrenia. *Psychiatry* **37**, 321–329.

Ruschena D, Mullen PE, Burgess P, et al. (1998) Sudden death in psychiatric patients. *Br J Psychiatry* **172**, 331–336.

Sacuzzo DP and Braff DL (1981) Early information processing deficit in schizophrenia: new findings using RDC, schizophrenic subgroups and manic controls. *Arch Gen Psychiatry* **38**, 175–179.

Salit SA, Kuhn EM, Hartz AJ, et al. (1998) Hospitalization costs associated with homelessness in New York city. *N Engl J Med* **338**, 1734–1740.

Salzman C (1980) The use of ECT in the treatment of schizophrenia. *Am J Psychiatry* **137**, 1032–1041.

Sanders RD and Mossman D (1999) An open trial of olanzapine in patients with treatment-refractory psychoses. *J Clin Psychopharmacol* **19**, 62–66.

Saykin AJ, Shtasel DL, Gur RE, et al. (1994) Neuropsychological deficits in neuroleptic-naive patients with first episode schizophrenia. *Arch Gen Psychiatry* **51**, 124–131.

Schizophrenia Collaborative Linkage Group for Chromosomes 3, 6, and 8 (1996) Additional support for schizophrenia linkage on chromosomes 6 and 8: a multicenter study. *Am J Med Gene* **67**, 580–594.

Schotte A, Janssen PF, Gommeren W, et al. (1996) Risperidone compared with new and reference antipsychotic drugs: *in vitro* and *in vivo* receptor binding. *Psychopharmacology (Berl)* **124**, 57–73.

Schulz R, Beach SR, Ives DG, et al. (2000) Association between depression and mortality in older adults: the cardiovascular health study. *Arch Intern Med* **160**, 1761–1768.

Seeman P, Corbett R, and Van Tol HH (1997) Atypical neuroleptics have low affinity for dopamine D_2 receptors or are selective for D_4 receptors. *Neuropsychopharmacology* **16**(2), 93–110.

Seidman LJ, Faraone SV, Goldstein JM, et al. (1997) Reduced subcortical brain volumes in nonpsychotic siblings of schizophrenic patients: a pilot magnetic resonance imaging study. *Am J Med Genet* **74**, 507–514.

Selten JP, Slaets JPJ, and Kahn R (1998) Prenatal exposure to influenza and schizophrenia in Surinamese and Dutch antillean immigrants to The Netherlands. *Schizophr Res* **30**, 101–103.

Serretti A, Lattuada E, Cusin C, et al. (1999) Factor analysis of delusional disorder symptomatology. *Compr Psychiatry* **40**, 143–147.

Sharpley MS, Hutchinson G, Murray RM, et al. (2001) Understanding the excess of psychosis among the African-Caribbean population in England. *Br J Psychiatry* **178**, S60–S68.

Shenton ME, Kikinis R, Jolesz FA, et al. (1992) Abnormalities of the left temporal lobe and thought disorder in schizophrenia: a quantitative magnetic resonance imaging study. *N Engl J Med* **327**, 604–611.

Shioiri T, Kato T, Inubushi T, et al. (1994) Correlations of phosphomonoesters measured by phosphorus-31 magnetic resonance spectroscopy in frontal lobes and negative symptoms in schizophrenia. *Psychiatr Res* **55**, 223–235.

Silverman C (1968) The epidemiology of depression: a review. *Am J Psychiatry* **124**, 883–891.

Siris SG (2000) Depression in schizophrenia: perspective in the era of "atypical" antipsychotic agents. *Am J Psychiatry* **157**, 1379–1389.

Slater E, Hare EH, and Price JS (1971) Marriage and fertility of psychiatric patients compared with national data. *Soc Biol* **18**(Suppl.), S60–S73.

Small JG, Hirsch SR, Aravantis LA, et al. (1997) Quetiapine in patients with schizophrenia: a high- and low-dose double-blind comparison with placebo. *Arch Gen Psychiatry* **54**, 549–557.

Small JG, Kellamus JJ, Milstein V, et al. (1975) A placebo controlled study of lithium combined with neuroleptics in chronic schizophrenic patients. *Am J Psychiatry* **132**, 1315–1317.

Smith GN, Kopala LC, Lapointe JS, et al. (1998) Obstetric complications, treatment response and brain morphology in adult onset and early-onset males with schizophrenia. *Psychol Med* **28**, 645–653.

Someya T, Masui A, Takahashi S, et al. (1987) Classification of paranoid disorders: a survey of 144 cases. *Jpn J Psychiatr Neurol* **41**, 162–163.

Stahl SM (2000) New drug discovery in the postgenomic era: from genomics to proteomics. *J Clin Psychiatry* **61**, 894–895.

Stanley JA, Williamson PC, Drost DJ, et al. (1995) An *in vivo* study of the prefrontal cortex of schizophrenic patients at different stages of illness via phosphorus magnetic resonance spectroscopy. *Arch Gen Psychiatry* **52**, 399–406.

Straub RE, MacLean CJ, Martin RB, et al. (1998) A schizophrenia locus may be located in region 10p15–p11. *Am J Med Genet* **81**, 296–301.

Straube ER and Oades RD (1992) *Schizophrenia: Empirical Research and Findings.* Academic Press, San Diego, CA.

Strauss JS, Carpenter WT Jr., and Bartko JJ (1974) The diagnosis and understanding of schizophrenia. Part III. Speculations on the processes that underlie schizophrenic symptoms and signs. *Schizophr Bull* **11**, 61–69.

Strakowski SM, Keck PE, Sax KW, et al. (1999) Twelve-month outcome of patients with DSM-III-R schizoaffective disorder: comparisons to matched patients with bipolar disorder. *Schizophr Res* **35**, 167–174.

Szeszko PR, Bilder RM, Lencz T, et al. (1999) Investigation of frontal lobe subregions in first-episode schizophrenia. *Psychiatr Res* **90**, 1–15.

Tamargo J (2000) Drug-induced torsades de pointes: from molecular biology to bedside. *Jpn J Pharmacol* **83**, 1–19.

Tamminga CA (1999) Glutamatergic aspects of schizophrenia. *Br J Psychiatry* **174**(Suppl. 37), 12–15.

Tamminga CA, Thaker GK, Moran M, et al. (1994) Clozapine in tardive dyskinesia: observations from human and animal model studies. *J Clin Psychiatry* **55**, 102–106.

Tandon R, Harrigan E, and Zorn SH (1997) Ziprasidone: a novel antipsychotic with unique pharmacology and therapeutic potential. *J Serotonin Res* **4**, 159–177.

Tarazi FI and Baldessarini RJ (2000) Dopamine D_4 receptors: neuropsychiatric implications. *TEN* **2**, 54–58.

Tauscher J, Kapur S, Verhoeff NPLG, et al. (2002) Brain serotonin 5-HT_{1A} receptor binding in schizophrenia measured by PET and [^{11}C]WAY-100635. *Arch Gen Psychiatry* **59**, 514–520.

Taylor MA (1992) Are schizophrenia and affective disorder related? A selective literature review. *Am J Psychiatry* **149**, 22–32.

Thakore JH, Mann JN, Vlahos I, et al. (2002) Increased visceral fat distribution in drug-naïve and drug-free patients with schizophrenia. *Int J Obstet Rel Metab Disord* **26**, 137–141.

Thomas SHL (1994) Drugs, QT interval abnormalities and ventricular arrhythmias. *Adverse Drug React Toxicol Rev* **13**, 77–102.

Thornley B and Adams CE (1998) Content and quality of 2000 controlled trials in schizophrenia over 50 years. *Br Med J* **317**, 1181–1184.

Tienari P (1991) Interaction between genetic vulnerability and family environment: the Finnish adoptive family study of schizophrenia. *Acta Psychiatr Scand* **84**, 460–465.

Tollefson GD, Beasley CM Jr., Tran PV, et al. (1997) Olanzapine versus haloperidol in the treatment of schizophrenia and schizoaffective and schizophreniform disorders: results of an international collaborative trial. *Am J Psychiatry* **154**, 457–465.

Tollefson GD, Birkett MA, Kiesler GM, et al. (2001) Double-blind comparison of olanzapine vs. clozapine in schizophrenic patients clinically eligible for treatment with clozapine. *Biol Psychiatry* **49**(1), 52–63.

Torrey EF (1980) *Schizophrenia and Civilization*. Aronson, New York.

Torrey EF, Bowler AE, and Clark K (1997) Urban birth and residence as risk factors for psychoses: an analysis of 1880 data. *Schizophr Res* **25**, 169–176.

Truffinet P, Tamminga CA, Fabre LF, et al. (1999) A placebo-controlled study of the D_4/5-HT_{2A} antagonist fananserin in the treatment of schizophrenia. *Am J Psychiatry* **156**, 419–425.

Tsai GE, Yang P, Chung LC, et al. (1998) D-Serine added to antipsychotics for the treatment of schizophrenia. *Biol Psychiatry* **44**, 1081–1089.

Tsuang MT, Stone WS, and Faraone SV (2001) Genes, environment and schizophrenia. *Br J Psychiatry* **178**(Suppl. 40), S18–S24.

van Kammen DP, Peters J, Yao J, et al. (1990) Norepinephrine in acute exacerbations of chronic schizophrenia. *Arch Gen Psychiatry* **47**, 161–168.

Van Petten C and Kutas M (1990) Interactions between sentence context and word frequency in event-related brain potentials. *Mem Cogn* **18**(4), 380–393.

Van Putten T, Marder SR, and Mintz J (1990) A controlled dose comparison of haloperidol in newly admitted schizophrenic patients. *Arch Gen Psychiatry* **47**, 754–758.

van Tol HHM, Pounzow JR, Guan HC, et al. (1991) Cloning of the gene for a human D_4 receptor with high affinity for the antipsychotic clozapine. *Nature* **350**, 610–614.

Velligan DI and Miller AL (1999) Cognitive dysfunction in schizophrenia and its importance to outcome: the place of atypical antipsychotic in treatment. *J Clin Psychiatry* **60**(Suppl. 23), 25–28.

Velligan DI, Bow-Thomas CC, Huntzinger C, et al. (2000) Randomized controlled trial of the use of compensatory strategies to enhance adaptive functioning in outpatients with schizophrenia. *Am J Psychiatry* **157**, 1317–1323.

Verdoux H, Geddes JR, Takei N, et al. (1997) Obstetric complications and age at onset in schizophrenia: an international collaborative meta-analysis of individual patient data. *Am J Psychiatry* **154**, 1220–1227.

Vieta E, Herraiz M, Fernandez A, et al. (2001) Efficacy and safety of risperidone in the treatment of schizoaffective disorder: initial results from a large, multicenter surveillance study. *J Clin Psychiatry* **62**, 623–630.

Vieweg V, Levenson J, Pandurangi A, et al. (1995) Medical disorders in the schizophrenic patients. *Int J Psychiatr Med* **25**, 137–172.

Vogel HP (1979) Fertility and sibship size in a psychiatric patient population: a comparison with national census data. *Acta Psychiatr Scand* **60**, 48–50.

Volavka J, Czobar P, Sheitman B, et al. (2002) Clozapine, olanzapine, risperidone, and haloperidol in the treatment of patients with chronic schizophrenia and schizoaffective disorder. *Am J Psychiatry* **159**, 255–262.

Waddington JL, Scully PJ, and O'Callighan E (1997) The new antipsychotics, and their potential for early intervention in schizophrenia. *Schizophr Res* **28**, 215–222.

Waddington JL, Youssef HA, and Kinsella A (1995) Sequential cross-sectional and 10-year prospective study of severe negative symptoms in relation to duration of initially untreated psychosis in chronic schizophrenia. *Psychol Med* **25**, 849–857.

Walker E (1981) Attentional and neuromotor functions of schizophrenics, schizoaffectives, and patients with other affective disorders. *Arch Gen Psychiatry* **38**, 1355–1358.

Wallace CJ, Nelson CJ, Liberman RP, et al. (1980) A review and critique of social skills training with schizophrenic patients. *Schizophr Bull* **6**, 42–63.

Waltrip RW, Buchanan RW, Carpenter WT, et al. (1997) Borna disease virus antibodies and the deficit syndrome of schizophrenia. *Schizophr Res* **23**, 253–257.

Warner JP, Barnes TRE, and Henry JA (1996) Electrocardiographic changes in patients receiving neuroleptic medication. *Acta Psychiatr Scand* **93**, 311–313.

Waxler NE (1979) Is outcome for schizophrenia better in nonindustrial societies? The case of Sri Lanka. *J Nerv Ment Dis* **167**, 144–158.

Weinberger DR (1987) Implications of normal brain development for the pathogenesis of schizophrenia. *Arch Gen Psychiatry* **44**, 660–669.

Weinberger DR and Berman KF (1988) Speculation of the meaning of cerebral metabolic "hypofrontality" in schizophrenia. *Schizophr Bull* **14**, 157–168.

Weinberger DR and Berman KF (1996) Prefrontal function in schizophrenia: confounds and controversies. *Philos T Roy Soc B* **351**, 1495–1503.

Weinberger DR and McClure RK (2002) Neurotoxicity, neuroplasticity, and MRI morphometry: what is happening in the schizophrenic brain? *Arch Gen Psychiatry* **59**, 553–558.

Weinberger DR, Egan MF, Bertolino A, et al. (2001) Prefrontal neurons and the genetics of schizophrenia. *Biol Psychiatry* **50**, 825–844.

Weiner DB (1992) Philippe Pinel's memoir on madness. *Am J Psychiatry* **149**, 725–732.

Wirshing DA, Marshall BD Jr., Green MF, et al. (1999) Risperidone in treatment-refractory schizophrenia. *Am J Psychiatry* **156**(9), 1374–1379.

Wirshing DA, Spellberg BJ, Erhart SM, et al. (1998) Novel antipsychotics and new onset diabetes. *Biol Psychiatry* **44**, 778–783.

Wolkin A, Rusinek H, Vaid G, et al. (1998) Structural magnetic resonance image averaging in schizophrenia. *Am J Psychiatry* **155**, 1064–1073.

Wolkowitz OM and Pickar D (1991) Benzodiazepines in the treatment of schizophrenia: a review and reappraisal. *Am J Psychiatry* **148**, 714–726.

Wolkowitz OM, Rapaport MH, and Pickar D (1990) Benzediazepine augmentation of neuroleptics. In *The Neuroleptic-Nonresponsive Patient: Characterization and Treatment*, Angrist B and Schulz SC (eds). American Psychiatric Press, Washington, DC, pp. 87–108.

Woods BT (1998) Is schizophrenia a progressive neurodevelopmental disorder? Toward a unitary pathogenetic mechanism. *Am J Psychiatry* **155**, 1661–1670.

World Health Organization (1973) *Report of the International Pilot Study of Schizophrenia*, Vol. 1. World Health Organization, Geneva.

World Health Organization (1979) *Schizophrenia: An International Follow-up Study*. John Wiley, New York.

Wright IC, Sharma T, Ellison ZR, et al. (1999) Supra-regional brain systems and the neuropathology of schizophrenia. *Cereb Cortex* **9**, 366–378.

Wyatt RJ (1991) Neuroleptics and the natural course of schizophrenia. *Schizophr Bull* **17**, 325–351.

Yamada N, Nakajima S, and Noguchi T (1998) Age at onset of delusional disorder is dependent on the delusional theme. *Acta Psychiatr Scand* **97**, 122–124.

Yap YG and Camm J (2000) Risk of Torsades de pointes with noncardiac drugs. *Br Med J* **320**, 1158–1159.

Zahn TP, Pickar D, and Haier RJ (1994) Effects of clozapine, fluphenazine, and placebo on reaction time measures of attention and sensory dominance in schizophrenia. *Schizophr Res* **13**, 133–144.

Zamani MG, De Hert M, Spaepen M, et al. (1994) Study of the possible association of HLA class II, CD_4 and CD_3 polymorphisms with schizophrenia. *Am J Med Genet* **54**, 372–377.

Zarate CA Jr. and Patel JK (2001) Sudden cardiac death and antipsychotic drugs: do we know enough? (Commentary) *Arch Gen Psychiatry* **58**, 1168–1171.

Zarate CA Jr., Tohen M, Banov MD, et al. (1995) Is clozapine a mood stabilizer? *J Clin Psychiatry* **56**, 108–112.

Zornberg GL, Buka SL, and Tsuang MT (2000) Hypoxic-ischemia-related fetal/neonatal complications and risk of schizophrenia and other nonaffective psychoses: a 19-year longitudinal study. *Am J Psychiatry* **157**, 196–202.

28 Mood Disorders: Depressive Disorders

Major depressive disorder (MDD), dysthymic disorder (DD), depressive disorder not otherwise specified (DDNOS) are the group of clinical conditions in the DSM-IV-TR characterized by depressive symptomatology. These conditions specifically exclude a history of manic, mixed or hypomanic episodes, and are not due to the physiologic effects of substances of abuse, other medications, or toxins. MDD is characterized by episodes of depression, each lasting at least 2 weeks. DD is characterized by at least 2 years of depressed mood accompanied by two or three depressive symptoms that fall short of threshold criteria for a major depressive episode. Depressive disorder not otherwise specified includes a set of conditions that do not meet criteria for MDD, DD, or adjustment disorder with depressed mood. These syndromes include premenstrual dysphoric disorder, minor depressive disorder, recurrent brief depressive disorder, and postpsychotic depressive disorder occurring during the residual phase of schizophrenia. In DSM-IV-TR, two other depressive disorders are diagnosed on the basis of etiology and include mood disorder due to a general medical condition and substance-induced mood disorder.

MAJOR DEPRESSIVE DISORDER

Diagnosis

The depressive disorders are characterized by lifelong vulnerability to episodes of disease, involving depressed mood or loss of interest and pleasure in activities. Individuals may demonstrate ongoing potential for cycling of mood from euthymia to depression to recovery and sometimes to hypomania or mania. When individuals cycle to hypomania or mania, then a diagnosis of bipolar II (in the case of hypomania) or bipolar I (in the case of mania) is made (see Chapter 30, page 797). When the mood disorder is severe, assessment for psychosis is essential.

The detection of major depressive episodes in both primary care settings and mental health settings requires the presence of mood disturbance or loss of interest and pleasure in activities for 2 weeks or more accompanied by at least four other symptoms of depression. There are problems in differential diagnosis because depressive experiences vary from individual to individual. One or more depressive episodes, occurring in the absence of a lifetime history of mania, hypomania, or intraepisode psychotic symptoms warranted a DSM-IV-TR diagnosis of Major Depressive Disorder. If the individual has had only one episode, then subtype "Single Episode" is noted (see DSM-IV-TR diagnostic criteria for Major Depressive Disorder, Single Episode below). Often, however, individuals suffer from multiple major depressive episodes during their lifetime. If the major depressive episodes have been recurrent, the subtype "Recurrent" is noted (see DSM-IV-TR diagnostic criteria for Major Depressive Disorder, Recurrent on page 738). Remission of depression requires a 2-month interval in which the full criteria are not met for a major depressive episode.

DSM-IV-TR Diagnostic Criteria

296.2x Major Depressive Disorder, Single Episode

A. Presence of a single Major Depressive Episode (see page 739).
B. The Major Depressive Episode is not better accounted for by Schizoaffective Disorder and is not superimposed on Schizophrenia, Schizophreniform Disorder, Delusional Disorder, or Psychotic Disorder Not Otherwise Specified.
C. There has never been a Manic Episode, a Mixed Episode, or a Hypomanic Episode.

Note: This exclusion does not apply if all of the manic-like, mixed-like, or hypomanic-like episodes are substance- or treatment-induced or are due to the direct physiological effects of a general medical condition.

If the full criteria are currently met for a Major Depressive Episode, specify its current clinical status and/or features:

Mild, Moderate, Severe Without Psychotic Features/Severe With Psychotic

Features

Chronic

With Catatonic Features

With Melancholic Features

With Atypical Features

With Postpartum Onset

If the full criteria are not currently met for a Major Depressive Episode, specify the current clinical status of the Major Depressive Disorder or features of the most recent episode:

In Partial Remission, In Full Remission (See linked section)

Chronic

With Catatonic Features

With Melancholic Features

With Atypical Features

With Postpartum Onset

DSM-IV-TR Diagnostic Criteria

296.3x Major Depressive Disorder, Recurrent

A. Presence of two or more Major Depressive Episodes (see page 739).

   Note: To be considered separate episodes, there must be an interval of at least 2 consecutive months in which criteria are not met for a Major Depressive Episode.

B. The Major Depressive Episodes are not better accounted for by Schizoaffective Disorder and are not superimposed on Schizophrenia, Schizophreniform Disorder, Delusional Disorder, or Psychotic Disorder Not Otherwise Specified.

C. There has never been a Manic Episode, a Mixed Episode, or a Hypomanic Episode.

   Note: This exclusion does not apply if all of the manic-like, mixed-like, or hypomanic-like episodes are substance- or treatment-induced or are due to the direct physiological effects of a general medical condition.

If the full criteria are currently met for a Major Depressive Episode, specify its current clinical status and/or features:

Mild, Moderate, Severe Without Psychotic Features/Severe With Psychotic Features

Chronic

With Catatonic Features

With Melancholic Features

With Atypical Features

With Postpartum Onset

If the full criteria are not currently met for a Major Depressive Episode, specify the current clinical status of the Major Depressive Disorder or features of the most recent episode:

In Partial Remission, In Full Remission

Chronic

With Catatonic Features
With Melancholic Features
With Atypical Features
With Postpartum Onset

Specify:
Longitudinal Course Specifiers (With and Without Interepisode Recovery)
With Seasonal Pattern

The core symptoms comprising a major depressive episode are illustrated in the DSM-IV-TR criteria. Each symptom is critical to evaluate in an individual with depressive symptomatology since each represents one of the essential features of a major depressive episode. Their persistence for much of the day, nearly every day for at least 2 weeks, is the criterion for diagnosis. The clinical syndrome is associated with significant psychological distress or impairment in psychosocial or work functioning.

DSM-IV-TR Diagnostic Criteria

Major Depressive Episode

A. Five (or more) of the following symptoms have been present during the same 2-week period and represent a change from previous functioning; at least one of the symptoms is either (1) depressed mood or (2) loss of interest or pleasure.

Note: Do not include symptoms that are clearly due to a general medical condition, or mood-incongruent delusions or hallucinations.

(1) Depressed mood most of the day, as indicated by either subjective report (e.g., feels sad or empty) or observation made by others (e.g., appears tearful).

Note: In children and adolescents, can be irritable mood.

(2) Markedly diminished interest or pleasure in all, or almost all, activities most of the day, nearly every day (as indicated by either subjective account or observation made by others).

(3) Significant weight loss when not dieting or weight gain (e.g., a change of more than 5% of body weight in a month), or decrease or increase in appetite nearly every day.

Note: In children, consider failure to make expected weight gains.

(4) Insomnia or hypersomnia nearly every day.

(5) Psychomotor agitation or retardation nearly every day (observable by others, not merely subjective feelings of restlessness or being slowed down).

(6) Fatigue or loss of energy nearly every day.

(7) Feelings of worthlessness or excessive or inappropriate guilt (which may be delusional) nearly every day (not merely self-reproach or guilt about being sick).
(8) Diminished ability to think or concentrate, or indecisiveness, nearly every day (either by subjective account or as observed by others).
(9) Recurrent thoughts of death (not just fear of dying), recurrent suicidal ideation without a specific plan, or a suicide attempt or a specific plan for committing suicide.

B. The symptoms do not meet criteria for a mixed episode.
C. The symptoms cause clinically significant distress or impairment in social, occupational, or other important areas of functioning.
D. The symptoms are not due to the direct physiological effects of a substance (e.g., a drug of abuse, a medication) or a general medical condition (e.g., hypothyroidism).
E. The symptoms are not better accounted for by bereavement, i.e., after the loss of a loved one, the symptoms persist for longer than 2 months or are characterized by marked functional impairment, morbid preoccupation with worthlessness, suicidal ideation, psychotic symptoms, or psychomotor retardation.

Reprinted with permission from the Diagnostic and Statistical Manual of Mental Disorders, Fourth Edition, Text Revision. Copyright 2000 American Psychiatric Association.

The clinical observation of mood reveals variations in presentation. An individual may have depressed symptomatology and experience typical sadness. Another individual may deny sadness and experience internal agitation and dysphoria. Another individual with depression may experience no feelings at all, and the depressed mood is inferred from the degree of psychological pain that is exhibited. Some individuals experience irritability, frustration, somatic preoccupation, and the sensation of being numb.

An equally important aspect of the depressive experience involves loss of interest or pleasure, when an individual feels no sense of enjoyment in activities that were previously considered pleasurable. There is associated reduction in all drives including energy and alteration in sleep, interest in food, and interest in sexual activity.

A common experience of insomnia or hypersomnia is noted in individuals with persistent depression. Observations of psychomotor activity include profound psychomotor retardation leading to stupor in more severe cases or alternatively significant agitation leading to inability to sit still and profound pacing in agitated forms of depression.

The complaint of guilt or guilty preoccupation is a common aspect of the depressive syndrome. Delusional forms of guilt are a common presentation of depressive disorder with psychotic features.

The loss of ability to concentrate, to focus attention, and to make decisions is a particularly distressing symptom for individuals. One may experience a loss of memory that simulates dementia. Loss of concentration is reflected in an inability to perform both complicated and simple tasks. The loss of ability to perform in school may be a symptom of a major depressive episode in children, and memory difficulties in the older adult may be mistaken for a primary dementia. In some older adults, a depressive episode with memory difficulties occurs in the early phase of an evolving dementia.

The most common psychiatric syndrome associated with thoughts of death, suicidal ideation, or completed suicide is a major depressive episode. The experience of hopelessness is commonly associated with suicidal ideation. The preoccupation with suicide in major depressive disorder requires that the assessment always includes careful monitoring of suicidality. Suicidality is the feature of depressive disorder that poses substantial risk of mortality in the disease. Prevention of suicide, more than any other treatment goal, requires immediate intervention and may require hospitalization. The risk for subsequent completed suicide for an individual hospitalized for an episode of severe MDD is estimated to be 15% (Coryell et al. 1982). To assess risk for suicide, one inquires about the presence of active suicidal ideation in relation to the current episode of depression and a history of prior suicide attempts. The occurrence of significant life events such as separation, divorce, and death of significant others may precipitate the episode. It is also necessary to review onsets of other medical conditions that may precipitate a new episode of depression. When alcohol or other drug use co-occurs with such significant life events, the risk of suicidal behavior during an episode of depression increases. The presence of a recent suicide attempt may suggest the need for immediate hospitalization and treatment.

Fawcett and colleagues (1990) looked at factors associated with suicide at different time points during the course of depression. Factors associated with suicide 1 year after assessment included severe anhedonia, insomnia, concentration difficulties, and comorbid panic attacks or substance abuse. Factors associated with suicide at 1 to 5 years after the assessment included prior suicide attempts, suicidal ideation, and hopelessness.

Familiarity with risk factors for major depressive disorder may help the clinician recognize or diagnose this common and serious psychiatric illness. Accordingly, The Depression Guideline Panel (1993a) enumerated the following 10 primary risk factors for depression: (1) history of prior episodes of depression; (2) family history of depressive disorder especially in first-degree relatives; (3) history of suicide attempts; (4) female gender; (5) age of onset before age 40; (6) postpartum period (7) comorbid medical illness; (8) absence of social support; (9) negative, stressful life events; (10) active alcohol or substance abuse.

The assessment of MDD involves the specific identification of 5 of 9 criterion symptoms that would constitute a diagnosis of MDD. A careful general medical assessment to ascertain the presence of an etiologic general medical condition is required. After the assessment for general medical conditions, one examines the individual for the presence of alcohol or drug dependence. Then the clinician is required to assess retrospectively the occurrence of prior episodes of mood disorder, either depression or mania. It is necessary to examine for other comorbid mental disorders as well. Depressive illnesses are very common and recurrent, but an individual with MDD may or may not recall prior episodes. It is therefore essential to interview a significant other or family member in addition to the individual with depression to identify prior manic, hypomanic, or prior depressive episodes. Family inquiry allows one to elicit the family history of addiction, anxiety, depressive disorder, mania, psychosis, trauma, or neurologic disorders in first-degree relatives.

The individual who presents for outpatient or hospital treatment for a primary depressive disorder will require general medical examination including a physical examination and laboratory testing to rule out an associated medical condition. Clinical assessment, including the cognitive mental status examination, will direct the extent of the general medical examination.

Traditional psychological testing may complement structured diagnostic instruments developed to ascertain the presence or absence of depressive disorders according to DSM-IV-TR criteria. Psychological testing such as the Rorschach Inkblot Test are sensitive to the degree of affective lability, intensity of suicidality, and impulse control in individuals with depression. In addition, inventories are commonly used in outpatient and inpatient settings to establish scores of clinical severity of depressive symptoms. Self-administered scales include the Beck Depression Inventory (Beck et al. 1961), the Zung Self-Rating Depression Scale (Zung 1965), and the Inventory for Depressive Symptomatology (self-report) (Rush et al. 1987). Clinician administered scales used for assessment of depressive symptoms include the Hamilton Rating Scale for Depression (Hamilton 1960), the Montgomery Asberg

Depression Rating Scale (Montgomery and Asberg 1979), and the Inventory for Depressive Symptomatology (clinician rated) (Rush et al. 1986). Structured diagnostic interviews that have been developed to confirm major psychiatric syndromes include the present state examination (Wing et al. 1967), the schedule for affective disorders, and schizophrenia (SADS) (Endicott and Spitzer 1978), and structured clinical interview for DSM-IV-TR Axis I disorders (SCID-I) (First et al. 1994). The use of these structured diagnostic interviews reliably assesses for the presence of an MDD. It is essential to recognize that a cross-sectional assessment is only one component of the total assessment. Corroborative family data and longitudinal assessment and reassessment of mood disorder symptoms are crucial in following the natural history and course of MDD.

Laboratory studies in the management of the individual with MDD includes complete blood count with differential, electrolytes, chemical screening for renal and liver function as well as thyroid function studies. More detailed evaluation will depend upon the nature of the clinical presentation as well as neuropsychological examination. These studies may identify cerebral vulnerability factors that would complicate the treatment for MDD.

When clinical signs suggest cognitive disruption or cognitive impairment, the clinician may also consider administering neuropsychological tests or conducting more focused neurologic examination to explore cognitive, behavioral, and neurological correlates of brain function. Neuropsychological assessment may help clarify the relative contribution of depression or another disease process to the individual's clinical presentation. Further, neuropsychological assessment will provide a functional analysis of the individual's cognitive and behavioral strengths and limitations. Neurological examination may reveal minor neurological abnormalities suggesting early neurodevelopmental vulnerability.

Individuals with MDD report health difficulties and actively use health services. Studies have indicated that as many as 23% of depressed individuals report health difficulties severe enough to keep them bedridden (Wells et al. 1988). A community sample of individuals with MDD demonstrated increased health care utilization in comparison to individuals in the general medical setting (Regier et al. 1988). The Medical Outcomes Study (Wells et al. 1989) examined role functioning, social functioning, and number of days in bed secondary to poor health, and compared the degree of impact of depression and other chronic medical conditions. Depression was associated with more impairment in occupational and interpersonal functioning, and more days in bed, in comparison to several common medical illnesses. individuals with MDD were shown to be as functionally impaired as individuals with serious, chronic medical conditions as well (Katon et al. 1990). individuals with MDD in a clinical sample evidence severely impaired occupational functioning, such as loss of work time (Wells et al. 1989). Further, long-term diminished activity has been shown to characterize a community sample of depressed individuals (Wells et al. 1988).

A significant relationship exists between MDD and mortality, characterized by suicide and accidents (Wells 1985). Therefore, an accurate diagnosis of MDD, early appropriate intervention, and specific assessment of suicidality is essential. Fifteen percent of individuals with MDD who require hospitalization owing to severe depression will die by committing suicide (Coryell et al. 1982). Approximately 10% of individuals with MDD who attempt suicide will eventually succeed in killing themselves. Roughly 50% of individuals who have successfully committed suicide carried a primary depressive diagnosis (Barklage 1991). individuals with MDD who were admitted to nursing homes were found to have a 59% greater likelihood of death within the first year of admission in comparison with nondepressed admissions. The epidemiologic catchment area (ECA) study indicated that individuals with MDD 55 years of age and older evidence a mortality rate over the next 15 months four times, higher than nondepressed controls matched for age.

Subtyping of MDD

The current subtyping of MDD is based on severity, cross-sectional features, and course features.

Severity/Psychotic/Remission   The rating of severity is based on a clinical judgment of the number of criteria present, the severity of the symptomatology, and the degree of functional distress. The ratings of current severity are classified as *mild, moderate, severe without psychotic features, severe with psychotic features, in partial remission*, or in *full remission* (see DSM-IV-TR diagnostic criteria below). The definition of "mild" refers to an episode that results in only mild impairment in occupational or psychosocial functioning or mild disability. "Moderate" implies a level of severity that is intermediate between mild and severe and is associated with moderate impairment in psychosocial functioning. The definition of "severe" describes an episode that meets several symptoms in excess of those required to make a diagnosis of major depressive episode and is associated with marked impairment in occupational or psychosocial functioning and definite disability characterized by inability to work or perform basic social functions. "Severe with psychotic features" indicates the presence of delusions or hallucinations, which occur in the context of the major depressive episode. Since the introduction of DSM-III, the categories of mood-congruent versus mood-incongruent psychotic features are made in the context of a psychotic depressive disorder. When the content of delusions or hallucinations is consistent with depressive themes, a mood-congruent psychotic diagnosis is made. When the psychotic features are not related to depressive themes or include symptoms such as thought insertion, broadcast, or withdrawal, the modifier of mood-incongruent psychotic features is used. A review by Kendler (1999) has suggested that mood-incongruent psychosis in MDD is associated with a poorer prognosis. For depression with psychotic features, whether they are mood-congruent or mood-incongruent, antipsychotic medication in combination with antidepressant medication or electroconvulsive therapy (ECT) is required to treat the disorder.

DSM-IV-TR Diagnostic Criteria

Severity/Psychotic/Remission Specifiers

Note: Code in fifth digit. Mild, Moderate, Severe Without Psychotic Features, and Severe With Psychotic Features can be applied only if the criteria are currently met for a Major Depressive Episode. In Partial Remission and In Full Remission can be applied to the most recent Major Depressive Episode in Major Depressive Disorder and to a Major Depressive Episode in Bipolar I or II Disorder only if it is the most recent type of mood episode.

.x1 — Mild: Few, if any, symptoms in excess of those required to make the diagnosis and symptoms result in only minor impairment in occupational functioning or in usual social activities or relationships with others.

.x2 — Moderate: Symptoms or functional impairment between "mild" and "severe."

.x3 — Severe Without Psychotic Features: Several symptoms in excess of those required to make the diagnosis, and symptoms markedly interfere with occupational functioning or with usual social activities or relationships with others.

.x4 — Severe With Psychotic Features: Delusions or hallucinations. If possible, specify whether the psychotic features are mood-congruent or mood-incongruent:

Mood-Congruent Psychotic Features: Delusions or hallucinations whose content is entirely consistent with the typical depressive themes of personal inadequacy, guilt, disease, death, nihilism, or deserved punishment.

Mood-Incongruent Psychotic Features: Delusions or hallucinations whose content does not involve typical depressive themes of personal inadequacy, guilt, disease, death, nihilism, or deserved punishment. Included are such symptoms as persecutory delusions (not directly related to depressive themes), thought insertion, thought broadcasting, and delusions of control.

.x5 — In Partial Remission: Symptoms of a Major Depressive Episode are present but full criteria are not met, or there is a period without any significant symptoms of a Major Depressive Episode lasting less than 2 months following the end of the Major Depressive Episode. (If the Major Depressive Episode was superimposed on Dysthymic Disorder, the diagnosis of Dysthymic Disorder alone is given once the full criteria for a Major Depressive Episode are no longer met.)

.x6 — In Full Remission: During the past 2 months, no significant signs or symptoms of the disturbance were present.

.x0 — Unspecified.

Reprinted with permission from the Diagnostic and Statistical Manual of Mental Disorders, Fourth Edition, Text Revision. Copyright 2000 American Psychiatric Association.

Partial remission indicates that the episode no longer meets full criteria for major depressive episode but that some symptoms are still present or the period of remission has been less than 2 months. In full remission, the individual has no significant symptoms of depression for a period of at least 2 months.

Cross-Sectional Features   The assessment of cross-sectional features involves the presence or absence of catatonic, melancholic, or atypical features during an episode of depression. The specifier *with catatonic features* is used when profound psychomotor retardation, prominent mutism, echolalia, echopraxia, or stupor dominates the clinical picture (see for DSM-IV-TR diagnostic criteria below). The presentation of catatonia requires a differential diagnosis that includes schizophrenia, catatonic type, bipolar I disorder, catatonic disorder due to a general medical condition, medication-induced movement disorder leading to catatonic features, or neuroleptic malignant syndrome.

DSM-IV-TR Diagnostic Criteria

With Catatonic Features

Specify if:

With Catatonic Features (can be applied to the current or most recent Major Depressive Episode, Manic Episode, or Mixed Episode in Major Depressive Disorder, Bipolar I Disorder, or Bipolar II Disorder)

The clinical picture is dominated by at least two of the following:

A. Motoric immobility as evidenced by catalepsy (including waxy flexibility) or stupor

B. Excessive motor activity (that is apparently purposeless and not influenced by external stimuli)

C. Extreme negativism (an apparently motiveless resistance to all instructions or maintenance of a rigid posture against attempts to be moved) or mutism

D. Peculiarities of voluntary movement as evidenced by posturing (voluntary assumption of inappropriate or bizarre postures), stereotyped movements, prominent mannerisms, or prominent grimacing

E. Echolalia or echopraxia

Reprinted with permission from the Diagnostic and Statistical Manual of Mental Disorders, Fourth Edition, Text Revision. Copyright 2000 American Psychiatric Association.

The specifier *with melancholic features* is applied when the depressive episode is characterized by profound loss of interest or pleasure in activities and lack of reactivity to external events as well as usual pleasurable stimuli (see DSM-IV-TR diagnostic criteria below). In addition, at least three of the following melancholic features must be present: depression is typically worse in the morning, early morning awakening, psychomotor change with marked retardation or agitation, significant weight loss, or profound and excessive guilt. A major depressive episode with melancholic features is particularly important to diagnose because of the prediction that it is more likely to respond to somatic treatment including electroconvulsive therapy. Individuals with melancholic features experience more recurrence of MDD. The findings of hypercortisolism following dexamethasone as well as reduced rapid eye movement (REM) latency is associated with the melancholic episodes of MDD (Rush et al. 1991).

DSM-IV-TR Diagnostic Criteria

With Melancholic Features

Specify if:

With Melancholic Features (can be applied to the current or most recent Major Depressive Episode in Major Depressive Disorder and to a Major Depressive Episode in Bipolar I or Bipolar II Disorder only if it is the most recent type of mood episode)

A. Either of the following, occurring during the most severe period of the current episode:

    (1) loss of pleasure in all, or almost all, activities

    (2) lack of reactivity to usually pleasurable stimuli (does not feel much better, even temporarily, when something good happens)

B. Three (or more) of the following:

    (1) distinct quality of depressed mood (i.e., the depressed mood is experienced as distinctly different from the kind of feeling experienced after the death of a loved one)

(2) depression regularly worse in the morning
(3) early morning awakening (at least 2 hours before usual time of awakening)
(4) marked psychomotor retardation or agitation
(5) significant anorexia or weight loss
(6) excessive or inappropriate guilt.

Reprinted with permission from the Diagnostic and Statistical Manual of Mental Disorders, Fourth Edition, Text Revision. Copyright 2000 American Psychiatric Association.

Finally, the category of major depressive episode *with atypical features* was previously called "atypical depression." This syndrome is characterized by prominent mood reactivity in which there is responsiveness of the depressed mood to external events and at least two of the following associated features: increased appetite or weight gain, hypersomnia, leaden paralysis (a feeling of profound anergia or heavy feeling), and interpersonal hypersensitivity (rejection sensitivity) (see DSM-IV-TR diagnostic criteria below). Depressive episodes with atypical features are also common in individuals with bipolar I or II disorder as well as seasonal affective disorder.

DSM-IV-TR Diagnostic Criteria

With Atypical Features

Specify if:

With Atypical Features (can be applied when these features predominate during the most recent 2 weeks of a current Major Depressive Episode in Major Depressive Disorder or in Bipolar I or Bipolar II Disorder when a current Major Depressive Episode is the most recent type of mood episode, or when these features predominate during the most recent 2 years of Dysthymic Disorder; if the Major Depressive Episode is not current, it applies if the feature predominates during any 2-week period)

A. Mood reactivity (i.e., mood brightens in response to actual or potential positive events)
B. Two (or more) of the following features:

    (1) significant weight gain or increase in appetite
    (2) hypersomnia
    (3) leaden paralysis (i.e., heavy, leaden feelings in arms or legs)
    (4) long-standing pattern of interpersonal rejection sensitivity (not limited to episodes of mood disturbance) that results in significant social or occupational impairment

C. Criteria are not met for With Melancholic Features or With Catatonic Features during the same episode.

Reprinted with permission from the Diagnostic and Statistical Manual of Mental Disorders, Fourth Edition, Text Revision. Copyright 2000 American Psychiatric Association.

Course Features MDD is diagnosed with certain course features such as postpartum onset, seasonal pattern, recurrent, chronic, and with or without full interepisode recovery. Depression *with postpartum onset* has been the subject of increasing attention in psychiatric consultation to obstetrics and gynecology. The specifier applies only to the current or most recent major depressive episode in MDD (or Bipolar Disorder) (see DSM-IV-TR diagnostic criteria below). The presence of a major depressive episode may occur from 2 weeks to 12 months after delivery, beyond the usual duration of postpartum "blues" (3–7 days). Postpartum blues are brief episodes of labile mood and tearfulness that occur in 50 to 80% of women within 5 days of delivery. However, depression is seen in 10 to 20% of women after childbirth (Miller 2002), which is higher than rates of depression found in matched controls. There is greater vulnerability in women with prior episodes of major mood disorder particularly bipolar disorder, and there is a high risk of recurrence with subsequent deliveries after an MDD with postpartum onset. The postpartum onset episodes can present either with or without psychosis. Postpartum psychotic episodes occur in 0.1 to 0.2% of deliveries. Depression in postpartum psychosis is associated with prominent guilt and may involve individuals with a prior history of bipolar I disorder. If an episode of postpartum psychosis occurs, there is a high risk of recurrence with subsequent deliveries. Heightened attention to identification of postpartum episodes is required because of potential risk of morbidity and mortality to mother and newborn child.

DSM-IV-TR Diagnostic Criteria

Postpartum Onset

Specify if:

With Postpartum Onset (can be applied to the current or most recent Major Depressive, Manic, or Mixed Episode in Major Depressive Disorder, Bipolar I Disorder, or Bipolar II Disorder; or to Brief Psychotic Disorder)

Onset of episode within 4 weeks postpartum.

Reprinted with permission from the Diagnostic and Statistical Manual of Mental Disorders, Fourth Edition, Text Revision. Copyright 2000 American Psychiatric Association.

The specifier *with seasonal pattern* is diagnosed when episodes of MDD occur regularly in fall and winter seasons and subsequently remit during spring and summer (see DSM-IV-TR diagnostic criteria on page 748). When the pattern of onset and remission occurs for the last 2 years, one diagnoses an MDD with seasonal pattern. Often, this pattern is characterized by atypical features including low energy, hypersomnia, weight gain, and carbohydrate craving. Although the predominant pattern is fall–winter depression, a minority of individuals show the reverse seasonal pattern with spring–summer depression. Specific forms of light therapy with 2500 lux exposure has been shown to be effective in MDD with seasonal pattern (Whirz-Justice 1993). Because seasonal depression has clinical features that are similar to atypical features, the risk of a possible bipolar II disorder must be considered since atypical features are more common in depressive episodes occurring as part of bipolar II. These individuals, when exposed to antidepressant medication or bright light therapy, may evolve a switch into hypomanic or manic episode.

DSM-IV-TR Diagnostic Criteria

Seasonal Pattern

Specify if:

With Seasonal Pattern (can be applied to the pattern of Major Depressive Episodes in Bipolar I Disorder, Bipolar II Disorder, or Major Depressive Disorder, Recurrent)

A. There has been a regular temporal relationship between the onset of Major Depressive Episodes in Bipolar I or Bipolar II Disorder or Major Depressive Disorder, Recurrent, and a particular time of the year (e.g., regular appearance of the Major Depressive Episode in the fall or winter). Note: Do not include cases in which there is an obvious effect of season-related psychosocial stressors (e.g., regularly being unemployed every winter).
B. Full remissions (or a change from depression to mania or hypomania) also occur at a characteristic time of the year (e.g., depression disappears in the spring).
C. In the last 2 years, two Major Depressive Episodes have occurred that demonstrate the temporal seasonal relationships defined in Criteria A and B, and no nonseasonal Major Depressive Episodes have occurred during that same period.
D. Seasonal Major Depressive Episodes (as described above) substantially outnumber the nonseasonal Major Depressive Episodes that may have occurred over the individual's lifetime.

Reprinted with permission from the Diagnostic and Statistical Manual of Mental Disorders, Fourth Edition, Text Revision. Copyright 2000 American Psychiatric Association.

Clinical and scientific attention to the course of MDD focuses upon the depiction of longitudinal course. Life charting of MDD involves the use of several course specifiers. Each episode is denoted with or without full recovery (see DSM-IV-TR diagnostic criteria below). The specifier chronic MDD involves the persistence of a major depressive episode continually, satisfying full MDD criteria for at least 2 years.

DSM-IV-TR Diagnostic Criteria

With and Without Interepisode Recovery

Specify if (can be applied to Recurrent Major Depressive Disorder or Bipolar I or II Disorder):

With Full Interepisode Recovery: if full remission is attained between the two most recent Mood Episodes

Without Full Interepisode Recovery: if full remission is not attained between the two most recent Mood Episodes

---

Reprinted with permission from the Diagnostic and Statistical Manual of Mental Disorders, Fourth Edition, Text Revision. Copyright 2000 American Psychiatric Association.

Epidemiology

The prevalence and incidence data on MDD vary to some degree due to methodological differences, nature of interview format, geographic location, and settings of the sample. Large-scale epidemiologic studies of mood disorders began in earnest in the early 1950s, culminating with a reanalysis of the NIMH epidemiologic catchment area (ECA) (Weissman et al. 1988b) study (probability sample of over 18,000 adults in five US communities) and more recently, results from the National Comorbidity Survey (NCS) (Kessler et al. 1994).

Across epidemiologic studies, MDD is found to be a common psychiatric disorder. The lifetime risk for MDD in community samples varies from 10 to 25% for women and 5 to 12% for men (American Psychiatric Association 2000). The point prevalence of MDD (proportion of the individuals that have the disorder being studied at a designated time) for adults in community samples has varied from 5 to 9% for women and from 2 to 3% for men (American Psychiatric Association 2000). The point prevalence of MDD in primary care outpatient settings ranges from 4.8 to 8.6% (Depression Guideline Panel 1993a). In hospitalized individuals for all medical conditions, more than 14% had MDD (Feldman et al. 1987). While the incidence rates of MDD in prepubertal boys and girls are equal, women over the course of their lifetime are 2 to 3 times more likely to have MDD after puberty (Kornstein 1997).

Whereas a strong relationship exists between low social class and schizophrenia, a weaker but nevertheless meaningful relationship may exist between low income status and the occurrence of MDD (Blazer et al. 1994). Analyses of the ECA data indicated that the lowest income group manifested twice the risk of MDD than the highest income group, while the NCS concluded that individuals with low socioeconomic status demonstrate higher risk for MDD than individuals who are economically well-off. The rates of MDD may also be influenced by childhood adversity including severe physical abuse, sexual abuse, neglect, and poor care (Harkness and Monroe 2002). The NCS identified the risk factors associated with having MDD comorbid with another mental disorder as opposed to MDD alone. These risk factors include younger age, lower level of education, and lower income.

For preschool children, the point prevalence is thought to be of 0.8% (Depression Guideline Panel 1993a). Point prevalences of major and minor depressive disorder of 1.8 and 2.5%, respectively, were found in a sample of 9-year-old children from the general population, based upon the use of a semistructured diagnostic instrument (Kashani et al. 1983). A semistructured diagnostic instrument was used to find a 4.7% point prevalence rate of major depressive disorder in a community sample of 150 adolescents. Those adolescents diagnosed with MDD had symptoms that met criteria for dysthymic disorder as well. A point prevalence rate of 3.3% was found for dysthymic disorder (Kashani et al. 1987). Weller and Weller (1990) have shown the prevalence of MDD in clinical samples of children and adolescents to be 58% in educational clinics, 28% in outpatient psychiatric clinics, and 40 to 60% in psychiatric hospitals. By comparison, a prevalence of 7% is found in hospitalized children. Emslie et al. (1990) assessed depressive symptoms by self-report in a large sample of high school students of mixed ethnic background in an urban school district. They found that Hispanic females reported more severe depression whereas white males reported the least severe scores of depression. For males and females, African-Americans and Hispanics reported significantly more depression than whites. Female gender, being behind in school, and nonwhite ethnicity predicted higher self-report scores of depressive symptoms.

Weissman and colleagues (1991) found a 1% prevalence of MDD in adults 65 years and older who lived in the community. The data indicate that a lower lifetime prevalence of MDD was found in the oldest age group ($\geq$age 65) in comparison to younger age groups. Women manifest an increased prevalence of MDD in comparison to men and no significant differences were found across racial or ethnic groups. However, other community samples of older adults were found to have a high prevalence (8–15%) of clinically significant depressive symptoms (but not a formal diagnosis of MDD). In a recent Stockholm group, the frequency of MDD was 5.9% and the rate of DD was 8.3% (Forsell et al. 1994).

In comparison with community settings, higher prevalence rates for MDD are found in treatment settings for older adults: 11% in hospitals, 5% in outpatient nonpsychiatric clinics, and 12% in long-term care settings (Blazer 1994). There is also a higher prevalence rate in treatment settings of clinically significant depression that is not severe enough to warrant a formal diagnosis of MDD: 25% prevalence in hospitals (Koenig et al. 1988) and 30.5% in long-term care facilities (Parmelee et al. 1989).

Klerman and Weissman (1989) as well as The Cross-National Collaborative Group (1992) called attention to a changing rate of MDD for recent birth cohorts found in North America, Puerto Rico, Western Europe, Middle East, Asia, and the Pacific Rim. Specifically, an earlier age of onset and increased rate of depression occur in individuals born in more recent decades. Historical, social, economic, or biological events most likely account for the variability in the rate of depression noted in different countries included in the study. However, an overall increase in the rate of depression was noted across many of the geographic locations.

Older adults continue to manifest a higher suicide rate than in younger age groups. However, suicide rates have increased in younger age groups as the changing rate of MDD is observed in younger cohorts. In keeping with the birth cohort effect, recurrences of MDD in late life may become a significant health concern as the population ages.

Course

The mean age of onset of major depression is 27 years of age (Weissman et al. 1988b), although an individual can experience the onset of MDD at any age. New symptoms of MDD often develop over several days to several weeks. Early manifestations of an episode of MDD include anxiety, sleeplessness, worry, and rumination prior to the experience of overt depression. Over a lifetime, the presence of one major depressive episode is associated with a 50% chance of a recurrent episode (Thase 1990). A history of two episodes is associated with a 70 to 80% risk of a future episode. Three or more episodes are associated with extremely high rates of recurrence (National Institute of Mental Health Consensus Development Conference Statement 1985). Because the majority of cases of MDD recur, continuation treatment and ongoing education regarding warning signs of relapse or recurrence are essential in ongoing clinical care.

In comparison to individuals who develop a single episode (many of whom return to premorbid functioning), individuals with recurrent episodes of depression are at greater risk to manifest bipolar disorder (Depression Guideline Panel 1993a). Individuals who experience several recurrent episodes of depression may develop a hypomanic or manic episode requiring rediagnosis to bipolar disorder. In children and adolescents, the transformation of a diagnosis of depression to a diagnosis of bipolar disorder is higher. Approximately 40% of adolescents who are depressed evolve into a bipolar course. Because bipolar disorder is initiated with a depressive episode in at least 4 of 5 cases (Goodwin and Jamison 1990), it is important to identify those individuals who are most likely to develop a bipolar disorder. Therefore, the clinician is confronted with significant diagnostic and treatment challenges when called upon to evaluate an individual, particularly an adolescent, who presents with depression and has no previous history of mania. Several risk factors have been identified (Akiskal 1983, Goodwin and Jamison 1990), which predict when a first episode of MDD will evolve into bipolar disorder: (1) the first episode of depression emerges during adolescence, (2) the depression is severe and includes psychotic features; (3) psychomotor retardation and hypersomnia are present, (4) a family history of bipolar disorder exists, particularly across two to three generations, and (5) the individual experiences hypomania induced by antidepressant medication.

Recurrent MDD requires longitudinal observation because of its highly variable course. Generally, complete remission of an episode of MDD heralds a return to premorbid levels of social, occupational, and interpersonal functioning. Therefore, the goal of treatment is in achieving full remission of depressive symptoms and recovery. Untreated episodes of depression last 6 to 24 months (Goodwin and Jamison 1990). Symptom remission and a return to premorbid level of functioning characterize approximately 66% of depressed individuals (Depression Guideline Panel 1993a). By comparison, roughly 5 to 10% of individuals continue to experience a full episode of depression for greater than 2 years and approximately 20 to 25% of individuals experience partial recovery between episodes. Furthermore, 25% of the individuals manifest "double depression," characterized by the development of MDD superimposed upon a mild, chronic dysthymic disorder (DD) (Keller and Shapiro 1982). Individuals with double depression often demonstrate poor interepisode recovery. The following four characteristics are seen in a partial remission of an episode (Depression Guideline Panel 1993a): (1) increased likelihood of a subsequent episode, (2) partial interepisode recovery following subsequent episodes, (3) possible requirement of longer-term treatment, and (4) treatment with a combination of pharmacotherapy and psychotherapy may be indicated.

Follow-up naturalistic studies have indicated that 40.3% of individuals with MDD carry the same diagnosis 1 year later, 2.6% evidence DD, 16.7% manifest incomplete recovery, and 40.5% do not meet criteria for MDD (Depression Guideline Panel 1993a). Keller and colleagues (1992) highlight the potential for chronicity in MDD. A 5-year follow-up study indicated that 50% of the 431 individuals showed recovery by 6 months but 12% of the sample continued to be depressed for the entire 5-year period. The authors noted that inadequate treatment may have contributed to the chronicity.

Poor outcome and likelihood of recurrent episodes is associated with comorbid conditions such as personality disorder, active substance or alcohol abuse, organicity, or medical illness. Recurrence and outcome may be affected by the rapidity of clinical intervention. Inadequate treatment (e.g., insufficient dosing or duration of pharmacotherapy) contributes to poor outcome, including chronic MDD. Several authors have asserted that early treatment intervention in an episode of MDD is considered to be relatively more effective than later intervention in an episode (Kupfer et al. 1989).

Depression in the Medically Ill

Whereas a 4 to 5% current prevalence rate of MDD exists in community samples, symptoms of depression are found in 12 to 36% of individuals with a general medical condition (Depression Guideline Panel 1993a). The rate of depression may be higher in individuals with a specific medical condition. MDD is identified as an independent condition and calls for specific treatment when it occurs in the presence of a general medical condition.

The Depression Guideline Panel (1993a) includes four possible relationships between depression and a general medical condition: (1) depression is biologically caused by the general medical condition, (2) an individual who carries a genetic vulnerability to MDD manifests the onset of depression triggered by the general medical condition, (3) depression is psychologically caused by the general medical condition, and (4) no causal relationship exists between the general medical condition and mood disorder. The first two cases warrant initial treatment directed at the general medical condition. Treatment is advocated for persistent depression upon stabilization of the general medical condition. When the general medical condition causes depression, specific treatment for the former condition is optimized, while psychiatric management, education, and antidepressant medication are administered to treat the depression. In cases where the two conditions are not etiologically related, appropriate treatment is indicated for each disorder.

Stroke   Some poststroke patients manifest depression owing to cerebrovascular disease related to cerebral infarction in left frontal and left subcortical brain regions. Mood disorder due to cerebrovascular disease is diagnosed when an individual manifests a recent stroke and has significant symptoms of depression. A point prevalence of mood disorder due to cerebrovascular disease in poststroke patients between 10 and 27% has been documented, with an average duration of depression lasting approximately 1 year (Depression Guideline Panel 1993). Case reports of mood disorder due to cerebrovascular disease in poststroke individuals suggest poor treatment compliance, irritability, and personality change (Ross and Rush 1981).

Alzheimer's Disease   According to DSM-IV-TR, when symptoms of clinically significant depressed mood accompany dementia of the Alzheimer's Type, and in the clinician's judgment, the depression is due to the direct physiological effects of the Alzheimer's disease, mood disorder due to Alzheimer's disease is diagnosed. When dementia consistent with cerebrovascular disease leads to prominent cognitive deficits, focal neurological signs and symptoms, significant impairment in functioning as well as predominant depressed mood, vascular dementia with depressed mood is diagnosed. The distinction between depressive disorders and dementia is often complicated because depression and dementia commonly co-occur. Treatment of co-occurring depressive features may relieve symptoms and improve overall quality of life.

Parkinson's Disease   Fifty percent of individuals with Parkinson's disease experience an MDD during the course of the illness. When depression occurs in this context, one diagnoses mood disorder due to Parkinson's disease. Active treatment of the depressive disorder may result in improvement in the signs and symptoms of depression without alleviation of the involuntary movement disorder or cognitive changes associated with subcortical brain disease. The underlying etiology of associated dementia and depressive disorder in Parkinson's disease appears to involve physiologic changes in subcortical brain regions.

Diabetes   It is estimated that the prevalence of depression in treated individuals with diabetes is three times as frequent than in the general population. Further, there is no difference in the prevalence rate of depression in individuals with insulin-dependent diabetes mellitus (Type I) in comparison with individuals with noninsulin-dependent mellitus (Type II). The symptomatic presentation of MDD in individuals with diabetes is similar to individuals without diabetes. Consequently, full assessment of and treatment for MDD is recommended in individuals who become depressed during the course of diabetes (Depression Guideline Panel 1993a). The relatively high point prevalence rate may be due to higher detection rate in this treated population having a chronic illness as well as metabolic and endocrine factors.

Coronary Artery Disease   When MDD is present, increased morbidity and mortality is reported in postmyocardial infarction patients as well as in individuals having coronary artery disease without myocardial infarction (MI). Therefore, treatment of MDD in individuals with coronary artery disease is indicated. Prevalence estimates of MDD in postmyocardial infarction range from 40 to 65%. Over a 15-month period, individuals 55 years or older who had mood disorder evidenced a mortality rate four times higher than expected, and coronary heart disease or stroke accounted for 63% of the deaths (Depression Guideline Panel 1993a). Depression may promote poor adherence to cardiac rehabilitation and worse outcome. During the first year following MI, depression is considered to be associated with a three- to fourfold increase in subsequent cardiovascular morbidity and mortality. Depression in individuals with coronary artery disease is associated with more social problems, functional impairment, and increased health care utilization (Musselman et al. 1998). Recent studies of erectile dysfunction, cardiovascular disease, and depression demonstrate that all three conditions share many of the same risk factors (Goldstein 2000).

Cancer   MDD occurs in 25% of individuals with cancer at some time during the illness. MDD should be assessed and treated as an independent disorder. The intense reaction in individuals diagnosed with cancer may lead to dysphoria and sadness without evolving a full syndrome of MDD. The consulting psychiatrist must evaluate the individual's response to chemotherapy, side effects of the treatment, and medication interactions in the overall assessment of the individual. Among individuals with cancer, MDD is typically characterized by heightened distress, impaired functioning, and decreased capacity to adhere to treatment. Treating comorbid MDD with psychotherapy or pharmacotherapy may improve the overall outcome in individuals with cancer and mitigate complications of MDD.

Chronic Fatigue Syndrome   Lifetime rates of MDD in individuals with chronic fatigue syndrome range from 46 to 75%. Comorbid anxiety and somatization disorders are also common in individuals with chronic fatigue. According to the Centers for Disease Control (CDC) criteria, the diagnosis of chronic fatigue syndrome is excluded in individuals whose symptoms meet criteria for a formal mental disorder, such as MDD or DD. Individuals whose symptoms meet criteria for both a mood disorder and a chronic fatigue syndrome should be maximally treated for the mood disorder with appropriate pharmacotherapy and cognitive–behavioral psychotherapy (Depression Guideline Panel 1993a). The etiological relationship between mood disorder and chronic fatigue syndrome is unclear.

Fibromyalgia   In comparison with other general medical conditions, little is known about the relationship between fibromyalgia and MDD. Two studies (Alfici et al. 1989, Hudson et al. 1985) have found higher lifetime rates of major mood disorder in fibromyalgia patients in comparison with rheumatoid arthritis patients.

Depression Due to Medications
If MDD is judged to be a direct physiologic effect of a medication, then substance-induced mood disorder is diagnosed. Medications reported to cause depression involve several drugs from the associated groups listed in Table 28-1.

Among antihypertensive treatment, beta-adrenergic blockers have been studied regarding the risk of depression. No significant differences are found between individuals treated with beta-blockers and those treated with other antihypertensives regarding the propensity to develop depressive symptoms. Lethargy is the most common side effect reported. No significant depressive complications are reported with calcium channel blockers or angiotensin converting enzyme (ACE) inhibitors.

Hormonal treatments, such as corticosteroids and anabolic steroids, can elicit depression, mania, or psychosis. Oral contraceptives require monitoring regarding the possible precipitation of depressive symptoms.

Because individuals with seizure disorders and Parkinson's disease are at high risk for concomitant MDD, it is difficult to establish a link between anticonvulsant or anti-Parkinsonian treatment and the precipitation of depression. Nevertheless, individuals require close monitoring and evaluation for evolution of depressive symptomatology.

Table 28-1	Medications Associated with Depression		
Cardiovascular Drugs	**Hormones**		**Psychotropics**
Methyldopa	Oral contraceptives		Benzodiazepines
Reserpine	Corticotropin and glucocorticoids		Neuroleptics
Propranolol	Anabolic steroids		
Guanethidine			
Clonidine			
Thiazide diuretics			
Digitalis			
Anticancer Agents	Anti-inflammatory and Anti-infective Agents		Others
Cycloserine	Nonsteroidal anti-inflammatory agents		Cocaine (withdrawal)
	Ethambutol		Amphetamines (withdrawal)
	Disulfiram		Levodopa
	Sulfonamides		Cimetidine
	Baclofen		Ranitidine
	Metoclopramide		

Comorbid Depression with Other Mental Disorders

More than 40% of individuals with MDD have additional symptoms that meet criteria during their lifetime for one or more additional mental disorders (Sargeant et al. 1990). In a recent community sample, assessing both pure and comorbid MDD based upon findings from the NCS, the current prevalence of major depression was 4.9% (Blazer et al. 1994). Of the sample with current MDD, 56.3% also had another mental disorder. The expression "comorbidity" comes from general medicine and denotes distinct but coexisting conditions. The multiaxial format of DSM-IV-TR requires delineation of multiple diagnoses on Axis I (clinical psychiatric syndromes), if present and specification of co-occurring syndromes on Axis I and II (personality disorders). The presence of a comorbid mental disorder may alter the course of major mood disorder in a dramatic fashion and is identified as a primary risk factor for poor treatment response. Therefore, proper assessment, preferably with the use of a semistructured diagnostic instruments, additional informants, and longitudinal observation, will identify comorbid conditions. In addition, specific guidelines are available to inform decision-making regarding which illness (MDD or other mental disorder) becomes the initial focus of treatment (Depression Guideline Panel 1993a).

Alcohol/Drug Dependence Results of family and twin studies in a population-based female sample are consistent with a modest correlation of the liability between alcohol dependence and MDD (Kendler et al. 1993a). It is common for individuals with alcohol dependence to evidence signs of depression or MDD, but alcoholism is not thought to be a common consequence of mood disorder. Between 10 and 30% of individuals with alcoholism manifest depression (Petty 1992), whereas alcoholism is thought to occur in under 5% of depressed individuals (Depression Guideline Panel 1993a).

Depressed women are more likely to self-medicate their mood disorder with alcohol than are depressed men (Depression Guideline Panel 1993a). The effect of comorbid alcoholism on the course of major mood disorder is unclear. Some evidence suggests that remission of depression occurs within the first month of sobriety (Brown and Schuckit 1988, Dorus et al. 1987). The effect of comorbid depression requires further attention in relation to the course of drug dependence. Drug dependence is often associated with major mood disorder and the presence of associated comorbid personality disorder.

Panic/Phobias/GAD The co-occurrence of symptoms of anxiety and depression is very common. Kendler et al. (1986) found very high genetic correlations between MDD and generalized anxiety disorder in contrast to a modest overlap between phobic disorders and MDD. Anxiety symptoms commonly appear in depressive syndromes and MDD is frequently comorbid with anxiety disorders. From a longitudinal perspective, either symptom constellation can be a precursor to the development of the other disorder. The combination of anxiety and depression predicts greater severity and impairment than the presence of each syndrome in isolation (Depression Guideline Panel 1993a). The association of severe panic and MDD is one of the predictors of suicidal risk. The clinician is advised to assess for symptoms of each disorder and to obtain a thorough family history. individuals with anxiety disorders often experience prior episodes of MDD or have relatives who suffer from mood disorder.

Ten to 20% of outpatients with MDD evidence comorbid panic disorder while 30 to 40% of depressed outpatients have had symptoms that met criteria for generalized anxiety disorder during the course of the mood disorder. In both cases, the anxiety disorder has preceded the major mood disorder about 50% of the time. An increased incidence of MDD is noted in individuals with anxiety disorders who are followed over time. For example, Munjack and Moss (1981) found that 91% of their agoraphobic individuals manifested an MDD within a 3-year period. MDD is a commonly manifested clinical outcome of a chronic anxiety state (Akiskal 1990).

The clinician is advised to evaluate three factors in order to determine treatment approaches when MDD co-occurs with panic disorder or social phobia: (1) the individual's family history, (2) the constellation of symptoms that were first evident in the current episode, and (3) the symptoms that cause the individual the most distress.

Recovery is less likely and symptomatology more severe in individuals with comorbid MDD and panic disorder than in cases with a single diagnosis. Lifetime suicide rate is twice as high for individuals with comorbid panic disorder and MDD than in panic disorder alone. It is imperative to assess for the presence of mood disorder and suicidality among individuals who present with symptoms of anxiety.

Obsessive-Compulsive Disorder The occurrence of symptoms of depression is very common in individuals with obsessive–compulsive disorder (OCD), although full symptom criteria may not be reached to warrant a formal diagnosis of MDD. Ten to 30% of individuals with OCD have mood symptoms that meet full criteria for MDD. The relationship between OCD and schizophrenia is less clear. Individuals with OCD are at an increased risk to develop MDD but not schizophrenia (Goodwin and Jamison 1990). It is important to distinguish between obsessive–compulsive personality features that can accompany and can exacerbate during an episode of depression and OCD itself. Symptoms of depression often diminish with successful initial treatment of OCD, since biological treatments typically involve use of selective serotonergic antidepressant medications such as clomipramine, fluoxetine, or fluvoxamine.

Posttraumatic Stress Disorder Individuals with PTSD often experience co-occurring depressive disorders, anxiety disorders, and substance use disorders. The range of reported rates of concurrent depressive disorder in individuals with PTSD is 30 to 50% (Bleich et al. 1997, Kessler et al. 1995) Many of the symptoms of PTSD overlap with signs and symptoms of depression such that both PTSD and MDD can be considered to be the result of traumatic events. In addition, depressive disorder may be associated with worse outcome in individuals with co-occurring PTSD (Shalev et al. 1998).

Somatization Disorder It is common for individuals with MDD to experience somatic symptoms including pain, although the intensity and frequency of the somatic complaints and the range of body systems affected do not usually meet criteria for somatization disorder.

Individuals who have mood symptoms that meet criteria for MDD evidence more complaints of pain, experience more physical, interpersonal, and occupational limitations, and perceive their overall health as worse than individuals with chronic medical illness (Wells et al. 1989). The clinician should carefully evaluate for the presence of MDD in cases where the individual reports unexplained pain. Typically, pain complaints are relieved upon successful treatment of the MDD. However, somatoform disorders, as outlined in DSM-IV-TR, may be associated with demoralization and depression.

Eating Disorders   There are little data available regarding prevalence of eating disorders in individuals with MDD. However, 33 to 50% of individuals with anorexia nervosa or bulimia nervosa experience a comorbid mood disorder. Between 50 and 75% of individuals with an eating disorder have a history of an MDD over a lifetime. Initial treatment is aimed at the eating disorder. If depression continues after proper nourishment has been re-established in anorexia nervosa, treatment is directed at the primary mood disorder.

Personality Disorders   High rates of personality disorders are found in depressed inpatients and outpatients. Most studies report a rate of co-occurrence between 30 and 40% in outpatients and 50 to 60% in inpatient samples (Shea et al. 1992). Several studies have found that individuals with comorbid MDD and personality disorder evidence an earlier age of onset for the first episode of depression, increased severity of depressive symptoms, more episodes, longer duration of episodes, poorer response to both pharmacotherapy and psychotherapy, and increased risk for self-injury (Black et al. 1988, Charney et al. 1981, Ionescu and Popescu 1989, Pfohl et al. 1984, Shea et al. 1987).

A particular relationship is noted for comorbid MDD and borderline personality disorder (BPD). In a general psychiatric population, depressed individuals show an estimated rate of 6% for co-occurring BPD (Depression Guideline Panel 1993). The link between BPD and MDD remains controversial. Gunderson and Phillips (1991) offered four possible relationships regarding the co-existence of MDD and BPD: (1) depression is primary and produces the symptoms of BPD, (2) BPD is primary and produces the symptoms of MDD, (3) MDD and BPD coexist but are unrelated, and (4) both disorders have nonspecific overlapping sources. For each hypothesis, the authors evaluated evidence from six areas: (1) comorbidity, (2) phenomenology, (3) family prevalence, (4) drug response, (5) biological factors, and (6) pathogenesis and outcome. The authors concluded that the evidence supports the notion that MDD and BPD coexist as independent disorders.

Grief and Bereavement   Depressive symptoms associated with normal grieving usually begin within 2 to 3 weeks of the loss and resolve spontaneously over 6 to 8 weeks. If full symptom criteria for MDD persist for more than 2 months beyond the death of a loved one, then an episode of MDD can be diagnosed. Specific treatment for a major depressive episode such as short-term psychotherapy focusing on unresolved grief or pharmacotherapy is indicated.

Depression in Children and Adolescents

In prepubertal children, MDD occurs equally among boys and girls (Depression Guideline Panel 1993a). MDD in childhood is considered to have high recurrence rates with up to 70% recurrence in 5 years. After puberty, girls experience an increased rate of depression as compared to boys. There is an increased risk of depressive disorder in children and adolescents when one or more of the parents are depressed. The earlier the age of onset of depression, the higher the familiar loading. In addition, a number of childhood psychosocial risk factors have been identified to be associated with juvenile-onset MDD. These risk factors include more perinatal insults, motor skill abnormalities, instability in caregivers, and psychopathology in the first-degree relatives (Jaffee et al. 2002). Adolescent-onset depression often takes on a more chronic course associated with dysthymic symptoms. In adolescence, MDD appears to be associated with greater fatigue, worthlessness, and more prominent vegetative signs, while DD has more prominent changes in mood, irritability, anger, and hopelessness. The signs and symptoms used for diagnosis in children and adolescents are identical to those used for diagnosis in adults except that irritable mood can substitute for depressed mood. The sequelae of depression in children and adolescents is often characterized by disruption in school performance, social withdrawal, increased behavioral disruption, and substance abuse. Differential diagnosis among children and adolescents with MDD include behavioral disorders such as conduct disorder, attention deficit hyperactivity disorder, and bipolar disorder.

Later-onset MDD in adolescents is also associated with decline in school performance, social withdrawal, or disruptive behavior. The critical differential diagnostic consideration in adolescents with MDD is the misdiagnosis of depression when the clinical presentation will evolve into a diagnosis of bipolar disorder. When depression occurs during adolescence, it often heralds a severe disorder with recurrent course and a family history of MDD is often noted. An additional psychosocial risk factor in later-onset depression in adolescence is childhood sexual abuse.

In a community sample of adolescents aged 14 to 18 years, onset of MDD was associated with female gender and suicidal ideation. The mean age of onset for the first episode of MDD was 14.9 years. Episodes of MDD were relatively longer in adolescents who had onset before the age of 15 (Lewinsohn et al. 1994).

Major Depressive Disorder in the Older Adult

Older adults with depression often experience cognitive impairment as part of the clinical syndrome. Symptoms of depression may simulate dementia with concentration difficulties, memory loss, and distractibility. Commonly, MDD and dementia co-occur. It is less frequent that findings of dementia are fully explained on the basis of depression (pseudodementia). The prevalence of MDD in older adults residing in nursing homes is estimated to be approximately 30% (Depression Guideline Panel 1993a). MDD in the elderly often co-occurs in the presence of medical conditions, which complicates the treatment for both the depression and the primary medical condition. Careful evaluation of medications may also reveal explanations for associated symptoms of depression. Older adults with first onset of depression must be carefully evaluated for co-occurring medical conditions. Among the common disorders to be considered are silent cerebral ischemic events, undiagnosed cancer, or complications of metabolic conditions such as adult-onset diabetes mellitus and thyroid dysfunction.

Etiology

Depressive disorders are common and recurrent, and associated with substantial psychosocial dysfunction as well as excess morbidity and mortality. Greater understanding of the underlying etiology and pathophysiology of MDD is the focus of genetic, neurobiologic, and psychosocial investigation.

Genetic Theories of Depression
Unipolar or nonbipolar MDD has been demonstrated to cluster in the first-degree relatives of individuals with depression. The observation that MDD is familial, however, does not address the issue whether the familial aggregation may be due to genetic or familial environmental factors. Multiple risk factors for MDD have been reported including gender, early parental loss, parental separation, rearing patterns, trauma and abuse, personality factors, prior major depression, low social class,

and stressful recent life events (Kendler et al. 1993b). While familial aggregation is largely due to genetic factors, the environmental risk factors that are not shared by relatives are clearly important in etiology.

Behavioral genetics involves the search for genetic transmission or mechanisms associated with environmental or cultural transmission of mental disorders. An understanding of the genetic liability to MDD will likely not yield identification of a single dominant gene responsible for this disorder because of substantial clinical heterogeneity, and probable genetic heterogeneity.

Twin studies provide methods for separating genetic and environmental contributions to the aggregation of depressive disorders in families. Several twin studies of MDD ascertained in clinical settings have reported higher concordance rates in monozygotic (MZ) than in dizygotic (DZ) twins, consistent with evidence of genetic liability to depression. A community-based twin study of major depression has confirmed the role of genetic factors in liability to adult depressive symptomatology (Kendler et al. 1992).

Kendler and colleagues (1992) estimated a 33 to 45% genetic liability to depression in women, depending on the criteria used to diagnose MDD. Moreover, a moderate role for individual specific environmental experiences was demonstrated to influence the risk for depression. A subsequent report on the prediction of major depression in women demonstrated an important etiologic role for the combination of genetic factors and specific individual environmental experiences in influencing vulnerability to depression. Given the estimated heritability in MDD, converging evidence supports the important role of environmental experiences in the etiology of major depression (Brown and Harris 1978). Kendler's work emphasizes individual specific life events including recent personal stressors rather than those that are shared by other family members.

Only one of three adoption studies of depression show significant clustering of unipolar disorder in biological relatives of adoptees with major depression, highlighting the significance of both genetic and environmental sources of the liability to depression. In the Danish Adoption Study of unipolar disorder, significantly higher rates of depression were found in the biological relatives of hospitalized adopted probands with depressive disorder compared with the biological relatives of control adoptees. No increased rate of depression was found in the adoptive-relatives of proband versus control adoptees, however, (Wender et al. 1986). The US adoption study demonstrated increased risk of depression in adoptees with a positive family history of depression in biological relatives, but this was short of statistical significance (Cadoret et al. 1990). Kendler and colleagues (1992) call for further research to examine the vulnerability within generations (the focus of twin studies) versus across generations (the focus of adoption studies).

The genetics of depressive temperament, a characterologic trait that may be predisposing to MDD, has not been the focus of empirical investigation. Family studies of clinical depression in childhood and adolescence demonstrate that early-onset depression, including depression in childhood, is more familial and likely to be associated with greater genetic liability (Orvaschel 1990).

All attempts to develop integrated etiologic models of depression have identified multiple psychosocial risk factors. In particular, female gender, limited social support, dependent, self-critical, and neurotic personality traits, and stressful life events appear to influence the vulnerability to MDD. Whether specific life events are as important later in the course of MDD as in the precipitation of initial episodes is the subject of ongoing investigation. Post (1992) argued that negative, stressful life events are associated with the initial or second episode of recurrent MDD whereas neurobiological factors are most relevant with subsequent recurrent episodes. Post asserted that sensitization to stressors and episodes may become encoded at the level of gene expression, underscoring the role of neurobiological factors in the progression of the illness.

Since genetic factors are operative in the etiology of MDD and prior depressive episodes place an individual at risk for future depression, indirect genetic factors operate in the vulnerability to lifetime risk. In summary, clinical and genetic epidemiologic studies suggest that MDD is a multifactorial disorder influenced by several genetic and environmental risk factors. The effectiveness of the individual's social support network in association with successful treatment may protect the individual from the vulnerability to recurrent MDD.

Neurobiological Theories of Depression   Biological mechanisms associated with the clinical syndrome of MDD emerge from animal models of depression and clinical research in humans informed by the contributions of neurochemistry and molecular biology. Animal models of depression in which typical antidepressant pharmacologic treatments reverse depression have substantiated the biological aspects of the depressive syndrome. In these animal models of depression, monkeys separated from their mothers show despair (Harlow and Harlow 1962). Antidepressant medications reverse these syndromes, and neurochemical changes associated with these interventions provide evidence for a direct pharmacologic effect of antidepressant treatment (McKinney 1988).

Nevertheless, the complex interrelation and interdependence of neurochemical systems involving critical neurotransmitters, synaptic regulation, nerve cell mediation and modulation, neuropeptides, and neuroendocrine systems are poorly understood. In the past four decades, explorations of these mechanisms have focused on simpler hypotheses derived from clinical observations of drug effects. The interaction of these multiple systems has been difficult to investigate in the laboratory.

In the early 1950s, the use of reserpine in hypertensive individuals, leading to depression in up to 15% of these individuals, predicted the association of amine depletion and MDD. This amine depletion effect of antihypertensives associated with the initial efficacy of monoamine oxidase inhibitors in depression contributed to the emerging hypothesis that catecholamine deficit was etiologic in major depression (Schildkraut 1965). The pharmacologic bridge asserted that clinical action of antidepressant drugs provided evidence supporting neurochemical hypotheses of MDD. Monoamine oxidase inhibitors (MAOIs) blocked the enzymatic metabolism of norepinephrine, dopamine, and serotonin, furthering evidence of catecholamine activity in MDD. Therapeutic benefits of tricyclic antidepressants (TCAs) and their pharmacologic activity provided further impetus to the biological hypotheses, which currently prevail. The development of selective serotonin reuptake inhibitors (SSRIs) that are effective treatments in MDD lends further support to the serotonergic hypotheses in MDD. The antidepressant–receptor activity reported by Goodwin and Jamison (1990) includes downregulation (decreasing the number) of postsynaptic beta-adrenergic receptors while enhancing response to serotonergic and alpha-adrenergic stimulation.

Neurotransmitters such as norepinephrine (NE), serotonin (5-HT), dopamine (DA), gamma-amino butyric acid (GABA), and acetylcholine (ACh) as well as their metabolites including 3-methoxy-4-hydroxyphenylglycol (MHPG), 5-hydroxy-indoleacetic acid (5-HIAA), dihydroxyphenyl acetic acid (DOPAC), vanillyl mandelic acid (VMA), and homovanillic acid (HVA) have been studied extensively in individuals with MDD, bipolar disorder, and controls. There are no consistent neurochemical findings distinguishing the two clinical syndromes (Goodwin and Jamison 1990). However, certain aspects of the depressive syndrome do appear to be significantly associated with certain neurotransmitter metabolite observations. The principal metabolite of serotonin, 5-HIAA, has been examined in postmortem studies of depressed individuals including suicide victims and deaths unrelated to suicide. Decreased cerebrospinal fluid 5-HIAA is present in those depressed individuals who have committed suicide (Goodwin and Jamison 1990). The data suggest that serotonergic system dysregulation is associated with suicide and associated impulsivity and aggressivity. Studies examining the principal metabolite of norepinephrine and dopamine, MHPG and HVA respectively, do not demonstrate consistent findings in relation to suicide or other clinical subtyping. In addition to cerebrospinal fluid studies, many observations of urinary and plasma levels of catecholamine metabolites have been performed in MDD. These studies do not provide consistent support for a straightforward catecholamine excess/deficit hypothesis of MDD.

Recent studies challenging the simpler paradigm of catecholamine deficit or excess in depression have focused upon neurotransmitter modulation of nerve cell regulation as well as effects of neurotransmitter systems on receptor sensitivity. Additional studies show that individuals with depression as well as those who have died by suicide are reported to have lower levels of the serotonin transporter (SERT) than in control subjects (Owens and Nemeroff 1998). As the pharmacology of the neurotransmitters and receptors is further explicated, receptor changes leading to effects on second messenger systems and the generation of new proteins affecting gene expression will become the focus of the neurobiology of MDD.

Specific abnormalities in sleep and circadian rhythms are among the most consistent findings in biological psychiatry. Clinical observations of insomnia and hypersomnia are commonly noted as a central feature of depressive disorder. Polysomnography (PSG) demonstrates that the progression of sleep from nonrapid eye movement (non-REM) stages 1 to 4 to rapid eye movement (REM) sleep is disrupted in MDD. EEG recordings demonstrate a shorter than normal onset of REM sleep termed *reduced or shortened REM latency*. The frequency of eye movements during REM sleep is greater, termed *increased REM density*. During the sleep laboratory evaluation, increased awakening during sleep leads to the reduction in total sleep time in MDD. Non-REM abnormalities include prolonged sleep latency, increased wakefulness, decreased arousal threshold, and early morning awakening (Kupfer and Thase 1983). Rush and colleagues (1986a) and Giles and colleagues (1989) have suggested that sleep EEG parameters are more trait-like and that some sleep EEG alterations may precede the onset of clinical depression.

Biological rhythm abnormalities include advances in the timing of daily rhythms such as REM sleep, cortisol, and body temperature. Endogenous processes within a day (approximately 25 hours) are *circadian rhythms*. Episodic recurrences of the illness over days, months, or years are called *infradian rhythms* (a period of more than 1 day). *Ultradian rhythms* are oscillations that occur more than once daily and occur at the cellular and neurohormonal level (Goodwin and Jamison 1990). Mechanisms that explain the alterations in oscillation of biological rhythms in depression are not well delineated. Clearly, homeostatic regulation of cellular, biochemical, and psychological phenomenon is necessary to maintain euthymia. The phase advance of a "strong oscillator" leading to depression has been suggested by Wehr and colleagues (1979). Seasonal variation in mood disorders represents the effect of change in light and temperature on the individual's biological vulnerability to depression. Treatments involving light manipulation have begun to address the impact of seasonal change on those individuals vulnerable to depression with seasonal pattern.

The contribution of endocrine system alterations in depression has been examined extensively in biological studies. Both hypothyroidism and hypercortisolism may result in depression.

Hypothalamic–pituitary–thyroid (HPT) axis abnormalities are commonly seen in individuals with bipolar disorder. Thyroid hormone has been used in antidepressant augmentation as well as in modulation of rapid cycling bipolar disorder (Bauer and Whydrow 1990, Goodwin et al. 1982). Neurotransmitters regulate hypothalamic functioning and initiate release of thyrotropin-releasing hormone (TRH) into the portal circulation. TRH is transported to the pituitary gland causing release of thyroid-stimulating hormone (TSH). TSH modulates synthesis and release of T_3 and T_4.

Thyroid studies in depression are not conclusive. There are more reports of slightly increased peripheral T_4 in major depression than a low T_4. Some individuals have mild or "sub-clinical" hypothyroidism as reflected in slight TSH abnormalities and associated antithyroid antibodies. The TRH stimulation test has provided suggestive findings: (1) blunted TSH response to TRH occurs in approximately 30% of depressed individuals, (2) a possible bipolar/unipolar difference has been reported with bipolar depression showing an augmented TSH response, while unipolar depression shows a blunted response (Goodwin and Jamison 1990), and (3) cerebrospinal fluid (CSF) TRH is found to be raised in some individuals with depression, possibly responsible for the blunted response of TSH to TRH, and lower levels of circulating T_3 and T_4. One implication of the suggested bipolar–unipolar distinction is that bipolar depressed individuals may demonstrate a false hypothyroidism, when their TSH response is consistent with the underlying bipolar disorder. Effective treatment of the bipolar disorder may reverse the TSH abnormality.

The hypothalamic–pituitary–adrenal axis (HPA) has been the subject of intensive investigation as well. The observation of elevated cortisol secretion from the adrenal glands has been replicated consistently in individuals with major depression. Corticotropin-releasing factor (CRF) is the hypothalamic hormone that regulates pituitary secretion of corticotropin (ACTH). CRF activity is influenced by multiple neurotransmitters such as 5HT, NE, ACh, and GABA. ACTH binds to cells in the adrenal cortex producing release of glucocorticoids, particularly cortisol. Cortisol inhibits secretion of ACTH at the anterior pituitary and CRF at the hypothalamus. Measurements of 24-hour urinary cortisol, cortisol in the CSF, and cortisol following dexamethasone suppression suggested increased cortisol secretion in MDD. The dexamethasone suppression test (DST) performed by offering dexamethasone at 11 p.m. is followed by serum cortisol at 8 a.m. and 4 p.m.

Psychosocial Theories of Depression The experience of depression elicits negative responses from others, including rejection from spouses, children, and other important individuals. In the social context, the persistence of depression, according to Coyne (1976), is associated with the continuing experience of negative responses from others over time. Behavioral treatments that involve social skills training and self-monitoring of mood attempt to alleviate behavioral consequences of depressive disorder. Lewinsohn (1974) suggested that individuals with depression have social skill deficits that make it difficult to obtain reinforcement from the social environment.

The cognitive or cognitive–behavioral perspective originally developed by Beck (1976) emphasizes a set of dysfunctional attitudes, cognitions, and images associated with depressive symptomatology. The cognitive–behavioral theory is the most empirically examined psychosocial theory in relation to the management and treatment of the depressed individual. In Beck's cognitive theory, cognitive distortions cause depression and are associated with maintenance of the disorder. The "cognitive triad" involves negative views of one's self, one's world and current situation, and the future. The cognitive theory delineates the importance of cognitive distortions, the "cognitive triad," and a conception of negative self-image that is called *negative self-schemas.*

The cognitive perspective is elaborated further by learned helplessness models, and hopelessness theory (Abramson 1989, Seligman 1975). In hopelessness theory, "depressogenic attributional style" leads individuals to regard stressful events as permanent rather than temporary, and affecting most of one's life rather than a specific aspect of one's life. Certain attributional styles lead to personal or internal, rather than global or external, explanations of the depressive disorder. The cognitive perspective as well as contributions from the helplessness–hopelessness models formed an empirical basis for cognitive–behavioral therapy

(CBT), initially developed by Beck and colleagues (1979). In CBT, education, behavioral assignments, and cognitive retraining form the active components of the psychotherapy (Beck et al. 1979). This cognitive therapy has been demonstrated to be an effective short-term psychotherapy for depression (DeRubeis et al. 1990).

Another current therapy called interpersonal therapy derives from a focus on difficulties in current interpersonal functioning. The relationship between psychological health and one's interpersonal environment has received substantial attention since 1940. Adolf Meyer articulated that psychological impairment was a consequence of the difficulty in adapting to the environment. Interpersonal approaches to the treatment of mental disorders are described by Harry Stack Sullivan, and Frieda Fromm-Reichmann as well. These authors highlighted the importance of one's current experience, functioning in social roles, interpersonal relationships, and adaptation to stress and environmental changes (Klerman et al. 1984).

The current iteration of the interpersonal approach is reflected in the development of a specific treatment for depression termed *interpersonal psychotherapy of depression* (IPT). IPT involves a formal diagnostic assessment, inventory of important current and past relationships, and definition of the current problem area. In IPT, four areas of focus that could relate to depressive symptoms are grief, interpersonal role disputes, role transitions, and interpersonal deficits.

An attempt at integration of biological and psychosocial theories of depression has focused on the disruption of biological rhythms associated with psychosocial stressors.

The loss of "social zeitgebers" has been proposed as a link between biological and psychosocial formulations (Ehlers 1988). The social zeitgebers theory suggests that social relationships, interpersonal continuity, and work tasks entrain biological rhythms. Disruptions of social rhythms due to loss of relationships interfere with biological rhythms that maintain homeostasis. This disruption leads to changes in neurobiological processes including alterations in neurotransmitter functions, neuroendocrine regulation, and neurophysiologic control of sleep/wake cycle and other normal circadian oscillations.

Treatment

The goals of treatment in MDD are full remission of symptoms of depression with restoration of optimal work and social functioning. During the course of treatment, ongoing education of the individual and family regarding remission, relapse, and recurrence is critical. This education alerts both those affected by the illness and their families to the early signs of relapse and can assist in prevention of recurrence. Improved social and work functioning following an episode of depression is an important associated goal of treatment. Many studies have demonstrated the benefit of depression-specific psychotherapy as an important aspect of maintaining remission and improving work and social functioning. The establishment of a collaborative working relationship among the individual with depression's, family, and the clinician is an essential aspect of recovery. The data that demonstrate efficacy in psychiatric management and treatment infers that a collaborative relationship is present.

All treatment, whether pharmacotherapy or psychotherapy or the integration of pharmacotherapy and psychotherapy, first requires a well-established diagnostic formulation in order to achieve optimal response to treatment. As the diagnostic process is undertaken, an ongoing therapeutic alliance must be established. In the treatment of MDD, an understanding of the clinical history of each individual's distress is necessary. As the clinical history is elicited, the appropriate target signs and symptoms of MDD are obtained and the individual is educated as to the nature of the symptom patterns that represent his or her unique form of depressive disorder.

The phases of treatment include

1. An acute phase directed at reduction and elimination of depressive signs and symptoms, and active restoration of psychosocial and work functioning.
2. A continuation phase directed at prevention of relapse and reduction of recurrence through ongoing education, pharmacotherapy, and depression-specific psychotherapy.
3. A maintenance phase of treatment directed at prevention of future episodes of depression based upon the individual's personal history of relapse and recurrence.

Acute phase treatment may involve all interventions that are directed toward decreasing signs and symptoms of depression and maintaining the individual's capacity to work and interact with others in a manner consistent with premorbid levels of social and work functioning. The acute phase treatments may include supportive psychotherapy focusing on resolution of current disputes. A form of supportive therapy may be combined with recommendations for pharmacotherapy. The standard pharmacotherapies that are available for treatment of depression have increased dramatically in the past two decades. In mild to moderate depressive disorder, more depression-specific forms of psychotherapy have been established including cognitive–behavioral psychotherapy, interpersonal psychotherapy, or short-term dynamic psychotherapy. In these forms of psychotherapy, which have been studied to address mild to moderate nonbipolar depressive disorder, the focus of the psychotherapy is very clearly explicated to the individual before the initiation of the psychotherapy. For severe depressive disorder with melancholic or psychotic features, these specific forms of short-term psychotherapy may not be as effective as focused pharmacotherapy. Pharmacotherapy, in these conditions, is associated with more rapid treatment response than is psychotherapy. During the acute phase of treatment for depressive disorder, the optimal treatment should result in resolution of depressive signs and symptoms anytime between week 8 and week 16 of treatment. If resolution of depressive signs and symptoms does not occur during the first 2 to 4 months, then the initial diagnostic formulation must be reviewed and alternative treatment strategies must be introduced. Some of the factors associated with lack of complete treatment response include the presence of co-occurring personality disorders, concurrent alcohol or substance abuse, a poor therapeutic alliance leading to lack of adherence to treatment recommendations, and persistent or unfavorable side effects of treatment.

When acute phase treatment does lead to remission of signs and symptoms, then the next phase of treatment begins. This phase of treatment is termed *continuation treatment* and its goal is prevention of relapse. It is often necessary to maintain ongoing pharmacotherapy for 6 to 12 months after an acute episode of depression during this continuation phase, because there is substantial vulnerability to relapse if medication treatment is prematurely interrupted. During the continuation phase, ongoing psychotherapy may be particularly important to address residual symptoms of depression and to alert the individual to a depressive response to subsequent traumatic circumstances; ongoing clinical interaction with significant others is required as well in order to address persisting interpersonal conflicts, and may promote even more complete recovery from the depressive episode. The continuation phase of treatment typically lasts 9 to 12 months to minimize the risk of recurrent episode. If this represents the initial episode of depression, then medication treatment may be carefully withdrawn at the end of the continuation phase. However, if this represents a history of recurrence of depression (particularly two or more episodes in the preceding 3 years), maintenance treatment may well be recommended. In addition, maintenance treatment is recommended if two prior episodes have occurred within one's lifetime.

Maintenance treatment of MDD is focused on prevention of future episodes of depression, after a recent recurrence of MDD and a prior history of two or more episodes of MDD. Often, the maintenance phase of treatment involves ongoing treatment with antidepressants or alternatively mood-stabilizing treatment (particularly lithium carbonate), or a combination to sustain recovery from depression. When there is early onset (adolescent onset) of depressive symptoms with associated psychosocial impairment, then ongoing maintenance treatment along with rehabilitative psychotherapy may be most critical. During maintenance treatment, continuing education of the individual and family, identification of prodromal symptoms, and continuing efforts at work and psychosocial rehabilitation are indicated. Often, the trials of maintenance pharmacotherapy in depression demonstrate the preventive benefit of maintenance medication. In the study quoted most often, recurrence rates of 20 to 25% were found in individuals maintained with full dose of imipramine, while the recurrence rate was 80 to 100% in those individuals treated with placebo. The advantage of ongoing maintenance medicine has also been demonstrated at 5 to 10 years. With tricyclic antidepressants, maintenance medication is likely more effective at full dose rather than lower doses. Limited data exists as to the dosing of SSRIs or other types of antidepressants in maintenance treatment.

The site of treatment for MDD is based upon the severity of the acute episode and the clinician's judgment of the individual's potential for suicide. Individuals with mild to moderate depression are often treated in primary care or specialty office settings. Acute phase pharmacotherapy involving antidepressant medication is often initiated by a primary care physician. However, the overall longitudinal care of MDD in primary care is the subject of increasing attention. Typically, individuals do not receive treatment for long-enough periods and there is limited attention to the domains of social or work functioning. The referral to a psychiatrist may include a request for more expertise regarding medication as well as the need for depression-specific psychotherapy. In addition, there has been a lack of focused attention to the role of integrated psychotherapy and pharmacotherapy in primary care. Inpatient treatment for depression is recommended when there is an immediate risk for suicide or recent suicide attempt. In these settings, safety of the individual is the primary concern and often, more intensive treatments including electroconvulsive therapy may be initiated. When there are comorbid general medical conditions and mental disorders, inpatient psychiatric hospitalization may be useful in stabilizing both the general medical condition as well as the associated mental disorder.

Pharmacotherapy and Other Somatic Treatment

Treatment during the acute phase with medication is highly efficacious in reducing signs and symptoms of MDD. Antidepressant medication has the most specific effect on reduction of symptoms and is often associated with improved psychosocial functioning. When symptoms of depression are mild to moderate, a course of depression-specific psychotherapy without medicine may also be effective. If symptoms of depression are moderate to severe, acute phase treatment with medications is often indicated. A wide variety of antidepressant medications have been documented as effective in moderate to severe MDD.

The range of treatments available in the United States has included the tricyclic antidepressants available since the 1960s, MAOIs available since the late 1950s, heterocyclic antidepressants available since the 1970s, and between 1989 and until the present, newer SSRIs have been available. In addition, antidepressants with both serotonergic and noradrenergic activity or noradrenergic activity alone have become available in the 1990s. Clearly, clinical trials comparing the efficacy of newer treatments with standard tricyclic antidepressants have shown equal efficacy with improvement in overall tolerance to side effects with newer treatments.

Antidepressant medications that are currently available for acute treatment of MDD are listed in the associated table (Table 28-2).

Table 28-2   **Antidepressant Medications Category**

Category			Side Effects			
Trade Name	Compound	Usual Therapeutic Dose (mg)	Sedation	Hypotension (Decreased Blood Pressure)	Anticholinergic (i.e., Dry Mouth Constipation)	Cardiac (Slowed Heart Rate)
Tricyclics						
Tertiary Amines						
Anafranil	Clomipramine	150–300	High	High	High	Yes
Elavil	Amitriptyline	150–300	High	High	High	Yes
Sinequan	Doxepin	150–300	High	Moderate	Moderate	Yes
Surmontil	Trimipramine	150–300	High	Moderate	Moderate	Yes
Tofranil	Imipramine	150–300	Moderate	High	Moderate	Yes
Norpramine	Desipramine	100–300	Low	High	Low	Yes
Pamelor	Nortriptyline	50–150	Moderate	Low	Low	Yes
Vivactil	Protriptyline	20–60	Low	Low	High	Yes
Monoamine Oxidase Inhibitors						
Marplan	Isocarboxazid	30–60	Low	Moderate	Low	Low
Nardil	Phenelzine	45–90	Low	Moderate	Low	Low
Parnate	Tranylcypromine	30–90	Low	Moderate	Low	Low
Atypical Agents						
Ascendin	Amoxapine	200–300	Low	Moderate	Low	Yes
Desyrel	Trazodone	300–600	High	High	Minimal	Low
Ludiomil	Maprotiline	150–200	Moderate	Moderate	Low	Low
Wellbutrin	Bupropion	150–450	Minimal	Low	Minimal	Yes
Selective Serotonin Reuptake Inhibitors						
Paxil	Paroxetine	20–50	Low	Minimal	Minimal	Low
Prozac	Fluoxetine	20–100	Minimal	Minimal	Minimal	Low
Zoloft	Sertraline	50–300	Minimal	Minimal	Minimal	Low
Luvox	Fluvoxamine	150–400	Low	Low	Low	Low
Celexa	Citalopram	20–50	Minimal	None	None	Minimal
Lexapro	Escitalopram	10–30	Minimal	None	None	Minimal
Serotonin/Norepinephrine Reuptake Inhibitors						
Effexor	Venlafaxine	75–450	Low	None	None	Minimal
Serotonin Transport Blocker and Antagonist						
Serzone	Nefazodone	200–600	Minimal	Low	Minimal	Minimal
Alpha-2-Adrenergic Antagonist						
Remeron	Mirtazapine	30–60	Moderate	Low	Minimal	Minimal

Choice of treatment with a specific antidepressant treatment in a given clinical situation is based on prior treatment response to medication, consideration of potential side effects, history of response in first-degree relatives to medicines, and the associated presence of co-occurring mental disorders that may lead to a more specific choice of antidepressant treatment. Table 28-3 illustrates an algorithm developed for pharmacotherapy of MDD, which includes a staged trial of newer medications (because of their superior side-effect profiles) followed by treatments with older medicines available for the treatment of MDD. The ultimate goal of pharmacotherapy is complete remission of symptoms during a standard 6- to 12-week course of treatment.

Table 28-3	Pharmacotherapy Algorithm in Major Depressive Disorder

Major Depressive Disorder, Single or Recurrent Episode, without Psychotic Features

Begin effective monotherapy with bupropion SR, citalopram, escitalopram, fluoxetine, nefazodone, paroxetine, sertraline, venlafaxine XR, or duloxetine (augment with lithium carbonate 600–900 mg).

or

Begin effective monotherapy with alternative antidepressant from list above (augment with bupropion SR, mirtazapine, or tricyclic antidepressant, either nortriptyline or desipramine, recognizing important drug interactions.

If ineffective, consider tranylcypromine, augmented with lithium carbonate, if necessary, for anergic features.

or

Consider phenelzine, augmented with lithium carbonate, if necessary, for anxious, dependent, and phobic features.

Augment with atypical antipsychotics for agitation, rumination, or suspicion.

or

Offer electroconvulsive therapy to remission (ECT).

Major Depressive Disorder, Single or Recurrent Episode, with Psychotic Features

Begin typical or atypical antipsychotic to adequate doses in order to interrupt delusional features, augmented with SSRI, venlafaxine XR, or tricyclic antidepressants, either nortriptyline or desipramine, recognizing important drug interactions.

or

Begin amoxapine as alternative.

or

Begin electroconvulsive therapy as alternative, in context of immediate suicide risk, physical deterioration, or prior response to electroconvulsive therapy

Major Depressive Disorder with Atypical Features

Begin SSRI starting at low dose to minimize early side effects.

or

Begin MAOI, either phenelzine or tranylcypromine, to therapeutic doses

Major Depressive Disorder with Catatonic Features

Begin lorazepam 1–3 mg/d, to interrupt catatonic symptoms; evaluate for presence of psychotic features or longitudinal history of bipolar disorder.

Add antipsychotic medication to therapeutic doses or lithium carbonate to therapeutic doses, if bipolar or schizoaffective disorder emerges from the longitudinal history.

Selective Serotonin Reuptake Inhibitors   The most commonly prescribed antidepressant medicines in the past 10 years are SSRIs. They are selectively active at serotonergic-neurochemical pathways and are effective in mild to moderate nonbipolar depression. They may also be particularly effective in MDD with atypical features as well as DD. Often, these treatments are well tolerated and involve single daily dosing for MDD. Because of selective serotonergic activity, these treatments have also been demonstrated to be effective with co-occurring OCD, panic disorder, generalized anxiety disorder, PTSD, premenstrual dysphoric disorder, bulimia nervosa, and social anxiety disorder as well as MDD. They tend to be reasonably well tolerated in individuals with comorbid medical conditions. There are particular medication-specific interactions based on inhibition of cytochrome P-450 liver enzyme systems that require attention if an individual is taking other medications for primary medical conditions or associated mental disorders. The currently available SSRIs in the United States include fluoxetine (Prozac), paroxetine (Paxil), sertraline (Zoloft), fluvoxamine (Luvox), citalopram (Celexa), and escitalopram (Lexapro).

Other Newer Antidepressants   In addition to SSRIs, greater attention has been brought to medicines with dual noradrenergic and serotonergic pathways including venlafaxine (Effexor XR) and duloxetine (Cymbalta). In addition, an alpha-2-adrenergic agonist, mirtazapine (Remeron) has become available as well as a serotonin transport blocker and antagonist nefazodone (Serzone). Recent concerns about hepatic complications associated with nefazodone have required liver function monitoring. A predominantly noradrenergic and dopaminergic agonist, bupropion (Wellbutrin), is also available in an immediate release and sustained release (SR) preparation.

Tricylic Antidepressants Tricyclic antidepressants have been best studied in individuals with MDD with melancholic features and with psychotic features. The combination of typical antipsychotic pharmacotherapy in association with tricyclic antidepressants has been recommended. The side-effect profile of tricyclic antidepressants has included moderate to severe sedation, anticholinergic effects including constipation and cardiac effects that has made these medicines less popular in typical primary care or psychiatric practice. Nevertheless, the secondary amines that are metabolites of imipramine and amitriptyline, specifically desipramine and nortriptyline, have continued to be useful agents in more refractory depression.

Monoamine Oxidase Inhibitors There continues to be a role for the use of MAOIs in individuals with MDD with atypical features. These agents may be particularly useful in intervention in depressive episodes with atypical features, characterized by prominent mood reactivity, reverse neurovegetative symptom patterns (i.e., overeating and oversleeping), and marked interpersonal rejection sensitivity. MAOIs continue to have a significant role in treatment of comorbid panic disorder, social phobia, and agoraphobia if individuals are not responsive to SSRIs. The ongoing prescription of phenelzine (Nardil) or tranylcypromine (Parnate) requires continued education of the individual regarding standard food interactions involving tyramine as well as specific drug–drug interactions involving sympathomimetic medications. These cautions regarding diet and drug interaction make MAO inhibitors less attractive to primary care physicians and most psychiatrists. However, they continue to be effective treatments that may be useful in depression with atypical features as well as anergic bipolar depression.

General Recommendations Increasingly, a trial of one class of antidepressants may be associated with incomplete response leading to a question of augmenting a treatment with another medicine versus switching from one medicine to another within the same class or to a different class altogether. Augmentation strategies with other medications, including adding lithium carbonate and other antidepressants, particularly those with a different mechanism of action, atypical antipsychotics, thyroid and stimulants, have been the focus of a number of reviews of treatment resistance (Thase and Rush 1995). A staging system for treatment-resistant depression (TRD) has been proposed and ranges from failure to respond to a single agent (Stage 1) to failure of multiple treatments and electroconvulsive therapy (Stage 5) as shown in Table 28-4.

All of the antidepressant medications used in the treatment of MDD must be prescribed in the context of an overall clinical relationship characterized by supportive interaction with the individual and family and ongoing education about the nature of the disorder and its treatment. Clinical management optimally involves careful monitoring of symptoms using standardized instruments and careful attention to side effects of medication in order to promote treatment adherence. Outpatient visits, which may be scheduled weekly at the outset of treatment, and subsequently biweekly encouragement and sustain collaborative treatment relationships. These office consultations allow the clinician to make dosage adjustments as indicated, monitor side effects, and measure clinical response to treatment.

For the majority of individuals with MDD, a course of 6 to 8 weeks of acute treatment with weekly outpatient visits is indicated. Subsequent office visits may be scheduled every

Table 28-4	Staging Criteria for Treatment-Resistant Depression
Stage	**Description**
1.	Failure of at least one adequate trial of an antidepressant
2.	Stage 1 resistance plus failure of adequate trial of an antidepressant from a distinctly different class than in Stage 1
3.	Stage 2 resistance plus failure of an adequate trial of a tricyclic antidepressant (TCA)
4.	Stage 3 resistance plus failure of an adequate trial of a monoamine oxidase inhibitor (MAOI)
5.	Stage 4 resistance plus failure of a course of bilateral electroconvulsive therapy (ECT).

2 to 4 weeks during the continuation phase of treatment. Appropriate adjustments of dose are determined by the psychiatrist as indicated by best clinical judgments of medication effect. Optimal dosing ranges of SSRIs, tricyclics, and MAOIs are noted in Table 28-2. Because of the early anxiety, agitation, and occasional insomnia associated with SSRIs, somewhat lower doses may be initiated early in the course before achieving the typical standard therapeutic dose.

Incomplete response, which entails the failure to respond to acute treatment with an antidepressant medication at 6 to 8 weeks, requires reassessment of diagnosis and determination of adequacy of dosing. Ongoing substance abuse, associated general medical condition, or concurrent mental disorder may partially explain a lack of complete response. If substance dependence is present, a full substance-free interval (preferably 4 weeks or longer) with appropriate detoxification and rehabilitation may be indicated. If a reassessment discloses an associated mental disorder, then more specific treatment of that associated disorder, whether it be bipolar disorder or concurrent posttraumatic disorder, is necessary. If the reassessment suggests an associated comorbid personality disorder, then appropriate and more specialized psychotherapy may be necessary in order to achieve a complete response to treatment. As indicated before, if the MDD has psychotic features, then antipsychotic pharmacotherapy to adequate doses must be initiated prior to initiating a course of standard tricyclic antidepressants or a combined serotonin norepinephrine uptake inhibitor such as venlafaxine (Effexor). If MDD is associated with severe personality disorder (e.g., borderline personality disorder), then adjunctive psychotherapy and low dose antipsychotic medications may be necessary. If the individual has severe melancholic, delusional, or catatonic features, a course of electroconvulsive therapy may be necessary to achieve remission of symptoms.

There is also evidence that continuation of treatment beyond 6 to 12 weeks may convert some partial responders to responders if drug treatment is increased to full doses. This time allows for evaluation of the role of focused psychotherapy to address residual interpersonal disputes, loss or grief, or ongoing social deficits. The associated augmentation strategies to standard treatments include lithium carbonate augmentation, tricyclic antidepressant augmentation of SSRIs, thyroid hormone augmentation, and bupropion augmentation of SSRIs.

Electroconvulsive Therapy   Electroconvulsive therapy (ECT) remains an effective treatment in individuals with severe MDD and those individuals with psychotic MDD. Many individuals who have responded to electroconvulsive therapy do not respond to pharmacotherapy. There is increased need for understanding the role of maintenance electroconvulsive therapy in those individuals who respond to electroconvulsive therapy because ongoing pharmacotherapy does not always prevent recurrence of depression after ECT is successful. ECT can be particularly useful in interrupting acute suicidality for those individuals who may require rapid resolution of symptoms. ECT may be indicated in older adults when lack of self-care and weight loss may represent a greater risk. The most common side effect associated with electroconvulsive therapy is amnesia for the period of treatment. There is no consistent evidence to suggest chronic cognitive or memory impairment as a result of ECT.

Other Somatic Treatments Light therapy investigators have continued to demonstrate benefit in individuals with seasonal MDD by providing greater than 2500 lux light therapy for 1 to 2 hours/day. Many of these individuals experience recurrent winter depression in the context of a recurrent MDD or bipolar II disorder. Bright light exposure has been associated with favorable response within 4 to 7 days. As with electroconvulsive therapy, light therapy is best prescribed by specialists who have experience in its use and can appropriately evaluate the indication for light therapy and monitor carefully the response to treatment.

Ongoing investigation of alternative brain stimulation techniques have been the subject of recent investigation. The use of a powerful magnet to provide transcranial magnetic stimulation has been the subject of several open trials. It is not yet determined whether the repetitive transcranial magnetic stimulation demonstrates its effectiveness through reduction of inhibitory neurotransmission or other mechanisms (George et al. 1999).

In addition, open clinical trials of vagus nerve stimulation (VNS), which has been found to be effective in epilepsy, has been the subject of attention in refractory MDD. Several sites of investigation have begun to reveal positive effects at 9 months using VNS implantation (Rush et al. 2000). This procedure requires the implantation of a stimulating device in the chest with the capacity to stimulate the vagus nerve at regular intervals through the course of the day.

Psychosocial Treatment

The past decade has also led to the development of more specific depression-based treatment for MDD. These treatments have included supportive psychiatric management techniques during pharmacotherapy, interpersonal psychotherapy, cognitive–behavioral therapy, brief dynamic psychotherapy, and marital and family therapy.

Clinical management and supportive psychotherapy is the standard in office practice. The clinician focuses on establishing a positive therapeutic relationship in the course of diagnosis and initiation of treatment of depression. The clinician is attentive to all signs and symptoms of the disorder, particularly suicidality. The clinician provides ongoing education, collaboration with the individual, and supportive feedback to the individual regarding ongoing response and prognosis. The supportive psychotherapeutic management of depression facilitates the ongoing pharmacologic response. Brief supportive psychotherapy in individuals with mild to moderate depression is indicated to improve medication compliance, to facilitate reduction of active depressive signs and symptoms, and to provide education regarding relapse and recurrence.

Interpersonal Psychotherapy Interpersonal psychotherapy in nonhospitalized individuals with nonbipolar MDD has been demonstrated to be effective in acute treatment trials. Interpersonal psychotherapy of depression addresses four areas of current interpersonal difficulties: 1) interpersonal loss or grieving; 2) role transitions; 3) interpersonal disputes; and 4) social deficits. This type of treatment, like other psychotherapies for depression, also involves education about the nature of MDD and the relationship between symptoms of depressive disorder and current interpersonal difficulties.

Prior studies demonstrated efficacy of interpersonal psychotherapy for outpatients with depression. Interpersonal psychotherapy, cognitive–behavioral psychotherapy, and medication treatment were comparable on several outcome measures and superior to placebo. (Elkin et al. 1989, Hollon et al. 1992). Medication treatment was associated with the most rapid response and was superior to both interpersonal psychotherapy and cognitive–behavioral therapy in more severely depressed individuals. Continuation studies with interpersonal psychotherapy (Thase et al. 1997) offered monthly as well as during maintenance treatment have demonstrated response in prevention of recurrence, and was superior to placebo treatment. Those individuals who received ongoing interpersonal psychotherapy and medication had the longest intervals without recurrence of depressive symptoms.

Cognitive-Behavioral Therapy   Cognitive–behavioral therapy for depression is a form of treatment aimed at symptom reduction through the identification and correction of cognitive distortions. These involve negative views of the self, one's current world, and the future. Several controlled studies have demonstrated the efficacy of cognitive therapy in resolution of MDD in adults (Depression Guideline Panel 1993b). Cognitive–behavioral therapy as well as interpersonal psychotherapy was somewhat less effective than medication treatment in moderate to severe MDD. However, other investigators (Hollon et al. 1992) have suggested a relatively equal response to cognitive–behavioral therapy and medication in more severely depressed outpatients.

Brief Dynamic Psychotherapy   Brief dynamic psychotherapy addresses current conflicts as manifestations of difficulty in early attachment and disruption of early object relationships. Brief dynamic psychotherapy was not specifically designed for treatment of MDD and is currently the subject of ongoing studies as well as controlled clinical trials in comparison with medication treatment. The results of these trials will allow us to address the appropriate role of brief dynamic psychotherapy in outpatients with mild to moderate depression. In addition, it will be important to understand whether dynamic psychotherapy may address demoralization or response to traumatic circumstances.

Martial and Family Therapy   It has been difficult to assess the specific efficacy of marital or family therapy in individuals with MDD based on current studies to date. There is substantial evidence that marital distress is a major event associated with the development of a depressive episode. Marital discord often will persist after the remission of depression and subsequent relapses are frequently associated with disruptions of marital relationships. There has been a single study (O'Leary and Beach 1990) focusing on efficacy of behaviorally oriented marital therapy in reducing symptoms of depression. There has been no controlled clinical trial of marital therapy in relation to other treatments for promoting the resolution of depressive signs and symptoms. Both acute and continuation phase treatment of MDD will require ongoing attention to marital and family issues to prevent recurrence of depression.

Factors Influencing Treatment Response

There are a number of factors that influence ultimate treatment response in MDD including individual characteristics, diagnostic issues, comorbidity, treatment-related complications including side effects, and demographic factors. Reevaluation of diagnosis, comorbidity, and the clinician–patient relationship itself is often critical.

Suicide Risk   individuals with MDD are often at increased risk for suicide. Suicidal risk assessment is especially indicated as individuals begin to recover from depression with increased energy and simultaneous continued despair. Persistent suicidal ideation coupled with increased energy can often lead to impulsive suicidal acts. The careful attention to the clinician–patient relationship can mediate suicidal urges through availability and accessibility. Outpatients and inpatients with MDD and melancholic features will often require antidepressant therapy addressing multiple neurotransmitter systems, or ECT as well.

Psychotic Features MDD with psychotic features requires careful assessment to rule out comorbid mental disorders. The combined treatment with antipsychotic as well as antidepressant medication is indicated. In addition, electroconvulsive therapy is an effective intervention in psychotic depression and may be considered as a first-line alternative.

Catatonic Features MDD with catatonic features can be associated with significant morbidity owing to the individual's refusal to eat or drink. Active treatment with a benzodiazepine such as lorazepam 1 to 3 mg daily may offer short-term treatment response. Subsequent treatment with lithium alone or in association with antidepressants may be indicated given the possible link between catatonic features and bipolar vulnerability (Hawkins et al. 1995). If psychosis is associated with catatonia, then atypical antipsychotic medication or a course of electroconvulsive therapy may be indicated as well (Bush et al. 1996).

Atypical Features Atypical features are associated with significant comorbid anxiety disorders, reverse neurovegetative symptoms such as hypersomnia, increased appetite and weight gain as well as fatigue and leaden paralysis. SSRIs are likely to be effective in individuals with MDD with atypical features as well as MAOIs. Conversely, tricyclic antidepressants, in particular, are unlikely to be effective in such individuals.

Severity Individuals with mild to moderate depression may be effectively treated with psychotherapy, pharmacotherapy, or the combination. Individuals with severe MDD almost always require somatic intervention with antidepressant medication or electroconvulsive therapy.

Recurrence Because MDD is a recurrent disorder, current treatment guidelines (Hirschfeld 1994) suggest maintenance antidepressant treatment at full therapeutic doses if there is a history of more than two prior episodes of MDD.

History of Hypomania or Mania Any of the antidepressant treatments including medication, electroconvulsive therapy, light therapy, or newer somatic interventions may induce hypomania or mania in individuals who are vulnerable to bipolar disorder. Individuals who may have a family history of bipolar disorder should be carefully evaluated for treatment with lithium carbonate or other anticonvulsant mood stabilizers before antidepressant treatment because they are at particular risk for antidepressant-induced mania. Attention to this history of prior hypomania or mania as well as family history may promote treatment response if such individuals have mood-stabilizing treatment offered initially.

Comorbidity with Alcohol or Substance Dependence The comorbidity of MDD and alcohol or other substance dependence requires careful attention to both diagnoses. The first priority in treatment is abstinence from alcohol or substance use. Co-occurring addiction will complicate depressive disorders and increases risk for suicide. If detoxification from alcohol or other substance abuse is required, this should be undertaken before initiation of any somatic antidepressant therapy. Individuals who have a family history of depression or bipolar disorder are likely to require early initiation of appropriate mood disorder treatment following detoxification.

Comorbidity with Obsessive-Compulsive Disorder In individuals with OCD, lifetime risk of MDD approaches 70%. The use of higher dose SSRI treatment is often indicated to treat both conditions. Alternatively, the tricyclic antidepressant, clomipramine

(Anafranil), may be effective for those individuals with both OCD and MDD who do not respond to SSRIs.

Comoribidty with Panic Disorder Lifetime risk of MDD approaches 50% in individuals with panic disorder. Because many of the SSRI and other antidepressants are effective treatments to treat panic as well as depression, these treatments have gained increasing popularity. One may continue to prescribe short-term courses of benzodiazepines, including lorazepam or clonazepam to alleviate acute symptoms of panic as low doses of antidepressant treatments are introduced into the treatment for comorbid panic and MDD. In addition, MAOIs continue to be effective treatments for both panic and MDD.

Refractory Major Depressive Disorder

A staging system for TRD has been proposed and ranges from failure to respond to a single agent (Stage 1) to failure of multiple treatments and electroconvulsive therapy (Stage 5; Thase and Rush 1995), and is presented in Table 28-4. The term refractory depression has been proposed to describe individuals who have Stage 5 treatment-resistant depression (Thase and Rush 1995).

Refractory MDD or Stage 5 in this table is estimated to occur in up to 20% of individuals (Thase and Howland 1994). A larger percentage of individuals with MDD, up to 30%, may show only partial improvement. The concept of treatment-resistant depression or refractory depression describes this lack of response to a number of clinical trials using optimal dosing and duration of antidepressant medication. One must typically offer the individual a rational series of treatment trials using optimal dosing and duration of each antidepressant. An individual is considered refractory if a course of three, four, or five treatments is offered without substantial clinical response. The standard approach to the management of refractory depression includes increasing the antidepressant dose and monitoring for a full 8- to 12-week course augmenting the treatment with several augmentation strategies using an adequate combination of antidepressant drug treatment and psychotherapy and switching to alternative somatic treatments including ECT when indicated.

Refractory MDD is ameliorated in the context of a caring and collaborative treatment relationship based on a favorable therapeutic alliance. Sometimes, individuals will undermine treatment through their own persistent use of substances such as alcohol or lack of adherence to specific pharmacotherapy recommendations. In this context, the attention to the therapeutic alliance is particularly critical. In assessing an individual with refractory symptoms, pharmacologic factors including pharmacokinetic considerations, drug–drug interactions, and extreme sensitivity to antidepressant drugs must be considered.

Despite many alternative strategies, substantial morbidity and occasional mortality are associated with refractory MDD. In addition, careful attention to psychosocial factors associated with refractoriness is critical. These psychosocial factors include early childhood adversity and abuse, early family dysfunction, increased neuroticism, and marked disruption in the development of a stable sense of self.

DYSTHYMIC DISORDER

Diagnosis

Dysthymic disorder is defined by the presence of chronic depressive symptoms most of the day, more days than not, for at least 2 years (see DSM-IV-TR diagnostic criteria for Dysthymic Disorder on page 773). While chronic depressive conditions were traditionally conceptualized as characterological and amenable to psychotherapy and resistant to pharmacotherapy, recent pharmacologic trials of antidepressants as well as depression-specific psychotherapy have demonstrated effectiveness in the overall treatment of DD. Both focused interpersonal and variations of cognitive–behavioral psychotherapy have demonstrated response in dysthymia. Individuals with DD have a substantial risk for the development of MDD. This highlights the importance of early assessment and treatment to minimize subsequent long-term complications.

DSM-IV-TR Diagnostic Criteria

300.4 Dysthymic Disorder

A. Depressed mood for most of the day, for more days than not, as indicated either by subjective account or by observation by others, for at least 2 years.

Note: In children and adolescents, mood can be irritable and duration must be at least 1 year.

B. Presence, while depressed, of two (or more) of the following:

   (1) poor appetite or overeating
   (2) insomnia or hypersomnia
   (3) low energy or fatigue
   (4) low self-esteem
   (5) poor concentration or difficulty making decisions
   (6) feelings of hopelessness

C. During the 2-year period (1 year for children or adolescents) of the disturbance, the person has never been without the symptoms in Criteria A and B for more than 2 months at a time.

D. No major depressive episode has been present during the first 2 years of the disturbance (1 year for children and adolescents); i.e., the disturbance is not better accounted for by chronic major depressive disorder or major depressive disorder, in partial remission.

Note: There may have been a previous major depressive episode provided there was a full remission (no significant signs or symptoms for 2 months) before development of the dysthymic disorder. In addition, after the initial 2 years (1 year in children or adolescents) of dysthymic disorder, there may be superimposed episodes of major depressive disorder, in which case both diagnoses may be given when the criteria are met for a major depressive episode.

E. There has never been a manic episode, a mixed episode, or a hypomanic episode, and criteria have never been met for cyclothymic disorder.

F. The disturbance does not occur exclusively during the course of a chronic psychotic disorder, such as schizophrenia or delusional disorder.

G. The symptoms are not due to the direct physiological effects of a substance (e.g., a drug of abuse, a medication) or a general medical condition (e.g., hypothyroidism).

H. The symptoms cause clinically significant distress or impairment in social, occupational, or other important areas of functioning.

Specify if:

Early onset: if onset is before age 21 years

Late onset: if onset is age 21 years or older *Specify* (for most recent 2 years of dysthymic disorder):

With atypical features

If signs and symptoms of DD follow an MDD, then a diagnosis of MDD, in partial remission, is made. A diagnosis of DD can be made if the individual develops full remission of MDD for 6 months and subsequently develops signs and symptoms of DD, which then last a minimum of 2 years. In contrast, the diagnosis of chronic MDD is made when an episode of MDD meets full criteria for MDD continuously for at least 2 years. If DD has been present for at least 2 years in adults (or 1 year in children and adolescents) and is subsequently followed by a superimposed MDD, then both DD and MDD are diagnosed, which is often referred to as "double depression." The following specifiers apply to DD as noted in DSM-IV-TR: *Early onset*—if the onset of dysthymic symptoms occurs before age 21; and *Late onset*—if the onset of dysthymic symptoms occurs at age 21 or older, and with atypical features.

Atypical features refer to a pattern of symptoms that include mood reactivity and two of the additional atypical symptoms (i.e., weight gain or increased appetite, hypersomnia, leaden paralysis, or interpersonal rejection sensitivity). Early-onset DD is usually associated with subsequent episodes of MDD. DD with atypical features may herald a bipolar I or II course.

The diagnosis of DD cannot be made if depressive symptoms occur during the course of a nonaffective psychosis such as schizophrenia, schizoaffective disorder, or delusional disorder. Diagnosis of depressive disorder NOS is made if there are symptoms that meet criteria for MDD during the residual phase of a psychotic disorder. If DD is determined to be etiologically related to a chronic medical condition, then one diagnoses mood disorder due to the general medical condition. If substance use is judged to be the etiologic factor, then a substance-induced mood disorder is diagnosed. Individuals with DD often have co-occurring personality disorders and in these situations, separate diagnoses on Axis I and II are made.

Ongoing studies have not completely clarified the distinction between DD and depressive personality disorder. Depressive temperaments may predispose an individual to a condition within the spectrum of Axis I mood disorders. However, it may not be specifically associated with MDD. This depressive temperament may also be associated with vulnerability to bipolar disorder.

Individuals with early-onset DD are at substantial risk for development of other mental disorders including alcohol or substance dependence, MDD, and personality disorders. Up to 15% of individuals with DD may also have a substance use pattern that meets criteria for comorbid alcohol or substance dependence diagnosis. The most common associated personality disorders include mixed, dependent, and borderline personality (Marin et al. 1993). Childhood and adolescent-onset DD is associated with a substantial risk for later occurrence of both MDD and bipolar disorder.

Epidemiology

A lifetime prevalence of 4.1% for women and 2.2% for men was reported for DD (Weissman et al. 1988a). In adults, DD is more common in women than in men. In children, DD occurs equally in both sexes. Across both women and men, DD has a 2.5% 12-month prevalence (Kessler et al. 1994).

Course

Dysthymic disorder often begins in late childhood or early adolescence and by definition takes a chronic course. The risk for development of MDD among children who have DD is significant because childhood onset of DD is an early marker for recurrent mood disorder, both recurrent MDD and bipolar disorder.

The course of DD suggests impairment in functional status including social and occupational and physical functioning. Individuals who have both DD and MDD have more severe functional impairment. Untreated DD contributes to significant occupational and financial burden. There is substantial reduction in activity, more days spent in bed, more complaints of poor general medical health, and more disability days than reported in the general population.

Etiology

Sleep abnormalities demonstrate reduced REM latency, increased REM density, reduced slow wave sleep, and impaired sleep continuity in 25 to 50% of individuals with DD. There are minimal data on cortisol or thyroid abnormalities in individuals with DD. Other neurobiological studies have not yielded consistent results.

Treatment

The treatment goals in DD are similar to those in MDD. They include full remission of symptoms and full psychosocial recovery. Many individuals who have been enrolled in clinical trials for MDD have an associated history of DD. Recent randomized controlled trials of pharmacotherapy (Keller et al. 2000) and cognitive–behavior therapy suggest a favorable response to active treatments. The most favorable response occurred in those individuals treated with both active medication and specific cognitive–behavioral treatments.

DEPRESSIVE DISORDER NOT OTHERWISE SPECIFIED

Depressive disorder NOS (DDNOS) refers to a variety of conditions listed in DSM-IV-TR that are distinguished from MDD, DD, adjustment disorder with depressed mood, or adjustment disorder with mixed anxiety and depressed mood. These conditions involve a large number of depressed individuals who do not meet formal criteria for MDD or DD. In the ECA study, 11% of subjects had DDNOS. In a primary care outpatient sample, the prevalence of DDNOS was 8.4 to 9.7%. DDNOS is associated with impairment in overall functioning and general health (Wells et al. 1989). Among the conditions listed as occurring within this category are premenstrual dysphoric disorder, minor depressive disorder, recurrent brief depressive disorder, postpsychotic depressive disorder of schizophrenia, and depressive episode superimposed on delusional disorder or other psychotic disorder.

PREMENSTRUAL DYSPHORIC DISORDER

Premenstrual dysphoric disorder (PMDD) is characterized by depressed mood, marked anxiety, affective lability, and decreased interest in activities, experienced during the last week of the luteal phase that remits during the follicular phase of the menstrual cycle. This pattern occurs for most months of the year. The severity of symptoms is comparable to MDD, but the duration is briefer by definition. The symptoms disappear with the onset of menses. Current criteria emphasize the disturbance in mood as well as impairment in social functioning associated with PMDD. Current assessments require that the typical cyclical patterns be confirmed by at least 2 months of prospective daily ratings. PMDD often worsens with increasing age, but then diminishes at menopause. PMDD appears to respond to standard SSRI treatments including fluoxetine (Prozac) as well as sertraline (Zoloft) but may not respond to other types of antidepressants, such as bupropion. This responsiveness to SSRIs suggests a premenstrual, serotonergic hypoactivity that may account for the premenstrual dysphoric symptomatology (Eriksson et al. 2002). For a more detailed discussion of PMDD, see the next chapter (Chapter 29).

MINOR DEPRESSIVE DISORDER

Minor depressive disorder is characterized by episodes lasting 2 weeks and characterized by at least two, but fewer than five, depressive symptoms (see DSM-IV-TR research criteria below). Minor depressive disorder is also associated with less psychosocial impairment than MDD. The prevalence of minor depressive disorder reported in primary care settings ranges from 3.4 to 4.7%. A number of general medical conditions have been associated with minor depressive disorder including stroke, cancer, and diabetes. Maier and colleagues (1992) report increased symptoms of minor depressive disorder in families in which a proband with MDD is present. In the differential diagnosis of minor depressive disorder, one must consider adjustment disorder with depressed mood and other experiences of sadness that may be part of grieving. Because of frequent co-occurrence with general medical condition, one must rule out a secondary mood disorder due to a general medical condition.

DSM-IV-TR Research Criteria

Minor Depressive Disorder

A. A mood disturbance, defined as follows:

(1) at least two (but less than five) of the following symptoms have been present during the same 2-week period and represent a change from previous functioning; at least one of the symptoms is either (a) or (b):

(a) depressed mood most of the day, nearly every day, as indicated by either subjective report (e.g., feels sad or empty) or observation made by others (e.g., appears tearful).

Note: In children and adolescents, can be irritable mood.

(b) markedly diminished interest or pleasure in all, or almost all, activities most of the day, nearly every day (as indicated by either subjective account or observation made by others)

(c) significant weight loss when not dieting or weight gain (e.g., a change of more than 5% of body weight in a month), or decrease or increase in appetite nearly every day.

Note: In children, consider failure to make expected weight gains.

(d) insomnia or hypersomnia nearly every day

    (e) psychomotor agitation or retardation nearly every day (observable by others, not merely subjective feelings of restlessness or being slowed down)

    (f) fatigue or loss of energy nearly every day

    (g) feelings of worthlessness or excessive or inappropriate guilt (which may be delusional) nearly every day (not merely self-reproach or guilt about being sick)

    (h) diminished ability to think or concentrate, or indecisiveness, nearly every day (either by subjective account or as observed by others)

    (i) recurrent thoughts of death (not just fear of dying), recurrent suicidal ideation without a specific plan, or a suicide attempt or a specific plan for committing suicide

(2) the symptoms cause clinically significant distress or impairment in social, occupational, or other important areas of functioning

(3) the symptoms are not due to the direct physiological effects of a substance (e.g., a drug of abuse, a medication) or a general medical condition (e.g., hypothyroidism)

(4) the symptoms are not better accounted for by Bereavement (i.e., a normal reaction to the death of a loved one)

B. There has never been a Major Depressive Episode (See linked section), and criteria are not met for Dysthymic Disorder.

C. There has never been a Manic Episode (See linked section), a Mixed Episode (See linked section), or a Hypomanic Episode (See linked section), and criteria are not met for Cyclothymic Disorder.

Note: This exclusion does not apply if all of the manic-, mixed-, or hypomanic-like episodes are substance or treatment induced.

D. The mood disturbance does not occur exclusively during Schizophrenia, Schizophreniform Disorder, Schizoaffective Disorder, Delusional Disorder, or Psychotic Disorder Not Otherwise Specified.

Reprinted with permission from the Diagnostic and Statistical Manual of Mental Disorders, Fourth Edition, Text Revision. Copyright 2000 American Psychiatric Association.

Minor depressive disorder tends to begin in late adolescence and probably affects men and women equally. Minor depressive disorder is often associated with greater impairment of routine activities in older adults. Consultation psychiatrists should pay careful attention to depressive symptoms in association with medical illness in order to establish the impact of depressive disorder on the overall course and recovery from general medical conditions (Cassem 1990).

RECURRENT BRIEF DEPRESSIVE DISORDER

Recurrent brief depressive disorder (RBDD) refers to brief episodes of recurrent depressive symptoms that last for at least 2 days but less than 2 weeks and meet full criteria (except duration) for MDD (see DSM-IV-TR research criteria below). These episodes typically occur monthly for 12 months, but are not specifically related to menstrual cycles. These depressive episodes typically cause clinically significant distress and impairment in social and occupational functioning. In some individuals, RBDD is associated with a high degree of suicidality (Maier et al. 1997).

DSM-IV-TR Research Criteria

Recurrent Brief Depressive Disorder

A. Criteria, except for duration, are met for a Major Depressive Episode
B. The depressive periods in Criterion A last at least 2 days but less than 2 weeks.
C. The depressive periods occur at least once a month for 12 consecutive months and are not associated with the menstrual cycle.
D. The periods of depressed mood cause clinically significant distress or impairment in social, occupational, or other important areas of functioning.
E. The symptoms are not due to the direct physiological effects of a substance (e.g., a drug of abuse, a medication) or a general medical condition (e.g., hypothyroidism).
F. There has never been a Major Depressive Episode, and criteria are not met for Dysthymic Disorder.
G. There has never been a Manic Episode, a Mixed Episode, or a Hypomanic Episode, and criteria are not met for Cyclothymic Disorder.

Note: This exclusion does not apply if all of the manic-, mixed-, or hypomanic-like episodes are substance- or treatment-induced.

H. The mood disturbance does not occur exclusively during Schizophrenia, Schizophreniform Disorder, Schizoaffective Disorder, Delusional Disorder, or Psychotic Disorder Not Otherwise Specified.

Reprinted with permission from the Diagnostic and Statistical Manual of Mental Disorders, Fourth Edition, Text Revision. Copyright 2000 American Psychiatric Association.

Associated clinical features may include comorbid substance dependence or anxiety disorders. By definition, recurrent brief depressive episodes are not associated with menstrual cycles and are as common among men as in women.

Up to 12 to 20% of first-degree relatives of individuals with recurrent brief depressive disorder have MDD. Ongoing research focusing on familial aggregation and associated comorbid conditions is important. It will be particularly important to address its association with personality characteristics and the overlap between personality disorder and the syndrome of RBDD.

MIXED ANXIETY–DEPRESSIVE DISORDER

The syndrome of mixed anxiety–depressive disorder is commonly diagnosed in outpatient medical practices internationally and it is included as a disorder in ICD-10. It is typically associated with dysphoric mood lasting at least 1 month and at least four associated clinical symptoms that are derived from both symptoms associated with MDD, DD, panic disorder, and generalized anxiety disorder (see DSM-IV-TR research criteria on page 779). These symptom characteristics include difficulty concentrating or mind going blank; sleep disturbance characterized by difficulty falling or staying asleep or restless; unsatisfying sleep; fatigue or low energy; irritability; worry; being easily moved to tears; hypervigilance; anticipating the worst; hopelessness and pessimism about the future; and low self-esteem or feelings of worthlessness. The symptoms cause significant impairment in social and occupational functioning or other aspects of functioning. These symptoms must not be due to the direct physiologic effects of a substance or a general medical condition. Finally, the symptoms are present in the absence of criteria being met for MDD, DD, panic disorder, or generalized anxiety disorder. The presence of these common mixed anxious and depressive symptoms is estimated to range from 1 to 2% in primary care settings.

DSM-IV-TR Research Criteria

Mixed Anxiety-Depressive Disorder

A. Persistent or recurrent dysphoric mood lasting at least 1 month.
B. The dysphoric mood is accompanied by at least 1 month of four (or more) of the following symptoms:

  (1) difficulty concentrating or mind going blank
  (2) sleep disturbance (difficulty falling or staying asleep, or restless, unsatis-fying sleep)
  (3) fatigue or low energy
  (4) irritability
  (5) worry
  (6) being easily moved to tears
  (7) hypervigilance
  (8) anticipating the worst
  (9) hopelessness (pervasive pessimism about the future)
  (10) low self-esteem or feelings of worthlessness

C. The symptoms cause clinically significant distress or impairment in social, occupa-tional, or other important areas of functioning.
D. The symptoms are not due to the direct physiological effects of a substance (e.g., a drug of abuse, a medication) or a general medical condition.
E. All of the following:

  (1) criteria have never been met for Major Depressive Disorder, Dysthymic Disorder, Panic Disorder, or Generalized Anxiety Disorder
  (2) criteria are not currently met for any other Anxiety or Mood Disorder (including an Anxiety or Mood Disorder, In Partial Remission)
  (3) the symptoms are not better accounted for by any other mental disorder.

POSTPSYCHOTIC DEPRESSIVE DISORDER OF SCHIZOPHRENIA

The diagnosis of postpsychotic depressive disorder of schizophrenia is intended to cover depressive episodes occurring during the residual phase of schizophrenia (see DSM-IV-TR research criteria on page 780). In the residual phase, there may be associated negative symptoms that can be difficult to differentiate from mood symptoms. The diagnosis should be made only if the full criteria are met for a major depressive episode and if the symptoms are not due to substance abuse, akinesia, or other antipsychotic medication effects.

DSM-IV-TR Research Criteria

Postpsychotic Depressive Disorder of Schizophrenia

A. Criteria are met for a Major Depressive Episode.

Note: The Major Depressive Episode must include Criterion A1: depressed mood. Do not include symptoms that are better accounted for as medication side effects or negative symptoms of Schizophrenia.

B. The Major Depressive Episode is superimposed on and occurs only during the residual phase of Schizophrenia.
C. The Major Depressive Episode is not due to the direct physiological effects of a substance or a general medical condition.

Features associated with the development of a postpsychotic depressive episode include limited social support, the impact of prior hospitalization, or the trauma of having a major mental illness. It is estimated that up to 25% of individuals with schizophrenia experience postpsychotic depressive disorder. There is no significant age of onset difference between men and women. Individuals who have a family history of MDD may be at higher risk for postpsychotic depression. Treatment studies have demonstrated the efficacy of standard antidepressive medication in the postpsychotic depressive disorder of schizophrenia.

Comparison of DSM-IV-TR/ICD-10 Diagnostic Criteria

The criteria for a major depressive episode in ICD-10 contains 10 items, in contrast to the nine DSM-IV-TR items (loss of self-esteem has been separated from inappropriate guilt). Furthermore, ICD-10 provides separate criteria sets for each level of severity of a major depressive episode: a threshold of 4 out of 10 symptoms defines mild, 6 out of 10 symptoms defines moderate, and 8 out of 10 symptoms defines severe. Furthermore, the ICD-10 diagnostic algorithm differs by requiring that there be at least two of the following three symptoms — depressed mood, loss of interest, and decreased energy — for mild and moderate depressive episodes and all three for severe episodes. ICD-10 episodes with psychotic features exclude first-rank symptoms and bizarre delusions, which if present would shift the diagnosis to schizoaffective disorder.

The ICD-10 Diagnostic Criteria for Research and DSM-IV-TR also differ on the threshold for defining when major depressive disorder is characterized as single episode versus recurrent. ICD-10 specifies that there be a period of at least two months free from any significant mood symptoms between mood episodes, whereas DSM-IV-TR requires an interval of at least two consecutive months in which full criteria for a major depressive episode have not been met.

The ICD-10 definition of dysthymic disorder specifies that three items from a list of 11 symptoms (which include five of the six DSM-IV-TR items) must accompany the depressed mood. Furthermore, ICD-10 restricts co-occurring major depressive episodes to "none or very few" and specifies that dysthymic disorder may follow a depressive episode without a period of full remission.

References

Abramson LY, Metalsky GI, and Alloy LB (1989) Hopelessness depression: a theory-based subtype of depression. *Psychol Rev* **96**, 358–372.

Alfici S, Sigal M, and Landau M (1989) Primary fibromyalgia syndrome—a variant of depressive disorder?. *Psychother Psychosom* **51**, 156–161.

Akiskal HS (1983) Dysthymic disorder: psychopathology of proposed chronic depressive subtypes. *Am J Psychiatry* **140**, 11–20.

Akiskal HS (1990) Toward a clinical understanding of the relationship of anxiety and depressive disorders. In *Comorbidity of Mood and Anxiety Disorders*, Maser JD and Cloninger CR (eds). American Psychiatric Press, Washington, DC, pp. 597–607.

American Psychiatric Association (1987) *Diagnostic and Statistical Manual of Mental Disorders*, 3rd ed., Rev. APA, Washington, DC.

American Psychiatric Association (2000) *Diagnostic and Statistical Manual of Mental Disorders*, 4th ed., Text Rev. APA, Washington, DC.

Barklage NE (1991) Evaluation and management of the suicidal patient. *Emerg Care Q* **7**, 9–17.

Bauer MS and Whydrow PC (1990) Rapid cycling bipolar affective disorder, II: treatment of refractory rapid cycling with high dose levothyroxine: a preliminary study. *Arch Gen Psychiatry* **47**, 435–440.

Beck AT (1976) *Cognitive Therapy and the Emotional Disorders*. International Universities Press, New York.

Beck AT, Rush AJ, and Shaw BF (1979) *Cognitive Therapy of Depression*. Guilford Press, New York.

Beck AT, Ward C, Mendelson M, et al. (1961) An inventory for measuring depression. *Arch Gen Psychiatry* **4**, 53–63.

Black DW, Bell S, and Hulbert J (1988) The importance of axis II in patients with major depression: a controlled study. *J Affect Disord* **14**, 115–122.

Blazer DG (1994) Epidemiology of late-life depression. In *Diagnosis and Treatment Depression in Late Life: Results of the NIH Consensus Development Conference*, Schneider LS, Reynolds CF, Lebowityz BD, et al. (eds). American Psychiatric Press, Washington, DC, pp. 9–19.

Blazer DG, Kessler RC, and McGonagle KA (1994) The prevalence and distribution of major depression in a national community sample: the national comorbidity survey. *Am J Psychiatry* **151**, 979–986.

Bleich A, Koslowsky, and Dolev A (1997) Posttraumatic stress disorder and depression. *Br J Psychiatry* **170**, 479–482.

Brown GW and Harris T (1978) *Social Origins of Depression: A Study of Psychiatric Disorder in Women*. Free Press, New York.

Brown SA and Schuckit MA (1988) Changes in depression among abstinent alcoholics. *J Stud Alcohol* **49**, 412–417.

Bush G, Fink M, Petrides G, et al. (1996) Catatonia, II: treatment with lorazepam and electroconvulsive therapy. *Acta Psychiatr Scand* **93**, 137–143.

Cadoret RD, O'Gorman TW, and Haywood E (1990) Genetic and environmental factors in major depression. *J Affect Disord* **19**, 23–29.

Cassem EH (1990) Depression and anxiety secondary to medical illness. *Psychiatr Clin North Am* **13**, 597–612.

Charney DS, Nelson JC, and Quinlan DM (1981) Personality traits and disorder in depression. *Am J Psychiatry* **138**, 1601–1604.

Coryell WR, Noyes R, and Clancy J (1982) Excess mortality in panic disorder: a comparison with primary unipolar depression. *Arch Gen Psychiatry* **39**, 701–703.

Coyne JC (1976) Toward an interactional description of depression. *Psychiatry* **39**, 28–40.

Cross-National Collaborative Group (1992) The changing rate of major depression: cross-national comparisons. *J Am Med Assoc* **268**, 3098–3105.

Depression Guideline Panel (1993a) *Depression in Primary Care: Vol. 1. Detection and Diagnosis, Clinical Practice Guideline*, AHCPR Publication No. 93-0550, No. 5. (April) U.S. Department of Health and Human Services, Public Health Agency, Agency for Health Care and Policy Research, Washington, DC.

Depression Guideline Panel (1993b) *Depression in Primary Care: Vol. 2. Treatment of Major Depression, Clinical Practice Guideline*, AHCPR Publication No. 93-0551, No. 5. (April) U.S. Department of Health and Human Services, Public Health Agency, Agency for Health Care and Policy Research, Washington, DC.

DeRubeis RJ, Hollon SD, Grove WM, et al. (1990) How does cognitive therapy work? cognitive change and symptom change in cognitive therapy and pharmacotherapy for depression. *J Consult Clin Psychiatry* **58**(6), 862–869.

Dorus W, Kennedy J, and Gibbons RD (1987) Symptoms and diagnosis of depression in alcoholics. *Alcohol: Clin Exp Res* **11**, 150–154.

Ehlers CL, Frank E, and Kupfer DJ (1988) Social zeitgebers and biological rhythms. *Arch Gen Psychiatry* **45**, 948–952.

Elkin I, Shea TM, and Watkins JT (1989) National institute of mental health treatment of depression collaborative research program. *Arch Gen Psychiatry* **46**, 971–982.

Emslie GE, Weinberg WA, and Rush JA (1990) Depressive symptoms by self-report in adolescent: phase I of the development of a questionnaire for depression by self-report. *J Child Neurol* **5**, 114–121.

Endicott J and Spitzer RL (1978) A diagnostic interview: the schedule for affective disorders and schizophrenia. *Arch Gen Psychiatry* **35**, 837–844.

Eriksson E, Andersch B, Ho HP, et al. (2002) Diagnosis and treatment of premenstrual dysphoria. *J Clin Psychiatry* **63**(Suppl. 7), 16–23.

Fawcett J, Scheftner WA, and Fogg L (1990) Time-related predictors of suicide in major affective disorder. *Am J Psychiatry* **147**, 1189–1194.

Feldman E, Hawton MR, and Arden M (1987) Psychiatric disorder in medical inpatients. *Q J Med* **63**, 405–412.

First MB, Spitzer RL, Gibbon M, et al. (1994) *Structured Clinical Interview for Axis I DSM-IV Disorders—Patient Edition (SCID-I/P, Version 2.0)*. Biometrics Research Department, New York State Psychiatric Institute, New York.

Forsell Y, Jorm AF, and Wonblad B (1994) Association of age, sex, cognitive dysfunction and disability with major depressive symptoms in an elderly sample. *Am J Psychiatry* **11**, 1600–1604.

George MS, Lisanby SH, and Sakeim HA (1999) Applications in neuropsychiatry. *Arch Gen Psychiatry* **56**, 300–311.

Giles DE, Jarret RB, and Roff HP (1989) Clinical predictors of recurrence in depression. *Am J Psychiatry* **146**, 764–767.

Goldstein I (2000) The mutually reinforcing triad of depressive symptoms, cardiovascular disease and erectile dysfunction. *Am J Cardiol* **86**(2A), 41F–45F.

Goodwin FK and Jamison KR (1990) *Manic–Depressive Illness*. Oxford University Press, New York.

Goodwin FK, Prange AJ, and Post RM (1982) Potentiation of antidepressant effects by L-triodothyconine in tricyclic nonresponders. *Am J Psychiatry* **139**, 34–38.

Gruenberg AM, Goldstein RD, and Bruss GS (1993) Co-occurrence of Major Mood Disorder and Personality Disorder. Poster Presented at Third International Congress on the Disorders of Personality. Cambridge, Massachusetts.

Gunderson JG and Phillips KA (1991) A current view of the interface between borderline personality disorder and depression. *Am J Psychiatry* **148**, 967–975.

Hamilton M (1960) A rating scale for depression. *J Neurol Neurosurg Psychiatry* **23**, 56–62.

Harkness KL and Monroe SM (2002) Childhood adversity and the endogenous versus nonendogenous distinction in women with major depression. *Am J Psychiatry* **159**, 387–393.

Harlow HF and Harlow HF (1962) Social deprivation in monkeys. *Sci Am* **207**, 136–146.

Hawkins JM, Archer KJ, Strakowski SM, et al. (1995) Somatic treatments of catatonia. *Int J Psychiatr Med* **25**, 345–369.

Hirschfeld RMA (1994) Guidelines for the long-term treatment of depression. *J Clin Psychiatry* **55**(Suppl), 61–69.

Hollon SD, DeRubeis RJ, and Evans MD (1992) Cognitive therapy and pharmacotherapy for depression: singly and in combination. *Arch Gen Psychiatry* **49**, 774–781.

Hudson JI, Hudson MS, and Pliner LF (1985) Fibromyalgia and major affective disorder: a controlled phenomenology and family history study. *Am J Psychiatry* **142**, 441–446.

Ionescu R and Popescu C (1989) Personality disorders in students with depressive pathology. *Neurol Psychiatr (Bucur)* **27**, 45–55.

Jaffee SR, Moffitt TE, Caspi A, et al. (2002) Differences in early childhood risk factors for juvenile-onset and adult-onset depression. *Arch Gen Psychiatry* **59**, 215–222.

Kashani JH, Carlson GA, and Beck NC (1987) Depression, depressive symptoms, and depressed mood among a community sample of adolescents. *Am J Psychiatry* **144**, 931–934.

Kashani JH, McGee RO, and Clarkson SE (1983) Depression in a sample of 9-year old children. *Arch Gen Psychiatry* **40**, 1217–1223.

Katon W, vonKorff M, and Lin E (1990) Distressed high utilizers of medical care: DSM-III-R diagnoses and treatment needs. *Gen Hosp Psychiatry* **12**, 355–362.

Keller MB, Lavori PW, and Mueller JI (1992) Time to recovery, chronicity and levels of psychopathology in major depression: a 5-year prospective follow-up of 431 subjects. *Arch Gen Psychiatry* **49**, 809–816.

Keller MB, McCullough JP, Klein DN, et al. (2000) A comparison of nefazodone, cognitive behavioral analysis system of psychotherapy and their combination for the treatment of chronic depression. *N Engl J Med* **342**, 1462–1470.

Keller M and Shapiro RW (1982) "Double depression": superimposition of acute depressive episodes on chronic depressive disorders. *Am J Psychiatry* **139**, 438–442.

Kendler KS (1991) Mood-incongruent psychotic affective illness: an historical and empirical review. *Arch Gen Psychiatry* **48**, 362–369.

Kendler KS, Heath AC, Martin AG, et al. (1986) Symptoms of anxiety and symptoms of depression: same genes, different environments?. *Arch Gen Psychiatry* **44**, 451–457.

Kendler KS, Heath AC, and Neale AC (1993a) Alcoholism and major depression in women: a twin study of the causes of comorbidity. *Arch Gen Psychiatry* **50**, 690–698.

Kendler KS, Kessler RC, and Neale MC (1993b) The prediction of major depression in women: toward an integrated etiologic model. *Am J Psychiatry* **150**, 1139–1147.

Kendler KS, Neale MC, and Kessler RC (1992) A population-based twin study of major depression in women. *Arch Gen Psychiatry* **49**, 257–266.

Kessler RC, McGonagle KA, and Zhao S (1994) Lifetime and 12-month prevalence of DSM-III-R psychiatric disorders in United States. *Arch Gen Psychiatry* **51**, 8–19.

Kessler RC, Somega A, and Bromet E (1995) Post–traumatic stress disorder in the National Comorbidity Survey. *Arch Gen Psychiatry* **52**, 1048–1060.

Klerman GI and Weissman MM (1989) Increasing rates of depression. *J Am Med Assoc* **261**, 2229–2235.

Klerman GI, Weissman MM, Rounsaville BJ, et al. (1984) *Interpersonal Psychotherapy of Depression*. Basic Books, New York.

Koenig HG, Meador KG, and Cohen HJ (1988) Depression in elderly hospitalized patients with medical illness. *Arch Intern Med* **148**, 1929–1936.

Kornstein SG (1997) Gender differences in depression: implications for treatment. *J Clin Psychiatry* **58**(Suppl. 15), 12–18.

Kupfer DJ, Frank E, and Perel JM (1989) The advantage of early treatment intervention in recurrent depression. *Arch Gen Psychiatry* **46**, 771–775.

Kupfer DJ and Thase ME (1983) The use of the sleep laboratory in the diagnosis of affective disorders. *Psychiatr Clin North Am* **6**, 3–25.

Lewinsohn PM (1974) A behavioral approach to depression. In *The Psychology of Depression: Contemporary Theory and Research*, Friedman RJ and Katz MM (eds). John Wiley, New York.

Lewinsohn PM, Clarke GN, and Seely JR (1994) Major depression in community adolescents: age at onset, episode duration, and time to recurrence. *J Am Acad Child Adolesc Psychiatry* **33**, 809–818.

Maier W, Gansicke M, and Weiffenbach O (1997) The relationship between major and subthreshold variants of unipolar depression. *J Affect Disord* **45**, 41–51.

Maier W, Lichteimann D, and Minges J (1992) The risk of minor depression in families of probands with major depression: sex differences and familiarity. *Eur Arch Psychiatr Clin Neurosci* **242**, 89–92.

Marin DB, Kocsis JH, and Frances AJ (1993) Personality disorders in dysthymia. *J Perspect Disord* **7**, 223–231.

McKinney WT (1988) *Models of Mental Disorders: A New Comparative Psychiatry*. Plenum Medical Book Company, New York.

Miller LJ (2002) Postpartum depression. *J Am Med Assoc* **287**(6), 762–765.

Montgomery SA and Asberg MC (1979) A new depression scale designed to be sensitive to change. *Br J Psychiatry* **134**, 382–389.

Munjack DJ and Moss HB (1981) Affective disorder and alcoholism. *Arch Gen Psychiatry* **38**, 869–871.

Musselman DL, Evans DL, and Nemeroff CB (1998) The relationship of depression to cardiovascular disease. *Arch Gen Psychiatry* **55**, 580–592.

National Institute of Mental Health Consensus Development Conference Statement (1985) Mood disorders: pharmacologic prevention of recurrences. *Am J Psychiatry* **142**, 469–476.

O'Leary KD and Beach SRH (1990) Marital therapy: a viable treatment for depression and marital discord. *Am J Psychiatry* **147**, 183–186.

Orvaschel H (1990) Early onset psychiatric disorder in high risk children and increased familial morbidity. *J Am Acad Child Adolesc Psychiatry* **29**, 184–188.

Owens MJ and Nemeroff CB (1998) The serotonin transporter and depression. *Depress Anxiety* **8**(Suppl. 1), 5–12.

Parmelee PA, Katz IR, and Lawton MP (1989) Depression among institutionalized aged: assessment and prevalence estimation. *J Gerontol* **44**(1), M22–M29.

Petty F (1992) The depressed alcoholic: clinical features and medical management. *Gen Hosp Psychiatry* **14**, 458–464.

Pfohl B, Stangl D, and Zimmerman M (1984) The implications of DSM-III personality disorders for patients with major depression. *J Affect Disord* **7**, 309–318.

Post RM (1992) Transduction of psychosocial stress into the neurobiology of recurrent affective disorder. *Am J Psychiatry* **149**, 999–1010.

Regier DA, Boyd JH, and Burke JD Jr. (1988) One-month prevalence of mental disorders in the United States: based on five epidemiologic catchment area sites. *Arch Gen Psychiatry* **145**, 1351–1357.

Ross ED and Rush AJ (1981) Diagnosis and neuroanatomical correlates of depression in brain-damaged patients: implications for a neurology of depression. *Arch Gen Psychiatry* **38**, 1344–1354.

Rush AJ, Cain JW, and Raese J (1991) Neurobiological bases for psychiatric disorders. In *Comprehensive Neurology*, Rosenberg RN (ed). Raven Press, New York, pp. 555–603.

Rush AJ, Erman MK, and Giles DE (1986a) Polysomnographic findings in recently drug-free and clinically remitted depressed patients. *Arch Gen Psychiatry* **43**, 878–884.

Rush AJ, George MS, and Sackeim HA (2000) Vagus nerve stimulation (VNS) for treatment-resistant depressions: a multicenter study. *Biol Psychiatry* **47**, 276–286.

Rush AJ, Hiser W, and Giles DE (1987) A comparison of self-reported versus clinician-rated symptoms in depression. *J Clin Res* **48**, 246–248.

Sargeant JK, Bruce ML, and Florio LP (1990) Factors associated with 1-year outcome of major depression in the community. *Arch Gen Psychiatry* **47**, 519–526.

Schildkraut JJ (1965) The catecholamine hypothesis of affective disorders: a review of supporting evidence. *Am J Psychiatry* **122**, 509–522.

Seligman MEP (1975) *Helplessness: On Depression, Development and Death*. WH Freeman, San Franciso.

Shalev AY, Feedman S, and Peri T (1998) Post-traumatic stress disorder and depression. *Am J Psychiatry* **155**, 630–637.

Shea MT, Glass DR, Pilkonis PA, et al. (1987) Frequency and implications of personality disorders in a sample of depressed outpatients. *J Perspect Disord* **1**, 27–42.

Shea MT, Widiger TA, and Klein MH (1992) Comorbidity of personality disorders and depression: implications for treatment. *J Consult Clin Psychol* **60**, 857–868.

Thase ME (1990) Relapse and recurrence in unipolar major depression: short-term and long-term approaches. *J Clin Psychiatry* **51**(Suppl. 6), 51–57.

Thase ME, Greenhouse JB, Frank E, et al. (1997) Treatment of major depression with psychotherapy or psychotherapy-pharmacotherapy combinations. *Arch Gen Psychiatry* **54**, 1009–1015.

Thase ME and Howland RH (1994) Refractory depression: relevance of psychosocial factors and therapies. *Psychiatr Ann* **24**, 232–240.

Thase ME and Rush AJ (1995) Treatment-resistant depression. In *Psychopharmacology: The Fourth Generation of Progress*, Bloom F and Kupfer DJ (eds). Raven Press, New York, pp. 1081–1097.

Wehr TA, Wirz-Justice A, and Goodwin FK (1979) Phase advance of the circadian sleep-wake cycle as an antidepressant. *Science* **206**, 710–713.

Weissman MM, Bruce ML, and Leaf PJ (1991) Affective disorders. In *Psychiatric Disorders in America*, Robins LN and Regier DA (eds). Free Press, New York, pp. 53–80.

Weissman MM, Leaf PJ, and Bruce ML (1988a) The epidemiology of dysthymia in five communities: rates, risks, comorbidity, and treatment. *Am J Psychiatry* **145**, 815–819.

Weissman MM, Leaf PJ, and Tischler GL (1988b) Affective disorders in five United States communities. *Psychol Med* **18**, 141–153.

Weller EB and Weller RA (1990) Depressive disorders in children and adolescents. In *Psychiatric Disorders in Children and Adolescents*, Garfinkle BD, Carlson GA, and Weller EB (eds). W. B. Saunders, Philadelphia, pp. 3–20.

Wells KB (1985) *Depression as a Tracer Condition for the National Study of Medical Care Outcomes-Background Review*. Rand, Santa Monica.

Wells KB, Golding JM, and Burnam MA (1988) Psychiatric disorder and limitations in physical functioning in a sample of the Los Angeles general population. *Am J Psychiatry* **145**, 712–717.

Wells KB, Stewart A, and Hays RD (1989) The functioning and well-being of depressed patients: results from the medical outcomes study. *J Am Med Assoc* **262**, 914–919.

Wender PH, Kety SS, and Rosenthal D (1986) Psychiatry disorders in the biological and adoptive families of adopted individuals with affective disorders. *Arch Gen Psychiatry* **46**, 923–929.

Whirz-Justice A, Graw P, and Kraucht K (1993) Light therapy in seasonal affective disorder is independent of time of day or circadian phase. *Arch Gen Psychiatry* **50**, 929–937.

Wing JK, Birley JLT, Cooper JE, et al. (1967) Reliability of a procedure for measuring and classifying "present psychiatric state.". *Br J Psychiatry* **111**, 499–515.

Zung WWK (1965) A self-rating depression scale. *Arch Gen Psychiatry* **12**, 63–70.

Mood Disorders: Premenstrual Dysphoric Disorder

Diagnosis

Premenstrual syndrome (PMS) is a combination of emotional, behavioral, and physical symptoms that occur in the premenstrual or luteal phase of the menstrual cycle. The term *premenstrual tension* appeared in the medical literature 70 years ago (Frank 1931) but widely accepted diagnostic criteria for PMS do not exist. Diagnostic criteria for PMS often require a minimum of one premenstrual symptom, such as the criteria proposed in the *American College of Obstetrics and Gynecology Practice Guidelines* (American College of Obstetrics and Gynecology 2000) or in the *International Classification of Diseases*, 10th Revision (World Health Organization 1993). Approximately 80% of women report at least mild premenstrual symptoms, 20 to 50% report moderate to severe premenstrual symptoms, and approximately 5% of women report severe symptoms for several days with impairment of role and social functioning (American Psychiatric Association 1994). The 5% of women with the severest form of PMS generally have symptoms that meet the diagnostic criteria for premenstrual dysphoric disorder (PMDD).

Research diagnostic criteria for PMDD are listed in the appendix of DSM-IV-TR (American Psychiatric Association 1994), and they are an updated version of the older DSM-III-R criteria for late luteal phase dysphoric disorder (American Psychiatric Association 1987) (see DSM-IV-TR Research Criteria on page 786). A clinician can indicate that a woman has symptoms that meet the diagnostic criteria for PMDD by recording the DSM-IV-TR diagnosis 311, depressive disorder not otherwise specified. To meet the PMDD criteria, at least five out of the eleven possible symptoms must be present in the premenstrual phase; these symptoms should be absent shortly following the onset of menses; and at least one of the five symptoms must be depressed mood, anxiety, lability, or irritability. The PMDD criteria require that role functioning be impaired as a result of the premenstrual symptoms. The functional impairment reported by women with PMDD is similar in severity to the impairment reported in major depressive disorder and dysthymic disorder (Pearlstein et al. 2000). Unlike the functional impairment reported in depressive disorders, women with severe PMS and PMDD report more disruption in their relationships and parenting roles than in their work roles (Campbell et al. 1997, Hylan et al. 1999, Robinson and Swindle 2000).

DSM-IV-TR Research Criteria

Premenstrual Dysphoric Disorder

A. In most menstrual cycles during the past year, five (or more) of the following symptoms were present for most of the time during the last week of the luteal phase, began to remit within a few days after the onset of the follicular phase, and were absent in the week postmenses, with at least one of the symptoms being either (1), (2), (3), or (4):

    (1) markedly depressed mood, feelings of hopelessness, or self-deprecating thoughts

    (2) marked anxiety, tension, feelings of being "keyed up," or "on edge"

    (3) marked affective lability (e.g., feeling suddenly sad or tearful or increased sensitivity to rejection)

    (4) persistent and marked anger or irritability or increased interpersonal conflicts

    (5) decreased interest in usual activities (e.g., work, school, friends, hobbies)

    (6) subjective sense of difficulty in concentrating

    (7) lethargy, easy fatigability, or marked lack of energy

    (8) marked change in appetite, overeating, or specific food cravings

    (9) hypersomnia or insomnia

    (10) a subjective sense of being overwhelmed or out of control

    (11) other physical symptoms, such as breast tenderness or swelling, headaches, joint or muscle pain, a sensation of "bloating," weight gain

B. The disturbance markedly interferes with work or school or with usual social activities and relationships (e.g., avoidance of social activities, decreased productivity and efficiency at work or school).

C. The disturbance is not merely an exacerbation of the symptoms of another disorder such as major depressive disorder, panic disorder, dysthymic disorder, or a personality disorder (although it may be superimposed on any of these disorders).

D. Criteria A, B, and C must be confirmed by prospective daily ratings during at least two consecutive symptomatic cycles. (The diagnosis may be made provisionally prior to this confirmation).

The PMDD criteria require that a woman prospectively rate her emotional, behavioral, and physical symptoms over two menstrual cycles to confirm the diagnosis. Several studies have reported that retrospective reports of premenstrual symptoms may inaccurately identify the timing or amplify the severity of symptoms compared to prospective reporting (Schnurr et al. 1994). Charting two menstrual cycles is advantageous, since some women have variability of symptom severity from cycle to cycle due to factors such as seasonal worsening, or a woman might have the unusual presence of follicular phase psychological symptoms due to a transient stressor. Studies conducted over the past two decades have used different instruments for daily ratings and various scoring methods to measure the premenstrual increase of symptoms (Schnurr et al. 1994). More recent studies tend to utilize visual analog scales, or Likert scale daily rating forms such as the Daily Record of Severity of Problems (Endicott and Harrison 1990), with a scoring method that compares the average of symptom scores during the premenstrual days to the average of symptom scores postmenses.

A woman presenting with PMS should ideally bring to her clinician two cycles of an established daily rating form, or alternatively ratings of her most problematic symptoms, rated with anchor points ranging from "not present" to "severe." The clinician should review the daily ratings to confirm that the symptoms are in fact confined largely to the premenstrual phase, with the relative absence of symptoms in the follicular phase, and the clinician should also assess premenstrual functional impairment (Figure 29-1). Ratings that demonstrate follicular symptoms with increased symptom severity in the premenstrual phase suggest "premenstrual exacerbation" of an underlying disorder rather than PMDD. The DSM-IV-TR PMDD criteria state that the premenstrual symptoms should not be an exacerbation of an underlying disorder, but that PMDD could be superimposed on another disorder, like panic disorder. No formal guidelines exist on how to apply this criterion clinically.

Epidemiology

Irritability has been identified as the most common premenstrual symptom in US and European samples (Endicott et al. 1999, Angst et al. 2001). Studies examining age, menstrual cycle characteristics, cognitive attributions, socioeconomic variables, lifestyle variables, and number of children have not yielded consistent conclusions (Endicott et al. 1999, Steiner and Born 2000). Studies have suggested some genetic liability for PMS, but the overlap

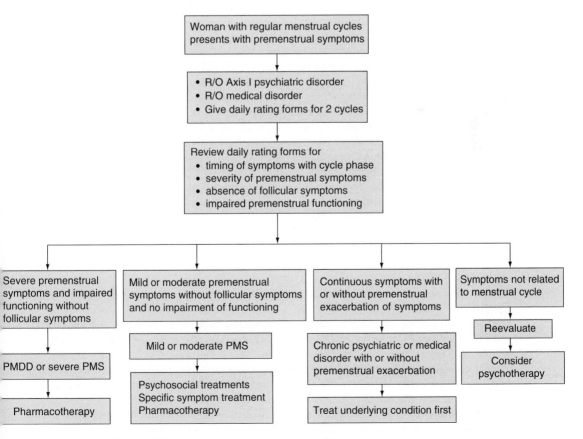

Figure 29-1 *Diagnosis and initial treatment algorithm of premenstrual symptoms.*

with genetic liability for major depression or personality characteristics has received mixed reports (Treloar et al. 2002). A polymorphism in the serotonin transporter promoter gene has been suggested in women who have both PMDD and seasonal affective disorder (Praschak-Rieder et al. 2002). Elevated lifetime prevalence of major depressive disorder in women with PMDD has been reported in several studies (Endicott 1994), as well as an elevated lifetime prevalence of postpartum depression (Critchlow et al. 2001). Even though premenstrual symptoms are described in women from menarche to menopause, it is unclear if symptoms remain stable or increase in severity with age (Endicott et al. 1999, Wittchen et al. 2002). PMS has been described in several countries and cultures and some cultures have a preponderance of somatic rather than emotional symptoms (Steiner and Born 2000).

Differential Diagnosis

Depression and anxiety disorders are the most common Axis I mental disorders that may be concurrent and exacerbated premenstrually, with less clear evidence for bipolar disorder, eating disorders, and substance abuse (Endicott 1994, Hendrick et al. 1996, Pearlstein and Stone 1998). Since most PMDD symptoms are affective or anxiety-related, "pure PMS" or PMDD is generally not diagnosed when an underlying depression or anxiety disorder is present; these women would be considered to have premenstrual exacerbation of their underlying depression or anxiety disorder. Personality disorders are not elevated in prevalence in women with PMDD (Critchlow et al. 2001), but women with PMDD and a personality disorder may demonstrate premenstrual phase amplification of personality dysfunction (Berlin et al. 2001). Schizophrenia may be an example of a disorder that does not have premenstrual exacerbation of psychotic symptoms but may have the superimposition of affective and anxiety symptoms of PMDD (Choi et al. 2001). The prevalence of premenstrually exacerbated disorders is unknown, but women with these conditions present frequently to their primary care clinician or gynecologist. Since most recent treatment studies have been conducted on women with PMS and PMDD without follicular symptomatology, this literature is not particularly informative on how to treat women with premenstrually exacerbated disorders. The general guideline is to treat the underlying disorder first and see if subsequent daily ratings suggest persistence of premenstrual symptoms that might meet the criteria for PMDD.

Several medical conditions should also be considered when evaluating a woman with premenstrual complaints. Symptoms of endometriosis, polycystic ovary disease, thyroid disorders, disorders of the adrenal system, hyperprolactinemia, and panhypopituitarism may mimic symptoms of PMS. Several general medical conditions may demonstrate a premenstrual increase in symptoms without accompanying emotional symptoms, such as migraines, asthma, epilepsy, irritable bowel syndrome, diabetes, allergies, and autoimmune disorders (Pearlstein and Stone 1998, Case and Reid 2001). It is presumed that the menstrual cycle fluctuations of gonadal hormones influence some of the symptoms of these medical conditions.

Etiology

There are several recent reviews of pathophysiologic hypotheses of PMS and PMDD and their evidence (Roca et al. 1996, Parry 1997, Yonkers 1997, Sundstrom et al. 1999, Steiner and Born 2000, Steiner and Pearlstein 2000). The majority of studies do not identify consistent abnormalities of hormones of the hypothalamic–pituitary–gonadal (HPG) axis, thyroid hormones, cortisol, prolactin, glucose, prostaglandins, vitamins, or electrolytes (Parry 1997). Decreased luteal phase peripheral beta-endorphin levels have been reported, but this may not reflect central opioid activity. Women with PMDD are more sensitive to the anxiolytic properties of carbon dioxide inhalation and lactate infusion, and increased adrenergic receptor binding may reflect abnormal noradrenergic function (Parry 1997,

Sundstrom et al. 1999, Steiner and Born 2000). Women with PMDD have abnormal melatonin secretion and other circadian system abnormalities (Parry and Newton 2001).

Since abnormalities in the HPG axis have not been identified, it is thought that premenstrual symptoms may occur due to a differential sensitivity to mood-perturbing effects of gonadal steroid fluctuations in women with PMS and PMDD (Schmidt et al. 1998). It is probable that the etiology of the "differential sensitivity" is multifactorial. The specific neurotransmitter, neuroendocrine, and neurosteroid abnormalities in women with PMS and PMDD are not known, but serotonin, norepinephrine, gamma-aminobutyric acid (GABA), allopregnanolone (an anxiolytic metabolite of progesterone that acts at the $GABA_A$ receptor), and factors involved in calcium homeostasis are all possibly involved.

A large number of studies have reported abnormalities in the serotonin system in women with PMS and PMDD. These include abnormal levels of whole blood serotonin, serotonin platelet uptake, and platelet tritiated imipramine binding; abnormal responses to serotonergic probes such as L-tryptophan, buspirone, meta-chlorophenylpiperazaine, and fenfluramine; and exacerbation of premenstrual symptoms after tryptophan depletion (Halbreich and Tworek 1993, Yonkers 1997, Sundstrom et al. 1999, Steiner and Pearlstein 2000, Parry 2001). Several studies have also suggested that women with PMDD have decreased luteal phase levels of GABA, abnormal allopregnanolone levels, and decreased sensitivity of the $GABA_A$ receptor as shown by flumazenil challenge, and the sedative and saccadic eye velocity responses to benzodiazepines (Sundstrom et al. 1999, Girdler et al. 2001). It is possible that the rapid efficacy of selective serotonin reuptake inhibitors (SSRIs) in PMDD may be due in part to their ability to increase allopregnanolone levels in the brain, thus enhancing GABA transmission as well as serotonin transmission (Guidotti and Costa 1998, Griffin and Mellon 1999).

Several factors that influence calcium and bone homeostasis fluctuate with the menstrual cycle and it is possible that some of these factors are abnormal in women with PMS and PMDD (Thys-Jacobs 2000). One study reported decreased bone mineral density in women with prospectively confirmed PMS (Thys-Jacobs et al. 1995); however, a later study in women with PMDD failed to find decreased bone mineral density compared to controls (Halbreich and Kahn 2001). Thys-Jacobs and colleagues reported that women with PMS had reduced periovulatory calcium levels and elevated parathyroid hormone levels compared to controls, perhaps secondary to elevated preovulatory estrogen levels, and these authors proposed that women with PMS may have a cyclical, transient secondary hyperparathyroidism (Thys-Jacobs and Alvir 1995). It has been reported that when calcium homeostasis is corrected in primary hyperparathyroidism, cerebrospinal fluid monoamine metabolites normalize and affective symptoms are reduced (Joborn et al. 1991). It is possible that the administration of supplemental calcium normalizes the periovulatory fluctuations in calcium and parathyroid hormone, thus regulating calcium effects on neurotransmitter synthesis and release, leading to symptom relief in women with PMS (Thys-Jacobs 2000).

Treatment

The treatment studies of SSRIs in PMDD have suggested a similar efficacy rate to treatment studies of SSRIs in major depressive disorder, with 60 to 70% of women responding to SSRIs compared to approximately 30% of women responding to placebo. In general, the effective SSRI doses are similar to the doses recommended for the treatment of major depressive disorder (Figure 29-2). A review of 15 randomized controlled trials (RCTs) of SSRIs reported that women with severe PMS or PMDD were approximately seven times more likely to respond to SSRIs compared to placebo (Dimmock et al. 2000). The efficacy of the continuous (daily) dosing and intermittent dosing (SSRI administered during the luteal phase only from ovulation to menses) RCTs was equivalent (Dimmock et al. 2000). There have not been reports of discontinuation symptoms from doses of fluoxetine (10 mg/day during luteal phase) and sertraline (50–100 mg/day during luteal phase) when they were abruptly stopped from the first day of menses. There are no published studies to date of the efficacy of "symptom onset" dosing of SSRIs, that is, administering SSRIs from the postovulatory day that premenstrual symptoms appear until menses. The efficacy of intermittent dosing, as well as the findings from most SSRI trials that efficacy is achieved by the first treatment cycle, has suggested a more rapid and different mechanism of action of SSRIs in PMDD compared to its effect in major depressive disorder that typically takes two to six weeks. As discussed above, it has been hypothesized that the rapid improvement of premenstrual symptoms by SSRIs may be due to an increase in allopregnanolone levels.

A large RCT with daily dosing of venlafaxine, an antidepressant with both serotonergic and noradrenergic action, reported that an average dose of 130 mg/day reduced emotional and physical symptoms of PMDD in 157 women (Freeman et al. 2001c). Smaller RCTs have reported efficacy with clomipramine, a tricyclic antidepressant with largely serotonergic action, in daily dosing (Sundblad et al. 1992) and luteal phase dosing (Sundblad et al. 1993). The doses of clomipramine reported to be effective for PMS (25–75 mg q.d.) are lower than expected effective doses for major depressive disorder (see Figure 29-2). One RCT reported that nefazodone was not superior to placebo in PMS (Landen et al. 2001); however, increasing nefazodone in the luteal phase was reported to improve premenstrual exacerbation

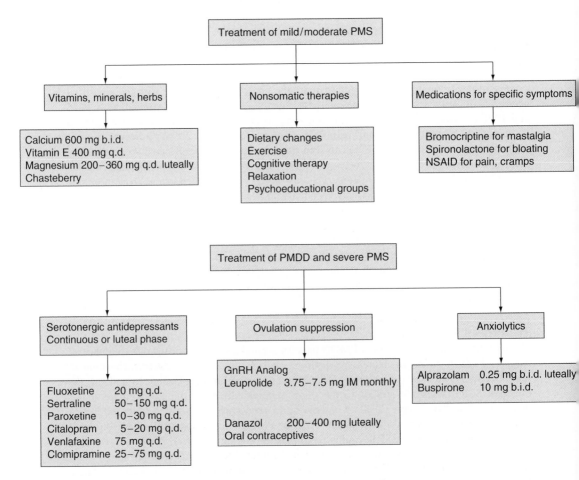

Figure 29-2 *Treatment algorithm of premenstrual symptoms.*

of major depressive disorder in a small crossover study (Miller et al. 2002). Three RCTs have compared SSRIs to nonserotonergic antidepressants and placebo, and each has reported specific efficacy of the SSRI over placebo and the nonserotonergic antidepressant. The selective superiority of serotonergic antidepressants for PMDD is compatible with the postulated serotonin dysfunction in PMDD.

Most SSRI trials have been six months or less in duration, so efficacy-based long-term treatment recommendations do not exist. Clinically, many women note the recurrence of premenstrual symptoms after SSRI discontinuation and many clinicians treat women over a long period of time. As reviewed, a few open studies report maintenance of SSRI efficacy over a couple of years (Yonkers 1997). Studies are needed to identify whether or not some women develop tolerance to the SSRI and need a higher dose over time and whether or not some women stay in remission for a period of time following SSRI discontinuation.

Gonadotropin releasing hormone (GnRH) agonists suppress ovulation by downregulating GnRH receptors in the hypothalamus, leading to decreased follicle-stimulating hormone and luteinizing hormone release from the pituitary, resulting in decreased estrogen and progesterone levels. GnRH agonists are administered parenterally (e.g., subcutaneous monthly injections of goserelin, intramuscular monthly injections of leuprolide, and daily intranasal buserelin) (see Figure 29-2). Ten double-blind, placebo-controlled studies of GnRH agonists in PMS and PMDD have been published to date, and GnRH agonists are reported to be superior to placebo in eight of these studies (Johnson 1998, Pearlstein and Steiner 2000). GnRH agonists lead to improvement in most emotional and physical premenstrual symptoms, with possible decreased efficacy for premenstrual dysphoria and severe premenstrual symptoms (Brown et al. 1994), or for the exacerbation of chronic depression (Freeman et al. 1997). After relief of PMS is achieved with a GnRH agonist, "add-back" hormone strategies have been investigated due to the undesirable medical consequences of the hypoestrogenic state resulting from prolonged anovulation. As reviewed, the addition of estrogen and progesterone to goserelin (Leather et al. 1999) and leuprolide (Schmidt et al. 1998) led to the reappearance of mood and anxiety symptoms (Pearlstein and Steiner 2000). Since women with severe PMS and PMDD have an abnormal response to normal hormonal fluctuations (Schmidt et al. 1998), it is not surprising that women in these studies had the induction of mood and anxiety symptoms from the addition of gonadal steroids, reducing the benefit of the replacement strategy.

Danazol, a synthetic steroid, alleviates premenstrual symptoms when administered at 200 to 400 mg q.d. doses that induce anovulation (Hahn et al. 1995). A recent study with danazol 200 mg/day administered during the luteal phase only, not causing anovulation, reported that breast tenderness but not other premenstrual symptoms were reduced (O'Brien and Abukhalil 1999). Prolonged anovulation with estrogen and progesterone administered most of the cycle or oophorectomy are not common treatments, largely due to the medical risks from the prolonged hypoestrogenic state, leading to the same long-term health issues as with GnRH agonists. Oophorectomy should be reserved for women with severe PMS and PMDD, unresponsive to antidepressants or hormonal treatment. In addition, the small literature with estrogen and progesterone administered most of the cycle has yielded mixed reports, (Johnson 1998, Epperson et al. 1999, Pearlstein and Steiner 2000).

Even though oral contraceptives (OCs) are a commonly prescribed treatment for PMS (Campbell et al. 1997, Hylan et al. 1999), there is minimal literature endorsing its efficacy. Anecdotally, women report that OCs may benefit, worsen, or not affect their premenstrual symptoms. As reviewed, the induction of dysphoria may be related to the type and dose of the progestin component, the androgenic properties of the progesterone, or to the estrogen/progestin ratio (Kahn and Halbreich 2001). A more recent RCT compared an oral contraceptive to placebo in 82 women with PMDD (Freeman et al. 2001a). Even though the OC containing ethinyl estradiol 30 μg and drospirenone 3 mg improved most premenstrual symptoms, due in large part to a placebo response rate of 40%, the OC was significantly more efficacious than placebo only in decreasing food cravings, increased appetite, and acne. Oral contraceptives have been reported to not alter the response to SSRIs in women with PMDD (Freeman et al. 2001b).

Alprazolam (administered during the luteal phase) has been reported to be superior to placebo in most studies (Smith et al. 1987, Harrison et al. 1990, Berger and Presser 1994, Freeman et al. 1995) but not all (Schmidt et al. 1993), and although it has a lower efficacy rate than SSRIs, it is effective for premenstrual emotional symptoms. Alprazolam should be tapered over the first few days of menses each cycle. An early (Rickels et al. 1989) and a more recent (Landen et al. 2001) study of buspirone 25 mg/day during the luteal weeks indicate some efficacy. Spironolactone has been reported to decrease premenstrual emotional and physical symptoms (Wang et al. 1995). Bromocriptine has been reported to decrease premenstrual breast tenderness (Andersch 1983). Previous studies reporting efficacy that deserve further study include nonsteroidal anti-inflammatory drugs (Mira et al. 1986), doxycycline (Toth et al. 1988), naltrexone (Chuong et al. 1988), and atenolol (Rausch et al. 1988).

A comprehensive review of 27 RCTs of complementary and alternative treatments in women with PMS reported that no treatment could be recommended on the basis of existent evidence (Stevinson and Ernst 2001). Since the review was published, a randomized controlled trial of *agnus catsups* fruit (chasteberry) in 170 women with PMS reported that chasteberry was superior to placebo in reducing irritability, mood alteration, anger, headache, and breast fullness (Schellenberg 2001). However, the method of diagnosis of PMS in the subjects was not clear in this study.

The largest treatment study to date in women with PMS has been a comparison of calcium 600 mg b.i.d. to placebo (Thys-Jacobs et al. 1998). Calcium was reported to have a 48% efficacy rate for reducing the emotional and physical symptoms of the PMDD diagnostic criteria, except for fatigue and insomnia, compared to 30% for placebo. However, women with concurrent psychiatric illness were not clearly excluded, and other treatments except for analgesics were allowed. The efficacy of calcium was somewhat less in women who were also taking OCs. The results of this study were notable, and calcium deserves further study. There is a study reporting efficacy with tryptophan in PMDD, which has not been available in the United States for a period of time (Steinberg et al. 1999).

Many lifestyle modifications and psychosocial treatments have been suggested for PMS. Lifestyle modifications are often suggested through self-help materials or in an individual or group psychoeducation format. A recent study reported that a weekly peer support and professional guidance group for four sessions was superior to waitlist control in terms of reducing premenstrual symptoms. The treatment consisted of diet and exercise regimens, self-monitoring and other cognitive techniques, and environment modification (Taylor 1999). Studies have not been conducted on individual lifestyle or psychosocial treatments to identify which components are most efficacious.

Dietary recommendations include decreased caffeine, frequent snacks or meals, reduction of refined sugar and artificial sweeteners, and increase in complex carbohydrates. As reviewed, premenstrual increased appetite and carbohydrate craving increases the availability of tryptophan in the brain, leading to increased serotonin synthesis (Pearlstein 1996). One controlled study reported that a drink containing simple and complex carbohydrates was superior to drinks that did not increase tryptophan availability for reducing premenstrual dysphoria, increased appetite, and decreased memory (Sayegh et al. 1995). Other than this study, there have been no published controlled trials of specific dietary regimens.

Exercise is likewise a frequently recommended treatment for PMS that has yet to be tested in a sample of women with prospectively confirmed PMS or PMDD. As reviewed, negative affect and other premenstrual symptoms improve with regular exercise in women in general (Pearlstein 1996, Scully et al. 1998). It is not clear if aerobic exercise is superior to nonaerobic exercise in terms of symptom relief. Cognitive therapy (CT) is reported to be a promising treatment for PMS. Two studies in women with prospectively confirmed PMS has reported superiority of individual CT over a waitlist control (Blake et al. 1998) and superiority of group CT over information-focused therapy for reducing symptoms (Christensen and Oei 1995). As reviewed, a few controlled studies conducted in women with less rigorously defined PMS indicate further support for CT and some support for relaxation therapy (Pearlstein 1996).

Although results of studies of light therapy have been equivocal, a recent crossover study reported that evening bright light for two premenstrual weeks decreased depression and tension (Lam et al. 1999). As reviewed, both light therapy and sleep deprivation may decrease premenstrual dysphoria by correcting abnormal circadian rhythms found in women with PMDD (Parry and Newton 2001). Preliminary controlled studies with massage (Hernandez-Reif et al. 2000), reflexology (Oleson and Flocco 1993), chiropractic manipulation (Walsh and Polus 1999), and biofeedback (Van Zak 1994) have suggested positive efficacy. Acupuncture has not been studied systematically.

Comparison of DSM-IV-TR/ICD-10 Diagnostic Criteria
Premenstrual Dysphoric Disorder is not included in ICD-10. A related condition "premenstrual tension syndrome" is included in Chapter 14 for diseases of the genitourinary system.

References

American College of Obstetrics and Gynecology (2000) *Premenstrual Syndrome. ACOG Practice Bulletin.* American College of Obstetrics and Gynecology, Washington, DC.

American Psychiatric Association (1987) *Diagnostic and Statistical Manual of Mental Disorders*, 3rd ed., Rev. APA, Washington, DC.

American Psychiatric Association (1994) *Diagnostic and Statistical Manual of Mental Disorders*, 4th ed. APA, Washington, DC.

Andersch B (1983) Bromocriptine and premenstrual symptoms: a survey of double-blind trials. *Obstet Gynecol Surv* **38**, 643–646.

Angst J, Sellaro R, Stolar M, et al. (2001) The epidemiology of perimenstrual psychological symptoms. *Acta Psychiatr Scand* **104**, 110–116.

Berger CP and Presser B (1994) Alprazolam in the treatment of two sub samples of patients with late luteal phase dysphoric disorder: a double-blind, placebo-controlled crossover study. *Obstet Gynecol* **84**, 379–385.

Berlin RE, Raju JD, Schmidt PJ, et al. (2001) Effects of the menstrual cycle on measures of personality in women with premenstrual syndrome: a preliminary study. *J Clin Psychiatry* **62**, 337–342.

Blake F, Salkovskis P, Gath D, et al. (1998) Cognitive therapy for premenstrual syndrome: a controlled trial. *J Psychosom Res* **45**, 307–318.

Brown CS, Ling FW, Andersen RN, et al. (1994) Efficacy of depot leuprolide in premenstrual syndrome: effect of symptom severity and type in a controlled trial. *Obstet Gynecol* **84**, 779–786.

Campbell EM, Peterkin D, O'Grady K, et al. (1997) Premenstrual symptoms in general practice patients. Prevalence and treatment. *J Reprod Med* **42**, 637–646.

Case AM and Reid RL (2001) Menstrual cycle effects on common medical conditions. *Compr Ther* **27**, 65–71.

Choi SH, Kang SB, and Joe SH (2001) Changes in premenstrual symptoms in women with schizophrenia: a prospective study. *Psychosom Med* **63**, 822–829.

Christensen AP and Oei TP (1995) The efficacy of cognitive behaviour therapy in treating premenstrual dysphoric changes. *J Affect Disord* **33**, 57–63.

Chuong CJ, Coulam CB, Bergstralh EJ, et al. (1988) Clinical trial of naltrexone in premenstrual syndrome. *Obstet Gynecol* **72**, 332–336.

Critchlow DG, Bond AJ, and Wingrove J (2001) Mood disorder history and personality assessment in premenstrual dysphoric disorder. *J Clin Psychiatry* **62**, 688–693.

Dimmock PW, Wyatt KM, Jones PW, et al. (2000) Efficacy of selective serotonin reuptake inhibitors in premenstrual syndrome: a systematic review. *Lancet* **356**, 1131–1136.

Endicott J (1994) Differential diagnoses and comorbidity. In *Premenstrual Dysphorias. Myths and Realities*, Gold JH and Severino SK (eds). American Psychiatric Press, Washington, DC, pp. 3–17.

Endicott J, Amsterdam J, Eriksson E, et al. (1999) Is premenstrual dysphoric disorder a distinct clinical entity? *J Women's Health Gender-Based Med* **8**, 663–679.

Endicott J and Harrison W (1990) *Daily Rating of Severity of Problems Form*. Department of Research Assessment and Training, New York State Psychiatric Institute, New York.

Epperson CN, Wisner KL, and Yamamoto B (1999) Gonadal steroids in the treatment of mood disorders. *Psychosom Med* **61**, 676–697.

Frank RT (1931) The hormonal causes of premenstrual tension. *Arch Neurol Psychiatry* **26**, 1053–1057.

Freeman EW, Kroll R, Rapkin A, et al. (2001a) Evaluation of a unique oral contraceptive in the treatment of premenstrual dysphoric disorder. *J Women's Health Gender-Based Med* **10**, 561–569.

Freeman EW, Rickels K, Sondheimer SJ, et al. (1995) A double-blind trial of oral progesterone, alprazolam, and placebo in treatment of severe premenstrual syndrome. *J Am Med Assoc* **274**, 51–57.

Freeman EW, Rickels K, and Sondheimer SJ (2001b) Concurrent use of oral contraceptives with antidepressants for premenstrual syndromes. *J Clin Psychopharmacol* **21**, 540–542.

Freeman EW, Rickels K, Yonkers KA, et al. (2001c) Venlafaxine in the treatment of premenstrual dysphoric disorder. *Obstet Gynecol* **98**, 737–744.

Freeman EW, Sondheimer SJ, and Rickels K (1997) Gonadotropin-releasing hormone agonist in the treatment of premenstrual symptoms with and without ongoing dysphoria: a controlled study. *Psychopharmacol Bull* **33**, 303–309.

Girdler SS, Straneva PA, Light KC, et al. (2001) Allopregnanolone levels and reactivity to mental stress in premenstrual dysphoric disorder. *Biol Psychiatry* **49**, 788–797.

Griffin LD and Mellon SH (1999) Selective serotonin reuptake inhibitors directly alter activity of neurosteroidogenic enzymes. *Proc Natl Acad Sci U S A* **96**, 13512–13517.

Guidotti A and Costa E (1998) Can the antidysphoric and anxiolytic profiles of selective serotonin reuptake inhibitors be related to their ability to increase brain 3-alpha-, 5-alpha-tetrahydroprogesterone (allopregnanolone) availability? *Biol Psychiatry* **44**, 865–873.

Hahn PM, Van Vugt DA, and Reid RL (1995) A randomized, placebo-controlled, crossover trial of danazol for the treatment of premenstrual syndrome. *Psychoneuroendocrinology* **20**, 193–209.

Halbreich U, Bergeron R, Yonkers KA, et al. (2002) Efficacy of intermittent, luteal phase sertraline treatment of premenstrual dysphoric disorder. *Obstet Gynecol* **100**, 1219–1229.

Halbreich U and Kahn LS (2001) Are women with premenstrual dysphoric disorder prone to osteoporosis? *Psychosom Med* **63**, 361–364.

Halbreich U and Tworek H (1993) Altered serotonergic activity in women with dysphoric premenstrual syndromes. *Int J Psychiatr Med* **23**, 1–27.

Harrison WM, Endicott J, and Nee J (1990) Treatment of premenstrual dysphoria with alprazolam. A controlled study. *Arch Gen Psychiatry* **47**, 270–275.

Hendrick V, Altshuler LL, and Burt VK (1996) Course of psychiatric disorders across the menstrual cycle. *Harv Rev Psychiatry* **4**, 200–207.

Hernandez-Reif M, Martinez A, Field T, et al. (2000) Premenstrual symptoms are relieved by massage therapy. *J Psychosom Obstetr Gynaecol* **21**, 9–15.

Hylan TR, Sundell K, and Judge R (1999) The impact of premenstrual symptomatology on functioning and treatment-seeking behavior: experience from the United States, United Kingdom, and France. *J Women's Health Gender-Based Med* **8**, 1043–1052.

Joborn C, Hetta J, Niklasson F, et al. (1991) Cerebrospinal fluid calcium, parathyroid hormone, and monoamine and purine metabolites and the blood-brain barrier function in primary hyperparathyroidism. *Psychoneuroendocrinology* **16**, 311–322.

Johnson SR (1998) Premenstrual syndrome therapy. *Clin Obstetr Gynecol* **41**, 405–421.

Kahn LS and Halbreich U (2001) Oral contraceptives and mood. *Expert Opin Pharmacother* **2**, 1367–1382.

Lam RW, Carter D, Misri S, et al. (1999) A controlled study of light therapy in women with late luteal phase dysphoric disorder. *Psychiatr Res* **86**, 185–192.

Landen M, Eriksson O, Sundblad C, et al. (2001) Compounds with affinity for serotonergic receptors in the treatment of premenstrual dysphoria: a comparison of buspirone, nefazodone and placebo. *Psychopharmacology* **155**, 292–298.

Leather AT, Studd JW, Watson NR, et al. (1999) The treatment of severe premenstrual syndrome with goserelin with and without 'add-back' estrogen therapy: a placebo-controlled study. *Gynecol Endocrinol* **13**, 48–55.

Miller MN, Miller BE, Chinouth R, et al. (2002) Increased premenstrual dosing of nefazodone relieves premenstrual magnification of depression. *Depress Anxiety* **15**, 48–51.

Mira M, McNeil D, Fraser IS, et al. (1986) Mefenamic acid in the treatment of premenstrual syndrome. *Obstet Gynecol* **68**, 395–398.

O'Brien PM and Abukhalil IE (1999) Randomized controlled trial of the management of premenstrual syndrome and premenstrual mastalgia using luteal phase-only danazol. *Am J Obstet Gynecol* **180**, 18–23.

Oleson T and Flocco W (1993) Randomized controlled study of premenstrual symptoms treated with ear, hand, and foot reflexology. *Obstet Gynecol* **82**, 906–911.

Parry BL (1997) Psychobiology of premenstrual dysphoric disorder. *Sem Reprod Endocrinol* **15**, 55–68.

Parry BL (2001) The role of central serotonergic dysfunction in the aetiology of premenstrual dysphoric disorder: therapeutic implications. *CNS Drugs* **15**, 277–285.

Parry BL and Newton RP (2001) Chronobiological basis of female-specific mood disorders. *Neuropsychopharmacology* **25**, S102–S108.

Pearlstein T (1996) Nonpharmacologic treatment of premenstrual syndrome. *Psychiatr Ann* **26**, 590–594.

Pearlstein TB, Halbreich U, Batzar ED, et al. (2000) Psychosocial functioning in women with premenstrual dysphoric disorder before and after treatment with sertraline or placebo. *J Clin Psychiatry* **61**, 101–109.

Pearlstein T and Steiner M (2000) Nonantidepressant treatment of premenstrual syndrome. *J Clin Psychiatry* **61**, 22–27.

Pearlstein T and Stone AB (1998) Premenstrual syndrome. *Psychiatr Clin North Am* **21**, 577–590.

Praschak-Rieder N, Willeit M, Winkler D, et al. (2002) Role of family history and 5-HTTLPR polymorphism in female seasonal affective disorder patients with and without premenstrual dysphoric disorder. *Eur Neuropsychopharmacol* **12**, 129–134.

Rausch JL, Janowsky DS, Golshan S, et al. (1988) Atenolol treatment of late luteal phase dysphoric disorder. *J Affect Disord* **15**, 141–147.

Rickels K, Freeman E, and Sondheimer S (1989) Buspirone in treatment of premenstrual syndrome. *Lancet* **1**, 777.

Robinson RL and Swindle RW (2000) Premenstrual symptom severity: impact on social functioning and treatment-seeking behaviors. *J Women's Health Gender-Based Med* **9**, 757–768.

Roca CA, Schmidt PJ, Bloch M, et al. (1996) Implications of endocrine studies of premenstrual syndrome. *Psychiatr Ann* **26**, 576–580.

Sayegh R, Schiff I, Wurtman J, et al. (1995) The effect of a carbohydrate-rich beverage on mood, appetite, and cognitive function in women with premenstrual syndrome. *Obstet Gynecol* **86**, 520–528.

Schellenberg R (2001) Treatment for the premenstrual syndrome with agnus castus fruit extract: prospective, randomised, placebo-controlled study. *Br Med J* **322**, 134–137.

Schmidt PJ, Grover GN, and Rubinow DR (1993) Alprazolam in the treatment of premenstrual syndrome. A double-blind, placebo-controlled trial. *Arch Gen Psychiatry* **50**, 467–473.

Schmidt PJ, Nieman LK, Danaceau MA, et al. (1998) Differential behavioral effects of gonadal steroids in women with and in those without premenstrual syndrome. *N Engl J Med* **338**, 209–216.

Schnurr PP, Hurt SW, and Stout AL (1994) Consequences of methodological decisions in the diagnosis of late luteal phase dysphoric disorder. In *Premenstrual Dysphorias. Myths and Realities*, Gold JH and Severino SK (eds). American Psychiatric Press, Washington, DC, pp. 19–46.

Scully D, Kremer J, Meade MM, et al. (1998) Physical exercise and psychological well being: a critical review. *Br J Sports Med* **32**, 111–120.

Smith S, Rinehart JS, Ruddock VE, et al. (1987) Treatment of premenstrual syndrome with alprazolam: results of a double-blind, placebo-controlled, randomized crossover clinical trial. *Obstet Gynecol* **70**, 37–43.

Steinberg S, Annable L, Young SN, et al. (1999) A placebo-controlled clinical trial of L-tryptophan in premenstrual dysphoria. *Biol Psychiatry* **45**, 313–320.

Steiner M and Born L (2000) Advances in the diagnosis and treatment of premenstrual dysphoria. *CNS Drugs* **13**, 287–304.

Steiner M and Pearlstein T (2000) Premenstrual dysphoria and the serotonin system: pathophysiology and treatment. *J Clin Psychiatry* **61**, 17–21.

Stevinson C and Ernst E (2001) Complementary/alternative therapies for premenstrual syndrome: a systematic review of randomized controlled trials. *Am J Obstet Gynecol* **185**, 227–235.

Sundblad C, Hedberg MA, and Eriksson E (1993) Clomipramine administered during the luteal phase reduces the symptoms of premenstrual syndrome: a placebo-controlled trial. *Neuropsychopharmacology* **9**, 133–145.

Sundblad C, Modigh K, Andersch B, et al. (1992) Clomipramine effectively reduces premenstrual irritability and dysphoria: a placebo-controlled trial. *Acta Psychiatr Scand* **85**, 39–47.

Sundstrom I, Backstrom T, Wang M, et al. (1999) Premenstrual syndrome, neuroactive steroids and the brain. *Gynecol Endocrinol* **13**, 206–220.

Taylor D (1999) Effectiveness of professional–peer group treatment: symptom management for women with PMS. *Res Nurs Health* **22**, 496–511.

Thys-Jacobs S (2000) Micronutrients and the premenstrual syndrome: the case for calcium. *J Am Coll Nutr* **19**, 220–227.

Thys-Jacobs S and Alvir JM (1995) Calcium-regulating hormones across the menstrual cycle: Evidence of a secondary hyperparathyroidism in women with PMS. *J Clin Endocrinol Metab* **80**, 2227–2232.

Thys-Jacobs S, Silverton M, Alvir J, et al. (1995) Reduced bone mass in women with premenstrual syndrome. *J Women's Health* **4**, 161–168.

Thys-Jacobs S, Starkey P, Bernstein D, et al. Premenstrual Syndrome Study Group (1998) Calcium carbonate and the premenstrual syndrome: effects on premenstrual and menstrual symptoms. *Am J Obstet Gynecol* **179**, 444–452.

Toth A, Lesser ML, Naus G, et al. (1988) Effect of doxycycline on premenstrual syndrome: a double-blind randomized clinical trial. *J Intern Med Res* **16**, 270–279.

Treloar SA, Heath AC, and Martin NG (2002) Genetic and environmental influences on premenstrual symptoms in an Australian twin sample. *Psychol Med* **32**, 25–38.

Van Zak DB (1994) Biofeedback treatments for premenstrual and premenstrual affective syndromes. *Int J Psychosom* **41**, 53–60.

Walsh MJ and Polus BI (1999) A randomized, placebo-controlled clinical trial on the efficacy of chiropractic therapy on premenstrual syndrome. *J Manip Physiol Ther* **22**, 582–585.

Wang M, Hammarback S, Lindhe BA, et al. (1995) Treatment of premenstrual syndrome by spironolactone: a double-blind, placebo-controlled study. *Acta Obstet Gynecol Scand* **74**, 803–808.

Wittchen HU, Becker E, Lieb R, et al. (2002) Prevalence, incidence and stability of premenstrual dysphoric disorder in the community. *Psychol Med* **32**, 119–132.

World Health Organization (1993) *International Classification of Diseases*, 10th Rev. World Health Organization, Geneva.

Yonkers KA (1997) Antidepressants in the treatment of premenstrual dysphoric disorder. *J Clin Psychiatry* **58**, 4–10.

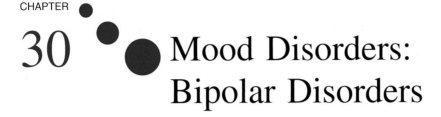

30 Mood Disorders: Bipolar Disorders

Diagnosis

The cardinal symptoms of bipolar disorder are discrete periods of abnormal mood and activation that define depressive and manic or hypomanic episodes. Diagnosis of such episodes is based exclusively on *phenomenology*, the descriptive appearance of the syndrome of interest. One may conceive of phenomenological data for the diagnosis of bipolar disorder as being of two types: *cross-sectional* and *longitudinal*. Cross-sectional data refer to descriptive aspects of a syndrome that occur at a particular point in time, such as the number and type of depressive symptoms that occur during an episode of depression. Longitudinal data refer to the course of symptoms over time, such as the timing, duration, and recurrence of depressive episodes. Both cross-sectional and longitudinal data are essential for the definition of mood disorders and the proper diagnosis of bipolar disorder. It is not infrequent that diagnostic errors occur when longitudinal data are neglected as the clinician focuses solely on cross-sectional presentation: "This must be bipolar disorder because the individual appears manic at the present time," or "This cannot be bipolar disorder because the individual is depressed now."

The DSM-based definition of bipolar disorder is built on the identification of individual mood *episodes* (Table 30-1). It is important to understand that the diagnosis of bipolar disorder derives from the occurrence of individual episodes over time. Persons who experience a manic, hypomanic, or mixed episode, virtually all of whom also have a history of one or more major depressive episodes (Winokur et al. 1969), are diagnosed with bipolar disorder. Those who experience major depressive and manic episodes are diagnosed with *bipolar I* disorder (see DSM-IV-TR diagnostic criteria on pages 798–801), and those with major depressive and hypomanic (milder manic) episodes are diagnosed with *bipolar II* disorder (see DSM-IV-TR diagnostic criteria on page 802).

Table 30-1	Summary of Mood Episodes and Mood Disorders	
Episode	**Disorder**
Major depressive episode	Major depressive disorder, single episode
Major depressive episode + major depressive episode	Major depressive disorder, recurrent
Major depressive episode + manic/mixed episode	Bipolar I disorder
Manic/mixed episode	Bipolar I disorder
Major depressive episode + hypomanic episode	Bipolar II disorder
Chronic subsyndromal depression	Dysthymic disorder
Chronic fluctuations between subsyndromal depression and hypomania	Cyclothymic disorder

DSM-IV-TR Diagnostic Criteria

296.0x Bipolar I Disorder, Single Manic Episode

A. Presence of only one Manic Episode and no past Major Depressive Episodes.

Note: Recurrence is defined as either a change in polarity from depression or an interval of at least 2 months without manic symptoms.

B. The Manic Episode is not better accounted for by Schizoaffective Disorder and is not superimposed on Schizophrenia, Schizophreniform Disorder, Delusional Disorder, or Psychotic Disorder Not Otherwise Specified.

Specify if:

Mixed: if symptoms meet criteria for a Mixed Episode

If the full criteria are currently met for a Manic, Mixed, or Major Depressive Episode, specify its current clinical status and/or features:

Mild, Moderate, Severe Without Psychotic Features/Severe With Psychotic Features
With Catatonic Features
With Postpartum Onset

If the full criteria are not currently met for a Manic, Mixed, or Major Depressive Episode, specify the current clinical status of the Bipolar I Disorder or features of the most recent episode:

In Partial Remission, In Full Remission
With Catatonic Features
With Postpartum Onset

DSM-IV-TR Diagnostic Criteria

296.40 Bipolar I Disorder, Most Recent Episode Hypomanic

A. Currently (or most recently) in a Hypomanic Episode.
B. There has previously been at least one Manic Episode or Mixed Episode.
C. The mood symptoms cause clinically significant distress or impairment in social, occupational, or other important areas of functioning.
D. The mood episodes in Criteria A and B are not better accounted for by Schizoaffective Disorder and are not superimposed on Schizophrenia, Schizophreniform Disorder, Delusional Disorder, or Psychotic Disorder Not Otherwise Specified.

Specify:

Longitudinal Course Specifiers (With and Without Interepisode Recovery)

With Seasonal Pattern (applies only to the pattern of Major Depressive Episodes)

With Rapid Cycling

Reprinted with permission from the Diagnostic and Statistical Manual of Mental Disorders, Fourth Edition, Text Revision. Copyright 2000 American Psychiatric Association.

DSM-IV-TR Diagnostic Criteria

296.4x Bipolar I Disorder, Most Recent Episode Manic

A. Currently (or most recently) in a Manic Episode.
B. There has previously been at least one Major Depressive Episode, Manic Episode, or Mixed Episode.
C. The mood episodes in Criteria A and B are not better accounted for by Schizoaffective Disorder and are not superimposed on Schizophrenia, Schizophreniform Disorder, Delusional Disorder, or Psychotic Disorder Not Otherwise Specified.

If the full criteria are currently met for a Manic Episode, specify its current clinical status and/or features:

Mild, Moderate, Severe Without Psychotic Features/Severe With Psychotic

Features
With Catatonic Features
With Postpartum Onset

If the full criteria are not currently met for a Manic Episode, specify the current clinical status of the Bipolar I Disorder and/or features of the most recent Manic Episode:

In Partial Remission, In Full Remission
With Catatonic Features
With Postpartum Onset

Specify:

Longitudinal Course Specifiers (With and Without Interepisode Recovery)

With Seasonal Pattern (applies only to the pattern of Major Depressive Episodes)

With Rapid Cycling

DSM-IV-TR Diagnostic Criteria

296.6x Bipolar I Disorder, Most Recent Episode Mixed

A. Currently (or most recently) in a Mixed Episode.
B. There has previously been at least one Major Depressive Episode, Manic Episode, or Mixed Episode.
C. The mood episodes in Criteria A and B are not better accounted for by Schizoaffective Disorder and are not superimposed on Schizophrenia, Schizophreniform Disorder, Delusional Disorder, or Psychotic Disorder Not Otherwise Specified.

If the full criteria are currently met for a Mixed Episode, specify its current clinical status and/or features:

Mild, Moderate, Severe Without Psychotic Features/Severe With Psychotic Features

With Catatonic Features

With Postpartum Onset

If the full criteria are not currently met for a Mixed Episode, specify the current clinical status of the Bipolar I Disorder and/or features of the most recent Mixed Episode:

In Partial Remission, In Full Remission

With Catatonic Features

With Postpartum Onset

Specify:

Longitudinal Course Specifiers (With and Without Interepisode Recovery)

With Seasonal Pattern (applies only to the pattern of Major Depressive Episodes)

With Rapid Cycling

DSM-IV-TR Diagnostic Criteria

296.5x Bipolar I Disorder, Most Recent Episode Depressed

A. Currently (or most recently) in a Major Depressive Episode.

B. There has previously been at least one Manic Episode or Mixed Episode.
C. The mood episodes in Criteria A and B are not better accounted for by Schizoaffective Disorder and are not superimposed on Schizophrenia, Schizophreniform Disorder, Delusional Disorder, or Psychotic Disorder Not Otherwise Specified.

If the full criteria are currently met for a Major Depressive Episode, specify its current clinical status and/or features:

Mild, Moderate, Severe Without Psychotic Features/Severe With Psychotic Features

Chronic

With Catatonic Features

With Melancholic Features

With Atypical Features

With Postpartum Onset

If the full criteria are not currently met for a Major Depressive Episode, specify the current clinical status of the Bipolar I Disorder and/or features of the most recent Major Depressive Episode:

In Partial Remission, In Full Remission

Chronic

With Catatonic Features

With Melancholic Features

With Atypical Features

With Postpartum Onset

Reprinted with permission from the Diagnostic and Statistical Manual of Mental Disorders, Fourth Edition, Text Revision. Copyright 2000 American Psychiatric Association.

DSM-IV-TR Diagnostic Criteria

296.7 Bipolar I Disorder, Most Recent Episode Unspecified

A. Criteria, except for duration, are currently (or most recently) met for a Manic, a Hypomanic, a Mixed, or a Major Depressive Episode.
B. There has previously been at least one Manic Episode or Mixed Episode.
C. The mood symptoms cause clinically significant distress or impairment in social, occupational, or other important areas of functioning.
D. The mood symptoms in Criteria A and B are not better accounted for by Schizoaffective Disorder and are not superimposed on Schizophrenia, Schizophreniform Disorder, Delusional Disorder, or Psychotic Disorder Not Otherwise Specified.
E. The mood symptoms in Criteria A and B are not due to the direct physiological effects of a substance (e.g., a drug of abuse, a medication, or other treatment) or a general medical condition (e.g., hyperthyroidism).

Specify:

Longitudinal Course Specifiers (With and Without Interepisode Recovery)

With Seasonal Pattern (applies only to the pattern of Major Depressive Episodes)

With Rapid Cycling

DSM-IV-TR Diagnostic Criteria

296.89 Bipolar II Disorder

A. Presence (or history) of one or more Major Depressive Episodes.
B. Presence (or history) of at least one Hypomanic Episode.
C. There has never been a Manic Episode or a Mixed Episode.
D. The mood symptoms in Criteria A and B are not better accounted for by Schizoaffective Disorder and are not superimposed on Schizophrenia, Schizophreniform Disorder, Delusional Disorder, or Psychotic Disorder Not Otherwise Specified.
E. The symptoms cause clinically significant distress or impairment in social, occupational, or other important areas of functioning.

Specify current or most recent episode:

Hypomanic: if currently (or most recently) in a Hypomanic Episode

Depressed: if currently (or most recently) in a Major Depressive Episode

If the full criteria are currently met for a Major Depressive Episode, specify its current clinical status and/or features:

Mild, Moderate, Severe Without Psychotic Features/Severe With Psychotic
Features
Chronic
With Catatonic Features
With Melancholic Features
With Atypical Features
With Postpartum Onset

If the full criteria are not currently met for a Hypomanic or Major Depressive Episode, specify the clinical status of the Bipolar II Disorder and/or features of the most recent Major Depressive Episode (only if it is the most recent type of mood episode):

In Partial Remission, In Full Remission
Chronic With Catatonic Features
With Melancholic Features
With Atypical Features
With Postpartum Onset

Specify:

Longitudinal Course Specifiers (With and Without Interepisode Recovery)

> **With Seasonal Pattern** (applies only to the pattern of Major Depressive Episodes)
>
> **With Rapid Cycling**

Reprinted with permission from the Diagnostic and Statistical Manual of Mental Disorders, Fourth Edition, Text Revision. Copyright 2000 American Psychiatric Association.

Not surprisingly, most data regarding bipolar disorder come from the study of the more severe end of the spectrum, primarily type I disorder. Throughout this chapter, data on bipolar disorder derive from studies of type I disorder unless otherwise noted. DSM-IV is the first version of the DSM series to include a specific category for bipolar II disorder. Previously, persons with depressive and hypomanic episodes were grouped under the broad "bipolar disorder not otherwise specified," which included a variety of unusual presentations. On the basis of evidence reviewed by Dunner (1993), the disorder was given separate categorical status.

This separation of type II from both type I and major depressive disorders was supported by several types of evidence. For instance, type II disorder occurs more frequently in families of persons with type II in comparison to families of persons with type I or major depressive disorder (Fieve et al. 1984, Coryell et al. 1984, Endicott et al. 1985). Study of the course over time of type II disorder indicated that persons with hypomania tended to have recurrent hypomanic episodes and did not convert into type I by developing mania (Coryell et al. 1995). In addition, persons with type II disorder may have more episodes over time than persons with type I (Dunner 1993), indicating that the course of type II differs from that of type I. However, biological differences between these bipolar types have not been reliably demonstrated (Dunner 1993). Nonetheless, it should not be construed that bipolar disorder type II is in all respects milder than type I, although hypomania is by definition less severe than mania. Specifically, the social and occupational function and quality of life for persons with type II disorder are similar to those for persons with type I disorder.

Persons who experience subsyndromal bipolar mood fluctuations over an extended period without major mood episodes are diagnosed with *cyclothymic disorder* (see DSM-IV-TR diagnostic criteria below). Much less is known about this milder disorder because afflicted persons present for medical attention less frequently than those with full-blown bipolar disorder. Cyclothymic disorder has been considered at various times a temperament, a personality disorder, and a disorder at the milder end of the bipolar spectrum (Akiskal 1981). Available data clearly indicate that cyclothymic disorder is related to the more severe bipolar disorders (Akiskal et al. 1977, Goodwin and Jamison 1990). However, it is not clear to what degree such categorical disorders may be related to underlying dimensional characteristics such as temperament (Akiskal and Akiskal 1988), however vaguely we presently define that construct.

DSM-IV-TR Diagnostic Criteria

301.13 Cyclothymic Disorder

A. For at least 2 years, the presence of numerous periods with hypomanic symptoms and numerous periods with depressive symptoms that do not meet criteria for a major depressive episode.

Note: In children and adolescents, the duration must be at least 1 year.

B. During the above 2-year period (1 year in children and adolescents), the person has not been without the symptoms in criterion A for more than 2 months at a time.
C. No major depressive episode, manic episode, or mixed episode has been present during the first 2 years of the disturbance.
D. The symptoms in criterion A are not better accounted for by schizoaffective disorder and are not superimposed on schizophrenia, schizophreniform disorder, delusional disorder, or psychotic disorder not otherwise specified.
E. The symptoms are not due to the direct physiological effects of a substance (e.g., a drug of abuse, a medication) or a general medical condition (e.g., hyperthyroidism).
F. The symptoms cause clinically significant distress or impairment in social, occupational, or other important areas of functioning.

Reprinted with permission from the Diagnostic and Statistical Manual of Mental Disorders, Fourth Edition, Text Revision. Copyright 2000 American Psychiatric Association.

Mood episodes are discrete periods of altered feeling, thought, and behavior. Typically, they have a distinct onset and offset, beginning over days or weeks and eventually ending gradually after several weeks or months. As noted earlier, bipolar disorder is defined by the occurrence of depressive plus manic, hypomanic, or mixed episodes, or the occurrence of only manic or mixed episodes.

Major depressive episodes are defined by discrete periods of depressed or blue mood or loss of interest or pleasure in life, which typically endures for weeks but must last for at least 2 weeks (see Chapter 28). These symptoms are often accompanied by changes in sleep, appetite, energy, cognition, and judgment. Depressive episodes in bipolar disorder are indistinguishable from those in major depressive disorder. About half of persons with bipolar disorder experience depressive episodes characterized by decreased sleep and appetite, whereas about half experience more "atypical" symptoms of increased sleep and appetite. Recall that the differential diagnosis between major depressive and bipolar disorders is made not by cross-sectional symptom analysis but by longitudinal course. The diagnostic decision tree for bipolar disorder is given in Figure 30-1.

Manic episodes are defined by discrete periods of abnormally elevated, expansive, or irritable mood accompanied by marked impairment in judgment and social and occupational function (see DSM-IV-TR diagnostic criteria below). These symptoms are frequently accompanied by unrealistic grandiosity, excess energy, and increases in goal-directed activity that frequently have a high potential for damaging consequences.

DSM-IV-TR Diagnostic Criteria

Manic Episode

A. A distinct period of abnormally and persistently elevated, expansive, or irritable mood, lasting at least 1 week (or any duration if hospitalization is necessary).
B. During the period of mood disturbance, three (or more) of the following symptoms have persisted (four if the mood is only irritable) and have been present to a significant degree:

  (1) inflated self-esteem or grandiosity
  (2) decreased need for sleep (e.g., feels rested after only 3 hours of sleep)

(3) more talkative than usual or pressure to keep talking

(4) flight of ideas or subjective experience that thoughts are racing

(5) distractibility (i.e., attention too easily drawn to unimportant or irrelevant external stimuli)

(6) increase in goal-directed activity (either socially, at work or school, or sexually) or psychomotor agitation

(7) excessive involvement in pleasurable activities that have a high potential for painful consequences (e.g., engaging in unrestrained buying sprees, sexual indiscretions, or foolish business investments)

C. The symptoms do not meet criteria for a mixed episode.

D. The mood disturbance is sufficiently severe to cause marked impairment in occupational functioning or in usual social activities or relationships with others, or to necessitate hospitalization to prevent harm to self or others, or there are psychotic features.

E. The symptoms are not due to the direct physiological effects of a substance (e.g., a drug of abuse, a medication, or other treatment) or a general medical condition (e.g., hyperthyroidism).

Note: Manic-like episodes that are clearly caused by somatic antidepressant treatment (e.g., medication, electroconvulsive therapy, light therapy) should not count toward a diagnosis of manic–depressive I disorder.

Reprinted with permission from the Diagnostic and Statistical Manual of Mental Disorders, Fourth Edition, Text Revision. Copyright 2000 American Psychiatric Association.

Hypomanic and manic symptoms may be identical, but hypomanic episodes are less severe (see DSM-IV-TR diagnostic criteria for hypomanic episode below). A person is "promoted" from hypomania to mania (type II to type I bipolar disorder) by the presence of one of three features: psychosis during the episode, sufficient severity to warrant hospitalization, or marked social or occupational role impairment. This is an imperfect set of criteria, however, because psychosis may or may not be an integral part of bipolar disorder (see below), because hospitalization may be due to social or personal factors or comorbidities not related to the disorder itself, and because the concept of marked role function impairment is not well operationalized (American Psychiatric Association 1994a, 2000). Overall, however, there is evidence that type II and type I bipolar disorders are separable. From time to time, individual authors propose additional subtypes of bipolar disorder, but these are not formally or consistently recognized.

DSM-IV-TR Diagnostic Criteria

Hypomanic Episode

A. A distinct period of persistently elevated, expansive, or irritable mood, lasting throughout at least 4 days, that is clearly different from the usual nondepressed mood.

B. During the period of mood disturbance, three (or more) of the following symptoms have persisted (four if the mood is only irritable) and have been present to a significant degree:

(1) inflated self-esteem or grandiosity
(2) decreased need for sleep (e.g., feels rested after only 3 hours of sleep)
(3) more talkative than usual or pressure to keep talking
(4) flight of ideas or subjective experience that thoughts are racing
(5) distractibility (i.e., attention too easily drawn to unimportant or irrelevant external stimuli)
(6) increase in goal-directed activity (either socially, at work or school, or sexually) or psychomotor agitation
(7) excessive involvement in pleasurable activities that have a high potential for painful consequences (e.g., the person engages in unrestrained buying sprees, sexual indiscretions, or foolish business investments)

C. The episode is associated with an unequivocal change in functioning that is uncharacteristic of the person when not symptomatic.
D. The disturbance in mood and the change in functioning are observable by others.
E. The episode is not severe enough to cause marked impairment in social or occupational functioning, or to necessitate hospitalization, and there are no psychotic features.
F. The symptoms are not due to the direct physiological effects of a substance (e.g., a drug of abuse, a medication, or other treatment) or a general medical condition (e.g., hyperthyroidism).

Note: Hypomanic-like episodes that are clearly caused by somatic antidepressant treatment (e.g., medication, electroconvulsive therapy, light therapy) should not count toward a diagnosis of manic–depressive II disorder.

Reprinted with permission from the Diagnostic and Statistical Manual of Mental Disorders, Fourth Edition, Text Revision. Copyright 2000 American Psychiatric Association.

It is important to note that the phenomenologic differentiation between hypomania and mania is not as cut-and-dried as one would hope—and as many genetic and biological studies assume. Of the three characteristics by which one is "promoted" from hypomania to mania, only the presence of psychosis is firmly grounded in the characteristics of the individual. The other two characteristics, marked social or occupational role impairment or hospitalization, clearly have components that are primarily external to the individual. If for instance, one individual has relatively mild manic symptoms but is living with a family who is unable to tolerate the behavior, he or she is more likely to be hospitalized. Similarly, the comorbid presence of a severe disorder is more likely to result in hospitalization and a "promotion" from type II to type I disorder. Contrarily, limited insurance benefits, or a more tolerant family increase the probability that a manic syndrome of a given severity will be managed without hospitalization and thus be diagnosed as "hypomania" rather than "mania." Genetic and biological investigators are thus well advised to keep these phenomenological issues in mind when designing studies—otherwise reifying what are psychosocial rather than genetic or biological distinctions may introduce unwarranted variability into their studies.

Classically, mania has been considered to be the opposite of depression: manic individuals were said to be cheery, optimistic, and self-confident. Hence the name bipolar disorder. However, in most descriptive studies, substantial proportions of hypomanic and manic individuals actually exhibit substantial dysphoric symptoms (Bauer et al. 1991, 1994a). Mixed episodes, defined as the simultaneous occurrence of full-blown manic and depressive episodes, are the most prominent example of dysphoria during mania (see DSM-IV-TR diagnostic criteria on page 807). Although it may have been suggested that dysphoric mania

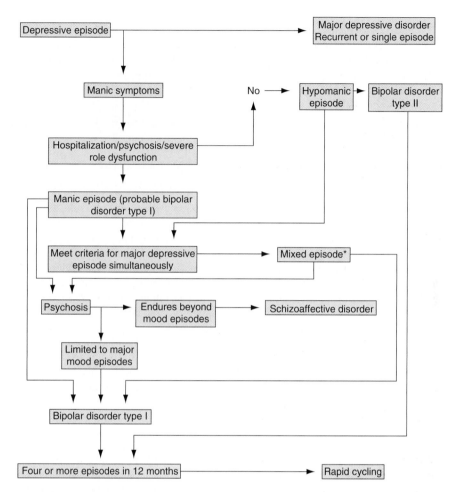

Figure 30-1 *Diagnostic decision tree for bipolar disorder. The building blocks for a diagnosis of bipolar disorder are individual episodes and their characteristics, as summarized in Table 30-1. This decision tree helps the psychiatrist through the steps that lead to diagnosis of manic–depressive disorder and identification of its subtypes. *Does not apply to hypomanic episode as per DSM-IV-TR. (Source: Bauer M, Whybrow P, Gyulai L, et al. [1994a] Testing definitions of dysphoric mania and hypomania: Prevalence, clinical characteristics, and Interepisode stability. J Affect Disord **32**, 201–211; McElroy S, Keck P, Pope H, et al. [1992] Clinical and research implications of the diagnosis of dysphoric or mixed mania or hypomania. Am J Psychiatr **149**, 1633–1644.)*

may constitute a separate subtype of mania (McElroy et al. 1992), the inclusion of this additional dichotomy is premature, and it may be of more use scientifically and clinically to consider dysphoric symptoms dimensionally rather than categorically (Bauer et al. 1994b).

DSM-IV-TR Diagnostic Criteria

Mixed Episode

A. The criteria are met both for a manic episode and for a major depressive episode (except for duration) nearly every day during at least a 1-week period.

B. The mood disturbance is sufficiently severe to cause marked impairment in occupational functioning or in usual social activities or relationships with others, or to necessitate hospitalization to prevent harm to self or others, or there are psychotic features.

C. The symptoms are not due to the direct physiological effects of a substance (e.g., a drug of abuse, a medication, or other treatment) or a general medical condition (e.g., hyperthyroidism).

Note: Mixed-like episodes that are clearly caused by somatic antidepressant treatment (e.g., medication, electroconvulsive therapy, light therapy) should not count toward a diagnosis of manic–depressive I disorder.

Further evidence that (hypo)mania is not the polar opposite of depression comes from investigation of self-reported quality of life in the various mood states of bipolar disorder (Vojta et al. 2001). Although classically thought to be a desirable state, individuals with mania or hypomania rate their preference for that state as equal to or less than their preference for euthymia, with depression and mixed states being rated less preferable. The ratings of quality of life for (hypo)mania were normally rather than bimodally distributed. Thus, the rating was not the average of two disparate groups; rather, (hypo)mania appears simply not to be a desirable state.

Rapid cycling is defined by the occurrence of four or more mood episodes within 12 months (see DSM-IV-TR diagnostic criteria below). It should be noted that, despite the name, the episodes are not necessarily or even commonly truly cyclical; the diagnosis is based simply on episode counting (American Psychiatric Association 1994a). This subcategory is of significance because it predicts a relatively poorer outcome and worse response to lithium and other treatments (Bauer and Whybrow 1993, Bauer et al. 1994c). Although rapid cycling has been considered by some to be an "end stage" of the disorder, empirical evidence indicates that it may have its onset at any time during the disorder (Bauer and Whybrow 1991, 1993, Bauer et al. 1994c) and may come and go during the course of illness (Coryell et al. 1992). Several specific risk factors may be associated with rapid cycling, each of which may give clues to its pathophysiology. These include female gender, antidepressant use, and prior or current hypothyroidism (Bauer and Whybrow 1993, Bauer et al. 1994c).

DSM-IV-TR Diagnostic Criteria

Rapid-Cycling Specifier

Specify if:

With rapid cycling (can be applied to manic–depressive I disorder or manic–depressive II disorder). At least four episodes of a mood disturbance in the previous 12 months that meet criteria for a major depressive, manic, mixed, or hypomanic episode.

Note: Episodes are demarcated by either partial or full remission for at least 2 months or a switch to an episode of opposite polarity (e.g., major depressive episode to manic episode).

Although the diagnosis of bipolar disorder is made on the basis of phenomenology, there are several reasons to conduct a thorough medical history and physical examination. First, there are several general medical or substance-related causes of mania and/or depression that, if treated, may lead to the resolution of the mood episode (see later). Similarly, mania may be the first sign of a general medical illness that will be progressive and serious in its own right. Second, medical evaluation is necessary before starting medications used in the treatment of bipolar disorder. Finally, for many individuals with mental disorders, particularly chronic or severe illnesses, their first contact with medical care as an adult is during the psychiatric interview—often under inpatient or even involuntary conditions. Because mental disorders are clearly not *protective* against medical illnesses, and since even common general medical illnesses may never have been screened for in the past, a thorough medical history and physical examination are necessary parts of the basic care of individuals with bipolar disorder.

Many textbooks recommend a history, physical examination, and laboratory testing for the routine evaluation of persons with mood disorders. Although the history and physical examination are commonsense medical procedures, the use of laboratory testing, particularly routine screening batteries, is supported by few data (Bauer et al. 1993, Agency for Health Care Policy and Research 1993). For instance, using screening for thyroid abnormalities in individuals presenting with depressed mood as an example, Briggs and coworkers (1993) found no evidence that the prevalence of thyroid disorders among ambulatory patients with depression exceeds that in the general population. It was therefore recommended to follow standard screening recommendations for the general population in individuals with depression.

The overall approach to evaluating persons with bipolar disorder for medical problems may be generalized as follows: Persons with mental disorders, including bipolar disorder, should have regular screening for disease detection and health maintenance purposes as recommended for the general population. However, it should also be kept in mind that individuals with bipolar disorder, by virtue of having an often severe and disabling behavioral disorder, are less likely than the general population *to have had adequate medical screening and treatment.* Thus, special care must be made to ensure that health problems are not overlooked and that appropriate treatment or referral is effected. Unfortunately, it is the exception rather than the rule to have well-integrated medical and mental health systems, so that the mental health provider can assume that some effort will need to be expended to ensure adequate care is delivered for individuals with bipolar disorder.

All newly identified individuals with bipolar disorder should undergo a history and if indicated a physical examination. If results of the history or physical examination reveal abnormalities, or if the individual has a mental disorder that is associated with a particular general medical condition, more intensive testing is warranted. A clear example of the last situation is when a person with bipolar disorder who has extensive exposure to lithium presents for treatment; such persons, particularly the elderly, require laboratory testing for renal and thyroid abnormalities that can be caused by lithium treatment.

Alcohol and drug abuse and dependence represent the most consistently described and most clinically important mental disorder comorbidities with bipolar disorder. Whereas rates of alcohol abuse combined with alcohol dependence are from 3 to 13% in the general population, lifetime rates for alcohol dependence from Epidemiological Catchment Area (ECA) data indicate that they are greater than 30% in persons with bipolar I disorder (Regier et al. 1990). Further, ECA lifetime rates for drug dependence in individuals with bipolar I disorder are greater than 25% and rates for any substance abuse or dependence are above 60%. Comparable rates for alcohol, drug, or any substance abuse or dependence in major depressive disorder in ECA data are, respectively, 12%, 11%, and 27%. Thus, bipolar disorder represents an enriched sample for substance use disorders, with substantially greater rates than for the general population or even those with unipolar depression.

The reasons for the co-occurrence of bipolar disorder and substance dependence are not clear. One hypothesis suggests that persons with bipolar disorder self-medicate with drugs or alcohol. According to this hypothesis, individuals blunt the painful symptoms of depression with drugs (McLellan et al. 1985); similarly, they may heighten the manic energy with stimulants (Weiss et al. 1988). Contrarily, they may also use substances to decrease manic symptoms, particularly if the symptoms are predominantly irritable or dysphoric. Alternatively, chronic substance use may convert otherwise unipolar depression into bipolar disorder by inducing substance-induced manic episodes (according to DSM-IV-TR, such persons would not be classified as having bipolar disorder but would be considered to have a substance-induced mood disorder) or by causing chronic central nervous system changes that change the course of the illness irreversibly, as Himmelhoch and colleagues (1976) proposed.

Finally, it is possible that some common genetic predisposition for mood instability is associated with both bipolar mood phenomenology and increased craving for substances, and the predominant phenotypic expression is then determined by other genetic or environmental factors. According to this hypothesis, some persons possessing the gene develop bipolar disorder, some develop substance dependence, and some develop both. Regardless of the mechanism, comorbid substance dependence represents an important clinical challenge for clinicians treating persons with bipolar disorder.

Among children and adolescents, the diagnosis of bipolar disorder is often complicated by less consistent mood and behavior baseline than that occurs in adults (Carlson and Kashani 1988). Little evidence is available regarding course and outcome in children. Available data indicate that, as with adults, mixed or cycling episodes predict more recurrences; unlike in adults, manic and mixed presentations may be associated with relatively shorter episodes compared to depressive presentations (Strober et al. 1995).

Epidemiology

Estimates of the lifetime risk for bipolar I disorder from epidemiological studies have ranged from 0.2 to 0.9% (Fremming 1951, Parsons 1965, James and Chapman 1975, Weissman and Myers 1978, Helgason 1979). The ECA study found a lifetime prevalence rate of 1.2% for combined type I and type II variants (Weissman et al. 1988); this agrees closely with the earlier study of Weissman and Myers (1978), which found 0.6% prevalence for each of the types individually. These rates are approximately tenfold greater than the prevalence rate for schizophrenia and about one-fifth that for major depressive disorder. Little is known regarding the prevalence of cyclothymic disorder.

Unlike major depressive disorder, bipolar disorder has an approximately equal gender distribution (Weissman et al. 1988). Few consistent data are available regarding differences in prevalence across ethnic, cultural, or rural–urban settings. However, one of the more intriguing puzzles is the tendency of bipolar disorder to occur in higher socioeconomic strata than schizophrenia, which tends to aggregate in lower socioeconomic strata. Although many theories have been advanced to explain this phenomenon (Goodwin and Jamison 1990, pp. 169–174), no certain mechanism has been identified. However, several issues are clear. First, the finding is most likely not exclusively due to diagnostic bias (i.e., overdiagnosing persons of lower socioeconomic class with schizophrenia more frequently than bipolar disorder and the converse in persons of higher socioeconomic class). Second, the upward socioeconomic "drift" is not due to highly impaired individuals "dragged" upward by higher functioning family members who are normal or who have adaptive subsyndromal bipolar spectrum characteristics; rather, individuals themselves, at least those with type II disorder, are in many cases highly successful and occupy higher socioeconomic levels (Coryell et al.

1989). Third, the findings are not limited to the United States but have been replicated in European samples as well (Lenzi et al. 1993).

Of particular interest in regard to the epidemiology of bipolar disorder is that the incidence of bipolar disorder (and depressive disorders) appears to have increased since the 1940s (Gershon et al. 1987). Reasons for this are not clear, although environmental factors, either physiological or psychosocial, may be responsible. For instance, exposure to increasingly severe social stressors, or the breakdown of cultural supports that may buffer stresses, may contribute; increases in exposure to putative environmental toxins might also be considered. In addition, in those families afflicted with bipolar disorder across generations, those in later generations tend to have earlier onset. This may be due to changes in genetic loading across generations or to environmental factors either within the family or in the wider environment (McInnis et al. 1993). Regardless of the cause, the increasing incidence and earlier onset of bipolar disorder indicate that this illness is not likely to decrease in importance as a clinical and public health issue.

Course

Outcome in bipolar disorder can be conceptualized according to three separate but inter-related domains: *clinical outcome, functional outcome*, and *illness costs*. Clinical outcome consists of parameters that measure the illness itself, such as symptom severity, episode number, and duration. Functional outcome consists of social and occupational status and subjective quality of life, areas of growing concern in both medical research (Stewart et al. 1989) and mental health research (Wells et al. 1989, Markowitz et al. 1989, Broadhead et al. 1990, National Institute of Mental Health 1992, Massion et al. 1993). Illness costs consist of both direct (treatment) costs and indirect illness costs, which include lost productivity, necessary nontreatment social supports, and nontreatment interventions such as jail and the legal system.

Bipolar disorder has its onset in most persons in adolescence and young adulthood, between the ages of 15 and 30. However, prepubertal mania and first-onset disease in the ninth decade of life are not unheard of. Once developed, multiple episodes are the rule. A review of the literature indicated that the majority of individuals with bipolar disorder have four or more episodes in a lifetime (Goodwin and Jamison 1990). Among rapid-cycling individuals, the basis for the diagnosis is four or more episodes in a year with an average of more than 50 lifetime episodes (Roy-Byrne et al. 1985). There is no typical pattern to episode recurrence, with some individuals having isolated manic, hypomanic, or depressive episodes, others switching from one pole to the other in linked episodes, and still others switching continually from one pole to the other in quasi-cyclical fashion. However, even among rapid-cycling individuals, episodes are rarely periodic. Rather, the pattern is more accurately described by chaotic dynamics (Angst 1981, Gottschalk et al. 1995).

Episode length typically ranges from 4 to 13 months, with depressive episodes typically longer than manic or hypomanic episodes (Goodwin and Jamison 1990, p. 40). Women appear to have more depressive relapses than manic ones, whereas men have a more even distribution (Angst 1978). Also women predominate among rapid-cycling individuals, representing 70 to 90% in most studies (Bauer and Whybrow 1993, Bauer et al. 1994c).

Early estimations of outcome in bipolar disorder were by and large optimistic, based on two types of data. First, bipolar disorder had been separated from *dementia praecox* (schizophrenia) by Kraepelin (1989) on the basis of relatively favorable outcome in terms of remitting versus chronic course of psychosis. Subsequent comparative studies, up until the present day, have found bipolar disorder to have better outcome than schizophrenia in terms of many parameters, including chronicity of symptoms, severity of impairment, and social and occupational function (Lundquist 1945, Petterson 1977, Tsuang et al. 1979,

Brockington et al. 1983, Williams and McGlashan 1987). Second, tremendous optimism accompanied the introduction of lithium treatment for bipolar disorder in the 1960s.

However, this relatively optimistic view, which derived primarily from experience in controlled clinical trials, contrasts with the overall guarded prognosis described by most longitudinal studies in the last three decades, which have been less controlled but more inclusive than formal clinical trials. In the early studies, 62% of bipolar individuals had equivocal to poor outcome (Levinstein et al. 1966) and 45% of manic individuals were chronically ill 6 years after hospitalization (Bratfos and Haug 1968). Another study found only 14.3% to be "well in every way" (Winokur et al. 1969) and another later study found only 24% in "full remission" during follow-up (Tohen et al. 1990).

Although these studies include data from the prelithium era, more recent studies from the lithium era are not terribly reassuring. Approximately 20 to 40% of individuals with bipolar disorder do not respond well to lithium (Prien and Gelenberg 1989), and that proportion may increase to as much as 80% for certain subgroups such as individuals who experience rapid-cycling pattern (Dunner and Fieve 1974, Maj et al. 1989) or mixed manic and depressive episodes (Keller et al. 1986a). When assessed 1.5 years after index hospitalization, between 7 and 32% of bipolar individuals remain chronically ill, depending on polarity of index episode (Keller et al. 1986a). Only 26% of one sample had good outcome after hospitalization for mania, whereas 40% had moderate and 34% had poor outcome (Harrow et al. 1990). The probability of remaining ill at 1, 2, 3, and 4 years after hospitalization for mania was, respectively, 51%, 44%, 33%, and 28% (Tohen et al. 1990). Sixty percent of an ambulatory sample of bipolar individuals had fair to poor outcome based on a global outcome score after 1-year follow-up (O'Connell et al. 1991).

Relatively little is known regarding clinical outcome in bipolar II individuals (Goodwin and Jamison 1990), although they appear to be at least as impaired in terms of relapse as bipolar I individuals. For instance, 70% of bipolar II individuals followed up for 5 years, experienced multiple relapses, whereas only 11% were episode free (Coryell et al. 1989).

Subsyndromal affective symptoms may remain in up to 13 to 34% (Harrow et al. 1990), and substantial interepisode morbidity may remain despite adequate treatment with lithium (Nilsson and Axelsson 1989). It is not clear whether such interepisode pathology represents incompletely resolved major affective episodes, medication side effects, demoralization due to functional impairment, or a combination of these factors (Welner et al. 1977, Nilsson and Axelsson 1989, Gitlin et al. 1989). It should be noted here that side effects are more than a trivial issue, as they may lead to medication discontinuation in 18 to 53%, a figure that is greater in lower socioeconomic classes (Goodwin and Jamison 1990). Thus, clinical outcome in bipolar disorder is heterogeneous, and lithium has not proved to be a panacea.

Substantial levels of functional impairment are also characteristic of bipolar disorder, even when major clinical indices have improved. The book-length study of bipolar individuals in the prelithium era by Winokur and colleagues (1969) documented their sample's functional impairment in detail. For instance, 79% of those employed before their index episode lost their jobs during that episode. Among those with incomplete remission during follow-up, 73% had long-term decrements in occupational status. Even more striking, 25% of those with complete remissions or only infrequent episodes developed similar occupational decrements. In another early study, 60% had less than satisfactory social recovery (Hastings 1958).

In a study of persons with bipolar disorder treated at the National Institute of Mental Health (NIMH), only 41% had returned to their jobs at 3 years of follow-up, and 15% were totally unemployed. Forty-five percent had normal family and social function, 21% evidenced "complete social withdrawal," and 11% "complete family disruption" (Carlson et al. 1974). On a global outcome assessment, 57% were judged recovered, 10% had intermittent episodes, and 28% were functionally impaired with moderate to severe affective symptoms. Dion and coworkers (1988) found that although 80% of their sample of bipolar individuals became symptom free by 6 months after an index major affective episode, only 43% were employed and only 21% were employed at preepisode levels. Harrow and colleagues (1990) found at 1.7 years of prospective follow-up after an index manic episode, that 23% of individuals were continuously unemployed, with 36% underemployed in comparison to preepisode levels. Occupational function was significantly worse than in a comparison group of depressive individuals without history of mania. In addition, 36% showed at least moderate impairment in social function. These deficits were unrelated to the presence of symptoms, with the exception of psychosis, which was associated with profound impairment. Tohen and coworkers (1990) found 28% of subjects unemployed after index hospitalization for mania. Bauwens and associates (1991) found that levels of functional disability correlated both with number of prior episodes and with residual interepisode psychopathology.

Five-year follow-up data from the NIMH Collaborative Program on the Psychobiology of Depression (Coryell et al. 1989) provide evidence that levels of impairment in bipolar type I and type II disorders are similar. This included similarly, fair to very poor work (in 30 and 42% of individuals with types I and II, respectively), marital (30 and 23%), social (45 and 45%), and recreational (45 and 48%) function; sense of satisfaction or contentment (57 and 62%); and overall social adjustment (68 and 62%). More recent analysis of that data set has revealed enduring deficits in educational and occupational status at 5 years of follow-up in a mixed group of bipolar and unipolar individuals, even in those who were recovered for 2 years (Coryell et al. 1993). This led the authors to comment succinctly: "Follow-up studies have usually defined recovery as the absence of symptoms. The present findings show that this convention may result in an overly benign portrayal of outcome" (Coryell et al. 1993, pp. 726).

Much less is known about which characteristics predict functional deficits in bipolar disorder, an issue of some importance in identifying high-risk groups for particular attention. A recent review (Bauer and Whybrow 2001) indicates, surprisingly, that baseline demographic and functional outcome do not predict future functional outcome. However, ongoing depressive symptoms, even to a mild degree, are strongly associated with ongoing functional deficits. The direction of causability is not clear, however. It is plausible that depressive symptoms render individuals less able to function in work and personal roles. It is equally plausible that unemployment, divorce, social isolation, and the like can cause or exacerbate depressive symptoms. In fact, both are likely. In any event, careful attention to functional deficits, depressive symptoms, and their interplay is important to optimizing care and hopefully outcome.

Although there are as yet few available data regarding direct and indirect illness costs for bipolar disorder, the direct treatment costs of bipolar disorder are substantial. Among the major mental disorders, the rate of hospitalization for bipolar disorder is exceeded only by that for schizophrenia (Klerman et al. 1992). If one can extrapolate to bipolar individuals from the data for aggregate mental illness costs (McGuire 1991), 55% of treatment costs derive from public sector services and 45% from the private sector.

It is also clear that substantial loss of productivity, in addition to personal suffering, may occur in bipolar disorder. In mental illness in general, functional impairment was responsible for 55% of the costs of nonaddictive mental illness in the United States in 1986 (Rice et al. 1990). In 1955, the figure was 39% (Fein 1958). Although these figures are derived from different methodologies and assumptions and may not be directly comparable (McGuire 1991), both studies indicate that functional impairment accounts for a substantial component of mental illness costs. It is even more striking that the functional impairment may be responsible for as much as 75% of the costs of affective illness (Stoudemire et al. 1986). Specifically in bipolar disorder, evidence indicates that costs from lost productivity are substantial as well. For instance, 19% of persons with bipolar disorder attempt suicide at some time in their lives (Klerman et al. 1992), thus placing almost one-fifth of persons with bipolar disorder at high risk of loss of life through this one cause alone. Without adequate treatment, a person with bipolar disorder from age 25 years can expect to lose 14 years of effective major activity (e.g., work, school, family role function) and 9 years of life (US Department of Health, Education, and Welfare Medical Practice Project 1979). The indirect costs of this disorder are also high, because 15% of persons with bipolar disorder are unemployed for at least 5 consecutive years and more than 25% of those younger than age 65 years receive disability payments (Klerman 1992). Therefore, it stands to reason that treatments targeted at reducing functional impairment, as well as clinical outcome, can have a substantial impact on the burden of mental illness costs to society and quality of life for the individual and her or his family (National Institute of Mental Health 1992).

Differential Diagnosis

Psychosis can occur in either pole of the disorder. If psychotic symptoms are limited to the major mood episode, the individual is considered to have bipolar disorder with psychotic features. On the other hand, if psychotic symptoms endure significantly into periods of normal mood, the diagnosis of schizoaffective disorder is made. For formal research diagnostic criteria and DSM definitions, 2 weeks of psychotic symptoms during normal mood is sufficient to convert a diagnosis of bipolar or major depressive disorder into schizoaffective disorder, because it is thought that such persons have a clinical course midway between individuals with mood disorders or schizophrenia. However, this cutoff point is fairly arbitrary, and its validity is not well established (Levitt and Tsuang 1988, Blacker and Tsuang 1992). For example, it may be that psychotic symptoms actually represent a separate, comorbid disorder, or they may be integral features of severe bipolar disorder that simply take longer to resolve. Identification of pathophysiological and genetic bases of psychosis and of bipolar disorder will certainly help resolve these issues.

Krauthammer and Klerman (1978) conceptualized secondary mania as mania occurring close on the heels of a specific known physiological insult, such as general medical illness or exposure to mania-inducing pharmacological agents. Which general medical illnesses may cause symptoms of bipolar disorder? Most medical illnesses that affect brain function have been described in case reports or small case series to cause one or another mental disorder. Several general medical illnesses have been associated with the development of bipolar disorder (Table 30-2), although none can be considered specific risk factors. Case reports or case series that propose that a putative causative medical illness is associated with bipolar disorder must be interpreted with caution. For instance, Josephson and MacKenzie (1979) described an association between hyperthyroidism and mania. However, almost all of these individuals had additional factors that most likely contributed to the development of mania, such as a preexisting mood disorder due to a general medical condition or a prior history of mood disorders. Too much thyroid hormone in and of itself is not

Table 30-2	Medical Disorders Commonly Associated with Mania	
Neurologic Disorders	**Endocrine**
Stroke	Hyperthyroidism (in those with preexisting manic–depressive disorder)
Head trauma	Postpartum status
Dementia	
Brain tumors	
Infection (including HIV)	
Multiple sclerosis	
Huntington's disease	

likely to cause mania (Bierwaltes and Ruff 1958). On the other hand, administration of medications has been observed frequently in clinical practice to be associated with the onset of mania, particularly in individuals with preexisting depression. Such medications are listed in Table 30-3. Depressive symptoms may also be associated with certain medical conditions (Table 30-4) and medications or drugs (Table 30-5).

Some controversies have been hotly debated, particularly regarding the role of antidepressants in causing mania and rapid cycling (Prien et al. 1973b, Lewis and Winokur 1982, Wehr et al. 1993, Altshuler et al. 1995). Of particular importance to clinical practice, all efficacious antidepressant treatments have been suspected to cause the induction of mania,

Table 30-3	Treatments and Drugs Commonly Associated with Mania

Antidepressants	**Dopaminergic Agents**
Medications	Levodopa
Bright visible spectrum light treatment	
Electroconvulsant therapy	**Drugs of Abuse**
	Alcohol
Adrenergic Agents	Cocaine
Decongestants	Hallucinogens
Bronchodilators	Amphetamines
Stimulants	Caffeine
Other Agents	
Isoniazid	
Corticosteroids	
Anabolic steroids	
Disulfiram	

Table 30-4	Medical Disorders Commonly Associated with Depression

Neurologic Disorders
Stroke
Head trauma
Dementia
Brain tumors
Infection (including HIV)
Multiple sclerosis
Parkinson's disease
Huntington's disease

Endocrine
Addison's disease
Cushing's disease
Hypothyroidism
Hyperthyroidism
Postpartum status

Cancers
Pancreatic

Metabolic
B_{12}, folate deficiencies
Any Medical Disease that Causes Significant Loss of
    Function or Self-esteem

Table 30-5	Treatments and Drugs Commonly Associated with Depression
High Blood Pressure Medications Alphamethyldopa Clonidine **Ulcer Medications** Cimetadine Ranitidine **Drugs of Abuse** Alcohol Sedatives Amphetamine (withdrawal) Cocaine (withdrawal) Nicotine (withdrawal)	**Hormones** Corticosteroids Oral contraceptives Anabolic steroids **Psychotropic Agents** Benzodiazepines Neuroleptics

with the exception of lithium and the possible exception of psychotherapy. Occasionally, when a new antidepressant is developed, hope is raised that it will be the agent that will not induce mania. Clinical experience has not borne out these early hopes. This caveat for antidepressants also includes nonpharmacological antidepressants such as light and electro-convulsive therapy (ECT). The latter effect is paradoxical, as ECT is also used successfully to treat mania.

Etiology

Dichotomous thinking has characterized the debate over the last decades regarding the causes and pathological bases of bipolar disorder and mental disorders in general. At one time, psychological and biological paradigms were consistently presented as mutually exclusive. Similarly, dichotomous thinking based on nature (genes) and nurture (environment) as the cause of bipolar disorder has at times shaped the approach to the issues. However, it is clear from current data that no single paradigm can explain the occurrence, and variability in course and severity of bipolar disorder. Rather, a more integrative approach to understanding the causes of bipolar disorder is needed, one which recognizes the contributions of varying degrees of importance from several sources.

The various hypotheses regarding the basis of bipolar disorder are presented below as if they were separate and mutually exclusive proposals, with outline and key references provided in Table 30-6. However, our approach to understanding the likely causes of bipolar disorder is not as reductionistic as it might appear. Rather, it derives from the statistical technique of logistic regression, albeit in a qualitative rather than quantitative fashion. That is, if the occurrence of bipolar disorder is the "dependent variable," there may be multiple "independent variables" that contribute to its occurrence. Some independent variables may have a very strong association (i.e., explain a large percentage of the variance), while others may be less important in predicting the dependent variable

Genetic and Congenital Hypotheses

Studies on the genetic basis of bipolar disorder, including both molecular and more traditional studies, are well summarized in two recent reviews (Craddock and Jones 1999, Potash and DePaulo 2000). Available evidence indicates that familial factors are important determinants of who will develop bipolar disorder. Numerous studies have shown that relatives of bipolar *probands* (identified cases) have higher rates of bipolar disorder than controls or unipolar probands (Table 30-7). Overall, rates of bipolar disorder in first-degree

Table 30-6	Major Hypotheses of the Pathophysiological Basis of Bipolar Disorder

Hypotheses	Key References*
Neurotransmitter	
Norepinephrine	Prange (1964)
	Schildkraut (1965)
	Bunney et al. (1972a, b, c)
Dopamine	Goodwin and Sack (1974)
	Crow and Deakin (1981)
Serotonin	Coppen et al. (1972)
	Goodwin and Jamison (1990)
Acetylcholine	Janowsky et al. (1973)
Second-messenger systems	Stahl (2000)
	Sassi and Soares (2002)
Neuroendocrine	
Various	Amsterdam et al. (1983)
Thyroid	Bauer and Whybrow (1990)
Neuroanatomical	Altshuler et al. (2000)
	Brambilla et al. (2001)
	Sassi and Soares (2002)
Cell Degeneration	Manji and Lenox (2000)
Physiological	
Membrane, electrolytes	Goodwin and Jamison (1990)
Biological rhythms, annual	Faedda et al. (1993)
Biological rhythms, circadian	*Wehr et al. (1982)
	Halaris (1987)
Kindling	Post et al. (1986a,b)
Psychosocial Hypotheses	
Stress	Johnson and Roberts (1995)
	Ellicott et al. (1990)
	Leverich (1990)
Psychoanalytic factors	Fenichel (1945)
	Cooper (1985)
	Kahn (1993)
Integrative biopsychosocial hypotheses	Johnson and Roberts (1995)
Hume et al. (1988)	

* The key references are either reviews or well-referenced primary data articles that will provide the reader with an entrance into the area.

relatives (parents, siblings, children) of probands with bipolar disorder are elevated 5 to 10 times over rates found in the general population. In the latter group, the rates are 0.5 to 1.5%, while in the former group, rates are 5 to 15% (Table 30-7).

Interestingly, rates of unipolar depression in first-degree relatives are about twofold elevated over those in the general population. Because of the rate of depression in the general population (5–20%), this means that a twofold increase is a rate of about 20%. Important for genetic counseling, this in turn means that the probability that a bipolar proband will have a unipolar child is greater than the probability that they will have a bipolar child (5–15% versus 20%); note that it is most likely that they will have neither (100 minus 25–35%).

Most genetic research has been done on bipolar I disorder. However, bipolar II disorder also appears to have a familial component. Bipolar II probands have more bipolar I disorder and more bipolar II disorder than unipolar depressives and less type I disorder than type I probands (Endicott et al. 1985, Simpson et al. 1993).

Table 30-7	Rates of Bipolar Disorder in First-Degree Relatives		
Study	**Proband is:**		
	Manic–Depressive	**Unipolar**	**Control**
Taylor et al. (1980)	4.8	4.1	—
Baron et al. (1982)	14.5	3.1	—
Gershon et al. (1982)	8.0	2.2	0.5
Coryell et al. (1985)	7.0	2.8	—
Tsuang et al. (1985)	3.9	2.2	0.2

Familial occurrence does not differentiate between inborn and environmental factors. Familial aggregation could be due to sharing genetic material, nongenetic congenital factors (e.g., similar inherited or acquired intrauterine factors, or exposure to similar perinatal risk factors), or physiologic or psychological environmental factors.

Data from other types of studies indicate that at least part of this risk is due to biological, and likely genetic factors. Twin studies indicate that *monozygotic* twins (derived from a single egg and sperm and therefore having an identical genome) have higher concordance rates for bipolar disorder than do *dizygotic* twins (derived from fertilization of two eggs)—60 to 80% for monozygotic twins versus 20 to 30% for dizygotic twins (Price 1968, Bertelsen 1979). Further, one adoption study showed that rates of bipolar disorder in persons adopted away from their biological families are closer to those in the biological families than the adoptive families (Price 1968, Mendlewicz and Rainer 1977). Finally, linkage studies, as summarized later, have suggested that in certain families bipolar disorder may be linked to specific genes. On the other hand, studies of monozygotic twins also indicate that only 40 to 70% are concordant for bipolar disorder. Thus, although there is clearly a genetic component to this illness, genetics is not destiny. More complex explanations must be sought (DePaolo et al. 1989).

Several *genetic loci*, or locations on chromosomes, have been proposed (Craddock and Jones 1999, Potash and DePaulo 2000) but independent confirmations have been lacking. Overall, the number of families in which a single gene has been associated with bipolar disorder is small. Further, no single locus has been replicated in multiple studies. The disparity in these findings may have several explanations. First, of course, is that the findings are falsely positive due to chance or to methodological problems. Alternatively, different genes may produce bipolar phenotype in different families. Finally, some studies indicate that bipolar disorder is polygenic, rather than due to a single gene (Gershon et al. 1982). It is also likely that genes may confer susceptibility to the disorder without actually determining that the disorder occurs. That is, to have the disorder one must have both the gene and another factor. This other factor may be a genetic (polygenic inheritance), change to the genome, or an environmental (intrauterine, postnatal physiologic, or psychosocial) stressor.

A related approach to investigating genetic contributions to bipolar disorder is to look for differences in genes that code for components of systems thought to be involved in the pathophysiology of the disorder. Chief among such candidate genes have been those responsible for dopamine and serotonin receptors, transporters, and metabolic enzymes (Potash and DePaulo 2000). The recent study by Mundo and coworkers (2001) is interesting in this regard. It showed that individuals who developed manic symptoms when treated with serotonin-active antidepressants had higher rates of the gene coding for a particular form of the serotonin transporter, compared to those similarly treated who did not develop manic symptoms. In addition, several studies have indicated that the gene coding for the norepinephrine-metabolizing enzyme catechol-*O*-methyl transferase (COMT) may be associated with the rapid-cycling form of bipolar disorder (Lachman et al. 1996, Kirov et al. 1998, Papolos et al. 1998).

In addition, though, recent evidence raises the possibility that the expression of a mental disorder that is coded genetically may not be due simply to the presence or absence of specific genes, but rather to modifying pieces of DNA in close proximity to important genes. Specifically, small sections of DNA, three base-pairs in length (called *trinucleotide repeats*), appear to be overrepresented in genetic disorders with prominent psychiatric symptoms, including fragile X syndrome and Huntington's disease. The disproportionate number of trinucleotide repeats are hypothesized to be responsible for over- or underexpression of the candidate gene, ultimately leading to neuropsychiatric symptoms (Petronis and Kennedy 1995). Recent evidence indicates that this may also be the case for bipolar disorder (Lindblad et al. 1998).

There has been little exploration of nongenetic congenital factors that may be responsible for bipolar disorder, although it is reasonable to suppose that intrauterine or perinatal factors that produce brain injury may lead to bipolar mood syndromes, just as head trauma in adult life may lead to mood disorders as well as cognitive impairment. Finally, nonbiologic familial factors have also been considered as etiologic in classic psychoanalytic descriptions such as anger turned inward contributing to depression and mania being a defense against depression (Abraham 1927). More recent work on environmental factors in the development of bipolar disorder has focused on effects of stress on the expression of episodes in already established bipolar disorder rather than on the development of the disorder itself (Post 1992).

It is intriguing in this regard that trinucleotide repeats, may actually change over the postconceptual period (i.e., during development), leading to changes in gene expression (Petronis and Kennedy 1995). This is contrary to classical Mendelian genetic theory, which assumes that genetic material is allocated during conception and cell division followed by the playing out of a genetically derived script, impervious to the impact of environmental factors. In contrast, data on these unstable regions of DNA provides the basis for hypothesizing that environment may actually alter genetic expression and perhaps transmission on to the next generation.

Neurotransmitter Hypotheses

A wide range of hypotheses have been put forward regarding the biological basis of bipolar and other mood disorders. The major hypotheses and their supporting evidence have been recounted in great detail in excellent and still reasonably current review by Goodwin and Jamison (1990). Stahl (2000) and Sassi and Soares (2002) have reviewed these issues in detail using the methodologies more recently available. To be specific, investigators have approached bipolar disorder from neurochemical, neuroendocrine, neuroanatomic, and neurophysiologic vantage points, in addition to the genetic and psychosocial orientations outlined above.

Each of these sets of methodologies has provided heuristically powerful conceptual models that have been tested, refined, and tested again. Each has something of value to contribute regarding the pathologic basis of bipolar disorder. Nonetheless, we do not yet have data to indicate whether the disorder is basically a disorder of a particular neurotransmitter, a particular neuroanatomic locus, or a particular physiologic system. Integration of these hypotheses awaits development of new methodologies for clinical neurobiologic investigations.

By extension from studies of depression and the actions of antidepressant medications, several neurotransmitter hypotheses have been proposed. Predominant among these has been the catecholamine hypothesis, articulated with regard to depression, by Prange (1964) and by Schildkraut (1965). Deficiency of norepinephrine or its effects was postulated to cause depression. A series of studies by Bunney and coworkers (1972a,b,c) explicitly extended these observations to bipolar disorder, proposing that changes in catecholamine function were responsible for the switch to mania.

Dopamine, which has been a prominent focus of schizophrenia research but relatively neglected in affective disorders until recently, has received attention specifically in the study of mania. Dopamine may underlie several of the prominent features of mania, including psychosis (Goodwin and Sack 1974), alterations in activity level (Goodwin and Sack 1974), and reward mechanisms (Crow and Deakin 1981). More recently, demonstration of prominent dopaminergic effects of the antidepressants nomifensine and bupropion have served to generate more attention for the role of dopamine in mood disorders (Kapur and Mann 1992). Serotonin has received somewhat more consistent attention as a substrate of mood disorders, particularly in Europe (Coppen et al. 1972). Attention to serotonin in the United States has increased recently when the relatively selective serotonin reuptake inhibitors fluoxetine, sertraline, and paroxetine were demonstrated to have antidepressant efficacy. A "permissive hypothesis" whereby serotonin alterations permit instability of catechol systems leading to manic and depressive episodes has been articulated in broad strokes by Goodwin and Jamison (1990, pp. 422–423) but has not been extensively developed.

Janowsky and coworkers (1973) proposed that acetylcholine deficits were associated with mania. As with the serotonin hypothesis, this posits that the cholinergic system also interacts with the catecholaminergic system to produce affective instability. Finally, recent evidence also suggests that plasma gamma-aminobutyric acid (GABA) may also be involved in the pathophysiology of bipolar disorder (Benes and Berretta 2001, Post et al. 1992, Petty et al. 1993, 1996).

Second-Messenger System Hypotheses

Much of the effort in investigating neurochemical systems involved in bipolar disorder has focused on the role of postreceptor intracellular mechanisms, known as second-messenger (and sometimes third- and fourth-messengers). This research is well summarized in the recent reviews by Stahl (2000) and by Sassi and Soares (2002). When neurotransmitters bind to postsynaptic neuronal receptors, a series of intracellular events are initiated that are mediated by chemical systems linked to those receptors. The so-called G-proteins link the receptors to second-messenger systems, which, in turn are linked to protein kinases that control the synthesis and operation of cellular components (Sassi and Soares 2002).

The cyclic AMP and phosphatidyl inositol systems are the most extensively studied of these second-messenger systems. Recent data have generated substantial interest in the phosphatidyl inositol system as a possible mediator of the clinical effects of lithium in bipolar disorder, particularly since this second-messenger system is linked to subtypes of adrenergic, serotonergic, dopaminergic, and cholinergic neurotransmitter systems. Specifically, lithium, at therapeutically relevant concentrations has been demonstrated to inhibit phosphatidyl inositol turnover in cultured cell lines and animal studies (el-Mallakh and Li 1993, Lenox and Watson 1994). In clinical studies, persons with bipolar disorder have demonstrated alterations in platelet phosphatidyl inositol levels (Brown et al. 1993) and responsiveness of neutrophil phosphoinositol accumulation (Greil et al. 1991). Cell lines derived from persons with bipolar disorder have been found to exhibit abnormalities of phosphatidyl inositol metabolism (Banks et al. 1990). In a magnetic resonance spectroscopy (MRS) study of persons with bipolar disorder, phosphomonoester levels were found to be higher when in the manic state than in remission or in normal controls (Kato et al. 1994, Deicken et al. 1995).

Neuroendocrine Hypotheses

Neuroendocrine hypotheses have sought to elucidate important mechanisms in the production and maintenance of symptoms rather than identify a specific etiologic agent in bipolar or other mood disorders. These hypotheses were developed from the literature on stress response in otherwise normal subjects (Mason 1975). Typical neuroendocrine studies investigate peripheral or cerebrospinal fluid abnormalities of a particular system in persons with mood disorders and in controls, and propose that either the neuroendocrine system itself or the neurotransmitter system that controls the hormone is in some way linked to the pathophysiology of the mood disorder of interest. Perhaps the most complete battery of neuroendocrine assessments in bipolar disorder was conducted by Amsterdam and colleagues (1983). Taken together, the literature does not identify particular endocrine findings as characteristic of bipolar disorder.

The thyroid axis may be of particular relevance to the pathophysiology of mood disorders (Bauer and Whybrow 2001), since it serves not only as a dependent variable that is studied as a function of mood (as most neuroendocrine systems have been), but because the thyroid axis has also been studied as an independent variable of some impact. Several studies have shown that thyroid hormone administration may actually ameliorate mood disorders in certain paradigms. Specifically, there is evidence that the thyroid hormone triiodothyronine (T_3) may speed the response of individuals with depression to antidepressant treatment and may convert nonresponders to responders (Joffe et al. 1993). Further, in the rapid cycling variant of bipolar disorder, evidence indicates that supplementation with high doses of the thyroid hormone thyroxine (T_4) may induce remission in persons who are refractory to standard pharmacotherapy (Bauer and Whybrow 1990). In both these types of studies, response to thyroid supplementation occur in subjects regardless of whether they had preexisting thyroid disease.

The mechanism for these effects has been the subject of much speculation. Various models posit that the brain is functionally hypothyroid either due to changes in hormone synthesis, transport, or metabolism, or due to increased demand; alternatively, other models propose that the brain has an excess of a thyroid-related substance, which is dimished by administration of exogenous thyroid hormone (Bauer and Whybrow 1990, 2001, Joffe et al. 1993).

Neuroanatomic Hypotheses

Two main types of studies have provided information on the possible neuroanatomic bases of bipolar disorder. In the first type, brains of persons with brain injuries who develop a phenomenologically bipolar picture have been analyzed, often neuropathologically, to determine sites of injury that may have produced the bipolar clinical picture. For example, lesions of the right side of the brain, particularly frontotemporal lesions, may be associated with manic-like syndromes (Starkstein et al. 1988).

In the second type of study, persons with bipolar disorder who do not have a known organic basis for their illness are studied either with *anatomic* (computerized tomography, magnetic resonance imaging [MRI]) or *functional* imaging (single photon or positron-emission tomography, or functional MRI or spectroscopy [MRS]) to identify regions of abnormality.

Among anatomic studies, abnormalities of computerized tomography (Nasrallah et al. 1989, Strakowski et al. 1993a,b) and subcortical (Jurjus et al. 1993a, Strakowski et al. 1993a,b) MRI have demonstrated abnormalities in persons with bipolar disorder. However, not all findings have been replicated (Jurjus et al. 1993b) and the findings may not be specific for bipolar disorder. Further, the degree to which anatomic abnormalities reflect pathogenic factors, as opposed to end organ damage or effects of chronic medication usage, has yet to be established.

MRI studies have been an area of intense interest over the past several years, with particular interest in the size of the temporal lobes, limbic system, basal ganglia, ventricles, and total brain volume. Unfortunately, no consistent findings have emerged (Altshuler et al. 2000, Brambilla et al. 2001, Hauser et al. 2000, Sassi and Soares 2002).

Among functional imaging studies, blood flow, glucose metabolism, and more recently functional MRI/MRS and neurotransmitter binding have been the major variables of interest. In studies using blood flow methodologies, frontal (Buchsbaum et al. 1986) and temporal (Post et al. 1987) cortical structures have been the site of abnormalities in bipolar disorder, while among subcortical areas the caudate has received the most attention (Baxter et al. 1985). Although no consistent evidence has emerged regarding a single neurotransmitter system or a single brain region, some promising results have recently emerged regarding serotonin 5-HT1A receptor levels in several brain regions (Drevets et al. 1999).

Cell Degeneration and Neuroprotective Effects of Medications

One of the most exciting areas of recent research focuses on the possibility that lithium and perhaps certain anticonvulsants such as valproate may actually exert a *neuroprotective* effect in bipolar disorder. Evidence indicates that these agents may protect nerve cells by stimulating production of protective proteins or by stimulating nerve growth (Manji and Lenox 2000). Interestingly, there is some clinical evidence from MRI that lithium treatment may actually increase total brain gray matter, although this will of course require replication (Manji and Lenox 2000). Thus, it is possible that cellular degeneration, albeit not as virulent as in Alzheimer's, may play a role in bipolar disorder.

Hypotheses Regarding Complex Physiologic Systems

Several complex systems, which for want of a better alternative are grouped together in this section as "physiologic" systems, have been postulated to play a pathogenic role in bipolar disorder. Classic theories of membrane and electrolyte balance (Goodwin and Jamison 1990, pp. 467–481) abnormalities have been extensively investigated in the past but appear, for the time being, to have passed out of favor. Two other hypotheses regarding complex systems have been of interest over the years: the biological rhythms and kindling theories.

Biological Rhythms

Two types of data indicate that biological rhythms may play a role in the pathogenesis of bipolar disorder. First, there are a large number of observational studies that have demonstrated seasonal peaks in the onset of affective episodes or hospitalizations for mood disorders. For bipolar disorder, the predominant seasons appear to be spring and fall (Goodwin and Jamison 1990, Kamo et al. 1993), although other patterns may occur with some consistency across years (Faedda et al. 1993). Seasonal affective disorder in which persons become depressed and remit at specific, regular times of year, has been codified in DSM-IV-TR by applying the course modifier "seasonal pattern" to recurrent mood disorders (Bauer and Dunner 1993). Although the relationship of seasonal affective disorder, particularly the winter depression variant, to bipolar disorder is not yet clear, there does appear to be some overlap. For instance, in most studies, a large percentage of persons with seasonal affective disorder have bipolar disorder. In addition, the clinical picture of winter depression is similar to the hypersomnolent, anergic, hyperphagic depression common in bipolar disorder (Bauer and Dunner 1993). Further, treatment with bright light has been shown to be efficacious in winter depression (Terman et al. 1989) and also appears to be an effective antidepressant in nonseasonal bipolars treated in the winter (Deltito et al. 1991) and perhaps in the summer (Bauer 1993); bright light also appears to be capable of inducing manic symptoms as do other antidepressants (Bauer et al. 1994b).

The second type of data, which may provide a mechanism for seasonal patterns is that persons with bipolar disorder often exhibit abnormalities of circadian or daily rhythms. Many rhythmic parameters have been studied in persons with bipolar and other mood disorders, with various abnormalities found regarding the *amplitude* (height of the rhythm) and *phase* (timing of the rhythm) (Halaris 1987). Among the most promising findings is that light sensitivity to suppression of the rhythmic hormone melatonin may be altered in persons with bipolar disorder (Lewy et al. 1980, 1985) and their relatives (Nurnberger et al. 1989).

One of the most prominent biological rhythms, sleep, has also been implicated in the pathogenesis of bipolar disorders. However, it should be noted that it is not clear whether it is the rhythmic aspects of sleep or its nonrhythmic, restorative components that are most relevant. One of the most striking findings in mania is the lack of need for sleep and there is evidence that sleep deprivation may be both antidepressant and promanic (Wehr et al. 1982). Thus, further exploration of sleep disturbance in bipolar disorder, both as a dependent and an independent variable, is warranted.

Kindling Models

The second major hypothesis involving complex physiologic systems proposes an analogy between the occurrence of episodes in bipolar disorder and seizures in animal models of epilepsy. Post and coworkers (1985, 1986a,b) have proposed that an autonomous pattern of affective episodes in bipolar disorder may develop from increasing sensitization of an individual to stressors. This process was proposed to be similar to kindling in animals and humans, in which subthreshold convulsant stimuli can decrease the threshold for seizures and eventually lead to spontaneous seizures. An analogy was also drawn between mood episodes in bipolar disorder and behavioral sensitization in animals, in which repeated exposure to pharmacological stimuli can decrease the threshold for specific behavioral responses.

There are several attractive aspects to this hypothesis. It is supported by the increased frequency of episodes over the course of bipolar disorder (Angst 1981) and the response of many persons with bipolar disorder to treatment with the anticonvulsants carbamazepine and valproate. However, the clinical data in support of this heuristically powerful conceptual paradigm are at this point quite limited (Bauer and Whybrow 1991). Thus, it is not clear whether the increase in episode frequency sometimes seen is due to accumulating damage from prior episodes, or is simply the unfolding over time of what was destined from the beginning to be a malignant case of the illness.

Stress and Bipolar Disorder

The possible association of stressful life events and the onset of depression has generated substantial interest among researchers from various theoretical backgrounds (Brown et al. 1977, 1989, Beck et al. 1979, Klerman et al. 1984, Perris 1984a,b,c, Paykel and Cooper 1992, Johnson and Roberts 1995). Most of the literature regarding analysis of the relationship between stressful life events and bipolar disorder has focused on the precipitation of episodes in established bipolar disorder rather than the onset of the disorder *de novo*.

Hall and coworkers (1977) in a prospective study of persons with bipolar I disorder found no difference in life events among those who became manic, those who became depressed, and those who remained well; the only exception was a somewhat increased incidence of work difficulties in those who developed manic symptoms. In a prospective study, Sclare and Creed (1990) found no difference in events prior to and subsequent to admission for mania. In contrast, a retrospective study by Kennedy and coworkers (1983) reported an increased rate in adverse life events not directly related to illness in the 4 months preceding admission to the hospital for mania compared to 4 months after. In a prospective study, Hunt and coworkers (1992) found a several fold increase in adverse life events the month prior to manic or depressive relapse, compared to baseline, without difference between manic and depressive relapses. In a prospective study, Ellicott and coworkers (1990) found that there were subgroups of persons with bipolar disorder who had varying thresholds of sensitivity to stress, and identified a significant association between stressful life events and the onset of mood disturbance. Of interest was that medication levels and compliance with treatment regimes did not account for any of the variance in outcome. Leverich (1990) also identified several factors, including stressful life events, associated with mood disturbance during the maintenance medication prophylaxis of mood disorders in general.

Thus, there are several studies that demonstrate a relationship between stressful life events and the onset of affective episodes in already established bipolar disorder. However, several studies failed to find meaningful associations. There are also several types of methodological problems that may make interpretation of the studies difficult, and comparison across studies impossible. Examples of such problems include recall bias in retrospective design, and in both retrospective and prospective studies sample heterogeneity, length of time window for identification of relevant events, definition of onset of mood episode, and choice of signal event (e.g., hospitalization versus onset of episode). Further, within prospective studies, differences in attribution and recall can be significantly different depending on whether a person is interviewed for life events prior to or after the index episode has commenced.

Thus, it is likely that adverse life events are associated with mood episodes, particularly those episodes that are sufficiently severe to warrant hospitalization. In this respect, such life events need to be attended to for clinical purposes. However, from a theoretical point of view it is not clear that such events actually play a pathogenic role.

Psychosocial Hypotheses

The psychological theories of mood disorders are broad in scope, and have included psychoanalytic, interpersonal, and cognitive–behavioral. These theories propose that the symptoms of mood disorders are produced by psychological factors, with biological components playing at most a secondary role in the expression of symptoms. Unfortunately, the bulk of theory regarding the psychological basis of mood disorders concerns depression, with little attention as yet to mania or bipolar disorder.

Psychobiological Hypotheses

Successful treatment of bipolar disorder with medications has made the biological basis of this disorder incontrovertible. Nonetheless, psychosocial factors may play prominent roles in the development of bipolar disorder and, once established, in its course. Several models that integrate psychological factors and biological mechanisms have been developed. These have been well reviewed recently by Johnson and Roberts (1995).

Several examples illustrate the diversity of these proposals. As described above, the kindling model proposes that discrete environmental stressors may be translated into enduring neurobiological changes that are responsible for mood episodes in bipolar disorder. Ehlers and coworkers (1988) have proposed that the regulation of biological rhythms in persons with bipolar disorder may be disrupted by changes in psychosocial events. Specifically, they propose that mood episodes cause disruptions in social rhythms (e.g., eating, sleeping, and other aspects of one's daily routine). They propose that these social rhythms are important regulators of biological circadian rhythms and without these regulators abnormalities of circadian develop, leading to the onset, worsening, or perpetuation of mood symptoms. Depue and colleagues (1985), Depue and Iacono (1989) have proposed that mood disordered individuals, including those with bipolar spectrum disorders, have deficits in the regulation of biological responses to stress. Thus, environmental stressors may cause disruptions of biological systems that cause mood symptoms in vulnerable individuals, even though similar stressors may not cause disruptions in those without mood disorders.

Hume and colleagues (1988) have proposed another stress-vulnerability model specifically for bipolar disorder in which the threshold for commencement of mood symptoms, particularly in bipolar disorder, is influenced by a combination of the "perception" one has of stressful life events and a vulnerable biochemical mood regulatory system. Thus, adverse life events, coupled with both psychological and biological vulnerability, are required to produce both the mood and the somatic symptoms of depression. Similar to cognitive theorists, Hume described attributions regarding the cause of adverse events, particularly one's control over events (Rotter 1966), as particularly important in producing the psychological vulnerability to depression and bipolar disorder. However, they do not describe specific mechanisms by which manic, as opposed to depressive, symptoms may be produced.

Treatment

Traditionally, treatment for bipolar disorder has been categorized as acute versus prophylaxis, or maintenance; that is, treatment geared toward resolution of a specific episode versus continued treatment to prevent further symptoms. Treatment can also be considered along several other lines (Table 30-8). For instance, interventions can be categorized as somatotherapy (pharmacotherapy, ECT, and light treatment) and psychotherapy. In addition, treatment can be categorized according to intensity. The division into inpatient versus outpatient treatment is becoming more and more blurred as partial or day hospital programs and intensive ambulatory treatment coupled with night hospital programs or respite beds become more popular.

In general, more structured treatment settings, such as full or partial hospitalization, are indicated if individuals are likely to endanger self or others, if bipolar disorder is complicated by other mental disorders or general medical conditions that make ambulatory management particularly dangerous, or if more aggressive management is desired than is easily available on an ambulatory basis (e.g., intensive psychosocial intervention or rapid dosage titration of psychotropic agents). In addition, although it is frequently an afterthought in textbooks, social factors play an important role in the decision to hospitalize in the real world. Such reasons may include lack of social support to ensure medication compliance during acute illness, social stresses aggravating symptoms and making treatment compliance difficult (e.g., manipulative or hostile living situation), or lack of transportation to accommodate frequent ambulatory appointments during acute illness. Unfortunately, it is sometimes the case, although less frequent in this era of managed care, that a

Table 30-8	Classification Schemata for Bipolar Disorder Treatment and Its Goals

1. Acute versus maintenance
2. Somatic versus psychotherapeutic
3. The intensity-of-care continuum*
   (a) Full hospitalization
   (b) Partial or day hospitalization
   (c) Night hospitalization or respite beds
   (d) Ambulatory care
4. Categorization by goal
   (a) Improve clinical outcome
   (b) Improve functional outcome
   (c) Improve host factors
     (i) Illness management skills
     (ii) Medical and psychiatric comorbidities

person's insurance plan covers inpatient but not ambulatory mental health treatment, forcing expensive inpatient care when less costly, time-limited, intensive ambulatory care would suffice.

Finally, treatment can be categorized according to its goals. Treatment can be focused on improving clinical outcome (episodes and symptoms) or functional outcome (social and occupational function and health-related quality of life). Although this categorization appears straightforward, clinical practice reveals many subtleties. For instance, it is erroneous to assume that clinical outcome is the domain of pharmacotherapy and that functional outcome is the domain of psychotherapy. In actuality, most psychotherapies by design focus on improving symptoms. Likewise, pharmacotherapeutic stabilization of symptoms clearly contributes to improved role function. Further, treatments that improve one domain may cause decrements in another. For instance, effective maintenance treatment with lithium may come at the cost of hand tremor, which interferes with work function and causes embarrassment in social situations.

Balancing the costs and benefits of various specific treatments—and every somatic and psychotherapeutic treatment has both costs and benefits—requires active participation of the person with bipolar disorder and, if available, his or her family (Bauer and McBride 2002). Compassionate psychoeducation and alliance building are integral goals of each form of treatment. In analogy to infectious disease treatment, attention to such host factors can often make the difference between success and failure of treatment.

Somatotherapy

The introduction of lithium for the treatment of bipolar disorder in the 1960s revolutionized management of the illness. Before that, bipolar disorder was managed with treatment targeted only toward resolution of individual episodes: antidepressants and ECT for depressive episodes, and neuroleptics and occasionally ECT for mania. In contrast, not only did lithium provide an additional treatment for acute mania and depression in bipolar disorder, it was also demonstrated to have substantial prophylactic, or preventive, effects on both manic and depressive episodes. An overview of efficacy and side effect data for mood stabilizers is provided here. The reader is also referred to an extensive summary in the book by Bauer and McBride (2002).

In evaluating the effectiveness of the various treatments for bipolar disorder, we have found it useful to propose an explicit definition for the term "mood stabilizer" and evaluate the role of various medications against this definition. The US Food and Drug Administration (FDA) does not formally define the term, but it stands to reason that an agent would be optimally useful for treatment of bipolar disorder if it had efficacy in four roles: (a) treatment of acute manic symptoms, (b) treatment of acute depressive symptoms, (c) prophylaxis of manic symptoms, and (d) prophylaxis of depressive symptoms. This approach leads to the conceptual 2×2 table illustrated in Table 30-9. Agents used in bipolar disorder can be listed in any or all of the four boxes in the table in which they have proven efficacy, and according to this schema, an agent may be categorized as a mood stabilizer if it can be listed as having efficacy in each of the four boxes.

We have reviewed the available peer-reviewed literature on treatment trials for four types in bipolar disorder published in December 2001, (Bauer and McBride 2002). Following the FDA lead of considering an agent to have efficacy with at least two such positive trials, we have listed the agents according to the revised 2×2 table in Table 30-9. Complete analysis to date can be found in Bauer and McBride (2002).

As can be seen, at least two placebo-controlled randomized controlled trials support the antimanic efficacy of lithium (Maggs 1963, Bunney et al. 1968, Goodwin et al. 1969, Stokes et al. 1971), carbamazepine (Ballenger 1978, 1980), valproate (Emrich et al. 1980, Pope et al. 1991, Bowden et al. 1994), olanzapine (Tohen 1999, 2000), and verapamil

Table 30-9	Summary of Efficacy Data from Randomized Controlled Trials for Treating the Various Phases of Bipolar Disorder* (At Least 2 Placebo-Controlled Trials)	
	Mania	**Depression**
Acute	Lithium	Lithium
	Carbamazepine	Lamotrigine
	Valproate	
	Olanzapine	
	Verapamil	
Prophylaxis	Lithium	Lithium

Source: Summarized from Bauer MS and McBride L (2002) *Structured group psychotherapy for manic–depressive disorder: The life goals program*, 2nd ed. F. A. Davis Company, New York.

(Giannini et al. 1984, Dubovsky 1986). There are additional randomized controlled trials (nonplacebo-controlled) that support efficacy for multiple older, typical neuroleptics as well as the benzodiazepines, lorazepam, and clonazepam.

In contrast to evidence regarding acute mania, evidence is scarce concerning efficacy of specific agents for acute depressive episodes. Most treatment is undertaken primarily by extension from treatment experience in unipolar depression. While a comprehensive discussion of evidence for efficacy of various antidepressants in unipolar depression is clearly beyond the scope of this chapter, it has been amply reviewed in several references (Gareri et al. 2000, Thase and Sachs 2000). Efficacy data from two or more randomized controlled studies exist only for lithium (Fieve et al. 1968, Goodwin et al. 1969, 1972, Baron et al. 1975, Mendels 1976) and lamotrigine (Calabrese et al. 1999, Bowden et al. 1999). Support for the efficacy of valproate and carbamazepine in acute depressive episodes in bipolar disorder is notably lacking.

In reviewing studies of agents for the prophylaxis of manic or depressive symptoms, we discovered that most of the studies reported recurrence rates without distinguishing between manic and depressive symptoms. For instance, some studies reported such statistics as time-to-first-episode without specifying whether the first episode was manic or depressed. Other studies reported summary statistics for affective symptoms without separating manic or depressive symptoms. We found that when studies did report specific polarity of symptoms during recurrence, it was infrequent that they reported impact of treatment on recurrence of depressive symptoms. Far and away, the most placebo-controlled support for any prophylactic agent comes from studies of lithium (Baastrup and Schou 1967, Coppen et al. 1971, Cundall et al. 1972, Stallone et al. 1973, Prien et al. 1973a,b, Fieve et al. 1976, Dunner et al. 1976) including studies of relapse prevention for depression (Fieve et al. 1976, Stallone et al. 1973, Kane et al. 1982), with support from controlled trials that are not placebo-controlled for carbamazepine and lamotrigine. The one prophylaxis study of valproate (Bowden et al. 2000) showed no difference from placebo (lithium was also found to be no different from placebo in this study, although the study was under-powered to make definitive conclusions about this comparison).

Thus, in summary, this standardized evidence-based review of available treatments for bipolar disorder indicates that, to date, only lithium fulfills the stringent definition of a mood stabilizer. It is hoped that additional agents soon take their place in the ranks based on high quality data.

It may be surprising that, given the paucity of data on treatment of acute depression and prophylaxis of bipolar disorder, we frequently encounter many other medications used chronically in this illness, sometimes as first-time agents, for instance, valproate and carbamazepine. Although neuroleptics have acute antimanic evidence, despite the fact that there is little evidence for prophylactic efficacy, they are often used chronically. This is because these agents are typically started during the course of an acute manic episode and clinicians are loathe to stop them and switch to a different agent such as lithium. In addition, many individuals have failed or have been intolerant of treatment with lithium and they are therefore treated using the "next best thing." This is not necessarily suboptimal treatment. However, it is important that the clinician recognize that data on long-term prophylactic efficacy is quite scanty for these agents—as it is for many other agents used in clinical practice.

Several additional issues in prophylaxis of bipolar disorder deserve comment. First, when is lifetime, or at least long-term, prophylaxis warranted? After one manic episode? One hypomanic episode? One depressive episode with a strong family history of bipolar disorder? There is insufficient empirical evidence with which to make strong recommendations, although a creative study by Zarin and Pass (1987) using computer-based modeling investigated tradeoffs of treatment versus observation based on costs and benefits of recurrence risks and drug side effects under several strategies. In clinical practice without clear guidelines, such decisions need to take into account the capability of the individual and family in reporting symptoms, rapidity of onset of episodes, episode severity, and associated morbidity. Clearly, the risks of a wait-and-see strategy would be different in a person who had a psychotic manic episode than in a person who had mild hypomania.

Second, can lithium ever be discontinued? Again, there are no solid data on which to base this decision. However, if lithium discontinuation is contemplated, there is evidence that rapid discontinuation (in less than 2 weeks) is more likely to result in relapse than slow taper (2–4 weeks), with relapse rates higher in type I individuals than in type II individuals (Faedda et al. 1993, Suppes et al. 1993). In type II individuals, relapse rates for rapid discontinuation versus slow taper were, respectively, 96 and 73%, whereas in type II individuals they were 91 and 33% (Faedda et al. 1993). There is some theoretical concern, based on a report of four individuals, that individuals in whom lithium has been discontinued may not be recaptured by resumption of lithium (Post et al. 1992), but these are preliminary observations on a sample from the NIMH that may not be representative of persons with bipolar disorder seen in general clinical practice.

Third, a set sequence of treatment for refractory bipolar disorder has yet to be established. In particular, persons with rapid cycling represent a treatment dilemma (Bauer 1994). Although antidepressants may induce rapid cycling, they often leave the person in a protracted, severe depression. Switching from one antimanic agent to another often results in resumption of cycling. Complex treatment strategies may be required, such as anticonvulsants plus lithium, combinations of anticonvulsants, or adjuvant treatment with high doses of the thyroid hormone thyroxine.

A treatment algorithm for refractory bipolar disorder, including strategies to deal with rapid cycling is found in Figure 30-2. It is derived from clinical practice guidelines from the US Veteran's Administration and, by design, primarily specifies drug classes rather than individual agents. The entry point for this algorithm is the occurrence of any major mood episode (depression, hypomania, mania, or mixed episode) in an unmedicated individual. Individuals with recurrence on medications may enter the algorithm at the appropriate point along the flow diagram. For simplicity of presentation, only depressive and cycling outcomes are illustrated. This is because depressive episodes are more common than manic or hypomanic episodes, and all but the most refractory of the latter episodes are relatively easily treated by the addition (or resumption) of lithium or anticonvulsants or the use of neuroleptics, as summarized above.

All psychotropic medications have side effects. Some are actually desirable (e.g., sedation with some antidepressants in persons with prominent insomnia), and specific

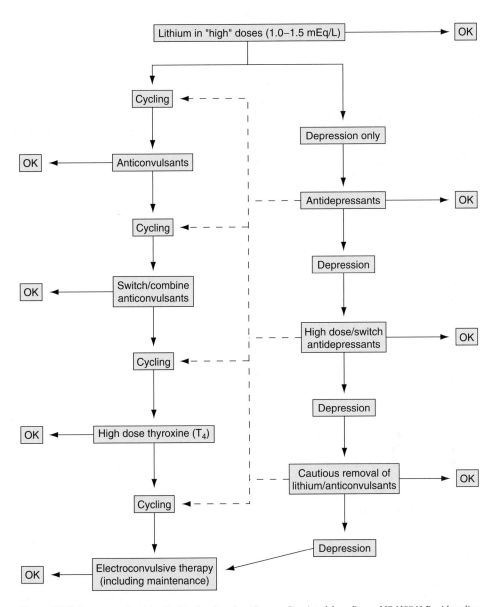

Figure 30-2 *Treatment algorithm for bipolar disorder. (Source: Reprinted from Bauer MS [1994] Rapid cycling. In Anticonvulsants in Mood Disorders, Joffe RT and Calabrese JR [eds]. Marcel Dekker, New York, pp. 1–26.) Note: Refractory mania is relatively rare. This general algorithm addresses the more common clinical scenarios of depression and rapid cycling. For a complete discussion of this topic, see Bauer and McBride 2002; of how to use various psychopharmacologic agents, see Bauer 2003.*

medications are often chosen on the basis of desired side effects. However, side effects usually represent factors that decrease an individual's quality of life and compromise compliance. Furthermore, all antidepressants can cause rapid cycling and mixed states in persons with bipolar disorder. These effects are not uncommonly encountered in clinical practice and should be watched for, even in persons taking mood-stabilizing agents.

Extensive reviews of side effects of the agents most commonly encountered in the treatment of bipolar disorder are available in books by Bauer and colleagues (Bauer and McBride 2002, Bauer 2003), Hyman and coworkers (1995), Schatzberg and coworkers (1997), and Ellsworth and coworkers (2001). It is also worth noting that electronic references are also proliferating, both for the desktop computer (www.Medscape.com) and for handheld devices (www.ePocrates.com). Several excellent review articles have summarized side effects of lithium (Gitlin et al. 1989, Goodwin and Jamison 1990, p. 701–709) and the various anticonvulsants (Swann 2001) including carbamazepine (Ketter and Post 1994), and sodium valproate (Keck et al. 1994), and lamotrigine (Botts and Raskind 1999) are also readily available.

A brief overview of the most frequent or important side effects of lithium, carbamazepine, and valproic acid can be found in Table 30-10a–c. Note that some side effects may be encountered at any serum level of the drug, even within the therapeutic range. Some side effects may be dose-related even within that range and may respond to dosage reduction. Others are more idiosyncratic and may need other management. Note that not all laboratory findings represent pathological processes that are associated with or presage morbidity for the individual; that is, not all are clinically significant.

Note also that the concept of the "therapeutic level" is not as straightforward as we would like to assume. The lower limit is usually established by the lowest level necessary for therapeutic effect, whereas the upper limit is set by the lowest level associated with regular, significant toxicity. This range is never established with complete precision. For some medications such as lithium, the therapeutic window is actually quite narrow, with toxic effects developing with some regularity after the upper limit of the therapeutic range is surpassed and with serious toxicity developing at only modestly higher serum levels. As a further complication, for many persons, the minimum level of lithium for good response may be substantially above the 0.5 to 0.8 mEq/L that is usually set as the lower therapeutic limit, but this is reached only at the cost of increased incidence of side effects (Gelenberg et al. 1989). On the other hand, experience with valproic acid, the upper limit of the therapeutic range for mood stabilization may actually be 125 mg/dL rather than the listed range of 100 mg/dL usually accepted for antiepileptic effect, and this level may be reached without undue side effects (Keck et al. 1994).

Thus, established therapeutic levels should be used as important guidelines, and exceeding therapeutic levels should be done only with careful monitoring. However, one must not be falsely reassured that reaching the lower level of a therapeutic range is equally effective for all individuals, while taking with a grain of salt the upper limits of the therapeutic range in drugs with a wider therapeutic window.

Another important issue to consider is drug–drug interactions that may lead to side effects (see Bauer 2003 for a comprehensive review). Such interactions are often associated with increases in serum levels of the drug of interest. For example, addition of thiazide diuretics, or nonsteroidal antiinflammatory agents, the latter available over the counter, is a common reason for increase in lithium level and development of toxicity. Drug–drug interactions for anticonvulsants have been reviewed in the references above. However, at other times the drug–drug interactions may not be reflected in an increased serum level if the main interaction is displacement of protein-bound drug. Because free drug concentrations are usually 1 to 10% of total serum drug, a displacement of even 50% of bound drug may be associated with negligible if any changes in total serum level. However, since both therapeutic and toxic effects are due to free, not bound, drug, unwanted side effects may develop despite total drug levels measured in the therapeutic range.

As noted previously, some side effects may be desirable. However, in many cases they are impediments to treatment, frequently of sufficient importance to lead to noncompliance

Table 30-10	Side Effects of Lithium and Commonly Used Anticonvulsants

Life-Threatening

| | At Therapeutic Levels | | At Toxic Levels |
	Idiopathic	Dose-Related	Dose-Related
Lithium			Renal failure Encephalopathy
CBZ	Agranulocytosis* Aplastic anemia* Stevens–Johnson*		
VPA	Hepatic necrosis	Thrombocytopenia	Thrombocytopenia
LMT	Stevens–Johnson*		

II: Clinically Significant Side Effects

	Lithium	CBZ	VPA	LMT
Neurologic/muscular	Lethargy Memory (anomia) Tremor† Myoclonus	Lethargy Blurred vision Ataxia†	Lethargy Depression Tremor† Ataxia	Lethargy Ataxia Blurred vision Headache
Endocrine/metabolic	Weight gain† Hypothyroidism		Weight gain†	
Cardiopulmonary				
Hematologic			Thrombocytopenia	
Renal	Polyuria			
Hepatic		Jaundice	Jaundice	
Gastrointestinal	Nausea† Diarrhea†	Nausea†	Nausea†	Nausea†
Dermatologic	Maculopapular rash Psoriasis Acne	Maculopapular rash Alopecia	Maculopapular rash	Maculopapular rash
Other			Back pain	

III: Subclinical Laboratory Abnormalities

	Lithium	CBZ	VPA	LMT
Neurologic/muscular				
Endocrine/metabolic	Increased TSH	Decreased FTI		
Cardiopulmonary	EKG T-wave depression			
Hematologic	Leukocytosis (to 20,000)	Leukopenia	Thrombocytopenia (OK > 20,000)	
Renal	Decreased urine specific gravity, GFR			
Hepatic		Increased LFTs	Increased LFTs	

†Typically during first 1–6 months of treatment.
*Most common reasons in our experience for noncompliance.

(Jamison et al. 1979). As clinicians, however, we might reframe the noncompliance issue more appropriately as "insufficient provider–patient cost-benefit analysis." Stressing compliance when a person suffers from significant side effects is usually much less effective than working to set appropriate expectations of the individual and to find a regimen of minimal toxicity. Goodwin and Jamison's (1990, p. 672) point that managing side effects is as much psychotherapeutic as medical is well taken in this regard.

Nonetheless, the astute clinician does have several strategies available to improve individuals' tolerance of medications. First, dose reduction may be achieved without compromising efficacy in some individuals. Some side effects, such as lithium-induced nausea, usually respond well to this, whereas others, such as lithium-induced memory loss, improve less reliably.

Second, simple changes in preparation may be helpful, such as using enteric-coated lithium. Uncoated valproic acid causes nausea so frequently that only the coated forms are routinely used; however, the pediatric "sprinkle" preparation may be of some benefit in persons with nausea even with enteric-coated valproic acid.

Third, changing the administration schedule may ameliorate side effects. Commonsense strategies such as taking nausea-inducing medications after a meal should not be overlooked. Single daily dosing of lithium, carbamazepine, or valproic acid may decrease daytime sedation without compromising efficacy. For more obscure reasons, single daily dosing of lithium appears to decrease polyuria quite effectively (Bowen et al. 1991).

Fourth, addition of medications to counteract side effects can sometimes be the only way to continue treatment. Addition of beta-blockers can reduce lithium- or valproic acid–induced tremors. Judicious use of thiazide diuretics, often in conjunction with potassium-sparing diuretics or potassium supplements, can reduce lithium-induced polyuria.

Finally, change to another drug may be the only alternative. This is clearly indicated in the case of serious allergic reactions. Polypharmacy should be avoided wherever possible.

Psychotherapies

One of the fastest moving areas of research in bipolar disorder has been psychotherapy. It is important to note that psychotherapy has been studied almost exclusively in the context of ongoing medication management, rather than as a substitute for, or alternative to, medication treatment. Rather, psychotherapy has been utilized as an adjuvant treatment to optimize outcome in the illness. Psychotherapy has been viewed as having one or more of several roles in the management of the disorder.

Recall that both somatic therapies and psychotherapies to date have been predominantly oriented toward improving clinical outcome. Under this conceptualization, psychotherapy has been thought to directly address symptoms, such as cognitive therapy for depressive symptoms. Less frequently has psychotherapy been developed with an explicit component geared toward addressing the functional deficits in bipolar disorder. However, functional outcome has often been measured in formal trials of various types of psychotherapy. A third conceptualization has been to use psychotherapy as a predominantly educative method to assist individuals in participating more effectively in treatment. In this latter regard, treatment is geared toward improving "host factors," that is, those factors not directly due to the disease but that have an impact on its course or treatment, through education, support, and problem solving. Such host factors include illness management skills, which may be improved through psychoeducation and attention to building the therapeutic alliance. Basics of education are summarized in Table 30-11.

An evidence-based review similar to that for somatotherapy has recently been done for psychotherapeutic interventions. This review (Bauer 2001b, Bauer and McBride 2002), identified five main types of psychotherapy that have been studied in bipolar disorder: couples–partners, group interpersonal or psychoeducative, cognitive–behavioral, family, and interpersonal and social rhythms. As summarized in Table 30-12, couples–partners, cognitive–behavioral, and family methods all have some randomized clinical trials data supporting a role in improving clinical outcome or functional outcome or the intermediate outcome variable of improving illness management skills. An additional finding in this review, which is quite striking, is the degree of convergent validity across interventions regarding agenda for disease management information and skills to be imparted.

Table 30-11	Basics of Education to Improve Disease Management Skills

1. Principles
A. Gear education to educational, cultural, motivational factors of individuals and their families.
B. Include both knowledge about the disorder in general and exploration of the individual's specific form of illness and how it affects their own life.
C. Pay close attention to opportunities for destigmatization and demystification.
D. Emphasize the role of the person in treatment and his/her family as comanagers of the illness, including judging costs and benefits of specific treatment options according to the individual's priorities.

2. Components of Psychoeducation
A. The disorder
  (1) Biological basis
    (a) Genetic factors (especially for persons of childbearing age)
    (b) Possible brain mechanisms
  (2) Environmental components
    (a) Psychosocial factors
    (b) Physical environmental factors
  (3) Course and outcome
    (a) Prevalence
    (b) Episode types and patterns
    (c) Potential triggers for episodes
    (d) Comorbidities and complications
B. Treatment
  (1) Somatic therapies: somatic and psychosocial
    (a) Goals
    (b) Side effect recognition and management
    (c) Costs and benefits of individual treatment options
  (2) Coping skills
    (a) Recognition of early warning signs of relapse
    (b) Avoidance/management of triggers for episodes
    (c) Activation of adaptive coping behaviors and avoidance of maladaptive responses

Specifically, imparting education, focusing on early warning symptoms and triggers of episodes, and developing detailed and individual-specific action plans are found across most of the other interventions as well. For instance, this core agenda is also an important part of such diverse approaches as the cognitive–behavioral interventions of Palmer and Williams (1995) and Lam and coworkers (2000); the psychoeducational interventions of Bauer and coworkers (1998), Perry and coworkers (1999), and Weiss and coworkers (2000); the interpersonal and social rhythms therapy (IPSRT) intervention of Frank and coworkers (1999); and the family intervention of Miklowitz and coworkers (1999). Whether or not the developers of these interventions came to this common agenda in isolation or as part of ongoing collaborations and discussions is less important than the impressive fact that the agenda has been identified and incorporated into each of these interventions. Thus, given the positive results most of these interventions with explicit disease management components (i.e., patient education, collaborative management strategies with the individual, inclusion of as wide a social support system as is available) have produced, it is likely that this basic approach will be critical. It will perhaps be more critical even than the specific type of intervention in which these disease management components are embedded.

Treatment of Bipolar Disorder across the Life Cycle

Although the somatotherapeutic and psychotherapeutic mainstays of treatment endure across the life cycle, several phases of life present particular challenges. There exist few data on treatment of bipolar disorder in childhood (Strober et al. 1995). Treatments are chosen by

Table 30-12   Patterns of Efficacy across Psychotherapy Type and Outcome Domaina*

Intervention	Clinical Outcome	Functional Outcome	Disease Management Skills
Couples/partners	+ Davenport et al. (1977) (C) − Clarkin et al. (1998) (A)	+ Davenport et al. (1977) (C) + Honig et al. (1997) (A/B) + Clarkin et al. (1998) (A)	+ Van Gent (1991) (A) − Clarkin et al. (1998) (A)
Group, interpersonal and/or psychoeducational	+ Volkmar et al. (1981) (C) + Kripke and Robinson (1985) (C) + Van Gent (1988) (C) + Van Gent and Zwart (1993) (C) + Cerbone et al. (1992) (C) − Weiss et al. (2000) (B)	+ Volkmar et al. (1981) (C) + Kripke and Robinson (1985) (C) + Cerbone et al. (1992) (C) + Bauer et al. (1998) (B)	+ Van Gent et al. (1988) (C) + Van Gent and Zwart (1993) (C) + Cerbone et al. (1992) (C) + Bauer et al. (1998) (B) + Weiss et al. (2000) (B)
Cognitive–behavioral	+/− Palmer and Williams (1995) (B) + Zaretsky et al. (1999) (B) + Lam et al. (2000) (A)	+/− Palmer and Williams (1995) (B) + Lam et al. (2000) (A)	+/− Cochran (1984) (A)
Family	+ Clarkin et al. (1990) (A) + Retzer et al. (1991) (C) + Miklowitz et al. (1999) (A)	+ Clarkin et al. (1990) (A)	− Miklowitz et al. (1999) (A)
Interpersonal/social rhythms	− Hlastala et al. (1997) (A) − Frank et al. (1999) (A)		
Individual psychoeducation	+ Perry et al. (1999) (A)	+ Perry et al. (1999) (A)	+ Peet and Harvey (1991) (A)
Other/eclectic	+ Benson (1975) (C)		

* Studies analyzed by type of intervention, positive (+), negative (−), or equivocal (+/−) impact on the outcome domain noted, and quality of evidence (A, B, or C). See text for detail.

extension from the adult literature, with the one caveat that there have been rare cases of liver failure in conjunction with valproic acid use in children younger than 10 years of age who have been exposed to multiple anticonvulsants (Dreifuss 1989).

In pregnancy, there is some evidence that lithium may be teratogenic, associated with increased rates of cardiac abnormalities (Weinstein and Goldfield 1975), although more recent data indicate that this risk may be overestimated (Cohen et al. 1994). Valproic acid and perhaps carbamazepine (Robert and Guiband 1983, Delgado-Escueta and Janz 1992, Scolnik et al. 1994) have been associated with neural tube defects (Robert and Guiband 1983), leaving the neuroleptics, antidepressants, and ECT as the preferable management strategies during pregnancy, particularly during the first trimester. Specific treatment strategies have been reviewed elsewhere (Sitland-Marken et al. 1989). It should be kept in mind, however, that treatment decisions are based on *risk*, not *certainty*. Risk of fetal malformation, parental attitude toward raising children with birth defects, severity of illness, and ease of management with alternative therapies all need to be considered in conjunction with the woman and her partner.

Aging also presents certain treatment concerns. Tricyclic antidepressants may be associated with clinically significant cardiac conduction abnormalities, hypotension, sedation, glaucoma, and urinary retention, particularly in the presence of prostatic hypertrophy. These are of even greater concern in the elderly. The risk of sedation due to neuroleptics and benzodiazepines, and of hypotension due to low-potency neuroleptics can also particularly complicate treatment of elderly persons with bipolar disorder. Such side effects can cause far-reaching and serious complications, such as hip fracture (Ray et al. 1987), which is not infrequently the initial event in a cascade of complications that can be terminal.

By contrast, lithium, carbamazepine, and valproic acid are relatively well tolerated in the elderly once attention is given to the slower clearance of drugs in general in this population group. The risk of clinically significant renal toxicity with appropriately dosed lithium is not great (Schou 1988, Gitlin 1993, Kehoe 1994). Although glomerular filtration rate decreases with age in persons treated with lithium, the rate of decline does not appear to be accelerated by lithium treatment (Lokkegaard et al. 1985, Vaamonde et al. 1986). Nonetheless, careful monitoring of renal function is needed in the elderly.

In addition, increasing age is clearly a risk factor for hypothyroidism (Bauer et al. 1993), as is lithium use (Bauer et al. 1990). Thus, elderly persons taking lithium should be followed up carefully for decrements in thyroid function, although hypothyroidism is not an indication for lithium discontinuation but rather simply for thyroid hormone supplementation.

Comparison of DSM-IV-TR/ICD-10 Diagnostic Criteria

The ICD-10 item set for a manic episode contains nine items in contrast to the seven items in the DSM-IV-TR criteria set, the two additional items being marked sexual energy or indiscretions and loss of normal social inhibitions. However, the number of items required by ICD-10 Diagnostic Criteria for Research remains the same as the number in DSM-IV-TR (i.e., three items if mood is euphoric, four items if mood is irritable), which is likely to result in a more inclusive diagnosis of a manic episode in ICD-10. Furthermore, the duration of mixed episodes differ, with DSM-IV-TR requiring a duration of 1 week (as is the case for a manic episode), whereas the ICD-10 Diagnostic Criteria for Research require a duration of at least 2 weeks.

The criteria sets for hypomanic episode differ as well. The ICD-10 Diagnostic Criteria for Research contain several additional items (increased sexual energy and increased sociability) and does not include the DSM-IV-TR items, inflated self-esteem and flight of ideas. Furthermore, ICD-10 does not require that the change in mood be observed by others.

Regarding the definition of bipolar I disorder, in addition to differences in the diagnostic criteria for a manic and major depressive episode, the ICD-10 definition of "Bipolar

Affective Disorder" (i.e., any combination of hypomanic, manic, mixed, and depressive episodes) does not distinguish between bipolar I and bipolar II disorder (i.e., cases of DSM-IV-TR Bipolar II Disorder are diagnosed as Bipolar Affective Disorder in ICD-10). However, ICD-10 Diagnostic Criteria for Research does include diagnostic criteria for bipolar II in its appendix, which are identical to the criteria set in DSM-IV-TR.

For cyclothymic disorder, the ICD-10 Diagnostic Criteria for Research provides list of symptoms that must be associated with the periods of depressed mood and hypomania, which differ from the ICD-10 item sets for dysthymic disorder and hypomania. In contrast, the DSM-IV-TR definition of cyclothymic disorder just refers to numerous periods of hypomania and depressive symptoms.

Acknowledgment

Portions of this chapter have been adapted with permission from Bauer MS and McBride L (2002) *Structured Group Psychotherapy for Manic–Depressive Disorder*, 2nd ed. F. A. Davis Company, New York.

References

Abraham K (1927) Notes on the psycho-analytical investigation and treatment of manic–depressive insanity and allied conditions (1911). In *Selected Papers of Karl* Abraham, MD, Bryan D, and Strachey A (trans). Hogarth Press, London, pp. 137–156.

AHCPR (Agency for Health Care Policy and Research) (1993) *Depression Panel Guideline Report*. US Government Printing Office, Washington, DC.

Akiskal HS (1981) Subaffective disorders: dysthymic, cyclothymic, and bipolar II disorders in the "borderline" realm. *Psychiatr Clin N Am* **4**, 25–46.

Akiskal HS and Akiskal K (1988) Reassessing the prevalence of bipolar disorders: clinical significance and artistic creativity. *Psychiatr Psychobiol* **3**, 29S–36S.

Akiskal HS, Djenderedjian AH, Rosenthal RH, et al. (1977) Cyclothymic disorder: validating criteria for inclusion in the bipolar affective group. *Am J Psychiatry* **134**, 1227–1233.

Altshuler LL, Bartzokis G, Grieder T, et al. (2000) An MRI study of temporal lobe structures in men with bipolar disorder or schizophrenia. *Biol Psychiatry* **48**(2), 147–162.

Altshuler LL, Curran J, Hauser P, et al. (1995) T2 hyperintensities in bipolar disorder: magnetic resonance imaging comparison and literature meta-analysis. *Am J Psychiatry* **152**(8), 1139–1144.

American Psychiatric Association (1994a) *Diagnostic and Statistical Manual of Mental Disorders*, 4th ed., APA, Washington, DC.

American Psychiatric Association Task Force for the Handbook of Psychiatric Measures (2000) *Handbook of Psychiatric Measures*. APA, Washington, DC.

Amsterdam JD, Winokur A, Lucki I, et al. (1983) A neuroendocrine test battery in bipolar patients and health subjects. *Arch Gen Psychiatry* **40**, 515–521.

Angst J (1978) The course of affective disorders: 2. typology of bipolar manic–depressive illness. *Arch Psychiatr Nervenkr* **226**, 65–73.

Angst J (1981) Course of affective disorders. In *Handbook of Biological Psychiatry*, van Praag (ed). Marcel Dekker, New York, pp. 225–242.

Baastrup P and Schou M (1967) Lithium as a prophylactic agent: its effect against recurrent depression and manic–depressive psychosis. *Arch Gen Psychiatry* **16**, 162–172.

Ballenger JC and Post RM (1978) Therapeutic effects of carbamazepine in affective illness: a preliminary report. *Commun Psychopharmacol* **2**, 159–175.

Ballenger JC and Post RM (1980) Carbamazepine in manic–depressive illness: a new treatment. *Am J Psychiatry* **137**(7), 782–790.

Banks R, Aiton J, Cramb G, et al. (1990) Incorporation of inositol into the phosphoinositides of lymphoblastoid cell lines established from bipolar manic–depressive patients. *J Affect Disord* **19**, 1–8.

Baron M, Gershon ES, Rudy V, et al. (1975) Lithium carbonate response in depression. *Arch Gen Psychiatry* **32**, 1107–1111.

Baron M, Gruen R, Asnis L, et al. (1982) Schizoaffective illness, schizophrenia, and affective disorders: morbidity risk and genetic transmission. *Acta Psychiatr Scand* **65**, 253–262.

Bauer MS (1993) Summertime bright-light treatment of bipolar major depressive episodes. *Biol Psychiatry* **33**, 663–665.

Bauer MS (1994) Rapid cycling. In *Anticonvulsants in Mood Disorders*, Joffe RT and Calabrese JR (eds). Marcel Dekker, New York, pp. 1–26.

Bauer MS (2001b) An evidence-based review of psychosocial interventions for bipolar disorder. *Psychopharmacol Bull* **35**, 109–134.

Bauer MS (2003) *Field Guide to Psychiatric Assessment and Treatment. Lippincott*, Williams & Wilkins, Philadelphia.

Bauer MS, Calabrese J, Dunner DL, et al. (1994b) Multisite data reanalysis of the validity of rapid cycling as a course modifier for bipolar disorder in DSM–IV. *Am J Psychiatry* **151**, 506–515.

Bauer MS, Crits-Christoph P, Ball W, et al. (1991) Independent assessment of manic and depressive symptoms by self-rating scale: characteristics and implications for the study of mania. *Arch Gen Psychiatry* **48**, 807–812.

Bauer MS and Dunner DL (1993) Validity of seasonal pattern as a modifier for recurrent mood disorders for DSM-IV. *Compr Psychiatry* **34**, 159–170.

Bauer M, Halpern L, and Schriger D (1993) Screening depressives for causative medical illness: the example of thyroid function testing. I. Literature review, meta-analysis, and hypothesis generation. *Depression* **1**, 210–219.

Bauer MS, Kurtz JW, Rubin LB, et al. (1994c) Mood and behavioral effects of four-week light treatment in winter depressives and controls. *J Psychiatr Res* **28**, 135–145.

Bauer MS and McBride L (2002) *Structured Group Psychotherapy for Manic–Depressive Disorder: The Life Goals Program*, 2nd ed., F. A. Davis Company, New York.

Bauer MS, McBride L, Chase C, et al. (1998) Manual-based group psychotherapy for bipolar disorder: a feasibility study. *J Clin Psychiatry* **59**, 449–455.

Bauer M and Whybrow P (1990) Rapid cycling bipolar affective disorder II. Adjuvant treatment of refractory rapid cycling with high dose thyroxine. *Arch Gen Psychiatry* **47**, 435–440.

Bauer MS and Whybrow PC (1991) Rapid cycling bipolar disorder: clinical features, treatment, and etiology. In *Advances in Neuropsychiatry and Psychopharmacology*, Vol. 2, Amsterdam JD (ed). Raven Press, New York, pp. 191–208.

Bauer MS and Whybrow P (1993) Validity of rapid cycling as a modifier for bipolar disorder in DSM-IV. *Depression* **1**, 11–19.

Bauer M and Whybrow PC (2001) Thyroid hormone, neural tissue, and mood modulation. *World J Biol Psychiatry* **2**, 59–69.

Bauer M, Whybrow P, Gyulai L, et al. (1994a) Testing definitions of dysphoric mania and hypomania: prevalence, clinical characteristics, and inter-episode stability. *J Affect Disord* **32**, 201–211.

Bauer M, Whybrow P, and Winokur A (1990) Rapid cycling bipolar affective disorder I: association with grade I hypothyroidism. *Arch Gen Psychiatry* **47**, 427–432.

Bauwens F, Tracy A, Pardoen D, et al. (1991) Social adjustment of remitted bipolar and unipolar out-patients. A comparison with age- and sex-matched controls. *Br J Psychiatry* **151**, 239–244.

Baxter LR Jr., Phelps ME, Mazziotta JC, et al. (1985) Cerebral metabolic rates for glucose in mood disorders: studies with positron emission tomography and fluorodeoxyglucose F 18. *Arch Gen Psychiatry* **42**, 441–447.

Beck AT, Rush AJ, Shaw B, et al. (1979) *Cognitive Therapy of Depression*. Guilford Press, New York.

Benes FM and Berretta S (2001) GABAergic interneurons: implications for understanding schizophrenia and bipolar disorder. *Neuropsychopharmacology* **25**,(1) 1–27.

Benson R (1975) The forgotten treatment modality in bipolar illness: psychotherapy. *Dis Nerv Syst* **36**, 634–638.

Bertelsen A (1979) A Danish twin study of manic–depressive disorders. In *Origin, Prevention, and Treatment of Affective Disorders*, Schou M and Stromgren E (eds). Academic Press, London, pp. 227–239.

Bierwaltes WH and Ruff GE (1958) Thyroxin and triiodothyronine in excessive dosage to euthyroid humans. *Arch Intern Med* **101**, 569–576.

Blacker D and Tsuang M (1992) Contested boundaries of bipolar disorder and the limits of categorical diagnosis in psychiatry. *Am J Psychiatry* **149**, 1473–1483.

Botts SR and Raskind J (1999) Gabapentin and lamotrigine in bipolar disorder. *Am J Health-Syst Pharm* **56**, 1939–1944.

Bowden C, Brugger A, Swann A, et al. (1994) Efficacy of divalproex vs lithium and placebo in the treatment of mania. *J Am Med Assoc* **271**, 918–924.

Bowden CL, Calabrese JR, McElroy SL, et al. (1999) The efficacy of lamotrigine in rapid cycling and non-rapid cycling patients with bipolar disorder. *Soc Biol Psych* **45**, 953–958.

Bowden CL, Calabrese JR, McElroy SL, et al. (2000) A randomized, placebo-controlled 12 month trial of divalproex and lithium in treatment of outpatients with bipolar I disorder. *Arch Gen Psychiatry* **57**, 481–489.

Bowen RC, Groff P, and Groff E (1991) Less frequent lithium administration and lower urine volume. *Am J Psychiatry* **148**, 189–192.

Brambilla P, Harenski K, Nicoletti M, et al. (2001) MRI study of posterior fossa structures and brain ventricles in bipolar patients. *J Psychiatr Res* **35**(6), 313–322.

Bratfos O and Haug J (1968) The course of manic–depressive psychosis. A follow-up investigation of 215 patients. *Acta Psychiatr Neurol Scand* **44**, 89–112.

Briggs J, McBride L, Hagino O, et al. (1993) Screening depressives for causative medical illness: the example of thyroid function testing II. Hypothesis testing in ambulatory depressives. *Depression* **1**, 220–224.

Broadhead WE, Blazer D, George L, et al. (1990) Depression, disability days, and days lost from work in a prospective epidemiologic survey. *JAMA* **264**, 2524–2528.

Brockington IF, Hillier V, Francis A, et al. (1983) Definitions of mania: concordance and prediction of outcome. *Am J Psychiatry* **140**, 435–439.

Brown G (1989) Life events and measurement. In *Life Events and Stress*, Brown G and Harris T (eds). Guilford Press, New York, pp. 3–45.

Brown G, Harris T, and Copeland J (1977) Depression and loss. *Br J Psychiatry* **130**, 1–18.

Brown A, Mallinger A, and Renbaum L (1993) Elevated platelet membrane phosphatidylinositol-4,5-bisphosphate in bipolar mania. *Am J Psychiatry* **150**, 1252–1254.

Buchsbaum MS, Wu J, DeLisi LE, et al. (1986) Frontal cortex and basal ganglia metabolic rates assessed by positron emission tomography with [^{18}F]2-deoxyglucose in affective illness. *J Affect Disord* **10**, 137–152.

Bunney WE, Goodwin FK, Davis JM, et al. (1968) A behavioral-biochemical study of lithium treatment. *Am J Psychiatry* **125**(5), 91–104.

Bunney WE Jr., Goodwin FK, and Murphy DL (1972a) The "switch process" in manic–depressive illness III. Theoretical implications. *Arch Gen Psychiatry* **27**, 312–317.

Bunney WE Jr., Goodwin FK, Murphy DL, et al. (1972b) The "switch process" in manic–depressive illness II. Relationship to catecholamines, REM sleep, and drugs. *Arch Gen Psychiatry* **27**, 304–309.

Bunney WE Jr., Murphy D, Goodwin FK, et al. (1972c) The "switch process" in manic–depressive illness I. A systematic study of sequential behavior change. *Arch Gen Psychiatry* **27**, 295–302.

Calabrese JR, Bowden CL, McElroy SL, et al. (1999) Spectrum of activity of lamotrigine in treatment-refractory bipolar disorder. *Am J Psychiatry* **156**(7), 1019–1023.

Carlson GA and Kashani JH (1988) Phenomenology of major depression from childhood through adulthood: analysis of three studies. *Am J Psychiatry* **145**, 1222–1225.

Carlson G, Kotin J, Davenport Y, et al. (1974) Follow-up of 53 bipolar manic–depressive patients. *Br J Psychiatry* **124**, 134–149.

Cerbone M, Mayo J, Cuthbertsone B, et al. (1992) Group therapy as an adjunct to medication in the management of bipolar disorder. *Group* **16**, 174–187.

Clarkin JF, Carpenter D, Hull J, et al. (1998) Effects of psychoeducational intervention for married patients with bipolar disorder and their spouses. *Psychiatr Serv* **49**, 531–533.

Clarkin JF, Glick I, Haas G, et al. (1990) A randomized clinical trial of inpatient family intervention. V. Results for affective disorder. *J Affect Disord* **18**, 17–28.

Cochran S (1984) Preventing medical noncompliance in the outpatient treatment of bipolar affective disorders. *J Consult Clin Psychol* **52**, 873–878.

Cohen LS, Friedman JM, and Jefferson JW (1994) A reevaluation of risk of *in utero* exposure to lithium. *JAMA* **271**, 146–150.

Cooper A (1985) Will neurobiology influence psychoanalysis? *Am J Psychiatry* **142**, 1395–1402.

Coppen A, Noguera R, Bailey J, et al. (1971) Prophylactic lithium in affective disorders: controlled trial. *Lancet* **2**, 275–279.

Coppen A, Prange AJ Jr., Whybrow PC, et al. (1972) Abnormalities of indolamines in affective disorders. *Arch Gen Psychiatry* **26**, 474–478.

Coryell W, Endicott J, Andreasen N, et al. (1985) Bipolar I, bipolar II, and nonbipolar major depression among the relatives of affectively ill probands. *Am J Psychiatry* **142**, 817–821.

Coryell W, Endicott J, Keller M, et al. (1989) Bipolar affective disorder and high achievement: a familial association. *Am J Psychiatry* **146**, 983–988.

Coryell W, Endicott J, and Keller M (1992) Rapidly cycling affective disorders: demographics, diagnosis, family history, and course. *Arch Gen Psychiatry* **49**, 126–131.

Coryell W, Endicott J, Maser J, et al. (1995) Long-term stability of polarity distinctions in affective disorders. *Am J Psychiatry* **152**, 385–390.

Coryell W, Endicott J, Reich T, et al. (1984) A family study of bipolar II disorder. *Br J Psychiatry* **145**, 49–54.

Coryell W, Scheftner W, Keller M, et al. (1993) The enduring psychosocial consequences of mania and depression. *Am J Psychiatry* **150**, 720–727.

Craddock N and Jones I (1999) Genetics of bipolar disorder. *J Med Gener* **36**, 585–594.

Crow T and Deakin J (1981) Affective change and the mechanisms of reward and punishment: a neurochemical hypothesis. In *Biological Psychiatry*, Perris C, Struwe G, and Jansson B (eds). Elsevier, Amsterdam, pp. 536–541.

Cundall RL, Brooks PW, and Murray LG (1972) A controlled evaluation of lithium prophylaxis in affective disorders. *Psychol Med* **2**, 308–311.

Davenport Y, Ebert M, Adland M, et al. (1977) Couples group therapy as an adjunct to lithium maintenance of the manic patient. *Am J Orthopsychiatry* **47**, 495–502.

Deicken RF, Calabrese G, Merrin EL, et al. (1995) Asymmetry of temporal lobe phosphorous metabolism in schizophrenia: A 31 phosphorous magnetic resonance spectroscopic imaging study. *Biol Psychiatry* **38**(5), 279–286.

Delgado-Escueta A and Janz D (1992) Consensus guidelines: preconception counseling, management, and care of the pregnant woman with epilepsy. *Neurology* **42**(Suppl. 5),, 149–160.

Deltito J, Moline M, Pollak C, et al. (1991) Effects of phototherapy on nonseasonal unipolar and bipolar depressive spectrum disorders. *J Affect Disord* **23**, 231–237.

DePaolo JR, Simpson SG, Folstein S, et al. (1989) The new genetics of bipolar affective disorder: clinical implications. *Clin Chem* **35/7(B)**, B28–B32.

Depue R and Iacono W (1989) Neurobiological aspects of affective disorders. *Annu Rev Psychol* **40**, 457–492.

Dion G, Tohen M, Anthony W, et al. (1988) Symptoms and functioning of patients with bipolar disorder six months after hospitalization. *Hosp Comm Psychiatry* **39**, 652–657.

Dreifuss FE (1989) Valproate toxicity. In *Antiepileptic Drugs*, 3rd ed., Levy R, Mattson RH, Meldrum B, et al. (eds). Raven Press, New York, pp. 643–651.

Drevets WC, Frank E, Price JC, et al. (1999) PET imaging of serotonin 1A receptor binding in depression. *Biol Psychiatry* **46**(10), 1375–1387.

Dubovsky SL, Franks RD, Allen S, et al. (1986) Calcium antagonists in mania: a double-blind study of verapamil. *Psychiatr Res* **18**, 309–320.

Dunner DL (1993) A review of the diagnostic status of "bipolar II" for the DSM-IV work group on mood disorders. *Depression* **1**, 2–10.

Dunner DL and Fieve RR (1974) Clinical factors in lithium prophylaxis failure. *Arch Gen Psychiatry* **30**, 229–233.

Dunner DL, Fleiss JL, and Fieve RR (1976) Lithium carbonate prophylaxis failure. *Br J Psychiatry* **129**, 40–44.

EBWG (Evidence-Based Working Group) (1992) A new approach to teaching the practice of medicine. *J Am Med Assoc* **268**, 2420–2425.

Ehlers C, Frank E, and Kupfer D (1988) Social zeitgebers and biological rhythms. *Arch Gen Psychiatry* **45**, 948–952.

Ellicott A, Hammen C, Gitlin M, et al. (1990) Life events and the course of bipolar disorder. *Am J Psychiatry* **147**(9), 1194–1198.

Ellsworth AJ, Witt DM, Dugdale DC, et al. (2001) *Mosby's 2001–02 Medical Drug Reference*. Mosby, St. Louis.

el-Mallakh R and Li R (1993) Is the Na$^+$-K$^+$-ATPase the link between phosphoinositide metabolism and bipolar disorder? *Rev J Neuropsychiatr Clin Neurosci* **5**, 361–368.

Emrich HM, Zerssen DV, Kissling W, et al. (1980) Effect of sodium valproate on mania: the GABA-hypothesis of affective disorders. *Arch Psychiatr Nervenkr* **229**, 1–16.

Endicott J, Nee J, Andreasen N, et al. (1985) Bipolar II: Combine or keep separate? *J Affect Disord* **8**, 17–28.

Faedda GL, Tondo L, Baldessarini RJ, et al. (1993) Outcome after rapid vs gradual discontinuation of lithium treatment in bipolar disorders. *Arch Gen Psychiatry* **50**, 448–455.

Fein R (1958) *Economics of Mental Illness*. Basic Books, New York.

Fenichel O (1945) *The Psychoanalytic Theory of Neuroses*. WW Norton, New York, p. 408.

Fieve R, Go R, Dunnere D, et al. (1984) Search for biological/genetic markers in a long-term epidemiological and morbid risk study of affective disorders. *J Psychiatr Res* **18**, 425–445.

Fieve RR, Kumbaraci R, and Dunner DL (1976) Lithium prophylaxis of depression in bipolar I, bipolar II, and unipolar patients. *Am J Psychiatry* **133**(8), 925–929.

Fieve RR, Platman SR, and Plutchik RR (1968) The use of lithium in affective disorders I: acute endogenous depression. *Am J Psychiatry* **125**, 487–491.

Frank E, Swartz H, Mallinger AG, et al. (1999) Adjunctive psychotherapy for bipolar disorder: effects of changing treatment modality. *J Abnorm Psychol* **108**, 579–587.

Fremming KH (1951) *The Expectation of Mental Infirmity in a Sample of the Danish Population*, No. 7, Occasional Papers in Eugenics. Cassell, London.

Gareri P, Falconi U, De Fazio P, et al. (2000) Conventional and new antidepressant drugs in the elderly. *Prog Neurobiol* **61**(4), 353–396.

Gelenberg AJ, Kane JM, Keller MB, et al. (1989) Comparison of standard and low serum levels of lithium for maintenance treatment of bipolar disorder. *N Engl J Med* **321**, 1489–1493.

Gershon ES, Hamovit J, Guroff JJ, et al. (1982) A family study of schizoaffective, bipolar I, bipolar II, unipolar, and normal control probands. *Arch Gen Psychiatry* **39**, 1157–1167.

Gershon ES, Hamovit JH, Guroff JJ, et al. (1987) Birth-cohort changes in manic and depressive disorders in relatives of bipolar and schizoaffective patients. *Arch Gen Psychiatry* **44**, 314–319.

Giannini AJ, Houser WL, Loiselle RH, et al. (1984) Antimanic effects of verapamil. *Am J Psychiatry* **141**(12), 1602–1603.

Gitlin M (1993) Lithium-induced renal insufficiency. *J Clin Psychopharmacol* **13**, 276–279.

Gitlin M, Cochran S, and Jamison K (1989) Maintenance lithium treatment: side effects and compliance. *J Clin Psychiatry* **50**, 127–131.

Goodwin FK and Jamison KR (1990) *Manic–Depressive Illness*. Oxford University Press, New York, pp. 369–596.

Goodwin FK, Murphy DL, and Bunney WF Jr. (1969) Lithium carbonate treatment in depression and mania: a longitudinal double-blind study. *Arch Gen Psychiatry* **21**, 486–496.

Goodwin FK, Murphy DL, Dunner DL, et al. (1972) Lithium response in unipolar versus bipolar depression. *Am J Psychiatry* **129**, 44–47.

Goodwin FK and Sack RL (1974) Behavioral effects of a new dopamine-beta-hydroxylase inhibitor (dusaric acid) in man. *J Psychiatr Res* **11**, 211–217.

Gottschalk A, Bauer M, and Whybrow P (1995) A chaotic attraction in bipolar disorder. *Arch Gen Psychiatry* **52**, 947–959.

Greil W, Steber R, and vanCalker D (1991) The agonist-stimulated accumulation of inositol phosphates is attenuated in neutrophils from male patients under chronic lithium therapy. *Biol Psychiatry* **30**, 443–451.

Halaris A (ed). (1987) *Chronobiology and Psychiatric Disorders.* Elsevier, New York.

Hall K, Dunner D, Zeller G, et al. (1977) Bipolar illness: a prospective study of life events. *Compr Psychiatry* **18**, 497–502.

Harrow M, Goldberg J, Grossman L, et al. (1990) Outcome in manic disorders. a naturalistic follow-up study. *Arch Gen Psychiatry* **47**, 665–671.

Hastings D (1958) Follow-up results in psychiatric illness. *Am J Psychiatry* **114**, 1057–1066.

Hauser P, Matochik J, Altshuler LL, et al. (2000) MRI-based measurements of temporal lobe and ventricular structures in patients with bipolar I and bipolar II disorders. *J Affect Disord* **60**(1), 25–32.

Helgason T (1979) Epidemiological investigations concerning affective disorders. In *Origin, Preventions, and Treatment of Affective Disorders*, Schou M and Stromgren E (eds). Academic Press, London, pp. 241–255.

Himmelhoch J, Mulla D, Neil JF, et al. (1976) Incidence and significance of mixed affective states in a bipolar population. *Arch Gen Psychiatry* **33**, 1062–1066.

Hlastala SA, Frank E, Mallinger AG, et al. (1997) Bipolar depression: an underestimated treatment challenge. *Depress Anxiety* **5**, 73–83.

Honig A, Hofman A, Rozendaal N, et al. (1997) Psycho-education in bipolar disorder: effect on expressed emotion. *Psychiatr Res* **72**, 17–22.

Hume AJA, Barker PJ, Robertson W, et al. (1988) Manic–depressive psychosis: an alternative therapeutic model of nursing. *J Adv Nursing* **13**, 93–98.

Hunt N, Bruce-Jones W, and Silverstone T (1992) Life events and relapse in bipolar affective disorder. *J Affect Dis* **25**, 13–20.

Hyman SE, Arana JW, and Rosenbaum JF (1995) *Handbook of Psychiatric Drug Therapy*, 3rd ed., Little Brown, Boston.

Institute of Medicine (1985) *Assessing Medical Technologies.* National Academy Press, Washington, DC.

James NM and Chapman CJ (1975) A genetic study of bipolar affective disorder. *Br J Psychiatry* **126**, 449–456.

Jamison KR, Gerner RH, and Goodwin FK (1979) Patient and physician attitudes toward lithium: relationship to compliance. *Arch Gen Psychiatry* **36**, 866–869.

Janowsky DS, El-Yousef MK, Davis JM, et al. (1973) Parasympathetic suppression of manic symptoms by physostigmine. *Arch Gen Psychiatry* **28**, 542–547.

Joffe R, Singer W, Levitt A, et al. (1993) A placebo-controlled comparison of lithium and triiodothyronine augmentation of tricyclic antidepressant in unipolar refractory affective depression. *Arch Gen Psychiatry* **50**, 387–393.

Johnson S and Roberts JR (1995) Life events and bipolar disorder: implications from biological theories. *Psychol Bull* **117**, 434–449.

Josephson AM and MacKenzie TB (1979) Appearance of manic psychosis following rapid normalization of thyroid status. *Am J Psychiatry* **136**, 846–847.

Jurjus GJ, Nasrallah HA, Brogan M, et al. (1993a) Developmental brain anomalies in schizophrenia and bipolar disorder: a controlled MRI study. *J Neuropsychiatr Clin Neurosci* **5**, 375–378.

Jurjus GJ, Nasrallah HA, Olson SC, et al. (1993b) Cavum septum pellucidum in schizophrenia, affective disorder, and health controls: a magnetic resonance imaging study. *Psychol Med* **23**, 319–322.

Kahn DA (1993) The use of psychodynamic psychotherapy in manic–depressive illness. *J Am Acad Psychoanal* **21**(3), 441–455.

Kamo J, Shin-ichiro T, Susumo N, et al. (1993) Season and mania. *Jpn J Psychiatr Neurol* **47**(2), 473–474.

Kane JM, Quitkin FM, Rifkin A, et al. (1982) Lithium carbonate and imipramine in the prophylaxis of unipolar and bipolar II illness: a prospective, placebo-controlled comparison. *Arch Gen Psychiatry* **39**(9), 1065–1069.

Kapur S and Mann JJ (1992) Role of the dopaminergic system in depression. *Biol Psychiatry* **32**, 1–17.

Kato T, Takahashi S, Shioiri T, et al. (1994) Reduction of brain phosphocreatine in bipolar II disorder detected by phosphorous-31 magnetic resonance spectroscopy. *J Affect Disord* **31**, 125–133.

Keck PE, McElroy SL, and Bennett JA (1994) Pharmacology and pharmacokinetics of valproic acid. In *Anticonvulsants in Mood Disorders*, Joffe RT and Calabrese JR (eds). Marcel Dekker, New York, pp. 27–42.

Kehoe RF (1994) A cross-sectional study of glomerular function in 740 unselected lithium patients. *Acta Psychiatr Scand* **89**, 68–71.

Keller M, Lavori P, Coryell W, et al. (1986a) Differential outcome of episodes of illness in bipolar patients: pure manic, mixed/cycling, and pure depressive. *JAMA* **255**, 3138–3142.

Kennedy S, Thompson R, Stancer HC, et al. (1983) Life events precipitating mania. *Br J Psychiatry* **142**, 398–403.

Ketter TA and Post RM (1994) Clinical pharmacology and pharmacokinetics of carbamazepine. In *Anticonvulsants in Mood Disorders*, Joffe RT and Calabrese JR (eds). Marcel Dekker, New York, pp. 147–188.

Kirov G, Murphy KC, Arranz MJ, et al. (1998) Low activity allele of catechol-O-methyltransferase gene associated with rapid cycling bipolar disorder. *Mol Psychiatry* **3**(4), 342–345.

Klerman G, Olfson M, Leon A, et al. (1992) Measuring the need for mental health care. *Health Affairs* **11**, 23–33. (Statistics from prepublication draft from Dr. A. Leon).

Klerman G, Weissman M, Rounsaville B, et al. (1984) *Interpersonal Psychotherapy of Depression.* Basic Books, New York.

Kraepelin E (1989) Manic–depressive insanity and paranoia. In *Classics of Psychiatry and Behavioral Science*, Barclay RM (trans) and Robertson GM (ed). Classics of Psychiatry and Behavioral Sciences Library Birmingham, AL. (Originally published in 1921, E&D Livingstone, Edinburgh.).

Krauthammer C and Klerman GL (1978) Secondary mania: manic syndromes associated with antecedent physical illness or drugs. *Arch Gen Psychiatry* **35**, 1333–1339.

Kripke DF and Robinson D (1985) Ten years with a lithium group. *McLean Hosp J* **10**, 1–11.

Lachman HM, Morrow B, Shprintzen R, et al. (1996) Association of codon 108/158 catechol-O-methyltransferase gene polymorphism with the psychiatric manifestations of velocardia-facial syndrome. *Am J Med Genet* **67**(5), 468–472.

Lam DH, Bright J, Jones S, et al. (2000) Cognitive therapy for bipolar illness—a pilot study of relapse prevention. *Cogn Ther Res* **24**, 503–520.

Lenox R and Watson D (1994) Lithium and the brain: a psychopharmacological strategy to a molecular basis for manic–depressive illness (review). *Clin Chem* **40**, L309–L314.

Lenzi A, Lazzerini F, Marazziti D, et al. (1993) Social class and mood disorders: clinical features. *Soc Psychiatr Epidemiol* **28**, 56–59.

Leverich M (1990) Factors associated with relapse during maintenance treatment of affective disorders. *Int J Clin Psychopharmacol* **5**, 135–156.

Levinstein S, Klein D, and Pollack M (1966) Follow-up study of formerly hospitalized voluntary psychiatric patients: the first two years. *Am J Psychiatr* **122**, 1102–1109.

Levitt J and Tsuang M (1988) The heterogeneity of schizoaffective disorders: implications for treatment. *Am J Psychiatry* **145**, 926–936.

Lewis JL and Winokur G (1982) The induction of mania: a natural history study with controls. *Arch Gen Psychiatry* **39**, 303–306.

Lewy A, Nurnberger J, Wehr T, et al. (1985) Supersensitivity to light: possible trait marker for manic–depressive illness. *Am J Psychiatry* **142**, 725–727.

Lewy A, Wehr T, Goodwin F, et al. (1980) Light suppresses melatonin secretion in humans. *Science* **210**, 1267–1269.

Lindblad K, Bylander PO, Zander C, et al. (1998) *Mol Psychiatry* **3**(5), 405–410.

Lokkegaard H, Andersen N, and Henriksen H (1985) Renal function in 153 manic–depressive patients treated with lithium for more than five years. *Acta Psychiatr Scand* **71**, 347–355.

Lundquist G (1945) Prognosis and course in manic–depressive psychosis. *Acta Psychiatr Neurol Scand* **35**(Suppl.), 1–96.

Maggs R (1963) Treatment of manic illness with lithium carbonate. *Br J Psychiatry* **150**, 863–864.

Maj M, Pirozzi R, and Starace F (1989) Previous pattern of course of the illness as a predictor of response to lithium prophylaxis in bipolar illness. *J Affect Disord* **17**, 237–241.

Manji HK and Lenox RH (2000) Signaling: cellular insights into the pathophysiology of bipolar disorder. *Biol Psychiatry* **48**(6), 518–530.

Markowitz J, Weissman M, Oulette R, et al. (1989) Quality of life in panic disorder. *Arch Gen Psychiatry* **46**, 984–992.

Mason J (1975) Emotion as reflected in patterns of endocrine integration. In *Emotions—Their Parameters and Measurement*, Levi L (ed). Raven Press, New York, pp. 143–181.

Massion A, Warshaw M, and Keller M (1993) Quality of life and psychiatric morbidity in panic disorder and generalized anxiety disorder. *Am J Psychiatry* **150**, 600–607.

McElroy S, Keck P, Pope H, et al. (1992) Clinical and research implications of the diagnosis of dysphoric or mixed mania or hypomania. *Am J Psychiatry* **149**, 1633–1644.

McGuire T (1991) Measuring the economic costs of schizophrenia. *Schizophr Bull* **17**, 375–388.

McInnis MG, McMahon FJ, Chase GA, et al. (1993) Anticipation in bipolar affective disorder. *Am J Hum Genet* **53**, 385–390.

McLellan AT, Childress AR, and Woody GE (1985) Drug abuse and psychiatric disorders: role of drug choice. In *Substance Abuse and Psychopathology*, Alterman AI (ed). Plenum Press, New York, pp. 137–172.

Mendels J (1976) Lithium in the treatment of depression. *Am J Psychiatry* **133**, 373–378.

Mendlewicz J and Rainer JD (1977) Adoption study supporting genetic transmission in manic–depressive illness. *Nature* **268**, 327–329.

Miklowitz DJ, Simoneau TL, George EL, et al. (1999) Family-focused treatment of bipolar disorder: 1-year effects of a psychoeducational program in conjunction with pharmacotherapy. *Biol Psychiatry* **48**, 582–592.

Mundo E, Walker M, Cate T, et al. (2001) The role of serotonin transporter protein gene in antidepressant-induced mania in bipolar disorder: preliminary findings. *Arch Gen Psychiatry* **58**(6), 539–544.

Nasrallah H, Coffman J, and Olson S (1989) Structural brain imaging findings in affective disorders: an overview. *J Neuropsychiatr Clin Neurosci* **1**, 21–26.

National Institute of Mental Health National Advisory Mental Health Council (1992) *Caring for People with Severe Mental Disorders. A National Plan of Research to Improve Services*, DHHS publication ADM91-1762, US Government Printing Office, Washington, DC.

Nilsson A and Axelsson R (1989) Psychopathology during long-term lithium treatment of patients with major affective disorders: a prospective study. *Acta Psychiatr Scand* **80**, 375–388.

Nurnberger J, Berrettini W, Tamarkin L, et al. (1989) Supersensitivity to melatonin suppression by light in young people at high risk for affective disorder: a preliminary report. *Neuropsychopharmacol* **1**, 217–223.

O'Connell R, Mayo J, Flatow L, et al. (1991) Outcome of bipolar disorder on long-term treatment with lithium. *Br J Psychiatry* **159**, 123–129.

Palmer AG and Williams H (1995) CBT in a group format for bipolar affective disorder. *Behav Cogn Psychother* **23**, 153–168.

Papolos DF, Veit S, Faedda GL, et al. (1998) Ultra-rapid cycling bipolar disorder is associated with low activity catecholamine-O-methyltransferase allele. *Mol Psychiatry* **3**(4), 346–349.

Parsons PL (1965) Mental health of Swansea's old folk. *Br J Prev Soc Med* **19**, 43–47.

Paykel E and Cooper Z (1992) Life events and social stress. In *Handbook of Affective Disorders*, Paykel E (ed). Guilford Press, New York, pp. 149–170.

Peet M and Harvey NS (1991) Lithium maintenance: 1. a standard education programme for patients. *Br J Psychiatry* **158**, 197–200.

Perris H (1984a) Life events and depression: Part 1. Effect of sex, age, and civil status. *J Affect Dis* **7**, 11–24.

Perry A, Tarrier N, Morriss R, et al. (1999) Randomised controlled trial of efficacy of teaching patients with bipolar disorder to identify early symptoms of relapse and obtain treatment. *Br Med J* **318**, 149–153.

Petronis A and Kennedy J (1995) Unstable genes—unstable mind? *Am J Psychiatry* **152**, 164–172.

Petterson WU (1977) Manic–depressive illness: a clinical, social, and genetic study. *Acta Psychiatr Scand (Suppl)* **269**.

Petty F, Kramer GL, Fulton M, et al. (1993) Low plasma GABA is a trait-like marker for bipolar illness. *Neuropsychopharmacol* **9**, 125–132.

Petty F, Rush J, Davis J, et al. (1996) Plasma gaba predicts acute response to divalproex in mania. *Biol Psychiatry* **39**, 278–284.

Pope H, McElroy S, Keck P, et al. (1991) Valproate in the treatment of acute mania. *Arch Gen Psychiatry* **48**, 62–68.

Post RM (1992) Transduction of psychosocial stress into the neurobiology of recurrent affective disorder. *Am J Psychiatry* **149**, 999–1010.

Post RM, DeLisi LE, Holcomb HH, et al. (1987) Glucose utilization in the temporal cortex of affectively ill patients: positron emission tomography. *Biol Psychiatry* **22**, 545–553.

Post RM, Leverich GS, Altshuler L, et al. (1992) Lithium-discontinuation-induced refractoriness: preliminary observations. *Am J Psychiatry* **149**, 1727–1729.

Post R, Rubinow D, and Ballenger J (1985) Conditioning, sensitization, and kindling: implications for the course of affective illness. In *Neurobiology of Mood Disorders*, Post R and Ballenger J (eds). Williams & Wilkins, Baltimore, pp. 432–466.

Post R, Rubinow D, and Ballenger J (1986a) Conditioning, sensitization, and the longitudinal course of affective illness. *Br J Psychiatry* **149**, 191–201.

Post RM, Uhde TW, Rubinow DR, et al. (1986b) Anti-manic effects of carbamazepine: mechanisms of action and implications for the biochemistry of manic–depressive illness. In *Mania: New Research and Treatment*, Swann A (ed). American Psychiatric Press, Washington, DC, pp. 95–176.

Potash JB and DePaulo JR (2000) Searching high and low: a review of the genetics of bipolar disorder. *Bipolar Disord* **2**, 8–26.

Prange AJ (1964) The pharmacology and biochemistry of depression. *Dis Nerv Syst* **25**, 217–221.

Price J (1968) Neurotic and endogenous depression: a phylogenetic view. *Br J Psychiatry* **114**, 119–120.

Prien R, Caffey E, and Klett CJ (1973a) Prophylactic efficacy of lithium carbonate in manic–depressive illness. Report of the veterans administration and national institute of mental health collaborative study group. *Arch Gen Psychiatry* **28**, 337–341.

Prien R and Gelenberg A (1989) Alternatives to lithium for the preventive treatment of bipolar disorder. *Am J Psychiatry* **146**, 840–848.

Prien RF, Klett CJ, and Caffey EM Jr. (1973b) Lithium carbonate and imipramine in prevention of affective episodes: a comparison in recurrent affective illness. *Arch Gen Psychiatry* **29**, 420–425.

Ray WA, Griffin MR, Schaffner W, et al. (1987) Psychotropic drug use and the risk of hip fracture. *N Engl J Med* **316**, 363–369.

Regier D, Farmer M, Rae D, et al. (1990) Comorbidity of mental disorders with alcohol and other drugs. Results from the epidemiological catchment area (ECA) study. *JAMA* **264**, 2511–2518.

Retzer A, Simon FB, Weber G, et al. (1991) A follow-up study of manic–depressive and schizoaffective psychoses after systemic family therapy. *Fam Process* **30**, 139–153.

Rice D, Kelman S, Miller L, et al. (1990) *The Economic Costs of Alcohol and Drug Abuse and Mental Illness: 1985*, DHHS publication (ADM) 90–1694, National Institute of Mental Health, Rockville, MD.

Robert E and Guiband P (1983) Maternal valproic acid and congenital neural tube defects. *Lancet* **2**, 937.

Rotter J (1966) Generalized expectancies for internal versus external control of reinforcement. *Psychol Monogr* **80**, 1–28.

Roy-Byrne P, Post R, Uhde T, et al. (1985) The longitudinal course of recurrent affective illness: life chart data from research patients at the NIMH. *Acta Psychiatr Scand* **71**(Suppl. 317),, 3–34.

Sassi RB and Soares JC (2002) Neural circuitry and signaling in bipolar disorder. In *Brain Circuitry in Psychiatry: Basic Science and Clinical Implications*, Kaplan GB and Hammer RP (eds). American Psychiatric Press, pp. 179–200.

Schatzberg AF, Cole JO, and DeBattista C (1997) *Manual of Clinical Psychopharmacology*, 3rd ed., American Psychiatric Press, Washington, DC.

Schildkraut J (1965) The catecholamine hypothesis of affective disorder: a review of supporting evidence. *Am J Psychiatr* **122**, 509–522.

Schou M (1988) Effects of long-term lithium treatment on kidney function: an overview. *J Psychiatr Res* **22**, 287–296.

Sclare P and Creed F (1990) Life events and the onset of mania. *Br J Psychiatry* **156**, 508–514.

Scolnik D, Nulman I, and Rovet J (1994) Neurodevelopment of children exposed in utero to phenytoin and carbamazepine monotherapy. *JAMA* **271**, 767–770.

Simpson SG, Folstein SE, Meyers DA, et al. (1993) Bipolar II: the most common bipolar phenotype? *Am J Psychiatry* **150**, 901–903.

Stahl SM (2000) Depression and bipolar disorders. *Essential Psychopharmacology*, 2nd ed., Ch. 5, Cambridge University Press, Cambridge, pp. 135–197.

Stallone F, Shelley E, Mendlewicz J, et al. (1973) The use of lithium in affective disorders III: a double-blind study of prophylaxis in bipolar illness. *Am J Psychiatry* **130**(9), 1006–1010.

Starkstein SE, Boston JD, and Robinson RGG (1988) Mechanisms of mania after brain injury: 12 case reports and review of the literature. *J Nerv Ment Dis* **176**, 87–100.

Stewart A, Greenfield S, Hays R, et al. (1989) Functional status and well-being of patients with chronic conditions. *JAMA* **262**, 907–913.

Stokes PE, Shamoian CA, Stoll PM, et al. (1971) Efficacy of lithium as acute treatment of manic–depressive illness. *Lancet* **1**, 1319–1325.

Stoudemire A, Frank R, Hedemark N, et al. (1986) The economic burden of depression. *Gen Hosp Psychiatry* **8**, 387–394.

Strakowski SM, Wilson DR, Tohen M, et al. (1993a) Structural brain abnormalities in first-episode mania. *Biol Psychiatry* **33**, 602–609.

Strober M, Schmidt-Lackner S, Freeman R, et al. (1995) Recovery and relapse in adolescents with bipolar affective illness: a five-year naturalistic, prospective follow-up. *J Am Acad Child Adolesc Psychiatry* **34**, 724–731.

Suppes T, Baldessarini RJ, Faedda GL, et al. (1993) Discontinuation of maintenance treatment in bipolar disorder: risks and implications. *Harv Rev Psychiatry* **1**, 131–144.

Swann AC (2001) Major system toxicities and side effects of anticonvulsants. *J Clin Psychiatry* **62**(Suppl. 14),, 16–21.

Taylor MA, Abrams R, and Hayman MA (1980) The classification of affective disorders: a reassessment of the bipolar–unipolar dichotomy: a clinical, laboratory, and family study. *J Affect Disord* **2**, 95–109.

Terman M, Terman J, Quitkin F, et al. (1989) Light therapy for seasonal affective disorder: a review of efficacy. *Neuropsychopharmacology* **2**, 1–22.

Thase ME and Sachs GS (2000) Bipolar depression: pharmacotherapy and related therapeutic strategies. *Biol Psychiatry* **48**(6), 558–572.

Tohen M, Jacobs TG, Grundy SL, et al. (2000) Efficacy of olanzapine in acute bipolar mania: a double-blind, placebo-controlled study. *Arch Gen Psychiatry* **57**, 841–849.

Tohen M, Sanger TM, McElroy SL, et al. (1999) Olanzapine versus placebo in the treatment of acute mania. *Am J Psychiatry* **156**(5), 702–709.

Tohen M, Waternaux C, and Tsuang M (1990) Outcome in mania: a 4-year prospective follow-up of 75 patients utilizing survival analysis. *Arch Gen Psychiatry* **47**, 1106–1111.

Tsuang MT, Faraone SV, and Fleming JA (1985) Familial transmission of major affective disorders: Is there evidence supporting the distinction between unipolar and bipolar disorders? *Br J Psychiatry* **146**, 268–271.

Tsuang M, Woolson R, and Fleming J (1979) Long-term outcome of major psychoses. *Arch Gen Psychiatry* **36**, 1295–1301.

US Department of Health, Education, and Welfare Medical Practice Project (1979) *A State-of-the-Science Report for the Office of the Assistant Secretary of the US Department of Health, Education, and Welfare, Policy Research*, Baltimore.

Vaamonde C, Milian N, Magrinat G, et al. (1986) Longitudinal evaluation of glomerular filtration rate during long-term lithium therapy. *Am J Kidney Dis* **7**, 213–216.

Van Gent E, Vida S, and Zwart F (1988) Group therapy in addition to lithium therapy in patients with bipolar disorders. *Acta Psychiatr Belg* **88**, 405–418.

Van Gent EM and Zwart F (1991) Psychoeducation of partners of bipolar-manic patients. *J Affect Disord* **21**, 15–18.

Van Gent EM and Zwart FM (1993) Five-year follow-up after educational group therapy added to lithium prophylaxis: five years after group added to lithium. *Depression* **1**, 225–226.

VHA (Veterans Health Administration) (1997) *Clinical Guidelines for Management of Persons with Psychoses*. Office of Performance Management, VHA Headquarters, Washington, DC.

Vojta C, Kinosian B, Glick H, et al. (2001) Self-reported quality of life across mood states in bipolar disorder. *Compr Psychiatry* **42**(3), 190–195.

Volkmar F, Shakir S, Bacon S, et al. (1981) Group therapy in the management of manic–depressive illness. *Am J Psychother* **35**, 226–234.

Wehr T, Goodwin F, Wirz-Justice A, et al. (1982) 48-hour sleep–wake cycles in manic–depressive illness: naturalistic observations and sleep deprivation experiments. *Arch Gen Psychiatry* **39**, 559–565.

Wehr T, Murdock R, Persad E, et al. (1993) Can antidepressants induce rapid cycling? (letters). *Arch Gen Psychiatr* **50**, 495–498.

Weinstein MR and Goldfield MD (1975) Cardiovascular malformations with lithium use during pregnancy. *Am J Psychiatry* **132**, 529–531.

Weiss RD, Griffin ML, Greenfield SF, et al. (2000) Group therapy for patients with bipolar disorder and substance dependence: results of a pilot study. *J Clin Psychiatry* **61**, 361–367.

Weiss RD, Mirin SM, Griffin ML, et al. (1988) Psychopathology in cocaine abusers: Changing trends. *J Nerv Ment Dis* **176**, 719–725.

Weissman MM, Leaf PJ, Tischler GL, et al. (1988) Affective disorders in five United States communities. *Psychol Med* **18**, 141–153.

Weissman MM and Myers JK (1978) Affective disorders in a US urban community: the use of research diagnostic criteria in an epidemiological survey. *Arch Gen Psychiatry* **35**, 1304–1311.

Wells K, Stewart A, Hays R, et al. (1989) The functioning and well-being of depressed patients. Results from the Medical Outcomes Study. *JAMA* **262**, 914–919.

Welner A, Welner Z, and Leonard A (1977) Bipolar manic–depressive disorder: a reassessment of course and outcome. *Compr Psychiatry* **18**, 327–332.

Williams P and McGlashan T (1987) Schizoaffective psychosis I. Comparative long-term outcome. *Arch Gen Psychiatry* **44**, 130–137.

Winokur G, Clayton PJ, and Reich T (1969) *Manic–Depressive Illness*. CV Mosby, St. Louis.

World Health Organization (1994) *International Statistical Classification of Diseases and Related Health Problems*, 10th Rev. World Health Organization, Geneva.

Zaretsky AE, Segal ZV, and Gemar M (1999) Cognitive therapy for bipolar depression: a pilot study. *Can J Psychiatry* **44**, 491–494.

Zarin DA and Pass TM (1987) Lithium and the single episode: when to begin long-term prophylaxis for bipolar disorder. *Med Care* **25**, S76–S84.

CHAPTER

31 Anxiety Disorders:
Panic Disorder with
and without
Agoraphobia

Diagnosis

According to the DSM-IV-TR, panic disorder is defined by recurrent and unexpected panic attacks. At least one of these attacks must be followed by 1 month or more of (1) persistent concern about having more attacks, (2) worry about the implications or consequences of the attack, or (3) changes to typical behavioral patterns (e.g., avoidance of work or school activities) as a result of the attack (see DSM-IV-TR diagnostic criteria below for Panic disorder with agoraphobia and page 846 for Panic disorder without agoraphobia). In addition, the panic attacks must not stem solely from the direct effects of illicit substance use, medication, or a general medical condition (e.g., hyperthyroidism, vestibular dysfunction) and are not better explained by another mental disorder (such as social phobia for attacks that occur only in social situations). A diagnosis of panic disorder with agoraphobia is warranted when the criteria for panic disorder are satisfied and accompanied by agoraphobia.

DSM-IV-TR Diagnostic Criteria

300.21 Panic Disorder with Agoraphobia

A. Both (1) and (2):

    (1) recurrent unexpected panic attacks
    (2) at least one of the attacks has been followed by one month (or more) of one (or more) of the following:

        (a) persistent concern about having additional attacks
        (b) worry about the implications of the attack or its consequences (e.g., losing control, having a heart attack, "going crazy")

B. The presence of agoraphobia.
C. The panic attacks are not due to the direct physiological effects of a substance (e.g., a drug of abuse, a medication) or a general medical condition (e.g., hyperthyroidism).
D. The panic attacks are not better accounted for by another mental disorder, such as social phobia (e.g., occurring on exposure to feared social situations), specific phobia (e.g., on exposure to a specific phobic situation), obsessive–compulsive disorder (e.g., on exposure to dirt in someone with an obsession about contamination), posttraumatic stress disorder (e.g., in response to stimuli associated with a severe stressor), or separation anxiety disorder (e.g., in response to being away from home or close relatives).

Reprinted with permission from the Diagnostic and Statistical Manual of Mental Disorders, Fourth Edition, Text Revision. Copyright 2000 American Psychiatric Association.

DSM-IV-TR Diagnostic Criteria

300.21 Panic Disorder without Agoraphobia

A. Both (1) and (2):

(1) recurrent unexpected panic attacks
(2) at least one of the attacks has been followed by 1 month (or more) of one (or more) of the following:

(a) persistent concern about having additional attacks
(b) worry about the implications of the attack or its consequences (e.g., losing control, having a heart attack, "going crazy")

B. Absence of agoraphobia.
C. The panic attacks are not due to the direct physiological effects of a substance (e.g., a drug of abuse, a medication) or a general medical condition (e.g., hyperthyroidism).
D. The panic attacks are not better accounted for by another mental disorder, such as social phobia (e.g., occurring on exposure to feared social situations), specific phobia (e.g., on exposure to a specific phobic situation), obsessive–compulsive disorder (e.g., on exposure to dirt in someone with an obsession about contamination), posttraumatic stress disorder (e.g., in response to stimuli associated with a severe stressor), or separation anxiety disorder (e.g., in response to being away from home or close relatives).

Reprinted with permission from the Diagnostic and Statistical Manual of Mental Disorders, Fourth Edition, Text Revision. Copyright 2000 American Psychiatric Association.

Although panic attacks are a cardinal feature of panic disorder and in combination with agoraphobia (i.e., anxiety about being in a place or a situation that is not easily escaped or where help is not easily accessible if panic occurs) are essential to a diagnosis of panic disorder with agoraphobia, the criteria sets for panic attacks (see DSM-IV-TR diagnostic criteria for Panic Attack on page 847) and for agoraphobia (see

DSM-IV-TR diagnostic criteria for Agoraphobia below) are listed separately as stand-alone, noncodable conditions that are referred to by the diagnostic criteria for panic disorder and agoraphobia without history of panic disorder. Notwithstanding, accurate diagnosis is difficult without a proficient understanding of these features. While the criteria for agoraphobia are generally straightforward, panic attacks can be difficult to understand.

DSM-IV-TR Diagnostic Criteria

Panic Attack

A panic attack is a discrete period of intense fear or discomfort in the absence of real danger that develops abruptly, reaches a peak within 10 min, and is accompanied by four (or more) of the following symptoms:

A. palpitations, pounding heart, or accelerated heart rate
B. sweating
C. trembling or shaking
D. sensations of shortness of breath or smothering
E. feeling of choking
F. chest pain or discomfort
G. nausea or abdominal distress
H. feeling dizzy, unsteady, light-headed, or faint
I. derealization (feelings of unreality) or depersonalization (being detached from oneself)
J. fear of losing control or going crazy
K. fear of dying
L. paresthesias (numbness or tingling sensations)
M. chills or hot flushes

Reprinted with permission from the Diagnostic and Statistical Manual of Mental Disorders, Fourth Edition, Text Revision. Copyright 2000 American Psychiatric Association.

DSM-IV-TR Diagnostic Criteria

Agoraphobia

A. Agoraphobia is characterized by anxiety about being in places or situations from which escape might be difficult (or embarrassing) or in which help may not be available in the event of having an unexpected or situationally predisposed panic attack or panic-like symptoms. Agoraphobic fears typically involve characteristic clusters of situations, such as being outside the home alone, being in a crowd, standing in a line, being on a bridge, or traveling in a motor vehicle.
B. The situations are avoided or are endured with marked distress or worry about having a panic attack or panic-like symptoms. Confronting situations is aided by the presence of a companion.

C. The anxiety or avoidance is not better accounted for by another mental disorder.

A number of investigations (Brown and Deagle 1992, Norton et al. 1999, Wilson et al. 1992) indicate that people report having what they consider to be a panic attack during or in association with actual physical threat (i.e., a true alarm situation). It is, however, important to distinguish between a fear reaction in response to actual threat and a panic attack. In an attempt to do so, the DSM-IV-TR has clarified that panic attacks occur "in the absence of real danger" (page 430). Such attacks involve a paroxysmal occurrence of intense fear or discomfort accompanied by a minimum of 4 of the 13 symptoms shown in diagnostic criteria for Panic Attack. The DSM-IV-TR recognizes three characteristic types of panic attacks, including those that are *unexpected* (i.e., not associated with an identifiable internal or external trigger and appear to occur "out of the blue"), *situationally bound* (i.e., almost invariably occur when exposed to a situational trigger or when anticipating it), and *situationally predisposed* (i.e., usually, but not necessarily, occur when exposed to a situational trigger or when anticipating it). The term *limited symptom attacks* is used to refer to panic-like episodes comprising fewer than four symptoms.

Although unexpected panic attacks are required for a diagnosis of panic disorder, not all panic attacks that occur in panic disorder are unexpected. The occurrence of unexpected attacks can wax and wane and over the developmental course of the disorder; they tend to become situationally bound or predisposed. Moreover, unexpected panic attacks as well as those that are situationally bound or predisposed can occur in the context of other mental disorders, including all of the other anxiety disorders (e.g., a person with social phobia might have an occasional unexpected panic attack without the other feature required to diagnose panic disorder; a dog phobic might panic whenever a large dog is encountered) (Barlow 1988) and some general medical conditions. A clear understanding of the distinction between types of panic attacks outlined in the DSM-IV-TR provides a foundation for diagnosis and differential diagnosis. As described by Taylor (2000), however, consideration of other characteristics of panic—including duration of attacks, frequency of attacks, number and intensity of symptoms, nature of catastrophic thinking, and mechanism responsible for termination of an attack—can be important in identifying, exacerbating, and controlling factors.

Panic disorder with or without agoraphobia is associated with impaired occupational and social functioning and poor overall quality of life (Katerndahl and Realini 1997, Leon et al. 1995). People with panic disorder, compared to people in the general population, report poorer physical health (Markowitz et al. 1989). Panic disorder is a leading reason for seeking emergency department consultations (Weissman 1991) and a leading cause for seeking mental health services, surpassing both schizophrenia and mood disorders (Boyd 1986). Panic disorder exceeds the economic costs associated with many other anxiety disorders such as social phobia, generalized anxiety disorder, and obsessive–compulsive disorder (Greenberg et al. 1999). The high medical costs are partly because individuals with panic disorder quite often present to their primary care physician or hospital emergency departments, thinking they are in imminent danger of dying or "going crazy" (Katerndahl and Realini 1995). In these settings, individuals may undergo a series of extensive medical tests before panic disorder is, if ever, finally diagnosed. Ruling out general medical conditions is good clinical practice but the process contributes substantially to the costs that panic disorder places on health care systems.

When assessing for the presence of panic disorder, the most comprehensive and accurate diagnostic information emerges when the clinician uses open-ended questions and empathic listening, combined with structured inquiry about specific events and symptoms (American Psychiatric Association 1995). Useful structured interviews include the *Structured Clinical Interview for DSM-IV* (SCID-IV) (First et al. 1996) and the *Anxiety Disorders Interview Schedule for DSM-IV* (ADIS-IV; Di Nardo et al. 1994). Diagnostic information can be usefully supplemented by short self-report questionnaires to assess the severity of symptoms and other variables (Taylor 2000) The *Beck Depression Inventory* (Beck and Steer 1987) and *Beck Anxiety Inventory* (Beck and Steer 1993) are quick, reliable, and valid measures that can be administered at the start of each treatment session to assess the severity of past-week general anxiety and depression. The *Anxiety Sensitivity Index* (Peterson and Reiss 1992) is another useful short questionnaire that can be used to gauge the severity of the individual's fear of bodily sensations. Scores on this scale can be used to assess whether treatment is altering the individual's tendency to catastrophically misinterpret bodily sensations. This scale has good reliability and validity, is sensitive to treatment-related effects, and its posttreatment scores predict who is likely to relapse after panic treatment (Taylor 1999).

To gain more detailed information on panic attacks, clinicians and clinical researchers are increasingly including some form of prospective monitoring in their assessment batteries (Shear and Maser 1994). The most widely used are the *panic attack records*. The individual is provided with a definition of a panic attack and then given a pad of panic attack records that can be readily carried in a purse or pocket. The individual is instructed to carry the records at all times and to complete one record (sheet) for each full-blown or limited symptom attack, soon after the attack occurs. Variants on the panic diaries developed by Barlow and colleagues (Barlow and Craske 1994, Rapee et al. 1990) are among the most informative and easy to use.

Consider the application of the panic attack record to the following case vignette. Sandra B. was a 20-year-old college student who presented to a student health clinic reporting recurrent panic attacks. Her first attack occurred seven months earlier while smoking marijuana at an end-of-term party. At the time, she felt depersonalized, dizzy, short of breath, and her heart was beating wildly. Sandra had an overwhelming fear that she was going crazy. Friends took her to a nearby hospital emergency department where she was given a brief medical evaluation, reassured that she was simply experiencing anxiety and given a prescription for lorazepam. In the following months, Sandra continued to experience unexpected panic attacks and became increasingly convinced that she was losing control of her mind. Most of her panics occurred unexpectedly during the day, although they sometimes also occurred at night, wrenching her out of a deep sleep. An example of how Sandra B. might complete the panic attack record for one of her panic attacks is shown in Figure 31-1. These records are then reviewed during treatment sessions to glean information about the links among beliefs, bodily sensations, and safety behaviors, and to assess treatment progress.

Sandra B. reported that the panic attack summarized in Figure 31-1 occurred when she was in a neighborhood supermarket. As she walked down the aisle, she looked at the long rows of fluorescent lights and then began to feel mildly depersonalized. Upon noticing this sensation, she began to increasingly worry that the depersonalization might become so intense that she would lose all contact with reality, to the point that she would be permanently insane. This greatly frightened her and led to an increase in the intensity of arousal sensations (as described in the cognitive model of panic). In an effort to reduce the intensity of the feared depersonalization, she averted her gaze from the lights and began studying the list of ingredients on cereal boxes. This distracting safety behavior calmed her down and reduced the feared depersonalization to the point that she was able to make her way to the express checkout counter and leave with the grocery items she had collected.

PANIC ATTACK RECORD

NAME: **Sandra.B.**

DATE: **Oct 2**   TIME: **4pm**   DURATION (min): **15**

WITH: SPOUSE _____   FRIEND _____   STRANGER _____   ALONE **✓**

STRESSFUL SITUATION: YES /(NO)   EXPECTED: YES /(NO)

MAXIMUM ANXIETY (CIRCLE)

0 -------- 1 -------- 2 -------- 3 -------- 4 --------(5)-------- 6 -------- 7 -------- 8
    NONE   MODERATE   EXTREME

SENSATIONS (CHECK):

POUNDING HEART	✓	SWEATING	✓	HOT/COLD FLASH	✓
TIGHT/PAINFUL CHEST	✓	CHOKING	___	FEAR OF DYING	___
BREATHLESS	✓	NAUSEA	___	FEAR OF GOING CRAZY	✓
DIZZY	✓	UNREALITY	✓	FEAR OF LOSING CONTROL	✓
TREMBLING	___	NUMB/TINGLE	✓		

THOUGHTS OR MENTAL IMAGES AT THE TIME (DESCRIBE):

I'm losing contact with reality

Figure 31-1 *A completed panic attack record for Sandra B.*

Lifetime comorbidity (i.e., the co-occurrence of two or more disorders at any point in a person's life, regardless of whether or not they overlap) in panic disorder is common, with over 90% of community-dwelling and treatment-seeking individuals having had symptoms meeting diagnostic threshold for at least one other disorder (Robins et al. 1991). The reader is referred to Taylor (2000) for detailed discussion of the various comorbidity models and how they account for the co-occurrence of other disorders with panic disorder.

Epidemiological studies indicate that major depressive disorder occurs in up to 65% of individuals with panic disorder at some point in their lives. In approximately two-thirds of these cases, the symptoms of depression develop along with, or secondary to, panic disorder (American Psychiatric Association 2000; Kessler et al. 1998). However, since depression precedes panic disorder in the remaining third (Breier et al. 1984), depressive symptoms co-occurring with panic disorder cannot be considered simply as a demoralized response to paroxysms of anxiety. While the risk of developing secondary depression appears to be more closely associated with the severity of agoraphobia than with the severity or frequency of panic attacks, this may be a confound of misdiagnosing of some behavioral manifestations of depression as agoraphobia (Taylor 2000). Panic disorder and depression do not appear to be identical disorders (Stein and Uhde 1990) and their co-occurrence may be due to a shared diathesis or mutual exacerbation of symptoms.

As illustrated in the case of Sandra B., panic disorder can be precipitated by the use of psychotropic drugs (Ballenger and Fyer 1996). Risk is higher with chronic use (Louie et al. 1996). Alcohol has been identified as playing a precipitating, maintaining, and aggravating role in panic disorder. The 6-month prevalence of alcohol abuse or dependence in panic disorder has been reported to be 40% in men and 13% in women (Leon et al. 1995). These rates are higher than those observed in people with other anxiety disorders and those with no anxiety disorder (Leon et al. 1995). Although alcohol problems have been reported to precede panic disorder in a majority of cases (Otto et al. 1992), most reports indicate that alcohol problems develop secondary to panic disorder, often as a means of self-medication (Bibb and Chambless 1986). Those having panic disorder with agoraphobia appear to be at greater risk for comorbid alcohol abuse or dependence than those without agoraphobia (Thyer et al. 1986).

Epidemiology

The 1-year prevalence for any panic attack, whether unexpected or situationally cued, is approximately 28% (Brown and Deagle 1992, Norton et al. 1992). Lifetime prevalence rates for unexpected panic attacks and agoraphobia are approximately 4 and 9% respectively (Wittchen et al. 1998). Investigations of unexpected panic attacks in college student samples using self-report methodology have revealed similar rates, ranging from approximately 5% (Norton et al. 1986, Wilson et al. 1991) to 11% (Asmundson and Norton 1993).

The National Comorbidity Study (Eaton et al. 1994) has reported the lifetime prevalence of panic disorder (with or without agoraphobia) in the general population to be 3.5%. However, despite uncertainty as to the reason, this rate is somewhat of an anomaly in the literature. Most epidemiological studies, including those based on Epidemiologic Catchment Area and other data sources have consistently shown lifetime rates between 1 and 2% (Eaton et al. 1991, Reed and Wittchen 1998, Weissman et al. 1997). Weissman and colleagues (1997) have demonstrated that despite some minor variation, lifetime prevalence rates are generally consistent around the world. One-year prevalence rates in the general community also vary slightly from lifetime rates, being between 0.2 and 1.7% (Weissman et al. 1997). In treatment-seeking individuals, the prevalence of panic disorder is considerably higher. Approximately 10% of individuals in mental health clinics and between 10 and 60% in various medical specialty clinics (e.g., cardiology, respiratory, vestibular) have panic disorder (Chignon et al. 1993, Rouillon 1997, Spinhoven et al. 1993, Stein et al. 1994). Panic disorder with agoraphobia is more common than panic disorder without agoraphobia in clinical samples (American Psychiatric Association 2000).

The clinical features of panic disorder such as number and severity of symptoms are much the same across the sexes (Oei et al. 1990). However, women are diagnosed with panic disorder more than twice as often as men (Weissman et al. 1997). Recent research indicates that women are more likely to have panic disorder with agoraphobia and that they are more likely to have recurrence of symptoms after remission of their panic attacks than are men (Yonkers et al. 1998). Men, on the other hand, are more likely to have panic disorder without agoraphobia (Yonkers et al. 1998) and are more likely to self medicate with alcohol than are women (Cox et al. 1993). The literature remains unclear as to why these sex differences exist but alludes to the possible role of biological and/or socialization factors (Bekker 1996, Yonkers 1994).

Course

Age of onset for panic disorder is distributed bimodally, typically developing between 15 and 19 or 25 and 30 years (Ballenger and Fyer 1996). Panic disorder symptoms may wax and wane but, if left untreated, the typical course is chronic (Keller et al. 1994, Uhde et al. 1985). Data from a sample of individuals assessed and treated through the Harvard/Brown Anxiety Disorders Research Program and followed prospectively over a 5-year period indicated remission rates in both men and women to be 39% (Yonkers et al. 1998). In general, among those receiving tertiary treatment, approximately 30% of individuals have symptoms that are in remission, 40 to 50% are improved but still have significant symptoms, and 20 to 30% are unimproved or worse at 6 to 10 years follow-up (American Psychiatric Association 2000).

Differential Diagnosis

A complete assessment for panic disorder includes a general medical evaluation (American Psychiatric Association 1995), consisting of a medical history, review of organ systems, physical examination, and blood tests. A general medical evaluation is important for identifying general medical conditions that mimic or exacerbate panic attacks or panic-like symptoms (e.g., seizure disorders, cardiac conditions, pheochromocytoma) (Goldberg 1988, Raj and Sheehan 1987). These disorders should be investigated and treated before contemplating a course of panic disorder treatment. It is also important to rule out the other anxiety disorders and major depressive disorder as primary factors in the person's panic attacks and avoidance prior to initiating treatment for panic disorder. See Figure 31-2 for a decision tree outlining the differential diagnosis for a panic attack.

Etiology

Cognitive Models—The Vicious Cycle

There are several contemporary cognitive models of panic disorder, which, for the most part, are based on variations of the "fear of anxiety" construct. Goldstein and Chambless (1978) proposed that fear of anxiety arises through the association of interoceptive cues with panic attacks. In other words, people with panic disorder are thought to learn to fear the recurrence of aversive panic episodes and thereby develop a fear of panic-related symptoms. Refuting the premise that fear of anxiety develops from the experience of panic attacks, Clark (1986) posited that panic attacks are the product of a tendency to *catastrophically misinterpret* autonomic arousal sensations that occur in the context of nonpathological anxiety (as well as physical illness, exercise, and ingestion of certain substances). Reiss and colleagues (Reiss 1999, Reiss and McNally 1985), incorporating components of the Goldstein and Chambless and Clark models, proposed that panic attacks arise as a consequence of both (1) a predispositional tendency to catastrophically misinterpret and respond with fear to the benign arousal sensations, and (2) a learned fear of anxiety that is maintained by the experience of panic episodes.

Most recently, Bouton, Mineka, and Barlow (2001) have described a variant of the original fear of anxiety model, suggesting that panic disorder develops when exposure to panic attacks conditions a person to respond with anticipatory anxiety (and sometimes with panic) to internal arousal and contextual cues. While each of these models has proven fruitful in research and treatment contexts, we focus below on the model of Clark (1986).

As described above, Clark (1986) proposes that panic attacks arise from the catastrophic misinterpretation of benign arousal sensations. To illustrate the cognitive processes proposed to underlie panic attacks, consider Sandra B.'s experience during one of her many attacks. In this instance, she had dizziness sensations stemming from influenza, perceived them as threatening, became aroused, misinterpreted the sensations as being indicative

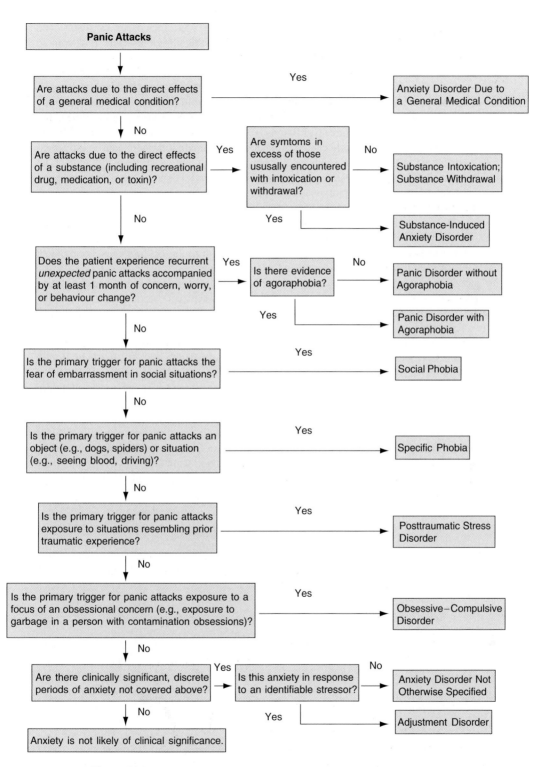

Figure 31-2 *A decision tree for assessment of patients presenting with panic attacks.*

that she was losing her mind, became further aroused with increasing dizziness, had further thoughts of going mad, and spiraled into panic. This vicious cycle is shown in Figure 31-3.

The vicious cycle model makes several assumptions. First, while recognizing that initial panic attacks may be caused by other factors (e.g., drug-related autonomic surges), it assumes that people prone to panic disorder have an enduring tendency to catastrophically misinterpret benign arousal sensations. Second, it assumes that misinterpretations can occur at the conscious and unconscious level (Clark 1988). Third, the cycle can be entered into at any point. For example, the cycle can be initiated by a contextual trigger, such as influenza-related dizziness in the case of Sandra B., or simply by having catastrophic thoughts about bodily sensations. Fourth, physiological changes are viewed as one of several components in a process, rather than as a pathogenic mechanism.

Cognitive models can also account for agoraphobia. Agoraphobia has long been regarded as a product of operant conditioning (Marks 1987). As noted above, it most often develops as a consequence of panic attacks. These attacks typically occur in particular situations (e.g., when in line at a shopping mall, when driving) and motivate the person to avoid or escape these situations. The avoidance and escape behaviors are negatively reinforced by the reduction of aversive autonomic arousal and other anxiety-related sensations. Cognitive factors such as expectations that an attack will be imminent and harmful and that coping will be ineffective play a significant role by influencing and maintaining avoidance behavior (Taylor and Rachman 1994).

A growing body of literature supports the vicious cycle model. Thoughts of imminent catastrophe have been identified as triggers of panic attacks (Hibbert 1984). Individuals with panic disorder relative to healthy and non-panic patient controls have been shown to be (1) characterized by strategic and automatic information processing (i.e., memory, attention) biases for physical threat cues (Logan and Goetsch 1993, McNally 1996); (2) more accurate, in some instances, at detecting body sensations (Ehlers and Breuer 1996); (3) more likely to report fear of somatic sensations and beliefs in their harmful consequences (Taylor 1999); and (4) more susceptible to the influence of instructional manipulations of control in response to pharmacological panic provocation challenges, panicking less often under the illusion of greater control in some (Rapee et al. 1986, Sanderson et al. 1989) but not all (Welkowitz et al. 1999) cases.

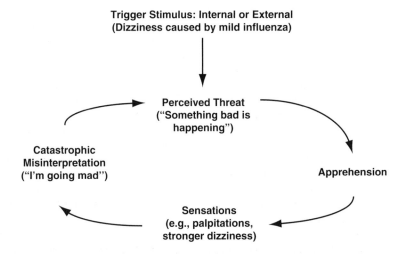

Figure 31-3 *Application of the cognitive model to illustrate one of Sandra B.'s panic attacks.*

Biological Models

Evidence suggests that several neurotransmitter systems, involving neurotransmitters or neuromodulators such as serotonin, noradrenalin, adenosine, gamma-aminobutyric acid, and cholecystokinin-4, play a role in panic disorder (McNally 1994). Various brain structures in the limbic system and associated regions have also been implicated. Contemporary biological models of panic, beginning with the pioneering work of Klein (1980), have grown in number and complexity in recent years in an effort to integrate and explain these findings. Recent emphasis has focused on the amygdala, a limbic structure that appears to be involved in coordinating the different neurotransmitters involved in anxiety disorders (Goddard and Charney 1997). Today, there is no single, leading biological model of panic. However, there are a number of useful models that guide research and clinical practice (Gorman et al. 2000, Klein 1993). Among the most promising is the neuroanatomical hypothesis recently revised by Gorman and colleagues (2000). This hypothesis is useful for several reasons. First, it integrates a wide range of findings, including animal research and studies of humans. Second, it provides a unifying framework for understanding why panic disorder is associated with so many biological dysregularities such as abnormalities in neurotransmitter systems and irregularities on various indices of autonomic functioning (Abelson et al. 2001, Cohen et al. 2000, Wilhelm et al. 2001, Yeragani et al. 2000). Third, the model accounts for treatment–outcome data, which show that both pharmacological and psychological therapies are effective treatments for panic disorder (as reviewed later in this chapter).

Gorman and colleagues (2000) have also developed a neuroanatomical hypothesis regarding the etiology and pathophysiology of panic disorder. They begin with the observation that there is a remarkable similarity between the physiological and behavioral consequences of panic attacks in humans and conditioned fear responses in animals. Similarities include autonomic arousal, fear evoked by specific cues (i.e., contextual fear), and avoidance of these cues. Animal research indicates that conditioned fear responses are mediated by a "fear network" in the brain, consisting of the amygdala and its afferent and efferent projections, particularly its connections with the hippocampus, medial prefrontal cortex, hypothalamus, and brainstem. Animal studies also show that activation of this network produces biological and behavioral reactions that are similar to those associated with panic attacks. Thus, Gorman and colleagues (2000) posit that a similar network is involved in panic disorder.

The fear network consists of a complex matrix of interconnections, implicating a number of brain structures and neurotransmitter systems. Sensory input passes through the anterior thalamus to the lateral nucleus of the amygdala. Input is then transferred to the central nucleus of the amygdala, which coordinates autonomic and behavioral responses (Davis 1992, LeDoux et al. 1988). Direct sensory input to the amygdala from brainstem structures and the sensory thalamus enables a rapid response to potentially threatening stimuli. The central nucleus of the amygdala projects to the following structures: (1) the parabrachial nucleus, producing an increase in respiratory rate; (2) the lateral nucleus of the hypothalamus, causing autonomic arousal and sympathetic discharge; (3) the locus coeruleus, leading to an increase in norepinephrine and to increases in blood pressure, heart rate, and behavioral fear responses (e.g., freezing); (4) the paraventricular nucleus of the hypothalamus, resulting in an increase in the release of adrenocorticoids; and (5) the periaqueductal gray region, leading to avoidance behaviors (Davis 1992, LeDoux et al. 1988). In addition, there are reciprocal connections between the amygdala and the sensory thalamus, prefrontal cortex, insula, and primary somatosensory cortex (de Olmos 1990).

According to Gorman and colleagues (2000), panic attacks arise from excessive activation of the fear network. In other words, the fear network becomes sensitized (conditioned) to respond to noxious stimuli such as internal (bodily sensations) and external (contexts or situations) that the person associates with panic. Sensitization of the network may be manifested by the strengthening of various projections from the central nucleus of the amygdala to brainstem sites (such as the locus ceruleus, periaqueductal gray region, and hypothalamus). The network could be over activated if brainstem inputs to the amygdala are dysregulated. However, autonomic activation (e.g., increased respiration and heart rate) and neuroendocrine activation (e.g., increased cortisol secretion) does not occur in all panic attacks. Moreover, a variety of biological agents with diverse physiological properties can trigger panic attacks in people with panic disorder (e.g., sodium lactate, yohimbine, CO_2, caffeine, cholecystokinin-4) (McNally 1994). It is, therefore, unlikely that a single brainstem dysregulation is responsible for panic or, in turn, that brainstem dysregulation is the only way of producing an overactive fear network (Gorman et al. 2000, McNally 1994).

Gorman and colleagues (2000) identify various other ways of activating the fear network. For example, the amygdala receives input from cortical regions involved in the processing and evaluation of sensory information. Therefore, a neurocognitive deficit in these cortico–amygdala pathways could result in the catastrophic misinterpretation of sensory information (i.e., misinterpretation of bodily sensations), leading to an inappropriate activation of the fear network. Notice that this pathway resembles the cognitive model of panic described earlier in this chapter. Thus, Gorman and colleagues (2000) model integrates the cognitive model and places it in a neuroanatomical context.

In addition to playing a role in panic disorder, the fear network is thought to play a role in other anxiety disorders and in mood disorders. This is consistent with the comorbidity between panic disorder and these disorders. Abnormalities in the fear network may vary from disorder to disorders. For example, the strength of various connections between components of the network may distinguish various disorders.

Medications, particularly selective serotonin re-uptake inhibitors (SSRIs), are thought to desensitize the fear network. This may happen in a number of ways. SSRIs increase serotonergic transmission in the brain (Blier et al. 1987). Serotonergic neurons originate in the brainstem raphe and project throughout the central nervous system (Tork and Hornung 1990). Some of these projections have inhibitory influences. For example, the greater the activity in the raphe, the greater the inhibition of noradrenergic neurons in the locus ceruleus, resulting in a reduction of cardiovascular symptoms associated with panic attacks, such as tachycardia (Aston-Jones et al. 1991). Similarly, the greater the activity in the raphe, the greater inhibition in the periaqueductal gray region, resulting in a reduction in avoidance behavior (Viana et al. 1997). Increased serotonergic activity also may reduce hypothalamic release of corticotropin-releasing factor, thereby resulting in a reduction of cortisol (Brady et al. 1992) and a reduction in activity of the locus ceruleus (Butler et al. 1990), thereby leading to a reduction in fear. SSRIs may also directly inhibit activity of the lateral nucleus of the amygdala (Stutzman and LeDoux 1999). Thus, there appear to be several ways in which SSRIs could desensitize the fear network. Effective psychological therapies are thought to reduce contextual fear and catastrophic misinterpretations at the level of the medial prefrontal cortex and hippocampus.

Gorman and colleagues' (2000) neuroanatomical hypothesis is elegant and comprehensive. However, it is a work in progress and will need to be modified as new findings emerge. Additional brain structures may need to be included in the fear network. For example, a growing body of research suggests that the bed nucleus of the stria terminalis (which is associated with the amygdala) plays an important role in fear (Rosen and Schulkin 1998) and, therefore, should also be included in the fear network.

The fear network is thought to be influenced by genetic factors and stressful life events, particularly events in early childhood (Gorman et al. 2000). The search for genetic markers and candidate genes for panic disorder has revealed several possible loci but, to date, none have been replicated across studies (van den Heuvel et al. 2000). Research with monozygotic and dizygotic twins show that panic disorder is moderately heritable, with 32 to 46% of variance in liability for panic being attributed to genetic factors (Kendler et al. 1993, Scherrer et al. 2000, van den Heuvel et al. 2000).

Vulnerability to panic disorder appears to result from a combination of disorder-specific and disorder-nonspecific factors (Kendler et al. 1995, Scherrer et al. 2000). The importance of nonspecific genetic factors is consistent with observation that panic disorder is often comorbid with other disorders. Twin studies suggest that nonspecific factors influence the vulnerability to several disorders, including panic disorder, bulimia nervosa, generalized anxiety disorder, and alcohol dependence (Kendler et al. 1995, Scherrer et al. 2000). Genetic factors specific to panic disorder may be those that influence the tendency to catastrophically misinterpret bodily sensations. This cognitive tendency is a distinguishing feature of panic disorder, as described above. Recent twin research indicates that it is moderately heritable in women but not men (Jang et al. 1999). Thus, some specific genetic factors in panic disorder appear to be sex linked.

Environmental events occurring during particular developmental phases such as separation from the primary caregiver during early childhood may activate the genes that modulate the fear network, thereby creating a vulnerability to panic disorder. Research suggests that later events, occurring during adolescence or early adulthood, then precipitate panic disorder in vulnerable individuals. These events may stress the individual at a psychological or physiological level. Events commonly associated with the onset of panic disorder include (1) separation, loss, or illness of a significant other; (2) being the victim of sexual assault or other forms of interpersonal violence, (3) financial or occupational stressors, and (4) intoxication with, or withdrawal from, a psychoactive substance such as marijuana, cocaine, or anesthetic (Taylor 2000).

Dynamic Models

The most promising psychodynamic models for understanding panic disorder are those that focus specifically on this disorder. Rather than review all the models, we will summarize the model developed by the Cornell Panic-Anxiety Study Group (Milrod et al. 1997, Shear et al. 1993) because it has led to a promising treatment. According to the Cornell group, people at risk for panic disorder have (1) a neurophysiological vulnerability to panic attacks, and/or (2) multiple experiences of developmental trauma. These factors lead the child to become frightened of unfamiliar situations and to become excessively dependent on the primary caregiver to provide a sense of safety. The caregiver is unable to provide support always, so the child develops a fearful dependency. This leads, in turn, to the development of unconscious conflicts about dependency (independence versus reliance on others) and anger (expression versus inhibition). The dependency conflict is said to express itself in a number of ways. Some panic-vulnerable people are sensitive to separation and overly reliant on others, while others are sensitive to suffocation and overly reliant on a sense of independence. These conflicts can activate conscious or unconscious fantasies of catastrophic danger, which can trigger panic attacks. In addition, the conflicts evoke aversive emotions, such as anxiety, anger, and guilt. The otherwise benign arousal sensations accompanying these emotions can become the focus of "conscious as well as unconscious cognitive catastrophizing" (Shear et al. 1993, p. 862), thereby leading to panic attacks.

Treatment

There are a number of approaches that can be taken in treating panic disorder with and without agoraphobia (see Figure 31-4).

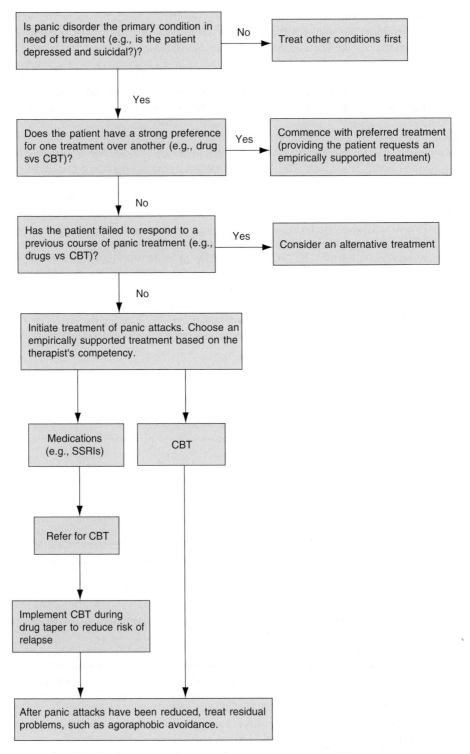

Figure 31-4 *A decision tree for treating panic disorder and agoraphobic avoidance.*

Somatic Treatment

Controlled studies show that effective antipanic medications include tricyclic antidepressants (e.g., imipramine), monoamine oxidase inhibitors (MAOIs; e.g., phenelzine), high-potency benzodiazepines (e.g., alprazolam), and SSRIs (e.g., fluvoxamine). These treatments have broadly similar efficacy, although there is some evidence that SSRIs tend to be most effective (Boyer 1995, Taylor 2000). The classes of medication differ in their side effects and their contraindications. Anticholinergic effects (e.g., blurred vision, dry mouth) are common problems with tricyclics. They are also contraindicated in individuals with particular comorbid cardiac disorders (Simon and Pollack 2000). Dietary restrictions (i.e., abstaining from foods containing tyramine) are a limitation of many MAOIs (Stein and Stahl 2000, Taylor 2000). Sedation, impaired motor coordination, and addiction are concerns with benzodiazepines (Barbone et al. 1998, Taylor 2000).

When efficacy and side effects are considered together, SSRIs emerge as the most promising drug treatments for panic disorder. However, even SSRIs have side effects, with the most problematic being a short-term increase in arousal-related sensations (Pohl et al. 1988). To overcome this problem, SSRIs can be started at a low dose (e.g., 5–10 mg/d for paroxetine; 12.5–25 mg/d for sertraline) and then increased gradually (e.g., up to 10–50 mg/d for paroxetine; up to 25–200 mg/d for sertraline). The choice of SSRI is determined on the basis of several factors, including side effects, individual preference, and the individual's history of responding (or not responding) to particular agents (Simon and Pollack 2000).

For drug refractory individuals, or individuals who are unable to tolerate SSRI side effects, combination medications are sometimes used. For example, SSRIs can be augmented with benzodiazepines (Uhlenhuth et al. 1999). The latter are used to dampen the side effects of SSRIs. Despite some positive preliminary reports supporting this strategy, its value in the treatment of panic disorder remains to be properly evaluated. An alternative strategy is to change the individual's medication. Some of the newer, non-SSRI antidepressants could be considered, such as venlafaxine, nefazodone, buproprion, or gabapentin (Simon and Pollack 2000). A concern with using these newer medications to treat panic disorder is that there are few data to guide the clinician. Another approach to the drug refractory individual is to use a psychosocial treatment such as cognitive–behavioral therapy (CBT), as an alternative or adjunctive intervention.

Psychosocial Treatments

CBT treatment packages include a number of components, such as psychoeducation (e.g., information about the cognitive model of panic), breathing retraining, cognitive restructuring, relaxation exercises, interoceptive exposure, and situational exposure (Taylor 2000). Breathing retraining involves teaching the individual to breathe with the diaphragm rather than with the chest muscles. Cognitive restructuring focuses on challenging individual's beliefs about the dangerousness of bodily sensations (e.g., challenging the belief that palpitations lead to heart attacks).

Interoceptive exposure involves inducing feared bodily sensations to further teach individuals that the sensations are harmless. For example, Sandra B.'s treatment involved interoceptive exposure exercises that induced depersonalization. Several tasks were used, including (1) staring at a ceiling fluorescent light for 1 minute, (2) staring at her reflection in the mirror for 2 minutes, and (3) staring at a spot on the wall for 3 minutes. Multiple tasks were used in order to promote the generalization of treatment effects (i.e., to help her learn that depersonalization was harmless regardless of how it arises).

Situational exposure involves activities that bring the individual into feared situations such as shopping malls, bridges, or tunnels. In Sandra B.'s case, situational and interoceptive exposure were combined. She was asked to visit a lighting store to spend time inspecting the various fluorescent lamps. Exposure exercises are often framed as "behavioral experiments" to test individuals' beliefs about the catastrophic consequences of arousal-related sensations. Sandra B.'s exposure exercises helped her test the belief that depersonalization leads to permanent insanity. The exercises were also used to help her test the alternative, noncatastrophic belief that depersonalization is an unpleasant but harmless experience.

A common practice in CBT is to encourage individuals to refrain from engaging in safety behaviors. Prior to treatment, Sandra B. typically engaged in distraction whenever she was exposed to depersonalization-inducing stimuli such as fluorescent lights. The CBT therapist encouraged her to refrain from distraction so she could learn that depersonalization is harmless, even when it becomes intense. Evidence suggests that reducing safety behaviors improves treatment efficacy (Taylor 2000). Despite the advantages of exposure exercises, they are medically contraindicated in some cases. For example, a hyperventilation exercise would not be used in an individual with severe asthma (Taylor 2000).

A large body of evidence shows that CBT is effective in reducing panic attacks, agoraphobia, and associated symptoms such as depression (Taylor 2000). However, not all CBT interventions may be necessary. Interoceptive exposure, situational exposure, and cognitive restructuring are the most widely used and supported interventions. Several studies suggest that breathing retraining reduces panic frequency. However, recent research casts doubt about the importance of hyperventilation in producing panic attacks. This suggests that breathing retraining may only be useful for a minority of individuals, for which chest breathing or hyperventilation plays a role in producing panic symptoms (Taylor 2001). Breathing retraining may be counterproductive if it prevents individuals from learning that their catastrophic beliefs are unfounded. Given these concerns, breathing retraining should be used sparingly in the treatment of panic disorder. If used at all, the clinician should ensure that the individual understands that breathing exercises are used to remove unpleasant but harmless sensations. Interoceptive exposure and cognitive restructuring are important for helping individuals learn that the sensations are not dangerous.

How effective is CBT compared to other therapies? A small but growing literature suggests that the efficacy of CBT is equal to or greater than that of alprazolam and imipramine at posttreatment (Barlow et al. 2000, Taylor 2000). Future research is needed to compare CBT to other pharmacotherapies, such as SSRIs. Preliminary evidence suggests that CBT is effective in treating individuals who have failed to respond to pharmacotherapies (Otto et al. 1999, Pollack et al. 1994). Follow-up studies suggest that CBT is effective in the long term and is likely to be more effective than short-term pharmacological treatment. It is not known whether drug treatments would be as effective as CBT if individuals remained on their medications. Any conclusions about the long-term efficacy of panic treatments are necessarily tentative because individuals sometimes seek additional treatment during the follow-up interval.

Several other approaches have been used in the treatment of panic disorder, including psychodynamic psychotherapies (Milrod et al. 2000, Wiborg and Dahl 1996), hypnosis (Delmonte 1995, Stafrace 1994), Eye Movement Desensitization and Reprocessing (EMDR) (Shapiro 1995), and mindfulness meditation (Kabat-Zinn 1990, Miller et al. 1995). Support for these treatments is limited largely to case studies and uncontrolled trials. Controlled studies (Feske and Goldstein 1997), although few in number, indicate that hypnosis and EMDR are of limited value in treating panic disorder. When used to treat this disorder, these treatments may be no better than placebo (Taylor 2000). Interventions that look more promising are mindfulness meditation (Miller et al. 1995) and psychodynamic psychotherapies modified to specifically focus on panic symptoms (Milrod et al. 2000, Wiborg and Dahl 1996). However, none have been extensively evaluated as panic treatments and none have been compared with empirically supported treatments such as CBT or SSRIs.

Combined Treatments

Many clinicians believe the optimal treatment consists of drugs combined with some form of psychosocial intervention (Alexander 1991, Fahy et al. 1992, Marriott et al. 1989). This view arose from observations that even the most effective drugs and the most effective psychosocial interventions do not eliminate panic disorder in all cases. It was thought that combination treatments might be a way to improve treatment outcome. The available evidence provides mixed support for this view. Evidence suggests that the efficacy of CBT is not improved when it is combined with either diazepam or alprazolam (Hafner and Marks 1976, Riley et al. 1995, Wardle et al. 1994). In fact, some studies have found that the efficacy of situational exposure is worsened when alprazolam is added (Echeburúa et al. 1993, Marks et al. 1993).

Several studies have compared CBT to CBT combined with imipramine. These results have also been mixed. Adding imipramine in the range of 150–300 mg/day to either situational exposure or CBT sometimes improves treatment outcome in the short-term, provided that individuals are able to tolerate the dose (Barlow et al. 2000, Taylor 2000). Any advantage of combined treatment tends to be lost at follow-up. Similarly, studies of combining CBT with SSRIs (fluvoxamine or paroxetine) have produced mixed results, with some studies finding the combination is no better than CBT alone (Sharp et al. 1996), others finding that the combination is most effective (de Beurs et al. 1995, Oehrberg et al. 1995), and yet others finding the combination to be most effective for some symptoms but not others (Stein et al. 2000). Methodological limitations of these studies might account for the inconsistent findings (Taylor 2000).

It remains unclear whether treatment outcome is enhanced by combining CBT with SSRIs. The previously discussed neuroanatomical model (Gorman et al. 2000) with its dual emphasis on cortical and serotonergic mechanisms suggests that this combined treatment might be superior to CBT alone and to SSRIs alone. On the other hand, pharmacotherapies such as SSRIs might undermine the individual's confidence in implementing CBT, particularly if they attribute their gains to medications rather than to their own efforts at using the skills learned in CBT (Basoglu et al. 1994, Brown and Barlow 1995). Large, well-designed studies are needed to explore these important issues.

A more promising type of combined therapy is a sequential approach, in which individuals are treated with pharmacotherapy during the acute phase, and then are treated with CBT as the medication is phased out. Several studies have shown that adding CBT during the tapering period for alprazolam and clonazepam reduces the relapse rate associated with these drugs (Abelson and Curtis 1993, Bruce et al. 1999, Hegel et al. 1994, Otto et al. 1993, Spiegel et al. 1994). It remains to be demonstrated that CBT can reduce relapse when individuals are tapered off other antipanic drugs such as SSRIs. However, there is no reason to expect that CBT would not be helpful in these cases.

Comparison of DSM-IV-TR/ICD-10 Diagnostic Criteria

The ICD-10 Diagnostic Criteria for Research for a panic attack are identical to the DSM-IV-TR criteria set except that ICD-10 includes an additional item (i.e., dry mouth). In contrast to the DSM-IV-TR algorithm, which does not give special weight to any particular symptom, the ICD-10 algorithm requires that at least one of the symptoms be palpitations, sweating, trembling, or dry mouth. Like DSM-IV-TR, ICD-10 requires recurrent panic attacks but, in contrast to DSM-IV-TR, it does not include a criterion requiring that the panic attacks be clinically significant.

The ICD-10 Diagnostic Criteria for Research for Agoraphobia differ markedly from the DSM-IV-TR criteria. The ICD-10 Diagnostic Criteria for Research specify that there be fear or avoidance of at least two of the following situations: crowds, public places, traveling alone, or traveling away from home. Furthermore, ICD-10 requires that at least two symptoms of anxiety (i.e., from the list of 14 panic symptoms) be present together on at least one occasion and that these anxiety symptoms be "restricted to, or predominate in, the feared situations or contemplation of the feared situations." In contrast, DSM-IV-TR Agoraphobia is defined in terms of "anxiety about being in places or situations from which escape might be difficult (or embarrassing) or in which help may not be available in the event of having an unexpected or situationally predisposed panic attack." No specific avoided situations or specific types of anxiety symptoms are required for a diagnosis.

References

Abelson JL and Curtis GC (1993) Discontinuation of alprazolam after successful treatment of panic disorder: a naturalistic follow-up study. *J Anxiety Disord* **7**, 107–117.

Abelson JL, Weg JG, Nesse RM, et al. (2001) Persistent respiratory irregularity in patients with panic disorder. *Biol Psychiatry* **49**, 588–595.

Alexander PE (1991) Management of panic disorders. *J Psychoact Drugs* **23**, 329–333.

American Psychiatric Association (1995) Practice guidelines for psychiatric evaluation of adults. *Am J Psychiatry* **152**(Suppl.), 63–80.

Asmundson GJG and Norton GR (1993) Anxiety sensitivity and spontaneous and cued panic attacks in college students. *Behav Res Ther* **31**, 199–201.

Aston-Jones G, Akaoka H, Charlety P, et al. (1991) Serotonin selectivity attenuates glutamate-evoked activation of noradrenergic locus coeruleus neurons. *J Neurosci* **11**, 760–769.

Ballenger JC and Fyer AJ (1996) Panic disorder and agoraphobia. In *DSM-IV Sourcebook*, Vol. 2, Widiger TA, Frances AJ, Pincus HA, et al. (eds). American Psychiatric Association, Washington, DC, pp. 411–471.

Barbone F, McMahon AD, and Davey PG (1998) Association of road-traffic accidents with benzodiazepine use. *Lancet* **352**, 1331–1336.

Barlow DH (1988) *Anxiety and Its Disorders*. Guilford Press, New York.

Barlow DH and Craske MG (1994) *Mastery of Your Anxiety and Panic II: Client Workbook*. Psychological Corporation, San Antonio, TX.

Barlow DH, Gorman JM, Shear MK, et al. (2000) Cognitive–behavioral therapy, imipramine, or their combination for panic disorder: a randomized controlled trial. *JAMA* **283**, 2529–2536.

Basoglu M, Marks IM, Kiliç C, et al. (1994) Alprazolam and exposure for panic disorder with agoraphobia: attribution of improvement to medication predicts subsequent relapse. *Br J Psychiatry* **164**, 652–659.

Beck AT and Steer RA (1987) *Manual for the Revised Beck Depression Inventory*. Psychological Corporation, San Antonio, TX.

Beck AT and Steer RA (1993) *Manual for the Beck Anxiety Inventory*. Psychological Corporation, San Antonio, TX.

Bekker MHJ (1996) Agoraphobia and gender: a review. *Clin Psychol Rev* **16**, 129–146.

Bibb J and Chambless DL (1986) Alcohol use and abuse among diagnosed agoraphobics. *Behav Res Ther* **24**, 49–58.

Blier P, DeMontigny C, and Chaput Y (1987) Modifications of the serotonin system by antidepressant treatments: implications for the therapeutic response in major depression. *J Clin Psychopharmacol* **7**, 24S–35S.

Bouton ME, Mineka S, and Barlow DH (2001) A modern learning theory perspective on the etiology of panic disorder. *Psychol Rev* **108**, 4–32.

Boyd JH (1986) Use of mental health services for the treatment of panic disorder. *Am J Psychiatry* **143**, 1569–1574.

Boyer W (1995) Serotonin uptake inhibitors are superior to imipramine and alprazolam in alleviating panic attacks: a meta-analysis. *Int Clin Psychopharmacol* **10**, 45–49.

Brady LS, Gold PW, Herkenham M, et al. (1992) The antidepressants fluoxetine, idazoxan and phenelzine alter corticotropin-releasing hormone and tyrosine hydroxylase mRNA levels in the rat brain: therapeutic implications. *Brain Res* **572**, 117–125.

Breier A, Charney DS, and Heninger GR (1984) Major depression in patients with agoraphobia and panic disorder. *Arch Gen Psychiatry* **41**, 1129–1135.

Brown TA and Barlow DH (1995) Long-term outcome in cognitive–behavioral treatment of panic disorder: clinical predictors and alternative strategies for assessment. *J Consult Clin Psychol* **63**, 754–765.

Brown TA and Deagle EA (1992) Structured interview assessment of nonclinical panic. *Behav Ther* **23**, 75–85.

Bruce TJ, Spiegel DA, and Hegel MT (1999) Cognitive–behavioral therapy helps prevent relapse and recurrence of panic disorder following alprazolam discontinuation: a long-term follow-up of the Peoria and Dartmouth studies. *J Consult Clin Psychol* **67**, 151–156.

Butler PD, Weiss JM, Stout JC, et al. (1990) Corticotropin-releasing factor produces fear-enhancing and behavioral activating effects following infusion into the locus coeruleus. *J Neurosci* **10**, 176–183.

Chignon JM, Lepine JP, and Ades J (1993) Panic Disorder in Cardiac Outpatients. *Am J Psychiatry* **150**, 780–785.

Clark DM (1986) A cognitive approach to panic. *Behav Res Ther* **24**, 461–470.

Clark DM (1988) A cognitive model of panic attacks. In *Panic: Psychological Perspectives*, Rachman S and Maser JD (eds). Lawrence Erlbaum, Hillsdale, NJ, pp. 71–89.

Cohen H, Benjamin J, Geva AB, et al. (2000) Autonomic dysregulation in panic disorder and in posttraumatic stress disorder: application of power spectrum analysis of heart rate variability at rest and in response to recollection of trauma or panic attacks. *Psychiatr Res* **96**, 1–13.

Cox BJ, Swinson RP, Shulman ID, et al. (1993) Gender effects and alcohol use in panic disorder with agoraphobia. *Behav Res Ther* **31**, 413–416.

Davis M (1992) The role of the amygdala in fear and anxiety. *Annu Rev Neurosci* **15**, 353–375.

de Beurs E, van Balkom AJLM, Lange A, et al. (1995) Treatment of panic disorder with agoraphobia: comparison of fluvoxamine, placebo, and psychological panic management combined with exposure and of exposure in vivo alone. *Am J Psychiatry* **152**, 683–691.

Delmonte MM (1995) The use of hypnotic regression with panic disorder: a case report. *Aust J Clin Hypnother Hypnosis* **16**, 69–73.

de Olmos J (1990) Amygdaloid nuclear gray complex. In *The Human Nervous System*, Paxinos G (ed). Academic Press, San Diego, pp. 583–610.

Di Nardo P, Brown TA, and Barlow DH (1994) *Anxiety Disorders Interview Schedule for DSM-IV*. Graywind, New York.

Eaton WW, Dryman A, and Weissman MM (1991) Panic and phobia: the diagnosis of panic disorder. In *Psychiatric Disorders in America: The Epidemiologic Catchment Area Study*, Robins LN and Reiger DA (eds). Free Press, New York, pp. 155–179.

Eaton WW, Kessler RC, Wittchen HU, et al. (1994) Panic and panic disorder in the United States. *Am J Psychiatry* **151**, 413–420.

Echeburúa E, De Corral P, Bajos EG, et al. (1993) Interactions between self-exposure and alprazolam in the treatment of agoraphobia without current panic: an exploratory study. *Behav Cogn Psychother* **21**, 219–238.

Ehlers A and Breuer P (1996) How good are patients with panic disorder at perceiving their heartbeats? *Biol Psychol* **42**, 165–182.

Fahy TJ, O'Rourke D, Brophy J, et al. (1992) The Galway study of panic disorder I. Clomipramine and lofepramine in DSM-III-R panic disorder: a placebo-controlled trial. *J Affect Disord* **25**, 63–76.

Feske U and Goldstein AJ (1997) Eye movement desensitization and reprocessing treatment for panic disorder: a controlled outcome and partial dismantling study. *J Consult Clin Psychol* **65**, 1026–1035.

First MB, Spitzer RL, Gibbon M, et al. (1996) *Structured Clinical Interview for DSM-IV Axis I—Patient*. Biometrics Research Department, New York State Psychiatric Institute, New York.

Goddard AW and Charney DS (1997) Toward an integrated neurobiology of panic disorder. *J Clin Psychiatry* **58**(Suppl. 2), 4–12.

Goldberg RJ (1988) Clinical presentations of panic-related disorders. *J Anxiety Disord* **2**, 61–75.

Goldstein AJ and Chambless DL (1978) A reanalysis of agoraphobia. *Behav Ther* **9**, 47–59.

Gorman J, Kent JM, Sullivan GM, et al. (2000) Neuroanatomical hypothesis of panic disorder. *Rev Am J Psychiatry* **157**, 493–505.

Greenberg PE, Sisitsky T, Kessler RC, et al. (1999) The economic burden of anxiety disorders in the 1990s. *J Clin Psychiatry* **60**, 427–435.

Hafner RJ and Marks IM (1976) Exposure in vivo of agoraphobics: contributions of diazepam, group exposure and anxiety evocation. *Psychol Med* **6**, 71–88.

Hegel MT, Ravaris CL, and Ahles TA (1994) Combined cognitive–behavioral and time-limited alprazolam treatment of panic disorder. *Behav Ther* **25**, 183–195.

Hibbert GA (1984) Ideational components of anxiety: their origin and content. *Br J Psychiatry* **144**, 618–624.

Jang KL, Stein MB, Taylor S, et al. (1999) Gender differences in the etiology of anxiety sensitivity: a twin study. *J Gender Specific Med* **2**, 39–44.

Kabat-Zinn J (1990) *Full Catastrophe Living*. Delta, New York.

Katerndahl DA and Realini JP (1995) Where do panic attack sufferers seek care? *J Fam Pract* **40**, 237–243.

Katerndahl DA and Realini JP (1997) Quality of life and panic-related work disability in subjects with infrequent panic and panic disorder. *J Clin Psychiatry* **58**, 153–158.

Keller MB, Yonkers KA, Warshaw MG, et al. (1994) Remission and relapse in subjects with panic disorder and panic with agoraphobia. *J Nerv Ment Disord* **182**, 290–296.

Kendler KS, Neale MC, Kessler RC, et al. (1993) Panic disorder in women: a population-based twin study. *Psychol Med* **23**, 397–406.

Kendler KS, Walters EE, Neale MC, et al. (1995) The structure of the genetic and environmental risk factors for six major psychiatric disorders in women: phobia, generalized anxiety disorder, panic disorder, bulimia, major depression and alcoholism. *Arch Gen Psychiatry* **52**, 374–383.

Kessler RC, Stang PE, Wittchen H-U, et al. (1998) Lifetime panic-depression comorbidity in the National Comorbidity Survey. *Arch Gen Psychiatry* **55**, 801–808.

Klein DF (1980) Anxiety reconceptualized. *Compr Psychiatry* **21**, 411–427.

Klein DF (1993) False suffocation alarms, spontaneous panics, and related conditions: an integrative hypothesis. *Arch Gen Psychiatry* **50**, 306–317.

LeDoux JE, Iwata J, Cicchetti P, et al. (1988) Different projections of the central amygdaloid nucleus mediate autonomic and behavioral correlates of conditioned fear. *J Neurosci* **8**, 2517–2519.

Leon AC, Portera L, and Weissman MM (1995) The social costs of anxiety disorders. *Br J Psychiatry* **166**(Suppl. 27), 19–22.

Logan AC and Goetsch VL (1993) Attention to external threat cues in anxiety states. *Clin Psychol Rev* **13**, 541–559.

Louie AK, Lannon RA, Ritzick EA, et al. (1996) Clinical features of cocaine-induced panic. *Biol Psychiatry* **40**, 938–940.

Markowitz JS, Weissman MM, Ouellette R, et al. (1989) Quality of life in panic disorder. *Arch Gen Psychiatry* **46**, 984–992.

Marks IM (1987) *Fears, Phobias, and Rituals.* Oxford University Press, New York.

Marks IM, Swinson RP, Basoglu M, et al. (1993) Alprazolam and exposure alone and combined in panic disorder with agoraphobia: a controlled study in London and Toronto. *Br J Psychiatry* **162**, 776–787.

Marriott P, Judd F, Jefferys D, et al. (1989) Panic and phobic disorders. Part I: problems associated with drug therapy. *Curr Ther* 107–121.

McNally RJ (1994) *Panic Disorder: A Critical Analysis.* Guilford Press, New York.

McNally RJ (1996) Cognitive bias in the anxiety disorders. In *Nebraska Symposium on Motivation, 1995: Perspectives on Anxiety, Panic, and Fear. Current Theory and Research in Motivation*, Vol. 43, Hope DA (ed). University of Nebraska Press, Lincoln, pp. 211–250.

Miller JJ, Fletcher K, and Kabat-Zinn J (1995) Three-year follow-up and clinical implications of a mindfulness meditation-based stress reduction intervention in the treatment of anxiety disorders. *Gen Hosp Psychiatry* **17**, 192–200.

Milrod BL, Busch FN, Cooper AM, et al. (1997) *Manual of Panic-Focused Psychodynamic Psychotherapy.* American Psychiatric Association, Washington, DC.

Milrod B, Busch F, Leon AC, et al. (2000) Open trial of psychodynamic psychotherapy for panic disorder: a pilot study. *Am J Psychiatry* **157**, 1878–1880.

Norton GR, Cox BJ, and Malan J (1992) Nonclinical panickers: a critical review. *Clin Psychol Rev* **12**, 121–139.

Norton GR, Dorward J, and Cox BJ (1986) Factors associated with panic attacks in nonclinical subjects. *Behav Ther* **17**, 239–252.

Norton GR, Pidlubny SR, and Norton PJ (1999) Predicting panic attacks and related variables. *Behav Ther* **30**, 319–330.

Oehrberg S, Christiansen PE, and Behnke K (1995) Paroxetine in the treatment of panic disorder: a randomized double-blind placebo-controlled study. *Br J Psychiatry* **167**, 374–379.

Oei TPS, Wanstall K, and Evans L (1990) Sex differences in panic disorder and agoraphobia. *J Anxiety Disord* **4**, 317–324.

Otto MW, Pollack MH, Penava SJ, et al. (1999) Group cognitive–behavior therapy for patients failing to respond to pharmacotherapy for panic disorder: a clinical case series. *Behav Res Ther* **37**, 763–770.

Otto MW, Pollack MH, Sachs GS, et al. (1992) Alcohol dependence in panic disorder patients. *J Psychiatr Res* **26**, 29–38.

Otto MW, Pollack MH, Sachs GS, et al. (1993) Discontinuation of benzodiazepine treatment: efficacy of cognitive–behavior therapy for patients with panic disorder. *Am J Psychiatry* **150**, 1485–1490.

Peterson RA and Reiss S (1992) *Anxiety Sensitivity Index Manual*, 2nd ed. International Diagnostic Systems, Worthington, OH.

Pohl R, Yergani V, Balon R, et al. (1988) The jitteriness syndrome in panic disorder patients treated with antidepressants. *J Clin Psychiatry* **49**, 100–104.

Pollack MH, Otto MW, Kaspi SP, et al. (1994) Cognitive–behavior therapy for treatment-refractory panic disorder. *J Clin Psychiatry* **55**, 200–205.

Raj A and Sheehan DV (1987) Medical evaluation of panic attacks. *J Clin Psychiatry* **48**, 309–313.

Rapee RM, Craske MG, and Barlow DH (1990) Subject-described features of panic attacks using self-monitoring. *J Anxiety Disord* **4**, 171–181.

Rapee R, Mattick R, and Murrell E (1986) Cognitive mediation in the affective component of spontaneous panic attacks. *J Behav Ther Exp Psychiatry* **17**, 245–254.

Reiss S (1999) The sensitivity theory of aberrant motivation. In *Anxiety Sensitivity: Theory, Research, and Treatment of the Fear of Anxiety*, Taylor S (ed). Lawrence Erlbaum, Mahwah, NJ, pp. 35–58.

Reiss S and McNally RJ (1985) The expectancy model of fear. In *Theoretical Issues in Behavior Therapy*, Reiss S and Bootzin RR (eds). Academic Press, New York, pp. 107–121.

Reed V and Wittchen HU (1998) DSM-IV panic attacks and panic disorder in a community sample of adolescents and young adults: How specific are panic attacks? *J Psychiatr Res* **32**, 335–345.

Riley WT, McCormick MGF, Simon EM, et al. (1995) Effects of alprazolam dose on the induction and habituation processes during behavioral panic induction treatment. *J Anxiety Disord* **9**, 217–227.

Robins LN, Locke BZ, and Reiger DA (1991) An overview of psychiatric disorders in America. In *Psychiatric Disorders in America: The Epidemiologic Catchment Area Study*, Robins LN and Reiger DA (eds). Free Press, New York, p. 328.

Rosen JB and Schulkin J (1998) From normal fear to pathological anxiety. *Psychol Rev* **105**, 325–350.

Rouillon F (1997) Epidemiology of Panic Disorder. *Hum Psychopharmacol* **12**, S7–S12.

Sanderson WC, Rapee RM, and Barlow DH (1989) The influence of an illusion of control on panic attacks induced via inhalation of 5.5% carbon dioxide-enriched air. *Arch Gen Psychiatry* **46**, 157–162.

Scherrer JF, True WR, Xian H, et al. (2000) Evidence for genetic influences common and specific to symptoms of generalized anxiety and panic. *J Affect Disord* **57**, 25–35.

Shapiro F (1995) *Eye Movement Desensitization and Reprocessing: Basic Principles, Protocols, and Procedures.* Guilford Press, New York.

Sharp DM, Power KG, Simpson RJ, et al. (1996) Fluvoxamine, placebo, and cognitive–behaviour therapy used alone and in combination in the treatment of panic disorder and agoraphobia. *J Anxiety Disord* **10**, 219–242.

Shear MK, Cooper AM, Klerman GL, et al. (1993) A psychodynamic model of panic disorder. *Am J Psychiatry* **150**, 859–866.

Shear MK and Maser JD (1994) Standardized assessment for panic disorder research: a conference report. *Arch Gen Psychiatry* **51**, 346–354.

Simon NM and Pollack MH (2000) The current status of the treatment of panic disorder: pharmacotherapy and cognitive–behavioral therapy. *Psychiatr Ann* **30**, 689–696.

Spiegel DA, Bruce TJ, Gregg SF, et al. (1994) Does cognitive–behavior therapy assist slow-taper alprazolam discontinuation in panic disorder? *Am J Psychiatry* **151**, 876–881.

Spinhoven P, Onstein EJ, Sterk PJ, et al. (1993) Hyperventilation and panic attacks in general hospital patients. *Gen Hosp Psychiatry* **15**, 148–154.

Stafrace S (1994) Hypnosis in the treatment of panic disorder with agoraphobia. *Aust J Clin Hypnosis* **22**, 73–86.

Stein MB, Asmundson GJG, Ireland D, et al. (1994) Panic disorder in patients attending a clinic for vestibular disorders. *Am J Psychiatry* **151**, 1697–1700.

Stein MB, Norton GR, Walker JR, et al. (2000) Do SSRIs enhance the efficacy of very brief cognitive–behavioral therapy for panic disorder? A pilot study. *Psychiatr Res* **94**, 191–200.

Stein DJ and Stahl S (2000) Serotonin and anxiety: current models. *Int Clin Psychopharmacol* **15**(Suppl. 2), S1–S6.

Stein MB and Uhde TW (1990) Panic disorder and major depression: lifetime relationship and biological markers. In *Clinical Aspects of Panic Disorder*, Ballenger JC (ed). John Wiley, New York, pp. 151–168.

Stutzman GE and LeDoux JE (1999) GABAergic antagonists block the inhibitory effects of serotonin in the lateral amygdala: a mechanism for modulation of sensory inputs related to fear conditioning. *J Neurosci* **19**, RC8.

Taylor S (1999) *Anxiety Sensitivity*. Lawrence Erlbaum, Mahwah, NJ.

Taylor S (2000) *Understanding and Treating Panic Disorder: Cognitive–Behavioral Approaches*. John Wiley, New York.

Taylor S (2001) Breathing retraining in the treatment of panic disorder: efficacy, caveats, and indications. *Scand J Behav Ther* **30**, 1–8.

Taylor S and Rachman S (1994) Stimulus estimation and overprediction of fear. *Br J Clin Psychol* **33**, 173–181.

Thyer BA, Parrish RT, Himle J, et al. (1986) Alcohol abuse among clinically anxious patients. *Behav Res Ther* **24**, 357–359.

Tork I and Hornung J-P (1990) Raphe nuclei and the serotonergic system. In *The Human Nervous System*, Paxinos G (ed). Academic Press, San Diego, pp. 1001–1022.

Uhde TW, Boulenger JP, Roy-Byrne PP, et al. (1985) Longitudinal course of panic disorder: clinical and biological considerations. *Prog Neuro-Psychopharmacol Biol Psychiatry* **9**, 39–51.

Uhlenhuth EH, Balter MB, Ban TA, et al. (1999) International study of expert judgment on therapeutic use of benzodiazepines and other psychotherapeutic medications. IV. Treatments in recommendations for the pharmacotherapy of anxiety disorders. *Depress Anxiety* **9**, 107–116.

van den Heuvel OA, van de Wetering BJM, Veltman DJ, et al. (2000) Genetic studies of panic disorder: a review. *J Clin Psychiatry* **61**, 756–766.

Viana MB, Graeff FG, and Loschmann PA (1997) Kainate microinjection into the dorsal raphe nucleus induces 5-HT release in the amygdala and periaqueductal gray. *Pharmacol Biochem Behav* **58**, 167–172.

Wardle J, Hayward P, Higgitt A, et al. (1994) Effects of concurrent diazepam treatment on the outcome of exposure therapy in agoraphobia. *Behav Res Ther* **32**, 203–215.

Weissman MM (1991) Panic disorder: impact on quality of life. *J Clin Psychiatry* **52**, 6–9.

Weissman MM, Bland RC, Canino GJ, et al. (1997) The cross-national epidemiology of panic disorder. *Arch Gen Psychiatry* **54**, 305–309.

Welkowitz LA, Papp L, Martinez J, et al. (1999) Instructional set and physiological response to CO_2 inhalation. *Am J Psychiatry* **156**, 745–748.

Wiborg IM and Dahl AA (1996) Does brief dynamic psychotherapy reduce the relapse rate of panic disorder? *Arch Gen Psychiatry* **53**, 689–694.

Wilhelm FH, Trabert W, and Roth WT (2001) Physiological instability in panic disorder and generalized anxiety disorder. *Biol Psychiatry* **49**, 596–605.

Wilson KG, Sandler LS, Asmundson GJG, et al. (1991) Effects of instructional set on self-reports of panic attacks. *J Anxiety Disord* **5**, 43–63.

Wilson KG, Sandler LS, Asmundson GJG, et al. (1992) Panic attacks in the nonclinical population: an empirical approach to case identification. *J Abnorm Psychol* **101**, 460–468.

Wittchen HU, Reed V, and Kessler RC (1998) The relationship of agoraphobia and panic in a community sample of adolescents and young adults. *Arch Gen Psychiatry* **55**, 1017–1024.

Yeragani VK, Pohl R, Jampala VC, et al. (2000) Increased QT variability in patients with panic disorder and depression. *Psychiatr Res* **93**, 225–235.

Yonkers KA (1994) Panic disorder in women. *J Women's Health* **3**, 481–486.

Yonkers KA, Zlotnick C, Allsworth J, et al. (1998) Is the course of panic disorder the same in women and men? *Am J Psychiatry* **155**, 596–602.

32 Anxiety Disorders: Social and Specific Phobias

Diagnosis

The experience of fear and the related emotion of anxiety are universal and familiar to everyone. Fear exists in all cultures and appears to exist across species. Presumably, the purpose of fear is to protect an organism from immediate threat and to mobilize the body for quick action to avoid danger. Emotion theorists consider fear to be an alarm response that fires in the presence of imminent threat or danger. The function of the primarily noradrenergic-mediated fear response is to facilitate immediate escape from threat (flight) or attack on the source of threat (fight) (Barlow 1991, 2002). Therefore, fear is often referred to as a fight-or-flight response (Cannon 1929). All the manifestations of fear are consistent with its protective function. For example, heart rate and breathing rate increase to meet the increased oxygen needs of the body, increased perspiration helps to cool the body to facilitate escape, and pupils dilate to enhance visual acuity.

Anxiety, on the other hand, is a future-oriented mood state in which the individual anticipates the possibility of threat and experiences a sense of uncontrollability focused on the upcoming negative event. In the DSM-IV-TR, anxiety is defined as "the apprehensive anticipation of future danger or misfortune accompanied by a feeling of dysphoria or somatic symptoms of tension" (American Psychiatric Association, 2000, p. 820). If one were to put anxiety into words, one might say, "Something bad might happen soon. I am not sure I can cope with it but I have to be ready to try." Anxiety is primarily mediated by the gamma-aminobutyric acid-benzodiazepine system (Barlow 1991, 2002).

Despite evidence that fear and anxiety are mediated by different brain systems, anxiety and fear are related, which makes sense ethologically. Experiencing anxiety after encountering signals of impending danger seems to lower the threshold for fear that is triggered when danger actually occurs (e.g., being attacked by a mugger or almost being hit by an automobile). Anxiety leads to a shift in attention toward the source of danger so that individuals become more vigilant for relevant threat cues and therefore are more likely to experience fear in the face of perceived immediate threat.

Fear and anxiety are not always adaptive, however. At times, the responses can occur in the absence of any realistic threat or it may be out of proportion to the actual danger. Almost everyone has situations that arouse anxiety and fear despite the fact that the actual risk is minimal. It is not unusual to become anxious before a job interview or a speech. Many individuals feel fearful when exposed to situations such as dental visits, seeing certain animals, or being at certain heights. For some people, these fears reach extreme levels and may cause significant distress or impairment in functioning. It is at this point that what we typically refer to as shyness and fearfulness might meet diagnostic criteria for social phobia or specific phobia respectively.

In the DSM-IV-TR, social phobia (also known as social anxiety disorder) is defined as a "marked and persistent fear of one or more social or performance situations in which the person is exposed to unfamiliar people or to possible scrutiny of others" (see DSM-IV-TR diagnostic criteria below). Typical situations feared by individuals with social phobia include meeting new people, interacting with others, attending parties or meetings, speaking formally, eating or writing in front of others, dealing with people in authority, and being assertive. Specific phobia is defined as a "marked and persistent fear that is excessive or unreasonable, cued by the presence or anticipation of a specific object or situation (e.g., flying, heights, animals, receiving an injection, seeing blood)" (see DSM-IV-TR diagnostic criteria on page 869).

DSM-IV-TR Diagnostic Criteria

300.23 Social Phobia (Social Anxiety Disorder)

A. A marked and persistent fear of one or more social or performance situations in which the person is exposed to unfamiliar people or to possible scrutiny by others. The individual fears that he or she will act in a way (or show anxiety symptoms) that will be humiliating or embarrassing. **Note:** In children, there must be evidence of the capacity for age-appropriate social relationships with familiar people and the anxiety must occur in peer settings, not just in interactions with adults.
B. Exposure to the feared social situation almost invariably provokes anxiety, which may take the form of a situationally bound or situationally predisposed panic attack. **Note:** In children, the anxiety may be expressed by crying, tantrums, freezing, or shrinking away from social situations with unfamiliar people.
C. The person recognizes that the fear is excessive or unreasonable. **Note:** In children, this feature may be absent.
D. The feared social or performance situations are avoided or else are endured with intense anxiety or distress.
E. The avoidance, anxious anticipation, or distress in the feared social or perfor- mance situation(s)
E. interferes significantly with the person's normal routine, occupational (or academic) functioning, or social activities or relationships, or there is marked distress about having the phobia.
F. In individuals under age 18 years, the duration is at least 6 months.
G. The fear or avoidance is not due to the direct physiological effects of a substance (e.g., a drug of abuse, a medication) or a general medical condition and is not better accounted for by another mental disorder (e.g., panic disorder with or without agoraphobia, separation-anxiety disorder, body dysmorphic disorder, a pervasive developmental disorder, or schizoid personality disorder).

H. If a general medical condition or another mental disorder is present, the fear in criterion A is unrelated to it, for example, the fear is not of stuttering, trembling in Parkinson's disease, exhibiting abnormal eating behavior in anorexia nervosa or bulimia nervosa.

Specify if:

Generalized: if the fears include most social situations (also consider the additional diagnosis of avoidant personality disorder)

DSM-IV-TR Diagnostic Criteria

300.29 Specific Phobia

A. Marked and persistent fear that is excessive or unreasonable, cued by the presence or anticipation of a specific object or situation (e.g., flying, heights, animals, receiving an injection, seeing blood).
B. Exposure to the phobic stimulus almost invariably provokes an immediate anxiety response, which may take the form of a situationally bound or situationally predisposed panic attack. **Note:** In children, the anxiety may be expressed by crying, tantrums, freezing, or clinging.
C. The person recognizes that the fear is excessive or unreasonable. **Note:** In children, this feature may be absent.
D. The phobic situation(s) is avoided or else is endured with intense anxiety or distress.
E. The avoidance, anxious anticipation, or distress in the feared situation(s) interferes significantly with the person's normal routine, occupational (or academic) functioning, or social activities or relationships, or there is marked distress about having the phobia.
F. In individuals under age 18 years, the duration is at least 6 months.
G. The anxiety, panic attacks, and phobic avoidance associated with the specific object or situation are not better accounted for by another mental disorder, such as obsessive–compulsive disorder (e.g., fear of dirt in someone with an obsession about contamination), posttraumatic stress disorder (e.g., avoidance of stimuli associated with a severe stressor), separation-anxiety disorder (e.g., avoidance of school), social phobia (e.g., avoidance of social situations because of fear of embarrassment), panic disorder with agoraphobia, or agoraphobia without history of panic disorder.

Specify type:

Animal type

Natural environment type (e.g., heights, storms, water)

Blood-injection-injury type

Situational type (e.g., airplanes, elevators, enclosed places)

Other type (e.g., fear of choking, vomiting, or contracting an illness; in children, fear of loud sounds or costumed characters)

The diagnostic criteria for specific and social phobias share many features. For both disorders, the phobic situation must almost invariably lead to an anxiety response (immediately, in the case of specific phobias), which may take the form of a panic attack. In addition, the individual must recognize that the fear is excessive or unreasonable (although this feature may be absent in children), avoid the phobic situation or endure it with intense distress, and experience marked distress or functional impairment as a result of the phobia. In the case of social phobia, the fear must not be related to another mental disorder or medical condition. For example, if an individual develops difficulties communicating after suffering a stroke, the fear must be unrelated to having other people notice one's problems in speaking. However, if the clinician judges that social anxiety is substantially in excess of what most individuals with this disability would experience, a diagnosis of anxiety disorder not otherwise specified may be appropriate.

Finally, for both disorders the fear must not be better accounted for by another problem. For example, an individual with obsessive–compulsive disorder who fears contamination from contact with injections would not receive an additional diagnosis of specific phobia unless there were additional concerns about injections that were unrelated to contamination (e.g., fear of fainting during an injection, fear of pain from the needle). Each diagnosis has specifiers and subtypes to allow for the provision of more specific diagnostic information. For social phobia, the clinician can specify whether the phobia is generalized (i.e., includes most social situations). For specific phobias, the clinician can indicate which one of five types best describes the focus of the phobia: animal, natural environment, blood-injection-injury, situational, or other.

DSM-IV-TR defines five main types of specific phobia: animal, natural environment, blood-injection-injury, situational, and other. These types were introduced on the basis of a series of reports to the DSM-IV Anxiety Disorders Work Group (Craske 1989, Curtis et al. 1990) showing that specific phobia types tend to differ on a variety of dimensions including age at onset, sex composition, patterns of covariation among phobias, focus of apprehension, timing and predictability of the phobic response, and type of physiological reaction during exposure to the phobic situation.

Although anxiety about physical sensations and the occurrence of panic is a feature typically associated with panic disorder, several studies have shown that panic-focused and symptom-focused apprehensions are not unique to panic disorder and agoraphobia. In fact, individuals with specific phobias score a full standard deviation above the mean for normal persons on the Anxiety Sensitivity Index (Reiss et al. 1986), a questionnaire that measures anxiety related to experiencing the physical sensations of fear. In other words, individuals with specific phobias tend to report anxiety about the sensations (e.g., racing heart, breathlessness, dizziness) typically associated with their fear. Also, there is evidence that in addition to fearing danger from the phobic object (e.g., a plane crash, being bitten by a dog), many individuals with specific phobias fear danger as a result of their reaction in the phobic situation (e.g., having a panic attack, losing control, being embarrassed) (Arntz et al. 1993, McNally and Steketee 1985). Also, the few relevant studies that have been conducted suggest that there may be differences in sensation-focused apprehension across specific phobia types.

Data are converging to indicate that individuals with phobias from the situational (e.g., claustrophobia) and blood-injury-injection types may be especially internally focused on their fear (Antony et al. 1997a, Hugdahl and Öst 1985). Whereas individuals with situational phobias tend to fear the possible consequences of panic, those with blood-injury-injection phobias seem uniquely concerned about sensations that indicate that fainting is imminent (e.g., lightheadedness, hot flashes).

Specific phobia types may differ with respect to timing and predictability of the phobic response as well. One study based on retrospective self-reports found that individuals with phobias of driving, enclosed places, and blood-injury were more likely to report that their fear was delayed in the phobic situation than were those with animal phobias (Craske et al. 1993). These data suggest that delayed and unpredictable panic attacks may be more characteristic of situational phobias than of other phobia types, consistent with the argument that situational phobias share more features with agoraphobia than do other specific phobia types.

Perhaps the most consistent difference among specific phobia types is the tendency for individuals with blood-injury-injection phobias to report a history of fainting in the phobic situation. Although all phobia types are associated with panic attacks in the phobic situation, only individuals with blood and injection phobias report fainting (Antony et al. 1997b). Specifically, individuals with blood-injury-injection phobias experience a diphasic physiological response, which includes an initial increase in arousal followed by a sharp drop in heart rate and blood pressure that can lead to fainting. This response occurs at times in approximately 70% of people with blood phobias and 56% of those with injection phobias and seems to be unique to situations involving blood and medical procedures (Öst 1992). In other words, people who faint in these situations still show the usual type of response (i.e., increased arousal) in other situations that they fear. Disgust has been identified as a potential mediator of faintness associated with blood-injury-injection stimuli (Page 2003).

The different responses experienced in different phobias have been explained from an evolutionary perspective. As mentioned earlier, the typical phobic responses of fear and panic are adaptive in that the increased arousal facilitates escape. In contrast, the most adaptive response during serious injury may be a drop in blood pressure to prevent excessive bleeding. It has been suggested that this response is mediated by an overactive sinoaortic baroreflex that is triggered by heightened arousal in situations involving blood or needles (Adler et al. 1991). Of course, in people with blood and injection phobias, the response is excessive and unwarranted, as there is typically no danger of excessive blood loss.

One of the variables considered by the DSM-IV Anxiety Disorders Work Group in its decision to classify specific phobias by types was the pattern of covariation observed among specific phobias within each of the four main types (Curtis et al. 1990). For example, about 70% of individuals with blood phobias tend to have injection phobias as well (Öst 1992). In addition, numerous factor analytical studies have found that blood-injection-injury phobias tend to cluster together as do animal phobias, natural environment phobias, and situational phobias (Arrindell 1980, Landy and Gaupp 1971, Liddell et al. 1991, Wilson and Priest 1968). In other words, having a phobia of one specific phobia type makes an individual more likely to have additional phobias of the same type than of other types. However, the clustering is not perfect; many studies show exceptions to this pattern (Curtis et al. 1998) and it has been argued that assigning specific phobias to types may not be diagnostically useful for a number of reasons (Antony et al. 1997b). The research on the classification of specific phobia types is inconsistent. For example, in several of these studies, height phobias tend to be associated with situational phobias (e.g., claustrophobia), despite height phobias being listed as an example of the natural environment type in DSM-IV-TR (Muris et al. 1999). Furthermore, it is not always clear where a particular phobia should be assigned. Is a phobia of dentists an example of a blood-injection-injury phobia or does it fall into the "other" type? Finally, it has been argued (Antony et al. 1997b) that simply naming the phobia (e.g., specific phobia, choking) is more informative and clinically useful than using the type classification "specific phobia, other type."

Specific phobias tend to co-occur with other specific phobias. One study found that 76% of a sample of 915 individuals with a lifetime history of specific phobias had one or more co-occurring specific phobias (Curtis et al. 1998). This finding is consistent with research showing that individuals with specific phobias often report multiple fears on a fear survey (Hofmann et al. 1997). However, other research indicates that comorbid phobias may not be as prevalent (Fredrikson et al. 1996) and that numbers in previous studies may have been inflated by a lack of discrimination between multiple phobias and fears of multiple situations that are accounted for by a single phobia. A recent methodologically rigorous study found that 15% of individuals with a principal diagnosis of specific phobia also met criteria for another type of specific phobia (Brown et al. 2001a).

For social phobia, DSM-IV-TR allows the clinician to specify whether it is "generalized," that is, it includes most social situations. In addition, a "discrete or circumscribed" subtype is often used by investigators to describe individuals with only one domain of social anxiety, usually involving performance-related situations (e.g., public speaking). Several studies have examined differences among these subtypes. Specifically, individuals with generalized social phobias tend to be younger, less educated, and less likely to be employed than are individuals with discrete social phobias. In addition, generalized social phobias are associated with more depression, anxiety, general distress, and concerns about negative evaluation from others (Heimberg et al. 1990, Turner et al. 1992). Discrete social phobias appear to be associated with greater cardiac reactivity.

As is the case with most disorders, a comprehensive assessment is important in helping the clinician to decide which treatment approach is most appropriate for a given individual. In the case of specific and social phobias, a thorough evaluation should include a structured or semistructured interview, self-report measures, and a behavioral assessment. Each of these measures provides different types of information that may be relevant to later treatment decisions.

During all parts of the initial evaluation, the clinician should be sensitive to several issues. First, for many individuals with phobias, even discussing the phobic object can provoke anxiety. For example, some individuals with spider phobias experience panic attacks when they discuss spiders. Some individuals with blood phobias faint when they discuss surgical procedures. Therefore, the clinician should ask the individual whether discussing the phobic object or situation will provoke anxiety. If the interview is likely to be a source of stress, the clinician should emphasize the importance of the information that is being collected, as well as the potential therapeutic value of discussing the feared object. As described later, exposure to the feared stimulus is an essential component of the treatment of most specific phobias. Of course, the interviewer should use his or her judgment when deciding how much to push the individual in the first session. For treatment to be effective, establishing trust in the clinician early in the course of treatment is essential.

With respect to social phobia, the assessment itself may be considered a phobic stimulus. Because individuals with social phobia fear the evaluation of others, a clinical interview may be especially frightening. Even completing self-report questionnaires in the waiting room may be difficult for individuals who fear writing in front of others. The clinician should be sensitive to this possibility and provide reassurance when appropriate.

Behavioral testing is an important part of any comprehensive evaluation for a phobic disorder. This is particularly the case if behavioral or cognitive–behavioral treatment is used. Because most individuals with phobias avoid the objects and situations that they fear, individuals may find it difficult to describe the subtle cues that affect their fear in the situation. In addition, it is not unusual for individuals to misjudge the amount of fear that they typically experience in the phobic situation. A behavioral approach test can be useful for identifying specific fear triggers as well as for assessing the intensity of the individual's fear in the actual situation.

To conduct a behavioral approach test, individuals should be instructed to enter the phobic situation for several minutes. For example, an individual with a snake phobia should be instructed to stand as close as possible to a live snake and note the specific cues that affect the fear (e.g., size of snake, color, movement) and the intensity of the fear (perhaps rating it on a 0–100 point scale). Individuals should pay special attention to their physical sensations (e.g., palpitations, sweating, blushing), negative thoughts (e.g., "I will fall from this balcony"), and anxious coping strategies (e.g., escape, avoidance, distraction).

Specific phobias tend to be more common among women than men. This finding seems to be strongest for phobias from the animal type, whereas sex differences are smaller for height phobias and blood-injury-injection phobias. In addition, social phobia tends to be slightly more prevalent among women than men, although these differences are relatively small (Antony and Swinson 2000a). One study examining sex differences and social phobia found significant gender differences in the presentation of social phobia (Turk et al. 1998). Whereas men were more fearful than women of urinating in public bathrooms and returning items to a store, women were more fearful than men of a number of situations including talking to people in authority, public speaking, being the center of attention, expressing disagreement, and throwing a party. Sex differences were not found in terms of comorbidity, social phobia subtypes, or duration of illness.

A variety of studies have shown that specific phobias, social phobia, and related conditions exist across cultures. For example, in Japan, a condition exists called *taijin kyôfu* in which individuals have an "obsession of shame." This condition has much overlap with social phobia in that it is often accompanied by fears of blushing, having improper facial expressions in the presence of others, looking at others, shaking, and perspiring in front of others (Takahashi 1989). In addition, studies have identified individuals with social and specific phobias in a variety of other non western countries including Saudi Arabia (Chaleby 1987), India (Raguram and Bhide 1985), Japan (Kleinknecht et al. 1997), and other East Asian countries (Chang 1997, Lee and Oh 1999). Interestingly, in some other cultures, the sex ratio for phobias tends to be reversed. For example, in studies from Saudi Arabia and India, up to 80% of individuals reporting for treatment of phobias were male. Similarly, in Japan about 60% of individuals with *taijin kyôfu* are male. In the case of phobias in India, it has been suggested that traditional gender roles may account for the difference in treatment seeking in Indian men and women (Raguram and Bhide 1985). Specifically, Indian women are often discouraged from leaving the house alone or conversing with others without the husband's permission. It is difficult to know how cultural expectations affect sex differences in phobias in other cultures.

Clinicians treating individuals from different cultures should be aware of cultural differences in presentation and response to treatment. In a review of culture-specific strategies in counseling, Sue (1990) summarized data on cultural differences in verbal communication styles, proxemics (i.e., use of interpersonal space), nonverbal communication, and other verbal cues (e.g., tone and loudness). Many cues that a clinician might use to aid in the diagnosis of social phobia in white Americans may not be useful for diagnosing the condition in other cultures. For example, although many clinicians interpret a lack of eye contact as indicating shyness or a lack of assertiveness, avoidance of eye contact among Japanese and Mexican-Americans is often viewed as a sign of respect, according to Sue (1990). In contrast to white Americans, Japanese are apparently more likely to view smiling as a sign of embarrassment or discomfort. Furthermore, cultural differences in tone and volume of speech may lead mental health professional to misinterpret their individuals. For example, whereas white Americans often are uncomfortable with silence in a conversation, British and Arab individuals may be more likely to use silence for privacy and other cultures use silence to indicate agreement among the parties or a sign of respect. In addition, Asian individuals have been reported to speak more quietly than white Americans, who in turn speak more quietly than those from Arab countries. Therefore, differences in the volume of speech should not be taken to imply differences in assertiveness or other indicators of social anxiety.

Among children, specific and social fears are common (Francis 1990, Straus and Last 1993). Because these fears may be transient, DSM-IV-TR has included a provision that social and specific phobias not be assigned in children unless they are present for more than 6 months. In addition, children may be less likely than adults to recognize that their phobia is excessive or unrealistic. The specific objects feared by children are often similar to those feared by adults, although children may be more likely to fear objects and situations that are not easily classified in the four main specific phobia types in DSM-IV-TR (e.g., balloons or costumed characters). In addition, children often report specific and social phobias having to do with school. Children with social phobia tend to avoid changing for gym class in front of others, eating in the cafeteria, or speaking in front of the class. They may stay home sick on days when frightening situations arise or may make frequent trips to the school nurse. Whereas some investigators have found that boys and girls are equally likely to present for treatment of phobias (Straus and Last 1993), others have found social phobia to be more common among girls than boys (Anderson et al. 1987). In one prospective study of childhood anxiety disorders, Last and colleagues (1996) found that almost 70% of children with a specific phobia were recovered over a 3- to 4-year period compared to a recovery rate of 86% for social phobia. Thus, almost a third of the clinical sample with specific phobia had symptoms that still met clinical criteria for specific phobia at the end of the follow-up period. This was the lowest recovery rate among the anxiety disorders that were studied. However, those in the clinical sample with specific phobia had the lowest rate of development of new mental disorders (15%) compared to the other anxiety disorders studied (e.g., the rate of development for new mental disorders was 22% for those in the clinical sample with social phobia).

Epidemiology

Phobias are among the most common mental disorders. Findings based on large community samples from five sites in the Epidemiological Catchment Area (ECA) study (Eaton et al. 1991) yielded lifetime prevalence estimates of 11.25% for specific phobias and 2.73% for social phobia. Estimates from the National Comorbidity Survey (NCS) (Kessler et al. 1994) were consistent with previous findings on specific phobias: a lifetime prevalence of 11.30% in a sample of more than 8000 individuals from across the United States. Table 32-1 lists lifetime prevalence rates for particular specific fears and phobias based on findings of the NCS (Curtis et al. 1998), with phobias of animals and heights being the most frequently diagnosed specific phobias. For social phobia, data from the NCS indicate a lifetime prevalence rate of 13.3%, much higher than that in the previously reported ECA study. This difference is likely due to methodological variations across the two studies (Antony and Swinson 2000a).

Course

The mean age at onset of social phobia is in the middle teens. The age at onset of specific phobias varies depending on the phobia type, with phobias of animals, blood, storms, and

Table 32-1	Lifetime Prevalence of Specific Fears with and without Specific Phobia					
Specific Fear	Lifetime Fears*		Lifetime Phobia Given Fear[†]		Lifetime Phobia with Specific Fear in Total Sample[‡]	
	%	s.e.	%	s.e.	%	s.e.
Height	20.4	0.7	26.2	1.8	5.3	0.5
Flying	13.2	0.7	26.9	2.4	3.5	0.3
Closed spaces	11.9	0.6	35.1	2.5	4.2	0.4
Being alone	7.3	0.6	40.7	3.3	3.1	0.4
Storms	8.7	0.5	33.1	3.4	2.9	0.4
Animals	22.2	1.1	25.8	1.2	5.7	0.4
Blood	13.9	0.7	32.8	2.1	4.5	0.3
Water	9.4	0.6	35.8	2.8	3.4	0.3
Any	49.5	1.2	22.7	1.1	11.3	0.6

revalence of lifetime fears in the total sample.
robability of specific phobia diagnosis in people endorsing each fear.
ercentage of people in total sample with specific phobia and each lifetime fear (i.e., 5.3% of total sample have lifetime specific phobia and
eight fear).
urce: Curtis GC, Magee WJ, Eaton WW, et al. (1998) Specific fears and phobias: Epidemiology and classification. *Br J Psychiatr* **173**,
2–217. Copyright 1998. The British Journal of Psychiatry.

water tending to begin in early childhood, phobias of heights beginning in the teens, and situational phobias beginning in the late teens to middle twenties. Although childhood fears are often transient (e.g., most children outgrow fear of the dark without treatment), fears that persist into adulthood usually have a chronic course unless treated.

Although many phobias begin after a traumatic event, many individuals do not recall the specific onset of their fear, and few empirical data have examined the initial period after the fear onset. Clinically, however, some individuals report a sudden onset of fear, whereas others report a more gradual onset. Studies examining the onset of phobias have tended to assess the onset of the *fear* rather than the onset of the *phobia* (i.e., the point at which the fear creates significant distress or functional impairment). A study by Antony and colleagues (1997b) suggests that the fear and phobia onset are often not the same. Individuals with specific phobias of heights, animals, blood-injection, or driving were asked to estimate the earliest age at which they could recall having their fear and the earliest age at which they could recall experiencing distress or functional impairment due to their fear. As shown in Table 32-2, phobias began at an average of 9 years after the fear onset. Anecdotally, the types of factors leading to the transition from fear to phobia included gradual increases in the intensity of fear, additional traumatic events (e.g., panic attacks, car accidents), increased life stress, and changes in living situation (e.g., starting a job that requires exposure to heights). Similarly, it is not unusual for individuals with social phobia to report having been shy as children, although their anxiety may not have reached phobic proportions until later.

Differential Diagnosis

Social anxiety is associated with a variety of DSM-IV-TR disorders. Similarly, several disorders other than specific phobia are associated with fear and avoidance of circumscribed stimuli. Therefore, accurate diagnosis of specific and social phobias depends on a thorough understanding of the DSM-IV-TR criteria and knowledge of how to distinguish these disorders from related conditions. Correct diagnosis depends on being able to evaluate the individual's focus of apprehension, reasons for avoidance, and range of situations feared.

| Table 32-2 | Mean Age of Onset (and Standard Deviations) for Specific Fears and Phobias and Agoraphobi |

| | Heights ($N = 15$) | Animals ($N = 15$) | Earliest Age of Recall (by Group) | | | | |
			Blood-Injection ($N = 15$)	Driving ($N = 15$)	PDA ($N = 15$)	F	η^2
Fear	20.47[ac]	10.80[ab]	7.93[b]	25.67[c]	28.14[c]	8.78***	0.3
	(17.53)	(8.37)	(3.71)	(11.84)	(11.95)		
Phobia	34.13[a]	20.00[bcd]	14.50[b]	32.20[acd]	29.07[ac]	6.95***	0.2
	(16.36)	(10.21)	(8.30)	(12.49)	(11.52)		
Difference	13.66[a]	9.2[ab]	6.50[ab]	6.53[ab]	0.93[b]	4.08**	0.
	(11.66)	(10.64)	(7.53)	(8.17)	(1.73)		

Note: PDA, panic disorder with agoraphobia. "Fear" refers to the age at which the fear began for individuals with specific phobias or the at which panic attacks began for individuals in the panic disorder with agoraphobia (PDA) group. "Phobia" refers to the age at which the f began to cause significant distress or functional impairment for the specific phobia groups or the age at which the individuals with PDA full criteria for the disorder. "Difference" was calculated by subtracting ages of onset for the fear from those for the phobia. Group me (across rows) sharing superscript letters do not differ at $P < 0.05$. **$P < 0.01$; ***$P < 0.001$.
Source: Antony MM, Brown TA, and Barlow DH (1997b) Heterogeneity among specific phobia types in DSM-IV-TR. *Behav Res Ther* 1089–1100. Copyright 1997 Elsevier Science.

Panic disorder with agoraphobia may easily be misdiagnosed as social phobia or a specific phobia (especially the situational type). For example, many individuals with panic disorder avoid a variety of social situations because of anxiety about having others notice their symptoms. In addition, some individuals with panic disorder may avoid circumscribed situations, such as flying, despite reporting no other significant avoidance. Four variables should be considered in making the differential diagnosis: (1) type and number of panic attacks, (2) focus of apprehension, (3) number of situations avoided, and (4) level of intercurrent anxiety.

Individuals with panic disorder experience unexpected panic attacks and heightened anxiety outside of the phobic situation, whereas those with specific and social phobias typically do not. In addition, individuals with panic disorder are more likely than those with specific and social phobias to report fear and avoidance of a broad range of situations typically associated with agoraphobia (e.g., flying, enclosed places, crowds, being alone, shopping malls). Finally, individuals with panic disorder are typically concerned only about the possibility of panicking in the phobic situation or about the consequences of panicking (e.g., being embarrassed by one's panic symptoms). In contrast, individuals with specific and social phobias are usually concerned about other aspects of the situation as well (e.g., being hit by another driver, saying something foolish).

Consider two examples in which the differential diagnosis with panic disorder might be especially difficult. First, individuals with claustrophobia are typically extremely concerned about being unable to escape from the phobic situation as well as being unable to breathe in the situation. Therefore, like individuals with panic disorder and agoraphobia, they usually report heightened anxiety about the possibility of panicking. The main variable to consider in such a case is the presence of panic attacks outside of claustrophobic situations. If panic attacks occur exclusively in enclosed places, a diagnosis of specific phobia might best describe the problem. In contrast, if the individual has unexpected or uncued panic attacks as well, a diagnosis of panic disorder might be more appropriate.

A second example is an individual who avoids a broad range of situations including shopping malls, supermarkets, walking on busy streets, and various social situations including parties, meetings, and public speaking. Without more information, this individual's problem might appear to meet criteria for social phobia, panic disorder with agoraphobia, or both diagnoses. As mentioned earlier, individuals with panic disorder often avoid social situations because of anxiety about panicking in public. In addition, individuals with social phobia might avoid situations that are typically avoided by individuals with agoraphobia for fear of seeing someone that they know or of being observed by strangers. To make the diagnosis in this case, it is necessary to assess the reasons for avoidance.

It may be difficult to distinguish among types of specific phobias. For example, is a bridge phobia best considered a situational type (i.e., driving) or a natural environment type (i.e., heights)? This decision should be based on the context of the bridge phobia. If the individual fears falling or fears other high places, a height phobia may be the appropriate diagnosis. In contrast, if bridges are one of many driving-related situations that the person fears, a driving phobia might be more appropriate.

Other diagnoses that should be considered before a diagnosis of specific phobia is assigned include posttraumatic stress disorder (PTSD) (if the fear follows a life-threatening trauma and is accompanied by other PTSD symptoms such as reexperiencing the trauma), obsessive–compulsive disorder (if the fear is related to an obsession, e.g., contamination), hypochondriasis (if the fear is related to a belief that he or she has some serious illness), separation-anxiety disorder (if the fear is of situations that might lead to separation from the family, for example, traveling on an airplane without one's parents), eating disorders (if the fear is of eating certain foods but not related to a fear of choking), and psychotic disorders (if the fear is related to a delusion).

Social phobia should not be diagnosed if the fear is related entirely to another disorder. For example, if an individual with obsessive–compulsive disorder avoids social situations only because of the embarrassment of having others notice her or his excessive hand washing, a diagnosis of social phobia would not be given. Furthermore, individuals with depression, schizoid personality disorder, or a pervasive developmental disorder may avoid social situations because of a lack of interest in spending time with others. To be considered social phobia, an individual must avoid these situations specifically because of anxiety about being evaluated negatively.

In the case of generalized social phobia, the diagnosis of avoidant personality disorder should be considered as well. Individuals with avoidant personality disorder tend to display more interpersonal sensitivity and have poorer social skills than social phobic individuals without avoidant personality disorder (Turner et al. 1986). Furthermore, most studies suggest that the differences between avoidant personality disorder and social phobia are more quantitative than qualitative and that the former may simply be a more severe form of the latter (Widiger 1992). Therefore, most individuals who meet criteria for avoidant personality disorder will meet criteria for social phobia as well.

Finally, social and specific phobias should be distinguished from normal states of fear and anxiety. Many individuals report mild fears of circumscribed situations or mild shyness in certain social situations. Others may report intense fears of public speaking or heights but insist that these situations rarely arise and that they have no interest in being in these situations. For the criteria for a specific or social phobia to be met, the individual must report significant distress about having the fear or must report significant impairment in functioning.

A variety of factors should be considered in deciding whether an individual's fear exceeds the threshold necessary for a diagnosis of specific or social phobia. To make the differential diagnosis between normal fears and clinical phobias, the clinician should consider the extent of the individual's avoidance, the frequency with which the phobic stimulus is encountered, and the degree to which the individual is bothered by having the fear. For example, an individual who fears seeing snakes in the wild but who lives in the city, never encounters snakes, and never even thinks about snakes would probably not be diagnosed with a specific phobia. In contrast, when an individual's fear of snakes leads to avoidance of walking through parks, camping, swimming, and watching certain television programs, despite having an interest in doing these things, a diagnosis of specific phobia would be appropriate.

Similar factors should be considered in deciding at what point normal shyness reaches an intensity that warrants a diagnosis of social phobia. An individual who is somewhat quiet in groups or when meeting new people but does not avoid these situations and is not especially distressed by his or her shyness would probably not receive a diagnosis of social phobia. In contrast, an individual who frequently refuses invitations to socialize because of anxiety, quits a job because of anxiety about having to talk to customers, or is distressed about her or his social anxiety would be likely to receive a diagnosis of social phobia.

Diagnostic decision trees for social and specific phobias are presented in Figures 32-1 and 32-2.

Etiology

Psychological Factors

Emotions are "contagious." That is, we learn to respond to stimuli, in part, by observing other people's responses and also by our own experiences in these situations. In other words, we come to fear dangerous situations easily. This is important from an ethological perspective because our ancestors who could learn to fear threatening objects or situations easily were more likely to survive and pass these genes to their offspring. This inherited tendency to learn to experience fear in particular situations is the basis of conditioning models of phobia development.

The two-stage model of Mowrer (1939) was a precursor to current conditioning models for phobia development. According to Mowrer, the first stage in the development of fear involves a classical conditioning process by which a previously neutral stimulus is associated with an aversive stimulus so that the neutral stimulus becomes a trigger for fear. For example, a fear of dogs might develop after an individual is bitten (an aversive stimulus) by a dog (a neutral stimulus). Mowrer's second stage relies on operant conditioning principles to explain the maintenance of phobias. According to Mowrer, phobias are maintained by negative reinforcement resulting from avoidance of the phobic object. In other words, avoidance prevents the uncomfortable symptoms that occur when one is frightened and thereby maintains the desire to avoid the phobic object and situation.

Despite the research interest generated by Mowrer's model, the model suffers from several problems. First, many individuals report no specific conditioning experiences that trigger their phobias. In fact, many individuals report having fears despite never even having encountered the phobic situation, let alone having experienced a trauma in the phobic situation. Second, Mowrer's theory does not explain why many individuals experience traumas but never develop fears. For example, one study found that although traumatic events were reported to be the cause of fear among 56% of individuals with fears of dogs, 66% of nonfearful subjects reported a history of traumatic experiences with dogs that did not lead to the development of fear (Di Nardo et al. 1988).

In response to these and other concerns with Mowrer's model, Rachman (1977) proposed three pathways to the development of fear. The first of these is *direct conditioning*, which typically involves the experience of being hurt or frightened by the phobic object or situation. Examples include being involved in an automobile accident, being humiliated in front of a group, falling or almost falling from a high place, or fainting at the sight of

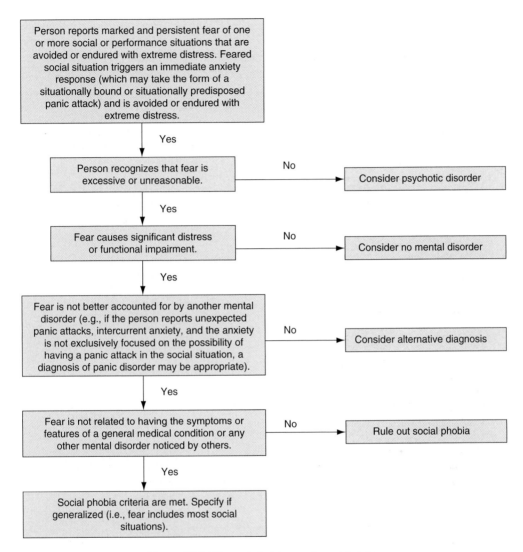

Figure 32-1 *Diagnostic decision tree for social phobia.*

blood. Rachman's second pathway is called *vicarious acquisition*, which involves witnessing some traumatic event or seeing someone behave fearfully in the presence of a phobic situation. For example, a child might develop a fear of snakes after seeing her father behave fearfully around snakes, or someone might develop a fear of public speaking after seeing another individual heckled by the audience during a presentation. For the third pathway, Rachman proposed that fears can develop through *informational and instructional pathways*. It is not surprising that individuals might develop flying phobias, given the frequency with which plane crashes are reported in the news. Similarly, a child might develop a fear of heights if his parents frequently warned him of the dangers of being near high places.

In addition to these pathways, Rachman acknowledged the role of biological constraints on the development of fear. Of particular relevance is the fact that fears are not randomly

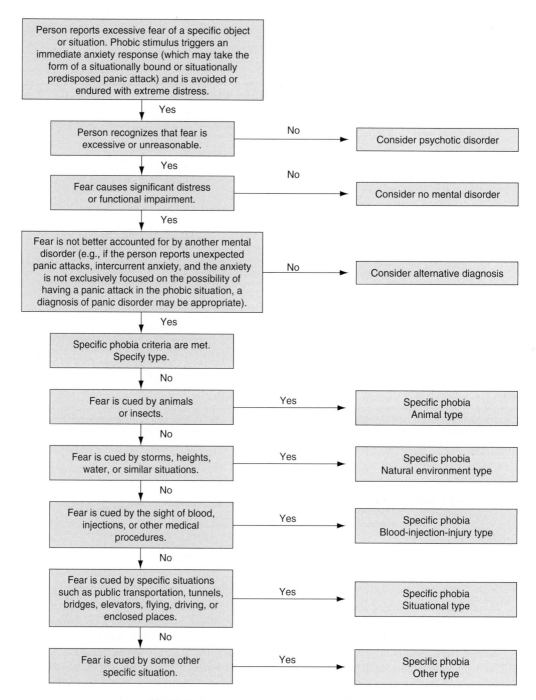

Figure 32-2 *Diagnostic decision tree for specific phobia.*

distributed. To explain this observation, Seligman (1971) proposed that organisms are predisposed to learn certain associations and not others. Seligman called his theory "preparedness" and hypothesized that individuals are "prepared" to develop some associations that lead to fear and not others. For example, an individual might be more likely to develop a fear of dogs after being bitten than to develop a fear of flowers after being pricked by a thorn. Seligman proposed that these associations evolved through natural selection processes to facilitate survival.

Evidence for the theory of preparedness is mixed. Although some authors have concluded that the studies to date do not support preparedness (McNally 1987), it may be argued that these studies have not adequately tested the theory. Most studies examining preparedness have attempted to associate dangerous objects (e.g., snakes) and nondangerous objects (e.g., flowers) with an aversive electrical shock and have found few differences in the subsequent development of fear. However, preparedness predicts that some "associations" are more difficult to establish than others, not that some "objects" are more easily feared than others. The theory does not necessarily predict that shock should be more easily associated with snakes than with flowers. A more appropriate experiment might be to compare the effects of a minor snakebite to the effects of being pricked by a thorny flower on the development of fear of each object. In any event, there is now strong evidence that conditioning processes play an important role in the development of phobic disorders (Bouton et al. 2001).

Numerous studies have examined the prevalence of Rachman's three pathways to fear development, as illustrated in Table 32-3. Most of these studies have focused on the development of specific phobias, although a few studies included social phobia groups. The majority of studies have found support for the model, indicating that both direct and

Table 32-3	Percentage of Individuals with Phobias Reporting Various Types of Onset*			
Study	Type of Fear	Direct Conditioning	Vicarious Conditioning	Information
McNally and Steketee (1985)	Animals	23	0	4
Menzies and Parker (2001)	Heights	19	15	7
Di Nardo et al. (1988)	Dogs	56	—	—
Merckelbach and Muris (1997)	Spiders	23	15	4
Merckelbach et al. (1992)	Spiders	66	59	34
Ehlers et al. (1994)	Driving	36	12	16
Merckelbach et al. (1996)	Spiders	41	18	5
Menzies and Clarke (1993b)	Heights	18	20	8
Öst (1991)	Blood	49	26	7
	Injection	57	21	5
Öst and Hugdahl (1985)	Blood	46	32	9
	Dentists	69	12	6
Kleinknecht (1994)	Blood-injury	76	20	3
Rimm et al. (1977)	Various	36	7	9
Hofmann et al. (1995a)	Public speaking	89	57	54
Muris et al. (1997)	Animals	45	0	29
Medical	44	0	11	
	Spiders	42	0	13
	Social (failure and criticism)	50	0	0
	All fears	40	1	27
Öst (1985)	Blood	50	25	2
	Animals	50	22	20
	Dentists	66	16	0
	Enclosed places	68	7	13
	Social	56	16	3
Antony (1994)	Heights	20	0	0
	Animals	20	7	7
	Blood-injections	27	0	7
	Driving	33	13	13

*Figures are rounded off to the nearest percent.

indirect forms of phobia acquisition occur frequently across a wide range of phobia types (McNally and Steketee 1985, Merckelbach and Muris 1997, Muris et al. 1997, Townend et al. 2000). However, numerous people report onsets that are unrelated to these pathways (e.g., "I have had this fear for as long as I can remember" or "I have always had this fear"). Overall, it appears that direct and indirect methods of fear development are relatively common, although the frequency of these onsets varies greatly across studies for a variety of reasons. First, studies have been inconsistent with respect to the populations studied (e.g., clinical groups, nonclinical subjects such as college students, individuals recruited through advertisements). In addition, some studies included mixed groups of individuals with a given fear (e.g., flying fears can be due to a specific phobia of flying, claustrophobia, or agoraphobia). Third, studies differed in the ways in which each pathway was defined. For example, an onset that followed an unexpected panic attack was included among the traumatic onsets in some studies but not others. Finally, some studies allowed subjects to list multiple causes, whereas other studies had subjects rate only the primary cause.

In addition to methodological differences, the inconsistency across studies may be partly explained by the lack of reliability of retrospective self-report. More recent studies have examined onset of phobias in children and included parental interviews to avoid problems associated with retrospective report (Merckelbach and Muris 1997, Poulton et al. 1999).

Despite the prevalence of direct and indirect conditioning events and informational onsets, it appears that they are not the whole story. In fact, studies have begun to include normal comparison groups and have found that these events are equally common in individuals who do not have phobias (Hofmann et al. 1995, Menzies and Parker 2001, Merckelbach et al. 1992). Ultimately, to answer the question of how phobias begin, we must discover the variables that lead only certain individuals to develop phobias after experiencing conditioning events or receiving information that leads to fear. For example, several investigators have found that a tendency to feel "disgust" in response to certain stimuli may be important in the development of some animal phobias and blood phobias (Davey et al. 1993, Merckelbach et al. 1993, Page 1994, Sawchuk et al. 2000, Woody and Teachman 2000). In addition, heightened disgust sensitivity in parents has been found to predict fear of disgust-relevant animals (e.g., snakes, mice, slugs, and cockroaches) in children (de Jong et al. 1997).

Several other variables have also been suggested as mediating factors in the development of fear. Stress at the time of the event may make individuals more likely to react fearfully. In addition, previous and subsequent exposure to the phobic object may protect an individual from the development of a phobia. For example, someone who grew up around dogs may be less likely to develop a phobia after being bitten than someone who has spent little time around dogs. The context of the event may also influence the reaction. For example, being with another supportive individual at the time of the trauma may protect an individual from developing fear. Finally, a number of individual difference variables such as perceived control, trait anxiety, and various personality factors may influence an individual's likelihood of developing a phobia after a conditioning event. In fact, there is evidence that personality factors and parenting styles may be especially relevant to the development of social phobia.

It has been proposed that a fourth nonassociative pathway be added to Rachman's three associative pathways to fear development (Poulton and Menzies 2002). Nonassociative fear models (Menzies and Clarke 1995) propose that a limited number of fears are not acquired by conditioning or other learning processes. Rather, these evolutionary adaptive fears are proposed to be innate or biologically determined. This is similar to preparedness theory; however, it maintains that fears are acquired through a learning or conditioning process and that some fears are more easily learned than others. According to Poulton and Menzies (2002), the nonassociative pathway to fear acquisition helps explain a number of research findings that run counter to associative models of fear development including the nonrandom distribution of common fears, and the emergence of some fears without any prior specific associative learning experiences (i.e., direct conditioning, vicarious conditioning, or informational transmission).

The work of Kagan and others (Kagan et al. 1984, Rosenbaum et al. 1991) has suggested that as early as 18 months of age, children differ with respect to their tendency to interact with other individuals, toys, and objects. Although about 70% of children are somewhat exploratory in these situations, about 15% of children are extremely exploratory, and the remaining 15% are quite shy and withdrawn. The behavior exhibited by the shy and withdrawn children has been called "behavioral inhibition" and has been proposed to be a predisposing factor in the development of social phobia and other anxiety disorders (Turner et al. 1996). One study found that the prevalence of social phobia was significantly greater (17%; $N = 64$) in children with behavioral inhibition than without (5%; $N = 152$) (Biederman et al. 2001). In addition, compared to nonanxious individuals, individuals with social phobia describe their parents as having (1) discouraged them from socializing, (2) placed undue importance on the opinions of others, and (3) used shame as a means of discipline (Bruch and Heimberg 1994). Other predictors of the development of social phobia include a childhood history of separation anxiety, self-consciousness or shyness in childhood and adolescence, and a low frequency of dating in adolescence (Bruch 1989, Bruch and Heimberg 1994).

Perfectionism is another personality variable that has been associated with social phobia (Antony et al. 1998a). Although several other anxiety disorders have also been associated with perfectionism, concern about making mistakes and a perception of having critical parents are highest among individuals with social phobia compared to individuals with other anxiety disorders (e.g., panic disorder, obsessive–compulsive disorder, or specific phobia).

Numerous studies have examined the role of cognitive variables in social and specific phobias and have consistently found that individuals with these disorders exhibit attentional and attributional biases regarding the phobic object or situation. In studies of information processing, people with social and specific phobias devote more attention to threat-related information than do nonphobic individuals (Kindt and Brosschot 1999, Mattia et al. 1993). They also show perceptual and cognitive distortions consistent with their phobias (Jones and Menzies 2000, Pauli et al. 1998, Purdon et al. 2001, Rapee 1997, Roth et al. 2001). For example, individuals with snake or spider phobias tend to overestimate the degree of activity in the feared animal before treatment but not after treatment (Rachman and Cuk 1992). Likewise, people with social phobia tend to rate their own performance during public speaking more critically than do nonphobic control subjects (Rapee and Lim 1992). Furthermore, the discrepancy between self-ratings and observer ratings is greater for people with social phobia than control subjects (Norton and Hope 2001). In addition, individuals with social phobia tend to report more negative self-evaluative thoughts and underestimate their performance when interacting with others relative to nonanxious subjects (Stopa and Clark 1993). More recent research has found that compared to nonanxious individuals, individuals with social phobia are more likely to experience negative imagery and to take an observer's point of view (i.e., see themselves from an external perspective) when exposed to feared social situations (Hackmann et al. 1998, Wells and Papageorgiou 1999). Other research has found that social phobia is associated with impaired thought suppression affecting both social phobia–related stimuli as well as nonsocial phobia–related stimuli (Fehm and Margraf 2002). Although it is clear that cognitive biases exist in individuals with phobias and that attentional and attributional biases improve after effective treatment, it is not known whether the cognitive biases exhibited by individuals contribute to the development of the fear or whether they are simply a manifestation of the fear.

Genetic and Familial Factors

Specific phobias and social phobia tend to run in families. It appears that being a first-degree relative of an individual with a specific phobia puts one at a greater risk for a specific phobia compared with first-degree relatives of never mentally ill controls (31% versus 11%). However, the particular phobia that is transmitted is usually different from that in the relative, although it is often from the same general type (e.g., animal, situational). Furthermore, relatives of people with specific phobias are not at increased risk for other types of anxiety disorders (including social phobia) or subclinical fears (Fyer et al. 1990). The heritability of blood and injection phobias may be even greater than that for other phobias. One study found that 61% of individuals with blood phobia and 29% of those with injection phobias reported having a first-degree relative with the same fear (Öst 1992). However, these findings should be interpreted with caution because relatives did not undergo independent interviews.

Findings for individuals with social phobia and their families show a similar pattern. In one study, 16% of first-degree relatives of subjects with social phobia had symptoms that met criteria for social phobia, whereas only 5% of first-degree relatives of never mentally ill control subjects had social phobia (Fyer et al. 1993). Furthermore, there is no increased risk among relatives of people with social phobia to develop other anxiety disorders. A more recent study found that in comparison to probands in a comparison group, the relative risk for generalized social phobia and avoidant personality disorder were tenfold for first-degree relatives of probands with social phobia (Stein et al. 1998).

Although the nature of the genetic contribution has yet to be specified (a low threshold for alarm reactions or vasovagal responses is one possibility), specific and social phobias may be related to personality factors that have been found to be highly heritable. Two traits that may be relevant are neuroticism (or emotionality) and extroversion (or sociability) (Plomin 1989). Average heritability estimates for these traits are about 50% across a wide range of genetic studies. Emotionality probably predisposes individuals to develop a range of anxiety and mood disorders, whereas sociability may be most relevant to social phobia. Furthermore, certain phobias may have other specific genetic contributions. Up to 70% of individuals with blood phobia report a history of fainting on exposure to blood (Öst 1992). It has been suggested that an inherited overactive baroreflex may contribute to the high rate of familial transmission of blood phobias (Adler et al. 1991).

Other Biological Factors

In contrast to the situation with other anxiety disorders, little is known about the physiological correlates of specific and social phobias. Only a few studies have examined physiological correlates of specific phobia. Research examining brain activity during the experience of phobic fear using positron emission tomography has yielded inconsistent results (Rauch et al. 1995, Wik et al. 1997), with some studies finding changes in cerebral blood flow associated with viewing phobia-relevant scenes and some studies finding no differences in cerebral blood flow between participants with and without phobias. Specific phobia may have been of less interest to researchers because no effective pharmacological treatments exist for this disorder. However, effective drug treatments have been identified for social phobia, leading to an increased interest in the biological factors underlying this disorder (Mathew et al. 2001).

Studies on the relationship between serotonin and social phobia have been mixed. Selective serotonin reuptake inhibitors (SSRIs) have been shown to be very effective in the treatment of social phobia. In addition, there is evidence of augmented cortisol response to fenfluramine in individuals with social phobia, suggesting an association between social phobia and selective supersensitivity in the serotonergic system (Tancer et al. 1994–1995). However, there is research showing that [3H] paroxetine binding (an indicator of serotonergic functioning) does not differ between social phobia individuals and nonanxious controls (Stein et al. 1995).

There has also been some evidence to suggest a relationship between dopamine and social phobia. Unlike panic disorder, which responds well to a variety of tricyclic antidepressants and monoamine oxidase inhibitors (MAOIs) (Buigues and Vallejo 1987, Schweizer et al. 1993), social phobia tends to have a positive response to MAOIs and show little response to tricyclic antidepressants (Levin et al. 1989). Whereas tricyclic antidepressants tend to act on noradrenergic and serotonergic systems, MAOIs affect noradrenergic, serotonergic, and dopaminergic systems (Cooper et al. 1983). This finding has led some investigators to suggest that the dopamine system is primarily involved in social phobia (Levin et al. 1989), which would explain why biological challenges that appear to affect noradrenergic activity (e.g., sodium lactate infusion, carbon dioxide inhalation) have little effect on individuals with social phobia, despite having panicogenic effects in individuals with panic disorder (Rapee et al. 1992). The dopamine hypothesis is consistent with findings that dopamine metabolite levels correlate with measures of extroversion (King et al. 1986) as well as findings that mice bred to be timid have been shown to be deficient in brain dopamine concentration (Lewis et al. 1989). In addition, a neuroimaging study found that striatal dopamine reuptake site densities were significantly lower in individuals with social phobia as compared to controls (Tiihonen et al. 1997).

With respect to neuroendocrine correlates in social phobia, studies of the hypothalamic–pituitary–thyroid and hypothalamic–pituitary–adrenal axes in social phobia have found few differences between individuals with social phobia and control persons. For example, research has found that individuals with social phobia and control subjects did not differ on tests of thyroid function (Tancer et al. 1990) or levels of urinary free cortisol (Potts et al. 1991). However, more recent studies have found evidence of cortisol differences associated with social anxiety. Some research has found that shy children have higher salivary cortisol than nonshy children (Schmidt et al. 1997). Other research has found that in comparison to control volunteers, social phobia individuals exhibited dichotomies in the distribution and magnitude of their cortisol response to a speech task (social phobia–related stress task), but not a physical exercise task (nonsocial phobia–related stress task) (Furlan et al. 2001).

Recent imaging studies have found a number of differences between social phobia individuals and controls. One study using functional magnetic resonance imaging (fMRI) found that conditioned aversive stimuli were associated with increased activation in the amygdala and hippocampus of social phobia individuals, whereas decreased activation in these areas was observed in normal controls (Schneider et al. 1999). Other research using repeat proton magnetic resonance spectroscopy has found significant differences between social phobics and controls in cortical gray matter. Specifically, Tupler and colleagues (1997) found that social phobia is associated with specific choline and myoinositol abnormalities in cortical and subcortical gray areas of the brain. Another study using single-photon emission computer tomography (SPECT) found that after an 8-week trial of citalopram, there was significantly decreased activity in the anterior and lateral part of the left temporal cortex, the left cingulum, and the anterior, lateral, and posterior part of the left midfrontal cortex in a small ($N = 15$) sample of social phobia individuals (Van der Linden et al. 2000a). Compared to treatment responders, treatment nonresponders had higher activity at baseline in the lateral left temporal cortex and the lateral left midfrontal regions. Further research is necessary to understand the significance of these imaging findings as well as their specificity to social phobia.

Finally, there may be good reason to consider different underlying mechanisms in individuals with performance-related phobias (e.g., public speaking) than in individuals with generalized social phobia (i.e., those who fear most social situations). Individuals with performance-related phobias tend to show more autonomic reactivity (e.g., rapid heart beat) in the phobic situation than do individuals with generalized social phobia (Levin et al. 1993). In addition, beta blockers such as atenolol may be useful for decreasing performance anxiety in normal individuals (Gorman and Gorman 1987), although they have little effect on individuals with generalized social phobia (Liebowitz et al. 1992). These facts have led some investigators to suggest that adrenergic hyperactivity may be involved in performance anxiety but not in generalized social phobia (Levin et al. 1989). However, it should be noted that despite limited evidence for the use of beta blockers in normal groups (e.g., musicians with performance anxiety), their utility for treating individuals with a diagnosis of social phobia (e.g., performance fears that lead to significant distress or impairment) has not been established.

Treatment

The main goal of treatment is to decrease fear and phobic avoidance to a level that no longer causes significant distress or functional impairment. In some cases, treatment includes strategies for improving specific skill deficits as well. For example, individuals with social phobia may lack adequate social skills and can sometimes benefit from social skills training. Likewise, some individuals with specific phobias of driving may have poor driving skills if their fear prevented them from learning how to drive properly. Typically, effective treatment for social phobia lasts several months, although treatment of discrete social phobias (e.g., public speaking) may take less time. Specific phobias can usually be treated relatively quickly. In fact, for certain phobias, the vast majority of individuals are able to achieve clinically significant, long-lasting improvement in as little as one session of behavioral treatment (Öst et al. 1991b, 1997a, 2001).

Effective treatments fall into one of two main categories: pharmacological treatment and cognitive–behavioral therapy (CBT). Pharmacological treatments have been used effectively for treating social phobia, although it is generally accepted that they are of limited utility for treating specific phobias. In contrast, CBT has been used with success for the treatment of specific and social phobias. Despite the existence of effective treatments, fewer than half of those who seek treatment in an anxiety disorders specialty clinic have previously received evidence-based treatments for their social anxiety (Rowa et al. 2000). Tables 32-4 and 32-5 summarize various treatments for social and specific phobias. Treatment decision trees for social and specific phobias are presented in Figures 32-3 and 32-4.

Somatic Treatments

Although pharmacotherapy is generally thought to be ineffective for specific phobias, it is not uncommon for phobic individuals occasionally to be prescribed low dosages of benzodiazepines to be taken in the phobic situation (e.g., while flying). Studies have been conducted that have examined the use of benzodiazepines and beta blockers alone or in combination with behavioral treatments for specific phobias and in general have found that drugs do not contribute much to the treatment of specific phobias (Antony and Barlow 2002). However, one problem with the research to date is that it has not taken into account differences among specific phobia types. For example, claustrophobia and other phobias of the situational type appear to share more features with panic disorder than with the other specific phobia types (Antony et al. 1997a). Therefore, medications that are effective for panic disorder (e.g., imipramine, alprazolam) may prove to be effective for situational phobias. Although there are few studies examining this hypothesis, preliminary data suggest that benzodiazepines may be helpful in the short term but lead to greater relapse in the long-term and possibly interfere with the therapeutic effects of exposure across sessions (Wilhelm and Roth 1996). For example, one study found that CBT and providing a benzodiazepine both led to fear reduction during dental surgery; however, whereas benzodiazepine treatment

Table 32-4	Treatments for Social Phobia		
Treatment	**Advantages**	**Disadvantages**	**Rating**
Cognitive–behavioral therapy (CBT) (e.g., exposure, cognitive restructuring, social skills training, education)	Good treatment response Brief course of treatment. Treatment gains maintained at follow-up. Considered first line.	May lead to temporary increases in discomfort or fear.	++++
SSRIs (e.g., paroxetine, fluvoxamine, sertraline)	Good treatment response Early response, relative to CBT Broad spectrum efficacy for comorbid disorders (i.e., depression) Lack of abuse potential Considered first line.	Side effects are common. Cost is a factor. May be a risk of relapse after discontinuation.	+++
Moclobemide	Good treatment response in some studies. Fewer side effects than phenelzine. Considered second line.	Side effects common. Does not separate from placebo in some studies. Potential exists for relapse after discontinuation.	++
Benzodiazepines (e.g., clonazepam, alprazolam)	Good treatment response. Considered adjunctive or second line.	Side effects and withdrawal occur. Potential for abuse. Relapse after discontinuation is likely. Does not treat certain comorbid conditions (i.e., depression).	++
MAOIs (e.g., phenelzine)	Good treatment response. Early response. Considered third line.	Relatively high rate of adverse effects. Dietary restrictions must be followed. Numerous drug interactions. Potential exists for relapse after discontinuation.	++
Gabapentin	Possibly beneficial. Considered third line.	Side effects are common. More research is needed.	++
β-blockers (e.g., atenolol)	Appears to be useful for "stage fright" in actors, musicians, and other performers.	Drugs are not effective for generalized social phobia. Benefits for discrete social phobias are questionable. Side effects occur. Potential exists for relapse after discontinuation.	+

++++ First treatment of choice. Helpful for most patients, with few side effects. Good long-term benefits.
+++ Helpful for most patients. Potential for relapse after treatment is discontinued.
++ More controlled research needed, although preliminary studies suggest potential benefit OR research has been mixed.
+ Not especially effective for generalized social phobia.

was associated with greater relapse during follow-up, CBT was associated with further improvements (Thom et al. 2000).

In contrast to specific phobias, social phobia has been treated successfully with a variety of pharmacological interventions including SSRIs such as sertraline (Blomhoff et al. 2001, Van Ameringen et al. 2001), fluvoxamine (Stein et al. 1999, van Vliet et al. 1994) and paroxetine (Allgulander and Nilsson, 2001, Liebowitz et al. 2002, Stein et al. 1998), benzodiazepines such as clonazepam (Davidson et al. 1993) and alprazolam (Reich and Yates 1988), traditional MAOIs such as phenelzine (Heimberg et al. 1998), and reversible

Table 32-5	Treatments for Specific Phobias		
Treatment	**Advantages**	**Disadvantages**	**Rating**
In vivo exposure	Highly effective Early response Treatment gains maintained at follow-up	May lead to temporary increases in discomfort or fear.	++++
Applied tension	Highly effective for individuals with blood-injection phobias who faint Early response Treatment gains maintained at follow-up	Treatment is relevant for a small percentage of individuals with specific phobias.	+++
Applied relaxation	May be effective for some individuals	Treatment has not been extensively researched for specific phobias	.++
Cognitive therapy	May help to reduce anxiety about conducting exposure exercises	Treatment has not been extensively researched for specific phobias. Treatment is probably not effective alone.	++
Benzodiazepines	May reduce anticipatory anxiety before individual enters phobic situation, and may reduce fear, particularly in situational specific phobias	Treatment has not been extensively researched for specific phobias. Treatment is probably not effective alone, in many cases. Side effects (e.g., sedation) occur Discontinuation of symptoms may undermine benefits of treatment.	++
SSRIs	May reduce panic sensations for individuals with situational phobias that are similar to panic disorder (e.g., claustrophobia)	Treatment has not been extensively researched for specific phobias. There are a few studies (primarily case reports) with promising results. Discontinuation of medication may result in a return of fear.	++

++++ Treatment of choice. Effective for almost all individuals.
+++ Very effective for a subset of individuals.
++ May be helpful for some individuals. More research needed.

inhibitors of monoamine oxidase A (RIMA) such as moclobemide (Versiani et al. 1992, 1996) and brofaromine (Lott et al. 1997).

Numerous controlled trials across a range of SSRIs including sertraline, fluvoxamine, and paroxetine have demonstrated their effectiveness in the treatment of social phobia, such that the SSRIs are currently considered the first-line medication treatment (for a meta-analysis of RCTs see Van der Linden et al. 2000b). Preliminary research indicates that paroxetine may be useful in the treatment of individuals with comorbid social phobia and alcohol use disorder (Randall et al. 2001). Owing to their tolerability and efficacy, the SSRIs have been referred to as "the new gold standard" in pharmacological treatment for social phobia (Van Ameringen et al. 1999b, 2000). Uncontrolled open trials and case series studies with citalopram (Bouwer and Stein 1998, Simon et al. 2001) and fluoxetine (Perugi et al. 1994–1995) suggest that these SSRIs may also be beneficial in the treatment of social phobia. Another benefit of SSRIs is their broad spectrum efficacy for common comorbid disorders such as depression and panic disorder.

Treatment of social phobia with other antidepressants (e.g., imipramine, nefazodone, venlafaxine) has been studied in a number of uncontrolled open trials. One study on 15

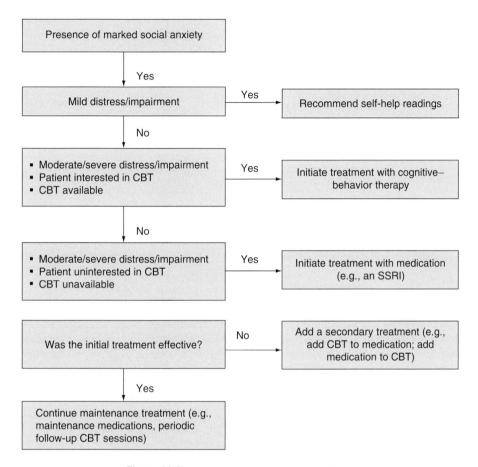

Figure 32-3 *Treatment decision tree for social phobia.*

individuals did not support the efficacy of imipramine for social phobia (Simpson et al. 1998). A number of studies examining the nonselective antidepressant nefazodone found it to be effective in 66 to 70% of individuals (Van Ameringen et al. 1999a). In addition, the serotonin and norepinephrine reuptake inhibitor venlafaxine has been found to be effective in reducing social phobia symptoms in two studies with small samples of individuals, the majority of whom did not respond to SSRIs (Altamura et al. 1999, Kelsey 1995).

Research on the use of anxiolytics for the treatment of social phobia have focused on high potency benzodiazepines (e.g., clonazepam, alprazolam) and the nonbenzodiazepine buspirone. Several studies have examined the utility of clonazepam for treating social phobia. In a placebo-controlled study, Davidson and colleagues (1993) found that 78% of individuals responded to clonazepam (mean dosage, 2.4 mg/day), whereas only 20% responded to placebo. One study comparing clonazepam to cognitive–behavioral group therapy found that individuals in both conditions improved significantly and no differences between treatment conditions were observed aside from greater improvement in the clonazepam group at 12 weeks of treatment (Otto et al. 2000). These results confirmed findings from smaller open trials and case studies supporting the use of clonazepam for social phobia (mean dosages, 2.1–2.75 mg/day) (Davidson et al. 1991a, Munjack et al. 1990). In addition, uncontrolled pilot studies have suggested that alprazolam (mean dosage, 2.9 mg/day) (Lydiard et al. 1988, Reich and Yates 1988) may be effective for social phobia,

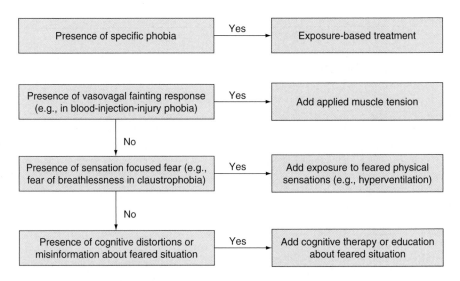

Figure 32-4 *Treatment decision tree for specific phobia.*

although more controlled clinical trials are needed. The findings on buspirone are mixed. A number of controlled trials have found no significant advantage of buspirone over placebo (Clark and Agras 1991, van Vliet et al. 1997). This is in contrast to previous uncontrolled studies that found some benefit to buspirone (Munjack et al. 1991, Schneier et al. 1993).

Owing to the potentially severe side effects of MAOIs as well as the necessity for certain dietary restrictions, they are not recommended as a first-line treatment. The findings from more recent trials involving RIMAs have been less encouraging than initial studies suggested. For example, a fixed dose study conducted over 12 weeks found that moclobemide did not have a significant benefit over placebo at five dosages ranging from 75 to 900 mg/day (Noyes et al. 1997). Other studies have also found poor responses to moclobemide (Oosterbaan et al. 2001, Schneier et al. 1998). Discontinuation of MAOIs and RIMAs have been associated with a tendency to relapse.

Research on beta blockers indicates that they are no better than placebo for most individuals with generalized social phobia (Liebowitz et al. 1992). Although beta blockers have been used to treat individuals from nonpatient samples with heightened performance anxiety (e.g., people with public speaking anxiety, musicians with stage fright) (Hartley et al. 1983, James et al. 1983), their efficacy for treating individuals with discrete social phobia has not been established. Nevertheless, beta blockers are often prescribed for discrete performance-related social phobias.

Preliminary findings suggest that gabapentin, a medication typically used in the treatment of partial seizures, may be effective in the treatment of social phobia. A placebo-controlled trial found that individuals taking gabapentin had significant reductions in social anxiety compared to the placebo group (Pande et al. 1999). However, more research is needed to confirm this finding.

Psychosocial Treatments

Numerous studies have shown that exposure-based treatments are effective for helping individuals to overcome a variety of specific phobias including fears of blood (Öst et al. 1984, 1991a), injections (Öst 1989), dentists (Jerremalm et al. 1986, Moore and Brødsgaard 1994), spiders (Hellström and Öst 1995, Muris et al. 1998, Öst 1996a, Öst et al. 1991b, 1997b), snakes (Gauthier and Marshall 1977, Hepner and Cauthen 1975), rats (Foa et al.

1977), enclosed places (Craske et al. 1995, Öst et al. 1982), thunder and lightning (Öst 1978), water (Menzies and Clarke 1993a), flying (Beckham et al. 1990, Howard et al. 1983, Öst et al. 1997b), heights (Baker et al. 1973), choking (Greenberg et al. 1988, McNally 1986), and balloons (Houlihan et al. 1993).

Furthermore, the way in which exposure is conducted may make a difference. Exposure-based treatments can vary on a variety of dimensions including the degree of therapist involvement, duration and intensity of exposure, frequency and number of sessions, and the degree to which the feared situation is confronted in imagination versus in real life. In addition, because individuals with certain specific phobias often report a fear of panicking in the feared situation, investigators (Antony and Swinson 2000a) have suggested that adding various panic management strategies (e.g., cognitive restructuring, exposure to feared sensations) may help increase the efficacy of behavioral treatments for specific phobias. It remains to be shown whether the addition of these strategies will improve the efficacy of treatments that include only exposure.

Several reviews have summarized the effects of the above-mentioned variables on exposure-based treatments (Antony and Barlow 1998, 2002, Antony and Swinson 2000a). Although some studies have led to contradictory results, the following generalizations are more or less accepted by the majority of investigators. First, exposure seems to work best when sessions are spaced close together. Second, prolonged exposure seems to be more effective than exposure of shorter duration. Third, during exposure sessions, individuals should be discouraged from engaging in subtle avoidance strategies (e.g., distraction) and overreliance on safety signals (e.g., being accompanied by one's spouse during exposure). Fourth, real-life exposure is more effective than exposure in imagination. Fifth, exposure with some degree of therapist involvement seems to be more effective than exposure that is exclusively conducted without the therapist present (Park et al. 2001). Exposure may be conducted gradually or quickly. Both approaches seem to work equally well, although individuals may be more compliant with a gradual approach. Finally, in the case of blood and injection phobias, the technique called applied muscle tension (Öst and Sterner 1987) should be considered as an alternative or addition to exposure therapy. Applied muscle tension involves having individuals repeatedly tense their muscles, which leads to a temporary increase in blood pressure and prevents fainting upon exposure to blood or medical procedures.

Cognitive strategies have also been used either alone or in conjunction with exposure for treating specific phobias (Craske and Rowe 1997). The evidence suggests that the addition of cognitive strategies to exposure may provide added benefit (Craske et al. 1995) for some individuals. For a detailed guide to integrating cognitive strategies with exposure see Antony and Swinson (2000a).

Specific phobias are among the most treatable of the anxiety disorders. For example, in as little as one session of guided exposure lasting 2 to 3 hours, the majority of individuals with animal or injection phobias are judged much improved or completely recovered (Antony et al. 2001a, Öst 1989, Öst et al. 1997b). A recent study demonstrated that one session of exposure treatment was effective in the treatment of children and adolescents with various specific phobias (Öst et al. 2001). Moreover, exposure conducted with a parent present was equally effective as exposure treatment conducted alone (Öst et al. 2001). However, despite how straightforward the concept of exposure may seem, many subtle clinical issues can lead to problems in implementing exposure-based treatments. For example, although an individual might be compliant with therapist-assisted exposure practices, he or she may refuse to attempt exposure practices alone between sessions. In such cases, involving a spouse or other family member as a coach during practices at home may help. In addition, gradually increasing the distance between therapist and individual during the therapist-assisted exposures will help the individual to feel comfortable when practicing alone.

However, to maintain the individual's trust and to maximize the effectiveness of behavioral interventions, it is important that exposure practices proceed in a predictable way, so that the individual is not surprised by unexpected events. Several self-help books and manuals for treating a range of specific phobias have been published in the past decade. Whereas some of these manuals were developed to be used with the assistance of a therapist (Bourne 1998, Antony et al. 1995, Craske et al. 1997), others were developed for self-administration (Brown 1996).

Recent developments in technology have started to have an impact on the treatment of specific phobias. Videotapes are commonly used to show feared stimuli to individuals during exposure. Computer-administered treatments have also been used (Smith et al. 1997). More recent is the use of virtual reality to expose individuals to simulated situations that are more difficult to replicate *in vivo* such as flying (Kahan et al. 2000) and heights (Rothbaum et al. 1995). Emerging data on the effectiveness of virtual reality is encouraging (Rothbaum et al. 2000). However, other preliminary studies indicate that *in vivo* exposure is still superior (Dewis et al. 2001).

Empirically validated psychosocial interventions for social phobia have primarily come from a cognitive–behavioral perspective and include four main types of treatment: (1) exposure-based strategies, (2) cognitive therapy, (3) social skills training, and (4) applied relaxation (Antony and Swinson 2000a, Turk et al. 1999). Exposure-based treatments involve repeatedly approaching fear-provoking situations until they no longer elicit fear. Through repeated exposure, individuals learn that their fearful predictions do not come true despite their having confronted the situation. Table 32-6 illustrates an example of an exposure hierarchy that might be used to structure an individual's exposure practices. An exposure hierarchy is a list of feared situations that are rank ordered by difficulty and used to guide exposure practices for phobic disorders including social phobia and specific phobia. The individual and the therapist generate a list of situations that the individual finds anxiety-provoking. Items are placed in descending order from most anxiety provoking to least anxiety provoking, and each item is rated with respect to how anxious the individual might be to practice the item. Exposure practices are designed to help the individual become more comfortable engaging in the activities from the hierarchy. Cognitive therapy helps individuals identify and change anxious thoughts (e.g., "Others will think I am stupid if I participate in a conversation at work") by teaching them to consider alternative ways of interpreting situations and to examine the evidence for their anxious beliefs. Social skills training is designed to help individuals become more socially competent when they interact with others. Treatment strategies may include modeling, behavioral rehearsal, corrective feedback, social reinforcement, and homework assignments. Finally, applied relaxation has been studied primarily by Öst and colleagues (1984) and involves learning to relax

Table 32-6	Exposure Hierarchy for Generalized Social Phobia	
Item	**Fear Rating (0–100)**
Have a party and invite everyone from work.	99
Go to work Christmas party for 1 h without drinking	90
Invite Cindy to have dinner and see a movie.	85
Go for a job interview	80
Ask boss for a day off from work	65
Ask questions in a meeting at work	65
Eat lunch with coworkers	60
Talk to a stranger on the bus	50
Talk to cousin on the telephone for 10 min	40
Ask for directions at the gas station.	35

one's muscles during rest, during movement, and eventually in anxiety-provoking social situations.

Although these methods are presented as four distinct treatment approaches, there is often overlap among the various treatments. Social skills training typically requires exposure to the phobic situation so that new skills may be practiced (e.g., behavioral rehearsal). The same may be said of applied relaxation, which includes learning to conduct relaxation exercises in the phobic situation. In fact, most treatments for social phobia involve some type of exposure to anxiety-provoking social interactions and performance-related tasks. Furthermore, many cognitive–behavioral therapists treat individuals using several different strategies delivered in a comprehensive package.

Studies demonstrating the efficacy of CBT for social phobia are too numerous to describe in detail, although several representative studies are reviewed here. In addition, studies that specifically compare cognitive–behavioral and medication treatments are described. For interested readers, more comprehensive reviews on CBT for social phobia have been written by Heimberg (2001) and Fresco and Heimberg (2001). Also, a clinical description of a cognitive–behavioral group treatment (CBGT) for social phobia is provided by Turk and colleagues (2001) and by Heimberg and Becker (2002).

Several studies have compared various cognitive–behavioral strategies and their combinations for treating social phobia. For example, Wlazlo and colleagues (1990) compared social skills training to exposure therapy conducted either individually or in groups. All three treatments led to significant improvements and there were no differences between treatments. However, exposure therapy conducted in groups tended to be more effective for the subset of individuals with social skills deficits, most likely by enabling those individuals with deficits to develop their skills through exposure to social situations and interactions in the group. Mattick and Peters (1988) found that guided exposure was more effective when cognitive therapy was included than when exposure was conducted without cognitive therapy. Scholing and Emmelkamp (1993) failed to replicate this finding and found that treatment was equally effective when exposure was conducted alone, it followed several sessions of cognitive therapy, or was integrated with cognitive therapy from the first session.

According to cognitive models of social phobia, one of the mechanisms by which CBT works is by causing a positive shift in an individual's self-representation (e.g., decreased negative self-focused thoughts and increased task-focused thoughts and positive self-focused thoughts). Indeed, there is evidence that following CBT, individuals report significantly fewer negative self-focused thoughts (Hofmann 2000). Similarly, cognitive biases are reduced following successful pharmacotherapy treatment as well and are related to the degree of symptomatic improvement in both psychological and pharmacological treatments (McManus et al. 2000).

In summary, it seems clear that effective psychosocial treatments and medications for social phobia exist. Although both types of treatments appear to be equally effective, each has advantages and disadvantages. Medication treatments may work more quickly and are less time-consuming for the individual and the therapist. In contrast, improvement after CBT appears to last longer. Owing to medication side effects, CBT may be more appropriate for some individuals. More studies are needed to examine the efficacy of combined medication and psychosocial treatments for social phobia. A meta-analysis of 24 studies examining cognitive–behavioral and medication treatments for social phobia found that both treatments were more effective than control conditions (Gould et al. 1997). In this study, the SSRIs and benzodiazepines tended to have the largest effect sizes among medications and treatments involving exposure either alone or with cognitive therapy had the largest effect sizes among CBT. Another meta-analytic study of 108 psychological and pharmacological treatment-outcome trials found that the pharmacotherapies (SSRIs, benzodiazepines, MAO inhibitors) were the most consistently effective treatments, with both SSRIs and benzodiazepine treatments equally effective and more effective than control groups (Fedoroff and Taylor 2001). Further, maintenance of treatment gains for CBT was moderate and continued during follow-up intervals. In comparison, the extent to which treatment gains for medication treatments are maintained following discontinuation is not known. Recent reviews of the efficacy of pharmacological and cognitive–behavioral treatments suggest that successful treatments may involve medication, CBT, or a combination of both (Scott and Heimberg 2000). The detailed application of cognitive–behavioral therapy to social phobia is now available in self-help format (Antony and Swinson 2000b). Self-help manuals may be used on their own or as a valuable tool in conjunction with therapy.

Treatment Nonresponse

Several variables may lead to an initially poor treatment response. Anticipating potential difficulties will help increase treatment efficacy. Possible reasons for a worse outcome include poor compliance, poor motivation, and poor understanding of the treatment procedures. In addition, interpersonal issues and other possible conflicts may interfere with the successful treatment of specific and social phobias.

Individuals fail to comply with treatment procedures for a variety of reasons. In the case of pharmacological treatments, individuals may avoid taking medications because of side effects, lack of confidence in efficacy, or preference for an alternative type of treatment. If individuals are not compliant with medications, the clinician should attempt to identify the reasons for poor compliance and to suggest methods of increasing compliance or changing to another type of treatment.

In the case of CBT, common reasons for poor compliance are anxiety about conforming to treatment, lack of time, and lack of motivation to conduct the treatment properly. Because CBT requires individuals to confront the situations they fear most, individuals often feel extreme anxiety about participating in the treatment. Individuals should be reassured that their anxiety is normal and that they will never be forced to do anything that they are unwilling to try. Furthermore, the difficulty of exposure tasks should be increased gradually to maximize treatment compliance. If individuals do not have the time or motivation to conduct treatment as suggested, therapists should be willing to find ways to make the treatment more accessible to the individual. For example, involvement of a friend or relative of the individual as a coach may allow the individual to conduct more practices without the therapist's assistance. The therapist could also explore the possibility that the individual consider beginning treatment later, when more time is available.

Poor motivation can lead to poor compliance with the treatment procedures. If an individual's symptoms are not especially severe, the distress and impairment created by the disorder may not be enough to motivate the individual to take medications regularly or to confront the phobic situation in a systematic way. Furthermore, as an individual improves in treatment, she or he may experience a decrease in motivation. Individuals should be encouraged to continue with treatment assignments even after improvement. More complete improvements may protect against a return of symptoms.

Finally, treatment procedures may be complicated for some individuals. This is especially the case for CBT. Individuals may fail to complete homework assignments (e.g., monitoring anxious cognitions) simply because the treatment rationale and the specifics of how to conduct the treatment procedures were not made clear. Therefore, therapists should continually assess the individual's understanding of the treatment procedures.

Comparison of DSM-IV-TR/ICD-10 Diagnostic Criteria

The ICD-10 Diagnostic Criteria for Research for Social Phobia specify that at least two symptoms of anxiety (i.e., from the list of 14 panic symptoms) be present together on at least one occasion along with at least one of the following anxiety symptoms: blushing or shaking, fear of vomiting, and urgency or fear of micturition or defecation. Furthermore, these anxiety symptoms must be "restricted to, or predominated in, the feared situations or contemplation of the feared situations." In contrast, the DSM-IV-TR criteria do not specify any particular types of anxiety symptoms nor is any restriction placed on whether anxiety can occur in situations other than social situations.

For specific phobia, the ICD-10 Diagnostic Criteria for Research also specify that the anxiety symptoms be "restricted to, or predominated in, the feared situations or contemplation of the feared situation." DSM-IV-TR again does not impose any such restriction.

References

Adler PSJ, France C, and Ditto B (1991) Baroreflex sensitivity at rest and during stress in individuals with a history of vasovagal syncope. *J Psychosom Res* **35**, 1–7.

Allgulander C and Nilsson B (2001) A prospective study of 86 new patients with social anxiety disorder. *Acta Psychiatr Scand* **103**, 447–452.

Altamura AC, Piolo R, Vitto M, et al. (1999) Venlafaxine in social phobia: a study in selective serotonin reuptake inhibitor non-responders. *Int Clin Psychopharmacol* **14**, 239–245.

American Psychiatric Association (2000) *Diagnostic and Statistical Manual of Mental Disorders*, 4th ed., Text Rev. APA, Washington, DC.

Anderson JC, Williams S, McGee R, et al. (1987) DSM-III disorders in preadolescent children. *Arch Gen Psychiatry* **44**, 69–76.

Antony MM (1994) *Heterogeneity among Specific Phobia Types Iin DSM-IV*. Unpublished doctoral dissertation. State University of New York, University at Albany, Albany, NY.

Antony MM and Barlow DH (1998) Specific phobia. In *Handbook of Cognitive and Behavioural Treatments for Psychological Disorders*, Caballo VE (ed). Pergamon, Oxford, UK, pp. 1–22.

Antony MM and Barlow DH (2002) Specific phobias. In *Anxiety and its Disorders: The Nature and Treatment of Anxiety and Panic*, 2nd ed., Barlow DH (ed). Guilford Press, New York.

Antony MM and Swinson RP (2000a) *Phobic Disorders and Panic in Adults: A Guide to Assessment and Treatment*. American Psychological Association, Washington, DC.

Antony MM and Swinson RP (2000b) *Shyness and Social Anxiety Workbook: Proven Techniques for Overcoming Fears*. New Harbinger, Oakland, CA.

Antony MM, Brown TA, and Barlow DH (1997a) Response to hyperventilation and 5.5% CO_2 inhalation of subjects with types of specific phobia, panic disorder, or no mental disorder. *Am J Psychiatry* **154**, 1089–1095.

Antony MM, Brown TA, and Barlow DH (1997b) Heterogeneity among specific phobia types in DSM-IV. *Behav Res Ther* **35**, 1089–1100.

Antony MM, Craske MG, and Barlow DH (1995) *Mastery of Your Specific Phobia*. The Psychological Corporation, San Antonio, TX.

Antony MM, McCabe RE, Leeuw I, et al. (2001a) Effect of exposure and coping style on *in vivo* exposure for specific phobia of spiders. *Behav Res Ther* **39**, 1137–1150.

Antony MM, Moras K, Meadows EA, et al. (1994) The diagnostic significance of the functional impairment and subjective distress criterion: an illustration with the DSM-III-R anxiety disorders. *J Psychopathol Behav Assess* **16**, 253–262.

Antony MM, Purdon CL, Huta V, et al. (1998a) Dimensions of perfectionism across the anxiety disorders. *Behav Res Ther* **36**, 1143–1154.

Arntz A, Lavy E, van den Berg G, et al. (1993) Negative beliefs of spider phobics: a psychometric evaluation of the spider phobia beliefs questionnaire. *Adv Behav Res Ther* **15**, 257–277.

Arrindell WA (1980) Dimensional structure and psychopathology correlates of the fear survey schedule (FSS-III) in a phobic population: a factorial definition of agoraphobia. *Behav Res Ther* **18**, 229–242.

Baker BL, Cohen DC, and Saunders JT (1973) Self-directed desensitization for acrophobia. *Behav Res Ther* **11**, 79–89.

Barlow DH (1991) Disorders of emotion. *Psychol Inq* **2**, 58–71.

Barlow DH (2002) *Anxiety and its Disorders: The Nature and Treatment of Anxiety and Panic*, 2nd ed., Guilford Press, New York.

Beckham JC, Vrana SR, May JG, et al. (1990) Emotional processing and fear measurement synchrony as indicators of treatment outcome in fear of flying. *J Behav Ther Exp Psychiatry* **21**, 153–162.

Biederman J, Hirshfeld-Becker DR, Rosenbaum JF, et al. (2001) Further evidence of association between behavioral inhibition and social anxiety in children. *Am J Psychiatry* **158**, 1673–1679.

Blomhoff S, Haug TT, Hellström K, et al. (2001) Randomised controlled general practice trial of sertraline, exposure therapy and combined treatment in generalised social phobia. *Br J Psychiatry* **179**, 23–30.

Bourne EJ (1998) *Overcoming Specific Phobia: A Hierarchy and Exposure-Based Protocol for the Treatment of all Specific Phobias (Therapist Protocol)*. New Harbinger, Oakland, CA.

Bouton ME, Mineka S, and Barlow DH (2001) A modern learning-theory perspective on the etiology of panic disorder. *Psychol Rev* **108**, 4–32.

Bouwer C and Stein DJ (1998) Use of the selective serotonin reuptake inhibitor citalopram in the treatment of generalized social phobia. *J Affect Disord* **49**, 79–82.

Brown D (1996) *Flying without Fear*. New Harbinger, Oakland, CA.

Brown TA, Campbell LA, Lehman CL, et al. (2001a) Current and lifetime comorbidity of the DSM-IV anxiety and mood disorders in a large clinical sample. *J Abnorm Psychol* **110**, 585–599.

Bruch MA (1989) Familial and developmental antecedents of social phobia: issues and findings. *Clin Psychol Rev* **9**, 37–47.

Bruch MA and Heimberg RG (1994) Differences in perceptions of parental and personal characteristics between generalized and nongeneralized social phobics. *J Anx Disord* **8**, 155–168.

Buigues J and Vallejo J (1987) Therapeutic response to phenelzine in patients with panic disorder and agoraphobia with panic attacks. *J Clin Psychiatry* **48**, 55–59.

Cannon WB (1929) Bodily changes in pain, hunger. In *Fear, and Rage*, 2nd ed., Appleton-Century-Crofts, New York.

Chaleby K (1987) Social phobias in Saudis. *Soc Psychiatry* **22**, 167–170.

Chang SC (1997) Social anxiety (phobia) and east Asian culture. *Depress Anx* **5**, 115–120.

Clark DB and Agras WS (1991) The assessment and treatment of performance anxiety in musicians. *Am J Psychiatry* **148**, 605–698.

Cooper JR, Bloom FE, and Roth RH (1983) *The Biochemical Basis of Neuropharmacology*. Oxford University Press, New York.

Craske MG (1989) The boundary between simple phobia and specific phobia. Report to the DSM-IV Anxiety Disorders Work Group. Phobia and Anxiety Disorders Clinic, Albany, New York.

Craske MG and Rowe MK (1997) A comparison of behavioral and cognitive treatments for phobias. In *Phobias: A Handbook of Theory, Research, and Treatment*, Davey GCL (ed). John Wiley, New York.

Craske MG, Antony MM, and Barlow DH (1997) *Mastery of your Specific Phobia: Therapist Guide*. Psychological Corporation/Graywind Publications, San Antonio, TX.

Craske MG, Mohlman J, Yi J, et al. (1995) Treatment of claustrophobia and snake/spider phobias: fear of arousal and fear of context. *Behav Res Ther* **33**, 197–203.

Craske MG, Zarate R, Burton T, et al. (1993) Specific fears and panic attacks: a survey of clinical and nonclinical samples. *J Anx Disord* **7**, 1–19.

Curtis GC, Hill EM, and Lewis JA Anxiety Disorders Work Group. (1990) *Heterogeneity of DSM-III-R Simple Phobia and the Simple Phobia/Agoraphobia Boundary: Evidence from the ECA Study*, Report to the DSM-IV. University of Michigan, Ann Arbor, MI.

Curtis GC, Magee WJ, Eaton WW, et al. (1998) Specific fears and phobias: epidemiology and classification. *Br J Psychiatry* **173**, 212–217.

Davey CL, Forster L, and Mayhew G (1993) Familial resemblances in disgust sensitivity and animal phobias. *Behav Res Ther* **31**, 41–50.

Davidson JRT, Ford SM, Smith RD, et al. (1991a) Long-term treatment of social phobia with clonazepam. *J Clin Psychiatry* **52**, 16–20.

Davidson JRT, Potts N, Richichi E, et al. (1993) Treatment of social phobia with clonazepam and placebo. *J Clin Psychopharmacol* **13**, 423–428.

de Jong PJ, Andrea H, and Muris P (1997) Spider phobia in children: disgust and fear before and after treatment. *Behav Res Ther* **35**, 559–562.

Dewis LM, Kirkby KC, Martin F, et al. (2001) Computer-aided vicarious exposure versus live graded exposure for spider phobia in children. *J Behav Ther Exp Psychiatry* **32**, 17–27.

Di Nardo PA, Guzy LT, Jenkins JA, et al. (1988) Etiology and maintenance of dog fears. *Behav Res Ther* **26**, 241–244.

Eaton WW, Dryman A, and Weissman MM (1991) Panic and phobia. In *Psychiatric Disorders in America: The Epidemiologic Catchment Area Study*, Robins LN and Regier DA (eds). Free Press, New York, pp. 155–179.

Ehlers A, Hofmann SG, Herda CA, et al. (1994) Clinical characteristics of driving phobia. *J Anx Disord* **8**, 323–337.

Fedoroff IC and Taylor S (2001) Psychological and pharmacological treatments for social phobia: a meta-analysis. *J Clin Psychopharmacol* **21**, 311–324.

Fehm L and Margraf J (2002) Thought suppression: specificity in agoraphobia versus broad impairment in social phobia? *Behav Res Ther* **40**, 57–66.

Foa EB, Blau JS, Prout M, et al. (1977) Is horror a necessary component of flooding (implosion)? *Behav Res Ther* **15**, 397–402.

Francis G (1990) Social phobia in childhood. In *Handbook of Child and Adult Psychopathology: A Longitudinal Perspective*, Hersen M and Last CG (eds). Pergamon Press, New York, pp. 163–168.

Fredrikson M, Annas P, Fischer H, et al. (1996) Gender and age differences in the prevalence of specific fears and phobias. *Behav Res Ther* **26**, 241–244.

Fresco DM and Heimberg RG (2001) Empirically supported psychological treatments for social phobia. *Psychiatr Ann* **31**, 489–496.

Furlan PM, DeMartinis N, Schweizer E, et al. (2001) Abnormal salivary cortisol levels in social phobic patients in response to acute psychological but not physical stress. *Biol Psychiatry* **50**, 254–259.

Fyer AJ, Mannuzza S, Chapman TF, et al. (1993) A direct interview family study of social phobia. *Arch Gen Psychiatry* **50**, 286–293.

Fyer AJ, Mannuzza S, Gallops MS, et al. (1990) Familial transmission of simple phobias and fears. *Arch Gen Psychiatry* **47**, 252–256.

Gauthier J and Marshall WL (1977) The determination of optimal exposure to phobic stimuli in flooding therapy. *Behav Res Ther* **15**, 403–410.

Gorman JM and Gorman LK (1987) Drug treatment of social phobia. *J Affect Disord* **13**, 183–192.

Gould RA, Buckminster S, Pollack MH, et al. (1997) Cognitive–behavioral and pharmacological treatment for social phobia: a meta-analysis. *Clin Psychol Sci Pract* **4**, 291–306.

Greenberg DB, Stern TA, and Weilburg JB (1988) The fear of choking: three successfully treated cases. *Psychosomatics* **29**, 126–129.

Hackmann A, Surawy C, and Clark DM, Hackmann A, Surawy C, and Clark DM (1998) Seeing yourself through others' eyes: Aa study of spontaneously occurring images in social phobia. *Behav Cogn Psychother* **26**, 3–12. Seeing yourself through others' eyes: A study of spontaneously occurring images in social phobia. *Behav Cogn Psychother* **26**, 3–12.

Hartley LR, Ungapen S, Dovie I, et al. (1983) The effect of beta-adrenergic blocking drugs on speakers' performance and memory. *Br J Psychiatry* **142**, 512–517.

Heimberg RG (2001) Current status of psychotherapeutic interventions for social phobia. *J Clin Psychiatry* **62**, 36–42.

Heimberg RG and Becker RE (2002) *Cognitive–Behavioral Group Treatment for Social Phobia*. Guilford Press, New York.

Heimberg RG, Dodge CS, Hope DA, et al. (1990) Cognitive–behavioral group treatment for social phobia: comparison with a credible placebo control. *Cog Ther Res* **14**, 1–23.

Heimberg RG, Liebowitz MR, Hope DA, et al. (1998) Cognitive–behavioral group therapy vs. phenelzine therapy for social phobia: 12-week outcome. *Arch Gen Psychiatry* **55**, 1133–1141.

Hellström K and Öst L-G (1995) One-session therapist directed exposure vs. two forms of manual directed self-exposure in the treatment of spider phobia. *Behav Res Ther* **33**, 959–965.

Hepner A and Cauthen NR (1975) Effect of subject control and graduated exposure on snake phobias. *J Consult Clin Psychol* **43**, 297–304.

Hofmann SG (2000) Self-focused attention before and after treatment of social phobia. *Behav Res Ther* **37**, 717–725.

Hofmann SG, Ehlers A, and Roth WT (1995) Conditioning theory: a model for the etiology of public speaking anxiety? *Behav Res Ther* **35**, 567–571.

Hofmann SG, Lehman CL, and Barlow DH (1997) How specific are specific phobias? *J Behav Ther Exp Psychiatry* **28**, 233–240.

Houlihan D, Schwartz C, Miltenberger R, et al. (1993) The rapid treatment of a young man's balloon (noise) phobia using in vivo flooding. *J Behav Ther Exp Psychiatry* **24**, 233–240.

Howard WA, Murphy SM, and Clarke JC (1983) The nature and treatment of fear of flying: a controlled investigation. *Behav Ther* **14**, 557–567.

Hugdahl K and Öst L-G (1985) Subjectively rated physiological and cognitive symptoms in six different clinical phobias. *Pers Individ Diff* **6**, 175–188.

James IM, Burgoyne W, and Savage IT (1983) Effect of pindolol on stress-related disturbances of musical performance: preliminary communication. *J Roy Soc Med* **76**, 194–196.

Jerremalm A, Jansson L, and Öst L-G (1986) Individual response patterns and the effects of different behavioral methods in the treatment of dental phobia. *Behav Res Ther* **24**, 587–596.

Jones MK and Menzies RG (2000) Danger expectancies, self-efficacy and insight in spider phobia. *Behav Res Ther* **38**, 585–600.

Kagan J, Reznick JS, Clarke C, et al. (1984) Behavioral inhibition to the unfamiliar. *Child Dev* **55**, 2212–2225.

Kahan M, Tanzer J, Darvin D, et al. (2000) Virtual reality-assisted cognitive-behavioral treatment for fear of flying: acute treatment and follow-up. *Cyber Psychol Behav* **3**, 387–392.

Kelsey JE (1995) Venlafaxine in social phobia. *Psychopharmacol Bull* **31**, 767–771.

Kessler RC, McGonagle KA, Zhao S, et al. (1994) Lifetime and 12-month prevalence of DSM-III-R psychiatric disorders in the United States: results from the national comorbidity survey. *Arch Gen Psychiatry* **51**, 8–19.

Kindt M and Brosschot JF (1999) Cognitive bias in spider-phobic children: comparison of a pictorial and a linguistic spider Stroop. *J Psychopathol Behav Assess* **21**, 207–220.

King RJ, Mefford IN, and Wang C (1986) CSF dopamine levels correlate with extraversion in depressed patients. *Psychiatr Res* **19**, 305–310.

Kleinknecht RA (1994) Acquisition of blood, injury, and needle fears and phobias. *Behav Res Ther* **32**, 817–823.

Kleinknecht RA, Dinnel DL, Kleinknecht EE, et al. (1997) Cultural factors in social anxiety: a comparison of social phobia symptoms and Taijin Kyofusho. *J Anx Disord* **11**, 157–177.

Landy FJ and Gaupp LA (1971) A factor analysis of the FSS-III. *Behav Res Ther* **9**, 89–93.

Last CG, Perrin S, Hersen M, et al. (1996) A prospective study of childhood anxiety disorders. *J Am Acad Child Adolesc Psychiatry* **35**, 1502–1510.

Lee SH and Oh KS (1999) Offensive type of social phobia: cross-cultural perspectives. *Int Med J* **6**, 271–279.

Levin AP, Saoud JB, Strauman T, et al. (1993) Responses of "generalized" and "discrete" social phobics during public speaking. *J Anx Disord* **7**, 207–221.

Levin AP, Schneier FR, and Liebowitz MR (1989) Social phobia: biology and pharmacology. *Clin Psychol Rev* **9**, 129–140.

Lewis MH, Gariepy J, and Devaud LL (1989) Dopamine and social behavior: a mouse model of 'timidity'. *Presented at the Meeting of the American College of Neuropsychopharmacology* (Dec), Maui, HI.

Liddell A, Locker D, and Burman D (1991) Self-reported fears (FSS-II) of subjects aged 50 years and over. *Behav Res Ther* **29**, 105–112.

Liebowitz MR, Schneier F, Campeas R, et al. (1992) Phenelzine vs. atenolol in social phobia: a placebo-controlled comparison. *Arch Gen Psychiatry* **49**, 290–300.

Liebowitz MR, Stein MB, Tancer M, et al. (2002) A randomized, double-blind, fixed-dose comparison of paroxetine and placebo in the treatment of generalized social anxiety disorder. *J Clin Psychiatry* **63**, 66–74.

Lott M, Greist JH, Jefferson JW, et al. (1997) Brofaromine for social phobia: a multicenter, placebo-controlled, double-blind study. *J Clin Psychopharmacol* **17**, 255–260.

Lydiard RB, Laraia MT, Howell EF, et al. (1988) Alprazolam in the treatment of social phobia. *J Clin Psychiatry* **49**, 17–19.

Mathew SJ, Coplan JD, and Gorman JM (2001) Neurobiological mechanisms of social anxiety disorder. *Am J Psychiatry* **158**, 1558–1567.

Mattia JI, Heimberg RG, and Hope DA (1993) The revised Stroop color-naming task in social phobics. *Behav Res Ther* **31**, 305–313.

Mattick RP and Peters L (1988) Treatment of severe social phobia: effects of guided exposure with and without cognitive restructuring. *J Consult Clin Psychol* **56**, 251–260.

McManus F, Clark DM, and Hackmann A (2000) Specificity of cognitive biases in social phobia and their role in recovery. *Behav Cogn Psychother* **28**, 201–209.

McNally RJ (1986) Behavioral treatment of choking phobia. *J Behav Ther Exp Psychiatry* **17**, 185–188.

McNally RJ (1987) Preparedness and phobias: a review. *Psychol Bull* **101**, 283–303.

McNally RJ and Steketee GS (1985) The etiology and maintenance of severe animal phobias. *Behav Res Ther* **23**, 431–435.

Menzies RG and Clarke JC (1993a) A comparison of *in vivo* and vicarious exposure in the treatment of childhood water phobia. *Behav Res Ther* **31**, 9–15.

Menzies RG and Clarke JC (1993b) The etiology of fear of heights and its relationship to severity and individual response patterns. *Behav Res Ther* **31**, 355–365.

Menzies RG and Clarke JC (1995) The etiology of phobias: a non-associative account. *Clin Psychol Rev* **15**, 23–48.

Menzies RG and Parker L (2001) The origins of height fear: an evaluation of neoconditioning explanations. *Behav Res Ther* **39**, 185–199.

Merckelbach H and Muris P (1997) The etiology of childhood spider phobia. *Behav Res Ther* **35**, 1031–1034.

Merckelbach H, Arntz A, Arrindell WA, et al. (1992) Pathways to spider phobia. *Behav Res Ther* **30**, 543–546.

Merckelbach H, de Jong PJ, Arntz A, et al. (1993) The role of evaluative learning and disgust sensitivity in the etiology and treatment of spider phobia. *Adv Behav Res Ther* **15**, 243–255.

Merckelbach H, Muris P, and Schouten E (1996) Pathways to fear in spider phobic children. *Behav Res Ther* **34**, 935–938.

Moore R and Brødsgaard I (1994) Group therapy compared with individual desensitization for dental anxiety. *Comm Dent Oral Epidemiol* **22**, 258–262.

Mowrer OH (1939) Stimulus response theory of anxiety. *Psychol Rev* **46**, 553–565.

Munjack DJ, Baltazar PL, Bohn PB, et al. (1990) Clonazepam in the treatment of social phobia: a pilot study. *J Clin Psychiatry* **51**, 35–40.

Munjack DJ, Bruns J, Baltazar PL, et al. (1991) A pilot study of buspirone in the treatment of social phobia. *J Anx Disord* **5**, 87–98.

Muris P, Mayer B, and Merckelbach H (1998) Trait anxiety as a predictor of behaviour therapy outcome in spider phobia. *Behav Cogn Psychother* **26**, 87–91.

Muris P, Merckelbach H, and Collaris R (1997) Common childhood fears and their origins. *Behav Res Ther* **35**, 929–937.

Muris P, Schmidt H, and Merckelbach H (1999) The structure of specific phobia symptoms among children and adolescents. *Behav Res Ther* **37**, 863–868.

Norton PJ and Hope DA (2001) Kernels of truth or distorted perceptions: self and observer ratings of social anxiety and performance. *Behav Ther* **32**, 765–786.

Noyes R, Moroz G, Davidson JRT, et al. (1997) Moclobemide in social phobia: a controlled dose-response trial. *J Clin Psychopharmacol* **17**, 247–254.

Oosterbaan DB, van Balkom AJLM, Spinoven P, et al. (2001) Cognitive therapy versus moclobemide in social phobia: a controlled study. *Clin Psychol Psychother* **8**, 263–273.

Öst L-G (1978) Behavioral treatment of thunder and lightning phobias. *Behav Res Ther* **16**, 197–207.

Öst L-G (1985) Ways of acquiring phobias and outcome of behavioral treatment. *Behav Res Ther* **23**, 683–689.

Öst L-G (1989) One-session treatment for specific phobias. *Behav Res Ther* **27**, 1–7.

Öst L-G (1991) Acquisition of blood and injection phobia and anxiety response patterns in clinical patients. *Behav Res Ther* **29**, 323–332.

Öst L-G (1992) Blood and injection phobia: background and cognitive, physiological, and behavioral variables. *J Abnorm Psychol* **101**, 68–74.

Öst L-G (1996a) One-session group treatment for spider phobia. *Behav Res Ther* **34**, 707–715.

Öst L-G and Hugdahl K (1985) Acquisition of blood and dental phobia and anxiety response patterns in clinical patients. *Behav Res Ther* **23**, 27–34.

Öst L-G and Sterner U (1987) Applied tension: a specific behavioral method for treatment of blood phobia. *Behav Res Ther* **25**, 25–29.

Öst L-G, Brandberg M, and Alm T (1997a) One versus five sessions of exposure in the treatment of flying phobia. *Behav Res Ther* **35**, 987–996.

Öst L-G, Fellenius J, and Sterner U (1991a) Applied tension, exposure in vivo, and tension-only in the treatment of blood phobia. *Behav Res Ther* **29**, 561–574.

Öst L-G, Ferebee I, and Furmark T (1997b) One-session group therapy of spider phobia: direct versus indirect treatments. *Behav Res Ther* **35**, 721–732.

Öst L-G, Johansson J, and Jerremalm A (1982) Individual response patterns and the effects of different behavioral methods in the treatment of claustrophobia. *Behav Res Ther* **20**, 445–460.

Öst L-G, Lindahl I-L, Sterner U, et al. (1984) Exposure in vivo vs. applied relaxation in the treatment of blood phobia. *Behav Res Ther* **22**, 205–216.

Öst L-G, Salkovskis PM, and Hellström K (1991b) One-session therapist directed exposure vs. self-exposure in the treatment of spider phobia. *Behav Ther* **22**, 407–422.

Öst L-G, Svensson L, Hellström K, et al. (2001) One-session treatment of specific phobias in youths: a randomized clinical trial. *J Consult Clin Psychol* **69**, 814–824.

Otto MW, Pollack MH, Gould RA, et al. (2000) A comparison of the efficacy of clonazepam and cognitive–behavioral group therapy for the treatment of social phobia. *J Anx Disord* **14**, 345–358.

Page AC (1994) Blood-injury phobia. *Clin Psychol Rev* **14**, 443–461.

Page AC (2003) The role of disgust in faintness elicited by blood and injection stimuli. *J Anx Disord.* **17**, 45–58.

Pande AC, Davidson JR, Jefferson JW, et al. (1999) Treatment of social phobia with gabapentin: a placebo-controlled study. *J Clin Psychopharmacol* **19**, 341–348.

Park J-M, Mataix-Cols D, Marks IM, et al. (2001) Two-year follow-up after a randomised controlled trial of self- and clinician-accompanied exposure for phobia/panic disorders. *Br J Psychiatry* **178**, 543–548.

Pauli P, Wiedemann G, and Montoya P (1998) Covariation bias in flight phobics. *J Anx Disord* **12**, 555–565.

Plomin R (1989) Environment and genes: determinants of behavior. *Am Psychol* **44**, 105–111.

Potts NLS, Davidson JRT, Krishnan KRR, et al. (1991) Levels of urinary free cortisol in social phobia. *J Clin Psychiatry* **52**, 41–42.

Poulton R and Menzies RG (2002) Non-associative fear acquisition: a review of the evidence from retrospective and longitudinal research. *Behav Res Ther* **40**, 127–149.

Poulton R, Menzies RG, Craske MG, et al. (1999) Water trauma and swimming experiences up to age 9 and fear of water at age 18: a longitudinal study. *Behav Res Ther* **37**, 39–48.

Purdon C, Antony MM, Monteiro S, et al. (2001) Social anxiety in college students. *J Anx Disord* **15**, 203–215.

Rachman S (1977) The conditioning theory of fear-acquisition: a critical examination. *Behav Res Ther* **15**, 375–387.

Rachman S and Cuk M (1992) Fearful distortions. *Behav Res Ther* **30**, 583–589.

Raguram R and Bhide AV (1985) Patterns of phobic neurosis: a retrospective study. *Br J Psychiatry* **147**, 557–560.

Randall CL, Johnson MR, Thevos AK, et al. (2001) Paroxetine for social anxiety disorder and alcohol use in dual-diagnosed patients. *Depress Anx* **14**, 255–262.

Rapee RM (1997) Perceived threat and perceived control as predictors of the degree of fear in physical and social situations. *J Anx Disord* **11**, 455–461.

Rapee RM and Lim L (1992) Discrepancy between self- and observer ratings of performance in social phobics. *J Abnorm Psychol* **101**, 728–731.

Rapee RM, Brown TA, Antony MM, et al. (1992) Response to hyperventilation and inhalation of 5.5% carbon dioxide-enriched air across the DSM-III-R anxiety disorders. *J Abnorm Psychol* **101**, 538–552.

Rauch SL, Savage CR, Alpert NM, et al. (1995) A positron emission tomographic study of simple phobic symptom provocation. *Arch Gen Psychiatry* **52**, 20–28.

Reich J and Yates W (1988) A pilot study of treatment of social phobia with alprazolam. *Am J Psychiatry* **145**, 590–594.

Reiss S, Peterson RA, Gursky DM, et al. (1986) Anxiety sensitivity, anxiety frequency, and the prediction of fearfulness. *Behav Res Ther* **24**, 1–8.

Rimm DC, Janda LH, Lancaster DW, et al. (1977) An exploratory investigation of the origin and maintenance of phobias. *Behav Res Ther* **15**, 231–238.

Rosenbaum JF, Biederman J, Hirshfeld DR, et al. (1991) Behavioral inhibition in children: A possible precursor to panic disorder or social phobia. *J Clin Psychiatry* **52**, 5–9.

Roth D, Antony MM, and Swinson RP (2001) Interpretations for anxiety symptoms in social phobia. *Behav Res Ther* **39**, 129–138.

Rothbaum BO, Hodges LF, Kooper R, et al. (1995) Effectiveness of computer-generated (virtual reality) graded exposure in the treatment of acrophobia. *Am J Psychiatry* **152**, 626–628.

Rothbaum BO, Hodges LF, Smith S, et al. (2000) A controlled study of virtual reality exposure therapy for the fear of flying. *J Consult Clin Psychol* **68**, 1020–1026.

Rowa K, Antony MM, Brar S, et al. (2000) Treatment histories of patients with three anxiety disorders. *Depress Anx* **12**, 92–98.

Sawchuk CN, Lohr JM, Tolin DF, et al. (2000) Disgust Sensitivity and contamination fears in spider and blood-injection-injury phobias. *Behav Res Ther* **38**, 753–762.

Schmidt LA, Fox NA, Rubin KH, et al. (1997) Behavioral and neuroendocrine responses in shy children. *Dev Psychobiol* **30**, 127–140.

Schneider F, Weiss U, Kessler C, et al. (1999) Subcortical correlates of differential classical conditioning of aversive emotional reactions in social phobia. *Biol Psychiatry* **45**, 863–871.

Schneier FR, Goetz D, Campeas R, et al. (1998) Placebo-controlled trial of moclobemide in social phobia. *Br J Psychiatry* **172**, 70–77.

Schneier FR, Saoud JB, Campeas R, et al. (1993) Buspirone in social phobia. *J Clin Psychopharmacol* **13**, 251–256.

Scholing A and Emmelkamp PMG (1993) Exposure with and without cognitive therapy for generalized social phobia: effects of individual and group treatment. *Behav Res Ther* **31**, 667–681.

Schweizer E, Rickels K, Weiss S, et al. (1993) Maintenance drug treatment of panic disorder: I. Results of a prospective, placebo-controlled comparison of alprazolam and imipramine. *Arch Gen Psychiatry* **50**, 51–60.

Scott EL and Heimberg RG (2000) Social phobia: an update on treatment. *Psychiatr Ann* **30**, 678–686.

Seligman MEP (1971) Phobias and preparedness. *Behav Ther* **2**, 307–320.

Simon NM, Sharma SG, Worthington JJ, et al. (2001) Citalopram for social phobia: a clinical case series. *Prog Neuro-Psychopharmacol Biol Psychiatry* **25**, 1469–1474.

Simpson HB, Schneier FR, Campeas RB, et al. (1998) Imipramine in the treatment of social phobia. *J Clin Psychopharmacol* **18**, 132–135.

Smith KL, Kirkby KC, Montgomery IM, et al. (1997) Computer-delivered modeling of exposure for spider phobia: relevant versus irrelevant exposure. *J Anx Disord* **11**, 489–497.

Stein MB, Chartier MJ, Hazen AL, et al. (1998) A direct-interview family study of generalized social phobia. *Am J Psychiatry* **155**, 90–97.

Stein MB, Delaney SM, Chartier MJ, et al. (1995) [^{3}H] paroxetine binding to platelets of patients with social phobia: comparison to patients with panic disorder and healthy volunteers. *Biol Psychiatry* **37**, 224–228.

Stein MB, Fyer AJ, Davidson JRT, et al. (1999) Fluvoxamine treatment of social phobia (social anxiety disorder): a double-blind, placebo-controlled study. *Am J Psychiatry* **156**, 756–760.

Stein MB, Liebowitz MR, Lydiard RB, et al. (1998) Paroxetine treatment of generalized social phobia (social anxiety disorder): a randomized controlled trial. *J Am Med Assoc* **380**, 708–713.

Stopa L and Clark DM (1993) Cognitive processes in social phobia. *Behav Res Ther* **31**, 255–267.

Straus CC and Last CG (1993) Social and simple phobias in children. *J Anx Disord* **7**, 141–152.

Sue DW (1990) Culture-specific strategies in counseling: a conceptual framework. *Prof Psychol Res Pract* **21**, 424–433.

Takahashi T (1989) Social phobia syndrome in Japan. *Compr Psychiatry* **30**, 45–52.

Tancer ME, Stein MB, Gelernter CS, et al. (1990) The hypothalamic-pituitary-thyroid axis in social phobia. *Am J Psychiatry* **147**, 929–933.

Tancer ME, Mailman RB, Stein MB, Tancer ME, Mailman RB, Stein MB, et al. (1994/1995) Neuroendocrine responsivity to monoaminergic system probes in generalized social phobia. *Anxiety* **1**, 216–223; Tancer ME, Stein MB, Gelernter CS, et al. (1990) The hypothalamic-pituitary-thyroid axis in social phobia. *Am J Psychiatry* **147**, 929–933.

Thom A, Sartory G, and Jöhren P (2000) Comparison between one-session psychological treatment and benzodiazepine in dental phobia. *J Consult Clin Psychol* **68**, 378–387.

Tiihonen J, Kuikka J, Bergstrom K, et al. (1997) Dopamine reuptake site densities in patients with social phobia. *Am J Psychiatry* **154**, 239–242.

Townend E, Dimigen G, and Fung D (2000) A clinical study of child dental anxiety. *Behav Res Ther* **38**, 31–46.

Tupler LA, Davidson JRT, Smith RD, et al. (1997) A repeat proton magnetic resonance spectroscopy study in social phobia. *Biol Psychiatry* **42**, 419–424.

Turk CL, Fresco DM, and Heimberg RG (1999) Social phobia: cognitive behavior therapy. In *Handbook of Comparative Treatments of Adult Disorders*, 2nd ed., Hersen M and Bellack AS (eds). John Wiley, New York.

Turk CL, Heimberg RG, and Hope DA (2001) Social anxiety disorder. In *Clinical Handbook of Psychological Disorders: A Step-by-Step Treatment Manual*, 3rd ed., Barlow DH (ed). Guilford Press, New York.

Turk CL, Heimberg RG, Orsillo SM, et al. (1998) An investigation of gender differences in social phobia. *J Anx Disord* **12**, 209–223.

Turner SM, Beidel DC, Dancu CV, et al. (1986) Psychopathology of social phobia and comparison with avoidant personality disorder. *J Abnorm Psychol* **95**, 389–394.

Turner SM, Beidel DC, and Townsley RM (1992) Social phobia: a comparison of specific and generalized subtype and avoidant personality disorder. *J Abnorm Psychol* **101**, 326–331.

Turner SM, Beidel DC, and Wolff PL (1996) Is behavioral inhibition related to the anxiety disorders? *Clin Psychol Rev* **16**, 157–172.

Van Ameringen M, Lane RG, Walker JR, et al. (2001) Sertraline treatment of generalized social phobia: a 20-week, double-blind, placebo-controlled study. *Am J Psychiatry* **158**, 275–281.

Van Ameringen M, Mancini C, and Oakman JM (1999a) Nefazodone in social phobia. *J Clin Psychiatry* **60**, 96–100.

Van Ameringen M, Mancini C, Oakman JM, et al. (1999b) Selective serotonin reuptake inhibitors in the treatment of social phobia: the emerging gold standard. *CNS Drugs* **11**, 307–315.

Van Ameringen M, Mancini C, Oakman JM, et al. (2000) Selective serotonin reuptake inhibitors in the treatment of social phobia: first line treatment at the turn of the century. In *Pharmacotherapy of Anxiety Disorders*, Palmer KJ (ed). Adis International Publications, Hong Kong, pp. 17–30.

Van der Linden GHH, Stein DJ, and van Balkom AJLM (2000b) The efficacy of the selective serotonin reuptake inhibitors for social anxiety disorder (social phobia): a meta-analysis of randomized controlled trials. *Int Clin Psychopharmacol* **15**(Suppl. 2), S15–S23.

van Vliet IM, den Boer JA, and Westenberg HGM (1994) Psychopharmacological treatment of social phobia: a double-blind placebo-controlled study with fluvoxamine. *Psychopharmacology* **115**, 128–134.

van Vliet IM, den Boer JA, Westenberg HGM, et al. (1997) Clinical effects of buspirone in social phobia: a double-blind placebo-controlled study. *J Clin Psychiatry* **58**, 164–168.

Versiani M, Nardi AE, Mundim FD, et al. (1992) Pharmacotherapy of social phobia: a controlled study with moclobemide and phenelzine. *Br J Psychiatry* **161**, 353–360.

Versiani M, Nardi AE, Mundim FD, et al. (1996) The long-term treatment of social phobia with moclobemide. *Int Clin Psychopharmacol* **11**(Suppl. 3), 83–88.

Wells A and Papageorgiou C (1999) The observer perspective: biased imagery in social phobia, agoraphobia, and blood/injury phobia. *Behav Res Ther* **37**, 653–658.

Widiger TA (1992) Generalized social phobia versus avoidant personality disorder: a commentary on three studies. *J Abnorm Psychol* **101**, 340–343.

Wik G, Fredrikson M, and Fischer H (1997) Evidence of altered cerebral blood-flow relationships in acute phobia. *Int J Neurosci* **91**, 253–263.

Wilhelm FH and Roth WT (1996) Acute and delayed effects of alprazolam on flight phobics during exposure. *Paper presented at the meeting of the Association for Advancement of Behavior Therapy* (Nov), New York.

Wilson GD and Priest HF (1968) The principal components of phobic stimuli. *J Clin Psychol* **24**, 191.

Wlazlo Z, Schroeder-Hartwig K, Hand I, et al. (1990) Exposure in vivo vs. social skills training for social phobia: long-term outcome and differential effects. *Behav Res Ther* **28**, 181–193.

Woody SR and Teachman BA (2000) Intersection of disgust and fear: normative and pathological views. *Clin Psychol Sci Pract* **7**, 291–311.

Anxiety Disorders: Obsessive-Compulsive Disorder

OBSESSIVE–COMPULSIVE DISORDER

Diagnosis

Obsessive–compulsive disorder (OCD) is an intriguing and often debilitating syndrome characterized by the presence of two distinct phenomena: obsessions and compulsions. Obsessions are intrusive, recurrent, unwanted ideas, thoughts, or impulses that are difficult to dismiss, despite their disturbing nature. Compulsions are repetitive behaviors, either observable or mental, that are intended to reduce the anxiety engendered by obsessions. Both obsessions and compulsions have been described in a wide variety of mental and neurological disorders (Jenike 1990). However, obsessions and compulsions that clearly interfere with the functioning and/or cause significant distress are the hallmark of OCD (see DSM-IV-TR diagnostic criteria below).

DSM-IV-TR Diagnostic Criteria

300.3 Obsessive–Compulsive Disorder

A. Either obsessions or compulsions:
   Obsessions as defined by (1), (2), (3), and (4):

   (1) recurrent and persistent thoughts, impulses, or images that are experienced, at some time during the disturbance, as intrusive and inappropriate and that cause marked anxiety or distress

---

(2) the thoughts, impulses, or images are not simply excessive worries about real-life problems

(3) the person attempts to ignore or suppress such thoughts, impulses, or images, or to neutralize them with some other thought or action

(4) the person recognizes that the obsessional thoughts, impulses, or images are a product of his or her own mind (not imposed from without as in thought insertion)

Compulsions as defined by (1) and (2):

(1) repetitive behaviors (e.g., hand washing, ordering, checking) or mental acts (e.g., praying, counting, repeating words silently) that the person feels driven to perform in response to an obsession, or according to rules that must be applied rigidly

(2) the behaviors or mental acts are aimed at preventing or reducing distress or preventing some dreaded event or situation; however, these behaviors or mental acts either are not connected in a realistic way with what they are designed to neutralize or prevent or are clearly excessive

B. At some point during the course of the disorder, the person has recognized that the obsessions or compulsions are excessive or unreasonable. Note: This does not apply to children.

C. The obsessions or compulsions cause marked distress, are time consuming (take more than 1 hour a day), or significantly interfere with the person's normal routine, occupational (or academic) functioning, or usual social activities or relationships.

D. If another Axis I disorder is present, the content of the obsessions or compulsions is not restricted to it (e.g., preoccupation with food in the presence of an eating disorder; hair pulling in the presence of trichotillomania; concern with appearance in the presence of body dysmorphic disorder (BDD); preoccupation with drugs in the presence of a substance use disorder; preoccupation with having a serious illness in the presence of hypochondriasis; preoccupation with sexual urges or fantasies in the presence of a paraphilia; or guilty ruminations in the presence of major depressive disorder).

E. The disturbance is not due to the direct physiological effects of a substance (e.g., a drug of abuse, a medication) or a general medical condition.

Specify if:

With poor insight: if, for most of the time during the current episode, the person does not recognize that the obsessions and compulsions are excessive or unreasonable

OCD's clinical presentation is characterized by phenomenological subtypes based on the content of the obsessions and corresponding compulsions. The list of subtypes in the Yale-Brown Obsessive–Compulsive Scale (Y-BOCS) (Table 33-1) was generated on the basis of clinical interviews with OCD patients in the 1980s (Goodman et al. 1989a). The basic types of obsessions and compulsions seem to be consistent across cultures (Rasmussen and Eisen 1992). The most common obsession is the fear of contamination, followed by pathological doubt, a need for symmetry, and aggressive obsessions. The most common compulsion is checking, which is followed by washing, symmetry, the need to ask or confess, and counting. Children with OCD present most

Table 33-1	Yale-Brown Obsessive–Compulsive Scale Symptom Checklist

Aggressive obsessions
  Fear might harm others
  Fear might harm self
  Violent or horrific images
  Fear of blurting out obsessions or insults
  Fear of doing something embarrassing
  Fear of acting on other impulses (e.g., robbing a bank, stealing groceries, overeating)
  Fear of being responsible for things going wrong (e.g., others will lose their job because of the patient)
  Fear something terrible might happen (e.g., fire, burglary)
  Other
Contamination obsessions
  Concerns or disgust with bodily waste (e.g., urine, feces, saliva)
  Concern with dirt or germs
  Excessive concern with environmental contaminants (e.g., asbestos, radiation, toxic wastes)
  Excessive concern with household items (e.g., cleansers, solvents, pets)
  Concerned will become ill
  Concerned will become ill (aggressive)
  Other
Sexual obsessions
  Forbidden or perverse sexual thoughts, images, or impulses
  Content involves children
  Content involves animals
  Content involves incest
  Content involves homosexuality
  Sexual behavior toward others (aggressive)
  Other
Hoarding or collecting obsessions
Religious obsessions

Obsession with need for symmetry or exactness
Miscellaneous obsessions
  Need to know or remember
  Fear of saying certain things
  Fear of not saying things just right
  Intrusive (neutral) images
  Intrusive nonsense sounds, words, or music
  Other
Somatic obsession–compulsion
Cleaning or washing compulsions
  Excessive or ritualized hand washing
  Excessive or ritualized showering, bathing, brushing the teeth, or\grooming
  Involves cleaning of household items or inanimate objects
  Other measures to prevent contact with contaminants
Counting compulsions
Checking compulsions
  Checking that did not or will not harm others
  Checking that did not or will not harm self
  Checking that nothing terrible did or will happen
  Checking for contaminants
  Other
Repeating rituals
Ordering or arranging compulsions
Miscellaneous compulsions
  Mental rituals (other than checking or counting)
  Need to tell, ask, or confess
  Need to touch
Measures to prevent
  Harm to self
  Harm to others
  Terrible consequences
Other

commonly with washing compulsions, which are followed by repeating rituals (Swedo et al. 1989a).

Most individuals with OCD have multiple obsessions and compulsions over time, with a particular fear or concern dominating the clinical picture at any one time. The presence of obsessions without compulsions, or compulsions without obsessions, is unusual. In the DSM-IV OCD field trial of 431 individuals, only 2% had predominantly obsessions and 2% had predominantly compulsions; the remaining 96% endorsed both obsessions and compulsions (Foa and Kozak 1995). Individuals who appear to have obsessions without compulsions frequently have unrecognized reassurance rituals or mental compulsions, such as repetitive, ritualized praying, in addition to their obsessions. Pure compulsions are also unusual in adults, although they do occur in children, especially in the young (e.g., 6 to 8 years of age; Swedo et al. 1989a). Most people have both mental and behavioral compulsions; in the DSM-IV field trial, 79.5% reported having both mental and behavioral compulsions, 20.3% had behavioral compulsions only, and 0.2% had only mental compulsions.

Contamination obsessions are the most frequently encountered obsessions in OCD. Such obsessions are usually characterized by a fear of dirt or germs. For example, a 38-year-old computer programmer was excessively preoccupied with the thought that her apartment would become dirty. She had never allowed a visitor into her apartment or worn a coat during the winter, because she feared that she would be unable to protect her apartment from dirt brought inside by either a visitor or a coat. Excessive washing is the compulsion most commonly associated with contamination obsessions. This behavior usually occurs after contact with the feared object; however, proximity to the feared stimulus is often sufficient to engender severe anxiety and washing compulsions, even though the contaminated object has not been touched. Most individuals with washing compulsions perform these rituals in response to a fear of contamination, but these behaviors occasionally occur in response to a drive for perfection or a need for symmetry. Some individuals, for example, repeatedly wash themselves in the shower until they feel "right" or must wash their right arm and then their left arm the same number of times.

Need for symmetry is a term that describes a drive to order or arrange things perfectly or to perform certain behaviors symmetrically or in a balanced way. Individuals describe an urge to repeat motor acts until they achieve a "just right" feeling that the act has been completed perfectly. Individuals with a prominent need for symmetry may have little anxiety but rather describe feeling unsettled or uneasy if they cannot repeat actions or order things to their satisfaction. Individuals with a need for symmetry frequently present with obsessional slowness, taking hours to perform acts such as grooming or brushing their teeth. A 23-year-old cook spent 2 hours a day brushing his teeth in a symmetrical fashion and as a result developed gingival erosion. He reported being exquisitely aware of exactly how the toothbrush touched each surface of each tooth and of how he placed the toothbrush and cup down after finishing. He was unable to describe any obsession or fear about not performing this task adequately but rather felt unable to stop until he had brushed completely, despite warnings from his dentist about the harm he was causing.

Individuals with somatic obsessions are worried about the possibility that they have or will contract an illness or disease. In the past, the most common somatic obsessions consisted of fears of cancer or venereal diseases. However, a fear of developing AIDS has become increasingly common. Checking compulsions consisting of checking and rechecking the body part of concern, as well as reassurance seeking, are commonly associated with this fear. For example, a 29-year-old firefighter spent 3 hours a day examining his throat in the mirror and palpating his lymph nodes to determine whether he had throat cancer.

People with sexual or aggressive obsessions are plagued by fears that they might harm others or commit a sexually unacceptable act such as molestation. Often, they are fearful not only that they will commit a dreadful act in the future but also that they have already committed the act. Individuals are usually horrified by the content of their obsessions and are reluctant to divulge them. It is striking that the content of these obsessions tends to consist of ideas that individuals find particularly abhorrent. A 32-year-old librarian who wanted to be a good mother had intrusive thoughts of stabbing her daughter. Individuals with these highly distressing obsessions frequently have checking and confession or reassurance rituals. They may report themselves to the police or repeatedly seek out priests to confess their imagined crimes. For example, a 29-year-old secretary constantly checked the local news to be certain that she had not murdered someone. An unsolved murder case caused her tremendous anxiety and led to extensive reassurance rituals.

Pathological doubt is a common feature of individuals with OCD who have a variety of different obsessions and compulsions. Individuals with pathological doubt are plagued by the concern that, as a result of their carelessness, they will be responsible for a dire event. They may worry, for example, that they will start a fire because they neglected to turn off the stove before leaving the house. Although many individuals report being fairly certain that they performed the act in question (e.g., locking the door, unplugging the hairdryer, paying the correct amount on a bill), they cannot dismiss the nagging doubt "What if?" Excessive doubt and associated feelings of excessive responsibility frequently lead to checking rituals.

For example, individuals may spend several hours checking their home before they leave. As with contamination obsessions, pathological doubt can lead to marked avoidance behavior. Some individuals become housebound to avoid the responsibility of potentially leaving the house unlocked.

There has been considerable interest in the role of insight, or awareness, in OCD. An ability to recognize the senselessness of the obsessions and the ability to resist obsessional ideas have been considered as the fundamental components of OCD (Jaspers 1923, Lewis 1936). However, research findings during the past decade have demonstrated a continuum of insight in this disorder, which ranges from excellent (i.e., complete awareness of the senselessness of the content of the obsessions), through poor insight, to delusional thinking (i.e., the obsessions are held with delusional conviction) (Insel and Akiskal 1986, Eisen and Rasmussen 1993, Kozak and Foa 1994, Lelliot et al. 1988, Foa and Kozak 1995). Combining data from a number of studies, 20 to 25% of individuals with OCD at some point during their illness are fairly convinced that their obsessions are realistic and that consequences other than anxiety would occur if they did not perform their compulsions. Nonetheless, most people with OCD are aware that other people think their symptoms are unrealistic and that the obsessions are caused by a mental disorder (Eisen et al. 1997a). To reflect the fact that many individuals lack insight, DSM-IV established a new OCD specifier, with poor insight. This specifier applies to "an individual who, for most of the time in the current episode, does not recognize that the obsessions or compulsions are excessive or unreasonable." DSM-IV-TR also acknowledges that the beliefs that underlie OCD obsessions can be delusional and notes that, in such cases, an additional diagnosis of delusional disorder or psychotic disorder not otherwise specified may be appropriate.

Women appear to develop OCD slightly more frequently than do men. A pooled sample from two studies with a total of 991 subjects found that 52% of the subjects were women (Foa and Kozak 1995, Rasmussen and Eisen 1992). However, a study that assessed the presence of comorbid disorders characterized by psychosis (schizophrenia, delusional disorder) or psychosis-like features (schizotypal personality disorder) in 475 individuals with OCD found a different sex ratio. Fifty-six percent of the individuals with OCD who did not have one of these comorbid disorders were women, whereas 85% of those with one of these comorbid disorders were men (Eisen and Rasmussen 1993). A predominance of males has also been observed in child and adolescent OCD population. In a study of 70 probands with OCD who were aged 6 to 18 years, 67% were males (Leonard et al. 1989). This finding may be due to the fact that males develop OCD at a younger age than females.

OCD frequently occurs in association with other Axis I disorders. In a study of 100 individuals with primary OCD, 67 had a lifetime history of major depressive disorder and 31 had symptoms that met criteria for current major depressive disorder (Rasmussen and Eisen 1991). Although it may be difficult to distinguish a primary from a secondary diagnosis, some individuals with OCD view their depressive symptoms as occurring secondary to the demoralization and hopelessness accompanying their OCD and report that they would not be depressed if they did not have OCD. However, others view their major depressive symptoms as occurring independently of their OCD symptoms, which may be less severe when they cycle into an episode of major depression, because they feel too apathetic to be as concerned with their obsessions and too fatigued to perform compulsions. Conversely, OCD symptoms may intensify during depressive episodes.

Although findings have varied, the generally accepted frequency of tic disorders in individuals with OCD is far higher than in the general population, with a rate of approximately 5 to 10% for Tourette's Disorder and 20% for any tic disorder (Leonard et al. 1992, Pitman et al. 1987). Conversely, individuals with Tourette's disorder have a high rate of comorbid OCD, with 30 to 40% reporting obsessive–compulsive symptoms (Lees et al. 1984, Robertson et al. 1988). The likelihood of childhood onset of OCD is greater in this group, and the presence of tics is associated with more severe OCD symptoms in children (Leonard et al. 1992). There is an increased rate of both OCD and tic disorders in the first-degree relatives of OCD probands with a family lifetime history of tics (Pauls et al. 1995, Nestadt et al. 2000) and an increased frequency of tic disorders in the first-degree relatives of OCD probands compared to controls (Grados et al. 2001).

Studies of individuals with schizophrenia or schizoaffective disorder have found rates of OCD ranging from 8 to 46% (Eisen et al. 1997a, Porto et al. 1997, Berman et al. 1995). This strikingly large range is most likely due to the OCD criteria used (i.e., subclinical OCD symptoms versus OCD symptoms severe enough to cause significant impairment or distress). Regardless, it is clear that a significant number of people with schizophrenia have OCD symptoms that require assessment, and may benefit from treatment.

The relationship between OCD and personality disorders, particularly obsessive–compulsive personality disorder (OCPD), has received considerable attention. Early observations noted the presence of OCPD traits in individuals with OCD (Lewis 1936). Systematic studies have yielded inconsistent findings. In a study of 96 subjects with OCD that used the Structured Clinical Interview for DSM-III personality disorders (SCID-II), 36 had a personality disturbance that met criteria for one or more personality disorders (Baer et al. 1990). Dependent ($N = 12$), histrionic ($N = 9$), and obsessive–compulsive ($N = 6$) personality disorders were most frequent. However, a study that used the DSM-III-R criteria found that OCPD was present in 25 of 59 subjects with OCD; the higher rate of OCPD found with the DSM-III-R criteria may reflect changes in the criteria set between DSM-III and DSM-III-R. A recent study of the rate of OCPD in first-degree relatives of OCD probands found a similar frequency of OCPD in people with OCD. OCPD occurred in 32% of the probands and was twice as frequent in the relatives of OCD probands as in relatives of control probands (Samuels et al. 2000), suggesting that OCPD may share a common familial etiology with OCD.

Epidemiology

Until the mid-1980s, OCD was considered extremely rare. This perception was based on studies from the 1950s and 1960s that examined the frequency of mental disorders in inpatient and outpatient settings. The results of a large epidemiological study, the national ECA survey, conducted in the United States in 1984, painted a different picture of OCD's prevalence. This study found that OCD was the fourth most common mental disorder (after the phobias, substance use disorders, and major depressive disorder), with a prevalence of 1.6% over 6 months and a lifetime prevalence of 2.5% (Myers et al. 1984, Robins et al. 1984). Although the ECA survey has been criticized as overestimating OCD's prevalence (Stein et al. 1997), a subsequent study in the United States and several epidemiological studies in other countries have supported its findings (Flament et al. 1988, Bland et al. 1988, Orley and Wing 1979, Zohar et al. 1992, Angst 1994, Yeh and Chang 1989).

Course

Age at onset usually refers to the age when OCD symptoms (obsessions and compulsions) reach a severity level, wherein they lead to impaired functioning or significant distress or are time consuming (i.e., meet DSM-IV-TR criteria for the disorder). Reported age at onset is usually during late adolescence. People with OCD, however, usually describe the onset of minor symptoms in childhood, well before the onset of symptoms meeting the full criteria for the disorder.

In several studies, earlier age at onset has been associated with an increased rate of OCD in first-degree relatives (Pauls et al. 1995, Nestadt et al. 2000). These data suggest that there is a familial type of OCD characterized by early onset. Age at onset of OCD may also be a predictor of course. The vast majority of individuals report a gradual worsening of obsessions and compulsions prior to the onset of full-criteria OCD, which is followed by a chronic course. However, Swedo and colleagues (1998) have described a subtype of OCD that begins before puberty and is characterized by an episodic course with intense exacerbations. Exacerbations of OCD symptoms in this subtype have been linked with Group A beta-hemolytic Streptococcal infections, which has led to the subtype designation of pediatric autoimmune neuropsychiatric disorders associated with streptococcal infections (PANDAS). In their study of 50 children with PANDAS, the average age of onset was 7.4 years. Whether the course of illness in individuals with PANDAS continues to be episodic into adulthood, or, as is the case with postpubertal onset, tends to be chronic, is not known.

The course of OCD is usually waxing and waning—that is, once an individual acquires OCD, obsessions or compulsions, or both, are present continuously, with varying degrees of intensity over time. Relatively few individuals have either a progressively deteriorating course or a truly episodic course (Rasmussen and Eisen 1991). A recent 2-year naturalistic prospective study of 65 adults with OCD, in which the effect of treatment was assessed, supports the earlier findings that OCD is usually chronic with fluctuations in symptom intensity but no lasting remission; it is notable that this course was most common even during an era when effective treatments were available. Although 50% of the subjects achieved partial remission in the first year of the study, the probability of subsequent relapse was 48%. Only 12% achieved full and sustained remission (Eisen et al. 1999). In contrast, a better outcome was found in a follow-up study of 144 people with OCD assessed in the 1950s and again in the 1990s (mean length of follow-up from illness onset was 47 years). Most subjects reported a significant decrease in OCD symptom severity, which varied from complete recovery (20%), to recovery with continued subclinical symptoms (28%), to continued OCD but with clear improvement (35%). Better outcome was associated with later age of onset and poorer social functioning at baseline (Skoog and Skoog 1999).

Differential Diagnosis

OCD is sometimes difficult to distinguish from certain other disorders. Obsessions and compulsions may appear in the context of other syndromes, which can raise the question whether the obsessions and compulsions are a symptom of another disorder or whether both OCD and another disorder are present. A general guideline is that if the content of the obsessions is not limited to the focus of concern of another disorder (e.g., an appearance concern, as in BDD, or food concerns, as in an eating disorder) and if the obsessions or compulsions are preoccupying as well as distressing or impairing, OCD should generally be diagnosed. Diagnostic dilemmas may also arise when it is unclear whether certain thoughts are obsessions or whether, instead, they are ordinary worries, ruminations, overvalued ideas, or delusions. In a similar vein, questions may develop about whether certain behaviors constitute true compulsions or whether they should instead be conceptualized as impulses, tics, or addictive behaviors.

Both OCD and the other anxiety disorders are characterized by the use of avoidance to manage anxiety. However, OCD is distinguished from these disorders by the presence of compulsions. For individuals with preoccupying fears or worries but no rituals, several other features may be useful in establishing the diagnosis of OCD. In social phobia and specific phobia, fears are circumscribed and related to specific triggers (in specific phobia) or social situations (in social phobia). As many as 60% of people with OCD experience full-blown panic symptoms. However, unlike panic disorder, in which panic attacks occur spontaneously, panic symptoms occur in OCD only during exposure to specific feared triggers such as contaminated objects. The worries that are present in generalized anxiety disorder (GAD) are more ego syntonic and involve an exaggeration of ordinary concerns, whereas the obsessional thinking of OCD is more intrusive, is limited to a specific set of concerns (e.g., contamination, blasphemy), and usually has an irrational, senseless, or unreasonable quality.

One question is how to differentiate OCD from psychotic disorders such as schizophrenia and delusional disorder. Another question is how to distinguish OCD with insight from OCD without insight (delusional OCD). One distinguishing feature between OCD and the psychotic disorders is that the latter are not characterized by prominent ritualistic behaviors. If compulsions are present in an individual with prominent psychotic symptoms, the possibility of a comorbid OCD diagnosis should be considered. Furthermore, although schizophrenia may be characterized by obsessional thinking, other characteristic features of the disorder, such as prominent hallucinations or thought disorder, are also present. With regard to delusional disorder, paranoid and grandiose concerns are generally not considered to fall under the OCD rubric. However, some other types of delusional disorder, such as the somatic and jealous types, seem to bear a close resemblance to OCD and are not always easily distinguished from it.

The second issue noted above—how to distinguish OCD with insight from OCD without insight—is complex. As previously discussed, insight in OCD is increasingly being recognized as spanning a spectrum from good to poor to absent. Both clinical observations and research findings indicate that some individuals hold their obsessional concerns with delusional intensity, and believe that their concerns are reasonable. In DSM-IV-TR, delusional OCD may be double coded as both OCD and delusional disorder or as both OCD and psychotic disorder not otherwise specified; in other words, individuals with delusional OCD would receive both diagnoses. This double coding reflects the fact that it is unclear whether OCD with insight and OCD without insight constitute the same or different disorders. Further research using validated scales to assess insight in OCD is needed to shed light on this question.

Differential diagnosis questions have been raised with regard to kleptomania, trichotillomania, pathological gambling, and other disorders involving impulsive behaviors. Several features have been said to distinguish these disorders from OCD. For example, compulsions—unlike behaviors of the impulse control disorders—generally have no gratifying element, although they do diminish anxiety. In addition, the affective state that drives the behaviors associated with these disorders may differ. In OCD, fear is frequently the underlying drive that leads to compulsions, which, in turn, decrease anxiety. In the impulse control disorders, individuals frequently describe heightened tension, but not fear, preceding an impulsive behavior. However, OCD and the impulse control disorders have some features in common (McElroy et al. 1993). Research is ongoing to explore the relationship between OCD and the impulse control disorders by examining similarities and differences in treatment response, biological markers, and familial transmission.

Complex motor tics of Tourette's disorder may be difficult to distinguish from OCD compulsions. Both tics and compulsions are preceded by an intrusive urge and are followed by feelings of relief. However, OCD compulsions are usually preceded by both anxiety and obsessional concerns, whereas, in Tourette's disorder, the urge to perform a tic is not preceded by an obsessional fear. This distinction breaks down to some extent when considering the "just right" perceptions of some individuals with OCD (Leckman et al. 1994). The "just right" perception refers to the need to perform a certain motor action, such as touching, tapping, checking, ordering, arranging, or counting, until it feels right. Determining when an action has been performed enough or perfectly may depend on tactile, visual, or auditory perceptions. In a study of individuals with Tourette's disorder and OCD symptoms, most individuals could distinguish between the mental urge to do something repeatedly until it felt right and a physical urge to perform a motor tic. However, it is sometimes difficult for mental health professionals to distinguish between complex tics and compulsions, especially when an individual has both disorders (Miguel et al. 1995).

Fears of illness that occur in OCD, referred to as somatic obsessions, may be difficult to distinguish from hypochondriasis. Usually, however, individuals with somatic obsessions have other current or past classic OCD obsessions unrelated to illness concerns. Individuals with OCD also often engage in classic OCD rituals, such as checking or reassurance seeking, in an attempt to diminish their illness concerns. Unlike individuals with OCD, individuals with hypochondriasis experience somatic and visceral sensations. Body dysmorphic disorder (BDD), a preoccupation with an imagined or slight defect in appearance (e.g., thinning hair, facial scarring, or a large nose), has many similarities to OCD (Phillips 1991). Individuals with BDD experience obsessional thinking about the supposed defect and usually engage in associated repetitive ritualistic behaviors, such as mirror checking and reassurance seeking. Preliminary evidence suggests that BDD also appears similar to OCD in terms of age of onset, course of illness, and other variables (Phillips et al. 1995). Nonetheless, emerging data suggest that there are some important differences between the two disorders (Phillips et al. 1998), and they are currently classified separately in DSM-IV-TR. Insight, for example, is more frequently impaired in BDD than in OCD (Eisen et al. 1997b). If the content of a individual's obsessions involves a concern about a supposed defect in appearance, BDD, rather than OCD, is the diagnosis that should be given.

Obsessive–compulsive personality disorder is a lifelong maladaptive personality style characterized by perfectionism, excessive attention to detail, indecisiveness, rigidity, excessive devotion to work, restricted affect, lack of generosity, and hoarding. OCD and OCPD have historically been considered variants of the same disorder on a continuum of severity, with OCD viewed as the more severe manifestation of illness. Contrary to this notion, studies using structured interviews to establish diagnosis have found that not all individuals with OCD also have OCPD. One reason for the perception that these disorders are linked lies in the frequency of several OCPD traits in individuals with OCD. In one study, the majority of 114 individuals with OCD had perfectionism and indecisiveness (82 and 70, respectively). In contrast, other OCPD traits, such as restricted affect, excessive devotion to work, and rigidity, were seen infrequently.

Although perfectionism and indecisiveness are relatively common traits in individuals with OCD, the distinction between OCD and OCPD is important, and several guidelines may be useful in distinguishing them. Unlike OCPD, OCD is characterized by distressing, time-consuming ego-dystonic obsessions and repetitive rituals aimed at diminishing the distress engendered by obsessional thinking. One of the hallmarks that has been traditionally used to distinguish OCD from OCPD is that, in contrast, OCPD features are considered egosyntonic. In addition, as previously noted, the traits of restricted affect, excessive devotion to work, and rigidity are generally characteristic of OCPD but not OCD. Although useful, these guidelines are not absolute, and some individuals defy easy categorization. Some individuals, for example, spend hours each day engaged in egosyntonic behaviors such as excessive cleaning; such individuals may seek treatment not because they are disturbed by their behaviors but because the behaviors cause problems in functioning or family friction. It is unclear whether some of these individuals should be diagnosed with OCPD or subthreshold OCD.

Etiology

Genetic Factors

A number of approaches have been used to evaluate the role of heredity in OCD. Twin studies have examined the rates of concordant monozygotic twins versus discordant monozygotic twins with OCD. A review of this literature reveals a concordance rate of

63% in monozygotic twins (Rasmussen and Tsuang 1986). Although these studies have methodological limitations (e.g., a lack of a comparison group consisting of dizygotic twins), the data do support the notion that genetic factors are implicated in the expression of OCD. Given the concordance rate of less than 100% in monozygotic twins, it is clear that environment also plays a role in OCD's phenotypic expression.

A second approach to examining the role of genetics in OCD has been to investigate the rate of OCD in family members of OCD probands. A number of studies before 1988 found increased frequency of OCD in family members (McKeon and Murray 1987). However, it is difficult to interpret these findings because the studies were hampered by several methodological limitations. Several subsequent studies that used considerably improved methodology (Pauls et al. 1995, Lenane et al. 1990, Fyer et al. 1993, Riddle et al. 1990, Black et al. 1992) interviewed first-degree relatives of adult OCD probands using structured interviews; a control group was used in two of these studies (Pauls et al. 1995, Black et al. 1992). Pauls and associates (1995), in their study of 446 first-degree relatives of 100 OCD probands, found that 10.3% of these subjects had full OCD, and 7.9% had subthreshold OCD. These rates were significantly higher than rates in control group relatives (1.9% had OCD, and 2% had subthreshold OCD). In two other family studies, an increased frequency of familial OCD was found in families in which the proband had an early age of OCD onset, before age 14 years (Bellodi et al. 1992) and 18 years (Nestadt et al. 2000).

Further evidence supporting familial transmission of OCD has been obtained by studying the frequency of OCD in relatives of individuals with Gilles de la Tourette's Syndrome (TS). In a number of studies of TS individuals, the frequency of obsessive–compulsive symptoms was much higher (40%) than that predicted by general population rates (Pauls et al. 1995). Family studies have similarly found higher rates of OCD symptoms among family members of TS individuals (Pauls et al. 1986) as well as higher rates of Tourette's disorder and tics in first-degree relatives of children with OCD (Leonard et al. 1992). In addition, as previously noted, there are differences in the types of OCD symptoms seen in individuals with TS plus OCD versus those with OCD alone. Moreover, it has been found that even among those OCD individuals who do not have TS, if they share the TS/OCD symptom cluster (checking and ordering), they are more likely to have a positive family history for OCD. This may imply that there are distinct subtypes of OCD, some of which are familial and some of which are not (Eapen et al. 1997). Taken together, the available data support familial transmission in some cases of OCD and suggest that genetic factors play an important role in its etiology, particularly in individuals with comorbid tic disorder. Thus, in recent years a molecular genetics approach has begun to be applied to OCD, although there have been not significant findings to date. Segregation analysis, which would help to establish patterns of disease transmission, has revealed only that it is unlikely that OCD is a single gene disease (Pauls 1999). Association studies with candidate genes have focused mostly on the serotonin and dopamine systems, since medications treating OCD and TS are known to involve these systems. However, these studies have not yielded any significant consistently positive results (Nicolini et al. 1999, Pato et al. 2002). Nonetheless, as the technology improves and a better understanding of OCD's etiology and subtypes is gained, these genetics analyses could prove more fruitful.

Neurobiological Factors
Brain-imaging techniques have advanced the search for abnormalities in brain functioning and/or structure in individuals with OCD. Numerous studies have now been done with both structural imaging—CT (computed tomography) and MRI (magnetic resonance imaging) (Szeszko et al. 1999, Robinson et al. 1995)—and functional imaging—PET (positron emission tomography), SPECT (single photon emission computed tomography), fMRI (functional magnetic resonance imaging), and MRS (magnetic resonance spectroscopy).

These techniques have demonstrated abnormalities in OCD individuals (Saxena et al. 1998, Cottraux and Gerard 1998). These abnormalities occur at rest and with symptom provocation (Rauch et al. 1994, Brieter et al. 1996), and they are "normalized" with effective treatment (Baxter et al. 1992, Benkelfat et al. 1990, Hoehn-Saric et al. 1991, Swedo et al. 1992).

While not all results are in agreement, a majority of these studies have implicated abnormalities in the orbitofrontal cortex, anterior cingulate cortex, and structures of the basal ganglia and thalamus. These structures are proposed to be linked in neuroanatomical circuits (Insel 1992, Baxter 1992). One well-articulated model by Saxena and colleagues (1998) proposes that OCD symptoms are mediated by hyperactivity in orbitofrontal–subcortical circuits, which might be due to an imbalance in tone between direct and indirect striato–pallidal pathways (Baxter et al. 1987, 1988, Nordahl et al. 1989, Swedo et al. 1989b, Saxena et al. 1998). Some studies have implicated a preferential role for right anterolateral orbitofrontal cortex in both OCD symptoms and symptom response.

Further indirect evidence implicating a role for basal ganglia dysfunction in OCD lies in the clinical relationship between neurological insults to the basal ganglia and the subsequent development of obsessions and compulsions. There is an association between OCD and Tourette's disorder, Sydenham's chorea, bilateral necrosis of the globus pallidus, and postencephalitic parkinsonian symptoms.

The hypothesis that OCD involves an abnormality in the serotonin neurotransmitter system has been called the serotonin hypothesis. Several different lines of investigation support this hypothesis: (1) therapeutic response of individuals to chronic administration of medication, (2) measurements of central and peripheral neurotransmitter or metabolite concentration, and (3) pharmacologic challenge paradigms that measure behavioral and neuroendocrine effects produced by acute administration of selective pharmacologic agents (Pigott 1996).

All the evidence from treatment studies point to a role for serotonin and speak of a need for prolonged administration to see a positive effect. All of the antidepressants that effectively treat OCD affect serotonin (Greist et al. 1995b). These antidepressants are potent inhibitors of the presynaptic reuptake of serotonin (i.e., serotonin reuptake inhibitors (SRIs)). Those antidepressants that primarily affect the noradrenergic system have not been found to have antiobsessional properties. Exactly how the SSRIs improve OCD symptoms remains unclear; while the immediate action of these agents may be to increase serotonin in the synapse, they undoubtably cause a cascade of changes, both presynaptically and postsynaptically. Decreased levels of cerebrospinal 5-hydroxyindoleacetic acid, a serotonin metabolite that is reduced with serotonin reuptake inhibition, have been correlated with clinical improvement after clomipramine treatment (Thoren et al. 1980). A decrease in platelet serotonin levels—an indirect measure of neuronal reuptake—has been highly correlated with clinical improvement with clomipramine ($r = 0.77$; Flament et al. 1987). These various studies—measures of plasma levels of SSRIs, metabolite concentration, and serotonin platelet concentration—generally support the association between the improvement of OCD with an SRI and acute alterations of serotonin in the brain and, in turn, support the serotonin hypothesis. Figure 33-1 shows a serotonin synapse with several of the possible sites of action for drugs that alter OCD symptoms.

Pharmacologic challenge studies constitute yet another line of evidence supporting the role of serotonin in the pathophysiology of OCD. The serotonin receptor partial agonist *m*-chlorophenylpiperazine has been shown to increase symptoms of OCD and anxiety in individuals with OCD but to have no effect in normal control subjects (Zohar et al. 1987, Hollander et al. 1992). The increase in obsessions can be blocked with pretreatment by the serotonin receptor antagonist metergoline (Pigott et al. 1991) or by chronic treatment with clomipramine (Zohar et al. 1988). Challenge studies with other serotonergic agents have not implicated serotonin in the pathophysiology of OCD. For example, no behavioral

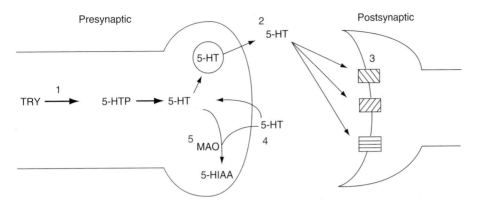

Figure 33-1 *Diagram of a serotonin (5-HT) synapse describes several of the possible sites of action for drugs that alter OCD symptoms. At (1) the rate-limiting step in serotonin synthesis, L-tryptophan (TRY) is hydroxylated to 5-hydroxytryptophan (5-HTP). After serotonin is formed, it is sequestered into vesicles that are released at the presynaptic cell membrane (2). Fenfluramine increases this release. Once released, serotonin can interact with a number of different postsynaptic receptors (3). Several selective agonists (buspirone, m-chlorophenylpiperazine) have been developed to activate each of these serotonin receptor subtypes. Metergoline is a nonselective antagonist, blocking serotonin effects at each of these sites. The inactivation of serotonin is mediated by reuptake (4), the step inhibited by clomipramine, fluvoxamine, and fluoxetine. Finally (5), serotonin is either metabolized to its metabolite, 5-hydroxyindoleacetic acid (5-HIAA), by the enzyme monoamine oxidase (MAO) or recycled back into vesicles for release. (Source: Reprinted from Insel TR and Winslow JT [1990] Neurobiology of obsessive–compulsive disorder. In Obsessive–Compulsive Disorders: Theory and Management, 2nd ed, Jenike MA, Baer L, and Minichiello WE [eds]. Mosby Year Book, St. Louis, Missouri, p. 118, Copyright 1990, with permission from Elsevier.)*

or neuroendocrine changes were found after administration of fenfluramine, a serotonin-releasing and reuptake-blocking agent (Hewlett and Martin 1993), or after administration of tryptophan, a serotonin precursor that increases serotonin synthesis (Barr et al. 1994), which differs from the findings in depression (Delgado and Moreno 1998). It is unclear whether these negative findings are attributable to methodological limitations or constitute evidence against the serotonin hypothesis.

Although available data are not entirely consistent, on balance there is now substantial evidence implicating serotonin in the pathophysiology of OCD. However, the exact role of this neurotransmitter and whether it is involved in the etiology, or is instead part of a final common pathway, of this disorder remains unclear.

The role of the dopamine system in OCD's pathophysiology has also been investigated (Goodman et al. 1990a). When added to the SRIs, dopamine antagonists (neuroleptic agents) decrease symptoms of OCD in individuals with OCD and comorbid tics as well as in individuals with OCD and comorbid schizotypal personality disorder. It has been hypothesized that some forms of OCD, particularly OCD plus Tourette's disorder, may involve an imbalance in activity between serotonergic and dopaminergic systems (Goodman et al. 1990a, Stein et al. 1997, Saxena et al. 1996, McDougle et al. 2000, Koran et al. 2000).

Psychological Factors

A model based on the psychological concept of conditioning has also been used to understand the development of obsessions and compulsions (Baer and Minichiello 1990). Compulsions, whether mental or observable, usually decrease the anxiety engendered by obsessional thoughts. Thus, if a person is preoccupied with fears of contamination from germs, repetitive hand washing usually decreases the anxiety caused by these fears. The compulsion becomes a conditioned response to anxiety. Because of the tension-reducing aspect of the compulsion, this learned behavior becomes reinforced and eventually fixed

(Rachman and Hodgson 1980). Compulsions, in turn, actually reinforce anxiety because they prevent habituation from occurring; that is, by performing a compulsion, contact with the fear-evoking stimulus (e.g., dirt) is not maintained, and habituation (a decrease in fear associated with the stimulus) does not occur. Thus, the vicious circle linking obsessions and compulsions is maintained (Figure 33-2). This learning-theory model of OCD has had a major influence on the way behavioral therapy is used in its treatment.

Recent theory has attempted to integrate the biology of OCD with psychological models by proposing a phylogenetic model based on systems theory. In this model, behavioral inhibition and harm-assessment systems, which develop early in human phylogeny, are disrupted. This disruption can occur at a hierarchically primary level of biological organization, resulting in neurobiologic disturbance, or at a hierarchically higher level of organization, leading to psychological disturbances. Such a model can help explain the diversity of symptoms seen in OCD, from the more primitive biologically based behaviors based on fight/flight and risk to more psychologically sophisticated behaviors involving morality and guilt. This model might also explain why neither biological nor psychological treatments alone always lead to complete remission of symptoms (Cohen et al. 1997).

Treatment

Both pharmacologic and behavioral therapies have proved effective for OCD. The majority of controlled treatment trials have been performed with adults aged 18 to 65 years. However, these therapies have been shown to be effective for individuals of all ages. In general, children and the elderly tolerate most of these medications well. For children, lower doses are indicated because of lower body mass (Leonard et al. 1989, 1991, Flament et al. 1985). For instance, the recommended dose for clomipramine in children is up to 150 mg/day (3 mg/kg/day) versus 250 mg/day in adults. Use of lower doses should also be considered in the elderly because their decreased ability to metabolize medications can increase the risk of side effects and toxicity (Pato and Steketee 1997, Pato and Zohar 2001). Behavioral therapy has also been used successfully in all age groups, although when treating children with this modality it is usually advisable to use a parent as a cotherapist. A flowchart that outlines treatment options for OCD is shown in Figure 33-3.

In general, the goals of treatment are to reduce the frequency and intensity of symptoms as much as possible and to minimize the amount of interference the symptoms cause. It should be noted that few individuals experience a cure or complete remission of symptoms. Instead, OCD should be viewed as a chronic illness with a waxing and waning course. Symptoms are often worse during times of psychosocial stress. Even when on medication, individuals with OCD are often upset when they experience even a mild symptom exacerbation, anticipating that their symptoms will revert to their worst, which is rarely the case. Anticipating with the individual that stress may make the symptoms worse can often be helpful in long-term treatment.

Somatic Treatments

The most extensively studied agents for OCD are medications that affect the serotonin system (see Figure 33-1). The principal pharmacologic agents used to treat OCD are

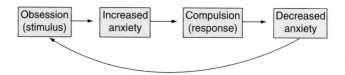

Figure 33-2 *Learning theory of OCD.*

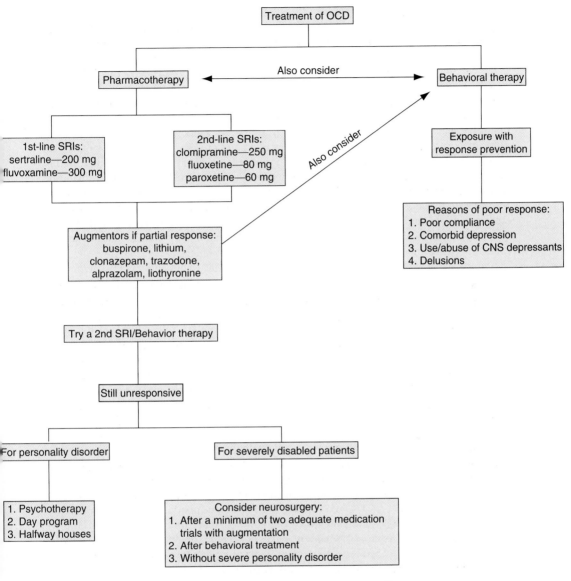

Figure 33-3 *Flowchart of treatment options for OCD.*

the SRIs, which include clomipramine, fluoxetine, fluvoxamine, sertraline, paroxetine, citalopram and escitalopram.

The tricyclic antidepressant clomipramine is among the most extensively studied pharmacological agents in OCD. This drug is unique among the antiobsessional agents in which in addition to its potency as an SRI, it has significant affinity for noradrenergic, dopaminergic, muscarinic, and histaminic receptors. An extensive review of all double-blind trials of clomipramine in OCD is included in the 1991 report of The Clomipramine Collaborative Study Group (1991). The most common side effects were those typical of the tricyclic antidepressants, including dry mouth, dizziness, tremor, fatigue, somnolence, constipation, nausea, increased sweating, headache, mental cloudiness, and sexual dysfunction. Previous data have indicated that at doses of 300 mg/day or more, the risk of seizures is 2.1% (DeVeaugh-Geiss et al. 1989), but at doses of 250 mg/day or less, the risk of seizures is low (0.48%) and comparable to that of other tricyclic antidepressants. It is therefore recommended that doses of 250 mg/day or less be used.

Recent studies of IV clomipramine have been particularly promising because it seems to have a quicker onset of action and fewer side effects than the oral form, and it may be effective even in individuals who do not respond to oral clomipramine. Oral clomipramine, like other SRIs, usually takes a minimum of 4 to 6 weeks to produce a clinically significant clinical response, but in at least one study by Koran, in which he used IV pulse dosing, individuals showed a response within 4.5 days (Koran et al. 1997, Fallon et al. 1998). The reasons for this unique response are not fully understood, but it is postulated that the IV preparation avoids first-pass hepatoenteric metabolism, leading to increased bioavailability of the parent compound clomipramine. This in turn may play a role in rapidly desensitizing serotonergic receptors or initiating changes in postsynaptic serotonergic neurons. Although studies of IV clomipramine for obsessional states date as far back as 1973 (Walter 1973), this preparation is still not FDA-approved for clinical use in the United States. Cardiac monitoring is recommended during the use of IV clomipramine.

Fluoxetine (as well as fluvoxamine, sertraline, paroxetine, citalopram and escitalopram) is often referred to as a selective serotonin reuptake inhibitor (SSRI) (Greist et al. 1995b) because it has a far more potent effect on serotonergic than on noradrenergic or other neurotransmitter systems. Despite their different chemical structures, all of the SSRIs appear to have similar efficacy in treating OCD (Greist et al. 1995b). Fluoxetine and the other SSRIs have fewer side effects than clomipramine, reflecting its more selective mechanism of action. The most common side effects are headache, nausea, insomnia, anorexia, dry mouth, somnolence, nervousness, tremor, and diarrhea. Side effects occur more frequently at higher doses (Tollefson et al. 1994b). Fluvoxamine is a unicyclic agent that differs from the other SSRIs in that it does not have an active metabolite. Sertraline is a naphthalenamine derivative with an active metabolite, *n*-desmethylsertraline. Paroxetine is a phenylpiperidine compound that is marketed as an antidepressant and that, like sertraline, shows promise in the treatment of OCD. Citalopram is a bicyclic phthaline derivative with S (active) and R (inactive) enantiomers; it is unique in its selectivity for serotonin reuptake compared to the other SSRIs. Since it has few significant secondary binding properties, its minimal effect on hepatic metabolism probably makes it safer to combine with other medications. Most studies of other medications for OCD have consisted of only case reports or small samples. One small trial suggested that venlafaxine, a medication which, like clomipramine, inhibits the re-uptake of both serotonin and norepinephrine, may hold some promise (Zajecka et al. 1990).

The efficacy of each SSRI—clomipramine, fluoxetine, fluvoxamine, sertraline, paroxetine, and citalopram—is supported by existing data. During the last 10 years, at least seven head-to-head SRI comparison studies have been done, six of which compared clomipramine to fluoxetine (Pigott et al. 1990, Lopez-Ibor et al. 1996), fluvoxamine (Freedman et al. 1994, Koran et al. 1996), paroxetine (Zohar and Judge 1996), or sertraline (Bisserbe et al. 1997); one study compared fluvoxamine to both paroxetine and citalopram (Mundo et al. 1997). All of the studies found that the agents studied were equally efficacious, although they may have been underpowered to detect differences among medications. However, several meta-analyses (Jenike et al. 1990a, Greist et al. 1995, Griest and Jefferson 1998) of OCD trials, which compared SRIs across large placebo-controlled multicenter trials, lend some support to the notion that clomipramine might be more effective than the more selective agents. However, like most meta-analyses, these studies are flawed by factors that include variations in the study protocol, sample size, and the number of treatment-resistant and treatment-naïve subjects. Nonetheless, as Griest and colleagues (1995) point out, these differences cannot explain the fact that the clomipramine trial had a lower drop out rate

(12% overall) (Griest and Jefferson 1998, Greist et al. 1995) than other trials, despite a higher rate of side effects (e.g., 97% for clomipramine versus 57% for fluoxetine [Jenike et al. 1990a]). In conclusion, these meta-analyses support a trial of clomipramine in all individuals who do not respond to SRIs, even though clomipramine tends to cause more side effects.

It is worth noting that the SSRIs, via their effect on the liver cytochrome system, can inhibit the metabolism of certain other drugs. Fluoxetine can elevate blood levels of a variety of coadministered drugs, including tricyclic antidepressants (such as clomipramine), carbamazepine, phenytoin, and trazodone (Devane 1994). However, the other SSRIs (with the exception of citalopram) can theoretically cause similar elevations, although fewer reports on such interactions are currently available. Some clinicians have taken advantage of these interactions by carefully combining fluvoxamine with clomipramine in order to block clomipramine's metabolism to desmethylclomipramine; this in turn favors serotonin reuptake inhibition provided by the parent compound rather than the norepinephrine reuptake inhibition provided by the metabolite. However, caution should be exercised with this approach since the elevation in clomipramine levels, and perhaps other compounds, can be nonlinear and quickly lead to dangerous toxicity (Szegedi et al. 1996); at the very least, clomipramine levels should be carefully monitored.

All of the SSRIs are generally well tolerated, with a relatively low percentage of individuals experiencing notable side effects or discontinuing them because of side effects. In addition, these compounds are unlikely to be lethal in overdose, except for clomipramine, which can lead to cardiac arrhythmias and death. All these agents can cause sexual side effects, ranging from anorgasmia to difficultly with ejaculatory function. However, such symptoms are not readily volunteered by the individual; thus it is important to ask. Should such symptoms be experienced, conservative measures may include dosage reduction, transient drug holidays for a special weekend or occasion, or switching to another SSRI since individuals may not have the same degree of dysfunction with a different agent. However, if the clinician feels that it is critical to continue with the same agent, various treatments have been reported in the literature. Usually taken within a few hours of sexual activity, no one agent has been shown to work consistently. Among those that have been tried are yohimbine, buspirone, cyproheptadine, buproprion, dextroamphetamine, methylphenidate, amantidine, and nefazodone, to name a few (Jenike et al. 1998, pp. 506–508).

If an individual has had only a partial response to an antiobsessional agent of adequate dose and duration, the next question is whether to change the SSRI or add an augmenting agent. Current clinical practice suggests that if there is no response at all to an SSRI, it may be best to change to another SSRI. However, if there has been some response to treatment, an augmentation trial of at least 2 to 8 weeks may be warranted (Jenike 1993, Goodman et al. 1993, March et al. 1997, Griest and Jefferson 1998). No augmentation agent has been firmly established as efficacious. Although many augmentation agents appeared promising in open trials, they failed to be effective in more systematic trials (Goodman et al. 1993), although some of the later studies did not report response to the SRI alone, leaving unanswered the question of whether some augmentation strategies may be effective in partial SSRI responders. Many questions about augmentation remain unanswered, including the optimal duration of augmentation, comparative efficacy of different agents, predictors of response, and mechanism of action (Jenike 1992, 1993). Nonetheless, these agents do help some individuals significantly, and thus their systematic use should be considered (see Table 33-2).

In individuals with severe symptoms or comorbid psychosis or tic disorder, pimozide 1 to 3 mg/day, haldol 2 to 10 mg/day, and other neuroleptic agents (risperidone 2–8 mg/day and olanzapine 2.5–10 mg/day) have been used with some success (Goodman et al. 1993, McDougle et al. 1990, 2000, Stein et al. 1997, Saxena et al. 1996, Koran et al. 2000).

Table 33-2	Potential Augmenting Agents for Treatment-Resistant Obsessive–Compulsive Disorder
Augmenting Agent	**Suggested Dosage Range***
Lithium	300–600 mg/day[†]
Clonazepam	1–3 mg/day
Tryptophan	2–10 g/day[‡]
Trazodone	100–200 mg/day
Buspirone	15–60 mg/day
Alprazolam	0.5–2 mg/day
Methylphenidate	10–30 mg/day
Haloperidol	2–10 mg/day
Pimozide	2–10 mg/day
Nifedipine	10 mg t.i.d
Liothyronine sodium	10–25 mg/day
Clonidine	0.1–0.6 mg/day
Fenfluramine	Up to 60 mg/day

*Add these to an ongoing trial of antidepressant medication. It should be noted that most of these dosages have not been tested with rigorous clinical trials but simply represent some of the reported doses tried in the current literature. Some would not recommend augmentation unless the initial treatment showed some response.

[†]*Use with caution*—there have been some reports of elevated lithium levels with ongoing fluoxetine treatment.

[‡]Because the use of l-tryptophan has been implicated in an increased incidence of eosinophilia, the authors advise against the prescribing and use of this agent until the issue is resolved.

Source: Jenike MA (1991) Management of patient with treatment-resistant obsessive–compulsive disorder. In Current Treatments of Obsessive–Compulsive Disorder, Pato MT and Zohar J (eds). American Psychiatric Press, Washington DC, p. 146.

However, the use of a neuroleptic agent should be considered carefully in light of the risk of extrapyramidal symptoms and side effects such as weight gain, lethargy, and tardive dyskinesia. Thus, when a neuroleptic drug is used, target symptoms should be established before beginning treatment and the medication discontinued within several months if target symptoms do not improve.

The use of lithium (300–600 mg/day) and buspirone (up to 60 mg/day) as augmentation agents has also been explored. Both agents looked promising in open trials (Jenike 1992, Jenike et al. 1991, Markovitz et al. 1990) but failed to be effective in more systematic trials (McDougle et al. 1991, 1993, Pigott et al. 1992a). Augmentation with fenfluramine (up to 60 mg/day), clonazepam (up to 5 mg/day), clonidine (0.1–0.6 mg/day), and trazodone (100–200 mg/day), as well as the combination of clomipramine with any of the SSRIs, has had anecdotal success but has not been evaluated in methodologically rigorous studies (Rasmussen et al. 1993, Pigott et al. 1992b). Some potential augmenting agents and their dosage ranges are presented in Table 33-2.

There are a number of studies on the long-term efficacy of pharmacotherapy for OCD. One study that included a follow-up period of 2 years for 38 individuals with OCD on sertraline showed continued efficacy with fewer side effects with longer-term treatment (Rasmussen et al. 1997). Another study assessed a larger group of individuals and attempted to answer important clinical questions not only about long-term efficacy but also about the effects of medication discontinuation after 1 year of treatment (Koran et al. 2002). The latter is an important question because few studies of systematic discontinuation have been done, and in those that have been done, relapse rates were quite high, above 90% (Pato et al. 1988, Leonard et al. 1991). This sertraline study (Koran et al. 2002) involved 223 individuals who had been successfully treated with single-blind sertraline for 52 weeks and were then randomized in a double-blind manner to continue treatment for another 6 months or placebo. One-third of the individuals in the placebo group relapsed; this was surprisingly lower than the percentage found in earlier studies. The authors offered several plausible explanations for this, which included the possibility that 1 year of effective treatment may provide sustained benefit for individuals, and that individuals may have engaged in self-directed behavior therapy, something that was not readily available at the time of the previous discontinuation studies. They also noted that while OCD symptom ratings did not worsen in the placebo-treated group as a whole, quality of life did significantly deteriorate. This finding points to the need for more sensitive measures of individual improvement and for further studies of long-term treatment efficacy.

Occasionally, even after receiving adequate pharmacotherapy (including augmentation), adequate behavioral therapy, and a combination of behavioral therapy and pharmacotherapy, individuals may still experience intractable OCD symptoms. Such individuals may be candidates for neurosurgery. Although criteria for who should receive neurosurgery vary, it has been suggested that failure to respond to at least 5 years of systematic treatment is a reasonable criterion (Mindus and Jenike 1992). The procedures that have been most successful interrupt tracts involved in the serotonin system. The surgical procedures used—anterior capsulotomy, cingulotomy, and limbic leukotomy—all aim to interrupt the connection between the cortex and the basal ganglia and related structures. Current stereotactic surgical techniques involve the creation of precise lesions, which are often only 10 to 20 mm, to specific tracts. These procedures have often been done with radio-frequency heated electrodes and more recently with gamma knife techniques. Postsurgical risks have been minimized, and in some cases cognitive function and personality traits improve along with symptoms of OCD (Jenike 1998).

Psychosocial Treatments

Behavioral therapy is effective for OCD both as a primary treatment and as an augmentation agent (Marks et al. 1988, 1980, Foa et al. 1985, Griest 1994). This form of therapy is based on the principle of exposure and response prevention. The individual is asked to endure, in a graduated manner, the anxiety that a specific obsessional fear provokes while refraining from compulsions that allay that anxiety. The principles behind the efficacy of behavioral treatment are explained to the individual in the following way. Although compulsions, either covert or overt, usually immediately relieve anxiety, this is only a short-term solution; the anxiety will ultimately return, requiring the performance of another compulsion. However, if the individual resists the anxiety and urge to ritualize, the anxiety will eventually decrease on its own (i.e., habituation will occur), and the need to perform the ritual will eventually disappear. Thus, behavioral therapy helps the individual habituate to the anxiety and extinguish the compulsions.

Compulsions, especially overt behaviors like washing rituals, are more successfully treated by behavioral therapy than are obsessions alone or covert rituals like mental checking. This is because covert rituals are harder to physically resist than are rituals like hand washing and checking a door. In fact, Jenike (1993) reported that washing rituals are the most amenable to behavioral treatment, followed by checking rituals and then mental rituals.

For rituals that do not constitute overt behaviors, techniques other than exposure and response prevention have been used in conjunction with exposure and response prevention. These approaches include imaginal flooding and thought stopping. In imaginal flooding, the anxiety provoked by the obsessions is evoked by continually repeating the thought, often with the help of a continuous-loop tape or the reading of a "script" composed by the individual and therapist, until the thought no longer provokes anxiety. In thought stopping, a compulsive mental ritual (e.g., continually repeating a short prayer in one's head) is stopped by simply shouting, making a loud noise, or snapping a rubber band on the wrist in an attempt to interrupt the thought.

In the early stages of treatment, a behavioral assessment is performed. During this assessment, the content, frequency, duration, amount of interference and distress, and attempts to resist or ignore the obsessions and compulsions are catalogued. An attempt is made to clarify the types of symptoms, any triggers that bring on the obsessions and compulsions, and the amount and type of avoidance used to deal with the symptoms. The individual, usually with the help of a therapist, then develops a hierarchy of situations according to the amount of anxiety they provoke. During treatment, individuals gradually engage in the anxiety-provoking situations included in their hierarchy without performing anxiety-reducing rituals.

Despite its efficacy, behavioral therapy has limitations. To begin with, about 15 to 25% of individuals refuse to engage in behavioral treatment initially or drop out early in treatment because it is so anxiety provoking (Griest 1994). Behavioral treatment fails in another 25% of individuals for a variety of other reasons (Griest 1994, Foa et al. 1983), including concomitant depression; the use of central nervous system depressants, which may inhibit the ability to habituate to anxiety; lack of insight; poor compliance with homework, resulting in inadequate exposure; and poor compliance on the part of the therapist in enforcing the behavioral paradigm (Griest 1994). Thus, overall, 50 to 70% of individuals are helped by this form of therapy.

Behavior therapy can be used as the sole treatment of OCD, particularly with individuals whose contamination fears or somatic obsessions make them resistant to taking medications. Behavioral treatment is also a powerful adjunct to pharmacotherapy. Some research appears to indicate that combined treatment may be more effective than pharmacotherapy or behavioral therapy alone, although these findings are still preliminary (Marks et al. 1980, Cottraux et al. 1990, Foa 1994, Simpson et al. 1999). Some studies have even suggested that adding pharmacotherapy to behavior therapy may be particularly helpful in reducing obsessions, while compulsions respond to behavior therapy (Hohagen et al. 1998, Direnfeld et al. 2000). From a clinical perspective, it may be useful to have individuals begin treatment with medication to reduce the intensity of their symptoms or comorbid depressive symptoms if present; individuals may then be more amenable to experiencing the anxiety that will be evoked by the behavioral challenges they perform.

The data on the discontinuation of behavioral therapy are encouraging. In summarizing data from several 1- to 6-year follow-up studies of behavioral therapy, O'Sullivan and Marks (1991) noted that overall about 75% of individuals continued to do well at follow-up. However, most studies also noted that few individuals were symptom free. One small study looked at the role of behavioral therapy in the context of medication discontinuation and was a bit less optimistic, finding that at least three of five individuals who discontinued medication while receiving behavioral therapy had a relapse of symptoms requiring medication reinitiation (Baer et al. 1994). A larger clinical trial is currently assessing this issue.

The use of psychotherapeutic techniques of either a psychoanalytic or a supportive nature has not been proved successful in treating the specific obsessions and compulsions that are a hallmark of OCD. However, the more characterological aspects that are part of OCPD may be helped by a more psychoanalytically oriented approach. The defense mechanisms of reaction formation, isolation, and undoing, as well as a pervasive sense of doubt and need to be in control, are hallmarks of the obsessive–compulsive character. Salzman (1983) and MacKinnon and Michels (1971) have written elegantly on how to approach the maladaptive aspects of this character style in therapy. In essence, the individual must be encouraged to take risks and learn to feel comfortable with, or at least less anxious about, making mistakes and to accept anxiety as a natural and normal part of human experience. Techniques for meeting such goals in treatment may include the therapist's being relatively active in therapy to ensure that the individual focuses on the present rather than getting lost in perfectly recounting the past, as well as the therapist's being willing to take risks and present herself or himself as less than perfect.

Comparison of DSM-IV-TR/ICD-10 Diagnostic Criteria

The ICD-10 Diagnostic Criteria for Research for Obsessive–Compulsive Disorder differentiate between obsessions and compulsions on the basis of whether they are thoughts, ideas, or images (obsessions) or acts (compulsions). In contrast, DSM-IV-TR distinguishes between obsessions and compulsions on the basis of whether the thought, idea, or image causes anxiety or distress or prevents or reduces it. Thus, in DSM-IV-TR, there can be cognitive compulsions that would be considered obsessions in ICD-10. In addition, ICD-10 sets a minimum duration of at least 2 weeks, whereas DSM-IV-TR has no minimum duration.

References

Angst A (1994) The epidemiology of obsessive–compulsive disorder. In *Current Insights in Obsessive Compulsive Disorder*, Hollander E, Zohar J, Marazziti D, et al. (eds). John Wiley, West Sussex, UK, pp. 93–104.

Baer L (1994) Factor analysis of symptom subtypes of obsessive–compulsive disorder and their relation to personality and tic disorders. *J Clin Psychiatry* **55**, 18–23.

Baer L, Jenike MA, Ricciardi JN, et al. (1990) Standardized assessment of personality disorders in obsessive–compulsive disorder. *Arch Gen Psychiatry* **47**, 826–830.

Baer L and Minichiello WE (1990) Behavior therapy for obsessive–compulsive disorder. In *Obsessive–Compulsive Disorders: Theory and Management*. Jenike MA, Baer L, and Minichiello WE (eds). Year Book Medical Publishers, St. Louis, Missouri.

Barr LL, Goodman WK, McDougle LJ, et al. (1994) Tryptophan depletion in patients with obsessive–compulsive disorder who respond to serotonin reuptake inhibitors. *Arch Gen Psychiatry* **51**, 309–317.

Baxter LR (1992) Neuroimaging studies of obsessive–compulsive disorder. *Psychiatr Clin North Am* **15**, 871–884.

Baxter LR, Phelps ME, Mazziotta JC, et al. (1987) Local cerebral glucose metabolic rates in obsessive–compulsive disorder. A comparison with rates in unipolar depression and in normal controls. *Arch Gen Psychiatry* **4**, 211–218.

Baxter LR, Schwartz JM, Bergman KS, et al. (1992) Caudate glucose metabolic rate changes with both drug and behavior therapy for obsessive–compulsive disorder. *Arch Gen Psychiatry* **49**, 681–689.

Baxter LR, Schwartz JM, Mazziotta JC, et al. (1988) Cerebral glucose metabolic rates in nondepressed patients with obsessive–compulsive disorder. *Am J Psychiatry* **145**, 1560–1563.

Bellodi L, Sciuto G, Diaferia G, et al. (1992) Psychiatric disorders in the families of patients with obsessive–compulsive disorder. *Psychiatr Res* **42**, 111–120.

Benkelfat C, Nordahl TE, Semple WE, et al. (1990) Local cerebral glucose metabolic rates in obsessive–compulsive disorder. Patients treated with clomipramine. *Arch Gen Psychiatry* **47**, 840–848.

Berman I, Kalinowski A, and Berman SM (1995) Obsessive and compulsive symptoms in chronic schizophrenia. *Compr Psychiatry* **36**(1), 6–10.

Bisserbe JC, Lane RM, and Flament MF (1997) A double-blind comparison of sertraline and clomipramine in outpatients with obsessive–compulsive disorder. *Eur Psychiatry* **12**, 82–93.

Black DW, Nayes R, Goldstein RB, et al. (1992) A family study of obsessive–compulsive disorder. *Arch Gen Psychiatry* **49**, 362–368.

Bland RC, Newman SC, and Orn H (1988) Lifetime prevalence of psychiatric disorders in Edmonton. *Acta Psychiatr Scand* **77**(Suppl.), 33–42.

Brieter HC, Rauch SL, Kwong KK, et al. (1996) Functioning magnetic resonance imaging of symptoms provocation in obsessive–compulsive disorder. *Arch Gen Psychiatry* **49**, 595–606.

Cohen LJ, Stein D, and Galykner I (1997) Towards an integration of psychological and biological models of obsessive–compulsive disorder: phylogenetics considerations. *CNS Spect* **2**(10), 26–44.

Cottraux J and Gerard D (1998) Neuroimaging and neuroanatomical issues in obsessive–compulsive disorder; toward and integrative model-perceived impulsivity. In *Obsessive–Compulsive Disorder: Theory Research and Treatment*, Swinson RP, Martin M, et al. (eds). Guilford Press, New York, pp. 154–180.

Cottraux J, Mollard E, Bouvard M, et al. (1990) A controlled study of fluvoxamine and exposure in obsessive–compulsive disorder. *Int Clin Psychopharmacol* **5**, 17–30.

Delgado PL and Moreno FA (1998) Different roles for serotonin in anti-obsessional drug action and the pathophysiology of obsessive–compulsive disorder. *Br J Psychiatry* **173**(Suppl. 35), 21–25.

Devane CL (1994) Pharmacogenetics and drug metabolism of newer antidepressant agents. *J Clin Psychiatry* **55**(Suppl.), 38–45.

DeVeaugh-Geiss J, Landau P, and Katz R (1989) Treatment of obsessive–compulsive disorder with clomipramine. *Psychiatr Ann* **19**, 97–101.

Direnfeld D, Pato MT, and Gunn S (2000) Behavior therapy as adjuvant treatment in OCD. *Poster Presentation, at APA Annual Meeting*, 14–18 May, Chicago, IL.

Eapen V, Robertson MM, Alsobrook JP, et al. (1997) Obsessive compulsive symptoms in Gilles de la Tourette's syndrome and obsessive compulsive disorder: differences by diagnosis and family history. *Am J Med Genet* **74**(4), 432–438.

Eisen JL, Beer DA, Pato MT, et al. (1997a) Obsessive–compulsive disorder in schizophrenia and schizoaffective disorders. *Am J Psychiatry* **154**, 271–273.

Eisen JL, Goodman W, Keller MB, et al. (1999) Patterns of remission and relapse in OCD: a 2-year prospective study. *J Clin Psychiatry* **60**, 346–351.

Eisen JL, Phillips KA, and Rasmussen SA (1997b) *Insight in Body Dysmorphic Disorder versus OCD. New Research Program and Abstracts*, American Psychiatric Association, 150th Annual Meeting. American Psychiatric Association, San Diego, CA.

Eisen JL and Rasmussen SA (1993) Obsessive–compulsive disorder with psychotic features. *J Clin Psychiatry* **54**, 373–379.

Fallon BA, Liebowitz MR, and Campeas R (1998) Intravenous clomipramine for obsessive–compulsive disorder refractory to oral clomipramine. *Arch Gen Psychiatry* **55**, 918–924.

Flament MF, Rapoport JL, Berg O, et al. (1985) Clomipramine treatment of childhood compulsive disorder. *Arch Gen Psychiatry* **42**, 977–983.

Flament MF, Rapoport JL, Murphy DL, et al. (1987) Biochemical changes during clomipramine treatment of childhood obsessive–compulsive disorder. *Arch Gen Psychiatry* **44**, 219–225.

Flament MF, Whitaker A, Rapoport JL, et al. (1988) Obsessive–compulsive disorder in adolescence: an epidemiologic study. *J Am Acad Child Adolesc Psychiatry* **27**, 764–771.

Foa EB (1994) Recent findings in the efficacy of behavioral therapy and clomipramine for obsessive–compulsive disorder (OCD). *Presented at the 14th National Conference of the Anxiety Disorders Association of America*, 20 March, Santa Monica, CA.

Foa EB, Grayson JB, Steketee GS, et al. (1983) Success and failure in the behavioral treatment of obsessive–compulsives. *J Consult Clin Psychol* **51**, 287–297.

Foa EB and Kozak MJ (1995) DSM-IV field trial: obsessive–compulsive disorder. *Am J Psychiatry* **152**, 90–96.

Foa EB, Steketee GS, and Ozarow BJ (1985) Behavior therapy with obsessive–compulsives: from theory to treatment. In *Obsessive-Compulsive Disorder: Psychological and Pharmacological Treatment*, Mavisskalian M, Turner SM, and Michelson L (eds). Plenum Press, New York, pp. 49–129.

Freedman CPL, Trimble MR, Deakin JFW, et al. (1994) Fluvoxamine versus clomipramine in the treatment of obsessive–compulsive disorder: a multicenter randomized double-blind parallel group comparison. *J Clin Psychiatry* **55**, 301–305.

Fyer A, Mannuzza S, Chapman TF, et al. (1993) Familial transmission of obsessive–compulsive disorder. *Presented, at the First International Obsessive–Compulsive Disorder Conference*, 12–13 March, Capri, Italy.

Goodman WK, McDougle CJ, Barr LC, et al. (1993) Biological approaches to treatment-resistant obsessive–compulsive disorder. *J Clin Psychiatry* **54**(Suppl.), 16–26.

Goodman WK, McDougle CJ, Lawrence HP, et al. (1990a) Beyond the serotonin hypothesis: a role for dopamine in some forms of obsessive–compulsive disorder. *J Clin Psychopharmacol* **51**(Suppl.), 36–43.

Goodman WK, Price LH, Delgado PL, et al. (1990b) Specificity of serotonin reuptake inhibitors in the treatment of obsessive–compulsive disorder. *Arch Gen Psychiatry* **47**, 577–585.

Goodman WK, Price LH, Rasmussen SA, et al. (1989a) The Yale-Brown obsessive–compulsive scale. Development, use, and reliability. *Arch Gen Psychiatry* **46**, 1006–1011.

Grados MA, Riddle MA, Samuels JF, et al. (2001) The familial phenotype of obsessive–compulsive disorder in relation to tic disorders: the Hopkins OCD family study. *Biol Psychiatry* **50**(8), 559–565.

Griest JH (1994) Behavior therapy for obsessive–compulsive disorder. *J Clin Psychiatry* **55**(Suppl.), 60–68.

Griest JH and Jefferson JW (1998) Pharmacotherapy for obsessive–compulsive disorder. *Br J Psychiatry* **173**(Suppl. 35), 64–70.

Greist JH, Jefferson JW, Kobak KA, et al. (1995) Efficacy and tolerability of serotonin transport inhibitors in obsessive–compulsive disorder. *Arch Gen Psychiatry* **52**, 53–60.

Hewlett WA and Martin K (1993) Fenfluramine challenges and serotonergic functioning in obsessive–compulsive disorder. *Presented at the First International Obsessive–Compulsive Disorder Congress*, 12–13 March, Capri, Italy.

Hoehn-Saric R, Pearlson G, Harris G, et al. (1991) Effects of fluoxetine on regional cerebral blood flow in obsessive–compulsive patients. *Am J Psychiatry* **148**, 1243–1245.

Hohagen F, Winkelmann G, Rasche-Rauchle H, et al. (1998) Combination of behavior therapy with fluvoxamine in comparison with behaviour therapy and placebo. *Br J Psychiatry* **173**(Suppl. 35), 71–78.

Hollander E, DeCaria C, Nitescu A, et al. (1992) Serotonergic function in obsessive–compulsive disorder: behavioral and neuroendocrine responses to oral *m*-chlorophenylpiperazine and fenfluramine in patients and healthy volunteers. *Arch Gen Psychiatry* **49**, 21–28.

Insel TR (1992) Toward a neuroanatomy of obsessive–compulsive disorder. *Arch Gen Psychiatry* **49**, 739–744.

Insel TR and Akiskal HS (1986) Obsessive–compulsive disorder with psychotic features: a phenomenological analysis. *Am J Psychiatry* **143**, 1527–1533.

Insel TR and Winslow JT (1990) Neurobiology of obsessive–compulsive disorder. In *Obsessive–Compulsive Disorders: Theory and Management*, 2nd ed., Jenike MA, Baer L, and Minichiello WE (eds). Mosby Year Book, St. Louis, Missouri, p. 118.

Jaspers K (1923) Hoeing J and Hamilton MW (trans) (1963) *General Psychopathology*. University of Chicago Press, Chicago. (Originally published in 1923.)

Jenike MA (1990) Theories of etiology. In *Obsessive–Compulsive Disorders: Theory and Management*, Jenike MA, Baer L, and Minichiello WE (eds). Mosby Year Book, St. Louis, Missouri.

Jenike MA (1991) Management of patients with treatment-resistant obsessive–compulsive disorder. In *Current Treatments of Obsessive–Compulsive Disorder*, Pato MT and Zohar J (eds). American Psychiatric Press, Washington, DC, p. 146.

Jenike MA (1992) Pharmacologic treatment of obsessive–compulsive disorders. *Psychiatr Clin North Am* **15**, 895–919.

Jenike MA (1993) Augmentation strategies for treatment-resistant obsessive–compulsive disorder. *Harv Rev Psychiatry* **1**, 17–26.

Jenike MA (1998) Neurosurgical treatment of obsessive–compulsive disorder. *Br J Psychiatry* **173**(Suppl. 35), 79–90.

Jenike MA, Baer L, and Griest JH (1990a) Clomipramine versus fluoxetine in obsessive–compulsive disorder: a retrospective comparison of side effects and efficacy. *J Clin Psychopharmacol* **10**, 122–124.

Jenike MA, Baer L, and Minichiello WE (1998) *Obsessive–Compulsive Disorder: Practical Management*. Mosby, St. Louis, Missouri.

Koran LM, Hackett E, Rubin A, et al. (2002) Efficacy of sertraline in the long term treatment of obsessive–compulsive disorder. *Am J Psychiatry* **159**, 88–95.

Koran LM, McElroy SL, Davison JRT, et al. (1996) Fluvoxamine versus clomipramine for obsessive–compulsive disorder: a double-blind comparison. *J Clin Psychopharmacol* **16**, 121–129.

Koran LM, Ringold AL, and Elliot MA (2000) Olanzapine augmentation for treatment resistant obsessive–compulsive disorder. *J Clin Psychiatry* **61**, 514–517.

Koran LM, Sallee FR, and Pallanti S (1997) Rapid benefit of intravenous pulse loading of clomipramine in obsessive–compulsive disorder. *Am J Psychiatry* **154**, 396–401.

Kozak MJ and Foa EB (1994) Obsessions, overvalued ideas, and delusions in obsessive–compulsive disorder. *Behav Res Ther* **32**, 343–353.

Leckman JL, Walker DE, Goodman WK, et al. (1994) "Just right" perceptions associated with compulsive behavior in Tourette's syndrome. *Am J Psychiatry* **151**, 675–680.

Lees AJ, Robertson M, Trimble MR, et al. (1984) A clinical study of Gilles de la Tourette syndrome in the United Kingdom. *J Neurol Neurosurg Psychiatry* **47**, 1–8.

Lelliot PT, Noshirvani HF, Basoglu M, et al. (1988) Obsessive–compulsive beliefs and treatment outcome. *Psychol Med* **18**, 697–702.

Lenane MC, Swedo SE, Leonard H, et al. (1990) Psychiatric disorders in first-degree relatives of children and adolescents with obsessive–compulsive disorder. *J Am Acad Child Adolesc Psychiatry* **29**, 407–412.

Leonard HL, Lenane MC, Swedo SE, et al. (1992) Tics and Tourette's disorder: a 2- to 7-year follow-up of 54 obsessive–compulsive children. *Am J Psychiatry* **149**, 1244–1251.

Leonard HL, Swedo SE, Lenane MD, et al. (1991) A double-blind desipramine substitution during long-term clomipramine treatment in children and adolescents with obsessive–compulsive disorder. *Arch Gen Psychiatry* **48**, 922–927.

Leonard HL, Swedo SE, Rapoport JL, et al. (1989) Treatment of childhood obsessive–compulsive disorder with clomipramine and desipramine: a double-blind crossover comparison. *Arch Gen Psychiatry* **46**, 1088–1092.

Lewis A (1936) Problems of obsessional illness. *Proc R Soc Med* **29**, 325–336.

Lopez-Ibor JJ, Saiz J, Cottraux J, et al. (1996) Double-blind comparison of fluoxetine versus clomipramine in the treatment of obsessive–compulsive disorder. *Eur Neuropsychopharmacol* **6**, 111–118.

MacKinnon RA and Michels R (1971) The obsessive patient. In *The Psychiatric Interview in Clinical Practice*, MacKinnon RA and Michels R (eds). W. B. Saunders, Philadelphia, pp. 89–109.

March JS, Frances A, Carpenter D, et al. (1997) The expert consensus guideline series: treatment of obsessive–compulsive disorder. *J Clin Psychiatry* **58**(Suppl. 4),.

Markovitz PJ, Stagnos J, and Calabresa JR (1990) Buspirone augmentation of fluoxetine on obsessive–compulsive disorder. *Am J Psychiatry* **147**, 798–800.

Marks I, Lelliot P, Basoglu M, et al. (1988) Clomipramine, self exposure and therapist-added exposure in obsessive–compulsive ritualizers. *Br J Psychiatry* **152**, 522–534.

Marks I, Stern A, Mawson D, et al. (1980) Clomipramine and exposure for obsessive–compulsive rituals. *Br J Psychiatry* **136**, 1–25.

McDougle CJ, Epperson CN, Pelton GH, et al. (2000) A double-blind, placebo-controlled study of risperidone addition in serotonin reuptake inhibitor refractory obsessive–compulsive disorder. *Arch Gen Psychiatry* **57**, 794–801.

McDougle CJ, Goodman WK, Leckman JF, et al. (1993) Limited therapeutic effect of addition of buspirone in fluvoxamine refractory obsessive–compulsive disorder. *Am J Psychiatry* **150**, 647–649.

McDougle CJ, Goodman WK, Price LH, et al. (1990) Neuroleptic addition in fluvoxamine refractory obsessive–compulsive disorder. *Am J Psychiatry* **147**, 652–654.

McDougle CJ, Price LH, Goodman WK, et al. (1991) A controlled trial of lithium augmentation in fluvoxamine refractory obsessive–compulsive disorder: lack of efficacy. *J Clin Psychopharmacol* **11**, 175–184.

McElroy SL, Hudson JI, Phillips KA, et al. (1993) Clinical and theoretical implications of a possible link between obsessive–compulsive and impulse control disorders. *Depression* **1**, 121–132.

McKeon P and Murray R (1987) Familial aspects of obsessive–compulsive neurosis. *Br J Psychiatry* **51**, 528–534.

Miguel EC, Coffey BJ, Baer L, et al. (1995) Phenomenology of intentional behaviors in obsessive-compulsive disorder and Tourette's disorder. *J Clin Psychiatry* **56**, 246–255.

Mindus P and Jenike MA (1992) Neurosurgical treatment of malignant obsessive–compulsive disorder. *Psychiatr Clin North Am* **15**, 921–938.

Mundo E, Bianchi L, and Bellodi L (1997) Efficacy of fluvoxamine, paroxetine and citalopram in the treatment of obsessive–compulsive disorder: a single-blind study. *J Clin Psychopharmacol* **17**, 267–271.

Myers JK, Weissman MM, Tischler GL, et al. (1984) Six–month prevalence of psychiatric disorders in three communities, 1980 to 1982. *Arch Gen Psychiatry* **41**, 949–958.

Nestadt G, Samuels J, Riddle M, et al. (2000) A family study of obsessive–compulsive disorder. *Arch Gen Psychiatry* **57**, 358–363.

Nicolini H, Cruz C, Camarena B, et al. (1999) Understanding the genetic basis of obsessive–compulsive disorder. *CNS Spect* **4**(5), 32–48.

Nordahl TE, Benkelfat C, Semple WE, et al. (1989) Cerebral glucose metabolic rates in obsessive–compulsive disorder. *Neuropsychopharmacology* **2**, 23–28.

Orley J and Wing JK (1979) Psychiatric disorders in two African villages. *Arch Gen Psychiatry* **36**, 513–520.

O'Sullivan G and Marks I (1991) Follow-up studies of behavioral treatment of phobia and obsessive–compulsive neurosis. *Psychiatr Ann* **21**, 368–373.

Pato MT, Pato CP, and Pauls DL (2002) Recent findings in the genetics of OCD. *J Clin Psychiatry* **63**(Suppl. 6), 30–33.

Pato MT and Steketee G (eds). (1997) *OCD Across the Life Cycle in American Psychiatric Press: Review of Psychiatry*, Vol. 16, American Psychiatric Press, Washington, DC.

Pato MT and Zohar J (eds). (2001) *Current Treatments of Obsessive–Compulsive Disorder*. American Psychiatric Press, Washington, DC.

Pato MT, Zohar-Kadouch R, Zohar J, et al. (1988) Return of symptoms after discontinuation of clomipramine in patients with obsessive–compulsive disorder. *Am J Psychiatry* **145**, 1521–1525.

Pauls DL (1999) Phenotypic variability in obsessive–compulsive disorder and its relationship to familial risk. *CNS Spect* **4**(6), 57–61.

Pauls DL, Alsobrook MP, Goodman W, et al. (1995) A family study of obsessive–compulsive disorder. *Am J Psychiatry* **152**, 76–84.

Pauls DL, Towbin KE, Leckman JF, et al. (1986) Gilles de la Tourette's syndrome and obsessive–compulsive disorder: evidence supporting a genetic relationship. *Arch Gen Psychiatry* **43**, 1180–1182.

Phillips KA (1991) Body dysmorphic disorder: the distress of imagined ugliness. *Am J Psychiatry* **148**, 1138–1149.

Phillips KA, McElroy SL, Hudson JI, et al. (1995) Body dysmorphic disorder: an OCD spectrum disorder, a form of affective spectrum disorder, or both? *J Clin Psychiatry* **56**(Suppl.), 41–51.

Pigott TA (1996) OCD: where the serotonin selective story begins. *J Clin Psychiatry* **57**(Suppl. 6), 11–20.

Pigott TA, L'Hereux F, Hill JL, et al. (1992a) A double-blind study of adjuvant buspirone hydrochloride in clomipramine-treated patients with obsessive–compulsive disorder. *J Clin Psychopharmacol* **12**, 11–18.

Pigott TA, Littenfer XF, Rubenstein CS, et al. (1992b) A double-blind, placebo-controlled study of trazodone in patients with obsessive–compulsive disorder. *J Clin Psychopharmacol* **12**, 156–162.

Pigott TA, Pato MT, Bernstein SE, et al. (1990) Controlled comparison of clomipramine and fluoxetine in the treatment of obsessive–compulsive disorder. *Arch Gen Psychiatry* **47**, 926–932.

Pigott TA, Zohar J, Hill JL, et al. (1991) Metergoline blocks the behavioral and neuroendocrine effects of orally administered *m*-chlorophenylpiperazine in patients with obsessive–compulsive disorder. *Biol Psychiatry* **29**, 418–426.

Pitman RK, Green RC, Jenike MA, et al. (1987) Clinical comparison of Tourette's disorder and obsessive–compulsive disorder. *Am J Psychiatry* **144**, 1166–1171.

Porto L, Bermanzohn PC, Pollack S, et al. (1997) A profile of obsessive–compulsive symptoms in schizophrenia. *CNS Spect* **2**, 21–25.

Rachman SJ and Hodgson RJ (1980) *Obsessions and Compulsions*. Prentice-Hall, Englewood Cliffs, NJ.

Rasmussen SA and Eisen JL (1991) Phenomenology of obsessive–compulsive disorder. In *Psychobiology of Obsessive–Compulsive Disorder*, Insel J, Rasmussen S (eds). Springer-Verlag, New York, pp. 743–758.

Rasmussen SA and Eisen JL (1992) The epidemiology and clinical features of OCD. *Psychiatr Clin North Am* **15**, 743–758.

Rasmussen SA, Eisen JL, and Pato MT (1993) Current issues in the pharmacologic management of obsessive–compulsive disorder. *J Clin Psychiatry* **54**(Suppl.), 4–9.

Rasmussen S, Hackett E, DuBoff E, et al. (1997) A 2-year study of sertraline in the treatment of obsessive–compulsive disorder. *Int Clin Psychopharmacol* **12**(6), 309–316.

Rasmussen SA and Tsuang MT (1986) Clinical characteristics and family history in DSM-III obsessive–compulsive disorder. *Am J Psychiatry* **143**, 317–322.

Rauch SL, Jenike MA, Alpert NM, et al. (1994) Regional cerebral blood flow measured during symptom provocation in obsessive–compulsive disorder using oxygen 15-labeled carbon dioxide and positron emission tomography. *Arch Gen Psychiatry* **51**, 62–70.

Riddle MA, Schaill L, King R, et al. (1990) Obsessive–compulsive disorder in children and adolescents: phenomenology and family history. *J Am Acad Child Adolesc Psychiatry* **29**, 766–772.

Robertson MM, Trimble MR, and Lees AJ (1988) The psychopathology of the Gilles de la Tourette syndrome: a phenomenological analysis. *Br J Psychiatry* **152**, 283–390.

Robins LN, Helzer JE, Weissman MM, et al. (1984) Lifetime prevalence of specific psychiatric disorders in three sites. *Arch Gen Psychiatry* **41**, 958–967.

Robinson D, Wu H, Munne RA, et al. (1995) Reduced caudate nucleus volume in obsessive–compulsive disorder. *Arch Gen Psychiatry* **52**, 393–398.

Salzman L (1983) Psychoanalytic therapy of the obsessional patient. *Curr Psychiatr Ther* **9**, 53–59.

Samuels J, Nestadt G, and Bienvenu OJ (2000) Personality disorders and normal personality dimensions in obsessive–compulsive disorder. *Br J Psychiatry* **177**, 457–462.

Saxena S, Brody AL, Schwartz JM, et al. (1998) Neuroimaging and frontal–subcortical circuitry in obsessive–compulsive disorder. *Br J Psychiatry* **173**(Suppl. 35), 26–37.

Saxena S, Wang D, Bystritsky A, et al. (1996) Risperidone augmentation of SRI treatment for refractory obsessive–compulsive disorder. *J Clin Psychiatry* **57**, 303–306.

Simpson HB, Gorfinkle KS, and Liebowitz MR (1999) Cognitive–behavioral therapy as an adjunct to serotonin reuptake inhibitors in obsessive–compulsive disorder: an open trial. *J Clin Psychiatry* **60**, 584–590.

Skoog G and Skoog I (1999) A 40-year follow-up of patients with obsessive–compulsive disorder. *Arch Gen Psychiatry* **56**, 121–127.

Stein DJ, Bouwer C, Hawkridge S, et al. (1997) Risperidone augmentation of serotonin reuptake inhibitors in obsessive–compulsive disorder and related disorders. *J Clin Psychiatry* **58**, 119–122.

Swedo SE, Leonard HL, Garvey M, et al. (1998) Pediatric autoimmune neuropsychiatric disorders associated with streptococcal infection: clinical description of the first 50 cases. *Am J Psychiatry* **155**, 264–271.

Swedo SE, Pietrini P, Leonard HL, et al. (1992) Cerebral glucose metabolism in childhood onset obsessive–compulsive disorder. Revisualization during pharmacology. *Arch Gen Psychiatry* **49**, 690–694.

Swedo SE, Rapoport JL, Leonard H, et al. (1989a) Obsessive–compulsive disorder in children and adolescents: clinical phenomenology of 70 consecutive cases. *Arch Gen Psychiatry* **46**, 335–341.

Swedo SE, Schapiro MB, Grady CL, et al. (1989b) Cerebral glucose metabolism in childhood-onset obsessive–compulsive disorder. *Arch Gen Psychiatry* **46**, 518–523.

Szegedi A, Wetzel H, Leal M, et al. (1996) Combination treatment with clomipramine and fluvoxamine: drug monitoring, safety and tolerability data. *J Clin Psychiatry* **57**, 257–264.

Szeszko PR, Robinson D, Alvir JMJ, et al. (1999) Orbital frontal and amygdala volume reductions in obsessive–compulsive disorder. *Arch Gen Psychiatry* **56**, 913–919.

The Clomipramine Collaborative Study Group (1991) Efficacy of clomipramine in OCD: results of a multicenter double-blind trial. *Arch Gen Psychiatry* **48**, 730–738.

Thoren P, Asberg M, Bertilsson L, et al. (1980) Clomipramine treatment of obsessive–compulsive disorder. II. Biochemical aspects. *Arch Gen Psychiatry* **37**, 1289–1294.

Tollefson GD, Rampey AH, Potvin JH, et al. (1994b) A multicenter investigation of fixed dose fluoxetine in the treatment of obsessive–compulsive disorder. *Arch Gen Psychiatry* **51**, 559–567.

Walter CS (1973) Clinical impression of treatment of obsessional states with intravenous clomipramine. *J Int Med* **1**, 413–416.

Yeh EH and Chang L (1989) Prevalence of psychiatric disorders in Taiwan. *Acta Psychiatr Scand* **79**, 136–147.

Zajecka JM, Fawcett J, and Guy C (1990) Co-existing major depression and obsessive–compulsive disorder treated with venlafaxine. *J Clin Psychopharmacol* **10**, 152–153.

Zohar J and Insel TR (1987) Obsessive–compulsive disorder: psychobiological approaches to diagnosis, treatment, and pathophysiology. *Biol Psychiatry* **22**, 667–687.

Zohar J, Insel TR, Zohar KR, et al. (1988) Serotonergic responsivity in obsessive–compulsive disorder. Effects of chronic clomipramine treatment. *Arch Gen Psychiatry* **45**, 167–172.

Zohar J and Judge R (1996) Paroxetine versus clomipramine in the treatment of obsessive–compulsive disorder. *Br J Psychiatry* **169**, 468–474.

Zohar AH, Ratoni G, Pauls DL, et al. (1992) An epidemiological study of obsessive–compulsive disorder and related disorders in Israeli adolescents. *J Am Acad Child Adolesc Psychiatry* **31**, 1057–1061.

34 ● Anxiety Disorders: Traumatic Stress Disorders

POSTTRAUMATIC STRESS DISORDER

Diagnosis

Posttraumatic stress disorder (PTSD) is defined in the DSM-IV-TR by six different criteria (see DSM-IV-TR diagnostic criteria on page 927). The diagnosis of PTSD is based on a history of exposure to a traumatic stressor, the simultaneous appearance of three different symptom clusters, a minimal duration, and the existence of functional disturbance. To qualify as traumatic, the event must have involved actual or threatened death or serious injury or a threat to the individual or others, and exposure to this event must arouse an intense affective response characterized by fear, helplessness, or horror. In children, disorganized or agitated behavior can be seen in lieu of an intense affective response. Symptomatically, there must be at least one of five possible intrusive-reexperiencing symptoms. These have the quality of obsessive, recurring, intrusive, and distressing recollections either in the form of imagery or thoughts or in the form of recurrent distressing dreams. Intense psychological distress or physiological reactivity on exposure to either an external reminder or an internal reminder of the trauma can also occur. The flashback experience, or reliving of the event, is less common.

DSM-IV-TR Diagnostic Criteria

309.81 Posttraumatic Stress Disorder

A. The person has been exposed to a traumatic event in which both of the following were present:

    (1) the person experienced, witnessed, or was confronted with an event or events that involved actual or threatened death or serious injury, or a threat to the physical integrity of self or others

    (2) the person's response involved intense fear, helplessness, or horror. **Note:** In children, this may be expressed instead by disorganized or agitated behavior

B. The traumatic event is persistently reexperienced in one (or more) of the following ways:

    (1) recurrent and intrusive distressing recollections of the event, including images, thoughts, or perceptions. **Note:** In young children, repetitive play may occur in which themes or aspects of the trauma are expressed

    (2) recurrent distressing dreams of the event. **Note:** In children, there may be frightening dreams without recognizable content

    (3) acting or feeling as if the traumatic event were recurring (includes a sense of reliving the experience, illusions, hallucinations, and dissociative flashback episodes, including those that occur on awakening or when intoxicated). **Note:** In young children, trauma-specific reenactment may occur

    (4) intense psychological distress at exposure to internal or external cues that symbolize or resemble an aspect of the traumatic event

    (5) physiological reactivity on exposure to internal or external cues that symbolize or resemble an aspect of the traumatic event

C. Persistent avoidance of stimuli associated with the trauma and numbing of general responsiveness (not present before the trauma), as indicated by three (or more) of the following:

    (1) efforts to avoid thoughts, feelings, or conversations associated with the trauma

    (2) efforts to avoid activities, places, or people that arouse recollections of the trauma

    (3) inability to recall an important aspect of the trauma

    (4) markedly diminished interest or participation in significant activities

    (5) feeling of detachment or estrangement from others

    (6) restricted range of affect (e.g., unable to have loving feelings)

    (7) sense of a foreshortened future (e.g., does not expect to have a career, marriage, children, or a normal life span)

D. Persistent symptoms of increased arousal (not present before the trauma), as indicated by two (or more) of the following:

    (1) difficulty falling or staying asleep

    (2) irritability or outbursts of anger

(3) difficulty concentrating
(4) hypervigilance
(5) exaggerated startle response

E. Duration of the disturbance (symptoms in criteria B, C, and D) is more than 1 month.
F. The disturbance causes clinically significant distress or impairment in social, occupational, or other important areas of functioning.

Specify if:

Acute: if duration of symptoms is less than 3 months

Chronic: if duration of symptoms is 3 months or more

Specify if:

With delayed onset: if onset of symptoms is at least 6 months after the stressor

---

Reprinted with permission from the Diagnostic and Statistical Manual of Mental Disorders, Fourth Edition, Text Revision. Copyright 2000 American Psychiatric Association.

Symptom cluster C in the DSM-IV-TR criteria in actuality embodies two somewhat different psychopathologies—namely, phobic avoidance and numbing or withdrawal. The phobic avoidance is expressed either in (1) efforts to avoid thoughts and feelings and conversations associated with the trauma or (2) in efforts to avoid activities, places, or people that arouse recollections of the trauma. (3) Psychogenic amnesia, a more dissociative symptom, also is in this symptom grouping, followed by (4) markedly diminished interest, (5) feeling detached or estranged, (6) having a restricted range of affect, and (7) having a sense of a foreshortened future. At least three of these seven symptoms must be present.

Hyperarousal symptoms, somewhat similar to those of generalized anxiety disorder, are also present in PTSD and at least one of five of the following symptoms is required: difficulty sleeping, irritability or anger, poor concentration, hypervigilance, and exaggerated startle response.

With regard to the symptoms as a whole, it is evident that they embody features of different psychiatric disorders, including obsessive–compulsive processes, generalized anxiety disorder, panic attacks, phobic avoidance, dissociation, and depression. Finally, it is necessary for symptoms to have lasted at least 1 month and for the disturbance to have caused clinically significant distress or impairment.

Epidemiology

Community-based studies conducted in the United States have documented a lifetime prevalence rate for PTSD of approximately 8% of the adult population (Kessler et al. 1995). General population female-to-male lifetime prevalence ratio is 2 : 1 (Breslau 2001). The highest rates of PTSD occurrence for particular traumatic exposures (occurring in one-third to three-fourths of those exposed) are among survivors of rape, military combat and captivity, graves registration (i.e., registering dead bodies through the morgue), and ethnically or politically motivated interment and genocide (Breslau 2001).

Epidemiological studies show that PTSD often remains chronic, with a significant number of people remaining symptomatic, several years after the initial event. In support of this view are epidemiological data that show that recovery does not occur frequently. For example, the National Vietnam Veterans Readjustment study (Kulka et al. 1990) found lifetime and current prevalence rates of PTSD to be, respectively, 30.9 and 15.2% in men and 26.9 and 8.5% in women. In a population of rape victims, Kilpatrick and colleagues (1987) found a lifetime prevalence rate of 75.8% and a current prevalence rate of 39.4%. In children, studies by Pynoos and associates (1987, 1993) revealed prevalence rates of 58.4% in children exposed to sniper attacks in the United States and 70.2% in those exposed to an earthquake in Armenia. In two of the Epidemiological Catchment Area (ECA) sites, Davidson and coworkers (1991) and Helzer and others (1987) found that 47 and 33%, respectively, retained the diagnosis of PTSD for more than 1 year. Kessler and colleagues (1995) documented that one-third of those diagnosed with PTSD fail to recover even after many years. Therefore, chronicity of PTSD is not limited to the more severe treatment-seeking samples.

Course

Immediately following traumatic exposure, a high percentage of individuals develop a mixed symptom picture, which includes disorganized behavior, dissociative symptoms, psychomotor change, and sometimes, paranoia. The diagnosis of Acute Stress Disorder accounts for many of these reactions. These reactions are generally short-lived, although by 1 month the symptom picture often settles into a more classic PTSD presentation. After rape, for example, as many as 90% of individuals may qualify for the diagnosis of PTSD. Approximately 50% of people with PTSD recover, and approximately 50% develop a persistent, chronic form of the illness still present 1 year following the traumatic event.

The longitudinal course of PTSD is variable (Blank 1993). Permanent recovery occurs in some people, whereas others show a relatively unchanging course with only mild fluctuation. Still others show a more obvious fluctuation with intermittent periods of well-being and recurrences of major symptoms. In a limited number of cases, the passage of time does not bring a resolution of symptoms, and the individual's condition tends to deteriorate with age. Particular symptoms that have been noted to increase with time in many people include startle response, nightmares, irritability, and depression. Clinicians, during World War II, also observed that the existence of marked startle response and hypervigilance in the acute aftermath of exposure to combat often represented a comparatively poor prognostic sign. In children, PTSD can be, and often is, chronic and debilitating (Nader et al. 1990).

General medical conditions may occur as a direct consequence of the trauma (e.g., head injury, burns). In addition, chronic PTSD may be associated with increased rates of adverse physical outcomes, including musculoskeletal problems and cardiovascular morbidity (Beckham et al. 1997, Boscarino 1997, Schnurr and Jankowski 1999).

Differential Diagnosis

PTSD symptoms may overlap with symptoms of a number of other disorders in the DSM-IV-TR. Both PTSD and adjustment disorder are etiologically related to stress exposure. PTSD may be distinguished from adjustment disorder by assessing whether the traumatic stress meets the severity criteria described earlier. Also, if there are an insufficient number of symptoms to qualify for the diagnosis, this might merit a diagnosis of adjustment disorder.

Specific phobias may arise after traumatic exposure. For example, after an automobile accident, victims may develop phobic avoidance of traveling, but without the intrusive or hyperarousal symptoms. In such cases, a diagnosis of specific phobia should be given instead of a diagnosis of PTSD.

The criteria set for generalized anxiety disorder include a list of six symptoms of hyperarousal, of which four are common to PTSD: being on edge, poor concentration, irritability, and sleep disturbance. PTSD requires the additional symptoms as described earlier, and the worry in PTSD is focused on concerns about reexperiencing the trauma. In contrast, the worry in generalized anxiety disorder is about a number of different situations and concerns. However, it is possible for the two conditions to coexist.

In obsessive–compulsive disorder, recurring and intrusive thoughts occur, but the individual recognizes these to be inappropriate and unrelated to any particular life experience. Obsessive–compulsive disorder is a common comorbid condition in PTSD and may develop with generalization (e.g., compulsive washing for months after a rape to reduce contamination feelings). It may also develop by activation of an underlying obsessive–compulsive disorder diathesis.

Autonomic hyperarousal is a cardinal part of panic attack, which may indicate a diagnosis of panic disorder. To distinguish between panic disorder and PTSD, the therapist needs to assess whether panic attacks are related to the trauma or reminders of the same (in which case they would be subsumed under a diagnosis of PTSD) or whether they occur unexpectedly and spontaneously (in which case a diagnosis of panic disorder would be justified).

Depression and PTSD share a significant overlap, including four of the criterion C cluster symptoms and three of the criterion D cluster symptoms. Thus, an individual who presents with reduced interest, estrangement, numbing, impaired concentration, insomnia, irritability, and sense of a foreshortened future may manifest either disorder. PTSD may give rise to depression as well, and it is possible for the two conditions to coexist. In a few instances, an individual with prior depression may be more vulnerable to developing PTSD. Reexperiencing symptoms are present only in PTSD.

Dissociative disorders also overlap with PTSD. In the early aftermath of serious trauma, the clinical picture may be predominantly one of the dissociative states (see the section on Acute Stress Disorder [ASD] on page 938). ASD differs from PTSD in that the symptom pattern occurs within the first few days after exposure to the trauma, lasts no longer than 4 weeks, and is typically accompanied by prominent dissociative symptoms.

More rarely, PTSD must be distinguished from other disorders producing perceptual alterations, such as schizophrenia and other psychotic disorders, delirium, substance use disorders, and general medical conditions producing psychosis (e.g., brain tumors).

The differential diagnosis is important but, notwithstanding, PTSD is unlikely to occur in isolation. Psychiatric comorbidity is the rule rather than the exception, and a number of studies have demonstrated that, in both clinical and epidemiological populations (Davidson et al. 1991, Davidson et al. 1985), a wide range of disorders is likely to occur at an increased probability. These include major depressive disorder, all of the anxiety disorders, alcohol and substance use disorders, somatization disorder, and schizophrenia and schizophreniform disorder. A few studies have documented the course of comorbid conditions. For example, Shalev and colleagues (1990) have shown that major depressive disorder co-occurs with PTSD, but can take a separate course. Several researchers have provided evidence that comorbid substance abuse tends to be a consequence rather than a precursor of PTSD (Breslau et al. 1991, Bremner et al. 1996).

Etiology

The Event

PTSD is defined in terms of etiology as much as phenomenology. The disorder cannot exist unless the individual has been exposed to a traumatic event with a particular set of properties. Community-based epidemiological studies suggest that 70% of individuals will experience at least one traumatic event meeting criterion A(1)—see table description of PTSD over the course of the lifetime (Norris 1992). The relative severity of the traumatic event, predisposing factors, and peritraumatic environmental factors must all be considered in understanding the etiology of PTSD. In most instances, occurrence of the disorder represents the outcome of an interaction among these three groups of factors.

The likelihood of developing PTSD with regard to the nature of the event was reviewed by March (1990, 1993). A consistent relationship occurred between magnitude of stress exposure and risk of developing PTSD. This association held up in many different trauma populations in adults and children.

In the St. Louis ECA study, PTSD rates were three times higher in wounded Vietnam veterans than in nonwounded veterans (Helzer et al. 1987). In the North Carolina ECA study, PTSD was much more likely to occur in sexual assault victims who were physically injured than in those who were noninjured (Winfield et al. 1990). Pynoos and colleagues (1987, 1993) showed that physical proximity to the stressful event was linearly related to the risk of PTSD symptoms in two different populations. Saigh (1991) revealed that PTSD could arise in children from direct, witnessed, or verbal exposure. Aspects of the symptom picture vary with stressor-specific factors (Nader et al. 1991, Kendall-Tackett et al. 1993).

March (1993) concluded that besides the objective event characteristics—namely, actual or threatened death or injury or threat to physical integrity—cognitive and affective responses to the stressor are also important in determining the likelihood that PTSD will develop. In particular, the experience of intense fear, helplessness, or horror is a determinant of a person's likelihood to develop PTSD. There are medical/surgical events (Shalev 1990) such as a cancer diagnosis or open-heart surgery that have been documented to meet criterion A (DSM-IV-TR criteria for PTSD) in some individuals. Medical events that are witnessed may also be considered traumatic if the witness's response involves intense fear, helplessness, and horror. For example, the spouse of an individual with diabetes who witnessed multiple medically indicated amputations in the individual can consider it a traumatic event.

Biological Factors

Identification of biological changes related to PTSD has provided hypotheses for understanding how some individuals develop PTSD in response to a traumatic event whereas others do not (Yehuda 2002). As summarized by Yehuda (2002), individuals with chronic PTSD have increased circulating levels of norepinephrine (Yehuda et al. 1998) and increased reactivity of the alpha-2-adrenergic receptors (Southwick et al. 1993). These changes have been hypothesized to possibly account for some of the somatic symptoms that occur in individuals with PTSD. Neuroanatomical studies have implicated alterations in the amygdala and hippocampus in individuals with PTSD (Rauch et al. 2000). Functional magnetic resonance imaging and positron-emission tomography have demonstrated increased reactivity of the amygdala and anterior paralimbic region to trauma-related stimuli (Lieberzon et al. 1999). Furthermore, in response to trauma-related stimuli, there is decreased reactivity of the anterior cingulate and orbitofrontal areas (Shin et al. 1999). These biological alterations suggest that there may be a neuroanatomical substrate for symptoms (intrusive recollections and other cognitive problems) that characterize PTSD (Schnuff et al. 2001, Vasterling et al. 1998). However, it is unknown whether these changes are preexisting, a result of traumatic exposure, or a result of having PTSD (Pitman 2001).

A meta-analytic review found a positive association between the diagnosis of PTSD and basal cardiovascular activity (Yehuda et al. 1998). Particularly, individuals with a current PTSD diagnosis had higher resting heart rate (HR) relative to both trauma-exposed individuals without a PTSD diagnosis and nontrauma-exposed controls. An additional analysis revealed that differences were greatest in studies with the most chronic PTSD samples (Buckley and Kaloupek 2001). Along with increased 24-hour urinary catecholamines, results suggest an increase in sympathetic tone (Pitman 1993). There has been repeated demonstration that there is heightened sympathetic arousal in individuals with PTSD when reexposed to the original trauma in controlled settings.

There is evidence of brain dysfunction in individuals with PTSD as evidenced by abnormalities in evoked potentials. For example, as reported by Pitman and colleagues (1999), electroencephalographic event-related potential (ERP) response abnormalities in PTSD include reduced P2 amplitude at high stimulus intensities, impaired P1 habituation, and attenuated P3 amplitude to target auditory stimuli. Larger P3 and N1 amplitude responses and shorter P3 and N1 latencies have been reported in PTSD subjects in response to trauma-related stimuli. On the basis of a review of these studies (Pitman et al. 1999), these ERP findings suggest that individuals with PTSD have increased cortical inhibition to high-intensity stimuli, impairments in memory and concentration, auditory gating deficits and heightened selective attention to trauma-related stimuli. However, whether these processing abnormalities are a precursor or a result of PTSD awaits further study.

The hypothalamic–pituitary–adrenal (HPA) axis has been the most extensively studied neuroendocrine system in PTSD, the findings of which were comprehensively reviewed by Yehuda and coworkers (1991). They summarized the principal findings as follows: reduced 24-hour urinary cortisol excretion, supersuppression of cortisol after low-dose dexamethasone administration, blunting of corticotropin in response to corticotropin-releasing hormone, and increased numbers of glucocorticoid receptors. Their interpretation of these findings suggested that chronic PTSD is accompanied by supersuppression of the emergency HPA response to acute stress. The authors speculated that this may result from the organism's attempt to protect itself from the potentially toxic effect of high levels of corticosteroids that might occur with repeated exposure to stress or from reminders of the trauma. In further support of the importance of HPA axis alteration in PTSD is the finding (Yehuda et al. 1991) that glucocorticoid receptor changes also correlate with the severity of PTSD symptoms, but not with the less specific anxiety and depressive symptoms measured on other rating scales. More recently, in a large sample of Vietnam veterans, combat-exposed veterans with current PTSD had lower cortisol compared to noncombat-exposed veterans without PTSD or combat-exposed veterans with lifetime PTSD but without current PTSD (Boscarino 1996).

Psychological Factors

Conditioning theory has been helpful in explaining the process through which stimuli that are associated with a traumatic event can alone elicit intense emotional responses in individuals who have PTSD. Cues (i.e., conditioned stimuli) that are present at the time of the trauma (the unconditioned stimulus) become associated with the unconditioned emotional response (fear, helplessness, or horror). Following the traumatic event, these cues alone can then repeatedly elicit the strong emotional response. For example, a woman who has been raped (unconditioned stimulus) in a dark alley (conditioned stimulus) by a man (conditioned stimulus) and has an intense fear response (unconditioned response) may demonstrate a fear response (now the conditioned response) when she sees a dark alley (conditioned stimulus) or is in the presence of a man (conditioned stimulus). Avoidance behaviors develop to decrease anxiety associated with the conditioned stimuli. For example, the woman who has been raped may avoid going outside when it is dark and also avoid being in the company of men. Behavioral treatments using exposure principles require confrontation with the feared situation and may ultimately lead to reduction of anxiety (Solomon et al. 1992).

Genetic-Familial Factors

Connor and Davidson (1997) reviewed many of the complexities involved in studying familial risk factors of PTSD. From the available literature, which is based on male combat veterans, general population surveys and rape-trauma-related PTSD, there is evidence to suggest that anxiety and depression in families is a risk factor for PTSD (Davidson et al. 1998). A twin study of Vietnam veterans concordant and discordant for combat exposure has shown that a significant part of the variance is explained on the basis of genetic factors with respect to all three symptom clusters (i.e., intrusive, avoidant, and hyperarousal symptoms) (True et al. 1993). McLeod and colleagues (2001) examined the role of genetic and environmental influences on the relationship between combat exposure, posttraumatic stress disorder symptoms, and alcohol use in 4072 male–male twin pairs; the authors tested three hypotheses: (1) alcohol use and PTSD may share an environmental risk factor (i.e., combat) that increases the possibility that they will occur together; (2) the relationship between PTSD and alcohol problems is that one may develop as a consequence of the other; and (3) PTSD and alcohol problems occur together because of a shared vulnerability that increases risk for both disorders. Their analyses supported hypothesis (3); the same additive genetic influences that affect the level of combat exposure also include the level of alcohol use and level of PTSD symptoms. These findings are most consistent with the shared vulnerability hypothesis in which combat exposure, PTSD symptoms, and alcohol use are associated because some portion of the genes that influence vulnerability to combat also influence vulnerability to PTSD symptoms and alcohol consumption. It is important to note, however, that specific unique environmental factors the twins did not share were more important than genetic factors for combat exposure and PTSD symptoms, whereas environmental influences appeared about equally important as genetic influences on alcohol use. Overall, the evidence suggests that psychiatric history, both personal or in family members, increases the likelihood of being exposed to a trauma and of developing PTSD once exposed (True and Lyons 1999, Hidalgo and Davidson 2000).

Other Factors

Although systematic research is scant, it may be that individuals exposed to repeated or continuous trauma, particularly of an interpersonal nature, may be more likely to develop PTSD. Trauma involving loss of community or support structures is likely to be particularly damaging. Because social support has been held to produce a buffering effect, lack of support might be considered an additional vulnerability factor. Women are at more risk than men for PTSD.

Treatment

A number of goals are common to all treatments of PTSD and can be summarized as follows: (1) to reduce intrusive symptoms; (2) to reduce avoidance symptoms; (3) to reduce numbing and withdrawal; (4) to dampen hyperarousal; (5) to reduce psychotic symptoms when present; and (6) to improve impulse control when this is a problem. By reducing troublesome symptoms, a number of other important goals can also be accomplished as follows: (1) to develop the capacity to interpret events more realistically with respect to their threat content; (2) to improve interpersonal work and leisure functioning; (3) to promote self-esteem, trust, and feelings of safety; (4) to explore and clarify meanings attributed to the event; (5) to promote access to memories that have been dissociated or repressed when judged to be clinically appropriate; (6) to strengthen social support systems; and (7) to move from identification as a victim to that of a survivor.

The three major treatment approaches, pharmacotherapeutic, cognitive–behavioral, and psychodynamic, all emphasize different aspects of the problem. Pharmacotherapy targets the underlying neurobiological alterations found in PTSD and attempts to control symptoms so that the above treatment goals can be more effectively accomplished. Cognitive–behavioral treatments emphasize the phobic avoidance and counterproductive reenactments that often occur, along with the identification of faulty beliefs that arise owing to the trauma, and replace them with more adaptive beliefs, usually in association with direct therapeutic exposure. The psychodynamic approach emphasizes the associations that arise from the trauma experience and that lead to unconscious and conscious representations. Defense mechanisms that lead to lack of memory, and the contributions from early development, are also brought into play in psychodynamic therapy.

General principles of treating PTSD involve explanation and destigmatization, which can be provided both to the individual and to family members. This often includes a description of the symptoms of PTSD and the way in which it can affect behaviors and relationships. Information can be given about general treatment principles, pointing out that sometimes cure is attainable but that at other times symptom containment is a more realistic treatment goal, particularly in chronic and severe PTSD. Regaining self-esteem and attaining greater control over impulses and affect are also desired in many instances. Information can be provided as to appropriate literature, local support groups and resources, and names and addresses of national advocacy organizations. If the therapist attends to these important issues early in treatment, the individual is able to more readily build trust and also to appreciate that the therapist shows a good understanding both of the condition and of the individual.

PTSD is sometimes comparatively straightforward to treat and at other times it is more complicated. However, treatment by a mental health clinician (rather than a primary care clinician) is almost always indicated. The initial history taking can evoke strong affect to a greater degree than is customarily found in other disorders. In fact, it may take several interviews for the details to emerge. A sensitive yet persistent approach is needed on the part of the interviewer. During treatment, although the mental health care clinician will clearly want to impart a sense of optimism to the individual, it is also a reflection of reality to point out early that recovery may be a slow process and that some symptoms (e.g., phobic avoidance, startle response) may persist. It is important for the mental health care clinician to be comfortable in hearing and tolerating unpleasant affect and often horrifying stories. All these must take place in a noncritical and accepting manner. Specific treatment approaches include the use of pharmacotherapy, psychotherapy, anxiety management, and attention to the general issues described earlier.

A stepwise sequence of approaches may be used in the treatment of PTSD but it must be said that there are no definitive guidelines currently in place. As a result, the particular order in which treatments are considered varies on the basis of individual circumstances. Also, no uniform definition exists as to what constitutes a good or poor response to treatment. In general, some symptoms of chronic PTSD persist, albeit at a considerably reduced level, in people who have undergone treatment. A summary of the limited information available for predicting response to pharmacotherapy and behavioral therapy in PTSD arising from combat trauma is given elsewhere (Davidson and Fairbank 1993).

Somatic Treatments

PTSD may be accompanied by enduring neurochemical and psychophysiological changes and can lead to substantial impairment and distress. Sometimes, the intensity of symptoms is severe enough to preclude the effective use of trauma-focused psychotherapy. In these situations, the use of medication should not be delayed unnecessarily. Initial studies showed benefit for the tricyclic antidepressant and monoamine oxidase inhibitor medications. However, the selective serotonin reuptake inhibitors (SSRIs) have now replaced these as first-line agents, based upon evidence from several placebo-controlled trials. The main groups of medications relevant to the treatment of PTSD along with dose ranges and chief side effects are listed in Table 34-1. A suggested sequencing of treatment is outlined in Table 34-2.

Table 34-1   Medications in Posttraumatic Stress Disorder: Dose Ranges and Side Effects

Drug Category	Dose Range (mg/day)	Common or Problematical Side Effects
Antidepressants		Gastrointestinal disturbance, sexual dysfunction, agitation
Selective serotonin reuptake inhibitors		
Fluoxetine	10–60	
Fluvoxamine	50–300	
Sertraline	50–200	Insomnia
Paroxetine	10–60	Tiredness
Nefazodone	50–600	Headache, dry mouth, nausea
Tricyclic antidepressants		Anticholinergic effects, cardiovascular symptoms, weight gain
Amitriptyline	50–300	Sexual dysfunction, sedation (for all tricyclic antidepressants)
Imipramine	50–300	
Monoamine oxidase inhibitors		
Phenelzine	15–90	Weight gain, dizziness, sleep disturbance, sexual dysfunction, hypertensive reactions, hyperpyretic states
Anticonvulsants		
Carbamazepine	200–1500	Hematological effects
Valproic acid	125–2000	Gastrointestinal disturbance, sedation
Lamotrigine	50–200	Rash, exfoliative dermatitis, Stevens–Johnson syndrome
Mood stabilizers		
Lithium carbonate	300–1200	Gastrointestinal disturbance, polyuria, headache
Antiadrenergic drugs		
Propranolol	20–160	Depression, hypertension, rebound hypertension
Clonidine	0.1–0.4	Memory problems, dizziness, tiredness
Prazosin	2–10	Dizziness, hypotension
Anxiolytics	0.5–6	
Benzodiazepines		
Clonazepam	0.5–6	
Alprazolam	0.25–4	Sedation, memory problems, incoordination, dependence
Diazepam	2–40	Withdrawal, rebound, disinhibition (for all benzodiazepines)
Chlordiazepoxide	5–40	
Others		
Azapirones	5–60	
Buspirone		Agitation, gastrointestinal disturbance, headaches
Neuroleptics		
Thioridazine	25–300	Extrapyramidal symptoms
Haloperidol	0.5–4	Sedation, anticholinergic effects
Others		

Several placebo-controlled trials have shown positive effects for the SSRI medications, including fluoxetine, sertraline (Davidson et al. 2001, Brady et al. 2000) and paroxetine (Marshall et al. 1998). Long-term use of sertraline is associated with a substantial reduction in relapse over a 15-month period (Frank et al. 1988). Data support positive effects for SSRI in men and women and in adults who have survived all major classes of trauma (e.g., combat, sexual violence, nonsexual violence, and accident). Each of these medications has broad-spectrum properties across the full symptom range of the disorder as well as improving function and, perhaps, resilience or stress coping (Connor et al. 1999). They also support the benefit of SSRI in those with and without comorbid major depression (Davidson et al. 2001, Brady et al. 2000, Marshall et al. 1998, Connor et al. 1999, van der Kolk et al. 1994, Davidson et al. in press).

At this point, the indications for antipsychotic and mood-stabilizing drugs are poorly defined, but clinical experience suggests that they continue to have a role in the pharmacologic treatment of PTSD. Antipsychotic medications can be useful in individuals with

Table 34-2	Pharmacotherapy Steps for Posttraumatic Stress Disorder

Step 1

Selective serotonin reuptake inhibitor (SSRI)
Adjunctive medications:
    If prominent hyperarousal: benzodiazepine or buspirone
    If prominent mood liability or explosiveness: anticonvulsant or lithium
    If prominent dissociation: valproic acid
    If persistent insomnia: trazodone
    If psychotic: atypical antipsychotic

Step 2

If no response or intolerance to SSRI:
    Dual action antidepressant, e.g., mirtazapine, venlafaxine
    Adjunctive medications as above

Step 3

If no response to Step 1 or 2:
    Monoamine oxidase inhibitor
    Adjunctive medications as above

Step 4

Other useful drugs:
    Propranolol—hyperarousal
    Clonidine—startle response
    Neuroleptics—psychosis, poor impulse control

poor impulse control or in those who manifest features of borderline personality disorder. Lithium and carbamazepine can also be useful in such individuals but might benefit individuals who are subject to mood swings and angry or explosive outbursts. The appropriate role for the use of benzodiazepines is not well defined. The antiphobic and antiarousal effects of the benzodiazepines should, in theory, be helpful in PTSD. However, withdrawal from short-acting benzodiazepines may also introduce an additional set of problems with intense symptom rebound. In individuals who have a propensity to abuse alcohol and other substances, benzodiazepines are not recommended.

Overall, the antidepressants, mood stabilizers, and anticonvulsants are the medication groups that are generally considered primary for treating PTSD; beta-blockers, alpha-2-agonists, and anxiolytics have a less clearly defined place. Often, individuals need a combination of drugs, but polypharmacy should be utilized in a carefully planned fashion. Also, since the time course of response may be slow, it is advisable to persist with a particular course of action for at least 8 weeks before deciding that it has been unhelpful. It is possible that avoidance and numbing symptoms respond more effectively to SSRI drugs.

Cognitive and Behavioral Therapies

Despite theoretical differences, most schools of psychotherapy recognize that cognitively oriented approaches to the treatment of anxiety must include an element of exposure (Marks 1987). Because PTSD involves aberrant and voluntary programs for the avoidance of danger that are conditioned by real experience, correction of these "fear structures" requires exposure to ensure habituation. Although a range of possible PTSD interventions has recently been reviewed (Foa et al. 2000) including group therapy, cognitive–behavioral therapy, eye movement desensitization and reprocessing, and psychodynamic therapy, the preponderance of current evidence suggests that the primary effective component of PTSD treatment is prolonged exposure (Rothbaum et al. 2000). Prolonged exposure depends on the fact that anxiety will be extinguished in the absence of real threat, given a sufficient duration of exposure *in vivo* or in imagination to traumatic stimuli. In PTSD, the individual retells the traumatic experience as if it were happening again, until doing so becomes a pedestrian exercise and anxiety decreases. Between sessions, individuals perform exposure homework, including listening to tapes of the flooding sessions and limited exposure *in vivo*. A review of 12 studies suggests that prolonged exposure is a component of the most well-controlled study designs and is associated with positive results (Rothbaum et al. 2000). However, not every individual may be a candidate for exposure. Owing to the high anxiety and temporarily increased symptoms associated with prolonged exposure, there are individuals who will be reluctant to confront traumatic reminders. Individuals in whom guilt or anger are primary emotional responses to the traumatic event (as opposed to anxiety) may not profit from prolonged exposure (Foa et al. 1995, Pitman et al. 1991). More empirical research is needed to evaluate how this efficacious treatment can be most effectively implemented in nonacademic settings. In addition, additional research is needed to identify methods to increase individual tolerability of the treatment.

Anxiety management techniques are designed to reduce anxiety by providing individuals with better skills for controlling worry and fear. Among such techniques are muscle relaxation, thought stopping, control of breathing and diaphragmatic breathing, communication skills, guided self-dialogue, and stress inoculation training (SIT). Although these interventions have less empirical evidence regarding treatment efficacy for PTSD, generally the results are positive and further controlled evaluation across trauma population samples is needed.

Further, cognitive approaches to the treatment of PTSD have also gained empirical support (Resick and Schnicke 1992). A cognitive approach to treatment includes training individuals in challenging problematic cognitions such as self-blame. In a recent comparison of cognitive therapy to imaginal exposure in the treatment of chronic PTSD, both treatments were associated with positive improvements at posttreatment and follow-up, with no differences in outcome between treatments (Tarrier et al. 1999). However, individuals who received imaginal exposure were more likely to experience an increase in PTSD symptoms during the treatment course, and those who did were more likely to miss treatment sessions, rate the therapy as less credible, and be rated as less motivated by the therapist.

Other recent approaches have focused on efficaciously treating one aspect of PTSD symptomatology, such as anger (Yehuda 1999), nightmares (Krakow et al. 2001), or authority problems (Lubin and Johnson 2000). There has also been a recent report of positive results using interventions to target both PTSD and a comorbid disorder. For example, Triffleman and colleagues (1999) reported individual improvement using a group intervention to simultaneously treat co-occurring substance abuse and PTSD. Falsetti and colleagues (2001) have reported an intervention entitled multiple channel exposure therapy (M-CET) to treat comorbid panic attacks and PTSD.

In contrast to the treatment-efficacy literature for adults with PTSD, the child-focused PTSD literature is limited to open trials and case reports (Ruggiero et al. 2001). Treatment practices for childhood PTSD have recently been surveyed (Cohen et al. 2001). However, in their review of the current literature, Ruggiero and colleagues (2001) underscore that adult treatment approaches need to be empirically evaluated for use in children with PTSD.

As no single treatment for PTSD has been shown to be curative, individual characteristics, characterization of the nature and range of stress responses of trauma victims (McFarlane and Yehuda 2000), partial response (Taylor et al. 2001), treatment combinations, sequencing of treatment approaches, and further well-controlled investigations of current approaches are all important empirical topics to be addressed. For example, in individuals unwilling to undergo exposure therapy, teaching of affect management skills may be helpful (Wolfsdorf and Zlotnick 2001).

Psychodynamic Therapy

Psychodynamically based approaches emphasize the interpretation of the traumatic event as being a critical determinant of symptoms. Treatment is geared to alter attributions, usually by means of slow exposure and through confrontation and awareness of the negative affect that have been generated by the trauma. Conflictual meanings begin to appear, and it is the task of treatment to reinterpret the experience in a more realistic and adaptive fashion. During such treatment, it is important to ensure that the affect intensity is not overwhelming or disorganizing. Obviously, support needs to be provided throughout, and sometimes other treatment approaches are used adjunctively. Excessive and maladaptive behaviors such as avoidance, use of alcohol or work, or risk taking may occur as a means of coping with the experience and these need to be identified and addressed.

ACUTE STRESS DISORDER

Diagnosis

It has long been recognized that clinically significant dissociative states are seen in the immediate aftermath of overwhelming trauma. In addition, many individuals may experience less clinically severe dissociative symptoms or alterations of attention and time sense. Because such syndromes, even when short-lasting, can produce major disruption of everyday activities, they may require clinical attention. During triage situations after a disaster, it can be important to recognize this clinical picture, which may require treatment intervention and which may also be predictive of later PTSD. As a result of these considerations, a decision was made to include in DSM-IV a new entity, acute stress disorder (ASD), grouped together with PTSD in the anxiety disorders section. Essentially, it represents the clinical features of PTSD along with conspicuous dissociative symptoms, of which at least three must be present (see DSM-IV-TR diagnostic criteria below). The possible dissociative symptoms in ASD are a subjective sense of numbing; detachment or absence of emotional response; reduced awareness of one's surroundings; derealization; depersonalization; and dissociative amnesia.

DSM-IV-TR Diagnostic Criteria

308.3 Acute Stress Disorder

A. The person has been exposed to a traumatic event in which both of the following were present:

    (1) the person experienced, witnessed, or was confronted with an event or events that involved actual or threatened death or serious injury, or a threat to the physical integrity of self or others

    (2) the person's response involved intense fear, helplessness, or horror

B. Either while experiencing or after experiencing the distressing event, the individual has three (or more) of the following dissociative symptoms:

(1) a subjective sense of numbing, detachment, or absence of emotional responsiveness
(2) a reduction in awareness of his or her surroundings (e.g., "being in a daze")
(3) derealization
(4) depersonalization
(5) dissociative amnesia (i.e., inability to recall an important aspect of the trauma)

C. The traumatic event is persistently reexperienced in at least one of the following ways: recurrent images, thoughts, dreams, illusions, flashback episodes, or a sense of reliving the experience; or distress on exposure to reminders of the traumatic event.
D. Marked avoidance of stimuli that arouse recollections of the trauma (e.g., thoughts, feelings, conversations, activities, places, people).
E. Marked symptoms of anxiety or increased arousal (e.g., difficulty sleeping, irritability, poor concentration, hypervigilance, exaggerated startle response, motor restlessness).
F. The disturbance causes clinically significant distress or impairment in social, occupational, or other important areas of functioning or impairs the individual's ability to pursue some necessary task, such as obtaining necessary assistance or mobilizing personal resources by telling family members about the traumatic experience.
G. The disturbance lasts for a minimum of 2 days and a maximum of 4 weeks and occurs within 4 weeks of the traumatic event.
H. The disturbance is not due to the direct physiological effects of a substance (e.g., a drug of abuse, a medication) or a general medical condition is not better accounted for by brief psychotic disorder, and is not merely an exacerbation of a preexisting Axis I or Axis II disorder.

Reprinted with permission from the Diagnostic and Statistical Manual of Mental Disorders, Fourth Edition, Text Revision. Copyright 2000 American Psychiatric Association.

However, there is a lack of empirical evidence for some of the assumptions inherent in the conceptualization of ASD, and there has been a call for empirical evidence of acutely traumatized individuals to address these assumptions (Bryant and Harvey 1997). The current emphasis placed on acute dissociative responses may be flawed in that there are multiple pathways to PTSD, and most trauma survivors who display severe acute stress reactions without dissociation can develop PTSD (Harvey and Bryant 1999). Reviews of these conceptual issues have recently been published (Bryant and Harvey 1997, Marshall et al. 1999).

Because ASD, by definition, cannot last longer than 1 month, if the clinical picture persists, a diagnosis of PTSD is appropriate. Some increased symptoms are expected in the great majority of subjects after exposure to major stress. These remit in most cases and only reach the level of clinical diagnosis if they are prolonged, exceed a tolerable quality, or interfere with everyday function. Resolution may be more difficult if there has been previous psychiatric morbidity, subsequent stress, and lack of social support.

Epidemiology

Little is known about the epidemiology of ASD as defined in DSM-IV-TR, but after events such as rape and criminal assault, the clinical picture of acute PTSD is found in 70 to 90% of individuals, although the frequency of the particular dissociative symptoms is unknown. One problem of most postdisaster surveys is that they evaluate subjects at points several months or years after the event. This makes any meaningful assessment of acute stress syndromes difficult. One exception was the self-report-based assessment of morbidity 2 months after an earthquake in Ecuador, which found a 45% rate of caseness (being a clinical case), with the most prominent symptoms being fear, nervousness, tenseness, worry, insomnia, and fatigue (Lima et al. 1989).

In a study by Koopman and colleagues (1994) of individuals who had been exposed to a firestorm, the participants showed a high incidence of dissociative symptoms, including time distortions, alterations in cognition and memory, and derealization. Most of these symptoms had lessened by a 4-month follow-up. A study by Bryan and Panasetis (2001) reported that 53% of participants reported panic attacks during their trauma, and those who had symptoms that met the criteria for ASD reported more peritraumatic panic symptoms. These data suggest that peritraumatic panic may be related to subsequent PTSD.

Retrospective reports of acute stress symptoms should be interpreted cautiously because of the influence of current symptoms on recall of acute symptoms. In a longitudinal study evaluating report of acute stress symptoms at 1 month and 2 years posttrauma, at least one of the four ASD diagnostic clusters was recalled inaccurately by 75% of individuals (Harvey and Bryant 2000).

Course

Although data do not exist on the course and natural history of ASD as now defined, studies by Koopman and coworkers (1994) indicated that dissociative and cognitive symptoms, which are so common in the immediate wake of trauma, improve spontaneously with time. However, they also found that the likelihood of developing PTSD symptoms at 7-month follow-up was more strongly related to the occurrence of dissociative symptoms than to anxiety symptoms immediately after exposure to the trauma. However, other studies have questioned the dissociative criteria as critical for the prediction of later PTSD (Marshall et al. 1999, Brewin et al. 1999).

Differential Diagnosis

ASD may need to be distinguished from several related disorders (Figure 34-1). Brief psychotic disorder may be a more appropriate diagnosis if the predominant symptoms are psychotic. It is possible that a major depressive disorder can develop posttraumatically and that there may be some overlap with ASD, in which case both disorders are appropriately diagnosed. When ASD-like symptoms are caused by direct physiological perturbation, the symptoms may be more appropriately diagnosed with reference to the etiological agent. Thus, an ASD-like picture that develops secondary to head injury is more appropriately diagnosed as mental disorder due to a general medical condition, whereas a clinical picture related to substance use (e.g., alcohol intoxication) is appropriately diagnosed as substance-induced disorder. Substance-related ASD is confined to the period of intoxication or withdrawal. Head injury–induced ASD needs substantiating by evidence from the history, physical examination, and laboratory testing that the symptoms are a direct physiological consequence of head trauma.

Etiology

Little is known about the etiology of ASD specifically, but it is likely that many of the same factors that apply to PTSD are relevant for ASD, that is, trauma intensity, preexisting psychopathology, family and genetic vulnerability, abnormal personality, lack of social supports at the time of the trauma, and physical injury are all likely to increase vulnerability for ASD.

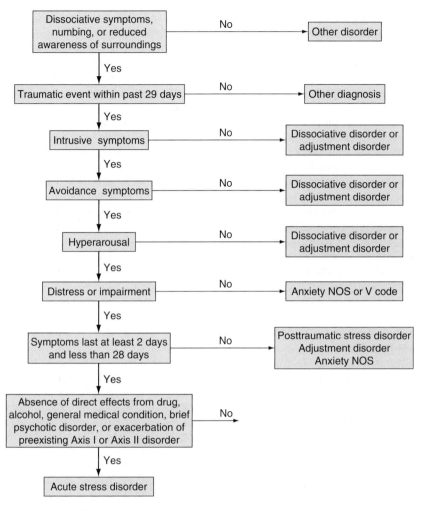

Figure 34-1 *Diagnostic decision tree for acute stress disorder.*

The role of acute arousal in the development of PTSD has been evaluated in one study (Bryant et al. 2000). Resting HR and ASD symptoms together were found to account for 36% of the variance in PTSD prediction (Bryant and Harvey 2000). Further, a formula using resting HR following the trauma exposure (HR > 90 beats/minute) and the diagnosis of ASD to predict PTSD development possessed strong sensitivity (88%) and specificity (85%) (Bryant et al. 2000).

Treatment

Lundin (1994) reviewed the treatment of acute traumatic stress states and pointed out the six general principles involved in administering any treatment immediately after trauma. These include principles of brevity, immediacy, centrality, expectancy, proximity, and simplicity. That is, treatment of acute trauma is generally aimed at being brief, provided immediately after the trauma whenever possible, administered in a centralized and coordinated fashion with the expectation of the person's return to normal function and as proximately as possible to the scene of the trauma, and not directed at any uncovering or explorative procedures but rather at maintaining a superficial, reintegrating approach.

People most highly at risk, and therefore perhaps most in need of treatment, are as follows: survivors with psychiatric disorders; traumatically bereaved people; children, especially when separated from their parents; individuals who are particularly dependent on psychosocial supports, such as the elderly, handicapped, and mentally retarded individuals; and traumatized survivors and body handlers.

Different components of treatment include providing information, psychological support, crisis intervention, and emotional first aid. Providing information about the trauma is important as it can enable the survivor to fully recognize and accept all the details of what happened. Information needs to be given in a way that conveys hope and the possibility that psychological pain and threat of loss may be coped with. Unrealistic hope needs to be balanced by the provision of realistic explanations as to what happened. Psychological support helps to strengthen coping mechanisms and promotes adaptive defenses. The survivor benefits if he or she recognizes the need to take responsibility for a successful outcome and is as actively involved with this as possible. Crisis intervention is often used after disasters and acts of violence or other serious traumas. It has been described by a number of investigators. Emotional first aid has been described by Caplan (1984) using the six principles presented earlier and is used to achieve any of the following: acceptance of feelings, symptoms, reality, and the need for help; recognition of psychologically distressing issues; identification of available resources; acceptance of responsibility and absence of blame; cultivation of an optimistic attitude; and efforts to resume activities of daily life as much as possible.

Civilian trauma survivors with ASD were found to engage in the cognitive strategies of punishment and worry more than survivors without ASD (Warda and Bryant 1998), and cognitive–behavioral therapy has been shown to reduce these strategies and increase the use of reappraisal and social control strategies (Bryant et al. 2001). However, the relation of these findings to the development of PTSD has not yet been determined.

There is little investigation as to whether early recognition and effective treatment of acute stress reactions prevent the development of PTSD, although it is safe to assume that they are likely to have beneficial effects in this regard. Nonetheless, as was recognized during World War II, rapid and effective treatment of acute combat stress did not always prevent veterans from developing subsequent chronicity. More recently, an intervention designed to prevent the development of PTSD and administered in the acute phase, critical incident stress debriefing (Mitchell and Everly 2000), has been found to be ineffective in preventing the development of PTSD (Carlier 2000, Carlier et al. 2000). However, there has been an initial study with motor vehicle accident survivors that suggested exposure therapy, and exposure therapy with anxiety management training may be effective in preventing PTSD (Bryant et al. 1999).

Comparison of DSM-IV-TR/ICD-10 Diagnostic Criteria

The ICD-10 Diagnostic Criteria for Research for Posttraumatic Stress Disorder provides a different stressor criterion: a situation or event "of exceptionally threatening or catastrophic nature, which would be likely to cause pervasive distress in almost everyone", which is similar to the DSM-III-R definition of a traumatic stressor. DSM-IV-TR instead defines a traumatic stressor as "an event or events that involved actual or threatened death or serious injury, or a threat to the physical integrity of self or others." Furthermore, the ICD-10 diagnostic algorithm differs from that specified in DSM-IV-TR in that the DSM-IV-TR criterion D (i.e., symptoms of increased arousal) is not required. In contrast to DSM-IV-TR, which requires that the symptoms persist for more than one month, the ICD-10 Diagnostic Criteria for Research do not specify a minimum duration.

For acute stress disorder, the ICD-10 Diagnostic Criteria for Research differs in several ways from the DSM-IV-TR criteria: (1) primarily anxiety symptoms are included; (2) it is required that the onset of the symptoms be within 1 hour of the stressor; and (3) the symptoms must begin to diminish after not more than 8 hours (for transient stressors) or 48 hours (for extended stressors). In contrast to DSM-IV-TR, the ICD-10 Diagnostic Criteria for Research does not require dissociative symptoms or that the event be persistently reexperienced.

References

Beckham JC, Crawford AL, Kirby AC, et al. (1997) Chronic posttraumatic stress disorder and chronic pain in Vietnam combat veterans. *J Psychosom Res* **43**, 379–389.

Blank AS (1993) The longitudinal course of posttraumatic stress disorder. In *Posttraumatic Stress Disorder: DSM-IV and Beyond*, Foa EB (ed). American Psychiatric Press, Washington, DC, pp. 3–22.

Boscarino JA (1996) Posttraumatic stress disorder, exposure to combat, and lower plasma cortisol among Vietnam veterans: findings and clinical implications. *J Consult Clin Psychol* **64**, 191–201.

Boscarino JA (1997) Diseases among men 20 years after exposure to severe stress: Implications for clinical research and medical care. *Psychosom Med* **59**, 605–614.

Brady K, Pearlstein T, Asnis GM, et al. (2000) Efficacy and safety of sertraline treatment of posttraumatic stress disorder: a randomized controlled trial. *J Am Med Assoc* **283**, 1837–1844.

Bremner JD, Southwick SM, Carnell A, et al. (1996) Chronic PTSD in Vietnam combat veterans: course of illness and substance abuse. *Am J Psychiatry* **153**, 369–375.

Breslau N (2001) The epidemiology of posttraumatic stress disorder: what is the extent of the problem? *J Clin Psychiatry* **62**, 16–22.

Breslau N, Davis GC, Andreski P, et al. (1991) Traumatic events and posttraumatic stress disorder in an urban population of young adults. *Arch Gen Psychiatry* **48**, 216–222.

Brewin CR, Andrews B, Rose S, et al. (1999) Acute stress disorder and posttraumatic stress disorder in victims of violent crimes. *Am J Psychiatry* **156**, 360–366.

Bryant RA and Harvey AG (1997) Acute stress disorder: a critical review of diagnostic issues. *Clin Psychol Rev* **17**, 757–773.

Bryant RA and Harvey AG (2000) *Acute Stress Disorder: A Handbook of Theory, Assessment, and Treatment*. American Psychological Association, Washington, DC.

Bryant RA and Panasetis P (2001) Panic symptoms during trauma and acute stress disorder. *Behav Res Ther* **39**, 961–966.

Bryant RA, Harvey AG, Guthrie R, et al. (2000) A prospective study of psychophysiological arousal, acute stress disorder, and posttraumatic stress disorder. *J Abnorm Psychol* **109**, 341–344.

Bryant RA, Sackville T, Dang ST, et al. (1999) Treating acute stress disorder: an evaluation of cognitive behavior therapy and supportive counseling techniques. *Am J Psychiatry* **156**, 1780–1786.

Buckley TC and Kaloupek DG (2001) A meta-analytic examination of basal cardiovascular activity in posttraumatic stress disorder. *Psychosom Med* **63**, 585–594.

Caplan G (1984) *Principles of Preventive Psychiatry*. Basic Books, New York.

Carlier IV (2000) Critical incident stress debriefing. In *International Handbook of Human Response to Trauma. The Plenum Series on Stress and Coping*, Yehuda R (ed). Kluwer Academic/Plenum Publishers, New York, pp. 379–387.

Carlier IV, Voerman AE, and Gersons BP (2000) The influence of occupational debriefing on posttraumatic stress symptomatology in traumatized police officers. *Br J Med Psychol* **73**, 87–98.

Cohen JA, Mannarino AP, and Rogal S (2001) Treatment practices for childhood posttraumatic stress disorder. *Child Abuse Neglect* **25**, 123–135.

Connor KM and Davidson JRT (1997) Familial risk factors in posttraumatic stress disorder. *Ann N Y Acad* **821**, 35–51.

Connor KM, Sutherland SM, Tupler LA, et al. (1999) Fluoxetine in posttraumatic stress disorder: Randomized double-blind study. *Br J Psychiatry* **175**, 17–22.

Davidson JRT and Fairbank JA (1993) The epidemiology of posttraumatic stress disorder. In *Posttraumatic Stress Disorder: DSM-IV and Beyond*, Foa EB (ed). American Psychiatric Press, Washington, DC, pp. 147–172.

Davidson JRT, Hughes GH, Blazer DG, et al. (1991) Posttraumatic stress disorder in the community: an epidemiologic study. *Psychol Med* **21**, 713–721.

Davidson JRT, Pearlstein T, Londborg P, et al. (2001) Efficacy of sertraline in preventing relapse of posttraumatic stress disorder: results of a 28-week double-blind placebo-controlled study. *Am J Psychiatry* **158**, 1974–1981.

Davidson JRT, Swartz M, Storck M, et al. (1985) A diagnostic and family study of posttraumatic stress disorder. *Am J Psychiatry* **142**, 90–93.

Davidson JRT, Tupler LA, Wilson WH, et al. (1998) A family study of chronic posttraumatic stress disorder following rape trauma. *J Psychiatr Res* **32**, 301–309.

Falsetti SA, Resnick HS, Davis J, et al. (2001) Treatment of posttraumatic stress disorder with comorbid panic attacks: combining cognitive processing therapy with panic control treatment techniques. *Group Dynamics* **5**, 252–260.

Foa EB, Keane TM, and Friedman MJ (2000) *Effective treatments for PTSD: Practice Guidelines from the International Society for Traumatic Stress Studies*. Guilford Press, New York.

Foa EB, Riggs DS, Massie ED, et al. (1995) The impact of fear activation and anger on the efficacy of exposure treatment for posttraumatic stress disorder. *Behav Ther* **26**, 487–499.

Frank JB, Giller ELJ, Kosten TB, et al. (1988) A randomized clinical trial of phenelzine and imipramine for posttraumatic stress disorder. *Am J Psychiatry* **145**, 1289–1291.

Harvey AG and Bryant RA (1999) Dissociative symptoms in acute stress disorder. *J Traum Stress* **12**, 573–680.

Harvey AG and Bryant RA (2000) Memory for acute stress disorder symptoms: a two year prospective study. *J Nerv Ment Dis* **188**, 602–607.

Helzer JE, Robins LN, and McEnvoy L (1987) Posttraumatic stress disorder in the general population. *N Eng J Med* **317**, 1630–1634.

Hidalgo RB and Davidson JRT (2000) Posttraumatic stress disorder: epidemiology and health-related considerations. *J Clin Psychiatry* **61**, 5–13.

Kendall-Tackett KA, Williams LM, and Finkelhor D (1993) Impact of sexual abuse on children: a review and synthesis of recent empirical studies. *Psychol Bull* **113**, 164–180.

Kessler RC, Sonnega A, Bromet E, et al. (1995) Posttraumatic stress disorder in the national comorbidity survey. *Arch Gen Psychiatry* **52**, 1048–1060.

Kilpatrick DB, Saunders BE, Veronen LJ, et al. (1987) Criminal victimization: lifetime prevalence, reporting to police, and psychological impact. *Crime Delinquency* **33**, 479–489.

Koopman C, Classen C, and Spiegel D (1994) Predictors of posttraumatic stress symptoms among survivors of the Oakland/Berkeley, California firestorm. *Am J Psychiatry* **151**, 888–894.

Krakow B, Hollifield M, Johnston L, et al. (2001) Imagery rehearsal therapy for chronic nightmares in sexual assault survivors with posttraumatic stress disorder: a randomized control trial. *J Am Med Assoc* **286**, 537–545.

Kulka RA, Schlenger WE, Fairbank JA, et al. (1990) *Trauma and the Vietnam War Generation: Report of Findings from the National Vietnam Veterans Readjustment Study*. Brunner/Mazel, New York.

Lieberzon I, Taylor SF, Amdur R, et al. (1999) Brain activation in PTSD in response to trauma-related stimuli. *Biol Psychiatry* **45**, 817–826.

Lima BR, Chavez H, Samniego N, et al. (1989) Disaster severity and emotional disturbance: Implications for primary mental health care in developing countries. *Acta Psychiatr Scand* **79**, 74–82.

Lubin H and Johnson DR (2000) Interactive psychoeducational group therapy in the treatment of authority problems in combat-related posttraumatic stress disorder. *Int J Psychophysiol* **50**, 277–296.

Lundin T (1994) The treatment of acute trauma: posttraumatic stress disorder prevention. *Psychiatr Clin North Am* **17**, 385–391.

March JS (1990) The nosology of posttraumatic stress disorder. *J Anx Disord* **4**, 61–82.

March JS (1993) What constitutes a stressor? In *Posttraumatic Stress Disorder: DSM-IV and Beyond*, Foa EB (ed). American Psychiatric Press, Washington, DC, pp. 37–54.

Marks IM (1987) *Fears, Phobias, and Rituals*. Oxford University Press, New York.

Marshall RD, Schneier FR, Fallon BA, et al. (1998) An open trial of paroxetine in patients with noncombat related, chronic posttraumatic stress disorder. *J Clin Psychopharmacol* **18**, 10–18.

Marshall RD, Spitzer R, and Liebowitz MR (1999) Review and critique of the new DSM-IV diagnosis of acute stress disorder. *Am J Psychiatry* **156**, 1677–1688.

McFarlane AC and Yehuda R (2000) Clinical treatment of posttraumatic stress disorder: conceptual challenges raised by recent research. *Aust N Z J Psychiatry* **34**, 940–953.

McLeod DS, Koenen KC, Meyer JM, et al. (2001) Genetic and environmental influences on the relationship among combat exposure, posttraumatic stress disorder symptoms, and alcohol use. *J Traum Stress* **14**, 259–275.

Mitchell JT and Everly GS (2000) Critical incident stress management and critical incident stress debriefings: evolution, effects, and outcomes. In *Psychological Debriefing: Theory, Practice, and Evidence*. Wilson JP (ed). Cambridge University Press, New York, pp. 71–90.

Nader K, Pynoos RS, Fairbanks L, et al. (1990) Children's PTSD reactions one year after a sniper attack at their school. *Am J Psychiatry* **147**, 1526–1530.

Nader K, Stuber M, and Pynoos RS (1991) Posttraumatic stress reactions in preschool children with catastrophic illness: assessment needs. *Compr Ment Health Care* **1**, 223–239.

Norris FH (1992) Epidemiology of trauma: frequency and impact of different potentially traumatic events on different demographic events. *J Consult Clin Psychol* **60**, 409–418.

Pitman RK (1993) Biological findings in posttraumatic stress disorder: implications for DSM-IV classification. In *Posttraumatic Stress Disorder: DSM-IV and Beyond*, Foa EB (ed). American Psychiatric Press, Washington, DC.

Pitman RK (2001) Hippocampal diminution in PTSD: More (or less?) than meets the eye. *Hippocampus* **11**, 73–74.

Pitman RK, Altman B, Greenwald E, et al. (1991) Psychiatric complications during flooding therapy for posttraumatic stress disorder. *J Clin Psychiatry* **52**, 17–20.

Pitman RK, Orr SP, Shalev A, et al. (1999) Psychophysiologic alterations in posttraumatic stress disorder. *Sem Clin Neuropsychiatr* **4**, 234–241.

Pynoos RS, Frederick CJ, Nader K, et al. (1987) Life threat and posttraumatic stress in school-age children. *Arch Gen Psychiatry* **44**, 1057–1063.

Pynoos RS, Goenjian A, Tashjian M, et al. (1993) Posttraumatic stress reactions in children after the 1988 American earthquake. *Br J Med Psychol* **163**, 239–247.

Rauch SL, Whalen PJ, Shin LM, et al. (2000) Exaggerated amygdala response to masked facial stimuli in posttraumatic stress disorder: a functional MRI study. *Biol Psychiatry* **47**, 769–776.

Resick PA and Schnicke MK (1992) Cognitive processing therapy for sexual assault victims. *J Consult Clin Psychol* **60**, 748–756.

Rothbaum BO, Meadows EA, Resick PA, et al. (2000) Cognitive–behavioral therapy. In *Effective Treatments for PTSD: Practice Guidelines from the International Society for Traumatic Stress Studies*, Friedman MJ (ed). Guilford Press, New York, pp. 320–325.

Ruggiero KJ, Morris TL, and Scotti JR (2001) Treatment for children with posttraumatic stress disorder: current status and future directions. *Clin Psychol-Sci Pract* **8**, 210–227.

Saigh PA (1991) The development of posttraumatic stress disorder following four different types of traumatization. *Behav Res Ther* **29**, 213–216.

Schnuff N, Neylan TC, Lenoci MA, et al. (2001) Decreased hippocampal N-acetylaspartate in the absence of atrophy in posttraumatic stress disorder. *Biol Psychiatry* **50**, 952–959.

Schnurr PP and Jankowski MK (1999) Physical health and posttraumatic stress disorder: review and synthesis. *Sem Clin Neuropsychiatr* **4**, 295–304.

Shalev A, Bleich A, and Ursano RJ (1990) Posttraumatic stress disorder: somatic comorbidity and effort tolerance. *Psychosom* **31**, 197–203.

Shin LM, McNally RJ, Kosslyn SM, et al. (1999) Regional cerebral blood flow during script-driven imagery in childhood sexual abuse-related PTSD: a PET investigation. *Am J Psychiatry* **156**, 575–584.

Solomon SD, Gerrity ET, and Muff AM (1992) Efficacy of treatments for posttraumatic stress disorder: an empirical review. *J Am Med Assoc* **268**, 633–638.

Southwick SM, Krystal JH, Morgan CA, et al. (1993) Abnormal noradrenergic function in posttraumatic stress disorder. *Arch Gen Psychiatry* **50**, 266–274.

Tarrier N, Pilgrim H, Sommerfield C, et al. (1999) A randomized trial of cognitive therapy and imaginal exposure in the treatment of chronic posttraumatic stress disorder. *J Consult Clin Psychol* **67**, 13–18.

Taylor S, Fedoroff IC, Koch WJ, et al. (2001) Posttraumatic stress disorder arising after road traffic collisions: patterns of response to cognitive–behavioral therapy. *J Consult Clin Psychol* **69**, 541–551.

Triffleman E, Carroll K, and Kellogg S (1999) Substance dependence posttraumatic stress disorder therapy: an integrated cognitive–behavioral approach. *J Subst Abuse* **17**, 3–14.

True WR and Lyons MJ (1999) Genetic risk factors for PTSD: a twin study. In *Risk Factors for Posttraumatic Stress Disorder*, Yehuda R (ed). American Psychiatric Press, Washington, DC, pp. 61–78.

True WR, Rice J, Eisen SA, et al. (1993) A twin study of genetic and environmental contributions to liability for posttraumatic stress symptoms. *Arch Gen Psychiatry* **50**, 257–265.

van der Kolk B, Dreyfuss D, Michaels M, et al. (1994) Fluoxetine in posttraumatic stress disorder. *J Clin Psychiatry* **55**, 517–522.

Vasterling JJ, Brailey K, Constans JI, et al. (1998) Attention and memory dysfunction in posttraumatic stress disorder. *Neuropsychology* **12**, 125–133.

Warda G and Bryant RA (1998) Thought control strategies in acute stress disorder. *Behav Res Ther* **36**, 1171–1175.

Winfield I, George LK, Swartz M, et al. (1990) Sexual assault and psychiatric disorders among a community sample of women. *Am J Psychiatry* **147**, 335–341.

Wolfsdorf BA and Zlotnick C (2001) Affect management in group therapy for women with posttraumatic stress disorder and histories of childhood sexual abuse. *J Clin Psychiatry* **57**, 169–181.

Yehuda R (1999) Managing anger and aggression in patients with posttraumatic stress disorder. *J Clin Psychiatry* **15**, 33–37.

Yehuda R (2002) Posttraumatic stress disorder. *N Engl J Med* **346**(2), 108–114.

Yehuda R, Giller ELJ, Southwick SM, et al. (1991) Hypothalamic–pituitary–adrenal dysfunction in posttraumatic stress disorder. *Biol Psychiatry* **30**, 266–274.

Yehuda R, Siever LJ, Teicher MH, et al. (1998) Plasma norepinephrine and 3-methoxy-4-hydroxyphenylglycol concentrations and severity of depression in combat posttraumatic stress disorder and major depressive disorder. *Biol Psychiatry* **44**, 56–63.

35 Anxiety Disorders: Generalized Anxiety Disorder

Diagnosis

Generalized Anxiety Disorder (GAD) is defined as excessive anxiety and worry (apprehensive expectation) occurring for a majority of days during at least a 6-month period, about a number of events or activities (such as work or school performance) (see DSM-IV-TR diagnostic criteria below). In individuals with GAD, the anxiety and worry are accompanied by at least three of six somatic symptoms (only one accompanying symptom is required in children), which include restlessness or feeling keyed up or on edge, being easily fatigued, difficulty concentrating or mind going blank, irritability, muscle tension, and sleep disturbance. In addition, the affected individual has difficulty controlling his/her worry, and the anxiety, worry, or somatic symptoms cause clinically significant distress or impairment in social, occupational, and/or other important areas of functioning. Further, the GAD symptoms should not be due to the direct physiological effects of a substance such as drugs or alcohol or a general medical condition, and should not occur exclusively during a mood disorder, psychotic disorder, or pervasive developmental disorder.

DSM-IV-TR Diagnostic Criteria

300.02 Generalized Anxiety Disorder

A. Excessive anxiety and worry (apprehensive expectation), occurring more days than not for at least 6 months, about a number of events or activities (such as work or school performance).
B. The person finds it difficult to control the worry.
C. The anxiety and worry are associated with three (or more) of the following six symptoms (with at least some symptoms present for more days than not for the past 6 months). **Note:** Only one item is required in children.

   (1) restlessness or feeling keyed up or on edge
   (2) being easily fatigued

(3) difficulty concentrating or mind going blank

(4) irritability

(5) muscle tension

(6) sleep disturbance (difficulty falling or staying asleep, or restless unsatisfying sleep)

D. The focus of anxiety and worry is not confined to features of an Axis I disorder, for example, the anxiety or worry is not about having a panic attack (as in panic disorder), being embarrassed in public (as in social phobia), being contaminated (as in obsessive–compulsive disorder), being away from home or close relatives (as in separation anxiety disorder), gaining weight (as in anorexia nervosa), having multiple physical complaints (as in somatization disorder), or having a serious illness (as in hypochondriasis), and the anxiety and worry do not occur exclusively during posttraumatic stress disorder.

E. The anxiety, worry, or physical symptoms cause clinically significant distress or impairment in social, occupational, or other important areas of functioning.

F. The disturbance is not due to the direct physiological effects of a substance (e.g., a drug of abuse, a medication) or a general medical condition (e.g., hyperthyroidism) and does not occur exclusively during a mood disorder, a psychotic disorder, or a pervasive developmental disorder.

Worry and anxiety are part of normal human behavior and it may be difficult to define a cutoff point distinguishing normal or trait anxiety (i.e., a relatively stable tendency to perceive various situations as threatening) from GAD. However, as described in the DSM-IV-TR definition of GAD, individuals suffering from a *disorder* exhibit significant distress and impairment in functioning as a result of their anxiety symptoms.

Individuals with GAD experience chronic anxiety and tension. They find the worry as being uncontrollable. However, some individuals intentionally initiate and maintain worry with an almost superstitious assumption that, by doing so, they can avert a negative event (Rapee 1991). Individuals tend to worry predominantly about family, personal finances, work, and illness (Sanderson and Barlow 1990). They are also likely to report worrying over minor matters, such as making a slight social *faux pas*. The majority report being anxious for at least 50% of the time during an average day (Sanderson and Barlow 1990). In children and adolescents, the worries often revolve around the quality of their performance in school or other competitive areas (American Psychiatric Association 1994). They may also worry about potential catastrophic events. They are concerned with their own physical or mental imperfections or inadequacies, and typically require excessive reassurance (Bernstein and Borchardt 1991). They often appear shy, overcompliant, perfectionistic, and frequently describe multiple physical complaints (Bernstein and Borchardt 1991). They may have an unusually mature and serious manner and appear older than their actual age (Bernstein and Borchardt 1991). These children are often the eldest in small, competitive, achievement-oriented families (Bernstein and Borchardt 1991).

Individuals with GAD commonly complain of feeling tense, jumpy, and irritable. They have difficulty falling or staying asleep, and tire easily during the day (Brawman-Mintzer et al. 1993). Particularly distressing to such individuals is the difficulty in concentrating and collecting their thoughts (Brawman-Mintzer et al. 1993). Cognitions appear to play a central role in GAD, as well as other anxiety disorders. Patterns of cognitions, however, appear to be disorder-specific. When the frequency of anxiety, worry, or panic attacks among individuals with GAD and panic disorder, as well as the severity of anxiety associated with each were examined (Breitholtz et al. 1999), 34% of GAD individuals' cognitions were found to center on interpersonal conflict or the issue of acceptance by others, while only 1.4% of panic disorder individuals reported such concerns. While individuals with GAD also had exaggerated worries over relatively minor matters, panic disorder individuals reported a significantly greater frequency of cognitions concerning physical dangers or catastrophes (e.g., accident, injury, death).

Individuals may present with complaints of muscular tension, especially in their neck and shoulders (Brawman-Mintzer et al. 1993). They may experience headaches, frequently described as frontal and occipital pressure or tension. They complain about sweaty palms, feel shaky and tremulous, complain of dryness of the mouth, and experience palpitations and difficulty in breathing (Brawman-Mintzer et al. 1993). Individuals may also experience gastrointestinal symptoms such as heartburn and epigastric fullness. Approximately 30% of individuals experience severe gastrointestinal symptoms of irritable bowel syndrome (Tollefson et al. 1991). The physical complaints frequently lead individuals to seek medical attention, and most will initially consult a primary care physician. Although they frequently complain of palpitations and breathing difficulty, studies suggest that individuals with GAD do not differ from normal comparison subjects on measures of respiration and heart rate (Kollai and Kollai 1992). Individuals with GAD may also present complaining of chest pain. Although chest pain is more frequently reported by individuals with panic disorder, Carter and Maddock (1992) observed that 34% of individuals with GAD without panic attacks experienced chest pain. They also found that these individuals were predominantly males and many had undergone extensive cardiac evaluations that revealed no demonstrable cardiac pathology.

Special laboratory and diagnostic evaluation of individuals with GAD may occasionally be required to exclude general medical conditions that mimic symptoms of generalized anxiety (see the section, Differential Diagnosis). An evaluation to identify these disorders includes a personal and family medical history, review of systems, and a careful physical examination including neurological examination. Laboratory evaluation should include an electrocardiogram, screening for abusable substances, urinalysis, complete blood count, serum electrolytes, liver and thyroid function tests, calcium, phosphorus, and blood urea nitrogen.

An examination of the relative frequencies of various comorbid diagnoses in individuals with GAD obtained from the available studies reveals that other anxiety and mood disorders frequently complicate the course of GAD (Sanderson and Barlow 1990, Brawman-Mintzer et al. 1993, Wittchen et al. 1994, see diagnostic decision tree for GAD). Angst (1993) evaluated psychiatric comorbidity in a longitudinal epidemiological study in Zurich, Switzerland. Strong associations between GAD and major depression and between GAD and dysthymia were found, but a relatively low association with panic disorder was found. A high comorbidity of GAD with hypomania was also found. Further, the presence of comorbidity was associated with a high suicide attempt risk. In addition, individuals with comorbid disorders were treated more frequently and endorsed more work impairment than GAD individuals without comorbid disorders.

Alcoholism also complicates the clinical course of GAD for some individuals; however, the available literature suggests that the diagnosis of alcohol abuse is not as prevalent in GAD as in other anxiety disorders, and the pattern of abuse is often a brief and nonpersistent one (Brawman-Mintzer et al. 1993). GAD onset is usually later than that of the alcohol use disorder (Kushner et al. 1999). Personality disorders have been observed to co-occur in approximately 50% of individuals with GAD (Emmanuel et al. 1992, Gasperini et al. 1990). For example, rates of GAD and personality disorders in clinical populations have ranged from 31 to 46% (Gasperini et al. 1990, Mauri et al. 1992, Mavissakalian et al. 1993,

Sanderson et al. 1991, Starcevic et al. 1995). Cluster C personality disorders, specifically avoidant personality disorder, dependent personality disorder, and obsessive–compulsive personality disorder are common (Mauri et al. 1992, Mavissakalian et al. 1993). Interestingly, Cluster A personality traits, in particular, suspiciousness and mistrust, may be prominent in GAD as well (Mavissakalian et al. 1993).

Epidemiology

Despite the shifting diagnostic criteria affecting the prevalence studies, current data indicate that GAD is probably one of the more common psychiatric disorders. Breslau and Davis (1985) reported a lifetime prevalence of 45% for GAD, according to DSM-III diagnostic criteria. However, when these researchers used the more stringent criteria outlined in the DSM-III-R, which required a duration of 6 months, the prevalence rate dropped dramatically to 9%. The Epidemiologic Catchment Area Study (ECA) (Blazer et al. 1991), a five-center epidemiological study of the prevalence of psychiatric disorders in the United States, reported a lifetime prevalence for DSM-III-defined GAD of 4.1 to 6.6% in the three sites that assessed for GAD. One of the most recent epidemiological surveys of DSM-III-R GAD was conducted as a part of the National Comorbidity Survey of psychiatric disorders in the United States by Kessler and colleagues (Kessler et al. 1994, Wittchen et al. 1994). Prevalence rates in the total sample ($N = 8098$) were 1.6% for current GAD (defined as the most recent 6-month period of anxiety), 3.1% for 12-month GAD, and 5.1% for lifetime GAD, with lifetime prevalence higher in females (6.6%) than males (3.6%).

Studies examining DSM-IV GAD prevalence rates have been conducted outside the United States. Wittchen and colleagues (1998) examined GAD in a sample of adolescents and adults in Munich, Germany and found a lifetime prevalence of 0.8% and a 12-month prevalence of 0.5%. Bhagwanjee and colleagues (1998) examined rates of GAD in a sample from South Africa and found current prevalence of GAD in a sample of adults to be 3.7%. In another German sample, Carter and colleagues (2001) reported a 12-month prevalence rate of 1.5%.

GAD appears at even higher rates in clinical settings, particularly in primary care settings. For example, Shear and colleagues (1994) found prevalence rates of GAD, using DSM-III-R criteria, reported by individuals at four primary care centers, to be twice as high as those reported in community samples (i.e., 10 versus 5.1%). Similarly, a collaborative study by the World Health Organization (WHO) across 15 international sites reported prevalence rates of GAD at approximately 8% in primary care settings (Maier et al. 2000, Sartorius et al. 1996).

Rates of GAD appear similar in special populations such as children and the elderly. GAD appears to be less prevalent in children than in adults. Data from the National Comorbidity Study indicate that for both lifetime and 12-month prevalence rates, GAD occurs at the lowest rate in younger ages and at the highest rate in older adults (Wittchen et al. 1994). Anderson and associates (1987) reported a 1-year prevalence rate of 2.9% for overanxious anxiety disorder, the DSM-III-R equivalent of GAD in children. In a community sample of 150 adolescents, Kashani and Orvaschel (1988) reported a 6-month prevalence rate of 7.3% for overanxious anxiety disorder. Finally, in a clinical setting the prevalence of childhood overanxious anxiety disorder was even higher, with up to 52% of the children seen having anxiety symptoms that met criteria for the disorder (Last et al. 1987). It should be mentioned that in DSM-IV, the diagnosis of childhood overanxious anxiety disorder was subsumed within the diagnosis of GAD. Epidemiological data on prevalence of GAD in childhood using DSM-IV-TR criteria are currently lacking. In the elderly, GAD appears to account for the majority of anxiety disorders, with prevalence rates ranging from 0.7 to 7.3% (Beekman et al. 1998, Flint 1994).

Course

GAD individuals frequently report that they have been anxious all their lives. Typically, they were moderately anxious during childhood, later developing full-blown GAD when their stress levels increased through activities such as attending college or starting work. Individuals with early onset of symptoms report experiencing significant anxiety and fears, social isolation, obsessionality, more academic difficulties, and disturbed home environment during their childhood. The social maladjustment and emotional overreactivity persist into adulthood. Epidemiological studies (Kendler et al. 1992a, Burke et al. 1991) and clinical studies (Barlow et al. 1986, Rogers et al. 1999) suggest that the onset of GAD typically begins between the late teens and late twenties. However, not all GAD individuals have a lifelong history of excessive anxiety. Some individuals develop their disorder at a later age, that is, in one's thirties or later. These individuals frequently report identifiable, precipitating stressful events, specifically unexpected, negative, important events in the year preceding development of GAD (Blazer et al. 1987, Hoehn-Saric et al. 1993).

Retrospective and prospective reports indicate that the typical course of GAD is chronic, nonremitting, and that it often persists for a decade or longer (Blazer et al. 1991, Angst and Vollrath 1991, Mancuso et al. 1993, Noyes et al. 1996). For example, Noyes and colleagues (1996) evaluated 112 individuals with anxiety neuroses (a DSM-II term that is roughly equivalent to GAD) 4 to 9 years after the onset of the disorder and found that only 12% of the individuals were symptom-free, while 48% had moderate to severe levels of anxiety symptoms. In addition, 25% of individuals reported moderate to marked impairment in functioning. Rickels and colleagues (1986) reported that two-thirds of individuals treated initially with diazepam relapsed within 1 year of discontinuation of treatment. Other studies utilizing criteria prior to the DSM-III-R for GAD found comparable levels of chronicity, with almost half the individuals reporting moderate symptoms at follow-up (Yonkers et al. 2000). Mancuso and associates (1993) evaluated 44 individuals with DSM-III-R-defined GAD approximately 16 months following discontinuation of successful treatment with the benzodiazepine adinazolam. The authors found that half of the subjects still had anxiety symptoms that met diagnostic criteria for GAD at follow-up. These individuals also reported significant feelings of dissatisfaction, as well as impairment in job performance.

Wittchen and coworkers (1994) found that approximately 80% of subjects with GAD reported substantial interference with their life, a high degree of professional help-seeking, and a high prevalence of taking medications because of their GAD symptoms. The disability associated with GAD was found to be similar to that found in individuals with panic disorder or major depression (Kessler et al. 1999).

Differential Diagnosis

Anxiety can be a prominent feature of many psychiatric disorders and a number of disorders should be considered in the differential diagnosis of GAD (Figure 35-1). Several symptom profiles discriminate between major depressive disorder or dysthymic disorder and GAD (Brown et al. 1994). Individuals with major depressive disorder exhibit higher rates of dysphoric mood, psychomotor retardation, suicidal ideation, guilt, hopelessness, and help-lessness, as well as more work impairment than individuals with GAD (Riskind et al. 1991). In contrast, individuals with GAD show higher rates of somatic symptoms, specif-ically, muscle tension and autonomic symptoms (e.g., respiratory or cardiac complaints) than depressed individuals.

Panic disorder is characterized by the presence of panic attacks; that is, recurrent, discrete episodes of intense anxiety or fear associated with a cluster of somatic symptoms reflecting autonomic hyperactivity such as rapid heartbeat, dizziness, numbness or tingling, trouble breathing or choking, and nausea or vomiting. In contrast, individuals with GAD predominantly experience symptoms of muscle tension and vigilance such as fatigue, muscle

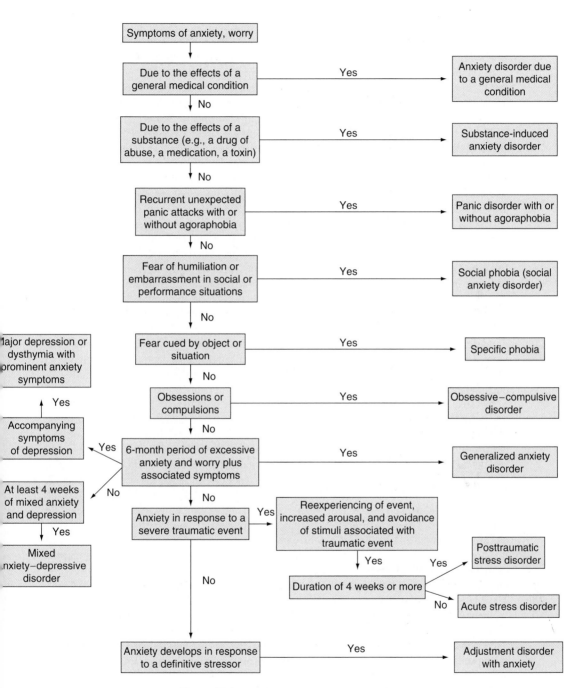

Figure 35-1 *Diagnostic decision tree for GAD.*

soreness, insomnia, difficulty in concentrating, restlessness, and irritability (Brawman-Mintzer et al. 1994). Anxiety is also a part of the clinical picture of obsessive–compulsive disorder (OCD) and may be a central factor in initiating and maintaining obsessions and compulsions. Obsessive thoughts are described as ego-dystonic intrusions that often take the form of urges, impulses, or images. They are often senseless and are frequently accompanied by time-consuming compulsions designed to reduce mounting anxiety. In contrast, the worries in GAD are about realistic concerns, such as health and finances.

In phobic disorders, the anxiety is characteristically associated with a specific phobic object or situation that is frequently avoided by the individual. Such is the case with social anxiety disorder as well, in which the individual is afraid of or avoids situations in which he or she may be the focus of potential scrutiny by others. Anxiety is also a characteristic part of the presentation of posttraumatic stress disorder (PTSD) and acute stress disorder. However, unlike in GAD, the principal symptoms experienced in PTSD and acute stress disorder follow exposure to a traumatic event and are characterized by avoidance of reminders of the event and persistent reexperiencing of the traumatic event (American Psychiatric Association 1994). Finally, in adjustment disorders, anxiety when present occurs in response to a specific life stressor or stressors and generally does not persist for more than 6 months (American Psychiatric Association 1994).

Many general medical conditions may present with prominent anxiety symptoms and must be considered in the differential diagnosis of generalized anxiety (see Table 35-1). Individuals with GAD may complain of palpitations, skipped heartbeats, and chest pain. In addition, many GAD individuals, especially males, fear having an acute myocardial infarction and often present to the emergency room for evaluation. However, most individuals with GAD without a concomitant cardiovascular disease do not experience severe chest pain. Following the controversial evidence suggesting an association between mitral valve prolapse (MVP) and panic disorder, researchers evaluated the prevalence of MVP in individuals with GAD (Dager et al. 1986) and found no evidence of increased prevalence in individuals with GAD. Nevertheless, individuals with anxiety symptoms associated with unexplained chest pain should be evaluated for possible cardiovascular disease.

Anxiety is a prominent feature of hyperthyroidism with some overlap in the symptomatology of thyrotoxicosis and GAD. Symptoms such as tachycardia, tremulousness, irritability, weakness, and fatigue are common to both disorders. In GAD, however, the peripheral manifestations of excessive concentrations of circulating thyroid hormones are absent, including symptoms such as weight loss, increased appetite, warm and moist skin, heat intolerance, and dyspnea on effort. Pheochromocytomas, also known as chromaffin tumors, produce, store, and secrete catecholamines. They are derived most often from the adrenal medulla, as well as the sympathetic ganglia, and occasionally from other sites. The clinical features of these tumors, most commonly hypertension and hypertensive paroxysms, are predominantly due to the release of catecholamines. Individuals may also experience diaphoresis, tachycardia, chest pain, flushing, nausea and vomiting, headache, and significant apprehension. Although the clinical presentation frequently mimics spontaneous panic attacks, pheochromocytomas should also be considered in the differential diagnosis of GAD. The diagnosis of pheochromocytoma can be confirmed by increased levels of catecholamines (epinephrine and norepinephrine) or catecholamine metabolites (metanephrines and vanillylmandelic acid) in a 24-hour urine collection.

Menopause is commonly referred to as the period that encompasses the transition between the reproductive years and beyond the last episode of menstrual bleeding. Frequently associated with significant anxiety, menopause should be considered in the differential diagnosis of GAD. However, other associated symptoms such as vasomotor instability, atrophy of urogenital epithelium and skin, and osteoporosis make the diagnosis of menopause probable. Another endocrinologic disorder, hyperparathyroidism, can present with anxiety symptoms, and the initial evaluation of serum calcium levels may be indicated. Finally, certain neurologic conditions such as complex partial seizures, intracranial tumors and strokes, and cerebral ischemic attacks may be associated with symptoms typically observed in anxiety disorders and may require appropriate evaluation.

Table 35-1	Medical Conditions and Drugs That May Cause Anxiety

Endocrine Disorders

Addison's disease
Cushing's syndrome
Hyperparathyroidism
Hyperthyroidism
Hypothyroidism
Carcinoid
Pheochromocytoma

Drug Side Effects

Anticonvulsants
Antidepressants
Antihistamines
Antihypertensive agents
Antiinflammatory agents
Antiparkinsonian agents
Caffeine
Digitalis
Sympathomimetics
Thyroid supplements

Substance Use Related
Cocaine
Hallucinogens
Amphetamines

Withdrawal Syndromes
Alcohol
Narcotics
Sedatives–hypnotics

Gastrointestinal Disorders
Peptic ulcer disease

Infectious Diseases
Miscellaneous viral and bacterial infections

Cardiovascular and Circulatory Disorders

Anemia
Congestive heart failure
Coronary insufficiency
Dysrhythmia e.g. atrial fibrillation
Hypovolemia
Myocardial infarction

Respiratory Disorders

Asthma
Chronic obstructive pulmonary disease
Pulmonary embolism
Pulmonary edema

Immunological, Collagen, and Vascular Disorders
Systemic lupus erythematosus
Temporal arteritis

Metabolic Conditions
Acidosis
Acute intermittent porphyria
Electrolyte abnormalities
Hypoglycemia

Neurological Disorders
Brain tumors
Cerebral syphilis
Cerebrovascular disorders
Encephalopathies
Epilepsy (especially temporal lobe epilepsy)
Postconcussive syndrome
Vertigo
Akathisia

Anxiety disorders can occur frequently in association with intoxication and withdrawal from several classes of substances (see Table 35-1). Excessive use of caffeine, especially in children and adolescents, may cause significant anxiety. Cocaine intoxication may be associated with anxiety, agitation, and hypervigilance. During cocaine withdrawal, individuals may also present with prominent anxiety, irritability, insomnia, fatigue, depression, and cocaine craving. Adverse reaction to marijuana includes extreme anxiety that usually lasts less than 24 hours. Mild opioid withdrawal presents with symptoms of anxiety and dysphoria. However, accompanying symptoms such as elevated blood pressure, tachycardia, pupilary dilation, rhinorrhea, piloerection, and lacrimation are rare in individuals with GAD.

The clinical phenomenology observed both in alcohol and sedative–hypnotic drug withdrawal and in GAD, although variable, may be highly similar. In both conditions, nervousness, tachycardia, tremulousness, sweating, nausea, and hyperventilation occur prominently. Additionally, the same drugs (i.e., benzodiazepines) can be used to treat anxiety symptoms, and some individuals may use alcohol in an attempt to alleviate anxiety. Thus, the symptoms of an underlying anxiety disorder may be difficult to differentiate from the withdrawal symptoms associated with the use of benzodiazepines or alcohol. The use of many commonly prescribed medications may produce side effects manifesting as anxiety (see Table 35-1).

Such medications include sympathomimetics or other bronchodilators such as theophylline, anticholinergics, antiparkinsonian preparations, corticosteroids, thyroid supplements, oral contraceptives, antihypertensive, and cardiovascular medications such as digitalis, insulin (secondary to hypoglycemia), and antipsychotic and antidepressant medications. Finally, heavy metals and toxins such as organophosphates, paint, and insecticides may also cause anxiety symptoms.

Etiology

Genetic Factors
Genetic transmission of a disorder suggests that certain gene-encoded changes in proteins and the resulting biological abnormalities may play a role in the pathophysiology of specific disorders. Skre and collaborators (1993) examined 20 monozygotic and 29 dizygotic twins with DSM-III-R-defined GAD. They found GAD to be diagnosed in 22% of first-degree relatives of 33 probands with anxiety disorders. In the largest twin study to date, which included 1033 female twin pairs, Kendler and associates (1992a) found that genetic factors play a significant, but not overwhelming role in the etiology of GAD, with the heritability of GAD estimated at around 30% in comparison to 70% heritability in major depressive disorder. In addition, the authors found that the vulnerability to GAD and major depressive disorder is influenced by the same genetic factors (Kendler et al. 1992b). Other studies have suggested that while genetic factors may predispose a person to GAD, unique and familial environmental factors play an important role in the development of GAD (Kendler et al. 1995, Scherrer et al. 2000). Others have found no support for the role of inheritance in GAD (Mendlewicz et al. 1993).

Other Biological Factors
Studies of the biological aspects of GAD have focused on the evaluation of catecholamine and autonomic responses, neuroendocrine measures, sleep, neuroanatomical/neuroimaging studies, infusion studies, and evaluation of other neurotransmitter systems (Table 35-2). Although there is limited evidence for abnormalities in catecholamine function in GAD individuals, however, current data do not support a strong association between abnormal catecholamine system function and GAD.

Since increases in plasma cortisol levels have been shown to be a critical component of normal stress responses (Curtis et al. 1970), researchers hypothesized that plasma baseline cortisol levels may be elevated in individuals with GAD. This hypothesis was not supported by studies measuring urinary free cortisol levels in GAD individuals when compared with normal controls (Rosenbaum et al. 1983). However, these findings do not exclude the possibility of hypothalamic–pituitary–adrenal (HPA) axis dysfunction in individuals with GAD. The test most commonly used to assess HPA function is the dexamethasone suppression test (DST). Indeed, some studies have shown a higher prevalence of an "escape" (nonsuppression) response in following dexamethasone administration (that was not attributable to the presence of depression) in GAD individuals when compared to normal comparison subjects (Avery et al. 1985). These data indicate that there may be dysregulation of the HPA axis in these individuals, as observed following dexamethasone suppression test, possibly associated with abnormal stress response in these individuals.

Consistent with the response pattern observed in HPA function studies are findings from studies evaluating peripheral markers of autonomic function such as electrodermal activity, skin conductance, respiration, and blood pressure. While these studies failed to demonstrate differences in measures of electrodermal activity, respiration, blood pressure, and heart interbeat interval at rest, researchers observed that females with GAD showed a significantly lower skin conductance response to stress provoking situations and a slower habituation to

Table 35-2	Generalized Anxiety Disorder: Biological Studies
Measure	**Results**
Catecholamine function	
Plasma catecholamine levels	Negative
Platelet α_2-adrenoreceptor binding sites	Decreased
Growth hormone response to clonidine stimulation	Blunted
Yohimbine stimulation	Negative
Levels of catecholamine degradation enzymes	Normal
Hypothalamic–pituitary–adrenal axis	
Urinary free cortisol	Normal
Dexamethasone suppression test	Nonsuppression
Thyroid function	Normal
Autonomic function	
Autonomic activity at rest	Normal
Autonomic response to stress (skin conductance)	Lower
Challenge studies	
Lactate infusion	Increased anxiety symptoms/not panic attacks
Neurotransmitter abnormalities	
Benzodiazepine-binding sites	Decreased
Serotoninergic activation via m-chlorophenylpiperazine administration	Anxiogenic

stress (Hoehn-Saric et al. 1989). These data suggest that individuals with GAD may have weaker autonomic responses to stress as well as a more prolonged time to recovery.

Challenge studies have become an increasingly important tool in the investigation of the phenomenology and biology of anxiety disorders. The interest in the lactate challenge model evolved from the observation that intravenous administration of sodium lactate provokes physiological and psychological symptoms of panic in individuals with panic disorder at a significantly higher rate than in normal comparison subjects (Cowley et al. 1988). Cowley and associates (1988) evaluated the response of individuals with GAD to the administration of sodium lactate. The authors found that individuals with GAD without current or prior panic attacks demonstrated a lower rate of lactate-induced panic attacks than individuals with panic disorder. However, they were significantly more likely to report increased anxiety symptoms than nonpsychiatric controls, suggesting some similarities with panic disorder.

Alterations in different neurotransmitter systems have been implicated in the pathophysiology of various anxiety disorders. It is generally accepted that anxiety disorders are not associated with abnormalities in only one neurotransmitter system; rather dynamic interactions among several different neurotransmitter systems are believed likely to underlie different anxiety states. Presently, there are data suggesting that the catecholamine (described earlier), serotonin, and GABA-benzodiazepine systems may be involved in the pathophysiology of anxiety disorders.

Benzodiazepines have been the treatment of choice for many individuals with GAD. They act at specific recognition sites in the brain, the benzodiazepine receptors, which are located in a subunit of a receptor for gamma-aminobutyric acid (GABA), the major inhibitory neurotransmitter in the brain. Several lines of evidence suggest that the GABA-benzodiazepine receptor complex may be involved in the mediation of anxiety responses. Studies with animals suggest a relationship between benzodiazepine receptors, and fear and anxiety. For example, studies examining response following exposure to stressful stimuli in animal models (e.g., cold swim) have shown a decrease in benzodiazepine receptor binding in the frontal cortex, hippocampus, and hypothalamus, which are areas related to fear and anxiety (Drugan et al. 1989). Models using gamma-2 knockout mice have shown a reduction in $GABA_A$ receptor clustering in the hippocampus and cerebral cortex along with behavioral inhibition to aversive stimuli and increased responsiveness in trace fear conditioning (Lesch 2001).

Research with humans also supports the role of benzodiazepine receptor problems in anxiety reactions (Dorow et al. 1987, Ferrarese et al. 1990, Rickels et al. 1988a, Rocca et al. 1998). The peripheral benzodiazepine receptors found on platelets and lymphocytes have been studied most extensively, and studies suggest that there is a decrease in the number of benzodiazepine-binding sites on platelets and lymphocytes of individuals with GAD (Rocca et al. 1998). Researchers have shown that low levels of peripheral lymphocyte benzodiazepine receptors are reversed with effective treatment. Following successful treatment with benzodiazepines, the number of binding sites increased (Ferrarese et al. 1990, Rocca et al. 1998). However, the peripheral benzodiazepine receptors are pharmacologically distinct from central benzodiazepine receptors, and, therefore, the significance of these results is unclear. Roy-Byrne and colleagues (1991), using the slowing of saccadic eye movements as a measure of central benzodiazepine effects, have shown a possible decrease in the sensitivity to diazepam in individuals with GAD. This suggests that benzodiazepine receptors may be different in individuals with GAD. Benzodiazepine-induced chemotaxis is also impaired in GAD individuals but is not restored with diazepam treatment (Sacerdote et al. 1999).

Alterations in serotonergic (5-HT) neurotransmission have been implicated in the mediation of fear and anxiety responses in animal models (Ramboz et al. 1998, Taylor et al. 1985) and in humans (Iny et al. 1994, Garvey et al. 1993, 1995, Kahn et al. 1991). Specifically, researchers hypothesize that anxiety may represent dysregulated serotonergic activity in critical brain areas. For example, serotonin receptor 1A ($5-HT_{1A}$) knockout mice show behaviors consistent with increased anxiety (Ramboz et al. 1998). Further, there is evidence suggesting that the reduction of serotonergic neurotransmission in animals, achieved by lesions of the serotonin system or serotonin receptor blockade, has anxiolytic effects in animal models (Eison 1990). This hypothesis is further supported by the observation that many anxiolytic agents affect serotonergic neurotransmission (Gray 1988). Specifically, drugs that affect serotonergic activity, such as the serotonin ($5-HT_{1A}$) receptor agonists buspirone, ipsapirone, and gepirone decrease the firing of serotonergic neurons and exert antianxiety effects in GAD individuals (Gray 1988). Finally, Germine et al. (1992) found that the administration of m-chlorophenylpiperazine (mCPP), a compound that activates the various serotonin receptors, causes greater anxiety responses in individuals with GAD than in normal individuals. Given the available data, whether overactivity or underactivity of the 5-HT system is the mechanism for GAD development remains unclear (Jetty et al. 2001, Nutt 2001).

Neuropeptides may also play a role in the pathogenesis of GAD and other anxiety disorders. The cholecystokinin (CCK) system is one of the neuropeptides implicated in anxiety in animal models (Harro et al. 1993, Lydiard 1994, Woodruff and Hughes 1991). CCK, a highly abundant neurotransmitter in the brain, has also been implicated in anxiety in humans (Bradwejn and Koszycki 1992, Brawman-Mintzer et al. 1997, Kennedy et al. 1999, Adams et al. 1995, Goddard et al. 1999). CCK may be possibly involved in the pathophysiology of panic disorder and may also play a role in the biology of GAD (Lydiard 1994). Corticotropin-releasing factor (CRF), a major physiological regulator of adrenocorticotropic hormone (ACTH), appears to be involved in stress and anxiety responses (Koob 1999, Chrousos and Gold 1992). Administration of CRF to various parts of animal brains has elicited anxiety and fear responses (e.g., suppression of exploratory behavior, shock-induced freezing) (Butler et al. 1990, Griebel 1999, Koob and Gold

1997). Interestingly, both these peptides are functionally antagonized by benzodiazepines. Neuropeptide Y (Britton et al. 1997, Widerlov et al. 1988, Boulenger et al. 1996, Stein et al. 1996) and tachykinins (Beresford et al. 1995) may play a role in anxiety. Further, research has suggested that glutamate may play a role in anxiety in both animal models and human studies (Trullas et al. 1989, Miserendino et al. 1990, Moghaddam et al. 1994).

Several potential neuroanatomic anxiogenic sites in the central nervous system (CNS) have been proposed based on brain imaging and neuroanatomic studies. The areas potentially involved in anxiety are the parts of the limbic system involving the hippocampus, prefrontal cortex, occipital lobes, basal ganglia and brain stem structures, specifically the locus coeruleus, nucleus paragigantocellularis, and periaqueductal gray (Gray 1988). These structures are rich in noradrenergic, GABAergic, and serotonergic receptors, which are believed to be involved in the pathophysiology of different anxiety states such as GAD.

Only a few imaging studies in GAD have appeared in the literature. In one study, individuals with GAD displayed decreases in cortical blood flow compared to control subjects. Significant negative correlations between state anxiety and cerebral blood flow in most brain regions were observed (Mathew et al. 1982b). Using magnetic resonance imaging (MRI) and single photon emission tomography (SPET), Tiihonen and colleagues (1997) found that those with GAD had decreased benzodiazepine receptor binding in the left temporal pole as compared to matched healthy controls. In a study using functional MRI in GAD individuals, Lorberbaum and colleagues (2001) found greater activity in the right cingulate, right medial prefrontal and orbitofrontal cortex, right temporal poles, and right dorsomedial thalamus, during periods of anticipatory anxiety, compared with rest periods, than matched control subjects. Further, only matched control subjects displayed increased activity in the medial prefrontal cortex.

Psychological Mechanisms

Psychological models, which emphasize the cognitive–behavioral processes involved in the onset and maintenance of GAD, have emerged in recent years. Individuals' thoughts and behaviors are thought to instigate and maintain episodes of anxiety. Such thoughts and behaviors may be triggered by life events. For example, Blazer and associates (1987) found evidence suggesting the importance of negative life events in the onset of GAD. Additionally, one's cognitive style may trigger anxiety.

In support of cognitive theories of GAD, anxious individuals with GAD were more likely to perceive ambiguous information as threatening and/or negative, and to perceive that they are more likely than others to experience threatening situations (Rapee 1991). Individuals with GAD also pay more attention to the detection of potentially threatening information and incorporate this information into highly elaborate cognitive schemas, thus lowering their threshold for activation of an anxiety response (Josephs 1994). The threatening information then elicits anxious affect, and the individual begins to worry in an attempt to further define the problem.

Barlow and colleagues also postulated that individuals with GAD are likely to be characterized by a perception of lack of control over threatening events (Rapee 1991). In addition, the authors found that individuals are likely to believe that they have little control over their emotions, especially their worrying, leading to further distress. It has been suggested that the interaction between perceived uncontrollability and a cognitive focus on negative/threatening stimuli may amplify the general worry to pathological levels (Rapee 1991). Finally, Borkovec and colleagues (1993) suggested that worrying may suppress emotional processing, and temporarily reduce anxiety. This may help maintain the pathological cognitive state (Rapee 1991).

Psychodynamic theories offer a different view of the origins of anxiety disorders. In his initial explanation of the origin of anxiety (called toxic theory of anxiety), Freud stated that an abnormal amount of undischarged sexual energy (or libido) can manifest itself as anxiety

(Josephs 1994). He believed that unexpressed/ungratified sexual wishes result in undis-charged libido that is experienced subjectively as anxiety. Freud described various examples of unexpressed sexual urges such as sexual trauma (for example, activation of sexual urges following seduction in childhood), unhealthy sexual practices (such as *coitus interruptus*), and repression (when the threatening sexual urge or wish is banished from consciousness).

In his later work, Freud abandoned the toxic model, and developed another conceptual framework for the understanding of anxiety called the *signal theory of anxiety* (Josephs 1994). The concept of signal anxiety followed the development of Freud's structural model of the mind, which proposes three interacting psychological functions: ego (which mediates between the demands of primitive drives, the social and parental prohibitions, and reality), superego (representing the internalized parental and social prohibitions), and id (representing the primitive drives and urges) (Josephs 1994). Freud believed that anxiety serves as a signal to the ego of a threat (in the form of an unconscious drive or wish arising from the id), which, if enacted, may be dangerous to the ego, signaling the potential punishment by the superego or the external world. According to this model, the ego can activate defense mechanisms, such as repression, and prevent the actualization of the forbidden urge either by preventing the expression of the wish or by avoiding the life situations in which the wish might be potentially expressed. Ideally, repression into the unconscious (i.e., out of subject's awareness) should successfully contain the drives. However, if the defenses fail, one may experience symptomatic anxiety and other distressing psychological symptoms. Implicit in this model is the concept that the individuals themselves are not consciously aware of these processes. Therefore, the promotion of subjects' insight into unconscious conflicts and the uncovering of the unconscious origins of anxiety through interpretation and other techniques is the primary goal (and method) of the psychoanalytic treatment approach.

Sullivan developed a theory of anxiety based on the importance of interpersonal relationships (Josephs 1994). He viewed affects (such as anxiety) as forms of interpersonal communication. According to this model, anxiety communicates the sense of insecurity in interpersonal relationships. For example, a mother who is insecure in her role may communicate her insecurity to the infant when she is anxious in her child's presence. The child in turn identifies her anxiety and expresses anxious affect herself. Another approach to the understanding of the origins of anxiety was offered by object relations theorists such as Klein and Bowlby. They believed that anxiety reflects a fear of the loss of the nurturing object or fear of being hurt by the antagonistic object (Josephs 1994).

Finally, self psychology theorists, such as Kohut, believed that the individual strives to achieve and maintain an integrated, cohesive sense of self (Josephs 1994). Beginning at an early age, the individual develops this sense of self through idealization of important others, such as important caregivers (called self-objects), and through a process of positive interaction with caregivers (called mirroring). He believed that inadequate provision of these experiences can lead to anxiety (fear of disintegration) and the loss of the cohesive self (Josephs 1994).

Treatment

Since GAD is a chronic, relapsing illness, most treatments do not cure the individual and when treatments are discontinued, symptoms may return. Each case must be considered individually according to the severity and chronicity of the disorder, the severity of somatic symptoms, the presence of stressors, and the presence of specific personality traits. The clinician may also need to work with the individual to determine how much improvement is sufficient. For example, a reduction in disability may occur without a marked change in symptoms. Symptoms may persist but occur less frequently, or their intensity may be reduced. All these variations have important treatment implications, including decisions regarding the need for long-term treatment. Individuals with milder forms of GAD may respond well to simple psychological interventions, and require no medication treatment. In more severe forms of GAD, it may become necessary to see the individual regularly and to provide both more specific psychological and pharmacological interventions. Figure 35-2 can be used as a guide to the treatment of GAD using, primarily, medications.

During the early (acute) phase of treatment, an attempt should be made to control the individual's symptomatology. It may take 3 to 6 months for an optimal response to be achieved. However, there may be a considerable variation in the length of the initial treatment phase. For example, clinical response to benzodiazepines occurs early in treatment. Response to other anxiolytic medications or to cognitive–behavioral or psychodynamic treatment generally requires longer periods of time. During the maintenance phase, treatment gains are consolidated. Unfortunately, studies suggesting how long treatment should be continued are limited. Routinely, pharmacological treatment is continued for a total of 6 to 12 months before attempting to discontinue medications. Recent data indicate that *maintenance* psychotherapeutic treatments such as cognitive–behavioral therapy may be helpful in maintaining treatment gains in individuals with anxiety disorders following the

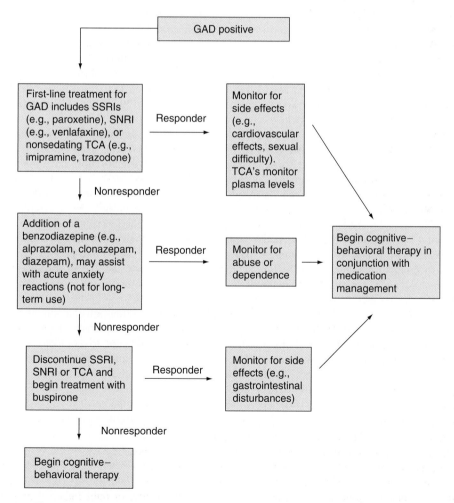

Figure 35-2 *Generalized anxiety disorder treatment flowchart emphasizing pharmacotherapy.*

discontinuation of pharmacotherapy (Spiegel et al. 1994). It is clear that many individuals may experience chronic and continuous symptoms that require years of long-term treatment.

The vast majority of individuals with GAD who present for treatment have been ill for many years and frequently have received a variety of treatments. Some individuals have been sent to psychiatrists for treatment as a "last resort" in order to learn how to cope with their various ill-defined somatic and emotional complaints. Individuals may feel shame and guilt over their inability to control symptoms. They are often demoralized and angry, and feel that their symptoms are not taken seriously. Thus, it is important to help the individual understand their illness and to conceptualize it as a health problem rather than a *personal weakness*. Once the burden of perceived responsibility is lifted from the individual, and they believe that effective treatment of their illness is possible, a working alliance with the treating physician can begin. The treatment plan should be outlined clearly, and the individual cautioned that recovery may have a gradual, variable course. Finally, during the critical early stages of treatment, the clinician should make a special effort to be available in person or by phone to answer questions and provide support.

Somatic Therapies

A number of anxiolytic agents are effective in the treatment of GAD (see Table 35-3). Benzodiazepines are commonly used for the treatment of GAD and are still considered by some clinicians to be the first-line treatment for GAD (Uhlenhuth et al. 1999). Several controlled studies have demonstrated the efficacy of different benzodiazepines such as diazepam, chlordiazepoxide, and alprazolam in the treatment of GAD. The available placebo-controlled studies found that diazepam, alprazolam, and lorazepam were effective in the treatment of GAD (Cohn and Wilcox 1984, Cutler et al. 1993, Ellie and Lamontagne 1984, Laakmann et al. 1998, Rickels et al. 1983, 1997, Ruiz 1983).

The benzodiazepines have a broad spectrum of effects including sedation, muscle relaxation, anxiety reduction, and decreased physiologic arousal (e.g., palpitations, tremulousness, etc.). Interestingly, available studies indicate that benzodiazepines have the most pronounced effect on hypervigilance and somatic symptoms of GAD, but exhibited fewer effects on psychic symptoms such as dysphoria, interpersonal sensitivity, and obsessionality (Hoehn-Saric et al. 1988). The main difference between individual benzodiazepines is potency and elimination half-life. These differences may have important treatment implications. For example, benzodiazepines with relatively short elimination half-lives such as alprazolam (range of 10–14 hours) may require dosing at least three to four times a day in order to avoid interdose symptom rebound. Conversely, the use of longer-acting compounds such as clonazepam (range of 20–50 hours) may minimize the risk of interdose symptom recurrence.

Benzodiazepines exert their therapeutic effects quickly, often after a single dose. However, concern has emerged over the use of benzodiazepines, particularly, long-term benzodiazepine use. Side effects of benzodiazepines, such as sedation, psychomotor impairment, and memory disruption were noted by treating clinicians, and confirmed in research studies (Lader 1999). Further, although it was suggested that the use pattern of benzodiazepines by individuals with anxiety disorders may not represent abuse, addiction, or drug dependence as typically understood (Romach et al. 1995), the chronic use of benzodiazepines in the treatment of GAD has been increasingly discouraged in recent years (Ballenger et al. 2001).

When initiating treatment with benzodiazepines, it is helpful for individuals to take an initial dose at home in the evening to see how it affects them. Gradual titration to an effective dose allows for limiting unwanted adverse effects. A final daily dosage of alprazolam between 2 and 4 mg/day, 1 and 2 mg/day for clonazepam, or 15 and 20 mg/day of diazepam, is usually sufficient for the majority of individuals. Upon treatment discontinuation, it is

able 35-3	Anxiolytic Agents		
Drug	Daily Dosage Range (mg)	Advantages	Disadvantages
Selective serotonin reuptake inhibitors			
Paroxetine	20–40	Efficacy with GAD	Gastrointestinal side effects
Fluoxetine	20–60	Efficacy with comorbid depression	Delayed onset
Sertraline	50–200		Sexual side effects
Citalopram	20–40	Favorable side effects profile compared with TCAs	
Fluvoxamine	100–300	Easy dosing schedule	
Serotonergic and noradrenergic reuptake inhibitors			
Venlafaxine extended release (XR)	75–225	Efficacy with GAD	Gastrointestinal side effects
		Efficacy with comorbid depression	Sexual side effects
			Potential for increased blood pressure
Benzodiazepines			
Alprazolam	2–6	Rapid onset of action	Sedation
Clonazepam	1–3	Favorable side effects profile	Multiple doses for shorter acting agents
Lorazepam	4–10		Physical dependence
Diazepam	15–20		Limited antidepressant effects
			Sexual side effects
Tricyclic antidepressants			
Imipramine	75–300	Once-daily dosage	Delayed onset
		Efficacy with comorbid depression	Need for titration
			Activation
			Anticholinergic effects
			Orthostatic hypotension
			Weight gain
			Toxicity in overdose
			Sexual side effects
Atypical antidepressants			
Trazodone	150–600	Once-daily dosage	Delayed onset
		Efficacy with comorbid depression	Orthostatic hypotension
			Weight gain
		Low anticholinergic effects	Sexual side effects
			Priapism (rare)
			Sedation
Azapirones			
Buspirone	30–60	No withdrawal symptoms	Multiple doses
		No physical dependence	
		Favorable side effects profile	

important to consider appropriate taper in order to avoid withdrawal symptoms. Possible factors that may contribute to the severity of withdrawal and the ultimate outcome of benzodiazepine taper include the dosage, duration of treatment, the benzodiazepine elimination half-life and potency, and the rate of benzodiazepine taper (gradual versus abrupt). Additionally, individual factors such as premorbid personality features have been implicated. It appears that a taper rate of 25% per week is probably too rapid for many individuals (Brawman-Mintzer and Lydiard 1994). A slow benzodiazepine taper of at least 4 to 8 weeks, with the final 50% of the taper conducted even more gradually, is recommended, with the individual decreasing the daily dose of the benzodiazepines during this period by the lowest possible percentage.

Clinical trials conducted in the early 1990s have confirmed that tricyclic antidepressants (TCAs) may also be effective in the treatment of GAD (Brawman-Mintzer and Lydiard 1994). Rickels and colleagues (1993) completed a placebo-controlled study which compared imipramine, trazodone, and diazepam in GAD individuals without comorbid depression or panic disorder. Data analysis revealed that the efficacy of imipramine and trazodone was comparable to diazepam. It should be noted that diazepam demonstrated greater efficacy than imipramine during the first 2 weeks of treatment with the greatest degree of response in the somatic and hyperarousal symptoms; however, imipramine and trazodone exhibited higher efficacy after 6 to 8 weeks of treatment with psychic symptoms of tension, apprehension, and worry being more responsive to the antidepressants. Owing, in part, to their side effect profile, need for dose titration, and importantly the emergence of new and effective agents (as described below), the use of TCAs in the treatment of GAD has been reserved for those resistant to these newer agents.

Selective serotonin reuptake inhibitors (SSRIs) are rapidly becoming a key tool in the treatment of GAD. Recent estimates suggest that 19% of experts recommend the use of SSRIs as first-line treatment for GAD, reflecting a 15% increase in 5 years (Uhlenhuth et al. 1999). Several controlled double-blind studies (Rocca et al. 1997, Bellew et al. 2000, Pollack et al. 1997) have demonstrated the efficacy of paroxetine in the treatment of GAD. The most problematic side effect associated with SSRI use is the interference with sexual function (e.g., delayed orgasm or abnormal ejaculation) in women and men (Michelson et al. 2000, Rosen et al. 1999). A variety of treatment strategies have been suggested for the management of SSRI-induced sexual dysfunction. Such strategies include waiting for tolerance to develop, dosage reduction, drug holidays, and various augmentation strategies with 5-hydroxytryptamine-2 (5-HT$_2$), 5-HT$_3$, and alpha-2-adrenergic receptor antagonists, 5-HT$_{1A}$ and dopamine receptor agonists, and phosphodiesterase (PDE5) enzyme inhibitors (Rosen et al. 1999).

The antidepressant venlafaxine extended release (XR) is an inhibitor of both 5-HT and NE reuptake, serotonergic and noradrenergic reuptake inhibitors (SNRI). Several large, placebo-controlled trials (Sheehan 1999, Allgulander et al. 2001, Davidson et al. 1999, Gelenberg et al. 2000)) have evaluated it in the treatment of individuals with DSM-IV-TR-diagnosed GAD. As a result, venlafaxine XR was the first antidepressant approved by the FDA for the treatment of GAD. The adverse events for GAD individuals treated with venlafaxine XR resembled those in depression trials. The most common adverse events included nausea, somnolence, dry mouth, dizziness, sweating, constipation, and anorexia.

Nefazodone is a phenylpiperazine compound chemically related to trazodone. The efficacy of nefazodone in the treatment of GAD has been evaluated in one open-label trial (Hedges et al. 1996). Of the 15 study completers ($N = 21$), 12 were rated as overall much or very much improved following treatment with nefazodone. More research, however, is required to further define the potential of nefazodone in treating individuals with GAD. Several other psychotherapeutic agents have been tested in the treatment of individuals with GAD. For example, the alpha-2-adrenoreceptor antagonist mirtazapine, which is also a 5-HT$_2$, 5-HT$_3$, and H(1) receptors antagonist, has been evaluated as a potential anxiolytic in the treatment of individuals with major depressive disorder and comorbid GAD in an 8-week, open-label study (Goodnick et al. 1999). Results suggest that this antidepressant may be useful in the treatment of anxiety symptoms.

The azapirone group of drugs was introduced in response to concerns over chronic benzodiazepine use in subjects with anxiety symptoms. Buspirone hydrochloride, the only currently marketed azapirone, was the first nonbenzodiazepine anxiolytic agent approved for the treatment of persistent anxiety by the FDA. Results have been mixed about the efficacy of buspirone over placebo and benzodiazepines (Spiegel et al. 1994, Pollack et al. 1997, Davidson et al. 1999, Delle Chiaie et al. 1995, Enklemann 1991, Rickels et al. 1988b,

1982, Bohm et al. 1990, Goldberg and Finnerty 1979, Lader and Scotto 1998, Pecknold et al. 1989, Wheatley 1982). For example, in four placebo-controlled studies that compared buspirone to a standard benzodiazepine, two showed no benefit for diazepam and buspirone over placebo, and two showed no benefit for buspirone over placebo (Olajide and Lader 1987, Pecknold et al. 1985, Ross and Matas 1987). Benzodiazepines may also be slightly more effective than buspirone in the treatment of somatic symptoms of anxiety but no significant differences appear to exist between buspirone and benzodiazepines in measures of psychic anxiety (Rickels et al. 1997). Buspirone, however, may be more effective in the treatment of anger/hostility symptoms than benzodiazepines (Rickels et al. 1997).

Side effects most frequently associated with buspirone use included gastrointestinal system-related side effects, such as appetite disturbances and abdominal complaints, and dizziness. Prior use of benzodiazepines may adversely affect the therapeutic response to buspirone (Schweizer et al. 1986). DeMartinis and colleagues (2000) found that buspirone treatment was less effective for individuals who had been taking benzodiazepines within 30 days of initiating buspirone treatment. Delle Chiaie and colleagues (1995) reported that a gradual 2-week taper of lorazepam with a simultaneous addition of buspirone for 6 weeks prevents the development of clinically significant rebound anxiety or benzodiazepine withdrawal. This approach was shown to provide clinically significant relief of anxiety symptoms in GAD individuals previously treated with benzodiazepines for 8 to 14 weeks. Perhaps the most significant problem with the use of buspirone has been that experts have advocated too low a dose to produce symptom reduction. In order to achieve optimal response, buspirone dosing in the range of at least 30 to 60 mg/day is currently recommended.

When faced with treatment resistance, clinician should evaluate whether an adequate treatment trial was complete. An attempt should be made to maintain the individual on medication for at least 6 weeks. Although there are no data suggesting that certain doses may be particularly effective in the treatment of GAD, it is advisable to titrate the medication up to maximally tolerated doses prior to discontinuing the medication for nonresponse. It is important to inquire about the presence of side effects such as sedation, anticholinergic effects, or sexual side effects, which may limit the attainment of a therapeutic dosage and reduce compliance. Additionally, many individuals with GAD fear that they may become *drug-dependent* and thus avoid dose increases. Some estimate of the individual's compliance may be helpful in determining whether a treatment was adequate, as indicated by blood plasma levels or pill counts. Drug plasma levels may also be useful to identify individuals who are rapid metabolizers. A careful evaluation for the presence of psychiatric comorbid conditions that may contribute to treatment refractoriness should follow. As mentioned, comorbidity which may reflect more severe loading for psychopathology is often associated with increased severity of illness and poorer response to treatment in comparison to individuals with an uncomplicated (i.e., single) disorder. Thus, treatment strategies in GAD individuals with a concurrent disorder may differ from those in an uncomplicated disorder, often requiring multiple drug therapy. The clinician should also be alert to the presence of underlying general medical conditions such as hyperthyroidism, which may present with refractory anxiety, or conditions/medications that may alter the effects of treatment, such as hepatic disease or medications (e.g., steroids) that affect hepatic clearance.

Psychosocial Therapies

Numerous studies have shown that psychological interventions are beneficial in the comprehensive management of anxiety disorders (Brown et al. 1993). However, data suggesting that specific psychotherapeutic techniques yield better results in the treatment of individuals with GAD are inconclusive, and more evidence is needed on the comparative efficacy and long-term effects of different psychological treatments.

In recent years, specific cognitive–behavioral therapy (CBT) interventions for the treatment of individuals with anxiety disorders have been developed. Components of CBT include teaching individuals to identify and label irrational thoughts and to replace them with positive self-statements or modify them by challenging their veracity. The cognitive modification approaches are combined with behavioral treatments such as exposure or relaxation training. There is currently evidence suggesting that CBT may be more effective in the treatment of GAD than other psychotherapeutic interventions, such as behavioral therapy alone or nonspecific supportive therapy (Chambless and Gillis 1993). For example, Barlow and colleagues (1984) showed significant improvement in clinical ratings and measures of anxiety in individuals with GAD treated with relaxation and CBT. A nontreatment (waiting list) control group remained unchanged. Six additional studies confirmed the efficacy of CBT compared with waiting list or pill placebo (Borkovec and Costello 1993). Further, Borkovec and colleagues (1993) observed that individuals tend to maintain improvement following CBT over 6 to 12 months of follow-up.

CBT targeting intolerance of uncertainty, erroneous beliefs about worry, poor problem orientation, and cognitive avoidance demonstrated effectiveness at posttreatment (no change in the delayed treatment control group) 6- and 12-month follow-up, with 77% of the treatment group no longer having symptoms meeting criteria for a GAD diagnosis (Ladouceur et al. 2000). Cognitive therapy was also compared to analytic psychotherapy, and was found to be significantly more effective (Borkovec and Costello 1993). Overall, two-thirds in the cognitive therapy group achieved clinically significant improvements and cognitive therapy was associated with significant reductions in medication usage.

Many individuals with milder forms of GAD will benefit from simple psychological interventions such as supportive psychotherapy. They may experience lessening of anxiety when given the opportunity to discuss their difficulties with a supportive clinician and to become better informed about their illness. Thus, basic supportive techniques such as reassurance, clarification of individual concerns, direct suggestions, and advice are often effective in reducing anxiety symptoms.

Relaxation techniques such as progressive muscle relaxation and biofeedback have also been utilized in the treatment of individuals with anxiety symptoms. Few controlled studies have examined their effectiveness. In a recent controlled study, Borkovec and Costello (1993) compared a comprehensive relaxation treatment and cognitive–behavioral therapy in the treatment of individuals with DSM-III-R-defined GAD. The authors found that both treatments were equally effective and superior to a nonspecific supportive treatment intervention. Biofeedback was also found to be effective in the treatment of individuals with GAD (Rice et al. 1993). It should be noted that relaxation may be associated with a paradoxical increase in anxiety and tension in individuals with GAD. However, with repeated training, specifically in the context of cognitive–behavioral therapy (see the section on cognitive–behavioral therapy), this phenomenon may be used to achieve habituation and anxiety extinction.

Combined Treatment

A meta-analytic review of controlled trials examining CBT and pharmacotherapy for GAD, which included 35 studies, demonstrated the robustness of CBT in the treatment of GAD (Gould et al. 1997). Overall, both modalities offered clear efficacy to individuals, with the effect size for CBT not being statistically different from psychopharmacological approaches. CBT demonstrated greater effects in reducing depression and was associated with clear maintenance of treatment gains, whereas long-term efficacy of pharmacologic treatment was attenuated following medication discontinuation.

Comparison of DSM-IV-TR/ICD-10 Diagnostic Criteria
The ICD-10 Diagnostic Criteria for Research specify that four symptoms from a list of 22 be present. In contrast, DSM-IV-TR requires three out of a list of six (of which five are included among the ICD-10 list of 22).

References

Adams JB, Pyke RE, Costa J, et al. (1995) A double-blind, placebo-controlled study of a CCK-B receptor antagonist, CI-988, in patients with generalized anxiety disorder. *J Clin Psychopharmacol* **15**(6), 428–434.

Allgulander C, Hackett D, and Salinas E (2001) Venlafaxine extended release (ER) in the treatment of generalized anxiety disorder. *Br J Psychiatry* **179**, 15–22.

American Psychiatric Association (1994) *Diagnostic and Statistical Manual of Mental Disorders*, 4th ed., APA, Washington, DC.

Anderson JC, Williams S, and McGee R (1987) DSM-III disorders in preadolescent children: prevalence in a large sample from the general population. *Arch Gen Psychiatry* **44**, 69–76.

Angst J (1993) Comorbidity of anxiety, phobia, compulsion, and depression. *Int J Clin Psychopharmacol* **8**(Suppl. 1), 21–25.

Angst J and Vollrath M (1991) The natural history of anxiety disorder and generalized anxiety disorder. *Acta Psychiatr Scand* **141**, 572–575.

Avery DH, Osgodd TB, Ishiki DM, et al. (1985) The DST in psychiatric outpatients with generalized anxiety disorder, panic disorder, or primary affective disorder. *Am J Psychiatry* **142**, 844–848.

Ballenger JC, Davidson JRT, Lecrubier Y, et al. (2001) Consensus statement on generalized anxiety disorder from the international consensus group on depression and anxiety. *J Clin Psychiatry* **62**(Suppl. 11), 53–58.

Barlow DH, Blanchard RB, Vermilyea JB, et al. (1986) Generalized anxiety and generalized anxiety disorder: description and reconceptualization. *Am J Psychiatry* **143**, 40–44.

Barlow DH, Cohen AS, and Waddell MT (1984) Panic and generalized anxiety disorders: nature and treatment. *Behav Ther* **15**, 431–449.

Beekman ATF, Bremmer MA, Deeg DJH, et al. (1998) Anxiety disorders in later life: a report from the longitudinal aging study, Amsterdam. *Int J Geriatr Psychiatry* **13**, 717–726.

Bellew KM, McCafferty JP, Iyengar M, et al. (2000) Paroxetine treatment of GAD: a double-blind, placebo-controlled trial. *American Psychiatric Association 2000 Annual Meeting* (May 13–18), Chicago, IL.

Beresford IJ, Sheldrick RL, Ball DI, et al. (1995) GR159897, a potent non-peptide antagonist at tachykinin NK2 receptors. *Eur J Psychopharmacol* **272**(2–3), 241–248.

Bernstein GA and Borchardt CM (1991) Anxiety disorders of childhood and adolescence: a critical review. *J Am Acad Child Adolesc Psychiatry* **30**(4), 519–532.

Bhagwanjee A, Parekh A, Paruk Z, et al. (1998) Prevalence of minor psychiatric disorders in an adult African rural community in South Africa. *Psychol Med* **28**, 1137–1147.

Blazer D, Hughes D, and George LK (1987) Stressful life events and the onset of a generalized anxiety syndrome. *Am J Psychiatry* **144**, 1178–1183.

Blazer DG, Hughes D, George LK, et al. (1991) Generalized anxiety disorder. In *Psychiatric Disorders in America: The Epidemiologic Catchment Area Study*, Robins LN and Regier DA (eds). Free Press, New York, pp. 180–203.

Bohm C, Placchi M, Stallone F, et al. (1990) A double-blind comparison of buspirone, clobazam, and placebo in patients with anxiety treated in a general practice setting. *J Clin Psychopharmacol* **10**(3 (Suppl.)), 38S–42S.

Borkovec TD and Costello E (1993) Efficacy of applied relaxation and cognitive–behavioral therapy in the treatment of generalized anxiety disorder. *J Consult Clin Psychol* **61**(4), 611–619.

Boulenger JP, Jerabek I, Jolicoeur FB, et al. (1996) Elevated plasma levels of neuropeptide Y in patients with panic disorders. *Am J Psychiatry* **153**(1), 114–116.

Bradwejn J and Koszycki D (1992) The cholecystokinin hypothesis of panic and anxiety disorders: a review. *Ann N Y Acad Sci* **713**, 273–282.

Brawman-Mintzer O and Lydiard RB (1994) Psychopharmacology of anxiety disorders. *Psychiatr Clin North Am* **1**, 51–79.

Brawman-Mintzer O, Lydiard RB, Bradwejn J, et al. (1997) Effects of the cholecystokinin agonist pentagastrin in patients with generalized anxiety disorder. *Am J Psychiatry* **154**(5), 700–702.

Brawman-Mintzer O, Lydiard RB, Crawford MM, et al. (1994) Somatic symptoms in generalized anxiety disorder with and without comorbid psychiatric disorders. *Am J Psychiatry* **151**, 930–932.

Brawman-Mintzer O, Lydiard RB, Emmanuel N, et al. (1993) Psychiatric comorbidity in patients with generalized anxiety disorder. *Am J Psychiatry* **150**, 1216–1218.

Breitholtz E, Johansson B, and Öst LG (1999) Cognitions in generalized anxiety disorder and panic disorder patients: a prospective approach. *Behav Res Ther* **37**, 533–544.

Breslau N and Davis GC (1985) DSM-III Generalized anxiety disorder: an empirical investigation of more stringent criteria. *Psychiatr Res* **14**, 231–238.

Britton KT, Southerland S, Van Uden E, et al. (1997) Anxiolytic activity of NPY receptor agonists in the conflict test. *Psychopharmacology* **132**(1), 6–13.

Brown TA, Barlow DH, and Liebowitz MR (1994) The empirical basis of generalized anxiety disorder. *Am J Psychiatry* **151**(9), 1272–1280.

Brown TA, O'Leary D, and Barlow DH (1993) Generalized anxiety disorder. In *Clinical Handbook of Psychological Disorders: A step-by-step Treatment Manual*, Barlow DH (ed). Guilford Press, New York, pp. 137–188.

Burke KC, Burke JD Jr., Rae DS, et al. (1991) Comparing age at onset of major depression and other psychiatric disorders by birth cohorts in five US community populations. *Arch Gen Psychiatry* **48**(9), 789–795.

Butler PD, Weiss JM, Stout JC, et al. (1990) Corticotropin-releasing factor produces fear-enhancing and behavioral activating effects following infusion into the locus coeruleus. *J Neurosci* **10**(1), 176–183.

Carter CS and Maddock RJ (1992) Chest pain in generalized anxiety disorder. *Int J Psychiatr Med* **22**(3), 291–298.

Carter RM, Wittchen HU, Pfister H, et al. (2001) One-year prevalence of sub-threshold and threshold DSM-IV generalized anxiety disorder in a nationally representative sample. *Depress Anx* **3**, 78–88.

Chambless DL and Gillis MM (1993) Cognitive therapy of anxiety disorders. *J Clin Consult Psychol* **61**(2), 248–260.

Chrousos GP and Gold PW (1992) The concepts of stress and stress disorders. Overview of physical and behavioral homeostasis. *JAMA* **267**(9), 1244–1252.

Cohn JB and Wilcox CS (1984) Long-term comparison of alprazolam, lorazepam, and placebo in patients with an anxiety disorder. *Psychopharmacology* **4**(2), 93–98.

Cowley DS, Dager SR, McClellan J, et al. (1988) Response to lactate infusion in generalized anxiety disorder. *Biol Psychiatry* **24**, 409–414.

Curtis G, Fogel M, McEvoy D, et al. (1970) Urine and plasma corticosteroids, psychological tests, and effectiveness of psychological defenses. *J Psychiatr Res* **7**, 237–247.

Cutler NR, Sramek JJ, Keppel Hesselink JM, et al. (1993) A double-blind, placebo-controlled study comparing the efficacy and safety of ipsapirone versus lorazepam in patients with generalized anxiety disorder: a prospective multicenter trial. *J Clin Psychopharmacol* **13**(6), 429–437.

Dager SR, Comess KA, and Dunner DL (1986) Differentiation of anxious patients by two-dimensional echocardiographic evaluation of the mitral valve. *Am J Psychiatry* **143**, 533–535.

Davidson JR, DuPont RL, Hedges D, et al. (1999) Efficacy, safety, and tolerability of venlafaxine extended release and buspirone in outpatients with generalized anxiety disorder. *J Clin Psychiatry* **60**(8), 528–535.

Delle Chiaie R, Pancheri P, Casacchia M, et al. (1995) Assessment of the efficacy of buspirone in patients affected by generalized anxiety disorder, shifting buspirone from prior treatment with lorazepam: a placebo-controlled, double-blind study. *J Clin Psychopharmacol* **15**(1), 12–19.

DeMartinis N, Rynn M, Rickels K, et al. (2000) Prior benzodiazepine use and buspirone response in the treatment of generalized anxiety disorder. *J Clin Psychiatry* **61**(2), 91–94.

Dorow R, Duka T, Holler L, et al. (1987) Clinical perspectives of beta- carbolines from first studies in humans. *Brain Res Bull* **19**(3), 319–326.

Drugan RC, Skolnick P, Paul SM, et al. (1989) A pretest procedure reliably predicts performance in two animal models of inescapable stress. *Pharmacol Biochem Behav* **33**(3), 649–654.

Eison MS (1990) Serotonin: a common neurobiologic substrate in anxiety and depression. *J Clin Psychopharmacol* **10**, 26S–30S.

Ellie R and Lamontagne Y (1984) Alprazolam and diazepam in the treatment of generalized anxiety. *J Clin Psychopharmacol* **4**(3), 125–129.

Emmanuel NP, Mintzer O, Lydiard RB, et al. (1992) Prevalence of personality disorders in general anxiety disorder. *Presented at the 12th National Conference of the Anxiety Disorders Association of America*, Houston, Texas.

Enklemann R (1991) Alprazolam versus buspirone in the treatment of outpatients with generalized anxiety disorder. *Psychopharmacology* **105**(3), 428–432.

Ferrarese C, Appollonio I, Frigo M, et al. (1990) Decreased density of benzodiazepine receptors in lymphocytes of anxious patients: reversal after chronic diazepam treatment. *Acta Psychiatr Scand* **82**(2), 169–173.

Flint AJ (1994) Epidemiology and comorbidity of anxiety disorders in the elderly. *Am J Psychiatry* **151**, 640–649.

Garvey MJ, Noyes R Jr., Woodman C, et al. (1993) A biological difference between panic disorder and generalized anxiety disorder. *Biol Psychiatry* **34**(8), 572–575.

Garvey MJ, Noyes R Jr., Woodman C, et al. (1995) Relationship of generalized anxiety symptoms to urinary 5-hydroxyindoleacetic acid and vanillylmandelic acid. *Psychiatr Res* **57**(1), 1–5.

Gasperini M, Battaglia M, Diaferia G, et al. (1990) Personality features related to generalized anxiety disorder. *Compr Psychiatry* **31**(4), 363–368.

Gelenberg AJ, Lydiard RB, Rudolph RL, et al. (2000) Efficacy of venlafaxine extended-release capsules in nondepressed outpatients with generalized anxiety disorder: a 6-month randomized controlled trial. *JAMA* **283**, 3082–3088.

Goddard AW, Woods SW, Money R, et al. (1999) Effects of the CCK antagonist CI-988 on responses to mCPP in generalized anxiety disorder. *Psychiatr Res* **85**, 225–240.

Goldberg HL and Finnerty RJ (1979) The comparative efficacy of buspirone and diazepam in the treatment of anxiety. *Am J Psychiatry* **136**(9), 1184–1187.

Goodnick PJ, Puig A, DeVane CL, et al. (1999) Mirtazapine in major depression with comorbid generalized anxiety disorder. *J Clin Psychiatry* **60**, 446–448.

Gould RA, Otto MA, Pollack MH, et al. (1997) Cognitive–behavioral and pharmacological treatment of generalized anxiety disorder: a preliminary meta-analysis. *Behav Ther* **28**(2), 285–305.

Gray JA (1988) The neuropsychological basis of anxiety. In *Handbook of Anxiety Disorders*, Last CG and Hersen M (eds). Pergamon Press, New York, pp. 10–37.

Griebel G (1999) Is there a future for neuropeptide receptor ligands in the treatment of anxiety disorders? *Pharmacol Ther* **82**(1), 1–61.

Harro J, Vasar E, and Bradwejn J (1993) CCK in animal and human research on anxiety. *TIPS* **14**, 244–249.

Hedges DW, Reimherr FW, Strong RE, et al. (1996) An open trial of nefazodone in adult patients with generalized anxiety disorder. *Psychopharmacol Bull* **32**(4), 671–676.

Hoehn-Saric R, Hazlett RL, and McLeod DR (1993) Generalized anxiety disorder with early and late onset of anxiety symptoms. *Compr Psychiatry* **34**(5), 291–298.

Hoehn-Saric R, McLeod DR, and Zimmerli WD (1988) Differential effects of alprazolam and imipramine in generalized anxiety disorder: somatic versus psychic symptoms. *J Clin Psychiatry* **49**, 293–301.

Hoehn-Saric R, McLeod DR, and Zimmerli WD (1989) Somatic manifestations in women with generalized anxiety disorder. *Arch Gen Psychiatry* **46**, 1113–1119.

Iny LJ, Pecknold J, Suranyi-Cadotte BE, et al. (1994) Studies of a neurochemical link between depression, anxiety, and stress from [3H]imipramine and [3H]paroxetine binding on human platelets. *Biol Psychiatry* **36**(5), 281–291.

Jetty PV, Charney DS, and Goodard AW (2001) Neurobiology of generalized anxiety disorder. *Psychiatr Clin North Am* **24**(1), 75–98.

Josephs L (1994) Psychoanalytic and related interpretations. In anxiety and related disorders. *A Handbook*, Wolman BB and Stricker G (eds). Wiley-Interscience, New York, pp. 11–29.

Kahn RS, Wetzler S, Asnis GM, et al. (1991) Pituitary hormone response to meta-chlorophenylpiperazine in panic disorder and healthy control subjects. *Psychiatr Res* **37**(1), 25–34.

Kashani JH and Orvaschel H (1988) Anxiety disorders in mid-adolescence: a community sample. *Am J Psychiatry* **145**, 960–964.

Kendler KS, Neale MC, Kessler RC, et al. (1992a) Generalized anxiety disorder in women. *Arch Gen Psychiatry* **49**, 267–272.

Kendler KS, Neale MC, Kessler RC, et al. (1992b) Major depression and generalized anxiety disorder. *Arch Gen Psychiatry* **49**, 716–722.

Kendler KS, Walters EE, Neale MC, et al. (1995) The structure of the genetic and environmental risk factors for six major psychiatric disorders in women: phobia, generalized anxiety disorder, panic disorder, bulimia, major depression, and alcoholism. *Arch Gen Psychiatry* **52**(5), 374–383.

Kennedy JL, Bradwejn J, Koszycki D, et al. (1999) Investigation of cholestokinin system genes in panic disorder. *Mol Psychiatry* **4**(3), 284–285.

Kessler RC, DuPont RL, Berglund P, et al. (1999) Impairment in pure and comorbid generalized anxiety disorder and major depression at 12 months in two national surveys. *Am J Psychiatry* **156**, 1915–1923.

Kollai M and Kollai B (1992) Cardiac vagal tone in generalized anxiety disorder. *Br J Psychiatry* **161**, 831–835.

Koob GF (1999) Corticotropin-releasing factor, norepinephrine, and stress. *Biol Psychiatry* **46**(9), 1167–1180.

Koob GF and Gold LH (1997) Molecular biological approaches in the behavioural pharmacology of anxiety and depression. *Behav Pharmacol* **8**, 652.

Kushner MG, Sher KJ, and Erickson DJ (1999) Prospective analysis of the relationship between DSM-III anxiety disorders and alcohol use disorders. *Am J Psychiatry* **156**(5), 723–732.

Laakmann G, Schule C, Lorkowski G, et al. (1998) Buspirone and lorazepam in the treatment of generalized anxiety disorder in outpatients. *Psychopharmacology* **136**(4), 357–366.

Lader MH (1999) Limitations on the use of benzodiazepines in anxiety and insomnia: Are they justified? *Eur Neuropsychopharmacol* **9**(Suppl. 6), S399–S405.

Lader M and Scotto JC (1998) A multicentre double-blind comparison of hydroxyzine, buspirone, and placebo in patients with generalized anxiety disorder. *Psychopharmacology* **139**(4), 402–406.

Ladouceur R, Dugas MJ, Freeston MH, et al. (2000) Efficacy of a cognitive–behavioral treatment for generalized anxiety disorder: evaluation in a controlled clinical trial. *J Clin Consult Psychol* **68**(6), 957–964.

Last CG, Hersen M, and Karzdin AE (1987) Comparison of DSM-III separation anxiety and overanxious disorders: demographic characteristics and patterns of comorbidity. *J Am Acad Child Adolesc Psychiatry* **4**, 527–531.

Lesch KP (2001) Genetic dissection of anxiety and related disorders. In *Anxiety Disorders*, Nutt D and Ballenger J (eds). Blackwell Science, Oxford.

Lorberbaum JP, Varon D, Brawman-Mintzer O, et al. (2001) The functional neuroanatomy of anticipatory anxiety in healthy adults and patients with generalized anxiety disorder. *Presented at the 21st National Conference of Anxiety Disorders Association of America*, Atlanta.

Lydiard RB (1994) Neuropeptides and anxiety: focus on cholecystokinin. *Clin Chem* **40**, 315–318.

Maier W, Gaeniscke M, Freyberger HJ, et al. (2000) Generalized anxiety disorder (ICD-10) in primary care from a cross-cultural perspective: a valid diagnostic entity? *Acta Psychiatr Scand* **101**, 29–36.

Mancuso DM, Townsend MH, and Mercante DE (1993) Long-term follow-up of generalized anxiety disorder. *Compr Psychiatry* **34**, 441–446.

Mathew RJ, Weinman ML, and Claghorn JL (1982b) Anxiety and cerebral blood flow. In *The Biology of Anxiety*, Mathew RJ (ed). Brunner/Mazel, New York.

Mathew RJ, Ho BT, Francis DJ, et al. (1982a) Catecholamines and anxiety. *Acta Psychiatr Scand* **65**, 142–147.

Mauri M, Sarno N, Rossi VM, et al. (1992) Personality disorders associated with generalized anxiety, panic, and recurrent depressive disorders. *J Perspect Disord* **6**, 162–167.

Mavissakalian MR, Hamann MS, Abou Haidar S, et al. (1993) DSM-III personality disorders in generalized anxiety, panic/agoraphobia, and obsessive–compulsive disorders. *Compr Psychiatry* **34**(4), 243–248.

Mendlewicz J, Papadimitriou G, and Wimotte J (1993) Family study of panic disorder: comparison to generalized anxiety disorder, major depression, and normal subjects. *Psychiatr Genet* **3**, 73–78.

Michelson D, Bancroft J, Targum S, et al. (2000) Female sexual dysfunction associated with antidepressant administration: a randomized, placebo-controlled study of pharmacologic intervention. *Am J Psychiatry* **157**, 239–243.

Miserendino MJ, Sananes CB, Melia KR, et al. (1990) Blocking of acquisition but not expression of conditioned fear-potentiated startle by NMDA antagonists in the amygdala. *Nature* **345**(6277), 716–718.

Moghaddam B, Bolinao ML, Stein-Behrens B, et al. (1994) Glucocorticoids mediate the stress-induced extracellular accumulation of glutamate. *Brain Res* **655**(1–2), 251–254.

Noyes R Jr., Holt CS, and Woodman CL (1996) Natural course of anxiety disorders. In *Long-term Treatments of Anxiety Disorders*, Mavissakalian MR and Prien RF (eds). American Psychiatric Press, Washington, DC.

Nutt DJ (2001) Neurobiological mechanisms in generalized anxiety disorder. *J Clin Psychiatry* **62**(Suppl. 11), 22–27.

Olajide D and Lader M (1987) A comparison of buspirone, diazepam, and placebo in patients with chronic anxiety states. *J Clin Psychopharmacol* **7**(3), 148–152.

Pecknold JC, Familamiri P, Chang H, et al. (1985) Buspirone: Anxiolytic? *Prog Neuropsychopharmacol Biol Psychiatry* **9**(5–6), 639–642.

Pecknold JC, Matas M, Howarth BG, et al. (1989) Evaluation of buspirone as an antianxiety agent: Buspirone and diazepam vs. placebo. *Can J Psychiatry* **34**(8), 766–771.

Pollack MH, Worthington JJ, Manfro GG, et al. (1997) Abecarnil for the treatment of generalized anxiety disorder: a placebo-controlled comparison of two dosage ranges of abecarnil and buspirone. *J Clin Psychiatry* **58**(Suppl. 1), 19–23.

Ramboz S, Oosting R, Amara DA, et al. (1998) Serotonin receptor 1A knockout: an animal model of anxiety-related disorder. *Proc Natl Acad Sci U S A* **95**(24), 14476–14481.

Rapee RM (1991) Generalized anxiety disorder: a review of clinical features and theoretical concepts. *Clin Psychol Rev* **11**, 419–440.

Rice KM, Blanchard EB, and Purcell M (1993) Biofeedback treatments of generalized anxiety disorder: preliminary results. *Biofeedback Self-Reg* **18**(2), 93–104.

Rickels K, Case WG, and Schweizer E (1988a) The drug treatment of anxiety and panic disorder. *Stress Med* **4**(4), 231–239.

Rickels K, Case WG, Downing RW, et al. (1986) One-year follow-up of anxious patients treated with diazepam. *J Clin Psychopharmacol* **6**, 32–36.

Rickels K, Csanalosi I, Greisman P, et al. (1983) A controlled clinical trial of alprazolam for the treatment of anxiety. *Am J Psychiatry* **140**(1), 82–85.

Rickels K, Downing R, Schweizer E, et al. (1993) Antidepressants for the treatment of generalized anxiety disorder. *Arch Gen Psychiatry* **50**, 884–895.

Rickels K, Schweizer R, Csanalosi I, et al. (1988b) Long-term treatment of anxiety and risk of withdrawal. Prospective comparison of clorazepate and buspirone. *Arch Gen Psychiatry* **45**(5), 444–450.

Rickels K, Schweizer E, DeMartinis N, et al. (1997) Gepirone and diazepam in generalized anxiety disorder: a placebo-controlled trial. *J Clin Psychopharmacol* **17**(4), 272–277.

Rickels K, Weisman K, Norstad N, et al. (1982) Buspirone and diazepam in anxiety: a controlled study. *J Clin Psychiatry* **43**,(12 Pt 2), 81–86.

Riskind JH, Moore R, Harman B, et al. (1991) The relation of generalized anxiety disorder to depression in general and dysthymic disorder in particular. In *Chronic Anxiety: Generalized Anxiety Disorder and Mixed Anxiety–Depression*, Rapee RM and Barlow DH (eds). Guilford Press, New York.

Rocca P, Beoni AM, Eva C, et al. (1998) Peripheral benzodiazepine receptor messenger RNA is decreased in lymphocytes of generalized anxiety disorder patients. *Biol Psychiatry* **43**(10), 767–773.

Rogers MP, Warshaw MG, Goisman RM, et al. (1999) Comparing primary and secondary generalized anxiety disorder in a long-term naturalistic study of anxiety disorder. *Depress Anx* **10**, 1–7.

Romach M, Busto U, Somer G, et al. (1995) Clinical aspects of chronic use of alprazolam and lorazepam. *Am J Psychiatry* **152**(8), 1161–1167.

Rosen RC, Lane RM, and Menza M (1999) Effects of SSRIs on sexual function: a critical review. *J Clin Psychopharmacol* **19**, 67–85.

Rosenbaum AH, Schatzberg AF, Jost FA, et al. (1983) Urinary free cortisol levels in anxiety. *Psychosomatics* **24**, 835–837.

Ross CA and Matas M (1987) A clinical trial of buspirone and diazepam in the treatment of anxiety. *J Clin Psychopharmacol* **19**, 67–85.

Roy-Byrne PP, Cowley DS, Hommer D, et al. (1991) Neuroendocrine effects of diazepam in panic and generalized anxiety disorders. *Biol Psychiatry* **30**, 73–80.

Ruiz AT (1983) A double-blind study of alprazolam and lorazepam in the treatment of anxiety. *J Clin Psychiatry* **44**(2), 60–62.

Sacerdote P, Panerai AE, Frattola L, et al. (1999) Benzodiazepine-induced chemotaxis is impaired in monocytes from patients with generalized anxiety disorder. *Psychoneuroendocrinology* **24**(2), 243–249.

Sanderson WC and Barlow DH (1990) A description of patients diagnosed with DSM-III-R generalized anxiety disorder. *J Nerv Ment Dis* **178**, 588–591.

Sanderson WC, Wetzler S, Beck AT, et al. (1991) Prevalence of personality disorders among patients with anxiety disorders. *Psychiatr Res* **51**(2), 167–174.

Sartorius N, Ustun B, Lecrubier Y, et al. (1996) Depression comorbid with anxiety: results from the WHO study on psychological disorders in primary health care. *Br J Psychiatry* **168**(Suppl. 30), 38–43.

Scherrer JF, True WR, Xian H, et al. (2000) Evidence for genetic influences common and specific to symptoms of generalized anxiety disorder and panic. *J Affect Disord* **57**(1–3), 25–35.

Schweizer E, Rickels K, and Lucki I (1986) Resistance to the anxiety effect of buspirone in patients with a history of benzodiazepine use. *N Engl J Med* **314**, 719–720.

Shear MK, Schulberg HC, and Madonia M (1994) Panic and generalized anxiety disorder in primary care. *Paper Presented at a Meeting of the Association for Primary Care*, Washington, DC.

Sheehan DV (1999) Venlafaxine extended release (XR) in the treatment of generalized anxiety disorder. *J Clin Psychiatry* **60**(Suppl. 22), 23–28.

Skre I, Torgersen S, Lygren S, et al. (1993) A twin study of DSM-III-R anxiety disorders. *Acta Psychiatr Scand* **88**, 85–92.

Spiegel DA, Bruce TJ, Gregg SF, et al. (1994) Does cognitive–behavior therapy assist slow-taper alprazolam discontinuation in panic disorder. *Am J Psychiatry* **151**, 876–881.

Starcevic V, Uhlenhuth EH, and Fallon S (1995) The tridimensional personality questionnaire as an instrument for screening personality disorders: use in patients with generalized anxiety disorder. *J Pers Disord* **9**, 247–253.

Stein MB, Hauger RL, Dhalla KS, et al. (1996) Plasma neuropeptide Y in anxiety disorders: findings in panic disorder and social phobia. *Psychiatr Res* **59**(3), 183–188.

Taylor DP, Eison MS, Riblet LA, et al. (1985) Pharmacological and clinical effects of buspirone. *Pharmacol Biochem Behav* **23**(4), 687–694.

Tiihonen J, Kuikka J, Rasanen P, et al. (1997) Cerebral benzodiazepine receptor binding and distribution in generalized anxiety disorder: a fractal analysis. *Mol Psychiatry* **2**(6), 463–471.

Tollefson GD, Luxenberg M, Valentine R, et al. (1991) An open label trial of alprazolam in comorbid irritable bowel syndrome and generalized anxiety disorder. *J Clin Psychiatry* **52**(12), 502–508.

Trullas RB, Jackson B, and Skolnick P (1989) Anxiolytic properties of 1-aminocyclopropanecarboxylic acid, a ligand at strychnine-insensitive glycine receptors. *Pharmacol Biochem Behav* **34**(2), 313–316.

Uhlenhuth EH, Balter MB, Ban TA, et al. (1999) International study of expert judgement on therapeutic use of benzodiazepines and other psychotherapeutic medications: VI. Trends in recommendations for the pharmacotherapy of anxiety disorders, 1992–1997. *Depress Anx* **9**, 107–116.

Wheatley D (1982) Buspirone: multicenter efficacy study. *J Clin Psychiatry* **42**, 92–94.

Widerlov E, Lindstrom LH, Wahlestedt C, et al. (1988) Neuropeptide Y and peptide YY as possible cerebrospinal fluid makers for major depression and schizophrenia, respectively. *J Psychiatr Res* **22**(1), 69–79.

Wittchen HU, Nelson CB, and Lachner G (1998) Prevalence of mental disorders and psychological impairments in adolescents and young adults. *Psychol Med* **28**, 109–126.

Wittchen HU, Zhao S, Kessler RC, et al. (1994) DSM-III-R generalized anxiety disorder in the National Comorbidity Survey. *Arch Gen Psychiatry* **51**, 355–364.

Woodruff GN and Hughes J (1991) Cholecystokinin antagonists. *Ann Rev Pharmacol Toxicol* **31**, 469–501.

Yonkers KA, Dyck IR, Warshaw M, et al. (2000) Factors predicting the clinical course of generalized anxiety disorder. *Br J Psychiatry* **176**, 544–549.

36

Somatoform Disorders

The somatoform disorders are characterized by physical symptoms suggestive of but not fully explained by a general medical condition or the direct effects of a substance. In this class, symptoms are not intentionally produced and are not attributable to another mental disorder. To warrant a diagnosis, symptoms must be clinically significant in terms of causing distress or impairment in important areas of functioning. The disorders included in this class are somatization disorder, undifferentiated somatoform disorder, conversion disorder, pain disorder, hypochondriasis, body dysmorphic disorder, and somatoform disorder not otherwise specified (NOS). This chapter begins with information about differential diagnosis, epidemiology and treatment as it applies to the diagnostic class as a whole, followed by individual sections covering each of the somatoform disorders.

The somatoform disorders class was created for clinical utility, not on the basis of an assumed common etiology or mechanism. In DSM-IV-TR terms, it was designed to facilitate the differential diagnosis of conditions in which the first diagnostic concern is the need to "exclude occult general medical conditions or substance-induced etiologies for the bodily symptoms." As shown in Figure 36-1, only after such explanations are reasonably excluded should somatoform disorders be considered.

The somatoform disorder concept should be distinguished from traditional concepts of "psychosomatic illness" and "somatization." The psychosomatic illnesses involved structural or physiological changes hypothesized as deriving from psychological factors. In the DSM-III, DSM-III-R, and DSM-IV somatoform disorders, such objective changes are generally not evident. The "classic" psychosomatic illnesses of Alexander (1950) included bronchial asthma, ulcerative colitis, thyrotoxicosis, essential hypertension, rheumatoid arthritis, neurodermatitis, and peptic ulcer. In DSM-IV-TR, most of these illnesses would be diagnosed as a general medical condition on Axis III, and in some cases with an additional designation of psychological factors affecting medical condition on Axis I. By definition, the diagnosis of "psychological factors affecting medical condition" is not a mental disorder, but it is included in DSM-IV-TR in the section for other conditions that may be a focus of clinical attention; it involves the presence of one or more specific psychological or behavioral factors that adversely affect a general medical condition (see Chapter 45 for more information).

The descriptive use of the term "somatization" in somatization disorder is not to be confused with theories that generally postulate a somatic expression of psychological distress (Lipowski 1988, Kellner 1990, Malt 1991). Steckel (Steckel et al. 1943), who coined the term, defined somatization, in 1943, as the process of a "bodily disorder" occurring as the expression of a "deep-seated neurosis." However, as argued by Kellner (1990), "empirical studies ... suggest that there is no single theory that can adequately explain somatization, which is not only multifactorially determined but is an exceedingly complex phenomenon." Furthermore, treatment strategies derived from somatization theories have not proven effective. For example, the postulation that individuals with somatoform disorders are alexithymic, that is, are unable to process emotions and psychological conflicts verbally and therefore do so somatically, suggested that teaching such individuals to "appreciate" and "verbalize" their emotions would circumvent the need to "somatize" them. Such treatment approaches have been ineffective (Cloninger 1987).

Differential Diagnosis of Somatoform Disorders

As shown in Figure 36-1, after it is determined that physical symptoms are not fully explained by a general medical condition or the direct effect of a substance, somatoform disorders must be differentiated from other mental conditions with physical symptoms. In contrast to malingering and factitious disorder, symptoms in somatoform disorders are not under voluntary control, that is, they are not intentionally produced or feigned. Determination of intentionality may be difficult and must be inferred from the context in which symptoms present. Somatic symptoms may also be involved in disorders in other diagnostic classes. However, in such instances, the overriding focus is on the primary symptom complex (i.e., anxiety, mood, or psychotic symptoms) rather than the physical

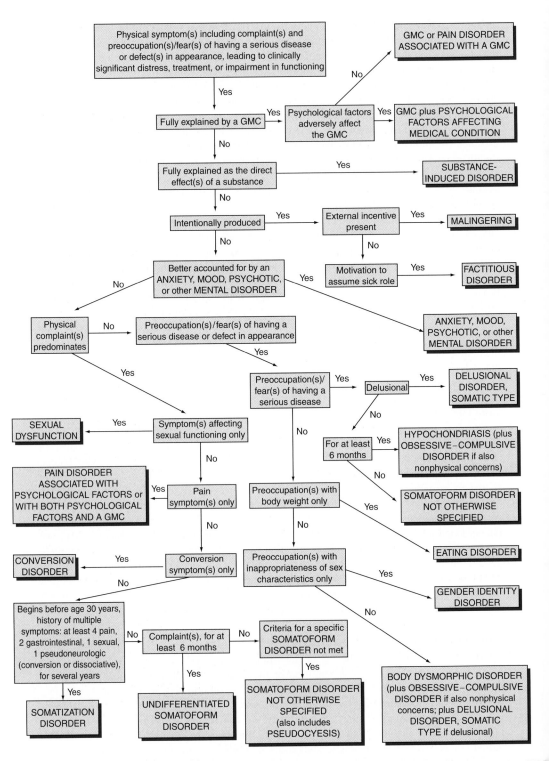

Figure 36-1 *Differential diagnosis of clinically significant physical symptoms. Shadowed boxes represent diagnostic categories; GMC general medical condition.*

symptoms. In panic disorder and in generalized anxiety disorder, physical symptoms such as chest pain, shortness of breath, palpitations, sweating, and tremulousness may occur. However, such somatic symptoms occur only in the context of fear or anxious foreboding. In general, there is a lack of a consistent physical focus. In mood disorders (particularly major depressive disorder) and in schizophrenia and other psychotic disorders, somatic preoccupations, fears, and even delusions and false perceptions may be evident. In the mood disorders, these are generally mood congruent (e.g., "I'm so worthless not even my organs work anymore"), whereas in the psychoses, bizarre and mood-incongruent beliefs are typical (e.g., "Half of my brain was removed by psychic neurosurgery").

Whereas it is assumed that the specific disorders in the somatoform grouping are heterogeneous in terms of pathogenesis and pathophysiology, they are also phenomenologically diverse (see Figure 36-1). In somatization disorder, undifferentiated somatoform disorder, conversion disorder, and pain disorder, the focus is on the physical complaints themselves, and thus on perceptions. In hypochondriasis and body dysmorphic disorder, emphasis is on physically related preoccupations or fears, and thus on cognitions. Somatization disorder and, to a lesser extent, undifferentiated somatoform disorder are characterized by multiple symptoms of different types; conversion disorder, pain disorder, hypochondriasis, and body dysmorphic disorder are defined on the basis of a single symptom or a few symptoms of a certain type (see Figure 36-1). Whereas somatization disorder, undifferentiated somatoform disorder, and hypochondriasis are, by definition, at least 6 months in duration, conversion disorder, pain disorder, body dysmorphic disorder, and somatoform disorder NOS may be of short duration as long as they are associated with clinically significant distress or impairment.

Epidemiology of Somatoform Disorders

In view of the vicissitudes of diagnostic approaches and the recency of the current somatoform disorder grouping, it is not surprising that estimates of the frequency of this group of disorders in the general population as well as in clinical settings are inconsistent if not nonexistent. Yet, existing data seem to indicate that such problems are indeed common and account for a major proportion of clinical services, especially in primary care settings. A World Health Organization study reported ICD-10 diagnoses of hypochondriasis in nearly 1% and of somatization disorder in nearly 3% of individuals in primary care clinics in 14 countries (Ormel et al. 1994). Another study using primary care sites found 14% of 1000 individuals to be suffering from some somatoform disorder: 8% with "multisomatoform disorder" (see the Undifferentiated Somatoform Disorder section), 4% with somatoform disorder NOS, 2% with hypochondriasis, and 1% with somatoform pain disorder (Spitzer et al. 1994).

Considering prevalence in nonclinic, community populations, Escobar and coworkers (1989) reported that nearly 20% of community respondents in Puerto Rico and 4.4% of comparable non-Hispanic Los Angeles residents fulfilled criteria for an "abridged somatization disorder," a construct with a lower threshold than somatization disorder that would generally correspond to a DSM-IV-TR diagnosis of either undifferentiated somatoform disorder or somatoform disorder NOS. In the Epidemiological Catchment Area community study (Robins et al. 1984), a low estimate of the frequency of somatization disorder (0.06–0.6%) was reported. Methodological problems may have led to a falsely low rate, as discussed in the somatization disorder section. Other studies have estimated much greater frequency, at least among women (Table 36-1).

The epidemiology of the specific somatoform disorders is discussed individually in following sections.

Table 36-1	Epidemiology and Natural History of the Somatoform Disorders		
Somatoform Disorder	**Prevalence and Incidence**	**Age at Onset**	**Course and Progress**
Somatization disorder	US women 0.2–2%; women/men = 10 : 1	First symptoms by adolescence, full criteria met by mid-20s, not after 30 year by definition	Chronic with fluctuations in severity Most active in early adulthood Full remissions rare
Undifferentiated somatoform disorder	"Abridged somatization disorder" type estimated as 11–15% of US adults, 20% in Puerto Rico Preponderance of women in US but not Puerto Rico	Variable	Variable conversion disorder
Conversion disorder	Conversion symptoms common, as high as 25% Treated conversion symptoms: 11–500 per 100,000 5–14% of general hospital admissions 5–24% of psychiatric outpatients 1–3% of psychiatric outpatient referrals 4% of neurological outpatient referrals 1% of neurological admissions	Late childhood to early adulthood, most before age 35 year If onset in middle or late life, neurological or general medical condition more likely	Individual conversion symptoms generally remit within days to weeks Relapse within 1 year in 20 to 25%
Pain disorder	10–15% of US adults with work disability owing to back pain yearly A predominant symptom in more than half of general hospital admissions Present in as many as 38% of psychiatric admissions, 18% of psychiatric outpatients	Any age	Good if less than 6 months in duration Unemployment, personality disorder, potential for compensation, and habituation to addictive drugs associated with poorer prognosis
Hypochondriasis	Perhaps 4–9% in general medical settings, but unclear whether full syndrome criteria are met Equal in both sexes	Early adulthood typical	10% recovery, two-thirds a chronic but fluctuating course, 25% do poorly Better prognosis if acute onset, absence of personality disorder, absence of secondary gain
Body dysmorphic disorder	Not routinely screened for in psychiatric or general population studies Perhaps 2% of patients seeking corrective cosmetic surgery	Adolescence or early adulthood Perhaps in women at menopause	Generally chronic, fluctuating severity In a lifetime, multiple defects perceived Incapacitating: one-third house-bound
Somatoform disorder NOS	Unknown	Variable	Variable

Treatment of Somatoform Disorders

Whereas specific somatoform disorders indicate specific treatment approaches, some general guidelines apply to the somatoform disorders as a whole (Table 36-2). By reorganizing and synthesizing the recommendations of Stoudemire (1988) and Kellner (1991) into three goals and three general strategies, the therapeutic goals include (1) as an overriding goal, prevention of the adoption of the sick role and chronic invalidism; (2) minimization of unnecessary costs and complications by avoiding unwarranted hospitalizations, diagnostic

Table 36-2	Treatment of DSM-IV-TR Somatoform Disorders		
Somatoform Disorder	**Treatment Goals**	**Psychotherapy and Psychosocial Strategies and Techniques**	**Pharmacological and Physical Strategies and Techniques***
Somatoform disorders, as a group	1. Prevent adoption of the sick role and chronic invalidism 2. Minimize unnecessary costs and complications by avoiding unwarranted hospitalizations, diagnostic and treatment procedures, and medications 3. Pharmacological control of comorbid syndromes	1. Consistent treatment, generally by same physician, coordinated if multiple 2. Supportive office visits, scheduled at regular intervals 3. Focus gradually shifted from symptoms to personal and social problems	1. Only as clearly indicated, or as time-limited empirical trial 2. Avoid drugs with abuse or addictive potential
Somatization disorder	1, 2, and 3; also • Instill, whenever possible, insight regarding temporal association between symptoms and personal, interpersonal, and situational problems	1, 2, and 3; also • Establish firm therapeutic alliance • Educate the individuals with somatization disorder regarding manifestations of somatization disorder (psychoeducative approach) • Consistent reassurance	1 and 2, also • Antianxiety and antidepressant drugs for comorbid anxiety or depressive disorders; if diagnosis unclear, consider empirical trial
Undifferentiated somatoform disorder	1, 2, and 3	1, 2, and 3	1 and 2
Conversion disorder	1, 2, and 3; also • Prompt removal of symptoms	Acute: • Reassurance, suggestion to remove symptom • Consider narcoanalysis (interview after drowsiness from amobarbital or other sedative–hypnotic, sometimes followed by methylphenidate or other stimulant), hypnotherapy, or behavioral therapy Chronic: 1, 2, and 3 • Exploration of various conflict areas, particularly interpersonal relationships • Long-term, intensive, insight-oriented dynamic psychotherapy recommended by some	1 and 2; also • Consider narcoanalysis as an interviewing or psychotherapy adjunct
Pain disorder	1, 2, and 3; also • Acute pain: Relieve symptom • Chronic pain: Maintain function and motility rather than focus on total pain relief	1, 2, and 3; also • Chronic pain: Consider physical and occupational therapy, operant conditioning, cognitive–behavioral therapy	1 and 2; also • Acute: Acetaminophen and NSAIDs alone or as adjuncts to opioids (if necessary) • Chronic: Tricyclic antidepressants, acetaminophen, and NSAIDs; if necessary, milder opioids or pure opioid agonists, but these only if tied to nonpain objectives (such as increasing activity) • Consider acupuncture, transcutaneous electrical nerve stimulation

(continued overleaf)

Table 36-2 (continued)			
Somatoform Disorder	Treatment Goals	Psychotherapy and Psychosocial Strategies and Techniques	Pharmacological and Physical Strategies and Techniques*
Hypochondriasis	1, 2, and 3; also • Pharmacological control of central syndrome itself	1, 2, and 3; also • Cognitive–behavioral therapy involving prevention of checking rituals and reassurance seeking	2; also • Attempt to decrease hypochondriacal symptoms with SSRIs at higher than antidepressant doses or clomipramine
Body dysmorphic disorder	1, 2, and 3, especially avoiding corrective surgery; also • Pharmacological control of central syndrome itself	1, 2, and 3; also • Cognitive–behavioral therapy involving prevention of checking rituals and reassurance seeking	2; also • Attempt to decrease hypochondriacal symptoms with SSRIs at higher than antidepressant doses or clomipramine
Somatoform disorder NOS	1, 2, and 3; also • Evaluate carefully for alternative general medical or other mental disorder to which the symptoms can be attributed	1, 2, and 3	1 and 2

*NSAIDs, Nonsteroidal antiinflammatory drugs; SSRIs, selective serotonin reuptake inhibitors.

and treatment procedures, and medications (especially those of an addictive potential); and (3) effective treatment of comorbid mental disorders, such as depressive and anxiety syndromes. The three general treatment strategies include (1) consistent treatment, generally by the same physician, with careful coordination if multiple physicians are involved; (2) supportive office visits, scheduled at regular intervals rather than in response to symptoms; and (3) a gradual shift in focus from symptoms to an emphasis on personal and interpersonal problems.

SOMATIZATION DISORDER

Diagnosis
Somatization disorder is a polysymptomatic somatoform disorder characterized by multiple recurring pains and gastrointestinal, sexual, and pseudoneurological symptoms occurring for a period of years with onset before age 30 years (see DSM-IV-TR diagnostic criteria below). The physical complaints are not intentionally produced and are not fully explained by a general medical condition or the direct effects of a substance. To warrant diagnosis, they must result in medical attention or significant impairment in social, occupational, or other important areas of functioning.

DSM-IV-TR Diagnostic Criteria

300.81 Somatization Disorder

A. A history of many physical complaints beginning before age 30 years that occur over a period of several years and result in treatment being sought or significant impairment in social, occupational, or other important areas of functioning.

B. Each of the following criteria must have been met, with individual symptoms occurring at any time during the course of the disturbance:

(1) *four pain symptoms*: a history of pain related to at least four different sites or functions (e.g., head, abdomen, back, joints, extremities, chest, rectum, during menstruation, during sexual intercourse, or during urination)

(2) *two gastrointestinal symptoms*: a history of at least two gastrointestinal symptoms other than pain (e.g., nausea, bloating, vomiting other than during pregnancy, diarrhea, or intolerance of several different foods)

(3) *one sexual symptom*: a history of at least one sexual or reproductive symptom other than pain (e.g., sexual indifference, erectile or ejaculatory dysfunction, irregular menses, excessive menstrual bleeding, vomiting throughout pregnancy)

(4) *one pseudoneurological symptom*: a history of at least one symptom or deficit suggesting a neurological condition not limited to pain (conversion symptoms such as impaired coordination or balance, paralysis or localized weakness, difficulty swallowing or lump in throat, aphonia, urinary retention, hallucinations, loss of touch or pain sensation, double vision, blindness, deafness, seizures; dissociative symptoms such as amnesia; or loss of consciousness other than fainting)

C. Either (1) or (2):

(1) After appropriate investigation, each of the symptoms in criterion B cannot be fully explained by a known general medical condition or the direct effects of a substance (e.g., a drug of abuse, a medication).

(2) When there is a related general medical condition, the physical complaints or resulting social or occupational impairment is in excess of what would be expected from the history, physical examination, or laboratory findings.

D. The symptoms are not intentionally produced or feigned (as in factitious disorder or malingering).

Reprinted with permission from the Diagnostic and Statistical Manual of Mental Disorders, Fourth Edition, Text Revision. Copyright 2000 American Psychiatric Association.

The concept and criteria for somatization disorder (historically referred to as hysteria or Briquet's syndrome) embraced by DSM-IV-TR are the distillation of a long and convoluted struggle to describe this complex, multifaceted syndrome (Martin 1988). As reviewed by Veith (1965), the origins of the concept can be traced to descriptions in the medical literature of the pre-Hippocratic Egyptians, who attributed otherwise unexplained physical symptoms to peregrinations of the uterus; this hypothesis probably derived from observations that such presentations were predominantly seen in women with onset during the reproductive years. In the fifth century AD, the Hippocratic literature formalized the concept, adopting the term *hysteria* from the Greek word for uterus. In time, belief in a uterine cause was abandoned, but use of the term hysteria continued.

In the mid-nineteenth century, Paul Briquet (1859) adopted the term hysteria for the syndrome he described in his monograph, *Traité Clinique et Thérapeutique à l'Hystérie*, as characterized by dramatic and excessive medical complaints without evidence of an organic cause. Ultimately, such a description would constitute the basis for somatization disorder, yet the medical complaint aspect of hysteria was overshadowed for many years by psychodynamic interpretations originating with observations by Breuer and Freud (1955). In fact, much of Freud's theory of the unconscious can be traced to his work with hysteria. According to psychodynamic theory, "psychic energy" was converted into physical symptoms, thereby the term *conversion*. Although conversion symptoms were eventually reserved for pseudoneurological complaints, the more general term somatization came to be used for any body symptoms explained as an expression of a neurosis (Lipowski 1988, Steckel et al. 1943). In time, the physical complaint aspect of hysteria was de-emphasized, with increased attention to intrapsychic, personality, or characterological features of hysteria. Meanwhile, in lay usage, hysteria came to signify excessive or histrionic emotional displays regardless of whether physical symptoms were involved. By the 1950s, the meaning had become so diffuse that the term hysteria, as attacked by Chodoff and Lyons (1958), had at least five connotations, only one of which related to physical complaints.

In 1951, Purtell and colleagues (1951) resurrected Briquet's formulation of a syndrome characterized by multiple medically unexplained somatic complaints, adding a quantitative perspective that required a given number of symptoms from a specified list for a diagnosis. This approach was refined in 1962 by Perley and Guze (1962) and again in 1972 by Feighner and colleagues (1972), who included hysteria among the 13 psychiatric diagnoses "canonized" as sufficiently studied to be considered valid and reliable psychiatric disorders. DSM-III recognized the need for inclusion of the syndrome characterized in the Feighner criteria but sought to make the diagnosis more usable. Somatization disorder was the term coined to escape the pejorative connotation of hysteria, yet avoiding the use of eponyms such as Briquet's syndrome. It also attempted to simplify the criteria of Feighner and colleagues by reducing the required number of symptoms to 14 in women and 12 (to prevent a possible sex bias) in men, from a list of 37 potential symptoms. In order to simplify the criteria set, a new diagnostic algorithm was developed for DSM-IV by Cloninger and colleagues from a reanalysis of an existing data set requiring four pain, two nonpain gastrointestinal, one sexual or reproductive, and one pseudoneurological symptom (either conversion or dissociative) (Cloninger and Yutzy 1993, Yutzy et al. 1992).

Whereas criteria require the onset of symptoms before the age of 30 years, most individuals would have had some symptoms at least by adolescence or early adulthood. Symptoms are often described in a dramatic yet imprecise way and may be reported inconsistently from interview to interview (Martin et al. 1979). The medical history is usually complicated with multiple medical investigations, procedures, and medication trials. If there have been symptoms for at least 6 months but the onset is later than at age 30 years, or if the required number and distribution of symptoms are not evident, undifferentiated somatoform disorder is diagnosed. If the duration has been less than 6 months, somatoform disorder NOS applies. In general, the greater the number and diversity of symptoms, and the longer they have been present without development of signs of an underlying general medical condition, the greater can be the confidence that a diagnosis of somatization disorder is correct.

Epidemiology

In the US, somatization disorder is found predominantly in women, with a female/male ratio of approximately 10 : 1 (see Table 36-1). This ratio is not as large in some other cultures (e.g., in Greeks and Puerto Ricans). Thus, gender- and culture-specific rates are more meaningful than generalized figures. The lifetime prevalence of somatization disorder in US women has been estimated to be between 0.2 and 2%. The magnitude of this discrepancy is attributable, at least in part, to methodological differences. The Epidemiological Catchment Area study (Robins et al. 1984), the most recent large-scale general population study in the US to include an assessment for somatization disorder, found a lifetime risk of somatization disorder of only 0.2 to 0.3% in US women. However, this study may have underestimated the prevalence of somatization disorder because nonphysician interviewers were used. It is argued that it is difficult for lay interviewers to critically assess whether somatic symptoms are fully explained by physical conditions. As a result, they may more readily accept individuals' general medical explanations of symptoms, resulting in fewer diagnoses of somatization disorder. With age and method of assessment taken into account, the lifetime risk for somatization disorder was estimated to be 2% in US women (Cloninger et al. 1975).

Course
Somatization disorder is rare in children younger than 9 years of age (Robins and O'Neal 1953) (see Table 36-1). Characteristic symptoms of somatization disorder usually begin during adolescence, and the criteria are met by the mid-twenties (Guze and Perley 1963). Somatization disorder is a chronic illness characterized by fluctuations in the frequency and diversity of symptoms (Guze et al. 1986). Full remissions occur rarely, if ever. Whereas the most active symptomatic phase is in early adulthood, aging does not appear to lead to total remission (Goodwin and Guze 1989). Pribor and colleagues (1994) found that women with somatization disorder older than 55 years did not differ from younger somatization individuals in the number of somatic symptoms. Longitudinal follow-up studies have confirmed that 80 to 90% of individuals initially diagnosed with somatization disorder will maintain a consistent clinical picture and be rediagnosed similarly after 6 to 8 years (Cloninger 1993, Cloninger et al. 1986). Women with somatization disorder seen in mental health treatment settings are at increased risk for attempted suicide, although such attempts are usually unsuccessful and may reflect manipulative gestures more than intent to die (Martin et al. 1985). It is not clear whether such risk is true for individuals with somatization disorder seen only in general medical settings.

Differential Diagnosis
As defined in DSM-IV-TR, somatization disorder is characterized by multiple recurring physical symptoms and, as will be described, often multiple psychiatric complaints (Wetzel et al. 1994). Thus, it is not surprising that somatization disorder may present in a manner suggestive of multiple general medical and, although too often forgotten, psychiatric disorders (see Table 36-3). Indeed, it can be said that an essential aspect of somatization disorder is its simulation of other syndromes. As described by Preskorn (1995), "Briquet's syndrome (i.e., somatization disorder) is fundamentally a syndrome of apparent syndromes" (see Table 36-3). Thus, the first task in the diagnosis of somatization disorder is the exclusion of other suggested medical and psychiatric conditions.

To help in this, Cloninger (1986) identified three features that generally characterize somatization disorder but rarely general medical disorders. Slightly restated, these are (1) involvement of multiple organ systems, (2) early onset and chronic course without development of physical signs or structural abnormalities, and (3) absence of laboratory abnormalities characteristic of the suggested physical disorders (Table 36-4). Another way of characterizing the distinction is the "reverse funnel effect" (Pinta 1995, personal communication). With most general medical conditions, the process of investigation "funnels down" to fewer and fewer specific diagnostic possibilities; in somatization disorder, the more extensive the investigation, the greater the number of suggested disorders.

Several general medical conditions may also fit this pattern and may be confused with somatization disorder. These include multiple sclerosis, other neuropathies, systemic lupus erythematosus, acute intermittent porphyria, other hepatic and hematopoietic porphyrias, hypercalcemia, certain chronic systemic infections such as brucellosis and trypanosomiasis, myopathies, and vasculitides. In general, such conditions begin with disseminated, nonspecific subjective symptoms and transient or equivocal physical signs or laboratory abnormalities.

Somatization disorder is characterized by excessive psychiatric as well as physical complaints (Wetzel et al. 1994). Thus, other mental disorders, including anxiety and mood disorders and schizophrenia, may be suggested. Although no specific exclusion criteria regarding other mental disorders are given, one must be careful in accepting "comorbidity" and critically evaluate whether suggested syndromes are truly additional syndromes or simply manifestations of somatization disorder (Preskorn 1995).

The overlap between somatization disorder and anxiety disorders may be a particular problem. Individuals with somatization disorder frequently complain of many of

Table 36-3	Somatoform Disorders: A Syndrome of Simulated Syndromes		
Symptom Examples	Examples of Simulated Neurological Conditions	Examples of Simulated Nonneurological General Medical Conditions	Examples of Simulated Psychiatric Conditions
Symptoms* of somatization disorder			
Pain			
Headache	Migraine	Temporal arteritis	Pain disorder
Abdomen	"Abdominal epilepsy"	Peptic ulcer disease	Pain disorder
Back	Lumbosacral radiculopathy	Ruptured disk	Pain disorder
Joints or extremities		Fibromyalgia	Pain disorder
Chest		Angina	Panic disorder
Menstruation, intercourse		Endometriosis	Dyspareunia, vaginismus
Urination	Neurogenic bladder	Urinary tract infection	
Gastrointestinal (nonpain)			
Difficulty swallowing	Myasthenia gravis	Esophageal motility disorder	Eating disorder
Nausea	Raised intracranial pressure	Meniere's disease	Eating disorder
Bloating		Galactase deficiency	Eating disorder
Vomiting (nonpregnancy)		Raised intracranial pressure	Eating disorder
Diarrhea		Irritable bowel syndrome	Eating disorder
Intolerance to several foods		Food allergy	Eating disorder
Sexual (nonpain)			
Loss of interest			Major depressive episode
Erectile–ejaculatory dysfunction	Diabetic neuropathy	Antihypertensive drug effect	
Menorrhagia		Leiomyofibroma	
Vomiting throughout pregnancy		Preeclampsia, eclampsia	
Pseudoneurological			
Conversion			
Sensory	Stroke (hemianesthesia)		Schizophrenia/(hallucinations)
Motor	Huntington's disease	Myopathy	Catatonia
Seizures	Epilepsy	Electrolyte imbalance	Catatonia
Mixed	Multiple sclerosis	Electrolyte imbalance	Catatonia
Dissociative			
Amnesia	Amnestic disorder	Anticholinergic drug effects	Dissociative identity disorder
Loss of consciousness (nonfainting)	Coma	Metabolic encephalopathy	Catatonia
Symptoms* often associated with somatization disorder			
Anxiety, panic		Pheochromocytoma	Generalized anxiety and panic disorders
Dysphoria, affective lability	Frontal lobe syndrome	Endocrinopathy	Major mood disorders
Cluster B personality features	Frontal lobe syndrome	Acute intermittent porphyria	Brief psychotic disorder

*All of these symptoms may be reported by patients with somatization disorder, without the clinical consistency and pathological findings t support the diagnosis of neurological, general medical, or psychiatric conditions separate from somatization disorder.
Developed in conjunction with Sheldon H. Preskorn.

able 36-4	Discrimination of Somatization Disorder from General Medical Conditions
'eatures Suggesting Somatization Disorder	**Features Suggesting a General Medical Condition**
nvolvement of multiple organ systems	Involvement of single or few organ systems
.arly onset and chronic course without development of physical signs or structural abnormalities	If early onset and chronic course, development of physical signs and structural abnormalities
Absence of laboratory abnormalities characteristic of the suggested general medical condition	Laboratory abnormalities evident

rce: Martin RL and Yutzy SH (1994) Somatoform disorders. In *The American Psychiatric Press Textbook of Psychiatry*, 2nd ed., Hales , Yudofsky SC, and Talbott JA (eds). American Psychiatric Press, Washington, DC, p. 600.

the same somatic symptoms as individuals with anxiety disorders, such as increased muscle tension, features of autonomic hyperactivity, and even discrete panic attacks. Likewise, individuals with anxiety disorder may report irrational disease concerns and such somatic complaints as those involving gastrointestinal function that are commonly seen in somatization disorder. However, individuals with anxiety disorders neither typically report sexual and menstrual complaints or conversion or dissociative symptoms as in somatization disorder, nor do they have the associated histrionic presentation and personal, marital, and social maladjustment common in individuals with somatization disorder (Cloninger 1993).

It must be remembered that an anxiety disorder may be comorbid with somatization disorder. Here, objective observation of the individual rather than reliance on the individual's report may facilitate an additional diagnosis. For example, individuals with somatization disorder may report that they are presently overwhelmed by anxiety while speaking calmly or even cheerfully about their symptoms, or they may be redirectable while in the midst of a reported panic attack.

Mood disorders (in particular, depression) frequently present with multiple somatic complaints, especially in certain cultures such as in India, where somatic but not mental complaints are acceptable. A longitudinal history identifying age at onset and course of illness may facilitate discrimination of a mood disorder from somatization disorder. In mood disorders, the age at onset of the somatic symptoms is generally later than in somatization disorder; their first appearance generally correlates discretely with the onset of mood symptoms, and a lengthy pattern of multiple recurring somatic complaints is not seen. Also, resolution of the underlying mood disorder will generally result in disappearance of the somatic complaints.

From the other perspective, individuals with somatization disorder often present with depressive complaints. In somatization disorder, a thorough investigation will reveal a multitude of somatic as well as "depressive" symptoms. Interestingly, somatization disorder individuals complaining of depression have been found to proffer greater depressive symptoms than individuals with major depression (DeSouza et al. 1988). As in anxiety disorders, major depressive episodes may occur in individuals with somatization disorder and must be differentiated from the tendency to have multiple complaints, which is characteristic of somatization disorder. As with anxiety disorders, in considering comorbidity with a depressive disorder, the individual's reports should be corroborated by collateral information or by direct observation. Thus, the veracity of the self-report of overwhelming depression and suicidal ideation should be doubted if the individual appears cheerful and charming, at least at times, when interviewed, or if the individual is reported to be actively involved in social activities on an inpatient psychiatric service.

Schizophrenia may present with generally single but occasionally multiple unexplained somatic complaints. Interview usually uncovers psychotic symptoms such as delusions, hallucinations, or disorganized thought. In some cases, the underlying psychosis cannot be identified initially, but in time, schizophrenia will become manifest (Goodwin and Guze 1989). Hallucinations are included as examples of conversion symptoms in DSM-IV-TR, as they were in the Purtell, Perley–Guze, and Feighner criteria, which may lead to diagnostic problems (Martin 1996). As discussed in the conversion disorder section, careful analysis of this symptom is warranted so that a misdiagnosis is not made, relegating an individual to long-term neuroleptic treatment on the basis of conversion hallucinations.

Individuals with histrionic, borderline, and antisocial personality disorders frequently have an excess of somatic complaints, at times presenting with somatization disorder. Cloninger and Guze (1979) and Cloninger and colleagues (1975) have identified that antisocial personality disorder and somatization disorder cluster in individuals and within families and may share common causes. Dissociative phenomena, in particular dissociative identity disorder, are commonly associated with somatization disorder (Martin 1996). Because dissociative symptoms are included in the diagnostic criteria for somatization, a separate diagnosis of a dissociative disorder is not made if such symptoms occur only in the course of somatization disorder.

Unlike that in hypochondriasis and body dysmorphic disorder, in which preoccupations and fears concerning the interpretation of symptoms predominate, the focus in somatization disorder is on the physical complaints themselves. Unlike that in pain disorder and conversion disorder, multiple complaints of different types are reported; by definition, in DSM-IV-TR, the history is of pain in at least four sites or functions (e.g., pain with intercourse, pain in swallowing), at least two nonpain gastrointestinal symptoms, at least one nonpain sexual or reproductive symptom, and at least one conversion or dissociative (i.e., pseudoneurological) symptom.

Etiology

Many theories on the cause of somatization disorder have been proposed since the early uterine hypothesis was dismissed. Yet, etiology remains unknown. Psychodynamic hypotheses regarding the physical expression of unconscious conflict by conversion or somatization have been influential. Even Freud assumed a "constitutional diathesis," as had Charcot before him. Evidence exists for both biological and psychosocial contributions.

Somatization disorder has been shown to be familial. It is observed that in 10 to 20% of female relatives of individuals affected by somatization disorder, there is a lifetime risk in US women 10 to 20 times greater than that of the general population (Guze et al. 1986). Yet, aggregation in families may be attributable to both genetic and environmental factors. A cross-fostering study of a Swedish population demonstrated that genetic background and postnatal influences contribute to the risk of somatization disorder independently (Bohman et al. 1984, Cloninger et al. 1984). Of additional interest are observations that male relatives of individuals with somatization disorder show increased rates of antisocial personality and alcoholism, suggesting an etiological link (Cloninger 1993).

Certain promising theories have focused on learning principles with possible organic underpinnings. Ford (1983) and later Quill (1985) postulated a social communication model based on learning theory to explain somatization disorder. Both hypothesized that individuals learn to somatize as a means of expressing their wants and needs and evoking care, nurturance, and support from family and caregivers. That different sex ratios may exist in different cultures suggests that such learning differs from culture to culture.

In the 1970s, impaired information-processing problems involving attention and memory were identified in experimental neuropsychological testing (Ludwig 1972, Bendefeldt et al. 1976). Such deficits may result in vague, nonspecific, and impressionistic description for experience. These may underlie a tendency for excessive somatic complaints and, together with tendencies for impulsiveness and monotony intolerance, may contribute to the often associated multiple personal and social problems (Cloninger 1993). In 1981, Flor-Henry and coworkers (1981) reported that the pattern of neuropsychological defects found in subjects with somatization disorder differed from that in normal control, schizophrenic, and psychotic depression comparison groups. Subjects with somatization disorder had greater bilateral, symmetrical patterns of frontal lobe dysfunction in comparison with normal control subjects and greater dominant hemisphere impairment than control and depressive subjects. Nondominant hemisphere dysfunction was also identified, with greater impairment in the anterior as opposed to posterior regions. However, subjects with somatization disorder had less nondominant hemisphere disorganization than schizophrenic subjects. Of interest, these findings were similar to findings in males with antisocial personality disorder, giving further support to an etiological link with this disorder.

Treatment

First, a "management" rather than a "curative" strategy is recommended for somatization disorder. With the current absence of an identified definitive treatment, a modest, practical, empirical approach should be taken. This should include efforts to minimize distress and functional impairments associated with the multiple somatic complaints; to avoid unwarranted diagnostic and therapeutic procedures and medications; and to prevent potential complications including chronic invalidism and drug dependence.

In this regard, the general recommendations outlined above for somatoform disorders should be followed (see Table 36-2). Consistent with these guidelines, Ford (1983) and Quill (1985) recommended that the individual be encouraged to see a single physician with an understanding of and, preferably, experience in treating somatization disorder. This helps limit the number of unnecessary evaluations and treatments. Both Smith and colleagues (1986) and Murphy (1982) advocated routine, brief, supportive office visits scheduled at regular intervals to provide reassurance and prevent individuals from "needing to develop" symptoms to obtain care and attention. This "medical" management can well be provided by a primary care physician, perhaps in consultation with a psychiatrist. The study by Smith and colleagues (1986) demonstrated that such a regimen led to markedly decreased health care costs, with no apparent decrements in health or satisfaction of individuals.

More ambitious goals have been proposed with the recommendation for multiple approaches including individual psychotherapy, nonfocused group therapy, and electro-convulsive therapy (Martin and Yutzy 1994). Whereas early observations indicated some promise with each of these approaches, studies have been generally uncontrolled and used small samples. Subsequent investigations have rarely attempted to replicate reported findings using sophisticated methodology.

Of note in the treatment of somatization disorder was the identification in 1935 by Luff and Garrod (1935) of a three-part approach. Scallet and coworkers (1976) subsequently endorsed this approach, which they called eclectic, recommending "reeducation, reassurance, and suggestion." This approach was further developed by multiple authors, such as Quill (1985), Cloninger (1986), Smith and colleagues (1986), and Murphy (1982), from whom three interrelated components emerge: (1) establishment of a strong relationship or bond between the clinician and the individual; (2) education of the individual regarding the nature of somatization disorder; and (3) provision of support and reassurance.

The first component, establishing a strong therapeutic bond, is important in the treatment of somatization disorder. Without it, it will be difficult for the individual to overcome skepticism deriving from past experience with many physicians and other therapists who "never seemed to help." In addition, trust must be strong enough to withstand the stress of withholding unwarranted diagnostic and therapeutic procedures that the individual may feel are indicated. The cornerstone of establishing a therapeutic relationship is laid when the clinician indicates an understanding of the individual's pain and suffering, legitimizing the symptoms as real. This demonstrates a willingness to provide direct compassionate assistance. A full investigation of the medical and psychosocial histories, including extensive record review, will illustrate to individuals the willingness of the clinician to gain the fullest understanding of them and their plight. This also provides another opportunity to evaluate for the presence of an underlying general medical condition and to obtain a fuller picture of psychosocial difficulties that may relate temporally to somatic symptoms.

Only after the diagnosis has been clearly established and the therapeutic alliance is firmly in place can the clinician confidently limit diagnostic evaluations and therapies to those performed on the basis of objective findings as opposed to merely subjective complaints. Of course, the clinician should remain aware that individuals with somatization disorder are still at risk for development of general medical illnesses so that a vigilant perspective should always be maintained.

The second component is education. This involves advising individuals that they suffer from a "medically sanctioned illness," that is, a condition recognized by the medical community and one about which a good deal is known. Ultimately, it may be possible to introduce the concept of somatization disorder, which can be described in a positive light (i.e., the individual does not have a progressive, deteriorating, or potentially fatal medical disorder, and the individual is not "going crazy" but has a condition by which many symptoms will be experienced). A realistic discussion of prognosis and treatment options can then follow.

The third component is reassurance. Individuals with somatization disorder often have control and insecurity issues, which often come to the forefront when they perceive that a particular physical complaint is not being adequately addressed. Explicit reassurance should be given that the appropriate inquiries and investigations are being performed and that the possibility of an underlying physical disorder as the explanation for symptoms is being reasonably considered.

In time, it may be appropriate to gradually shift emphasis away from somatic symptoms to consideration of personal and interpersonal issues. In some individuals, it may be appropriate to posit a causal theory between somatic symptoms and "stress," that is, that there may be a temporal association between symptoms and personal, interpersonal, and even occupational problems. In individuals for whom such "insight" is difficult, behavioral techniques may be useful.

Even following such therapeutic guidelines, individuals with somatization disorder are often difficult to treat. Attention-seeking behavior, demands, and manipulation are common, necessitating firm limits and careful attention to boundary issues. This, again, is a management rather than a curative approach. Thus, such behaviors should generally be dealt with directively rather than interpreted to the individual.

No effective somatic treatments for somatization disorder itself have been identified. In the 1960s, Wheatley (1962) reported that low doses of anxiolytic drugs provided symptom amelioration in double-blind clinical trials using general practitioners. He also noted that whereas chlordiazepoxide was recommended for reasons of effectiveness, preference of the individuals, safety, and symptom relief, the best results were obtained by optimistic physicians using low doses of any anxiolytic medication. Surprisingly little systematic study of the pharmacological management of somatization disorder has been done since.

Individuals with somatization disorder may complain of anxiety and depression, suggesting readily treatable comorbid mental disorders. As previously discussed, it is often difficult to distinguish actual comorbid conditions from aspects of somatoform disorder itself. Pharmacological interventions are likely to be helpful in the former but not in the latter. At times, such discrimination will be impossible, and an empirical trial of such treatments may be indicated. Individuals with somatization disorder are often inconsistent and erratic in their use of medications. They will often report unusual side effects that may not be explained pharmacologically. This makes evaluation of treatment response difficult. In addition, drug dependence and suicide gestures and attempts are not uncommon.

UNDIFFERENTIATED SOMATOFORM DISORDER

Diagnosis

As defined in DSM-IV-TR, this category includes disturbances of at least 6 months' duration, with one or more unintentional, clinically significant, medically unexplained physical complaints (see DSM-IV-TR diagnostic criteria below). In a sense, it is a residual category, subsuming syndromes with somatic complaints that do not meet criteria for any of the "differentiated" somatoform disorders, yet are not better accounted for by any other mental disorder. On the other hand, it is a less residual category than somatoform disorder NOS, in that the disturbance must last at least 6 months (see Figure 36-1). Virtually any unintentional, medically unexplained physical symptoms causing clinically significant distress or impairment can be considered. In effect, this category serves to capture syndromes that resemble somatization disorder but do not meet full criteria.

DSM-IV-TR Diagnostic Criteria

300.81 Undifferentiated Somatoform Disorder

A. One or more physical complaints (e.g., fatigue, loss of appetite, gastrointestinal or urinary complaints).
B. Either (1) or (2):

   (1) After appropriate investigation, the symptoms cannot be fully explained by a known general medical condition or the direct effects of a substance (e.g., a drug of abuse, a medication).
   (2) When there is a related general medical condition, the physical complaints or resulting social or occupational impairment is in excess of what would be expected from the history, physical examination, or laboratory findings.

C. The symptoms cause clinically significant distress or impairment in social, occupational, or other important areas of functioning.
D. Duration of the disturbance is at least 6 months.
E. The disturbance is not better accounted for by another mental disorder (e.g., another somatoform disorder, sexual dysfunction, mood disorder, anxiety disorder, sleep disorder, or psychotic disorder).
F. The symptom is not intentionally produced or feigned (as in factitious disorder or malingering).

Reprinted with permission from the Diagnostic and Statistical Manual of Mental Disorders, Fourth Edition, Text Revision. Copyright 2000 American Psychiatric Association.

The term undifferentiated somatoform disorder was introduced in 1987 with DSM-III-R, replacing the atypical somatoform disorder of DSM-III. However, the category has not been well used, not only by mental health professionals but also by primary care physicians for whom identification of such a syndrome could be useful. Terms that have been used in a similar manner include *subsyndromal, forme fruste,* or *abridged* somatization disorder (Kirmayer and Robbins 1991). Escobar and coworkers (1989), defining an abridged syndrome as requiring at least six significant unexplained somatic symptoms for women and four for men, argued that especially in primary care settings, such a condition was much more common than a full somatization disorder and it predicted disability and future use of medical services. This group also argued that this construct met many of the suggested requirements for validity as a mental disorder, although adequate follow-up and family studies have not yet been done.

Owing to this as well as the underuse of such a construct, perhaps attributable, at least in part, to the ambiguity of designation as undifferentiated, consideration was given to differentiating an abridged somatization syndrome as "multisomatoform disorder" in DSM-IV. However, owing to uncertainties about the nature of such an entity, especially as to overlap with other syndromes such as anxiety and depressive disorders, and because the few data available suggested a variable course (Cloninger 1996), unlike somatization disorder, such a syndrome was left under the undifferentiated somatoform disorder rubric in DSM-IV. A more specific designation could have proved misleading clinically, promoting a false sense of security, with a tendency to preclude efforts to uncover a general medical or substance-related explanation for symptoms or to identify another mental disorder better accounting for the symptoms.

In addition to the range of symptoms specified in the other somatoform disorders, individuals with undifferentiated somatoform disorder, complaining primarily of fatigue (chronic fatigue syndrome), bowel problems (irritable bowel syndrome), or multiple muscle aches/weakness (fibromyalgia) can be considered for undifferentiated somatoform disorder. Substantial controversy exists regarding the etiology of such syndromes. Even if an explanation on the basis of a known pathophysiological mechanism cannot be established, many argue that the syndromes should be considered general medical conditions. However, for the time being, these syndromes could be considered in a highly tentative manner under the undifferentiated somatoform disorder rubric. Careful reconsideration of the undifferentiated somatoform label should be undertaken at regular intervals if the symptoms persist. The clinician should remain ever vigilant to the emergence of another general medical condition or mental disorder. Noteworthy is also the fact, when individuals are diagnosed with chronic fatigue syndrome, that careful evaluation procedures as recommended by an international study group should be followed (Fukuda et al. 1994).

Epidemiology

Some have argued that undifferentiated somatoform disorder is the most common somatoform disorder. Escobar and coworkers (1991), using an abridged somatization disorder construct requiring six somatic symptoms for women and four for men, reported that 11% of non-Hispanic US whites and Hispanics, 15% of US blacks, and 20% of Puerto Ricans in Puerto Rico fulfilled criteria. A preponderance of women was evident in all groups except the Puerto Rican sample (see Table 36-1). According to Escobar, such an abridged somatoform syndrome is 100 times more prevalent than a full somatization disorder.

Course

As shown in Table 36-1, it appears that the course and prognosis of undifferentiated somatoform disorder are highly variable. This is not surprising, because the definition of this disorder allows a great deal of heterogeneity.

Differential Diagnosis

In comparison to the situation when the full criteria for the well-validated somatization disorder are met, exclusion of an as-yet-undiscovered general medical or substance-induced explanation for physical symptoms is far less certain when the less stringent criteria for undifferentiated somatoform disorder are met. Thus, the diagnosis of undifferentiated somatoform disorder should remain tentative, and new symptoms should be carefully investigated.

Because undifferentiated somatoform disorder represents a somewhat residual category, the major diagnostic process, once occult general medical conditions and substance-induced explanations have been considered, is one of exclusion. As shown in Figure 36-1, whether the somatic symptoms are intentionally produced as in malingering and factitious disorder must be addressed. Here, motivation for external rewards (for malingering) and a pervasive intent to assume the sick role (for factitious disorder) must be assessed. The next consideration is whether the somatic symptoms are the manifestation of another mental disorder. Anxiety and mood disorders commonly present with somatic symptoms; high rates of anxiety and major depressive disorders are reported in individuals with somatic complaints attending family medicine clinics (Kirmayer et al. 1993). Of course, undifferentiated somatoform disorder could be diagnosed in addition to one of these disorders, so long as the symptoms are not accounted for by the other mental disorder. Crucial in this determination is whether the symptoms are present during periods in which the anxiety or mood disorders are not actively present.

Next, other somatoform disorders must be considered. In general, undifferentiated somatoform disorders are characterized by unexplained somatic complaints; the most common according to Escobar and coworkers (Escobar et al. 1989) are female reproductive symptoms, excessive gas, abdominal pain, chest pain, joint pain, palpitations, and fainting, rather than preoccupations or fears as in hypochondriasis or body dysmorphic disorder. However, an individual with some manifestations of these two disorders but not meeting full criteria could conceivably receive a diagnosis of undifferentiated somatoform disorder. An example is an individual with recurrent yet shifting hypochondriacal concerns that do respond to medical reassurance. If symptoms are restricted to those affecting the domains of sexual dysfunction, pain, or pseudoneurological symptoms, and the specific criteria for a sexual dysfunction, pain disorder, and/or conversion disorder are met, the specific disorder or disorders should be diagnosed. If other types of symptoms or symptoms of more than one of these disorders have been present for at least 6 months, yet criteria for somatization disorder are not met, undifferentiated somatoform disorder should be diagnosed. By definition, undifferentiated somatoform disorder requires a duration of 6 months. If this criterion is not met, a diagnosis of somatoform disorder NOS should be considered.

Individuals with an apparent undifferentiated somatoform disorder should be carefully evaluated for somatization disorder. Typically, individuals with somatization disorder are inconsistent historians, at one evaluation reporting a large number of symptoms fulfilling criteria for the full syndrome and at another time endorsing fewer symptoms (Martin et al. 1979). In addition, with follow-up, additional symptoms may become evident, and criteria for somatization disorder will be satisfied. Individuals with multiple somatic complaints not diagnosed with somatization disorder because of a reported onset later than 30 years of age may be inaccurately reporting a later age at onset. If the late age at onset is accurate, the individual should be carefully scrutinized for an occult general medical condition.

Etiology

Theories of etiology involving the concept of somatization have been posited by some. As reviewed by Kirmayer and Robbins (1991), somatization can be viewed as "a pattern of illness behavior by which bodily idioms of distress may serve as symbolic means of social regulation as well as protest or contestation." However, as previously discussed, such hypotheses have defied verification.

If it is assumed that undifferentiated somatoform disorder is simply an abridged form of somatization disorder, etiological theories reviewed under that diagnosis should apply. An intriguing research question is why the syndrome is fully expressed in some and only partially expressed in others.

Treatment

In view of the broad inclusion and minimal exclusion criteria for undifferentiated somatoform disorder, it is difficult to make treatment recommendations beyond the generic guidelines outlined for the somatoform disorders in general. More definitive recommendations await a more extensive empirical database. A substantial proportion of individuals with undifferentiated somatoform disorders improve or recover with no formal therapy. However, appropriate psychotherapy and pharmacological intervention may accelerate the process.

Kellner (1991) outlined some recommendations for individuals with symptoms of headache, fibromyalgia, and chronic fatigue syndrome, conditions that some would include under undifferentiated somatoform disorder. Generally recommended are brief psychotherapy of a supportive and educative nature. As with somatization disorder, the physician–patient relationship is of great importance. Judicious use of pharmacotherapy may be of benefit also, particularly if the somatoform syndrome is intertwined with an anxiety or depressive syndrome. Here, usual antianxiety and antidepressant medications are recommended. Individuals with unexplained pains may benefit from pain management strategies as outlined in the pain disorder section.

CONVERSION DISORDER

Diagnosis

As defined in DSM-IV-TR, conversion disorders are characterized by symptoms or deficits affecting voluntary, motor, or sensory function that are suggestive of, yet are not fully explained by, a neurological or other general medical condition or the direct effects of a substance (see Table 36-1 and DSM-IV-TR diagnostic criteria below). The diagnosis is not made if the presentation is explained as a culturally sanctioned behavior or experience, such as bizarre behaviors resembling a seizure during a religious ceremony. Symptoms are not intentionally produced or feigned, that is, the person does not consciously contrive a symptom for external rewards, as in malingering, or for the intrapsychic rewards of assuming the sick role, as in factitious disorder.

DSM-IV-TR Diagnostic Criteria

300.11 Conversion Disorder

A. One or more symptoms or deficits affecting voluntary motor or sensory function that suggest a neurological or other general medical condition.
B. Psychological factors are judged to be associated with the symptom or deficit because the initiation or exacerbation of the symptom or deficit is preceded by conflicts or other stressors.
C. The symptom or deficit is not intentionally produced or feigned (as in factitious disorder or malingering).

D. The symptom or deficit cannot, after appropriate investigation, be fully explained by a general medical condition, or by the direct effects of a substance, or as a culturally sanctioned behavior or experience.

E. The symptom or deficit causes clinically significant distress or impairment in social, occupational, or other important areas of functioning or warrants medical evaluation.

F. The symptom or deficit is not limited to pain or sexual dysfunction, does not occur exclusively during the course of somatization disorder, and is not better accounted for by another mental disorder.

Specify type of symptom or deficit:

With motor symptom or deficit (e.g., impaired coordination or balance, paralysis or localized weakness, difficulty swallowing or lump in throat, aphonia, and urinary retention)

With sensory symptom or deficit (e.g., loss of touch or pain sensation, double vision, blindness, deafness, and hallucinations)

With seizures or convulsions (includes seizures or convulsions with voluntary sensory components)

With mixed presentation (if symptoms of more than one category are evident).

Reprinted with permission from the Diagnostic and Statistical Manual of Mental Disorders, Fourth Edition, Text Revision. Copyright 2000 American Psychiatric Association.

Four subtypes with specific examples of symptoms are defined: with motor symptom or deficit (e.g., impaired coordination or balance, paralysis or localized weakness, difficulty swallowing or lump in throat, aphonia, and urinary retention); with sensory symptom or deficit (e.g., loss of touch or pain sensation, double vision, blindness, deafness, and hallucinations); with seizures or convulsions; and with mixed presentation (i.e., has symptoms of more than one of the other subtypes). The list of examples is also contained among the pseudoneurological symptoms listed in the diagnostic criteria for somatization disorder. Although determination is highly subjective and of questionable reliability and validity, association with psychological factors is required.

To a great extent, the concept of a conversion disorder derived from the work of neurologists such as Charcot, Breuer, and Freud (1893–1895) in the late nineteenth and early twentieth centuries and more recently of Ziegler and Paul (1954) and Marsden (1986). Conversion disorder was called conversion reaction in DSM-I and hysterical neurosis, conversion type in DSM-II. In both DSM-I and DSM-II, the conversion process was restricted to symptoms affecting the voluntary motor and sensory nervous systems. Symptoms for which there was some physiological understanding (generally involving the autonomic nervous system) were subsumed under the psychophysiological disorders.

Unfortunately, conversion disorder or conversion hysteria came to be equated, at least by some, with hysteria, a term used by others to describe a more pervasive, chronic, and polysymptomatic disorder, denoted as somatization disorder in DSM-III, DSM-III-R, and DSM-IV. Whereas conversion symptoms are among its most dramatic symptoms, somatization disorder is characterized by multiple unexplained symptoms in many organ systems; in conversion disorder, even a single symptom affecting voluntary motor or sensory function may suffice. Such nosological inconsistencies have resulted in a great deal of confusion, both in research and in clinical practice.

To add to the confusion, DSM-III and DSM-III-R used a broadened definition of conversion, including disorders characterized by symptoms involving any "loss or alteration in physical functioning suggesting a physical disorder," as long as the mechanism of conversion was evident, that is, the symptom was "an expression of a psychological conflict or need." Thus, disparate symptoms, including those involving primarily the autonomic or endocrine system, for example, "psychogenic" vomiting (assumedly expressing revulsion and disgust) and "pseudocyesis" (interpreted as representing unconscious conflict regarding pregnancy), were included as examples of conversion symptoms. In DSM-IV, conversion disorder was again restricted to symptoms affecting the voluntary motor and sensory systems. This change was consistent with the symptomatic, epidemiological, and prognostic differences between the pseudoneurological conversion symptoms and other types of symptoms involving "function."

The relationship of conversion disorder to the dissociative disorders warrants comment (Martin 1996). Long recognized as related, they were subsumed as subtypes of hysterical neurosis in DSM-II: conversion involving voluntary motor and sensory functioning, and dissociation affecting memory and identity. They are unified in one category in ICD-10: dissociative (conversion) disorders. DSM-IV retained the basic organization of DSM-III and DSM-III-R, classifying conversion disorder with the somatoform disorders; the dissociative disorders compose their own major grouping. However, the DSM-IV-TR text acknowledges the symptomatic, epidemiological, and probable pathogenetic similarities between conversion and dissociative symptoms. Such symptoms have been attributed to similar psychological mechanisms, and they often occur in the same individual, sometimes during the same episode of illness. DSM-IV-TR does suggest that individuals with conversion disorder be carefully scrutinized for dissociative symptoms.

Hallucinations are included among the sensory nervous symptoms in DSM-IV-TR. Whereas the concept of conversion hallucinations has a long tradition (Martin 1996), DSM-III and DSM-III-R noted hallucinations as a manifestation of only two nonpsychotic disorders: posttraumatic stress disorder, in which a traumatic event is reexperienced; and multiple personality disorder (dissociative identity disorder in DSM-IV-TR), wherein one or more personalities hear the voice of, talk with, or engage in activities with one or more of the other personalities. Inclusion of hallucinations as a conversion symptom was supported by the somatization disorder field trial, in which one third of a large sample of nonpsychotic women with evidence of unexplained somatic complaints reported a history of hallucinations. Among the 40% who had symptoms that met criteria for somatization disorder, more than half reported hallucinations (Martin 1995, unpublished data). Women with other conversion symptoms were more likely to report hallucinations than were those with no other conversion symptoms.

In general, conversion hallucinations (referred to by some as pseudohallucinations) differ in several ways from those in psychotic conditions. Conversion hallucinations typically occur in the absence of other psychotic symptoms, insight that the hallucinations are not real may be retained, and they often involve more than one sensory modality, whereas hallucinations in psychoses generally involve a single sensory modality, usually auditory. Conversion hallucinations also often have a naive, fantastic, or childish content, as if they are part of a fairy tale, and are described eagerly, sometimes even provocatively, as an interesting story (e.g., "I was driving downtown and a flying saucer flew over my car and I saw you [the psychiatrist] in a window and I heard your voice calling to me"). They often bear some understandable psychological purpose, although the individual may not be aware of intent. In the example given, the "sighting" was reported at the time that no further sessions were scheduled.

Epidemiology

Vastly different estimates of the incidence and prevalence of conversion disorder have been reported. Much of this difference may be attributable to methodological differences from study to study, including the changing definition of conversion disorder, ascertainment procedures, and populations studied. General population estimates have generally been derived indirectly, extrapolating from clinic or hospital samples.

Conversion symptoms themselves may be common; it was reported that 25% of normal postpartum and medically ill women had a history of conversion symptoms at some time during their life (Cloninger 1993), yet in some instances, there may have been no resulting clinically significant distress or impairment. Lifetime prevalence rates of treated conversion symptoms in general populations are much more modest, ranging from 11 to 500 per 100,000 (Martin 1996) (see Table 36-1). About 5 to 24% of psychiatric outpatients, 5 to 14% of general hospital patients, and 1 to 3% of outpatient psychiatric referrals reported a history of conversion symptoms (Cloninger 1993, Ford and Folks 1985, Toone 1990), although their current treatment was not necessarily for conversion symptoms. A rate of nearly 4% of outpatient neurological referrals (Perkin 1989) and 1% of neurological admissions (Ziegler and Paul 1954) involved conversion disorder. In virtually all studies, an excess (to the extent of 2 : 1 to 10 : 1) of women reported conversion symptoms relative to men (Ljunberg 1957, Stefansson et al. 1976, Raskin et al. 1966). In part, this may relate to the simple fact that women seek medical evaluation more often than men do, but it is unlikely that this fully accounts for the sex difference. There is a predilection for lower socioeconomic status; less educated, less psychologically sophisticated, and rural populations are overrepresented (Veith 1965, Weinstein et al. 1969, Lazare 1981, Folks et al. 1984). Consistent with this, higher rates (nearly 10%) of outpatient psychiatric referrals are for conversion symptoms in "developing" countries (Stafanis et al. 1976). As countries develop, there may be a declining incidence in time, which may relate to increasing levels of education, and medical and psychological sophistication (Nandi et al. 1992).

Course

Age at onset is typically from late childhood to early adulthood. Onset is rare before the age of 10 (Maloney 1980) and after 35, but cases with an onset as late as the ninth decade have been reported (Weddington 1979). The likelihood of a neurological or other medical condition is increased when the age at onset is in middle or late life. Development is generally acute, but symptoms may develop gradually as well. The course of individual conversion symptoms is generally short; half (Folks et al. 1984) to nearly all (Carter 1949) symptoms remit by the time of hospital discharge. However, symptoms relapse within one year in one-fifth to one-fourth of individuals. Typically, one symptom is present in a single episode, but multiple symptoms are generally involved longitudinally. Factors associated with good prognosis include acute onset, clearly identifiable precipitants, a short interval between onset and institution of treatment, and good intelligence (Toone 1990). Conversion blindness, aphonia, and paralysis are associated with relatively good prognosis, whereas individuals with seizures and tremor do more poorly. Some individuals diagnosed initially with conversion disorder will have a presentation that meets the criteria for somatization disorder when they are observed longitudinally (Kent et al. 1995).

Individual conversion symptoms are generally self-limited and do not lead to physical changes or disabilities. Rarely, physical sequelae such as atrophy may occur. Marital and occupational problems are not as frequent in individuals with conversion disorder as they are in those with somatization disorder (Tomasson et al. 1991, Coryell and House 1984). In a long-term follow-up study, excess mortality by unnatural causes was observed (Coryell and House 1984). However, the reason for this was unclear in that none of the deaths was by suicide.

Differential Diagnosis

As shown in Figure 36-1, the first consideration is whether the conversion symptoms are explained on the basis of a general medical condition. Because conversion symptoms by definition affect voluntary, motor, or sensory function (thus pseudoneurological), neurological conditions are usually suggested, but other general medical conditions may be implicated as well. Neurologists are generally first consulted by primary care physicians for conversion symptoms; mental health clinicians become involved only after neurological or general medical conditions have been reasonably excluded. Nonetheless, mental health clinician should have a good appreciation of the process of making such exclusions. More than 13% of actual neurological cases are diagnosed as functional before the elucidation of a neurological illness (Perkin 1989). Even after referral, vigilance for an emerging general medical condition should continue. A significant percentage—21% (Gatfield and Guze 1962) to 50% (Slater and Glithero 1965)—of individuals diagnosed with conversion symptoms are found to have neurological illness on follow-up.

Apparent conversion symptoms mandate a thorough evaluation for possible underlying physical explanation. This evaluation must include a thorough medical history; physical (especially neurological) examination; and radiographical, blood, urine, and other tests as clinically indicated. Reliance should not be placed on determination of whether psychological factors explain the symptom. As reviewed by Cloninger (1987), such determinations are unreliable except, perhaps, in cases in which there is a clear and immediate temporal relationship between a psychosocial stressor and the symptom, or in cases in which similar situations led to conversion symptoms in the past. A history of previous conversion or other unexplained symptoms, particularly if somatization disorder is diagnosable, lessens the probability that an occult medical condition will be identified (Cloninger 1993). Although conversion symptoms may occur at any age, symptoms are most often first manifested in late adolescence or early adulthood. Conversion symptoms first occurring in middle age or later should increase suspicion of an occult physical illness.

Symptoms of many neurological illnesses may appear inconsistent with known neurophysiological or neuropathological processes, suggesting conversion and posing diagnostic problems. These illnesses include multiple sclerosis, in which blindness due to optic neuritis may initially present with normal fundi; myasthenia gravis, periodic paralysis, myoglobinuric myopathy, polymyositis, and other acquired myopathies, in which marked weakness in the presence of normal deep tendon reflexes may occur; and Guillain–Barré syndrome, in which early extremity weakness may be inconsistent (Cloninger 1993).

Complicating diagnosis is the fact that physical illness and conversion or other apparent psychiatric overlay are not mutually exclusive. Individuals with physical illnesses that are incapacitating and frightening may appear to be exaggerating symptoms. Also, individuals with actual neurological illness will also have "pseudo" symptoms. For example, individuals with actual seizures may have pseudoseizures as well (Desai et al. 1982). Considering these observations, psychiatrists should avoid a rash and hasty diagnosis of conversion disorder when faced with symptoms that are difficult to interpret.

As with the other somatoform disorders, symptoms of conversion disorder are not intentionally produced, in distinction to malingering or factitious disorder. To a large part, this determination is based on assessment of the motivation for external rewards (as in malingering) or for the assumption of the sick role (as in factitious disorder). The setting is often an important consideration. For example, conversion-like symptoms are frequent in military or forensic settings, in which obvious potential rewards make malingering a serious consideration.

A diagnosis of conversion disorder should not be made if a conversion symptom is fully accounted for by a mood disorder or by schizophrenia (e.g., disordered motility as part of a catatonic syndrome of a psychotic mood disorder or schizophrenia). If the symptom is a hallucination, it must be remembered that the descriptors differentiating conversion from psychotic hallucinations should be seen only as rules of thumb. Differentiation should be based on a comprehensive assessment of the illness. In the case of hallucinations, posttraumatic stress disorder and dissociative identity disorder (multiple personality disorder) must also be excluded. If the conversion symptom cannot be fully accounted for by the other mental disorders, conversion disorder should be diagnosed in addition to the other disorder if it meets criteria (e.g., an episode of unexplained blindness in an individual with a major depressive episode). In hypochondriasis, neurological illness may be feared ("I have strange feelings in my head; it must be a brain tumor"), but the focus here is on preoccupation with fear of having the illness rather than on the symptom itself as in conversion disorder.

By definition, if symptoms are limited to sexual dysfunction or pain, conversion disorder is not diagnosed. Criteria for somatization disorder require multiple symptoms in multiple organ systems and functions, including symptoms affecting motor or sensory function (conversion symptoms) or memory or identity (dissociative symptoms). Thus, it would be superfluous to make an additional diagnosis of conversion disorder in the context of a somatization disorder.

A last consideration is whether the symptom is a culturally sanctioned behavior or experience. Conversion disorder should not be diagnosed if symptoms are clearly sanctioned or even expected, are appropriate to the sociocultural context, and are not associated with distress or impairment. Seizure-like episodes, such as those that occur in conjunction with certain religious ceremonies, and culturally expected responses, such as women "swooning" in response to excitement in Victorian times, qualify as examples of these symptoms.

Etiology

The term conversion implies etiology because it is derived from a hypothesized mechanism of converting psychological conflicts into somatic symptoms, often symbolically (e.g., repressed rage is converted into paralysis of an arm that could be used to strike). A number of psychological factors have been promoted as part of such an etiological process, but evidence for their essential involvement is scanty at best. Theoretically, anxiety is reduced by keeping an internal conflict or need out of awareness by symbolic expression of an unconscious wish as a conversion symptom (primary gain). However, individuals with active conversion symptoms often continue to show marked anxiety, especially on psychological tests (Lader and Sartorius 1968, Mears and Horvath 1972). Symbolism is infrequently evident, and its evaluation involves highly inferential and unreliable judgments (Raskin et al. 1966). Overinterpretation of symbolism in persons with occult medical disorder may contribute to misdiagnosis. Secondary gain, whereby conversion symptoms allow avoidance of noxious activities or the procurement of otherwise unavailable support, may also occur in persons with medical conditions, who may take advantage of such benefits (Raskin et al. 1966, Watson and Buranen 1979).

Individuals with conversion disorder may show a lack of concern out of keeping with the nature or implications of the symptom (the so-called *la belle indifférence*). However, indifference to symptoms is not invariably present in conversion disorder (Lewis and Berman 1965) and is also seen in individuals with general medical conditions (Weinstein et al. 1969), on the basis of denial or stoicism (Pincus 1982). Conversion symptoms may present in a dramatic or histrionic fashion and may be highly suggestible. A dramatic presentation is also seen in distressed individuals with medical conditions. Even symptoms based on an underlying medical condition may respond to suggestion, at least temporarily (Gatfield and Guze 1962). In many instances, preexisting personality disorders (in particular histrionic personality disorder) are evident and may predispose to conversion disorder. Persons with conversion disorder may often have a history of disturbed sexuality (Lewis 1974) many (one-third) report a history of sexual abuse, especially incestuous. Thus, two-thirds may not report such a history. Individuals with conversion disorder are often reported to be the youngest or the youngest of a sex in sibling order, but this is not a consistent finding (Ziegler et al. 1960, Stephens and Kamp 1962).

If not directly etiological, many psychosocial factors have been suggested as predisposing to conversion disorder. At a minimum, many persons with conversion disorder are in chaotic, domestic, and occupational situations. As previously mentioned, individuals from rural backgrounds and those who are psychologically and medically unsophisticated appear to be predisposed, as are those with existing neurological disorders. In the last case, a tendency to conversion symptoms has been attributed to "modeling," that is, individuals with neurological disorders are likely to have observed in others, as well as in themselves, various neurological symptoms, which they then may simulate as conversion symptoms.

Available data suggest a genetic contribution. Conversion symptoms are more frequent in relatives of individuals with conversion disorder (Toone 1990). In a nonblinded study, rates of conversion disorder were found to be elevated tenfold in female (fivefold in male) relatives of individuals with conversion disorder (Ljunberg 1957). Accumulated data from available twin studies show 9 concordant and 33 discordant, monozygotic pairs and no concordant but 43 discordant dizygotic pairs (Inouye 1972). Nongenetic familial factors, particularly incestuous childhood sexual abuse, may also be involved in some. Nearly one-third of individuals with medically unexplained seizures reported childhood sexual abuse, compared with less than 10% of those with complex partial epilepsy (Alper et al. 1993). Data looking specifically at abuse history in other well-defined conversion disorder cases are not available.

Treatment

Reports of the treatment of conversion disorder date from those of Charcot, which generally involved symptom removal by suggestion or hypnosis. Breuer and Freud, using such psychoanalytic techniques as free association and abreaction of repressed affects, had more ambitious objectives in their treatment of Anna O., including the resolution of unconscious conflicts. To date, whereas some recommend long-term, intensive, insight-oriented psychodynamic psychotherapy in pursuit of such goals (Ford 1995), most mental health clinicians advocate a more pragmatic approach, especially for acute cases.

Therapeutic approaches vary according to whether the conversion symptom is acute or chronic. Whichever the case, direct confrontation is not recommended. Such a communication may cause an individual to feel even more isolated. An undiscovered physical illness may also underlie the presentation.

In acute cases, the most frequent initial aim is removal of the symptom. The pressure behind accomplishing this depends on the distress and disability associated with the symptom (Ford 1995). If the individual is not in great distress and the need to regain function is not immediate, a conservative approach of reassurance, relaxation, and suggestion is recommended (Ford 1983). With this technique, the individual is reassured that on the basis of evaluation the symptom will disappear completely and, in fact, is already beginning to do so. The individual can then be encouraged to ventilate about recent events and feelings, without any causal relationships being suggested. This is in contrast to attempts at abreaction, by which repressed material, particularly regarding a painful experience or a conflict, is brought back to consciousness.

If symptoms do not resolve with such conservative approaches, a number of other techniques for symptom resolution may be instituted. It does appear that prompt resolution of conversion symptoms is important because the duration of conversion symptoms is associated with a greater risk of recurrence and chronic disability (Cloninger 1993). The other techniques include narcoanalysis (e.g., amobarbital interview), hypnosis, and behavioral therapy (Ford 1995). In narcoanalysis, amobarbital or another sedative–hypnotic medication such as lorazepam is given intravenously to the point of drowsiness. Sometimes this is followed by administration of a stimulant medication, such as methamphetamine. The individual is then encouraged to discuss stressors and conflicts. This technique may be effective acutely, leading to at least temporary symptom relief as well as expansion of the information known about the individual. This technique has not been shown to be especially effective with more chronic conversion symptoms. In hypnotherapy, symptoms may be removed with the suggestion that the symptoms will gradually improve posthypnotically. Information regarding stressors and conflicts may be explored as well. Formal behavioral therapy, including relaxation training and even aversive therapy, has been proposed and reported by some to be effective. In addition, simply manipulating the environment to interrupt reinforcement of the conversion symptom is recommended.

Anecdotally, somatic treatments including phenothiazines, lithium, and electroconvulsive therapy have been reported effective. However, in many cases, this may be attributable to simple suggestion. In other cases, resolution of another psychiatric disorder, such as a psychotic disorder or a mood disorder, may have led to the symptom's removal. It should be evident from the preceding discussion that in acute conversion disorders, it may be not the particular technique but the influence of suggestion that is specifically associated with symptom relief. It is likely that in various rituals, such as exorcism and other religious ceremonies, immediate "cures" are based on suggestion. Suggestion seems to play a major role in the resolution of "mass hysteria," in which a group of individuals who believe that they have been exposed to some noxious influence such as a "toxin" or even a "spell," experience similar symptoms that do not appear to have any organic basis. Often, the epidemic can be contained if affected individuals are segregated. Simple announcements that no such factor has been identified and that symptoms experienced by the group have been linked to mass hysteria have been effective.

Thus far, this discussion has centered on acute treatment primarily for symptom removal. Longer-term approaches include strategies previously discussed for somatization disorder—a pragmatic, conservative approach involving support and exploration of various conflict areas, particularly of interpersonal relationships. A certain degree of insight may be attained, at least in terms of appreciating relationships between various conflicts and stressors and the development of symptoms. Others advocate long-term, intensive, insight-oriented, dynamic psychotherapy.

PAIN DISORDER

Diagnosis

As defined in DSM-IV-TR, the essential feature of pain disorder is pain with which psychological factors "have an important role in the onset, severity, exacerbation, or maintenance" (see Table 36-1 and DSM-IV-TR diagnostic criteria on page 996). Pain disorder is subtyped as pain disorder associated with psychological factors and pain disorder associated with both psychological factors and a general medical condition. The third possibility, pain disorder associated with a general medical condition, is not considered to be a mental disorder, because the requirement is not met that psychological factors play an important role. Thus, the DSM-IV-TR concept of pain disorder as a mental disorder was broadened and allowed the clinician much greater specificity in considering etiological factors and a more useful schema for differential diagnosis. The focus is placed on the presence of psychological factors rather than the exasperating determination of whether the pain is attributable to organic disease.

DSM-IV-TR Diagnostic Criteria

307.xx Pain Disorder

A. Pain in one or more anatomical sites is the predominant focus of the clinical presentation and is of sufficient severity to warrant clinical attention.
B. The pain causes clinically significant distress or impairment in social, occupational, or other important areas of functioning.
C. Psychological factors are judged to have an important role in the onset, severity, exacerbation, or maintenance of the pain.
D. The symptom or deficit is not intentionally produced or feigned (as in factitious disorder or malingering).
E. The pain is not better accounted for by a mood, anxiety, or psychotic disorder and does not meet criteria for dyspareunia.

Code as follows:

307.80 Pain Disorder Associated with Psychological Factors: Psychological factors are judged to have the major role in the onset, severity, exacerbation, or maintenance of the pain. (If a general medical condition is present, it does not have a major role in the onset, severity, exacerbation, or maintenance of the pain.) This type of pain disorder is not diagnosed if criteria are also met for somatization disorder.

Specify if:

Acute: Duration of less than 6 months
Chronic: Duration of 6 months or longer

307.89 Pain Disorder Associated with both Psychological Factors and a General Medical Condition: Both psychological factors and a general medical condition are judged to have important roles in the onset, severity, exacerbation, or maintenance of the pain. The associated general medical condition or anatomical site of the pain (see below) is coded on Axis III.

Specify if:

Acute: Duration of less than 6 months
Chronic: Duration of 6 months or longer

Note: The following is not considered to be a mental disorder and is included here to facilitate differential diagnosis.

Pain Disorder Associated with a General Medical Condition: A general medical condition has a major role in the onset, severity, exacerbation, or maintenance of the pain. (If psychological factors are present, they are not judged to have a major role in the onset, severity, exacerbation, or maintenance of the pain.) The diagnostic code for the pain is selected based on the associated general medical condition if one has been established or on the anatomical location of the pain if the underlying general medical condition is not yet clearly established—for example, low back (724.2), sciatic (724.3), pelvic (625.9), headache (784.0), facial (784.0), chest (786.50), joint (719.4), bone (733.90), abdominal (789.0), breast (611.71), renal (788.0), ear (388.70), eye (379.91), throat (784.1), tooth (525.9), and urinary (788.0).

A diagnosis of pain disorder requires that the pain be of sufficient severity to warrant clinical attention, that is, it causes clinically significant distress or impairment. A number of instruments have been developed to assess the degree of distress associated with the pain. Such measures include the numerical rating scale and visual analog scale as described by Scott and Huskisson (1976), the McGill Pain Questionnaire, and the West Haven–Yale Multidimensional Pain Inventory (Osterweis et al. 1987).

DSM-IV-TR includes a number of exclusionary conventions. By definition, if pain is restricted to pain with sexual intercourse, the sexual disorder, dyspareunia, not pain disorder, is diagnosed. If pain occurs in the context of a mood, anxiety, or psychotic disorder, pain disorder is diagnosed only if it is an independent focus of clinical attention and is not better accounted for by the other disorder, a highly subjective judgment.

If pain occurs exclusively during the course of somatization disorder, pain disorder is not diagnosed because pain symptoms are part of the criteria for somatization disorder and are thereby subsumed under the more comprehensive diagnosis. Because somatization disorder is virtually a lifelong condition, this exclusion generally applies in someone with somatization disorder by history. Important here is that in addition to pain, somatization disorder involves multiple symptoms of the gastrointestinal system, the reproductive system, and the central and peripheral nervous systems; whereas in pain disorder, the focus is on pain symptoms only.

Specification of acute versus chronic pain disorder on the basis of whether the duration is less than or greater than 6 months is an important distinction. Whereas acute pain, in most cases, will be linked with physical disorders, when pain remains unexplained after 6 months, psychological factors are often involved (Cloninger 1993). However, the psychiatrist must remember that a significant minority (in one study 19%) of individuals with chronic pain of no apparent physical origin will ultimately be found to have occult organic disease (Cloninger 1993).

In individuals with unexplained pelvic pain, clinicians should be warned about cavalier conclusions regarding the absence of physical disease. With laparoscopy, a high frequency of occult organic disease has been identified in several studies. Thus, laparoscopy may be indicated in individuals with pelvic pain. Electromyography may be helpful in distinguishing muscle contraction headaches. Failure to show coronary artery spasm with provocative procedures and failure to respond to nitroglycerin may be useful in distinguishing individuals with pain disorder from those in whom the pain is attributable to coronary artery disease.

Epidemiology

Given the fact that diagnostic criteria for pain have significantly changed across the various editions of the DSMs, only estimates can be made for the epidemiological parameters of pain disorder. As to pain itself, some empirical studies suggest that it is common. Perhaps as indirect evidence of this is the proliferation of pain clinics nationally. Of course, many individuals attending these clinics fall into the category of pain disorder associated with a general medical condition, but undoubtedly, some also have involvement of psychological factors as required for a diagnosis of pain disorder as a mental disorder. The same would apply to the 10 to 15% of adults in the United States in any given year who have work disability because of back pain (Osterweis et al. 1987). Pain has been found to be a predominant symptom in 75% of consecutive general medical patients, with 75% of these (thus 50% overall) judged as having no identifiable physical cause (King 1994). As reviewed by Stoudemire (1988), no apparent physical basis is found in 40 to 50% of individuals presenting with nonspecific abdominal pain. At least half of such individuals show major personality problems in addition, with such aberrations associated with poor outcome. Whereas primary care and other nonpsychiatric physicians probably see most pain patients, 38% of psychiatric inpatient admissions (Delaplaine et al. 1978) and 18% attending a psychiatric outpatient clinic (Chaturvedi 1987) report pain as a significant problem.

Course

Given the heterogeneity of conditions subsumed under the pain disorder rubric, course and prognosis vary widely. The subtyping at 6 months is of significance. The prognosis for total remission is good for pain disorders of less than 6 months' duration. However, for syndromes of greater than 6 months' duration, chronicity is common. The site of the pain may be another factor. As described by Stoudemire and Sandhu (1987), certain anatomically differentiated pain syndromes can be distinguished, and each has its own characteristic pattern. These include syndromes characterized primarily by headache, facial pain, chest pain, abdominal pain, and pelvic pain. In such syndromes, symptoms tend to be recurrent, with relapses occurring in association with stress. A high rate of depression has been observed among individuals with unexplained facial pain. Facial pain is often alleviated by antidepressant medication. This effect has been observed in both individuals with depressive symptoms and those without.

Other factors affecting course and prognosis include associated mental disorders and external reinforcement. Employment at the outset of treatment predicts improvement (Martin 1995). Chronicity is more likely in the presence of certain personality diagnoses or traits, such as pronounced passivity and dependency. External reinforcement includes litigation involving potential financial compensation or disability. Continuation of the pain disorder may prove more lucrative than its resolution and return to work. Level of activity, which is generally associated with improvement, is discouraged by fears of losing compensation. Thus, although outright malingering may be rare (Leavitt and Sweet 1986), pain behaviors are often reinforced and maintained. Habituation with addictive drugs is associated with greater chronicity.

Differential Diagnosis

As shown in Figure 36-1, the differential diagnosis begins with an assessment of whether the presentation is fully explained by a general medical condition. If not, it may be assumed that psychological factors play a major role. If it is judged that psychological factors do not play a major role, a diagnosis of pain disorder associated with a general medical condition may apply. As previously mentioned, this does not have a mental disorder code.

If psychological factors are involved, the first consideration is whether the pain is feigned. If so, either malingering or factitious disorder is diagnosed, depending on whether external incentives or assumption of the sick role is the motivation. Evidence of malingering includes consideration of external rewards relative to the chronology of the development and maintenance of the pain. In factitious disorder, a pattern of successive hospitalizations and medical evaluations is evident. Inconsistency in presentation, lack of correspondence to known anatomical pathways or disease patterns, and lack of associated sensory or motor function changes suggest malingering or factitious disorder, but pain disorder associated with psychological factors may show this pattern as well. The key question is whether the individual is experiencing rather than feigning the pain.

Determination of the relative contributions of psychological and general medical factors is difficult. Of course, careful assessment of the nature and severity of the potential underlying medical condition and the nature and degree of pain that would be expected should be made. Traditionally, the so-called conversion V or neurotic triad (consisting of elevation of the hypochondriasis and hysteria scales with a lower score on the depression scale) on the Minnesota Multiphasic Personality Inventory has been purported to indicate emotional indifference to the somatic concerns as might be expected if the symptom is attributable to psychological factors rather than organic disease. However, evidence indicates that this configuration may also occur as an adjustment to chronic illness.

Etiology

In considering the etiology of pain disorder, possible mechanisms of pain itself must be considered. As reviewed by King (1994), the definition of pain sanctioned by the International Association for the Study of Pain Subcommittee on Taxonomy is "an unpleasant sensory and emotional experience associated with actual or potential tissue damage." It goes on to acknowledge that pain is not simply "activity induced in the nociceptor and nociceptive pathways by a noxious stimulus" but "is always a psychological state...." Thus, it accepts the hypothesis that pain involves psychological as well as physical factors.

Many theories of the etiology and pathophysiology of pain involving both biological and psychological factors have been proposed. It is known that a neuropathway descends from the cerebral cortex and medulla, which inhibits the firing of pain transmission neurons when it is activated (Cloninger 1993). This system is apparently mediated by the endogenous opiate-like compounds, endorphins, and by serotonin. Indeed, metabolites of both of these neurotransmitters may be reduced in the cerebrospinal fluid of individuals with chronic pain (von Knorring and Attkisson 1979).

The gate control theory developed by Melzack and Wall (1983), as reviewed by King (1994), links biological and psychological factors. It hypothesizes a gatelike mechanism involving the dorsal horn of the spinal cord by which large A-beta fibers as well as small A-delta and C fibers carry impulses from the periphery to the substantia gelatinosa and T-cells in the spinal cord. Activation of the large fibers inhibits, whereas activation of the small fibers facilitates transmission to the T-cells. In addition, impulses descending from the brain, influenced by cognitive processes, may either inhibit or facilitate transmission of pain impulses. Such a mechanism may explain how psychological processes affect pain perception.

By definition, both pain disorder associated with psychological factors and pain disorder associated with both psychological factors and a general medical condition involve psychological factors. In the case of the former, it is presumed that there is little contribution from general medical conditions; in the latter, both physical and psychological factors contribute. A plethora of not necessarily mutually exclusive theories has been proposed to explain how this takes place.

As reviewed by Cloninger (1993), psychological constructs involving learning theories, both operant and classical conditioning, may apply. In operant paradigms, pain-related complaints are reinforced by increased attention, relief from obligations, monetary compensation, and the pleasurable effects of analgesics. In classical conditioning, originally neutral settings such as a workplace or bedroom where pain was experienced come to evoke pain-related behavior. Social and cultural attitudes may also have effects. Individuals with unexplained pain are more likely than others to have close relatives with chronic pain. Although findings have differed from study to study, ethnic differences may also have effects, such as greater pain tolerance in Irish and Anglo-Saxon groups in comparison to southern Mediterranean groups.

Treatment

Treatment of pain overall has been well summarized by King (1994). An overriding guideline is that the clinician not do anything that will actually perpetuate and even promote "pain-related behavior." Thus, a major goal is to encourage activity. Other guidelines include avoidance of sedative–antianxiety drugs, judicious use of analgesics on a fixed interval schedule so as not to reinforce pain-related behaviors, avoidance of opioids, and consideration of alternative treatment approaches such as relaxation therapy. Depression should be treated with appropriate antidepressant drugs, not sedative–antianxiety medications. The difficulties in managing individuals with pain disorder have resulted in the establishment of many clinics and programs especially designed for pain. Referral to such a service may be indicated. Intervention should best be provided early in the course of the syndrome, before pain-related behaviors become entrenched. Once continuing disability compensation is established, therapeutic efforts become much more difficult.

The preceding general guidelines apply whether or not a general medical basis for the pain is involved. Of course, if only pain disorder associated with psychological factors is involved, psychological management will be the mainstay. For individuals with pain associated with general medical factors (not a mental disorder) in which psychological factors do not play a major role, efforts should be made to prevent the development of psychological problems in response to the resulting distress, isolation and loss of function, and iatrogenic effects such as exposure to potentially addicting drugs.

In acute pain, the major goal is to relieve the pain (Osterweis et al. 1987). Thus, pharmacological agents generally play a more significant role than in chronic syndromes. Whereas the risk of developing opioid dependence appears to be surprisingly low (4 per 12,000) among individuals without a prior history of dependence (Porter and Jick 1980), nonopioid agents should be used whenever they can be expected to be effective. As discussed for chronic pain, these include, in particular, acetaminophen and the nonsteroidal antiinflammatory drugs (NSAIDs), of which aspirin is considered a member. Even if an opioid analgesic is employed, these drugs should be continued as adjuncts; often, they lessen the required dose of the opioid.

It is with the chronic syndromes that proper management is crucial to ease distress and prevent the development of additional problems. As advised by King (1994), the overriding goal is to maintain function, because total relief of the pain may not be possible. Physical and occupational therapy may play a major role. There may be resistance to the involvement of a mental health professional as an indication that the pain is not seen as real. Such issues must first be resolved. An attempt should be made to ascertain the roles that psychological and general medical factors play in the maintenance of the pain.

A large variety of psychotherapies including individual, group, and family strategies have been employed. Two techniques that warrant special attention are operant conditioning and cognitive–behavioral therapy. In operant conditioning, the pattern of reinforcement of pain behavior by medication, attention, and excuse from responsibilities is to be interrupted and reinforcement shifted to usual daily activities. To assess the role of operant conditioning, it may be necessary to have individuals keep a diary and to interview family members to identify any conditioning patterns. In cognitive–behavioral therapies, the goal is the identification and correction of attitudes, beliefs, and expectations. Biofeedback and relaxation techniques may be used to minimize muscle tension that may aggravate if not cause pain. Hypnosis may also be used to achieve muscle relaxation and to help the individual "dissociate" from the pain.

Pharmacological intervention may also be useful in chronic syndromes. Effort should be made to avoid opioids if possible. Agents to be tried first include antidepressants, acetaminophen, NSAIDs (including aspirin), and anticonvulsants such as carbamazepine. Antidepressants seem particularly useful for neuropathic pain, headache, facial pain, fibrositis, and arthritis (including rheumatoid arthritis). Analgesic action seems to be independent of antidepressant effects. Most work has been done with the tricyclic antidepressants; other classes, such as the monoamine oxidase inhibitors (MAOIs) and the selective serotonin reuptake inhibitors (SSRIs), may be effective as well. Although it was thought that the action is mediated by serotoninergic effects, agents such as desipramine with predominantly noradrenergic activity seem to be effective as well. NSAIDs, of which aspirin, ibuprofen, naproxen, and piroxicam are commonly used examples, may alleviate pain through inhibition of prostaglandin synthesis. Unfortunately, this effect may also contribute to side effects, such as aggravation of peptic or duodenal ulcers and interference with renal function. For individuals unable to tolerate NSAIDs, acetaminophen should be tried.

If opioid analgesics are used, it is recommended that use be tied to objectives such as increasing level of activity rather than simply pain alleviation (King 1994). Milder opioids, such as codeine, oxycodone, and hydrocodone, should be implemented first. The once widely used propoxyphene has less analgesic effect than these drugs; it is not devoid of abuse potential as once thought and is not recommended. Pure opioid agonists such as morphine, methadone, and hydromorphone should be tried next. Meperidine, also in this class, is contraindicated for prolonged use because accumulation of the toxic metabolite, normeperidine, a cerebral irritant, may result in anxiety, psychosis, or seizures. Meperidine may also have a lethal interaction with MAOIs. There are no advantages to mixed opioid agonist–antagonists. The commonly used pentazocine should be avoided because it has abuse potential and psychotomimetic effects in some individuals. It remains to be seen whether newer agents (buprenorphine, butonphanol, and nalbuphine) have lower abuse potential as claimed. Above all, psychiatrists should be judicious in the use of opioid analgesics, considering not only their abuse potential but their large number of side effects including constipation, nausea and vomiting, excessive sedation, and, in higher doses, respiratory depression that may be fatal (King 1994).

In addition to pharmacotherapy, a number of other "physical" techniques have been used, such as acupuncture and transcutaneous electrical nerve stimulation. These carry little risk of adverse effects or aggravation of the pain disorder. Other procedures such as trigger point injections, nerve blocks, and surgical ablation may be recommended if specifically indicated by an underlying general medical disorder.

HYPOCHONDRIASIS

Diagnosis

As defined in DSM-IV-TR, the essential feature in hypochondriasis is preoccupation with fears or the idea of having a serious disease based on the "misinterpretation of bodily symptoms" (see DSM-IV-TR diagnostic criteria on page 1002). This is in contrast to somatization disorder, conversion disorder, and pain disorder, in which the symptoms themselves are the predominant focus (see Table 36-1). There was some debate in the development of DSM-IV as to whether it was necessary that a body complaint be present. On the basis of empirical data, however, it was determined that this requirement was a valid one and helped to distinguish the "disease conviction" of hypochondriasis from "disease fear" as in phobic disorder (Cote et al. 1996). Bodily symptoms may be interpreted broadly to include misinterpretation of normal body functions. In hypochondriasis, the preoccupation persists despite reassurance from physicians and the accumulation of evidence to the contrary. As in the other somatoform disorders, symptoms must result in clinically significant distress or impairment in important areas of functioning. The duration must be at least 6 months. Hypochondriasis is not diagnosed if the hypochondriacal concerns are better accounted for by another mental disorder, such as major depressive episodes or various psychotic disorders with somatic delusions.

DSM-IV-TR Diagnostic Criteria

300.7 Hypochondriasis

A. Preoccupation with fears of having, or the idea that one has, a serious disease based on the person's misinterpretation of bodily symptoms.
B. The preoccupation persists despite appropriate medical evaluation and reassurance.
C. The belief in criterion A is not of delusional intensity (as in delusional disorder, somatic type) and is not restricted to a circumscribed concern about appearance (as in body dysmorphic disorder).
D. The preoccupation causes clinically significant distress or impairment in social, occupational, or other important areas of functioning.
E. The duration of the disturbance is at least 6 months.
F. The preoccupation is not better accounted for by generalized anxiety disorder, obsessive–compulsive disorder, panic disorder, a major depressive episode, separation anxiety, or another somatoform disorder.

Specify if:

With poor insight: If, for most of the time during the current episode, the person does not recognize that the concern about having a serious illness is excessive or unreasonable

In the development of DSM-IV, owing to observations that the disease conviction resembled disease phobia or the incorrigible ideas of obsessive–compulsive disorder, placement of hypochondriasis with the anxiety disorders was considered (Cote et al. 1996). Similarly, a case can be made that disease conviction is on a continuum with somatic delusions of disease, suggesting inclusion with the delusional disorders. In the end, such considerations were resolved by keeping hypochondriasis with the somatoform disorders, defining it in terms of an idea that one already has a particular illness rather than fears of acquiring one to distinguish it from a disease phobia, and by excluding cases in which the idea was of delusional proportions to differentiate hypochondriasis from delusional disorder, somatic type.

Epidemiology

Some degree of preoccupation with disease is apparently common. As reviewed by Kellner (1991), 10 to 20% of "normal" and 45% of "neurotic" persons have intermittent unfounded worries about illness, with 9% of individuals doubting reassurances given by physicians. In another review, Kellner (1985) estimated that 50% of all individuals attending physicians' offices "suffer either primary hypochondriacal symptoms or have minor somatic disorders with hypochondriacal overlay." How these relate to hypochondriasis as a disorder is difficult to assess because these estimates do not appear to distinguish between a focus on the symptoms themselves (as in somatization disorder) and preoccupation with the implications of the symptoms (as in hypochondriasis). The Epidemiological Catchment Area study (Robins et al. 1984) did not consider hypochondriasis. A 1965 study reported prevalence figures ranging from 3 to 13% in different cultures (Kenyon 1965), but it is not clear whether this represents a syndrome comparable to the current definition or just hypochondriacal symptoms. As already noted, many individuals manifest some hypochondriacal symptoms as part of other mental disorders, and others have transient hypochondriacal symptoms in response to stresses such as serious physical illness yet never fulfill the inclusion criteria for DSM-IV-TR hypochondriasis. Assessment of the incidence and prevalence of hypochondriasis undoubtedly requires study of general or primary care rather than psychiatric populations, because individuals with hypochondriasis are convinced that they suffer from some physical illness. To date, study of such populations suggests that 4 to 9% of individuals in general medical settings suffer from hypochondriasis (Fallon et al. 1993).

It does appear that hypochondriasis is equally common in males and females. Data concerning socioeconomic class are conflicting.

Course

Data are conflicting, but it appears that the most common age at onset is in early adulthood. Available data suggest that approximately 25% of individuals with a diagnosis of hypochondriasis do poorly, 65% show a chronic but fluctuating course, and 10% recover. This pertains to the full syndrome. A much more variable course is seen in individuals with just some hypochondriacal concerns. It appears that acute onset, absence of a personality disorder, and absence of secondary gain are favorable prognostically.

Differential Diagnosis

As shown in Figure 36-1, the first step in approaching individuals with distressing or impairing preoccupation with or fears of having a serious disease is to exclude the possibility of explanation on the basis of a general medical condition. Fears that may seem excessive may also occur in individuals with general medical conditions with vague and subjective symptoms early in their disease course. These include neurological diseases, such as myasthenia gravis and multiple sclerosis; endocrine diseases; systemic diseases that affect several organ systems, such as systemic lupus erythematosus; and occult malignant neoplasms (Kellner 1991). The disease conviction of hypochondriasis may actually be less amenable to medical reassurance than the fears of individuals, with general medical illnesses, who may at least temporally accept such encouragement. Hypochondriacal complaints are not often intentionally produced such that differentiation from malingering and factitious disorder is seldom a problem.

Exclusion is made if the preoccupation is better accounted for by another mental disorder. DSM-IV-TR lists generalized anxiety disorder, obsessive–compulsive disorder, panic disorder, a major depressive episode, separation anxiety, or another somatoform disorder as candidates. Chronology will be of utmost importance in such discriminations. Hypochondriacal concerns occurring exclusively during episodes of another disturbance, such as an anxiety or depressive disorder, do not warrant an additional diagnosis of hypochondriasis. The presence of symptoms of another mental disorder will also be helpful. For example, an individual with hypochondriacal complaints as part of a major depressive episode will show other symptoms of depression, such as sleep and appetite disturbance, feelings of worthlessness, and self-reproach, although depressed elderly individuals may deny sadness or other expressions of depressed mood. A confounding factor is that individuals with hypochondriasis often have comorbid anxiety or depressive syndromes (Kenyon 1965). Again, characterizing the symptoms by chronology will be useful. Treatment trials may also have diagnostic significance. Depressed individuals who are hypochondriacal may respond to non-SSRI antidepressant medications or electroconvulsive therapy (often necessary to reverse a depressive state of sufficient severity to lead to such profound symptoms), with resolution of the hypochondriacal as well as the depressive symptoms.

Hypochondriasis is differentiated from other somatoform disorders such as pain, conversion, and somatization disorders by its predominant feature of preoccupation with and fears of having an underlying illness based on the misinterpretation of body symptoms, rather than the physical symptoms themselves. Individuals with these other somatoform disorders at times are concerned with the possibility of underlying illness, but this will generally be overshadowed by a focus on the symptoms themselves.

The next consideration is whether the belief is of delusional proportions. Individuals with hypochondriasis, although preoccupied, generally acknowledge the possibility that their concerns are unfounded. Delusional individuals do not. Somatic delusions of serious illness are seen in some cases of schizophrenia and in delusional disorder, somatic type. In general, individuals with schizophrenia who have such delusions also show other signs of schizophrenia, such as disorganized speech, peculiarities of thought and behavior, hallucinations, and other delusions. Belief that an underlying illness is being caused by some bizarre process may also be seen (e.g., "I'm trying not to defecate because it will cause my brain to turn to jelly"). Schizophrenic individuals may also show improvement with neuroleptic treatment, at least in the "active" symptoms of their illness, under which somatic delusions are included.

Differentiation from delusional disorder, somatic type, may be more difficult. It is often a thin line between preoccupation and fear that is a conviction and that which is a delusion. Often, the distinction is made on the basis of whether the individual can consider the possibility that the conviction is erroneous. Yet, individuals with hypochondriasis vary in the extent to which they can do this. DSM-IV-TR acknowledges this by its inclusion of the specifier with poor insight. In the past, some argued that differentiation could be made on the basis of response to neuroleptics, especially pimozide; individuals with delusional disorder, but not hypochondriasis, respond. Interestingly, there is now at least one report of successful treatment of a syndrome corresponding to delusional disorder, somatic type, in a nondepressed individual with the SSRI paroxetine (Brophy 1994). As with hypochondriasis, response was obtained only when the dose was raised beyond an antidepressant dose (to 60 mg/day).

If it is concluded that the preoccupations are not delusional, the next consideration is whether the duration requirement of 6 months has been met (see Figure 36-1). Syndromes of less than 6 months' duration are diagnosed under either somatoform disorder NOS or adjustment disorder if the symptoms are an abnormal response to a stressful life event. The reason to make such a distinction is to distinguish hypochondriasis from transient syndromes, the longitudinal course of which have been shown to be more variable, suggesting heterogeneity (Barsky et al. 1993).

Other diagnostic considerations include whether the preoccupations or fears are restricted to preoccupations with being overweight, as in anorexia nervosa; with the inappropriateness of one's sex characteristics, as in a gender identity disorder; or with defects in appearance, as in body dysmorphic disorder. The preoccupations of hypochondriasis resemble the obsessions, and the health checking and efforts to obtain reassurance resemble the compulsions of obsessive–compulsive disorder. However, if such manifestations are health centered only, obsessive–compulsive disorder is not diagnosed. If, on the other hand, nonhealth related obsessions and compulsions are present, obsessive–compulsive disorder may be diagnosed in addition to hypochondriasis.

Etiology

Until recently, psychoanalytic hypotheses of etiology predominated. Freud hypothesized that hypochondriasis represented "the return of object libido onto the ego with cathexis of the body" (Viederman 1985). Subsequently, the cathexis to the body hypothesis was elaborated on to include interpretations involving disturbed object relations—displacement of repressed hostility to the body to communicate anger indirectly to others. Dynamic mechanisms involving masochism, guilt, conflicted dependency needs, and a need to suffer and be loved at the same time have also been suggested (Stoudemire 1988). The presence of such "narcissistic" mechanisms has been suggested as the reason that individuals with hypochondriasis were "unanalyzable." Other psychological theories involve defense against feelings of low self-esteem and inadequacy, perceptual and cognitive abnormalities, and operant conditioning involving reinforcement for assumption of the sick role.

Biological theories have been suggested as well. Hypochondriacal ideas have been attributed to a hypervigilance to insult, including overperception of physical problems (Barsky and Klerman 1983). This has been posited in particular in reference to hypochondriasis as an aspect of depression or anxiety disorders. Hypochondriasis has been included by some in the posited obsessive–compulsive spectrum disorders along with obsessive–compulsive and body dysmorphic disorders, anorexia nervosa, Tourette's disorder, trichotillomania, pathological gambling, and other impulsive disorders (Hollender 1993). All these disorders involve repetitive thoughts or behaviors that individuals are unable to delay or inhibit without great difficulty. Evidence for this clustering includes observations of clinical improvement with SSRIs such as fluoxetine even in nondepressed individuals with hypochondriasis, body dysmorphic disorder, obsessive–compulsive disorder, and anorexia nervosa. Because such a response is not evident with non-SSRI antidepressants, some type of common serotonin dysregulation is suggested for these disorders.

Treatment

Until recently, it appeared that individuals with hypochondriasis as a primary condition benefited, but only modestly, from psychiatric intervention. Individuals referred early for psychiatric evaluation and treatment showed a slightly better prognosis than those continuing with only medical evaluations and treatments (Kellner 1983). Of course, the first step in treatment is getting the individual to a mental health clinician. Individuals with hypochondriasis generally present initially to nonpsychiatric physicians and are often reluctant to see a mental health clinician. Referral should be done sensitively, with the referring physician stressing to the individual that his or her distress is real and that psychiatric evaluation will be a supplement to, not a replacement for, continued medical care.

Initially, the generic techniques outlined for the somatoform disorders in general should be followed. However, it has not been demonstrated that a specific psychotherapy for hypochondriasis is available. As reviewed by Fallon and colleagues (1993), dynamic psychotherapy is of minimal effectiveness; supportive–educative psychotherapy as described by Kellner (1991) is only somewhat helpful, and primarily for those with syndromes of less than 3 years' duration; and cognitive–behavioral therapy, especially response prevention of checking rituals and reassurance seeking, is of only moderate effectiveness at best. All of these techniques seem to lack definitive effects on hypochondriasis itself.

Until recently, this could be said of pharmacological approaches also. Pharmacotherapy of comorbid depressive or anxiety syndromes was often effective, and control of such syndromes aided in general management, yet hypochondriasis itself was not ameliorated. Although controlled trials are lacking, anecdotal and open-label studies suggest that serotoninergic agents such as clomipramine and the SSRI fluoxetine may be effective in ameliorating hypochondriasis. Similar effects are expected from the other SSRIs. Response to fluoxetine has been reported with doses recommended for obsessive–compulsive disorder, rather than usual antidepressant doses (i.e., 60–80 mg rather than 20–40 mg/day). Such pharmacotherapy is best combined with the generic psychotherapy recommendations for somatoform disorders, as well as with cognitive–behavioral techniques to disrupt the counterproductive checking and reassurance-seeking behaviors.

BODY DYSMORPHIC DISORDER

Diagnosis

As defined in DSM-IV-TR, the essential feature of this disorder is preoccupation with an imagined defect in appearance or a markedly excessive concern with a minor anomaly (see DSM-IV-TR diagnostic criteria below). In body dysmorphic disorder, a person can be preoccupied with an imagined defect while she or he actually has some other anomaly and is not appearing normal. To exclude conditions with trivial or minor symptoms, the preoccupation must cause clinically significant distress or impairment. By definition, body dysmorphic disorder is not diagnosed if symptoms are limited to preoccupation with body weight, as in anorexia nervosa or bulimia nervosa, or to perceived inappropriateness of sex characteristics, as in gender identity disorder.

DSM-IV-TR Diagnostic Criteria

300.7 Body Dysmorphic Disorder

A. Preoccupation with an imagined defect in appearance. If a slight physical anomaly is present, the person's concern is markedly excessive.
B. The preoccupation causes clinically significant distress or impairment in social, occupational, or other important areas of functioning.
C. The preoccupation is not better accounted for by another mental disorder (e.g., dissatisfaction with body shape and size in anorexia nervosa).

Reprinted with permission from the Diagnostic and Statistical Manual of Mental Disorders, Fourth Edition, Text Revision. Copyright 2000 American Psychiatric Association.

According to De Leon and coworkers (1989), preoccupations most often involve the nose, ears, face, or sexual organs. Common complaints include a diversity of imagined flaws of the face or head, including defects in the hair (e.g., too much or too little), skin (e.g., blemishes), and shape or symmetry of the face or facial features (e.g., nose is too large and deformed). However, any body part may be the focus, including genitals, breasts, buttocks, extremities, shoulders, and even overall body size.

In terms of its relationship to the psychotic disorders, DSM-IV dropped the DSM-III-R exclusionary rule that body dysmorphic disorder not be diagnosed if the preoccupation was of delusional intensity (i.e., the individual totally lacked insight or the ability to consider the possibility that the concern was unjustified). This exclusion remains in ICD-10. As De Leon and colleagues (1989) pointed out, it is extremely difficult to determine whether a dysmorphic concern is delusional in that with body dysmorphic disorder, a continuum exists from clearly nondelusional preoccupations to unequivocal delusions such that defining a discrete boundary between the two ends of the spectrum would be artificial. Furthermore, some individuals seem to move back and forth along this continuum. Support for rejecting the exclusion is preliminary evidence that dysmorphic preoccupations may respond to the same pharmacotherapy (SSRIs), regardless of whether the concerns are delusional (Hollander et al. 1993). Perhaps as a reflection of the state of knowledge at this point, both body dysmorphic disorder and delusional disorder, somatic type, can be diagnosed on the basis of the same symptoms, in the same individual, at the same time. Thus, the definition of body dysmorphic disorder differs from hypochondriasis, which is not diagnosed if hypochondriacal concerns are determined to be delusional.

Epidemiology

Knowledge of such parameters is still incomplete. In general, individuals with body dysmorphic disorder first present to nonpsychiatric physicians such as plastic surgeons, dermatologists, and internists because of the nature of their complaints and are not seen psychiatrically until they are referred (De Leon et al. 1989). Many resist or refuse referral because they do not see their problem as psychiatric; thus, study of psychiatric clinic populations may underestimate the prevalence of the disorder. It has been estimated that 2% of individuals seeking corrective cosmetic surgery suffer from this disorder (Andreasen and Bardach 1977). Although women outnumber men in this population, it is not known whether this sex distribution holds true in the general population.

Course

Age at onset appears to peak in adolescence or early adulthood (Phillips 1991). Body dysmorphic disorder is generally a chronic condition, with a waxing and waning of intensity but rarely full remission (Phillips et al. 1993). In a lifetime, multiple preoccupations are typical; in one study, the average was four (Phillips et al. 1993). In some, the same preoccupation remains unchanged. In others, new perceived defects are added to the original ones. In still others, symptoms remit, only to be replaced by others. The disorder is often highly incapacitating, with many individuals showing marked impairment in social and occupational activities. Perhaps a third becomes housebound. Most attribute their limitations to embarrassment concerning their perceived defect, but the attention and time-consuming nature of the preoccupations and attempts to investigate and rectify defects also contribute. The extent to which individuals with body dysmorphic disorder receive surgery or medical treatments is unknown. Superimposed depressive episodes are common, as are suicidal ideation and suicide attempts. Actual suicide risk is unknown.

In view of the nature of the defects with which individuals are preoccupied, it is not surprising that they are found most commonly among individuals seeking cosmetic surgery. Preoccupations persist despite reassurance that there is no defect to surgically correct. Surgery or other corrective procedures rarely if ever lead to satisfaction and may even lead to greater distress with the perception of new defects attributed to the surgery.

Differential Diagnosis

The preoccupations of body dysmorphic disorder must first be differentiated from usual concerns with grooming and appearance. Attention to appearance and grooming is universal and socially sanctioned. However, diagnosis of body dysmorphic disorder requires that the preoccupation cause clinically significant distress or impairment. In addition, in body dysmorphic disorder, concerns focus on an imaginary or exaggerated defect, often of something, such as a small blemish, that would warrant scant attention even if it were present. Persons with histrionic personality disorder may be vain and excessively concerned with appearance. However, the focus in this disorder is on maintaining a good or even exceptional appearance, rather than preoccupation with a defect. Such concerns are probably unrelated to body dysmorphic disorder. In addition, by nature, the preoccupations in body dysmorphic disorder are essentially unamenable to reassurance from friends or family or consultation with physicians, cosmetologists, or other professionals.

Next, the possibility of an explanation by a general medical condition must be considered (see Figure 36-1). As mentioned, individuals with this disorder often first present to plastic surgeons, oral surgeons, and others, seeking correction of defects. By the time a mental health professional is consulted, it has generally been ascertained that there is no physical basis for the degree of concern. As with other syndromes involving somatic preoccupations (or delusions), such as olfactory reference syndrome and delusional parasitosis (both included under delusional disorder, somatic type), occult medical disorders, such as an endocrine disturbance or a brain tumor, must be excluded.

In terms of explanation on the basis of another mental disorder, there is little likelihood that symptoms of body dysmorphic disorder will be intentionally produced as in malingering or factitious disorder. Unlike in other somatoform disorders, such as pain, conversion, and somatization disorders, preoccupation with appearance predominates. Somatic preoccupations may occur as part of an anxiety or mood disorder. However, these preoccupations are generally not the predominant focus and lack the specificity of dysmorphic symptoms. Because individuals with body dysmorphic disorder often become isolative, social phobia may be suspected. However, in social phobia, the person may feel self-conscious generally but will not focus on a specific imagined defect. Indeed, the two conditions may coexist, warranting both diagnoses. Diagnostic problems may present with the mood-congruent ruminations of major depression, which sometimes involve concern with an unattractive appearance in association with poor self-esteem. Such preoccupations generally lack the focus on a particular body part that is seen in body dysmorphic disorder. On the other hand, individuals with body dysmorphic disorder commonly have dysphoric affects described by them variously as anxiety or depression. In some cases, these affects can be subsumed under body dysmorphic disorder; but in other instances, comorbid diagnoses of anxiety or mood disorders are warranted.

Differentiation from schizophrenia must also be made. At times, a dysmorphic concern will seem so unusual that such a psychosis may be considered. Furthermore, individuals with this disorder may show ideas of reference in regard to defects in their appearance, which may lead to the consideration of schizophrenia. However, other bizarre delusions, particularly of persecution or grandiosity, and prominent hallucinations are not seen in body dysmorphic disorder. From the other perspective, schizophrenia with somatic delusions generally lacks the focus on a particular body part and defect. Also in schizophrenia, bizarre interpretations and explanations for symptoms are often present, such as "this blemish was a sign from Jesus that I am to protect the world from Satan." Other signs of schizophrenia, such as hallucinations and disorganization of thought, are also absent in body dysmorphic disorder. As previously mentioned, the preoccupations in body dysmorphic disorder appear to be on a continuum from full insight to delusional intensity whereby the individual cannot even consider the possibility that the preoccupation is groundless. In such instances, both body dysmorphic disorder and delusional disorder, somatic type, are to be diagnosed.

Body dysmorphic disorder is not to be diagnosed if the concern with appearance is better accounted for by another mental disorder. Anorexia nervosa, in which there is dissatisfaction with body shape and size, is specifically mentioned in the criteria as an example of such an exclusion. DSM-III-R also mentioned transsexualism (gender identity disorder in DSM-IV-TR) as such a disorder. Although not specifically mentioned in DSM-IV-TR, if a preoccupation is limited to discomfort or a sense of inappropriateness of one's primary and secondary sex characteristics, coupled with a strong and persistent cross-gender identification, body dysmorphic disorder is not diagnosed.

The preoccupations of body dysmorphic disorder may resemble obsessions and ruminations as seen in obsessive–compulsive disorder. Unlike the obsessions of obsessive–compulsive disorder, the preoccupations of body dysmorphic disorder focus on concerns with appearance. Compulsions are limited to checking and investigating the perceived physical defect and attempting to obtain reassurance from others regarding it. Still, the phenomenology is similar, and the two disorders are often comorbid. If additional obsessions and compulsions not related to the defect are present, obsessive–compulsive disorder can be diagnosed in addition to body dysmorphic disorder.

Etiology

A number of sociological, psychological, and neurobiological theories have been proposed. Body dysmorphic disorder has been explained, at least in part, as an exaggerated incorporation of societal ideals of physical perfection and acceptance of cosmetic plastic surgery to attain such goals. A high frequency of insecure, sensitive, obsessional, schizoid, anxious, narcissistic, introverted, and hypochondriacal personality traits in body dysmorphic individuals have been described (Phillips 1991). Various psychodynamic mechanisms and symbolic meanings of dysmorphic symptoms have been suggested (Phillips 1991), going back to Freud's case of the Wolfman who had dysmorphic preoccupations regarding his nose.

Some interesting neurobiological possibilities have emerged, particularly concerning observations that hypochondriasis, body dysmorphic disorder, and a number of other conditions involving compelling repetitive thoughts or behaviors may respond preferentially to SSRIs, not to other antidepressant drugs. An obsessive–compulsive spectrum disorders grouping, the pathological process of which is mediated by serotoninergic dysregulation, has been suggested. As further evidence, symptoms of body dysmorphic disorder as well as those of obsessive–compulsive disorder may be aggravated by the partial serotonin agonist *m*-chlorophenylpiperazine (Hollander et al. 1992).

Treatment

First, the generic goals and treatments as outlined for the somatoform disorders overall should be instituted. These are beneficial in interrupting an unending procession of repeated evaluations and the possibility of needless surgery, which may lead to additional perceptions that surgery has resulted in further disfigurement.

Traditional insight-oriented therapies have not generally proved to be effective. Results with traditional behavioral techniques, such as systematic desensitization and exposure therapy, have been mixed. At least without amelioration with effective pharmacotherapy, the preoccupations do not extinguish as would be expected with phobias. A cognitive–behavioral approach similar to what was recommended for hypochondriasis may be more effective. This includes response prevention techniques whereby the individual is not permitted to repetitively check the perceived defect in mirrors. In addition, individuals are advised not to seek reassurance from family and friends, and these persons are instructed not to respond to such inquiries. Some individuals adopt such behaviors spontaneously, avoiding mirrors and other reflecting surfaces, refusing even to allude to their perceived defects to others. Such "self-techniques" may be encouraged and refined.

Biological treatments have long been used but until recently were of limited benefit to individuals with body dysmorphic disorder. Approaches have included electroconvulsive therapy, tricyclic and MAOI antidepressants, and neuroleptics (particularly pimozide) (Andreasen and Bardach 1977). In most reports of positive response to tricyclic or MAOI antidepressant drugs, it is unclear whether response was truly in terms of the dysmorphic syndrome or simply represented improvement in comorbid depressive or anxiety syndromes. Response to neuroleptic treatment has been suggested as a diagnostic test to distinguish body dysmorphic disorder from delusional disorder, somatic type (Riding and Munro 1975). The delusional syndromes often respond to neuroleptics; body dysmorphic disorders, even when the body preoccupations are psychotic, generally do not. Pimozide has been singled out as a neuroleptic with specific effectiveness for somatic delusions, but this specificity does not appear to apply to body dysmorphic disorder.

An exception to this uninspiring picture is the observation of a possible preferential response to antidepressant drugs with serotonin reuptake blocking effects, such as clomipramine, or SSRIs, such as fluoxetine and fluvoxamine (Hollander et al. 1992). Phillips and coworkers (1993) reported that more than 50% of individuals with body dysmorphic disorder showed a partial or complete remission with either clomipramine or fluoxetine, a response not predicted on the basis of coexisting major depressive or obsessive–compulsive disorder. As with hypochondriasis, effectiveness is generally achieved at levels recommended for obsessive–compulsive disorder rather than for depression (e.g., 60 to 80 mg rather than 20 to 40 mg/day of fluoxetine). The SSRIs appear to ameliorate delusional as well as nondelusional dysmorphic preoccupations. Successful augmentation of clomipramine or SSRI therapy has been suggested with buspirone, another drug with serotoninergic effects. Neuroleptics, particularly pimozide, may also be helpful adjuncts, particularly if delusions of reference are present. Little seems to be gained with the addition of anticonvulsants, or benzodiazepines to the SSRI therapy.

SOMATOFORM DISORDER NOT OTHERWISE SPECIFIED

Somatoform disorder NOS is the true residual category for this diagnostic class. By definition, disorders considered under this category are characterized by somatic symptoms, but criteria for any of the specific somatoform disorders are not met. Several examples are given, but syndromes potentially included under this category are not limited to these. Unlike for undifferentiated somatoform disorder, no minimal duration is required (see DSM-I-TR description of Somatoform Disorder NOS below). DSM-IV-TR lists as examples pseudocyesis, disorders involving hypochondriacal complaints but of less than 6 months' duration, and disorders involving unexplained physical complaints, such as fatigue or body weakness not due to another mental disorder and again of less than 6 months' duration. This last syndrome would seem to resemble neurasthenia of short duration, a syndrome with a long historical tradition with inclusion in DSM-II, ICD-9, and ICD-10. Neurasthenia was considered for inclusion as a separate DSM-IV somatoform disorder. Reasons that it was not included in DSM-IV include difficulties in delineating it from depressive and anxiety disorders and from other somatoform disorders. If included, neurasthenia could have become a clinical "wastebasket" that could facilitate premature closure of diagnostic inquiry, such that underlying general medical conditions as well as other mental disorders would more likely be overlooked.

DSM-IV-TR description

300.81 Somatoform Disorder Not Otherwise Specified

This category includes disorders with somatoform symptoms that do not meet criteria for any specific somatoform disorder. Examples include:

A. Pseudocyesis: a false belief of being pregnant that is associated with objective signs of pregnancy, which may include abdominal enlargement (although the umbilicus does not become everted), reduced menstrual flow, amenorrhea, subjective sensation of fetal movement, nausea, breast engorgement and secretions, and labor pains at the expected date of delivery. Endocrine changes may be present, but the syndrome cannot be explained by a general medical condition that causes endocrine changes (e.g., a hormone-secreting tumor).

B. A disorder involving nonpsychotic hypochondriacal symptoms of less than 6 months' duration.
C. A disorder involving unexplained physical symptoms (e.g., fatigue or body weakness) of less than 6 months' duration that are not due to another mental disorder.

Reprinted with permission from the Diagnostic and Statistical Manual of Mental Disorders, Fourth Edition, Text Revision. Copyright 2000 American Psychiatric Association.

Inclusion of pseudocyesis as an example of Somatoform Disorder NOS deserves special mention. This syndrome, not mentioned at all in DSM-II, was included in DSM-III and DSM-III-R as an example of a conversion symptom under the broadened definition of conversion, on the basis that it represented a somatic expression of a psychological conflict or need, in this case involving ambivalence toward pregnancy. The resulting conflict was resolved somatically as a false pregnancy, lessening anxiety (primary gain) and leading to unconsciously needed environmental support (secondary gain). With the restriction of conversion in DSM-IV to include only symptoms affecting voluntary motor and sensory function, pseudocyesis was excluded from the conversion disorder definition. In a sense, it is placed in the somatoform disorder NOS category for lack of a more appropriate place. Pseudocyesis is a reasonably discrete syndrome for which specific criteria as listed in DSM-IV-TR can be delineated. These criteria were derived from a review of the existing literature (Lipowski 1988). However, given its rarity, it is not listed as a specified somatoform disorder. Whelan and Stewart (1990) reported six cases in 20 years of consulting to a unit in which 2500 women delivered per year. It could also be described as a psychophysiological endocrine disorder. On the basis of a literature review (Lipowski 1988), in many cases, a neuroendocrine change accompanies and at times may antedate the false belief of pregnancy. This approaches inclusion as a medical condition, which would lend itself to consideration of psychological factors affecting medical condition. However, in most instances, a discrete general medical condition (such as a hormone-secreting tumor) cannot be identified.

Comparison of DSM-IV-TR/ICD-10 Diagnostic Criteria
The ICD-10 Diagnostic Criteria for Research for Somatization Disorder has both a different item set and algorithm. Six symptoms are required out of a list of 14 symptoms, which are broken down into the following groups: 6 gastrointestinal symptoms, 2 cardiovascular symptoms, 3 genitourinary symptoms, and 3 "skin and pain" symptoms. It is specified that the symptoms occur in at least two groups. In contrast, DSM-IV-TR requires 4 pain symptoms, 2 gastrointestinal symptoms, 1 sexual symptom and 1 pseudoneurological symptom. Furthermore, the ICD-10 Diagnostic Criteria for Research specify that there must be "persistent refusal to accept medical reassurance that there is no adequate physical cause for the physical symptoms." DSM-IV-TR only requires that the symptoms result in treatment being sought or significant impairment in social, occupational, or other important areas of functioning and that the symptoms cannot be fully explained by a known general medical condition or substance. For Undifferentiated Somatoform Disorder, the ICD-10 Diagnostic Criteria for Research and the DSM-IV-TR criteria are almost identical.

Regarding conversion disorder, ICD-10 considers conversion a type of dissociative disorder and includes separate criteria sets for dissociative motor disorders, dissociative convulsions, and dissociative anesthesia and sensory loss in a section that also includes dissociative amnesia and dissociative fugue.

For pain disorder, the ICD-10 Diagnostic Criteria for Research require that the pain last at least 6 months and that it not be "explained adequately by evidence of a physiological process or a physical disorder." In contrast, DSM-IV-TR does not force the clinician to make this inherently impossible judgment and instead requires the contribution of psychological factors. Furthermore, DSM-IV-TR includes both acute (duration less than 6 months) and chronic pain (more than 6 months). This disorder is referred to in ICD-10 as "Persistent Somatoform Pain Disorder."

ICD-10 provides a single criteria set that applies to both the DSM-IV-TR categories of hypochondriasis and body dysmorphic disorder. The ICD-10 Diagnostic Criteria for Research for Hypochondriasis specifies that the belief is of a "maximum of two serious physical diseases" and requires that at least one be specifically named by the individual with the disorder. The DSM-IV-TR has no such requirement.

References

Alexander F (1950) *Psychosomatic Medicine*. WW Norton, New York.

Alper K, Devinsky O, Vasquez B, et al. (1993) Nonepileptic seizures and childhood sexual and physical abuse. *Neurology* **43**, 1950–1953.

American Psychiatric Association (2000) *Diagnostic and Statistical Manual of Mental Disorders*, 4th ed., Text Rev. APA, Washington, DC.

Andreasen NC and Bardach J (1977) Dysmorphophobia: symptom or disease. *Am J Psychiatry* **134**, 673–676.

Barsky AJ and Klerman GL (1983) Overview: hypochondriasis, bodily complaints, and somatic styles. *Am J Psychiatry* **140**, 273–282.

Barsky AJ, Cleary PD, Sarnie MK, et al. (1993) The course of transient hypochondriasis. *Am J Psychiatry* **150**, 484–488.

Bendefeldt F, Miller LL, and Ludwig AM (1976) Cognitive hysteria. *Arch Gen Psychiatry* **33**, 1250–1254.

Bohman M, Cloninger CR, von Knorring A-L, et al. (1984) An adoption study of somatoform disorders III. Cross-fostering analysis and genetic relationship to alcoholism and criminality. *Arch Gen Psychiatry* **41**, 872–878.

Breuer J and Freud S (1955) Studies on hysteria. In *The Standard Edition of the Complete Psychological Works of Sigmund Freud*, Vol. 2, Strachey J (trans-ed). Hogarth Press, London. Originally published in 1893–1895.

Briquet P (1859) *Traité Clinique et Thérapeutique à l'Hystérie*. J-B Baillière & Fils, Paris.

Brophy JJ (1994) Monosymptomatic hypochondriacal psychosis treated with paroxetine: a case report. *Ir J Psychol Med* **11**, 21–22.

Carter AB (1949) The prognosis of certain hysterical symptoms. *Br Med J* **1**, 1076–1079.

Chaturvedi SK (1987) Prevalence of chronic pain in psychiatric patients. *Pain* **19**, 231–237.

Chodoff P and Lyons H (1958) Hysteria, the hysterical personality and "hysterical conversion". *Am J Psychiatry* **131**, 734–740.

Cloninger CR (1986) Somatoform and dissociative disorders. In *Medical Basis of Psychiatry*, Winokur G and Clayton PJ (eds). W. B. Saunders, Philadelphia, pp. 123–151.

Cloninger CR (1987) Diagnosis of somatoform disorders: a critique of DSM-III. In *Diagnosis and Classification in Psychiatry: A Critical Appraisal of DSM-III*, Tischler GL (ed). Cambridge University Press, New York, pp. 243–259.

Cloninger CR (1993) Somatoform and dissociative disorders. In *Medical Basis of Psychiatry*, 2nd ed., Winokur G and Clayton PJ (eds). W. B. Saunders, Philadelphia, pp. 169–192.

Cloninger CR (1996) Somatization disorder. In *DSM-IV Sourcebook*, Vol. 2, Widiger TA, Frances AJ, Pincus HA, et al. (eds). American Psychiatric Association, Washington, DC, pp. 885–892.

Cloninger CR and Guze SB (1979) Psychiatric illness and female criminality: the role of sociopathy and hysteria in the antisocial woman. *Am J Psychiatry* **127**, 303–311.

Cloninger CR, Martin RL, Guze SB, et al. (1986) A prospective follow-up and family study of somatization in men and women. *Am J Psychiatry* **143**, 873–878.

Cloninger CR, Reich T, and Guze SB (1975) The multifactorial model of disease transmission III. Familial relationship between sociopathy and hysteria (Briquet's syndrome). *Br J Psychiatry* **127**, 23–32.

Cloninger CR, Sigvardsson S, von Knorring A-L, et al. (1984) An adoption study of somatoform disorders II. Identification of two discrete somatoform disorders. *Arch Gen Psychiatry* **41**, 863–871.

Cloninger CR and Yutzy S (1993) Somatoform and dissociative disorders: a summary of changes for DSM-IV. In *Current Psychiatric Therapy*, Dunner DL (ed). W. B. Saunders, Philadelphia, pp. 310–313.

Coryell W and House D (1984) The validity of broadly defined hysteria and DSM-III conversion disorder: outcome, family history, and mortality. *J Clin Psychiatry* **45**, 252–256.

Cote G, O'Leary T, Barlow DH, et al. (1996) Hypochondriasis. In *DSM-IV Sourcebook*, Vol. 2, Widiger TA, Frances AJ, Pincus HA, et al. (eds). American Psychiatric Association, Washington, DC, pp. 933–948.

De Leon J, Bott A, and Simpson G (1989) Dysmorphophobia: body dysmorphic disorder or delusional disorder, somatic subtype. *Compr Psychiatry* **30**, 457–472.

Delaplaine R, Ifabumuyi OI, Merskey H, et al. (1978) Significance of pain in psychiatric hospital patients. *Pain* **4**, 143–152.

Desai BT, Porter RJ, and Penry K (1982) Psychogenic seizures. A study of 42 attacks in six patients, with intensive monitoring. *Arch Neurol* **39**, 202–209.

DeSouza C, Othmer E, Gabrielli W, et al. (1988) Major depression and somatization disorder: the overlooked differential diagnosis. *Psychiatr Ann* **18**, 340–348.

Escobar JI, Rubio-Stipec M, Canino G, et al. (1989) Somatic Symptom Index (SSI): a new and abridged somatization construct: prevalence and epidemiological correlates in two large community samples. *J Nerv Ment Dis* **177**, 140–146.

Escobar JI, Swartz M, Rubio-Stipec M, et al. (1991) Medically unexplained symptoms: distribution, risk factors, and comorbidity. In *Current Concepts of Somatization: Research and Clinical Perspectives*, Kirmayer LJ and Robbins JM (eds). American Psychiatric Press, Washington, DC, pp. 63–68.

Fallon BA, Klein BW, and Liebowitz MR (1993) Hypochondriasis: treatment strategies. *Psychiatr Ann* **23**, 374–381.

Feighner JP, Robins E, Guze SB, et al. (1972) Diagnostic criteria for use in psychiatric research. *Arch Gen Psychiatry* **26**, 57–63.

Flor-Henry P, Fromm-Auch D, Tapper M, et al. (1981) A neuropsychological study of the stable syndrome of hysteria. *Biol Psychiatry* **16**, 601–626.

Folks DG, Ford CV, and Regan WM (1984) Conversion symptoms in a general hospital. *Psychosomatics* **25**, 285–295.

Ford CV (1983) *The Somatizing Disorders: Illness as a Way of Life.* Elsevier Scientific, New York.

Ford CV (1995) Conversion disorder and somatoform disorder not otherwise specified. In *Treatments of Psychiatric Disorders*, Vol. 2, 2nd ed., Gabbard GO (ed). American Psychiatric Association, Washington, DC, pp. 1735–1753.

Ford CV and Folks DG (1985) Conversion disorders: an overview. *Psychosomatics* **26**, 371–383.

Fukuda K, Straus SE, Hickie I, et al. (1994) The chronic fatigue syndrome: a comprehensive approach to its definition and study. *Ann Intern Med* **121**, 953–959.

Gatfield PD and Guze SB (1962) Prognosis and differential diagnosis of conversion reactions (a follow-up study). *Dis Nerv Syst* **23**, 1–8.

Goodwin DW and Guze SB (1989) *Psychiatric Diagnosis*, 4th ed. Oxford University Press, New York.

Guze SB, Cloninger CR, Martin RL, et al. (1986) A follow-up and family study of Briquet's syndrome. *Br J Psychiatry* **149**, 17–23.

Guze SB, Cloninger CR, Martin RL, et al. (1986) A follow-up and family study of Briquet's syndrome. *Br J Psychiatry* **149**, 17–23.

Guze SB and Perley MJ (1963) Observations on the natural history of hysteria. *Am J Psychiatry* **19**, 960–965.

Hollender E (1993) Obsessive–compulsive spectrum disorders: an overview. *Psychiatr Ann* **23**, 355–358.

Hollander E, Cohen LJ, and Simeon D (1993) Body dysmorphic disorder. *Psychiatr Ann* **23**, 359–364.

Hollander E, DeCaria CM, Nitescu A, et al. (1992) Serotonergic function in obsessive–compulsive disorder. Behavioral and neuroendocrine responses to oral *m*-chlorophenylpiperazine and fenfluramine in patients and healthy volunteers. *Arch Gen Psychiatry* **49**, 21–28.

Inouye E (1972) Genetic aspects of neurosis. *Int J Ment Health* **1**, 176–189.

Kellner R (1983) The prognosis of treated hypochondriasis: a clinical study. *Acta Psychiatr Scand* **67**, 69–79.

Kellner R (1985) Functional somatic symptoms and hypochondriasis. A survey of empirical studies. *Arch Gen Psychiatry* **42**, 821–832.

Kellner R (1990) Somatization: theories and research. *J Nerv Ment Dis* **178**, 150–160.

Kellner R (1991) *Psychosomatic Syndromes and Somatic Symptoms.* American Psychiatric Press, Washington, DC.

Kent D, Tomasson K, and Coryell W (1995) Course and outcome of conversion and somatization disorders: a four-year follow-up. *Psychosomatics* **36**, 138–144.

Kenyon FE (1965) Hypochondriasis: a survey of some historical, clinical, and social aspects. *Br J Psychiatry* **138**, 117–133.

King SA (1994) Pain disorders. In *The American Psychiatric Press Textbook of Psychiatry*, 2nd ed., Hales RE, Yudofsky SC, and Talbott JA (eds). American Psychiatric Press, Washington, DC, pp. 591–622.

Kirmayer LJ and Robbins JM (1991) Introduction: concepts of somatization. In *Current Concepts of Somatization: Research and Clinical Perspectives*, Kirmayer LJ and Robbins JM (eds). American Psychiatric Press, Washington, DC, pp. 1–19.

Kirmayer LJ, Robbins JM, Dworkin M, et al. (1993) Somatization and the recognition of depression and anxiety in primary care. *Am J Psychiatry* **150**, 734–741.

Lader M and Sartorious N (1968) Anxiety in patients with hysterical conversion symptoms. *J Neurol Neurosurg Psychiatry* **31**, 490–495.

Lazare A (1981) Conversion symptoms. *N Engl J Med* **305**, 745–748.

Leavitt F and Sweet JJ (1986) Characteristics and frequency of malingering among patients with low back pain. *Pain* **25**, 357–374.

Lewis WC (1974) Hysteria: the consultant's dilemma: 20th century demonology, pejorative epithet, or useful diagnosis. *Arch Gen Psychiatry* **30**, 145–151.

Lewis WC and Berman M (1965) Studies of conversion hysteria. I. Operational study of diagnosis. *Arch Gen Psychiatry* **13**, 275–282.

Lipowski ZJ (1988) Somatization: the concept and its clinical application. *Am J Psychiatry* **145**, 1358–1368.

Ljunberg L (1957) Hysteria: clinical, prognostic and genetic study. *Acta Psychiatr Scand* **32**(Suppl.),, 1–162.

Ludwig AM (1972) Hysteria. A neurobiological theory. *Arch Gen Psychiatry* **27**, 771–777.

Luff MC and Garrod M (1935) The after-results of psychotherapy in 500 adult cases. *Br Med J* **2**, 54–59.

Maloney MJ (1980) Diagnosing hysterical conversion disorders in children. *J Pediatr* **97**, 1016–1020.

Malt UF (1991) Somatization: an old disorder in new bottles. *Psychiatr Fenn* **22**, 1–13.

Marsden CD (1986) Hysteria—a neurologist's view. *Psychol Med* **16**, 277–288.

Martin RL (1988) Problems in the diagnosis of somatization disorder: effects on research and clinical practice. *Psychiatr Ann* **18**, 357–362.

Martin RL (1995) DSM-IV changes for the somatoform disorders. *Psychiatr Ann* **25**, 29–39.

Martin RL (1996) Conversion disorder, proposed autonomic arousal disorder, and pseudocyesis. In *DSM-IV Sourcebook*, Vol. 2, Widiger TA, Frances AJ, Pincus HA, et al. (eds). American Psychiatric Association, Washington, DC, pp. 893–914.

Martin RL, Cloninger CR, and Guze SB (1979) The evaluation of diagnostic concordance in follow-up studies, II: A blind prospective follow-up of female criminals. *J Psychiatr Res* **15**, 107–125.

Martin RL, Cloninger CR, Guze SB, et al. (1985) Mortality in a follow-up of 500 psychiatric outpatients. *Arch Gen Psychiatry* **42**, 58–66.

Martin RL and Yutzy SH (1994) Somatoform disorders. In *The American Psychiatric Press Textbook of Psychiatry*, 2nd ed., Hales RE, Yudofsky SC, and Talbott JA (eds). American Psychiatric Press, Washington, DC, pp. 591–622.

Mears R and Horvath TB (1972) "Acute" and "chronic" hysteria. *Br J Psychiatry* **121**, 653–657.

Melzack R and Wall PD (1983) *The Challenge of Pain*. Basic Books, New York.

Murphy GE (1982) The clinical management of hysteria. *JAMA* **247**, 2559–2564.

Nandi DN, Banerjee G, Nandi S, et al. (1992) Is hysteria on the wane? A community survey in West Bengal, India. *Br J Psychiatry* **160**, 87–91.

Ormel J, VonKorff M, Ustun B, et al. (1994) Common mental disorders and disability across cultures: results from the WHO collaborative study on psychological problems in general health care. *JAMA* **272**, 1741–1748.

Osterweis M, Kleinman A, Mechanic D (eds) (1987) *Pain and Disability*. National Academy Press, Washington, DC.

Perkin GD (1989) An analysis of 7836 successive new outpatient referrals. *J Neurol Neurosurg Psychiatry* **52**, 447–448.

Perley M and Guze SB (1962) Hysteria: the stability and usefulness of clinical criteria. A quantitative study based upon a 6–8 year follow-up of 39 patients. *N Engl J Med* **266**, 421–426.

Phillips KA (1991) Body dysmorphic disorder: the distress of imagined ugliness. *Am J Psychiatry* **148**, 1138–1149.

Phillips KA, McElroy S, Keck PE, et al. (1993) Body dysmorphic disorder: 30 cases of imagined ugliness. *Am J Psychiatry* **150**, 302–308.

Pincus J (1982) Hysteria presenting to a neurologist. In *Hysteria*, Roy A (ed). John Wiley, Chichester, UK, pp. 131–144.

Porter J and Jick H (1980) Addiction rare in patients treated with narcotics [letter]. *N Engl J Med* **302**, 303.

Preskorn SH (1995) Beyond DSM-IV: what is the cart and what is the horse. *Psychiatr Ann* **25**, 53–62.

Pribor EF, Smith DS, and Yutzy SH (1994) Somatization disorder in elderly patients. *Am J Geriatr Psychiatry* **2**, 109–117.

Purtell JJ, Robins E, and Cohen ME (1951) Observations on clinical aspects of hysteria. A quantitative study of 50 hysteria patients and 156 control subjects. *JAMA* **146**, 902–909.

Quill TE (1985) Somatization disorder. One of medicine's blind spots. *JAMA* **254**, 3075–3079.

Raskin M, Talbott JA, and Meyerson AT (1966) Diagnosis of conversion reactions: predictive value of psychiatric criteria. *JAMA* **197**, 530–534.

Riding J and Munro A (1975) Pimozide in the treatment of monosymptomatic hypochondriacal psychosis. *Acta Psychiatr Scand* **52**, 23–30.

Robins LN, Helzer JE, Weissman MM, et al. (1984) Lifetime prevalence of specific psychiatric disorders in three sites. *Arch Gen Psychiatry* **41**, 949–958.

Robins E and O'Neal P (1953) Clinical features of hysteria in children. *Nerv Child* **10**, 246–271.

Scallet A, Cloninger CR, and Othmer E (1976) The management of chronic hysteria: a review and double-blind trial of electrosleep and other relaxation methods. *Dis Nerv Syst* **37**, 347–353.

Scott J and Huskisson EC (1976) Graphic representation of pain. *Pain* **2**, 175–184.

Slater ETO and Glithero C (1965) A follow-up of patients diagnosed as suffering from "hysteria". *J Psychosom Res* **9**, 9–13.

Smith GR Jr., Monson RA, and Ray DC (1986) Psychiatric consultation in somatization disorder. A randomized controlled study. *N Engl J Med* **314**, 1407–1413.

Spitzer RL, Williams JBW, Kroenke K, et al. (1994) Utility of a new procedure for diagnosing mental disorders in primary care: the PRIME-MD 1000 Study. *JAMA* **272**, 1749–1756.

Stafanis C, Markidis M, and Christodoulou G (1976) Observations on the evolution of the hysterical symptomatology. *Br J Psychiatry* **128**, 269–275.

Steckel W, Paul E, and Paul C (trans) (1943) *The Interpretation of Dreams: New Developments and Technique*. Liveright, New York.

Stefansson JH, Messina JA, and Meyerowitz S (1976) Hysterical neurosis, conversion type: clinical and epidemiological considerations. *Acta Psychiatr Scand* **59**, 119–138.

Stephens JH and Kamp M (1962) On some aspects of hysteria: a clinical study. *J Nerv Ment Dis* **13**, 275–282.

Stoudemire GA (1988) Somatoform disorders, factitious disorders, and malingering. In *Textbook of Psychiatry*, Talbott JA, Hales RE, and Yudofsky SC (eds). American Psychiatric Press, Washington, DC, pp. 533–556.

Stoudemire A and Sandhu J (1987) Psychogenic/idiopathic pain syndromes. *Gen Hosp Psychiatr* **9**, 79–86.

Tomasson K, Kent D, and Coryell W (1991) Somatization and conversion disorders: comorbidity and demographics at presentation. *Acta Psychiatr Scand* **84**, 288–293.

Toone BK (1990) Disorders of hysterical conversion. In *Physical Symptoms and Psychological Illness*, Bass C (ed). Blackwell Scientific Publications, London, pp. 207–234.

Veith I (1965) *Hysteria: The History of a Disease*. University of Chicago Press, Chicago.

Viederman M (1985) Somatoform and factitious disorders. In *Psychiatry*, Vol. 1, Cavenar JO (ed). JB Lippincott, Philadelphia, pp. 1–20.

von Knorring L and Attkisson CC (1979) Endorphins in CSF of chronic pain patients, in relation to augmenting–reducing response in visual averaged evoked response. *Neuropsychobiology* **5**, 322–326.

Watson CG and Buranen C (1979) The frequency and identification of false positive conversion reactions. *J Nerv Ment Dis* **167**, 243–247.

Weddington WW (1979) Conversion reaction in an 82-year-old man. *J Nerv Ment Dis* **167**, 368–369.

Weinstein EA, Eck RA, and Lyerly OG (1969) Conversion hysteria in Appalachia. *Psychiatry* **32**, 334–341.

Wetzel RD, Guze SB, Cloninger CR, et al. (1994) Briquet's syndrome (hysteria) is both a somatoform and a "psychoform" illness: an MMPI study. *Psychosom Med* **56**, 564–569.

Wheatley D (1962) Evaluation of psychotherapeutic drugs in general practice. *Psychopharmacol Bull* **2**, 25–32.

Whelan CI and Stewart DE (1990) Pseudocyesis—a review and report of six cases. *Int J Psychiatr* **20**, 97–108.

Yutzy SH, Pribor EF, Cloninger CR, et al. (1992) Reconsidering the criteria for somatization disorder. *Hosp Comm Psychiatr* **43**, 1075–1076. 1149.

Ziegler FJ, Imboden JB, and Meyer E (1960) Contemporary conversion reactions: a clinical study. *Am J Psychiatry* **116**, 901–910.

Ziegler DK and Paul N (1954) On the natural history of hysteria in women. *Dis Nerv Syst* **15**, 3–8.

37 Factitious Disorders

Diagnosis

An individual with a factitious disorder consciously induces or feigns illness in order to obtain a psychological benefit by being in the sick role. It is the conscious awareness of the production of symptoms that differentiates factitious disorder from the somatoform disorders in which the individual unconsciously produces symptoms for an unconscious psychological benefit. It is the underlying motivation to produce symptoms that separates factitious disorders from malingering. Individuals who malinger consciously feign or induce illness in order to obtain some external benefit such as money, narcotics, or excuse from duties. While the distinctions among these disorders appear satisfyingly clear, in practice, individuals often blur the boundaries. Individuals with somatoform disorders will sometimes consciously exaggerate symptoms that they have unconsciously produced, and it is a rare individual who consciously creates illness and yet receives no external gain at all, be it disability benefits, excuse from work, or even food and shelter.

Talcott Parsons described the "sick role" in 1951 and noted that in our society there are four aspects of this role. First, the individual is not able to will himself or herself back to health but instead must "be taken care of." Second, the individual in the sick role must regard the sickness as undesirable and want to get better. Third, the sick individual is obliged to seek medical care and cooperate with his or her medical treatment. Finally, the sick individual is exempted from the normal responsibilities of his or her social role (Parsons 1951).

Individuals with factitious disorders seek, often desperately, the sick role. They usually have little insight into the motivations of their behaviors but are still powerfully driven to appear ill to others. In many cases, they endanger their own health and life in search of this role. Individuals with this disorder will often induce serious illness or undergo numerous unnecessary, invasive procedures. As most people avoid sickness, the actions of these individuals appear to run counter to human nature. Also, since entry into the "sick role" requires that the sick person should try to get better, individuals with factitious disorders must conceal the voluntary origin of their symptoms. The inexplicability of their actions combined with their deceptive behavior stir up both intense interest and intense (usually negative) countertransference in health care providers.

While physicians have known about the feigning of illness since the time of ancient Greece (Feldman 2000), it is likely that Richard Asher's 1951 article in *Lancet* brought the concept of factitious illness into general medical knowledge. Asher coined the term *Munchausen's syndrome* referring to the Baron von Munchausen, a character in German literature who was known for greatly exaggerating the tales of his exploits. (The use of this term may be somewhat unfair to the baron. Apparently, Rudolf Raspe, his unauthorized biographer, may have greatly overstated both the Baron's exploits and his tendency to exaggerate (Guziec et al. 1994)). Asher described Munchausen's syndrome as a severe, chronic factitious disorder combined with antisocial behavior including wandering from hospital to hospital (peregrination). However, his memorable term has often been used interchangeably with "factitious disorder" and incorrectly applied to individuals with less severe forms of the disease.

Individuals have been known to create or feign numerous illnesses, both acute and chronic, in all of the medical specialties. These illnesses can be either physical or psychological. It appears that the only limit is the creativity and knowledge of a given individual. In fact, there is at least one case report of an individual who feigned factitious disorder itself (Gurwith and Langston 1980). The individual claimed to have Munchausen's syndrome and to have undergone numerous unnecessary procedures and operations, and, as a result, claimed that he required immediate hospitalization. He displayed his abdomen, which appeared to have numerous surgical scars and hinted that searches of his hospital room would be fruitful. However, collateral information revealed that the physicians and hospitals he had reported had never treated the individual, and his "scars" washed off with soap and water. Individuals with a factitious disorder are often quite medically sophisticated. Even though acquired immune deficiency syndrome was not described until the early 1980s, the first factitious cases followed shortly thereafter, at least as early as 1986 (Miller et al. 1986).

For a diagnosis of factitious disorder (see DSM-IV-TR diagnostic criteria below) to be justified, a person must be intentionally producing an illness; his or her motivation is to occupy the sick role, and there must not be external incentives for the behavior. The diagnosis is further subclassified, depending on whether the factitious symptoms are predominantly physical, psychological, or a combination of both. The DSM also includes a category for individuals with factitious symptoms who do not meet the listed criteria. The most common example of factitious disorder not otherwise specified is factitious disorder by proxy (see page 1020), in which the individual creates symptoms in another person, usually a dependent, in order to occupy the sick role. Individuals who readily admit to inducing symptoms, such as self-mutilating individuals, are not diagnosed with factitious disorder as they are not using their symptoms to occupy the sick role.

DSM-IV-TR Diagnostic Criteria

Factitious Disorder

A. Intentional production or feigning of physical or psychological signs or symptoms.
B. The motivation for the behavior is to assume the sick role.
C. External incentives for the behavior (such as economic gain, avoiding legal responsibility, or improving physical well-being, as in malingering) are absent.

Code based on type

300.16 With Predominantly Psychological Signs and Symptoms: if psychological signs and symptoms predominate in the clinical presentation

300.19 With Predominantly Physical Signs and Symptoms: if physical signs and symptoms predominate in the clinical presentation

> **300.19 With Combined Psychological and Physical Signs and Symptoms:** if both psychological and physical signs and symptoms are present and neither predominates in the clinical presentation.

Reprinted with permission from the Diagnostic and Statistical Manual of Mental Disorders, Fourth Edition, Text Revision. Copyright 2000 American Psychiatric Association.

Individuals with Factitious Disorder with Predominantly Physical Signs and Symptoms present with physical signs and symptoms. The three main methods that individuals use to create illness are (1) giving a false history, (2) faking clinical and laboratory findings, and (3) inducing illness (e.g., by surreptitious medication use, inducing infection, or preventing wound healing) (Eisendrath 1994). There are reports of factitious illnesses in all of the medical specialties. Particularly common presentations include fever, self-induced infection, gastrointestinal symptoms, impaired wound healing, cancer, renal disease (especially hematuria and nephrolithiasis), endocrine diseases, anemia, bleeding disorders, and epilepsy (Wise and Ford 1999). True Munchausen's syndrome fits within this subclass and is the most severe form of the illness. According to the DSM-IV-TR, individuals with Munchausen's syndrome have a chronic factitious disorder with physical signs and symptoms, and in addition, have a history of recurrent hospitalization, peregrination, and *pseudologia fantastica*—dramatic, untrue, and extremely improbable tales of their past experiences (American Psychiatric Association 2000).

Another subtype of factitious disorder includes individuals who present feigning psychological illness. They both report and mimic psychiatric symptoms. These individuals can be particularly difficult to diagnose as psychiatric diagnosis depends greatly on the individual's report. There are reports of factitious psychosis, posttraumatic stress disorder, and bereavement (Pope et al. 1982, Sparr and Pankratz 1983, Snowdon et al. 1978). In addition, there are reports of psychological distress due to false claims of being a victim of stalking, rape, or sexual harassment (Pathe et al. 1999, Feldman et al. 1994, Feldman-Schorrig 1996), and these cases are often diagnosed with a factitious psychological disorder such as posttraumatic stress disorder. While individuals with factitious psychological symptoms feign psychiatric illness, they also often suffer from true comorbid psychiatric disorders, particularly Axis II disorders and substance abuse (Pope et al. 1982, Popli et al. 1992). Case reports suggest that individuals with psychological factitious disorder have a high rate of suicide and a poor prognosis (Eisendrath 2001, Pope et al. 1982, Popli et al. 1992). While Munchausen's syndrome is considered a subset of physical factitious disorder, there are case reports of individuals presenting with psychological symptoms who also have some of the key features of Munchausen's (pathological lying, wandering, and recurrent hospitalizations) (Merrin et al. 1986, Popli et al. 1992).

DSM-III separated factitious disorder into two disorders, based on whether the symptoms were physical or psychological. However, case reports clarified that this distinction was often artificial (Merrin et al. 1986, Parker 1993). Some individuals present with simultaneous psychological and physical factitious symptoms, and some individuals move between physical and psychological presentations over time. For example, an individual who presented with a factitious posttraumatic stress disorder, when confronted about the nature of his symptoms, began complaining of physical symptoms. DSM-IV was revised to account for individuals who present with both psychological signs and symptoms, adding a subtype for Combined Psychological and Physical Signs and Symptoms, though this category of individuals is the least studied.

Numerous reports (Carney and Brown 1983, Reich and Gottfried 1983, Wise and Ford 1999) in the literature describe two different subclasses of factitious individuals. The first type fits with the classic Munchausen's syndrome diagnosis: they have chronic factitious symptoms associated with antisocial traits, pathological lying, minimal social supports, wandering from hospital to hospital, and very poor work and relationship functioning. They are often very familiar with hospital procedure and use this knowledge to present dramatically during off-hours or at house-officer transition times when the factitious nature of their symptoms is least likely to be discovered. Males comprise the majority of these cases. Individuals with Munchausen's syndrome appear to have an extremely poor prognosis (Eisendrath 2001, Carney and Brown 1983). Fortunately, this most severe class of individuals makes up the minority of factitious individuals, probably fewer than 10%.

The second, and more typical, type of individual does not display pathological lying or wandering. Their recurrent presentations are usually within the same community, and they become well-known within the local health care system. They often have stable social supports and employment, and a history of a medically related job. This larger class of factitious individuals is mostly made up of women, and is more likely to accept psychiatric treatment and to show improvement. Plassmann (1994a) reviewed 1070 cases of individuals with factitious, but not Munchausen's disorder. He found that 78% of the individuals were women and 58% had a medically related job. Finally, there are individuals who may have an episode of factitious disorder in reaction to a life stressor, but may return to premorbid functioning after the stressor is resolved (Goldstein 1998).

All types of factitious disease show a strong association with substance abuse (Kent 1994), as well as borderline and narcissistic personality disorders. In a case series by Ehlers and Plassmann (1994), 9 of 18 individuals had personality features that met criteria for borderline personality disorder, and another 6 of 18 had personality features that met criteria for narcissistic personality disorder. Factitious individuals span a broad age range. Reports in the literature show individuals ranging from 4 to 85 years (Croft and Jervis 1989, Davis and Small 1985). Of note, a 4-year-old child with factitious disorder reported that he had been coached by his mother and may be better diagnosed as a victim of factitious disorder by proxy (Croft and Jervis 1989). The next youngest case found was 8 years old (Absolut de la Gastine et al. 1998, Libow 2000). Ethnicity is frequently not reported in case studies and series, so it is difficult to determine if there are any ethnic differences in the prevalence or presentation of factitious disorder.

The diagnosis of factitious disorder is made in several ways (see Figure 37-1). Factitious disorder is occasionally diagnosed accidentally when the individual is discovered in the act of creating symptoms. A history of inconsistent or unexplainable signs and symptoms or failure to respond to appropriate treatment can prompt health care providers to probe for evidence of the disorder, as can evidence of peregrination or pathological lying. In some cases, it is a diagnosis of exclusion in an otherwise inexplicable case.

If there is suspicion of a factitious disorder, confirmation can be difficult. Laboratory examination can confirm some factitious diagnoses such as exogenous insulin or thyroid hormone administration. Collateral information from family members or previous health care providers can also be extremely helpful. Factitious disorder with psychological signs and symptoms can be particularly difficult to diagnose, as so much of psychiatric diagnosis relies on the individual's report. However, there is some evidence that neuropsychological testing may be helpful in making the diagnosis. Both McCaffrey and Bellamy-Campbell (1989) and Fairbank and colleagues (1985) report the ability to detect over 90% of cases of factitious posttraumatic stress disorder using the MMPI. However, Perconte (Perconte and Goreczny 1990) was unsuccessful in attempting to replicate the findings. In addition, there is a report of MMPI test results being used to support a diagnosis of factitious disorder with psychological features in a woman thought to be feigning symptoms of multiple personality disorder (Coons 1993).

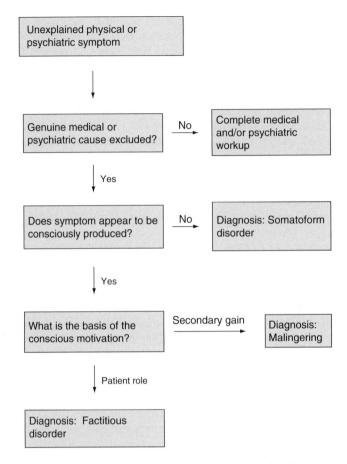

Figure 37-1 *Diagnostic decision tree for factitious disorder.*

The course of untreated factitious disorder is variable. While individuals with factitious disorder commonly suffer a great deal of morbidity, fatal cases appear to be less common. One survey of 41 cases noted only one fatality, though many of the other cases were life-threatening (Reich and Gottfried 1983). However, individuals with psychological signs and symptoms are reported to have a high rate of suicide and a poor prognosis (Pope et al. 1982, Popli et al. 1992).

In factitious disorder by proxy, one person creates or feigns illness in another person, usually a child, though occasionally the victim is an elder or developmentally delayed adult (see DSM-IV-TR Research Criteria on page 1021). The veterinary literature even reports cases of factitious disorder by proxy in which the victim is a pet (Munro and Thrusfield 2001). Factitious disorder by proxy is not defined as a specific disorder in DSM-IV-TR, but instead is listed under the "not otherwise specified" heading with research criteria included. While rare instances of fathers perpetrating factitious disorder by proxy have been reported (Meadow 1998), the perpetrator is usually the mother (Rosenberg 1987). Usually, the victim is a preverbal child (McClure et al. 1996). While numerous symptoms have been reported, common presentations include apnea, seizures, and gastrointestinal problems. The mothers appear extremely caring and attentive when observed, but appear indifferent to the child when they are not aware of being observed (Eisendrath 2001).

DSM-IV-TR Research Criteria

Factitious Disorder by Proxy

A. Intentional production of or feigning of physical or psychological signs or symptoms in another person who is under the individual's care.
B. The motivation for the perpetrator's behavior is to assume the sick role by proxy.
C. External incentives for the behavior (such as economic gain) are absent.
D. The behavior is no better accounted for by another mental disorder.

Reprinted with permission from the Diagnostic and Statistical Manual of Mental Disorders, Fourth Edition, Text Revision. Copyright 2000 American Psychiatric Association.

The diagnosis of factitious disorder by proxy is usually made by having an index of suspicion in a child with unexplained illnesses. The diagnosis is supported if symptoms occur only in the parent's presence and resolve with separation. Covert video surveillance has been used to diagnose this condition, though it raises questions of invasion of privacy. In general, it has been felt that the welfare of the child overrides the parent's right to privacy.

As counterintuitive as it is to comprehend why anyone would induce illness in oneself, it can be even more difficult to understand inducing illness in one's own child. The perpetrator in factitious disorder by proxy appears to seek not the "sick role" but the "parent to the sick child" role. This role is similar to the sick role in that it provides structure, attention from others, caring, and relief from usual responsibilities. The parent also receives some psychological benefit from inducing illness in his or her child. On the basis of case reports, the parent often has a comorbid personality disorder and a history of family dysfunction (Bools et al. 1994).

Epidemiology

The nature of factitious disorder makes it difficult to determine how common it is within the population. Individuals attempt to conceal themselves, thereby artificially lowering the prevalence. The tendency of individuals to present themselves several times at different facilities, however, may artificially raise the prevalence. Most estimates of the prevalence of the disease, therefore, rely on the number of factitious individuals within a given inpatient population. Such attempts have generated estimates that 0.5 to 3% of medical and psychiatric inpatients suffer from factitious disorder. Of 1288 individuals referred for psychiatric consultation at a Toronto general hospital, 10 (0.8%) were diagnosed with factitious disorder. A prospective examination of all 1538 individuals hospitalized in a Berlin neurology department over 5 years found five (0.3%) cases of factitious disorder (Bauer and Boegner 1996). An examination of 506 individuals with fever of unknown origin (FUO) revealed that 2.2% of the fevers were of factitious origin (Rumans and Vosti 1978), and a review of 199 Belgian individuals with FUO found 7 out of 199 (3.5%) to be factitious (Knockaert et al. 1992). A similar study of individuals with FUO at the National Institutes of Health (NIH) revealed that 9.3% of the fevers were factitious (Aduan et al. 1979). The increased prevalence found at the NIH may be due to the fact that the study was undertaken in a more tertiary setting, and it is a reminder that the prevalence of factitious disorder likely varies widely depending on the population and the setting. Gault and colleagues (1988) examined 3300 renal stones brought in by individuals and found that 2.6% of these stones were mineral and felt to be submitted by factitious or malingering individuals. There is much less data on the prevalence of factitious disorder with psychological features. A study of psychiatric inpatients showed a prevalence of 0.5% of admissions determined to be the result of a factitious psychological condition (Bhugra 1988). There are few data about the prevalence of factitious disorder in an outpatient population. Because factitious individuals do not readily identify themselves in large community surveys, it is not currently possible to determine the prevalence of the disorder in the general population.

As in factitious disorder, the exact prevalence of factitious disorder by proxy is unknown. There have been studies of the annual incidence of factitious disorder by proxy in the general population in both the UK and New Zealand. In New Zealand, the annual incidence of factitious disorder by proxy in children less than 16 years was found to be 2.0/100,000 (18 total cases) (Denny et al. 2001). In the United Kingdom, the annual incidence in children under 16 was 0.5/100,000 (128 total cases) (McClure et al. 1996). As for the incidence within clinical populations, an Argentinean survey of 113 children with FUO found four (3.5%) cases of factitious fever (Chantada et al. 1994). A survey of 20,090 children brought in with apnea found 54 (0.27%) to be victims of factitious disorder by proxy (Kravitz and Wilmott 1990). Finally, a review of children brought in for the treatment of acute, life-threatening episodes of diverse etiologies ranging from seizure disorders to electrolyte abnormalities found 1.5% to be factitious (Rahilly 1991). Factitious disorder by proxy appears to have a much higher mortality rate than self-inflicted factitious disorder. In Rosenberg's survey of 117 victims, there was a 9% mortality rate (Rosenberg 1987), and of the 54 victims of the disorder in the apnea survey, 3 index cases and 5 siblings were dead at the follow-up (Kravitz and Wilmott 1990). More recently, McClure found that 8 of 128 index cases in the United Kingdom were fatal (6.25%) (McClure et al. 1996) while Denny reported no fatalities in 18 index cases (Denny et al. 2001).

Differential Diagnosis
The differential diagnosis of factitious disorder includes rare or complex physical illness, somatoform disorders, malingering, other psychiatric disorders, and substance abuse (McKane and Anderson 1997). It is especially important to rule out genuine physical illness since individuals with a factitious disorder often induce real physical illness. Furthermore, it is always important to remember that individuals with factitious disorders are certainly not immune to the physical illnesses that plague the general population.

Etiology
Both psychological and biological factors have been postulated to play a role in the etiology of factitious disorder. Although numerous case reports have generated speculation that a factitious disorder may run in families, this could be explained by environmental factors, genetic factors, or both. The presence of central nervous system (CNS) abnormalities in some individuals with factitious disorders have led some to hypothesize that underlying brain dysfunction contributes to a factitious disorder. One review of factitious individuals with *pseudologia fantastica* found CNS abnormalities (such as EEG abnormality, head injury, imaging abnormalities, or neurological findings) in 40% of the individuals (King and Ford 1988). There have been case reports of MRI (Fenelon et al. 1991) and SPECT (Mountz et al. 1996) abnormalities, but it is unknown if these abnormalities were related to the disorder.

In addition, childhood developmental disturbances are thought to contribute to factitious disorder. Predisposing factors are thought to include (1) serious childhood illness or illness in a family member during childhood, especially if the illness was associated with attention and nurturing in an otherwise distant family, (2) past anger with the medical profession, (3) past significant relationship with a health care provider, and (4) factitious disorder in a parent (McKane and Anderson 1997).

Individuals with factitious disorder create illness in pursuit of the sick role. For these individuals, being in the sick role allows them to compensate for an underlying psychological deficit. Most authors identify several common psychodynamic motivations for factitious disorder (Feldman 2000, Eisendrath 2001, Guziec et al. 1994, Folks 1995, Hyler and Sussman 1981). First, individuals with little sense of self may seek the sick role in order to provide a well-defined identity around which to structure themselves. Others may seek the sick role in order to meet dependency needs that have gone unmet elsewhere. As an individual, they receive the attention, caring, and nurturing of the health care environment and are relieved of many of their responsibilities. In addition, some individuals may engage in factitious behaviors for masochistic reasons. They feel they deserve punishment for some forbidden feelings and thus they should suffer at the hands of their physicians. Other individuals may be motivated by anger at physicians and dupe them in retaliation. Individuals with a history of childhood illness or abuse may attempt to master past traumas by creating a situation over which they have control. Finally, some authors have speculated that some individuals may be enacting suicidal wishes through their factitious behavior (Schoenfeld et al. 1987, Roy and Roy 1995).

Treatment

The goals in treating individuals with a factitious disorder are twofold; first to minimize the damage done by the disorder to both the individual's own health and the health care system. The second goal is to help individuals recover, at least partially, from the disorder. These goals are furthered by treating comorbid medical illnesses, avoiding unnecessary procedures, encouraging individuals to seek psychiatric treatment, and providing support for health care clinicians. Because the literature is based exclusively on case reports and series, determining treatment effectiveness is difficult. As mentioned before, individuals with true Munchausen's syndrome (including antisocial traits, pathological lying, wandering, and poor social support) are felt to be refractory to treatment. While factitious disorder is extremely difficult to cure, effective techniques exist to minimize morbidity, and some individuals are able to benefit greatly from psychiatric intervention.

Soon after Asher's (1951) article was published, many individuals with a factitious disorder were vigorously confronted once the nature of their illness was discovered. Unfortunately, most individuals would deny their involvement and seek another clinician who was unaware of their diagnosis (Eisendrath 2001). In addition, the idea of "blacklists" was proposed in order to aid detection of these individuals. However, issues regarding an individual's confidentiality as well as concerns about cursory medical evaluations that might miss genuine physical illness prevented this idea from being adopted (Eisendrath 2001). Although aggressive confrontation is usually unsuccessful, supportive, nonpunitive confrontation may be helpful for some. In one case series, 33 individuals were confronted with the factitious nature of their illness. While only 13 admitted feigning illness, most of the individuals' illnesses subsequently improved, at least in the short term (Reich and Gottfried 1983).

Eisendrath suggested three alternatives to confrontation that he found effective. First is inexact interpretation, in which the clinician interprets the psychodynamics thought to be underlying the individual's behavior without explicitly identifying the factitious behavior. He gave the example of an individual suspected of having factitious disorder who developed septicemia after her boyfriend proposed marriage. The consultant suggested that the individual might feel a need to punish herself when good things happened to her. She agreed, and soon after, admitted that she had injected a contaminant intravenously (Eisendrath 2001). The second technique is the therapeutic double-blind. The clinician presents the individual with a new medical intervention to treat his or her illness. The individual is told that one possibility is that the individual's illness has a factitious origin, and that, if so, the treatment would not be expected to work while, if the illness is biological, the treatment will work and the individual will improve. The individual must decide to give up the factitious illness or admit it. A third technique is to provide the individual with a face-saving way, such as hypnosis or biofeedback, of giving up his or her symptoms without admitting that they are not genuine. Eisendrath (2001) points out that in emergent situations, there may not be time for nonconfrontational techniques, and more directly confrontational means may be necessary.

Another important component in the treatment of individuals with factitious disorder is the coordination of health care among all clinicians. This allows for fewer unnecessary interventions, minimizes splitting among the health care team, and allows the health care team to vent and process the strong emotions that arise when caring for factitious individuals. This decreases both the negative impact on the clinicians and the chance that anger will be acted out on the individual.

There are no clear data supporting the effectiveness of medications in treating factitious disorder. There is a case report of effective pimozide treatment in an individual thought to have delusional symptoms (Prior and Gordon 1997), as well as a case report of a factitious individual with comorbid depression improving when treated with an antidepressant in addition to intensive psychotherapy (Earle and Folks 1986).

While many individuals with factitious disorder are hesitant to pursue mental health treatment, there are numerous case reports of successful treatment of the disorder with long-term psychotherapy. In many of these cases, the therapy lasted several years, including one individual who received treatment while imprisoned for over 10 years (Miller et al. 1985). Plassmann reports a case series of 24 factitious individuals. Twelve of these individuals accepted psychotherapy and 10 continued with long-term treatment, lasting up to four and a half years. He reports "significant, or at least marked, improvement" in those 10 individuals (Plassmann 1994b). These case reports support the idea that treatment of individuals with factitious disorder is not impossible, and these individuals can improve. However, expectations must be realistic as improvement in the disorder itself can take several years. Techniques that target short-term reduction in the production of factitious symptoms can be effective more quickly. See Figure 37-2 for a treatment flowchart for factitious disorder.

Treating individuals with factitious disorder often raises ethical questions including those regarding confidentiality, privacy, and medical decision-making, and it is important to be alert to these issues. Often, individuals with factious disorder will want to keep their diagnosis confidential, even when to do so may harm the individual or others. For example, although a consulting clinician may diagnose an individual with factitious disorder, the individual may refuse consent to reveal this information to the referring physician. If the consultant does inform the referring physician, she has violated the individual's confidentiality, but if she does not, the referring physician is likely to continue to treat the individual for the incorrect diagnosis. Dilemmas regarding the individual's privacy also arise with factitious individuals. For example, hospital room searches could often help clarify the diagnosis or remove materials the individual is using to harm himself, but these searches also violate the individual's privacy. Dilemmas surrounding medical decision-making can arise when an individual with factitious disorder refuses treatment or requests potentially harmful treatments. It can often be difficult to resolve these ethical dilemmas. In general, even though the factitious individual is deceptive within the relationship between the clinician and the individual, the clinician is not released from his or her responsibilities within that relationship, and the individual retains his or her rights of confidentiality, privacy, and autonomy. As with all such individuals, emergency situations require different ethical guidelines. Often, an ethics consultation can be very helpful in sorting through the difficult issues of care of the individual in the setting of factitious disorder.

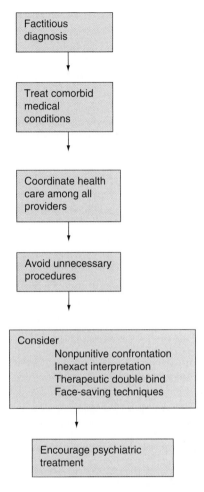

Figure 37-2 *Treatment flowchart for factitious disorder.*

Owing to the high morbidity and mortality, treatment of Factitious Disorder By Proxy requires at least temporary separation from the parent and notification of local child protective agencies. The perpetrators often face criminal charges of child abuse. There is high psychiatric morbidity in the children—many go on to develop factitious disorder or other psychiatric illnesses themselves. Psychiatric intervention is necessary to ameliorate this morbidity as much as possible in these children (McGuire and Feldman 1989). In this disorder, there are some case reports of successful psychotherapeutic treatments of the parents (Rand and Feldman, 2001).

Comparison of DSM-IV/ICD-10 Diagnostic Criteria
The ICD-10 Diagnostic Criteria for Research and the DSM-IV-TR criteria sets are almost identical.

References

Absolut de la Gastine G, Penniello MJ, Le Treust M, et al. (1998) Urinary calculi and Munchausen's syndrome. *Arch Pediatr* **5**(5), 517–520.

Aduan RP, Fauci AS, Dale DC, et al. (1979) Factitious fever and self-induced infection: a report of 32 cases and review of the literature. *Ann Int Med* **90**(2), 230–242.

American Psychiatric Association (2000) *Diagnostic and Statistical Manual of Mental Disorders*, 4th ed., Text Rev. APA, Washington, DC.

Asher R (1951) Munchausen's syndrome. *Lancet* **1**, 339–341.

Bauer M and Boegner F (1996) Neurological syndromes in factitious disorder. *J Nerv Ment Dis* **184**(5), 281–288.

Bhugra D (1988) Psychiatric Munchausen's syndrome. Literature review with case reports. *Acta Psychiatr Scand* **77**(5), 497–503.

Bools C, Neale B, and Meadow R. (1994) Munchausen syndrome by proxy: a study of psychopathology. *Child Abuse Negl* **18**(9), 773–788.

Carney MW and Brown JP (1983) Clinical features and motives among 42 artifactual illness patients. *Br J Med Psychol* **56**(Pt 1), 57–66.

Chantada G, Casak S, Plata JD, et al. (1994) Children with fever of unknown origin in Argentina: an analysis of 113 cases. *Pediatr Infect Dis J* **13**(4), 260–263.

Coons PM (1993) Use of the MMPI to distinguish genuine from factitious multiple personality disorder. *Psychol Rep* **73**(2), 401–402.

Croft RD and Jervis M (1989) Munchausen's syndrome in a 4-year-old. *Arch Dis Child* **64**(5), 740–741.

Davis JW and Small GW (1985) Munchausen's syndrome in an 85-year-old man. *J Am Geriatr Soc* **33**(2), 154–155.

Denny SJ, Grant CC, and Pinnock R (2001) Epidemiology of Munchausen syndrome by proxy in New Zealand. *J Paediatr Child Health* **37**(3), 240–243.

Earle JR Jr. and Folks DG (1986) Factitious disorder and coexisting depression: a report of successful psychiatric consultation and case management. *Gen Hosp Psychiatry* **8**(6), 448–450.

Ehlers W and Plassmann R (1994) Diagnosis of narcissistic self-esteem regulation in patients with factitious illness (Munchausen syndrome). *Psychother Psychosom* **62**(1–2), 69–77.

Eisendrath SJ (1994) Factitious physical disorders. *West J Med* **160**(2), 177–179.

Eisendrath SJ (2001) Factitious disorders and malingering. In *Treatment of Psychiatric Disorders*, 3rd ed., Gabbard GO (ed). American Psychiatric Publishing, Washington, DC, pp. 1825–1844.

Fairbank JA, McCaffrey RJ, and Keane TM (1985) Psychometric detection of fabricated symptoms of posttraumatic stress disorder. *Am J Psychiatry* **142**(4), 501–503.

Feldman M (2000) Factitious disorders. In *Comprehensive Textbook of Psychiatry*, 7th ed., Sadock B and Sadock V (eds). Lippincott, Williams & Wilkins, Philadelphia, pp. 1533–1544.

Feldman MD, Ford CV, and Stone T. (1994) Deceiving others/deceiving oneself: four cases of factitious rape. *S Med J* **87**(7), 736–738.

Feldman-Schorrig S (1996) Factitious sexual harassment. *Bull Am Acad Psychiatry Law* **24**(3), 387–392.

Fenelon G, Mahieux F, Roullet E, et al. (1991) Munchausen's syndrome and abnormalities on magnetic resonance imaging of the brain. *BMJ* **302**(6783), 996–997.

Folks DG (1995) Munchausen's syndrome and other factitious disorders. *Neurol Clin* **13**(2), 267–281.

Gault MH, Campbell NR, and Aksu AE. (1988) Spurious stones. *Nephron* **48**(4), 274–279.

Goldstein AB (1998) Identification and classification of factitious disorders: an analysis of cases reported during a ten-year period. *Int J Psychiatry Med* **28**(2), 221–241.

Gurwith M and Langston C (1980) Factitious Munchausen's syndrome. *N Engl J Med* **302**(26), 1483–1484.

Guziec J, Lazarus A, and Harding JJ. (1994) Case of a 29-year-old nurse with factitious disorder. The utility of psychiatric intervention on a general medical floor. *Gen Hosp Psychiatry* **16**(1), 47–53.

Hyler SE and Sussman N (1981) Chronic factitious disorder with physical symptoms (the Munchausen syndrome). *Psychiatry Clin North Am* **4**(2), 365–377.

Kent JD (1994) Munchausen's syndrome and substance abuse. *J F Subst Abuse Treat* **11**(3), 247–251.

King BH and Ford CV (1988) Pseudologia fantastica. *Acta Psychiatr Scand* **77**(1), 1–6.

Knockaert DC, Vanneste LJ, Vanneste SB, et al. (1992) Fever of unknown origin in the 1980s. An update of the diagnostic spectrum. *Arch Int Med* **152**(1), 51–55.

Kravitz RM and Wilmott RW (1990) Munchausen syndrome by proxy presenting as factitious apnea. *Clin Pediatr (Phila)* **29**(10), 587–592.

Libow JA (2000) Child and adolescent illness falsification. *Pediatrics* **105**(2), 336–342.

McCaffrey RJ and Bellamy-Campbell R (1989) Psychometric detection of fabricated symptoms of combat-related post-traumatic stress disorder: a systematic replication. *J Clin Psychol* **45**(1), 76–79.

McClure RJ, Davis PM, Meadow SR, et al. (1996) Epidemiology of Munchausen syndrome by proxy, nonaccidental poisoning, and non-accidental suffocation. *Arch Dis Child* **75**(1), 57–61.

McGuire TL and Feldman KW (1989) Psychologic morbidity of children subjected to Munchausen's syndrome by proxy. *Pediatrics* **83**(2), 289–292.

McKane JP and Anderson J (1997) Munchausen's syndrome: rule breakers and risk takers. *Br J Hosp Med* **58**(4), 150–153.

Meadow R (1998) Munchausen syndrome by proxy abuse perpetrated by men. *Arch Dis Child* **78**(3), 210–216.

Merrin EL, Van Dyke C, Cohen S, et al. (1986) Dual factitious disorder. *Gen Hosp Psychiatry* **8**(4), 246–250.

Miller RD, Blancke FW, Doren DM, et al. (1985) The Munchausen patient in a forensic facility. *Psychiatry Q* **57**(1), 72–76.

Miller F, Weiden P, Sacks M, et al. (1986) Two cases of factitious acquired immune deficiency syndrome. *Am J Psychiatry* **143**(11), 1483.

Mountz JM, Parker PE, Liu HG, et al. (1996) Tc-99m HMPAO brain SPECT scanning in Munchausen syndrome. *J Psychiatr Neurosci* **21**(1), 49–52.

Munro HM and Thrusfield MV (2001) 'Battered pets': Munchausen's syndrome by proxy (factitious illness by proxy). *J Small Anim Pract* **42**(8), 385–389.

Parker PE (1993) A case report of Munchausen syndrome with mixed psychological features. *Psychosomatics* **34**(4), 360–364.

Parsons T (1951) *The Social Structure*. Free Press, Glencoe, IL, pp 436–439.

Pathe M, Mullen PE, and Purcell R (1999) Stalking: false claims of victimisation. *Br J Psychiatry* **174**, 170–172.

Perconte ST and Goreczny AJ (1990) Failure to detect fabricated posttraumatic stress disorders with the use of the MMPI in a clinical population. *Am J Psychiatry* **147**(8), 1057–1060.

Plassmann R (1994a) Munchausen's syndrome and factitious diseases. *Psychother Psychosom* **62**(1–2), 7–26.

Plassmann R (1994b) Inpatient and outpatient long-term psychotherapy of patients suffering from factitious disorders. *Psychother Psychosom* **62**(1–2), 96–107.

Pope HG Jr., Jonas JM, and Jones B (1982) Factitious psychosis: phenomenology, family history, and long-term outcome of nine patients. *Am J Psychiatry* **139**(11), 1480–1483.

Popli AP, Masand PS, and Dewan MJ (1992) Factitious disorders with psychological symptoms. *J Clin Psychiatry* **53**(9), 315–318.

Prior TI and Gordon A (1997) Treatment of factitious disorder with pimozide. *Can J Psychiatry* **42**(5), 532.

Rahilly PM (1991) The pneumographic and medical investigation of infants suffering apparent life threatening episodes. *J Paediatr Child Health* **27**(6), 349–353.

Rand DC and Feldman MD (2001) An explanatory model for Munchausen by proxy abuse. *Int J Psychiatr Med* **31**(2), 113–126.

Reich P and Gottfried LA (1983) Factitious disorders in a teaching hospital. *Ann Int Med* **99**(2), 240–247.

Rosenberg DA (1987) Web of deceit: a literature review of Munchausen syndrome by proxy. *Child Abuse Negl* **11**(4), 547–563.

Roy M and Roy A (1995) Factitious hypoglycemia. An 11-year follow-up. *Psychosomatics* **36**(1), 64–65.

Rumans LW and Vosti KL (1978) Factitious and fraudulent fever. *Am J Med* **65**(5), 745–755.

Schoenfeld H, Margolin J, and Baum S (1987) Munchausen syndrome as a suicide equivalent: abolition of syndrome by psychotherapy. *Am J Psychother* **41**(4), 604–612.

Snowdon J, Solomons R, and Druce H (1978) Feigned bereavement: twelve cases. *Br J Psychiatry* **133**, 15–19.

Sparr L and Pankratz LD (1983) Factitious posttraumatic stress disorder. *Am J Psychiatry* **140**(8), 1016–1019.

Wise MG and Ford CV (1999) Factitious disorders. *Prim Care* **26**(2), 315–326.

38 Dissociative Disorders

Dissociative phenomena are best understood through the term *désagrégation* (disaggregation) originally given by Janet (1920). Events normally experienced as connected to one another on a smooth continuum are isolated from the other mental processes with which they would ordinarily be associated. The dissociative disorders are a disturbance in the organization of identity, memory, perception, or consciousness. When memories are separated from access to consciousness, the disorder is dissociative amnesia. Fragmentation of identity results in dissociative fugue or dissociative identity disorder (DID; formerly multiple personality disorder). Disintegrated perception is characteristic of depersonalization disorder. Dissociation of aspects of consciousness produces acute stress disorder and various dissociative trance and possession states. Numbing and amnesia are diagnostic components of posttraumatic stress disorder (PTSD), both of which are described in Chapter 34. These dissociative and related disorders are more a disturbance in the organization or structure of mental contents than in the contents themselves. Memories in dissociative amnesia are not so much distorted or bizarre as they are segregated from one another. The identities lost in dissociative fugue or fragmented in DID are two-dimensional aspects of an overall personality structure. In this sense, individuals with DID suffer not from having more than one personality but rather from having less than one personality. The problem involves information processing: the failure of integration of elements rather than the contents of the fragments.

The dissociative disorders have a long history in classical psychopathology, being the foundation on which Freud began his explorations of the unconscious (Breuer and Freud 1955) and Janet (1920) developed dissociation theory. Although much attention in psychiatry has shifted to diagnosis and treatment of mood, anxiety, and thought disorders, dissociative phenomena are sufficiently persistent and interesting that they have elicited growing attention from both professionals and the public. There are at least four reasons for this:

1. They are fascinating phenomena in and of themselves, involving the loss of or change in identity, or memory, or a feeling of detachment from extreme and traumatic physical events.
2. Dissociative disorders seem to arise in response to traumatic stress.
3. Dissociative disorders remain an area of psychopathology for which the best treatment is psychotherapy, although adjunctive pharmacological interventions can be helpful.
4. Dissociation as a phenomenon has much to teach us about information processing in the brain.

Etiology

Dissociation may seem like a historical aberration, a throwback to earlier and more primitive models of the mind. Yet, these disorders are surprisingly congruent with information processing–based theories of mental function. For example, connectionist and parallel distributed processing models (Rumelhart and McClelland 1986) take a bottom-up rather than a top-down approach to cognitive organization. Traditional models emphasize a supraordinate structure in which broad categories of information structure the processing of specific examples of those categories, that is, the category "sweet" must exist to make sense of "sugar," "candy," and "jelly." In the parallel distributed processing models, subunits or neural nets process information through patterns of co-occurrence of input stimuli that lead to activation patterns in these neural nets, which produce pattern recognition. The output of one neuronal system becomes the input to another, thereby gradually building up integrated and complex patterns of activation and inhibition. A bottom-up processing model system has the advantage of accounting for the processing of vast amounts of information and the ability to recognize patterns with approximate information. Nevertheless, such models make the classification and integration of information problematical.

Information seems to be processed on the basis of the co-occurrence of patterns of activation rather than its appearance in a predefined category. Therefore, in parallel distributed processing system models, failures in integration of mental contents are theoretically likely to occur. Inappropriate but apparent similarities may appear when activation patterns are similar, and conversely, no two pieces of information are necessarily connected. There have been models created to explain psychotic, dissociative, and mood disorders, based on abnormal or defective neuronal association network patterns (Li and Spiegel 1992, Hoffman 1987). These neural models assumed that when there are problems with the processing of input information (a model for traumatic input), the brain is more likely to have difficulty achieving a coherent and balanced output. This could then lead to the development of dissociation of information and data manifested in the subject's inability to process smoothly all of the incoming information.

There are two broad categories of memory known as *explicit and implicit* (Schacter 1992), *declarative and procedural* (Squire 1987), or *episodic and semantic* (Tulving 1983).

These two basic memory systems serve different functions. *Explicit* or *episodic memory* involves recall of personal experience identified with the self, for example, "I went dancing last night." The second type is known as *implicit* or *procedural memory*. This involves the execution of routine operations, such as driving a car, or typing on a keyboard. Most of these rather automatic operations could be carried out with little conscious awareness, but yet with a high degree of proficiency. These two types of memory seem to reside in different cerebral anatomical localizations. Episodic memory seems to be primarily associated with limbic system function, primarily involving the hippocampal formation and mamillary bodies. On the other hand, procedural memory appears to be a function of basal ganglia and cortical functioning (Kosslyn and Koenig 1992).

The fact that there are separate memory systems may account for certain types of dissociative phenomena (Spiegel et al. 1993). For example, the automaticity observed in certain types of dissociative disorders reflect the separation of self-identification associated with explicit memory from routine activity in implicit or procedural memory. It is thus not at all foreign to our mental processing to act in an automatic way devoid of explicit self-identification. Future research on the neurobiology of memory may well provide insights into the functional disintegration of memory, perception, identity, and consciousness seen in dissociative disorders (Zola-Morgan et al. 1982, Zola-Morgan and Squire 1985).

One of the important developments in the modern understanding of dissociative disorders is the establishment of a clearer link between trauma and dissociation (Spiegel and Cardeña 1991, Spiegel and Spiegel 1978). Although the role of traumatic stress in eliciting dissociative symptoms was a part of Janet's early thinking (Van der Hart et al. 1989) as well as that of Breuer and Freud (1955), more attention was paid to the symptoms, developmental issues, and personality features than to the role of traumatic stressors themselves. Later work has examined in more detail the proximate role of trauma in eliciting dissociative symptoms.

Trauma can be understood as the experience of being made into an object, a thing, the victim of someone else's rage or of nature's indifference. Trauma represents the ultimate experience of helplessness: loss of control over one's own body. There is growing clinical evidence that dissociation occurs as a defense during traumatic experiences, constituting an attempt to maintain mental control at the moment when physical control has been lost (Spiegel et al. 1988, Putnam 1985, Kluft 1984a, Spiegel 1984). Many assault victims report floating above their body, feeling sorry for the person being assaulted beneath them. Individuals, victims of childhood abuse, have reported "taking themselves elsewhere" where they could "safely play," by themselves or with imaginary friends, while their bodies were brutally abused by a perpetrator. In fact, there is evidence (Terr 1991) that children exposed to multiple traumas as opposed to single-blow traumas are more likely to use dissociative defense mechanisms, which include spontaneous trance episodes and amnesia.

As noted in the section on DID, there is an accumulating literature suggesting a connection between a history of childhood physical and sexual abuse and the development of dissociative symptoms (Coons and Milstein 1986, Kluft 1984a, 1985, Spiegel 1984). Similarly, dissociative symptoms have been found to be more prevalent in individuals with Axis II disorders, such as borderline personality disorder, when there has been a history of childhood abuse (Herman et al. 1989, Chu and Dill 1990).

Epidemiology of Dissociative Disorders

Dissociative disorders are not among the more common psychiatric illnesses but are not rare. Few good epidemiological studies have been performed. Some estimate the prevalence at only 1 per 10,000 in the population (Coons 1984), but far higher proportions are reported among populations of those with mental disorders. In fact, the prevalence of the disorder seems to be associated to the specific population under study. For example, data from the general population suggest that the numbers are higher than initially described by Coons

(Kluft 1991), as high as 1% (Ross 1991, Ross et al. 1991b, Vanderlinden et al. 1991). On the other hand, the data seem to indicate that the numbers are even higher in specialized inpatient populations, as high as 3% (Kluft 1991, Ross 1991, Ross et al. 1991a).

There has been a rise in reported cases, which may be attributed to greater awareness of the diagnosis among mental health professionals, to the availability of specific criteria, and to previous misdiagnosis of DID as schizophrenia or borderline personality disorder. Some experts attribute possible underdiagnosis to family disavowal of sexual and physical abuse. However, there is also controversy about possible overdiagnosis of the syndrome, while others propose that the increase is the result of hypnotic suggestion and inadequate handling by therapists (Brenner 1994, 1996, Frankel 1990, Ganaway 1989, 1995, McHugh 1995a, 1995b, Spanos et al. 1985, 1986). Individuals who most commonly have the disorder are highly hypnotizable and therefore especially sensitive to suggestion or cultural influences. Although therapists' expectations amplified with hypnosis may account for some cases, they cannot account for many individuals diagnosed without benefit of hypnosis or by "skeptical" therapists.

Women make up the majority of cases, accounting for 90% of the cases or more, in some studies (Putnam et al. 1986, Coons et al. 1988, Schultz et al. 1989). Strangely, the most common dissociative disorder diagnosis falls into the "not otherwise specified" category, both in the United States (Mezzich et al. 1989, Saxe et al. 1993) and in non-Western countries, where dissociative trance and possession trance are the most common dissociative disorder diagnoses (Adityanjee et al. 1989, Saxena and Prasad 1989). Dissociative disorders are ubiquitous around the world, although the structure of the symptoms varies across cultures (Adityanjee et al. 1989, Berger et al. 1994, Boe et al. 1993, Brown et al. 1999, Coons and Milstein 1986, Draijer and Langeland 1999, Eriksson and Lundin 1996, Friedl and Draijer 2000, Horen et al. 1995, Modestin et al. 1996, Putnam 1989, Ronquillo 1991, Sar et al. 2000, Wittkower 1970). Indeed, the symptomatology reflects cultural biases. In Western cultures, which emphasize the importance of the individual, dissociation often takes the form of dissociated elements of individual personality, while in Eastern cultures, which are more sociocentric, possession trance, in which individuals feel themselves to be taken over by an outside entity or entities, is more common.

DISSOCIATIVE AMNESIA

Diagnosis
This is the classical functional disorder of episodic memory (see DSM-IV-TR diagnostic criteria on page 1032). It does not involve procedural memory or problems in memory storage, as in Wernicke–Korsakoff syndrome. Furthermore, unlike dementing illnesses, dissociative amnesia is reversible (Janet 1920), for example, by using hypnosis or narcoanalysis. It has three primary characteristics:

1. Type of memory lost: The memory loss is episodic. The first-person recollection of certain events, rather than knowledge of procedures, is lost.
2. Temporal structure: The memory loss is for one or more discrete time periods, ranging from minutes to years. It is not vagueness or inefficient retrieval of memories but rather a dense unavailability of memories that were encoded and stored. Unlike the situation in amnestic disorders, for example, resulting from damage to the medial temporal lobe in surgery (the case of H.M. [Milner 1959]), in Wernicke–Korsakoff syndrome, or in Alzheimer's dementia, there is usually no difficulty in learning new episodic information. Thus, the amnesia of dissociative disorders is typically retrograde rather than anterograde (Loewenstein 1991). However, a dissociative syndrome of continuous

difficulty in incorporating new information that mimics organic amnestic syndromes has been observed (Schacter 1995).

3. Type of events forgotten: The memory loss is usually for events of a traumatic or stressful nature. This fact has been noted in the language of the DSM-IV-TR diagnostic criteria. In one study (Coons and Milstein 1986), the majority of cases involved child abuse (60%), but disavowed behaviors such as marital problems, sexual activity, suicide attempts, criminal activity, and the death of a relative have also been reported as precipitants.

DSM-IV-TR Diagnostic Criteria

308.12 Dissociative Amnesia

A. The predominant disturbance is one or more episodes of inability to recall important personal information, usually of a traumatic or stressful nature, that is too extensive to be explained by ordinary forgetfulness.

B. The disturbance does not occur exclusively during the course of dissociative identity disorder, dissociative fugue, posttraumatic stress disorder, acute stress disorder, or somatization disorder and is not due to the direct physiological effects of a substance (e.g., a drug of abuse, a medication) or a neurological or other general medical condition (e.g., amnestic disorder due to head trauma).

C. The symptoms cause clinically significant distress or impairment in social, occupational, or other important areas of functioning.

Reprinted with permission from the Diagnostic and Statistical Manual of Mental Disorders, Fourth Edition, Text Revision. Copyright 2000 American Psychiatric Association.

Dissociative amnesia most frequently occurs after an episode of trauma, and its onset may be gradual or sudden. It occurs most often in the third and fourth decades of life (Coons and Milstein 1986, Ross 1989, Putnam 1989). It usually involves one episode, but multiple periods of lost memory are not uncommon (Coons and Milstein 1986). Comorbidity with conversion disorder, bulimia nervosa, alcohol abuse, and depression are common, and Axis II diagnoses of histrionic, dependent, or borderline personality disorders occur in a substantial minority of such individuals (Coons and Milstein 1986).

Individuals with Dissociative Amnesia typically demonstrate not vagueness or spotty memory but rather a loss of any episodic memory for a finite period. They may not initially be aware of the memory loss; that is, they do not remember that they do not remember. They often report being told that they have done or said things that they cannot remember.

Some individuals do suffer from episodes of selective amnesia, usually for specific traumatic incidents, which may be interwoven with periods of intact memory. In these cases, the amnesia is for a type of material remembered rather than for a discrete time period (Loewenstein 1991).

Although information is kept out of consciousness in dissociative amnesia, it may well exert an influence on consciousness: out of sight does not mean out of mind. For example, a rape victim with no conscious recollection of an assault nonetheless behaves like someone who has been sexually victimized. Such individuals often suffer detachment and demoralization, are unable to enjoy intimate relationships, and show hyperarousal to stimuli reminiscent of the trauma. This loss of explicit memory with retention of implicit knowledge is similar to priming in memory research. Individuals who have read a word in a list complete a word stem (a partial word such as "pre" for "present") more quickly if they have seen that word minutes or even hours earlier. This priming effect occurs despite the fact that they cannot consciously recall having read the word, or even the list in which it occurred. When asked in a free recall format to list the word they have seen, they cannot name it, yet they act as though they have seen it and do remember it. Similarly, individuals instructed in hypnosis to forget having seen a list of words nonetheless demonstrate priming effects of the hypnotically suppressed list (Kihlstrom 1987). It is the essence of dissociative amnesia that material kept out of conscious awareness is nonetheless active and may influence consciousness indirectly (Van der Hart 2001).

Individuals with dissociative amnesia generally do not suffer disturbances of identity, except to the extent that their identity is influenced by the warded-off memory. It is not uncommon for such individuals to develop depressive symptoms as well, especially when the amnesia occurs in the wake of a traumatic stressor.

Treatment

Often, individuals suffering from dissociative amnesia experience spontaneous recovery when they are removed from the stressful or threatening situation, when they feel safe, and/or when exposed to personal cues from their past (i.e., home, pets, family members) (Kardiner and Spiegel 1947, Loewenstein 1991, Maldonado et al. 2000, Maldonado and Spiegel 2002, Reither and Stoudemire 1988). Cases in which exposure to a safe environment is not enough to restore normal memory functioning, pharmacologically facilitated interviews may prove useful (Baron and Nagy 1988, Naples and Hackett 1978, Perry and Jacobs 1982).

Most individuals with dissociative disorders are highly hypnotizable on formal testing and are therefore easily able to make use of hypnotic techniques such as age regression (Spiegel and Spiegel 1978). Hypnosis can enable such individuals to reorient temporally and therefore achieve access to otherwise dissociated and unavailable memories.

If there is traumatic content to the warded-off memory, individuals may abreact, that is, express strong emotion as these memories are elicited. Such abreactions are rarely damaging in themselves but are not intrinsically therapeutic either. They may be experienced by the individual as a reinflicting of the traumatic stressor. Such individuals need psychotherapeutic help in integrating these warded-off memories and the associated affect into consciousness, thereby gaining a sense of mastery over them.

One technique that can help bring such memories into consciousness while modulating the affective response to them is a projective technique known as "the screen technique" (Spiegel 1981). While using hypnosis, such individuals are taught to recall the traumatic event as if they were watching it on an imaginary movie or television screen. This technique is often helpful for individuals who are unable to remember the event as if it were occurring in the present, either because for some highly hypnotizable individuals that approach is too emotionally taxing or because others are not sufficiently hypnotizable to be able to engage in such hypnotic age regression. The screen can be employed to facilitate cognitive restructuring of the traumatic memory, for example, by picturing on the left side of the screen some component of the traumatic experience, and on the right side something they did to protect themselves or someone else during it. This makes the memory both more complex and more bearable.

A particularly useful feature of this technique is that it allows for the recollection of traumatic events without triggering an uncontrolled reliving of the trauma, as is the case of traumatic flashbacks. The screen technique provides a "controlled dissociation" between the psychological and somatic aspects of memory retrieval. Individuals can be put into self-hypnosis and instructed to get their body into a state of floating comfort and safety. They can do this by imagining that they are somewhere safe and comfortable: "Imagine that you are floating in a bath, a lake, a hot tub, or just floating in space." They are reminded that no matter what they see on the screen their bodies are safe and comfortable: "Do the work on your imaginary screen, not in your body." In this way, the tendency for physiological arousal to accompany and intensify the working through of traumatic memories can be controlled, facilitating the psychotherapeutic work.

The psychotherapy of dissociative amnesia involves accessing the dissociated memories, working through affectively loaded aspects of these memories, and supporting the individual through the process of integrating these memories into consciousness.

DISSOCIATIVE FUGUE

Diagnosis

Dissociative fugue combines failure of integration of certain aspects of personal memory with loss of customary identity and automatisms of motor behavior (see DSM-IV-TR diagnostic criteria below). It involves one or more episodes of sudden, unexpected, purposeful travel away from home, coupled with an inability to recall portions or all of one's past, and a loss of identity or the assumption of a new identity. The onset is usually sudden, and it frequently occurs after a traumatic experience or bereavement. A single episode is not uncommon, and spontaneous remission of symptoms can occur without treatment.

DSM-IV-TR Diagnostic Criteria

308.13 Dissociative Fugue

A. The predominant disturbance is sudden, unexpected travel away from home or one's customary place of work, with inability to recall one's past.
B. Confusion about personal identity or assumption of new identity (partial or complete).
C. The disturbance does not occur exclusively during the course of dissociative identity disorder and is not due to the direct physiological effects of a substance (e.g., a drug of abuse, a medication) or a general medical condition (e.g., temporal lobe epilepsy).
D. The symptoms cause clinically significant distress or impairment in social, occupational, or other important areas of functioning.

It was originally thought that the assumption of a new identity, as in the classical case of the Reverend Ansel Bourne (James 1984), was typical of dissociative fugue. However, a review of the literature (Reither and Stoudemire 1988) shows that in the majority of cases there is loss of personal identity but no clear assumption of a new identity.

Many cases of dissociative fugue remit spontaneously. Again, hypnosis can be useful in accessing dissociated material. Not infrequently, fugue episodes represent dissociated but purposeful activity.

Treatment

Hypnosis can be helpful in treating dissociative fugue by accessing otherwise unavailable components of memory and identity. The approach used is similar to that for dissociative amnesia. Hypnotic age regression can be used as the framework for accessing information available at a previous time. Demonstrating to individuals that such information can be made available to consciousness enhances their sense of control over this material and facilitates therapeutic working through of emotionally laden aspects of it.

Once reorientation is established and the overt identity and memory loss of the fugue have been resolved, it is important to work through interpersonal or intrapsychic issues that underlie the dissociative defenses. Such individuals are often relatively unaware of their reactions to stress because they can so effectively dissociate them (Spiegel 1974). Thus, effective psychotherapy is anticipatory, helping individuals to recognize and modify their tendency to set aside their own feelings in favor of those of others. Individuals with dissociative fugue may be helped with a psychotherapeutic approach that facilitates conscious integration of dissociated memories and motivations for behavior previously experienced as automatic and unwilled. It is often helpful to address current psychosocial stressors, such as marital conflict, with the involved individuals. To the extent that current psychosocial stress triggers fugue, resolution of that stress can help resolve it and reduce the likelihood of recurrence. Highly hypnotizable individuals prone to these extreme dissociative symptoms (Spiegel and Spiegel 1978, Spiegel 1974, Spiegel et al. 1988) often have great difficulty in asserting their own point of view in a personal relationship. Rather, they interact with others as though they were undergoing a spontaneous trance experience. One such individual described herself as a "disciple in search of a teacher." Psychotherapy can help such individuals recognize and modify their tendency to unthinking compliance with others, and extreme sensitivity to rejection and disapproval.

In the past, medication-facilitated interviews were used to reverse dissociative amnesia or fugue. However, such techniques offer no advantage over hypnosis and are not especially effective (Perry and Jacobs 1982). Not infrequently, the ceremony of injecting the drug elicits spontaneous hypnotic phenomena before the pharmacological effect is felt, and sedation, respiratory depression, and other side effects can be troublesome. It also promotes dependency on the therapist. On the contrary, when hypnosis is used, individuals are trained on self-hypnotic techniques, promoting the use of hypnosis instead of spontaneous dissociation. This enhances the individuals' level of control while enhancing a sense of mastery and self-control.

DEPERSONALIZATION DISORDER

Diagnosis

This dissociative disorder involves lack of integration of one or more components of perception (see DSM-IV-TR diagnostic criteria on page 1036). The essential feature of depersonalization disorder is the occurrence of persistent feelings of unreality, detachment, or estrangement from oneself or one's body, usually with the feeling that one is an outside observer of one's own mental processes (Steinberg 1991). Individuals suffering depersonalization are distressed by it. They are aware of some distortion in their perceptual experience and therefore are not hallucinating or delusional. Affected individuals often fear that they are "going crazy." The symptom is not infrequently transient.

DSM-IV-TR Diagnostic Criteria

300.6 Depersonalization Disorder

A. Persistent or recurrent experiences of feeling detached from, and as if one is an outside observer of, one's mental processes or body (e.g., feeling like one is in a dream).
B. During the depersonalization experience, reality testing remains intact.
C. The depersonalization causes clinically significant distress or impairment in social, occupational, or other important areas of functioning.
D. The depersonalization experience does not occur exclusively during the course of another mental disorder, such as schizophrenia, panic disorder, acute stress disorder, or another dissociative disorder, and is not due to the direct physiological effects of a substance (e.g., a drug of abuse, a medication) or a general medical condition (e.g., temporal lobe epilepsy).

Reprinted with permission from the Diagnostic and Statistical Manual of Mental Disorders, Fourth Edition, Text Revision. Copyright 2000 American Psychiatric Association.

Derealization, in which affected individuals notice an altered perception of their surroundings, resulting in the world seeming unreal or dream-like, frequently occurs as well. Such individuals often ruminate anxiously about this symptom and are preoccupied with their own somatic and mental functioning.

Depersonalization frequently co-occurs with a variety of other symptoms, especially anxiety, panic, or phobic symptoms. It is often a symptom of PTSD and also occurs as a symptom of alcohol and drug abuse, as a side effect of the use of prescription medication, and during stress and sensory deprivation. The symptom of depersonalization is also commonly seen in the course of a number of other neurological and psychiatric disorders (Pies 1991). It is considered a disorder when it is a persistent and predominant symptom. The phenomenology of the disorder involves both the initial symptoms themselves and the reactive anxiety caused by them.

Treatment

Depersonalization is most often transient and may remit without formal treatment. Recurrent or persistent depersonalization should be thought of both as a symptom in itself and as a component of other syndromes requiring treatment, such as anxiety disorders and schizophrenia.

The symptom itself may respond to training in self-hypnosis. Paradoxically, induction or deliberate worsening of symptoms may provide relief by teaching a method of controlling them. For example, a hypnotic induction may induce transient depersonalization symptoms, such as a sense of detachment from part of the body, in such individuals. This is a useful exercise, in that by having a structure for inducing the symptoms, one provides the individual with a context for understanding and controlling them. They are presented as a spontaneous form of hypnotic dissociation that can be modified. Such individuals can be taught to induce a pleasant sense of floating lightness or heaviness in place of the anxiety-related somatic detachment. The use of an imaginary screen to picture problems in a way that detaches them from the typical somatic response is also helpful (Spiegel and Spiegel 1978). Other relaxation techniques such as systematic desensitization, progressive muscle relaxation, and biofeedback may also be of help. Psychotherapy aimed at working through emotional responses to any traumatic or other stressors that tend to elicit the depersonalization is also helpful.

Pharmacological approaches involve balancing therapeutic benefit and risk. Antianxiety medications are most commonly used and may be helpful in reducing the amplification of depersonalization caused by anxiety. However, depersonalization and derealization are also side effects of antianxiety drugs, so their use should be carefully monitored. Increasing dosage, a standard technique when there is lack of therapeutic response, may also increase symptoms, leading to a spiral of increasing symptoms and drug dosage but without therapeutic benefit.

However, appropriate pharmacological treatment for comorbid disorders is an important part of treatment. Use of antianxiety medications for generalized anxiety or phobic disorders (Stein and Uhde 1989) or of antipsychotic medications (Nuller 1982) for psychotic disorders is often beneficial in conditions in which there is contributory comorbidity.

DISSOCIATIVE IDENTITY DISORDER (MULTIPLE PERSONALITY DISORDER)

Diagnosis

Dissociative identity disorder (DID) is a rare but real disorder that is the most widely discussed of the dissociative disorders. It involves the "presence of two or more distinct identities or personality states (each with its own relatively enduring pattern of perceiving, relating to, and thinking about the environment and self)" (American Psychiatric Association 2000) (see DSM-IV-TR diagnostic criteria below). The diagnostic criteria also require that "At least two of these identities or personality states recurrently take control of the person's behavior" (American Psychiatric Association 2000), and that there be amnesia: "Inability to recall important personal information that is too extensive to be explained by ordinary forgetfulness" (American Psychiatric Association 2000). It is a failure of integration of various aspects of identity and personality structure. Often different relationship styles (dependent versus assertive/aggressive) and mood states (depressed versus hostile) segregate with different identities and personal memories. Such individuals may be mystified by events that occurred in another "state," or by responses of others to them for behavior that occurred in a different "state." This fragmentation of personality often occurs in response to trauma in childhood, and is perceived by the individual as protective, allowing him or her to tolerate and partially evade chronic abuse. These individuals thus view treatment ambivalently as an attempt to deprive them of a defense against attack. They also tend to see others as irrational and unfair, since response to one aspect of their personality frequently reflects experience with other aspects. One DID individual (prior to diagnosis) reported puzzlement about accusations by friends and acquaintances that she had made hostile comments for which she had no memory. She would find people angry at her for no reason. Thus, their personality fragmentation renders them vulnerable to interpersonal problems, yet gives them the belief that they are relatively protected from them.

DSM-IV-TR Diagnostic Criteria

308.14 Dissociative Identity Disorder

A. The presence of two or more distinct identities or personality states (each with its own relatively enduring pattern of perceiving, relating to, and thinking about the environment and self).

B. At least two of these identities or personality states recurrently take control of the person's behavior.

C. Inability to recall important personal information that is too extensive to be explained by ordinary forgetfulness.

D. The disturbance is not due to the direct physiological effects of a substance (e.g., blackouts or chaotic behavior during alcohol intoxication) or a general medical condition (e.g., complex partial seizures).

Note: In children, the symptoms are not attributable to imaginary playmates or other fantasy play.

The diagnosis can be facilitated by psychological testing. Scales of trait dissociation have been developed (Bernstein and Putnam 1986, Ross 1989, Carlson et al. 1993), and individuals with DID score extremely high on these scales, in contrast to normal populations and other groups of individuals (Ross et al. 1990, Steinberg et al. 1990). Those with DID score far higher than normal individuals on standard measures of hypnotizability, whereas schizophrenic individuals tend to have lower than normal scores or the absence of high hypnotizability (Spiegel et al. 1982, Spiegel and Fink 1979, Lavoie and Sabourin 1980, Pettinati 1982, Pettinati et al. 1990, Van der Hart and Spiegel 1993). Thus, there is comparatively little overlap in the hypnotizability scores of individuals with schizophrenia and those with DID. Form level on the Rorschach test is usually within the normal range, but there are frequent emotionally dramatic responses, often involving mutilation (especially with the color cards) of a type that is often seen in histrionic personality disorder as well (Scroppo et al. 1998). Form level is an assessment of the match between the percept (what the subject reports seeing) and the inkblot structure. Good form level involves relatively little distortion of the image to match percept to inkblot. Good form level is useful in distinguishing individuals with DID (formerly multiple personality disorder (American Psychiatric Association 1994)) from those with schizophrenia, who have poor form level.

DID is more frequently recognized during childhood (Kluft 1984a) but typically emerges between adolescence and the third decade of life; it rarely presents as a new disorder after age 40 years, but there is often considerable delay between initial symptom presentation and diagnosis (Putnam et al. 1986).

Untreated, it is a chronic and recurrent disorder. It rarely remits spontaneously, but the symptoms may not be evident for certain time periods (Kluft 1985). DID has been called *a disease of hiddenness* (Schacter 1995). The dissociation itself hampers self-monitoring and accurate reporting of symptoms and history. Many individuals with the disorder are not fully aware of the extent of their dissociative symptoms. They may be reluctant to bring up symptoms because of confusion or shame about the illness or because they encountered previous skepticism. Furthermore, because the majority of individuals report histories of sexual and physical abuse (Kluft 1985, 1991, Coons and Milstein 1986, Spiegel 1984, Braun and Sachs 1985), the shame associated with that and fear of retribution may inhibit reporting of symptoms as well.

There are no convincing studies of the absolute prevalence of DID, although there is widespread agreement that the number of diagnosed cases has increased considerably in the United States and some European countries in the past 2 decades (Boon and Draijer 1993). Two studies have estimated the prevalence as approximately 1% of psychiatric inpatients (Saxe et al. 1993, Ross et al. 1991a). Factors that may account for the increase in the number of true reported cases include (1) more general awareness of the diagnosis among mental health professionals, (2) the availability of specific diagnostic criteria starting with DSM-III, and (3) reduced misdiagnosis of DID as schizophrenia or borderline personality disorder.

Other authors attribute the increase in reported cases to social contagion, hypnotic suggestion, and misdiagnosis (Frankel 1990, Ganaway 1995, McHugh 1995a, 1995b, Spanos et al. 1986). Proponents of this point of view argue that these individuals are highly hypnotizable and therefore quite suggestible. They would therefore be especially vulnerable to direct or implicit hypnotic suggestion. They note that not infrequently a few specialist clinicians make the vast majority of diagnoses. However, it has been observed that the symptoms of individuals diagnosed by specialists in dissociation do not differ from those of individuals diagnosed by psychiatrists, psychologists, and physicians in more general practice who diagnose one or two cases a year. Furthermore, such individuals have been noted to persist in presenting symptoms for an average of 6.5 years before attaining the diagnosis (Putnam 1985). They encounter many clinicians who are convinced that they do not have DID and that they have some other disorder, such as schizophrenia. Were they so easily suggestible, it seems likely that they would accept a suggestion that they have other disorders as well, such as schizophrenia or borderline personality disorder.

Nonetheless, because these individuals are indeed highly hypnotizable and therefore suggestible (Spiegel 1974, Frischholz 1985), care must be taken in the manner in which the illness is presented to them. However, it is unlikely that the increased number of cases currently reported is accounted for by suggestion alone. Reduction in previous misdiagnosis and increased recognition of the prevalence and sequelae of physical and sexual abuse in childhood (Kluft 1984a, 1991, Frischholz 1985, Spiegel 1984, Terr 1991, Herman et al. 1989) are also reasonable explanations.

The major comorbid mental disorders are the depressive disorders, substance use disorders, and borderline personality disorder. Sexual, eating, and sleep disorders co-occur less commonly. Such individuals frequently display self-mutilative behavior, impulsiveness, and overvaluing and devaluing of relationships. Indeed, approximately a third of individuals with DID have symptoms that fit criteria for borderline personality disorder as well. Such individuals are also more frequently depressed (Horevitz and Braun 1984). Conversely, research shows dissociative symptoms in many individuals with borderline personality disorder, especially those who report histories of physical and sexual abuse (Chu and Dill 1990, Ogata et al. 1990). Indeed, the impulsiveness, splitting, hostility, and fear of abandonment, frequently seen in certain personality states, are similar to the presentation of many individuals with borderline personality disorder (Breuer and Freud 1955, pp. 706–710). Many such individuals also have symptoms that meet criteria for PTSD, with intrusive flashbacks, recurrent dreams of physical and sexual abuse, avoidance of and loss of pleasure in usually pleasurable activities, and symptoms of hyperarousal, especially when exposed to reminders of childhood trauma (Breuer and Freud 1955, pp. 463–468, Kluft 1985, 1991, Spiegel and Cardeñã 1990).

Thus, comorbidity is a complex issue. In addition, these individuals are not infrequently misdiagnosed as having schizophrenia (Kluft 1987). This diagnostic confusion is understandable in that they have an apparent delusion that their bodies are occupied by more than one person. In addition, they frequently have auditory hallucinations when one personality state speaks to or comments on the activities of another. When misdiagnosed as schizophrenic, individuals with DID are frequently given neuroleptics, which results in a poor therapeutic response and a flattening of affect that tends to confirm the misdiagnosis (since flat affect is characteristic of schizophrenia).

Individuals with DID commonly report somatic or conversion symptoms (Ross et al. 1990) and other psychosomatic symptoms, such as migraine headaches (Spiegel 1987). Studies have shown that approximately a third of these individuals have complex partial seizures (Schenk and Bear 1981), although later studies did not show seizure rates that high. Furthermore, the studies did not show substantial elevations in scores on Dissociative Experiences Scale in individuals with complex partial seizures as compared with those of other neurological individuals (Loewenstein and Putnam 1988). However, there is sufficient comorbidity that individuals recently diagnosed with DID should be evaluated for the possibility of a seizure disorder.

Treatment

Psychosocial Treatment

It is possible to help individuals with DID gain control over the dissociative process underlying their symptoms in several ways (Maldonado et al. 2000, Maldonado and Spiegel 2002). The fundamental psychotherapeutic stance should involve meeting persons undergoing treatment halfway, a form of structured empathy in which their experience of themselves as fragmented is acknowledged while the reality that the fundamental problem is a failure of integration of disparate memories and aspects of the self is kept in view. In this sense, such individuals suffer from having less than one personality rather than more than one. Therefore, the goal in therapy is to facilitate integration of disparate elements. This can be done in a variety of ways.

Secrets are frequently a problem with such individuals who attempt to use the clinician to reinforce a dissociative strategy of withholding relevant information from certain personality states. Such individuals often like to confide in the clinician with the idea that the information is to be kept from other parts of the self, for example, traumatic memories or plans for self-destructive activities.

Clear limit setting and commitment on the part of the clinician to helping all portions of the individual's personality structure learn about warded-off information are important. It is wise to clarify explicitly that the clinician will not become involved in secret collusion. Furthermore, when important agreements are negotiated, such as commitments on the part of individuals to seek medical help before acting on a thought to harm themselves or others, it is useful to discuss with the individuals that this is an "all-points bulletin," requiring attention from all the relevant personality states. The excuse that certain personality states were "not aware" of the agreement should not be accepted.

Hypnosis can be helpful in facilitating psychotherapy as well as establishing the diagnosis (Spiegel and Spiegel 1978, Braun 1984, Kluft 1982, Maldonado et al. 2000). First of all, the simple structure of hypnotic induction may elicit dissociative phenomena. Hypnosis can be particularly helpful in facilitating access to dissociated personalities. They may simply occur spontaneously during hypnotic induction. An alternative strategy is to hypnotize the individual and use age regression to reorient to a time when a different personality state was manifest. An instruction later to change times back to the present usually elicits a return to the other personality state. This then becomes a means of teaching such an individual how to control the dissociative process.

Alternatively, entering the state of hypnosis may make it possible simply to address and elicit different identities or personality states. Individuals can be taught a simple self-hypnosis exercise for this purpose. For example, the individual can be told to count to herself or himself from one to three, as was previously described in Clinical Vignette 6. After some formal exercises such as this, it is often possible to ask the individual to speak with a given alter personality, without the formal use of hypnosis. Merely asking to talk with a given identity usually suffices after a while.

Because the loss of memory in DID is complex and chronic (Charcot 1890), its retrieval is likewise a more extended and integral part of the psychotherapeutic process. The therapy becomes an integrating experience of information sharing among disparate personality elements. Conceptualizing DID as a chronic PTSD, the psychotherapeutic strategy involves a focus on working through traumatic memories in addition to controlling the dissociation.

Controlled access to memories greatly facilitates psychotherapy. As with dissociative amnesia, a variety of strategies can be employed to help individuals with DID break down amnesic barriers. Eliciting various identities or personality states can facilitate access to memories previously unavailable to consciousness. While so-called *pseudomemories* can occur (Charcot 1890), previously dissociated traumatic memories are often accurate (Janet 1920).

Once these memories of earlier traumatic experience have been brought into consciousness, it is crucial to help the individual work through the painful affect, inappropriate self-blame, and other reactions to these memories (Spiegel et al. 1982, Lindemann 1944). It may be useful to have individuals visualize the memories rather than relive them as a means of making their intensity more manageable. It can also be useful to have individuals divide the memories, for example, picturing on one side of an imaginary screen something an abuser did to them and on the other side how they tried to protect themselves from the abuse. Such techniques can help make the traumatic memories more bearable by placing them in a broader perspective, one in which trauma victims can also identify adaptive aspects of their response to the trauma.

This and similar approaches can help these individuals work through traumatic memories, enabling them to bear them in consciousness and therefore reducing the need for dissociation as a means of keeping such memories and associated painful affect out of consciousness. Although these techniques can be helpful and often result in reduced fragmentation and integration (Spiegel 1984, 1986a, Kluft 1986), a number of complications can occur in the psychotherapy of these individuals.

The therapeutic process can be thought of as a kind of grief work (Lindemann 1944) in which information retrieved from memory is reviewed, traumatic memories are put into perspective, and emotional expression is encouraged and worked through, thereby making it more possible to endure and disseminate the information as widely as possible among various parts of the individual's personality structure. Instructions to other alter personalities to *listen* while a given one is talking and reviewing previously dissociated material can be helpful.

The psychotherapy of DID can be a time-consuming and emotionally taxing process. The rule of thirds (Kluft 1991, Schacter 1995) is a helpful guideline. Spend the first third of the psychotherapy session assessing the individual's current mental state and life problems and defining a problem area that might benefit from retrieval into conscious memory and working through. Spend the second third of the session accessing and working through this memory. Allow a final third for helping the individual assimilate the information, regulate and modulate emotional responses, and discuss any responses to the psychiatrist and plans for the immediate future. The clinician may resist doing this because the intense abreactive materials are often so compelling and interesting. The individual may also resist sharing information across personalities. Nonetheless, the clinician can be helpful in imposing structure on often chaotic memories and identity states.

Given the intensity of the material that often emerges involving memories of sexual and physical abuse and sudden shifts in mental state accompanied by amnesia, the clinician is called on to take a clear and structured role in managing the psychotherapy. Appropriate limits must be set concerning self-destructive or threatening behavior, agreements must be made regarding physical safety and treatment compliance, and other matters must be presented to the individual in such a way that dissociative ignorance is not an acceptable explanation for failure to live up to the agreements.

Transference applies with special meaning to individuals who have been physically and sexually abused, especially in childhood. They have experienced individuals who are presumed to be caretakers acting instead in an exploitative and sometimes sadistic fashion. They thus expect similar betrayal from mental health clinicians. Although their reality testing is good enough that they can perceive genuine caring, they often unconsciously expect psychiatrists to exploit them. They may experience working through of traumatic memories as a reinflicting of the trauma, with the clinician taking sadistic pleasure in their suffering. They may expect excessive passivity on the part of the clinician identifying the psychiatrist with some uncaring family figure who knew that abuse was occurring but did little or nothing to stop it. It is important in managing the therapy to keep these issues in mind and make them frequent topics of discussion. This can diffuse, if not eliminate, such traumatic transference distortions of the therapeutic relationship (Spiegel 1988).

The ultimate goal of psychotherapy is integration of the individual's multiple ego states. It is often the case that one or more of the personality states may exert considerable resistance to the process of integration, particularly early in the process of therapy. Also, individuals may experience efforts of integration as an attempt on the part of the therapist to "kill" personalities. These fears must be worked through and the individual needs to understand that the goal is to learn how to control the episodes of dissociation. This gives individuals a sense of gradually being able to control their dissociative processes in order to work through the traumatic memories. In order to enhance mastery and control, the process of the psychotherapy must help individuals minimize rather than reinforce the content of traumatic memories, which often involves reexperiencing a sense of helplessness in a symbolic reenactment of the trauma (Freud 1958a, Maldonado et al. 2000).

At the same time, the dissociative defense represents an internalization of the abusive people in the individual's past, a kind of identification with the aggressor, which makes the individual feel powerful rather than helpless. Setting aside the defense also means acknowledging and bearing the helplessness of having been victimized and working through the irrational self-blame that gave such individuals a fantasy of control over events during which they were helpless. Yet, difficult as it is, ultimately the goal of psychotherapy is mastery over the dissociative process, controlled access to dissociative states, integration of warded-off painful memories and material, and a more integrated continuum of identity, memory, and consciousness. Although there have been no controlled trials of the outcome of psychotherapy for this disorder, case series reports indicate a positive outcome in a majority of cases (Kluft 1984b, 1986, 1991).

The stages of therapy are presented in Table 38-1.

Somatic Treatment

As with other dissociative disorders, there is little evidence that psychoactive drugs are of great help in reversing dissociative symptoms (Maldonado et al. 2000). In the past,

Table 38-1	Stages of Therapy
Stage	**Technique**
Establishing treatment	Education, atmosphere of safety, instill confidence
Preliminary interventions	Confirm diagnosis, set limits, access dissociation with hypnosis
History gathering	Explore components of dissociative structure
Working through trauma	Grief work
Move toward integration	Enhance communication across dissociative states
Integration–resolution	Encourage development of integrated self
Learning coping skills	Help with life decisions and relationships
Solidification of gains	Transference examination
Follow-up	Maintenance

Source: Kluft RP (1991) Multiple personality disorder. In *American Psychiatric press Review of Psychiatry*, Vol. 10, Tasman A and Goldfinger SM (eds). American Psychiatric Press, Washington, DC.

short-acting barbiturates such as sodium amobarbital were used intravenously to reverse functional amnesia, but this technique is no longer employed, largely because of poor results (Perry and Jacobs 1982). Research data provide no evidence suggesting that any medication regimen has any significant therapeutic effect on the dissociative process manifested by DID individuals (Loewenstein 1991, Markowitz and Gill 1996, Putnam 1989). To date, pharmacological treatment has been limited to symptom control or the management of comorbid conditions (e.g., depression).

Of all available classes of psychotropic agents, antidepressants are the most useful class for the treatment of individuals with DID. That is because individuals suffering from dissociation frequently experience comorbid dysthymic or major depressive disorder. Selective serotonin reuptake inhibitors (SSRIs) are particularly useful, given their high level of effectiveness, low side effect profile, and even lower danger in overdose, compared to tricyclic antidepressants and monoamine oxidase inhibitors. Nevertheless, medication compliance may be a problem with dissociative individuals because dissociated personality states may interfere with medication taking or may take the medication in an overdose attempt.

Benzodiazepines have mostly been used to facilitate recall by controlling secondary anxiety associated with retrieval of traumatic memories (i.e., medication-facilitated interviews). Nevertheless, despite their short-term usefulness, CNS-depressant agents may cause sudden mental state transitions, which may in turn increase rather than decrease amnesic barriers. Therefore, as useful as they could be on a short-term basis (i.e., acute management of a panic attack), the long term of these agents may, in fact, contribute rather than treat dissociative episodes.

There are several uses for anticonvulsant agents. We know that seizures disorders have a high rate of comorbidity with DID. Thus, anticonvulsant agents may help control the dissociation associated with epileptogenic activity. On the other hand, anticonvulsant agents have proven to be effective in the management of mood disorders, as well as the impulsiveness associated with personality disorders and brain injury. Also, despite their effectiveness, these agents produce less amnestic side effects than the benzodiazepines and thus may be preferred. On the other hand, the need for closer monitoring due to potential toxicity, particularly in overdoses, makes their use less desirable than the newer SSRIs.

Of all pharmacological agents available, antipsychotics may be the less desirable. First, they are rarely useful in reducing dissociative symptoms. In fact, there have been reports of increased levels of dissociation and an increased incidence of side effects when used in individuals suffering from dissociative disorders.

DISSOCIATIVE TRANCE DISORDER

Diagnosis

Dissociative-like phenomena have been described in virtually every culture (Lewis-Fernandez 1994, Katz 1982, Kirmayer 1994). Yet they appear to be more prevalent in the less-heavily industrialized Second and Third World countries. Studies on the prevalence of dissociative disorders in India have suggested that the 1-year prevalence of dissociative trance disorder is approximately 3.5% of all psychiatric hospitalizations, making it a highly frequent mental disorder (Adityanjee et al. 1989, Saxena and Prasad 1989). Trance and possession syndromes are by far the most common type of dissociative disorders seen around the world. On the other hand, DID, which is relatively more common in the United States, is virtually never diagnosed in underdeveloped countries. This difference in prevalence and distribution of dissociative disorder across different populations may be mediated by cultural, as well as biological factors. For example, Eastern culture is far more sociocentric than Western culture. Thus, being "possessed" by an outside entity would be more culturally comprehensible and acceptable in the East. On the other hand, an apparent proliferation of individual identities would fit better with the Western preoccupation with individualism. Nonetheless, the underlying dissociative mechanism inhibiting integration of perception, memory, and identity may suggest a common underlying mechanism amongst these dissociative syndromes.

Trance and possession episodes are usually understood as an idiom of distress and yet they are not viewed as normal. That is, they are not a generally accepted part of cultural and religious practice, which often does involve normal trance phenomena, such as trance dancing in the Balinese Hindu culture. Trance dancers enjoy the remarkable privilege of being the only portion of this socially rigid society able to elevate their social status. The way they are able to do that is by developing the ability to enter trance states. During these altered states of consciousness, which usually occur within the context of a socially acceptable ceremony setting, they dance over hot coals, hold a sword at their throat, or in other ways exhibit supernormal powers of concentration and physical prowess. The mechanism mediating these phenomena is not fully understood, but there is evidence of elevations in plasma noradrenaline, dopamine, and beta-endorphin among Balinese trance dancers during trance states. This form of trance is considered socially normal and even exalted.

By contrast, disordered trance and possession trance are viewed by the local community as an aberrant form of behavior that requires intervention. Such symptoms often arise in the context of family or social distress, for example, discomfort in a new family environment. Thus, cultural informants make it clear that people with dissociative trance disorder are abnormal.

Differences in culture clearly influence almost all mental disorders (Table 38-2). Delusional content of a schizophrenic individual is often dramatically different in a Hindu versus a Christian. Similarly, the manifestations of major depressive disorder may take a different form in China, where it looks more like what used to be called neurasthenia, where it may present with far more somatic symptoms, compared with predominantly guilty ruminations, seen in Western individuals (Kleinman 1977). Similarly, variations in the form and presentation of the various dissociative disorders, depending on the population under study, only underscore the ubiquity of the mechanism of dissociation. The DSM-IV task force voted to include dissociative trance disorder in the DSM-IV Appendix for Criteria Sets Provided For Further Study to stimulate further research on the question of whether it should be a separate Axis I disorder or whether it should be included as a subtype in the category of dissociative disorders not otherwise specified.

Dissociative trance disorder has been divided into two broad categories, dissociative trance and possession trance (American Psychiatric Association 2000) (see DSM-IV-TR research criteria for Dissociative Trance Disorder on page 1045). Dissociative trance phenomena are characterized by a sudden alteration in consciousness, not accompanied by distinct alternative identities. In this form, the dissociative symptom involves an alteration in consciousness rather than identity. Also, in dissociative trance, the activities performed

Table 38-2	Characteristics of Dissociation in Western and Eastern Cultures	
Dissociative Phenomenon	Western	Eastern
Splitting of consciousness	Depersonalization	Dissociative trance
Splitting of identity	DID (multiple personality disorder): multiple internal identities	Possession trance: control by external identities
Splitting of memory	Dissociative amnesia	Secondary in dissociative trance, more common in possession trance
Loss of somatic control	Conversion disorder	Dissociative trance, e.g., *lata, ataque de nervios*
Treatment	Therapist induces dissociation in subject, often with hypnosis	Healer enters trance or dissociative state to take on offending spirit

are rather simple, usually involving sudden collapse, immobilization, dizziness, shrieking, screaming, or crying. Memory is rarely affected, and if there is amnesia, it is fragmented.

DSM-IV-TR Research Criteria

Dissociative Trance Disorder

A. Either (1) or (2):

   (1) trance, i.e., temporary marked alteration in the state of consciousness or loss of customary sense of personal identity without replacement by an alternate identity, associated with at least one of the following:

      (a) narrowing of awareness of immediate surroundings, or unusually narrow and selective focusing on environmental stimuli
      (b) stereotyped behaviors or movements that are experienced as being beyond one's control

   (2) possession trance, a single or episodic alteration in the state of consciousness characterized by the replacement of customary sense of personal identity by a new identity. This is attributed to the influence of a spirit, power, deity, or other person, as evidenced by one (or more) of the following:

      (a) stereotyped and culturally determined behaviors or movements that are experienced as being controlled by the possessing agent
      (b) full or partial amnesia for the event

B. The trance or possession trance state is not accepted as a normal part of a collective cultural or religious practice.
C. The trance or possession trance state causes clinically significant distress or impairment in social, occupational, or other important areas of functioning.
D. The trance or possession trance state does not occur exclusively during the course of a psychotic disorder (including mood disorder with psychotic features and brief psychotic disorder) or dissociative identity disorder, and is not due to the direct physiological effects of a substance or a general medical condition.

Dissociative trance phenomena frequently involve sudden, extreme changes in sensory and motor control. A classic example is the *ataque de nervios*, prevalent in Latin-American countries. For example, this phenomenon is estimated to have a 12% lifetime prevalence rate in Puerto Rico (Lewis-Fernandez 1994). A typical episode involves a sudden feeling of anxiety, followed by total body shakes, which may mimic convulsions. This is then followed by hyperventilation, unintelligible screaming, agitation, and often violent bodily movements. Often, this is followed by collapse and probably transient loss of consciousness. After the episode is over, subjects complain of fatigue and having been confused, although this behavior is dramatically different from classic postictal states. Some subjects may experience amnesia at least to some aspects of the event (Lewis-Fernandez 1994).

Other examples include lata and "falling out." Lata represents the Malay version of trance disorder. In these episodes, afflicted individuals usually experience a sudden vision, mostly of a threatening spirit. The observable behavior includes screaming or crying and physical manifestation of overtly violent behavior that often requires the sufferer to be physically restrained. Individuals often report episodes of amnesia, but there is no clear possession by the offending spirit (Lewis-Fernandez 1994). On the other hand, "falling out" more commonly occurs among African-Americans in the southern United States. Similar to other trance episodes, the affected individual may enter a trance state, followed by bodily collapse, the inability to see or speak, despite the fact that they are fully conscious. Temporary confusion may be observed, although subjects are not usually amnesic to what occurred during the episode (Lewis-Fernandez 1994).

In contrast to dissociative trance episodes, possession trance involves the assumption of a distinct alternative identity. The new identity is presumed to be that of a deity, ancestor, or spirit who has transiently taken possession of the subject's mind and body. Different from dissociative trance episodes, which are characterized by rather crude, simplistic, regressive-like behaviors, possession trance victims often exhibit rather complex behavior. During these episodes, subjects may, for example, express otherwise forbidden thoughts or needs, engage in unusual and uncharacteristic aggressive behavior (e.g., verbal or physical expressions of aggression), or may attempt to negotiate for change in family or social status. Also, in contrast to dissociative trance episodes, possession trance episodes are often followed by dense amnesia for a large portion of the episode during which the spirit identity was in control of the subject's behavior.

Treatment

Treatment of these disorders varies from culture to culture. Rubbing the body with special potions, negotiating to change the affected person's social circumstances, and physical restraint are often used. Ceremonies to remove or appease the invading spirit are also employed.

Comparison of DSM-IV-TR/ICD-10 Diagnostic Criteria

The ICD-10 Diagnostic Criteria for Research for dissociative amnesia specify that there be a "convincing association in time between the onset of symptoms of the disorder and stressful events, problems, or needs." In DSM-IV-TR, the criteria set notes that the forgotten information is usually of a stressful or traumatic nature.

For dissociative fugue, in contrast to DSM-IV-TR, the ICD-10 Diagnostic Criteria for Research specify "amnesia for the journey." Furthermore, in contrast to DSM-IV-TR, the ICD-10 Diagnostic Criteria for Research do not indicate that there is an inability to recall one's past during the fugue or that there be confusion about personal identity.

Dissociative identity disorder is included in ICD-10 as an example of an "other dissociative (conversion) disorder" under the rubric "multiple personality disorder." The ICD-10 Diagnostic Criteria for Research and the DSM-IV-TR criteria are almost identical.

Finally, ICD-10 has a single category "depersonalization–derealization syndrome" for presentations characterized by either depersonalization or derealization. In contrast, the DSM-IV-TR category includes only depersonalization and mentions derealization as an associated feature. Furthermore, unlike DSM-IV-TR that includes this category in the dissociative disorders section, ICD-10 includes the category within the "other neurotic disorders" grouping.

References

Adityanjee R, Raju GSP, and Khandelwal SK (1989) Current status of multiple personality disorder in India. *Am J Psychiatry* **146**, 1607–1610.

American Psychiatric Association (1994) *Diagnostic and Statistical Manual of Mental Disorders.* 4th ed., APA, Washington, DC.

American Psychiatric Association (2000) *Diagnostic and Statistical Manual of Mental Disorders.* 4th ed., Text Rev. APA, Washington, DC.

Baron DA and Nagy R (1988) The amobarbital interview in a general hospital setting, friend or foe: a case report. *Gen Hosp Psychiatry* **10**, 220–222.

Berger D, Saito S, Ono Y, et al. (1994) Dissociation and child abuse histories in an eating disorder cohort in Japan. *Acta Psychiatr Scand* **90**, 274–280.

Bernstein EM and Putnam FW (1986) Development, reliability, and validity of a dissociation scale. *J Nerv Ment Dis* **174**, 727–735.

Boe T, Haslerud J, and Knudsen H (1993) Multiple personality: a phenomenon also in Norway? *Tidsskr Nor Laegeforen* **113**, 3230–3232.

Boon S and Draijer N (1993) Multiple personality disorder in the Netherlands: a clinical investigation of 71 patients. *Am J Psychiatry* **150**, 489–494.

Braun BG (1984) Uses of hypnosis with multiple personality. *Psychiatr Ann* **14**, 34–40.

Braun BG and Sachs RG (1985) The development of multiple personality predisposing, precipitating, and perpetuating factors. In *Childhood Antecedents of Multiple Personality.* Kluft RP (ed.). American Psychiatric Press, Washington, DC, pp. 37–64.

Brenner I (1994) The dissociative character: a reconsideration of "multiple personality". *J Am Psychoanal Assoc* **42**, 819–846.

Brenner I (1996) The characterological basis of multiple personality. *Am J Psychother* **50**, 154–166.

Breuer J and Freud S (1955) Studies on hysteria. In *The Standard Edition of the Complete Psychological Works of Sigmund Freud*, Vol. 2, Strachey J (trans-ed). Hogarth Press, London, pp. 183–251. (Originally published in 1895).

Brown L, Russell J, Thornton C, et al. (1999) Dissociation, abuse and the eating disorders: evidence from an Australian population. *Aust N Z J Psychiatry* **33**(4), 521–528.

Carlson EB, Putnam FW, Ross CA, et al. (1993) Validity of the dissociative experiences scale in screening for multiple personality disorder: a multicenter study. *Am J Psychiatr* **150**, 1030–1036.

Charcot JM (1890) *Oeuvres Complets de JM Charcot*, Vol. 11, Lecrosnier et Babe, Paris.

Chu JA and Dill DL (1990) Dissociative symptoms in relation to childhood physical and sexual abuse. *Am J Psychiatry* **147**, 887–892.

Coons PM (1984) The differential diagnosis of multiple personality. *Psychiatr Clin North Am* **12**, 51–67.

Coons PM and Milstein V (1986) Psychosexual disturbances in multiple personality: characteristics, etiology, treatment. *J Clin Psychiatry* **47**, 106–110.

Coons PM, Bowman ES, and Milstein V (1988) Multiple personality disorder: a clinical investigation of 50 cases. *J Nerv Ment Dis* **176**, 519–527.

Draijer N and Langeland W (1999) Childhood trauma and perceived parental dysfunction in the etiology of dissociative symptoms in psychiatric inpatients. *Am J Psychiatry* **156**(3), 379–385.

Eriksson NG and Lundin T (1996) Early traumatic stress reactions among Swedish survivors of the Estonia disaster. *Br J Psychiatry* **169**, 713–716.

Frankel FH (1990) Hypnotizability and dissociation. *Am J Psychiatry* **147**, 823–829.

Freud S (1958a) Psycho-analytic notes on an autobiographical account of a case of paranoia (dementia paranoides). In *The Standard Edition of the Complete Psychological Works of Sigmund Freud*, Vol. 12, Strachey J (trans-ed). Hogarth Press, London, pp. 3–82. (Originally published in 1911).

Friedl MC and Draijer N (2000) Dissociative disorders in Dutch psychiatric inpatients. *Am J Psychiatry* **157**(6), 1012–1013.

Frischholz EJ (1985) The relationship among dissociation, hypnosis, and child abuse in the development of multiple personality. In *Childhood Antecedents of Multiple Personality*, Kluft RP (ed.). American Psychiatric Press, Washington, DC, pp. 100–126.

Ganaway GK (1989) Historical versus narrative truth: clarifying the role of exogenous trauma in the etiology of MPD and its variants. *Dissociation* **2**, 205–220.

Ganaway GK (1995) Hypnosis, childhood trauma, and dissociative identity disorder: toward an integrative theory. *Int J Clin Exp Hypn* **43**, 127–144.

Herman JL, Perry JC, and Van der Kolk BA (1989) Childhood trauma in borderline personality disorder. *Am J Psychiatry* **146**, 490–495.

Hoffman RE (1987) Computer simulations of neural information processing and the schizophrenia/mania dichotomy. *Arch Gen Psychiatry* **44**, 178–187.

Horen SA, Leichner PP, and Lawson JS (1995) Prevalence of dissociative symptoms and disorders in an adult psychiatric inpatient population in Canada. *Can J Psychiatry* **40**, 185–191.

Horevitz RP and Braun BG (1984) Are multiple personalities borderline? *Psychiatr Clin North Am* **7**, 69–87.

James W (1984) *William James on Exceptional Mental States. The 1896 Lowell Lectures*, Taylor E (ed.). The University of Massachusetts Press, Amherst, MA.

Janet P (1920) *The Major Symptoms of Hysteria*. Macmillan, New York, p. 332.

Kardiner A and Spiegel H (1947) *War, Stress, and Neurotic Illness*. Hoeber, New York.

Katz R (1982) *Boiling Energy: Community Healing Among the Kalahari Kung*. Harvard University Press, Cambridge, MA.

Kihlstrom JF (1987) The cognitive unconscious. *Science* **237**, 1445–1452.

Kirmayer KJ (1994) Pacing the void: social and cultural dimensions of dissociation. In *Dissociation: Culture, Mind and Body*, Spiegel D (ed.). American Psychiatric Press, Washington, DC, pp. 91–122.

Kleinman A (1977) Depression, somatization and the "new cross-cultural psychiatry". *Soc Sci Med* **11**, 3–10.

Kluft RP (1982) Varieties of hypnotic intervention in the treatment of multiple personality. *Am J Clin Hypn* **24**, 230–240.

Kluft RP (1984a) Multiple personality in childhood. *Psychiatr Clin North Am* **7**, 121–134.

Kluft RP (1984b) Treatment of multiple personality disorder: a study of 33 cases. *Psychiatr Clin North Am* **7**, 9–29.

Kluft RP (1985) The natural history of multiple personality disorder. In *Childhood Antecedents of Multiple Personality*. Kluft RP (ed.). American Psychiatric Press, Washington, DC, pp. 197–238.

Kluft RP (1986) Personality unification in multiple personality disorder: a follow-up study. In *Treatment of Multiple Personality Disorder*. Braun BG (ed.). American Psychiatric Press, Washington, DC, pp. 29–60.

Kluft RP (1987) First rank symptoms as diagnostic indicators of multiple personality disorder. *Am J Psychiatry* **144**, 293–298.

Kluft RP (1991) Multiple personality disorder. In *American Psychiatric Press Review of Psychiatry*, Vol. 10, Tasman A and Goldfinger SM (eds). American Psychiatric Press, Washington, DC, pp. 161–188.

Kosslyn SM and Koenig O (1992) *Wet Mind: The New Cognitive Neuroscience*. Free Press, New York.

Lavoie G and Sabourin M (1980) Hypnosis and schizophrenia: a review of experimental and clinical studies. In *Handbook of Hypnosis and Psychosomatic Medicine*. Burrows GD and Dennerstein L (eds). Elsevier/North-Holland Biomedical Press, New York, pp. 377–419.

Lewis-Fernandez R (1994) Culture and dissociation: A comparison of ataque de nervios among Puerto Ricans and "possession syndrome" in India. In *Dissociation: Culture, Mind and Body*, Spiegel D (ed.). American Psychiatric Press, Washington, DC, pp. 123–167.

Li D and Spiegel D (1992) A neural network model of dissociative disorders. *Psychiatr Ann* **22**, 144–147.

Lindemann E (1944) Symptomatology and management of acute grief. *Am J Psychiatry* **101**, 141–148.

Loewenstein RJ (1991) Psychogenic amnesia and psychogenic fugue: a comprehensive review. In *American Psychiatric Press Review of Psychiatry*, Vol. 10, Tasman A and Goldfinger SM (eds). American Psychiatric Press, Washington, DC, pp. 189–222.

Loewenstein RJ and Putnam FW (1988) A comparative study of dissociative symptoms in patients with complex partial seizures, multiple personality disorder, and posttraumatic stress disorder. *Dissociation* **1**, 17–23.

Maldonado JR and Spiegel D (2003) Dissociative disorders. In *The American Psychiatric Publishing Textbook of Clinical Psychiatry*, 4th edition, Hales RE and Yudofsky SC (eds). American Psychiatric Press, Washington, DC, pp. 709–742.

Maldonado JR, Butler LD, and Spiegel D (2000) Treatment of dissociative disorders. In *Treatments that Work*. Nathan P and Gorman JM (eds). Oxford University Press, New York, pp. 463–496.

Markowitz JS and Gill HS (1996) Pharmacotherapy of dissociative identity disorder. *Ann Pharmacother* **30**, 1498–1499.

McHugh PR (1995a) Dissociative identity disorder as a socially constructed artifact. *J Pract Psychiatr Behav Health* **1**, 158–166.

McHugh PR (1995b) Witches, multiple personalities, and other psychiatric artifacts. *Nat Med* **1**, 110–114.

Mezzich JE, Fabrega H, Coffman GA, et al. (1989) DSM-III disorders in a large sample of psychiatric patients: frequency and specificity of diagnoses. *Am J Psychiatry* **146**, 212–219.

Milner B (1959) The memory defect in bilateral hippocampal lesions. *Psychiatr Res Rep* **11**, 42–52.

Modestin J, Ebner G, Junghan M, et al. (1996) Dissociative experiences and dissociative disorders in acute psychiatric inpatients. *Compr Psychiatr* **37**(5), 355–361.

Naples M and Hackett T (1978) The Amytal interview: history and current uses. *Psychosomatics* **19**, 98–105.

Nuller YL (1982) Depersonalization: symptoms, meaning, therapy. *Acta Psychiatr Scand* **66**, 451–458.

Ogata S, Silk K, Goodrich S, et al. (1990) Childhood sexual and physical abuse in adult patients with borderline personality disorder. *Am J Psychiatr* **147**, 1008–1013.

Perry JC and Jacobs DJ (1982) Overview: clinical applications of the Amytal interview in psychiatry emergency settings. *Am J Psychiatr* **139**, 552–559.

Pettinati HM (1982) Measuring hypnotizability in psychotic patients. *Int J Clin Exp Hypn* **30**, 404–416.

Pettinati HM, Kogan LG, Evans FJ, et al. (1990) Hypnotizability of psychiatric inpatients according to two different scales. *Am J Psychiatr* **147**, 69–75.

Pies R (1991) Depersonalization's many faces. *Psychiatr Times* **8**(4), 27–28.

Putnam FW (1985) Dissociation as a response to extreme trauma. In *Childhood Antecedents of Multiple Personality*, Kluft RP (ed.). American Psychiatric Press, Washington, DC, pp. 65–97.

Putnam FW (1989) *Diagnosis and Treatment of Multiple Personality Disorder*. Guilford Press, New York.

Putnam FW, Guroff JJ, Silberman ED, et al. (1986) The clinical phenomenology of multiple personality disorder: review of 100 recent cases. *J Clin Psychiatr* **47**, 285–293.

Reither AM and Stoudemire A (1988) Psychogenic fugue states: a review. *South Med J* **81**, 568–571.

Ronquillo EB (1991) The influence of "espiritismo" on a case of multiple personality disorder. *Dissociation* **4**, 39–45.

Ross CA (1989) *Multiple Personality Disorder: Diagnosis, Clinical Features, and Treatment*. John Wiley, New York.

Ross CA (1991) Epidemiology of multiple personality disorder and dissociation. *Psychiatr Clin North Am* **14**, 503–518.

Ross CA, Anderson G, Fleisher WP, et al. (1991a) The frequency of multiple personality disorder among psychiatry inpatients. *Am J Psychiatry* **148**, 1717–1720.

Ross CA, Joshi S, and Currie R (1991b) Dissociative experiences in the general population: a factor analysis. *Hosp Comm Psychiatry* **42**, 297–301.

Ross CA, Miller SD, Reagor P, et al. (1990) Structured interview data on 102 cases of multiple personality disorder from four centers. *Am J Psychiatr* **147**, 596–601.

Rumelhart DE and McClelland JL (1986) *Parallel Distributed Processing: Explorations in the Microstructure of Cognition*. The MIT Press, Cambridge, MA.

Sar V, Tutkun H, Alyanak B, et al. (2000) Frequency of dissociative disorders among psychiatric outpatients in Turkey. *Compr Psychiatry* **41**(3), 216–222.

Saxe GN, van der Kolk BA, Berkowitz R, et al. (1993) Dissociative disorders in psychiatric patients. *Am J Psychiatry* **150**, 1037–1042.

Saxena S and Prasad K (1989) DSM-III subclassification of dissociative disorders applied to psychiatric outpatients in India. *Am J Psychiatry* **146**, 261–262.

Schacter D (1992) Understanding implicit memory: a cognitive neuroscience approach. *Am Psychol* **47**, 559–569.

Schacter DL (1995) Memory distortion: History and current status. In *Memory Distortion: How Minds, Brains, and Societies Reconstruct the Past*. Schacter DL (ed.). Harvard University Press, Cambridge, MA, pp. 1–42.

Schenk L and Bear D (1981) Multiple personality and related dissociative phenomena in patients with temporal lobe epilepsy. *Am J Psychiatry* **138**, 1311–1316.

Schultz R, Braun BG, and Kluft RP (1989) Multiple personality disorder: phenomenology of selected variables in comparison to major depression. *Dissociation* **2**, 45–51.

Scroppo JC, Drob SL, Weinberger JL, et al. (1998) Identifying dissociative identity disorder: a self-report and projective study. *J Abnorm Psychol* **107**(2), 272–284.

Spanos NP, Weekes JR, and Bertrand LD (1985) Multiple personality: a social psychological perspective. *J Abnorm Psychol* **94**, 362–376.

Spanos NP, Weekes JR, Menary E, et al. (1986) Hypnotic interview and age regression procedures in elicitation of multiple personality symptoms: a simulation study. *Psychiatry* **49**, 298–311.

Spiegel D (1981) Vietnam grief work using hypnosis. *Am J Clin Hypn* **24**, 33–40.

Spiegel D (1984) Multiple personality as a posttraumatic stress disorder. *Psychiatr Clin North Am* **7**, 101–110.

Spiegel D (1986a) Dissociating damage. *Am J Clin Hypn* **29**, 123–131.

Spiegel D (1987) Chronic pain masks depression, multiple personality disorder. *Hosp Comm Psychiatry* **38**, 933–935.

Spiegel D (1988) The treatment accorded those who treat patients with multiple personality disorder. *J Nerv Ment Dis* **176**, 535–536.

Spiegel D and Cardenã E (1990) New uses of hypnosis in the treatment of posttraumatic stress disorder. *J Clin Psychiatry* **51**(Suppl.), 39–43.

Spiegel D and Cardenã E (1991) Disintegrated experience: the dissociative disorders revisited. *J Abnorm Psychol* **100**, 366–378.

Spiegel D and Fink R (1979) Hysterical psychosis and hypnotizability. *Am J Psychiatry* **136**, 777–781.

Spiegel D, Detrick D, and Frischholz EJ (1982) Hypnotizability and psychopathology. *Am J Psychiatry* **139**, 431–437.

Spiegel D, Frischholz EJ, and Spira J (1993) Functional Disorders of Memory. In *American Psychiatric Press Review of Psychiatry*, Vol. 12, Oldham JM, Riba MB, and Tasman A (eds). American Psychiatric Press, Washington, DC, pp. 747–782.

Spiegel D, Hunt T, and Dondershine H (1988) Dissociation and hypnotizability in posttraumatic stress disorder. *Am J Psychiatry* **145**, 301–305.

Spiegel H (1974) The grade 5 syndrome: the highly hypnotizable person. *Int J Clin Exp Hypn* **22**, 303–319.

Spiegel H and Spiegel D (1978) *Trance and Treatment: Clinical Uses of Hypnosis*. Basic Books, New York, pp. 13–14; Copyright 1978 HarperCollins Publishers. Reprinted 1987. American Psychiatric Press., Washington DC.

Squire LR (1987) *Memory and Brain*. Oxford University Press, New York.

Stein MB and Uhde TW (1989) Depersonalization disorder: effects of caffeine and response to pharmacotherapy. *Biol Psychiatry* **26**, 315–320.

Steinberg M (1991) The spectrum of depersonalization: Assessment and treatment. In *American Psychiatric Press Review of Psychiatry*, Vol. 10, Tasman A and Goldfinger SM (eds). American Psychiatric Press, Washington, DC, pp. 223–247.

Steinberg M, Rounsaville B, and Ciucchetti D (1990) The structured clinical interview for DSM-III-R dissociative disorders: preliminary report on a new diagnostic instrument. *Am J Psychiatry* **147**, 76–81.

Terr LC (1991) Childhood traumas: an outline and overview. *Am J Psychiatry* **148**, 10–20.

Tulving E (1983) *Elements of Episodic Memory*. Clarendon Press, Oxford.

Van der Hart O (2001) Generalized dissociative amnesia: episodic, semantic and procedural memories lost and found. *Aust. N Z J Psychiatry* **35**, 589–600.

Van der Hart O and Spiegel D (1993) Hypnotic assessment and treatment of trauma-induced psychoses. *Int J Clin Exp Hypn* **41**, 191–209.

Van der Hart O, Brown P, and Van der Kolk BA (1989) Pierre Janet's treatment of posttraumatic stress. *J Traum Stress* **2**, 379–396.

Vanderlinden J, Van Dyck R, Vandereycken W, et al. (1991) Dissociative experiences in the general population of the Netherlands and Belgium: a study with the dissociative questionnaire (DIS-Q). *Dissociation* **4**, 180–184.

Wittkower ED (1970) Transcultural psychiatry in the Caribbean: past, present and future. *Am J Psychiatry* **127**, 162–166.

Zola-Morgan S and Squire LR (1985) Medial temporal lesions in monkeys impair memory in a variety of tasks sensitive to human amnesia. *Behav Neurosci* **99**, 22–34.

Zola-Morgan S, Squire LR, and Mishkin M (1982) The neuroanatomy of amnesia: Amygdala-hippocampus vs. temporal stem. *Science* **218**, 1337–1339.

An adult's sexuality has seven components—gender identity, orientation, intention (what one wants to do with a partner's body and have done with one's body during sexual behavior), desire, arousal, orgasm, and emotional satisfaction (Levine 1989). The first three components constitute our sexual identity. The second three comprise our sexual function. The seventh, emotional satisfaction, is based on our personal reflections on the first six. The DSM-IV-TR designates impairments of five of these components as pathologies. Variations in orientation and the failure to find ordinary sexual experience emotionally satisfying, although problems for some, are not designated as *disorders* (see Figure 39-1 for a diagnostic decision tree covering the sexual disorders).

While the psychological foundations for a healthy sexual life are laid down during childhood through parent–child relationships, each subsequent phase of life—adolescence, young adulthood, middle-life, and older age—has inherent developmental challenges and potentials. The normal tasks of sexual development at each phase provide the clinician with an understanding of age-related etiologies of sexual disorders (Levine 1992). Adolescent sexual troubles often reflect difficulties consolidating a personally acceptable sexual identity. Young adult dysfunctions often indicate the presence of psychological obstacles to growing comfortable as a sexual pleasure-seeking, pleasure-giving person while integrating sex into the larger context of human attachment. Middle-life disorders often represent failures to maintain psychological intimacy and to diplomatically negotiate tensions within an increasingly complex interpersonal relationship. The dysfunctions of older persons often represent failures to preserve sexual function in the face of biological assaults of menopause, aging, illness, medications, radiation, and surgery. Most etiologic factors can operate in another epoch as well. For instance, a young person's new indifference to sexual behavior may be due to an SSRI or an older person's new marriage may expose previously avoided personal discomfort with receiving and giving sexual pleasure.

THE SEXUAL DYSFUNCTIONS

While sex is widely thought of as recreation, psychiatrists recognize it as an important means of establishing and reaffirming emotional attachments. Sexual competence—the ability to desire a partner, become aroused, and attain orgasm in a cooperative manner

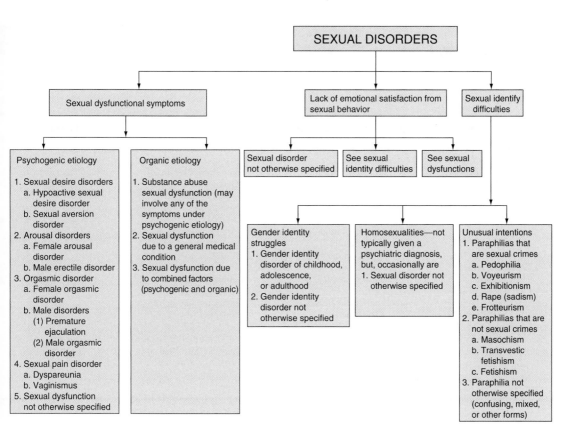

Figure 39-1 *Diagnostic decision tree for sexual disorders.*

when together—is a valuable developmental accomplishment because it enables a person to experience the physical expressions and emotional complexities of love. Mutually pleasurable sexual behavior tends to recur far more often in couples than unilaterally satisfying behavior. Mutually pleasurable sexual behavior allows both partners to be comforted and stabilized by loving and feeling loved. The dysfunctions are symptomatic deficits in the quest for these widespread ideals: sexual competence, fun, and stabilization of the self.

DSM-IV-TR specifies three criteria for each sexual dysfunction (American Psychiatric Association 1994). The first criterion describes the psychophysiologic impairment—for example, absence of sexual desire, arousal, or orgasm. The second and third criteria are the same for each impairment: the dysfunction causes marked distress or interpersonal difficulty and the dysfunction is not better accounted for by another Axis I diagnosis or not due exclusively to the direct physiological effects of a substance (e.g., a drug of abuse, a medication) or a general medical condition. Table 39-1 lists the first criterion of each of the 12 sexual dysfunction diagnoses. DSM-IV-TR gives the clinician additional latitude for deciding when a person who meets the first criterion qualifies for a disorder. The clinician is asked to consider the effects of the individual's age, experience, ethnicity and cultural background, the degree of subjective distress, adequacy of sexual stimulation, and symptom frequency. No instructions are provided about how to exercise this judgment. In this way, DSM-IV-TR makes it clear that understanding sexual life requires more than counting symptoms; it requires judgment.

Table 39-1   **Delineating Criteria of 12 Sexual Dysfunction Diagnoses**

Sexual Desire Disorders	Sexual Arousal Disorders	Orgasmic Disorders	Sexual Pain Disorders
Hypoactive sexual desire disorder: persistently or recurrently deficient (or absent) sexual fantasies and desire for sexual activity	Female sexual arousal disorder: persistent or recurrent inability to attain, or to maintain until completion of the sexual activity, an adequate lubrication–swelling response of sexual excitement	Female orgasmic disorder: persistent or recurrent delay in, or absence of, orgasm after a normal sexual excitement phase	Dyspareunia: recurrent or persistent genital pain associated with sexual intercourse in either a male or a female
Sexual aversion disorder: persistent or recurrent extreme aversion to, and avoidance of, all (or almost all) genital sexual contact with a sexual partner	Male erectile disorder: persistent or recurrent inability to attain, or to maintain until completion of the sexual activity, an adequate erection	Male orgasmic disorder: persistent or recurrent delay in, or absence of, orgasm after a normal sexual excitement phase during sexual activity	Vaginismus: recurrent or persistent involuntary spasm of the musculature of the outer third of the vagina that interferes with sexual intercourse
Sexual Dysfunction Due to a General Medical Condition Any of the above-mentioned diagnoses must be judged to be exclusively due to the direct physiological effects of a medical condition	**Substance-Induced Sexual Dysfunction** A sexual dysfunction that is fully explained by substance use in that it develops within a month of substance intoxication	Premature ejaculation: persistent or recurrent ejaculation with a minimal sexual stimulation before, on, or shortly after penetration and before the person wishes it	
		Sexual Dysfunction Not Otherwise Specified For problems that do not meet the categories just described	

Epidemiology

Numerous attempts to describe the prevalence of sexual dysfunction have been made in the past 25 years. These range from attempts to define the frequency of a particular dysfunction, for instance male erectile disorder, to attempts to estimate the prevalence of a series of separate dysfunction—for example, desire, arousal, and orgasmic disorders of women. All such efforts quickly confront methodological influences of sampling, means of obtaining the information, definition of each dysfunction, purpose of the study, and perspective of its authors (Laumann and Michael 2001). These data not surprisingly, therefore, demonstrate a range of prevalence depending on the problem studied. Gender identity disorders are relatively rare (<1–2%). Lifelong sexual desire disorders among women may involve 15% but are less frequent among men. Acquired desire disorders among older individuals are probably three times as common. Perhaps more than half of women at age 55 years have recognized a deterioration in their sexual function. Perhaps 25% of women in their twenties have difficulty having orgasm and 33% of men less than age 40 claim to ejaculate too rapidly. The majority of men by age 70 years are likely to be having erection problems. The recent careful epidemiologic study, designed by sociologists, successfully generated a representative sample of the US (Laumann et al. 1994a). They interviewed men and women between age 18 and 59 years and found that sexual dysfunction is common, particularly among young women and older men. This is noteworthy for psychiatrists because our studies of sexual dysfunction caused by medications or acquired psychiatric disorders tend to assume that individuals are generally functionally intact prior to becoming ill or taking medications. This assumption is not tenable on the basis of a generation of epidemiologic studies.

Etiology

Etiologic ideas about sexual dysfunction are a relatively simple conceptual challenge involving notions about the individual's psychology and his or her cultural expectations. In contrast, for couples, they involve two individual psychologies, their interpersonal impact on one another, and their cultures. The clinician must be wary when one coupled person is presented as having a sexual dysfunction and the partner is presented as *normal*. Sexual dysfunction in a couple is a two-person problem in terms of immediate effects and often in terms of cause as well. How a partner regards the sexual characteristics of the other is a subtle ingredient of sexual comfort, competence, and dysfunction. For instance, a young woman's new inability to attain orgasm with her husband may be traced to her embarrassment at sharing her excitation with him because she perceives him to be generally critical of her. Similarly, the origin of a husband's erectile dysfunction may be traced to the emergence of his wife's negative regard for him, which stemmed from something other than his sexual behavior. This *ordinary* connectivity of a couple's sexual function is referred to as the couple's sexual equilibrium (Levine 1998a). The sexual equilibrium explains five observations: (1) improvement and deterioration of sexual function can rapidly occur; (2) when a couple's nonsexual relationship is good, their sexual life may not be; (3) individual psychotherapy is often insufficient to help coupled individuals improve their sexual life; (4) a negative attitude from the partner can block improvement in a couple's sexual life regardless of the therapy format and therapist skill; and (5) a conversation with a therapist who is attuned to the emotional meanings of a couple's interaction can shift a dysfunctional equilibrium back to mutually satisfying sexual behavior.

The Problems of Sexual Desire

Sexual desire manifestations are diverse: erotic fantasies, sexual dreams, initiation of sexual behavior, receptivity to partner-initiated sexual behavior, masturbation, genital sensations, heightened responsivity to erotic environmental cues, and sincere statements about wanting to behave sexually. For most of the twentieth century, these have been referred to as manifestations of libido. Psychiatrists spoke of libido as if it was a homogeneous instinctive force. Clinicians will find it far more useful to conceptualize that the diverse and changeable desire manifestations are produced by the intersection of three mental forces: drive (biology), motive (psychology), and wish (culture).

Drive   By only partially understood psychoneuroendocrine mechanisms, the preoptic area of the anterior-medial hypothalamus and the limbic system periodically produce sexual drive. *Drive* is recognized by genital tingling, heightened responsivity to erotic environmental cues, plans for self or partner sexual behavior, nocturnal orgasm, and increased erotic preoccupations. These are often spontaneous. Although people can become aroused and attain orgasm without evident drive, it propels the entire sexual psychophysiological process. Without drive, the sexual response system is far less efficient and capable. While men as a group seem to have significantly more drive than women as a group, in both sexes, drive requires the presence of a modest amount of testosterone. Drive is frequently dampened by medications that act within the central nervous system, substances of abuse, psychiatric illness, systemic physical illness, despair, and aging. It is heightened by low doses of a few often-abused substances such as alcohol or amphetamine, manic mechanisms, falling in love, joy, and some dopaminergic compounds such as those used to treat Parkinson's disease.

Motive   The psychological aspect of desire is referred to as *motive* and is recognized by willingness to bring one's body to the partner for sexual behavior either through initiation or receptivity. Motive often directly stems from the person's perception of the context of the nonsexual and sexual relationship. Sexual desire diagnoses are often made in persons who have adequate drive manifestations. Most sexual desire problems in physically healthy adults are simply generated by one partner's *unwillingness* to engage in sexual behavior. This is often a secret, however. Sexual motives are originally programmed by social and cultural experiences. Children and adolescents acquire values, beliefs, expectations, and rules for sexual expression. Young people have to find a way to negotiate their way through the fact that their early motives to behave sexually frequently coexist with their motives *not* to engage in sexual behavior. Conflicted motives often persist throughout life but the reasons for the conflict evolve. A teenager possessed of considerable drive and motive to make love may inhibit all sexual activities because of moral considerations emanating from religious education or the sense that he or she is just not developmentally ready yet.

Wish   An 80-year-old man who had no drive manifestations and had avoided all sexual contact with his wife for a decade because he could not get an erection, passionately answered a doctor's query about his sexual desire, "Of course, I have sexual desire! I am a red-blooded American male! Why do you think I am here?" In fact, he was only speaking about his wish to be sexually capable now that an effective treatment for erectile problems existed. The doctor asked an imprecise question. The doctor should have separately explored his drive manifestations, his sexual motivation to exchange sexual pleasure with his wife in recent years, and his wish for sexual rejuvenation.

The appearance and disappearance of sexual desire is often enigmatic to an individual, but its ebb and flow result from the ever-changing intensities of its components, biological *drive*, psychological *motive*, and socially acquired concepts, *wish* (Table 39-2) (Levine 2002). In women, this interplay is generally more difficult to delineate because drive and motive are sometimes inseparable (Basson 2003).

Sexual Desire Diagnoses

Two official diagnoses are given to men and women whose desires for partner sexual behavior are deficient: hypoactive sexual desire disorder (HSDD) (see DSM-IV-TR diagnostic criteria on page 1057) and sexual aversion disorder (SAD) (see DSM-IV-TR diagnostic

Table 39-2	Three Interactive Components of Sexual Desire

Sexual Drive — Biological Component
Evolves over time, decreasing with increasing age
Diminished by many psychotropic and antihypertensive medications
Manifested by the internally stimulated genital sensations and thoughts of sexual behavior that
  occur within a person's privacy

Sexual Motivation — Psychological Component
Highly contextual in terms of relationship status
The most socially and psychologically responsive of the three components
Evolves over time but not predictably
Manifested by a person's willingness to bring his or her body to a specific person for sexual
  behavior

Sexual Wish — Social Component
Expectations for sexual behavior based on membership in various subcultural groups such as
  family, religion, gender, region, and nation
These expectations begin as cognitions of what is right and wrong and what a person is entitled to
  sexually and are influenced by what people think others in their cohort are experiencing
Often clinically difficult to distinguish from motivation, which wishes influence

criteria on page 1057). The differences between the two revolve around the emotional intensity with which the individual avoids sexual behavior. When visceral anxiety, fear, or disgust is routinely felt as sexual behavior becomes a possibility, sexual aversion is diagnosed. HSDD is far more frequently encountered. It is present in at least twice as many women than men; female to male ratio for aversion is far higher (Kaplan 1987). Like all sexual dysfunctions, the desire diagnoses may be lifelong or may have been acquired after a period of ordinary fluctuations of sexual desire. Acquired disorders may be partner specific (*situational*) or may occur with all subsequent partners (*generalized*).

DSM-IV-TR Diagnostic Criteria

302.71 Hypoactive Sexual Desire Disorder

A. Persistently or recurrently deficient (or absent) sexual fantasies and desire for sexual activity. The judgment of deficiency or absence is made by the clinician, taking into account factors that affect sexual functioning, such as age and the context of the person's life.
B. The disturbance causes marked distress or interpersonal difficulty.
C. The sexual dysfunction is not better accounted for by another Axis I disorder (except another sexual dysfunction) and is not due exclusively to the direct physiological effects of a substance (e.g., a drug of abuse, a medication) or a general medical condition.

Specify type:

Lifelong type

Acquired type

Specify type:

Generalized type

Situational type

Specify:

Due to psychological factors

Due to combined factors

Reprinted with permission from the Diagnostic and Statistical Manual of Mental Disorders, Fourth Edition, Text Revision. Copyright 2000 American Psychiatric Association.

DSM-IV-TR Diagnostic Criteria

302.79 Sexual Aversion Disorder

A. Persistent or recurrent extreme aversion to, and avoidance of, all (or almost all) genital sexual contact with a sexual partner.

B. The disturbance causes marked distress or interpersonal difficulty.

C. The sexual dysfunction is not better accounted for by another Axis I disorder (except another sexual dysfunction).

Specify type:

Lifelong type

Acquired type

Specify type:

Generalized type

Situational type

Specify:

Due to psychological factors

Due to combined factors

When the clinician concludes that the individual's acquired generalized HSDD is either due to a medical condition, a medication, or a substance of abuse, the diagnosis is further elaborated to sexual dysfunction due to general medical condition (for instance, HSDD due to multiple sclerosis). The frequency of the specific etiologies are heavily dependent on the clinical setting. In oncology settings, medical causes occur in high frequency; in drug rehabilitation programs, methadone maintenance will be a common cause. In marital therapy clinics, anger and loss of respect for the partner, hidden incompatibility of sexual identity between the self and the partner because of covert homosexuality or paraphilia, an affair, or childhood sexual abuse will commonly be the basis. In general mental health settings, medication side effects will often be the top layer of several causes. When a major depression disorder is diagnosed, for instance, the desire disorder is often assumed to be a symptom of the depression. This usually is incorrect. The desire disorder often preceded the decompensation into depression.

Those with *lifelong* deficiencies of sexual desire are often perceived to be struggling with either: (1) sexual identity issues involving gender identity, orientation, or a paraphilia; (2) having failed to grow comfortable as a sexual person due to extremely conservative cultural backgrounds, developmental misfortunes, or abuses. Occasionally the etiology is enigmatic, raising the important question whether it is possible to never have any sexual drive manifestations on a biological basis. (Theoretically, the answer is yes.) Both acquired and lifelong desire disorders are often associated with past or chronic mood disorders. Disorders of desire are often listed as "of unknown etiology" (Rosen and Leiblum 1995), but clinicians should be skeptical of this idea because: (1) the individual may not tell the clinician the truth early in the relationship; (2) the individual may have strong defenses against knowing the truth; (3) the individual may not be able to speak freely in front of the partner; (4) the individual may not know what is occurring in the partner's life, despite being influenced negatively by it; (5) the clinician may not realize the usual causes of the problem; or (6) the clinician may not believe in developmental influences on the organization of adult sexual function.

Sexual aversion should strongly suggest three possibilities to the clinician: (1) that a remote traumatic experience is being relived by the partner's expression of interest in sexual behavior; (2) that without the symptom the individual feels powerless to say "no" to sexual advances; or (3) that the individual feels guilty about her own sexual behavior with another person.

The clinician's attention should focus on the individual's sexual development as a child, adolescent, and young adult when the aversion is lifelong, whereas when it is *acquired*, the focus of the history should be on the period immediately prior to the onset of the symptom.

Desire disorders require the clinician to think both in terms of development and personal meanings of sex to the individuals under their care (Table 39-3). Because all explanations are speculative, they should at least make compelling sense of the individuals' life experiences. Some explanations are based on the influence of remote developmental processes. The term *madonna–whore complex* misleads us into thinking this is only a male pattern. The syndrome is manifested by normal sexual capacity with anyone but the fiancé or spouse. Freud interpreted this as a sign of incomplete resolution of the oedipal complex (Freud 1912). The man was thought to be unable to sexually desire his beloved because he had unconsciously made her into his mother. He withdrew his sexual interest from her to protect himself from symbolic incest. Some women are comparably unable to sexually enjoy their partners because they unconsciously confuse their beloved with their father. Another form can be seen among individuals whose parents were grossly inadequate caregivers. When these men and women find a reliable, kind, supportive person to marry, they quickly discover a strong motive to avoid sexual behavior with their fiancé. The individual makes the partner into a good-enough parent, experiences anxiety as an unconscious threat of incest associated with the possibility of sex, and becomes skillful at avoiding sexual opportunities (Levine 1998b).

Most sexual desire disorders are difficult to quickly overcome. Brief treatment generally should not be undertaken. Serious individual or couple issues frequently underlie these diagnoses. They have to be afforded time to emerge and to be worked through. However, clinicians need not be pessimistic about all of these conditions. For example, helping a couple resolve a marital dispute may return them to their usual normal sexual desire manifestations. For many individuals and couples, therapy assists the couple to more calmly accept the profound implications of continuing marital discord, infidelity, homosexuality, or other contributing factors. Some treatment failures lead to divorce and the creation of a relationship with a new partner. There is then no further sign of the desire problem. Problems rooted in early developmental experiences are particularly difficult to overcome. While DSM-IV-TR asks the clinician to make many distinctions among the desire disorders, no follow-up study has been published in which either the subtypes (lifelong, acquired, situational, and generalized) or etiologic organizers (relationship deterioration with and

Table 39-3	Obstacles to Discovering the Psychological Contributants to a Sexual Desire Disorder

Obstacles That Reside in the patient
The patient may not tell the psychiatrist the truth about life circumstances
The patient may have strong defenses against knowing the truth
The patient may be unable to tell the truth in front of the partner
The patient may not actually know what is occurring in the partner's life, although she or he is reactive to it

Obstacles That Reside in the Psychiatrist
The psychiatrist may not realize the psychological factors that usually cause these problems
The psychiatrist may not believe that developmental influences can organize an adult sexual function such as sexual motivation
The psychiatrist may not like to deal with the murky complexity of nonbiological developmental and interpersonal issues when thinking about etiology

without extramarital affairs, sexual identity incompatibilities, parental, and medical) are separated into good and poor prognosis categories (O'Carroll 1991).

Developmental and identity matters are typically approached in long-term individual psychotherapy. In these sessions, women often discuss the development of their femininity from adolescence to young womanhood, focusing on issues of body image, beauty, social worth to others, moral sensibilities, social awkwardness, and whether they consider themselves deserving of personal physical pleasure. Men often discuss similar issues in terms of masculinity.

Anger, loss of respect, marital discord, and extramarital affairs may be approached in either individual or conjoint formats. In either setting, individuals often formulate the etiology as having fallen out of love with the partner. Those whose cultural backgrounds limit their ease in being a sexual person are often encouraged in educational and cultural experiences that might help them outgrow their earliest notions about what is proper sexual behavior.

The Problems of Sexual Arousal

The emotion interchangeably referred to as sexual arousal or sexual excitement generates changes in respiration, pulse, and muscular tension as well as an increased blood flow to the genitals. Genital vasocongestion creates vaginal lubrication, clitoral tumescence, labial color changes; and penile erection, testicular elevation, and penile color changes (Masters and Johnson 1966). How arousal is centrally coordinated in either sex remains mysterious. During lovemaking, men and women do not necessarily maintain or progressively increase their arousal; rather often there is a fluctuating intensity of arousal which is reflected in variations in vaginal wetness and penile turgidity and nongenital signs of arousal.

FEMALE SEXUAL AROUSAL DISORDER

The specificity and validity of this disorder is unclear. In women, it is far more difficult to separate arousal and desire problems than in men. The perimenopausal period is now recognized as generating complaints about decreased drive, motivation, lubrication, and arousal in at least 35 to 50% of women (Dennerstein et al. 2000). However, it is unclear whether to label the problem as primarily of desire or arousal. It is assumed to be endocrine in origin even though estrogen, progesterone, and testosterone replacement do not reliably reverse the pattern. Even in younger regularly menstruating women, however, diminished motivation and dampened drive makes it difficult to sustain arousal. Many have called into question the accepted notions that desire necessarily precedes arousal and that they are separate physiological processes (Basson 2001). Female sexual arousal disorder implies that drive and motivation are relatively intact although arousal is difficult (see DSM-IV-TR diagnostic criteria on page 1061). The disorder is usually an *acquired* diagnosis. Premenopausal women who have this disorder focus on the lack of moisture in the vagina or their failure to be excited by the behaviors that previously reliably brought pleasure. They have drive and motive and wish, but enigmatically are unable to sustain arousal. Some mental factor arises to distract them from their excitement during lovemaking. Therapy is focused, therefore, on the meaning of what preoccupies them. This often involves the dynamics of their current individual or partnered life or the influence of their past relationships on their present. With therapy, the diagnosis often is changed to an HSDD.

DSM-IV-TR Diagnostic Criteria

302.72 Female Sexual Arousal Disorder

A. Persistent or recurrent inability to attain, or to maintain until completion of the sexual activity, an adequate lubrication-swelling response of sexual excitement.
B. The disturbance causes marked distress or interpersonal difficulty.
C. The sexual dysfunction is not better accounted for by another Axis I disorder (except another sexual dysfunction) and is not due exclusively to the direct physiological effects of a substance (e.g., a drug of abuse, a medication) or a general medical condition.

Specify type:

Lifelong type

Acquired type

Specify type:

Generalized type

Situational type

Specify:

Due to psychological factors

Due to combined factors

In peri- and postmenopausal women, arousal problems are more often focused on the body as a whole rather than just genital moisture deficiencies. Skin insensitivity, often a euphemism for decreased pleasure in response to oral and manual nipple, breast, and vulvar stimulation, is often initially treated as a symptom of "estrogen" deficiency. Early in the menopause, a small minority of women have an increase in drive due to changing testosterone–estrogen ratios. Yet, they may still subjectively experience arousal as different than it used to be. Therapy often focuses on the women's concerns about estrogen replacement and the consequences of menopause in terms of body image, attractiveness, fears of partner infidelity, loss of health and vigor, and aging.

Aging of the female arousal mechanisms, whether simply due to shifts in ovarian endocrine production or systemic aging mechanisms, occurs earlier than deterioration of orgasmic physiology. Women with decreasing arousal are often, therefore, still reliably orgasmic with the use of vaginal lubricants well into old age. Women who have been treated with chemotherapy for breast cancer are a particularly problematic group to offer assistance to for their new arousal problems. Fear of stimulating the remaining cancerous cells makes systemic estrogen replacement contraindicated.

In 1999, a renewed interest in female arousal disorder sometimes casually called *female sexual dysfunction* (Berman and Goldstein 2001) surfaced in response to the efficacy of Viagra for men's arousal problems. It was reasoned that since the penis and clitoris are embryologic homologs with comparable adult histology, the drug would improve women's arousal. An open-labeled study concluded that Viagra was highly effective (Berman et al. 2001) but when placebo-controlled trials were concluded, the drug did not improve arousal any more than placebo (Basson et al. 2002).

MALE ERECTILE DISORDER

The mechanisms of erection—the sequestering and maintaining arterial blood within the corpora cavernosa—are being elucidated by urological research. Their research has led to a diminishing emphasis on "psychogenic impotence" diagnosis (Krane et al. 1989). Urologists may refer to male erectile disorders (ED) of a psychogenic origin as "adrenergic" ED, a reference to the preponderance of sympathetic tone on the corporal mechanisms that maintain flaccidity. Adrenergic dominance of the penile arterial tone is created by a mind that perceives the sexual context as a dangerous, frightening, or as unwanted (see DSM-IV-TR diagnostic criteria below).

DSM-IV-TR Diagnostic Criteria

302.72 Male Erectile Disorder

A. Persistent or recurrent inability to attain, or to maintain until completion of the sexual activity, an adequate erection.
B. The disturbance causes marked distress or interpersonal difficulty.
C. The erectile dysfunction is not better accounted for by another Axis I disorder (other than a sexual dysfunction) and is not due exclusively to the direct physiological effects of a substance (e.g., a drug of abuse, a medication) or a general medical condition.

Specify type:

Lifelong type

Acquired type

Specify type:

Generalized type

Situational type

Specify:

Due to psychological factors

Due to combined factors

Reprinted with permission from the Diagnostic and Statistical Manual of Mental Disorders, Fourth Edition, Text Revision. Copyright 2000 American Psychiatric Association.

The prevalence of ED rises dramatically in the sixth decade of life from less than 10 to 30%; it increases further during the seventh decade (Feldman et al. 1994). Aging, medical conditions such as diabetes, prostatic cancer, hypertension, and cardiovascular risk factors predict the most common pattern of ED due to a medical condition in this age group. While medication-induced, neurological, endocrine, metabolic, radiation, and surgical causes of erectile dysfunction also exist, in population studies, diabetes, hypertension, smoking, lipid abnormalities, obesity, and lack of exercise are correlated with the progressive deterioration of erectile functioning in the sixth and seventh decades (Althof and Seftel 1995). These factors are thought to create a relative penile anoxemia, which stimulates the conversion of corporal smooth muscle cells into fibrocytes. The gradual loss of elasticity of the corpora interferes with filling and sequestering of arterial blood (Carrier et al. 1993). Erections at first become unreliable and finally impossible to obtain or sustain.

At every age, *selectivity* of erectile failure is the single most important diagnostic feature of primary erectile dysfunction. Clinicians should inquire about the relative firmness and duration of erections under each of these circumstances: masturbation, sex other than intercourse, sex with other female or male partners, upon stimulation with explicit media materials, in the middle of the night, and upon awakening. If under some circumstances the erection is firm and lasting, the clinician can usually assume that the man's neural, endocrine, and vascular physiology is sufficiently normal and that the problem is psychogenic in origin. This is true even for men in their fifties and older. Clinicians often feel more certain about this diagnosis when no diseases thought to lead to erectile dysfunction are present (O'Keefe and Hunt 1995).

Lifelong male ED typically is psychogenic and involves either a sexual identity dilemma—such as transvestism, gender identity disorder, a homoerotic orientation, a paraphilia, or another diagnosis that expresses the individual's fear of being sexually close to a partner. Sexual identity problems are often initially denied unless the clinician is nonjudgmental and thorough during the inquiry. However, obsessive–compulsive disorder, schizoid personality, a psychotic disorder, or severe character disorders may be present. Occasionally, a reasonably normal young man with an unusually persistent fear of sexual intercourse seeks attention. These good prognosis cases are sometimes informally referred to as anxious beginners (Table 39-4). With that exception, men with lifelong male arousal disorder (MAD), when taken into individual therapy, are usually perceived as having a strong motive to avoid sexual behavior and while dysfunctional with a partner during much of their therapy, might equally be diagnosed as having HSDD with normal drive but a motive to avoid partner sex. The prognosis with older men with lifelong erectile dysfunction is poor even with modern erectogenic agents. Long-term therapy, even if it does not enable regular intercourse, may enable more emotional and sexual closeness to a partner. Some reasonably masculine-appearing men with mild gender identity problems can quickly become potent if they can reveal their need during sexual relationship to cross-dress (use a fetish article of clothing) to a partner who calmly accepts his requirement. However, most of these men have inordinate fears of sexually bonding to any woman, and, in therapy, become preoccupied with basic developmental issues. Some of them marry and form companionate relationships that are rarely or never consummated.

In dramatic contrast, men with long-established good potency who have recently lost their erectile capacities with their partner—acquired psychogenic ED—have a far better prognosis (Table 39-5). They may be treated in individual or couples format, depending on the precipitants of the sexual problem and the status of their relationship with their partner. Many of these therapies become focused on resentments that have not been identified, discussed, and worked through by the couple. Such distressed couples are most efficiently helped in a conjoint format. When extramarital affairs are part of the relationship deterioration and cannot be discussed, most clinicians simply work with one spouse. Potency is frequently lost following a separation or divorce. Impaired potency after a spouse's death is either about unresolved grief or problems that exist prior to the wife's terminal illness. Men also often get worried about their potency when their financial or vocational lives crumble, when they have a serious new physical illness such as a myocardial infarction or stroke, or when their wives become seriously ill. The esthetics of lovemaking require a

Table 39-4	What the Clinician Should Expect to Encounter Among Men Who Have Never Been Able to Have Intercourse with a Woman

Unconventional Sexual Identity
Gender identity problem
   Wish to be a woman
   A history of cross-dressing in women's clothing in private and/or public
   Suspected by psychiatrist but information initially withheld
Homoeroticism
   Without sexual behavior with men
   With sexual behavior with men but not known to the female partner
   With sexual behavior with men and known to the female partner
Paraphilia
   One or more of a wide range of paraphilic patterns
   Preference for prepubertal or young adolescents often initially denied unless thoroughly, systematically, and nonjudgmentally questioned
   Compulsivity with or without obvious paraphilic imagery confined to masturbation with the help of pornographic images for stimulation

Serious Character Disorders (Men Have Strong Fear of Closeness to Women)
Obsessive–compulsive
Schizotypal
Schizoid
Avoidant
Past history of psychotic decompensation

Anxious Beginners
Psychiatrically normal young men with inordinate anxiety and shyness that quickly respond to psychiatrist's encouragement and optimism and partner warmth and patience

Table 39-5	Apparent Precipitants of Recently Acquired Psychogenic Erectile Disorder and Their Associated Private Emotions*

Deterioration of marital relationship: anger, guilt, disdain, sadness
Divorce: abandonment, anger, guilt, sadness, shame
Deterioration of personal or spousal health: sadness, anxiety, anger, shame
Death of spouse (*widower's impotence*): sadness, longing, guilt
Threat of or actual unemployment: anxiety, worthlessness, guilt, anger, shame
Financial reversal: shame, guilt, anxiety
Surreptitious extramarital affair: guilt
Reunited marriage after extramarital affair: shame, anxiety

*These short lists of simple emotions are a mere introduction to what transpires within the man's mind as a result of the meanings that the sexual behavior has for him. Although incomplete and oversimplified, they are listed to remind the psychiatrist that what the man feels about his life competes with sexual arousal during sexual behavior to generate the psychogenic erectile dysfunction.

context of reasonable physical health; when one spouse becomes chronically ill or disfigured by illness or surgery, either one of the couple may lose their willingness to be sexual. This may be reflected in impaired erections or sexual avoidance.

Regardless of the precipitating factors, men with arousal disorders have performance anxiety. They anticipate erectile failure before sex begins and vigilantly monitor their state of tumescence during sex (Masters and Johnson 1970). Performance anxiety is present in almost all impotent men. Performance anxiety is efficiently therapeutically addressed by identifying it to the individual and asking him to make love without trying intercourse on several occasions to demonstrate to himself how different lovemaking can feel for him when he is not risking failure. This enables many to relax, concentrate on sensation, and return to previous states of sensual abandon during lovemaking. This technique is known as *sensate focus*.

The psychological treatment of acquired arousal disorders is often highly satisfying for the professional because many of the men are anxious for help. Motivation to behave sexually is often present, fear can be allayed, and men can learn to appreciate the emotional complexity of their lives. They can be shown how their minds prevented intercourse until they could acknowledge what has been transpiring within and around them. Many recently separated men, for example, are grieving, angry, guilty, uncertain, and worried about their finances. Yet, they may propel themselves into a new relationship. Two characteristics seem to predispose to erectile problems at key life transitions: (1) the pursuit of the masculine standard that men ought to be able to perform intercourse with anyone, anywhere, under any circumstances; (2) the inability to readily grasp the nature and significance of his inner experiences. "Yes, my schizophrenic daughter became homeless in another city, my wife was depressed and began drinking to excess in response, and I had a financially costly affair with my secretary. What do these have to do with my loss of potency?" (Table 39-6).

Sildenafil revolutionized the treatment of erectile dysfunction in 1998. This phosphodiesterase type-5 inhibitor maintains corporal vasodilation by preventing the degradation of cGMP. Sexual arousal leads to the corporal secretion of nitric oxide, which is converted by an enzyme into cGMP. Sildenafil is increasingly effective as the dose is increased from 25 to 50 up to 100 mg. The drug must not be used when any organic nitrate is being taken because it dangerously potentiates the hypotensive effect of the nitrates, risking brain and myocardial infarction (Goldstein et al. 1998). Sildenafil is dramatically underutilized by psychiatrists.

Prior to sildenafil, urologists argued that most erectile dysfunction was organic in origin, but since the drug works at about the same rate regardless of the pretreatment etiology, most erectile dysfunction is now recognized to be of mixed—organic and psychosocial—origin (Lue 2000). Three conditions have unique response profiles: after prostatectomy the response rate is approximately 34%, among diabetics it is approximately 43%, and among the spinal cord injured, it is approximately 80%, the same rate seems to improve psychogenic ED. Other medical interventions are also effective in varying degrees for largely organic erectile dysfunction: vacuum pump, the intracavernosal injection of vasodilating substances,

Table 39-6	Pathogenesis Model for Acquired Erectile Dysfunction

Functional cognitive predispositions
  A normal (or real, adequate, or competent) man is able to have intercourse with anyone under any circumstances
  Feelings are a womanly intrusion on my reason; I am disinterested and relatively unaware of them.
Precipitating events (See Table 39-5)
        ↓
One episode of erectile failure
        ↓
Performance anxiety
        ↓
Another episode of erectile failure
        ↓
More performance anxiety
        ↓
Decreased frequency of sexual initiation
        ↓
Changes in the sexual equilibrium
        ↓
Established pattern of impotence with partner

intraurethral alprostadil, the surgical implantation of a penile prosthesis (Ohl 1994), and outside the United States, sublingual apomorphine. Because sildenafil's rate of improving erections is significantly higher than the restoration of a mutually satisfactory sexual equilibrium (approximately 44%), psychological ED that persists after medication should be treated by a mental health professional (Pallas et al. 2000).

PROBLEMS WITH ORGASM

FEMALE ORGASMIC DISORDER

Diagnosis

The attainment of reasonably regular orgasms with a partner is a crucial personal developmental step for young women. This task of adult sexual development rests upon a subtle interplay of physiology, individual psychology, and culture. Reliable orgasmic attainment is usually highly valued by the woman and is often reflected in enhanced self-esteem, confidence in her femininity, relationship satisfaction, and the motive to continue to behave sexually.

Orgasm is the reflexive culmination of arousal. It is manifested by rhythmic vaginal wall contractions and the release of muscular tension and pelvic vasocongestion, accompanied by varying degrees of pleasurable body sensations. Its accomplishment requires: (1) the physiologic apparatus to augment and sustain arousal; (2) the psychological willingness to be swept away by excitement; and (3) tenacious focus on the required physical work of augmenting arousal. The diagnosis of female orgasmic disorder (FOD) is made when the woman's psychology persistently interferes with her body's natural progression through arousal (see DSM-IV-TR diagnostic criteria below).

DSM-IV-TR Diagnostic Criteria

302.73 Female Orgasmic Disorder

A. Persistent or recurrent delay in, or absence of, orgasm following a normal sexual excitement phase. Women exhibit wide variability in the type or intensity of stimulation that triggers orgasm. The diagnosis of female orgasmic disorder should be based on the clinician's judgment that the woman's orgasmic capacity is less than would be reasonable for her age, sexual experience, and the adequacy of sexual stimulation she receives.

B. The disturbance causes marked distress or interpersonal difficulty.

C. The orgasmic dysfunction is not better accounted for by another Axis I disorder (except another sexual dysfunction) and is not due exclusively to the direct physiological effects of a substance (e.g., a drug of abuse, a medication) or a general medical condition.

Specify type:

Lifelong type

Acquired type

Specify type:

Generalized type

Situational type

Specify:

Due to psychological factors

Due to combined factors

Reprinted with permission from the Diagnostic and Statistical Manual of Mental Disorders, Fourth Edition, Text Revision. Copyright 2000 American Psychiatric Association.

Estimates of prevalence of both lifelong and acquired psychological FOD range from 10 to 30% (Laumann et al. 1994b). Some of this variability is due to the different definitions of anorgasmia. It remains a difficult scientific judgment, however, where to draw the line between dysfunction and normality—for example, is it normal to attain orgasms during one-third of partner sexual experiences? (Tiefer 1998). Few women are always orgasmic.

While assessing for the presence of this disorder, the doctor should determine the answers to the following questions. Does the individual have orgasms under any of the following sexual circumstances: solitary masturbation, partner manual genital stimulation, oral–genital stimulation, vibratory stimulation, any other means? Does she have orgasms with a partner different than her significant other? How are they stimulated? Does a particular fantasy make orgasmic attainment easier or possible? Under what conditions has she ever been orgasmic? Has she had an orgasm during her sleep?

The lifelong *generalized* variety of the disorder is recognized when a woman has never been able to attain orgasm alone or with a partner by any means, although she regularly is aroused. When a woman can only readily attain orgasm during masturbation, she is diagnosed as having a lifelong *situational* type. Women with any form of lifelong FOD more clearly have conflicts about personal sexual expression due to fear, guilt, ignorance, or obedience to tradition than those with the acquired variety. Women who can masturbate to orgasm often feel fear and embarrassment about sharing their private arousal with any other person.

The acquired varieties of this disorder are more common and are characterized by both complete anorgasmia, too-infrequent orgasms, and too-difficult orgasmic attainment. The most common cause of this problem are serotonergic compounds. Prospective studies of various antidepressants have demonstrated up to 70% incidence of this disorder among those treated with serotonergic antidepressants. Bupropion and nefazodone do not cause this problem (Segraves 1998). When medications are not the cause of an acquired FOD, the clinician needs to carefully assess the meaning of the changes in her life prior to the onset of the disorder. Some of these women are in the midst of making a transition to a new partner after many years in another relationship. Some seem to suffer from memories of earlier shame-ridden behaviors such as incest.

Etiology

During most of the twentieth century, psychoanalysts thought that almost 90% of women were orgasmically dysfunctional. Prior to 1970, the accepted concept of normality required a woman to be brought to orgasm by penile thrusting. Orgasmic fulfillment through solitary masturbation or partner manual or oral stimulation was viewed as signifying the presence of a neurotic obstacle to mature femininity. This paternalistic idea has weakened considerably in the last generation.

The biologic potential for orgasmic attainment is an inborn endowment of nearly all physically healthy women. The cultural and psychological factors that influence orgasmic attainment are usually fundamental to the etiology of FOD. Centuries-old beliefs that sexual knowledge, behavior, and sexual pleasure were not the prerogative of "good girls" powerfully affect some women's sexual adjustment. These beliefs cause young women to be uninformed about the location and role of their clitoris and ashamed of their erotic desires and sexual sensations. For women with FOD, modern concepts of equality of sexual expression are insufficient to overcome these traditional beliefs. These emotionally powerful beliefs often lie behind their classic dysfunctional pattern: the women can become aroused to a personal plateau beyond which they cannot progress; thereafter, their excitement dissipates. After numerous repetitions, they begin to lose motivation to participate in sex with their partner. They may eventually meet the criteria for Hypoactive Sexual Disorder.

Treatment

When a clinician applies a label of disorder to a relatively anorgasmic woman, the woman often privately interprets the diagnosis as meaning that she has a serious and difficult problem to overcome. Clinicians need to be careful about this because some women are relatively easy to help. It must be realized that many women gradually undo the effects of their culture on their own and grow to be increasingly responsive sexually with time and growing trust of their partners. Clinicians can do many women a great service by offering education and reassurance. Giving an inhibited woman new-to-her information in an encouraging manner can subdue her anxiety and foster her optimism. On the other hand, some women with this disorder are profoundly entrenched in not being too excited, and treatments fail. The ideal era to begin treatment is young adulthood (Killman et al. 1986).

Four formats are known to be of help. Individual therapy is the most commonly employed. In lifelong varieties of the disorder, therapy focuses on the cultural sources of sexual inhibition and how and when they impacted upon the individual. In the situational varieties, the therapist focuses on the meaning of the life changes that preceded the onset of the disorder. Group therapy is highly effective in helping women reliably masturbate to orgasm and be moderately effective in overcoming partner inhibition. It is typically done with college and graduate students in campus settings, not older women. Couple therapy may be useful to assist the couple with the subtleties of their sexual equilibrium. The personal and interpersonal dimensions of orgasmic attainment can be stressed. Often, other issues then come to the fore that initially seemed to have little to do with orgasmic attainment. The most cost-effective treatment is bibliotherapy. Female orgasmic attainment has been widely written about in the popular press since the early 1970s. It is widely believed that these articles and books, which strongly encourage knowledge of her genital anatomy, masturbation, and active pursuit of orgasm, have enabled many women to grow more comfortable and competent in sexual expression.

MALE ORGASMIC DISORDER

When a man can readily attain a lasting erection with a partner, yet is consistently unable to attain orgasm in the body of the partner, he is diagnosed with male orgasmic disorder (MOD) (see DSM-IV-TR diagnostic criteria on page 1069). The disorder has three levels of severity: (1) the most common form is characterized by the *ability* to attain orgasm with a partner outside of her or his body, either through oral, manual, or personal masturbation; (2) the more severe form is characterized by the man's inability to ejaculate in his partner's presence; and (3) the rarest form is characterized by the inability to ejaculate when awake. The disorder is usually lifelong and not partner specific. These men cannot allow themselves to be swept away in arousal by another person. They are sexually vigilant to not allow themselves to be controlled by the partner's power to convey them to orgasm. This power would provide the partner with personal pleasure and the man with this disorder, while initially appearing to be a sexual superman, ultimately disappoints the partner. Their psychological dysfunction represents a capacity to use a mental mechanism, which other men would love to possess in smaller degrees. Both the partners and the therapists of these men tend to describe them as controlling, unemotional, untrusting, hostile, obsessive–compulsive, or paranoid. Some of these men get better with psychotherapy, others improve spontaneously with time, and, for others, the dysfunction leads to the cessation of the aspiration for sex with a partner. One controlled study of individuals with numerous sexual dysfunctions suggested that bupropion 300 to 450 mg/day may improve the capacity to ejaculate in a minority of individuals. Another controlled study found that 150 mg/day was insufficient (Masand et al. 2001).

DSM-IV-TR Diagnostic Criteria

302.74 Male Orgasmic Disorder

A. Persistent or recurrent delay in, or absence of, orgasm following a normal sexual excitement phase during sexual activity that the clinician, taking into account the person's age, judges to be adequate in focus, intensity, and duration.
B. The disturbance causes marked distress or interpersonal difficulty.
C. The orgasmic dysfunction is not better accounted for by another Axis I disorder (except another Sexual Dysfunction) and is not due exclusively to the direct physiological effects of a substance (e.g., a drug of abuse, a medication) or a general medical condition.

Specify type:
Lifelong Type
Acquired Type

Specify type:
Generalized Type
Situational Type

Specify:
Due to Psychological Factors
Due to Combined Factors

Reprinted with permission from the Diagnostic and Statistical Manual of Mental Disorders, Fourth Edition, Text Revision. Copyright 2000 American Psychiatric Association.

PREMATURE EJACULATION

Diagnosis

Premature ejaculation is a high-prevalence (25–40%) (Frank et al. 1978) disorder seen primarily in heterosexuals characterized by an untamably low threshold for the reflex sequence of orgasm (see DSM-IV-TR diagnostic criteria on page 1070). The problem, a physiological *efficiency* of sperm delivery, causes social and psychological distress. In failing to develop a sense of control over the timing of his orgasm in the vagina, the man fails to meet his standards of being a satisfying sexual partner. However, his partner does not explicitly or implicitly object, and his rapidity is not likely to cause him to seek medical attention. The range of intravaginal containment times among self-diagnosed individuals extends from immediately before or upon vaginal entry (rare), to less than a minute (usual), to less than the man and his partner desire (not infrequent). Time alone is a misleading indicator, however. The essence of the self-diagnosis is an emotionally unsatisfying sexual equilibrium apparently due to the man's inability to temper his arousal. Most men sometimes ejaculate before they wish to, but not persistently.

DSM-IV-TR Diagnostic Criteria

302.75 Premature Ejaculation

A. Persistent or recurrent ejaculation with minimal sexual stimulation before, on, or shortly after penetration and before the person wishes it. The clinician must take into account factors that affect duration of the excitement phase, such as age, novelty of the sexual partner or situation, and recent frequency of sexual activity.
B. The disturbance causes marked distress or interpersonal difficulty.
C. The premature ejaculation is not due exclusively to the direct effects of a substance (e.g., withdrawal from opioids).

Specify type:

Lifelong type

Acquired type

Specify type:

Generalized type

Situational type

Specify:

Due to psychological factors

Due to combined factors

The history should clarify the answers to following questions: why is he seeking therapy now? Is the individual a sexual beginner or a beginner with a particular partner? Does he have inordinately high expectations for intravaginal containment time for a man his age and experience? Is he desperate about losing the partner because of the rapid ejaculation? Is the relationship in jeopardy for another reason? Does his partner have a sexual dysfunction? Does she have orgasms with him other than through intercourse? Is he requesting help in order to cover his infidelity? Is his partner now blaming the man's sexual inadequacy for her infidelity? Is his new symptom a reflection of his fear about having a serious physical problem during sex such as angina, a stroke, or another myocardial infarction? The answers will enable the clinician to classify the rapid ejaculation into an acquired or lifelong and specific or general pattern, to sense the larger context in which his sexual behavior is conducted, and to plan treatment.

Premature ejaculation reflects to the man's sense that his contribution to the sexual equilibrium is deficient. It implies that he considers that he is far behind most men in his vaginal containment time and that he wants to provide his partner with a better opportunity to be nurtured during lovemaking through prolonged intercourse. Typically, he aspires to "bring" his partner to orgasm during intercourse. If anxiety lowers the ejaculatory threshold and keeps it from its natural evolution to a higher level over time, then premature ejaculation is a self-perpetuating pattern. Premature ejaculation may last a lifetime.

Treatment

There are three efficient approaches to this dysfunction. The first is simply to refuse to confirm the individual's self-diagnosis. Some anxious beginners, men with reasonable intravaginal containment times of 2 or more minutes, and those with exaggerated notions of sexual performance can be calmed down by a few visits. When they no longer think of themselves as dysfunctional, their intravaginal containment times improve. The second is the use of serotonergic medications. In a study of 15 carefully selected stable couples, daily administration of clomipramine 25 and 50 mg increased intravaginal containment times on average of 249 and 517% over baseline observations (Althof et al. 1995). At these dosage levels, there were few side effects. Numerous similar reports testify to the fact that various serotonergic reuptake inhibitors can significantly lengthen the duration of intercourse (Waldinger et al. 1994). Clinicians need to determine with each individual whether the medication can be taken within hours or days of anticipated intercourse. Improvement is not sustained after medication is stopped. Serotonergic medications are the most common treatment of rapid ejaculation because they are so quickly effective in over 90% of men. The third approach is behaviorally oriented sex therapy that trains the man to focus his attention on his penile sensations during vaginal containment and to signal his partner to cease movement or to apply a firm squeeze of the glans/shaft area to interrupt the escalation of arousal. This requires an increase in communication and full cooperation of the partner, which in themselves can go a long way in improving their sexual equilibrium.

Rapid ejaculation in some men reflects mere inexperience; for others it is stubborn physiological efficiency; for others it reflects fear of personal harm, which is either related to physical illness or to unresolved fears of closeness to a woman; and yet for others it reflects a partnership with a profoundly inhibited blaming partner. If the psychodynamic question is asked of men with persistent rapid ejaculation "Why does this man want to finish intercourse so quickly?" the answers vary from, "It is not a relevant question!" to "I'm afraid of her!" to "I'm afraid of what will happen to me." For instance, a large percentage of men ejaculate quickly for the first months after a myocardial infarction.

The advantages of costlier couple psychotherapy are to allow the man and his partner to understand their lives better, to address both of their sexual anxieties, and to deal with other important nonsexual issues in their relationship. Effective psychotherapy allows the man to become positioned to continue the usual biological evolution that occurs during the life cycle from rapid ejaculation, which is true for many young men, to occasional difficulty in ejaculating, which is true for many men in their sixties.

SEXUAL PAIN DISORDERS

The clinician needs to consider a series of questions when dealing with a woman who reports painful intercourse. Does she have a known gynecologic abnormality that is generally associated with pain? Is there anything about her complaint of pain that indicates a remarkably low pain threshold? Does she now have an aversion to sexual intercourse? At what level of physical discomfort did she develop the aversion? Does her private view of her current relationship affect her willingness to be sexual and her experience of pain? Does her partner's sexual style cause her physical or mental discomfort—for example, is he overly aggressive or does he stimulate memories of former abuse? What has been the partner's response to her pain? What role does her anticipation of pain play in her experience of pain?

These clinical questions are typical biopsychosocial ones. Sex-limiting pain often is the result of the subtle interplay of personal and relational, cognitive and affective, and fundamental biological processes that are inherent in other human sexual struggles that operate to produce these confusing disorders (Meana and Binik 1994).

The DSM-IV-TR presents dyspareunia and vaginismus as distinct entities. However, they have been viewed as inextricably connected in much of the modern sexuality literature—vaginismus is known to create dyspareunia and dyspareunia has been known to create vaginismus.

DYSPAREUNIA

Diagnosis

Recurrent uncomfortable or painful intercourse in either gender is known as dyspareunia (see DSM-IV-TR diagnostic criteria below). Women's dyspareunia varies from discomfort at intromission, to severe unsparing pain during penile thrusting, to vaginal irritation following intercourse. In both sexes, recurring coital pain leads to inhibited arousal and sexual avoidance. *Dyspareunia* is used as both a symptom and a diagnosis. When coital pain is caused solely by defined physical pathology, dyspareunia due to a medical condition is diagnosed. When coital pain is due to vaginismus, insufficient lubrication, or other presumably psychogenic factors, dyspareunia not due to a medical condition diagnosis is made. Psychogenic etiologies may include a CNS pain perception problem raising the question, "What do we mean by psychogenic?" This arena's nomenclature will undoubtably change when a breakthrough in understanding the causes of coital pain occurs.

DSM-IV-TR Diagnostic Criteria

302.76 Dyspareunia

A. Recurrent or persistent genital pain associated with sexual intercourse in either a male or a female.
B. The disturbance causes marked distress or interpersonal difficulty.
C. The disturbance is not caused exclusively by vaginismus or lack of lubrication, is not better accounted for by another Axis I disorder (except another sexual dysfunction), and is not due exclusively to the direct physiological effects of a substance (e.g., a drug of abuse, a medication) or a general medical condition.

Specify type:

Lifelong type

Acquired type

Specify type:

Generalized type

Situational type

Specify:
Due to psychological factors
Due to combined factors

Because the *symptom* dyspareunia is produced by numerous organic conditions, the clinician should be certain that the individual has had a pelvic examination by a person equipped to assess a broad range of regional pathology (McKay 1992). Vulvovestibulitis is diagnosed by pain in response to cotton swab touching in a normal appearing vulvar vestibule. A fundamental question remains unanswered about this often devastating problem: "Is the disorder of local or central origin?" In these individuals and some others, the pain cannot be classified with certainty as a *symptom* or a *disorder*. Pain upon penile or digital insertion may be due to an intact hymen or remnants of the hymenal ring, vaginitis, cervicitis, episiotomy scars, endometriosis, fibroids, ovarian cysts, and so on. Postcoital dyspareunia often begins at orgasm when uterine contractions occur. Fibroids, endometriosis, and pelvic inflammatory disease should be considered. Postmenopausal pain, particularly if the woman has had many years without intercourse, is often a result of thinning of the vaginal mucosa, loss of elasticity of the labia and vaginal outlet, and decreased lubrication. Normal menopause, however, is often associated with mild pain due to inadequate lubrication (in both partners).

Dyspareunia in men is usually due to a medical condition. Herpes, gonorrhea, prostatitis, and Peyronie's disease cause pain during intercourse. Remote trauma to the penis may cause penile chordee or bowing which makes intercourse mechanically difficult and sometimes painful. Pain experienced upon ejaculation can be a side effect of trazodone.

Etiology

Pain associated with intercourse may have purely subjective or psychologic origin. Couple dynamics are often relevant, but the pain may be seen as a means of not allowing painful memories of childhood sexual abuse into clear focus. Fear of or helplessness about negotiating interpersonal conflicts may eventually lead to pain becoming a solution for avoiding unwanted sexual behaviors. While clinicians tend to assume that pain has unconscious origins, sometimes it is merely faked; more often the individual is quite aware of its developmental origins but is too embarrassed to quickly communicate it to the doctor.

Personal psychological origins of painful intercourse pass through the common denominator of anxiety. Such anxiety may take the forms of dread of physical damage, worry about the psychological dependence that might result from physical union, fear of a first or another pregnancy, or a sexually transmitted disease. Intense anxiety, the psychological source of her pain, may lead to involuntary contraction of vaginal muscles, which is the mechanical source of her pain. Thus, dyspareunia and vaginismus reinforce each other. Both situational and acquired dyspareunia may reflect a woman's conscious or unconscious motivation to avoid sex with a particular partner; it may be her only means to express her despair about their nonsexual relationship. *Lifelong* dyspareunia draws the clinician's attention to developmental experiences.

VAGINISMUS

Diagnosis

Vaginismus is an involuntary spasm of the musculature of the outer third layer of the vagina, which makes penile penetration difficult or impossible (see DSM-IV-TR diagnostic criteria below). The diagnosis is not made if an organic cause is known. Although a woman with vaginismus may wish to have intercourse, her symptom prevents the penis from entering her body. It is as though her vagina says, "No!" In lifelong vaginismus, the anticipation of pain at the first intercourse causes muscle spasm. Pain reinforces the fear and on occasion, the partner's response gives her good reason to dread a second opportunity to have intercourse. Early episodic vaginismus may be common among women, but most of the cases that are brought to medical attention are chronic. Lifelong vaginismus is relatively rare. The clinician needs to focus attention on what may have made the idea of intercourse so overwhelming to her: parental intrusiveness, sexual trauma, childhood genital injury, illnesses whose therapy involved orifice penetration, and surgery.

DSM-IV-TR Diagnostic Criteria

302.51 Vaginismus

A. Recurrent or persistent involuntary spasm of the musculature of the outer third of the vagina that interferes with sexual intercourse.
B. The disturbance causes marked distress or interpersonal difficulty.
C. The disturbance is not better accounted for by another Axis I disorder (e.g., somatization disorder) and is not due exclusively to the direct physiological effects of a general medical condition.

Specify type:

Lifelong type

Acquired type

Specify type:

Generalized type

Situational type

Specify:

Due to psychological factors

Due to combined factors

Reprinted with permission from the Diagnostic and Statistical Manual of Mental Disorders, Fourth Edition, Text Revision. Copyright 2000 American Psychiatric Association.

The woman with lifelong vaginismus not only has a history of unsuccessful attempts at penetration but displays an avoidance of finger and tampon penetration. The most dramatic aspect of her history, however, is her inability to endure a speculum examination of her vagina. Vaginismus is a phobia of vaginal entrance.

TREATMENT OF DYSPAREUNIA AND VAGINISMUS

While vaginismus has the reputation of being readily treatable by gynecologists by pairing relaxation techniques with progressively larger vaginal dilators, the mental health professional typically approaches the problem differently. The psychological approach to both vaginismus and dyspareunia is attuned to the role that her symptom plays in her life. The therapy, therefore, does not begin with a cavalier, optimistic attempt to remove the symptom, which only frightens some individuals. Rather, it begins with a patient exploration of the developmental and interpersonal meanings of the need for the symptom. "I wonder how this problem originally got started? Can you tell me a bit more about your life?" In the course of assisting women with these problems, a variety of techniques may be utilized including relaxation techniques, sensate focus, dilatation, marital therapy, and medication. Short-term therapies should not be expected to have lasting good results because once the symptom is relieved, other problematic aspects of the individual's sexual equilibrium and nonsexual relationship often come into focus. Clinicians have developed an impression that women with a diagnosis of dyspareunia are particularly difficult to help permanently. However, this is a largely unstudied topic.

SEXUAL DYSFUNCTION DUE TO A GENERAL MEDICAL CONDITION

Many general medical conditions can cause sexual dysfunction, including neurological conditions (e.g., multiple sclerosis, spinal cord lesions, neuropathy, temporal lobe lesions), endocrine conditions (e.g., diabetes mellitus, hypothyroidism, hyper- and hypoadrenocorticism, hyperprolactinemia, hypogonadal states, pituitary dysfunction), vascular conditions, and genitourinary conditions (e.g., testicular disease, Peyronie's disease, urethral infections, postprostatectomy complications, genital injury, atrophic vaginitis, infections of the vagina and external genitalia, postsurgical complications such as episiotomy scars, shortened vagina, cystitis, endometriosis, uterine prolapse, pelvic infections, neoplasms).

The diagnosis of Sexual Dysfunction due to a General Medical Condition applies when the sexual dysfunction is judged to be exclusively due to the direct physiological effects of the general medical condition (see DSM-IV-TR diagnostic criteria below). This determination is based on history (e.g., impaired erectile functioning during masturbation), physical examination (e.g., evidence of neuropathy), and laboratory findings (e.g., nocturnal penile tumescence, pulse wave assessments, ultrasound studies, intracorporeal pharmacological testing or angiography). If both a primary sexual dysfunction and a general medical condition are present, then the primary diagnosis with the subtype "With Combined Factors" should be used (e.g., Male Erectile Dysfunction With Combined Factors).

DSM-IV-TR Diagnostic Criteria

Sexual Dysfunction due to ... [Indicate the General Medical Condition]

A. Clinically significant sexual dysfunction that results in marked distress or interpersonal difficulty predominates in the clinical picture.
B. There is evidence from the history, physical examination, or laboratory findings that the sexual dysfunction is fully explained by the direct physiological effects of a general medical condition.

C. The disturbance is not better accounted for by another mental disorder (e.g., major depressive disorder).

Select code and term based on the predominant sexual dysfunction:

625.8 Female hypoactive sexual desire disorder due to... [indicate the general medical condition]: if deficient or absent, sexual desire is the predominant feature

608.89 Male hypoactive sexual desire disorder due to ... [indicate the general medical condition]: if deficient or absent, sexual desire is the predominant feature

607.84 Male erectile disorder due to ... [indicate the general medical condition]: if male erectile dysfunction is the predominant feature

625.0 Female dyspareunia due to ... [indicate the general medical condition]: if pain associated with intercourse is the predominant feature

608.89 Male dyspareunia due to ... [indicate the general medical condition]: if pain associated with intercourse is the predominant feature

625.8 Other female sexual dysfunction due to ... [indicate the general medical condition]: if some other feature is predominant (e.g., orgasmic disorder) or no feature predominates

608.89 Other male sexual dysfunction due to ... [indicate the general medical condition]: if some other feature is predominant (e.g., orgasmic disorder) or no feature predominates

Coding note: Include the name of the general medical condition on Axis I, e.g., 607.84 male erectile disorder due to diabetes mellitus; also code the general medical condition on Axis III.

SUBSTANCE-INDUCED SEXUAL DYSFUNCTION

The diagnosis of Substance-Induced Sexual Dysfunction applies when a clinically significant sexual dysfunction is judged to be exclusively due to the direct physiological effects of a medication or drug of abuse (see DSM-IV-TR diagnostic criteria on page 1077). Sexual dysfunctions can occur in association with intoxication with the following classes of substances: alcohol, amphetamines and related substances, cocaine, opioids, sedatives, hypnotics, and anxiolytics. Acute intoxication with or chronic abuse of substances of abuse has been reported to decrease sexual interest and cause arousal problems in both sexes. A decrease in sexual interest, arousal disorders, and orgasmic disorders may also be caused by prescribed medications, including antihypertensives, histamine H_2 receptor antagonists, antidepressants, neuroleptics, anxiolytics, anabolic steroids, and antiepileptics. Painful orgasm has been reported with the use of fluphenazine, thioridazine, and amoxapine. Priapim has been reported with use of chlorpromazine, trazodone, closapine, and following penile injections of papaverine or prostaglandin. Serotonin reuptake inhibitors may close decreased sexual desire, arousal, or orgasmic disorders.

DSM-IV-TR Diagnostic Criteria

292.89 Substance-Induced Sexual Dysfunction

A. Clinically significant sexual dysfunction that results in marked distress or interpersonal difficulty predominates in the clinical picture.
B. There is evidence from the history, physical examination, or laboratory findings that the sexual dysfunction is fully explained by substance use as manifested by either (1) or (2):

   (1) the symptoms in criterion A developed during, or within a month of, substance intoxication
   (2) medication use is etiologically related to the disturbance

C. The disturbance is not better accounted for by a sexual dysfunction that is not substance induced. Evidence that the symptoms are better accounted for by a sexual dysfunction that is not substance induced might include the following: the symptoms precede the onset of the substance use or dependence (or medication use); the symptoms persist for a substantial period of time (e.g., about a month) after the cessation of intoxication, or are substantially in excess of what would be expected given the type or amount of the substance used or the duration of use; or there is other evidence that suggests the existence of an independent non-substance-induced sexual

dysfunction (e.g., a history of recurrent non-substance-related episodes).

Note: This diagnosis should be made instead of a diagnosis of substance intoxication only when the sexual dysfunction is in excess of that usually associated with the intoxication syndrome and when the dysfunction is sufficiently severe to warrant independent clinical attention.

Code [specific substance]-induced sexual dysfunction:
(291.8 Alcohol; 292.89 Amphetamine [or Amphetamine-like Substance]; 292.89 Cocaine; 292.89 Opioid; 292.89 Sedative, Hypnotic, or Anxiolytic; 292.89 Other [or Unknown] Substance)

Specify if:

With impaired desire

With impaired arousal

With impaired orgasm

With sexual pain

Specify if:

With onset during intoxication: if the criteria are met for intoxication with the substance and the symptoms develop during the intoxication syndrome

SEXUAL DYSFUNCTION NOT OTHERWISE SPECIFIED (NOS)

This diagnosis is reserved for circumstances that leave the clinician uncertain as to how to diagnose the individual. This may occur when the individual has too many fluctuating dysfunctional symptoms without a clear pattern of prominence of anyone of them. Sometimes, the clinician is unable to determine whether the dysfunction is the basic complaint or whether the sexual complaints are secondary to marital dysfunction. At other times the etiology is the uncertain: psychogenic, due to a general medical condition, or substance induced. When the individual does not emphasize the dysfunction as the problem but emphasizes instead the lack of emotional satisfaction from sex, the psychiatrist may temporarily provide this not otherwise specified (NOS) diagnosis. It is usually possible to find a better dysfunction diagnosis after therapy begins.

GENDER IDENTITY DISORDER

The organization of a stable gender identity is the first component of sexual identity to emerge during childhood. The processes that enable this accomplishment are so subtle that when a daughter consistently acts as though she realizes that "I am a girl and that is all right," or when a son's behavior announces that "I am a boy and that is all right," families rarely even remember their children's confusion and behaviors to the contrary. Adolescent and adult gender problems are not rare. They are, however, commonly hidden from social view, sometimes long enough to developmentally evolve into other less-dramatic forms of sexual identity.

Early Forms: Extremely Feminine Young Boys

Although occasionally the parents of a feminine son have a convincing anecdote about persistent feminine interests dating from early in the second year of life, boyhood femininity is more typically only apparent by the third year. By the fourth year, playmate preferences become obvious. Same-sex playmate preference is a typical characteristic of young children. Cross-gender-identified children consistently demonstrate the opposite sex playmate preference (Maccoby and Jacklin 1987). The avoidance of other boys has serious consequences in terms of social rejection and loneliness throughout the school years. The peer problems of feminine boys cause some of their behavioral and emotional problems, which are in evidence by middle-to-late childhood (Zucker 1990). However, psychometric studies support clinical impressions that feminine boys have emotional problems even before peer relationships become a factor—that is, something more basic about being cross-gender-identified creates problems. Young feminine boys have been shown to be depressed and have difficulties with separation anxiety (Coates and Person 1985).

Speculations about the origin of boyhood femininity generally suggest converging cumulative forces. Any child's cross-gender identifications are likely to involve a host of factors: constitutional forces, problematic interactions with parents, problematic internal processing of life experiences, and family misfortune—financial, reproductive, physical disease, emotional illness, or death of vital persons. These factors are sometimes restated as temperament, disturbed family functioning, separation–individuation problems, and trauma.

Temperament is a dual phenomenon being both the child's predisposition to respond to the world in a certain way and the aspects of the child to which others respond. The common temperamental factors of feminine boys have been described as: a sense of body fragility and vulnerability that leads to the avoidance of rough-and-tumble play; timidity and fearfulness in the face of new situations; a vulnerability to separation and loss; an unusual capacity for positive emotional connection to others; an ability to imitate; sensitivities to sound, color, texture, odor, temperature, and pain (Coates et al. 1992).

The development of boyhood femininity *may* occur within the mind of the toddler in response to a loss of emotional availability of the nurturant mother. The child creates a maternal (feminine) self through imitation and fantasy in order to make up for the mother's emotional unavailability. This occurs beyond the family's awareness, and is left in place by the family either ignoring what has transpired in the son or valuing it. The problem for the effeminate boy is that reality—the social expectations of other people—is unyielding on gender issues; the adaptive early life solution becomes progressively more maladaptive with time.

The answer to the question whether boyhood femininity is entirely constitutional, an adaptive solution, or due to a combination that includes some other process is not known. A few reports of femininity giving way to psychotherapeutic interventions with young boys and their families are of heuristic value but limited in follow-up duration (Zucker 1995).

Green prospectively studied a large well-matched group of feminine boys for over a decade and discovered that boyhood effeminacy was a frequent precursor of adolescent homoeroticism and homosexual behavior rather than gender identity disorders. He observed, as had others before, that without therapy feminine gender role behaviors give rise to more masculine behavioral styles as adolescence emerges (Green 1987).

Early Forms: Masculine Girls (Tomboys)

The masculinity of girls may become apparent as early as age 2 years. The number of girls brought to clinical attention for cross-gendered behaviors, self-statements, and aspirations is consistently less than boys by a factor of 1 : 5 at any age of childhood in Western countries (except Poland). It is not known whether this reflects a genuine difference in incidence of childhood gender disorders, cultural perceptions of femininity as a negative in boys versus the neutral-to-positive perception of boy-like behaviors in girls, the broader range of cross-gender expression permitted to girls but not to boys, or an intuitive understanding that cross-gender identity more accurately predicts homosexuality in boys than girls.

The distinction between tomboys and gender-disordered girls is often difficult to make. Tomboys are thought of as not as deeply unhappy about their femaleness, not as impossible to occasionally dress in stereotypic female clothing, and not thought to have a profound aversion to their girlish and future womanly physiologic transformations. Tomboys are able to enjoy some feminine activities along with their obvious pleasures in masculine-identified toys and games and the company of boys. Girls who are diagnosed as gender-disordered generally seem to have a relentless intensity about their masculine preoccupations and an insistence about their future. The onset of their cross-gendered identifications is early in life. Although most lesbians have a history of tomboyish behaviors, most tomboys develop a heterosexual orientation.

Diagnosis

Adults who permanently change their bodies to deal with their gender dilemmas represent the far end of the spectrum of adaptations to gender problems (Devor 1999). Even the lives of those who reject bodily change, however, have considerable pain because the images of a better gendered self may recur throughout life, becoming more powerful whenever life becomes strained or disappointing.

The diagnosis of the extreme end of the gender identity disorder spectrum is clinically obvious. The challenging diagnostic task for clinicians is to suspect a gender problem and inquire about gender identity and its evolution in those whose manner suggest a unisexed or cross-gendered appearance, those with dissociative gender identity disorder (GID), severe forms of character pathology, and those who seem unusual in some undefinable manner.

DSM-IV-TR provides the clinician with two Axis I gender diagnoses: Gender Identity Disorder, and Gender Identity Disorder Not Otherwise Specified (GIDNOS). To qualify for GID, an individual of any age must meet four criteria (see DSM-IV-TR diagnostic criteria on page 1080).

DSM-IV-TR Diagnostic Criteria

Gender Identity Disorder

A. A strong and persistent cross-gender identification (not merely a desire for any perceived cultural advantages of being the other sex). In children, the disturbance is manifested by four (or more) of the following:

   (1) repeatedly stated desire to be, or insistence that he or she is, the other sex
   (2) in boys, preference for cross-dressing or simulating female attire; in girls, insistence on wearing only stereotypical masculine clothing
   (3) strong and persistent preferences for cross-sex roles in make-believe play or persistent fantasies of being the other sex
   (4) intense desire to participate in the stereotypical games and pastimes of the other sex
   (5) strong preference for playmates of the other sex

In adolescents and adults, the disturbance is manifested by symptoms such as a stated desire to be the other sex, frequent passing as the other sex, desire to live or be treated as the other sex, or the conviction that he or she has the typical feelings and reactions of the other sex. Persistent discomfort with his or her sex or sense of inappropriateness in the gender role of that sex.

In children, the disturbance is manifested by any of the following: in boys, assertion that his penis or testes are disgusting or will disappear or assertion that it would be better not to have a penis, or aversion toward rough-and-tumble play and rejection of male stereotypical toys, games, and activities; in girls, rejection of urinating in a sitting position, assertion that she has or will grow a penis, or assertion that she does not want to grow breasts or menstruate, or marked aversion toward normative feminine clothing.

B. In adolescents and adults, the disturbance is manifested by symptoms such as preoccupation with getting rid of primary and secondary sex characteristics (e.g., request for hormones, surgery, or other procedures to physically alter sexual characteristics to simulate the other sex) or belief that he or she was born the wrong sex.

C. The disturbance is not concurrent with a physical intersex condition.

D. The disturbance causes clinically significant distress or impairment in social, occupational, or other important areas of functioning.

Code based on current age:

302.6 Gender identity disorder in children

302.85 Gender identity disorder in adolescents or adults
Specify (for sexually mature individuals):

Sexually attracted to males

Sexually attracted to females

Sexually attracted to both

Sexually attracted to neither

Criterion A: Strong, Persistent Cross-Gender Identification Because young children may not verbalize enough about their inner experiences for the clinician to be certain that this criterion is met, at least four of five manifestations of cross-gender identification must be present: (1) repeatedly stated desire to be, or insistence that he or she is, the opposite sex; (2) in boys, preference for cross-dressing or simulating female attire; in girls, insistence on wearing stereotypical masculine clothing; (3) strong and persistent preferences for cross-gender roles in fantasy play or persistent fantasies of being the opposite sex; (4) intense desire to participate in the games and pastimes of the opposite sex; (5) strong preference for playmates of the opposite sex.

In adolescence and adulthood, this criterion is fulfilled when the individual states the desire to be the opposite sex, has frequent social forays into appearing as the opposite sex, desires to live or be treated as the opposite sex, or has the conviction that his or her feelings and reactions are those typical of the opposite sex.

Criterion B: Persistent Discomfort with One's Gender or the Sense of Inappropriateness in a Gender Role This criterion is fulfilled in boys who assert that their penis or testicles are disgusting or will disappear or that it would be better not to have these organs; or who demonstrate an aversion toward rough-and-tumble play and rejection of male stereotypical toys, games, and activities. In girls, rejection of urinating in a sitting position or assertion that they do not want to grow breasts or menstruate, or marked aversion towards normative feminine clothing fulfill this criterion.

Among adolescents and adults, this criterion is fulfilled by the individuals' exhibiting the following characteristics: preoccupation with getting rid of primary and secondary sex characteristics; preoccupation with thoughts about hormones, surgery, or other alterations of the body to enhance the capacity to pass as a member of the opposite sex such as electrolysis for beard removal, cricoid cartilage shave to minimize the Adam's apple, breast augmentation; or preoccupation with the belief that one was born into the wrong sex.

Criterion C: Not Due to an Intersex Condition In the vast majority of clinical circumstances, the individual possesses normal genital anatomy and sexual physiology. When an individual with a gender identity disorder and an accompanying intersex condition such as congenital adrenal hyperplasia, an anomaly of the genitalia, or a chromosomal abnormality is encountered, the clinician will be uncertain whether the intersex condition is the cause of the GID. The clinician may either diagnose GIDNOS or classify the individual as having a GID and list the physical factor on Axis III as a comorbid condition. The relationship between GID and intersex conditions is a controversial topic that may get clarified with further research being done in Germany.

Criterion D: Significant Distress and Impairment It is likely that many children, adolescents, and adults struggle for a while to consolidate their gender identity but eventually find an adaptation that does not impair their capacities to function socially, academically, or vocationally as a member of their sex. These persons do *not* qualify for GID nor do those who simply are not stereotypic in how they portray their gender roles. Mental health professionals occasionally encounter parents who are disturbed by their adolescent child's gender roles. Parental distress is not the point of criterion D; this criterion refers to distress of the individual.

Children, teenagers, and adults exist who rue the day they were born to their biological sex and who long for the opportunity to simply live their lives in a manner befitting the other gender. They repudiate the possibility of finding happiness within the broad framework of roles given to members of their sex by their society. Their repudiation is not motivated by an intellectual attack on sexism, homophobia, or any other injustice imbedded in cultural mores. A gender-disordered person literally repudiates his or her body, repudiates the self in that body, and rejects performing roles expected of people with that body. It is a subtle, usually self-contained rebellion against the need of others to designate them in terms of their biological sex.

The repudiation and rebellion may first occur as a subjective internal drama of fantasy, as behavioral expression in play, or a preference for the company of others. Regardless of when and how it is displayed, the drama of the gender-disordered involves the relentless feeling that "life would be better—easier, fuller, more enjoyable—if I and others could experience me as a member of the opposite sex."

By mid-adolescence, the extremely gender-disordered have often envisioned the solution for their paralyzing self-consciousness: to live as a member of the opposite gender, to transform their bodies to the extent possible by modern medicine, and to be accepted by all others as the opposite sex. Most people with these cross-gender preoccupations, however, do not go beyond the fantasy or private cross-dressing. Those that do, eventually come to psychiatric attention. When a clinician is called in, the family has one set of hopes, the individual another. The clinician has many tasks, one of which is to mediate between the ambitions of the gender-disordered person and society and see what can be done to help the individual. Negative countertransference may steer the clinician to deal with the opportunity expeditiously: "Obviously the patient is sick, maybe psychotic, and needs help. I don't take care of people who do these things. Refer *it* out!" With a little supervisory encouragement to perform a thorough evaluation, therapists soon find that these individuals possess many of the ordinary aspects of life and one unusual ambition—they often want to be the opposite sex so badly that they are willing to make it a priority over family, friends, vocation, and material acquisition.

The usual clarity of distinctions between heterosexual, bisexual, and homosexual orientations rests upon the assumption that the biological sex and psychological gender of the person and the partner are known. A woman who designates herself as a lesbian is understood to mean she is erotically attracted to other women. *Lesbian* loses its meaning if the woman says she feels she *is* a man and lives as one. She insists, "I am a heterosexual man; men are attracted to women as am I!" The baffled clinician may erroneously think, "You are a female therefore you are a lesbian!" DSM-IV-TR suggests that adults with GIDs should be subgrouped according to which sex the individual is currently sexually attracted: males, females, both, or neither. This makes sense for most individuals with GID because it is their gender identity that is most important to them. Some are rigid about the sex of those to whom they are attracted because it supports their idea about their gender, others are bierotic and are not too concerned with their orientation, still others have not had enough experiences to overcome their uncertainty about their orientation. A few individuals with GID find all partners too complicated and are only interested in themselves (Blanchard 1989).

If an accurate community-based study of the gender impaired could be conducted, most cases would be diagnosed as Gender Identity Disorder Not Otherwise Specified (GIDNOS). The diagnostician needs to understand that gender identity development is a dynamic evolutionary process and clinicians get to see people at crisis points in their lives. At any given time, although it is clear that the individual has some form of GID, it may not be that which is described in DSM-IV-TR as GID. Here is one example: an adult female calls herself a "neuter." She wants her breasts removed because she hates to be perceived as a woman. For 2 years she has been exploring "neuterdom" and "I am definitely not interested in being a man!" If in 2 years, she evolves to meet criterion 1, her current GIDNOS diagnosis will change.

GIDNOS is a large category designed to be inclusive of those with unusual genders who do not clearly fit the criteria of GID. There is no implication that if an individual is labeled GIDNOS that his or her label cannot change in the future. GIDNOS would contain the many forms of transvestism—masculine-appearing boys and teenagers with persistent cross-dressing (former fetishistic transvestites) who are evolving toward GID, socially isolated men who want to become a woman shortly after their wives or mothers die (secondary transvestites) but express considerable ambivalence about the very matter they passionately desired at their last visit, extremely feminized homosexuals including those with careers as "drag queens" who seem to want to change their sex when depressed, and so on. GIDNOS would also capture men who want to be rid of their genitals without being feminized, unisexual females who imagine themselves as males but who are terrified of any social expression of their masculine gender identity, hypermasculine lesbians in periodic turmoil over their gender, and those women who strongly identify with both male and female who lately want mastectomies. In using gender identity diagnoses, clinicians need to remember that extremely masculine women or extremely feminine men are not to be dismissed as homosexual. "Lesbian" or "gay" is only a description of orientation. They are more aptly described as also cross-gendered.

Treatment

The treatment of these conditions, although not as well based on scientific evidence as some psychiatric disorders, has been carefully scrutinized by multidisciplinary committees of specialists within the Harry Benjamin International Gender Dysphoria Association for over 20 years. For more details in managing an individual, please consult its "Standards of Care" (Meyer et al. 2001). The treatment of any GID begins after a careful evaluation, including parents, other family members, spouses, psychometric testing, and occasionally physical and laboratory examination. The details will depend on the age of the individual. It is possible, of course, to have a GID as well as mental retardation, a psychosis, dysthymia, severe character pathology, or any other psychiatric diagnosis (Table 39-7).

Psychotherapy

No one knows how to cure an adult's gender problem. People who have long lived with profound cross-gender identifications do not get insight—either behaviorally modified or medicated—and find that they subsequently have a conventional gender identity.

Table 39-7	Steps in Evaluation of the Profoundly Gender Disordered

Formal evaluation and diagnosis—gender identity disorder or gender identity disorder NOS. Can the patient be referred to a gender program? Is another treatable psychiatric or physical disorder present?

Individual psychotherapy within the gender program or with an interested professional. Do the diagnoses remain the same? If yes, does the patient consistently want to
Discuss his (or her) situation but make no changes?
Increase cross-dressing toward crossliving?
Prepare the family for the real-life test?
Obtain permission to proceed with hormones?

Approval for hormones from a gender committee or on written recommendation from the psychiatrist to an endocrinologist. Individual or group psychotherapy should continue.

Real-life test of living and working full time in the aspired-to-gender role for at least 1 year. Does the patient want to continue to surgery?

Gender committee approval for surgery. Many patients have cosmetic surgery other than that listed with only ordinary patient–surgeon consent. This most often involves breast augmentation but may include numerous other attempts to improve ability to pass as opposite sex and be attractive.
Men—genital reconstruction
Women—mastectomy, hysterectomy, genital reconstruction; Most patients will not complete all of these steps.

Psychotherapy is useful, nonetheless (Lothstein et al. 1981). If the individual is able to trust a therapist, there can be much to talk about—family relationships are often painful, barriers to relationship intimacy are profound, work poses many difficult issues, and the individual has to make monumental decisions. The central one is, "How am I going to live my life? Should I go through with cross-gender living, hormone therapy, mastectomy, or genital surgery?" The therapist can help the individual recognize the drawbacks and advantages of the various available options and to respect the initially unrecognized or unstated ambivalence. Completion of the gender transformation process usually takes longer than the individual desires, and the therapist can be an important source of support during and after these changes.

Group Therapy

Group therapy for gender-disordered people has the advantages of allowing individuals to know others with gender problems, of decreasing their social isolation, and of being among people who do not experience their cross-gender aspirations and their past behaviors as weird (Keller et al. 1982). Group members can provide help with grooming and more convincing public appearances. The success of these groups depends on the therapist's skills in selection of the individuals and using the group process. Groups are generally only available in a few specialized treatment programs.

Living in the aspired-to-gender role—working, relating, conducting the activities of daily living—is a vital process that enables one of three decisions: to abandon the quest, to simply live in this new role, or to proceed with breast or genital surgery (Petersen and Dickey 1995). Some clinicians use the real-life test as a criterion for recommending hormones but this varies because some individuals' abilities to present themselves in a new way is definitely enhanced by prior administration of cross-sex hormones. The reason for the real-life test is to give the individual, who created a transsexual solution in fantasy, an opportunity to experience the solution in social reality. Passing the real-life test is expected to be associated with improved psychological function (Blanchard et al. 1985).

Hormone Therapy

Ideally, hormones should be administered by endocrinologists who have a working relationship with a mental health team dealing with gender problems. The effects of administration of estrogen to a biological male are: breast development, testicular atrophy, decreased sexual drive, decreased semen volume and fertility, softening of skin, fat redistribution in a female pattern, and decrease in spontaneous erections. Breast development is often the highest concern to the individual. Because hair growth is not affected by estrogens, electrolysis is often used to remove beard growth. Side effects within recommended doses are minimal but hypertension, hyperglycemia, lipid abnormalities, thrombophlebitis, and hepatic dysfunction have been described. The most dramatic effect of hormones is on the sense of well-being. Individuals report feeling calmer, happier knowing that their bodies are being demasculinized and feminized. All results derive from open-labeled studies.

The administration of androgen to females results in an increased sexual drive, clitoral tingling and growth, weight gain, and amenorrhea and hoarseness. An increase in muscle mass may be apparent if weight training is undertaken simultaneously. Hair growth depends on the individual's genetic potential. Androgens are administrated intramuscularly 200 to 300 mg/month and are generally safe. It is prudent, however, to periodically monitor hepatic, lipid, and thyroid functioning. Most individuals are delighted with their bodily changes, although some are disappointed that they remain short, wide-hipped, relatively hairless men with breasts that do not significantly regress.

Surgical Therapy

Surgical intervention is the final external step. It should not occur without a mental health professional's input, even when the individual provides a heartfelt convincing set of reasons to bypass the real-life test, hormones, and therapeutic relationship. Genital surgery is expensive, time consuming, at times painful, and has frequent anatomic complications and functional disappointments. Surgery can be expected to add further improvements in the lives of individuals (Mate-Kole et al. 1990)—more social activities with friends and family, more activity in sports, more partner sexual activity, and improved vocational status.

Males Surgery consists of penectomy, orchiectomy, vaginoplasty, and fashioning of a labia. The procedures used for the creation of a neovagina have evolved over the years. Postoperatively, the individual must maintain the patency of the neovagina by initially constantly wearing and then periodically using a vaginal dilator. Vaginal stenosis or shortening is a frequent complication (McEwan et al. 1986). The quest for an unmistakable feminine shape leads many young adult individuals to augmentation mammoplasty and the shaving of their cricoid cartilage.

Females The creation of a male-appearing chest through mastectomies and contouring of the chest wall requires only a brief hospital stay. Individuals are usually immediately delighted with their newfound freedom, but their fantasies of going shirtless are often not fulfilled due to the presence of two noticeable horizontal chest scars. The creation of a neophallus that can become erect, contain a functional urethra throughout its length (enabling urination while standing), and pass as an unremarkable penis in a locker room has been a significant surgical challenge. It is far from perfected (Gilbert et al. 1988). The surgery is, however, the most time-consuming, technically difficult, and expensive of all the sex-reassignment procedures. Erection is made possible by a penile prosthesis. Many prudent individuals consider themselves reassigned when they have a hysterectomy, oophorectomy, and mastectomy. Some just have a mastectomy. They find a partner who understands the situation and supports the idea of living with, and loving with, female genitals.

THE PARAPHILIAS

Diagnosis

A paraphilia is a disorder of intention, the final component of sexual identity to develop in children and adolescents. Intention refers to what individuals want to do with a sexual partner and what they want the partner to do with them during sexual behavior. Normally, the images and the behaviors of intention fall within ranges of peaceable mutuality. The disorders of intention are recognized by unusual eroticism (images) and often socially destructive behaviors such as sex with children, rape, exhibitionism, voyeurism, masochism, obscene phone calling, or sexual touching of strangers. While 5% of the diagnoses of paraphilia are given to women, etiologic speculations refer to male sexual identity development gone awry. This raises the important question about what happens to girls who have the same developmental misfortunes that are speculated to create male paraphilia (Beier 2000). Accounts of paraphilic behaviors have been in the nonmedical literatures for centuries, but they have been of psychiatric interest only since 1905 (Freud 1905). Freud thought of the paraphilias as deviations in the aim of the sexual instinct. He coined the term by combining the Greek words for "along the side" (para) and "love" (philia). In 1905, paraphilia denoted those fixed preferences for sexual behaviors that led to forms of orgasmic attainment other than the uniting of penis and vagina.

Now it is apparent that paraphilias occur among individuals of all orientations and among those with conventional and unconventional gender identities. A homosexual sadist is paraphilic only on the basis of sexual cruelty. A transsexual who desires to be beaten during arousal is paraphilic only on the basis of masochism.

Erotic intentions that are *not* longstanding, unusual, and highly arousing may be problematic in some way but they are not clearly paraphilic. The *sine qua non* of the diagnosis of paraphilia is unusual, often hostile, dehumanized eroticism that has preoccupied the individual for most of his adolescent and adult life. The paraphilic fantasy is often associated with this preoccupying arousal when it occurs in daydreams and masturbation reveries or is encountered in explicit films or magazines. The specific imagery varies from one paraphilic individual to the next, but both the imagined behavior and its implied relationship to the partner are unusual in that they are preoccupied with aggression. Images of rape, obscene phone calling, exhibitionism, and touching of strangers, for example, are rehearsals of victimization. In masochistic images, the aggression is directed at the self—for instance, autoerotic strangulation, slavery, torture, and spanking. In others, the aggression is well disguised as *love* of children or teenagers. In some, such as simple clothing fetishism, the aggression may be absent. Aggression is so apparent in most paraphilic content, however, that when none seems to exist, the clinician needs to wonder whether it is actually absent or being hidden from the doctor. Paraphilic fantasies often rely heavily upon the image of a partner who does not possess "personhood." Some imagery in fact has no pretense of a human partner at all; clothing, animals, or excretory products are the focus. Other themes such as preoccupation with feet or hair, combine both human and inanimate interests. Paraphilic images are usually devoid of any pretense of caring or human attachment. The hatred, anger, fear, vengeance, or worthlessness expressed in them require no familiarity with the partner. Paraphilic images are conscious—clearly known to the individual. They should not be confused with speculations about "unconscious" aggression or sadomasochism that some assume are part of all sexual behavior (Kernberg 1991). Clinicians should expect to occasionally see paraphilic individuals whose preoccupations are not hostile to others.

An individual's paraphilic themes often change in intensity or seem to change in content from time to time. The stimuli for these changes often remain unclear. It is a moot point whether changes should be considered a shift to a different disorder, a new paraphilia, or a natural evolution of the basic problem. The shifts from imagining talking "dirty" on the phone in order to scare a woman to imagining raping can be considered an intensification of sadism. Switches between sadism and masochism or voyeurism and exhibitionism are common. Changes from voyeurism to pedophilia or from pedophilia to rape, however, raise the question whether a new disorder has developed. The most socially significant shifts are from erotic imagery to sexual behavior. In most instances, it is reasonable to consider that paraphilia is a basic developmental disorder in which particular erotic and sexual manifestations are shaped by the individuality of the person's history.

Most paraphilic adults can trace their fantasy themes to puberty and many can remember these images from earlier years. When adolescent rapists or incest offenders are evaluated, they often are able to report prepubertal aggressive erotic preoccupations. Men who report periodic paraphilic imagery interspersed with more usual eroticism have had their paraphilic themes from childhood or early adolescence. To make a diagnosis of paraphilia, the individual must evidence at least 6 months of the unusual erotic preoccupation. Duration is usually not in question, even among adolescents, however (Shaw 1999).

To be paraphilic means that the erotic imagery exerts a pressure to play out the often imagined scene. In its milder forms, the pressure results merely in a preoccupation with a behavior. For instance, a man who prefers to be spoken to harshly and dominated by his wife during sex thinks about his masochistic images primarily around their sexual behaviors. He does not spend hours daydreaming of his erotic preferences. In its more intense forms, paraphilias create a *drivenness* to act out the fantasy in sexual behavior—usually in masturbation. Frequent masturbation, often more than once daily, continues long after adolescence. In the most severe situations, the need to attend to the fantasy and masturbate is so overpowering that life's ordinary activities cannot efficiently occur. Masturbation and sometimes partner-seeking behavior—such as finding a woman to shock through exhibiting an erection—is experienced as driven. The individual reports either that he cannot control his behavior or he controls it with such great effort that his work, study, parenting, and relationships are disrupted. This pressure to behave sexually often leads the man to believe he has a high sex drive. Some severe paraphilics describe their masturbation-to-orgasm frequencies as 10/day. Even when the individual's estimate of his frequency of orgasm strains credulity less, the return of sexual drive manifestations so soon after orgasm suggests that either something is wrong with the individual's sexual drive generator, their satiety mechanisms, or that their existential anxiety overpowers their other defense mechanisms.

Paraphilic men often report collecting and viewing pornography, visiting sexual book stores to see explicit videos or peep shows, frequenting prostitutes for their special sexual behaviors, downloading explicit images from the Internet, or extensively using telephone sex services or strip clubs. Victimization of others, the public health problem, is the least common form of sexual acting out but it is by no means rare (Abel et al. 1987). When the behavioral diagnosis of exhibitionism, pedophilia, or sadism is made, the clinician should assume that the numbers of victims far exceed the number stated in the criminal charges.

Two other conditions, compulsive sexual behavior and sexual addiction, not part of the DSM-IV-TR, are informally and synonymously used to refer to heterosexual and homosexual men and women who display an intense drivenness to behave sexually without paraphilic imagery. The personal, interpersonal, and medical consequences of paraphilic and nonparaphilic sexual compulsivity seem indistinguishable as do their usual psychiatric comorbidities: depression, anxiety disorders, substance abuse, and attention deficit disorders (Kafka and Prentky 1998).

A severe sexual dysfunction involving desire, arousal, or orgasm with a partner, although not invariably, is often present among paraphilics (Pawlak 1991). The wives of paraphilics tell stories with these themes: "He is not interested in sex with me." "He never initiates." "He doesn't seem to enjoy our sexual life together except when.... " "He is usually not potent." "Even when we do make love, he rarely ejaculates." Some paraphilic men, however, are able to function well without paraphilic fantasies, but others are either able to primarily function when their partners are willing to meet their special requirements for arousal or when they fantasize about their paraphilic script (Abel 1989).

THE SPECIFIC PARAPHILIAS
CRIMINAL SEX-OFFENDING BEHAVIORS
EXHIBITIONISM

Exhibitionism generally involves teenagers and men displaying their penises so that the witness will be shocked or (in the paraphilic's fantasy) sexually interested (see DSM-IV-TR diagnostic criteria on page 1088). They may or may not masturbate during or immediately following this act of victimization. This diagnosis is not usually made when a man is arrested for "public indecency" and his penile exposures are motivated to arrange homosexual contact in a public place generally unseen by heterosexuals. Penile display in parks is one way to make anonymous contact. The presence or absence of exhibitionistic imagery allows the clinician to make the distinction between paraphilia and homosexual courting.

DSM-IV-TR Diagnostic Criteria

302.4 Exhibitionism

A. Over a period of at least 6 months, recurrent, intense sexually arousing fantasies, sexual urges, or behaviors involving the exposure of one's genitals to an unsuspecting stranger.

B. The person has acted on these sexual urges, or the sexual urges or fantasies cause marked distress or interpersonal difficulty

Reprinted with permission from the Diagnostic and Statistical Manual of Mental Disorders, Fourth Edition, Text Revision. Copyright 2000 American Psychiatric Association.

PEDOPHILIA

Pedophilia is the most widely and intensely socially repudiated of the paraphilias (see DSM-IV-TR diagnostic criteria below). Pedophiles are men who erotically and romantically prefer children or young adolescents. They are grouped into categories depending upon their erotic preferences for boys or girls and for infant, young, or pubertal children. Some pedophiles have highly age- and sex-specific tastes, others are less discriminating. Since the diagnosis of pedophilia requires, over a period of at least 6 months, recurrent, intense sexually arousing fantasies, sexual urges, or behaviors involving sexual activity with a prepubescent child or children the disorder should not be expected to be present in every person who is guilty of child molestation. Some intrafamilial child abuse occurs over a shorter time interval and results from combinations of deteriorated marriages, sexual deprivation, sociopathy, and substance abuse. Child molestation, whether paraphilic or not, is a crime, however. Child molesters show several patterns of erectile responses to visual stimulation in the laboratory. Some have their largest arousal to children of a specific age and others respond to both children and adults (Barbaree and Marshall 1995). Others respond with their greatest arousal to aggressive cues.

DSM-IV-TR Diagnostic Criteria

302.2 Pedophilia

A. Over a period of at least 6 months, recurrent, intense sexually arousing fantasies, sexual urges, or behaviors involving sexual activity with a prepubescent child or children (generally age 13 years or younger).

B. The person has acted on these sexual urges, or the sexual urges or fantasies cause marked distress or interpersonal difficulty.

C. The person is at least age 16 years and at least 5 years older than the child or children in Criterion A.

Note: Do not include an individual in late adolescence involved in an ongoing sexual relationship with a 12- or 13-year-old.

Specify if:

Sexually Attracted to Males

Sexually Attracted to Females

Sexually Attracted to Both

Specify if:

Limited to Incest

Specify type:

Exclusive Type (attracted only to children)

Nonexclusive Type

VOYEURISM

Men whose sexual life consists of watching homosexual or heterosexual videos in sexual book stores occasionally come to psychiatric attention after being charged with a crime following a police raid (see DSM-IV-TR diagnostic criteria below). They may or may not qualify for this diagnosis. The voyeurs who are more problematic for society are those who watch women through windows or break into their dwellings for this purpose. Some of these crimes result in rape or nonsexual violence, but many are motivated by pure voyeuristic intent (which is subtly aggressive).

DSM-IV-TR Diagnostic Criteria

302.82 Voyeurism

A. Over a period of at least 6 months, recurrent, intense sexually arousing fantasies, sexual urges, or behaviors involving the act of observing an unsuspecting person who is naked, in the process of disrobing, or engaging in sexual activity.
B. The person has acted on these sexual urges, or the sexual urges or fantasies cause marked distress or interpersonal difficulty

SEXUAL SADISM

While rape is an extreme variety of sadism, paraphilic sadism is present only in a minority of rapists (see DSM-IV-TR diagnostic criteria on page 1090). It is defined by the rapist's prior use of erotic scripts that involve a partner's fear, pain, humiliation, and suffering. Rapists are highly dangerous men whose antisocial behaviors are generally thought to be unresponsive to ordinary psychiatric methods. Their violence potential often makes psychiatric therapy outside of institutions imprudent. Noncriminal paraphilic sadism—that is, arousal to images of harming another that has not crossed into the behavioral realm, can be treated in outpatient settings.

DSM-IV-TR Diagnostic Criteria

302.84 Sexual Sadism

A. Over a period of at least 6 months, recurrent, intense sexually arousing fantasies, sexual urges, or behaviors involving acts (real, not simulated) in which the psychological or physical suffering (including humiliation) of the victim is sexually exciting to the person.
B. The person has acted on these sexual urges with a nonconsenting person, or the sexual urges or fantasies cause marked distress or interpersonal difficulty

---

Reprinted with permission from the Diagnostic and Statistical Manual of Mental Disorders, Fourth Edition, Text Revision. Copyright 2000 American Psychiatric Association.

FROTTEURISM

Frotteurism, the need to touch and rub against nonconsenting persons, although delineated as a criminal act, is probably better understood as a less malignant form of paraphilic sadism (see DSM-IV-TR diagnostic criteria below). Frotteurism often occurs in socially isolated men who become sexually driven to act out. They often are unaware of how frightening they can be.

DSM-IV-TR Diagnostic Criteria

302.89 Frotteurism

A. Over a period of at least 6 months, recurrent, intense sexually arousing fantasies, sexual urges, or behaviors involving touching and rubbing against a nonconsenting person.
B. The person has acted on these sexual urges, or the sexual urges or fantasies cause marked distress or interpersonal difficulty

---

Reprinted with permission from the Diagnostic and Statistical Manual of Mental Disorders, Fourth Edition, Text Revision. Copyright 2000 American Psychiatric Association.

NONCRIMINAL FORMS OF PARAPHILIA

Because the individual manifestations of paraphilia depend on the particular individual life history of the affected, over 40 paraphilic categories have been identified (Money 1986), although only a few are listed in the DSM-IV-TR. Most of these are unusual means of attaining arousal during masturbation or consenting partner behaviors. Each of the themes identified below demonstrate a wide range of manifestations from the bizarre to the more "reasonable" and from the common to the unique. They often subtly combine elements of more than one paraphilia.

FETISHISM/TRANSVESTIC FETISHISM

Fetishism, the pairing of arousal with wearing or holding an article of clothing or inanimate object such as an inflatable doll, has a range of manifestations from infantilism in which a person dresses up in diapers to pretend he is a baby to the far more common use of a female undergarment for arousal purposes (see DSM-IV-TR diagnostic criteria below). Fetishism when confined to one garment for decades is classified as a paraphilia, but many cases involve more complex varieties of cross-dressing and overlap with gender identity disorders, usually GIDNOS. Fetishistic transvestism is the diagnosis used when it is apparent that the urges to use the clothing of the opposite sex is part of a larger mental preoccupation with that sex (see DSM-IV-TR diagnostic criteria below).

DSM-IV-TR Diagnostic Criteria

302.81 Fetishism

A. Over a period of at least 6 months, recurrent, intense sexually arousing fantasies, sexual urges, or behaviors involving the use of nonliving objects (e.g., female undergarments).
B. The fantasies, sexual urges, or behaviors cause clinically significant distress or impairment in social, occupational, or other important areas of functioning.
C. The fetish objects are not limited to articles of female clothing used in cross-dressing (as in transvestic fetishism) or devices designed for the purpose of tactile genital stimulation (e.g., a vibrator).

Reprinted with permission from the Diagnostic and Statistical Manual of Mental Disorders, Fourth Edition, Text Revision. Copyright 2000 American Psychiatric Association.

DSM-IV-TR Diagnostic Criteria

302.03 Transvestic Fetishism

A. Over a period of at least 6 months, in a heterosexual male, recurrent intense sexually arousing fantasies, sexual urges, or behaviors involving cross-dressing.
B. The fantasies, sexual urges, or behaviors cause clinically significant distress or impairment in social, occupational, or other important areas of functioning.

Specify if:

With gender dysphoria: if the person has persistent discomfort with gender role or identity

---

Reprinted with permission from the Diagnostic and Statistical Manual of Mental Disorders, Fourth Edition, Text Revision. Copyright 2000 American Psychiatric Association.

SEXUAL MASOCHISM

Sexual masochism is diagnosed over a range of behaviors from the sometimes fatal need to nearly asphyxiate oneself to the request to be spanked by the partner in order to be excited (see DSM-IV-TR diagnostic criteria below). Masochism may be the most commonly reported or acknowledged form of female paraphilia, although it is more common among men. Sadists and masochists sometimes find one another and work out arrangement to act out their fantasies and occasionally reverse roles.

DSM-IV-TR Diagnostic Criteria

302.83 Sexual Masochism

A. Over a period of at least 6 months, recurrent, intense sexually arousing fantasies, sexual urges, or behaviors involving the act (real, not simulated) of being humiliated, beaten, bound, or otherwise made to suffer.
B. The fantasies, sexual urges, or behaviors cause clinically significant distress or impairment in social, occupational, or other important areas of functioning.

Reprinted with permission from the Diagnostic and Statistical Manual of Mental Disorders, Fourth Edition, Text Revision. Copyright 2000 American Psychiatric Association.

PARAPHILIA NOT OTHERWISE SPECIFIED

Paraphilia not otherwise specified is a DSM-IV-TR category for other endpoints of abnormal sexual development that lead to preoccupations with amputated body parts, feces, urine, sexualized enemas, and sex with animals.

Etiology

Paraphilia has been considered in 15 somewhat different ways, depending on era, ideology, and region: (1) an impairment in the bonding function of sexuality; (2) a courtship disorder; (3) the erotic form of hatred motivated by the need for revenge for childhood trauma; (4) a fixation to childhood misunderstandings that women had penises and that men could lose theirs during sex (castration anxiety); (5) the unsuccessful repair of early life passive, helpless experiences with a terrifying, malignant, malicious preoedipal mother; (6) a strategy to stabilize a conventional masculine or feminine gender identity; (7) a strategy to deny the differences between the sexes and the generations of child and parent; (8) an outcome of childhood sexual abuse; (9) a consequence of far less than ideal parent–child relationships; (10) a soft neurological sign of a neural wiring defect; (11) a released behavior due to cerebral pathology—for example, temporal lobe dysfunction, or substance abuse; (12) the sexual face of an addiction disorder; (13) an unusual manifestation of an affective disorder; (14) an obsessive–compulsive spectrum disorder; (15) a defective self-system requiring a patch—that is, a sexual preoccupation—to shore up the private, carefully-hidden-from-others sense of inadequate subjective masculinity.

Whatever its ultimate etiologies and nature, the paraphilias are sexual identity disorders that generally make normal erotic and sexual loving unattainable. Culture asks us to have some image of attachment, some ability to neutralize anger toward others, some ability to contain the anxiety over closeness, and some psychological motive to simultaneously enhance the self and the partner through sexual contact. Ordinary intentions aim for peaceable mutuality between real people; paraphilic ones aim at aggressive one-sidedness. This sexual identity disorder could be referred to as a disorder of self, specifically of that part of the self that maintains a sense of masculinity. Paraphilics often bear an enigmatic paradox between what they want to be and what they are. They often hunger for a behavior that feels uncontrollable or sick and which robs them of autonomy. This is why the behaviors are often thought of as addictions and are often associated with other forms of substance abuse, obsessive–compulsive phenomena, and affective symptoms. Relative to the dynamic fluctuations of sexual dysfunctions, intention disorders are tenacious throughout life.

Treatment

Four general approaches are employed to treat the paraphilias: evaluation only, psychotherapy, medications, and external controls. The treatments are not mutually exclusive; rather, they are often multimodal in application.

Evaluation only is often selected when the evaluator concludes that the paraphilia is benign in terms of society, the individual will be resistant to the other approaches, and does not suffer greatly in terms of social and vocational functioning in ways that might be improved. Often, these are isolated men with private paraphilic sexual pleasures, such as telephone sex with a masochistic scenario.

What constitutes psychotherapy for paraphilia heavily depends on the therapist training rather than strident declarations of treatment of choice. Little optimism exists that any form of therapy can permanently change the nature of a long-established paraphilic erotic script, even among teenage sex offenders. Individual psychodynamic psychotherapy can be highly useful in diminishing paraphilic intensifications and gradually teaching the individual better management techniques of the situations that have triggered acting out. Well-described cognitive–behavioral interventions exist for interrupting paraphilic arousal via pairing masturbatory excitement with either aversive imagery or aversive stimuli. Comprehensive behavioral treatment involves social skills training, assertiveness training, and confrontation with the rationalizations that are used to minimize awareness of the victims of sexual crimes, and marital therapy (Abel 1995). The self-help movement has created 12-step programs for sexual addictions to which many individuals now belong. Group psychotherapy is offered by trained therapists as well. When the lives of paraphilics are illuminated in various therapies, it becomes apparent that the emotional pain of the individuals is thought to be great; the sexual acting out is often perceived as a defense against recurrent unpleasant emotions from any source. These often, however, involve self-esteem and primitive anxiety.

In the early 1980s, depo-medroxyprogesterone (Provera) was first used to treat those who were constantly masturbating, seeking out personally dangerous sexual outlets, or committing sex crimes. The weekly 400- to 600-mg injections often led to the men being able to work, study, or participate in activities that were previously beyond them because of concentration or attention difficulties (Gijs and Gooren 1996). In the late 1980s, the use of oral Provera, 20 to 120 mg/day led to similar results: the drug enabled these men to leave their former state in which their sexual needs took priority over other life demands—and they did not have depo-Provera's side effect profile: weight gain, hypertension, muscle cramps, and gynecomastia. Today, gonadotrophin-releasing blockers are occasionally used for this purpose (Kreuger and Kaplan 2001). The possible side effects are similar to oral Provera. Despite the fact that the clinical results are among the most powerful effected by any psychopharmacologic treatment, many clinicians cannot overcome their disinclination about giving a "female" hormone to a man or working with individuals who victimize others sexually. Serotonergic agents are now more commonly used as a first line of treatment and their administration, of course, creates fewer countertransference obstacles

(Risen and Althof 1995). While these studies are not as methodologically sophisticated as they need to be, the SSRIs are in widespread use for compulsive sexual behaviors and sexual obsessions. Their efficacy is the source of the speculation that some of the paraphilias may be an obsessive–compulsive spectrum disorder.

Sexual advantage-taking, whether it be by a paraphilic clinician with the individuals under his care, by a pedophilic mentally retarded man in the neighborhood, or of a grandfather who has abused several generations of his offspring, can often be stopped by making it *impossible* for these behaviors to be unknown to most people in his life. The clinician's staff can be told, the neighbors can know, the family can meet to discuss the current crisis and review who has been abused over the years and plan to never allow the grandfather alone with any child in or outside the family. The concept of external control is taken over by the judicial system when sex crimes are highly repugnant or heinous. The offender is removed from society for punishment and the protection of the public. Increasing pressure exists to criminalize sexual advantage-taking by clinicians who are even more susceptible to losing their licenses at least for several years.

Clinicians need to be realistic about the limitations of various therapeutic ventures. Sexual acting out may readily continue during therapy beyond the awareness of the therapist (Travin 1995). The more violent and destructive the paraphilic behavior to others, the less the therapist should risk ambulatory treatment. Since paraphilia occurs in individuals with other mental disorders, the clinician needs to remain vigilant that the treatment program is comprehensive and does not lose sight of the paraphilia just because the depressive or compulsive symptoms are improved. Paraphilia may be improved by medications and psychotherapy, but the clinician should expect that the intention disorder is the individual's lasting vulnerability.

SEXUAL DISORDER NOT OTHERWISE SPECIFIED

If the clinician is uncertain about how to categorize a person's problem, it is more reasonable to use this diagnosis than one that does not encompass the range of the individual's suffering. Sexual disorder not otherwise specified can be used when the therapist perceives a dramatic interplay between issues of sexual identity and sexual dysfunction, or when "everything" seems to be amiss. DSM-IV-TR, however, encourages the clinician to make multiple sexual diagnoses involving, for instance, a gender identity disorder, a desire disorder, erectile, and orgasmic disorder.

DSM-IV-TR provides two examples when it would be appropriate to use the diagnosis sexual disorder NOS: (1) nonparaphilic compulsive sexual behaviors—that is, relentless pursuit of masturbatory or heterosexual or homosexual partner experiences without evidence of paraphilic imagery; (2) complicated or exaggerated struggles to manage homosexual urges. Despite the removal of homosexuality from the DSM in 1974 (Bayer 1981), men (particularly) and women still generate symptoms in their struggle to balance the demands of their homoeroticism with their ambitions to participate in conventional family life. This ongoing struggle can generate a variety of anxiety, depressive, compulsive, substance abusing, and suicidal states.

Comparison of DSM-IV-TR/ICD-10 Diagnostic Criteria
For hypoactive sexual desire disorder, the ICD-10 Diagnostic Criteria for Research and the DSM-IV-TR criteria are essentially identical except that ICD-10 specifies a minimum duration of at least 6 months (DSM-IV-TR has no minimum duration).

The ICD-10 Diagnostic Criteria for Research for Sexual Aversion Disorder differs from the DSM-IV-TR criteria in several ways. In contrast to DSM-IV-TR, which restricts the condition to the aversion to, and avoidance of, sexual genital contact, ICD-10 also includes presentations characterized by sexual activity resulting in "strong negative feelings and an inability to experience any pleasure." Furthermore, ICD-10 excludes cases in which the aversion is due to performance anxiety. Finally, ICD-10 specifies a minimum duration of at least 6 month whereas DSM-IV-TR does not specify any minimum duration.

For female sexual arousal disorder and male erectile disorder, the ICD-10 Diagnostic Criteria for Research and the DSM-IV-TR criteria are essentially equivalent except that ICD-10 specifies a minimum duration of at least 6 months. ICD-10 includes a single category ("Failure of Genital Response") with two separate criteria sets by gender. In contrast, DSM-IV-TR includes two separate categories.

For female and male orgasmic disorders, the ICD-10 Diagnostic Criteria for Research and the DSM-IV-TR criteria are essentially equivalent except that ICD-10 specifies a minimum duration of at least 6 months. In contrast to DSM-IV-TR, which has male and female versions defined separately, ICD-10 has a single category that applies to both genders.

For premature ejaculation, the ICD-10 Diagnostic Criteria for Research and the DSM-IV-TR criteria are essentially equivalent except that ICD-10 specifies a minimum duration of at least 6 months. Similarly, the ICD-10 Diagnostic Criteria for Research and the DSM-IV-TR criteria for Dyspareunia and Vaginismus are essentially equivalent except that ICD-10 specifies a minimum duration of at least 6 months. Furthermore, these conditions are referred to in ICD-10 as "Nonorganic Dyspareunia" and "Nonorganic Vaginismus."

The definition of a paraphilia is essentially the same in DSM-IV-TR and ICD-10. However, ICD-10 does not include a separate category for Frotteurism and has a combined "Sadomasochism" category.

For gender identity disorder, ICD-10 defines three separate disorders: "Gender Identity Disorder of Childhood," "Dual-role Transvestism," and "Transsexualism" all of which are included under the single DSM-IV-TR category Gender Identity Disorder.

References

Abel GG (1989) Paraphilias. In *Comprehensive Textbook of Psychiatry*, Vol. V. Kaplan and Sadock (eds). Williams & Wilkins, Baltimore, pp. 1069–1085.

Abel GG and Osborn CA (1995) Behavioral therapy treatment for sex offenders. In *Sexual Deviation*, 3rd ed., Rosen I (ed). Oxford University Press, London.

Abel GG, Becker JV, Mittelman MS, et al. (1987) Self-reported sex crimes of non-incarcerated paraphiliacs. *J Interpers Viol* **2**, 3.

Althof SE and Seftel AD (1995) The evaluation and management of erectile dysfunction. *Psychiatr Clin North Am* **18**(1), 177–192.

Althof SE, Levine SB, Corty E, et al. (1995) Double-blind crossover study of clomipramine for rapid ejaculation in 15 couples. *J Clin Psychiatry* **56**(9), 402–407.

American Psychiatric Association (1994) *Diagnostic and Statistical Manual*, 4th ed. APA, Washington, DC.

Basson R (2001) Using a different model for female sexual response to address women's problematic low sexual desire. *J Sex Marit Ther* **27**, 395–403.

Basson R (2003) Women's difficulties with low desire and sexual avoidance. In *Handbook of Clinical Sexuality for Mental Health Professionals*, Levine SB, Risen CB, and Althof SE (eds). Brunner/Routledge, New York.

Basson R, McInnes R, Smith MD, et al. (2002) Efficacy and safety of sildenafil citrate in women with sexual dysfunction associated with female sexual arousal disorder. *J Women's Health Gender-Based Stud* **11**(4), 367–377.

Bayer R (1981) *Homosexuality and American Psychiatry: The Politics of Diagnosis*. Basic Books, New York.

Beier KM (2000) Female analogies to perversion. *J Sex Marit Ther* **26**, 79–91.

Berman JR and Goldstein I (2001) Female sexual dysfunction. *Urol Clin North Am* **28**(2), 405–416.

Berman JR, Berman LA, Lin H, et al. (2001) Effect of sildenafil on subjective and physiologic parameters of female sexual response in women with sexual arousal disorder. *J Sex Marit Ther* **27**, 411–420.

Blanchard R (1989) The concept of autogynephilia and the typology of male gender dysphoria. *J Nerv Ment Dis* **177**, 616–623.

Blanchard R, Steiner BW, and Clemmensen LH (1985) Gender dysphoria, gender reorientation, and the clinical management of transsexualism. *J Consult Clin Psychol* **53**, 295–304.

Carrier S, Brock G, Kour NW, et al. (1993) Pathophysiology of erectile dysfunction. *Urology* **42**(4), 468–481.

Coates S and Person E (1985) Extreme boyhood femininity: isolated behavior or pervasive disorder? *J Am Acad Child Psychiatry* **24**, 702–709.

Coates S, Friedman RC, and Wolfe S (1992) The etiology of boyhood gender identity disorder: A model for integrating psychodynamics, temperament, and development. *Psychoanal Dialogues* **1**, 481–523.

Dennerstein L, Dudley EC, Hopper JL, et al. (2000) A prospective population-based study of menopausal symptoms. *Obstet Gynecol* **96**(3), 351–358.

Devor H (1999) *FTM: Female to Male Transsexualism.* Indiana University Press, Bloomington, Ind.

Feldman HA, Goldstein I, Hatzichristou DG, et al. (1994) Impotence and its medical and psychosocial correlates: results of the Massachusetts male aging study. *J Urol* **151**(1), 54–61.

Frank E, Anderson C, and Rubinstein D (1978) Frequency of sexual dysfunction in "normal" couples. *N Engl J Med* **299**, 111–113.

Freud S (1905) Three essays on the theory of sexuality. In *The Standard Edition of the Complete Works of Sigmund Freud*, Strachy J (ed). Hogarth Press, London, pp. 125–243.

Freud S (1912) On the universal tendency to debasement in the sphere of love (Contributions to the Psychology of Love II). In *Standard Edition of the Complete Works of Sigmund Freud*, Vol. 11. Strachey L (ed). Hogarth Press, London, pp. 179–190.

Gijs L and Gooren L (1996) Hormonal and psychopharmacological interventions in the treatment of paraphilias: an update. *J Sex Res* **33**, 273–290.

Gilbert DA, Winslow BH, Gilbert DM, et al. (1988) Transsexual surgery in the genetic female. *Clin Plas Surg* **15**(3), 471–487.

Goldstein I, Lue TF, Padma-Nathan H, et al. (1998) Oral sildenafil in the treatment of erectile dysfunction. Sildenafil study group. *N Engl J Med* **338**(20), 1397–1404.

Green R (1987) *"Sissy Boy Syndrome" and the Development of Male Homosexuality.* Yale University Press, New Haven.

Kafka MP and Prentky RA (1998) Attention-deficit/hyperactivity disorder in males with paraphilia and paraphilia-related disorder: a comorbidity study. *J Clin Psychiatry* **59**(7), 388–396.

Kaplan HS (1987) *Sexual Aversion, Sexual Phobias, and Panic Disorder.* Brunner/Mazel New York.

Keller AC, Althof SE, and Lothstein LM (1982) Group psychotherapy with gender identity patients—a four year study. *Am J Psychother* **36**, 223–228.

Kernberg OF (1991) Aggression and love in the relationship of a couple. In *Perversions and Near-Perversions in Clinical Practice: New Psychoanalytic Perspectives*, Fogel GI and Myers WA (eds). Yale University Press, New Haven.

Killman PR, Mills KH, Caid C, et al. (1986) Treatment of secondary orgasmic dysfunction: an outcome study. *Arch Sex Behav* **15**, 211–229.

Krane RJ, Goldstein I, and Saenz de Tejada I (1989) Impotence. *N Engl J Med* **321**, 1648–1659.

Kreuger RB and Kaplan MS (2001) Depot-leuprolide acetate for treatment of paraphilias: a report of twelve cases. *Arch Sex Behav* **30**(4), 409–422.

Laumann EO and Michael RT (eds) (2001) *Sex, Love, and Health in America: Private Choices and Public Policies.* University of Chicago Press, Chicago.

Laumann EO, Gagnon J, and Michael RT (1994a) *Sex in America.* University of Chicago Press, Chicago.

Laumann EO, Gagnon JH, Michael RT, et al. (1994b) *The Social Organization of Sexuality.* University of Chicago Press, Chicago.

Levine SB (1989) *Sex is not Simple.* Ohio Psychology Publications, Columbus.

Levine SB (1992) *Sexual Life: AA Clinician's Guide.* Plenum Press, New York.

Levine SB (1998a) *The Nature of Love in Sexuality in Mid-Life.* Kluwer Academic/Plenum Publishers, New York, pp. 1–22.

Levine SB (1998b) *Sexuality in Mid-life.* Kluwer Academic/Plenum Publishers, New York.

Levine SB (2002) Re-exploring the concept of sexual desire. *J Sex Marit Ther* **28**(1), 39–51.

Lothstein LM and Levine SB (1981) Expressive psychotherapy with gender dysphoric patients. *Arch Gen Psychiatry* **38**, 924–929.

Lue TF (2000) Erectile dysfunction. *N Engl J Med* **342**(24), 1802–1813.

Maccoby EE and Jacklin CN (1987) Gender segregation in childhood. *Adv Child Dev Behav* **20**, 239–287.

Masand PS, Ashton AK, Gupta S, et al. (2001) Sustained-release bupropion for selective serotonin reuptake inhibitor-induced sexual dysfunction: a randomized, double-blind, placebo-controlled, parallel-group study. *Am J Psychiatry* **158**(5), 805–807.

Masters WH and Johnson V (1966) *Human Sexual Response.* Little, Brown & Co, Boston.

Masters WH and Johnson V (1970) *Human Sexual Inadequacy.* Little, Brown & Co, Boston.

Mate-Kole C, Freschi M, and Robin A (1990) A controlled study of psychological and social change after surgical gender reassignment in selected male transsexuals. *Br J Psychiatry* **157**, 261–264.

McEwan L, Ceber S, and Davis J (1986) Male-to-female surgical genital reassignment. In *Transsexualism and Sex Reassignment*, Walters WAW and Ross MJ (eds). Oxford University Press, New York.

McKay M (1992) Vulvodynia: diagnostic patterns. *Dermatol Clin North Am* **10**, 423–433.

Meana M and Binik YM (1994) Painful coitus: a review of female dyspareunia. *J Nerv Ment Dis* **182**(5), 264–272.

Meyer W (Chairman), Bockting WO, Cohen-Kettenis P, et al. (2001) *Harry Benjamin International Gender Dysphoria Association's the Standard of Care for Gender Identity Disorders*, Sixth Version, 6th Rev. Symposion Publishing, Dusseldorf.

Money J (1986) *Lovemaps: Clinical Concepts of Sexual/Erotic Health and Pathology, Paraphilia, and Gender Transpositions in Childhood, Adolescence, and Maturity*. Irvington Publishers, New York.

O'Carroll R (1991) Sexual desire disorders: a review of controlled treatment studies. *J Sex Res* **28**, 607–624.

Ohl DA (1994) Treatments for erectile dysfunction. In *Sexual Dysfunction Neurologic, Urologic, and Gynecologic Aspects*, Lechtenberg R and Ohl DA (eds). Lea and Febiger, Philadelphia, pp. 292–361.

O'Keefe M and Hunt DK (1995) Assessment and treatment of impotence. *Med Clin North Am* **79**(2), 415–434.

Pallas J, Levine SB, Althof SE, et al. (2000) A study using Viagra in a mental health practice. *J Sex Marit Ther* **26**(1), 41–50.

Pawlak AE, Boulet JR, and Bradford JMW (1991) Discriminant analysis of a sexual-function inventory with intrafamilial and extrafamilial child molesters. *Arch Sex Behav* **20**(1), 27–34.

Petersen ME and Dickey R (1995) Surgical sex reassignment: a comparative survey of international centers. *Arch Sex Behav* **24**(2), 135–156.

Risen CB and Althof SE (1995) A case of a paraphilia. In *Case Studies in Sex Therapy*, Rosen RC and Leiblum SR (eds). Guilford Press, New York.

Rosen RC and Leiblum SR (1995) Hypoactive sexual desire. *Psychiatr Clin North Am* **18**(1), 107–121.

Segraves RT (1998) Antidepressant-induced sexual dysfunction. *J Clin Psychiatry* **59**(Suppl. 4), 48–54.

Shaw J (ed) (1999) *Sexual Aggression*. American Psychiatric Press, Washington, DC.

Tiefer L (1998) A feminist critique of the sexual dysfunction nomenclature. *Women Ther* **7**, 3–21.

Travin S (1995) Compulsive sexual behaviors. *Psychiatr Clin North Am* **18**(1), 155–169.

Waldinger MD, Hengeveld MW, and Zwinderman AH (1994) Paroxetine treatment of premature ejaculation: a double-blind, randomized, placebo-controlled study. *Am J Psychiatry* **151**(9), 1377–1379.

Zucker KJ (1990) Psychosocial and erotic development in cross-gender identified children. *Can J Psychol* **35**(6), 487–495.

Zucker KJ (1995) Treatment of cross-gender identified children. *A Presentation at the Society for Sexual Therapy and Research Meeting* (Mar), New York.

40 Eating Disorders

In the current diagnostic nomenclature of the *Diagnostic and Statistical Manual of Mental Disorders*, Fourth Edition (DSM-IV-TR), eating disorders consist of two clearly defined syndromes: anorexia nervosa and bulimia nervosa. Many individuals presenting for treatment of an eating disorder fail to meet the formal criteria for either anorexia nervosa or bulimia nervosa, which raises an important theoretical and practical question: what is an eating disorder? Although this topic has received surprisingly little attention, it has been suggested that a working definition of an eating disorder might be "a persistent disturbance of eating behavior or behavior intended to control weight, which significantly impairs physical health or psychosocial functioning" (Fairburn and Walsh 2002). This definition clearly encompasses the recognized disorders, anorexia nervosa and bulimia nervosa. In addition, it provides a basis for viewing eating disorders as clinically significant problems that do not meet criteria for anorexia nervosa or bulimia nervosa. The term *atypical eating disorder* is often applied to such problems, even though the number of individuals suffering from them may well outnumber those with "typical" eating disorders. One example of an atypical eating disorder is that of women who are overly concerned about their weight, have dieted to a below-normal weight, but have not ceased menstruating and, therefore, do not meet full criteria for anorexia nervosa. Another is that of individuals who binge and vomit regularly, but at less than the twice-a-week frequency required for bulimia nervosa.

An additional example of a clinically important atypical eating disorder is the occurrence of frequent binge-eating that is not followed by the self-induced vomiting or other inappropriate attempts to compensate that are characteristic of bulimia nervosa. This disturbance, for which the name *binge-eating disorder* has been proposed (DSM-IV-TR appendix B) (Yanovski 1993), is a common behavioral pattern among obese individuals who present for treatment at weight-loss clinics.

At present, obesity is not considered an eating disorder. Obesity refers to an excess of body fat and is viewed as a general medical, not a psychiatric, condition. At this stage of our knowledge, obesity is conceived as an etiologically heterogeneous condition. Obese individuals are at increased risk for a number of serious medical problems and are subject to significant social stigmatization and its psychological sequelae. However, the widely held assumption that obesity is the result of a psychiatric disorder in which eating is used as a coping mechanism for depression or anxiety has not been substantiated by empirical research. Studies of obese and normal-weight subjects from the general population have found no more psychiatric disturbance in those who are overweight than in those who are of normal weight (Seidell and Thjhuis 2002). Therefore, it seems appropriate at present to describe as having an eating disorder only those obese individuals who manifest a clear behavioral abnormality that impairs health or psychosocial functioning.

ANOREXIA NERVOSA

Diagnosis

The DSM-IV-TR criteria for Anorexia Nervosa require the individual to be significantly underweight for age and height (see DSM-IV-TR diagnostic criteria below). Although it is not possible to set a single weight-loss standard that applies equally to all individuals, DSM-IV-TR provides a benchmark of 85% of the weight considered normal for age and height as a guideline. Despite being of an abnormally low body weight, individuals with anorexia nervosa are intensely afraid of gaining weight and becoming fat, and remarkably, this fear typically intensifies as the weight falls.

DSM-IV-TR Diagnostic Criteria

307.1 Anorexia Nervosa

A. Refusal to maintain body weight at or above a minimally normal weight for age and height (e.g., weight loss leading to maintenance of body weight less than 85% of that expected; or failure to make expected weight gain during period of growth, leading to body weight less than 85% of that expected).
B. Intense fear of gaining weight or becoming fat, even though underweight.
C. Disturbance in the way in which one's body weight or shape is experienced, undue influence of body weight or shape on self-evaluation, or denial of the seriousness of the current low body weight.
D. In postmenarcheal females, amenorrhea, i.e., the absence of at least three consecutive menstrual cycles. (A woman is considered to have amenorrhea if her periods occur only following hormone, e.g., estrogen, administration.)

Specify type:

Restricting type: during the current episode of anorexia nervosa, the person has not regularly engaged in binge-eating or purging behavior (i.e., self-induced vomiting or the misuse of laxatives, diuretics, or enemas).

> **Binge-eating/purging type**: during the current episode of anorexia nervosa, the person has regularly engaged in binge-eating or purging behavior (i.e., self-induced vomiting or the misuse of laxatives, diuretics, or enemas).

Reprinted with permission from the Diagnostic and Statistical Manual of Mental Disorders, Fourth Edition, Text Revision. Copyright 2000 American Psychiatric Association.

DSM-IV-TR criterion C requires a disturbance in the person's judgment about his or her weight or shape. For example, despite being underweight, individuals with anorexia nervosa often view themselves or a part of their body as being too heavy. Typically, they deny the grave medical risks engendered by their semistarvation and place enormous psychological importance on whether they have gained or lost weight. For example, someone with anorexia nervosa may feel intensely distressed if her or his weight increases by half a pound. Finally, criterion D requires that women with anorexia nervosa be amenorrheic.

DSM-IV-TR suggests that individuals with anorexia nervosa be classed as having one of two variants, either the binge-eating/purging type or the restricting type. Individuals with the restricting type of anorexia nervosa do not engage regularly in either binge-eating or purging, and compared with individuals with the binge-eating/purging form of the disorder, are not as likely to abuse alcohol and other drugs, exhibit less mood lability, and are less active sexually. There are also indications that the two subtypes may differ in their response to pharmacological intervention (Halmi et al. 1986).

Anorexia nervosa often begins innocently. Typically, an adolescent girl or young woman who is of normal weight or, perhaps, a few pounds overweight decides to diet. This decision may be prompted by an important but not extraordinary life event, such as leaving home for camp, attending a new school, or a casual unflattering remark by a friend or family member. Initially, the dieting seems no different from that pursued by many young women, but as weight falls, the dieting intensifies. The restrictions become broader and more rigid; for example, desserts may first be eliminated, then meat, then any food that is thought to contain fat. The person becomes increasingly uncomfortable if she is seen eating and avoids meals with others. Food seems to assume a moral quality so that, for example, vegetables are viewed as "good" and anything with fat is "bad." The individual has idiosyncratic rules about how much exercise she must do, and when, where, and how she can eat.

Food avoidance and weight loss are accompanied by a deep and reassuring sense of accomplishment, and weight gain is viewed as a failure and a sign of weakness. Physical activity, such as running or aerobic exercise, often increases as the dieting and weight loss develop. Inactivity and complaints of weakness usually occur only when emaciation has become extreme. The person becomes more serious and devotes little effort to anything but work, dieting, and exercise. She may become depressed and emotionally labile, socially withdrawn, and secretive, and she may lie about her eating and her weight. Despite the profound disturbances in her view of her weight and of her calorie needs, reality testing in other spheres is intact, and the person may continue to function well in school or at work. Symptoms usually persist for months or years until, typically at the insistence of friends or family, the person reluctantly agrees to see a physician.

Course

The course of anorexia nervosa is enormously variable. Some individuals have mild and brief illnesses and either never come to medical attention or are seen only briefly by their pediatrician or general medical physician. It is difficult to estimate the frequency of this phenomenon because such individuals are rarely studied. Most of the literature on course and outcome is based on individuals who have been hospitalized for anorexia nervosa. Although such individuals presumably have a relatively severe illness and adverse outcomes, a substantial fraction, probably between one-third and one-half, make full and complete psychological and physical recoveries. On the other hand, anorexia nervosa is also associated with an impressive long-term mortality. The best data currently available suggest that 10 to 20% of individuals who have been hospitalized for anorexia nervosa will, in the next 10 to 30 years, die as a result of their illness. Much of the mortality is due to severe and chronic starvation, which eventually terminates in sudden death. In addition, a significant fraction of individuals commit suicide.

Between these two extremes are a large number of individuals whose lives are impaired by persistent difficulties with eating. Some are severely affected maintaining a chronic state of semistarvation, bizarre eating rituals, and social isolation; others may gain weight but struggle with bulimia nervosa and strict rules about food and eating; and still others may recover initially but then relapse into another full episode. There is a high frequency of depression among individuals who have had anorexia nervosa and a significant frequency of drug and alcohol abuse, but psychotic disorders develop only rarely. Thus, in general, individuals either recover or continue to struggle with psychological and behavioral problems that are directly related to the eating disorder. It is of note that it is rare for individuals who have had anorexia nervosa to become obese.

In assessing individuals who may have anorexia nervosa, it is important to obtain a weight history including the individual's highest and lowest weights and the weight he or she would like to be now. For women, it is useful to know the weight at which menstruation last occurred, because it provides an indication of what weight is normal for that individual. Probably the greatest problem in the assessment of individuals with anorexia nervosa is their denial of the illness and their reluctance to participate in an evaluation. A straightforward but supportive and nonconfrontational style is probably the most useful approach, but it is likely that the individual will not acknowledge significant difficulties in eating or with weight and will rationalize unusual eating or exercise habits. It is therefore helpful to obtain information from other sources such as the individual's family.

An impressive array of physical disturbances has been documented in anorexia nervosa, and the physiological bases of many are understood (Walsh 2001) (Table 40-1). Most of these physical disturbances appear to be secondary consequences of starvation, and it is not clear whether or how the physiological disturbances described here contribute to the development and maintenance of the psychological and behavioral abnormalities characteristic of anorexia nervosa. The central nervous system is clearly affected. Computed tomography has demonstrated that individuals with anorexia nervosa have enlarged ventricles, an abnormality that improves with weight gain. The cerebrospinal fluid concentrations of a variety of neurotransmitters and their metabolites are altered in underweight individuals with anorexia nervosa and tend to normalize as weight is restored. An intriguing exception may be the serotonin metabolite 5-hydroxyindoleacetic acid, which has been reported to be elevated in the cerebrospinal fluid of individuals with anorexia nervosa after they have achieved a normal or near-normal weight. Kaye (1997) has suggested that the elevated 5-hydroxyindoleacetic acid levels may reflect a serotoninergic abnormality that is tied to the obsessional traits often observed in anorexia nervosa.

Some of the most striking physiological alterations in anorexia nervosa are those of the hypothalamic–pituitary–gonadal axis. In women, estrogen secretion from the ovaries is markedly reduced, accounting for the occurrence of amenorrhea. In analogous fashion, testosterone production is diminished in men with anorexia nervosa. The decrease in gonadal steroid production is due to a reduction in the pituitary's secretion of the gonadotropins luteinizing hormone and follicle-stimulating hormone, which in turn is secondary to diminished release of gonadotropin-releasing hormone from the hypothalamus.

Table 40-1	Medical Problems Commonly Associated with Anorexia Nervosa

Skin
  Lanugo
Cardiovascular system
  Hypotension
  Bradycardia
  Arrhythmias
Hematopoietic system
  Normochromic, normocytic anemia
  Leukopenia
    Diminished polymorphonuclear leukocytes
Fluid and electrolyte balance
  Elevated blood urea nitrogen and creatinine concentrations
  Hypokalemia
  Hyponatremia
  Hypochloremia
  Alkalosis
Gastrointestinal system
  Elevated serum concentration of liver enzymes
  Delayed gastric emptying
  Constipation
Endocrine system
  Diminished thyroxine level with normal thyroid-stimulating hormone level
  Elevated plasma cortisol level
  Diminished secretion of luteinizing hormone, follicle-stimulating hormone, estrogen, or testosterone
Bone
  Osteoporosis

Therefore, the amenorrhea of anorexia nervosa is properly viewed as a type of hypothalamic amenorrhea. It is of interest that in a significant minority, amenorrhea begins before substantial weight loss has occurred, suggesting that factors other than malnutrition, such as psychological distress, contribute significantly to the disruption of the reproductive endocrine system.

In an adult with anorexia nervosa, the status of the hypothalamic–pituitary–gonadal axis resembles that of a pubertal or prepubertal child—the secretion of estrogen or testosterone, of luteinizing hormone and follicle-stimulating hormone, and of gonadotropin-releasing hormone is reduced. This endocrinological picture may be contrasted with that of post-menopausal women who have a similar reduction in estrogen secretion but who, unlike women with anorexia nervosa, show increased pituitary gonadotropin secretion. Further-more, even the circadian patterns of luteinizing hormone and follicle-stimulating hormone secretion in adult women with anorexia nervosa closely resemble the patterns normally seen in pubertal and prepubertal girls (Figure 40-1). Although similar abnormalities are also seen in other forms of hypothalamic amenorrhea and are therefore not specific to anorexia nervosa, it is nonetheless striking that this syndrome is accompanied by a physiological arrest or regression of the reproductive endocrine system.

The functioning of other hormonal systems is also disrupted in anorexia nervosa, although typically not as profoundly as is the reproductive axis. Presumably as part of the metabolic response to semistarvation, the activity of the thyroid gland is reduced. Plasma thyroxine levels are somewhat diminished, but the plasma level of the pituitary hormone and thyroid-stimulating hormone is not elevated. The activity of the hypothalamic–pituitary–adrenal axis is increased, as indicated by elevated plasma levels of cortisol and by resistance to dexamethasone suppression. The regulation of vasopressin (antidiuretic hormone) secretion from the posterior pituitary is disturbed, contributing to the development of partial diabetes insipidus in some individuals.

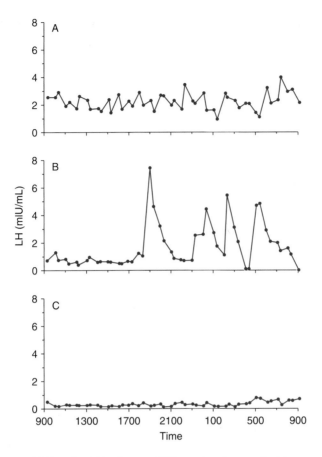

Figure 40-1 *Patterns of 24-hour luteinizing hormone (LH) secretion of a normal adult woman (A), of a woman with anorexia nervosa showing a pattern normally seen in adolescence (B), and of a woman with anorexia nervosa showing a pattern normally seen before puberty (C).*

Anorexia nervosa is often associated with the development of leukopenia and of a normochromic, normocytic anemia of mild to moderate severity. Surprisingly, leukopenia does not appear to result in a high vulnerability to infectious illnesses. Serum levels of liver enzymes are sometimes elevated, particularly during the early phases of refeeding, but the synthetic function of the liver is rarely seriously impaired so that the serum albumin concentration and the prothrombin time are usually within normal limits. Serum cholesterol levels are sometimes elevated in anorexia nervosa, although the basis of this abnormality remains obscure. In some individuals, self-imposed fluid restriction and excessive exercise produce dehydration and elevations of serum creatinine and blood urea nitrogen. In others, water loading may lead to hyponatremia. The status of serum electrolytes is a reflection of the individual's salt and water intake and the nature and the severity of the purging behavior. A common pattern is hypokalemia, hypochloremia, and mild alkalosis resulting from frequent and persistent self-induced vomiting.

It has become clear that individuals with anorexia nervosa have decreased bone density compared with age- and sex-matched peers and, as a result, are at increased risk for fractures. Low levels of estrogen, high levels of cortisol, and poor nutrition have been cited as risk factors for the development of reduced bone density in anorexia nervosa.

Theoretically, estrogen treatment might reduce the risk of osteoporosis in women who are chronically amenorrheic because of anorexia nervosa, but controlled studies indicate that this intervention is of limited, if any, benefit.

Abnormalities of cardiac function include bradycardia and hypotension, which are rarely symptomatic. The pump function of the heart is compromised, and congestive heart failure occasionally develops in individuals during overly rapid refeeding. The electrocardiogram shows sinus bradycardia and a number of nonspecific abnormalities. Arrhythmias may develop, often in association with fluid and electrolyte disturbances. It has been suggested that significant prolongation of the QT interval may be a harbinger of life-threatening arrhythmias in some individuals with anorexia nervosa, but this has not been conclusively demonstrated.

The motility of the gastrointestinal tract is diminished, leading to delayed gastric emptying and contributing to complaints of bloating and constipation. Rare cases of acute gastric dilatation or gastric rupture, which is often fatal, have been reported in individuals with anorexia nervosa who consumed large amounts of food when binge-eating.

Epidemiology

Anorexia nervosa is a relatively rare illness. Even among high-risk groups, such as adolescent girls and young women, the prevalence of strictly defined anorexia nervosa is only about 0.5%. The prevalence rates of partial syndromes are substantially higher (Van Hoeken et al. 1998). Despite the infrequent occurrence of anorexia nervosa, most studies suggest that its incidence has increased significantly during the last 50 years, a phenomenon usually attributed to changes in cultural norms regarding desirable body shape and weight.

Anorexia nervosa usually affects women; the ratio of men to women is approximately 1 : 10 to 1 : 20. Anorexia nervosa occurs primarily in industrialized and affluent countries and some data suggest that even within those countries, anorexia nervosa is more common among the higher socioeconomic classes. Some occupations, such as ballet dancing and fashion modeling, appear to confer a particularly high risk for the development of anorexia nervosa. Thus, anorexia nervosa appears more likely to develop in an environment in which food is readily available but in which, for women, being thin is somehow equated with higher or special achievement.

Differential Diagnosis

Although depression, schizophrenia, and obsessive–compulsive disorder may be associated with disturbed eating and weight loss, it is rarely difficult to differentiate these disorders from anorexia nervosa. Individuals with major depression may lose significant amounts of weight but do not exhibit the relentless drive for thinness characteristic of anorexia nervosa. In schizophrenia, starvation may occur because of delusions about food, for example, that it is poisoned. Individuals with obsessive–compulsive disorder may describe irrational concerns about food and develop rituals related to meal preparation and eating but do not describe the intense fear of gaining weight and the pervasive wish to be thin that characterize anorexia nervosa.

A wide variety of medical problems cause serious weight loss in young people and may at times be confused with anorexia nervosa. Examples of such problems include gastric outlet obstruction, Crohn's disease, and brain tumors. Individuals whose weight loss is due to a general medical illness generally do not show the drive for thinness, the fear of gaining weight, and the increased physical activity characteristic of anorexia nervosa. However, the clinician is well advised to consider any chronic medical illness associated with weight loss, especially when evaluating individuals with unusual clinical presentations such as late age at onset or prominent physical complaints, for example, pain and gastrointestinal cramping while eating.

Etiology

The syndrome of anorexia nervosa was clearly recognized and, in fact, named in the late nineteenth century. Almost simultaneously, Sir William Gull in England and Charles Lasègue in France described series of cases of young women with impressive weight loss and psychological disturbance. Gull termed this illness *anorexia nervosa* and Lasègue—*anorexie hystérique*. Anorexia nervosa's long history suggests that although changing cultural norms for what is viewed as esthetically desirable may have played a role in increasing the frequency of anorexia nervosa, they do not fully explain the occurrence of the syndrome.

At present, the etiology of anorexia nervosa is fundamentally unknown. However, it is possible to identify risk factors whose presence increases the likelihood of anorexia nervosa. It is also possible to describe the course and complications of the syndrome and to suggest interactions between features of the disorder, for example, between malnutrition and psychiatric illness. Thus, as indicated in Figure 40-2, the difficulties that lead to the development of anorexia nervosa may be distinct from the forces that intensify the symptoms and perpetuate the illness once it has begun.

Anorexia nervosa occurs more frequently in biological relatives of individuals who present with the disorder. The prevalence rate of anorexia nervosa among sisters of such individuals is estimated to be approximately 6%; the morbid risk among other relatives ranges from 2 to 4%. Some evidence for a genetic component in the etiology of anorexia nervosa comes from twin studies, which reported substantially higher concordance rates for monozygotic than for dizygotic twin pairs (Klump et al. 2001). However, conclusive data for genetic transmission of the disorder are not yet available.

Individual mental disorder in parents, dysfunctional family relationships, and impaired family interaction patterns have been implicated in the etiology of anorexia nervosa. Mothers of individuals with anorexia nervosa are often described as overprotective, intrusive, perfectionistic, and fearful of separation; fathers are described as withdrawn, passive, emotionally constricted, obsessional, moody, and ineffectual. Family systems theorists have suggested that impaired family interactions such as pathological enmeshment, rigidity,

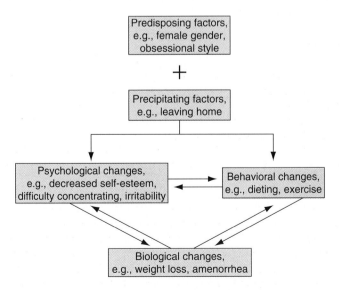

Figure 40-2 *Schematic diagram illustrating how an interplay of factors may lead to the initiation and persistence of anorexia nervosa.*

overprotectiveness, and difficulties confronting and resolving conflicts are central features of anorexic pathology (Minuchin et al. 1978). However, few empirical studies have been conducted to date, particularly studies that also examine psychiatrically or medically ill comparison groups. Therefore, the precise role of the family in the development and course of anorexia nervosa, although undoubtedly important, has not been clearly delineated.

The increased prevalence of anorexia nervosa has been connected to the current emphasis in contemporary Western society on an unrealistically thin appearance in women (Hsu 1996). There is substantial evidence that a desire to be slim is common among middle- and upper-class white women and that this emphasis on slimness has increased significantly during the past several decades. In the United States, anorexia nervosa develops much more frequently in white adolescents than in adolescents from other racial groups. It has been suggested that a variety of characteristics may protect African–American girls from having eating disorders, including more acceptance of being overweight, more satisfaction with their body image, and less social pressure regarding weight (Striegel-Moore et al. 2000).

It has also been suggested that the emphasis of contemporary Western society on achievement and performance in women, which is a shift from the more traditional emphasis on deference, compliance, and unassertiveness, has left many young women vulnerable to the development of eating disorders such as anorexia nervosa. These multiple and contradictory role demands are embodied within the modern concept of a superwoman who performs all of the expected roles (e.g., is competent, ambitious, and achieving, yet also feminine, nurturing, and sexual) and, in addition, devotes considerable attention to her appearance (Gordon 1990). Various psychoanalytic theories have also been postulated (e.g., defense against fantasies of oral impregnation; underlying deficits in the development of object relations; deficits in self-structure), but such hypotheses are difficult to verify. Bruch (1973, 1982) suggested that anorexia nervosa stems from failures in early attachment, attempts to cope with underlying feelings of ineffectiveness and inadequacy, and an inability to meet the demands of adolescence and young adulthood. These ideas, as well as her conceptualization that the single-minded focus on losing weight in anorexia nervosa is the concrete manifestation of a struggle to achieve a sense of identity, purpose, specialness, and control, are compelling and clinically useful. Cognitive–behavioral theories emphasize the distortions and dysfunctional thoughts (e.g., dichotomous thinking) that may stem from various causal factors, all of which eventually focus on the belief that it is essential to be thin.

Although the existence of a specific predisposing personality style has not been conclusively documented, certain traits have commonly been reported among women with anorexia nervosa. Women hospitalized for anorexia nervosa have greater self-discipline, conscientiousness, and emotional caution than women hospitalized for bulimia nervosa and women with no eating disorders (Casper et al. 1992). In addition, even after they have recovered from their illness, women who have had anorexia nervosa tend to avoid risks and to exhibit high levels of caution in emotional expression and strong compliance with rules and moral standards (Srinivasagam et al. 1995).

Because anorexia nervosa typically begins during adolescence, developmental issues are thought to play an important etiological role. Critical challenges at this time of life include the need to establish independence, a well-defined personal identity, fulfilling relationships, and clear values and principles to govern one's life. Family struggles, conflicts regarding sexuality, and pressures regarding increased heterosexual contact are also common. However, it is not clear that difficulties over these issues are more salient for individuals who will develop anorexia nervosa than for other adolescents. Depression has been implicated as a nonspecific risk factor, and higher levels of depressive symptoms as well as insecurity, anxiety, and self-consciousness have been documented in adolescent girls in comparison with adolescent boys. Similarly, the progression of physical and sexual maturation and the concomitant increase in women's percentage of body fat may have a substantial impact on the self-image of adolescent girls, particularly because the relationship between self-esteem and satisfaction with physical appearance and body characteristics is stronger in women than in men.

Treatment

The first goal of treatment is to engage the individual and her or his family. For most individuals with anorexia nervosa, this is challenging. Individuals usually minimize their symptoms and suggest that the concerns of the family and friends, who have often been instrumental in arranging the consultation, are greatly exaggerated. It is helpful to identify a problem that the individual can acknowledge, such as weakness, irritability, difficulty concentrating, or trouble with binge-eating. The clinician may then attempt to educate the individual regarding the pervasive physical and psychological effects of semistarvation and about the need for weight gain if the acknowledged problem is to be successfully addressed.

A second goal of treatment is to assess and address acute medical problems, such as fluid and electrolyte disturbances and cardiac arrhythmias. Depending on the severity of illness, this may require the involvement of a general medical physician. The additional but most difficult and time-consuming goals are the restoration of normal body weight, the normalization of eating, and the resolution of the associated psychological disturbances. The final goal is the prevention of relapse.

As already noted, virtually all of the physiological abnormalities described in individuals with anorexia nervosa are also seen in other forms of starvation, and most improve or disappear as weight returns to normal. Therefore, weight restoration is essential for physiological recovery. More surprisingly, perhaps, weight restoration is believed to be essential for psychological recovery as well. Accounts of human starvation amply document the profound impact of starvation on mental health. Starving individuals lose their sense of humor, their interest in friends and family fades, and mood generally becomes depressed. They may develop peculiar behavior similar to that of individuals with anorexia nervosa, such as hoarding food or concocting bizarre food combinations. If starvation disrupts psychological and behavioral functioning in normal individuals, it presumably does so as well in those with anorexia nervosa. Thus, correction of starvation is a prerequisite for the restoration of both physical and psychological health.

A common major impediment to the treatment of individuals with anorexia nervosa is their disagreement with the goals of treatment; many of the features of their illness are simply not viewed by these individuals as a problem. In addition, this may be compounded by a variety of concerns of the individual, such as basic mistrust of relationships, feelings of vulnerability and inferiority, and sensitivity to perceived coercion. Such concerns may be expressed through considerable resistance, defiance, or pseudocompliance with the clinician's interventions and contribute to the power struggles that often characterize the treatment process. The clinician must try to avoid colluding with the individual's attempts to minimize problems but at the same time allow the individual enough independence to maintain the alliance. Dealing with such dilemmas is challenging and requires an active approach on the part of the clinician. In most instances, it is possible to preserve the alliance while nonetheless adhering to established limits and the need for change.

The initial stage of treatment should be aimed at reversing the nutritional and behavioral abnormalities (Figure 40-3). The intensity of the treatment required and the need for partial or full hospitalization should be determined by the current weight, the rapidity of weight loss, and the severity of associated medical and behavioral problems and of other symptoms such as depression. In general, individuals whose weights are less than 75% of the expected weight should be viewed as medically precarious and require intensive treatment, such as hospitalization.

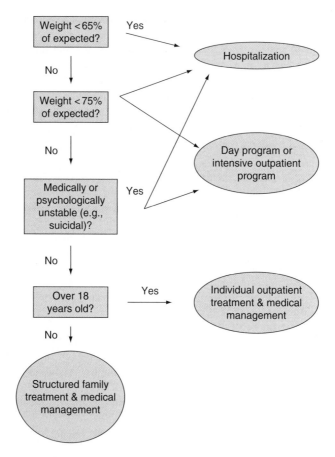

Figure 40-3 *Algorithm for choice of initial treatment of anorexia nervosa.*

Most inpatient or day treatment units experienced in the care of individuals with anorexia nervosa use a structured treatment approach that relies heavily on supervision of calorie intake by the staff. Individuals are initially expected to consume sufficient calories to maintain weight, usually requiring 1500 to 2000 kcal/day in four to six meals. After the initial medical assessment has been completed and weight has stabilized, calorie intake is gradually increased to an amount necessary to gain 2 to 5 lb/week. Because the consumption of approximately 4000 kcal beyond maintenance requirements is needed for each pound of weight gain, the daily calorie requirements become impressive, often in the range of 4000 kcal/day. Some eating disorder units provide only food while others rely on nutritional supplements. During this phase of treatment, it is necessary to monitor individuals carefully; many will resort to throwing food away or vomiting after meals. Careful supervision is also required to obtain accurate weights; individuals may consume large amounts of fluid before being weighed or hide heavy articles under their clothing.

During the weight restoration phase of treatment, individuals require substantial emotional support. It is probably best to address fears of weight gain with education about the dangers of semistarvation and with the reassurance that individuals will not be allowed to gain "too much" weight. Most eating-disorder units impose behavioral restrictions, such as limits on physical activity, during the early phase of treatment. Some units use an explicit behavior modification regimen in which weight gain is tied to increased privileges and failure to gain weight results in bed rest.

A consistent and structured treatment approach, with or without an explicit behavior modification program, is generally successful in promoting weight recovery but requires substantial energy and coordination to maintain a supportive and nonpunitive treatment environment. In most experienced treatment units, parenteral methods of nutrition, such as nasogastric feeding or intravenous hyperalimentation, are only rarely needed. Nutritional counseling and behavioral approaches can also be effective in helping individuals expand their dietary repertoire to include foods they have been frightened of consuming.

As weight increases, individual, group, and family psychotherapy can begin to address other issues in addition to the distress engendered by gaining weight (Garner and Garfinkel 1997). For example, it is typically important for individuals to recognize that they have come to base much of their self-esteem on dieting and weight control and are likely to judge themselves according to harsh and unforgiving standards. Similarly, individuals should be helped to see how the eating disorder has interfered with the achievement of personal goals such as education, sports, or making friends.

There is, at present, no general agreement about the most useful type of psychotherapy or the specific topics that need to be addressed. Most eating disorders programs employ a variety of psychotherapeutic interventions. A number of experts recommend the use of individual and group psychotherapy using cognitive–behavioral techniques to modify the irrational overemphasis on weight. Although most authorities see little role for traditional psychoanalytic therapy, individual and group psychodynamic therapy can address such problems as insecure attachment, separation and individuation, sexual relationships, and other interpersonal concerns. There is good evidence supporting the involvement of the family in the treatment of younger individuals with anorexia nervosa. Family therapy can be helpful in addressing family members' fears about the illness; interventions typically emphasize parental cooperation, mutual support and consistency, and establishing boundaries regarding the individual's symptoms and other aspects of his or her life (Lock et al. 2000).

Despite the multiple physiological disturbances associated with anorexia nervosa, there is no clearly established role for medication (Zhu and Walsh 2002). The earliest systematic medication trials in anorexia nervosa focused on the use of neuroleptics. Theoretically, such agents might help to promote weight gain, to reduce physical activity, and to diminish the distorted thinking about shape and weight, which often reaches nearly delusional proportions. Early work in the late 1950s and 1960s using chlorpromazine led to substantial enthusiasm, but two placebo-controlled trials of the neuroleptics, sulpiride and pimozide, were unable to establish significant benefits. In recent years, interest has grown in taking advantage of the impressive weight gain associated with some atypical antipsychotics (e.g., olanzapine); however, no controlled data supporting this intervention have yet appeared.

Four controlled studies, three of tricyclic antidepressants and one of fluoxetine, have examined the use of antidepressants in the treatment of anorexia nervosa. The benefits of the antidepressants compared to placebo were small and of uncertain clinical significance. Therefore, despite the frequency of depression among individuals with anorexia nervosa, there is no good evidence supporting the use of antidepressant medication in their treatment.

One of the more interesting pharmacological interventions examined in controlled trials of anorexia nervosa is the use of cyproheptadine. Cyproheptadine is an antihistamine used in the treatment of a variety of allergic conditions that has been associated with weight gain. The weight gain is thought to be related to cyproheptadine's potency as a serotonin antagonist because animal studies suggest that decreases in hypothalamic serotonin are usually associated with increases in food consumption. Unfortunately, although controlled trials have provided some evidence of benefit, the impact of cyproheptadine in anorexia nervosa appears limited.

A large percentage of individuals with anorexia nervosa remain chronically ill; 30 to 50% of individuals successfully treated in the hospital require rehospitalization within 1 year of discharge. Therefore, posthospitalization outpatient treatments are recommended to prevent relapse and improve overall short- and long-term functioning. Several studies have attempted to evaluate the efficacy of various outpatient treatments for anorexia nervosa including behavioral, cognitive–behavioral, and supportive psychotherapy, as well as a variety of nutritional counseling interventions. Although most of these treatments seem to be helpful, the clearest findings to date support two interventions. For individuals whose anorexia nervosa started before age 18 years and who have had the disorder for less than 3 years, family therapy is effective, and for adult individuals, cognitive–behavioral therapy reduces the rate of relapse. Preliminary information suggests that fluoxetine treatment may reduce the risk of relapse among individuals with anorexia nervosa who have gained weight, but additional controlled data are required to document the usefulness of this intervention.

BULIMIA NERVOSA

Diagnosis

The salient behavioral disturbance of bulimia nervosa is the occurrence of episodes of binge-eating (see DSM-IV-TR diagnostic criteria below). During these episodes, the individual consumes an amount of food that is unusually large considering the circumstances under which it was eaten. Although this is a useful definition and conceptually reasonably clear, it can be operationally difficult to distinguish normal overeating from a small episode of binge-eating. Indeed, the available data do not suggest that there is a sharp dividing line between the size of binge-eating episodes and the size of other meals. On the other hand, while the border between normal and abnormal eating may not be a sharp one, both individual reports and laboratory studies of eating behavior clearly indicate that, when binge-eating, individuals with bulimia nervosa do indeed consume larger than normal amounts of food (Walsh et al. 1992).

DSM-IV-TR Diagnostic Criteria

307.51 Bulimia Nervosa

A. Recurrent episodes of binge-eating. An episode of binge-eating is characterized by both of the following:

   (1) eating, in a discrete period of time (e.g., within any 2-hour period), an amount of food that is definitely larger than most people would eat during a similar period of time and under similar circumstances.

   (2) a sense of lack of control over eating during the episode (e.g., a feeling that one cannot stop eating or control what or how much one is eating).

B. Recurrent inappropriate compensatory behavior in order to prevent weight gain, such as self-induced vomiting; misuse of laxatives, diuretics, enemas, or other medications; fasting; or excessive exercise.

C. The binge-eating and inappropriate compensatory behaviors both occur, on average, at least twice a week for 3 months.

D. Self-evaluation is unduly influenced by body shape and weight.

E. The disturbance does not occur exclusively during episodes of anorexia nervosa.

Specify type:

Purging type: during the current episode of bulimia nervosa, the person has regularly engaged in self-induced vomiting or the misuse of laxatives, diuretics, or enemas.

Nonpurging type: during the current episode of bulimia nervosa, the person has used other inappropriate compensatory behaviors, such as fasting or excessive exercise, but has not regularly engaged in self-induced vomiting or the misuse of laxatives, diuretics, or enemas.

Reprinted with permission from the Diagnostic and Statistical Manual of Mental Disorders, Fourth Edition, Text Revision. Copyright 2000 American Psychiatric Association.

Episodes of binge-eating are associated, by definition, with a sense of loss of control. Once the eating has begun, the individual feels unable to stop until an excessive amount has been consumed. This loss of control is only subjective, in that most individuals with bulimia nervosa will abruptly stop eating in the midst of a binge episode if interrupted, for example, by the unexpected arrival of a roommate.

After overeating, individuals with bulimia nervosa engage in some form of inappropriate behavior in an attempt to avoid weight gain. Most individuals who present to eating disorders clinics with this syndrome report self-induced vomiting or the abuse of laxatives. Other methods include misusing diuretics, fasting for long periods, and exercising extensively after eating binges.

The DSM-IV-TR criteria require that the overeating episodes and the compensatory behaviors both occur at least twice a week for 3 months to merit a diagnosis of bulimia nervosa. This criterion, although useful in preventing the diagnostic label from being applied to individuals who only rarely have difficulty with binge-eating, is clearly an arbitrary one.

Criterion D in the DSM-IV-TR definition of bulimia nervosa requires that individuals with bulimia nervosa exhibit an overconcern with body shape and weight. That is, they tend to base much of their self-esteem on how much they weigh and how slim they look.

Finally, in the DSM-IV-TR nomenclature, the diagnosis of bulimia nervosa is not given to individuals with anorexia nervosa. Individuals with anorexia nervosa who recurrently engage in binge-eating or purging behavior should be given the diagnosis of anorexia nervosa, binge-eating/purging subtype, rather than an additional diagnosis of bulimia nervosa.

In DSM-IV-TR, a subtyping scheme was introduced for bulimia nervosa in which individuals are classed as having either the purging or the nonpurging type of bulimia nervosa. This scheme was introduced for several reasons. First, those individuals who purge are at greater risk for the development of fluid and electrolyte disturbances such as hypokalemia. Second, data suggest that individuals with the nonpurging type of bulimia nervosa weigh more and have fewer mental disorders compared with those with the purging type. Finally, most of the published literature on the treatment of bulimia nervosa has been based on studies of individuals with the purging type of this disorder.

Bulimia nervosa typically begins after a young woman who sees herself as somewhat overweight starts a diet and, after some initial success, begins to overeat. Distressed by her lack of control and by her fear of gaining weight, she decides to compensate for the overeating by inducing vomiting or taking laxatives, methods she has heard about from friends or seen in media reports about eating disorders. After discovering that she can successfully purge, the individual may, for a time, feel pleased in that she can eat large amounts of food and not gain weight. However, the episodes of binge-eating usually increase in size and in frequency and occur after a variety of stimuli, such as transient depression or anxiety or a sense that she has begun to overeat. Individuals often describe themselves as "numb" while they are binge-eating, suggesting that the eating may serve to avoid uncomfortable emotional states. Individuals usually feel intensely ashamed of their "disgusting" habit and may become depressed by their lack of control over their eating.

The binge-eating tends to occur in the late afternoon or evening and almost always while the individual is alone. The typical individual presenting to eating disorders clinics has been binge-eating and inducing vomiting 5 to 10 times weekly for 3 to 10 years. Although there is substantial variation, binges tend to contain 1000 or more calories and to consist of sweet, high-fat foods that are normally consumed as dessert, such as ice cream, cookies, and cake. Although individuals complain of "carbohydrate craving," they only rarely binge-eat foods that are pure carbohydrates, such as fruits. Individuals usually induce vomiting or use their characteristic compensatory behavior immediately after the binge and feel substantial relief that the calories are "gone." In reality, it appears that vomiting is the only purging method capable of disposing of a significant number of ingested calories. The weight loss associated with the misuse of laxatives and diuretics is primarily due to the loss of fluid and electrolytes, not calories.

When not binge-eating, individuals with bulimia nervosa tend to restrict their calorie intake and to avoid the foods usually consumed during episodes of binge-eating. Although there is some phenomenological resemblance between binge-eating and substance abuse, there is no evidence that physiological addiction plays any role in bulimia nervosa.

Among individuals with bulimia nervosa who are seen at eating disorders clinics, there is an increased frequency of anxiety and mood disorders, especially major depressive disorder and dysthymic disorder, of drug and alcohol abuse, and of personality disorders. It is not certain whether this comorbidity is also observed in community samples or whether it is a characteristic of individuals who seek treatment.

In a small fraction of individuals, bulimia nervosa is associated with the development of fluid and electrolyte abnormalities that result from the self-induced vomiting or the misuse of laxatives or diuretics. The most common electrolyte disturbances are hypokalemia, hyponatremia, and hypochloremia. Individuals who lose substantial amounts of stomach acid through vomiting may become slightly alkalotic; those who abuse laxatives may become slightly acidotic.

There is an increased frequency of menstrual disturbances such as oligomenorrhea among women with bulimia nervosa. Several studies suggest that the hypothalamic–pituitary–gonadal axis is subject to the same type of disruption as is seen in anorexia nervosa but that the abnormalities are much less frequent and severe.

Individuals who induce vomiting for many years may develop dental erosion, especially of the upper front teeth. The mechanism appears to be that stomach acid softens the enamel, which in time gradually disappears so that the teeth chip more easily and can become reduced in size. Some individuals develop painless salivary gland enlargement, which is thought to represent hypertrophy resulting from the repeated episodes of binge-eating and vomiting. The serum level of amylase is sometimes mildly elevated in individuals with bulimia nervosa because of increased amounts of salivary amylase.

Most individuals with bulimia nervosa have surprisingly few gastrointestinal abnormalities. Potentially life-threatening complications such as an esophageal tear or gastric rupture occur, but fortunately, rarely. The long-standing use of syrup of ipecac to induce vomiting can lead to absorption of some of the alkaloids and cause permanent damage to nerve and muscle.

Over time, the symptoms of bulimia nervosa tend to improve although a substantial fraction of individuals continue to engage in binge-eating and purging (Keel et al. 1999). On the other hand, some controlled clinical trials have reported that structured forms of psychotherapy have the potential to yield substantial and sustained recovery in a significant fraction of individuals who complete treatment (Fairburn et al. 1993, Pyle et al. 1990). It is not clear what factors are most predictive of good outcome, but those individuals who cease binge-eating and purging completely during treatment are least likely to relapse (Olmstead et al. 1994).

Epidemiology

Soon after bulimia nervosa was recognized as a distinct disorder, surveys indicated that many young women reported problems with binge-eating, and it was suggested that the syndrome of bulimia nervosa was occurring in epidemic proportions. Later careful studies have found that although binge-eating is frequent, the full-blown disorder of bulimia nervosa is much less common, probably affecting 1 to 2% of young women in the United States (Fairburn and Beglin 1990). Although sufficient research data do not exist to pinpoint specific epidemiological trends in the occurrence of bulimia nervosa, research suggests that women born after 1960 have a higher risk for the illness than those born before 1960 (Kendler et al. 1991).

Bulimia nervosa primarily affects women; the ratio of men to women is approximately 1 : 10. It also occurs more frequently in certain occupations (e.g., modeling) and sports (e.g., wrestling, running).

Differential Diagnosis

Bulimia nervosa is not difficult to recognize if a full history is available. The binge-eating/purging type of anorexia nervosa has much in common with bulimia nervosa, but is distinguished by the characteristic low body weight and, in women, amenorrhea. Some individuals with atypical forms of depression overeat when depressed; if the overeating meets the definition of a binge described previously (i.e., a large amount of food is consumed with a sense of loss of control), and if the binge-eating is followed by inappropriate compensatory behavior, occurs sufficiently frequently, and is associated with overconcern regarding body shape and weight, an additional diagnosis of bulimia nervosa may be warranted. Some individuals become nauseated and vomit when upset; this and similar problems are probably not closely related to bulimia nervosa and should be viewed as a somatoform disorder.

Many individuals who believe they have bulimia nervosa have a symptom pattern that fails to meet full diagnostic criteria because the frequency of their binge-eating is less than twice a week or because what they view as a binge does not contain an abnormally large amount of food. Individuals with these characteristics fall into the broad and heterogeneous category of atypical eating disorders. Binge-eating disorder (see section on binge-eating disorder on page 1116), a category currently included in the DSM-IV-TR appendix B for categories that need additional research, is characterized by recurrent binge-eating similar to that seen in bulimia nervosa but without the regular occurrence of inappropriate compensatory behavior.

Etiology

As in the case of anorexia nervosa, the etiology of bulimia nervosa is uncertain. Several factors clearly predispose individuals to the development of bulimia nervosa, including being an adolescent girl or young adult woman. A personal or family history of obesity and of mood disturbance also appears to increase risk. Twin studies have suggested that inherited factors are related to the risk of developing bulimia nervosa, but what these factors are and how they operate are unclear.

Many of the same psychosocial factors related to the development of anorexia nervosa are also applicable to bulimia nervosa, including the influence of cultural esthetic ideals of thinness and physical fitness. Evidence also suggests an important role of sociocultural influences in the development of bulimia nervosa. For example, the frequency of the disorder has been reported to be increasing among immigrants to the United States and United Kingdom from non western countries (Hsu 1990). Although the rate of the disorder appears to be lower among nonwhite and non western cultures, the frequency of bulimia nervosa has been reported to be increasing among these groups, especially among the higher socioeconomic classes. Surprisingly, several epidemiological and clinical studies in the United States found no relationship between bulimia nervosa and social class (Kendler et al. 1991).

Although not proven, it seems likely that several factors serve to perpetuate the binge-eating once it has begun (Figure 40-4). First, most individuals with bulimia nervosa, because of both their concern regarding weight and their worry about the effect of the binge-eating, attempt to restrict their food intake when they are not binge-eating. The psychological and physiological restraint that is thereby entailed presumably makes additional binge-eating more likely. Second, even if mood disturbance is not present at the outset, individuals become distressed about their inability to control their eating, and the resultant lowering of self-esteem contributes to disturbances of mood and to a reduced ability to control impulses to overeat. In addition, cognitive–behavioral theories emphasize the role of rigid rules regarding food and eating, and the distorted and dysfunctional thoughts that are similar to those seen in anorexia nervosa. Interpersonal theories also implicate interpersonal stressors as a primary factor in triggering binge-eating. There is no evidence to suggest that a particular personality structure is characteristic of women with bulimia nervosa (Wonderlich 2002).

There are also indications that bulimia nervosa is accompanied by physiological disturbances that disrupt the development of satiety during a meal and therefore increase the likelihood of binge-eating. These disturbances include an enlarged stomach capacity, a delay in stomach emptying, and a reduction in the release of cholecystokinin, a peptide hormone secreted by the small intestine during a meal that normally plays a role in terminating eating behavior (Geracioti and Liddle 1988, Geliebter et al. 1992). All these abnormalities appear to predispose the individual to overeat and therefore to perpetuate the cycle of binge-eating.

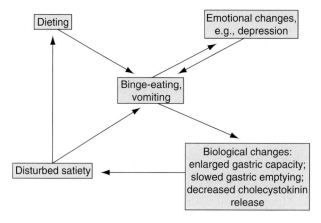

Figure 40-4 *Diagram illustrating factors that may perpetuate bulimia nervosa.*

It has been suggested that childhood sexual abuse is a specific risk factor for the development of bulimia nervosa. Scientific support for this hypothesis is weak. The best studies to date have found that compared with women without psychiatric illness, women with bulimia nervosa do indeed report increased frequencies of sexual abuse. However, the rates of abuse are similar to those found in other mental disorders and occur in a minority of women with bulimia nervosa. Thus, while early abuse may predispose an individual to psychiatric problems generally, it does not appear to lead specifically to an eating disorder, and most individuals with bulimia nervosa do not have histories of sexual abuse (Welch and Fairburn 1994).

Treatment

The power struggles that often complicate the treatment process in anorexia nervosa occur much less frequently in the treatment of individuals with bulimia nervosa. This is largely because the critical behavioral disturbances, binge-eating and purging, are less ego-syntonic and are more distressing to these individuals. Most bulimia nervosa individuals who pursue treatment agree with the primary treatment goals, and wish to give up the core behavioral features of their illness.

The treatment of bulimia nervosa has received considerable attention in recent years and the efficacies of both psychotherapy and medication have been explored in numerous controlled studies (Figure 40-5). The form of psychotherapy that has been examined most intensively is cognitive–behavioral therapy, modeled on the therapy of the same type for depression (Agras 1993). Cognitive–behavioral therapy for bulimia nervosa concentrates on

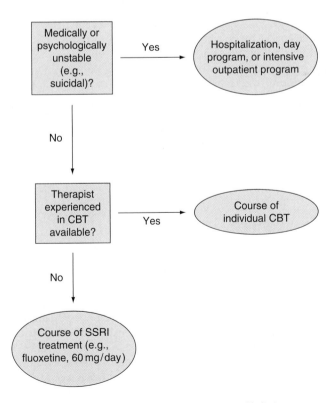

Figure 40-5 *Algorithm for choice of initial treatment of bulimia nervosa.*

the distorted ideas about weight and shape, on the rigid rules regarding food consumption and the pressure to diet, and on the events that trigger episodes of binge-eating. The therapy is focused and highly structured and is usually conducted in 3 to 6 months. Approximately 25 to 50% of individuals with bulimia nervosa achieve abstinence from binge-eating and purging during a course of cognitive–behavioral therapy, and in most, this improvement appears to be sustained. The most common mode of cognitive–behavioral therapy is individual treatment, although it can be given in either individual or group format. The effect of cognitive–behavioral therapy is greater than that of supportive psychotherapy and of interpersonal therapy, indicating that cognitive–behavioral therapy should be the treatment of choice for bulimia nervosa.

The other commonly used mode of treatment that has been examined in bulimia nervosa is the use of antidepressant medication (Zhu and Walsh 2002). This intervention was initially prompted by the high rates of depression among individuals with bulimia nervosa and has now been tested in more than a dozen double-blind, placebo-controlled studies using a wide variety of antidepressant medications. Active medication has been consistently found to be superior to placebo, and although there have been no large "head-to-head" comparisons between different antidepressants, most antidepressants appear to possess roughly similar antibulimic potency (Figure 40-6). Fluoxetine at a dose of 60 mg/day is favored by many investigators because it has been studied in several large trials and appears to be at least as effective as, and better tolerated than, most other alternatives. It is notable that it has not been possible to link the effectiveness of antidepressant treatment for bulimia nervosa to the pretreatment level of depression. Depressed and nondepressed individuals with bulimia nervosa respond equally well in terms of their eating behavior to antidepressant medication.

Although antidepressant medication is clearly superior to placebo in the treatment of bulimia nervosa, several studies suggest that a course of a single antidepressant medication is generally inferior to a course of cognitive–behavioral therapy. However, individuals who fail to respond adequately to, or who relapse following a trial of psychotherapy, may still respond to antidepressant medication.

A major factor influencing the treatment of bulimia nervosa is the presence of other significant psychiatric or medical illness. For example, it can be difficult for individuals who are currently abusing drugs or alcohol to use the treatment methods described, and many experts suggest that the substance abuse needs to be addressed before the eating disorder can be effectively treated. Other examples include the treatment of individuals with bulimia nervosa and serious personality disturbance and those with insulin-dependent diabetes mellitus who "purge" by omitting insulin doses. In treating such individuals, the clinician must decide which of the multiple problems must be first addressed, and may elect to tolerate a significant level of eating disorder to confront more pressing disturbances.

BINGE-EATING DISORDER

Diagnosis

As noted earlier, binge-eating disorder is a proposed diagnostic category related to, but quite distinct from, bulimia nervosa. The phenomenon of binge-eating without purging among the obese was clearly described by Stunkard (1959), 20 years before bulimia nervosa was recognized. Yet binge-eating disorder has been the focus of sustained attention only in the last decade. Suggested diagnostic criteria for binge-eating disorder are included in an appendix of DSM-IV-TR, which provides criteria sets for further study (see DSM-IV-TR research criteria on page 1118). These criteria require recurrent episodes of binge-eating, which are defined just as for bulimia nervosa. The major difference from bulimia nervosa is that individuals with binge-eating disorder do not regularly use inappropriate compensatory behavior, although the precise meaning of "regularly" is not specified. Other differences

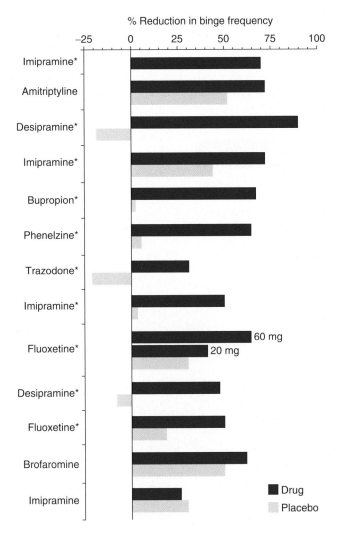

Figure 40-6 *Results of controlled trials of antidepressants in bulimia nervosa. (*indicates a statistically significant difference between the active medication and placebo; Source: Reprinted from Child Adolesc Psychiatr Clin N Am* **4***, Walsh BT and Devlin MJ, Eating disorders, 343–357, Copyright 1995 with permission from Elsevier.)*

from the definition of bulimia nervosa relate to the frequency of binge-eating: individuals with bulimia nervosa must binge-eat, on average, at least two times per week over the last 3 months, whereas individuals with binge-eating disorder must binge-eat at least 2 days per week over the last 6 months. A major reason for the difference in the criteria is that the end of a binge episode in bulimia nervosa is usually clearly marked by the occurrence of inappropriate compensatory behavior, such as purging, whereas in binge-eating disorder, the end of a binge episode may be more difficult to identify precisely. The criteria attempt to deal with this definitional difficulty by requiring the frequency of binge-eating to be measured in terms of the number of days per week on which episodes occur, and, because of the potential difficulty in distinguishing "normal" overeating from binge-eating, to require a 6-month duration, rather than 3 months for bulimia nervosa. In addition, the suggested DSM-IV-TR criteria for binge-eating disorder require that individuals report behavioral evidence of a sense of loss of control over eating, such as eating large amounts of food when not physically hungry. Finally, while there is some evidence that individuals with binge-eating disorder tend to be more concerned about body image than individuals of similar weight, the criteria for binge-eating disorder require only that there is marked distress over the binge-eating. Thus, the criteria for binge-eating disorder do not require that self-evaluation be overly influenced by concerns regarding body weight and shape, as is required for bulimia nervosa.

DSM-IV-TR Research Criteria

Binge Eating Disorder

A. Recurrent episodes of binge eating. An episode of binge eating is characterized by both of the following:

1. eating, in a discrete period of time (e.g., within any 2-hour period), an amount of food that is definitely larger than most people would eat in a similar period of time under similar circumstances
2. a sense of lack of control over eating during the episode (e.g., a feeling that one cannot stop eating or control what or how much one is eating)

B. The binge-eating episodes are associated with three (or more) of the following:

1. eating much more rapidly than normal
2. eating until feeling uncomfortably full
3. eating large amounts of food when not feeling physically hungry
4. eating alone because of being embarrassed by how much one is eating
5. feeling disgusted with oneself, depressed, or very guilty after overeating

C. Marked distress regarding binge eating is present.
D. The binge eating occurs, on average, at least 2 days a week for 6 months.

Note: The method of determining frequency differs from that used for

Bulimia Nervosa; future research should address whether the preferred method of setting a frequency threshold is counting the number of days on which binges occur or counting the number of episodes of binge eating.

E. The binge eating is not associated with the regular use of inappropriate compensatory behaviors (e.g., purging, fasting, excessive exercise) and does not occur exclusively during the course of Anorexia Nervosa or Bulimia Nervosa.

In theory, binge-eating disorder should be easy to recognize on the basis of individual self-report: the individual describes the frequent consumption of large amounts of food in a discrete period of time about which he or she feels distressed and unable to control. Difficulties arise, however, because of uncertainty about what precisely constitutes a "large amount of food," especially for an obese individual, and regarding what constitutes a discrete period of time. Many individuals describe eating continuously during the day or evening, thereby consuming a large amount of food, but it is not clear whether such behavior is best viewed as binge-eating.

Individuals who meet the proposed definition of binge-eating disorder clearly have increased complaints of depression and anxiety compared to individuals of similar weight without binge-eating disorder.

Individuals with binge-eating disorder who are obese should be followed by a primary care physician for assessment and treatment of the complications of obesity. There is no evidence suggesting that the behavioral disturbances characteristic of binge-eating disorder add to the physical risks of obesity. Whether the presence of binge-eating disorder affects the natural history of obesity is an intriguing but unanswered question.

Epidemiology

The epidemiology of binge-eating disorder is uncertain. Cross-sectional studies suggest that the prevalence of binge-eating disorder among adults is a few percent and that the prevalence is higher among obese individuals in the community and among obese individuals who attend weight-loss clinics. Similarly, the frequency of binge-eating disorder increases with the degree of obesity. In contrast to anorexia nervosa and bulimia nervosa, individuals with binge-eating disorder are more likely to be men (the female to male ratio is roughly 1.5 : 1 compared to approximately 10 : 1 for anorexia nervosa and bulimia nervosa), from minority ethnic groups, and middle-aged (Yanovski 1993).

Differential Diagnosis

As noted above, the most difficult issue in the diagnostic assessment of binge-eating disorder is determining whether the eating pattern of concern to the individual meets the proposed definition of binge-eating. There are numerous varieties of unhealthy eating, such as the consumption of high-fat foods, and the nosology of these patterns of eating is poorly worked out. Some individuals with atypical depression binge-eat when depressed; if the individual meets criteria for both binge-eating disorder and an atypical depression, both diagnoses should be made.

Etiology

Very little is known about the etiology of binge-eating disorder. Binge-eating disorder is clearly associated with obesity, but it is uncertain to what degree the binge-eating is a contributor to, and to what degree a consequence of, the obesity.

Treatment

For most individuals with binge-eating disorder, there are three related goals. One is behavioral, to cease binge-eating. A second focuses on improving symptoms of mood and anxiety disturbance, which are frequently associated with binge-eating disorder. The third is weight loss for individuals who are also obese.

Treatment approaches to binge-eating disorder are currently under active study. There is good evidence that psychological (e.g., CBT) and pharmacological (e.g., SSRI) interventions that are effective for bulimia nervosa are also useful in reducing the binge frequency of individuals with binge-eating disorder and in alleviating mood disturbance. However, it is not clear how helpful these approaches are in facilitating weight loss. Standard behavioral weight-loss interventions employing caloric restriction appear useful in helping individuals control binge-eating, but the benefits of such treatment have not been compared to those of more psychologically oriented treatments, such as CBT.

Comparison of DSM-IV-TR/ICD-10 Diagnostic Criteria

The ICD-10 Diagnostic Criteria for Research and the DSM-IV-TR criteria for anorexia nervosa differ in several ways. ICD-10 specifically requires that the weight loss be self-induced by the avoidance of "fattening foods" and that in men there be a loss of sexual interest and potency (corresponding to the amenorrhea requirement in women). Finally, in contrast to DSM-IV-TR, which gives anorexia nervosa precedence over bulimia nervosa, ICD-10 excludes a diagnosis of anorexia nervosa if regular binge-eating has been present.

For bulimia nervosa, the ICD-10 Diagnostic Criteria for Research and the DSM-IV-TR criteria for bulimia nervosa are similar except that ICD-10 requires a "persistent preoccupation with eating and a strong desire or sense of compulsion to eat." Furthermore, whereas the ICD-10 definition requires a self-perception of being too fat (identical to an item in anorexia nervosa), the DSM-IV-TR criteria set requires instead that "self-evaluation is unduly influenced by body shape and weight."

Both DSM-IV-TR and ICD-10 include categories unique to their systems. DSM-IV-TR has a category for "Binge-Eating Disorder" in its appendix of research categories whereas ICD-10 has categories for "Overeating associated with other psychological disturbances" and "Vomiting associated with other psychological disturbances."

References

Agras WS (1993) Short-term psychological treatments for binge-eating. In *Binge Eating: Nature, Assessment, and Treatment*. Fairburn CG and Wilson GT (eds). Guilford Press, New York, p. 270.

Bruch H (1973) *Eating Disorders. Obesity, Anorexia Nervosa, and the Person Within*. Basic Books, New York.

Bruch H (1982) Anorexia nervosa: Therapy and theory. *Am J Psychiatry* **132**, 1531.

Casper RC, Hedeker D, and McClough JF (1992) Personality dimensions in eating disorders and their relevance for subtyping. *J Am Acad Child Adolesc Psychiatry* **31**, 830.

Fairburn CG and Beglin SJ (1990) Studies of the epidemiology of bulimia nervosa. *Am J Psychiatry* **147**, 401.

Fairburn CG, Jones R, Peveler RC, et al. (1993) Psychotherapy and bulimia nervosa: Longer-term effects of interpersonal psychotherapy, behavior therapy and cognitive behavior therapy. *Arch Gen Psychiatry* **50**, 419.

Fairburn CG and Walsh BT (2002) Atypical eating disorders. In *Eating Disorders and Obesity: A Comprehensive Textbook*, 2nd ed. Brownell KD and Fairburn CG (eds). Guilford Press, New York, p. 171.

Garner DM and Garfinkel PE (eds) (1997) *Handbook of Psychotherapy for Anorexia Nervosa and Bulimia*, 2nd ed. Guilford Press, New York.

Geliebter A, Melton P, McCray RS, et al. (1992) Gastric capacity, gastric emptying, and test-meal intake in normal and bulimic women. *Am J Clin Nutr* **56**, 656.

Geracioti TD and Liddle RA (1988) Impaired cholecystokinin secretion in bulimia nervosa. *N Engl J Med* **319**, 683.

Gordon RA (1990) *Anorexia and Bulimia: Anatomy of a Social Epidemic*. Basil Blackwell, Cambridge, MA.

Halmi KA, Eckert ED, LaDu TJ, et al. (1986) Anorexia nervosa: treatment efficacy of cyproheptadine and amitriptyline. *Arch Gen Psychiatry* **43**, 177.

Hsu KL (1990) *Eating Disorders*. Guilford Press, New York.

Hsu LK (1996) Epidemiology of the eating disorders. *Psychiatr Clin North Am* **19**, 681.

Kaye WH (1997) Anorexia nervosa, obsessional behavior, and serotonin. *Psychopharmacol Bull* **33**, 335.

Keel PK, Mitchell JE, Miller KB, et al. (1999) Long-term outcome of bulimia nervosa. *Arch Gen Psychiatry* **56**, 63.

Kendler KS, Maclean C, Neale M, et al. (1991) The genetic epidemiology of bulimia nervosa. *Am J Psychiatry* **148**, 1627.

Klump KL, Kaye W, and Strober M (2001) The evolving genetic foundations of eating disorders. *Psychiatr Clin North Am* **24**, 215.

Lock J, le Grange D, Agras WS, et al. (2000) *Treatment Manual for Anorexia Nervosa*. Guilford Press, New York.

Minuchin S, Rosman BL, and Baker L (1978) *Psychosomatic Families. Anorexia Nervosa in Context*. Harvard University Press, Cambridge, MA.

Olmstead MP, Kaplan AS, and Rockert W (1994) Rate and prediction of relapse in bulimia nervosa. *Am J Psychiatry* **151**, 738.

Pyle RL, Mitchell JE, Eckert ED, et al. (1990) Maintenance treatment and 6-month outcome for bulimic patients who respond to initial treatment. *Am J Psychiatry* **147**, 871.

Seidell JC and Thjhuis MAR (2002) Obesity and quality of life. In *Eating Disorders and Obesity: A Comprehensive Textbook*, 2nd ed., Brownell KD and Fairburn CG (eds). Guilford Press, New York, p. 388.

Srinivasagam NM, Kaye WH, Plotnicov KH, et al. (1995) Persistent perfectionism, symmetry, and exactness after long-term recovery from anorexia nervosa. *Am J Psychiatry* **152**, 1630.

Striegel-Moore RH, Schreiber GB, Lo A, et al. (2000) Eating disorder symptoms in a cohort of 11- to 16-year-old black and white girls: the NHLBI growth and health study. *Int J Eat Disord* **27**, 49.

Stunkard AJ (1959) Eating patterns and obesity. *Psychiatry Q* **33**, 284.

Van Hoeken D, Lucas AR, and Hoek HW (1998) Epidemiology. In *Neurobiology in the Treatment of Eating Disorders*, Hoek HW, Treasure JL, and Katzman MA (eds). John Wiley, Chichester, pp. 97.

Walsh BT (2001) Eating disorders. In *Harrison's Principles of Internal Medicine*, 15th ed., Braunwald E, Fauci AS, Kasper DL, et al. (eds). McGraw-Hill, New York, p. 486.

Walsh BT, Hadigan CM, Kissileff HR, et al. (1992) Bulimia nervosa: A syndrome of feast and famine. In *The Biology of Feast and Famine: Relevance to Eating Disorders*. Anderson GH and Kennedy SH (eds) Academic Press, Orlando, p. 3.

Welch SL and Fairburn CG (1994) Sexual abuse and bulimia nervosa: three integrated case control comparisons. *Am J Psychiatry* **151**, 402.

Wonderlich SA (2002) Personality and eating disorders. In *Eating Disorders and Obesity: A Comprehensive Textbook*, 2nd ed., Brownell KD and Fairburn CG (eds). Guilford Press, New York, p. 204.

Yanovski SZ (1993) Binge eating disorder: Current knowledge and future directions. *Obes Res* **1**, 306.

Zhu AJ and Walsh BT (2002) Pharmacological treatment of eating disorders. *Can J Psychiatry* **47**, 227.

41 ● Sleep and Sleep-Wake Disorders

Phenomenology and Organization of Sleep

Physiological Regulation of Sleep and Wakefulness

Before discussing the various disorders of sleep, it makes sense to begin with a discussion of the normal physiological regulation of sleep and wakefulness. Three physiological processes regulate sleep and wakefulness (Borbely and Ackermann 1992).

Ultradian Rhythm of Rapid Eye Movement (REM) and Non-Rapid Eye Movement (Non-REM) Sleep

Sleep consists of two major processes, REM (rapid eye movement) and non-REM sleep, which alternate throughout the sleep period (Kryger et al. 2000). Sleep normally begins in the adult with non-REM sleep and is followed after about 70 to 90 minutes by the first REM period. Thereafter, non-REM sleep and REM sleep oscillate with a cycle length (the interval between onset of each non-REM or REM period) of about 80 to 110 minutes. This cycle of REM and non-REM sleep is an example of an ultradian rhythm, a biological rhythm with a cycle length considerably less than 24 hours (Figure 41-1).

On the basis of electroencephalographical (EEG) characteristics, non-REM sleep in humans is further divided into four stages: stage 1, a brief transitional stage between wakefulness and sleep; stage 2, which occupies the greatest amount of time during sleep; and stages 3 and 4, sometimes called delta sleep because of the characteristic high-amplitude slow EEG waves (delta waves) (Table 41-1). The amount of ocular activity per minute of REM sleep is quantified as REM density; this can be measured by either visual scoring (e.g., on an analog scale from 0 to 8 per minute) or by computer analysis. Dreaming is commonly reported and is usually vivid when subjects are awakened from REM sleep but also occurs during non-REM sleep, especially at sleep onset during stage 1 sleep.

Circadian (24-Hour) Rhythm of Sleep and Wakefulness The rest–activity or sleep–wake cycle is an example of a circadian rhythm (Table 41-2). Other examples

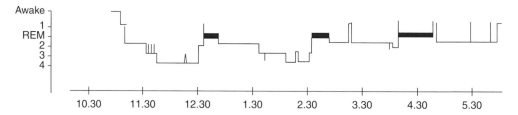

Figure 41-1 *All-night polygraphic sleep stages in a normal young volunteer.*

Table 41-1	Commonly Used Terms in Human Sleep Studies
Term	**Definition**
Delta wave	Electroencephalographic pattern conventionally defined as ≤75 mV, ≤0.5 Hz or cycles per second wave; the amplitude tends to decrease with normal aging
Non-REM sleep	Stages 1, 2, 3, and 4 sleep
Total sleep time	Non-REM and REM sleep time
REM latency	Time from onset of sleep to onset of REM sleep; declines from about 70–100 minutes in the 20 s to 55–70 minutes in the elderly, short REM latency associated with narcolepsy, depression, and a variety of clinical conditions
REM sleep	Rapid eye movement sleep; characterized by low-voltage, relatively fast frequency EEG, bursts of rapid eye movements, and loss of tone (atonia) in the major antigravity muscles; associated with dreaming
Sleep efficiency	Percentage of time in bed spent in sleep; usually above 90% in the young, falls somewhat with age
Sleep latency	Time from "lights out" to onset of sleep
Stage 1 sleep	A brief transitional state of sleep between wakefulness and sleep, characterized by low-voltage, mixed-frequency EEG, and slow eye movements; about 5% of total sleep time
Stage 2 sleep	Characterized by K complexes and sleep spindles (12–14 per cycle rhythms) in the EEG; usually about 45–75% of total sleep time
Stages 3 and 4 sleep	Sometimes referred to as delta sleep, based on amount of sleep delta waves in EEG, 20–50% of an epoch (i.e., 30 or 60 s) for stage 3, more than 50% for stage 4; amount per night declining from about 20–25% of total sleep time in the teens to nearly zero in the elderly
WASO	Wake time sleep onset
REM density	A measure of amount of ocular activity per minute of REM sleep

Table 41-2	Commonly Used Terms in Chronobiology
Term	**Definition**
Acrophase	The time, at which the maximal point of a circadian rhythm occurs, that is, maximal secretion of cortisol normally occurs at midmorning in humans.
Circadian rhythm	Refers to biological rhythms having a cycle length of about 24 hours, derived from Latin *circa dies*, "about 1 d"; examples include the sleep–wake cycle in humans, temperature, cortisol, and psychological variation in the 24-hour day; characterized by exact cycle length (tau), amplitude, and phase position.
Constant routine	An experimental method used to estimate amplitude and phase position of circadian temperature and neuroendocrine rhythms; the subject remains awake for about 36 hours under dim light, with head elevated slightly, eating frequent equal-calorie meals, while blood samples are withdrawn unobtrusively every 20–30 minutes and rectal temperature is measured about once a minute.
Dim light melatonin onset (DLMO)	An experimental method for estimating the phase of melatonin onset; under dim light conditions starting in late afternoon, blood samples are withdrawn every 20–30 minutes to determine when melatonin secretion begins.
Nadir	Time when the minimal point of a circadian rhythm occurs.
Phase position	Temporal relationship between rhythms or between one rhythm and the environment; for example, maximal daily temperature peak (acrophase) usually occurs in the late afternoon.
Phase-advanced rhythm	Phase position of biological rhythm occurs earlier than reference, that is, the individual retires and arises early.
Phase-delayed rhythm	Phase position of biological rhythm occurs later than reference, that is, the individual retires and arises late.
Phase-response curve	Graph showing the magnitude and direction of change in phase position of circadian rhythm depending upon timing of Zeitgeber with reference to the endogenous oscillator.
Tau	Cycle length, that is, from one acrophase to the next.
Zeitgebers	Time cues, such as social activities, meals, and bright lights, that influence phase position of rhythm.

include the hypothalamic–pituitary–adrenal axis, thyroid-stimulating hormone, and core body temperature. (Circadian rhythms can be characterized by three difference measures: (a) cycle length (*tau*) (e.g., the time between two peaks of the ~24 hour temperature curve); (b) amplitude (e.g., the difference between the minimum value of the cycle (*nadir*) and maximum value (*acrophase*), for example, the difference between the lowest and highest points in the ~24 hour temperature curve; and (c) phase position of the rhythm (e.g., the time of day when the acrophase occurred)) (Kryger et al. 2000, Moore-Ede et al. 1982).

The propensity for sleep and wakefulness varies in a circadian fashion, at least after infancy, and is modulated in part by one or more biological clocks. The suprachiasmatic nucleus (SCN) in the anterior hypothalamus plays a decisive role in the regulation of most circadian rhythms in humans and animals. The endogenous activity rhythms of the SCN are synchronized with the environment primarily by ambient light. Information regarding light reaching the retina is conveyed to the SCN directly through the retinohypothalamic tract and indirectly through the intergeniculate leaflet of the lateral geniculate body. Changes in light intensity, especially at dawn and dusk, are particularly important in synchronizing endogenous oscillators controlling rhythms of sleep–wake, cortisol, melatonin, and core body temperature with one another and with the outside world.

If humans are allowed to choose their sleep–wake cycles in the absence of time cues such as daily light–dark signals or clocks, they usually show, as most mammalian species do, a sleep–wake cycle longer than 24 hours. The self-selected rest–activity cycle is typically about 24.5 to 25 hours in length, although it may increase, for example, to 36 hours (24 hours awake and 12 hours asleep). These observations imply that neurons within the SCN have an inherent rhythmicity of approximately 24.5 to 25 hours. Subjects in a time-free environment are said to be "free-running" because endogenous processes, such as a circadian oscillator, rather than environmental cues, determine their sleep–wake, endocrine, and other rhythms.

The propensity for character and duration of sleep are closely related to the phase position of the underlying circadian oscillator. If the daily temperature curve is used to index the phase position of the biological clock, sleep in general and REM sleep in particular, occur most commonly near the nadir of the temperature rhythm. Thus, in persons who live a conventional sleep schedule (11 P.M.–7 A.M.), REM sleep is more common in the last half of the night when core body temperature is lowest than in the first half and more likely in morning naps than in afternoon naps. Furthermore, subjects tend to awaken on the rising phase of the temperature rhythm.

Appropriate exposure to light and darkness can change the phase position of the underlying biological oscillator or, in some circumstances, the amplitude of circadian rhythms (Czeisler et al. 1989). Bright light at the beginning of the subjective evening, in conjunction with dark during the subjective morning, delays and resets the phase position of the temperature, cortisol, melatonin, and sleep–wake rhythms; dark in the subjective evening and bright light in the subjective morning have the opposite effect. The magnitude and direction of the changes induced by bright light or other Zeitgebers ("timegivers") at any particular time form the *phase–response curve*.

The phase position of the circadian oscillator can also be estimated in humans by the 24-hour rhythms of cortisol or melatonin secretion. Because these rhythms can be affected by exercise, meals, light, and so forth, the conditions under which they are measured should be controlled. For example, clinical investigators may use a "constant routine" condition in which the subjects are kept awake in bed for 36 hours under constant low-intensity light (Minors and Waterhouse 1984). An alternative is to determine the onset of melatonin secretion under dark conditions (dim light melatonin onset) (Lewy and Sack 1989). As discussed later, various strategies are under experimental development with the hope that appropriate administration of light–dark cycles, melatonin, vitamin B_{12}, or specific medications will "nudge" and "squash" the circadian oscillator correctly to better manage the clinical disorders of sleep–wakefulness, such as jet lag, delayed sleep syndrome, and shift-work problems (Lewy and Sack 1989, Czeisler et al. 1990). In addition, bright light has been shown to have antidepressant effects in individuals with winter depression, some individuals with major depressive disorder, and individuals with premenstrual dysphoric disorder.

If animals suffer lesions of the SCN, they no longer exhibit circadian rhythms of temperature, cortisol secretion, eating, drinking, or sleep–wakefulness. Sleep and wakefulness, for example, are taken in brief bouts throughout the 24-hour day. Total sleep time, however, may increase under these circumstances. Although no selective lesion of the human SCN has been documented, a case report has been published of a 34-year-old woman who suffered damage to the anterior hypothalamus, presumably ablating the SCN, and who exhibited a polyphasic sleep–wake cycle (Cohen and Albers 1993).

Homeostatic Regulation of Sleep–Wakefulness   Common experience suggests that the longer one is awake, the more likely one is to fall asleep. Furthermore, sleep reverses the sleepiness and other consequences of wakefulness. Thus, sleep can be said to perform a homeostatic function; it is a time of rest and restoration that overcomes the "ravages of wakefulness" (Daan et al. 1984). Consistent with the hypothesis, sleep deprivation usually decreases sleep latency and increases sleep efficiency and delta sleep on recovery nights.

The precise regulation of sleep and wakefulness remains an area of intense investigation and theory. Two of the current theories of sleep–wake regulation include the two-process model (Daan et al. 1984) and the opponent process model (Edgar et al. 1993). The first postulates that sleep and wakefulness are regulated by a circadian process (process C), which sets the circadian thresholds for sleep and wakefulness, and a homeostatic process (process S), in which sleep propensity builds up with wakefulness and dissipates during non-REM sleep, especially delta sleep. The opponent process model postulates that the SCN promotes alertness and that duration of wakefulness facilitates sleep.

Normal Age-Related Changes in Sleep and Wakefulness

The newborn spends nearly 50% of total sleep time in REM sleep. Because infants may sleep up to 16 hours a day, the infant may spend 8 hours in REM sleep per day. Often, to the consternation of the parents, the newborn has a polyphasic sleep–wake pattern, with short bouts of sleep and wakefulness throughout the 24-hour day, until several months of age when the child eventually sleeps through the night. Daytime napping, however, often persists until the age of 4 to 6 years. Stages 3 and 4 sleep increase in the early years. Maximal "depth" of sleep may occur during the prepubertal period, when children are often difficult to awake at night. Adolescents often still need at least 10 hours of sleep. Yet, during adolescence, stages 3 and 4 sleep decline and daytime sleepiness increases, partially in association with the normal Tanner stages of pubertal development (Carskadon et al. 1980). Teenagers are also phase-delayed, which means that they may not get sleepy until the early morning hours (e.g., 2–3 A.M.) and do not naturally wake up until the later morning hours. Early school start times and social pressures may produce mild sleep deprivation during weekdays, with some catch-up on weekends.

As adults enter middle age and old age, sleep often becomes more shallow, fragmented, and variable in duration and circadian timing compared with that of young adults. Stages 1 and 2 and wake time after sleep onset tend to increase; REM latency and stages 3 and 4 decline, probably at an earlier age in men than in women and possibly related to changes in brain structure and metabolism (Feinberg 1974, Feinberg et al. 1990). Daytime sleepiness and napping usually increase with age, often as a function of disturbed nocturnal sleep. The elderly frequently choose an "early-to-bed, early-to-rise" pattern reflecting, in part, an apparent phase advance of the circadian clock. Even when they retire at the same time that they did when they were young, they still tend to wake up early, thus sleep-depriving themselves. This can lead to daytime sleepiness and napping. Although average total sleep time actually increases slightly after age 65 years, greater numbers of persons fall into either long-sleeping (>8 hours) or short-sleeping (<7 hours) subgroups. Psychiatrists should always consider the role of chronobiological factors when evaluating individuals with sleep disorders, especially the elderly, who have more sleep–wake complaints than younger persons. The sleep–wake patterns and the early bedtimes of the elderly, short REM latency, sleep fragmentation at night, and napping during the day may reflect a phase advance and reduced amplitude of the circadian oscillator (Duffy and Czeisler 2002, Duffy et al. 2002).

Factors that could contribute to these age-related patterns include loss of influence from Zeitgebers (light, work schedules, social demands, physical exercise) and a weaker signal from the circadian oscillator to effector systems. Indoor living conditions or loss of hearing and sight may deprive individuals of cues that synchronize the circadian system. In a significant number of totally blind persons, for example, the circadian oscillator free-runs in the normal environment, with resulting regular periods of insomnia and hypersomnia every 3 weeks as the circadian oscillator delays by about 45 minutes each 24 hours while the subject tries to maintain a normal sleep period (11 P.M.–7 A.M.). In a study of normally sighted elderly individuals in San Diego, California, exposure to self-selected bright light averaged 45 minutes and 90 minutes per day for healthy women and men, respectively; 30 minutes per day for individuals with Alzheimer's disease living at home; and 2 minutes for chronically ill, institutionalized individuals (Campbell et al. 1988, Jacobs et al. 1989). Perhaps not surprisingly, the elderly in one nursing home study never spent more than an hour in either consolidated sleep or wakefulness throughout a 24-hour period (Jacobs et al. 1989, Ancoli-Israel et al. 1989).

Neurophysiology and Neurochemistry of Sleep

The non-REM sleep cycle is regulated within the brain stem (Steriade and McCarley 1990). The so-called pontine preparation, made by a transection at the pontomesencephalic junction in the cat, blocks input to the pons from the forebrain. The isolated brain stem generates periodic episodes of rapid eye movements and muscle atonia, the physiological signatures of REM sleep. In contrast, the forebrain of this preparation generates alternating periods of EEG slow waves and EEG arousal, suggestive of non-REM sleep and wakefulness, respectively.

Consistent with the concept that the brain stem regulates REM sleep, an Israeli soldier ceased having REM sleep after suffering a shrapnel wound to the brain stem (Lavie et al. 1984). Some antidepressant medications, notably monoamine oxidase inhibitors (MAOIs), completely eliminate REM sleep when they are taken at high clinical doses for more than 2 weeks (Landolt et al. 2001). No specific deleterious effects have been attributed to the loss of REM sleep in these individuals. These observations underscore the mystery about the fundamental functions of REM sleep in particular, and sleep in general.

Lesions of the locus subcoeruleus in the cat result in REM sleep without atonia, in which the animal appears to act out dreams (i.e., fighting, stalking, or playing while still in REM sleep) (Hendricks et al. 1982). A clinical analog of REM sleep without atonia is the REM sleep behavior disorder (Mahowald and Schenck 1992). Individuals with this disorder maintain muscle tone during REM sleep and act out the content of dreams (e.g., a man ran across his bedroom and crashed into a dresser as he dreamed that he was a linebacker in a football game).

At least five anatomical sites have been implicated in non-REM sleep: the basal forebrain area, thalamus, hypothalamus, dorsal raphe nucleus, and solitary nucleus (Steriade and McCarley 1990). Thalamocortical and corticothalamic loops play an especially important role in the generation of the EEG patterns that define wakefulness, non-REM sleep, and REM sleep (Steriade et al. 1994). Cholinergic, aminergic, histaminergic, and other projections to the thalamus determine the membrane potential of thalamocortical cells. As these cells progressively hyperpolarize, they develop bursting patterns of firing that drive assemblies of cortical cells at the frequencies of the spindle wave (12–14 Hz) and the delta wave (0.3–2.0 Hz).

No specific "sleep neurotransmitter" has been identified that is responsible for the induction or maintenance of sleep, but many different types of neurochemicals (neurotransmitters, neuromodulators, neuropeptides, immune modulators) have been implicated. Adenosine is a potential sleep promoting neurotransmitter; its concentration in basal forebrain increases with prolonged wakefulness. Caffeine probably promotes alertness by blocking the adenosine A_1-receptor. Of particular importance to psychiatry, acetylcholine, released from neurons originating in the dorsal tegmentum, induces REM sleep and cortical activation. Serotonin and norepinephrine, on the other hand, inhibit REM sleep, possibly by inhibition of cholinergic neurons responsible for REM sleep. These physiological mechanisms may be involved in both depression and the sleep disturbances associated with depression and other neuropsychiatric disorders, such as short REM latency (see later). For example, depression may be associated with a functional serotonin deficiency. The suppression of REM sleep during treatment with antidepressants may reflect either enhanced serotoninergic or noradrenergic neurotransmission or anticholinergic effects.

In addition, considerable current research suggests that sleep and immunological processes are intimately related. Several neuroimmunomodulators, such as specific interleukins or tumor necrosis factor, may promote sleep (Kapas et al. 1993). In contrast, sleep deprivation may alter immune function, for example, reducing activity of natural killer cells (Irwin et al. 1992).

Sleep Disorders

Sleep disorders can be divided into four major categories based on the type of sleep disturbance: (1) insomnias, disorders associated with complaints of insufficient, disturbed, or nonrestorative sleep; (2) hypersomnias, disorders of excessive sleepiness; (3) disturbances of the circadian sleep–wake cycle; and (4) parasomnias, abnormal behaviors or abnormal physiological events in sleep (American Psychiatric Association 1994, Kryger et al. 2000). By definition, the DSM-IV-TR limits itself to chronic disorders (at least 1 month in duration). On the other hand, the *International Classification of Sleep Disorders* includes sleep disorders of short-term and intermediate duration, which in fact are more common than chronic disorders (Diagnostic Classification Steering Committee Thorpy MJC 1990).

Sleep disorders can also be categorized according to presumed etiology. According to DSM-IV-TR, primary sleep disorders are presumed to arise from endogenous abnormalities in sleep–wake-generating mechanisms, timing mechanisms, sleep hygiene, or conditioning, rather than occurring secondary to medical or psychiatric disorders. Two types of primary sleep disorders are defined: *dyssomnias* (abnormalities in the amount, quality, or timing of sleep) and *parasomnias* (abnormal behaviors associated with sleep, such as nightmares or sleepwalking). Three other etiologic types of sleep disorders are included in DSM-IV-TR: sleep disorders related to other mental disorders, sleep disorders due to a general medical condition, and substance-induced sleep disorders.

Disorders of sleep and wakefulness are common. Insomnia complaints are reported by about one-third of adult Americans during a 1-year period; clinically significant obstructive sleep apnea may be seen in as many as 10% of working, middle-aged men; and sleepiness is an underrecognized cause of dysphoria, automobile accidents, and mismanagement of individuals by sleep-deprived physicians. Nearly all physicians will hear complaints of sleep problems. Psychiatrists may be even more likely than other medical specialists to receive these complaints. Of particular importance for mental disorders, prospective epidemiological studies suggest that persistent complaints of either insomnia (Ford and Kamerow 1989, Livingston et al. 1993) or hypersomnia (Ford and Kamerow 1989) are risk factors for the later onset of depression, anxiety disorders, and substance abuse.

To assist the individual with a sleep complaint, one needs to have a diagnostic framework with which one can obtain the information needed about both the individual as a person and his or her disorder. Two issues are particularly important: (i) How long has the individual had the sleep complaint? Transient insomnia and short-term insomnia, for example, usually occur in persons undergoing acute stress or other disruptions, such as admission to a hospital, jet lag, bereavement, or change in medications. Chronic sleep disorders, on the other hand, are often multidetermined and multifaceted. (ii) Does the individual suffer from any preexisting or comorbid disorders? Does another condition cause the sleep complaint, modify a sleep complaint, or affect possible treatments? In general, because common sleep disorders are frequently secondary to underlying causes, treatment should be directed at underlying medical, mental, pharmacological, psychosocial, or other disorders.

A detailed history of the complaint and attendant symptoms must be obtained (Tables 41-3 and 41-4). Special attention should be given to the timing of sleep and wakefulness; qualitative and quantitative subjective measures of sleep and wakefulness; abnormal sleep-related behaviors; respiratory difficulties; medications or other substances affecting sleep, wakefulness or arousal; expectations, concerns, attitudes about sleep, and efforts used by the individual to control symptoms; and the sleep–wake environment. The clinician must be

Table 41-3	Office Evaluation of Chronic Sleep Complaints

A detailed history and review of the sleep complaint: predisposing, precipitating, and perpetuating factors
Review of difficulties falling asleep, maintaining sleep, and awakening early
The timing of sleep and wakefulness in the 24-hour day
Evidence of excessive daytime sleepiness and fatigue
Bedtime routines, sleep setting, physical security, preoccupations, anxiety, beliefs about sleep and sleep loss, fears about consequences of sleep loss
Medical and neurological history and examination, routine laboratory examinations: look for obesity, short fat neck, enlarged tonsils, narrow upper oral airway, foreshortened jaw (retrognathia), and hypertension
Psychiatric history and present symptomatology
Use of prescription and nonprescription medications, alcohol, stimulants, toxins, insecticides, and other substances
Evidence of sleep-related breathing disorders: snoring, orthopnea, dyspnea, headaches, falling out of bed, nocturia
Abnormal movements or behaviors associated with sleep disorders: "jerky legs," leg movements, myoclonus, restless legs, leg cramps, cold feet, nightmares, enuresis, sleepwalking, epilepsy, bruxism, sleep paralysis, hypnagogic hallucinations, cataplexy, night sweats, and so on
Social and occupational history, marital status, living conditions, financial and security concerns, physical activity
Sleep–wake diary for 2 weeks
Interview with bed partners or persons who observe individual during sleep
Tape-recording of respiratory sounds during sleep to screen for sleep apnea

Table 41-4	Selected Disorders and Terms Used in Clinical Sleep Disorders Medicine

Term	Definition
Apnea index	Number of apneic events per hour of sleep; usually is considered pathological if ≥ 5.
Cataplexy	Sudden, brief loss of muscle tone in the waking stage, usually triggered by emotional arousal (laughing, anger, surprise), involving either a few muscle groups (i.e., facial) or most of major antigravity muscles of the body; may be related to muscle atonia normally occurring during REM sleep; is associated with narcolepsy.
Hypopnea	50% or more reduction in respiratory depth for 10 seconds or more during sleep.
Multiple Sleep Latency Test	An objective method for determining daytime sleepiness; sleep latency and REM latency are determined for four or five naps (i.e., a 20-min opportunity to sleep every 2 hours between 10 A.M. and 6 P.M.); normal mean values are above 15 minutes.
Periodic limb movements in sleep index	Number of leg kicks per hour of sleep; usually is considered pathological if ≥ 5.
Polysomnography	Describes detailed, sleep laboratory-based, clinical evaluation of individual with sleep disorder; may include electroencephalographical measures, eye movements, muscle tone at chin and limbs, respiratory movements of chest and abdomen, oxygen saturation, electrocardiogram, nocturnal penile tumescence, esophageal pH, as indicated.
Respiratory disturbance index	Number of apneas and hypopneas per hour of sleep.
Sleep apnea	Sleep-related breathing disorder characterized by at least five episodes of apnea per hour of sleep, each longer than 10 seconds in duration.

alert to the possibility that sleep complaints are somatic symptoms, which reflect individual ways of experiencing, expressing, and coping with psychosocial distress, stress, or psychiatric disorders.

Sleep disorders vary with age and gender and, possibly, with culture and social class. As mentioned previously, the circadian timing of rest–activity, duration of sleep at night, and daytime napping and sleepiness vary with age and gender. In addition, parasomnias are most common in boys, Kleine–Levin syndrome in adolescent boys, delayed sleep phase syndrome in adolescents and young adults, insomnia in middle-aged and elderly women, REM sleep behavior disorder and sleep-related breathing disorders in middle-aged men, and advanced sleep phase syndrome in the elderly. Sleep–wake patterns are also influenced by cultural or geographical factors, such as the siesta and late bedtime commonly associated with tropical climates, or the winter hypersomnia and summer hyposomnia said to occur near the arctic circle. Insomnia is more common in lower than in middle and upper socioeconomic classes, perhaps reflecting the stress of poverty, crowding and lack of privacy, poor medical care, drugs and alcohol, lack of physical security, and so forth.

One approach to the differential diagnosis of persistent sleep disorders is suggested in the algorithm in Figure 41-2. First, determine whether the sleep complaint is due to another medical, psychiatric, or substance abuse disorder. Second, consider the role of circadian rhythm disturbances and sleep disorders associated with abnormal events predominantly during sleep. Finally, evaluate in greater detail the complaints of insomnia (difficulty initiating or maintaining sleep) and excessive sleepiness.

Clinicians can usually diagnose most sleep disorders by traditional, simple but systematic clinical methods. Referral to a specialized sleep disorders center, however, should be considered in individuals suspected of having severe intractable insomnia, persistent excessive daytime sleepiness, and sleep disorders due to a general medical condition (such as narcolepsy, REM sleep behavior disorder, sleep apnea, periodic limb movements in sleep [PLMS], or sleep-related epilepsy). Specialists in sleep disorders medicine will evaluate the individual and, if necessary, arrange for sleep laboratory or ambulatory diagnostic procedures.

One of the most important and common laboratory examinations is all-night polysomnography, which typically records the EEG activity's eye movements with the electrooculogram, and muscle tone with the electromyogram from the chin (submental) muscles. These measures are used to determine sleep stages visually scored as 20- or 30-second epochs by a sleep technician. To evaluate sleep-related respiration and cardiovascular function, measures are made of nasal and oral air flow with a thermistor; of sounds of breathing and snoring with a small microphone near the mouth; of respiratory movements of the chest and abdominal walls; of heart rate with the electrocardiogram; and of blood-oxygen saturation with finger oximetry. To evaluate PLMS, an electromyogram from the shin (anterior tibial) muscles is obtained. Other more specialized tests include intraesophageal pressures, which increase during the upper airway resistance syndrome if respiration is impeded, nocturnal penile tumescence in the evaluation of impotence, and core body temperature (usually rectal or tympanic membrane).

Daytime sleepiness can be evaluated in the sleep laboratory with the Multiple Sleep Latency Test, which measures sleep latency during opportunities for napping during the day (see Table 41-4). In addition, subjective sleepiness can be assessed by a questionnaire, the Stanford Sleepiness Scale, in which the subject rates sleepiness on a 7-point scale at set intervals throughout the day.

Two research laboratory procedures have been developed for experimental measurement of circadian phase in humans: the constant routine method for temperature and neuroendocrine secretions, and the dim light melatonin onset method for melatonin (see Table 41-2).

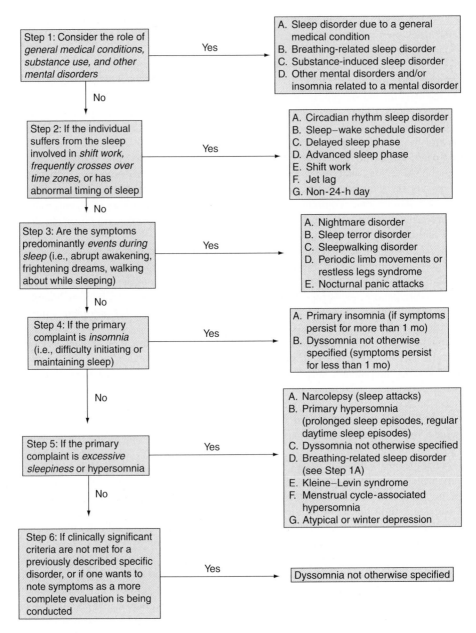

Figure 41-2 *An algorithm for the differential diagnosis of persistent sleep disorder complaints.*

DYSSOMNIAS

PRIMARY INSOMNIA

Diagnosis

Primary insomnia is a subjective complaint of poor, insufficient, or nonrestorative sleep lasting more than a month; associated with significant distress or impairment; and without obvious relationships to another sleep, medical or mental disorder, or physiological effects of a substance (see DSM-IV-TR diagnostic criteria below). Primary insomnia is similar to some insomnia diagnoses in the International Classification of Sleep Disorders, including psychophysiological insomnia, which is often ascribed to conditioned arousal factors; sleep state misperception, in which the magnitude of the subjective complaint often exceeds that of the objective abnormality; and idiopathic insomnia, with a childhood onset and lifelong course.

DSM-IV-TR Diagnostic Criteria

307.42 Primary Insomnia

A. The predominant complaint is difficulty initiating or maintaining sleep, or nonrestorative sleep, for at least 1 month.
B. The sleep disturbance (or associated daytime fatigue) causes clinically significant distress or impairment in social, occupational, or other important areas of functioning.
C. The sleep disturbance does not occur exclusively during the course of narcolepsy, breathing-related sleep disorder, circadian rhythm sleep disorder, or a parasomnia.
D. The disturbance does not occur exclusively during the course of another mental disorder (e.g., major depressive disorder, generalized anxiety disorder, a delirium).
E. The disturbance is not due to the direct physiological effects of a substance (e.g., a drug of abuse, a medication) or a general medical condition.

Reprinted with permission from the Diagnostic and Statistical Manual of Mental Disorders, Fourth Edition, Text Revision. Copyright 2000 American Psychiatric Association.

In general surveys of the prevalence of insomnia in the population, about 1 in 3 people reported "insomnia" during the previous year, about 1 in 6 described it as "serious," and about 1 in 12 called it "chronic" (Ancoli-Israel and Roth 1999). The rates of insomnia are higher in women than in men, in the elderly than in the young, and in the lower than in the higher socioeconomic classes. In a survey conducted by the Gallup Poll for the National Sleep Foundation (Ancoli-Israel and Roth 1999, Roth and Ancoli-Israel 1999), the most common complaint of insomniacs is waking up feeling drowsy rather than specific complaints about sleep, implying that the sleepiness insomniacs experience could be associated with some morbidity. Compared with transient insomniacs or normal control subjects, chronic insomniacs reported greater difficulty enjoying family and social relationships, greater difficulty concentrating, more problems with memory, greater frequency of falling asleep while visiting friends, and more automobile accidents due to sleepiness. Nevertheless, only about 5% of individuals with chronic insomnia ever sought medical attention specifically for insomnia. Only a minority of individuals have ever used prescription sleeping pills. On the other hand, most mental health professionals do not routinely inquire about difficulties with sleep and wakefulness. If these individuals with chronic or serious insomnia are to be helped, mental health professionals must be proactive and ask specific questions about sleep and its disorders.

Diagnosis and treatment of chronic insomnia are often challenging and difficult (Hauri 1991). Both the clinician and the individual must be forbearing and realistic as they jointly explore the evolution, causes, manifestations, and ramifications of the sleep complaint. In part, the diagnosis of primary insomnia is reached by exclusion after a careful differential diagnosis of other causes. Simple answers and simple solutions are rare. Even if insomnia is initially precipitated by a single event or condition, chronic insomnia is usually maintained by various predisposing and perpetuating factors. For example, a business woman in her early thirties had insomnia during a period of intense stress in her business, but it continued long after the stress had been satisfactorily resolved. Factors that contributed to chronicity included her lifelong somewhat obsessive, anxious personality structure and after the onset of her insomnia, her gradually escalating concerns about her insomnia; these resulted in advanced sleep phase as she tried to spend more time in bed for "rest" and the use of wine and sleeping pills at bedtime to sleep. If all these factors can be properly sorted out and dealt with, both the clinician and the individual will be gratified.

Etiology
The etiology of primary insomnia is unclear, but it may be dependent more on the factors that perpetuate it than on those that precipitate it.

Treatment
Treatment of insomnia should, insofar as possible, be directed at identifiable causes, or those factors that perpetuate the disorders, such as temperament and lifestyle, ineffective coping and defense mechanisms, inappropriate use of alcohol or other substances, maladaptive sleep–wake schedules, and excessive worry about poor sleep. The harder these individuals try to sleep, the worse it is. They keep themselves awake by their apprehensions: "If I don't get to sleep right now, I'll make a bad impression tomorrow." Cognitive–behavioral therapy (CBT) therefore is very effective, as shown by Morin and colleagues (1993). An 8-week group intervention aimed at changing maladaptive sleep habits and altering dysfunctional beliefs and attitudes about sleeplessness was effective in reducing sleep latency, waking up after sleep onset, and early morning awakening, and in increasing sleep efficiency. In a second study, Morin and colleagues (1999) found that CBT and pharmacological approaches were both effective for the short-term management of insomnia, but that improvement was better sustained over time with the behavioral treatment.

Clinical management is often multidimensional, involving psychosocial, behavioral, and pharmacological approaches. The relationship with the treating clinician can often be important since many insomniac individuals are skeptical that they can be helped overtly. They are focused on the symptom rather than the underlying causes, and are not psychologically minded. Behavioral treatments, in combination with addressing sleep hygiene, may be helpful in treating psychophysiological and other insomnias. Relaxation training (progressive relaxation, autogenic training, meditation, deep breathing) can be effective if overtaught to become automatic. Two other behavioral therapies have been shown to be effective for insomnia: stimulus control and sleep restriction therapy (Bootzin and Nicassio 1978, Spielman et al. 1987, Morin et al. 1994).

The aim of stimulus control therapy is to break the negative associations of being in bed unable to sleep (Table 41-5). It is especially helpful for individuals with sleep-onset insomnia and prolonged awakenings. Sleep restriction therapy (Table 41-6) is based on the observation that more time spent in bed leads to more fragmented sleep. Both therapies may take 3 to 4 weeks or longer to be effective.

A wide variety of sedating medications have commonly been used as sleeping pills including benzodiazepines, imidazopyridines (zolpidem), pyrazolopyrimidines (zaleplon), chloral hydrate, antihistamines (diphenhydramine, hydroxyzine, doxylamine), certain antidepressants (amitriptyline, doxepin, trimipramine, and trazodone), barbiturates, and over-the-counter medications. However, they do vary in their pharmacokinetic properties and side effects (Table 41-7). The ideal sleeping pill would shorten latency to sleep; maintain normal physiological sleep all night without blocking normal behavioral responses to the

Table 41-5	Sleep Hygiene and Stimulus Control Rules

Curtail time spent awake while in bed.
Go to bed only when sleepy.
Do not remain in bed for more than 20–30 minutes while awake.
Get up at the same time each day.
Avoid looking at the bedroom clock.
Avoid caffeine, alcohol, and tobacco near bedtime.
Exercise during the morning or afternoon.
Eat a light snack before bed.
Adjust sleeping environment for optimal temperature, sound, and darkness.
Do not worry right before and in bed. Use the bed for sleeping.
Do not nap during the day.

Table 41-6	Sleep Restriction Therapy

Stay in bed for the amount of time you think you sleep each night, plus 15 minutes.
Get up at the same time each day.
Do not nap during the day.
When sleep efficiency is 85% (i.e., sleeping for 85% of the time in bed), go to bed 15 minutes earlier.
Repeat this process until you are sleeping for 8 hours or the desired amount of time.
Example: if you report sleeping only 5 hours a night and you normally get up at 6 A.M., you are
  allowed to be in bed from 12:45 A.M. until 6 A.M.

Table 41-7	Clinical Characteristics of Sedative–Hypnotics

Name	Dose (mg)	Absorption	Active Metabolite	Half-Life
Chlordiazepoxide (Librium)	5–10	Intermediate	Yes	2–4 d
Diazepam (Valium)	2–10	Fast	Yes	2–4 d
Estazolam (ProSom)*	0.5–2.0	Intermediate	Yes	17 h
Flurazepam (Dalmane)*	7.5–30	Intermediate to fast	Yes	2–4 d
Clorazepate (Tranxene)	7.5–15	Fast	Yes	2–4 d
Clonazepam (Klonopin)	0.5–1.0	Intermediate	Yes	2–3 d
Quazepam (Doral)*	7.5–15	Intermediate	Yes	2–4 d
Oxazepam (Serax)	10–15	Slow	No	8–12 h
Lorazepam (Ativan)	0.5–4.0	Intermediate	No	10–20 h
Temazepam (Restoril)*	7.5–15	Slow	No	10–20 h
Alprazolam (Xanax)	0.25–2	Intermediate	No	14 h
Zoplicone[†]	7.5–15	Fast	Yes	4–6.5 h
Triazolam (Halcion)*	0.125–0.5	Intermediate	No	2–5 h
Zolpidem (Ambien)*	5–10	Fast	No	2–5 h
Zaleplon (Sonata)*	5–10	Fast	No	1 h

*Marketed as a sleeping pill in the United States.
[†]Not yet marketed in the United States.

crying baby or the alarm clock; leave neither hangover nor withdrawal effects the next day; and be devoid of tolerance and side effects such as impairment of breathing, cognition, ambulation, and coordination (Gillin and Byerley 1990). Furthermore, sleeping pills should not be habit-forming or addictive. Unfortunately, the ideal sleeping pill has not yet been found. Sleeping pills, if given in appropriate doses, are effective compared to placebo at least from a few days to a few weeks. More recently developed sleeping pills (such as zaleplon) have demonstrated their superiority after 1 year in double-blind studies with a parallel placebo group. The question, however, is what the lowest adequate dose is for an individual, that is, the dose that will promote sleep with the least number of side effects.

The duration of action of these medications is important for several reasons (Table 41-8). Drugs with long half-life metabolites may have next-day hangover effects and tend to accumulate with repeated nightly administration, especially in the elderly, who metabolize and excrete the drugs more slowly than the young do. In addition, long half-life metabolites may act addictively or synergistically the next day with alcohol, with drugs with sedative side effects, or during periods of decreased alertness, such as the afternoon dip in arousal levels. Because the elderly are more sensitive to both the benefits and the side effects at a given dose than are younger individuals, a dose for the elderly and debilitated individual should normally be about half of that for young and middle-aged individuals.

Short half-life hypnotics usually produce less daytime sedation than long half-life drugs, but they often result in more rebound insomnia when they are discontinued (Gillin et al. 1989). Whereas nearly all hypnotics and sedatives can produce amnesia, the problem may be more common with some short half-life drugs, especially for material that is learned during the periods of peak concentrations of drugs, for example, if the subject is awakened during the middle of the night. Administration of zaleplon 4 hours or more before arising in the morning does not appear to be associated with impairment in motor performance (Vermeeren et al. 2002).

Individuals should be educated about the anticipated benefits and limitations of sleeping pills, side effects, and appropriate use, and should be followed up by office visits or phone calls regularly if prescriptions are renewed. Although hypnotics are usually prescribed for relatively short periods of time (2–6 weeks at most), about 0.5 to 1% of the population uses a hypnotic nearly every night for months or years. Whether this practice is good, useless, or bad remains controversial. Treatment of these individuals should focus on the lowest possible effective dose—intermittently if possible—for the treatment of insomnia.

Hypnotics are relatively contraindicated in individuals with sleep-disordered breathing; during pregnancy; in substance abusers, particularly alcohol abusers; and in those individuals who may need to be alert during their sleep period (e.g., physicians on call). In addition, caution should be used in prescribing hypnotics to individuals who snore loudly; to individuals who have renal, hepatic, or pulmonary disease; and to the elderly.

Melatonin received enormous coverage in the popular press in the mid-1990s, with extravagant claims that it can prevent all ills from aging to cancer and treat everything from jet lag and insomnia to depression and acquired immunodeficiency syndrome (AIDS). The scientific reality is still far removed from most of these claims at the present time. What is known is that melatonin is synthesized and released from the pineal gland under dark ambient conditions at a time that is determined by the individual's internal biological clock

Table 41-8	Comparison of Long and Short Half-Life Hypnotics	
Measure	**Half-Life**	
	Short	**Long**
Sedative hangover effects	+	++++
Accumulation with consecutive nightly use	0	+++
Tolerance	+++	+
Withdrawal insomnia	+++	+
Anxiolytic effects next day	0	+++
Amnesia	+++	++
Full benefits the first night	+++	++

Note: Although zaleplon is short acting, research suggests that it does not have some of the problems of other short-acting hypnotics, such as tolerance or withdrawal insomnia.

located within the SCN at the anterior portion of the hypothalamus. For individuals who are synchronized with the local light–dark environment, melatonin is usually secreted at night. The duration of secretion is approximately 8 to 12 hours, depending partially on age, season of the year, and lighting conditions. Bright light prevents or terminates secretion of melatonin. For these reasons, melatonin has sometimes been called the hormone of the night or of sleep. In addition, nocturnal melatonin secretion appears to be blunted with normal aging, with administration of beta-adrenergic blockers (propranolol, pindolol, metoprolol), and in some populations of individual (including individuals with mood disorders, premenstrual depression, and panic disorder).

The functions of melatonin in humans are poorly understood, although in animals it has been implicated in seasonal behaviors, breeding, reproductive physiology, and timing of adolescence.

The limited database available suggests that melatonin may eventually have a role in the prevention and treatment of circadian and sleep disturbances. Some evidence suggests that it has intrinsic hypnotic effects. Laboratory studies suggest that people are more likely to sleep during the period of endogenous melatonin secretion than during periods of the day without melatonin secretion. Furthermore, some, but not all, studies suggest that melatonin (0.3–10.0 mg) may induce and maintain sleep when administered to normal subjects or, in a few studies, to individuals with insomnia, jet lag, or other circadian rhythm disturbances. In addition, it is possible that melatonin administration can shift the phase position of the underlying biological clock. The entraining effects of a dose of 0.5 mg melatonin act like a "dark pulse," that is, the phase-response curve is nearly opposite that of light. Melatonin induced phase-advanced rhythms when administered in the late afternoon or early evening, and it delayed the circadian clock when administered in the early morning. Future research is needed to fulfill the promise that melatonin can be used to prevent or treat some forms of insomnia or other sleep disorders, especially in the elderly, or in cases associated with circadian rhythm disorders (jet lag, shift work, the non-24-hour-day syndrome, phase displacement), neurological disorders, or psychiatric disorders.

The scientific clinical database for the use of melatonin in humans is limited at this time (Brown 1995). Few well-designed clinical trials exist to establish clinical benefits or risks in specific disorders or conditions. Little is known about optimal doses, timing of melatonin administration, duration of treatment, drug interactions, or populations at risk, if any. The safety of melatonin, especially melatonin available in health food stores, is unknown. Melatonin is currently treated by the US Food and Drug Administration as a nutritional supplement rather than a medication. Therefore, purity of the product, safety, efficacy, and claims by manufacturers are not carefully regulated in the United States. Physicians are advised to maintain a watchful eye at this time and to be prudently cautious about recommendations to individuals and the public about the uses and benefits of melatonin.

PRIMARY HYPERSOMNIA

Diagnosis

A specific diagnostic category for primary hypersomnia exists in DSM-IV-TR, defining a disorder characterized by clinically significant excessive sleepiness of at least 1 month's duration, with significant distress or impairment (see DSM-IV-TR diagnostic criteria on page 1138). The hypersomnia is not caused by another primary sleep disorder, a mental disorder, a general medical condition, or a substance. Individuals with primary hypersomnia usually present with complaints of long and nonrestorative nocturnal sleep, difficulty awakening ("sleep drunkenness"), daytime sleepiness, and intellectual dysfunction; do not experience the accessory symptoms of narcolepsy such as cataplexy, sleep paralysis, and hypnagogic hallucinations; and often report frequent headaches and Raynaud's phenomena.

307.44 Primary Hypersomnia

A. The predominant complaint is excessive sleepiness for at least 1 month (or less if recurrent) as evidenced by either prolonged sleep episodes or daytime sleep episodes that occur almost daily.
B. The excessive sleepiness causes clinically significant distress or impairment in social, occupational, or other important areas of functioning.
C. The excessive sleepiness is not better accounted for by insomnia and does not occur exclusively during the course of another sleep disorder (e.g., narcolepsy, breathing-related sleep disorder, circadian rhythm sleep disorder, or a parasomnia) and cannot be accounted for by an inadequate amount of sleep.
D. The disturbance does not occur exclusively during the course of another mental disorder.
E. The disturbance is not due to the direct physiological effects of a substance (e.g., a drug of abuse, a medication) or a general medical condition.

Specify if:

Recurrent: if there are periods of excessive sleepiness that last at least 3 days occurring several times a year for at least 2 years

Previously called non-REM narcolepsy, this relatively rare disorder is represented by perhaps 5 to 10% of individuals presenting to sleep disorders centers for evaluation of hypersomnia. The diagnosis must be made on the basis of polysomnographic confirmation of hypersomnia; subjective complaints of excessive sleepiness are not adequate. A family history of excessive sleepiness may be present.

Although usually seen as a persistent complaint, primary hypersomnia includes recurrent forms, well defined with periods of excessive sleepiness of at least 3 days' duration occurring several times a year for at least 2 years. Among the recurrent or intermittent hypersomnia disorders are Kleine–Levin syndrome, usually seen in adolescent boys, and menstrual cycle–associated hypersomnia syndrome. In addition to hypersomnia (up to 18 hours per day), individuals with Kleine–Levin syndrome often demonstrate aggressive or inappropriate sexuality, compulsive overeating, and other bizarre behaviors. The rare nature of this syndrome and its unusual behaviors may be mistaken for psychosis, malingering, or a personality disorder (Waller et al. 1984).

Another syndrome, idiopathic recurring stupor, has been described and may be confused with hypersomnia (Rothstein et al. 1992). Individuals experience attacks of stupor or coma as infrequently as once or twice a year to as often as once a week. The duration of each episode varies from 2 hours to 4 days. Unlike individuals with hypersomnia, these individuals are in a stuporous coma-like state and cannot be easily aroused or awakened. Furthermore, unlike the EEG of hypersomnia with its sleep spindles and K complexes, the EEG during stupor is characterized by diffuse activity at 13 to 18 Hz. Because the episode can be promptly but temporarily reversed by administration of flumazenil, a benzodiazepine receptor antagonist, a search was made for an endogenous ligand for the benzodiazepine receptor in plasma and cerebrospinal fluid. The investigators discovered significantly increased levels of "endozepine 4" in blood and cerebrospinal fluid during periods of coma or stupor, suggesting that this syndrome is caused by this endogenous benzodiazepine-like compound. The syndrome occurs predominantly in men; mean age at onset is age 47 years (range, age 22–67 years). The cause is unknown.

Aside from associated general medical conditions and mental disorders, the frequency and importance of hypersomnia and daytime sleepiness in otherwise healthy individuals have been increasingly recognized. Sleepiness, for example, as a result of sleep deprivation, disrupted sleep, or circadian dyssynchronization, probably plays a major role in mistakes and accidents in sleepy drivers, interns and medical staff, and industrial workers. Mental health professionals have an obligation to recognize and advise individuals under their care about the dangers inherent in acute or chronic sleepiness.

Treatment

Clinical management is controversial owing to the lack of controlled studies. As in narcolepsy, the stimulant compounds are the most widely used and most often successful of the treatment options available. However, some individuals are intolerant of stimulants or report no significant therapeutic effects. For individuals intolerant of, or insensitive to, stimulants, some success has been obtained with the use of stimulating antidepressants, both of the MAOI and the selective serotonin reuptake inhibitor (SSRI) classes. Methysergide, a serotonin receptor antagonist, may be effective in some treatment-resistant cases but must be used with caution in view of the possibility of pleural and retroperitoneal fibrosis with persistent, uninterrupted use. Careful documentation should be maintained of interruption of drug use at regular intervals and of physical examinations that find the absence of obvious side effects of any sort.

NARCOLEPSY

Diagnosis

Narcolepsy is associated with a pentad of symptoms: (1) excessive daytime sleepiness, characterized by irresistible "attacks" of sleep in inappropriate situations such as driving a car, talking to a supervisor, or social events; (2) cataplexy, which is sudden bilateral loss of muscle tone, usually lasting seconds to minutes, generally precipitated by strong emotions such as laughter, anger, or surprise; (3) poor or disturbed nocturnal sleep; (4) hypnagogic hallucinations, varied dreams at sleep onset; and (5) sleep paralysis, a brief period of paralysis associated with the transitions into, and out of, sleep (see DSM-IV-TR diagnostic criteria below).

DSM-IV-TR Diagnostic Criteria

347. Narcolepsy

A. Irresistible attacks of unrefreshing sleep that occur daily for at least 3 months.
B. The presence of one or both of the following:

    (1) cataplexy (i.e., brief episodes of sudden bilateral loss of muscle tone, most often in association with intense emotion)

> (2) recurrent intrusions of elements of REM sleep into the transition between sleep and wakefulness, as manifested by either hypnopompic or hypnagogic hallucinations or sleep paralysis at the beginning or end of sleep episodes
>
> C. The disturbance is not due to the direct physiological effects of a substance (e.g., a drug of abuse, a medication) or another general medical condition.

Reprinted with permission from the Diagnostic and Statistical Manual of Mental Disorders, Fourth Edition, Text Revision. Copyright 2000 American Psychiatric Association.

Narcolepsy is lifelong. The first symptom is usually excessive sleepiness, typically developing during the late teens and early twenties. The full syndrome of cataplexy and other symptoms unfolds in several years.

Observers may mistake classic sleepiness in its mild form as withdrawal, poor motivation, negativism, and hostility. The hypnagogic imagery and sleep paralysis symptoms, alone and in combination, may resemble bizarre psychiatric illness. Like many medical disorders, narcolepsy presents a wide range of severity, from mild to cases so severe that employment is functionally impossible. Partial remissions and exacerbations occur. Sleep paralysis and hypnagogic imagery may be seen without cataplexy; cataplexy may present in isolation without other REM-associated phenomena. The presence of REM sleep onset at night or during daytime naps, an important sleep laboratory parameter, remains the most valid and reliable method available for diagnosing narcolepsy. Because of the seriousness of the disorder and likelihood that amphetamine or other stimulants will be used to treat the individual at some time, it is important that the diagnosis of narcolepsy be objectively verified as soon as possible. Furthermore, stimulant abusers have been known to feign symptoms of narcolepsy to obtain prescriptions.

Narcolepsy is not a rare disease; the prevalence rate of 0.03 to 0.16% approximates that of multiple sclerosis. Narcolepsy is associated with significant social and financial impairment for affected individuals and their families (Broughton and Ghanem 1976). For example, automobile accidents may result from either sleepiness or cataplexy. Most states prohibit narcoleptic individuals from driving, at least as long as they are symptomatic.

Etiology

Narcolepsy is now understood as an inherited, physiological disturbance of REM sleep regulation (Mignot et al. 1991, 1993a). It is also seen in dogs and other mammals. Genetic markers in humans (Mignot et al. 1991, 1993a) and basic neurochemical and neurophysiological studies in canine narcolepsy (Siegel et al. 1992, Mignot et al. 1993b) may clarify the basic pathophysiological process of human narcolepsy. Narcoleptic individuals often enter REM sleep right after sleep onset (the "sleep-onset REM periods"), reflecting an abnormally short or even nonexistent first non-REM sleep period (Figure 41-3). Several of the core symptoms of narcolepsy can be understood as abnormal physiological representations of normal REM sleep. For example, cataplexy can be understood as an abrupt presentation during wakefulness of the paralysis normally seen in REM sleep. Cataplexy is usually triggered by an emotional stimulus. Sleep-onset REM periods may be subjectively appreciated as hypnagogic hallucinations, which may be accompanied by sleep paralysis. Dissociated REM sleep inhibition of the voluntary musculature may lead to complaints of cataplexy and sleep paralysis.

A strong association between narcolepsy and the human leukocyte antigen HLA-DR2 phenotype has been demonstrated (Honda et al. 1986, Rosenthal et al. 1991). Studies to

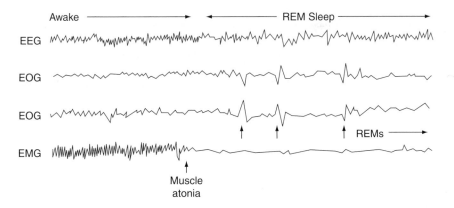

Figure 41-3 *REM-onset sleep in an individual with narcolepsy. EEG, electroencephalogram; EOG, electrooculogram; EMG, electromyogram; REMs, rapid eye movements.*

date suggest that between 90 and 100% of Asian and white narcoleptics have the HLA-DR2 and DQw1 phenotype, versus 20 to 40% of nonnarcoleptic control subjects. The frequent occurrence of this trait in "normal" populations limits the utility of this test for diagnostic purposes.

In recent years, a potential biochemical abnormality has been identified in both canine and human narcolepsy. Narcoleptic dogs appear to have a nonfunctional receptor (OX2R) for orexin (hypocretin), a peptide neurotransmitter that has also been associated with feeding and energy metabolism. "Knockout" mice, which no longer make this peptide, appear to have a narcoleptic-like syndrome. Levels of orexin/hypocretin have been reported to be low in both autopsied brains and spinal fluid in human narcoleptics.

Treatment

The major goals of treatment of narcolepsy include (a) to improve quality of life, (b) to reduce excessive daytime sleepiness (EDS), and (c) to prevent cataplectic attacks. The major wake-promoting medications are: modafinil, amphetamine, dextroamphetamine, and methylphenidate. Modafinil is preferred on grounds of efficacy, safety, availability, and low risk of abuse and diversion. Pemoline is helpful but it carries the rare risk of hepatic toxicity, which can be fatal. The pharmacological treatment of cataplexy, sleep paralysis, and hypnagogic hallucinations includes administration of activating SSRIs such as fluoxetine and tricyclic antidepressants such as protriptyline. Another new drug, sodium oxybate xyrem, appears to be well-tolerated and beneficial for the treatment of cataplexy, daytime sleepiness, and inadvertent sleep attacks (Littner et al. 2001, US Xyrem Multicenter Study Group 2002).

BREATHING-RELATED SLEEP DISORDER

Diagnosis

The essential feature of breathing-related sleep disorder (BRSD) is sleep disruption resulting from sleep apnea or alveolar hypoventilation, leading to complaints of insomnia or, more commonly, excessive sleepiness (see DSM-IV-TR diagnostic criteria on page 1142). The disorder is not accounted for by other medical or psychiatric disorders or by medications or other substances. Breathing-related sleep disorder (BRSD) was first described in 1877, yet it was recognized as a serious problem only about 30 years ago.

DSM-IV-TR Diagnostic Criteria

780.59 Breathing-Related Sleep Disorder

A. Sleep disruption, leading to excessive sleepiness or insomnia, that is judged to be due to a sleep-related breathing condition (e.g., obstructive or central sleep apnea syndrome or central alveolar hypoventilation syndrome).

B. The disturbance is not better accounted for by another mental disorder and is not due to the direct physiological effects of a substance (e.g., a drug of abuse, a medication) or another general medical condition (other than a breathing-related disorder).

Coding note: Also code sleep-related breathing disorder on Axis III.

The major diagnostic criterion for sleep apnea is cessation of breathing lasting at least 10 seconds and an apnea index (number of apneic events per hour of sleep) of 5 or more (Figure 41-4). Most apneic episodes are terminated by transient arousals. Hypopneas (50% decrease in respiration) may also produce arousal or hypoxia even when complete apneas do not occur. Therefore, rather than just the apnea index, a respiratory disturbance index (number of respiratory events, or number of apneas plus hypopneas per hour of sleep) is used. Whereas the criterion for the respiratory disturbance index has not been fully established, many clinician use a respiratory disturbance index of 10 or greater for purposes of diagnosis. Each time respiration ceases, the individual must awaken to start breathing again. Once the person goes back to sleep, breathing stops again. This pattern continues throughout the night. Clinically, however, it is not unusual to see individuals who stop breathing for 60 to 120 seconds with each event and experience hundreds of events per night. Many individuals with BRSD cannot sleep and breathe at the same time and therefore spend most of the night not breathing and not sleeping. In contrast, the central alveolar hypoventilation syndrome is not associated with either apneas or hypopneas, but impaired ventilatory control or hypoventilation results in hypoxemia. It is most common in morbid obesity.

Sleep apnea is characterized by repetitive episodes of upper airway obstruction that occur during sleep, resulting in numerous interruptions of sleep continuity, hypoxemia, hypercapnia, bradytachycardia, and pulmonary and systemic hypertension (Shepard 1992). It may be associated with snoring, morning headaches, dry mouth on awakening, excessive movements during the night, falling out of bed, enuresis, cognitive decline and personality changes, and complaints of either insomnia or, more frequently, hypersomnia and excessive daytime sleepiness (Guilleminault et al. 1973, Roehrs et al. 1985, Aldrich and Chauncey 1990). The typical individual with clinical sleep apnea is a middle-aged man who is overweight or who has anatomical conditions narrowing his upper airway.

The lifetime prevalence of BRSD in adults has been estimated to be 9% in men and 4% in women (Young et al. 1993). The prevalence does increase with age, particularly in postmenopausal women. The prevalence in the elderly has been estimated to be 28% in men and 19% in women (Ancoli-Israel et al. 1991c).

During apneas and hypopneas, the blood-oxygen level often drops to precarious levels. In addition, one often sees cardiac arrhythmias and nocturnal hypertension in association with the respiratory disturbances. The cardiac arrhythmias include bradycardia during the events

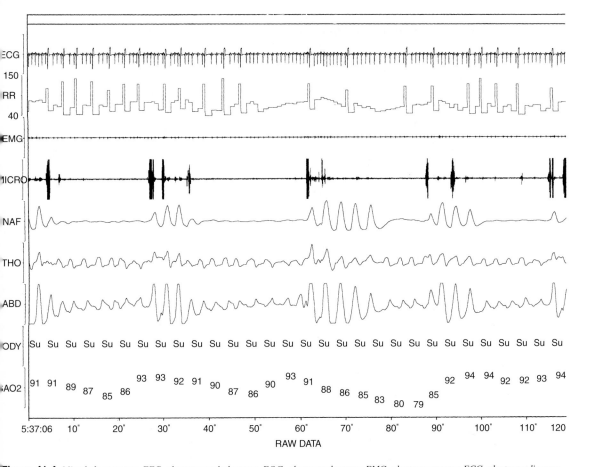

Figure 41-4 *Mixed sleep apnea. EEG, electroencephalogram; EOG, electrooculogram; EMG, electromyogram; ECG, electrocardiogram.*

and tachycardia after the end of the events. It is not unusual to see premature ventricular contractions, trigeminy and bigeminy, asystole, second-degree atrioventricular block, atrial tachycardia, sinus bradycardia, and ventricular tachycardia. However, the electrocardiogram taken during the waking state might be normal. It is only during the respiratory events during sleep that the abnormalities appear.

BRSD, especially central sleep apnea, is commonly seen in individuals with congestive heart failure (Findley et al. 1985). Cor pulmonale may also be a consequence of long-standing BRSD and is seen in both sleep apnea syndrome and primary hypoventilation. Individuals may present with unexplained respiratory failure, polycythemia, right ventricular failure, and nocturnal hypertension. About 50% of individuals with BRSD have hypertension, and about one-third of all hypertensive individuals have BRSD. In the large cross-sectional study, it was found that both systolic and diastolic blood pressure (SDB) as well as the prevalence of hypertension increased significantly with increasing SDB (Nieto et al. 2000). It has also been shown that there is a dose–response association between SDB at baseline and hypertension 4 years later suggesting that SDB may be a risk factor for hypertension and consequent cardiovascular morbidity (Peppard et al. 2000).

The most common symptoms of BRSD include excessive daytime sleepiness and snoring. The excessive daytime sleepiness probably results from sleep fragmentation caused by the frequent nocturnal arousals occurring at the end of the apneas, and possibly from hypoxemia.

The excessive daytime sleepiness is associated with lethargy, poor concentration, decreased motivation and performance, and inappropriate and inadvertent attacks of sleep. Sometimes the individuals do not realize they have fallen asleep until they awaken.

The second complaint is loud snoring, sometimes noisy enough to be heard throughout or even outside the house. Often the wife has complained for years about the snoring and has threatened to sleep elsewhere if she has not moved out already. Bed partners describe a characteristic pattern of loud snoring interrupted by periods of silence, which are then terminated by snorting sounds. Snoring results from a partial narrowing of the airway caused by multiple factors, such as inadequate muscle tone, large tonsils and adenoids, long soft palate, flaccid tissue, acromegaly, hypothyroidism, or congenital narrowing of the oral pharynx (Fairbanks 1987). Snoring has been implicated not only in sleep apnea but also in angina pectoris, stroke, ischemic heart disease, and cerebral infarction, even in the absence of complete sleep apneas (Koskenvuo et al. 1985, Partinen and Palomaki 1985). Because the prevalence of snoring increases with age, especially in women (Kripke et al. 1990), and because snoring can have serious medical consequences, the psychiatrist must give serious attention to complaints of loud snoring. Snoring is not always a symptom of BRSD. Approximately 25% of men and 15% of women are habitual snorers.

Individuals with BRSD are frequently overweight. In some individuals, a weight gain of 20 to 30 lb might bring on episodes of BRSD. The same fatty tissue seen on the outside is also present on the inside, making the airway even more narrow. Because obstructive sleep apnea is always caused by the collapse of the airway, in individuals of normal weight, anatomical abnormalities (such as large tonsils, long uvula) must be considered.

Other symptoms of BRSD include unexplained morning headaches, nocturnal confusion, automatic behavior, dysfunction of the autonomic nervous system, or night sweats. The severity of BRSD will depend on the severity of the cardiac arrhythmias, hypertension, excessive daytime sleepiness, respiratory disturbance index, amount of sleep fragmentation, and amount of oxygen desaturation.

Mild to moderate sleep-related breathing disturbances increase with age, even in elderly subjects without major complaints about their sleep. The frequency is higher in men than in women, at least until the age of menopause, after which the rate in women increases and may approach that of men. With use of the apnea index of 5 or more apneic episodes per hour as a cutoff criterion, prevalence rates range from 27 to 75% for older men and from 0 to 32% for older women (Ancoli-Israel 1989). In general, the severity of apnea in these older persons is mild (an average apnea index of about 13) compared with that seen in individuals with clinical sleep apnea. However, older men and women with mild apnea have been reported to fall asleep at inappropriate times significantly more often than older persons without apnea. Furthermore, the frequency of sleep apnea and other BRSDs is higher in individuals with hypertension, congestive heart failure, obesity, dementia, and other medical conditions.

Increased mortality rates have been noted in excessively long sleepers (Kripke et al. 1990); therefore sleep apnea may account for some of these excess deaths (Kripke 1983). This is also consistent with evidence that excess deaths from all causes increase between 2 and 8 A.M., specifically deaths related to ischemic heart disease in individuals older than 65 years (Mitler et al. 1987). There have been several studies suggesting that untreated sleep apnea in the elderly may lead to shorter survival (Bliwise et al. 1988, Fleury 1992, Ancoli-Israel et al. 1996).

The clinical significance of relatively mild "subclinical" sleep apneas is not fully understood yet. Mental health clinicians should be aware, however, that such disturbances might be associated with either insomnia or excessive daytime sleepiness. Furthermore, for some individuals with sleep apnea, administration of hypnotics, alcohol, or other sedating medications is relatively contraindicated. The risk is not yet known, but reports indicate that benzodiazepines as well as alcohol may increase the severity of mild sleep apnea (Mendelson et al. 1981, Block et al. 1983). Therefore, clinicians should inquire about snoring, gasping, and other signs and symptoms of sleep apnea before administering a sleeping pill. If individuals have excessive sleepiness or morning hangover effects while taking benzodiazepines, major tranquilizers, or other sedating medications, the psychiatrist should consider the possibility of an iatrogenic BRSD due to medications.

The diagnosis of BRSD must be differentiated from other disorders of excessive sleepiness such as narcolepsy. Individuals with BRSD will not have cataplexy, sleep-onset paralysis, or sleep-onset hallucination. Narcolepsy is not usually associated with loud snoring or sleep apneas. In laboratory recordings, individuals with BRSD do not usually have sleep-onset REM periods either at night or in multiple naps on the Multiple Sleep Latency Test. However, one must be aware that both BRSD and narcolepsy can be found in the same individual. BRSD must also be distinguished from other hypersomnias, such as those related to major depressive disorder or circadian rhythm disturbances.

Etiology

There are three types of apnea, based on differences in the underlying etiology. The first is obstructive sleep apnea, which involves the collapse of the pharyngeal airway during inspiration, with partial or complete blockage of airflow. The person still attempts to breathe, and one can observe the diaphragm moving, but the airway is blocked and therefore there is no air exchange. It can be caused by bagginess or excessive pharyngeal mucosa and a large uvula, fatty infiltration at the base of the tongue, or collapse of the pharyngeal walls. The resulting decreased air passage compromises alveolar ventilation and causes blood-oxygen desaturation and strenuous attempts at inspiration through the narrowed airway, all of which lighten and disrupt sleep. Hypercapnia, which results either from obstructive sleep apnea or from lung disease, reduces breathing without the presence of disruptive inspiratory efforts.

The second type is central sleep apnea, which results from failure of the respiratory neurons to activate the phrenic and intercostal motor neurons that mediate respiratory movements. There is no attempt to breathe, and although the airway is not collapsed, there is no respiration. This type of apnea is more commonly associated with heart disease (Olson and Strohl 1986).

The third type is mixed sleep apnea, which is a combination, generally beginning with a central component and ending with an obstructive component.

Treatment

Sleep apnea is sometimes alleviated by weight loss, avoidance of sedatives, use of tongue-retaining devices, and breathing air under positive pressure through a face mask (continuous positive airway pressure [CPAP]) (Guilleminault and Stoohs 1990, Aubert 1992). Oxygen breathed at night may alleviate insomnia associated with apnea that is not accompanied by impeded inspiration. Surgery may be helpful, for example, to correct enlarged tonsils, a long uvula, a short mandible, or morbid obesity. Pharyngoplasty, which tightens the pharyngeal mucosa and may also reduce the size of the uvula, or the use of a cervical collar to extend the neck, may relieve heavy snoring (Rodenstein 1992). Although tricyclic antidepressants are sometimes used in the treatment of clinical sleep apnea in young adults, they may cause considerable toxic effects in older people. The newer shorter-acting nonbenzodiazepine hypnotics seem to be safer in these individuals and may be considered in those individuals who snore.

CIRCADIAN RHYTHM SLEEP DISORDER (SLEEP–WAKE SCHEDULE DISORDERS)

Circadian rhythm disturbances result from a mismatch between the internal or endogenous circadian sleep–wake system and the external or exogenous demands on the sleep–wake system (see DSM-IV-TR diagnostic criteria below). The individual's tendency to sleep–wakefulness does not match that of her or his social circumstances or of the light–dark cycle. Although some individuals do not find this mismatch to be a problem, for others the circadian rhythm disturbance interferes with the ability to function properly at times when alertness or sleepiness is desired or required. For those individuals, insomnia, hypersomnia, sleepiness, and fatigue result in significant discomfort and impairment. The circadian rhythm disturbances include delayed sleep phase, advanced sleep phase, shift work, jet lag, and a non-24-hour-day syndrome.

DSM-IV-TR Diagnostic Criteria

307.45 Circadian Rhythm Sleep Disorder

A. A persistent or recurrent pattern of sleep disruption leading to excessive sleepiness or insomnia that is due to a mismatch between the sleep–wake schedule required by a person's environment and his or her circadian sleep–wake pattern.
B. The sleep disturbance causes clinically significant distress or impairment in social, occupational, or other important areas of functioning.
C. The disturbance does not occur exclusively during the course of another sleep disorder or other mental disorder.
D. The disturbance is not due to the direct physiological effects of a substance (e.g., a drug of abuse, a medication) or a general medical condition.

Specify type:

Delayed sleep phase type: a persistent pattern of late-sleep onset and late awakening times, with an inability to fall asleep and awaken at a desired earlier time

Jet lag type: sleepiness and alertness that occur at an inappropriate time of day relative to local time, occurring after repeated travel across more than one time zone

Shift work type: insomnia during the major sleep period or excessive sleepiness during the major awake period associated with night shift work or frequently changing shift work

Unspecified type

The diagnosis of circadian rhythm sleep disorder is based on a careful review of the history and circadian patterns of sleep–wakefulness, napping, alertness, and behavior. The diagnosis of circadian rhythm sleep disorder requires significant social or occupational impairment or marked distress related to the sleep disturbance. It is often useful for individuals with chronic complaints to keep a sleep–wake diary covering the entire

24-hour day each day for several weeks. If possible, an ambulatory device that measures rest–activity, such as a wrist actigraph, might supplement the sleep–wake diary. Wrist actigraphs record acceleration of the wrist at frequent intervals, such as every minute, and save it for later display. Because the wrist is mostly at rest during sleep, the record of wrist rest–activity provides a fairly accurate estimate of the timing and duration of sleep–wakefulness. In addition, some commercial wrist activity devices have a built-in photometer, which provides a record of ambient light–darkness against which the rest–activity pattern can be compared.

The prevalence of circadian rhythm disturbances has not been established. Approximately two-thirds of shift workers have difficulty with their schedules. Circadian rhythm disturbances must be differentiated from sleep-onset insomnia due to other causes (such as pain, caffeine consumption), early morning insomnia due to depression or alcohol use, and changes in sleep patterns due to lifestyle or lifestyle changes.

DELAYED SLEEP PHASE TYPE

Diagnosis

In the delayed sleep phase type, there is a delay in the circadian rhythm in the sleep–wake cycle (Vignau et al. 1993). These individuals are generally not sleepy until several hours after "normal" bedtime (i.e., 2–3 A.M.). If allowed to sleep undisturbed, they will sleep for 7 or 8 hours, which means they awaken around 10 to 11 A.M. People with delayed sleep phase are considered extreme "owls." They may or may not complain of sleep-onset insomnia. They usually enjoy their alertness in the evening and night and have little desire to sleep beginning at 10 P.M. or midnight. Their problem is trying to wake up at normal times (i.e., 6–7 A.M.). In essence, their rhythm is shifted to a later clock time relative to conventional rest–activity patterns.

Individuals with delayed sleep phase often choose careers that allow them to set their own schedules, such as freelance writers. Delayed sleep phase occurs commonly in late adolescence and young adulthood, such as in college students. As many of these individuals age, however, their endogenous sleep–wake rhythm advances and they eventually are able to conform themselves to a normal rest period at night.

For others, however, this phase shift of the endogenous oscillator may lead at a later age to the advanced sleep phase (Richardson 1990). In this condition, individuals become sleepy earlier in the evening (e.g., 7–8 P.M.). They will also sleep for 7 to 8 hours, but that means they awaken around 2 to 3 A.M. These individuals are "larks," being most alert in the morning. They complain of sleep maintenance insomnia, that is, they cannot stay asleep all night long. This condition is more prevalent in the elderly than in the young.

Etiology

The etiology of extreme "night owls" and "larks" is probably multifaceted but, in some cases, appears to reflect genetic factors. Jones and colleagues (1999) described a family in which extreme phase advance (bedtime about 7 P.M.) appeared to be consistent with an autosomal dominant trait. One member of the family was studied in a temporal isolation facility; as predicted, her endogenous sleep–wake cycle averaged less than 24 hours, clearly different from most subjects who average about 24.2 to 24.5 hours. Members of this family appear to have a mutation of one of the "clock genes" (Jones et al. 1999). In addition, Ancoli-Israel and colleagues (2001) identified a pedigree of one family with phase delay.

Treatment

Clinical management includes chronobiological strategies to shift the phase position of the endogenous circadian oscillator in the appropriate direction. For example, exposure to bright light in the morning advances the delayed sleep phase, that is, individuals will become sleepy earlier in the evening (Rosenthal et al. 1990). On the other hand, administration of bright light in the evening acts to delay the circadian rhythm, that is, individuals will get sleepy later in the evening. Light is usually administered in doses of 2500 lux for a period of 2 hours per day, although the ideal intensity and duration are yet to be determined. For some individuals, spending more time outdoors in bright sunlight may be sufficient to treat the sleep phase. For example, individuals with delayed sleep phase should be encouraged to remove blinds and curtains from their windows, which would allow the sunlight to pour into their bedrooms in the morning when they should arise. In addition, gradual adjustments of the timing of the sleep–wake cycle may be used to readjust the phase position of the circadian oscillator. For example, individuals with delayed phase disorder can be advised to delay the onset of sleep by 2 to 3 hours each day (i.e., from 4 to 7 to 10 A.M., and so on) until the appropriate bedtime. After that, they should maintain regular sleep–wake patterns, with exposure to bright light in the morning.

SHIFT-WORK TYPE

Diagnosis

Shift-work problems occur when the circadian sleep–wake rhythm is in conflict with the rest–activity cycle imposed by the externally determined work schedule (Akerstedt 1991). Nearly a quarter of all American employees have jobs that require them to work outside the conventional 8 A.M. to 5 P.M. schedule. Different patterns include rotating schedules and more or less permanent evening and night schedules. Rotating schedules, particularly rapidly shifting schedules, are difficult because constant readjustment of the endogenous circadian oscillator to the imposed sleep–wake cycle is necessary. In both rotating and shift-work schedules, further difficulties are encountered because the worker is usually expected to readjust to a normal sleep–wake cycle on weekends and holidays. Even if the worker can adjust his or her circadian system to the work schedule, he or she is then out of synchrony with the rhythm of family and friends during off-duty hours. These individuals, therefore, are constantly sleep deprived and constantly sleepy. They endure impaired performance and increased risk of accidents, somatic complaints, and poor morale; hypnotics, stimulants, and alcohol are used excessively in relationship to unusual or shifting work schedules (Moore-Ede 1986, Akerstedt 1991, Czeisler et al. 1990). Shift-work schedules may have played a role in human errors that contributed to the Three Mile Island and Chernobyl accidents and the Challenger disaster.

Treatment

No totally satisfactory methods currently exist for managing shift-work problems. Because people vary in their ability to adjust to these schedules, self-selection or survival of the fittest may be involved for those who can find other employment or work schedules. Older individuals appear to be less flexible than younger persons in adjusting to shift work. Some experiments suggest that the principles of chronobiology may be useful in reducing the human costs of shift work. For example, because the endogenous pacemaker has a cycle length (tau) longer than 24 hours, rotating shift workers do better when their schedules move in a clockwise direction (i.e., morning to evening to night) rather than in the other direction. Appropriate exposure to bright lights and darkness may push the circadian pacemaker in the correct direction and help stabilize its phase position, especially in association with the use of dark glasses outside and blackout curtains at home to maintain darkness at the appropriate times for promotion of sleep and shifting of the circadian pacemaker (Czeisler et al. 1990). Naps may also be useful in reducing sleep loss. Modest amounts of coffee may maintain alertness early in the shift but should be avoided near the end of the shift.

JET LAG TYPE

Diagnosis

Jet lag occurs when individuals travel across several time zones. Traveling east advances the sleep–wake cycle and is typically more difficult than traveling west (which delays the cycle). Jet lag may be associated with difficulty initiating or maintaining sleep or with daytime sleepiness, impaired performance, and gastrointestinal disturbance after rapid transmeridian flights (Moore-Ede 1986). Individuals older than 50 years appear to be more vulnerable to jet lag than are younger persons.

Treatment

Considerable research and theorizing are underway to better prevent and manage the problems associated with jet lag. Some efforts before departure may be useful to prevent or ameliorate these problems. For persons who plan to readjust their circadian clock to the new location, it may be possible to move the sleep–wake and light–dark schedules appropriately before departure. In addition, good sleep hygiene principles should be respected before, during, and after the trip. For example, many people are sleep deprived or in alcohol withdrawal when they step on the plane because of last-minute preparations or farewell parties. Whereas adequate fluid intake on the plane is necessary to avoid dehydration, alcohol consumption should be avoided or minimized because it causes diuresis and may disrupt sleep maintenance.

On arriving at the destination, it may be preferable to try to maintain a schedule coinciding with actual home time if the trip is going to be short. For example, the individual should try to sleep at times that correspond to the usual bedtime or with the normal midafternoon dip in alertness. If, on the other hand, the trip will be longer and it is desirable to synchronize the biological clock with local time, exposure to appropriate schedules of bright light and darkness may be helpful, at least theoretically. Unfortunately, the exact protocols have not been established in all instances yet and require further research and experimentation. In addition, some of these protocols require avoidance of bright light at certain times, necessitating wearing dark goggles, for example, when traveling.

In addition to synchronizing the clock with the new environment, sleep and rest should be promoted by good sleep hygiene principles, by avoidance of excessive caffeine and alcohol, and, possibly, by administration of short-duration hypnotics. Care should be taken, however, to avoid hangover effects or amnesia associated with hypnotics. Because individual responses to sleeping pills vary considerably from person to person, it is often helpful to develop experience with specific compounds and doses before departure.

OTHER TYPE (NON-24-HOUR-DAY SYNDROME)

The non-24-hour-day (or "hypernyctohemeral") syndrome is characterized by free-running in the natural environment, that is, the subject goes to bed and arises about 45 minutes later each day. The average duration of the sleep–wake cycle is about 24.5 to 25.0 hours. During the course of about 3 weeks, the subject's sleep–wake cycle "goes around the clock" as the timing of the sleep period gradually delays. The lengthened sleep–wake cycle of these individuals in the natural environment is similar to that of normal subjects living in a time-free environment. The disorder appears to be relatively common in individuals with total blindness, because they no longer perceive visual Zeitgebers. In many cases, the cause is unknown, but it is sometimes observed in individuals who are socially or linguistically isolated. Management may include bright light therapy in the morning to entrain the endogenous oscillator. Administration of vitamin B_{12} may be helpful, perhaps by enhancing the effectiveness of Zeitgebers (Kamgar-Parsi et al. 1983).

PERIODIC LIMB MOVEMENTS IN SLEEP

Diagnosis

Periodic limb movements in sleep (PLMS), previously called nocturnal myoclonus, is a disorder in which repetitive, brief, and stereotyped limb movements occur during sleep, usually about every 20 to 40 seconds. Dorsiflexions of the big toe, ankle, knee, and sometimes the hip are involved (Ancoli-Israel et al. 1991b, Chesson et al. 1999) (Table 41-9 and Figure 41-5).

Questioning of the individual or bed partner often yields reports of restlessness, kicking, unusually cold or hot feet, disrupted and torn bedclothes, unrefreshing sleep, insomnia, or excessive daytime sleepiness. Individuals may be unaware of these pathological leg movements or arousals, although their bed partners may be all too aware of the kicking, frequent movements, and restlessness (Coleman et al. 1983, Ancoli-Israel et al. 1986). If these disorders are strongly suspected, the individual should probably be referred to a sleep disorders laboratory for evaluation and an overnight polysomnogram with tibial electromyograms. These disorders are often associated with transient arousals in the EEG recording. Diagnosis is made when the periodic limb movement index (number of leg jerks per hour of sleep) is 5 or greater, accompanied by arousals. The jerks occur primarily in the legs but may also appear in less severe forms in the arms. The movements can be bilateral or unilateral and occur in stage 1 and stage 2 sleep. Individuals often have reduced deep sleep because the jerks continually awaken them.

A related disturbance, restless legs syndrome, is associated with disagreeable sensations in the lower legs, feet, or thighs that occur in a recumbent or resting position and cause an almost irresistible urge to move the legs (Walters et al. 1995). Whereas almost all individuals with restless legs syndrome have PLMS, not all individuals with PLMS have restless legs syndrome. Restless legs syndrome may be frequent in individuals with uremia and rheumatoid arthritis or in pregnant women.

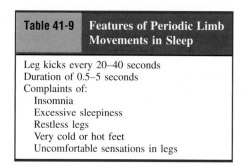

Table 41-9	Features of Periodic Limb Movements in Sleep

Leg kicks every 20–40 seconds
Duration of 0.5–5 seconds
Complaints of:
  Insomnia
  Excessive sleepiness
  Restless legs
  Very cold or hot feet
  Uncomfortable sensations in legs	

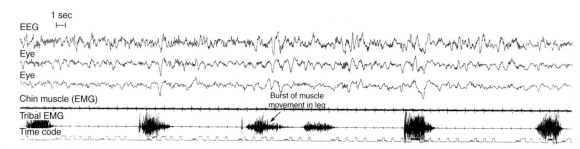

Figure 41-5 *Periodic limb movements in sleep. Time scale: 1 cm = 1 s. EEG, electroencephalogram; EMG, electromyogram.*

Both PLMS and restless legs syndrome usually occur in middle-aged people, but many individuals report having had the same sensations as adolescents and even as children. It has been suggested that both conditions are familial, perhaps due to an autosomal dominant gene.

Individuals with PLMS are reported to sleep about an hour less per night than control subjects without PLMS (Ancoli-Israel et al. 1991b). Interestingly, the prevalence of PLMS is not higher in insomniac individuals than in those without insomnia. Complaints of excessive daytime sleepiness increase in individuals with PLMS, probably consequent to the numerous sleep interruptions. The psychiatrist may find it useful to talk with a bed partner, who will often describe kicking and leg twitches during sleep in individuals with PLMS.

The myoclonic movements are not related to seizure disorder but should be distinguished from seizures. Because complaints of insomnia and daytime sleepiness are not uncommon, other insomnias, sleep apnea, and narcolepsy should be ruled out.

Prevalence of PLMS in young and middle-aged adults has not been fully established. In sleep disorders clinic populations, about 11% of those complaining of insomnia are diagnosed with PLMS. In the elderly, however, this condition is extremely common; more than 45% have at least five leg kicks per hour of sleep (Ancoli-Israel et al. 1985, 1991b).

Treatment

Because the pathogenesis of PLMS is usually unknown, treatment is often symptomatic (Table 41-10). Some studies suggest that the movements arise subcortically from the brain or spinal cord; others suggest subclinical peripheral neuropathy. At the present time, dopaminergic agents such as levodopa (L-dopa), pergolide, or pramipexole generally provide the most effective treatment for both PLMS and restless legs syndrome (Walters et al. 1988, Chesson et al. 1999, Heninger et al. 1999, Montplaisir et al. 2000, 2002). Opiates, such as oxycodone and propoxyphene, have also been demonstrated to be effective in the treatment of PLMS and restless legs syndrome. Anticonvulsants, such as carbamazepine and gabapentin, have been shown to be effective in treatment of restless legs syndrome. Clonazepam, a benzodiazepine anticonvulsant, is effective in the treatment of PLMS and possibly for restless legs syndrome. Other benzodiazepines have also been used to treat

Table 41-10 Pharmacologic Treatment Options in RLS/PLMS

Medication	Dosage Range	Side Effects	Advantages	Disadvantages
L-dopa/carbidopa	25/100–100/400/D	Dyskinesia Nausea Hallucinations	Low cost	Breakthrough restlessness Loss of efficacy
Pergolide	0.05–1 mg	Dyskinesia Nausea Rhinitis Dizziness	High rate of response	Frequent side effects
Pramipexole	0.25–0.875 mg	Orthostasis Dizziness Sedation	High rate of response Good tolerance	Expense
Anticonvulsants	Variable	Sedation	Low cost Sleep promotion	Variable response
Opiates	Variable	Nausea Constipation	Low cost	Variable response Abuse potential
Clonazepam	0.5–2 mg	Sedation Dizziness	Sleep promotion	Variable response Abuse potential

these conditions, as they will decrease some of the awakenings but may have no effect on the number of leg movements (Chesson et al. 1999, Heninger et al. 1999).

PARASOMNIAS

The parasomnias are a group of disorders characterized by disturbances of either physiological processes or behavior associated with sleep, but not necessarily causing disturbances of sleep or wakefulness.

NIGHTMARE DISORDER

Diagnosis

The essential feature of this disorder is the repeated occurrence of frightening dreams that lead to full awakenings from sleep (Hartmann 1991, 1994) (see DSM-IV-TR diagnostic criteria below). The dreams or awakenings cause the individual significant distress or dysfunction. By definition, the disorder is excluded if the nightmare occurs in the course of another mental or medical disorder or as a direct result of a medication or substance. Many, but not all, nightmares occur during REM sleep; REM nightmares take place most often during the last half of the night when REM sleep is most common (see nightmares in posttraumatic stress disorder).

DSM-IV-TR Diagnostic Criteria

307.47 Nightmare Disorder

A. Repeated awakenings from the major sleep period or naps with detailed recall of extended and extremely frightening dreams, usually involving threats to survival, security, or self-esteem. The awakenings generally occur during the second half of the sleep period.

B. On awakening from the frightening dreams, the person rapidly becomes oriented and alert (in contrast to the confusion and disorientation seen in sleep terror disorder and some forms of epilepsy).

C. The dream experience, or the sleep disturbance resulting from the awakening, causes clinically significant distress or impairment in social, occupational, or other important areas of functioning.

D. The nightmares do not occur exclusively during the course of another mental disorder (e.g., a delirium, posttraumatic stress disorder) and are not due to the direct physiological effects of a substance (e.g., a drug of abuse, a medication) or a general medical condition.

Reprinted with permission from the Diagnostic and Statistical Manual of Mental Disorders, Fourth Edition, Text Revision. Copyright 2000 American Psychiatric Association.

Whereas more than half of the adult population probably experiences an occasional nightmare, nightmares start more commonly in children between the ages of 3 and 6 years. The exact prevalence is unknown.

Treatment

The disorder is usually self-limited in children but can be helped sometimes with psychotherapy, desensitization, or rehearsal instructions (Bakwin 1970). Secondary nightmares, as in posttraumatic stress disorder (PTSD), can be difficult to treat.

SLEEP TERROR DISORDER

Diagnosis

This disorder is defined as repeated abrupt awakenings from sleep characterized by intense fear, panicky screams, autonomic arousal (tachycardia, rapid breathing, and sweating), absence of detailed dream recall, amnesia for the episode, and relative unresponsiveness to attempts to comfort the person (Kales et al. 1980, Gordon 1992) (see DSM-IV-TR diagnostic criteria below). Because sleep terrors occur primarily during delta sleep, they usually take place during the first third of the night. These episodes may cause distress or impairment, especially for caretakers who witness the event. Sleep terrors may also be called night terrors, *pavor nocturnus*, or incubus.

DSM-IV-TR Diagnostic Criteria

307.46 Sleep Terror Disorder

A. Recurrent episodes of abrupt awakening from sleep, usually occurring during the first third of the major sleep episode and beginning with a panicky scream.
B. Intense fear and signs of autonomic arousal, such as tachycardia, rapid breathing, and sweating, during each episode.
C. Relative unresponsiveness to efforts of others to comfort the person during the episode.
D. No detailed dream is recalled and there is amnesia for the episode.
E. The episodes cause clinically significant distress or impairment in social, occupational, or other important areas of functioning.
F. The disturbance is not due to the direct physiological effects of a substance (e.g., a drug of abuse, a medication) or a general medical condition.

Reprinted with permission from the Diagnostic and Statistical Manual of Mental Disorders, Fourth Edition, Text Revision. Copyright 2000 American Psychiatric Association.

The prevalence of the disorder is estimated to be about 1 to 6% in children and less than 1% in adults. In children, it usually begins between the ages of 4 and 12 years and resolves spontaneously during adolescence. It is more common in boys than in girls. It does not appear to be associated with psychiatric illness in children. In adults, it usually begins between 20 and 30 years of age, has a chronic undulating course, is equally common in men and women, and may be associated with mental disorders, such as PTSD, generalized anxiety disorder, borderline personality disorder, and others. An increased frequency of enuresis and somnambulism has been reported in the first-degree relatives of individuals with night terrors.

Treatment

Nocturnal administration of benzodiazepines has been reported to be beneficial, perhaps because these drugs suppress delta sleep, the stage of sleep during which sleep terrors typically occur.

SLEEPWALKING DISORDER

Diagnosis

This disorder is characterized by repeated episodes of motor behavior initiated in sleep, usually during delta sleep in the first third of the night (see DSM-IV-TR diagnostic criteria below). While sleepwalking, the individual has a blank staring face, is relatively unresponsive to others, and may be confused or disoriented initially on being aroused from the episode. Although the person may be alert after several minutes of awakening, complete amnesia for the episode is common the next day. Sleepwalking may cause considerable distress, for example, if a child cannot sleep away from home or go to camp because of it. By definition, pure sleepwalking is excluded if it occurs as a result of a medication or substance or is due to a medical disorder. However, sleepwalking may be an idiosyncratic reaction to specific drugs, including tranquilizers and sleeping pills (Glassman et al. 1986).

DSM-IV-TR Diagnostic Criteria

307.46 Sleepwalking Disorder

A. Repeated episodes of rising from bed during sleep and walking about, usually occurring during the first third of the major sleep episode.
B. While sleepwalking, the person has a blank, staring face, is relatively unresponsive to the efforts of others to communicate with him or her, and can be awakened only with great difficulty.
C. On awakening (either from the sleepwalking episode or the next morning), the person has amnesia for the episode.
D. Within several minutes after awakening from the sleepwalking episode, there is no impairment of mental activity or behavior (although there may initially be a short period of confusion or disorientation).
E. The sleepwalking causes clinically significant distress or impairment in social, occupational, or other important areas of functioning.
F. The disturbance is not due to the direct physiological effects of a substance (e.g., a drug of abuse, a medication) or a general medical condition.

Reprinted with permission from the Diagnostic and Statistical Manual of Mental Disorders, Fourth Edition, Text Revision. Copyright 2000 American Psychiatric Association.

Most behaviors during sleepwalking are routine and of low-level intensity, such as sitting up, picking the sheets, or walking around the bedroom. More complicated behaviors may also occur, however, such as urinating in a closet, leaving the house, running, eating, talking, driving, or even committing murder (Luchins et al. 1978). A real danger is that the individual will be injured by going through a window or falling from a height.

Whereas about 10 to 30% of children have at least one sleepwalking episode, only about 1 to 5% have repeated episodes. The disorder most commonly begins between the ages of 4 and 8 years and usually resolves spontaneously during adolescence. Genetic factors may be involved, because sleepwalkers are reported to have a higher than expected frequency of first-degree relatives with either sleepwalking or sleep terrors (Bakwin 1970). Sleepwalking may be precipitated in affected individuals by gently sitting them up during sleep, by fever, or by sleep deprivation. Adult onset of sleepwalking should prompt the search for possible medical, neurological, psychiatric, pharmacological, or other underlying causes, such as nocturnal epilepsy.

Treatment
No treatment for sleepwalking is established, but some individuals respond to administration of benzodiazepines or sedating antidepressants at bedtime. The major concern should be the safety of the sleepwalker, who may injure herself or himself or someone else during an episode.

REM SLEEP BEHAVIOR DISORDER

Diagnosis
First described in 1986, this disorder, like sleepwalking, is associated with complicated behaviors during sleep such as walking, running, singing, and talking (Schenk et al. 1986). In contrast to sleepwalking, which occurs during the first third of the night during delta sleep, REM sleep behavior disorder usually occurs during the second half of the night during REM sleep. It apparently results from an intermittent loss of the muscle atonia that normally accompanies REM sleep, thus allowing the individual to act out her or his dream. Also, in contrast to sleepwalking, memory for the dream content is usually good. Furthermore, the idiopathic form typically occurs in men during the sixth or seventh decade of life. The cause or causes remain unknown. It has been reported in a variety of neurological disorders and during withdrawal from sedatives or alcohol; during treatment with tricyclic antidepressants or biperiden (Akineton); and in various neurological disorders including dementia, subarachnoid hemorrhage, and degenerative neurological disorders.

Treatment
Nocturnal administration of clonazepam, 0.5 to 1 mg, is usually remarkably successful in controlling the symptoms of this disorder. Individuals and their families should be educated about the nature of the disorder and warned to take precautions about injuring themselves or others.

NOCTURNAL PANIC ATTACKS

The typical daytime panic attack, as bizarre and frightening as it may seem to the individual experiencing it, is often fairly obvious to the assessing clinician. Symptoms of anxiety, sweating, tremor, dizziness, chest pain, and palpitations occur "out of the blue" with or without specific behavioral or associational stimuli. Once it has been diagnosed, treatment options may include pharmacotherapy with one of several classes of drugs, behavioral therapy, or a combined approach.

When these symptoms occur at night, the task of the assessing clinician is greatly complicated. The individual may assume that the cause is a nightmare or a night terror and may be resistant to the diagnosis of an anxiety disorder, particularly if the symptoms are absent or mild during the daytime. Individuals with panic disorder often have not only disturbed subjective sleep but also panic attacks during sleep (Stein et al. 1993, Koenigsberg et al. 1994). Clinician should remember that panic attacks could occur exclusively during sleep, without daytime symptoms, in some individuals.

Conversely, a report of "awakening in a state of panic" may be associated with a variety of other disorders including obstructive sleep apnea, gastroesophageal reflux, nocturnal angina, orthopnea, nightmares, night terrors, and others.

SLEEP-RELATED EPILEPSY

Some forms of epilepsy occur more commonly during sleep than during wakefulness and may be associated with parasomnia disorders. Nocturnal seizures may at times be confused with sleep terror, REM sleep behavior disorder, paroxysmal hypnogenic dystonia, or nocturnal panic attacks (Culebras 1992). They may take the form of generalized convulsions or may be partial seizures with complex symptoms. Nocturnal seizures are most common at two times: the first 2 hours of sleep, and around 4 to 6 A.M. They are more common in children than in adults. The chief complaint may be only disturbed sleep, torn up bedsheets and blankets, morning drowsiness (a postictal state), and muscle aches. Some individuals never realize that they suffer from nocturnal epilepsy until they share a bedroom or bed with someone who observes a convulsion.

SLEEP DISTURBANCES RELATED TO OTHER MENTAL DISORDERS

Diagnosis

Subjective and objective disturbances of sleep are common features of many mental disorders. General abnormalities include dyssomnias (such as insomnia and hypersomnia), parasomnias (such as nightmares, night terrors, and nocturnal panic attacks), and circadian rhythm disturbances (early morning awakening). Before assuming that a significant sleep complaint invariably signals a diagnosis of a mental disorder mental health specialists should go through a careful differential diagnostic procedure to rule out medical, pharmacological, or other causes. Even if the sleep complaint is primarily related to an underlying mental disorder, sleep disorders in the mentally ill may be exacerbated by many other factors, such as increasing age; comorbid, mental, sleep, and medical diagnoses; alcohol and substance abuse; effects of psychotropic or other medications; use of caffeinated beverages, nicotine, or other substances; lifestyle; past episodes of psychiatric illness (persisting "scars"); and cognitive, conditioned, and coping characteristics such as anticipatory anxiety about sleep as bedtime nears. Some features of these sleep disorders may persist during periods of clinical remission of the mental disorder and may be influenced by genetic factors. Finally, even if the sleep complaint is precipitated by a nonpsychiatric factor, psychiatric and psychosocial skills may be useful in ferreting out predisposing and perpetuating factors involved in chronic sleep complaints.

Although signs and symptoms of sleep disturbance are common in most mental disorders, an additional diagnosis of insomnia or hypersomnia related to another mental disorder is made according to DSM-IV-TR criteria only when the sleep disturbance is a predominant complaint and is sufficiently severe to warrant independent clinical attention (see DSM-IV-TR diagnostic criteria for Insomnia and Hypersomnia on page 1157). Many of the individuals with this type of sleep disorder diagnosis focus on the sleep complaints to the exclusion of other symptoms related to the primary mental disorder. For example, they may seek professional help with complaints of insomnia or oversleeping when they should be at work, excessive fatigue, or desire for sleeping pills, but initially, they minimize or strongly deny signs and symptoms related to poor mood, anxiety, obsessive rumination, alcohol abuse, or a personality disorder.

▰ DSM-IV-TR Diagnostic Criteria

307.42 Insomnia Related to... [Indicate the Axis I or Axis II Disorder]

A. The predominant complaint is difficulty initiating or maintaining sleep, or nonrestorative sleep, for at least 1 month that is associated with daytime fatigue or impaired daytime functioning.

B. The sleep disturbance (or daytime sequelae) causes clinically significant distress or impairment in social, occupational, or other important areas of functioning.

C. The insomnia is judged to be related to another Axis I or Axis II disorder (e.g., Major Depressive Disorder, Generalized Anxiety Disorder, Adjustment Disorder With Anxiety) but is sufficiently severe to warrant independent clinical attention.

D. The disturbance is not better accounted for by another Sleep Disorder (e.g., Narcolepsy, Breathing-Related Sleep Disorder, a Parasomnia).

E. The disturbance is not due to the direct physiological effects of a substance (e.g., a drug of abuse, a medication) or a general medical condition.

▰ DSM-IV-TR Diagnostic Criteria

307.44 Hypersomnia Related to... [Indicate the Axis I or Axis II Disorder]

A. The predominant complaint is excessive sleepiness for at least 1 month as evidenced by either prolonged sleep episodes or daytime sleep episodes that occur almost daily.

B. The excessive sleepiness causes clinically significant distress or impairment in social, occupational, or other important areas of functioning.

C. The hypersomnia is judged to be related to another Axis I or Axis II disorder (e.g., Major Depressive Disorder, Dysthymic Disorder) but is sufficiently severe to warrant independent clinical attention.

D. The disturbance is not better accounted for by another Sleep Disorder (e.g., Narcolepsy, Breathing-Related Sleep Disorder, a Parasomnia) or by an inadequate amount of sleep.

E. The disturbance is not due to the direct physiological effects of a substance (e.g., a drug of abuse, a medication) or a general medical condition.

Whereas insomnia is probably the most common sleep complaint in most mental disorders, hypersomnia is not infrequently reported, especially in association with the following: bipolar mood disorder during depressed periods; major depressive disorder with atypical features (i.e., hypersomniac, hyperphagic individuals with "leaden paralysis" and loss of energy); seasonal (winter) depression; stimulant abusers during withdrawal; some individuals with personality disorders; and individuals who are heavily sedated with anxiolytic, antipsychotic, or antidepressant medications, among other disorders (Table 41-11).

Polygraph recordings have now been obtained in most mental disorders, especially during episodes of illness rather than remission (Benca et al. 1992, Gillin et al. 1993). As summarized in Table 41-12, no single measure or constellation of measures has yet been found to be diagnostically pathognomonic for any specific disorder. Most diagnostic disorders are associated with insomnia, characterized by increased sleep latency and reduced total sleep, sleep efficiency, and delta sleep. Whereas short REM latency was once proposed as a biological marker for depression, studies suggest that it may also be associated with schizophrenia and some eating disorders.

Table 41-11 Selected Disorders of Apparent Hypersomnia or Excessive Daytime Sleepiness

Disorder	Sex	Hyperphagia	Depression	Hypersomnia	Excessive Daytime Sleepiness	Seasonality	Light Therapy
Atypical depression	F > M	++	+++	++	+	−	−
Seasonal affective disorder	F > M	++	+++	++	++	+++	+++
Bipolar depression	F = M	±	+++	+	+	+	+
Delayed sleep phase	M > F	−	±	−	AM	−	++
Kleine–Levin syndrome	M > F	++	+	+++	+++	−	−
Non-24-hour-day syndrome	M = F	−	−	−	−	−	+
Narcolepsy	M = F	−	±	+	+++	−	−
Sleep drunkenness	M = F	−	±	+++	AM	−	−
Sleep apnea	M > F	+	±	++	+++	−	−
Withdrawal from stimulants	M > F	++	+	++	++	−	−

Table 41-12 Generalized Polygraphic Sleep Features of Individuals with Mental Disorders*

Disorder	Total Sleep Time	Sleep Efficiency	Sleep Latency	REM Latency	Delta %	REM %	REM Density
Depression	↓↓	↓↓	↑↑	↓↓	↓↓	↓↓	↑
Alcoholism	↓	↓/=	↑	=	↓	↑	↑=
Panic disorder	↓/=	↓↓	↑↑	=	=	=	=
Generalized anxiety disorder	=	=	↑	=	=	=	=
Posttraumatic stress disorder	↓↓	↓↓	=	↑/=	=	↓↑	↑/=
Borderline disorder	↓/=	↓/=	↑/=	↓/=	=	=	=
Eating disorders	↓/=	↓/=	=	↓/=	=	=	↓/=
Schizophrenia	↓↓	↓↓	↑↑	↓↓	↓/=	=	↓
Insomnia	↓↓	↓↓	↑↑	=	↓↓	=	=
Narcolepsy	=	↓	↓↓	↓↓	=	=	=

*Two arrows (↑↑ or ↓↓) signify predominance of evidence; one arrow (↑ or ↓) signifies weak evidence, and (−) signifies weak evidence; equal sign (=) means no difference; ↓/= or ↑/= means mixed results.
Source: Data from Benca RM, Obermeyer WH, Thisted RA, et al. (1992) Sleep and psychiatric disorders: A meta-analysis. *Arch Gen Psych* **49**, 651–668; Gillin JC, Dow BM, Thompson P, et al. (1993) Sleep in depression and other psychiatric disorders. *Clin Neurosci* **1**, 90–; Dow BM, Kelsoe JRJ, and Gillin JC (1996) Sleep and dreams in Vietnam PTSD and depression. *Biol Psychiatr* **39**, 42–50.

More studies of sleep and sleep-related phenomenology have been conducted in *depression* than in any other disorder (Table 41-13 and Figure 41-6). Despite the common clinical impression that early morning wakefulness is a predominant symptom in depression, most of the objective measures in recent years have implicated abnormalities occurring at sleep onset and during the first non-REM and REM periods: prolonged sleep latency; reduced stages 3 and 4 sleep; increased duration and REM density of the first REM period; and associated neuroendocrine abnormalities, including growth hormone, thyroid-stimulating hormone, and melatonin. Furthermore, some studies have suggested that short REM latency (Giles et al. 1988) or reduced delta sleep ratio (amount of delta waves in first non-REM periods compared to second non-REM periods) (Kupfer et al. 1990) may predict relapse in depressed individuals. Some of these sleep-related abnormalities appear to persist during periods of clinical remission, such as short REM latency, loss of stages 3 and 4 sleep, and blunted nocturnal growth hormone release. Genetic factors may influence some of these measures, including short REM latency. Preliminary data suggest that short REM latency may be a genetic marker for depression in first-degree relatives of individuals with mood disorders (Mendlewicz et al. 1989).

Given the prevalence of sleep disturbance in depression, one puzzle is the well-established observation that sleep deprivation and some other manipulations of sleep have antidepressant effects in about half of depressed individuals (Table 41-14). Total and partial

Table 41-13	Sleep-Related Characteristics Associated with Depression

Short REM latency (state, possibly trait)
Reduced amounts of stages 3 and 4 sleep (state and trait)
Difficulties initiating and maintaining sleep
Increased amounts of ocular movement during REM sleep (REM density), especially during the first REM period
A redistribution of REM sleep toward the beginning of sleep: increased duration of the first REM period
Low arousal thresholds to auditory stimulation
Elevated core body temperature during sleep
Blunted or reduced levels of plasma growth hormone (state and trait)
Elevated levels of plasma cortisol, increased number of pulses, and earlier onset of the morning rise in cortisol levels
Reduced levels of plasma testosterone
Blunted levels of thyroid-stimulating hormone at sleep onset
Reduced nocturnal levels of plasma melatonin
Longer but flattened periods of prolactin release
Elevated cerebral glucose metabolic rate during the first non-REM period
Faster induction of REM sleep after administration of cholinergic agonists
Antidepressant effect of total and partial sleep deprivation and, possibly, selective REM sleep deprivation

Table 41-14	"Sleep Therapies" for Depression		
Sleep Manipulation	**Duration**	**Response Rate**	**Comment**
Total sleep deprivation	All night	25–60%	Temporary benefits Well documented
Partial sleep deprivation	First or second half of night	25–60%	Same Well documented
REM sleep deprivation	2–3 weeks	50%	Long-term benefits Only one study
Advance of sleep period (i.e., 5 P.M.–2 A.M.)	1–2 weeks	25–50%	Only a few studies

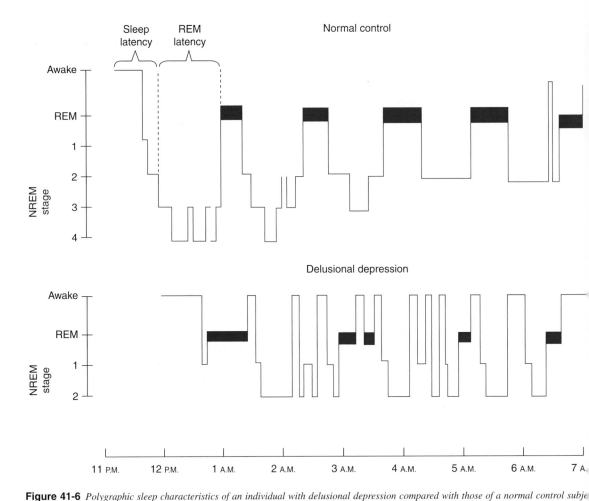

Figure 41-6 *Polygraphic sleep characteristics of an individual with delusional depression compared with those of a normal control subje*

sleep deprivation for one night has the best-documented benefits but, unfortunately, has not gained widespread clinical utility because most individuals usually wake up depressed again after napping or sleeping. One exception may be premenstrual depression: partial sleep deprivation for one night at the onset of symptoms often aborts the symptoms for that month.

Even though the polygraphic sleep findings in depression do not appear to be diagnostically specific, they remain among the best-documented biological abnormalities of any psychiatric disorder at this time. One challenge is to understand their pathophysiological mechanism. Because of the shallow, fragmented sleep and response to sleep deprivation, the sleep of individuals with depression has been described as "overaroused." For instance, the antidepressant response of sleep deprivation may "dampen down" an overly aroused limbic system in a subgroup of individuals. Several studies have shown that responders to sleep deprivation differ from nonresponders at baseline assessment before sleep deprivation by having a higher level of metabolic activity in the cingulate gyrus and that this overactivity approaches normality with clinical improvement (Wu et al. 1992, Ebert et al. 1994, Gillin et al. 2001a). Consistent with the overarousal hypothesis, a preliminary study using positron emission tomography to measure cerebral glucose metabolism suggested that depressed individuals are more metabolically active during the first non-REM period of the night than are normal control subjects (Ho et al. 1996). Because cholinergic projections from brain stem and basal forebrain are involved in central physiological arousal mechanisms, it is not surprising that depressed individuals are more likely than control subjects to awaken to an intravenous infusion of physostigmine (a cholinesterase inhibitor that facilitates cholinergic neurotransmission) during the first non-REM period (Berger et al. 1983). Moreover, depressed individuals enter REM sleep more rapidly after administration of cholinergic agonists, whether they are given orally before bed (Berger et al. 1983) or during non-REM sleep (Gillin et al. 1991).

The sleep disturbances of individuals with *schizophrenia* are often similar to those of depressed individuals, including short REM latency and reduced delta sleep, total sleep time, and sleep efficiency. Interestingly, while making nightly "sleep checks" on hospitalized individuals, nurses are more accurate in judging sleep time in schizophrenic individuals than in depressive individuals, who often appear to be asleep when they are actually awake.

Although less well studied, the sleep of individuals with *anxiety* disorders, such as generalized anxiety disorder, panic disorder, obsessive–compulsive disorder, acute stress disorder, and PTSD, is often disturbed (Uhde 1994). *Panic* attacks, for example, may occur occasionally during sleep itself, usually at the transition between stage 2 and delta sleep. Individuals with panic disorders during sleep are also likely to experience panic attacks during wakefulness either with relaxation or after sleep deprivation.

Individuals with *obsessive–compulsive* disorder frequently endure difficulties in the initiation and maintenance of sleep. They often have elaborate compulsive rituals before going to bed, for example, concerns about "germs" may necessitate long showers and fresh, clean "sterilized" pajamas and sheets each night. Polysomnographic features are sometimes similar to those described in major depressive disorder, even though the individuals do not have symptoms that meet full diagnostic criteria for major depressive disorder.

Classic symptoms of *posttraumatic stress disorder* include nightmares, night terrors, and violent thrashing about during sleep. These individuals are easily aroused. Combat survivors with PTSD sometimes seek a physically "secure" sleeping environment in which to sleep and wake up frequently during the night to "check the perimeter." These sleep problems in Vietnam veterans who suffer from PTSD are often complicated by chronic conditioning, alcohol and substance abuse, depression, anxiety, and significant interpersonal and social problems. Total sleep time is usually reduced with variable and inconsistent disturbances of REM sleep (Dow et al. 1996). Successful treatment of the disorder and the sleep complaints has been traditionally difficult. The nightmares of PTSD appear to occur in both non-REM and REM sleep. While SSRIs are often recommended in the treatment of PTSD, some of the activating antidepressants appear to worsen subjective complaints of sleep. Nefazodone, a sedative antidepressant, slowly improved subjective sleep quality, mood, and the number of reported nightmares during a 12-week open label study (Gillin et al. 2001b). Phenelzine and other MAOIs have also been reported to improve sleep and nightmares, but the possibility of serious drug interactions, alcoholism, and poor compliance limit their usefulness.

More recently, Raskin and colleagues have reported a significant reduction in nightmares and overall improvement in combat veterans with PTSD who were treated with prazosin, an alpha-1-adrenergic receptor antagonist (Taylor and Raskin 2002).

Changes in sleep patterns may occur in individuals with eating disorders (Blois et al. 1981). Night bingeing and increased sleep after eating are commonly reported in bulimic individuals, who are also reported to eat and shop for food while sleepwalking. The individual frequently does not remember these nocturnal episodes; they often become known from family or friends who have observed the behavior or from physical evidence of shopping or eating behaviors. Individuals with anorexia are often hyperactive, needing little sleep. Given the degree of physical and psychic stress associated with eating disorders, it is surprising how limited the objective sleep disturbances associated with these disorders are.

Treatment

The sleep complaint in the individual with an apparent mental disorder deserves the same careful diagnostic and therapeutic attention that it does in any individual. Just because an individual is depressed does not mean that the complaint of insomnia or hypersomnia can be explained away as a symptom of depression. Too many individuals with depression have been found to have a BRSD; too many individuals with panic disorder to have insomnia secondary to caffeinism. Chronic sleep complaints are multidetermined and multifaceted, even in many individuals with mental disorder. Differential diagnosis remains the first obligation of the clinician before definitive treatment, which should be aimed at the underlying cause or causes.

Nonspecific treatments, such as use of sleep hygiene principles, are often helpful for both the sleep complaints and the underlying mental disorders. In particular, bipolar disorder individuals and individuals whose daily activities are poorly organized (like individuals with chronic schizophrenia and individuals with certain personality disorders) may benefit from fairly rigid sleep–wake and light–dark schedules to synchronize circadian rhythms and impose structure on their behavior. Physical exercise, meditation, relaxation methods, sleep restriction therapy, and cognitive psychotherapy may help individuals manage anxiety, rumination, and conditioned psychophysiological insomnia that often cause sleeplessness at night and fatigue during the day. Partial or total sleep deprivation may be like "paradoxical intention" therapy in the treatment of major depressive disorder or premenstrual dysphoric disorder but should probably be avoided in bipolar depression.

Medications may either help or hurt. Whether the individual should have drugs with sedating or activating properties should be considered. Timing and dose are important considerations in the context of pharmacokinetic and pharmacodynamic properties of drugs. Nighttime administration of sedating drugs may improve sleep and reduce daytime oversedation. Clinically significant drug side effects such as oversedation or activation may be more likely early in treatment than later, after tolerance has developed. On the other hand, some sedating medications, even short half-life sleeping aids, may have disinhibiting effects, even late into the next day, especially in elderly and cognitively impaired individuals. Doses of sleeping pills and other medications should usually be reduced by about half in the elderly compared with the dose for a young adult.

In general, avoid polypharmacy. Sleeping pills should be prescribed reluctantly to individuals who receive adequate doses of antidepressants. Although coadministration of a benzodiazepine may improve sleep during the first week of antidepressant therapy, a low dose of zolpidem, zaleplon, trazodone, or any other sedating antidepressant at night in addition to the antidepressant may be less likely to produce tolerance and may have additive antidepressant benefits. Antipsychotic medications should not be administered as sleeping aids unless the individual is psychotic or otherwise unresponsive to other medications.

SLEEP DISORDER DUE TO A GENERAL MEDICAL CONDITION

A sleep disorder due to a general medical condition is defined in DSM-IV-TR as a prominent disturbance in sleep severe enough to warrant independent clinical attention. Subtypes include insomnia, hypersomnia, parasomnia, and mixed types (see DSM-IV-TR diagnostic criteria on page 1163).

DSM-IV-TR Diagnostic Criteria

780.xx Sleep Disorder due to a General Medical Condition

A. A prominent disturbance in sleep that is sufficiently severe to warrant independent clinical attention.
B. There is evidence from the history, physical examination, or laboratory findings that the sleep disturbance is the direct physiological consequence of a general medical condition.
C. The disturbance is not better accounted for by another mental disorder (e.g., an Adjustment Disorder in which the stressor is a serious medical illness).
D. The disturbance does not occur exclusively during the course of a delirium.
E. The disturbance does not meet the criteria for Breathing-Related Sleep Disorder or Narcolepsy.
F. The sleep disturbance causes clinically significant distress or impairment in social, occupational, or other important areas of functioning.

Specify type:

.52 Insomnia Type: if the predominant sleep disturbance is insomnia

.54 Hypersomnia Type: if the predominant sleep disturbance is hypersomnia

.59 Parasomnia Type: if the predominant sleep disturbance is a Parasomnia

.59 Mixed Type: if more than one sleep disturbance is present and none predominates

Coding note: Include the name of the general medical condition on Axis I, for example, 780.52 Sleep Disorder Due to Chronic Obstructive Pulmonary Disease, Insomnia Type; also code the general medical condition on Axis III.

As a general rule, any disease or disorder that causes pain, discomfort, or a heightened state of arousal in the waking state is capable of disrupting or interfering with sleep. Examples of this phenomenon include pain syndromes of any sort, arthritic and other rheumatological disorders, prostatism and other causes of urinary frequency or urgency, chronic obstructive lung disease, and other pulmonary conditions. Many of these conditions increase in prevalence with advancing age, suggesting at least one reason that sleep disorders are more likely to be seen in senior populations. A few examples of sleep disorders due to general medical conditions follow.

Rheumatological Disorders

Rheumatological disorders often cause disturbances of sleep depth and continuity. The pain and discomfort associated with flares of rheumatoid arthritis lead to markedly disrupted sleep, with complaints of increased pain and stiffness the following day (Hirsch et al. 1994). Similar (although somewhat less intense) complaints are seen in association with untreated (or insufficiently treated) osteoarthritis. In both disorders, normal movements associated with shifts in position and stage in sleep may trigger awakenings from which return to sleep may be difficult or impossible. Similar problems may be seen with injuries to, or inflammation of, the back or ribs, with a report of awakening with pain associated with all shifts of position while asleep.

Fibromyalgia

Fibromyalgia is typically associated with complaints of chronic, relapsing fatigue with shallow, unrefreshing sleep and localized tenderness in different muscle groups ("trigger points") (Jennum et al. 1993). No laboratory evidence of articular, nonarticular, musculoskeletal, or metabolic disease exists. Onset usually begins in young women. Although increased amounts of alpha-wave intrusion and disruption of other sleep stages have been described in some individuals with fibromyalgia, this is not a uniform finding and is probably not important in the pathophysiological process (Saskin et al. 1986, Manu et al. 1994).

Pulmonary Conditions

Chronic obstructive pulmonary disease, asthma, cough, and other respiratory conditions are often associated with complaints of light and disturbed sleep. The basis for these complaints is physiological and transparent. In sleep, minute ventilation decreases. Variability in ventilation is also greater in REM sleep than in non-REM sleep, with decreases in hypoxic and hypercapnic ventilatory drive in REM. Thus, individuals with mild chronic obstructive pulmonary disease may report awakenings every few hours in sleep (in REM), whereas individuals with more severe lung disease may report repetitive arousals throughout the night and difficulty sustaining sleep for any protracted period. Nocturnal oximetry studies demonstrate the problem, and appropriate use of supplemental oxygen at night will diminish the severity of the complaint.

Cough is a good example of the impact of breathing disturbance on sleep. Because it is impossible to cough while asleep, the irritation of the lungs or oral mucosa that leads to cough necessitates an arousal of at least transient duration to recruit and coordinate the muscles needed to expel the rush of air that generates the cough. Chronic cough may be exacerbated in sleep. In addition, two occult causes for nocturnal coughing are nocturnal gastroesophageal reflux and occult obstructive sleep apnea. Sleep apnea may also lead to the presentation or exacerbation of asthmatic episodes in sleep. Administration of theophylline may be helpful (Mulloy and McNicholas 1993).

Congestive Heart Failure and Other Cardiac Disorders

Paroxysmal nocturnal dyspnea, orthopnea, and nocturia are classic symptoms of congestive heart failure but may be associated with or confused with sleep apnea, sleep terrors, or nocturnal panic disorder (Shepard 1992). Nocturnal angina may also lead to awakenings, with the possibility of exacerbation in REM sleep (as may be the case for some types of cardiac arrhythmias).

Gastrointestinal Conditions

Sleep disturbance is particularly associated with peptic ulcer disease and gastroesophageal reflux (Orr et al. 1983), and rectal urgency in individuals with colitis or ileitis. Individuals with a colostomy may find sleep disrupted as a consequence of short transit time through remaining gut.

Cerebral Degenerative Disorders

Sleep disturbances are common in individuals with Parkinson's disease, Huntington's chorea, advanced Alzheimer's disease, hereditary progressive dystonia, and other similar disorders.

Sleep in Elderly with Alzheimer's Disease

The sleep of older adults with Alzheimer's disease is extremely disturbed, with severely fragmented sleep, often to the extent that there is not a single hour in a 24-hour day that is spent fully awake or asleep (Jacobs et al. 1989). Individuals with mild to moderate dementia have extremely fragmented sleep at night, while those with severe dementia are extremely sleepy during both the day and night (Pat-Horenczyk et al. 1998). Sleep stages also change with dementia, with significantly lower amounts of stages 3, 4, and REM sleep, and significantly more awakenings, as well as more time spent awake during the night (Prinz et al. 1982a). This results in increased stage 1 sleep and decreased sleep efficiency (Bliwise 1994). It has also been shown that there is a high prevalence of sleep apnea in individuals with dementia, with as many as 80% having symptoms that meet the criteria for diagnosis (Ancoli-Israel et al. 1991a, 1997, Bliwise 1996). The sleep changes and disruption seen are likely due to the neuronal degeneration found in Alzheimer's disease.

Neuronal structures damaged in individuals with dementia include the basal forebrain and the reticular formation of the brain stem, the same structures implicated in sleep regulation (Prinz et al. 1982b).

The nocturnal awakenings seen in individuals with dementia are often accompanied by agitation, confusion, and wandering. These behaviors have been referred to as "sundowning" as it was believed that they typically occurred as the sun set. A recent study (Martin et al. 2000) challenged the idea of sundowning by showing that peak levels of agitation occur during various times of the day, but more often in the afternoon, rather than in the evening or night.

It has been suggested that agitation or sundowning may be a circadian rhythm disorder (Bliwise et al. 1993, Martin et al. 2000). These authors found an association between circadian rhythms of activity, agitation and light exposure, indicating that sleep disruption in demented individuals may be amenable to treatment using bright light exposure. Others have tested this theory by exposing individuals with dementia to bright light. The results have been mixed, but in general support the theory that increased light exposure, whether during the morning or evening, will improve both sleep and behavior to some extent (Satlin et al. 1992, Mishima et al. 1994, Ancoli-Israel et al. 2002).

Parkinson's Disease

Sleep difficulties are particularly common in individuals with Parkinson's disease with over half complaining of difficulty falling asleep and almost 90% complaining of difficulty staying asleep (Factor et al. 1990). Sleep recordings confirm that these individuals do in fact have a prolonged sleep latency and are awake about one-third of the night (Kales et al. 1971). The sleep disruption may be secondary to the Parkinson's disease itself or to the medication used to treat the disease. Neurochemical changes caused by the disease include reductions in serotonergic, noradrenergic, and cholinergic neurons, all of which are involved in sleep regulating mechanisms (Jellinger 1986). Dopaminergic agonists used to treat the disease affect sleep–wake patterns (Aldrich 1994). Motor activity, including tremors, muscle contractions, increased muscle tone, vocalizations, and PLMS all disrupt sleep. Respiratory disorders, most common in individuals with autonomic disturbance (Apps et al. 1985), are likely to contribute to sleep fragmentation. Finally, sleep–wake schedules are easily disrupted, either due to the medications, or to circadian rhythm abnormalities such as advanced or delayed sleep phase (Aldrich 1994). Sleep disruption often increases with the progression of the disease.

Sleep hygiene education may improve sleep in individuals with Parkinson's disease. For example, since individuals often complain of difficulty getting to the bathroom at night, having a commode available at the bedside may be extremely helpful (Shochat et al. 2001). The spouse or bed partner might consider sleeping in a different bed since the individual's disrupted sleep may impact the sleep of the bed partner. Since the bed partner is often also the caregiver, this sleep disruption may lead to early institutionalization. In addition to behavioral treatment of sleep problems, adjusting the time and dose of the dopaminergic medications used for treating Parkinson's disease may improve the problem. Low doses in the evening may prevent insomnia but may not sufficiently control nocturnal rigidity. Higher evening doses will promote sleep by minimizing nocturnal rigidity, however, this may cause sleep-onset insomnia. Withdrawal from dopamine agonists may lead to severe akinesia, which is associated with sleep disruption (Shochat et al. 2001). Some of the intermediate-acting sedative–hypnotics, such as clonazepam or temazepam, may improve the insomnia caused by nocturnal dyskinesia (Shochat et al. 2001). The shorter-acting benzodiazepines, such as zolpidem or zaleplon, are also indicated to help stabilize the sleep–wake schedule. Sedating tricyclic antidepressants such as amitriptyline may improve both sleep-onset insomnia and some daytime parkinsonian symptoms. However, since they can cause nocturnal delirium, they are contraindicated for cognitively impaired individuals.

Dopaminergic agents taken in the evening can cause sleep-onset insomnia. Chronic use of L-dopa causes vivid dreams, nightmares, and night terrors, particularly with demented individuals (Scharf et al. 1978). Therefore, for Parkinson's disease individuals with dementia suffering from nocturnal hallucinations and confusion, only very small doses of L-dopa can be used, and the sleep disruption is particularly difficult to manage.

SUBSTANCE-INDUCED SLEEP DISORDER

An important aspect of the evaluation of any individual, particularly those with sleep disorders, is the review of medications and other substances (including prescription, over-the-counter and recreational drugs, as well as alcohol, stimulants, narcotics, coffee and caffeine, and nicotine) and exposure to toxins, heavy metals, and so forth (Gillin and Drummond 2000). These substances may affect sleep and wakefulness during either ingestion or withdrawal, causing most commonly insomnia, hypersomnia, or, less frequently, parasomnia or mixed types of difficulties. On the basis of DSM-IV-TR criteria, a diagnosis of substance-induced sleep disorder may be made if the disturbance of sleep is sufficiently severe to warrant independent clinical attention and is judged to result from the direct physiological effects of a substance (see DSM-IV-TR diagnostic criteria below). Substance-induced sleep disorder cannot result from mental disorder or occur during delirium. If appropriate, the context for the development of sleep symptoms may be indicated by specifying with onset during intoxication or with onset during withdrawal.

DSM-IV-TR Diagnostic Criteria for

Substance-Induced Sleep Disorder

A. A prominent disturbance in sleep that is sufficiently severe to warrant independent clinical attention.
B. There is evidence from the history, physical examination, or laboratory findings of either (1) or (2):

    (1) the symptoms in criterion A developed during, or within a month of, substance intoxication or withdrawal
    (2) medication use is etiologically related to the sleep disturbance

C. The disturbance is not better accounted for by a sleep disorder that is not substance induced. Evidence that the symptoms are better accounted for by a sleep disorder that is not substance induced might include the following: the symptoms precede the onset of the substance use (or medication use); the symptoms persist for a substantial period of time (e.g., about a month) after the cessation of acute withdrawal or severe intoxication, or are substantially in excess of what would be expected given the type or amount of the substance used or the duration of use; or there is other evidence that suggests the existence of an independent non-substance-induced sleep disorder (e.g., a history of recurrent non-substance-related episodes).

D. The disturbance does not occur exclusively during the course of a delirium.

E. The sleep disturbance causes clinically significant distress or impairment in social, occupational, or other important areas of functioning.

Note: This diagnosis should be made instead of a diagnosis of substance intoxication or substance withdrawal only when the sleep symptoms are in excess of those usually associated with the intoxication or withdrawal syndrome, and when the symptoms are sufficiently severe to warrant independent clinical attention.

Code

[specific substance]–induced sleep disorder:
(291.8 alcohol; 292.89 amphetamine; 292.89 caffeine; 292.89 cocaine; 292.89 opioid; 292.89 sedative, hypnotic, or anxiolytic; 292.89 other [or unknown] substance)

Specify type:

Insomnia type: if the predominant sleep disturbance is insomnia

Hypersomnia type: if the predominant sleep disturbance is hypersomnia

Parasomnia type: if the predominant sleep disturbance is a parasomnia

Mixed type: if more than one sleep disturbance is present and none predominates

Specify if:

With onset during intoxication: if criteria are met for intoxication with the substance and the symptoms develop during the intoxication syndrome

With onset during withdrawal: if criteria are met for withdrawal from the substance and the symptoms develop during, or shortly after, a withdrawal syndrome

---

The recognition of substance-related sleep disturbances usually depends on active searching by the clinician, beginning with a careful history, physical examination, laboratory and toxicological testing, and information (with permission) from former health care providers or friends and relatives. Individuals may not know what prescription medications they are taking or the doses, and may forget to mention over-the-counter medications, coffee, occupational or environmental toxins, and so forth. In the case of alcohol and drugs of abuse, they may deny to themselves and others their use, or quantity, or frequency of use. Substance dependence and abuse is often associated with other psychiatric diagnoses or symptoms. When comorbidity does exist, it is important to establish, if possible, whether the sleep disturbance is primary or secondary, that is, whether the sleep disturbance is substance-induced (secondary) or whether the substance use functions as a form of "self-medication" for sleep disturbance, in which the sleep disturbance would be considered primary. Many individuals with alcoholism experience secondary depression during the first few weeks of withdrawal from alcohol and exhibit short REM latency and other sleep changes similar to those reported in primary depression (Moeller et al. 1993). This secondary depression usually remits spontaneously. Likewise, about one-third of individuals with unipolar depression and about three-fifths of individuals with bipolar disorder, manic type, have a substance use pattern that meets diagnostic criteria for alcoholism or substance abuse at some point. Prognosis and treatment may be altered in comorbid states, depending on whether the sleep disturbance is primary or secondary. In general, treatment should be aimed at the primary diagnosis after management of any acute withdrawal condition that may exist.

Alcohol

Alcohol is probably the most commonly self-administered "sleeping aid." Although it may be sedating, especially in middle-aged or elderly or sleep-deprived persons, its usefulness as a hypnotic is limited by potential disinhibiting and arousing effects, gastric irritation, falling blood-alcohol levels in the early part of the night with mild withdrawal symptoms and sleep fragmentation at the end of the night, morning headaches and hangover effects, tolerance with repeated use, and exacerbation of BRSDs such as apnea.

Virtually any type of sleep disturbance has been attributed to the effects of alcohol or alcohol withdrawal in individuals with alcohol abuse or dependence. Insomnia may occur during episodes of drinking and acute and chronic withdrawal. Complaints of insomnia and objective disruption of sleep continuity and stages 3 and 4 sleep have been reported for up to several years in some abstinent individuals. Hypersomnia may occur during heavy bouts of drinking, sometimes with peripheral compression neuropathies, or as "terminal hypersomnia" after delirium tremens. Circadian sleep disturbances may also occur during bouts of drinking, including periods of short polyphasic sleep–wake episodes. Parasomnias include sleepwalking and enuresis.

Because alcohol may temporarily improve the poor sleep of the chronic alcoholic individual, sleep disturbance may be a factor in relapse (Landolt and Gillin 2001). Treatment of the sleep disturbances of the chronic but abstinent alcoholic individual is difficult. Nonpharmacological approaches include sleep hygiene and sleep restriction, as well as attention to general nutrition, physical health, and psychosocial supports. Use of benzodiazepines or other hypnotics is not generally recommended because of cross-tolerance or deliberate or inadvertent overdose. In a preliminary report, Brower and colleagues (Karam-Hage and Brower 2000) reported that the sleep of abstinent alcoholic individuals improved when treated with gabapentin. It has been reported that increased REM percentage and short REM latency at admission to an inpatient alcohol treatment program are risk factors for relapse in primary alcoholic individuals without depression (Gillin et al. 1994).

Nicotine

Aside from medical complications, such as coughing that may interfere with sleep, smoking has been associated with both difficulty in falling asleep and getting up in the morning (Wetter and Young 1994), suggesting that nicotine may phase-delay the circadian oscillator. Furthermore, compared with nonsmokers, men who smoked reported more nightmares—women who smoked reported more daytime sleepiness. Furthermore, as blood-nicotine levels fall during the night, smokers go into relative withdrawal and start craving a cigarette. One of the best measures of nicotine dependence is how long the smoker can wait in the morning for the first smoke. Abstinence from smoking is associated with lighter and more fragmented sleep, daytime sleepiness on the Multiple Sleep Latency Test, irritability, craving, and other subjective emotional distress (Prosise et al. 1994).

Amphetamines and Cocaine
Stimulants initially prolong sleep onset and reduce REM sleep, sleep continuity, and sleep duration, but tolerance usually develops. During acute withdrawal, hypersomnia and excessive REM sleep occur for the first week or so but may be followed by a few days of insomnia (Weddington et al. 1990, Watson et al. 1992).

Caffeine
Like the stimulants, caffeine usually promotes arousal and delays sleep, but withdrawal may be associated with hypersomnia. It is probably the most commonly self-administered stimulant (Walsh et al. 1990), for example, the morning cup of coffee to "get going." Caffeine has some benefits as a mild stimulant to overcome sleepiness.

Opiates
Short-term use of opiates may increase sleep and subjective sleep quality and reduce REM sleep, especially in individuals who need an analgesic for relief of pain, but these drugs may also disrupt sleep. Tolerance usually develops with repeated administration. Withdrawal may be associated with hypersomnia or the "nods."

Sedatives, Hypnotics, and Anxiolytics
Tolerance usually develops with repeated administration of the sedating effects of barbiturates, chloral hydrate, and even benzodiazepines. This is true especially with short half-life agents, with the possible exception of zaleplon. As mentioned earlier, 1 or 2 days of withdrawal insomnia may occur after a few days of administration of short half-life benzodiazepines, such as triazolam (Gillin et al. 1989), but not with the newer nonbenzodiazepine hypnotics, such as zolpidem and zaleplon.

Potential side effects associated with sedating medications during the sleep period include falls and fractures, difficulty arousing to the telephone or the crying infant, amnesia, impairment of cognitive and motor skills, drug-induced sleepwalking, and possibly, BRSDs.

Other Substances
Many medications produce sleep disturbance, including those with central or autonomic nervous system effects, like adrenergic agonists and antagonists, dopamine agonists and antagonists, cholinergic agonists and antagonists, antihistamines, and steroids. Among the prescription drugs associated frequently with sleep disorders are the SSRIs, which have been connected with overarousal and insomnia in some individuals and, more commonly, sedation in other individuals (Beasley et al. 1991). Coadministration of trazodone at night has been shown, in a double-blind, placebo-controlled study, to be effective in managing fluoxetine-induced insomnia in depressed individuals (Nierenberg et al. 1994). Additional sleep-related disturbances occasionally associated with the SSRIs include sleepwalking, REM sleep behavior disorder, and rapid eye movements during non-REM sleep.

Comparison of DSM-IV-TR/ICD-10 Diagnostic Criteria
For primary insomnia, the ICD-10 Diagnostic Criteria for Research and the DSM-IV-TR criteria are almost identical except that ICD-10 requires a frequency of at least three times a week for at least a month, whereas DSM-IV-TR does not specify a required frequency. For primary hypersomnia, the ICD-10 Diagnostic Criteria for Research and the DSM-IV-TR criteria are almost identical except that ICD-10 also counts sleep drunkenness as a

presenting symptom. Furthermore, ICD-10 requires that the problems occur nearly every day for at least 1 month (or recurrently for shorter periods of time).

Since narcolepsy and breathing-related sleep disorder are included in Chapter VI (Diseases of the Nervous System) in ICD-10, there are no diagnostic criteria provided for these conditions.

For circadian rhythm sleep disorder, the ICD-10 Diagnostic Criteria for Research and the DSM-IV-TR criteria are almost identical except that ICD-10 specifies that the problems occur nearly every day for at least 1 month (or recurrently for shorter periods of time) (DSM-IV-TR has no specified duration). This condition is referred to in ICD-10 as "Nonorganic disorder of the sleep–wake cycle."

The ICD-10 Diagnostic Criteria for Research and the DSM-IV-TR criteria for nightmare disorder and sleepwalking disorder are essentially identical. The ICD-10 Diagnostic Criteria for Research and the DSM-IV-TR criteria sets for sleep terror disorder are almost identical except that ICD-10 explicitly limits the duration of the episode to less than 10 minutes.

References

Akerstedt T (1991) Shift work and sleep disturbances. In *Sleep and Health Risk*, Peter JH, Penzel T, Podszus T, et al. (eds). Springer-Verlag, New York, pp. 265–278.

Aldrich MS (1994) Parkinsonism. In *Principles and Practice of Sleep Medicine*, Kryger MH, Roth T, and Dement WC (eds). W. B. Saunders, Philadelphia, pp. 783–789.

Aldrich MS and Chauncey JB (1990) Are morning headaches part of obstructive sleep apnea syndrome? *Arch Intern Med* **150**, 1265–1267.

American Psychiatric Association (1994) *Diagnostic and Statistical Manual of Mental Disorders*. APA, Washington, DC.

Ancoli-Israel S (1989) Epidemiology of sleep disorders. In *Clinics in Geriatric Medicine*, Roth TR and Roehrs TA (eds). W. B. Saunders, Philadelphia, pp. 347–362.

Ancoli-Israel S and Roth T (1999) Characteristics of insomnia in the United States: I. Results of the 1991 National Sleep Foundation Survey. *Sleep* **22**, S347–S353.

Ancoli-Israel S, Klauber MR, Butters N, et al. (1991a) Dementia in institutionalized elderly: relation to sleep apnea. *Am Geriatr Soc* **39**, 258–263.

Ancoli-Israel S, Kripke DF, Klauber MR, et al. (1991b) Periodic limb movements in sleep in community-dwelling elderly. *Sleep* **14**(6), 496–500.

Ancoli-Israel S, Kripke DF, Klauber MR, et al. (1991c) Sleep disordered breathing in community-dwelling elderly. *Sleep* **14**(6), 486–495.

Ancoli-Israel S, Kripke DF, Klauber MR, et al. (1996) Morbidity, mortality, and sleep disordered breathing in community dwelling elderly. *Sleep* **19**, 277–282.

Ancoli-Israel S, Kripke DF, Mason W, et al. (1985) Sleep apnea and periodic movements in an aging sample. *J Gerontol* **40**, 419–425.

Ancoli-Israel S, Martin JL, Kripke DF, et al. (2002) Effect of light treatment on sleep and circadian rhythms in demented nursing home patients. *Am Geriatr Soc* **50**, 282–289.

Ancoli-Israel S, Parker L, Sinaee R, et al. (1989) Sleep fragmentation in patients from a nursing home. *J Gerontol* **44**, M18–M21.

Ancoli-Israel S, Poceta JS, Stepnowsky C, et al. (1997) Identification and treatment of sleep problems in the elderly. *Sleep Med Rev* **1**, 3–17.

Ancoli-Israel S, Schnierow B, Kelsoe J, et al. (2001) A pedigree of one family with delayed sleep phase syndrome. *Chronobiol Int* **18**, 831–841.

Ancoli-Israel S, Seifert AR, and Lemon M (1986) Thermal biofeedback and periodic movements in sleep: patient's subjective reports and a case study. *Biofeedback Self-Reg* **11**, 177–188.

Apps MCP, Sheaff PC, Ingram DA, et al. (1985) Respiration and sleep in Parkinson's disease. *J Neurol Neurosurg Psychiatry* **48**, 1240–1245.

Aubert G (1992) Alternative therapeutic approaches in sleep apnea syndrome. *Sleep* **15**, S69–S72.

Bakwin H (1970) Sleepwalking in twins. *Lancet* **2**, 446–447.

Beasley CM Jr., Sayler ME, Bosomworth JC, et al. (1991) High-dose fluoxetine efficacy and activating-sedating effects in agitated and retarded depression. *J Clin Psychopharmacol* **11**(3), 166–174.

Benca RM, Obermeyer WH, Thisted RA, et al. (1992) Sleep and psychiatric disorders: a meta-analysis. *Arch Gen Psychiatry* **49**, 651–668.

Berger M, Lund R, Bronisch T, et al. (1983) REM latency in neurotic and endogenous depression and the cholinergic REM induction test. *Psychiatr Res* **10**, 113–123.

Bliwise DL (1994) Sleep in dementing illness. *Annu Rev Psychiatry* **13**, 757–777.

Bliwise DL (1996) Is sleep apnea a cause of reversible dementia in old age? *J Am Geriatr Soc* **44**, 1407–1409.

Bliwise DL, Bliwise NG, Partinen M, et al. (1988) Sleep apnea and mortality in an aged cohort. *Am J Pub Health* **78**(5), 544–547.

Bliwise DL, Carroll JS, Lee KA, et al. (1993) Sleep and "sundowning" in nursing home patients with dementia. *Psychiatr Res* **48**, 277–292.

Block AJ, Dolly FR, and Slayton PC (1983) Does flurazepam ingestion affect breathing and oxygenation during sleep in patients with chronic obstructive lung disease? *Am Rev Respir Dis* **129**, 230–233.

Blois R, Monnier M, Tissot R, et al. (1981) Effect of DSIP on diurnal and nocturnal sleep in man. In *Sleep 1980*, Koella WP (ed.). S. Karger, Basel, pp. 301–303.

Bootzin RR and Nicassio PM (1978) Behavioral treatments for insomnia. In *Progress in Behavior Modification*, Hersen M, Eisler RM, and Miller PM (eds). Academic Press, New York, pp. 1–45.

Borbely AA and Ackermann P (1992) Concepts and models of sleep regulation: an overview. *J Sleep Res* **1**, 63–79.

Broughton R and Ghanem Q (1976) The impact on compound narcolepsy in the life of the patient. In *Narcolepsy, Advances in Sleep Research*, Guilleminault C, Dement W, Passant P, et al. (eds). Spectrum Publications, Hollingswood, New York, pp. 201–220.

Brown GM (1995) Melatonin in psychiatric and sleep disorders. *CNS Drugs* **3**, 209–226.

Campbell SS, Kripke DF, Gillin JC, et al. (1988) Exposure to light in healthy elderly subjects and Alzheimer's patients. *Physiol Behav* **42**, 141–144.

Carskadon MA, Harvey K, Duke P, et al. (1980) Pubertal changes in daytime sleepiness. *Sleep* **2**, 453–460.

Chesson AL Jr., Wise M, Davila D, et al. (1999) Practice parameters for the treatment of restless legs syndrome and periodic limb movement disorder. An American Academy of Sleep Medicine Report. Standards of Practice Committee of the American Academy of Sleep Medicine. *Sleep* **22**, 961–968.

Cohen RA and Albers HE (1993) Disruption of human circadian and cognitive regulation following a discreet hypothalamic lesion: a case study. *Neurology* **41**, 726–729.

Coleman R, Bliwise DL, Sajben N, et al. (1983) Epidemiology of periodic movements during sleep. In *Sleep/Wake Disorders: Natural History, Epidemiology, and Long-Term Evolution*, Guilleminault C and Lugaresi E (eds). Raven Press, New York, pp. 217–229.

Culebras A (1992) Neuroanatomic and neurologic correlates of sleep disturbances. *Neurology* **42**(Suppl. 6), 19–27.

Czeisler CA, Johnson MP, Duffy JF, et al. (1990) Exposure to bright light and darkness to treat physiologic maladaption to night work. *N Engl J Med* **322**(18), 1253–1259.

Czeisler CA, Kronauer RE, Allan JS, et al. (1989) Bright light induction of strong (type 0) resetting of the human circadian pacemaker. *Science* **244**, 1328–1332.

Daan S, Beersma DGM, and Borbely AA (1984) Timing of human sleep: recovery process gated by a circadian pacemaker. *Am J Physiol* **246**, R161–R183.

Diagnostic Classification Steering Committee, Thorpy MJ (Chair) (1990) *International Classification of Sleep Disorders: Diagnostic and Coding Manual*, Rev. American Academy of Sleep Medicine, Rochester.

Dow BM, Kelsoe JRJ, and Gillin JC (1996) Sleep and dreams in Vietnam PTSD and depression. *Biol Psychiatry* **39**, 42–50.

Duffy J and Czeisler CA (2002) Age-related change in the relationship between circadian period, circadian phase, and diurnal preference in humans. *Neurosci Lett* **318**, 117–120.

Duffy J, Zeitzer JM, Rimmer DW, et al. (2002) Peak of circadian melatonin rhythm occurs later within the sleep of older subjects. *Am J Physiol Endocrinol Metab* **282**, E297–E303.

Ebert D, Feistel H, Barocka A, et al. (1994) Increased limbic blood flow and total sleep deprivation in major depression with melancholia. *Psychiatr Res Neuroimag* **55**, 101–109.

Edgar DM, Dement WC, and Fuller CA (1993) Effect of SCN lesions on sleep in squirrel monkeys: evidence for opponent processes in sleep-wake regulation. *J Neurosci* **13**(3), 1065–1079.

Factor SA, McAlarney T, Sanchez-Ramos JR, et al. (1990) Sleep disorders and sleep effect in Parkinson's disease. *Movt Disord* **5**, 280–285.

Fairbanks DNF (1987) Snoring: an overview with historical perspectives. In *Snoring and Obstructive Sleep Apnea*, Fairbanks DNF, Fujita S, Ikematsu T, et al. (eds). Raven Press, New York, pp. 1–18.

Feinberg I (1974) Changes in sleep cycle patterns with age. *J Psychiatr Res* **10**, 283–306.

Feinberg I, Thode HC Jr., Chugani HT, et al. (1990) Gamma distribution model describes maturational curves for delta wave amplitude, cortical metabolic rate, and synoptic density. *J Theoret Biol* **142**, 149–161.

Findley LJ, Zwillich CW, Ancoli-Israel S, et al. (1985) Cheyne-Stokes breathing during sleep in patients with left ventricular heart failure. *South Med J* **78**, 11–15.

Fleury B (1992) Sleep apnea syndrome in the elderly. *Sleep* **16**(6), S39–S41.

Ford DE and Kamerow DB (1989) Epidemiologic study of sleep disturbance and psychiatric disorders: an opportunity for prevention? *JAMA* **262**, 1479–1484.

Giles DE, Jarrett RB, Roffwarg HP, et al. (1988) Reduced REM latency: a predictor of recurrence in depression. *Neuropsychopharmacology* **1**, 33–39.

Gillin JC and Byerley WF (1990) The diagnosis and management of insomnia. *N Engl J Med* **322**, 239–248.

Gillin JC and Drummond SPA (2000) Medication and substance abuse. In *Principles and Practice of Sleep Medicine*, Kryger MH, Roth T, and Dement WC (eds). W. B. Saunders, Philadelphia, pp. 1176–1195.

Gillin JC, Buchsbaum M, Wu J, et al. (2001a) Sleep deprivation as a model experimental antidepressant treatment: findings from functional brain imaging. *Depress Anxiety* **14**, 37–49.

Gillin JC, Dow BM, Thompson P, et al. (1993) Sleep in depression and other psychiatric disorders. *Clin Neurosci* **1**, 90–96.

Gillin JC, Smith TL, Irwin M, et al. (1994) Increased pressure for rapid eye movement sleep at time of hospital admission predicts relapse in nondepressed patients with primary alcoholism at 3-month follow-up. *Arch Gen Psychiatry* **51**, 189–197.

Gillin JC, Smith-Vaniz A, Schnierow B, et al. (2001b) An open-label, 12 week clinical and sleep EEG study of nefazodone in chronic combat-related posttraumatic stress disorder. *J Clin Psychiatry* **62**, 789–796.

Gillin JC, Spinweber CL, and Johnson LC (1989) Rebound insomnia: a critical review. *J Clin Psychopharmacol* **9**, 161–172.

Gillin JC, Sutton L, Ruiz C, et al. (1991) The cholinergic rapid eye movement induction test with are coline in depression. *Arch Gen Psychiatry* **48**, 264–270.

Glassman JN, Darko DF, and Gillin JC (1986) Medication-induced somnambulism in a patient with schizoaffective illness. *J Clin Psychiatry* **47**, 523–524.

Gordon N (1992) The more unusual sleep disturbances of childhood. *Brain Dev* **14**, 182–184.

Guilleminault C and Stoohs R (1990) Obstructive sleep apnea syndrome: Whom to treat and how to treat. In *Sleep and Respiration*, Issa FG, Suratt PM, and Remmers JE (eds). Wiley-Liss, New York, pp. 417–426.

Guilleminault C, Eldridge F, and Dement W (1973) Insomnia with sleep apnea: a new syndrome. *Science* **181**, 856–858.

Hartmann E (1991) *Boundaries in the Mind*. Basic Books, New York.

Hartmann E (1994) Nightmares and other dreams. In *Principles and Practice of Sleep Medicine*, Kryger M, Roth T, and Dement W (eds). W. B. Saunders, Philadelphia, pp. 407–410.

Hauri PJ (1991) *Case Studies in Insomnia*. Plenum Medical Book Publishers, New York.

Hendricks JC, Morrison AR, and Mann GL (1982) Different behaviors during paradoxical sleep without atonia depend on pontine lesion site. *Brain Res* **239**, 81–105.

Heninger W, Allen R, Earley C, et al. (1999) The treatment of restless legs syndrome and periodic limb movement disorder (Review). *Sleep* **22**, 970–999.

Hirsch M, Carlander B, Vergé M, et al. (1994) Objective and subjective sleep disturbances in patients with rheumatoid arthritis: a reappraisal. *Arthritis Rheum* **37**, 41–49.

Ho AP, Gillin JC, Buchsbaum MS, et al. (1996) Brain glucose metabolism during non-rapid eye movement sleep in major depression. A positron emission tomography study. *Arch Gen Psychiatry* **53**, 645–652.

Honda Y, Juji T, Matsuki K, et al. (1986) HLA-DR2 and Dw2 in narcolepsy and in other disorders of excessive somnolence without cataplexy. *Sleep* **9**, 133–142.

Irwin M, Smith TL, and Gillin JC (1992) Electroencephalographic sleep and natural cytotoxicity in depressed patients and control subjects. *Sleep Res* **6**, 128.

Jacobs D, Ancoli-Israel S, Parker L, et al. (1989) 24-hour sleep/wake patterns in a nursing home population. *Psychol Aging* **4**(3), 352–356.

Jellinger K (1986) Pathology of parkinsonism. In *Recent Developments in Parkinson's Disease*, Fahn S, Marsden CD, Jenner P, et al. (eds). Raven Press, New York, pp. 33–66.

Jennum P, Drewes AM, Andreasen A, et al. (1993) Sleep and other symptoms in primary fibromyalgia and in healthy controls. *J Rheumatol* **20**, 1756–1759.

Jones CR, Campbell SS, Zone SE, et al. (1999) Familial advanced sleep-phase syndrome: a short-period circadian rhythm variant in humans. *Nat Med* **5**, 1062–1065.

Kales A, Ansel RD, Markham CH, et al. (1971) Sleep in patients with Parkinson's disease and normal subjects prior to and following levodopa administration. *Clin Pharm Ther* **12**, 397–406.

Kales JD, Kales A, Soldatos CR, et al. (1980) Night terrors. *Arch Gen Psychiatry* **37**, 1413–1417.

Kamgar-Parsi B, Wehr TA, and Gillin JC (1983) Successful treatment of human non-24-hour sleep-wake syndrome. *Sleep* **6**, 257–264.

Kapas L, Obal F, and Krueger JM (1993) Humoral regulation of sleep. *Int Rev Neurobiol* **36**, 131–160.

Karam-Hage M and Brower KJ (2000) Gabapentin treatment for insomnia associated with alcohol dependence (letter). *Am J Psychiatry* **157**, 151.

Koenigsberg HW, Pollak CP, Fine J, et al. (1994) Cardiac and respiratory activity in panic disorder: effects of sleep and sleep lactate infusions. *Am J Psychiatry* **151**, 1148–1152.

Koskenvuo M, Kaprio J, Partinen M, et al. (1985) Snoring as a risk factor for hypertension and angina pectoris. *Lancet* **1**(8434), 893–896.

Kripke DF (1983) Epidemiology of sleep apnea among the aged: Is sleep apnea a fatal disorder? In *Sleep Wake Disorders: Natural History, Epidemiology, and Long-Term Evolution*, Guilleminault C and Lugaresi E (eds). Raven Press, New York, pp. 137–142.

Kripke DF, Ancoli-Israel S, Mason WJ, et al. (1990) Sleep apnea: association with deviant sleep durations and increased mortality. In *Obstructive Sleep Apnea Syndrome*, Guilleminault C and Partinen M (eds). Raven Press, New York, pp. 9–14.

Kryger MH, Roth T, and Dement WC (2000) *Principles and Practice of Sleep Medicine*. W. B. Saunders, Philadelphia.

Kupfer DJ, Frank E, McEachran AB, et al. (1990) Delta sleep ratio: a biological correlate of early recurrence in unipolar affective disorder. *Arch Gen Psychiatry* **47**, 1100–1105.

Landolt HP and Gillin JC (2001) Sleep abnormalities during abstinence in alcohol-dependent patients. Aetiology and management. *CNS Drugs* **15**, 413–425.

Landolt HP, Raimo EB, Schnierow BJ, et al. (2001) Sleep and sleep electroencephalogram in depressed patients treated with phenelzine. *Arch Gen Psychiatry* **58**, 268–276.

Lavie P, Pratt H, Scharf B, et al. (1984) Localized pontine lesion: nearly total absence of REM sleep. *Neurology* **34**, 118–120.

Lewy AJ and Sack RL (1989) The dim light melatonin onset as a marker for circadian phase position. *Chronobiol Int* **6**, 93–102.

Littner M, Johnson SF, McCall WV, et al. (2001) Practice parameters for the treatment of narcolepsy: an update for 2000. *Sleep* **24**, 451–466.

Livingston G, Blizard B, and Mann A (1993) Does sleep disturbance predict depression in elderly people? *Br J Gen Pract* **43**, 445–448.

Luchins DJ, Sherwood PM, Gillin JC, et al. (1978) Filicide during psychotropic-induced somnambulism: a case report. *Am J Psychiatry* **135**, 1404–1405.

Mahowald MW and Schenck CH (1992) Dissociated states of wakefulness and sleep. *Neurology* **42**(Suppl. 6), 44–52.

Manu P, Lane TJ, Matthews DA, et al. (1994) Alpha-delta sleep in patients with a chief complaint of chronic fatigue. *South Med J* **87**, 465–470.

Martin J, Marler M, Shochat T, et al. (2000) Circadian rhythms of agitation in institutionalized Alzheimer's disease patients. *Chronobiol Int* **17**, 405–418.

Mendelson WB, Garnett D, and Gillin JC (1981) Single case study: flurazepam-induced respiratory changes. *J Nerv Ment Dis* **169**, 261–264.

Mendlewicz J, Sevy S, and de Maertelaer V (1989) REM sleep latency and morbidity risk of affective disorders in depressive illness. *Neuropsychobiology* **22**(1), 14–17.

Mignot E, Nishino S, Hunt Sharp L, et al. (1993a) Heterozygosity at the *canarc-1* locus can confer susceptibility for narcolepsy: induction of cataplexy in heterozygous asymptomatic dogs after administration of a combination of drugs acting on monoaminergic and cholinergic systems. *J Neurosci* **13**, 1057–1064.

Mignot E, Renaud A, Nishino S, et al. (1993b) Canine cataplexy is preferentially controlled by adrenergic mechanisms: evidence using monoamine selective uptake inhibitors and release enhancers. *Psychopharmacology (Berl)* **113**, 76–82.

Mignot E, Wang C, Rattazzi C, et al. (1991) Genetic linkage of autosomal recessive canine narcolepsy with a μ immunoglobulin heavy-chain switch-like segment. *Proc Natl Acad Sci U S A* **88**, 3475–3478.

Minors DS and Waterhouse JM (1984) The use of the constant routine in unmasking the endogeneous component of human circadian rhythms. *Chronobiol Int* **1**, 205–216.

Mishima K, Okawa M, Hishikawa Y, et al. (1994) Morning bright light therapy for sleep and behavior disorders in elderly patients with dementia. *Acta Psychiatr Scand* **89**, 1–7.

Mitler MM, Hajdukovic RM, Shafor R, et al. (1987) When people die. Cause of death versus time of death. *Am J Med* **82**, 266–274.

Moeller FG, Gillin JC, Irwin M, et al. (1993) A comparison of sleep EEGs in patients with primary major depression and major depression secondary to alcoholism. *J Affect Disord* **27**, 39–42.

Montplaisir J, Denesle R, and Petit D (2000) Pramipexole in the treatment of restless legs syndrome: a follow-up study. *Eur J Neurol* **7**(Suppl.), 27–31.

Montplaisir J, Nicolas A, Denesle R, et al. (2002) Restless legs syndrome improved by pramipexole: a double-blind randomized trial. *Neurology* **52**, 938–943.

Moore-Ede MC (1986) Jet lag, shift work, and maladaption. *NIPS* **1**, 156–160.

Moore-Ede MC, Sulzman FM, and Fuller CA (1982) *The Clocks That Time Us: Physiology of the Circadian Timing System*. Harvard University Press, Cambridge.

Morin CM, Colecchi C, Stone J, et al. (1999) Behavioral and pharmacological therapies for late life insomnia. *JAMA* **281**, 991–999.

Morin CM, Culbert JP, and Schwartz SM (1994) Nonpharmacological interventions for insomnia: a meta-analysis of treatment efficacy. *Am J Psychiatry* **151**, 1172–1180.

Morin CM, Kowatch RA, Barry T, et al. (1993) Cognitive–behavior therapy for late-life insomnia. *J Consult Clin Psychol* **61**, 137–146.

Mulloy E and McNicholas WT (1993) Theophylline improves gas exchange during rest, exercise, and sleep in severe chronic obstructive pulmonary disease. *Am J Respir Crit Care Med* **148**, 1030–1036.

Nierenberg AA, Adler LA, Peselow E, et al. (1994) Trazodone for antidepressant-associated insomnia. *Am J Psychiatry* **151**, 1069–1072.

Nieto FJ, Young T, Lind B, et al. (2000) Sleep-disordered breathing, sleep apnea, and hypertension in a large community-based study. *JAMA* **283**, 1829–1836.

Olson LG and Strohl KP (1986) Pathophysiology and treatment of central sleep apnea. *Chest* **90**, 154–155.

Orr W, Lackey C, Robinson M, et al. (1983) Acid reflux and clearance in sleep in Barrett's esophagus. *Gastroenterology* **84**, 1265.

Partinen M and Palomaki H (1985) Snoring and cerebral infarction. *Lancet* **2**, 1325–1326.

Pat-Horenczyk R, Klauber MR, Shochat T, et al. (1998) Hourly profiles of sleep and wakefulness in severely versus mild-moderately demented nursing home patients. *Aging Clin Exp Res* **10**, 308–315.

Peppard P, Young T, Palta M, et al. (2000) Prospective study of the association between sleep-disordered breathing and hypertension. *N Engl J Med* **342**, 1378–1384.

Prinz PN, Peskind E, Raskind MA, et al. (1982a) Changes in sleep and waking EEG in nondemented and demented elderly. *J Am Geriatr Soc* **30**, 86–93.

Prinz PN, Vitaliano PP, Vitiello MV, et al. (1982b) Sleep, EEG, and mental function changes in senile dementia of the Alzheimer's type. *Neurobiol Aging* **3**, 361–370.

Prosise GL, Bonnet MH, Berry RB, et al. (1994) Effects of abstinence from smoking on sleep and daytime sleepiness. *Chest* **105**, 1136–1141.

Richardson GS (1990) Circadian rhythms and aging. *Biol Aging* **13**, 275–305.

Rodenstein DO (1992) Assessment of uvulopalatopharyngoplasty for the treatment of sleep apnea syndrome. *Sleep* **15**(6), S56–S62.

Roehrs T, Conway W, Wittig R, et al. (1985) Sleep–wake complaints in patients with sleep-related respiratory disturbances. *Am Rev Respir Dis* **132**, 520–523.

Rosenthal L, Roehrs TA, Hayashi H, et al. (1991) HLA DR2 in narcolepsy with sleep-onset REM periods but not cataplexy. *Biol Psychiatry* **30**, 830–836.

Rosenthal NE, Joseph-Vanderpool JR, Levendosky A, et al. (1990) Phase-shifting effects of bright morning light as treatment for delayed sleep phase syndrome. *Sleep* **13**(4), 354–361.

Roth T and Ancoli-Israel S (1999) Daytime consequences and correlates of insomnia in the United States: II. Results of the 1991 National Sleep Foundation Survey. *Sleep* (Suppl. 2), S354–S358.

Rothstein JD, Guidotti A, Tinuper P, et al. (1992) Endogenous benzodiazepine receptor ligands in idiopathic recurring stupor. *Lancet* **340**, 1002–1004.

Saskin P, Moldofsky H, and Lue FA (1986) Sleep and post-traumatic rheumatic pain modulation disorder (fibrositis syndrome). *Psychosom Med* **48**, 319–323.

Satlin A, Volicer L, Ross V, et al. (1992) Bright light treatment of behavioral and sleep disturbances in patients with Alzheimer's disease. *Am J Psychiatry* **149**, 1028–1032.

Scharf B, Moskovitz C, Lupton MD, et al. (1978) Dream phenomena induced by chronic levodopa therapy. *J Neural Transm* **43**, 143–151.

Schenk C, Bundlie S, Ettinger M, et al. (1986) Chronic behavioral disorders of human REM sleep: a new category of parasomnia. *Sleep* **9**, 293–308.

Shepard JW Jr. (1992) Hypertension, cardiac arythmias, myocardial infarction, and stroke in relation to obstructive sleep apnea. *Clin Chest Med* **13**(3), 437–458.

Shochat T, Loredo JS, and Ancoli-Israel S (2001) Sleep disorders in the elderly. *Curr Treat Opt Neurol* **3**, 19–36.

Siegel JM, Nienhuis R, Fahringer HM, et al. (1992) Activity of medial mesopontine units during cataplexy and sleep-waking states in the narcoleptic dog. *J Neurosci* **12**, 1640–1646.

Spielman AJ, Saskin P, and Thorpy MJ (1987) Treatment of chronic insomnia by restriction of time in bed. *Sleep* **10**, 45–56.

Stein MB, Chartier M, and Walker JR (1993) Sleep in nondepressed patients with panic disorder: I. Systematic assessment of subjective sleep quality and sleep disturbance. *Sleep* **16**, 724–726.

Steriade M and McCarley RW (1990) *Brainstem Control of Wakefulness and Sleep*. Plenum Press, New York.

Steriade M, Contreras D, and Amzica F (1994) Synchronized sleep oscillations and their paroxysmal developments. *Trends Neurosci* **17**, 199–208.

Taylor F and Raskind MA (2002) The alpha-1-adrenergic antagonist prazosin improves sleep and nightmares in civilian trauma posttraumatic stress disorder. *J Clin Psychopharmacol* **1**, 82–85.

Uhde TH (1994) The anxiety disorders. In *Principles and Practise of Sleep Medicine*, Kryger M, Roth T, and Dement WC (eds). W. B. Saunders, Philadelphia, pp. 871–898.

US Xyrem Multicenter Study Group (2002) A randomized, double-blind, placebo-controlled multicenter trial comparing the effects of three doses of orally administered sodium oxybate with placebo for the treatment of narcolepsy. *Sleep* **25**, 42–49.

Vermeeren A, Riedel WJ, van Boxtel MP, et al. (2002) Differential residual effects of zaleplon and zopiclone on actual driving: a comparison with a low dose of alcohol. *Sleep* **25**, 224–231.

Vignau J, Dahlitz M, Arendt J, et al. (1993) Biological rhythms and sleep disorders in man: the delayed sleep phase syndrome. In *Light and Biological Rhythms in Man*, Wettering L (ed.). Pergamon Press, Stockholm, pp. 261–271.

Waller D, Jarriel S, Erman M, et al. (1984) Recognizing and managing the adolescent with Kleine–Levin syndrome. *J Adolesc Health* **5**, 139–141.

Walsh JK, Muehlbach MJ, Humm TM, et al. (1990) Effect of caffeine on physiological sleep tendency and ability to sustain wakefulness at night. *Psychopharmacology* **101**, 271–273.

Walters AS, Aldrich MS, Allen R, et al. (1995) Toward a better definition of the restless legs syndrome. *Movt Disord* **10**, 634–642.

Walters AS, Hening WA, Kavey N, et al. (1988) A double-blind randomized crossover trial of bromocriptine and placebo in restless legs syndrome. *Ann Neurol* **24**, 455–458.

Watson R, Bakos L, Compton P, et al. (1992) Cocaine use and withdrawal: the effect on sleep and mood. *Am J Drug Alcohol Abuse* **18**, 21–28.

Weddington WW, Brown BS, Haertzen CA, et al. (1990) Changes in mood, craving, and sleep during short-term abstinence reported by male cocaine addicts. *Arch Gen Psychiatry* **47**, 861–868.

Wetter DW and Young TB (1994) The relationship between cigarette smoking and sleep disturbance. *Prev Med* **23**, 328–334.

Wu JC, Gillin JC, Buchsbaum MS, et al. (1992) Effect of sleep deprivation on brain metabolism of depressed patients. *Am J Psychiatry* **149**, 538–543.

Young T, Palta M, Dempsey J, et al. (1993) The occurrence of sleep-disordered breathing among middle-aged adults. *N Engl J Med* **328**, 1230–1235.

Impulse Control Disorders

Although dissimilar in behavioral expressions, the disorders in this chapter share the feature of impulse dyscontrol. Individuals who experience such dyscontrol are overwhelmed by the urge to commit certain acts that are often apparently illogical or harmful (McElroy et al. 1992). The outcome of each of these behaviors is often harmful, either for the afflicted individual (trichotillomania, pathological gambling) or for others (intermittent explosive disorder, pyromania, kleptomania). Trichotillomania, pyromania, and pathological gambling may involve episodes in which a sudden desire to commit the act of hair-pulling, fire-setting, or gambling is followed by rapid expression of the behavior. But in these conditions, the individual may spend considerable amounts of time fighting off the urge, trying not to carry out the impulse. The inability to resist the impulse is the common core of these disorders, rather than the rapid transduction of thought to action.

Because of the limited body of systematically collected data, the following sections largely reflect accumulated clinical experience. Therefore, the practicing psychiatrist should be particularly careful to consider the exigencies of individual subjects in applying treatment recommendations.

INTERMITTENT EXPLOSIVE DISORDER

Diagnosis

Individuals with intermittent explosive disorder have a problem with their temper (see DSM-IV-TR diagnostic criteria below). This definition highlights the centrality of impulsive aggression in intermittent explosive disorder. Impulsive aggression, however, is not specific to intermittent explosive disorder. It is a key feature of several mental disorders and nonpsychiatric conditions, and may emerge during the course of other mental disorders. Therefore, the definition of intermittent explosive disorder as formulated in the DSM-IV-TR is essentially a diagnosis of exclusion. As described in Criterion C, a diagnosis of intermittent explosive disorder is made only after other mental disorders that might account for episodes of aggressive behavior have been ruled out. The individual may describe the aggressive episodes as "spells" or "attacks." The symptoms appear within minutes to hours and, regardless of the duration of the episode, may remit almost as quickly. As in other impulse control disorders, the explosive behavior may be preceded by a sense of tension or arousal and is followed immediately by a sense of relief or release of tension.

DSM-IV-TR Diagnostic Criteria

312.34 Intermittent Explosive Disorder

A. Several discrete episodes of failure to resist aggressive impulses that result in serious assaultive acts or destruction of property.
B. The degree of aggressiveness expressed during the episodes is grossly out of proportion to any precipitating psychosocial stressors.
C. The aggressive episodes are not better accounted for by another mental disorder (e.g., antisocial personality disorder, borderline personality disorder, a psychotic disorder, a manic episode, conduct disorder, or attention-deficit/hyperactivity disorder) and are not due to the direct physiological effects of a substance (e.g., a drug of abuse, a medication) or a general medical condition (e.g., head trauma, Alzheimer's disease).

Reprinted with permission from the Diagnostic and Statistical Manual of Mental Disorders, Fourth Edition, Text Revision. Copyright 2000 American Psychiatric Association.

Episodes of violent behavior appear in several common psychiatric disorders such as antisocial personality disorder, borderline personality disorder, and substance use disorders and need to be distinguished from the violent episodes of individuals with intermittent explosive disorder, which are apparently rare. The study of Felthous and coworkers (1991) in which 15 men with rigorously diagnosed DSM-III-R intermittent explosive disorder were identified from among a group of 443 men who complained of violence, permitted some systematic observations about the "typical violent episode" as reported by individuals with intermittent explosive disorder. In the vast majority of instances, the subjects with intermittent explosive disorder identified their spouse, lover, or girlfriend or boyfriend as a provocateur of their violent episodes. Only one was provoked by a stranger. For most, the reactions occurred immediately and without a noticeable prodromal period. Only one subject stated that the outburst occurred between 1 and 24 hours after the perceived provocation. All subjects with intermittent explosive disorder denied that they intended the outburst to occur in advance. Most subjects remained well oriented during the outbursts, although two claimed to lose track of where they were. None lost control of urine or bowel function during the episode. Subjects reported various degrees of subjective feelings of behavioral dyscontrol. Only four felt that they completely lost control. Six had good recollection of the event afterward, eight had partial recollection, and one lost memory of the event afterward. Most subjects with intermittent explosive disorder attempted to help or comfort the victim afterward.

Although not explicitly stated in the DSM-IV-TR definition of intermittent explosive disorder, impulsive aggressive behavior may have many motivations that are not meant to be included within this diagnosis. Intermittent explosive disorder should not be diagnosed when the purpose of the aggression is monetary gain, vengeance, self-defense, social dominance, or expressing a political statement or when it occurs as a part of gang behavior. Typically, the aggressive behavior is ego-dystonic to individuals with intermittent explosive disorder, who feel genuinely upset, remorseful, regretful, bewildered, or embarrassed about their impulsive aggressive acts.

The physical and laboratory findings relevant to the diagnosis of intermittent explosive disorder and the differential diagnosis of impulsive aggression may be divided into two main groups: those associated with episodic impulsive aggression but not diagnostic of a particular disorder and those that suggest the diagnosis of a psychiatric or medical disorder other than intermittent explosive disorder. No laboratory or physical findings are specific for intermittent explosive disorder.

The first group of findings that are associated with impulsive aggression across a spectrum of disorders includes soft neurological signs such as subtle impairments in hand–eye coordination and minor reflex asymmetries. These signs may be elicited by a comprehensive neurological examination and simple pencil-and-paper tests such as parts A and B of the Trail Making Test. Measures of central serotonergic function such as CSF 5-HIAA levels, the fenfluramine challenge test, and positron emission tomography of prefrontal metabolism also belong to this group. Although these measures advanced our neurobiological understanding of impulsive aggression, their utility in the diagnosis of individual cases of intermittent explosive disorder and other disorders with impulsive aggression is yet to be demonstrated.

The second group of physical and laboratory findings is useful in the diagnosis of causes of impulsive aggression other than intermittent explosive disorder. The smell of alcohol in an individual's breath or a positive alcohol reading with a breathalyzer may help reveal alcohol intoxication. Blood and urine toxicology screens may reveal the use of other substances, and track marks on the forearms may suggest intravenous drug use. Partial complex seizures and focal brain lesions may be evaluated by use of the EEG and brain imaging. In cases without a grossly abnormal neurological examination, magnetic resonance imaging may be more useful than computed tomography of the head. Magnetic resonance imaging can reveal mesiotemporal scarring, which may be the only evidence for a latent seizure disorder, sometimes in the presence of a normal or inconclusive EEG. Diffuse slowing on the EEG is a nonspecific finding that is probably more common in, but not diagnostic of, individuals with impulsive aggression. Hypoglycemia, a rare cause of impulsive aggression, may be detected by blood chemistry screens.

In contrast to the more restrictive DSM-III and DSM-III-R criteria, the DSM-IV-TR definition of intermittent explosive disorder allows signs of generalized impulsivity or aggressiveness to be present between episodes. It also allows the clinician to give an additional diagnosis of intermittent explosive disorder in the presence of another disorder if the episodes are not better accounted for by the other disorder. These changes were deemed necessary because the clinical reality is that most individuals who have intermittent episodes of aggressive behavior also have some impulsivity between episodes and often present with other past or current mental disorders. There is minimal research-based data available regarding comorbidity. But the literature on the comorbidity of impulsive aggressive episodes suggests that it often occurs with three classes of disorders:

(1) Personality disorders, especially antisocial personality disorder and borderline personality disorder. By definition, antisocial personality disorder and borderline personality disorder are chronic and include impulsive aggression as an essential feature. Therefore, their diagnosis effectively excludes the diagnosis of intermittent explosive disorder.

(2) A history of substance-use disorders, especially alcohol abuse. A concurrent diagnosis of substance intoxication excludes the diagnosis of intermittent explosive disorder. However, many individuals with intermittent explosive disorder report past or family histories of substance abuse, and in particular alcohol abuse. In light of evidence linking personal and family history of alcohol abuse with impulsive aggression (Linnoila et al. 1989) and the evidence (reviewed later) linking both with low central serotonergic function, this connection may be clinically relevant. Therefore, when there is evidence suggesting that alcohol abuse may be present, a systematic evaluation of intermittent explosive disorder is warranted, and vice versa.

(3) Neurological disorders, especially severe head trauma, partial complex seizures, dementias, and inborn errors of metabolism. Intermittent explosive disorder is not diagnosed if the aggressive episodes are a direct physiological consequence of a general medical condition. Such cases would be diagnosed as personality change due to a general medical condition, delirium, or dementia. However, individuals with intermittent explosive disorder often have nonspecific findings on neurological examination, such as reflex asymmetries, mild hand–eye coordination deficits, and childhood histories of head trauma with or without loss of consciousness. Their EEGs may show nonspecific changes. Such isolated findings are compatible with the diagnosis of intermittent explosive disorder and preempt the diagnosis only when they are indicative of a definitely diagnosable general medical or neurological condition. Such "soft" neurological signs may be diagnosed by a full neurological examination and neuropsychological testing.

Some children with Tourette's disorder may be prone to rage attacks (Budman et al. 1998, 2000). The clinical manifestation of these rage attacks are similar to intermittent explosive disorder (IED) and may be more common among children with Tourette's who have comorbid mood disorders. On the basis of these observations, the rage attacks of these children may flow from an underlying dysregulation of brain function (Budman et al. 1998, 2000).

Epidemiology

Intermittent explosive disorder has been subjected to little systematic study. Episodic behavioral disorders are quite common and exist across a continuum between ictal causes (excessive neuronal discharges) and purely motivational causes (psychogenic). Temper proneness is also a relatively common clinical syndrome that is associated with a wide variety of mental disorders, and is usually found in individuals with central nervous system dysfunction, character disorders, and psychoactive substance abuse. "Pure" intermittent explosive disorder, on the other hand, as formulated in DSM-IV-TR, is probably a rare disorder.

Intermittent explosive disorder is assumed to be more common in men than in women, and men with the disorder are more likely to be encountered in forensic settings, whereas women with the disorder are more likely to be found in mental health settings. This difference in presentation may reflect the reduced severity of the aggressive acts committed by women with intermittent explosive disorder. Given the rarity of pure intermittent explosive disorder, reliable information about age at onset and course is lacking. Anecdotal case reports suggest that the disorder usually appears by the second or third decade of life and persists into middle life. It may become attenuated or remit completely as the individual ages. However, cognitive impairment caused by Alzheimer's disease and other age-related causes of dementia may result in the reappearance of impulsive aggressive behavior. The mode of onset of intermittent explosive disorder may be abrupt and without a prodromal period.

In one of the few studies of the prevalence of DSM-III-R intermittent explosive disorder among violent men, Felthous and colleagues (1991) found that of 443 subjects who complained of violence, only 15 (3.4%) met criteria for intermittent explosive disorder. The DSM-III-R definition of intermittent explosive disorder was more restrictive than the current DSM-IV-TR diagnosis because it required the absence of signs of generalized impulsivity or aggressiveness between episodes. The mean age of the 15 subjects who met these strict diagnostic criteria was 31.1 years. By design, they were all men. Most were white, with only one black and one Hispanic subject included. Seven (47%) were married, five (33%) were single, and three (20%) were divorced. Most (8, or 53%) were employed full time and 80% were employed either full time or part time. Most (10, or 67%) graduated from high school. Their estimated level of intellectual functioning ranged from intelligence quotients (IQs) of 75 to 125 with a mean of 102.5. The EEGs of 13 of the men with intermittent explosive disorder were normal; two showed excessive slowing.

Course

Little systematic study has been done on the course of intermittent explosive disorder. The onset of the disorder appears to be from late adolescence to the third decade of life, and it may be abrupt and without a prodromal period. Intermittent explosive disorder is apparently chronic and may persist well into middle life unless treated successfully. In some cases, it may decrease in severity or remit completely with old age.

Differential Diagnosis

The DSM-IV-TR diagnosis of intermittent explosive disorder is essentially a diagnosis of exclusion, and the clinician should evaluate and carefully rule out more common diagnoses that are associated with impulsive violence. The lifelong nonremitting history of impulsive aggression associated with antisocial personality disorder and borderline personality disorder, together with other features of antisocial behavior (in antisocial personality disorder) or impulsive behaviors in other spheres (in borderline personality disorder) may distinguish them from intermittent explosive disorder, in which baseline behavior and functioning are in marked contrast to the violent outbursts. Other features of borderline personality disorder such as unstable and intense interpersonal relationships, frantic efforts to avoid abandonment, and identity disturbance may also be elicited by a careful history. More than in most psychiatric diagnoses, collateral information from an independent historian may be extremely helpful. This is especially true in forensic settings. Of note, individuals with intermittent explosive disorder are usually genuinely distressed by their impulsive aggressive outbursts and may voluntarily seek psychiatric help to control them. In contrast, individuals with antisocial personality disorder do not feel true remorse for their actions and view them as a problem only insofar as they suffer their consequences, such as incarceration and fines. Although individuals with borderline personality disorder, like individuals with intermittent explosive disorder, are often distressed by their impulsive actions, the rapid development of intense and unstable transference toward the clinician during the evaluation period of individuals with borderline personality disorder may be helpful in distinguishing it from intermittent explosive disorder.

Other causes of episodic impulsive aggression are substance-use disorders, in particular alcohol abuse and intoxication. When the episodic impulsive aggression is associated only with intoxication, intermittent explosive disorder is ruled out. However, as discussed earlier, intermittent explosive disorder and alcohol abuse may be related, and the diagnosis of one should lead the clinician to search for the other.

Neurological conditions such as dementias, focal frontal lesions, partial complex seizures, and postconcussion syndrome after recent head trauma may all present as episodic impulsive aggression and need to be differentiated from intermittent explosive disorder. Other neurological causes of impulsive aggression include encephalitis, brain abscess, normal-pressure hydrocephalus, subarachnoid hemorrhage, and stroke. In these instances, the diagnosis would be personality change due to a general medical condition, aggressive type, and it may be made with a careful history and the characteristic physical and laboratory findings.

Chronic impulsivity and aggression may occur as part of disorders first diagnosed during childhood and adolescence such as conduct disorder, oppositional defiant disorder, attention-deficit/hyperactivity disorder, and mental retardation. In addition, impulsive aggression may appear during the course of a mood disorder, especially during a manic episode, which precludes the diagnosis of intermittent explosive disorder, and during the course of an agitated depressive episode. Impulsive aggression may also be an associated feature of schizophrenia, in which it may occur in response to hallucinations or delusions. Impulsive aggression may also appear in variants of obsessive–compulsive disorder (OCD), which may present with concurrent impulsive and compulsive symptoms.

A special problem in the differential diagnosis of impulsive aggression, which may arise in forensic settings, is that it may represent purposeful behavior. Purposeful behavior is distinguished from intermittent explosive disorder by the presence of motivation and gain in the aggressive act, such as monetary gain, vengeance, or social dominance. Another diagnostic problem in forensic settings is malingering, in which individuals may claim to have intermittent explosive disorder to avoid legal responsibility for their acts.

Common disorders that should be excluded before intermittent explosive disorder is diagnosed and features that may be helpful in the differential diagnosis are summarized in Table 42-1.

Table 42-1 | **Differential Diagnosis of Intermittent Explosive Disorder**

Intermittent Explosive Disorder Must Be Differentiated from Aggressive Behavior in	In Contrast to Intermittent Explosive Disorder, the Other Condition
Substance intoxication or withdrawal	Is due to the direct physiological effects of a substance
Delirium or dementia (substance induced or due to a general medical condition)	Includes characteristic symptoms (e.g., memory impairment, impaired attention)
	Requires the presence of an etiological general medical condition or substance use
Personality change due to a general medical condition, aggressive type	Requires presence of an etiological general medical condition
Conduct disorder or antisocial personality disorder	Is characterized by more general pattern of antisocial behavior
Other mental disorders (schizophrenia, manic episode, oppositional defiant disorder, borderline personality disorder)	Includes the characteristic symptoms of the other mental disorder

Source: First M and Frances A (eds) (1995) *DSM-IV Handbook of Differential Diagnosis*. American Psychiatric Press, Washington, DC, p. 200.

Etiology

Theories about the etiology of impulsive aggressive outbursts and intermittent explosive disorder have been part of psychiatry from its origins. Possession by spirits, humoral imbalances, and "moral weakness" were all suggested to play a role. Since the second half of the nineteenth century, two main lines of explanation, which are to a large extent complementary, have been developed to account for the existence of individuals with episodic impulsive aggression. One line of explanation viewed the etiology of impulsive aggression as stemming from the effects of early childhood experiences and possibly childhood trauma on the development of self-control, frustration tolerance, planning ability, and gratification delay, which are all important for self-prevention of impulsive aggressive outbursts. Early experiences with "good-enough" mothering that fosters phase-appropriate delay of gratification and the development of the potential for imitation and identification with the mother are considered important for normal development. Too much or too little frustration as well as overgratification or undergratification may impair the normal development of the ability to anticipate frustration and delay gratification (Khantzian and Mack 1983).

A second line of explanation, which has yielded numerous positive findings during the past 15 years, views impulsive aggression as the result of variations in brain mechanisms that mediate behavioral arousal and behavioral inhibition. A rapidly growing body of evidence has shown that impulsive aggression may be related to defects in the brain serotonergic system, which acts as an inhibitor of motor activity (Kavoussi et al. 1997, Staner and Mendlewicz 1998). Animal studies suggest that serotonergic neurons play a role in behavioral inhibition and thus provide an impetus to explore the role of serotonin in human impulsivity. Although the majority of the human studies involved individuals who suffered from impulsive aggression in the context of disorders other than intermittent explosive disorder, their findings may be relevant to the behavioral dimension of impulsive aggression, of which intermittent explosive disorder is a "pure" form. Siever and colleagues (1991) and Stein and colleagues (1993) have confirmed a relationship between levels of 5-hydroxyindoleacetic acid (5-HIAA) in the CSF and impulsive or aggressive behaviors. Linnoila and coworkers (1989) who divided aggressive behaviors into impulsive and nonimpulsive forms, found that reduced CSF 5-HIAA levels were correlated with impulsive aggression only. Pharmacological challenge studies of the serotonergic system have also demonstrated that low serotonergic responsiveness (as measured by the neuroendocrine response to serotonergic agonists) correlates with scores of impulsive aggression. Studies of impulsive aggression among alcoholics have further defined a probable relationship between such behaviors and diminished serotonergic function (Virkkunen et al. 1995, Virkkunen and Linnoila 1993).

The literature on serotonin and suicide, which may be viewed as an extreme form of self-directed aggression, suggests another link between serotonin and aggression. Postmortem studies found that brain stem levels of serotonin were decreased in suicide victims, and reduced imipramine binding, which is thought to be associated with reduced presynaptic serotonergic binding sites, was found in the brains of suicide completers. Furthermore, an increase in postsynaptic 5-hydroxytryptamine ($5-HT_2$) receptors was found in the brains of suicide completers, and this finding was confirmed in subsequent studies. An increase in $5-HT_2$ receptors, which are thought to be mostly postsynaptic, may reflect the brain's reaction to a decrease in functional serotonergic neurons, with consequent upregulation of postsynaptic serotonin binding sites (Stanley and Mann 1988).

Another line of neurobiological evidence links impulsive aggression with dysfunction of the prefrontal cortex. Studies of neuropsychiatric patients with localized structural brain lesions have demonstrated that some bilateral lesions in the prefrontal cortex may be specifically associated with a chronic pattern of impulsive aggressive behaviors. Neurological studies suggest that the prefrontal cortical regions associated with impulsive aggression syndromes are involved in the processing of affective information and the inhibition of motor responsiveness, both of which are impaired in individuals with impulsive aggression. Interictal episodes of aggression may occur among some individuals with epilepsy. In a quantitative MRI study of such episodes among individuals with temporal lobe epilepsy (TLE) (Woermann et al. 2000), three groups (24 TLE individuals with aggressive behavior, 24 TLE individuals without such behavior and 35 nonpatient controls) were compared. The researchers concluded that the aggressive behavior was associated with a reduction of frontal neocortical gray matter.

Further evidence linking the prefrontal cortex with the serotonergic system and impulsive aggression comes from postmortem and animal studies suggesting that the prefrontal cortex is rich in excitatory $5-HT_2$ receptors, whose number is increased in suicide victims and correlated with aggressive social behavior in primates. Lower levels of CSF 5-HIAA were found in neurological patients who suffered frontal brain injuries than in individuals with injuries in other brain regions. Furthermore, the fenfluramine challenge test, a neuroendocrine challenge to the serotonergic system, was found to increase cerebral prefrontal glucose metabolism in normal control subjects. Brain imaging studies with positron emission tomography have found selective reductions in glucose metabolism in the prefrontal and frontal cortex of individuals with impulsive aggression. The regional reductions in glucose metabolism in impulsive aggressive individuals were more significant during the continuous performance task, whose performance was impaired in neurological patients with frontal lesions and was found to increase frontal glucose metabolism in normal subjects (Raine et al. 1994).

Thus, biological studies implicate the serotonergic system and the prefrontal cortex in the pathogenesis of impulsive aggression. The diagnosis of intermittent explosive disorder is sometimes considered in forensic settings; the biological correlates of impulsive aggression focus attention on, but do not solve, the complicated problem of personal responsibility for impulsive violent acts that are correlated with objective biological findings.

Data from a study of visual-evoked potentials and EEGs in a large group of children and adolescents who demonstrated aggressive behavior also suggest that such behavior may be associated with altered innate characteristics of central nervous system function (Bars et al. 2001).

Treatment

Given the rarity of pure intermittent explosive disorder, it is not surprising that few systematic data are available on its response to treatment and that some of the recommended treatment approaches to intermittent explosive disorder are based on treatment studies of impulsivity and aggression in the setting of other mental disorders and general medical conditions. Thus, no standard regimen for the treatment of intermittent explosive disorder can be recommended at this time. Both psychological and somatic therapies have been utilized in the treatment of intermittent explosive disorder. A prerequisite for both modalities is the willingness of the individual to acknowledge some responsibility for the behavior and participate in attempts to control it.

Psychosocial Treatments

Lion (1992) has described the major psychotherapeutic task of teaching individuals with intermittent explosive disorder how to recognize their own feeling states and especially the affective state of rage. Lack of awareness of their own mounting anger is presumed to lead to the buildup of intolerable rage that is then discharged suddenly and inappropriately in a temper outburst. Individuals with intermittent explosive disorder are therefore taught how to first recognize and then verbalize their anger appropriately. In addition, during the course of insight-oriented psychotherapy, they are encouraged to identify and express the fantasies surrounding their rage. Group psychotherapy for temper-prone individuals has also been described. The cognitive–behavioral model of psychological treatment may be usefully applied to problems with anger and rage management.

Somatic Treatments

Several classes of medications have been used to treat intermittent explosive disorder. The same medications have also been used to treat impulsive aggression in the context of other disorders. These included beta-blockers (propranolol and metoprolol), anticonvulsants (carbamazepine and valproic acid), lithium, antidepressants (tricyclic antidepressants and serotonin reuptake inhibitors), and antianxiety agents (lorazepam, alprazolam, and buspirone). Mattes (1990) compared the effectiveness of two commonly used agents, carbamazepine and propranolol, for the treatment of rage outbursts in a heterogeneous group of individuals. He found that although carbamazepine and propranolol were overall equally effective, carbamazepine was more effective in individuals with intermittent explosive disorder and propranolol was more effective in individuals with attention-deficit/hyperactivity disorder. A substantial body of evidence supports the use of propranolol—often in high doses—for impulsive aggression in individuals with chronic psychotic disorders and mental retardation. Lithium has been shown to have antiaggressive properties and may be used to control temper outbursts. In individuals with comorbid major depressive disorder, OCD, or cluster B and C personality disorders, SSRIs may be useful. Overall, in the absence of more controlled clinical trials, the best approach may be to tailor the psychopharmacological agent to coexisting psychiatric comorbidity. In the absence of comorbid disorders, carbamazepine, titrated to antiepileptic blood levels, may be used empirically.

KLEPTOMANIA

Diagnosis

Kleptomania shares with all other impulse control disorders the recurrent failure to resist impulses (see DSM-IV-TR diagnostic criteria below). Unfortunately, in the absence of epidemiological studies, little is known about kleptomania. Clinical case series and case reports are limited. Family, neurobiological, and genetic investigations are not available. There are no established treatments of choice. Therefore, in reading this section, the reader must keep in mind that much of what is described is based on limited data or on anecdotal information.

DSM-IV-TR Diagnostic Criteria

312.32 Kleptomania

A. Recurrent failure to resist impulses to steal objects that are not needed for personal use or for their monetary value.
B. Increasing sense of tension immediately before committing the theft.
C. Pleasure, gratification, or relief at the time of committing the theft.
D. The stealing is not committed to express anger or vengeance and is not in response to a delusion or a hallucination.

E. The stealing is not better accounted for by conduct disorder, a manic episode, or antisocial personality disorder.

At presentation, the typical individual suffering from kleptomania is a 35-year-old woman who has been stealing for about 15 years and may not mention kleptomania as the presenting complaint or in the initial history (Goldman 1991, McElroy et al. 1991a). The individual may complain instead of anxiety, depression, lability, dysphoria, or manifestations of character pathology. There is often a history of a tumultuous childhood and poor parenting, and in addition, acute stressors may be present, such as marital or sexual conflicts. The individual experiences the urge to steal as irresistible, and the thefts are commonly associated with a thrill, a high, a sense of relief, or gratification. Generally, the behavior has been hard to control and has often gone undetected by others. Kleptomania may be restricted to specific settings or types of objects, and the individual may or may not be able to describe rationales for these preferences. Quite often, the objects taken are of inherently little financial value, or have meaningless financial value relative to the income of the person who has taken the object. Additionally, the object may never actually be used. These factors often help distinguish theft from kleptomania. The theft is followed by feelings of guilt or shame and, sometimes, attempts at atonement. The frequency of stealing episodes may greatly fluctuate in concordance with the degree of depression, anxiety, or stress. There may be periods of complete abstinence. The individual may have a past history of psychiatric treatments including hospitalizations or of arrests and convictions, whose impact on future kleptomanic behavior can vary.

Although the typical subject may be a 35-year-old woman, it is important to remember that men, children, and elderly persons may present with or engage in kleptomania. Interestingly, Goldman's review (1991) suggested that men may first present for evaluation 15 years later than women. Kleptomania occurs transculturally and has been described in various Western and Eastern cultures. Asian observers have also noted an overlap with eating disorders (Lee 1994). Atypical presentations should raise a greater suspicion of an organic etiology, and a medical evaluation is then indicated. Medical conditions that have been associated with kleptomania include cortical atrophy, dementia, intracranial mass lesions, encephalitis, normal-pressure hydrocephalus, benzodiazepine withdrawal, and temporal lobe epilepsy. A complete evaluation when such suspicions are present includes a physical and neurological examination, general serum chemistry and hematological panels, and an EEG with temporal leads or computed tomography of the brain (Chiswick 1976, Khan and Martin 1977, Mendez 1988, Wood and Garralda 1990, Coid 1984, McIntyre 1990).

Among individuals with kleptomania who present for treatment, there is a high incidence of comorbid mood, anxiety, and eating disorders, when compared to rates in the general population. In reviewing 26 case reports of kleptomania, Goldman (1991) reported mention of histories of depression in 13 individuals (50%), anxiety in 8 individuals (31%), and bulimia nervosa in 3 individuals (12%). Similar percentages are noted by McElroy and colleagues (1991b) in the review of 56 individuals with probable kleptomania: 57% with mood disorder symptoms, 34% with anxiety disorder symptoms, and 11% with bulimic symptoms. Comorbidity patterns among individuals who present for treatment may be greater than among random samples. More reliable comorbidity rates can be found in a prospective investigation of 20 individuals with kleptomania conducted by McElroy and coworkers (1991a). Lifetime DSM-III-R comorbidity rates were 40% major depressive disorder, 50% substance abuse, 40% panic disorder, 40% social phobia, 45% OCD,

30% anorexia nervosa, 60% bulimia nervosa, and 40% other impulse control disorders. Dissociative symptoms, significant character pathology, and trauma histories are commonly encountered among this group (Goldman 1991, McElroy et al. 1991b). Unfortunately, Axis I dissociative pathology and Axis II pathology have not yet been systematically investigated in these individuals.

Epidemiology

No epidemiological studies of kleptomania have been conducted, and thus its prevalence can be calculated only grossly and indirectly. In a thorough review of the existing literature, Goldman (1991) found that in a series of shoplifters, the estimate of kleptomania ranged from 0 to 24%. The frequency of kleptomania may be indirectly extrapolated from incidence rates of kleptomania in comorbid disorders with known prevalence, such as bulimia nervosa. Such speculations suggest at least a 0.6% prevalence of kleptomania in the general population (Goldman 1991). However, given that people who shoplift are often not caught, this is almost certainly an underestimate. Its presence may be further obscured because the behavior is often shameful and, consequently, treatment may not be sought. In addition, studies examining comorbidity of other disorders may neglect to inquire about kleptomania.

Despite the lack of valid epidemiological data, there is general agreement that kleptomania is more common among women than among men. In a retrospective review of 56 cases that appeared to fulfill DSM-III-R criteria for kleptomania, McElroy and colleagues (1991b) found that 77% were women. Similarly, in a prospective series of 20 individuals with DSM-III-R kleptomania, 75% were women (McElroy 1991a). However, women generally seek treatment more frequently than men, whereas men are more likely to become involved with the penal system. Consequently, this may not reflect true gender distribution.

Course

In two separate studies, the mean age at onset of kleptomania was reported to be 20 years (Goldman 1991, McElroy et al. 1991a). The subjects included individuals who had begun stealing as early as 5 to 7 years of age. The disorder appears to be chronic, lasting for decades, albeit with varying intensity. Fifteen or 16 years may elapse before treatment is sought (Goldman 1991, McElroy et al. 1991a). Onset in and beyond the fifth decade of life appears to be unusual, and in some of these cases, remote histories of past kleptomania can be elicited (Goldman 1991). At peak frequency, McElroy and colleagues (1991a) found a mean of 27 episodes a month, essentially daily stealing, with one individual reporting four acts daily. The majority of individuals may eventually be apprehended for stealing once or more, and a minority may even be imprisoned; more often than not these repercussions do not result in more than a temporary remission of the behavior. Individuals with kleptomania may also have extensive histories of mental health treatments, including hospitalization for other conditions, most commonly depression or eating disorders. Because of the unavailability of longitudinal studies, the prognosis is not known. It appears, however, that without treatment, the behavior may be likely to persist for decades, sometimes with significant associated morbidity. There may be transient periods of remission.

Differential Diagnosis

Generally, the diagnosis of kleptomania is not a complicated one to make. However, kleptomania may frequently go undetected because the individual may not mention it spontaneously and the clinician may fail to inquire about it as part of the routine history. The index of suspicion should rise in the presence of commonly associated symptoms such as chronic depression, other impulsive or compulsive behaviors, tumultuous backgrounds, or unexplained legal troubles. It could convincingly be argued that a cursory review of compulsivity and impulsivity, citing multiple examples for the individual, should be a part of any thorough and complete mental health evaluation. In addition, it is important to do a careful differential diagnosis and pay attention to the various exclusion criteria before diagnosing theft as kleptomania. Possible diagnoses of sociopathy, mania, or psychosis should be carefully considered. In this regard, the clinician must inquire about the affective state of the individual during the episodes, the presence of delusions or hallucinations associated with the occurrence of the behavior, the motivation behind the stealing, and the fate and subsequent use of the objects.

Etiology

The etiology of kleptomania is essentially unknown, although various models have been proposed in an effort to conceptualize the disorder. At present, the available empirical data are insufficient to substantiate any of these models.

With the exception of scant information on family history, data regarding possible familial or genetic transmission of a kleptomania diathesis are unavailable. One study found the risk for major mood disorders in first-degree relatives of probands with kleptomania to be 0.31—similar to the familial risk for probands with major depressive disorder (McElroy et al. 1991a). In the same study, 7% of first-degree relatives of individuals with kleptomania had histories of OCD. These findings, combined with other lines of evidence, might suggest that kleptomania shares a common biological diathesis with mood disorders or OCD.

The affective spectrum model suggests that kleptomania and other impulse control disorders may share a common underlying biological diathesis with other disorders, such as depression, panic disorder, OCD, and bulimia nervosa (McElroy et al. 1992, 1991b, Hudson and Pope 1990). The apparent high comorbidity of kleptomania with depression and bulimia nervosa has already been noted. As early as 1911, Janet (1911) recognized the alleviation of depressive symptoms on the commission of kleptomanic acts. In some individuals, kleptomania responds to treatment with thymoleptic agents or electroconvulsive therapy. These observations are cited as support for an affective spectrum model.

Although the affective spectrum has been claimed to encompass obsessive–compulsive pathology (Hudson and Pope 1990), there exists a more specific model conceptualizing kleptomania and other impulse disorders as obsessive–compulsive spectrum disorders (McElroy et al. 1993). Several lines of evidence support this model. First, there are phenomenological similarities between the classical obsessions and compulsions of OCD and the irresistible impulses and repetitive actions characteristic of kleptomania. In addition, there appears to be a greater than chance occurrence of OCD in probands with kleptomania and in their relatives. In addition, both conditions have significant comorbidity with mood, anxiety, substance use, and eating disorders. However, OCD rituals are more clearly associated with relief of anxiety and harm avoidance, whereas kleptomanic acts seem to be associated with gratification or pleasure. In addition, OCD is associated with a clear preferential response to SSRIs as opposed to general thymoleptics. The limited treatment literature does not support a similar response pattern in kleptomania. Unfortunately, the role of the serotonergic or of any other neurotransmitter system has not been investigated in kleptomania. Interestingly, a large study found subjects with mixed anorexia and bulimia nervosa to have a higher lifetime prevalence of kleptomania than those with either anorexia or bulimia nervosa alone (Herzog et al. 1992). This could suggest a relationship between kleptomania and both the obsessive–compulsive (anorexic) and affective (bulimic) spectrum.

Alternatively, kleptomania could be conceptualized as an addictive disorder. The irresistible impulse to steal is reminiscent of the urge and the high associated with drinking or using drugs (McElroy et al. 1992). Marks (1990) has proposed a constellation of behavioral (i.e., nonchemical) addictions encompassing OCD, compulsive spending, gambling, binging, hypersexuality, and kleptomania. This model postulates certain concepts thought to be common in all these disorders, such as craving, mounting tension, "quick fixing," withdrawal, external cuing, and habituation. These components have not yet been well investigated in kleptomania.

It should be emphasized that the lack of neurobiological or prospective pharmacological treatment data for kleptomania limits any conclusions that can be drawn with regard to biological models.

In addition to the foregoing theories, numerous psychological formulations of kleptomania have been postulated over the years. A frequent theme, reported by numerous authors and reviewed by Goldman (1991) and McElroy and coworkers (1991b) is that of kleptomania as an acting out aimed at alleviating depressive symptoms. Fishbain (1987) has carefully described the case of a woman whose kleptomanic episodes were closely related to depressive bouts and who experienced an apparent antidepressant effect from the thrill and excitement of her risk-taking behavior.

From a psychodynamic point of view, kleptomania has been viewed over the decades as a manifestation of a variety of unconscious conflicts, with sexual conflicts figuring prominently in the literature. Case reports have described conscious sexual gratification, sometimes accompanied by frank masturbation or orgasm during kleptomanic acts (Fishbain 1987, Fenichel 1945). Thus, it has been suggested, kleptomanic behavior serves to discharge a sexual drive that may have forbidden connotations similar to those of masturbation, and the stolen object itself may have unconscious symbolic or overt fetishistic significance. Although no systematic studies exist, there has long been an implication in the literature on kleptomania that those afflicted with kleptomania suffer disproportionately from a variety of sexual dysfunctions. Turnbull (1987) described six individuals with a primary diagnosis of kleptomania, all of whom had dysfunctional sexual relationships with their partners, compulsive promiscuity, or anorgasmia.

Other cases of kleptomania have been understood as reflecting conflictual infantile needs and attempts at oral gratification, masochistic wishes to be caught and punished related to a harsh guilt-inducing superego or primitive aggressive strivings, penis envy or castration anxiety with the stolen object representing a penis, a defense against unwelcome passive homosexual longings, restitution of the self in the presence of narcissistic injuries, or the acquisition of transitional objects (Beldoch 1991). These various formulations are presented in more detail in Goldman's review (1991). One should probably conclude that the psychodynamics associated with kleptomania ought to be carefully tailored to the individual subject. The literature on kleptomania has frequently implicated disturbed childhoods, inadequate parenting, and significant character disturbances in kleptomanic individuals. From this perspective, kleptomania can be more effectively understood in the context of an individual's overall character. Unfortunately, no clinical studies exist that systematically explore Axis II psychopathology in these individuals.

Treatment

The general goal of treatment is the eradication of kleptomanic behavior. Treatment typically occurs in the outpatient setting, unless comorbid conditions such as severe depression, eating disturbances, or more dangerous impulsive behaviors dictate hospitalization. In the initial contact with the clinician, as described earlier, it is important that the appropriate differential diagnoses be considered. The interview must be conducted in a respectful climate that ensures confidentiality. Individuals not only may experience considerable guilt or shame for stealing but also may be unrevealing because of the fear of legal repercussions. In the acute treatment phase, the aim is to decrease significantly or, ideally, eradicate episodes of stealing during a period of weeks to months. Concurrent conditions may compound the problem and require independently targeted treatment.

The acute treatment of kleptomania has not been, to date, systematically investigated. Recommendations are based on retrospective reviews, case reports, and small case series. Maintenance treatment for kleptomania has not been investigated either, and only anecdotal data exist for individuals who have been followed up for significant periods after initial remission.

As with any condition that may be associated with intense guilt or shame, kleptomania must be approached respectfully by the clinician. Individuals can be reassured, and their negative feelings alleviated to some degree with proper initial psychoeducation. The treatment alliance can be strengthened by consistently maintaining a nonjudgmental and supportive stance. In addition, individuals' fears regarding breaks of confidentiality and criminal repercussions must be addressed.

No treatments have been systematically shown to be effective for kleptomania. These treatment recommendations are supported by case reports and retrospective reviews only. In general, it appears that thymoleptic medications and behavioral therapy may be the most efficacious treatments for the short term, whereas long-term psychodynamic psychotherapy may be indicated and have good results for selected individuals.

Somatic Treatments

Mixed results have been reported regarding the pharmacological treatment of kleptomania. In a literature review of 56 cases of kleptomania, McElroy and coworkers (1991b) noted that somatic treatments were described for eight individuals. Significant improvement was reported for seven of these. Treatment included antidepressants alone, antidepressants combined with antipsychotics or stimulants, electroconvulsive therapy alone, or electroconvulsive therapy with antidepressants. The medications most commonly used to treat kleptomania are the antidepressants. In a series of 20 individuals fulfilling DSM-III-R criteria for kleptomania, McElroy and colleagues (1991a) found that 18 had received antidepressants and of those 56 individuals, 10 had partial or complete remission of both kleptomanic urges and behavior. It has been suspected that kleptomania may respond selectively to SSRIs because of the anticompulsive and antiimpulsive properties of these compounds. Of these 18 individuals, 10 were administered fluoxetine alone and only 2 had a full response and 1 had a partial response. These data are not suggestive of a high response rate to SSRIs, but dose and duration of treatment were not explicitly stated. In a report on three individuals with concurrent DSM-III-R kleptomania and bulimia nervosa treated with serotonergic antidepressants, two received high-dose fluoxetine and one trazodone; all three showed significant improvement in kleptomania, independent of the course of bulimia nervosa and depression (McElroy et al. 1989). It is still unclear whether kleptomania responds preferentially to serotonergic antidepressants, and this question awaits further study. Other agents reported to have treated kleptomania successfully include nortriptyline (McElroy et al. 1991b) and amitriptyline (Fishbain 1987). In addition, it remains unclear if the antikleptomanic effect of thymoleptics is dependent on or independent of their antidepressant effect.

A number of other medications have been employed to treat kleptomania. These include antipsychotics (McElroy et al. 1991b, Fishbain 1987), stimulants (McElroy et al. 1991b), valproic acid (McElroy et al. 1991a), carbamazepine (McElroy et al. 1991a), clonazepam (McElroy et al. 1991a), and lithium (McElroy et al. 1991a, Monopolis and Lion 1983). Lithium augmentation may be of benefit when kleptomania does not respond to an antidepressant alone (Burstein 1992). Finally, there have been some reports of successful treatment of kleptomania with electroconvulsive therapy, which may have been administered for a concurrent mood disorder (McElroy et al. 1991b).

Although little is known about maintenance pharmacological treatment for kleptomania, there is a suggestion in the literature that symptoms tend to recur with cessation of thymoleptic treatment and again remit when treatment is reinstituted (McElroy et al. 1991a, Fishbain 1987).

Psychosocial Treatments

Formal studies of psychosocial interventions for kleptomania have not been performed. However, a number of clinical reports have supported behavioral therapy for kleptomania. The available clinical literature suggests that for most individuals, this may be a more efficacious approach than insight-oriented psychotherapy. Different behavioral techniques have been employed with some success, including aversive conditioning (Guidry 1969, Keutzer 1972), systematic desensitization (Marzagao 1972), covert sensitization (Gauthier and Pellerin 1982, Glover 1985), and behavior modification (Fishbain 1987, Wetzel 1966). In their review of 56 reported cases of kleptomania, McElroy and colleagues (1991a) noted that the eight individuals who were treated with behavioral therapy—mostly aversive conditioning—showed significant improvement. We give here some specific examples of behavioral techniques that have been successfully employed and described. One individual was taught to hold her breath as a negative reinforcer whenever she experienced an impulse to steal (Keutzer 1972). Another individual was taught to use systematic desensitization techniques to control the mounting anxiety associated with the impulse to steal (Marzagao 1972). An individual treated by covert sensitization learned to associate images of nausea and vomiting with the desire to steal (Glover 1985). A woman who experienced sexual excitement associated with shoplifting and would masturbate at the site of the act was instructed to practice masturbation at home, while fantasizing kleptomanic acts (Fishbain 1987). There is a suggestion in the literature that these techniques remain effective over the long term (Gauthier and Pellerin 1982, Glover 1985).

Finally, it appears that the most effective behavioral treatment of all may be complete abstinence, that is, the individual should no longer visit any of the stores or settings where kleptomanic acts occur. A number of individuals who never come to psychiatric attention apparently employ this technique successfully, and it may be an appropriate treatment goal if it does not result in excessive restrictions of activity and lifestyle.

The psychodynamic treatment of kleptomania centers on the exploration and working through of the underlying conflict or conflicts. In a review of 26 case reports, McElroy and associates (1991b) reported that four of five individuals had a good response to psychoanalysis or related therapy. However, in another review of 20 cases (meeting DSM-III-R criteria) McElroy and coworkers (1991a) reported that of 11 individuals treated with psychotherapy, none showed improvement. There are case reports in the literature of successful psychodynamic treatment of kleptomania (Schwartz 1992). Such treatment, possibly in combination with other approaches, may be indicated for individuals for whom a clear conflictual basis for the behavior can be formulated, who also have the needed insight and motivation to undertake this type of treatment. In proposing such treatments, which may be long term, the clinician should consider whether there are immediate risks that must be addressed, such as a high risk of legal consequences.

PYROMANIA AND FIRE-SETTING BEHAVIOR

Diagnosis

The primary characteristics of pyromania are recurrent, deliberate fire-setting, the experience of tension or affective arousal before the fire-setting, an attraction or fascination with fire and its contexts, and a feeling of gratification or relief associated with the setting of a fire or its aftermath (see DSM-IV-TR diagnostic criteria on page 1191).

DSM-IV-TR Diagnostic Criteria

312.33 Pyromania

A. Deliberate and purposeful fire-setting on more than one occasion.
B. Tension or affective arousal before the act.
C. Fascination with, interest in, curiosity about, or attraction to fire and its situational contexts (e.g., paraphernalia, uses, consequences).
D. Pleasure, gratification, or relief when setting fires, or when witnessing or participating in their aftermath.
E. The fire-setting is not done for monetary gain, as an expression of sociopathic ideology, to conceal criminal activity, to express anger or vengeance, to improve one's living circumstances, in response to a delusion or hallucination, or as a result of impaired judgment (e.g., in dementia, mental retardation, substance intoxication).
F. The fire-setting is not better accounted for by conduct disorder, a manic episode, or antisocial personality disorder

True pyromania is present in only a small subset of fire setters. Multiple motivations are cited as causes for fire-setting behavior. These include arson for profit, crime concealment, revenge, vandalism, and political expression. In addition, fire-setting may be associated with other psychiatric diagnoses. Fire-setting behavior may be a focus of clinical attention, even when criteria for pyromania are not present. Because the large majority of fire-setting events are not associated with true pyromania, this section also addresses fire-setting behavior in general.

Prins and colleagues (1985) have suggested the following motivations for intentional arson: financial reward, to conceal another crime, for political purposes, as a means of revenge, as a symptom of other (nonpyromania) psychiatric conditions (e.g., in response to a delusional belief), as attention-seeking behavior, as a means of deriving sexual satisfaction, and as an act of curiosity when committed by children. Revenge and anger appear to be the most common motivations for fire-setting (O'Sullivan and Kelleher 1987).

The diagnosis of pyromania emphasizes the affective arousal, thrill, or tension preceding the act, as well as the feeling of tension relief or pleasure in witnessing the outcome. This is useful in distinguishing between pyromania and fire-setting elicited by other motives (i.e., financial gain, concealment of other crimes, political, arson related to other mental illness, revenge, attention seeking, erotic pleasure, part of conduct disorder).

The onset of pyromania has been reported to occur as early as age 3 years, but the condition may initially present in adulthood. Because of the legal implications of fire-setting, individuals may not admit previous events, which may result in biased perceptions of the common age at onset. Men greatly outnumber women with the disorder.

In children and adolescents, the most common elements are excitation caused by fires, enjoyment produced by fires, relief of frustration by fire-setting, and expression of anger through fire-setting (Brandford and Dimock 1986).

Fire-setting behavior may be common among more impaired psychiatric individuals. In a study of 191 nongeriatric individuals in a psychiatric hospital who were admitted for other reasons, 26 had some form of fire-setting behavior (including threats). Of these, 70% had actually set fires. None had a diagnosis of true pyromania (Soltys 1992).

Epidemiology

No data are available on the prevalence or incidence of pyromania, but it is apparently uncommon. Although pyromania is a rare event, fire-setting behavior is common in the histories of psychiatric patients. Geller and Bertsch (1985) found that 26 of 191 nongeriatric state hospital individuals had histories of some form of fire-setting behavior. Unlike pyromania, which is rare among women, fire-setting behavior was common in the histories of female individuals (22%) as well as male individuals (28.8%).

Among children with mental disorders, fire-setting behavior is apparently quite common. Kolko and Kazdin (1988) found that among a sample of children attending an outpatient psychiatry clinic, approximately 20 had histories of fire-setting. For a sample of inpatient children, the rate was approximately 35% (Kolko and Kazdin 1988).

Course

There are no data regarding the course of and prognosis for pyromania. However, the impulsive nature of the disorder suggests a repetitive pattern. Again, because legal consequences may occur, the individual may be motivated to represent the index episode as a unique event. Fire-setting for nonpsychiatric reasons may be more likely to be a single event.

Differential Diagnosis

Other causes of fire-setting must be ruled out. Fire-setting behavior may be motivated by circumstances unrelated to mental disorders. Such motivations include profit, crime concealment, revenge, vandalism, and political statement or action (Geller 1987, Lowenstein 1989). Furthermore, fire-setting may be a part of ritual, cultural, or religious practices in some cultures.

Fire-setting may occur in the presence of other mental disorders. A diagnosis of fire-setting is not made when the behavior occurs as a part of conduct disorder, antisocial personality disorder, or a manic episode or if it occurs in response to a delusion or hallucination. The diagnosis is also not given if the individual suffers from impaired judgment associated with mental retardation, dementia, or substance intoxication.

Etiology

Because pyromania is rare, there is little reliable scientific literature available regarding individuals who fit the diagnostic criteria. But because of the morbid impact that arson has on society, fire-setting behavior (which often does not fulfill criteria for pyromania) has been the focus of scientific investigation and literature.

Arson has been the subject of several investigations of altered neuroamine function. These findings include the observation that platelet monoamine oxidase is negatively correlated with fire-setting behavior of adults who had been diagnosed with attention-deficit disorder in childhood (Kuperman et al. 1988).

Investigation of the function of serotonergic neurotransmission in individuals with aggressive and violent behaviors has included studies of CSF concentrations of 5-HIAA in individuals with a history of fire-setting. 5-HIAA is the primary metabolite of serotonin, and its concentration in the CSF is a valid marker of serotonin function in the brain. Virkkunnen and colleagues (1987, 1994) demonstrated that impulsive fire-setting was associated with low CSF concentrations of 5-HIAA. This finding was consistent with other observations associating impulsive behaviors with low CSF 5-HIAA levels (such as impulsive violence and impulsive suicidal behavior). A history of suicide attempt strongly predicts recidivism of arson (DeJong et al. 1992).

Treatment

Because of the danger inherent in fire-setting behavior, the primary goal is elimination of the behavior. The treatment literature does not distinguish between pyromania and fire-setting behavior of other causes.

Much of the literature is focused on controlling fire-setting behavior in children and adolescents.

Pharmacotherapy

There are no reports of pharmacological treatment of pyromania. Because fire-setting may be frequently embedded in the context of other mental disorders, therapeutic attention may be directed primarily to the underlying disorder. However, the dangerous nature of fire-setting requires that the behavior be controlled. Much in the same fashion that one would seek to educate impaired individuals about the functional risks associated with their symptoms—and to establish boundaries of acceptable behavior—the fire-setting behavior must be directly addressed, even if it is not a core symptom of the associated disorder.

Psychosocial Treatments

It has been estimated that up to 60% of childhood fire-setting is motivated by curiosity. Such behavior often responds to direct educational efforts. In children and adolescents, focus on interpersonal problems in the family and clarification of events preceding the behavior may help control the behavior (Lowenstein 1989). The treatments described for fire-setting are largely behavioral or focused on intervening in family or intrapersonal stresses that may precipitate the episode of fire-setting.

One technique combines overcorrection, satiation, and negative practice with corrective consequences. The child is supervised in constructing a controlled, small fire in a safe location. The fire is then extinguished by the child. Throughout the process, the parent verbally instructs the child in safety techniques.

The graphing technique has been used as the basis of several intervention programs with fire setters. The clinician and the individual agree on a goal of stopping the fire-setting behavior. The clinician and the individual construct a graph that details the events, feelings, and behaviors associated with fire-setting episodes. These factors are described on a chronological line graph. The graph is utilized to help the individual see the cause-and-effect relationships between personal events, feelings, and subsequent behaviors. The specific intent is to educate individuals so that they are able to identify the events that put them at risk for fire-setting. Then the individuals are equipped to label the feelings as a signal that may allow them to use alternative modes for discharging their feelings. This technique may help the individual curtail other maladaptive behaviors as well. Follow-up reports suggest that individuals who have successfully completed a graphing intervention may be at substantially lower risk for future fire-setting.

Relaxation training may be used (or added to graphing techniques) to assist in the development of alternative modes of dealing with the stress that may precede fire-setting.

Principles of cognitive–behavioral therapy have been recently applied to childhood fire-setting (Kolko 2001).

PATHOLOGICAL GAMBLING

Diagnosis

Gambling as a behavior is common. Current estimates suggest that approximately 80% of the adult population in the United States gamble. The amount of money wagered legally in the United States grew from $17 billion in 1974 to $210 billion in 1988, an increase of more than

1200%, making gambling the fastest-growing industry in America (Lesieur and Rosenthal 1991). DSM-IV-TR, like DSM-III-R before it, covertly recognized the ubiquity of gambling behavior and the desire to gamble by the careful wording of Criterion A for pathological gambling: "Persistent and recurrent maladaptive gambling behavior as indicated by five (or more) of the following." This definition of pathological gambling differs from some other definitions of impulse control disorders not elsewhere classified, which are worded as "Failure to resist an impulse to." This difference implies that neither gambling behavior nor failure to resist an impulse to engage in it is viewed as pathological in and of itself. Rather, the maladaptive nature of the gambling behavior is the essential feature of pathological gambling and defines it as a disorder (see DSM-IV-TR diagnostic criteria below).

DSM-IV-TR Diagnostic Criteria

312.31 Pathological Gambling

A. Persistent and recurrent maladaptive gambling behavior as indicated by five (or more) of the following:

   (1) is preoccupied with gambling (e.g., preoccupied with reliving past gambling experiences, handicapping or planning the next venture, or thinking of ways to get money with which to gamble)

   (2) needs to gamble with increasing amounts of money in order to achieve the desired excitement

   (3) has repeated unsuccessful efforts to control, cut back, or stop gambling

   (4) is restless or irritable when attempting to cut down or stop gambling

   (5) gambles as a way of escaping from problems or of relieving a dysphoric mood (e.g., feelings of helplessness, guilt, anxiety, depression)

   (6) after losing money gambling, often returns another day to get even ("chasing" one's losses)

   (7) lies to family members, therapist, or others to conceal the extent of involvement with gambling

   (8) has committed illegal acts such as forgery, fraud, theft, or embezzlement to finance gambling

   (9) has jeopardized or lost a significant relationship, job, or educational or career opportunity because of gambling

   (10) relies on others to provide money to relieve a desperate financial situation caused by gambling

B. The gambling behavior is not better accounted for by a manic episode.

It is not difficult to diagnose pathological gambling once one has the facts. It is much more of a challenge to elicit the facts, because the vast majority of individuals with pathological gambling view their gambling behavior and gambling impulses as ego syntonic, and may often lie about the extent of their gambling (Criterion A7). Individuals with pathological gambling may first seek medical or psychological attention because of comorbid disorders.

Given the high prevalence of addictive disorders in pathological gambling and the increased prevalence of pathological gambling in those with alcoholism and other substance abuse, an investigation of gambling patterns and their consequences is warranted for any individual who presents with a substance abuse problem. Likewise, the high rates of comorbidity with mood disorders suggest the utility of investigating gambling patterns of individuals presenting with an affective episode.

The spouses and the significant others of individuals with pathological gambling deserve special attention. Individuals with pathological gambling usually feel entitled to their behavior and often rely on their families to bail them out (Criterion A10). As a consequence, it is often the spouse of the individual with pathological gambling who first realizes the need for treatment and who bears the consequences of the disorder. Lorenz (1981) conducted a survey of 103 wives of pathological gamblers who attended Gam-Anon meetings (for family members of individuals with pathological gambling). She found that most spouses had to borrow money and were harassed or threatened by bill collectors. Most spouses physically assaulted the gambler, verbally abused their children, and experienced murderous or destructive impulses toward the gambler. Although the gamblers themselves appeared less violent than the general population norms, their spouses were more violent, possibly because of desperation and anger. Eleven percent of the spouses of individuals with pathological gambling admitted to having attempted suicide, and this result was replicated in a later study. These findings have two main implications for the assessment of pathological gambling: first, the spouse may be a valuable and motivated informant who should be questioned about the individual's behavior, and second, spouses should be specifically asked about the effects of the individual's illness on their own well-being and functioning and about suicidal ideation and attempts and the control of their own impulsivity.

An important and understudied area is the clinical presentation of pathological gambling in women. Women constitute a third of all individuals with pathological gambling in epidemiological studies. However, they are extremely underrepresented in treatment populations, and most psychoanalytic theories of pathological gambling ignore them completely. Part of this bias may be due to the fact that gambling carries a greater social stigma for women, that women gamblers are more likely to live and to gamble alone, and that treatment programs for pathological gambling in the United States were first pioneered in Veterans Hospitals. Compared to men with pathological gambling, women with pathological gambling are more likely to be depressed and to gamble as an escape rather than because of a craving for action and excitement. Pathological gambling begins at a later age in female than in male gamblers, often after adult roles have been established. Big winning is usually less important than the need to impress. Women typically play less competitive forms of gambling in which luck is more important than skill, and they play alone. Their progression into the disorder is often more rapid, and the time between the onset of the disorder and the time they present for treatment is usually much shorter than for men (3 years compared to 20 years). The shorter duration makes for a better prognosis in treatment, but, unfortunately, few of the women with pathological gambling ever come to treatment.

The choice of gambling activities is dictated by local availability and cultural norms. Horseracing, cockfights, roulette, slot machines, casino card games, state-sponsored lotteries, and the stock market may all be used by the pathological gambler. Likewise, the extent of gambling considered normal varies across cultures. DSM-IV-TR approaches this issue by concentrating on the consequences of gambling rather than on its frequency and type.

Overall, individuals with pathological gambling have high rates of comorbidity with several other psychiatric disorders and conditions. Individuals presenting for clinical treatment of pathological gambling apparently have impressive rates of comorbidity. Ibanez and coworkers (2001) reported 62.3% of one group seeking treatment had a comorbid psychiatric disorder. The most frequent diagnosis they found were personality disorders (42%), alcohol abuse or dependence (33.3%), and adjustment disorders (17.4%).

There is also evidence for extensive comorbidity of pathological gambling with major depressive disorder and with bipolar disorder. In several surveys, between 70 and 80% of all individuals with pathological gambling also had mood symptoms that met criteria for a major depressive episode, a manic episode, or a hypomanic episode at some point in their life. More than 50% had recurrent major depressive episodes (Lesieur and Rosenthal 1991). A complicating factor is that recovering pathological gamblers may experience depressive episodes after cessation of gambling. In addition, some individuals with pathological gambling may gamble to relieve feelings of depression (Criterion A5). Despite Criterion B for pathological gambling, which essentially precludes the diagnosis of pathological gambling if the behavior occurs exclusively during the course of a manic episode, many individuals have a disturbance that meets criteria for both disorders because they gamble both during and between manic and hypomanic episodes. Between 32 and 46% of individuals with pathological gambling were reported to also have mood symptoms that meet criteria for bipolar disorder, bipolar II disorder, or cyclothymic disorder (McElroy et al. 1992).

Although data is not yet conclusive, a meaningful association between problem gambling and suicidal behavior and/or ideation appears to exist. Phillips and coworkers (1997) conclude that "Las Vegas, the premier US gambling setting, displays the highest levels of suicide in the nation, both for residents of Las Vegas and for visitors to that setting. In general, visitors to and residents of major gaming communities experience significantly elevated suicide levels. In Atlantic City, abnormally high suicide levels for visitors and residents appeared only after gambling casinos were opened. The findings do not seem to result merely because gaming settings attract suicidal individuals." In other reports, between 12 and 24% of individuals with pathological gambling in various settings have had a history of at least one suicide attempt. In one study, 80% of individuals with pathological gambling had a history of either suicide attempts or suicidal ideation (Lesieur and Rosenthal 1991).

Epidemiology

Pathological gambling is considered to be the most common of the impulse control disorders not elsewhere classified. The number of people whose gambling behavior meets criteria for pathological gambling in the United States is estimated to be between 2 and 6 million (Volberg 1988). The prevalence of pathological gambling in several communities in the United States has been assessed. Surveys conducted between 1986 and 1990 in Maryland, Massachusetts, New York, New Jersey, and California estimated the prevalence of "probable pathological gamblers" among the adult population to be between 1.2 and 2.3%. These states have a broad range of legal wagering opportunities and a heterogeneous population. Similar surveys in Minnesota and Iowa, states with limited legal wagering opportunities and more homogeneous populations, yielded prevalence rates of 0.9 and 0.1%, respectively (Rosenthal 1992). It thus appears that availability of gambling opportunities as well as demographic makeup may influence the prevalence of pathological gambling. A 1998 study of national prevalence, using DSM-IV criteria, determined that the prevalence of pathological gambling was 1.2% (1.7% for men and 0.8% for women). In addition to these individuals who fulfilled DSM-IV criteria, the researchers classified an additional 1.5% as "problem gamblers." The combined total of "pathological gamblers" and "problem gamblers" is 5.5 million adult Americans (Gerstein et al. 1999). During the past 20 years, many states have turned to lotteries as a way of increasing their revenues without increasing taxes. At this time, some form of gambling is legal in 47 of the 50 states as well as in more than 90 countries worldwide. From 1975 to 1999, revenues from legal gambling in the United States has risen from $3 to 58 billion (Volberg 2002). (Given the dramatic increase in the amounts of money wagered in legal gambling activities during the past 20 years, the prevalence and incidence of pathological gambling are expected to increase.)

It is estimated that women make up to one-third of all Americans with pathological gambling. Nevertheless, they are underrepresented in Gamblers Anonymous, in which only 2 to 4% of the members are women. This pattern is echoed in England and Australia, where women make up 7 and 10% of Gamblers Anonymous members respectively. The reason for this discrepancy was postulated to be the greater social stigma attached to pathological gambling in women and the characteristic pattern of solitary gambling in women. Nonwhites and those with less than a high school education are more highly represented among pathological gamblers than in the general population. The demographic makeup of individuals in treatment for pathological gambling differs substantially from the demographics of all individuals with pathological gambling. Jewish persons are overrepresented in treatment settings and in Gamblers Anonymous, whereas women, minorities, and those younger than age 30 years are underrepresented in Gamblers Anonymous and in treatment (Lesieur and Rosenthal 1991).

Course

Pathological gambling usually begins in adolescence in men and later in life in women. The onset is usually insidious, although some individuals may be "hooked" by their first bet. There may be years of social gambling with minimal or no impairment followed by an abrupt onset of pathological gambling that may be precipitated by greater exposure to gambling or by a psychosocial stressor. The gambling pattern may be regular or episodic, and the course of the disorder tends to be chronic. Over time, there is usually a progression in the frequency of gambling, the amounts wagered, and the preoccupation with gambling and with obtaining money with which to gamble. The urge to gamble and gambling activity generally increase during periods of stress or depression, as an attempted escape or relief (Criterion A5). Rosenthal (1992) described four typical phases in the course of a typical male individual with pathological gambling: winning, losing, desperation, and hopelessness (Linnoila et al. 1989).

There are four typical phases in the course of pathological gambling.

Winning Many male gamblers become involved with gambling because they are good at it and receive recognition for their early successes. Women with pathological gambling are less likely to have a winning phase. Traits that foster a winning phase and are typical of male individuals with pathological gambling are competitiveness, high energy, ability with numbers, and interest in the strategy of games. The early winnings lead to a state in which a large proportion of the gambler's self-esteem derives from gambling, with accompanying fantasies of winning and spectacular success.

Losing A string of bad luck or a feeling that losing is intolerable may be the precipitant of chasing behavior; previous gambling strategies are abandoned as the gambler attempts to win back everything all at once. The gambler experiences a state of urgency, and bets become more frequent and heavy. Debts accumulate, and only the most essential are paid. Covering up and lying about gambling become more frequent. As this is discovered, relationships with family members deteriorate. Losing gamblers use their own and their family's money, go through savings, take out loans, and finally exhaust all legitimate sources. Eventually, they cannot borrow any more, and faced with threats from creditors or loss of a job or marriage, they go to their family and finally confess. This results in the "bailout": debts are paid in return for a promise to stop or cut down gambling. Any remission, if achieved at all, is short-lived. After the bailout there is an upsurge of omnipotence; the gambler believes that it is possible to get away with anything, bets more heavily, and loses control altogether.

Desperation   This stage is reached when the gambler begins to do things that would previously be inconceivable: writing bad checks, stealing from an employer, or other illegal activities. Done once, these behaviors are much more likely to be repeated. The behavior is rationalized as a short-term loan with an intention to pay it back as soon as the winning streak arrives. The gambler feels just one step away from winning and solving all the problems. Attention is increasingly taken up with illegal loans and various scams to make money. The gambler becomes irritable and quick tempered. When reminded of responsibilities or put in touch with guilt feelings, the gambler responds with anger and projective blame. Appetite and sleep deteriorate and life holds little pleasure. A common fantasy at this stage is of starting life over with a new name and identity, the ultimate "clean slate."

Hopelessness   For some gamblers, there is a fourth stage in which they suddenly realize that they can never get even, but they no longer care. This is often a revelation, and the precise moment when it occurred is often remembered. From this point on, just playing is all that matters. Gamblers often acknowledge knowing in advance that they will lose and play sloppily so that they lose even if they have the right horse or a winning hand. They seek action or excitement for its own sake and gamble to the point of exhaustion.

Few gamblers seek help in the winning phase. Most seek help only during the later phases and only after a friend, family member, or employer has intervened. Two-thirds of the gamblers have committed illegal activities by then, and the risk of suicide increases as the gambler progresses through the phases of the illness.

Without treatment, the prognosis of pathological gambling is poor. It tends to run a chronic course with increasing morbidity and comorbidity, gradual disruption of family and work roles and relationships, depletion of financial reserves, entanglement with criminals and the criminal justice system, and, often, suicide attempts. In the hands of an experienced psychiatrist, it is an "extremely treatable disorder" with a favorable prognosis (Rosenthal 1992). The difference between a poor and a good prognosis depends on treatment, and treatment depends on a diagnosis. As noted earlier, the diagnosis of pathological gambling is often missed in clinical settings because mental health professionals do not think to ask about it. Because most individuals with pathological gambling do not see themselves as having a disorder and many of them do not even consider themselves as having a problem with gambling, collateral information from a family member may be extremely helpful.

Differential Diagnosis

The differential diagnosis of pathological gambling is relatively straightforward (Table 42-2). Pathological gambling should be differentiated from professional gambling, social gambling, and a manic episode. Social gambling, engaged in by the vast majority of adult Americans, typically occurs with friends or colleagues, lasts for a specified time, and is limited by predetermined acceptable losses. Professional gambling is practiced by highly skilled and disciplined individuals, and involves carefully limited risks. Many individuals with pathological gambling may feel that they are actually professional gamblers. Chasing behavior and unplanned losses distinguish the pathological gamblers. Individuals in a manic episode may exhibit a loss of judgment and excessive gambling resulting in financial disasters. A diagnosis of pathological gambling should be given only if a history of maladaptive gambling behavior exists at times other than during a manic episode. Problems with gambling may also occur in individuals with antisocial personality disorder. If criteria are met for both disorders, both can be diagnosed.

Etiology

Pathological gambling has been included in DSM-III, DSM-III-R, DSM-IV, and DSM-IV-TR as a disorder of impulse control. Pathological gambling can also be viewed as an

Table 42-2	Differential Diagnosis of Pathological Gambling
Pathological Gambling Must Be Differentiated From	**In Contrast to Pathological Gambling, the Other Condition**
Professional gambling	Is characterized by discipline and limited risk taking
	Is intended to be a source of income
Social gambling	Usually occurs among friends
	Is characterized by limited time spent on gambling and limited risk taking
Manic episode	Involves episodes of characteristic symptoms (e.g., flight of ideas)
	Is characterized by symptoms that persist at times when individual is not gambling

Source: First M and Frances A (eds) (1995) *DSM-IV Handbook of Differential Diagnosis*. American Psychiatric Press, Washington, DC, pp. 196–197.

addictive disorder (Murray 1993), an affective spectrum disorder (McElroy et al. 1992), and an obsessive–compulsive spectrum disorder (Hollander et al. 1992) DSM-IV-TR maintains a close relationship between pathological gambling and addictive disorders in that several of the diagnostic criteria for pathological gambling were intentionally made to resemble criteria for substance dependence (Table 42-3).

The parallels between pathological gambling and addictive disorders are manifold. Pathological gambling has been viewed as the "pure" addiction, because it involves several aspects of addictive behavior without the use of a chemical substance. The parallels between substance dependence, in particular alcohol dependence, and pathological gambling have led to the successful adoption of the self-help group model of Alcoholics Anonymous to Gamblers Anonymous. Patterns of comorbidity also suggest a possible link between pathological gambling and addictions, in particular alcoholism. In addition to the comorbidity of pathological gambling and substance use disorders, family studies have demonstrated a familial clustering of alcoholism and pathological gambling. Ramirez and colleagues (1983) found that 50% of individuals with pathological gambling had a parent with alcoholism; other studies have also found high rates of a family history of substance dependence in individuals with pathological gambling. There is also a greater prevalence of pathological gambling in parents of individuals with pathological gambling.

The links between pathological gambling and affective disorders are also supported by family studies that demonstrate high rates of affective disorders in first-degree relatives of individuals with pathological gambling (McElroy et al. 1992), as well as by high rates of comorbidity of pathological gambling and affective disorders. In addition, as noted by many authors and incorporated in the DSM-IV-TR criteria for pathological gambling, many individuals with pathological gambling gamble as a way of relieving dysphoric moods (criterion A5), and cessation of gambling may be associated with depressive episodes in the majority of recovering gamblers (Linden 1986).

The links between pathological gambling and obsessive spectrum disorders are less clear. Although a popular name for pathological gambling is compulsive gambling, the vast majority of individuals with pathological gambling do not experience the urge to gamble as ego-dystonic until late in the course of their illness, after they have suffered some of its consequences. The rates of comorbidity of pathological gambling and OCD and obsessive–compulsive personality disorder are not nearly as high as the rates of comorbidity of pathological gambling and affective and addictive disorders. Nevertheless, pathological gambling shares several characteristics with compulsions: it is repetitive, often has ritualized aspects, and is meant to relieve or reduce distress. Moreover, sporadic reports on the

Table 42-3	Comparison of DSM-IV-TR Criteria for Pathological Gambling and Substance Dependence
Pathological Gambling	**Substance Dependence**
A. Persistent and recurrent maladaptive gambling behavior as indicated by at least five (or more) of the following:	A maladaptive pattern of substance use, leading to clinically significant impairment or distress, as manifested by three (or more) of the following:
A1. Is preoccupied with gambling (e.g., preoccupied with reliving past gambling experiences, handicapping or planning the next venture, or thinking of ways to get money with which to gamble)	5. A great deal of time is spent in activities necessary to obtain the substance or recover from its effects
A2. Needs to gamble with increasing amounts of money to achieve the desired excitement	1. (tolerance) (a). A need for markedly increased amounts of the substance to achieve intoxication or desired effect or (b). markedly diminished effect with continued use of the same amount of substance
A3. Has repeated unsuccessful efforts to control, cut back, or stop gambling	4. There is a persistent desire or unsuccessful attempts to cut down or control substance use
A4. Is restless or irritable when attempting to cut down or stop gambling	2. (withdrawal) (a). The characteristic withdrawal syndrome for the substance
A5. Gambles as a way of escaping from problems or relieving a dysphoric mood	
A6. After losing money gambling, often returns another day to get even ("chasing" one's losses)	2. (withdrawal) (b). The same substance is taken to relieve or avoid withdrawal symptoms
	3. The substance is often taken in larger amounts or over a longer period than was intended
A7. Lies to family members, therapist, or others to conceal the extent of involvement with gambling	
A8. Has committed illegal activities such as forgery, fraud, theft, or embezzlement to finance gambling	
A9. Has jeopardized or lost a significant relationship, job, or educational opportunity because of gambling	6. Important social, occupational, or recreational activities are given up or reduced because of substance use
A10. Relies on others to provide money to relieve a desperate financial situation caused by gambling	
B. The gambling behavior is not better accounted for by a manic episode	
	7. The substance use is continued despite knowledge of having a persistent or recurrent physical or psychological problem that is likely to have been caused or exacerbated by the substance

Source: Adapted from American Psychiatric Association (2000) *Diagnostic and Statistical Manual of Mental Disorders*, 4th ed., Text Rev. APA, Washington, DC.

effectiveness of SSRIs in the treatment of pathological gambling suggest a possible link to obsessive spectrum disorders (Hollander et al. 1992).

The association between altered function of the serotonin neurotransmitter system and impulsive behaviors has focused attention on a potential role for serotonin function in the neurophysiology of pathological gambling. Several studies have provided data supporting such a link. These findings include blunted prolactin response after intravenous administration of the serotonin reuptake inhibitor, clomipramine (Moreno et al. 1991), increased prolactin response after the administration of a serotonin agonist, m-CPP (DeCaria et al. 1996), low platelet MAO-B activity (a correlate central nervous system concentrations of the serotonin metabolite 5-HIAA) (Blanco et al. 1996, Carrasco et al. 1994). However, direct measure of cerebrospinal fluid 5-HIAA in pathological gamblers has yielded mixed results (Roy et al. 1988, Bergh et al. 1997, Ibanez et al. 2002). Preliminary data supports potential utility of serotonin reuptake inhibitor medications in the treatment of pathological gambling (Hollander et al. 1998, 2000, Ibanez et al. 2002). A potential role for noradrenergic function has been explored as well. In preliminary support for such a role, pathological gamblers have been shown to have higher urinary and cerebrospinal fluid concentrations of noradrenaline and metabolites (Roy et al. 1988, Bergh et al. 1997). In addition, increased growth hormone secretion, a measure of noradrenergic reactivity, has been found in response to oral administration of clonidine, an alpha-2-adrenergic agonist (Ibanez et al. 2002).

Because of the "addictive" aspects of pathological gambling—and the role that dopaminergic function plays in chemical addictions—attention has been directed at dopamine function among pathological gamblers. Two available studies have yielded contradictory data (Roy et al. 1988, Bergh et al. 1997).

The incidence of pathological gambling among first-degree family members of pathological gamblers appears to be approximately 20% (Ibanez et al. 2002). Inherited factors may explain 62% of variance in the diagnosis (Eisen et al. 1998) and some of these genetic factors may also contribute to the risk for conduct disorder, antisocial personality disorder, and alcohol abuse (Eisen et al. 2001). At this time, early molecular genetics studies of pathological gamblers point to possible associated polymorphisms in genes that code for both serotonergic and dopaminergic factors (Ibanez et al. 2002).

Psychoanalytic theories of gambling were the first systematic attempts to account for pathological gambling. Erotization of the fear, tension, and aggression involved in gambling behavior, as well as themes of grandiosity and exhibitionism, were explored by several authors during the first quarter of the twentieth century. Freud (1961) in his influential essay on Dostoevsky suggested that the pathological gambler actually gambled to lose, not to win, and traced the roots of the disorder to the ambivalence felt by the young man toward his father. The father, the object of his love, is not only loved but also hated, and this results in unconscious guilt. The gambler then loses to punish himself, in what Freud labeled "moral masochism." Freud also spoke of "feminine masochism" in which losing is a way of gaining love from the father, who will somehow reward the loser for loyalty. To lose is to suffer, and for the feminine masochist, suffering equals love. Interestingly, in the later spirit of DSM-IV-TR, Freud also conceptualized pathological gambling as an addiction and included it in a triad with alcoholism and drug dependence. He saw all three as manifestations of that primary addiction, masturbation, or at least masturbatory fantasies. Like most researchers after him, Freud focused only on male gamblers.

Bergler, a psychoanalyst who actually treated many individuals with pathological gambling, expanded on Freud's idea that the pathological gambler gambles to lose (Lesieur and Rosenthal 1991). He traced the roots of this desire to lose to the rebellion of gamblers against the authority of their parents and against the parents' intrusive introduction of the reality principle into their lives. The rebellion causes guilt, and the guilt creates the need for self-punishment. Bergler thought that the gambler's characteristic aggression is actually pseudoaggression, a craving for defeat and rejection. He saw the gambler as one who perpetuates an adversarial relationship with the world. The dealer in the casino, the gambler's opponents at the card table, the stock exchange, and the roulette wheel are all unconsciously identified with the refusing mother or the rejecting father. Overall, psychoanalytic approaches to pathological gambling (Lesieur and Rosenthal 1991) generally conceptualized it as either a compulsive neurosis (Freud, Bergler, Rosenthal) or an impulse disorder (Fenichel). Fenichel focused on the gambler's entitlement and intense need to "get the stuff," an oral fixation. Several published case reports documented the successful treatment of pathological gambling by psychoanalysis.

Learning theories of pathological gambling focus on the learned and conditioned aspects of gambling and use the quantifiable nature of the behavior to test specific hypotheses. One hypothesis was that individuals with pathological gambling crave the excitement and tension associated with their gambling, as evidenced by the fact that they are much more likely to place last-second wagers than are low-frequency gamblers, to prolong their excitement. Higher wagers placed by individuals with pathological gambling also produce greater excitement, and greater amounts of money are required to achieve the same "buzz" over time, an observation incorporated in the diagnostic criteria for pathological gambling (Criterion A2).

Treatment

The goals of treatment of an individual with pathological gambling are the achievement of abstinence from gambling, rehabilitation of the damaged family and work roles and relationships, treatment of comorbid disorders, and relapse prevention. This approach echoes the goals of treatment of an individual with substance dependence. There are many similarities and several important differences between the treatment of pathological gambling and the treatment of substance dependence. For most individuals without severe acute psychiatric comorbidity, such as major depressive disorder with suicidal ideation or alcohol dependence with a history of delirium tremens, treatment may be given on an outpatient basis. Inpatient treatment in specialized programs may be considered if the gambler is unable to stop gambling, lacks significant family or peer support, or is suicidal, acutely depressed, multiply addicted, or contemplating some dangerous activity.

No standard treatment of pathological gambling has emerged. Despite many reports of behavioral and cognitive interventions for pathological gambling, there are minimal data available from well-designed or clearly detailed treatment studies (Petry 2002). Pharmacologic treatments (described further below) offer promise, but research-guided approaches are still insufficient to offer a standardized approach. Therefore, general approaches, based in clinical experience and available resources (such as Gamblers Anonymous or other support groups) should be considered.

The treatment of pathological gambling may consist of participation in Gamblers Anonymous, individual therapy, family therapy, treatment of comorbid disorders, and medication treatment. As is the case for substance dependence, the gambler needs to be abstinent to be accessible to any or all of these treatment modalities. For many gamblers, participation in Gamblers Anonymous is sufficient, and it is an essential part of most treatment plans. Gamblers Anonymous is a 12-step group built on the same principles as Alcoholics Anonymous. It utilizes empathic confrontation by peers who struggle with the same impulses and a group approach. Gam-Anon is a peer support group for family members of individuals with pathological gambling. Extensive data are lacking, but overall, Gamblers Anonymous appears somewhat less effective than Alcoholics Anonymous in achieving and maintaining abstinence.

Individual therapy is often useful as an adjunct to Gamblers Anonymous. Rosenthal (1992) stressed that to maintain abstinence and use Gamblers Anonymous successfully, many gamblers need to understand why they gamble. Therapy involves confronting and teasing out the vicissitudes of the individual's sense of omnipotence and dealing with the various self-deceptions, the defensive aspects of the individual's lying, boundary issues, and problems involving magical thinking and reality. Relapse prevention involves knowledge and avoidance of specific triggers. In addition to psychodynamic therapy, behavioral treatment of pathological gambling has been proposed, with imagined desensitization achieving better rates of remission than aversive conditioning.

The greatest differences between the treatment of pathological gambling and other addictions are in the area of family therapy. Because relapse may be difficult to detect (there is no substance to be smelled on the individual's breath, no dilated or constricted pupils, no slurred speech or staggered gait) and because of a long history of exploitative behavior by the individual, the spouse and the other family members tend to be more suspicious of, and angry at, the individual with pathological gambling compared with families of alcoholic individuals. Frequent family sessions are often essential to offer the gambler an opportunity to make amends, learn communication skills, and deal with preexisting intimacy problems. In addition, the spouse and other family members have often acquired their own psychiatric illnesses during the course of the individual's pathological gambling and need individualized treatment to recover.

Although research reports of the pharmacological treatment of pathological gambling have begun to emerge, there are still as yet insufficient data to come to any conclusions about the utility of medication. The effectiveness of selective serotonin reuptake inhibitors has been examined in a limited number of double-blind trials, but do show promise. The opiate antagonist, naltrexone, has also shown preliminary evidence of efficacy. Doses at the higher end of the usual treatment range should be considered with both these classes of agents. The use of mood stabilizers (lithium and carbamazepine) has been the subject of a limited number of reports. At this time, no clear guidelines for pharmacologic treatment have emerged (Grant and Kim 2002, Haller and Hinterhuber 1994, Hollander et al. 2000, Kim and Grant 2001, Kim et al. 2001).

TRICHOTILLOMANIA

Diagnosis

The essential feature of trichotillomania is the recurrent failure to resist impulses to pull out one's own hair. Resulting hair loss may range in severity from mild (hair loss may be negligible) to severe (complete baldness and involving multiple sites on the scalp or body) (see DSM-IV-TR diagnostic criteria below). Individuals with this condition do not want to engage in the behavior, but attempts to resist the urge result in great tension. Thus, hair-pulling is motivated by a desire to reduce this dysphoric state. In some cases, the hair-pulling results in a pleasurable sensation, in addition to the relief of tension. Tension may precede the act or may occur when attempting to stop. Distress over the symptom and the resultant hair loss may be severe.

DSM-IV-TR Diagnostic Criteria

312.39 Trichotillomania

A. Recurrent pulling out of one's hair resulting in noticeable hair loss.
B. An increasing sense of tension immediately before pulling out the hair or when attempting to resist the behavior.
C. Pleasure, gratification, or relief when pulling out the hair.
D. The disturbance is not better accounted for by another mental disorder and is not due to a general medical condition (e.g., a dermatological condition).
E. The disturbance causes clinically significant distress or impairment in social, occupational, or other important areas of functioning.

Typically, the person complaining of unwanted hair-pulling is a young adult or the parent of a child who has been seen pulling out hair (Winchel 1992). Hair-pulling tends to occur in small bursts that may last minutes to hours. Such episodes may occur once or many times each day. Hairs are pulled out individually and may be pulled out rapidly and indiscriminately. Often, however, the hand of the individual may roam the afflicted area of scalp or body, searching for a shaft of hair that may feel particularly coarse or thick. Satisfaction with having pulled out a complete hair (shaft and root) is frequently expressed. Occasionally the experience of hair-pulling is described as quite pleasurable. Some individuals experience an itch-like sensation in the scalp that is eased by the act of pulling. The person may then toss away the hair shaft or inspect it. A substantial number of people then chew or consume (trichophagia) the hair. Hair-pulling is most commonly limited to the eyebrows and eyelashes. The scalp is the next most frequently afflicted site. However, hairs in any location of the body may be the focus of hair-pulling urges, including facial, axillary, chest, pubic, and even perineal hairs.

Anxiety is almost always associated with the act of hair-pulling. Such anxiety may occur in advance of the hair-pulling behavior. A state of tension may occur spontaneously—driving the person to pull out hair in an attempt to reduce dysphoric feelings. Varying lengths of time must pass before the tension abates. Consequently, the amount of hair that may be extracted in an episode varies from episode to episode and from person to person. Frequently, hair-pulling begins automatically and without conscious awareness. In such circumstances, individuals discover themselves pulling out hairs after some have already been pulled out. In these situations, dysphoric tension is associated with the attempt to stop the behavior.

Circumstances that seem to predispose to episodes of hair-pulling include both states of stress and, paradoxically, moments of particular relaxation. Frequently, hair-pulling occurs when at-risk individuals are engaged in a relaxing activity that promotes distraction and ease (e.g., watching television, reading, talking on the phone).

It is common for hair pullers to report that the behavior does not occur in the presence of other people. A frequent exception may be that many pull hair in the presence of members of the nuclear family.

Some individuals have urges to pull hairs from other people and may sometimes try to find opportunities to do so surreptitiously (such as initiating bouts of play fighting). There have been reports of affected individuals pulling hairs from pets, dolls, and other fibrous materials, such as sweaters or carpets (Tabatabai 1981).

The distress that usually accompanies trichotillomania varies in severity. Concerns tend to focus on the social and vocational consequences of the behavior. Themes of worry include fear of exposure, a feeling that "something is wrong with me," anxiety about intimate relationships, and sometimes inability to pursue a vocation. Because certain kinds of work, such as reading and writing at a desk, seem to precipitate episodes of hair-pulling, some afflicted individuals make career choices based on the avoidance of deskwork. Leisure activities that may involve a risk of exposure (ranging from gymnastics class to sexual intimacy) may be avoided.

Patterns of hair-pulling behavior among children are less well described. Usually, the parent observes a child pulling out hair and may note patches of hair loss. Children may sometimes be unaware of the behavior or may, at times, deny it. Childhood trichotillomania has been reported to be frequently associated with thumb sucking or nail biting (Friman 1987). It has been suggested that trichotillomania with onset in early childhood may occur frequently with spontaneous remissions. Consequently, some have recommended that trichotillomania in early childhood may be considered a benign habit with a self-limited course. However, many individuals who present with chronic trichotillomania in adulthood report onset in early childhood (Reeve et al. 1992).

Individuals with trichotillomania have increased risk for mood disorders (major depressive disorder, dysthymic disorder) and anxiety symptoms. The frequency of specific anxiety disorders (such as generalized anxiety disorder and panic disorders as well as OCD) may be increased as well. Although it has been suggested that trichotillomania in childhood or adolescence is associated with schizophrenia or severe disruptions of the family system, no systematically collected data support such conclusions.

In general, the diagnosis of trichotillomania is not complicated. The essential symptom—recurrently pulling out hair in response to unwanted urges—is easily described by the individual. When the individual acknowledges the hair-pulling behavior and areas of patchy hair loss are evident, the diagnosis is not usually in doubt. Problems in diagnosis may arise when the diagnosis is suspected but the individual denies it. Such denial may occur in younger individuals and some adults. When the problem is suspected but denied by the individual, a skin biopsy from the affected area may aid in making the diagnosis.

Areas of hair loss can be marked by complete alopecia or can appear diffusely thinned or "ratty." Altered scalp appearance can range from small areas of thinned hair to complete baldness. For unclear reasons, several patterns of scalp loss are typical. Frequently, coin-sized areas of alopecia are noted at the vertex or at temporal or occipital regions. Among more severely afflicted people a peculiar pattern, so-called *tonsure trichotillomania*, may appear: a completely bald head except for a narrow, circular fringe circumscribing the outer boundary of the scalp, producing a look reminiscent of medieval friars.

Despite the hair loss, most individuals with this condition have no overtly unusual appearance on cursory inspection. If the hair loss is not covered by clothing or accessories, artful combing of hair or use of eyeliner and false eyelashes may easily hide it. The ease with which the condition may often be hidden may explain the general underappreciation of its apparent frequency and potential associated distress.

Histological findings are considered characteristic and may aid diagnosis when it is suspected despite denial by the individual. Biopsy samples from involved areas may have the following features. Short and broken hairs are present. The surface of the scalp usually shows no evidence of excoriation. On histological examination, normal and damaged follicles are found in the same area, as well as an increased number of catagen (i.e., nongrowing) hairs. Inflammation is usually minimal or absent. Some hair follicles may show signs of trauma (wrinkling of the outer root sheath). Involved follicles may be empty or contain a deeply pigmented keratinous material. The absence of inflammation distinguishes trichotillomania-induced alopecia from alopecia areata, the principal condition in the differential diagnosis (Mehregan 1970, Muller 1990).

Epidemiology

Trichotillomania was long thought to be an uncommon condition, often accompanied by other psychiatric conditions. Although definitive studies of frequency rates in the general population are still lacking, three surveys of college-age samples support the emerging view that trichotillomania is quite common. In two of these samples, totaling approximately 3000 undergraduate students, a lifetime incidence of self-identified trichotillomania (reaching full symptom criteria as described in DSM-III-R) was present in about 1% of the respondents. Some features of the condition—but not meeting full criteria—were identified in an additional 1 to 2% (Rothbaum et al. 1993, Christenson et al. 1991a).

These may be underestimates of the lifetime incidence of the disorder. Had these studies applied DSM-IV-TR criteria, which have become slightly less restrictive than DSM-III-R criteria, the rates might have been higher. In addition, because onset may occur later in life than the mean ages of individuals in these groups, the true lifetime incidence would probably be higher. Moreover, these samples consist of a selected population—largely first-year college students—and may not reflect the general population. Nonetheless, these studies indicate that the condition is likely to be far more common than previously assumed. But definitive, controlled studies of the prevalence of the condition have not yet been performed.

Reliable data regarding sex ratio in the general population are not yet available. It has long been suggested that women greatly outnumber men. But, as noted above, surveys of college students suggest that the true ratio may be near parity. Although the apparent preponderance of women presenting for treatment may reflect the true sex ratio, it may alternatively reflect self-selection for presentation for treatment. Self-selection may reflect gender-related, culturally based attitudes regarding appearance, as well as an acceptance of normative hair loss among men. Because such gender-related distinctions may not be made by parents who are concerned about hair-pulling habits in their children, the apparent equal presentation of male and female children may more accurately reflect the true sex ratio.

Course

The age at onset typically ranges from early childhood to young adulthood. Peak ages at presentation may be bimodal, with an earlier peak about age 5 to 8 years among children in whom it has a self-limited course, whereas among individuals who present to clinicians in adulthood, the mean age at onset is approximately 13 years (Rothbaum et al. 1993, Winchel 1992, Swedo et al. 1989). Initial onset after young adulthood is apparently uncommon. There have been reports of onset as early as 14 months of age and as late as 61 years.

Trichotillomania may be one of the earliest occurring conditions in psychiatry. Some parents insist that their child began pulling hair before 1 year of age. When trichotillomania begins before age 6 years, it tends to be a milder condition. It often responds to simple interventions and may be self-limited, with a duration of several weeks to several months, even if not treated. It often occurs in association with thumb sucking. In some cases, it remits spontaneously when therapeutic attention is directed at concurrent, severe thumb sucking (Watson and Allen 1993). It has been suggested that trichotillomania in childhood may be associated with severe intrapsychic or familial mental disorder. But there is no reliable evidence that supports such a conclusion. Indeed, some have suggested that because it may be common and frequently self-limiting, it should be considered a normal behavior among young children.

Some individuals have continuous symptoms for decades. For others, the disorder may come and go for weeks, months, or years at a time. Sites of hair-pulling may vary over time. Circumscribed periods of hair-pulling (weeks to months) followed by complete remission are reported among children.

Progression of the condition appears to be unpredictable. Waxing and waning of the severity of hair-pulling and number of hair-pulling sites occur in most individuals. It is not known which factors may predict a protracted and unremitting course.

Because of the unavailability of longitudinal studies of trichotillomania, generalizations about prognosis cannot be made. Individuals who present in research clinics typically have histories of many years (up to decades) of hair-pulling. Presentation after age 40 years appears to be far less common than in the previous three decades of life, suggesting that the condition may eventually remit spontaneously, even when untreated. It is likely that the persistent cases seen in research environments reflect the more severe end of the spectrum. As noted earlier, trichotillomania in children may often be a time-limited phenomenon.

Differential Diagnosis

Among individuals presenting with alopecia who complain of hair-pulling urges, the diagnosis is not usually in doubt. When individuals deny hair-pulling, other (dermatological) causes of alopecia should be considered. These include alopecia areata, male pattern hair loss, chronic discoid lupus erythematosus, lichen planopilaris, folliculitis decalvans, pseudopelade, and alopecia mucinosa.

Trichotillomania is not diagnosed when hair-pulling occurs in response to a delusion or hallucination.

Many people twist and play with their hair. This may be exacerbated in states of heightened anxiety but does not qualify for a diagnosis of trichotillomania.

Some individuals may present with features of trichotillomania but hair damage may be so slight as to be virtually undetectable, even under close examination. In such conditions, the disorder should be diagnosed only if it results in significant distress to the individual.

Trichotillomania may have a short, self-limited course among children and may be considered a temporary habit. Therefore, among children, the diagnosis should be reserved for situations in which the behavior has persisted during several months.

Etiology

The etiology of trichotillomania is unknown. The phenomenological similarities between trichotillomania and OCD have prompted speculations that the pathophysiology of the two conditions may be related. The apparent association between altered serotonergic function and OCD has guided attention toward the possible role of serotonergic function in the underlying cause of trichotillomania. Thus, interest has been spurred in examining serotonergic function in individuals with trichotillomania. As yet, however, only limited laboratory investigations have emerged.

Ninan and coworkers (1992) obtained CSF from eight individuals with trichotillomania and measured concentrations of the primary serotonin metabolite 5-HIAA. Baseline concentrations of 5-HIAA did not differ from those of control subjects, nor was there a relationship between the baseline 5-HIAA concentration and the severity of trichotillomania symptoms. However, seven of these individuals were then treated with SSRIs (fluoxetine and clomipramine). The researchers found a negative correlation between baseline CSF 5-HIAA concentration and the degree of improvement after treatment. This observation does not, however, directly support a conclusion that altered serotonin function is etiologically related to trichotillomania.

Swedo and associates (1991) used positron emission tomography to measure regional brain glucose in three groups: individuals with trichotillomania, individuals with OCD, and normal control subjects. Like the individuals with OCD, those with trichotillomania had altered patterns of glucose utilization compared with normal control subjects. However, the regional patterns of altered glucose utilization were not the same in the trichotillomania and OCD groups.

A morphometric MRI study compared volumes of brain structures in 10 female subjects with trichotillomania versus 10 normal controls. Left putamen volume was found to be significantly smaller in trichotillomania subjects as compared with normal matched controls (O'Sullivan et al. 1997).

Performance on particular neuropsychological tests may offer an additional basis for defining the underlying neuropathological process in individuals with trichotillomania. In addition, because impaired performance on such tests may indicate altered function in particular brain regions, they may help localize brain regions in which altered function may be associated with trichotillomania.

On the basis of such tests, Rettew and colleagues (1991) have suggested that individuals with trichotillomania may have deficits in spatial processing. Patterns of deficits on such tests may provide further support for a relationship between trichotillomania and other psychiatric conditions. Rettew and coworkers found similarities between subjects with trichotillomania and subjects with OCD.

Keuthen and colleagues (1996) also speculated that individuals with trichotillomania would demonstrate alterations in neuropsychological function similar to individuals with OCD, who have been shown to have impairments in executive, visual–spatial and nonverbal memory function. In a study of 20 subjects with trichotillomania and 20 matched healthy controls, they demonstrated the presence of impaired performance on two of these three parameters (nonverbal memory and executive function). These results were interpreted as supporting the presumed relationship between trichotillomania and OCD.

However, Stanley and colleagues (1997), in their study of 21 trichotillomania subjects (compared with 17 healthy controls) did not find evidence of deficits in visual–spatial ability, motor function, or executive function. But, differences were found on measures of divided attention, leading to the suggestion that trichotillomania might be more properly conceptualized as an affective or anxiety-based disorder, and that any demonstrated similarities with OCD may be related to their shared overlap with anxiety/affective disorders.

Additional support for a possible relationship between trichotillomania and OCD may come from family history studies. In a preliminary investigation of psychiatric diagnoses among first-degree relatives of probands with trichotillomania, Lenane and associates (1992) found increased frequencies (compared with normal control subjects) of OCD, as well as mood and anxiety disorders. Bienvenu and Colleagues (2000) examined 300 first-degree relatives of 343 individuals with OCD, and found increased rates of "grooming" conditions (e.g., nail biting, skin picking, trichotillomania), and other impulse control disorders (e.g., kleptomania, pathological gambling, pyromania).

In summary, few data are available to support any particular model of the etiological pathophysiology of trichotillomania. Early studies point to some alteration of brain activity. Inconsistent support has been found in these early explorations for a relationship with OCD.

Treatment

Treatment of trichotillomania typically occurs in an outpatient setting. Eradication of hair-pulling behavior is the general focus of treatment. Distress, avoidant behaviors, and cosmetic impairment are secondary to the hair-pulling behavior and would be likely to remit if the hair-pulling behavior is controlled. However, if sufficient control of hair-pulling cannot be attained, treatment goals should emphasize these associated problems as well. Even if hair-pulling persists, therapeutic interventions may be targeted at reducing secondary avoidance and diminishing distress.

Treatment may be considered in three phases:

Initial Contact   The diagnosis is made and the individual and clinician agree on a strategy that may incorporate both pharmacological and psychological interventions. If distress is severe, supportive interventions should be immediately considered in anticipation of incomplete treatment response or of a delay of weeks to months before interventions may be beneficial.

Acute Treatment   Even when treatment of hair-pulling behavior is optimally successful, there may be a delay of several weeks to months before adequate control is attained. Therefore, the acute treatment phase may be prolonged.

Maintenance   It is not known how long individuals must maintain active treatment interventions to prevent relapse. It should be anticipated that a substantial number of individuals require ongoing treatment for an extended time. Pharmacological treatments may need to be maintained for open-ended periods. Behavioral or hypnotic intervention may require periodic "booster shots" to support continuation of benefits.

A variety of treatment approaches have been advocated for trichotillomania. However, there have, as yet, been few controlled studies of the efficacy of any treatment approach. A number of investigations of the use of antidepressants with specific inhibition of serotonin reuptake (i.e., fluoxetine and clomipramine) have yielded mixed results (Rothbaum et al. 1993, Winchel et al. 1992, Swedo et al. 1989, Stein et al. 1997, Jaspers 1996). A multimodal approach, simultaneously utilizing several complementary treatment options, may turn out to be the most effective approach for most individuals.

While a number of treatment options can be currently offered to individuals with trichotillomania, the durability of long-term outcomes is unclear. Keuthen and colleagues (1998, 2001) followed a group of hair pullers who had "naturalistic" treatment in the community. Treatments were pharmacologic, behavioral, or both. Among those who had benefits, improvements were often lost over time, and persistent treatment and ongoing treatment was common over the course of several years.

Stress Management

Before embarking on a course of treatment, the clinician and the individual should first consider the course and severity of the condition. Because early remission may occur in cases of recent onset, mild trichotillomania of short duration does not necessarily require immediate intervention. In particular, if the hair-pulling first occurred during a period of stress, the behavior may spontaneously diminish as the stressful circumstances abate. In such circumstances, therapeutic attention may best be directed toward examining and seeking to diminish the basis for stress. Teaching alternative stress reduction methods may be useful in reducing recent-onset trichotillomania. However, when individuals with trichotillomania present to the clinician, it is often likely to have been a persistent condition and may have been present for many years or decades. Among such individuals, stress reduction may also be useful in reducing trichotillomania but complete remission is less likely.

Pharmacotherapy

A variety of medications have been used in the treatment of trichotillomania. In 1989, initial reports appeared demonstrating the apparent benefits of fluoxetine and clomipramine. Clomipramine was found to be superior to desipramine (Swedo et al. 1989). Fluoxetine was reported beneficial in open treatment (Winchel et al. 1992). Although reports for more than 60 individuals have subsequently added support for the use of these medications, the two double-blind studies in which fluoxetine has been compared with placebo did not demonstrate any improvement compared to placebo (Christenson et al. 1991b, Streichenwein and Thornby 1995). Fluvoxamine (Stanley et al. 1997b), citalopram (Stein et al. 1997), and venlafaxine (Ninan et al. 1998) have been reported to be efficacious in open trials. Although further controlled studies of SSRIs are needed, the use of such medications would be a prudent first step if a pharmacological approach has been agreed upon.

Initial evidence of improvement is usually first reported by the individual as greater awareness of the inclination to pull hair. This is usually followed by an ability to abort hair-pulling episodes more quickly than in the past. The ability to resist the urge follows. In cases with a good outcome, the inclination to pull diminishes and may eventually disappear. Individuals who pull from several sites may find that the rate of improvement varies from site to site.

There have been conflicting reports of early relapse of symptoms in some individuals treated with clomipramine or fluoxetine. Although good maintenance of benefit has been reported for some individuals 6 months and longer after the initiation of treatment, early relapse after several weeks to months has been reported as well. Keuthen and coworkers (2001) have provided long-term data on maintenance of response over time. Following a group of individuals who had varying forms of treatment (pharmacologic and psychological) for several years after an index evaluation, the authors concluded that initial improvement was common, but over time there was an increase in symptom scores and self-esteem scores worsened in the group over time. This problem remains to be further evaluated in long-term treatment studies. If early relapse does turn out to be common, it would distinguish trichotillomania from depression and OCD, in which, once established, medication benefits are often well maintained as long as medication is continued. Optimal duration of treatment for well-treated individuals is also still unknown. In accordance with standards developed for the treatment of other conditions, it would be reasonable to continue medication for at least 6 months before tapering. Reinitiation of treatment may be necessary.

Other Medications

Christenson and coworkers (1991c) have reported successful treatment with lithium. This observation awaits replication.

Because trichotillomania is often accompanied by other manifestations of anxiety—and for many individuals is exacerbated by stressful conditions—attempts at treatment with anxiolytic agents may be useful. There are no published reports of such treatments.

Adjunctive treatment with pimozide, a neuroleptic agent, has been advocated for some individuals who are refractory to other medications (Stein and Hollander 1992). The potential benefits of neuroleptics has been reported now by several authors (Potenza et al. 1998, Gabriel 2001, Gupta and Gupta 2000, Epperson et al. 1999). Most of these reports describe individuals for whom SSRIs provided insufficient benefits. The addition of atypical neuroleptics much improved their outcomes. The greater margin of safety and tolerability associated with atypical neuroleptics have made this a more viable treatment option.

Van Ameringen and colleagues (1999) described the use of haloperidol in nine individuals with trichotillomania. Six had previously failed treatment with SSRIs. Eight of nine individuals responded to the haloperidol. The possible superiority of neuroleptics prompted these authors to speculate that trichotillomania may be similar to Tourette's syndrome (TS), which responds preferentially to neuroleptics.

Psychosocial Treatments

Various behavioral techniques have been tried (Diefenbach et al. 2000). The most successful technique, habit reversal, is based on designing competitive behaviors that should inhibit the behavior of hair-pulling (Azrin and Nunn 1977, Azrin et al. 1980, Rosenbaum and Ayllon 1981). For example, if hair-pulling requires raising the arm to the scalp and contracting the muscles of the hand to grasp a hair, the behaviorist may design a behavioral program in which the individual is taught to lower the arm and extend the muscles of the hand. As with behavioral techniques in general, these interventions are most successful when the individual is strongly motivated and compliant. In addition, the treating psychiatrist should be experienced in the use of such techniques. If necessary, a referral should be made to such an experienced individual. Modified behavioral approaches have been described for children and adolescents (Vitulano et al. 1992, Rapp et al. 1998).

Cognitive–behavioral therapy (CBT) has been developed for, and applied to, individuals with trichotillomania. At this time, the potential for the efficacy of this treatment approach appears good. Ninan and colleagues (2000) compared CBT to clomipramine in the treatment of trichotillomania. The authors reported that CBT had a dramatic effect in reducing symptoms of trichotillomania and was significantly more effective than clomipramine ($P = 0.016$) or placebo ($P = 0.026$). Clomipramine resulted in symptom reduction greater than that with placebo, but the difference fell short of statistical significance. Placebo response was minimal.

There are no formal studies of the use of hypnosis for trichotillomania, but there are many published reports of beneficial treatment (Barabasz 1987, Cohen et al. 1999, Fabbri and Dy 1974, Kohen 1996, Rowen 1981, Zalsman et al. 2001). Benefits may be variable. Some individuals may have dramatic improvement. For some who improve, the benefits may be short-lived. As with behavioral interventions, the benefits of this approach are sometimes dependent on a highly motivated individual who can regularly carry out self-hypnotic measures as instructed by the therapist. Some individuals who have obtained partial benefits from either hypnosis or medication do well when both treatments are combined. Successful use of hypnotherapy for children with trichotillomania has also been reported (Cohen et al. 1999).

Many psychoanalytically oriented descriptions of individuals with trichotillomania have been published. These reports generally describe the psychodynamic formulations of individual cases, and should not be the basis for generalizations about most individuals with trichotillomania. Although individuals with trichotillomania may benefit from exploration and attempts to reduce intrapsychic conflict, the literature does not provide persuasive evidence of the efficacy of this approach in reducing hair-pulling.

Self-help groups for individuals with trichotillomania have appeared. Some are based in the structure of other 12-step programs. Some individuals appear to experience meaningful reduction in hair-pulling symptoms after beginning participation in such a group. Although the efficacy of such groups in reducing symptoms remains to be established, most individuals with trichotillomania can benefit from meeting other individuals with similar symptoms. Because of the lack of general awareness of trichotillomania, these individuals frequently believe that they are "oddball" individuals with a behavior that is unique. Many have experienced parental condemnation for the behavior and have been frequently castigated for a "habit" that may be viewed by others as under their voluntary control. The experience of meeting others with the condition is extremely supportive for such individuals and may help reduce the attendant stress while supporting self-esteem. Where programs specifically oriented toward trichotillomania may not be generally available, these individuals may benefit from groups oriented toward OCD.

Comparison of DSM-IV-TR/ICD-10 Diagnostic Criteria

The ICD-10 Diagnostic Criteria for Research do not include diagnostic criteria for intermittent explosive disorder. It is included in ICD-10 as an "other habit and Impulse Control Disorder."

The ICD-10 Diagnostic Criteria for Research and the DSM-IV-TR criteria for kleptomania, pyromania, and trichotillomania are essentially equivalent.

Finally, the ICD-10 Diagnostic Criteria for Research for pathological gambling are monothetic (i.e., A plus B plus C plus D are required) whereas the DSM-IV-TR criteria set is polythetic (i.e., 5 out of 10 required) with different items. Furthermore, the ICD-10 criteria specify "two or more episodes of gambling over a period of at least 1 year," whereas DSM-IV-TR does not specify a duration.

References

American Psychiatric Association (2000) *Diagnostic and Statistical Manual of Mental Disorders*, 4th ed., Text Rev. APA, Washington, DC.

Azrin NA and Nunn R (1977) *Habit Control in a Day*. Simon & Schuster, New York.

Azrin NS, Nunn RG, and Frantz SE (1980) Treatment of hair-pulling (trichotillomania): a comparitive study of habit reversal and negative practice training. *J Behav Ther Exp Psychiatry* **11**, 13–20.

Barabasz M (1987) Trichotillomania: a new treatment. *Int J Clin Exp Hypn* **35**, 146–154.

Bars DR, Heyrend FL, Simpson CD, et al. (2001) Use of visual evoked-potential studies and EEG data to classify aggressive, explosive behavior of youths. *Psychiatr Serv* **52**, 81–86.

Beldoch M (1991) Stolen objects as transitional objects. *Am J Psychiatry* **148**, 1754.

Bergh C, Eklund T, Sodersten P, et al. (1997) Altered dopamine function in pathological gambling. *Psychol Med* **27**, 473–475.

Bienvenu OJ, Samuels JF, Riddle MA, et al. (2000) The relationship of obsessive–compulsive disorder to possible spectrum disorders: results from a family study. *Biol Psychiatry* **48**, 287–293.

Blanco C, Orensanz-Munoz L, Blanco-Jerez C, et al. (1996) Pathological gambling and platelet MAO activity: a psychobiological study. *Am J Psychiatry* **153**, 119–121.

Brandford J and Dimock J (1986) A comparative study of adolescents and adults who wilfully set fires. Psychiatr. *J Univ Ottawa* **11**, 228–234.

Budman CL, Bruun RD, Park KS, et al. (1998) Rage attacks in children and adolescents with Tourette's disorder: a pilot study. *J Clin Psychiatry* **59**, 576–580.

Budman CL, Bruun RD, Park KS, et al. (2000) Explosive outbursts in children with Tourette's disorder. *J Am Acad Child Adolesc Psychiatry* **39**, 1270–1276.

Burstein A (1992) Fluoxetine-lithium treatment for kleptomania. *J Clin Psychiatry* **53**, 28–129.

Carrasco JL, Saiz-Ruiz J, Hollander E, et al. (1994) Low platelet monoamine oxidase activity in pathological gambling. *Acta Psychiatr Scand* **90**, 427–431.

Chiswick D (1976) Shoplifting, depression and an unusual intracranial lesion (a case report). *Med Sci Law* **16**, 266–268.

Christenson GA, Mackenzie TB, and Mitchell JE (1991a) Characteristics of 60 adult chronic hair pullers. *Am J Psychiatry* **148**, 365–370.

Christenson GA, Mackenzie TB, Mitchell JE, et al. (1991b) A placebo-controlled, double-blind crossover study of fluoxetine in trichotillomania. *Am J Psychiatry* **148**, 1566–1571.

Christenson GA, Popkin MK, Mackenzie TB, et al. (1991c) Lithium treatment of chronic hair-pulling. *J Clin Psychiatry* **52**, 116–120.

Cohen HA, Barzilai A, and Lahat E (1999) Hypnotherapy: an effective treatment modality for trichotillomania. *Acta Paediatr* **88**, 407–410.

Coid J (1984) Relief of diazepam-withdrawal syndrome by shoplifting. *Br J Psychiatry* **145**, 552–554.

DeCaria CM, Hollander E, Grossman R, et al. (1996) Diagnosis, neurobiology, and treatment of pathological gambling. *J Clin Psychiatry* **57**, 80–83. Discussion 83–84.

DeJong J, Virkkunen M, and Linnoila M (1992) Factors associated with recidivism in a criminal population. *J Nerv Ment Dis* **180**, 543–550.

Diefenbach GJ, Reitman D, and Williamson DA (2000) Trichotillomania: a challenge to research and practice. *Clin Psychol Rev* **20**, 289–309.

Eisen SA, Lin N, Lyons MJ, et al. (1998) Familial influences on gambling behaviour: an analysis of 3359 twin pairs. *Addiction* **93**, 1375–1384.

Eisen SA, Slutske WS, Lyons MJ, et al. (2001) The genetics of pathological gambling. *Semin Clin Neuropsychiatry* **6**, 195–204.

Epperson CN, Fasula D, Wasylink S, et al. (1999) Risperidone addition in serotonin reuptake inhibitor-resistant trichotillomania: Three cases. *J Child Adolesc Psychopharmacol* **9**, 43–49.

Fabbri R Jr. and Dy AJ (1974) Hypnotic treatment of trichotillomania: two cases. *Int J Clin Exp Hypn* **22**, 210–215.

Felthous AR, Bryant SG, Wingerter CB, et al. (1991) The diagnosis of intermittent explosive disorder in violent men. *Bull Am Acad Psychiatr Law* **19**, 71–79.

Fenichel O (1945) *The Psychoanalytic Theory of Neurosis*. WW Norton, New York.

First M and Frances A (eds). (1995) *DSM-IV Handbook of Differential Diagnosis*. American Psychiatric Press, Washington, DC, pp. 196–197.

Fishbain DA (1987) Kleptomania as risk-taking behavior in response to depression. *Am J Psychother* **41**, 598–603.

Freud S (1961) Dostoevsky and parricide. In *The Standard Edition of the Complete Psychological Works of Sigmund Freud*, Vol. 21, Strachey J (ed). Hogarth Press, London, 175–198.

Friman PC and Hove G (1987) Apparent covariation between child habit disorders: effects of successful treatment for thumb-sucking on untargeted chronic hair-pulling. *J Appl Behav Anal* **20**, 421–425.

Gabriel A (2001) A case of resistant trichotillomania treated with risperidone-augmented fluvoxamine. *Can J Psychiatry* **46**, 285–286.

Gauthier J and Pellerin D (1982) Management of compulsive shoplifting through covert sensitization. *J Behav Ther Exp Psychiatry* **13**, 73–75.

Geller JL (1987) Firesetting in the adult psychiatric population. *Hosp Comm Psychiatry* **38**, 501–506.

Geller JL and Bertsch G (1985) Fire-setting behavior in the histories of a state hospital population. *Am J Psychiatry* **142**, 464–468.

Gerstein DR, Volberg RA, Harwood R, et al. (1999) *Gambling Impact And Behavior Study: Report to the National Gambling Impact Study Commission*. National Opinion Research Center at the University of Chicago, Chicago, IL.

Glover JH (1985) A case of kleptomania treated by covert sensitization. *Br J Clin Psychol* **24**, 213–214.

Goldman MJ (1991) Kleptomania: making sense of the nonsensical. *Am J Psychiatry* **148**, 986–996.

Grant JE and Kim SW (2002) Pharmacotherapy of pathological gambling. *Psychiatr Ann* **32**, 186–191.

Guidry LS (1969) Use of a covert punishing contingency in compulsive stealing. *J Behav Ther Exp Psychiatry* **6**, 169.

Gupta MA and Gupta AK (2000) Olanzapine is effective in the management of some self-induced dermatoses: three case reports. *Cutis* **66**, 143–146.

Haller R and Hinterhuber H (1994) Treatment of pathological gambling with carbamazepine. *Pharmacopsychiatry* **27**, 129.

Herzog DB, Keller MB, Sacks NR, et al. (1992) Psychiatric comorbidity in treatment-seeking anorexics and bulimics. *J Am Acad Child Adolesc Psychiatry* **31**, 810–818.

Hollander E, DeCaria CM, Finkell JN, et al. (2000) A randomized double-blind fluvoxamine/placebo crossover trial in pathologic gambling. *Biol Psychiatry* **47**, 813–817.

Hollander E, DeCaria CM, Mari E, et al. (1998) Short-term single-blind fluvoxamine treatment of pathological gambling. *Am J Psychiatry* **155**, 1781–1783.

Hollander E, Frenkel M, Decaria C, et al. (1992) Treatment of pathological gambling with clomipramine. *Am J Psychiatry* **149**, 710–711.

Hudson JI and Pope HG (1990) Affective spectrum disorder: Does antidepressant response identify a family of disorders with a common pathophysiology? *Am J Psychiatry* **147**, 552–564.

Ibanez A, Blanco C, Donahue E, et al. (2001) Psychiatric comorbidity in pathological gamblers seeking treatment. *Am J Psychiatry* **158**, 1733–1735.

Ibanez A, Blanco C, and Saiz-Ruiz J (2002) Neurobiology and genetics of pathological gambling. *Psychiatr Ann* **32**, 181–185.

Janet P, La Kleptomanie, et al. (1911) Depression mentale. *J Psychol Norm Pathol* **8**, 97–103.

Jaspers JP (1996) The diagnosis and psychopharmacological treatment of trichotillomania: a review. *Pharmacopsychiatry* **29**, 115–120.

Kavoussi R, Armstead P, and Coccaro E (1997) The neurobiology of impulsive aggression. *Psychiatr Clin North Am* **20**, 395–403.

Keuthen NJ, Fraim C, Deckersbach T, et al. (2001) Longitudinal follow-up of naturalistic treatment outcome in patients with trichotillomania. *J Clin Psychiatry* **62**, 101–107.

Keuthen NJ, O'Sullivan RL, Goodchild P, et al. (1998) Retrospective review of treatment outcome for 63 patients with trichotillomania. *Am J Psychiatry* **155**, 560–561.

Keuthen NJ, Savage CR, O'Sullivan RL, et al. (1996) Neuropsychological functioning in trichotillomania. *Biol Psychiatry* **39**, 747–749.

Keutzer CS (1972) Kleptomania: a direct approach to treatment. *Br J Med Psychol* **45**, 159–163.

Khan K and Martin IC (1977) Kleptomania as a presenting feature of cortical atrophy. *Acta Psychiatr Scand* **56**, 168–172.

Khantzian EJ and Mack JE (1983) Self-preservation and the care of the self. Ego instincts reconsidered. *Psychoanal Stud Child* **38**, 209–232.

Kim SW and Grant JE (2001) The psychopharmacology of pathological gambling. *Semin Clin Neuropsychiatry* **6**, 184–194.

Kim SW, Grant JE, Adson DE, et al. (2001) Double-blind naltrexone and placebo comparison study in the treatment of pathological gambling. *Biol Psychiatry* **49**, 914–921.

Kohen DP (1996) Hypnotherapeutic management of pediatric and adolescent trichotillomania. *J Dev Behav Pediatr* **17**, 328–334.

Kolko DJ (2001) Efficacy of cognitive–behavioral treatment and fire safety education for children who set fires: initial and follow-up outcomes. *J Child Psychol Psychiatry* **42**, 359–369.

Kolko DJ and Kazdin AE (1988) Parent–child correspondence in identification of firesetting among child psychiatric patients. *J Child Psychol Psychiatry* **29**, 175–184.

Kuperman S, Kramer J, and Loney J (1988) Enzyme activity and behavior in hyperactive children grown up. *Biol Psychiatry* **24**, 375–383.

Lee S (1994) The heterogeneity of stealing behaviors in Chinese patients with anorexia nervosa in Hong Kong. *J Nerv Ment Dis* **182**, 304–307.

Lenane MC, Swedo SE, Rapoport JL, et al. (1992) Rates of obsessive–compulsive disorder in first degree relatives of patients with trichotillomania: a research note. *J Child Psychol Psychiatry* **33**, 925–933.

Lesieur HR and Rosenthal RJ (1991) Pathological gambling: a review of the literature. *J Gambling Stud* **7**, 5–39.

Linden RD, Pope HG Jr., and Jonas JM (1986) Pathological gambling and major affective disorder: preliminary findings. *J Clin Psychiatry* **47**, 201–203.

Linnoila M, De Jong J, and Virkkunen M (1989) Family history of alcoholism in violent offenders and impulsive fire setters. *Arch Gen Psychiatry* **46**, 613–616.

Lion JR (1992) The intermittent explosive disorder. *Psychiatr Ann* **2**, 64–66.

Lorenz V (1981) Differences found among Catholic, Protestant, and Jewish families of pathological gamblers. In *Fifth National Conference on Gambling and Risk Taking*. Lake Tahoe, CA.

Lowenstein LF (1989) The etiology, diagnosis and treatment of the fire-setting behaviour of children. *Child Psychiatr Hum Dev* **19**, 186–194.

Marks I (1990) Behavioural (non-chemical) addictions. *Br J Addict* **85**, 1389–1394.

Marzagao LR (1972) Systemic desensitization treatment of kleptomania. *J Behav Ther Exp Psychiatry* **3**, 327–328.

Mattes JA (1990) Comparative effectiveness of carbamazepine and propranolol for rage outbursts. *J Neuropsychiatr Clin Neurosci* **2**, 159–164.

McElroy SL, Hudson JI, Phillips KA, et al. (1993) Clinical and theoretical implications of a possible link between obsessive–compulsive and impulse control disorders. *Depression* **1**, 121–132.

McElroy SL, Hudson JI, Pope HG, et al. (1991a) Kleptomania: clinical characteristics and associated psychopathology. *Psychol Med* **21**, 93–108.

McElroy SL, Hudson JI, Pope HG Jr., et al. (1992) The DSM-III-R impulse control disorders not elsewhere classified: Clinical characteristics and relationship to other psychiatric disorders. *Am J Psychiatry* **149**, 318–327.

McElroy SL, Keck PE Jr., Pope HG Jr., et al. (1989) Pharmacological treatment of kleptomania and bulimia nervosa. *J Clin Psychopharmacol* **9**, 358–360.

McElroy SL, Pope HG Jr., Hudson JI, et al. (1991b) Kleptomania: a report of 20 cases. *Am J Psychiatry* **148**, 652–657.

McIntyre AW and Emsley RA (1990) Shoplifting associated with normal-pressure hydrocephalus: report of a case. *J Geriatr Psychiatr Neurol* **3**, 229–230.

Mehregan AH (1970) Trichotillomania. A clinicopathologic study. *Arch Dermatol* **102**, 129–133.

Mendez MF (1988) Pathological stealing in dementia. *J Am Geriatr Soc* **36**, 825–826.

Monopolis S and Lion JR (1983) Problems in the diagnosis of intermittent explosive disorder. *Am J Psychiatry* **140**, 1200–1202.

Moreno I, Saiz-Ruiz J, and Lopez-Ibor JJ (1991) Serotonin and gambling dependence. *Hum Psychopharmacol Clin Exp* **6**, 9–12.

Muller SA (1990) Trichotillomania: a histopathologic study in sixty-six patients. *J Am Acad Dermatol* **23**, 56–62.

Murray JB (1993) Review of research on pathological gambling. *Psychol Rep* **72**, 791–810.

Ninan PT, Knight B, Kirk L, et al. (1998) A controlled trial of venlafaxine in trichotillomania: interim phase I results. *Psychopharmacol Bull* **34**, 221–224.

Ninan PT, Rothbaum BO, Marsteller FA, et al. (2000) A placebo-controlled trial of cognitive–behavioral therapy and clomipramine in trichotillomania. *J Clin Psychiatry* **61**, 47–50.

Ninan PT, Rothbaum BO, Stipetic M, et al. (1992) CSF 5-HIAA as a predictor of treatment response in trichotillomania. *Psychopharmacol Bull* **28**, 451–455.

O'Sullivan GH and Kelleher MJ (1987) A study of fire-setters in the southwest of Ireland. *Br J Psychiatry* **151**, 818–823.

O'Sullivan RL, Rauch SL, Breiter HC, et al. (1997) Reduced basal ganglia volumes in trichotillomania measured via morphometric magnetic resonance imaging. *Biol Psychiatry* **42**, 39–45.

Petry NM (2002) Psychosocial treatments for pathological gambling: current status and future directions. *Psychiatr Ann* **32**, 192–196.

Phillips DP, Welty WR, and Smith MM (1997) Elevated suicide levels associated with legalized gambling. *Suicide Life-Threat Behav* **27**, 373–378.

Potenza MN, Wasylink S, Epperson CN, et al. (1998) Olanzapine augmentation of fluoxetine in the treatment of trichotillomania. *Am J Psychiatry* **155**, 1299–3000.

Prins H, Tennent G, and Trick K (1985) Motives for arson (fire raising). *Med Sci Law* **25**, 275–278.

Raine A, Buchsbaum MS, Stanley J, et al. (1994) Selective reductions in prefrontal glucose metabolism in murderers. *Biol Psychiatry* **36**, 365–373.

Ramirez LF, McCormick RA, Russo AM, et al. (1983) Patterns of substance abuse in pathological gamblers undergoing treatment. *Addict Behav* **8**, 425–428.

Rapp JT, Miltenberger RG, Long ES, et al. (1998) Simplified habit reversal treatment for chronic hair-pulling in three adolescents: a clinical replication with direct observation. *J Appl Behav Anal* **31**, 299–302.

Reeve EA, Bernstein GA, and Christenson GA (1992) Clinical characteristics and psychiatric comorbidity in children with trichotillomania. *J Am Acad Child Adolesc Psychiatry* **31**, 132–138.

Rettew DC, Cheslow DL, Rapoport JL, et al. (1991) Neuropsychological test performance in trichotillomania: a further link with obsessive–compulsive disorder. *J Anxiety Disord* **5**, 225–235.

Rosenbaum MS and Ayllon T (1981) The habit-reversal technique in treating trichotillomania. *Behav Ther* **12**, 473–481.

Rosenthal RJ (1992) Pathological gambling. *Psychiatr Ann* **22**, 72–78.

Rothbaum BO, Shaw L, Morris R, et al. (1993) Prevalence of trichotillomania in a college freshman population. *J Clin Psychiatry* **54**, 72–73.

Rowen R (1981) Hypnotic age regression in the treatment of a self-destructive habit: trichotillomania. *Am J Clin Hypn* **23**, 195–197.

Roy A, Adinoff B, Roehrich L, et al. (1988) Pathological gambling. A psychobiological study. *Arch Gen Psychiatry* **45**, 369–373.

Schwartz HJ (1992) Psychoanalytic psychotherapy for a woman with diagnoses of kleptomania and bulimia. *Hosp Comm Psychiatry* **43**, 109–110.

Siever LJ, Kahn RS, Lawlor BA, et al. (1991) Critical issues in defining the role of serotonin in psychiatric disorders. *Pharmacol Rev* **43**, 509–525.

Soltys SM (1992) Pyromania and firesetting behaviors. *Psychiatr Ann* **22**, 79–83.

Staner L and Mendlewicz J (1998) Heredity and role of serotonin in aggressive impulsive behavior. *Encephale* **24**, 355–364.

Stanley MA, Hannay HJ, and Breckenridge JK (1997b) The neuropsychology of trichotillomania. *J Anxiety Disord* **11**, 473–488.

Stanley M and Mann JJ (1988) Biological factors associated with suicide. In *Review of Psychiatry*, Vol. 7, Frances AJ and Hales RE (eds). American Psychiatric Press, Washington, DC.

Stein DJ, Bouwer C, and Maud CM (1997) Use of the selective serotonin reuptake inhibitor citalopram in treatment of trichotillomania. *Eur Arch Psychiatr Clin Neurosci* **247**, 234–236.

Stein DJ and Hollander E (1992) Low-dose pimozide augmentation of serotonin reuptake blockers in the treatment of trichotillomania. *J Clin Psychiatry* **53**, 123–126.

Stein DJ, Hollander E, and Liebowitz MR (1993) Neurobiology of impulsivity and the impulse control disorders. *J Neuropsychiatr Clin Neurosci* **5**, 9–17.

Streichenwein SM and Thornby JI (1995) A long-term, double-blind, placebo-controlled crossover trial of the efficacy of fluoxetine for trichotillomania. *Am J Psychiatry* **152**, 1192–1196.

Swedo SE, Leonard HL, Rapoport JL, et al. (1989) A double-blind comparison of clomipramine and desipramine in the treatment of trichotillomania (hair-pulling). *N Engl J Med* **321**, 497–501.

Swedo SE, Rapoport JL, Leonard HL, et al. (1991) Regional cerebral glucose metabolism of women with trichotillomania. *Arch Gen Psychiatry* **48**, 828–833.

Tabatabai SE and Salari-Lak M (1981) Alopecia in dolls! *Cutis* **28**, 206.

Turnbull JM (1987) Sexual relationships of patients with kleptomania. *South Med J* **80**, 995–998.

Van Ameringen M, Mancini C, Oakman JM, et al. (1999) The potential role of haloperidol in the treatment of trichotillomania. *J Affect Disord* **56**, 219–226.

Virkkunen M, Goldman D, Nielsen DA, et al. (1995) Low brain serotonin turnover rate (low CSF 5-HIAA) and impulsive violence. *J Psychiatr Neurosci* **20**, 271–275.

Virkkunen M and Linnoila M (1993) Brain serotonin, type II alcoholism and impulsive violence. *J Stud Alcohol* (Suppl. 11), 163–169.

Vitulano LA, King RA, Scahill L, et al. (1992) Behavioral treatment of children and adolescents with trichotillomania. *J Am Acad Child Adolesc Psychiatry* **31**, 139–146.

Volberg RA (2002) The epidemiology of pathological gambling. *Psychiatr Ann* **32**, 171–178.

Volberg RA and Steadman HJ (1988) Refining prevalence estimates of pathological gambling. *Am J Psychiatry* **145**, 502–505.

Watson TS and Allen KD (1993) Elimination of thumb-sucking as a treatment for severe trichotillomania. *J Am Acad Child Adolesc Psychiatry* **32**, 830–834.

Wetzel R (1966) Use of behavior techniques in a case of compulsive stealing. *J Consult Psychol* **5**, 367–374.

Winchel RM (1992) Trichotillomania: Presentation and treatment. *Psychiatr Ann* **22**, 8–89.

Winchel RM, Jones JS, Stanley B, et al. (1992) Clinical characteristics of trichotillomania and its response to fluoxetine. *J Clin Psychiatry* **53**, 304–308.

Woermann FG, van Elst LT, Koepp MJ, et al. (2000) Reduction of frontal neocortical grey matter associated with affective aggression in patients with temporal lobe epilepsy: an objective voxel by voxel analysis of automatically segmented MRI. *J Neurol Neurosurg Psychiatry* **68**, 162–169.

Wood A and Garralda ME (1990) Kleptomania in a 13-year-old boy. A sequel of a "lethargic" encephalitic/depressive process? *Br J Psychiatry* **157**, 770–772.

Zalsman G, Hermesh H, and Sever J (2001) Hypnotherapy in adolescents with trichotillomania: three cases. *Am J Clin Hypn* **44**, 63–68.

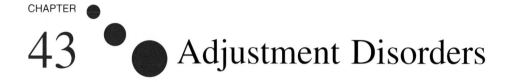

CHAPTER

43 Adjustment Disorders

Diagnosis

The essential feature of adjustment disorder (AD) is the development of clinically significant emotional or behavioral symptoms in response to an identifiable psychosocial stressor (see DSM-IV-TR diagnostic criteria below). The symptoms must develop within 3 months after the onset of the stressor (criterion A). The clinical significance of the reaction is indicated either by marked distress that is in excess of what would be expected given the nature of the stressor or by significant impairment in social or occupational (academic) functioning (criterion B). This disorder should not be used if the emotional and cognitive disturbances meet the criteria for *another* specific Axis I disorder (e.g., a specific anxiety or mood disorder) or are merely an exacerbation of a preexisting Axis I or Axis II disorder (criterion C). AD may be diagnosed if other Axis I or II disorders are present, but do not account for the pattern of symptoms that have occurred in response to the stressor. The diagnosis of AD does not apply when the symptoms represent bereavement (criterion D). By definition, AD must resolve within 6 months of the termination of the stressor or its consequences (criterion E). However, the symptoms may persist for a prolonged period (i.e., longer than 6 months) if they occur in response to a chronic stressor (e.g., a chronic, disabling general medical condition) or to a stressor that has enduring consequences (e.g., the financial and emotional difficulties resulting from a divorce).

DSM-IV-TR Diagnostic Criteria

309.xx Adjustment Disorders

A. The development of emotional or behavioral symptoms in response to an identifiable stressor(s) occurring within 3 months of the onset of the stressor(s).

B. These symptoms or behaviors are clinically significant as evidenced by either of the following:

(1) marked distress that is in excess of what would be expected from exposure to the stressor

(2) significant impairment in social or occupational (academic) functioning

C. The stress-related disturbance does not meet the criteria for another specific Axis I disorder and is not merely an exacerbation of a preexisting Axis I or Axis II disorder.

D. The symptoms do not represent bereavement.

E. Once the stressor (or its consequences) has terminated, the symptoms do not persist for more than an additional 6 months.

Specify if:

Acute: if the disturbance lasts less than 6 months

Chronic: if the disturbance lasts for 6 months or longer

Adjustment disorders are coded based on the subtype, which is selected according to the predominant symptoms. The specific stressor(s) can be specified on Axis IV.

309.0 With Depressed Mood

309.24 With Anxiety

309.28 With Mixed Anxiety and Depressed Mood

309.3 With Disturbance of Conduct

309.4 With Mixed Disturbance of Emotions and Conduct

309.9 Unspecified

The symptoms of AD are defined in terms of their being a maladaptive response to a psychosocial stressor. There are, in fact, no specific symptoms of AD; any combination of behavioral or emotional symptoms that occur in association with a stressor may qualify. The nature of the symptomatology is described by a variety of possible "subtypes", including With Depressed Mood, With Mixed Anxiety and Depressed Mood, With Disturbance of Conduct, With Mixed Disturbance of Emotions and Conduct, and Unspecified.

Although this diagnosis lacks rigorous specificity, its treatment is no less challenging or less important. AD's lack of a designated symptom profile results in this diagnosis having insufficient specificity. However, it is this lack of specificity, which permits the psychiatrist to have a "diagnosis" to use when the individual is presenting with early, vague, nonconcrete symptomatology, which should be noted, identified, and followed. This is similar to the situation with early fever, or fever of unknown origin, which, by the way, may never go on to a specific medical diagnosis, but be at discharge simply diagnosed as a "fever of unknown origin." Unspecified chest pain is another example where the individual may never have a specific diagnosis even over time. Spitzer has described the ADs as a "wild card" in the psychiatric lexicon, that allows a place for an uncertain, early, not completely developed diagnosis to be housed until it disappears, develops into a full blown category, persists in a subsyndromal state, or disappears. As said above, this is not uncommon with physical or mental subsyndromal states.

No criteria or guidelines are offered in DSM-IV-TR to quantify the degree of stress required for the diagnosis of AD or assess its effect or meaning for a particular individual at a given time. Many of the statements regarding the problem of assessing maladaptation described above apply equally well to the assessment of stressors (Woolston 1988, Zilberg et al. 1982, Perris 1984). Mezzich and coworkers (1981) attempted to classify and quantify the psychosocial stressors in 13 domains (i.e., health, bereavement, love and marriage, parental, family stressors for children and adolescents, other familial relationships, work, school, financial, legal, housing, and miscellaneous). The measurement of the severity of the stressor and its temporal and causal relationship to demonstrable symptoms are often uncertain.

According to DSM-IV-TR, even if a specific and presumably causal stressor is identified, if enough symptoms develop so that diagnostic criteria are met for a specific disorder, then that diagnosis should be made instead of a diagnosis of AD (American Psychiatric Association 1980, 1987, 2000). Therefore, the presence of stressors does not automatically signify a diagnosis of AD, and conversely, a diagnosis of a specific disorder (e.g., major depressive or anxiety disorder) does not imply the absence of concomitant or concurrent stressful events (Setterberg et al. 1991).

Although the diagnosis of AD requires evidence of maladaption, it is notable that no specific requirement for functional impairment has been included (e.g., there is no requirement for a certain decrement in the Global Assessment of Functioning Scale score in order to make the diagnosis). Fabrega and colleagues (1986) stated that both subjective symptoms and decrement in social function can be considered maladaptive and that the severity of either of these is subject to great individual variation. However, they could not conclude that the level of severity of psychiatric illness observed correlates with impaired functioning in three areas: occupational status, family, or other individuals.

The clinician needs to examine the individual's behavior to see whether it is beyond what is expected in a particular situation, and for that individual. In order to do this, the clinician needs to take into account the individual's cultural beliefs and practices, his or her developmental age, and the transient nature of the behavior. If the behavior lasts a few moments or is an impulsive outburst, it would not qualify for a maladaptive response to justify the diagnosis of AD. The behavior in question should be maladaptive for that individual, in his/her culture, and sufficiently persistent to qualify for the maladaptation attribute of the AD diagnosis.

The criterion and predictive validity of the diagnosis of AD in 92 children who had new onset insulin-dependent diabetes mellitus were examined. DSM-III criteria were employed, plus requiring four clinically significant signs or symptoms, and the time frame extended to 6 months (instead of the 3 months specified in the definition) after the diagnosis of diabetes. Thirty-three percent of the cohort developed AD (mean 29 days after the medical diagnosis) and the average episode length was 3 months with a recovery rate of 100%. The 5-year cumulative probability of a new psychiatric disorder was 0.48 in comparison to 0.16 for the non-AD subjects. The findings support the criterion validity of the AD diagnosis using the criterion of predicting the future development of psychiatric disorder.

Construct validity was also observed in a retrospective data study comparing outpatients with single-episode major depressive disorder, recurrent major depressive disorder, dysthymic disorder, depressive disorder NOS, and AD with depressed mood with or without mixed anxiety (Jones et al. 1999). The Medical Outcomes Study 36-item Short Form Health Status Survey (SF-36) was completed before and 6 months after treatment. The diagnostic categories were significantly different at baseline, but did not differ with regard to outcome at follow-up. Females were significantly more likely to be diagnosed with major depressive disorder or dysthymic disorder than with AD. Females were also more likely to score lower on the Mental Component Summary scales of the SF-36 scales at admission. Individuals with AD scored higher on all SF-36 scales, as did the other diagnostic groups at baseline and again at follow-up. There was no significant difference among diagnostic groups with regard to treatment outcome. The authors concluded that the results support the construct validity of the AD diagnostic category (Jones et al. 1999).

Significant occurrence of comorbidity has been reported in studies of AD using structured diagnostic instruments. In a cohort of children, adolescents, and adults, approximately 70% of individuals with AD had at least one additional Axis I diagnosis (Fabrega et al. 1987). In the study of correlates of depressive disorders in children, 45% of those with AD with depressed mood had another disorder (Kovacs et al. 1984). However, comorbidity in AD was less than in dysthymic disorder or major depressive disorder, suggesting a "purer" or a more encapsulated disturbance in AD.

Several studies reported an association of suicidal behavior in adolescents and young adults with AD. One study found that 56% of those hospitalized for suicidal behavior in an urban hospital setting met the DSM-II criteria for transient situational disturbance (an earlier diagnostic label for what came to be called AD) (Minnaar et al. 1980). A retrospective review of 325 consecutive hospital admissions for deliberate self-poisoning revealed that 58% of all cases met criteria for AD with depressed mood, the majority of whom were women aged 15 to 24 years (McGrath 1989). In a Scandinavian sample of 58 consecutive suicide victims aged 15 to 29 years, 14% were classified as AD with depressed mood (Runeson 1989); in a US population, 9% of suicide victims aged 10 to 29 years were reported to have AD (Fowler et al. 1986). These studies underscore the seriousness of AD in a subset of individuals and suggest that although the diagnosis may be subthreshold, its morbidity can be serious and at times even fatal.

The issue of boundaries between the specific mood and anxiety disorders, depressive disorder or anxiety disorder NOS, and the AD remains problematic. The specific mood and anxiety disorders are often associated with, and even precipitated by, stress. Therefore, it is not always possible to say one group of diagnoses is accompanied by stress (the AD) and another (e.g., major depressive disorder) is not. Stress may accompany many of the mental disorder but it is not an essential component to make certain diagnoses (e.g., major depressive disorder). More research is needed to carefully demarcate the boundaries or the meaning of these boundaries among the problem-level, subthreshold, and threshold disorders, in particular with regard to the role of stressors as etiological precipitants, concomitants, or factors essentially unrelated to the occurrence of a particular psychiatric diagnosis. Furthermore, serial and ongoing observation of the clinical course is required to ascertain whether the AD is a transitory remitting event, the prodromal state of a more serious and developing disorder, or an intermittent chronic state of a low-level mood disorder. There is considerable evidence indicating that major depressive disorder is a highly recurrent, often chronic condition that is frequently associated with low-grade symptoms prior to, and between, major episodes (Keller et al. 1995). Thus, the differential diagnoses of depressed mood must be linked to ongoing assessment, not cross-sectional evaluation, which is so often the case; it is essential to maintain a longitudinal view of the subthreshold disorders to know their place in an individual's affective history. Keller and coworkers (1995) described the need for a longitudinal taxonomy, a "course-based classification system."

In reviewing the diagnosis of AD for DSM-IV, one issue emerges as fundamental. The effect of the imprecision of this diagnosis on reliability and validity, because of the lack of behavioral or operational criteria, must be determined. One study (Aoki et al. 1995), however, found three psychological tests, Zung's Self-Rating Anxiety Scale (Zung 1971), Zung's Self-Rating Depression Scale (Zung 1965), and Profile of Mood States (McNair et al. 1971), to be useful tools for AD diagnosis among physical rehabilitation individuals. Although Aoki and colleagues (1995) succeeded in reliably differentiating individuals with AD from healthy individuals, they did not distinguish them from individuals with major depression or posttraumatic stress disorder (PTSD).

Course

Andreasen and Hoenk (1982) demonstrated at a 5-year follow-up that there were important differences in adolescents and adults with regard to prognosis. It would be important to extend this long-term observation to cohorts of the elderly and the "old elderly" (those older than 75 years). Although the prognosis was favorable and most adult individuals with AD were symptom free at 5 years (71% were completely well, 8% had an intervening problem, and 21% had a major depressive disorder or alcoholism), adolescents had a far different outcome. At a 5-year follow-up, 43% had a major psychiatric disorder (e.g., schizophrenia, schizoaffective disorder, major depressive disorder, substance abuse disorder, and personality disorder); 13% had an intervening mental disorder; and 44% had no mental disorder (Andreasen and Hoenk 1982). In adolescents, behavioral symptoms and the chronicity of the morbidity were the major predictors for psychopathological disorders at the 5-year follow-up. This was not so with the adults in the study, and raises the question of whether these adolescents were diagnosed as having AD as part of a prodrome of another more serious disorder.

Kovacs and associates (1994) reported a much different set of findings. The authors report that children who were older at the time of onset of AD recovered faster, and there was a trend for subjects with the depressed mood subtype to recover faster than subjects with other symptoms. The researchers concluded that among young, school-aged, clinic-based individuals, AD has clinical information value, and is associated with a favorable short-term prognosis, but is often associated with comorbid mental disorders, which complicates assessment. When effects of comorbidity were controlled for, there was no compelling evidence for a negative long-term prognosis during a follow-up period of 7 to 8 years specifically attributable to the earlier AD (Andreasen and Hoenk 1982).

Thus, even if AD is properly diagnosed, the negative prognosis that has been reported could be attributable to comorbid disorders such as depressive, anxiety, or conduct disorders that were not recognized (Andreasen and Hoenk 1982). Kovacs and colleagues (1994) furthermore reported that comorbid psychiatric disorders had no discernible effect on the speed of recovery from AD. Among both individuals with AD and the control subjects, similar rates of dysfunction were detected during the follow-up, probably attributable to the specific mental disorder that were present initially.

Snyder and Strain (1989) observed that in the acute care inpatient hospital setting, many of the individuals initially thought to have an AD did not maintain that diagnosis at the time of discharge. These same authors also observed that many individuals initially diagnosed as having major depressive disorder were reclassified to AD at discharge. It remains to be seen if either the major depressive disorder or the AD diagnosis is significantly altered at a 6-week follow-up and, in particular, when the individual has left the hospital. This evolution of psychiatric morbidity within the acute care general medical setting cautions the clinician to go slowly with treatment until there is a level of certainty to justify an intervention, in particular with a chemotherapeutic modality.

Epidemiology

AD has principally been studied in clinical samples. Epidemiological data in adults are not available. The AD diagnosis was not included in the Epidemiologic Catchment Area Study conducted in five disparate sites throughout the US, and there are only a few studies in children and adolescents. Andreasen and Wasek (1980) reported that 5% of an inpatient and outpatient sample were labeled AD. Fabrega and coworkers (1987) observed that 2.3% of a sample of individuals presenting to a walk-in diagnostic and evaluation center clinic met criteria for AD with no other Axis I or Axis II diagnoses. When individuals with other Axis I diagnoses (Axis I comorbidities) were also included, 20% had the diagnosis of AD. Of a sample of more than 11,000 individuals (all ages), 10% were found to have AD (Table 43-1), making it the second-largest diagnostic category (Fabrega et al. 1986, 1987, Mezzich et al. 1989). In the Pittsburgh sample studied, 16% of the children and adolescents younger than 18 years were diagnosed with AD (Fabrega et al. 1986). In adults, women predominated over men by approximately 2 : 1. The sex ratio was more equal in children and adolescents, although there was still a slight excess of women.

Table 43-1	Prevalence of Adjustment Disorder			
Study	**Sample Type**	**Sample Size**	**Assessment Method**	**Prevalence**
Bird et al. (1988)	Epidemiological, general population	Probability estimate of 2036 households	Structured rating scales; clinical interview	7.6% (CGAS* < Ld70) 4.2% (CGAS < Ld60)
Weiner and DelGaudio (1976)	Epidemiological, clinical services	1344	Clinical diagnosis	27% of all cases
Mezzich et al. (1989)	Clinical screening evaluation (all services)	11,282	Semistructured assessment instrument	10% (all ages) 16% (<Ld18 yr)
Faulstich et al. (1986)	Clinical (adolescent inpatient)	392	Chart review, clinical diagnosis	12.5%
Hillard et al. (1987)	Clinical (emergency room department)	100 adolescents 100 adults (random)	Chart review, clinical diagnosis	42% of adolescents 13% of adults
Doan and Petti (1989)	Clinical (partial hospital)	796	Chart review, clinical diagnosis	7%
Jacobson et al. (1980)	Clinical (four outpatient pediatric clinics)	20,000 pediatric patients	Clinical diagnosis	25–65% of cases with psychiatric diagnosis

Oxman and coworkers (1994) observed that 50.7% of elderly individuals (aged 55+ years) receiving elective surgery for coronary artery disease developed AD related to the stress of surgery. Thirty percent had symptomatic and functional impairment 6 months following surgery. It is reported that 27% of elderly individuals examined 5 to 9 days following a cerebral vascular accident had symptoms that fulfilled the criteria for AD (Kellermann et al. 1994). Spiegel (1996) observed that half of all individuals with cancer have a psychiatric disorder, usually an AD with depression. Since individuals treated for their mental states had longer survival time, treatment of depression in individuals with cancer should be considered integral to their medical treatment. AD is a frequently made diagnosis in individuals with head and neck surgery (16.8%) (Kugaya et al. 2000), individuals with HIV dementia (73%) (Pozzi et al. 1999), individuals with cancer from a multicenter survey of consultation–liaison psychiatry in oncology (27%) (Grassi et al. 2000), individuals with dermatological problems (29% of the 9% who had psychiatric diagnosis) (Pulimood et al. 1996), and suicide attempters (22%) examined in an emergency room (Schnyder and Valach 1997). Other studies include diagnosis of AD in more than 60% of inpatients being treated for severe burns (Perez-Jimenez et al. 1994), 20% of individuals in early stages of multiple sclerosis (Sullivan et al. 1995), and 40% of poststroke individuals (Shima et al. 1994).

There are two published epidemiological studies in populations of children and adolescents that included AD. One, conducted in Puerto Rico, employed a two-stage screening process using standardized rating scales as well as structured and unstructured clinical interviews (Bird et al. 1988, 1989). The prevalence rate of AD was determined to be 7.6% if an upper limit of 70 on the Children's Global Assessment Scale (CGAS) is applied (Shaffer et al. 1983). However, if an upper limit of 60 is imposed (corresponding to "moderate" impairment on the CGAS), the prevalence of AD dropped to 4.2%. This indicates that up to 40% of AD diagnosed individuals have only mild impairment, more than for any other diagnosis. A recent study conducted in a very large birth registry in Finland found that AD with mixed disturbance of emotions and conduct was the most frequent AD diagnosis, and occurred in 3.4% of the population at the time of the assessment (Almqvist et al. 1999). Other studies conducted in children who presented with psychiatric disturbance from four different clinics indicated rates of AD across the clinics ranging from 25 to 65% (Jacobson et al. 1980). The prevalence of AD in children and adolescents may be somewhat higher than it is in adults, but varies considerably according to the population studied.

Etiology

By definition, the ADs are stress-related phenomena in which a psychosocial stressor results in the development of maladaptive states and psychiatric symptoms. The condition is presumed to be time limited, that is, a transitory reaction; symptoms recede when the stressor is removed or a new state of adaptation is defined. There are also other stress-related disorders in DSM-IV-TR, such as PTSD and acute stress disorder, those stress reactions that follow a disaster or cataclysmic personal event (American Psychiatric Association 2000). These stress disorders are among the few conditions in DSM-IV-TR, along with substance-induced disorders and mental disorders due to a general medical condition, with a *known cause* and for which the etiological agent is *essential* to establishing the diagnosis. For the most part, the DSM-IV-TR is relatively atheoretical with regard to etiology and is instead phenomenologically driven in its definitions of disorders (Feighner et al. 1972). However, the DSM-IV-TR stress-induced disorders, including the AD, require the diagnostician to impute etiological significance to a life event—a stressor—and relate its effect in clinical terms to the individual, his/her symptoms, and his/her behavior.

That the relationship between stress and the occurrence of a mental disorder is both complex and uncertain has caused many to question the theoretical basis of AD (Rutter 1981, Weiner and Del Gaudio 1976, Holmes and Rahe 1967). The linear model of stress–disease interaction, which serves as the model for AD has been questioned (Woolston 1988, Paykel et al. 1971). The linear model presupposes that a direct and clearly identifiable pathological reaction may follow a stressful event, a scenario that no doubt occurs in some individuals with AD but may not accurately characterize others. For example, there may be multiple stressors, insidious or chronic, as opposed to discrete events. Furthermore, relatively minor precipitating events may generate a disturbance in an individual who has previously been sensitized to stress.

Several authors have criticized the stressor criterion in AD because stressors are difficult to specify and measure, and their clinical implications and impact are uncertain (Fabrega and Mezzich 1987). Questions pertain to whether individuals with AD are unusually sensitive to psychosocial events not likely to cause disturbance in others. Are there individuals who have been exposed to high levels of stress, the severity or accumulation of which would probably produce negative consequences in most people?

Diverse variables and modifiers are involved in the presentation of AD after exposure to a stress. Cohen (1981) argued that acute stresses are different from chronic ones in both psychological and physiological terms; that the meaning of the stress is affected by "modifiers"—ego strengths, support systems, prior mastery—and that one must differentiate manifest and latent meaning of the stressors (e.g., loss of a job may be a relief or a catastrophe). An objectively overwhelming stress could have little impact on one individual, whereas another individual could regard a minor one as cataclysmic. A recent minor stress superimposed on a previous underlying (major) stress (which had no observable effect on its own) may have a significant impact, not operating independently but by its additive effect—the concatenation of events (Hamburg, personal communication).

Treatment

Appropriate and timely treatment is essential for individuals with AD so that their symptoms do not worsen; do not further impair their important relationships; and do not compromise their capacity to work, study, or be active in their interpersonal pursuits. Treatment must attempt to forestall further erosion of the individual's capacity to function that could ultimately have grave and untoward consequences.

There are two approaches to treatment. One is based on the understanding that this disorder emanates from a psychological reaction to a stressor. The stressor needs to be identified, described, and shared with the individual; plans must be made to mitigate it, if possible. The abnormal response may be attenuated if the stressor can be eliminated or reduced. Popkin and coworkers (1990) have shown that in the medically ill, the most common stressor is the medical illness itself; and the AD may remit when the medical illness improves or a new level of adaptation is reached. The other approach to treatment is to provide intervention for the symptomatic presentation, despite the fact that it does not reach the threshold level for a specific disorder, on the premise that it is associated with impairment and that treatments that are effective for more pronounced presentations of similar pathology are likely to be effective. This may include psychotherapy, pharmacotherapy, or a combination of the two (Schatzberg 1990).

Psychosocial Treatments

Psychotherapeutic intervention in AD is intended to reduce the effects of the stressor, enhance coping to the stressor that cannot be reduced or removed, and establish a mental state and support system to maximize adaptation. Psychotherapy can involve any one of several approaches: cognitive–behavioral treatment, interpersonal therapy, psychodynamic efforts, or counseling.

The first goal of these psychotherapies is to analyze the nature of the stressors affecting the individual to see whether they may be avoided or minimized. It is necessary to clarify and interpret the meaning of the stressor for the individual. For example, an amputation of the leg may have devastated an individual's feelings about himself or herself, especially if the individual was a runner. It is necessary to clarify that the individual still has enormous residual capacity; that he or she can engage in much meaningful work, does not have to lose valued relationships, and can still be sexually active; and that it does not necessarily mean that further body parts will be lost. (However, it will also involve redirecting the physical activity to another pastime.) Otherwise, the individual's pernicious fantasies ("all is lost") may take over in response to the stressor (i.e., amputation), make the individual dysfunctional (at work, sex), and precipitate a painful dysphoria or anxiety reaction.

Some stressors may elicit an overreaction (e.g., the individual's attempted suicide or homicide after abandonment by a lover). In such instances of overreaction with feelings, emotions, or behaviors, the therapist would help the individual put his or her feelings and rage into words rather than into destructive actions and gain some perspective. The role of verbalization and the joining of affects and conflicts cannot be overestimated in an attempt to reduce the pressure of the stressor and enhance coping. Drugs and alcohol are to be discouraged.

Psychotherapy, medical crisis counseling, crisis intervention, family therapy, group treatment, cognitive–behavioral treatment, and interpersonal therapy all encourage the individual to express affects, fears, anxiety, rage, helplessness, and hopelessness to the stressors imposed (Pollin and Holland 1992). They also assist the individual to reassess reality in the service of adaptation. Following the example given above, the loss of a leg is not the loss of one's life. But it is a major loss. Sifneos (1989) believed that individuals with AD could profit most from brief psychotherapy. The psychotherapy should attempt to reframe the meaning of the stress, find ways to minimize it, and diminish the psychological deficit due to its occurrence. The treatment should expose the concerns and conflicts that the individual is experiencing; help the individual gain perspective on the adversity; and encourage the individual to establish relationships and to attend support groups or self-help groups for assistance in the management of the stressor and the self.

Wise (1988), drawing from his experience in military psychiatry, emphasized the variables of brevity, immediacy, centrality, expectance, proximity, and simplicity (BICEPS principles). The treatment structure encompasses a simple straightforward approach dealing with the immediate situation at hand that is troubling the individual. The treatment approach is brief, usually no more than 72 hours (True and Benway 1992).

In another sample, interpersonal psychotherapy was applied to depressed outpatients with human immunodeficiency virus (HIV) infection and was found to be useful (Markowitz et al. 1992). Some of the attributes of interpersonal psychotherapy are psychoeducation regarding the sick role; using a here-and-now framework; formulation of the problems from an interpersonal perspective; exploration of options for changing dysfunctional behavior patterns; and identification of focused interpersonal problem areas. Lazarus (1992) described a seven-pronged approach in the treatment of minor depression. The therapy includes assertiveness training, enjoyable events, coping, imagery, time projection, cognitive disputation, role-playing, desensitization, family therapy, and biological prophylaxis.

Support groups have been demonstrated to help individuals adjust and enhance their coping mechanisms, and they may prolong life as well. Spiegel and coworkers (1989) showed that women with stage IV breast cancer lived longer after ongoing group therapy than those with standard cancer care. However, these findings on group psychological intervention and mortality have not been confirmed in at least two replication trials reported to date (Goodwin et al. 2001, Cunningham et al. 1998).

Stewart and colleagues (1992) emphasized the need to consider psychopharmacological interventions as well as psychotherapy for the treatment of minor depression, and this recommendation might be extrapolated to other subthreshold disorders. This group recommends antidepressant therapy if there is no benefit from 3 months of psychotherapy or other supportive measures. Although psychotherapy is the first choice treatment, psychotherapy combined with benzodiazepines may be helpful, especially for individuals with severe life stress(es) and a significant anxious component (Uhlenhuth et al. 1995, Shaner 2000). Tricyclic antidepressants or buspirone were recommended in place of benzodiazepines for individuals with current or past heavy alcohol use because of the greater risk of dependence in these individuals (Uhlenhuth et al. 1995).

Pharmacological Treatments

Psychotropic medication has been used in the medically ill, in the terminally ill, and in individuals who have been refractory to verbal therapies. Rosenberg and associates (1991) described that, in the medically ill with depressive disorders (the type of depression was unspecified), 16 of 29 individuals (55%) improved within 2 days of treatment with the maximal dose of amphetamine derivatives. The presence of delirium was associated with a decreased response. Whether methylphenidate is similarly useful in AD with depressed mood remains to be examined. Reynolds (1992), reviewing randomized controlled trials, concluded that bereavement-related syndromal depression also appears to respond to antidepressant medication. The medication chosen should reflect the nature of the predominant mood that accompanies the AD (e.g., benzodiazepines for AD with anxious mood; antidepressants for AD with depressed mood). For example, Schatzberg (1990) recommended that the therapist consider both psychotherapy and pharmacotherapy in the AD with anxious mood and that the psychiatrist prescribe anxiolytics as part of the treatment.

Other authors have begun to examine the effect of homeopathic treatments. From a 25-week multicenter randomized placebo-controlled double-blind trial, a special extract from kava kava was reported to be effective in AD with anxiety and without the adverse side-effect profile associated with tricyclics and benzodiazepines (Volz and Kieser 1997). Tianeptine, alprazolam, and mianserin were found to be equally effective in symptom improvement in individuals with AD and anxious mood (Ansseau et al. 1996). In a random double-blind study, trazodone was more effective than clorazepate in individuals with cancer for the relief of anxious and depressed symptoms (Razavi et al. 1999). Similar findings were observed in HIV-positive individuals with AD (DeWit et al. 1999).

Those individuals who do not respond to counseling or the various modes of psychotherapy that have been outlined and to a trial of antidepressant or anxiolytic medications should be regarded as treatment nonresponders. It is essential to reevaluate the individual to ensure that the diagnostic impression has not altered and, in particular, that the individual has not developed a major mental disorder, which would require a more aggressive treatment, often biological. The clinician must also consider that an Axis II disorder might be interfering with the individual's resolution of the AD. Finally, if the stressor continues and cannot be removed (e.g., the continuation of a seriously impairing chronic illness), additional support and management strategies need to be employed to assist the individual in optimally adapting to the stressor.

Comparison of DSM-IV-TR/ICD-10 Diagnostic Criteria

In contrast to DSM-IV-TR (which requires the onset of symptoms within 3 months of the stressor), the ICD-10 Diagnostic Criteria for Research specify an onset within 1 month. Furthermore, ICD-10 excludes stressors of "unusual or catastrophic type." In contrast, DSM-IV-TR allows extreme stressors so long as the criteria are not met for posttraumatic or acute stress disorder. ICD-10 also provides for several different subtypes, including "brief depressive reaction" (depressive state lasting 1 month or less), "prolonged depressive reaction" (depressive state lasting up to 2 years).

References

American Psychiatric Association (1980) *Diagnostic and Statistical Manual of Mental Disorders*, 3rd ed. APA, Washington, DC.

American Psychiatric Association (1987) *Diagnostic and Statistical Manual of Mental Disorders*, 3rd ed., Rev. APA Washington, DC.

American Psychiatric Association (2000) *Diagnostic and Statistical Manual of Mental Disorders*, 4th ed., Text Rev. APA, Washington, DC.

Andreasen NC and Hoenk PR (1982) The predictive value of adjustment disorders: a follow-up study. *Am J Psychiatry* **139**, 584–590.

Andreasen NC and Wasek P (1980) Adjustment disorders in adolescents and adults. *Arch Gen Psychiatry* **37**, 1166–1170.

Ansseau M, Bataille M, Briole G, et al. (1996) Controlled comparison of tianeptine, alprazolam and mianserin in the treatment of adjustment disorders with anxiety and depression. *Hum Psychopharmacol Clin Exp* **11**, 293–298.

Aoki T, Hosaka T, and Ishida A (1995) Psychiatric evaluation of physical rehabilitation patients. *Gen Hosp Psychiatry* **17**, 440–443.

Bird HR, Canino G, Rubio-Stipec M, et al. (1988) Estimates of the prevalence of childhood maladjustment in a community survey in Puerto Rico. *Arch Gen Psychiatry* **45**, 1120–1126.

Bird HR, Gould MS, Yager T, et al. (1989) Risk factors for maladjustment in Puerto Rican children. *J Am Acad Child Adolesc Psychiatry* **28**, 847–850.

Cohen F (1981) Stress and bodily illness. *Psychiatr Clin North Am* **4**, 269–286.

Cunningham AJ, Edmonds CV, Jenkins GP, et al. (1998) A randomized controlled trial of the effects of group psychological therapy on survival in women with metastatic breast cancer. *Psychooncology* **7**, 508–517.

DeWit S, Cremers L, Hirsch D, et al. (1999) Efficacy of trazodone versus clorazepate in the treatment of HIV-positive subjects with adjustment disorder: a pilot study. *J Int Med Res* **27**, 223–232.

Doan RJ and Petti TA (1989) Clinical and demographic characteristics of child and adolescent partial hospital patients. *J Am Acad Child Adolesc Psychiatry* **28**(1), 66–69.

Fabrega H Jr. and Mezzich J (1987) Adjustment disorder and psychiatric practice: cultural and historical aspects. *Psychiatry* **50**, 31–49.

Fabrega H Jr., Mezzich J, Mezzich AC, et al. (1986) Descriptive validity of DSM-I. II. depressions. *J Nerv Ment Dis* **174**, 573–584.

Fabrega H Jr., Mezzich JE, Mezzich AC, et al. (1987) Adjustment disorder as a marginal or transitional illness category in DSM-III. *Arch Gen Psychiatry* **44**, 567–572.

Faulstich ME, Moore JR, Carey MP, et al. (1986) Prevalence of DSM-III conduct and adjustment disorders for adolescent psychiatric inpatients. *Adolescence* **21**, 333–337.

Feighner JP, Robins E, Guze SB, et al. (1972) Diagnostic criteria for use in psychiatric research. *Arch Gen Psychiatry* **26**, 57–63.

Fowler RC, Rich CL, and Young D (1986) San Diego suicide study II. substance abuse in young cases. *Arch Gen Psychiatry* **43**, 962–965.

Goodwin PJ, Leszcz M, Ennis M, et al. (2001) The effect of group psychosocial support on survival in metastatic breast cancer. *N Engl J Med* **345**, 1719–1726.

Grassi L, Gritti P, Rigatelli M, et al. (2000) Psychosocial problems secondary to cancer: an Italian multicenter survey of consultation-liaison psychiatry in oncology. Italian consultation liaison group. *Eur J Cancer* **36**, 579–585.

Hillard JR, Slomowitz M, and Levi LS (1987) A retrospective study of adolescents' visits to a general hospital psychiatric emergency service. *Am J Psychiatry* **144**, 432–436.

Holmes TH and Rahe RH (1967) The social readjustment rating scale. *J Psychosom Res* **11**, 213–218.

Jacobson AM, Goldberg ID, Burns BJ, et al. (1980) Diagnosed mental disorder in children and use of health services in four organized health care settings. *Am J Psychiatry* **137**, 559–565.

Jones R, Yates WR, Williams S, et al. (1999) Outcome for adjustment disorder with depressed mood: comparison with other mood disorders. *J Affect Disord* **55**, 55–61.

Keller M, Klein DN, Hirschfeld RMA, et al. (1995) Results of the DSM-IV mood disorders field trial. *Am J Psychiatry* **152**, 843–849.

Kellerman M, Jehete I, Gesztelyi R, et al. (1994) Screening for depressive symptoms in acute phase of a stroke. *Gen Hosp Psychiatry* **21**, 116–121.

Kovacs M, Feinberg TL, Crouse-Novak MA, et al. (1984) Depressive disorders in childhood. I. A longitudinal prospective study of characteristics and recovery. *Arch Gen Psychiatry* **41**, 643–649.

Kovacs M, Gatsonis C, Pollock M, et al. (1994) A controlled prospective study of DSM-III adjustment disorder in childhood. *Arch Gen Psychiatry* **51**, 535–541.

Kugaya A, Akechi T, Okuyama T, et al. (2000) Prevalence, predictive factors, and screening for psychological distress in patients with newly diagnosed head and neck cancers. *Cancer* **88**, 2817–2823.

Lazarus AA (1992) The multimodal approach to the treatment of minor depression. *Am J Psychother* **46**, 50–57.

Markowitz JC, Klerman GL, and Perry SW (1992) Interpersonal psychotherapy of depressed HIV-positive outpatients. *Hosp Comm Psychiatry* **43**, 885–890.

McGrath J (1989) A survey of deliberate self-poisoning. *Med J Aust* **150**, 317–318.

McNair DM, Lorr M, and Doppelman LF (eds) (1971) *Manual for the Profile of Mood States.* Educational and Industrial Testing Service, San Diego, CA.

Mezzich JE, Dow JT, Rich CL, et al. (1981) Developing an efficient clinical information system for a comprehensive psychiatric institute. II. Initial evaluation form. *Behav Res Methods Instrum* **13**, 464–478.

Mezzich JE, Fabrega H Jr., Coffman GA, et al. (1989) DSM-III disorders in a large sample of psychiatric patients: frequency and specificity of diagnoses. *Am J Psychiatry* **146**, 212–219.

Minnaar GK, Schlebusch L, and Levin A (1980) A current study of parasuicide in Durban. *S Afr Med J* **57**, 204–207.

Oxman TE, Barrett JE, Freeman DH, et al. (1994) Frequency and correlates of adjustment disorder relates to cardiac surgery in older patients. *Psychosomatics* **35**, 557–568.

Paykel ES, Prusoff BA, and Uhlenhuth EH (1971) Scaling of life events. *Arch Gen Psychiatry* **25**, 340–347.

Perez-Jimenez JP, Gomez-Bajo GJ, LopezCatillo JJ, et al. (1994) Psychiatric consultation and posttraumatic stress disorder in burned patients. *Burns* **20**, 532–536.

Perris H, von Knorring L, Oreland L, et al. (1984) Life events and biological vulnerability: a study of life events and platelet MAO activity in depressed patients. *Psychiatr Res* **12**, 111–120.

Pollin IS and Holland J (1992) A model for counseling the medically ill: the Linda Pollin Foundation approach. *Gen Hosp Psychiatry* **14**(Suppl. 6), 15–25.

Popkin MK, Callies AL, Colon EA, et al. (1990) Adjustment disorders in medically ill patients referred for consultation in a university hospital. *Psychosomatics* **31**, 410–414.

Pozzi G, Del Borgo C, Del Forna A, et al. (1999) Psychological discomfort and mental illness in patients with AIDS: implications for home care. *STDS* **13**, 555–564.

Pulimood S, Rajagopalan B, Rajagopalan M, et al. (1996) Psychiatric morbidity among dermatology inpatients. *Nat Med J India* **9**, 208–210.

Razavi D, Kormoss N, Collard A, et al. (1999) Comparative study of the efficacy and safety of trazodone versus clorazepate in the treatment of adjustment disorders in cancer patients: a pilot study. *J Int Med Res* **27**, 280–287.

Reynolds CF (1992) Treatment of depression in special populations. *J Clin Psychiatry* **53**(Suppl.), 45–53.

Rosenberg PB, Ahmed I, and Hurwitz S (1991) Methylphenidate in depressed medically ill patients. *J Clin Psychiatry* **52**, 263–267.

Runeson B (1989) Mental disorder in youth suicide: DSM-III-R axes I and II. *Acta Psychiatr Scand* **79**, 490–497.

Rutter M (1981) Stress, coping and development: some issues and some questions. *J Child Psychol Psychiatry* **22**, 323–356.

Schatzberg AF (1990) Anxiety and adjustment disorder: a treatment approach. *J Clin Psychiatry* **51**(Suppl.), 20–24.

Schnyder U and Valach L (1997) Suicide attempters in a psychiatric emergency room population. *Gen Hosp Psychiatry* **19**, 119–129.

Setterberg SR, Ernst M, Rao U, et al. (1991) Child psychiatrists' views of DSM-III-R: survey of usage and opinions. *J Am Acad Child Adolesc Psychiatry* **30**, 652–658.

Shaffer D, Gould MS, Brasic J, et al. (1983) A children's global assessment scale (CGAS). *Arch Gen Psychiatry* **40**, 1228–1231.

Shaner R (2000) Benzodiazepines in psychiatric emergency settings. *Psychiatr Ann* **30**, 268–289.

Shima S, Kitagawa Y, Kitamura T, et al. (1994) Poststroke depression. *Gen Hosp Psychiatry* **16**, 286–289.

Sifneos PE (1989) Brief dynamic and crisis therapy. In *Comprehensive Textbook of Psychiatry*, Vol. 2, 5th ed., Kaplan HI and Sadock BJ (eds). Williams & Wilkins, Baltimore, pp. 1562–1567.

Snyder S and Strain JJ (1989) Differentiation of major depression and adjustment disorder with depressed mood in the medical setting. *Gen Hosp Psychiatry* **12**, 159–165.

Spiegel D (1996) Cancer and depression. *Br J Psychiatry* **168**(Suppl. 30), 109–116.

Spiegel D, Bloom JR, Kraemer HC, et al. (1989) Effect of psychosocial treatment on survival in breast cancer. *Lancet* **1**, 888–891.

Stewart JW, Quitkin FM, and Klein DF (1992) The pharmacotherapy of minor depression. *Am J Psychother* **46**, 23–36.

Sullivan MJ, Winshenker B, and Mikail S (1995) Screening for major depression in the early stages of multiple sclerosis. *Can J Neurol Sci* **22**, 228–231.

True PK and Benway MW (1992) Treatment of stress reaction prior to combat using the "BICEPS" model. *Mil Med* **157**, 380–381.

Uhlenhuth EH, Balter MB, Ban TA, et al. (1995) International study of expert judgment on therapeutic use of benzodiazepines and other psychotherapeutic medications. III. Clinical features affecting experts' therapeutic recommendations in anxiety disorders. *Psychopharmacol Bull* **31**, 289–296.

Volz HP and Kieser M (1997) Kava-kava extract WS 1490 versus placebo in anxiety disorders: a randomized placebo-controlled 25-week outpatient trial. *Pharmacopsychiatry* **30**, 1–5.

Weiner IB and Del Gaudio AC (1976) Psychopathology in adolescence: an epidemiological study. *Arch Gen Psychiatry* **33**, 187–193.

Wise MG (1988) Adjustment disorders and impulse control disorders not otherwise classified. In *Textbook of Psychiatry*, Talbot JA, Hales R, and Yodofsky SC (eds). American Psychiatric Press, Washington, DC, pp. 605–620.

Woolston JL (1988) Theoretical considerations of the adjustment disorders. *J Am Acad Child Adolesc Psychiatry* **27**, 280–287.

Zilberg NJ, Weiss DS, and Horowitz MJ (1982) Impact of event scale: a cross-validation study and some empirical evidence supporting a conceptual model of stress response syndromes. *J Consult Clin Psychol* **50**, 407–414.

Zung W (1965) A self-rating depression scale. *Arch Gen Psychiatry* **12**, 63–70.

Zung W (1971) A rating instrument for anxiety disorders. *Psychosomatics* **12**, 371–379.

Everybody has a personality, or a characteristic manner of thinking, feeling, behaving, and relating to others. Some persons are typically introverted and withdrawn, others are more extraverted and outgoing. Some persons are invariably conscientious and efficient, whereas other persons might be consistently undependable and negligent. Some persons are characteristically anxious and apprehensive, whereas others are typically relaxed and unconcerned. These personality traits are often felt to be integral to each person's sense of self, as they involve what persons value, what they do, and their innate tendencies and preferences.

It is "when personality traits are inflexible and maladaptive and cause significant functional impairment or subjective distress [that] they constitute Personality Disorders" (American Psychiatric Association 2000, page 686). The DSM-IV-TR provides the diagnostic criteria for 10 personality disorders. Two additional diagnoses are placed within an appendix to DSM-IV-TR for criteria sets provided for further study (passive–aggressive and depressive). This chapter begins with a discussion of the diagnosis, etiology, and treatment of personality disorders in general, followed by a discussion of these issues for the 12 individual personality disorders.

PERSONALITY DISORDER

Diagnosis
A personality disorder is defined in DSM-IV-TR as "an enduring pattern of inner experience and behavior that deviates markedly from the expectations of the individual's culture, is pervasive and inflexible, has an onset in adolescence or early adulthood, is stable over time, and leads to distress or impairment" (American Psychiatric Association 2000, page 686). The DSM-IV-TR general diagnostic criteria for a personality disorder is provided below.

DSM-IV-TR General Diagnostic Criteria

Personality Disorder

A. An enduring pattern of inner experience and behavior that deviates markedly from the expectations of the individual's culture. This pattern is manifested in two (or more) of the following areas:

   (1) cognition (i.e., ways of perceiving and interpreting self, other people, and events)
   (2) affectivity (i.e., the range, intensity, lability, and appropriateness of emotional response)
   (3) interpersonal functioning
   (4) impulse control

B. The enduring pattern is inflexible and pervasive across a broad range of personal and social situations.
C. The enduring pattern leads to clinically significant distress or impairment in social, occupational, or other important areas of functioning.
D. The pattern is stable and of long duration and its onset can be traced back at least to adolescence or early adulthood.
E. The enduring pattern is not better accounted for as a manifestation or consequence of another mental disorder.
F. The enduring pattern is not due to the direct physiological effects of a substance (e.g., a drug of abuse, a medication) or a general medical condition (e.g., head trauma).

Personality disorder is the only class of mental disorders in DSM-IV-TR for which an explicit definition and criterion set are provided. A general definition and criterion set can be useful to clinicians because the most common personality disorder diagnosis in clinical practice is often the diagnosis "not otherwise specified" (NOS) (Clark et al. 1995). Clinicians provide the NOS diagnosis when they determine that a personality disorder is present but the symptomatology fails to meet the criterion set for one of the 10 specific personality disorders. A general definition of what is meant by a personality disorder is therefore helpful when determining whether the NOS diagnosis should in fact be provided. Points worth emphasizing with respect to the general criterion set are presented in the following discussion of the assessment, differential diagnosis, epidemiology, and course of personality disorders.

Assessment instruments are available to help clinicians obtain reliable and valid personality disorder diagnoses. Semistructured interviews will obtain reliable diagnoses of personality disorders and are therefore the preferred method for the assessment of personality disorders in clinical research (Kaye and Shea 2000, Widiger and Coker 2002, Zimmerman 1994). Semistructured interviews provide a researched set of required and recommended interview queries and observations to assess each of the personality disorder diagnostic criteria. Clinicians can find the administration of a semistructured interview to be constraining (Westen 1997), but a major strength of semistructured interviews is their assurance through an explicit structure that each relevant diagnostic criterion has in fact been systematically assessed. Idiosyncratic and subjective interviewing techniques are much more likely to result in gender- and culturally biased assessments relative to unstructured clinical interviews (Garb 1997, Widiger 1998). The manuals that accompany a semistructured interview also provide useful information for understanding the rationale of each diagnostic criterion, for interpreting vague or inconsistent symptomatology, and for resolving diagnostic ambiguities. There are currently five semistructured interviews for the assessment of the DSM-IV-TR (American Psychiatric Association 2000) personality disorder diagnostic criteria: (1) Diagnostic Interview for Personality Disorders (Zanarini et al. 1995); (2) International Personality Disorder Examination (Loranger 1999); (3) Personality Disorder Interview-IV (Widiger et al. 1995); (4) Structured Clinical Interview for DSM-IV-TR Axis II Personality Disorders (First et al. 1997); and (5) Structured Interview for DSM-IV-TR Personality Disorders (Pfohl et al. 1997). The particular advantages and disadvantages of each particular interview have been discussed extensively (Clark and Harrison 2001, Kaye and Shea 2000, Widiger and Coker 2002, Zimmerman 1994).

The administration of an entire personality disorder semistructured interview can take 2 hours, an amount of time that is impractical for routine clinical practice. However, this time can be reduced substantially by first administering a self-report questionnaire that screens for the presence of the DSM-IV-TR personality disorders (Widiger and Coker 2002). A clinician can then confine the interview to the few personality disorders that the self-report inventory suggested would be present. Self-report inventories are useful in ensuring that all of the personality disorders were systematically considered and in alerting the clinician to the presence of maladaptive personality traits that might otherwise have been missed. There are a number of alternative self-report inventories that can be used and the advantages and disadvantages of each of them have been discussed extensively (Clark and Harrison 2001, Kaye and Shea 2000, Millon et al. 1996, Widiger and Coker 2002).

Gender and cultural biases are one potential source of inaccurate personality disorder diagnosis that are worth noting in particular (Alarcon 1996, Garb 1997, Widiger 1998). One of the general diagnostic criteria for personality disorder is that the personality trait must deviate markedly from the expectations of a person's culture (see DSM-IV-TR general diagnostic criteria for Personality Disorder on page 1230). The purpose of this cultural deviation requirement is to compel clinicians to consider the cultural background of the individual. A behavior pattern that appears to be aberrant from the perspective of one's own culture (e.g., submissiveness or emotionality) could be quite normative and adaptive within another culture. The cultural expectations or norms of the clinician might not be relevant or applicable to an individual from a different cultural background. However, one should not infer from this requirement that a personality disorder is primarily or simply a deviation from a cultural norm. Deviation from the expectations of one's culture is not necessarily maladaptive, nor is conformity to one's culture necessarily healthy. Many of the personality disorders may even represent (in part) extreme or excessive variants of behavior patterns that are valued or encouraged within a particular culture. For example, it is usually adaptive to be confident but not to be arrogant, to be agreeable but not to be submissive, or to be conscientious but not to be perfectionistic. Gender and cultural biases of particular relevance to individual personality disorders will be discussed further in the chapter.

Alternative dimensional models of personality disorder are being developed. One such model, based on a theory of temperament and character, consists of seven dimensions. Cloninger (2000) proposes that there are four temperaments (reward dependence, harm avoidance, novelty seeking, and persistence), each governed by a particular neurotransmitter system, and three character dimensions (self-directedness, cooperativeness, and self-transcendence). The presence of a personality disorder is said to be determined primarily by the four temperaments and the particular form or manner of the personality disorder by the three character dimensions.

Another approach has been to apply the predominant model of general personality functioning to the study of personality disorders. Five broad domains of personality functioning have been identified empirically through the study of the languages of a number of different cultures (Hogan et al. 1997, Pervin and John 1999). Language can be understood as a sedimentary deposit of the observations of persons over the thousands of years of the language's development and transformation. The most important domains of personality functioning would be those with the greatest number of terms to describe and differentiate their various manifestations and nuances, and the structure of personality will be evident by the empirical relationship among the trait terms. Such lexical analyses of languages have typically identified five fundamental dimensions of personality: neuroticism (or negative affectivity) versus emotional stability, introversion versus extraversion, conscientiousness versus undependability, antagonism versus agreeableness, and closedness versus openness to experience (Costa and McCrae 1992). Each of these five broad domains can be differentiated further in terms of underlying facets. For example, the facets of antagonism versus agreeableness include suspiciousness versus trusting gullibility, tough-mindedness versus tender-mindedness, confidence and arrogance versus modesty and meekness, exploitation versus altruism and sacrifice, oppositionalism and aggression versus compliance, and deception and manipulation versus straightforwardness and honesty (Costa and McCrae 1992). Each of the DSM-IV-TR personality disorders can be understood as maladaptive variants of these personality traits that are evident in all persons to varying degrees (Widiger et al. 2002).

Table 44-1 provides a description of the DSM-IV-TR personality disorders in terms of this five-factor model. For example, the schizoid personality disorder (SZPD) may represent an extreme variant of introversion, avoidant may represent extreme neuroticism and introversion, and antisocial personality disorder (ASPD) may represent an extreme variant of antagonism and undependability. Advantages of understanding personality disorders in terms of this dimensional model are the provision of more specific descriptions of each of the individuals (including adaptive as well as maladaptive personality functioning) and the avoidance of arbitrary categorical distinctions. An additional factor is the ability to bring to bear on an understanding of personality disorders the extensive amount of research on

| Table 44-1 | DSM-IV-TR Personality Disorders from the Perspective of the Five-Factor Model of General Personality Functioning | | | | | | | | | |

	PRN	SZD	SZT	ATS	BDL	HST	NCS	AVD	DPD	OCP
Neuroticism										
Anxiousness			High		High			High	High	
Angry hostility	High			High	High		High			
Depressiveness					High	High		High		
Self-consciousness						High	High	High	High	
Impulsivity					High					
Vulnerability					High			High	High	
Extraversion										
Warmth		Low	Low			High			High	
Gregariousness		Low	Low			High		Low		
Assertiveness								Low	Low	High
Activity										
Excitement seeking				High		High		Low		
Positive emotionality		Low	Low			High				
Openness										
Fantasy			High			High	High			
Aesthetics										
Feelings		Low				High				
Actions			High							
Ideas			High							
Values										Low
Agreeableness										
Trust	Low		Low		Low	High			High	
Straightforwardness	Low			Low						
Altruism					Low		Low		High	
Compliance				Low	Low				High	Low
Modesty							Low		High	
Tender-mindedness				Low			Low			
Conscientiousness										
Competence					Low					High
Order										High
Dutifulness				Low						High
Achievement-striving							High			High
Self-discipline				Low						
Deliberation				Low						

the heritability, temperament, development, and course of general personality functioning (Costa and Widiger 2002).

Epidemiology

Estimates of the prevalence of personality disorder within clinical settings is typically above 50% (Mattia and Zimmerman 2001). As many as 60% of inpatients within some clinical settings would be diagnosed with borderline personality disorder (BPD) (American Psychiatric Association 2000, Gunderson 2001) and as many as 50% of inmates within a correctional setting could be diagnosed with ASPD (Widiger and Corbitt 1995). Although the comorbid presence of a personality disorder is likely to have an important impact on the course and treatment of an Axis I disorder (Dolan-Sewell et al. 2001), the prevalence of personality disorder is generally underestimated in clinical practice owing in part to the failure to provide systematic or comprehensive assessments of personality disorder symptomatology and perhaps as well to the lack of funding for the treatment of personality disorders (Zimmerman and Mattia, 1999).

According to the best available estimates, approximately 10 to 15% of the general population would be diagnosed with one of the 10 DSM-IV-TR personality disorders, excluding personality disorder not otherwise specified (PDNOS) (Mattia and Zimmerman 2001, Torgersen et al. 2001). Table 44-2 provides prevalence data reported by the best available studies to date for estimating the prevalence of individual personality disorders within a community population. All of these studies have important limitations, though, that qualify their results. For example, many of the studies sampled persons who would probably have less personality disorder pathology than a randomly selected sample (e.g., some studies have sampled persons without any history of Axis I psychopathology) and the studies have used either the DSM-III (American Psychiatric Association 1980) or DSM-III-R (American Psychiatric Association 1987) criterion sets rather than DSM-IV-TR (American Psychiatric Association 2000). Nevertheless, the prevalence estimates are generally close to those provided in DSM-IV-TR. Prevalence rates for individual personality disorders will be discussed later in this chapter.

There is also considerable personality disorder diagnostic co-occurrence (Bornstein 1998, Lilienfeld et al. 1994, Oldham et al. 1992, Widiger and Trull 1998). Individuals who meet the DSM-IV-TR diagnostic criteria for one personality disorder are likely to meet the diagnostic criteria for another. DSM-IV-TR instructs clinicians that all diagnoses should be recorded because it can be important to consider, for example, the presence of antisocial traits in someone with a BPD or the presence of paranoid traits in someone with a dependent personality disorder (DPD). However, the extent of diagnostic co-occurrence is at times so extensive that most researchers prefer a more dimensional description of personality (Cloninger 2000, Livesley 1998, Oldham and Skodol 2000, Widiger 2000). Diagnostic categories provide clear, vivid descriptions of discrete personality types, but the personality structure of actual individuals might be more accurately described by a constellation of maladaptive personality traits.

Course

Personality disorders must be evident since adolescence or young adulthood and have been relatively chronic and stable throughout adult life (see DSM-IV-TR general diagnostic criteria for personality disorder on page 1230). The World Health Organization's (WHO) *International Classification of Diseases*, 10th Revision (ICD-10, World Health Organization 1992) does recognize the existence of personality change secondary to catastrophic experiences and to brain injury or disease, but only the latter is included within DSM-IV-TR (American Psychiatric Association 2000). A 75-year-old man can be diagnosed with a DSM-IV-TR DPD, but the symptoms must have been present throughout the duration of his adulthood (e.g., since the age of 18 years), unless the dependent behavior was a direct, explicit expression of a neurochemical disease or lesion.

The requirement that a personality disorder be evident since late adolescence and be relatively chronic thereafter has been a traditional means by which to distinguish a personality disorder from an Axis I disorder (Millon et al. 1996, Spitzer et al. 1980). Mood, anxiety, psychotic, sexual, and other mental disorders have traditionally been conceptualized as conditions that arise at some point during a person's life and that are relatively limited or circumscribed in their expression and duration. Personality disorders, in contrast, are conditions that are evident as early as late adolescence (and in some instances prior to that time), are evident in everyday functioning, and are stable throughout adulthood. However, the consistency of this distinction across disorders in the classification has been decreasing with each edition of the DSM, as early-onset and chronic variants of Axis I disorders are being added to the diagnostic manual (e.g., early-onset dysthymia and generalized social phobia). Some researchers have in fact suggested abandoning the concept of personality disorders and replacing them with early-onset and chronic variants of existing Axis I disorders. For example, avoidant personality disorder could become generalized social

Table 44-2	Epidemiology of Personality Disorders														
	Sample	N	Int	DSM	PRN	SZD	STP	ATS	BDL	HST	NCS	AVD	DPD	OCP	PAG
Black et al. (1993)	R-HN	127	SIDP	III	1.6	0.0	3.9	0.0	5.5	3.9	0.0	3.2	2.4	7.9	12.6
Black et al. (1993)	R-OCD	120	SIDP	III	1.7	0.0	2.5	0.8	0.8	2.5	0.0	0.8	0.8	10.8	8.3
Coryell et al. (1989)	R-HN	185	SIDP	III	0.5	1.6	2.2	1.6	1.1	1.6	0.0	1.6	0.5	3.2	2.2
Drake et al. (1998)	Men(47)	369	Clinical	III	1.1	4.1	2.4	0.8	0.5	3.8	3.5	1.6	10.3	0.5	7.8
Klein et al. (1995)	R-DP	258	PDE	III-R	1.7	0.9	0.0	2.2	1.7	1.7	3.9	5.2	0.4	2.6	1.7
Lenzenweger et al. (1997)	Stdts	1646	PDE	III-R	0.4	0.4	0.0	0.8	0.0	1.9	1.2	0.4	0.4	0.0	0.0
Maier et al. (1992)	Comm	452	SCID-II	III-R	1.8	0.4	0.7	0.2	1.1	1.3	0.0	1.1	1.5	2.2	1.8
Moldin et al. (1994)	HN	302	PDE	III-R	0.0	0.0	0.7	2.6	2.0	0.3	0.0	0.7	1.0	0.7	1.7
Samuels et al. (1994)	Comm	762	Clinical	III	0.0	0.0	0.1	1.5	0.4	2.1	0.0	0.0	0.1	1.7	0.1
Torgersen et al. (2001)	Comm	2053	SIDP-R	III-R	2.4	1.7	0.6	0.7	0.7	2.0	0.8	5.0	1.5	2.0	1.7
Median					1.4	0.4	0.7	0.8	1.0	2.0	0.0	1.4	0.9	2.1	1.7
DSM-IV estimates					.5–2.5	uncm	3.0	2.0	2.0	2–3	<1	.5–1	—	1.0	

Note: N, number of persons in study; Int, interview that was used; DSM, Edition of Diagnostic and Statistical Manual that was used (DSM-III or DSM-III-R); PRN, paranoid; SZD, schizoid; STP, schizotypal; ATS, antisocial; BDL, borderline; HST, histrionic; NCS, narcissistic; AVD, avoidant; DPD, dependent; OCP, obsessive–compulsive; PAG, passive–aggressive; R-HN, relatives of hyper-normal (persons without history of mental disorder); R-OCD, relatives of persons with obsessive–compulsive anxiety disorder; Men(47), males of approximate age of 47 years; R-DP, relatives of persons with depression; Stdts, students; Comm, community; SIDP, Structured Interview for Personality Disorder (Pfohl B, Blum N, and Zimmerman M (1997) *Structured Interview for DSM-IV-TR Personality Disorder*. American Psychiatric Press, Washington, DC.); SCID-II, Structured Clinical Interview for DSM personality disorder (First M, Gibbon M, Spitzer RL, et al. (1997) *User's Guide for the Structured Clinical Interview for DSM-IV-TR Axis II Personality Disorders*. American Psychiatric Press, Washington, DC.); Clinical, unstructured or unspecified semistructured interview; PDE, Personality Disorder Examination; uncm, uncommon.

phobia, obsessive–compulsive personality disorder (OCPD) could become an early-onset variant of obsessive–compulsive anxiety disorder (OCAD), and BPD could become an early-onset and chronic mood dyscontrol. A precedent for this revision of the diagnostic manual is that ICD-10 currently does not include a diagnosis of schizotypal personality disorder (STPD), including instead a diagnosis of schizotypal disorder that is an early-onset and chronic variant of schizophrenia (World Health Organization 1992).

Etiology

A primary purpose of a diagnosis is to lead to scientific knowledge concerning the etiology for an individual's condition and the identification of a specific pathology for which a particular treatment (e.g., medication) would ameliorate the condition (Frances et al. 1995). However, many of the mental disorders in DSM-IV-TR, including the personality disorders, may not in fact have single etiologies or even specific pathologies. The DSM-IV-TR personality disorders might be, for the most part, constellations of maladaptive personality traits that are the result of multiple genetic dispositions interacting with a variety of detrimental environmental experiences (Clark and Watson 1999, Widiger and Sankis 2000). The DSM-IV-TR personality disorder diagnoses do provide the clinician with a substantial amount of important information concerning the etiology and pathology for an individual's particular personality syndrome, but there are likely to be alternative pathways to the development of maladaptive personality traits and alternative neurophysiological, cognitive–behavioral, interpersonal, and psychodynamic models for their pathology (Livesley 2001).

Treatment

One of the mistaken assumptions or expectations of Axis II is that personality disorders are untreatable. In fact, maladaptive personality traits are often the focus of clinical treatment (Beck and Freeman 1990, Benjamin 1993, Gabbard 2000, Gunderson and Gabbard 2000, Millon et al. 1996, Markovitz 2001, Paris 1998, Stone 1993). Personality disorders are among the more difficult of mental disorders to treat as they involve entrenched behavior patterns, some of which will be integral to an individual's self-image (Millon et al. 1996, Stone 1993). Nevertheless, there is compelling empirical support to indicate that meaningful responsivity to psychosocial and pharmacologic treatment does occur (Markovitz 2001, Perry et al. 1999, Sanislow and McGlashan 1998). Treatment of a personality disorder is unlikely to result in the development of a fully healthy or ideal personality structure, but clinically and socially meaningful change to personality structure and functioning does occur. In fact, given the considerable social, occupational, medical, and other costs that are engendered by such personality disorders as the antisocial and borderline, even marginal reductions in symptomatology can represent quite significant and meaningful public health care, social, and clinical benefits (Linehan 1993, 2000).

Specific DSM-IV-TR Personality Disorders

DSM-IV-TR includes 10 individual personality disorder diagnoses that are organized into three clusters: (a) paranoid, schizoid, and schizotypal (placed within an odd–eccentric cluster); (b) antisocial, borderline, histrionic, and narcissistic (dramatic–emotional–erratic cluster); and (c) avoidant, dependent, and obsessive–compulsive (anxious–fearful cluster) (American Psychiatric Association 2000). Each of these personality disorders, along with the two that are included in the appendix to DSM-IV-TR for disorders needing further study (i.e., passive–aggressive and depressive), will be discussed in turn.

CLUSTER A

PARANOID PERSONALITY DISORDER

Diagnosis

Paranoid personality disorder (PPD) involves a pervasive and continuous distrust and suspiciousness of the motives of others (American Psychiatric Association 2000), but the disorder is more than just suspiciousness. Persons with this disorder are also hypersensitive to criticism, they respond with anger to threats to their autonomy, they incessantly seek out confirmations of their suspicions, and they tend to be quite rigid in their beliefs and perceptions of others (Millon et al. 1996, Widiger et al. 1995). The presence of PPD is indicated by four or more of the seven diagnostic criteria presented in the DSM-IV-TR criteria for PPD (see below).

DSM-IV-TR Diagnostic Criteria

301.0 Paranoid Personality Disorder

A. A pervasive distrust and suspiciousness of others such that their motives are interpreted as malevolent, beginning by early adulthood, and present in a variety of contexts, as indicated by four (or more) of the following:

   (1) suspects, without sufficient basis, that others are exploiting, harming, or deceiving him or her
   (2) is preoccupied with unjustified doubts about the loyalty or trustworthiness of friends or associates
   (3) is reluctant to confide in others because of unwarranted fear that the information will be used maliciously against him or her
   (4) reads hidden demeaning or threatening meanings into benign remarks or events
   (5) persistently bears grudges, i.e. is unforgiving of insults, injuries, or slights
   (6) perceives attacks on his or her character or reputation that are not apparent to others and is quick to react angrily or to counterattack
   (7) has recurrent suspicions, without justification, regarding fidelity of spouse or sexual partner.

B. Does not occur exclusively during the course of schizophrenia, a mood disorder with psychotic features, or another psychotic disorder, and is not due to the direct physiological effects of a general medical condition.

Note: if criteria are met prior to the onset of schizophrenia, add "premorbid," e.g., paranoid personality disorder (premorbid).

Epidemiology

Trust versus mistrust is a fundamental personality trait along which all persons vary (Pervin and John 1999). Thirteen percent of the adult male population and 6% of the adult female population may be characteristically mistrustful of others (Costa and McCrae

1992). However, only 0.5 to 2.5% of the population are likely to meet the DSM-IV-TR diagnostic criteria for a PPD. It is suggested in DSM-IV-TR that approximately 10 to 30% of persons within inpatient settings and 2 to 10% within outpatient settings have this disorder (American Psychiatric Association 2000), but the lower end of these rates may represent the more accurate estimate. It does appear that more males than females have the disorder (Corbitt and Widiger 1995).

Course

Premorbid traits of PPD may be evident prior to adolescence in the form of social isolation, hypersensitivity, hypervigilance, social anxiety, peculiar thoughts, angry hostility, and idiosyncratic fantasies (American Psychiatric Association 2000). As children, they may appear odd and peculiar to their peers and they may not have achieved to their capacity in school. Their adjustment as adults is particularly poor with respect to interpersonal relationships. They may become socially isolated or fanatic members of groups that encourage or at least accept their paranoid ideation. They might maintain a steady employment but are difficult coworkers, as they tend to be rigid, controlling, critical, blaming, and prejudicial. They are likely to become involved in lengthy, acrimonious, and litigious disputes that are difficult, if not impossible, to resolve (Millon et al. 1996, Stone 1993).

Differential Diagnosis

PPD paranoid ideation is inconsistent with reality and is resistant to contrary evidence, but the ideation is not psychotic, absurd, inconceivable, or bizarre. PPD also lacks other features of psychotic and delusional disorders (e.g., hallucinations) and is evident since early adulthood, whereas a psychotic disorder becomes evident later within a person's life or remits after a much briefer period of time. Persons with PPD can develop psychotic disorders but to diagnose PPD in such cases, the paranoid personality traits must be evident prior to and persist after the psychotic episode. If PPD precedes the onset of schizophrenia, then it should be noted that it is premorbid to the schizophrenia (American Psychiatric Association 2000). However, it may not be meaningful to diagnose a person with both PPD and schizophrenia, as the premorbid paranoid traits may in some cases have simply represented a prodromal phase of the schizophrenic pathology.

Paranoid personality traits are evident in other personality disorders. Persons with avoidant personality disorder are socially withdrawn and apprehensive of others; borderline, antisocial, and narcissistic persons may be impatient, irritable, and antagonistic; and schizotypal persons may display paranoid ideation. The diagnosis of PPD often co-occurs with these other personality disorder diagnoses. Persons with PPD are prone to develop a variety of Axis I disorders, including substance-related, obsessive–compulsive anxiety, agoraphobia, and depressive disorders (American Psychiatric Association 2000).

Etiology

Research has indicated a genetic contribution to the development of suspiciousness and mistrust (Jang et al. 1998, Nigg and Goldsmith 1994, Plomin and Caspi 1999). There is some support for a genetic relationship of PPD with schizophrenia, but these findings have not always been replicated and the findings may have been due to the overlap of PPD with the STPD (Siever 1992). There is only limited support for a genetic relationship with delusional disorder, persecutory type (Nigg and Goldsmith 1994).

There are no systematic studies on possible psychosocial contributions to the development of PPD. There is some support for the contribution of excessive parental criticism and rejection but there has not yet been adequate prospective longitudinal studies (Miller et al. 2001). Paranoid belief systems could develop through parental modeling, a history of discriminatory exploitation or abandonment, or the projection of anger, resentment, and bitterness onto a group that is external to, and distinct from, oneself. Mistrust and suspicion is often evident in members of minority groups, immigrants, refugees, and other groups for whom such distrust can be a realistic and appropriate response to the social environment. It is conceivable that a comparably sustained experience through childhood and adolescence could contribute to the development of excessive paranoid beliefs that are eventually applied inflexibly and inappropriately to a wide variety of persons, but it can be very difficult to determine what is excessive or unrealistic suspicion and mistrust within a member of an oppressed minority (Alarcon and Foulks 1997). Paranoid suspiciousness could in fact be more closely associated with prejudicial attitudes, wherein a particular minority group in society becomes the inappropriate target of one's anger, blame, and resentment.

There has been little consideration given to the neurophysiological concomitants of nonpsychotic paranoid personality traits. More attention has been given to cognitive, interpersonal, and object-relational models of pathology. Paranoid beliefs do appear to have a self-perpetuating tendency resulting from the narrow and limited focus on signs and evidence for malicious intentions (Beck and Freeman 1990). The pathology of PPD, from this perspective, is inherent to the irrationality of the person's belief systems and is sustained by the biased information processing. There may also be an underlying motivation or need to perceive threats in others and to externalize blame that help sustain the accusations and distortions (Gabbard 2000, Millon et al. 1996).

Treatment

Persons with PPD rarely seek treatment for their feelings of suspiciousness and distrust. They experience these traits as simply accurate perceptions of a malevolent and dangerous world (i.e., ego-syntonic). They may not consider the paranoid attributions to be at all problematic, disruptive, or maladaptive. They are not delusional but they also fail to be reflective, insightful, or self-critical. They may recognize only that they have difficulty controlling their anger and getting along with others. They might be in treatment for an anxiety, mood, or substance-related disorder or for various marital, familial, occupational, or social (or legal) conflicts that are secondary to their personality disorder, but they also externalize the responsibility for their problems and have substantial difficulty recognizing their own contribution to their internal dysphoria and external conflicts. They consider their problems to be due to what others are doing to them, not to how they perceive, react, or relate to others.

The presence of paranoid personality traits complicate the treatment of an Axis I disorder or a relationship problem (Dolan-Sewell et al. 2001). Trust is central to the development of an adequate therapeutic alliance, yet it is precisely the absence of trust that is central to this disorder (Gabbard 2000, Stone 1993). It can be tempting to be less than forthright and open in the treatment of excessively suspicious persons because they distort, exaggerate, or escalate minor errors, misunderstandings, or inconsistent statements. However, therapists find that they weave an increasingly tangled web as they walk gingerly around the truth. Also, persons with PPD seize upon any kernel of deception to confirm their suspicion that the therapist is not to be trusted. It is preferable to be especially forthright and precise with paranoid individuals. Details that are inconsequential and of no interest to most individuals can be important to provide to persons with PPD so that they are ensured that nothing is being withheld or hidden from them.

Clinicians agree on several general principles in the treatment of paranoid personality traits (Beck and Freeman 1990, Gabbard 2000, Millon et al. 1996, Stone 1993). It is usually pointless and often harmful to rapport or to confront (or argue with) the paranoid beliefs. Such efforts may only alienate the individual and confirm his or her suspicions. The therapist should maintain a sincere and consistent respect for their autonomy and for their right to make their own decisions. However, one should not attempt to ingratiate oneself by being overly acquiescent and compliant. This can appear to be obviously patronizing, insincere, or manipulative. The goal is to develop, in a nonthreatening way, more self-reflection and self-awareness (e.g., recognition of the contribution of the paranoid traits and behaviors to the difficulties they are experiencing within their lives). A useful approach can be to communicate a sincere and respectful willingness to explore the implications, logic, and reality of the suspicions (Beck and Freeman 1990). Whenever one appears to be endangering rapport by moving too quickly, one should retreat to a more neutral and accepting position.

One must also be careful to avoid defensive reactions to the inevitable accusations. Any one of the conflicts they have had with others can develop within the therapeutic relationship (Benjamin 1993, Gabbard 2000) and persons with PPD have a tendency to be contentious, rigid, accusatory, suspicious, and litigious that can tax the empathy and patience of the therapist. One must attempt to maintain an empathic concern for their feelings of betrayal, and reassure them in an understanding, forthright manner that is neither patronizing nor disrespectful. Termination of treatment may at times be necessary if continuation would only result in further acrimony.

The suspicions, accusations, and acrimony often makes the person with PPD a poor candidate for group therapies. There is the potential to learn much about themselves within a group, but it is usually very difficult for them to develop the feelings of trust, respect, and security that are necessary for successful group therapy. Their propensity to make unfair hostile accusations alienate them from other group members, and they may quickly become a scapegoat for difficulties and conflicts that develop within the group.

There have been a variety of studies on the pharmacologic treatment of psychotic paranoid ideation and of STPD (which often includes paranoid personality traits) but little to no research on the pharmacologic responsivity of the nonpsychotic suspiciousness and ego-syntonic paranoid ideation of PPD (Markovitz 2001, Perry et al. 1999). Persons with PPD may also perceive the use of a medication to represent an effort to simply suppress or control their accusations and suspicions rather than to respectfully consider and address them. However, they may be receptive and responsive to the benefits of a medication to help control feelings of anxiousness or depression that are secondary to their personality disorder.

SCHIZOID PERSONALITY DISORDER

Diagnosis

The schizoid personality disorder (SZPD) is a pervasive pattern of social detachment and restricted emotional expression. Introversion (versus extraversion) is one of the fundamental dimensions of general personality functioning (Pervin and John 1999). Facets of introversion include low warmth (e.g., cold, detached, impersonal), low gregariousness (socially isolated, withdrawn), and low positive emotions (reserved, constricted or flat affect, anhedonic), which define well the central symptoms of SZPD (Widiger et al. 2002; see Table 44-1). The presence of SZPD is indicated by four or more of the seven diagnostic criteria presented in the DSM-IV-TR criteria for SZPD (see below).

DSM-IV-TR Diagnostic Criteria

301.20 Schizoid Personality Disorder

A. A pervasive pattern of detachment from social relationships and a restricted range of expression of emotions in interpersonal settings, beginning by early adulthood and present in a variety of contexts, as indicated by four (or more) of the following:

(1) neither desires nor enjoys close relationships, including being part of a family
(2) almost always chooses solitary activities
(3) has little, if any, interest in having sexual experiences with another person
(4) takes pleasure in few, if any, activities
(5) lacks close friends or confidants other than first-degree relatives
(6) appears indifferent to the praise or criticism of others
(7) emotional coldness, detachment, or flattened affectivity

B. Does not occur exclusively during the course of schizophrenia, a mood disorder with psychotic features, another psychotic disorder, or a pervasive developmental disorder, and is not due to the direct physiological effects of a general medical condition.

Note: if criteria are met prior to the onset of schizophrenia, add "premorbid," e.g., schizoid personality disorder (premorbid).

Reprinted with permission from the Diagnostic and Statistical Manual of Mental Disorders, Fourth Edition, Text Revision. Copyright 2000 American Psychiatric Association.

Epidemiology

Approximately half of the general population will exhibit an introversion within the normal range of functioning. However, only a small minority of the population would be diagnosed with an SZPD (Mattia and Zimmerman 2001). Estimates of the prevalence of SZPD within the general population have been less than 1% (see Table 44-2), and SZPD is among the least frequently diagnosed personality disorders within clinical settings. Many of the persons who were diagnosed with SZPD prior to DSM-III are probably now diagnosed with either the avoidant or the schizotypal personality disorders (Widiger et al. 1988), and prototypic (pure) cases of SZPD are likely to be quite rare within the population.

Course

Persons with SZPD would have been socially isolated and withdrawn as children. They may not have been accepted well by their peers, and may have even borne the brunt of some ostracism (American Psychiatric Association 2000). As adults, they have few friendships. The friendships that do occur are likely to be initiated by their peers or colleagues. They have few sexual relationships and may never marry. Relationships fail to the extent to which the other person desires or needs emotional support, warmth, and intimacy. Persons with SZPD may do well and even excel within an occupation, as long as substantial social interaction is not required. They prefer to work in isolation. They may eventually find employment and a relationship that is relatively comfortable, but they could also drift from one job to another and remain isolated throughout much of their life. If they do eventually become a parent, they have considerable difficulty providing warmth and emotional support, and they may appear neglectful, detached, and disinterested.

Differential Diagnosis

SZPD can be confused with the schizotypal and avoidant personality disorders as both involve social isolation and withdrawal (Kalus et al. 1993, Widiger et al. 1995). Schizotypal personality disorder, however, also includes an intense social anxiety and cognitive–perceptual aberrations. The major distinction with avoidant personality disorder is the absence of an intense desire for intimate social relationships. Avoidant persons will also exhibit substantial insecurity and inhibition, whereas the schizoid person is largely indifferent toward the reactions or opinions of others (Widiger et al. 1995).

The presence of premorbid schizoid traits can have prognostic significance for the course and treatment of schizophrenia (Siever 1992), but more importantly, it might not be meaningful to suggest that a person has an SZPD that is independent of or unrelated to a comorbid schizophrenia. The negative, prodromal, and residual symptoms of schizophrenia resemble closely the features of SZPD. Once a person develops schizophrenia, a diagnosis of SZPD can become rather pointless as all of the schizoid symptoms can then be understood as (prodromal or residual) symptoms of schizophrenia.

Etiology

A fundamental distinction for schizophrenic symptomatology is between positive and negative symptoms. Positive symptoms include hallucinations, delusions, inappropriate affect, and loose associations; negative symptoms include flattened affect, alogia, anhedonia, and avolition. SZPD has been conceptualized as representing subthreshold negative symptoms, comparable to the subthreshold positive symptoms (cognitive–perceptual aberrations) that predominate STPD. However, a genetic link of SZPD to schizophrenia that cannot be accounted for by comorbid STPD symptomatology has not been well established (Miller et al. 2001). Research has supported heritability for the personality dimension of introversion–extraversion (Jang et al. 1998, Jang and Vernon 2001, Plomin and Caspi 1999) and for the association of SZPD with introversion (Costa and Widiger 2002). The central pathology of SZPD does appear to be anhedonic deficits, or an excessively low ability to experience positive affect (Kalus et al. 1993, Rothbart and Ahadi 1994). Psychosocial models for the etiology of SZPD are lacking. It is possible that a sustained history of isolation during infancy and childhood, with an encouragement and modeling by parental figures of interpersonal withdrawal, indifference, and detachment could contribute to the development of schizoid personality traits (Bernstein and Travaglini 1999).

Treatment

Prototypic cases of SZPD rarely present for treatment, whether it is for their schizoid traits or a concomitant Axis I disorder. They feel little need for treatment, as their isolation is often ego-syntonic. Their social isolation is of more concern to their relatives, colleagues, or friends than to themselves. Their disinterest in and withdrawal from intimate or intense interpersonal contact is also a substantial barrier to treatment. They at times appear depressed but one must be careful not to confuse their anhedonic detachment, withdrawal, and flat affect with symptoms of depression.

If persons with SZPD are seen for treatment for a concomitant Axis I disorder (e.g., a sexual arousal disorder or a substance dependence), it is advisable to work within the confines and limitations of the schizoid personality traits (Beck and Freeman 1990, Stone 1993). Charismatic, engaging, emotional, or intimate therapists can be very uncomfortable, foreign, and even threatening to persons with SZPD. A more business-like approach can be more successful (Beck and Freeman 1990).

It is also important not to presume that persons with SZPD are simply inhibited, shy, or insecure. Such persons are more appropriately diagnosed with the avoidant personality disorder. Persons with SZPD are perhaps best treated with a supportive psychotherapy that emphasizes education and feedback concerning interpersonal skills and communication (Stone 1993). One may not be able to increase the desire for social involvements but one can increase the ability to relate to, communicate with, and get along with others. Persons with SZPD may not want to develop intimate relationships but they will often want to interact and relate more effectively and comfortably with others. The use of role playing and videotaped interactions can at times be useful in this respect. Persons with SZPD can have tremendous difficulty understanding how they are perceived by others or how their behavior is unresponsive to and perceived as rejecting by others.

Group therapy is often useful as a setting in which the individual can gradually develop self-disclosure, experience the interest of others, and practice social interactions with immediate and supportive feedback (Beck and Freeman 1990, Gabbard 2000). However, persons with SZPD are prone to being rejected by a group because of their detachment, flat affect, and indifference to the feelings of others. If the group is patient and accepting, they can benefit from the experience.

There have been many studies on the pharmacologic treatment of the schizotypal PD but no comparable studies on SZPD (Markovitz 2001, Perry et al. 1999). The schizotypal and schizoid PDs share many features, but the responsivity of the schizotypal PD to pharmacotherapy will usually reflect schizotypal social anxiety and cognitive–perceptual aberrations that are not seen in prototypic, pure cases of SZPD.

SCHIZOTYPAL PERSONALITY DISORDER

Diagnosis

Schizotypal PD (STPD) is a pervasive pattern of interpersonal deficits, cognitive and perceptual aberrations, and eccentricities of behavior (American Psychiatric Association 2000). The interpersonal deficits are characterized in large part by an acute discomfort with and reduced capacity for close relationships. The symptomatology of STPD has been differentiated further into components of positive (cognitive, perceptual aberrations) and negative (social aversion and withdrawal) symptoms comparable to the distinctions made for schizophrenia (Squires-Wheeler et al. 1997). The presence of STPD is indicated by five or more of the nine diagnostic criteria listed in the DSM-IV-TR criteria for STPD (see below).

DSM-IV-TR Diagnostic Criteria

301.22 Schizotypal Personality Disorder

A. A pervasive pattern of social and interpersonal deficits marked by acute discomfort with, and reduced capacity for, close relationships as well as by cognitive or perceptual distortions and eccentricities of behavior, beginning by early adulthood, and present in a variety of contexts, as indicated by five (or more) of the following:

    (1) ideas of reference (excluding delusions of reference)
    (2) odd beliefs or magical thinking that influences behavior and is inconsistent with subcultural norms (e.g., superstitiousness, belief in clairvoyance, telepathy, or "sixth sense"; in children and adolescents, bizarre fantasies or preoccupations)
    (3) unusual perceptual experiences, including bodily illusions
    (4) odd thinking and speech (e.g., vague, circumstantial, metaphorical, overelaborate, or stereotyped)
    (5) suspiciousness or paranoid ideation
    (6) inappropriate or constricted affect
    (7) behavior or appearance that is odd, eccentric, or peculiar
    (8) lacks close friends or confidants other than first-degree relatives
    (9) excessive social anxiety that does not diminish with familiarity and tends to be associated with paranoid fears rather than negative judgments about self

B. Does not occur exclusively during the course of schizophrenia, a mood disorder with psychotic features, another psychotic disorder, or a pervasive developmental disorder.

Note: if criteria are met prior to the onset of schizophrenia, add "premorbid," e.g., schizotypal personality disorder (premorbid).

Epidemiology

STPD may occur in as much as 3% of the general population although most studies with semistructured interviews have suggested a somewhat lower percent (see Table 44-2). STPD might occur somewhat more often in males (Corbitt and Widiger 1995, Raine et al. 1995). STPD co-occurs most often with the schizoid, borderline, avoidant, and paranoid personality disorders. Common Axis I disorders are major depressive disorder, brief psychotic disorder, and generalized social phobia (Miller et al. 2001).

Course

STPD is classified within the same diagnostic grouping as schizophrenia in ICD-10 (World Health Organization 1992) because of its close relationship in phenomenology, etiology, and pathology (Raine et al. 1995). However, it is classified as a personality disorder in DSM-IV-TR (American Psychiatric Association 2000) because its course and phenomenology are more consistent with a disorder of personality (i.e., early onset, evident in everyday functioning, characteristic of long-term functioning, and ego-syntonic). Persons with STPD are likely to be rather isolated in childhood. They may have appeared peculiar and odd to their peers, and may have been teased or ostracized. Achievement in school is usually impaired, and they may have been heavily involved in esoteric fantasies and peculiar interests, particularly those that do not involve peers. As adults, they may drift toward esoteric–fringe groups that support their magical thinking and aberrant beliefs. These activities can provide structure for some persons with STPD, but they can also contribute to a further loosening and deterioration if there is an encouragement of aberrant experiences. Only a small proportion of persons with STPD develop schizophrenia (Raine et al. 1995). The symptomatology of STPD does not appear to remit with age (Siever 1992). The course appears to be relatively stable, with some proportion of schizotypal persons remaining marginally employed, withdrawn, and transient throughout their lives.

Differential Diagnosis

Avoidant personality disorder and STPD share the features of social anxiety and introversion, but the social anxiety of STPD does not diminish with familiarity, whereas the anxiety of avoidant personality disorder (AVPD) is concerned primarily with the initiation of a relationship (Widiger et al. 1995). STPD is also a more severe disorder that includes a variety of cognitive and perceptual aberrations that are not seen in persons with AVPD.

An initial concern of many clinicians when confronted with a person with STPD is whether the more appropriate diagnosis is schizophrenia. Persons with STPD closely resemble persons within the prodromal or residual phases of schizophrenia. This differentiation is determined largely by the absence of a deterioration in functioning. It is indicated in DSM-IV-TR that one should note that STPD is "premorbid" if the schizotypal symptoms were present prior to the onset of schizophrenia (American Psychiatric Association 2000). Premorbid schizotypal traits will have prognostic significance for the course and treatment of schizophrenia and such traits should then be noted (Siever 1992). However, as discussed for SZPD, in most of these cases the schizotypal PD symptoms could then be readily understood as prodromal symptoms of schizophrenia.

Etiology

There is substantial empirical support for a genetic association of STPD with schizophrenia (Jang and Vernon 2001, Nigg and Goldsmith 1994, Siever 1992), which is not surprising given that the diagnostic criteria were obtained from the observations of biological relatives of persons with schizophrenia. Research has indicated further that the positive and negative symptoms may even have a distinct genetic relationship with the comparable symptoms of schizophrenia (Fanous et al. 2001). This suggests that the influence of familial etiological factors determining the expression of these symptom dimensions reaches across the boundary of psychotic illness to phenomena currently classified under the rubric of personality (Fanous et al. 2001, p. 672).

A predominant model for the psychopathology of STPD is deficits or defects in the attention and selection processes that organize a person's cognitive–perceptual evaluation of and relatedness to his or her environment (Raine et al. 1995). These defects may lead to discomfort within social situations, misperceptions and suspicions, and to a coping strategy of social isolation. Correlates of central nervous system dysfunction seen in persons with schizophrenia have been observed in laboratory tests of persons with STPD, including performance on tests of visual and auditory attention (e.g., backward masking and sensory gating tests) and smooth pursuit eye movement (Raine et al. 1997, Roitman et al. 1997). This dysfunction may be the result of dysregulation along dopaminergic pathways, which could be serving to modulate the expression of an underlying schizotypal genotype (Raine et al. 1995).

Treatment

Persons with STPD may seek treatment for their feelings of anxiousness, perceptual disturbances, or depression. Treatment of persons with STPD should be cognitive, behavioral, supportive, and/or pharmacologic, as they will often find the intimacy and emotionality of reflective, exploratory psychotherapy to be too stressful and they have the potential for psychotic decompensation.

Persons with STPD will often fail to consider their social isolation and aberrant cognitions and perceptions to be particularly problematic or maladaptive. They may consider themselves to be simply eccentric, creative, or nonconformist. Rapport can be difficult to develop as increasing familiarity and intimacy may only increase their level of discomfort and anxiety (Siever 1992). They are unlikely to be responsive to informality or playful humor. The sessions should be well-structured to avoid loose and tangential ideation.

Practical advice is usually helpful and often necessary (Beck and Freeman 1990). The therapist should serve as the individual's counselor, guide, or "auxiliary ego" to more adaptive decisions with respect to everyday problems (e.g., finding an apartment, interviewing for a job, and personal appearance). Persons with STPD should also receive social skills training directed at their awkward and odd behavior, mannerisms, dress, and speech. Specific, concrete discussions on what to expect and do in various social situations (e.g., formal meetings, casual encounters, and dates) should be provided. The rate of progress will tend to be slow, and it is helpful if there remains a continuity in the therapeutic relationship (Stone 1993).

Most of the systematic empirical research on the treatment of STPD has been confined to pharmacologic interventions. Low doses of neuroleptic medications (e.g., thiothixene) have shown some effectiveness in the treatment of schizotypal symptoms, particularly the perceptual aberrations and social anxiousness (Markovitz 2001, Siever 1992). Group therapy has also been recommended for persons with STPD but only when the group is highly structured and supportive (Millon et al. 1996). The emotional intensity and intimacy of unstructured groups will usually be too stressful. Schizotypal individuals with predominant paranoid symptoms may even have difficulty in highly structured groups.

CLUSTER B

ANTISOCIAL PERSONALITY DISORDER

Diagnosis

Antisocial personality disorder (ASPD) is a pervasive pattern of disregard for and violation of the rights of others (American Psychiatric Association 2000). Persons with ASPD will also be irresponsible and exploitative in their sexual relationships, and irresponsible as employees and parents. They may display a lack of empathy, an inflated or arrogant self-appraisal, a callous, cynical, and contemptuous response to the suffering of others, and a glib, superficial charm (Hare et al. 1991). This disorder has also been referred to as psychopathy (Hare et al. 1991), sociopathy, or dissocial (World Health Organization 1992) personality disorder. The presence of ASPD is indicated by the occurrence of a conduct disorder prior to age 15 years and by three of the seven adult diagnostic criteria presented in DSM-IV-TR Criteria for ASPD (see below).

DSM-IV-TR Diagnostic Criteria

301.7 Antisocial Personality Disorder

A. There is a pervasive pattern of disregard for and violation of the rights of others (occurring since age 15 years), as indicated by three (or more) of the following:

  (1) failure to conform to social norms with respect to lawful behaviors as indicated by repeatedly performing acts that are grounds for arrest
  (2) deceitfulness, as indicated by repeated lying, use of aliases, or conning others for personal profit or pleasure
  (3) impulsivity or failure to plan ahead
  (4) irritability and aggressiveness, as indicated by repeated physical fights or assaults
  (5) reckless disregard for safety of self or others
  (6) consistent irresponsibility, as indicated by repeated failure to sustain consistent work behavior or honor financial obligations
  (7) lack of remorse, as indicated by being indifferent to or rationalizing having hurt, mistreated, or stolen from another

B. The individual is at least age 18 years.
C. Evidence of conduct disorder with onset before age 15 years.
D. The occurrence of antisocial behavior is not exclusively during the course of schizophrenia or a manic episode.

Reprinted with permission from the Diagnostic and Statistical Manual of Mental Disorders, Fourth Edition, Text Revision. Copyright 2000 American Psychiatric Association.

All of the DSM-IV-TR assessment instruments described earlier include the assessment of ASPD. However, an instrument that is focused on the assessment of ASPD is the Psychopathy Checklist—Revised (PCL-R, Hare 1991). The PCL-R is commonly used within forensic and prison settings and is particularly well suited for the assessment of this disorder within settings that are heavily populated by persons with a criminal history (Kaye and Shea

2000, Widiger and Coker 2002). The PCL-R includes the assessment of psychopathic traits that are relatively more specific to ASPD within prison settings, such as lack of empathy, glib charm, and arrogance (Widiger et al. 1996). However, as suggested by its title, it is perhaps better described as a checklist than as a semistructured interview. Many of its items are scored primarily (if not solely) on the basis of a person's legal, criminal record rather than on the basis of interview questions. The availability of a detailed criminal history within prison settings has contributed to the PCL-R's excellent interrater reliability and predictive validity, but an application of the PCL-R within most other clinical settings will need to rely more heavily on PCL-R interview questions, the administration and scoring of which will be unclear for some PCL-R items (Lilienfeld 1994, Widiger and Coker 2002).

Persons with ASPD are at a high risk for developing substance-related and impulse dyscontrol disorders (Stoff et al. 1997, Sutker and Allain 2001). They are also likely to display borderline, narcissistic, and paranoid personality traits. Females with ASPD will also display histrionic personality traits (Hamburger et al. 1996, Widiger 1998).

Epidemiology

The National Institute of Mental Health Epidemiologic Catchment Area (ECA) study indicated that approximately 3% of males and 1% of females have ASPD (Robins et al. 1991). This rate has been replicated in subsequent studies, but it has also been suggested that the ECA finding may have underestimated the prevalence in males because of the failure to consider the full range of ASPD features. Other estimates have been as high as 6% in males (Kessler et al. 1994, Robins et al. 1991). The rate of ASPD within prison and forensic settings has been estimated at 50% (Hare et al. 1991, Robins et al. 1991) but the ASPD criteria may exaggerate the rate within such settings because of the emphasis given to overt acts of criminality, delinquency, and irresponsibility that are common to the persons within these settings (Sutker and Allain 2001, Widiger et al. 1996). More specific criteria for psychopathy provide a more conservative estimate of 20 to 30% of male prisoners with ASPD (Hare et al. 1991).

ASPD is much more common in males than in females (Corbitt and Widiger 1995, Robins et al. 1991). A sociobiological explanation for the differential sex prevalence is the presence of a genetic advantage for social irresponsibility, infidelity, superficial charm, and deceit in males that contributes to a higher likelihood of developing features of ASPD (Stoff et al. 1997, Sutker and Allain 2001). It has also been suggested that ASPD and histrionic personality disorder (HPD) share a biogenetic disposition (perhaps towards impulsivity or sensation-seeking) that is mediated by gender-specific biogenetic and sociological factors toward respective gender variants (Hamburger et al. 1996, Lilienfeld and Hess 2001).

Course

ASPD is evident in childhood in the form of a conduct disorder (Lynam 1996). Evidence of a conduct disorder prior to the age of 15 years is in fact required for a DSM-IV-TR ASPD diagnosis (American Psychiatric Association 2000). The continuation into adulthood is particularly likely to occur if multiple delinquent behaviors are evident prior to the age of 10 years (Lynam 1996, Moffitt 1993, Moffitt et al. 1996). As adults, persons with ASPD are unlikely to maintain steady employment and they may even become impoverished, homeless, or spend years within penal institutions (Robins et al. 1991). However, some persons with ASPD characterized by high rather than low levels of conscientiousness may express their psychopathic tendencies within a socially acceptable or at least legitimate profession (Hare 1991, Widiger and Lynam 1998). They may in fact be quite successful as long as their tendency to bend or violate the norms or rules of their profession and exploit, deceive, and manipulate others, contribute to a career advancement. Their success, however, may at some point unravel when their psychopathic behaviors become problematic or evident to others. The same pattern may also occur within sexual and marital relationships. They may at first appear to be charming, engaging, and sincere, but most relationships will end because of a lack of empathy, responsibility, and fidelity.

There does tend to be a gradual remission of antisocial behaviors, particularly overt criminal acts, as the person ages (Stoff et al. 1997, Sutker and Allain 2001). Persons with ASPD, however, are more likely than the general population to have died prematurely by violent means (e.g., accidents or homicides) and to engage in quite dangerous, high-risk behavior (Stoff et al. 1997).

Differential Diagnosis

ASPD will at times be difficult to differentiate from a substance dependence disorder in young adults because many persons with ASPD develop a substance-related disorder and many persons with a substance dependence engage in antisocial acts. The requirement that the ASPD features be evident prior to the age of 15 years will usually assure the onset of ASPD prior to the onset of a substance-related disorder. If both are evident prior to the age of 15 years, then it is likely that both disorders are in fact present and both diagnoses should then be made. ASPD and substance dependence will often interact, exacerbating and escalating each other's development (Myers et al. 1998, Sher and Trull 1994, Stoff et al. 1997, Sutker and Allain 2001).

Antisocial acts will also be evident in the histrionic and borderline personality disorders, as persons with these disorders will display impulsivity, sensation-seeking, self-centeredness, manipulativeness, and a low frustration tolerance. Females with ASPD are often misdiagnosed with HPD (Widiger 1998). Prototypic cases of ASPD might be distinguished from other personality disorders by the presence of the childhood history of conduct disorder and the cold, calculated exploitation, abuse, and aggression (Millon et al. 1996, Widiger et al. 1995). Persons with narcissistic personality disorder (NPD) are also characterized by a lack of empathy and may often exploit and use others. In fact, many of the traits of NPD are evident in psychopathy, including a lack of empathy, glib and superficial charm, and arrogant self-appraisal (Widiger et al. 1996).

Etiology

There is considerable support from twin, family, and adoption studies for a genetic contribution to the etiology of the criminal, delinquent tendencies of persons with ASPD (Nigg and Goldsmith 1994, Stoff et al. 1997). The genetic disposition may be somewhat stronger in ASPD females, perhaps because of greater social pressure on females against aggressive, exploitative, and criminal behavior (Hare et al. 1991). What is inherited by persons with ASPD, however, is unclear; it could be impulsivity, antagonistic callousness, or abnormally low anxiousness.

A predominant theory for the etiology of ASPD is that it results from abnormally low levels of behavioral inhibition and high levels of behavioral activation systems (BASs) that are important for normal, adaptive functioning (Fowles 2001, Widiger and Lynam 1998). The behavioral inhibition system (BIS) is responsible for inhibiting behavior in response to punishment and acts in opposition to the BAS that activates behavior in response to reward. The BIS has input into the reticular activating system providing experiences of anxiety or arousal. The clinical symptoms of ASPD might be manifestations of a weak or deficient BIS in combination with a normal or strong BAS that reduce normal sensitivity and anxiety in response to threatening and stressful situations. Activities that the average person would find stimulating, antisocial persons would find dull, impelling them to engage in risky, reckless, prohibited, and impulsive activities. Low arousal would also help minimize feelings of anxiety, guilt, or remorse and help resist aversive conditioning. Studies have indicated an electrodermal response hyporeactivity in psychopathic persons

(Fowles 2001, Stoff et al. 1997). This hyporeactivity may be particularly associated with a deficit in anticipatory anxiety and worrying, while not impairing the alarm reactions of flight versus fight. Abnormally low levels of behavioral inhibition may be mediated by the septohippocampal system (and the neurotransmitter serotonin). Deficiencies in response modulation (difficulties suspending a dominant set in response to negative feedback) are apparent in animals with septohippocampal dysfunction (Newman and Wallace 1993).

There are also substantial data to support the contribution of family, peer, and other environmental factors (Stoff et al. 1997). No single environmental factor appears to be specific to its development. Modeling by parental figures and peers, excessively harsh, lenient, or erratic discipline, and a tough, harsh environment in which feelings of empathy and warmth are discouraged (if not punished) and tough-mindedness, aggressiveness, and exploitation are encouraged (if not rewarded) have all been associated with the development of ASPD (Sutker and Allain 2001). For example, ASPD in some cases could be the result of an interaction of early experiences of physical or sexual abuse, exposure to aggressive parental models, and erratic discipline that develop a view of the world as a hostile environment, which is further affirmed over time through selective attention on cues for antagonism, encouragement and modeling of aggression by peers, and the immediate benefits that result from aggressive, exploitative behavior (Dodge et al. 1990). Persons with ASPD may have had their feelings of anxiety, guilt, and remorse extinguished through progressive and cumulative experiences of harsh aggression, violence, abuse, and exploitation.

The development of adequate guilt, conscience, and shame may also require a degree of distress-proneness (anxiousness or neuroticism) and attentional self-regulation (constraint). Normal levels of neuroticism will promote the internalization of a conscience (the introjection of the family's moral values) by associating distress and anxiety with wrongdoing, and the temperament of self-regulation will help modulate impulses into a socially acceptable manner (Clark et al. 2000, Fowles and Kochanska 2000, Kochanska and Murray 2000, Rothbart and Ahadi 1994). Studies have indicated that high levels of arousal at age 15 years serve as a protective factor against criminal activities at age 30 years in persons at high risk for becoming criminals (Raine et al. 1995, 1998). Additional factors may also help avoid the development of ASPD, such as high intelligence, which may contribute to the availability of alternative life paths, while other factors may exacerbate or escalate its development, such as drug or alcohol dependence (Sher and Trull 1994). In sum, ASPD appears to be the result of a constellation of factors, including genetic predisposition, experiences within the family, and sociological factors, coupled with the absence of preventive factors (Stoff et al. 1997, Sutker and Allain 2001).

Treatment

The presence of ASPD is important to recognize in the treatment of any Axis I disorder, as their tendency to be manipulative, dishonest, exploitative, aggressive, and irresponsible will often disrupt and sabotage treatment. It is also very easy to be seduced by psychopathic charm. Persons with ASPD can be seductive in their engaging friendliness, expressions of remorse, avowed commitment to change, and apparent response to or even fascination with the success, skills, and talents of the therapist, none of which will be sincere or reliable.

The extent to which ASPD is untreatable has at times been overstated and exaggerated (Salekin 2002). Nevertheless, ASPD is the most difficult personality disorder to treat (Gunderson and Gabbard 2000, Stone 1993, Stoff et al. 1997). Persons with ASPD will often lack a motivation or commitment to change. They might see only the advantages of their antisocial traits and not the costs (e.g., risks of arrest and failure to sustain lasting or meaningful relationships). They are prone to manipulate, abuse, or exploit their fellow individuals and the staff (Gabbard 2000). The immediate motivation for treatment is often provided by an external source, such as a court order or the demands of an employer or relative. Motivation may last only as long as an external pressure remains.

The most effective treatment is likely to be prevention through an identification and intervention early in childhood (Lynam 1996, Stoff et al. 1997). In adulthood, the most effective treatment may at times be simply some form of sustained incarceration (e.g., imprisonment), as many antisocial behaviors do tend to dissipate (or burn out) with time (Robins et al. 1991, Sutker and Allain 2001). The tendency to rationalize irresponsibility, minimize the consequences of acts, and manipulate others needs to be confronted on a daily and immediate basis. Community residential or wilderness programs that provide a firm structure, close supervision, and intense confrontation by peers have been recommended (Gabbard 2000). The involvement of family members in the treatment has been shown to be helpful, but there are also data to suggest that interventions with little professional input are less successful and are at times counterproductive (Salekin 2002).

There is some research to suggest that the ability to form a therapeutic alliance is an important indicator of treatment success. Factors to consider are the demographic similarity of the therapist and individual, the quality of the individual's past relationships, and the therapist's positive regard for the individual (Stoff et al. 1997, Sutker and Allain 2001). Many clinicians may also experience strong feelings of animosity and distaste for antisocial persons who have a history of abusive and exploitative acts (Gunderson and Gabbard 2000). Rational, utilitarian approaches that help the person consider the long-term consequences of behavior can be helpful (Beck and Freeman 1990, Salekin 2002). This approach does not attempt to develop a sense of conscience, guilt, or even regret for past actions, but focuses instead on the material value and future advantages to be gained by a more prosocial behavior pattern. There are data to suggest the use of pharmacotherapy in the treatment of impulsive aggression but it is unclear whether these findings would generalize to the full spectrum of ASPD psychopathology (Markovitz 2001).

BORDERLINE PERSONALITY DISORDER

Diagnosis

Borderline personality disorder (BPD) is a pervasive pattern of impulsivity and instability in interpersonal relationships and self-image (American Psychiatric Association 2000). A broad domain of general personality functioning is neuroticism (or emotional instability; Pervin and John 1999), characterized by facets of angry hostility, anxiousness, depressiveness, impulsivity, and vulnerability; BPD is essentially the most extreme and highly maladaptive variant of emotional instability (Widiger et al. 2002). This disorder is indicated by the presence of five or more of the nine diagnostic criteria presented in the DSM-IV-TR criteria for BPD (see below).

DSM-IV-TR Diagnostic Criteria

301.83 Borderline Personality Disorder

A. A pervasive pattern of instability of interpersonal relationships, self-image, and affects, and marked impulsivity beginning by early adulthood and present in a variety of contexts, as indicated by five (or more) of the following:

   (1) frantic efforts to avoid real or imagined abandonment. **Note:** do not include suicidal or self-mutilating behavior covered in criterion 5

(2) a pattern of unstable and intense interpersonal relationships characterized by alternating between extremes of idealization and devaluation

(3) identity disturbance: markedly and persistently unstable self-image or sense of self

(4) impulsivity in at least two areas that are potentially self-damaging (e.g., spending, sex, substance abuse, reckless driving, binge eating). **Note:** do not include suicidal or self-mutilating behavior covered in criterion 5

(5) recurrent suicidal behavior, gestures, or threats, or self-mutilating behavior

(6) affective instability due to a marked reactivity of mood (e.g., intense episodic dysphoria, irritability, or anxiety usually lasting a few hours and only rarely more than a few days)

(7) chronic feelings of emptiness

(8) inappropriate, intense anger or difficulty controlling anger (e.g., frequent displays of temper, constant anger, recurrent physical fights)

(9) transient, stress-related paranoid ideation or severe dissociative symptoms.

Reprinted with permission from the Diagnostic and Statistical Manual of Mental Disorders, Fourth Edition, Text Revision. Copyright 2000 American Psychiatric Association.

All of the DSM-IV-TR assessment instruments described earlier include the assessment of BPD. However, an instrument that is focused on the assessment of BPD is the Diagnostic Interview for Borderlines-Revised (DIB-R; Zanarini et al. 1989). The DIB-R provides a more thorough assessment of components of BPD (e.g., impulsivity, affective dysregulation, and cognitive–perceptual aberrations) than is provided by more general DSM-IV-TR personality disorder semistructured interviews, but clinicians might find it impractical to devote up to 2 hours to assess one particular personality disorder, especially when it is likely that other maladaptive personality traits not covered by the DIB-R are also likely to be present (Kaye and Shea 2000, Widiger and Coker 2002, Zanarini et al. 1998b).

Axis I Disorders are commonly comorbid with BPD. The range of potential Axis I comorbid psychopathology includes mood (major depressive disorder), anxiety (posttraumatic stress disorder), eating (bulimia nervosa), substance (alcohol dependence), dissociative (dissociative identity disorder), and psychotic (brief psychotic) disorders (Gunderson 2001, Links et al. 1998, Zanarini et al. 1998a). Persons with BPD also meet DSM-IV-TR criteria for at least one other personality disorder, particularly histrionic, dependent, antisocial, schizotypal, or passive–aggressive Links et al. 1998, Zanarini et al. 1998b). Researchers and clinicians have at times responded to this extensive co-occurrence by imposing a diagnostic hierarchy whereby other disorders are not diagnosed in the presence of BPD because BPD is generally the most severely dysfunctional disorder (Gunderson et al. 2000). A potential limitation of this approach is that it resolves the complexity of personality by largely ignoring it. This approach may fail to recognize the presence of maladaptive personality traits that could be important for understanding an individual's dysfunctions and for developing an optimal treatment plan (Zimmerman and Mattia 1999).

Epidemiology

Approximately 1 to 2% of the general population would meet the DSM-IV-TR criteria for BPD (see Table 44-2). BPD is the most prevalent personality disorder within hospital clinical settings. Approximately 15% of all inpatients (51% of inpatients with a personality disorder) and 8% of all outpatients (27% of outpatients with a personality disorder) have a BPD. Approximately 75% of persons with BPD will be female (Corbitt and Widiger

1995, Gunderson 2001). Persons with BPD meet DSM-IV-TR criteria for at least one Axis I disorder.

Course

As children, persons with BPD are likely to have been emotionally unstable, impulsive, and angry or hostile. Their chaotic impulsivity and intense affectivity may contribute to involvement within rebellious groups as a child or adolescent, along with a variety of Axis I disorders, including eating, substance use, and mood disorders. BPD is often diagnosed in children and adolescents, but considerable caution should be used when doing so as some of the symptoms of BPD (e.g., identity disturbance and unstable relationships) could be confused with a normal adolescent rebellion or identity crisis (Ad-Dab'bagh and Greenfield 2001, Gunderson 2001). As adults, persons with BPD may require numerous hospitalizations due to their affect and impulse dyscontrol, psychotic-like and dissociative symptomatology, and risk of suicide (Gunderson 2001, Zanarini et al. 1998a). Minor problems quickly become crises as the intensity of affect and impulsivity result in disastrous decisions. They are at a high risk for developing depressive, substance-related, bulimic, and posttraumatic stress disorders. The potential for suicide increases with a comorbid mood and substance-related disorder. Approximately 3 to 10% commit suicide by the age of 30 years (Gunderson 2001). Relationships tend to be very unstable and explosive, and employment history is poor (Daley et al. 2000, Stone 2001). Affectivity and impulsivity, however, may begin to diminish as the person reaches the age of 30 years, or earlier if the person becomes involved with a supportive and patient sexual partner (Stone 2001). Some, however, may obtain stability by abandoning the effort to obtain a relationship, opting instead for a lonelier but less volatile life. The mellowing of the symptomatology, however, can be easily disrupted by the occurrence of a severe stressor (e.g., divorce by or death of a significant other) that results in a brief psychotic, dissociative, or mood disorder episode.

Differential Diagnosis

Most persons with BPD develop mood disorders (Links et al. 1998) and it is at times difficult to differentiate BPD from a mood disorder if the assessment is confined to the current symptomatology (Gunderson 2001, Widiger and Coker 2002). A diagnosis of BPD requires that the borderline symptomatology be evident since adolescence, which should differentiate BPD from a mood disorder in all cases other than a chronic mood disorder. If there is a chronic mood disorder, then the additional features of transient, stress-related paranoid ideation, dissociative experiences, impulsivity, and anger dyscontrol that are evident in BPD should be emphasized in the diagnosis (Gunderson 2001, Widiger et al. 1995).

Etiology

There are studies to indicate that BPD may breed true, but most research has suggested an association with mood and impulse dyscontrol disorders (Silk 2000, Torgersen 2000). There is also consistent empirical support for a childhood history of physical and/or sexual abuse, as well as parental conflict, loss, and neglect (Johnson et al. 1999, Zanarini 2000). It appears that past traumatic events are important in many, if not in most, cases of BPD, contributing to the overlap and association with posttraumatic stress and dissociative disorders (Brodsky et al. 1995, Gunderson 2001, Heffernan and Cloitre 2000), but the nature and age at which these events have occurred will vary. BPD may involve the interaction of a genetic disposition towards dyscontrol of mood and impulses (i.e., emotionally unstable temperament), with a cumulative and evolving series of intensely pathogenic relationships (Gunderson 2001, Morey and Zanarini 2000).

There are numerous theories regarding the pathogenic mechanisms of BPD, most concern issues regarding abandonment, separation, and/or exploitative abuse, which is one of the reasons that frantic efforts to avoid abandonment is the first item in the DSM-IV-TR diagnostic criterion set (Gunderson et al. 1991, Zanarini et al. 1997). Persons with BPD have quite intense, disturbed, and/or abusive relationships with the significant persons of their past, including their parents (Gunderson 2001), contributing to the development of malevolent perceptions and expectations of others (Ornduff 2000). These expectations, along with an impairment in the ability to regulate affect and impulses (Linehan 1993), may contribute to the perpetuation of intense, angry, and unstable relationships. Neurochemical dysregulation is evident in persons with BPD but it is unclear whether this dysregulation is a result, cause, or correlate of prior interpersonal traumas (Gunderson 2001, Silk 2000).

Treatment

Persons with BPD often develop intense, dependent, hostile, unstable, and manipulative relationships with their therapists as they do with their peers. At one time they might be very compliant, responsive, and even idealizing, but later angry, accusatory, and devaluing. Their tendency to be manipulatively as well as impulsively self-destructive is often very stressful and difficult to treat (Stone 2000).

Persons with BPD are often highly motivated for treatment. Psychotherapeutic approaches tend to be both supportive and exploratory (Gabbard 2001, Gunderson 2001, Stone 1993, 2000). Therapists should provide a safe, secure environment in which anger can be expressed and actively addressed without destroying the therapeutic relationship. The historical roots of current bitterness, anger, and depression within past familial relationships should eventually be explored, but immediate, current issues and conflicts must also be explicitly addressed. Suicidal behavior should be confronted and contained, by hospitalization when necessary. Individuals with BPD can be very difficult to treat because the focus of the individual's love and wrath will often be shifted toward the therapist, and the treatment may itself become the individual's latest unstable, intense relationship. Immediate and ongoing consultation with colleagues is often necessary, as it is not unusual for therapists to be unaware of the extent to which they are developing or expressing feelings of anger, attraction, annoyance, or intolerance toward the individual with BPD.

A particular form of cognitive–behavioral therapy, dialectical behavior therapy, has been shown empirically to be effective in the treatment of BPD (Linehan 1993, 2000). Part of the strategy entails keeping individuals focused initially on the priorities of reducing suicidal threats and gestures, behaviors that can disrupt or resist treatment, and behaviors that affect the immediate quality of life (e.g., bulimia, substance abuse, or unemployment). Once these goals are achieved, the focus can then shift to a mastery of new coping skills, management of reactions to stress, and other individualized goals. Individual therapy is augmented by skills-training groups that may be highly structured (e.g., comparable to a classroom format). Individuals are taught skills for coping with identity diffusion, tolerating distress, improving interpersonal relationships, controlling emotions, and resolving interpersonal crises. Individuals are given homework assignments to practice these skills that are further addressed and reinforced within individual sessions. Negative affect is also addressed through a mindful meditation that contributes to an acceptance and tolerance of past abusive experiences and current stress. The dialectical component of the therapy is that "the dialectical therapist helps the individual achieve synthesis of oppositions, rather than focusing on verifying either side of an oppositional argument" (Linehan 1993, p. 204). An illustrative list of dialectical strategies is presented in Table 44-3.

Dialectical behavior therapy (DBT), however, also includes more general principles of treatment that are important to emphasize in all forms of therapy for BPD (Linehan 1993, Stone 1993, 2000), some of which are presented in Table 44-4. For example, exasperated therapists may unjustly experience and even accuse borderline individuals of being unmotivated or unwilling to work. It is important to appreciate that they do want to

Table 44-3	**Dialectical Behavior Therapy Strategies**

Alternate between acceptance and change strategies
Balance nurturing with demands for self-help
Balance persistence and stability with flexibility
Balance capabilities with limitations and deficits
Move with speed, keeping the patient slightly off balance
Take positions whole-heartedly
Look for what is not included in patient's own points of view
Provide developmental descriptions of change
Question intransigence of boundary conditions of the problem
Highlight importance of interrelationships in identity
Advocate a middle path
Highlight paradoxical contradictions in the patient's own behavior, in the therapeutic process, and in life in general
Speak in metaphors and tell parables and stories
Play the devil's advocate
Extend the seriousness or implications of the patient's statements
Add intuitive knowing to emotional experience and logical analysis
Turn problems into assets
Allow natural changes in therapy
Assess the individual, therapist, and process dialectically

Source: Reprinted from *Cognitive–Behavioral Treatment of Borderline Personality Disorder*, Linehan MM, Basic Propositions of BPD Treatment from DBT, 206, Copyright (1993) with permission from Guilford Press.

Table 44-4	**Basic Propositions of BPD Treatment from DBT**

1. Patients are doing the best they can.
2. Patients want to improve.
3. Patients need to do better, try harder, and be more motivated to change.
4. Patients may not have caused all of their own problems, but they have to solve them anyway.
5. The lives of suicidal, borderline individuals are unbearable as they are currently being lived.
6. Patients must learn new behaviors in all relevant contexts.
7. Patients cannot fail in therapy.
8. Therapists treating patients with BPD need support.

Source: Reprinted from *Cognitive–Behavioral Treatment of Borderline Personality Disorder*, Linehan MM, Basic Propositions of BPD Treatment from DBT, 106–108, Copyright (1993) with permission from Guilford Press.

improve and are doing the best that they can. One should not make the therapy personal, but instead identify the sources of the inhibition or interference to their motivation to change. One should take seriously their complaints that their lives are indeed unbearable but not absolve them of their responsibility to solve their own problems. They are unlikely to change simply through a passive reception of insight, nurturance, support, and medication. They will need to actively work on changing their lives. Therapists will often be tempted to rescue the individuals under their care, particularly when they are within a crisis. However, it is precisely at such times that there will be the best opportunity to develop and learn new coping strategies. Failures can occur, and it is a failure of the therapy that should be conscientiously and effectively addressed by the therapist. Finally, therapists need to honestly recognize their own limitations. All therapists have their own flaws and limits and individuals with BPD invariably strain and overwhelm these limits. Therapists need to be open and receptive to outside support, advice, and criticism.

Pharmacologic treatment of individuals with BPD is varied, as it depends primarily on the predominant Axis I symptomatology (Markovitz 2001, Soloff 2000). Persons with BPD can display a wide variety of Axis I symptoms, including anxiety, depression, hallucinations, delusions, and dissociations. It is important in their pharmacologic treatment not to be unduly influenced by transient symptoms or by symptoms that are readily addressed through exploratory or supportive techniques. On the other hand, it is equally important to be flexible in the use of medications and not to be unduly resistant to their use. Relying solely upon one's own psychotherapeutic skills can be unnecessary and even irresponsible.

HISTRIONIC PERSONALITY DISORDER

Diagnosis

Histrionic personality disorder (HPD) is a pervasive pattern of excessive emotionality and attention-seeking (American Psychiatric Association 2000). Histrionic persons tend to be emotionally manipulative and intolerant of delayed gratification (American Psychiatric Association 1980, 1987, Bornstein 1999). HPD is indicated by the presence of five or more of the eight diagnostic criteria presented in DSM-IV-TR criteria for HPD (see below).

DSM-IV-TR Diagnostic Criteria

301.50 Histrionic Personality Disorder

A pervasive pattern of excessive emotionality and attention-seeking, beginning by early adulthood and present in a variety of contexts, as indicated by five (or more) of the following:

A. is uncomfortable in situations in which he or she is not the center of attention
B. interaction with others is often characterized by inappropriate sexually seductive or provocative behavior
C. displays rapidly shifting and shallow expression of emotions
D. consistently uses physical appearance to draw attention to self
F. has a style of speech that is excessively impressionistic and lacking in detail
G. shows self-dramatization, theatricality, and exaggerated expression of emotion
H. is suggestible, i.e. easily influenced by others or circumstances
I. considers relationships to be more intimate than they actually are.

Reprinted with permission from the Diagnostic and Statistical Manual of Mental Disorders, Fourth Edition, Text Revision. Copyright 2000 American Psychiatric Association.

Epidemiology

Approximately 1 to 3% of the general population may be diagnosed with HPD (see Table 44-2; Mattia and Zimmerman 2001, Torgersen et al. 2001). A controversial issue is its differential sex prevalence (Bornstein 1999, Sprock et al. 1990, Widiger 1998). It is stated in DSM-IV-TR that the sex ratio for HPD is "not significantly different than the sex ratio of females within the respective clinical setting" (American Psychiatric Association 2000, p. 712). However, this should not be interpreted as indicating that the prevalence is the same for males and females. It has typically been found that at least two-thirds of persons with HPD are female, although there have been a few exceptions (Corbitt and Widiger 1995). Whether or not the rate will be significantly higher than the rate of women within a particular clinical setting depends upon many factors that are independent of the differential sex prevalence for HPD (Widiger 1998).

Course

Little is known about the premorbid behavior pattern of persons with HPD (Bornstein 1999). During adolescence, they are likely to be flamboyant, flirtatious, and attention-seeking. As adults, persons with HPD readily form new relationships but have difficulty sustaining them. They may fall in love quite quickly, but just as rapidly become attracted to another person. They are unlikely to be reliable or responsible. Relationships with persons of the same sexual orientation are often strained because of their competitive sexual flirtatiousness. Employment history is likely to be erratic, and may be complicated by the tendency to become romantically or sexually involved with colleagues, by their affective instability, and by their suggestibility. Persons with HPD may become devoted converts to faddish belief systems. They have a tendency to make impulsive decisions that will have a dramatic (or melodramatic) effect on their lives. The severity of the symptomatology may diminish somewhat as the person ages.

Differential Diagnosis

HPD involves to some extent maladaptive variants of stereotypically feminine traits (Sprock et al. 1990). The DSM-IV-TR diagnostic criteria for HPD are sufficiently stringent severe that a normal woman would not meet these criteria, but studies have indicated that clinicians will at times diagnose HPD in females who in fact have antisocial traits (Widiger 1998). Both of these disorders can involve impulsivity, sensation-seeking, low frustration tolerance, and manipulativeness, and the presence of a female gender may at times contribute to a false presumption of HPD. It is therefore important to adhere closely to the DSM-IV-TR diagnostic criteria when confronted with histrionic and antisocial symptoms in females.

Persons with HPD will often have borderline, dependent, or narcissistic personality traits. Prototypic cases of HPD can be distinguished from other personality disorders (Widiger et al. 1995, 2002). For example, the prototypic narcissistic person ultimately desires admiration whereas the histrionic person desires whatever attention, interest, or concern can be obtained. As a result, the histrionic person will at times seek attention through melodramatic helplessness and emotional outbursts that could be experienced as denigrating and humiliating to the narcissistic person. However, most cases will not be prototypic and the most accurate description of an individual's constellation of maladaptive personality traits will be the provision of multiple diagnoses (Oldham et al. 1992, Oldham and Skodol 2000).

Etiology

There is little research on the etiology of HPD. There is a suggestion that HPD may share a genetic disposition toward impulsivity or sensation-seeking with the ASPD (Hamburger et al. 1996, Lilienfeld and Hess 2001). It has also been suggested that HPD is (in part) a severe, maladaptive variant of the personality dimensions of extraversion and neuroticism (Widiger et al. 2002). Extraversion includes the facets of excitement-seeking, gregariousness, and positive emotionality, and neuroticism includes the facets of angry hostility, self-consciousness, and vulnerability (Costa and McCrae 1992) that are all characteristic of persons with HPD (Trull et al. 1998) and there is considerable empirical support for the heritability of these personality dimensions (Jang et al. 1998, Jang and Vernon 2001, Nigg and Goldsmith 1994, Plomin and Caspi 1999).

Environmental and social–cultural factors, however, may also play a significant role in the development of HPD (Bornstein 1999). Kernberg (1991a), for example, speculates that the fathers of females with HPD combine early sexual seductiveness with subsequent authoritarian puritanical attitudes, while the mother tends to be domineering, controlling, and intrusive. Such a history may indeed occur in some cases of HPD but there is unlikely to be a specific, common pattern to all cases. The tendency of a family to emphasize, value, or reinforce attention-seeking in a person with a genetic disposition toward emotionality may represent a more general pathway toward HPD (Cooper and Ronningstam 1992).

Affective instability is an important feature of HPD, which may be associated with a hyperresponsiveness of the noradrenergic system. This instability in the catecholamine functioning may contribute to a pronounced emotional reactivity to rejection and loss (Markovitz 2001). However, the attention-seeking of HPD can be as important to the disorder as the emotionality. The purpose of the exaggerated emotionality is often to evoke the attention and maintain the interest of others (Bornstein 1999, Gunderson and Gabbard 2000, Stone 1993). Persons with HPD are intensely insecure regarding the extent to which others appreciate, desire, or want their company. They need to be the center of attention to reassure themselves that they are valued, desired, attractive, or wanted.

Treatment

Persons with HPD readily develop rapport but it is often superficial and unreliable. Therapists may also fail to appreciate the extent of influence they can have on the highly suggestible individual with HPD (Bornstein 1999, Horowitz 1997). Persons with HPD can readily become converts to whatever the therapist may suggest or encourage. The transformation to the theoretical model or belief system of the clinician is unlikely to be sustained.

A key task in treating the individual with HPD is countering their global and diffuse cognitive style by insisting on attending to structure and detail within sessions and to the practical, immediate problems encountered in daily life (Beck and Freeman 1990, Gunderson and Gabbard 2000, Horowitz 1997, Stone 1993). It is also important to explore within treatment the historical source for their needs for attention and involvement. Persons with HPD are prone to superficial and transient insights but they will benefit from a carefully reasoned and documented exploration of their current and past relationships.

Many clinicians recommend the use of group therapy for persons with HPD (Beck and Freeman 1990, Gabbard 2000, Millon et al. 1996). It is quite easy for them to become involved within a group, which may then be very useful in helping them recognize and explore their attention-seeking, suggestibility, and manipulation, as well as develop alternative ways to develop more meaningful and sustained relationships. However, it is also important to closely monitor their involvements within the group, as they are prone to dominate and control sessions and they may escalate their attention-seeking to the point of suicidal gestures. The intense affectivity of persons with HPD may also be responsive to antidepressant treatment, particularly those individuals with substantial mood reactivity, hypersomnia, and rejection sensitivity (Markovitz 2001).

NARCISSISTIC PERSONALITY DISORDER

Diagnosis

Narcissistic personality disorder (NPD) is a pervasive pattern of grandiosity, need for admiration, and lack of empathy (American Psychiatric Association 2000). Persons with NPD can be very vulnerable to threats to their self-esteem. They may react defensively with rage, disdain, or indifference but are in fact struggling with feelings of shock, humiliation, and shame. NPD is indicated by the presence of five or more of the nine diagnostic criteria presented in the DSM-IV-TR Criteria for NPD (see page 1258).

> ## DSM-IV-TR Diagnostic Criteria
>
> ### 301.81 Narcissistic Personality Disorder
>
> A pervasive pattern of grandiosity (in fantasy or behavior), need for admiration, and lack of empathy, beginning by early adulthood and present in a variety of contexts, as indicated by five (or more) of the following:
>
> A. has a grandiose sense of self-importance (e.g. exaggerates achievements and talents, expects to be recognized as superior without commensurate achievements)
> B. is preoccupied with fantasies of unlimited success, power, brilliance, beauty, or ideal love
> C. believes that he or she is "special" and unique and can only be understood by, or should associate with, other special or high-status people (or institutions)
> D. requires excessive admiration
> E. has a sense of entitlement, i.e. unreasonable expectations of especially favorable treatment or automatic compliance with his or her expectations
> F. is interpersonally exploitative, i.e., takes advantage of others to achieve his or her own ends
> G. lacks empathy: is unwilling to recognize or identify with the feelings and needs of others
> H. is often envious of others or believes that others are envious of him or her
> I. shows arrogant, haughty behaviors or attitudes.

All of the semistructured interviews and self-report inventories described earlier include scales for the assessment of NPD. There is also a semistructured interview devoted to the assessment of narcissism (Diagnostic Interview for Narcissism (DIN); Gunderson et al. 1990), the research that was highly influential in the development of the DSM-IV-TR diagnostic criteria (Gunderson et al. 1991). There are also a number of self-report inventories devoted to the assessment of narcissistic personality traits, including the Narcissistic Personality Inventory (NPI) that has been used in a number of informative personality and social–psychological studies of narcissism (Rhodewalt and Morf 1995). The DIN and NPI have the useful feature of subscales for the assessment of various components of narcissism (e.g., NPI scales for superiority, vanity, leadership, authority, entitlement, exploitativeness, and exhibitionism).

Persons with NPD are considered to be prone to mood disorders, as well as anorexia and substance-related disorders, especially cocaine (American Psychiatric Association 2000, Cooper and Ronningstam 1992). Persons with NPD are likely to have comorbid antisocial (psychopathic), histrionic, paranoid, and borderline personality traits.

Epidemiology

Approximately 18% of males and 6% of females may be characterized as being excessively immodest (i.e., arrogant or conceited; Costa and McCrae 1992) but only a small percent of these persons would be diagnosed with NPD. In fact, the median prevalence rate obtained across 10 community data collections was zero (see Table 44-2). The absence of any cases within community studies, however, may reflect inadequacies within the diagnostic criteria or limitations of semistructured interview assessments of narcissism (Hilsenroth et al. 1996, Westen 1997). NPD is observed within clinical settings (approximately 2 to 20% of individuals) although it is also among the least frequently diagnosed personality disorders (American Psychiatric Association 2000, Gunderson et al. 1991).

Course

Little is known about the premorbid behavior pattern of NPD, other than through retrospective reports of persons diagnosed when adults (Cooper and Ronningstam 1992, Kernberg 1991b, Kohut 1977, Mattia and Zimmerman 2001). As adolescents, persons with NPD are likely to be self-centered, assertive, gregarious, dominant, and perhaps arrogant. They may have achieved well in school or within some other activity. As adults, many persons with NPD will have experienced high levels of achievement (Ronningstam and Gunderson 1990). However, their relationships with colleagues, peers, and staff will eventually become strained as their exploitative use of others and self-centered egotism become evident. Success may also be impaired by their difficulty in acknowledging or resolving criticism, deficits, and setbacks. Interpersonal and sexual relationships are usually easy for them to develop but difficult to sustain owing to their low empathy, self-centeredness, and need for admiration. Persons who are deferential and obsequious, or who share a mutual need for status and recognition, may help sustain a relationship. As parents, persons with NPD may attempt to live through their children, valuing them as long as they are a source of pride. Their personal sense of adjustment may be fine for as long as they continue to experience or anticipate success. Some may not recognize the maladaptivity of their narcissism until middle-age, when the emphasis given to achievement and status may begin to wane.

Differential Diagnosis

Individuals with NPD may often appear relatively high functioning. Exaggerated self-confidence may in fact contribute to success in a variety of professions and narcissistic traits will at times be seen in highly successful persons (Kernberg 1991b, Ronningstam and Gunderson 1990, Widiger et al. 1995). A diagnosis of NPD requires the additional presence of interpersonal exploitation, lack of empathy, a sense of entitlement, and other symptoms beyond simply arrogance and grandiosity.

Both narcissistic and antisocial persons may exploit, deceive, and manipulate others for personal gain, and both may demonstrate a lack of empathy or remorse. As indicated above, many of the traits of narcissism, such as arrogance and glib charm, are seen in psychopathic persons (Hare et al. 1991, Widiger et al. 1996). Prototypic cases can be distinguished, as the motivation for the narcissistic person will be for recognition, status, and other signs of success, whereas the prototypic antisocial person would be motivated more for material gain or for the subjugation of others (Widiger et al. 1995). Antisocial persons will also display an impulsivity, recklessness, and lax irresponsibility that may not be seen in narcissistic persons.

Etiology

There are no data on the heritability of the NPD (Jang and Vernon 2001, Nigg and Goldsmith 1994), although there are data on the heritability of arrogance, modesty, and conceit (Jang et al. 1998, Plomin and Caspi 1999). The etiological theories have been primarily sociological, psychodynamic, and interpersonal. For example, it has been suggested that current Western society has become overly self-centered with the decreasing importance of familial bonds, traditional social, religious, and political values or ideals, and rising materialism (Cooper and Ronningstam 1992, Millon et al. 1996).

Narcissism may also develop through unempathic, neglectful, and/or devaluing parental figures (Kernberg 1991b). The child may develop the belief that a sense of worth, value, or meaning is contingent upon accomplishment or achievement. Kohut (1977) has suggested that the parents failed to adequately mirror an infant's natural need for idealization. Benjamin (1993) and Millon and colleagues (1996) suggest that narcissistic persons received excessive idealization by parental figures, which they incorporated into their self-image. The irrationality of this idealization, or its being coupled with inconsistent indications of an actual disinterest and devaluation, may contribute to the eventual difficulties and conflicts surrounding self-image.

Conflicts and deficits with respect to self-esteem have been shown empirically to be central to the pathology of NPD (Raskin et al. 1991, Rhodewalt et al. 1998). Narcissistic persons must continually seek and obtain signs and symbols of recognition to compensate for feelings of inadequacy (Cooper and Ronningstam 1992, Stone 1993, Gabbard 2000). They are not persons who feel valued for their own sake. Value is contingent upon a success, accomplishment, or status. Their feelings of insecurity may be masked by a disdainful indifference towards rebuke and by overt expressions of arrogance, conceit, and even grandiosity. However, the psychopathology is still evident in such cases by the excessive reliance and importance that is continually placed upon status and recognition. Some narcissistic persons may in fact envy those who are truly indifferent to success and who can enjoy a modest, simple, and unassuming life.

Treatment

Persons with narcissistic personality traits seek treatment for feelings of depression, substance-related disorders, and occupational or relational problems that are secondary to their narcissism. Their self-centeredness and lack of empathy are particularly problematic within marital, occupational, and other social relationships, and they usually lack an appreciation of the contribution of their conflicts regarding self-esteem, status, and recognition (Gunderson and Gabbard 2000, Stone 1993). It is difficult for them even to admit that they have a psychological problem or that they need help, as this admission is itself an injury to their self-esteem. In addition, one of the characteristics of NPD is the belief that they can only be understood by persons of a comparably high social status or recognition. They may be unable to accept advice or insight from persons they consider less intelligent, talented, or insightful than themselves, which may eventually effectively eliminate most other persons.

When they are involved in treatment, persons with NPD will often require some indication that their therapist is among the best or at least worth their time. They are prone to idealizing their therapists (to affirm that he or she is indeed of sufficient status or quality) or to devalue them (to affirm that they are of greater intelligence, capacity, or quality than their therapist, to reject the insights that they have failed to identify, and to indicate that they warrant or deserve an even better therapist). How best to respond is often unclear. It may at times be preferable to simply accept the praise or criticism, particularly when exploration will likely be unsuccessful, whereas at other times it is preferable to confront and discuss the motivation for the devaluation (or the idealization).

Psychodynamic approaches to the treatment of NPD vary in the extent to which emphasis is given to an interpretation of underlying anger and bitterness, or to the provision of empathy and a reflection (or mirroring) of a positive regard and self-esteem (Cooper and Ronningstam 1992, Kernberg 1991b, Kohut 1977, Gabbard 2000). It does appear to be important to identify the current extent and historical source of the conflicts and sensitivities regarding self-esteem. Active confrontation may at times be useful, particularly when the therapeutic alliance is strong, but at other times the vulnerability of the individual may require a more unconditional support (Stone 1993). Cognitive–behavior approaches to NPD emphasize increasing awareness of the impact of narcissistic behaviors and statements on interpersonal relationships (Beck and Freeman 1990). The idealization and devaluation can be responsive to role playing and rational introspection, an intellectual approach that may itself be valued by some persons with NPD. However, therapists must be careful not to become embroiled within intellectual conflicts (or competitions). This approach may not work well with the narcissistic person who is motivated to defeat or humiliate the therapist (Kernberg 1991b).

Group therapy can be useful for increasing awareness of the grandiosity, lack of empathy, and devaluation of others. However, these traits not only interfere with the narcissistic person's ability to sustain membership within groups (and within individual therapy) but also may become quite harmful and destructive to the rapport of the entire group. There is no accepted pharmacologic approach to the treatment of narcissism (Markovitz 2001).

CLUSTER C

AVOIDANT PERSONALITY DISORDER

Diagnosis

Avoidant personality disorder (AVPD) is a pervasive pattern of timidity, inhibition, inadequacy, and social hypersensitivity (American Psychiatric Association 2000). Persons with AVPD may have a strong desire to develop close, personal relationships but feel too insecure to approach others or to express their feelings. AVPD is indicated by the presence of four or more of the seven diagnostic criteria presented in the DSM criteria for AVPD (see below).

DSM-IV-TR Diagnostic Criteria

301.82 Avoidant Personality Disorder

A pervasive pattern of social inhibition, feelings of inadequacy, and hypersensitivity to negative evaluation, beginning by early adulthood and present in a variety of contexts, as indicated by four (or more) of the following:

A. avoids occupational activities that involve significant interpersonal contact, because of fears of criticism, disapproval, or rejection
B. is unwilling to get involved with people unless certain of being liked
C. shows restraint within intimate relationships because of the fear of being shamed or ridiculed
D. is preoccupied with thoughts of being criticized or rejected in social situations
E. is inhibited in new interpersonal situations because of feelings of inadequacy
F. views self as socially inept, personally unappealing, or inferior to others
G. is unusually reluctant to take personal risks or to engage in any new activities because they may prove embarrassing

Reprinted with permission from the Diagnostic and Statistical Manual of Mental Disorders, Fourth Edition, Text Revision. Copyright 2000 American Psychiatric Association.

Epidemiology

Timidity, shyness, and social insecurity are not uncommon problems (Crozier and Alden 2001) and AVPD is one of the more prevalent personality disorders within clinical settings, occurring in 5 to 25% of all individuals presenting with personality disorders (American Psychiatric Association 2000, Mattia and Zimmerman 2001). However, AVPD may be diagnosed in only 1 to 2% of the general population (see Table 44-2). It appears to occur equally among males and females, with some studies reporting more males and others reporting more females (Corbitt and Widiger 1995).

Course

Persons with AVPD are shy, timid, and anxious as children (Bernstein and Travaglini 1999). Many are diagnosed with a social phobia during childhood. Adolescence is a particularly difficult developmental period due to the importance at this time of attractiveness, dating, and popularity. Occupational success may not be significantly impaired, as long as there is little demand for public performance. Persons with AVPD may in fact find considerable gratification and esteem through a job or career that they are unable to find within their relationships. The job may serve as a distraction from intense feelings of loneliness. Their avoidance of social situations will impair their ability to develop adequate social skills, and this will then further handicap any eventual efforts to develop relationships. As parents, they may be very responsible, empathic, and affectionate, but may unwittingly impart feelings of social anxiousness and awkwardness. Severity of the AVPD symptomatology diminishes as the person becomes older.

Differential Diagnosis

The most difficult differential diagnosis for AVPD is with generalized social phobia (Tillfors et al. 2001, van Velzen et al. 2000, Widiger 2001). Both involve an avoidance of social situations, social anxiety, and timidity, and both may be evident since late childhood or adolescence. Many persons with AVPD in fact seek treatment for a social phobia. To the extent that the behavior pattern pervades the person's everyday functioning and has been evident since childhood, the diagnosis of a personality disorder would be more descriptive. There are arguments to subsume all cases of AVPD into the diagnosis of generalized social phobia (as was done for schizoid disorder of childhood in DSM-IV-TR), but there is considerable empirical support for the existence of the personality dimensions of introversion and neuroticism and for an understanding of AVPD as a maladaptive variant of these personality traits (Costa and Widiger 2002, Trull et al. 1998, Widiger 2001).

Many persons with AVPD may also meet the criteria for DPD. This might at first glance seem unusual, given that AVPD involves social withdrawal whereas DPD involves excessive social attachment. However, once a person with AVPD is able to obtain a relationship, he or she will often cling to this relationship in a dependent manner. Both disorders include feelings of inadequacy, needs for reassurance, and hypersensitivity to criticism and neglect (i.e., abnormally high levels of anxiousness, self-consciousness, and vulnerability). A distinction between AVPD and DPD is best made when the person is seeking a relationship (Widiger et al. 1995). Avoidant persons tend to be very shy, inhibited, and timid (and are therefore slow to get involved with someone) whereas dependent persons urgently seek another relationship as soon as one ends (i.e., avoidant persons are high in introversion whereas dependent persons are high in extraversion). Avoidant persons may also be reluctant to express their feelings whereas dependent persons can drive others away by continuous expressions of neediness. The differentiation of AVPD from the schizoid, paranoid, and schizotypal personality disorders was discussed in previous sections.

Etiology

AVPD appears to be an extreme variant of the fundamental personality traits of introversion and neuroticism (Widiger et al. 2002). Introversion includes facets such as passivity, social withdrawal, and inhibition, while neuroticism includes self-consciousness, vulnerability, and anxiousness (Costa and McCrae 1992). The personality dimensions of neuroticism and introversion have substantial heritability, as do the more specific traits of social anxiousness, shyness, and inhibition (Jang et al. 1998, Jang and Vernon 2001, Nigg and Goldsmith 1994, Plomin and Caspi 1999).

In childhood, neuroticism appears as a distress-prone or inhibited temperament (Rothbart and Ahadi 1994). Shyness, timidity, and interpersonal insecurity might be exacerbated further in childhood through overprotection and excessive cautiousness (Schmidt et al. 2001). Parental behavior coupled with a distress-prone temperament has been shown to result in social inhibition and timidity (Burgess et al. 2001, Rothbart and Ahadi 1994). Most children and adolescents will have many experiences of interpersonal embarrassment, rejection, or humiliation, but these will be particularly devastating to the person who is already lacking in self-confidence or is temperamentally passive, inhibited, or introverted.

AVPD may involve elevated peripheral sympathetic activity and adrenocortical responsiveness, resulting in excessive autonomic arousal, fearfulness, and inhibition (Siever and Davis 1991). Just as ASPD may involve deficits in the functioning of a BIS, AVPD may involve excessive functioning of this same system (Depue and Lenzenweger 2001). The pathology of AVPD, however, may also be more psychological than neurochemical, with the timidity, shyness, and insecurity being a natural result of a cumulative history of denigrating, embarrassing, and devaluing experiences (Schmidt et al. 2001). Underlying AVPD may be excessive self-consciousness, feelings of inadequacy or inferiority, and irrational cognitive schemas that perpetuate introverted, avoidant behavior (Beck and Freeman 1990, Clark 2001, Dreessen et al. 1999).

Treatment

Persons with AVPD seek treatment for their avoidant personality traits, although many initially seek treatment for symptoms of anxiety, particularly social phobia (generalized subtype). It is important in such cases to recognize that the shyness is not due simply to a dysregulation or dyscontrol of anxiousness. There is instead a more pervasive and fundamental psychopathology, involving feelings of interpersonal insecurity, low self-esteem, and inadequacy (Millon et al. 1996, Stone 1993, Widiger 2001).

Social skills training, systematic desensitization, and a graded hierarchy of *in vivo* exposure to feared social situations have been shown to be useful in the treatment of AVPD (Beck and Freeman 1990, Clark 2001, Millon et al. 1996). However, it is also important to discuss the underlying fears and insecurities regarding attractiveness, desirability, rejection, or intimacy (Stone 1993, Gabbard 2000, Gunderson and Gabbard 2000). Persons with AVPD are at times reluctant to discuss such feelings, as they may feel embarrassed, they may fear being ridiculed, or they may not want to "waste the time" of the therapist with such "foolish" insecurities. They may prefer a less revealing or involved form of treatment. It is important to be understanding, patient, and accepting, and to proceed at a pace that is comfortable for the individual. Insecurities and fears can at times be addressed through cognitive techniques as the irrationality is usually readily apparent (Beck and Freeman 1990, Clark 2001). It remains useful though to identify the historical source of their development, as this understanding will help the individual appreciate the irrationality or irrelevance of their expectations and perceptions for their current relationships.

Persons with AVPD often find group therapies to be helpful. Exploratory and supportive groups can provide them with an understanding environment in which to discuss their social insecurities, to explore and practice more assertive behaviors, and to develop an increased self-confidence in approaching others and developing relationships outside of the group. Focused and specialized social skills-training groups would be preferable to unstructured groups that might be predominated by much more assertive and extraverted members.

Many persons with AVPD will respond to anxiolytic medications, and at times to antidepressants, particularly monoamine oxidase inhibitors such as phenelzine (Markovitz 2001). Normal and abnormal feelings of anxiousness can be suppressed or diminished through pharmacologic interventions (Widiger 2001). This approach may in fact be necessary to overcome initial feelings of intense social anxiety that are markedly disruptive to current functioning (e.g., inability to give required presentations at work or to talk to new acquaintances). However, it is also important to monitor closely a reliance on medications. Persons with AVPD could be prone to rely excessively on substances to control their feelings of anxiousness, whereas their more general feelings of insecurity and inadequacy would require a more comprehensive treatment.

DEPENDENT PERSONALITY DISORDER

Diagnosis

Dependent personality disorder (DPD) involves a pervasive and excessive need to be taken care of, which leads to submissiveness, clinging, and fears of separation (American Psychiatric Association 2000, Bornstein 1999, Pincus and Wilson 2001). Persons with DPD will also have low self-esteem, and will often be self-critical and self-denigrating. DPD is indicated by the presence of five or more of the eight diagnostic criteria presented in DSM-IV-TR Criteria for DPD (see below).

DSM-IV-TR Diagnostic Criteria

301.6 Dependent Personality Disorder

A pervasive and excessive need to be taken care of that leads to submissive and clinging behavior and fears of separation, beginning by early adulthood and present in a variety of contexts, as indicated by five (or more) of the following:

A. has difficulty making everyday decisions without an excessive amount of advice and reassurance from others.
B. needs others to assume responsibility for most major areas of his or her life.
C. has difficulty expressing disagreement with others because of fear of loss of support or approval (**Note:** Do not include realistic fears of retribution).
D. has difficulty initiating projects or doing things on his or her own (because of a lack of self-confidence in judgment or abilities rather than to a lack of motivation or energy).
E. goes to excessive lengths to obtain nurturance and support from others, to the point of volunteering to do things that are unpleasant.
F. feels uncomfortable or helpless when alone, because of exaggerated fears of being unable to care for himself or herself.
G. urgently seeks another relationship as a source of care and support when a close relationship ends.
H. is unrealistically preoccupied with fears of being left to take care of himself or herself.

Epidemiology

DPD is among the most prevalent of the personality disorders (American Psychiatric Association 2000), occurring in 5 to 30% of individuals presenting with personality disorders and 2 to 4% of the general community (Mattia and Zimmerman 2001). A controversial issue is its differential sex prevalence (Bornstein 1999, Widiger 1998). DPD is diagnosed more frequently in females but there is some concern that there might be a failure to recognize adequately the extent of dependent personality traits within males (Bornstein 1999, Corbitt and Widiger 1995).

Course

Persons with DPD are likely to have been excessively submissive as children and adolescents, and some may have had a chronic physical illness or a separation anxiety disorder during childhood (American Psychiatric Association 2000). Persons with DPD fear intensely a loss of concern, care, and support from others, particularly the person with whom they have an emotional attachment (Bornstein 1999, Stone 1993). They are unable to be by themselves, as their sense of self-worth, value, or meaning is obtained by or through the presence of a relationship. They have few other sources of self-esteem. Along with the need for emotional support are perpetual doubts and insecurities regarding the current source of support. Persons with DPD constantly require reassurance and reaffirmation that any particular relationship will continue, because they anticipate or fear that at some point they may again be alone (Overholser 1996). Because of their intense fear of being alone, they may become quickly attached to persons who are unreliable, unempathic, and even exploitative or abusive. More desirable or reliable partners are at times driven away by their excessive clinging and continued demands for reassurance. Occupational functioning is impaired to the extent that independent responsibility and initiative are required. Persons with DPD are prone to mood disorders, particularly major depressive disorder and dysthymic disorder, and to anxiety disorders, particularly agoraphobia, social phobia, and perhaps panic disorder. However, the severity of the symptomatology tends to decrease with age, particularly if the person has obtained a reliable, dependable, and empathic partner.

Differential Diagnosis

Excessive dependency will often be seen in persons who have developed debilitating mental and general medical disorders such as agoraphobia, schizophrenia, mental retardation, severe injuries, and dementia. However, a diagnosis of DPD requires the presence of the dependent traits since late childhood or adolescence (American Psychiatric Association 2000). One can diagnose the presence of a personality disorder at any age during a person's lifetime, but if, for example, a DPD diagnosis is given to a person at the age of 75 years, this presumes that the dependent behavior was evident since the age of approximately 18 years (i.e., predates the onset of a comorbid mental or physical disorder).

Deference, politeness, and passivity will also vary substantially across cultural groups. It is important not to confuse differences in personality that are due to different cultural norms with the presence of a personality disorder (Alarcon 1996, Alarcon and Foulks 1997, Bornstein 1999). The diagnosis of DPD requires that the dependent behavior be maladaptive, resulting in clinically significant functional impairment or distress.

Many persons with DPD will also meet the criteria for HPD and BPD. Persons with DPD and HPD may both display strong needs for reassurance, attention, and approval. However, persons with DPD tend to be more self-effacing, docile, and altruistic, whereas persons with HPD tend to be more flamboyant, assertive, and self-centered, and persons with BPD will tend to be much more dysfunctional and emotionally dysregulated (Bornstein 1999, Widiger et al. 1995).

Etiology

Central to the etiology and pathology of DPD is an insecure interpersonal attachment (Bornstein 1999, Pincus and Wilson 2001, Stone 1993). Insecure attachment and helplessness may be generated through a parent–child relationship, perhaps by a clinging parent or a continued infantilization during a time in which individuation and separation normally occurs (Gabbard 2000, Thompson and Zuroff 1998). However, DPD may also represent an interaction of an anxious–inhibited temperament with inconsistent or overprotective parenting (Bornstein 1999, O'Neill and Kendler 1998, Rothbart and Ahadi 1994). Dependent persons may turn to a parental figure to provide a reassurance, security, and confidence that they are unable to generate for themselves. They may eventually believe that their self-worth is contingent upon the worth or importance they have to another person (Beck and Freeman 1990).

Treatment

Persons with DPD are often in treatment for one or more Axis I disorders, particularly a mood (depressive) or an anxiety disorder. They tend to be very agreeable, compliant, and grateful individuals, at times to excess. An important issue in the treatment of persons with DPD is not letting the relationship with the therapist become an end in itself (Stone 1993). Many persons with DPD find the therapeutic relationship satisfying their need for support, concern, and involvement. The therapist can be perceived as a nurturing, caring, and dependable partner who is always available for as long as the individual desires. Successful treatment can in fact be feared because it suggests the termination of the relationship, an outcome that is at times avoided at all costs. As a result, they be may be excessively compliant, submissive, agreeable, and cooperative in order to be the individual that the therapist would want to retain. Therapists need to be careful not to unwittingly encourage or exploit this submissiveness, nor to commit the opposite error of rejecting and abandoning them to be rid of their needy and clinging dependency. Such responses are common in the interpersonal (marital and sexual) history of persons with DPD, and are at times experienced as well within therapeutic relationships. Persons with DPD tend to have unrealistic expectations regarding their therapist. They may attempt to have the therapist take control of their lives, and may make unrealistic requests or demands for their therapist's time, involvement, and availability.

Exploration of the breadth and source of the need for care and support is often an important component of treatment (Gunderson and Gabbard 2000). Persons with DPD often have a history of exploitative, rejecting, and perhaps even abusive relationships that have contributed to their current feelings of insecurity and inadequacy (Bornstein 1999). Cognitive–behavioral techniques are useful in addressing the feelings of inadequacy, incompetence, and helplessness (Beck and Freeman 1990). Social skills, problem-solving, and assertiveness training also makes important contributions.

Persons with DPD may also benefit from group therapy. A supportive group is useful in diffusing the feelings of dependency onto a variety of persons, in providing feedback regarding their manner of relating to others, and in providing practice and role models for more assertive and autonomous interpersonal functioning. There is no known pharmacologic treatment for DPD (Markovitz 2001).

OBSESSIVE–COMPULSIVE PERSONALITY DISORDER

Diagnosis

Obsessive–compulsive personality disorder (OCPD) includes a preoccupation with orderliness, perfectionism, and mental and interpersonal control (American Psychiatric Association 2000). OCPD is indicated by the presence of four or more of the eight diagnostic criteria presented in DSM criteria for OCPD (see page 1267).

DSM-IV-TR Diagnostic Criteria

301.4 Obsessive–Compulsive Personality Disorder

A pervasive pattern of preoccupation with orderliness, perfectionism, and mental and interpersonal control at the expense of flexibility, openness, and efficiency, beginning by early adulthood and present in a variety of contexts, as indicated by four (or more) of the following:

A. is preoccupied with details, rules, lists, order, organization, or schedules to the extent that the major point of the activity is lost
B. shows perfectionism that interferes with task completion (e.g., is unable to complete a project because his or her own overly strict standards are not met)
C. excessive devotion to work and productivity to the exclusion of leisure activities and friendships (not accounted for by obvious economic necessity)
D. is overconscientious, scrupulous, and inflexible about matters of morality, ethics, or values (not accounted for by cultural or religious identification)
E. is unable to discard worn-out or worthless objects even when they have no sentimental value
F. is reluctant to delegate tasks or to work with others unless they submit to exactly his or her way of doing things
G. adopts a miserly spending style toward both self and others; money is viewed as something to be hoarded for future catastrophes
H. shows rigidity and stubbornness.

Reprinted with permission from the Diagnostic and Statistical Manual of Mental Disorders, Fourth Edition, Text Revision. Copyright 2000 American Psychiatric Association.

Epidemiology

Conscientiousness is one of the fundamental dimensions of personality (Hogan et al. 1997, Pervin and John 1999), characterized by the tendency to emphasize duty, order, deliberation, discipline, competence, and achievement (Costa and McCrae 1992). Persons who are excessively organized, ordered, deliberate, dutiful, and disciplined would be characterized as having OCPD (Widiger et al. 2002). Only 1 to 2% of the general community may meet the diagnostic criteria for the disorder (see Table 44-2), but this could be an underestimation (Oldham and Frosch 1991). Up to 10% of the population has been estimated to be maladaptively stubborn, 4% excessively devoted to work, and 8% excessively perfectionistic (Nestadt et al. 1991). OCPD is one of the less frequently diagnosed personality disorders within inpatient settings, occurring in approximately 3 to 10% of individuals (American Psychiatric Association 2000), but its prevalence may be much higher within private practice settings. This disorder does appear to occur more often in males than in females but exceptions to this finding have been reported (Corbitt and Widiger 1995).

Course

As children, some persons with OCPD may have appeared to be relatively well-behaved, responsible, and conscientious. However, they may have also been overly serious, rigid, and constrained (Rothbart and Ahadi 1994). As adults, many will obtain good to excellent success within a job or career. They can be excellent workers to the point of excess, sacrificing their social and leisure activities, marriage, and family for their job (Oldham and Frosch 1991, Stone 1993). Relationships with spouse and children are likely to be strained because of their tendency to be detached and uninvolved, yet authoritarian and domineering with respect to decisions. A spouse may complain of a lack of affection, tenderness, and warmth. Relationships with colleagues at work may be equally strained by the excessive perfectionism, domination, indecision, worrying, and anger. Jobs that require flexibility, openness, creativity, or diplomacy may be particularly difficult. Persons with OCPD may be prone to various anxiety and physical disorders that are secondary to their worrying, indecision, and stress. Those with concomitant traits of angry hostility and competitiveness may be prone to cardiovascular disorders. Mood disorders may not develop until the person recognizes the sacrifices that have been made by their devotion to work and productivity, which may at times not occur until middle age. However, most will experience early employment or career difficulties, or even failures that may result in depression.

Differential Diagnosis

Devotion to work and productivity will vary substantially across cultural groups. One should be careful not to confuse normal cultural variation in conscientiousness with the presence of this personality disorder. A diagnosis of OCPD requires that the devotion to work be maladaptive or to the exclusion of leisure activities and friendships (American Psychiatric Association 2000).

OCPD resembles to some extent the obsessive–compulsive disorder (OCD). However, many persons with OCD fail to develop OCD, and vice versa (Pfohl and Blum 1991). OCD involves intrusive obsessions or circumscribed and repetitively performed rituals whose purpose is to reduce or control feelings of anxiety (American Psychiatric Association 2000). OCPD, in contrast, involves rigid, inhibited, and authoritarian behavior patterns that are more ego-syntonic. If both behavior patterns are present, both diagnoses should be given as these disorders are sufficiently distinct that it is likely that in such cases two different disorders are in fact present (Widiger et al. 1995).

OCPD may at times resemble narcissistic PD, as both disorders can involve assertiveness, domination, achievement, and a professed perfectionism. However, the emphasis in OCPD will be on work for its own sake, whereas narcissistic persons will work only to achieve status and recognition (Widiger et al. 1995). Persons with OCPD will also be troubled by doubts, worries, and self-criticism, whereas the narcissistic person will tend to be overly self-assured.

Etiology

A variety of studies have indicated heritability for the trait of obsessionality (Nigg and Goldsmith 1994). OCPD may also relate to the adult personality trait of conscientiousness–constraint (Costa and McCrae 1992, Widiger et al. 2002) and the childhood temperament of attentional self-regulation, both of which have demonstrated substantial heritability (Jang and Vernon 2001, Plomin and Caspi 1999, Rothbart and Ahadi 1994).

Early psychoanalytic theories regarding OCPD concerned issues of unconscious guilt or shame (Gunderson and Gabbard 2000). A variety of underlying conflicts have since been proposed, including a need to maintain an illusion of infallibility to defend against feelings of insecurity, an identification with authoritarian parents, or an excessive, rigid control of feelings and impulses (Gabbard 2000, Oldham and Frosch 1991, Stone 1993). Any one or more of these conflicts might be relevant for a particular person with OCPD, but there is quite limited empirical support for these particular models of etiology and pathology. OCPD includes personality traits that are highly valued within most cultures (e.g., conscientiousness) and some instances of OCPD may reflect exaggerated or excessive responses to the expectations of or pressures by parental figures.

Treatment

Persons with OCPD may fail to seek treatment for the OCPD symptomatology. They may seek treatment instead for disorders and problems that are secondary to their OCPD traits, including anxiety disorders, health problems (e.g., cardiovascular disorders), and problems within various relationships (e.g., marital, familial, and occupational). Treatment will be complicated by their inability to appreciate the contribution of their personality to these problems and disorders (Gunderson and Gabbard 2000, Oldham and Frosch 1991, Stone 1993). It is not unusual for persons with OCPD to perceive themselves as being simply conscientious, dutiful, moral, and responsible, rather than perfectionistic, stubborn, rigid, domineering, and unavailable. Their understanding is complicated further by the contribution of their traits to various achievements and successes (e.g., career advancement) and to the control of negative affect (e.g., ability to control feelings of dysphoria during a crisis). The OCPD traits are not invariably or always maladaptive, and persons with this disorder may not appreciate the disorder's cost to their physical health, psychological well-being, and personal relationships.

Cognitive–behavioral techniques that address the irrationality of excessive conscientiousness, moralism, perfectionism, devotion to work, and stubbornness can be effective in the treatment of OCPD (Beck and Freeman 1990). Persons with OCPD may in fact appreciate the rational approach to treatment provided by cognitive–behavioral therapy. A common difficulty though is the tendency to drift into lengthy and unproductive ruminations and intellectualized speculations (Beck and Freeman 1990, Gunderson and Gabbard 2000, Stone 1993). Therapeutic techniques that emphasize the acknowledgment, recognition, and acceptance of feelings will therefore be useful (Gabbard 2000). Gestalt techniques that focus upon and confront feeling states will often feel threatening to persons with OCPD, but precisely for this reason, they can also be quite revealing and useful. Persons with OCPD will attempt to control therapeutic sessions, and techniques that encourage uncontrolled, freely expressed associations to explore historical motivations for control, perfectionism, and workaholism are often helpful.

Persons with OCPD can be problematic in groups. They will tend to be domineering, constricted, and judgmental. There is no accepted pharmacologic treatment for OCPD (Markovitz 2001). Some persons with OCPD will benefit from anxiolytic or antidepressant medications, but this will typically reflect the presence of associated features or comorbid disorders. The core traits of OCPD might not be affected by pharmacologic interventions.

Personality Disorder Not Otherwise Specified

As indicated earlier, DSM-IV-TR includes a diagnostic category, personality disorder not otherwise specified (PDNOS), for persons with a personality disorder who do not meet the diagnostic criteria for any one of the 10 officially recognized diagnoses (see DSM-IV-TR definition of PDNOS on page 1270). PDNOS has in fact been the single most commonly used personality disorder diagnosis in almost every study in which it has been considered (Clark et al. 1995, Widiger and Coker 2002). It would not, of course, be possible to discuss the etiology, pathology, course, or treatment of the PDNOS disorder as the diagnosis refers to a wide variety of personality types. However, one usage of PDNOS is for the two personality disorders presented in the appendix to DSM-IV-TR for criterion sets provided for further study, the passive–aggressive and the depressive (American Psychiatric Association 2000).

DSM-IV-TR Definition

301.9 Personality Disorder Not Otherwise Specified

This category is for disorders of personality functioning (refer to the general diagnostic criteria for a Personality Disorder) that do not meet criteria for any specific Personality Disorder. An example is the presence of features of more than one specific Personality Disorder that do not meet the full criteria for any one Personality Disorder ("mixed personality"), but that together cause clinically significant distress or impairment in one or more important areas of functioning (e.g., social or occupational). This category can also be used when the clinician judges that a specific Personality Disorder that is not included in the Classification is appropriate. Examples include depressive personality disorder (DPPD) and passive-aggressive personality disorder.

PASSIVE–AGGRESSIVE (NEGATIVISTIC) PERSONALITY DISORDER

Diagnosis

Passive–aggressive personality disorder (PAPD) is a pervasive pattern of negativistic attitudes and passive resistance to authority, demands, responsibilities, or obligations (American Psychiatric Association 2000) (see DSM-IV-TR research criteria for PAPD, below). PAPD would be diagnosed by the presence of four or more of the seven criteria presented in DSM-IV-TR criteria for PAPD. Most of the DSM-IV-TR semistructured interviews include items for the assessment of PAPD (First et al. 1997, Pfohl et al. 1997, Widiger et al. 1995, Zanarini et al. 1995).

DSM-IV-TR Research Criteria

Passive–Aggressive Personality Disorder

A. A pervasive pattern of negativistic attitudes and passive resistance to demands for adequate performance, beginning by early adulthood and present in a variety of contexts, as indicated by four (or more) of the following:

   (1) passively resists fulfilling routine social and occupational tasks
   (2) complains of being misunderstood and unappreciated by others
   (3) is sullen and argumentative
   (4) unreasonably criticizes and scorns authority
   (5) expresses envy and resentment toward those apparently more fortunate
   (6) voices exaggerated and persistent complaints of personal misfortune
   (7) alternates between hostile defiance and contrition

B. Does not occur exclusively during major depressive episodes and is not better accounted for by dysthymic disorder.

PAPD was an officially recognized diagnosis in DSM-III-R (American Psychiatric Association 1987). It is in the appendix of DSM-IV-TR because there has been little research to support its validity. There was concern that the DSM-III-R diagnosis described a situational reaction rather than a pervasive and chronic personality disorder, and the criteria were revised substantially for DSM-IV to describe a more general and pervasive negativism (Gunderson 1998, Widiger et al. 1995). Compelling objections were raised in response to the decision to downgrade the recognition of this longstanding diagnosis (Wetzler and Morey 1999) and the new criteria may eventually prove to have more validity and clinical utility than the DSM-III-R version (McCann 1988, Millon 1993), but this additional research needs to be conducted in order for the diagnosis to be given an official recognition.

Epidemiology

Approximately 1 to 2% of the community will meet the DSM-III-R criteria for PAPD (see Table 44-2). Up to 5% of individuals were being diagnosed with PAPD earlier (McCann 1988, Millon 1993, Wetzler and Morey 1999). The rate was higher when semistructured interviews were used but still low compared to most other personality disorders. The prevalence rate with the DSM-IV-TR criteria are likely to be higher, given the expansion of the disorder from simply a passive resistance to demands for adequate performance to a more general negativism (Millon 1993). An approximately equal prevalence of males and females have traits that met the criteria for the disorder based upon the DSM-III and DSM-III-R criteria (Corbitt and Widiger 1995). However, the broader formulation of negativism resembles closely the general trait of oppositionalism (characterized by the tendency to be complaining, discontented, grumbling, whining, and argumentative), which does appear to occur more often in males than in females (Costa and McCrae 1992).

Course

Many persons with PAPD may have met the criteria for an oppositional defiant disorder during childhood, which is also characterized by the tendency to be irritable, complaining, oppositional, argumentative, and negativistic (American Psychiatric Association 1980). As adults, impairment is likely to be most evident with respect to employment. Persons with PAPD are irresponsible, lax, and negligent employees, as well as resistant, oppositional, and even hostile. Resolution of interpersonal conflicts is difficult due to the tendency of the passive–aggressive person to blame others. They are argumentative, sullen, and critical of their peers and friends, who may not tolerate their antagonism.

Differential Diagnosis

It is particularly important when assessing for PAPD to recognize that passive–aggressive behavior might be confined to settings in which persons have lost freedom, responsibility, or decision-making authority that was previously available to them and overt expressions of assertiveness or opposition are being discouraged. For example, it would not be surprising to observe passive–aggressive behavior within the military, prison, or some inpatient hospitals. It is important in such settings to verify that the negativistic behavior was evident earlier and is currently evident within other situations.

Etiology

Central to the psychopathology of PAPD appears to be bitter resentment (Millon et al. 1996). Passive–aggressive persons have a hostile, angry, and bitter attitude towards the world. There are no data on its heritability or psychosocial etiology. It has been suggested that passive–aggressive behavior is due in part to conflicts concerning dependency and resentment, or a history of mistreatment and neglect (McCann 1988). One might find a history of being exploited, neglected, mistreated, or abused by persons upon whom the person with PAPD relied. Negativistic traits may also be modeled by parental figures.

Treatment

Persons with PAPD rarely enter treatment to make effective changes to their personality or behavior. They are more likely to seek treatment for Axis I disorders (e.g., depression, anxiety, or somatoform disorder), or for marital, family, or occupational problems. The initiation of treatment is often at the insistence of a spouse, relative, or employer (Gabbard 2000, Stone 1993). They can be very difficult individuals to treat due to their tendency to be blaming, argumentative, pessimistic, and passively resistant (Millon et al. 1996). It is important for the therapist to remain supportive and empathic, carefully and benignly offering observations, suggestions, and reflections on the individual's tendency to be their own worst enemy. Cognitive treatment can be useful to directly address the false perceptions, assumptions, and attributions (Beck and Freeman 1990) as long as the therapist is not drawn into unproductive disagreements and arguments. It is common for therapists to become frustrated, impatient, and defensive in response to the negativism, criticism, and complaints. Periodic consultation with colleagues are advisable. Group therapy is often helpful once the individual has developed a commitment to the group, as the various members can provide consistent and confirmatory feedback regarding the negativistic and passive–aggressive behavior. There is no known pharmacologic treatment for PAPD (Markovitz 2001).

DEPRESSIVE PERSONALITY DISORDER

Diagnosis

Depressive personality disorder (DPPD) is a pervasive pattern of depressive cognitions and behaviors that have been evident since adolescence and characteristic of everyday functioning (American Psychiatric Association 2000). These are persons who characteristically display a gloominess, cheerlessness, pessimism, brooding, rumination, and dejection. DPPD would be diagnosed by the presence of five or more of the seven criteria presented in the DSM criteria for DPPD (see below).

DSM-IV-TR Research Criteria

Depressive Personality Disorder

A. A pervasive pattern of depressive cognitions and behaviors beginning by early adulthood and present in a variety of contexts, as indicated by five (or more) of the following:

    (1) usual mood is dominated by dejection, gloominess, cheerlessness, joylessness, unhappiness

    (2) self-concept centers around beliefs of inadequacy, worthlessness, and low self-esteem

    (3) is critical, blaming, and derogatory toward self

    (4) is brooding and given to worry

    (5) is negativistic, critical, and judgmental toward others

    (6) is pessimistic

    (7) is prone to feeling guilty or remorseful

B. Does not occur exclusively during major depressive episodes and is not better accounted for by dysthymic disorder.

DPPD was proposed for inclusion in DSM-III and DSM-III-R, but there were concerns that it may not be adequately distinguished from the mood disorder of dysthymia (Klein 1999, Phillips et al. 1995, 1998, Ryder and Bagby 1999, Widiger 1999). However, a field trial by the DSM-IV Mood Disorders Work Group indicated that many persons do meet diagnostic criteria for DPPD rather than early-onset dysthymia (Phillips et al. 1995, Widiger 1999). In addition, many persons diagnosed with early-onset dysthymia may not be adequately described as having a disorder that is confined to the regulation or control of their mood (Klein 1999, Phillips et al. 1998). However, the DSM-IV-TR diagnostic criteria for DPPD lack sufficient empirical support to warrant full recognition (Gunderson 1998).

Most of the DSM-IV-TR semistructured interviews include items for the assessment of DPPD (First et al. 1997, Pfohl et al. 1997, Widiger et al. 1995, Zanarini et al. 1995), and a semistructured interview that is devoted to its assessment is also available—the Diagnostic Interview for Depressive Personality (Gunderson et al. 1994).

Epidemiology
There are not yet published data on the prevalence of DPPD within the general population. DPPD is likely to be comorbid with early-onset dysthymia, although not all cases of DPPD will meet the DSM-IV-TR criteria for dysthymia (Klein 1999, Phillips et al. 1995).

Course
As children, persons with DPPD are pessimistic, gloomy, passive, and withdrawn. Performance in school is often inadequate to poor. This behavior pattern continues essentially unchanged into and through adulthood. Some, however, may eventually become good workers, exhibiting tremendous discipline and devotion to their work (Phillips et al. 1995). Relationships with peers and sexual partners, however, are invariably problematic. They are gloomy and irritable company, and have difficulty finding pleasure, joy, or satisfaction in leisure activities (Millon et al. 1996). They may also be quite withdrawn and lonely, but lack an apparent motivation or energy to seek or maintain relationships.

Differential Diagnosis
DPPD overlaps substantially with early-onset dysthymia. Early-onset dysthymia was in fact conceptualized previously as depressive personality or a characterologic depression prior to DSM-III-R (Keller 1989), and the alternative criteria for dysthymia that were placed in the appendix to DSM-IV-TR were developed in part on research on DPPD (Phillips et al. 1995, Widiger 1999). It is in fact noted in DSM-IV-TR that there may not be a meaningful distinction between these diagnoses (American Psychiatric Association 2000). Some may prefer to use the diagnosis of early-onset dysthymia, but a dysregulation in mood may not adequately explain why some persons are characterized by chronic attitudes of pessimism, negativism, hopelessness, and dejection.

Etiology
DPPD may represent a characterologic variant of mood disorder, in the same manner that STPD is perhaps a characterologic variant of schizophrenia. Support for this hypothesis

is provided by recent family history and biogenetic studies (Klein 1999). Trait depression is also a facet of the personality trait of neuroticism or negative affectivity, which has demonstrated substantial heritability within the general population (Jang et al. 1998, Jang and Vernon 2001, Pervin and John 1999). A characteristically low self-esteem, self-criticism, pessimism, brooding, and guilt may also result from continued, sustained criticism, derogation, and discouragement by a significant parental figure which is accepted and incorporated by the child (Stone 1993).

Treatment

Many persons with DPD are referred or seek treatment for a depressive mood disorder. It is important in such cases to recognize the extent to which the depressed mood reflects their fundamental view of themselves and the world. Their pessimism involves more than simply a dysregulation of mood. Cognitive–behavioral techniques have demonstrated efficacy in the treatment of depressive personality traits (Beck and Freeman 1990). The depressive individual's pessimistic view of themselves and their future should be systematically challenged. Explorations of the faulty reasoning, arbitrary inferences, selective perceptions, and misattributions can be influential in overcoming the pessimistic, gloomy, critical, and negativistic attitudes. Audio- or videotaped role playing is useful in helping the person recognize the occurrence and pervasiveness of the depressive cognitions, and in generating, developing, and rehearsing more realistic and accurate reasoning. However, exploration of the source for, and historical development of, self-defeating behaviors may also be helpful, not only to undermine their credibility and validity within current relationships and situations but also to address any motivation for their perpetuation (Stone 1993). Persons with DPPD will also be responsive to antidepressant pharmacotherapy, particularly tricyclic antidepressants (Klein 1999, Markovitz 2001, Widiger 1999).

Comparison of DSM-IV-TR/ICD-10 Diagnostic Criteria

The items sets for paranoid, schizoid, schizotypal, antisocial, histrionic, avoidant, dependent, and obsessive–compulsive personality disorders in the ICD-10 Diagnostic Criteria for Research and the DSM-IV-TR criteria differ but define essentially the same condition. Furthermore, ICD-10 does not consider schizotypal to be a personality disorder and instead includes this condition in the section containing schizophrenia and other psychotic disorders. ICD-10 also refers to several of the DSM-IV-TR disorders by different names: antisocial is called "dissocial," borderline is called "emotionally unstable personality disorder, borderline type," and obsessive–compulsive is called "anankastic."

ICD-10 includes an "emotionally unstable personality disorder" with two subtypes: impulsive type and borderline type; criteria are provided for each subtype but not for emotionally unstable personality disorder. Neither of these subtypes by themselves correspond to the DSM-IV-TR BPD, which includes some items from each of these subtypes. Narcissistic personality disorder in DSM-IV-TR is not included in ICD-10 as a specific personality disorder, although the DSM-IV-TR criteria set is included in Annex I of ICD-10 (i.e., "provisional criteria for selected disorders").

References

Ad-Dab'bagh Y and Greenfield B (2001) Multiple complex developmental disorder: the "multiple and complex" evolution of the "childhood borderline syndrome" construct. *J Am Acad Child Adolesc Psychiatry* **40**, 954–964.

Alarcon RD (1996) Personality disorders and culture in DSM-IV: A critique. *J Personal Disord* **10**, 260–270.

Alarcon RD and Foulks EF (1997) Cultural factors and personality disorders: a review of the literature. In *DSM-IV Sourcebook*, Vol. 3, Widiger TA, Frances AJ, Pincus HA, et al. (eds). American Psychiatric Association, Washington, DC, pp. 975–982.

American Psychiatric Association (1980) *Diagnostic and Statistical Manual of Mental Disorders*, 3rd ed., APA, Washington, DC.

American Psychiatric Association (1987) *Diagnostic and Statistical Manual of Mental Disorders*, 3rd ed., Rev. APA, Washington, DC.

American Psychiatric Association (2000) *Diagnostic and Statistical Manual of Mental Disorders*, 4th ed., Text Rev. APA, Washington, DC.

Beck AT and Freeman A (1990) *Cognitive Therapy of Personality Disorders*. Guilford Press, New York.

Benjamin LS (1993) *Interpersonal Diagnosis and Treatment of Personality Disorders*. Guilford Press, New York.

Bernstein DP and Travaglini L (1999) Schizoid and avoidant personality disorders. In *Oxford Textbook of Psychopathology*, Millon T, Blaney PH, and Davis RD (eds). Oxford University Press, New York, pp. 523–534.

Black DW, Noyes R, Pfohl B, et al. (1993) Personality disorder in obsessive–compulsive volunteers, well comparison subjects, and their first degree relatives. *Am J Psychiatry* **150**, 1226–1232.

Bornstein RF (1998) Reconceptualizing personality disorder diagnosis in the DSM-V: the discriminant validity challenge. *Clin Psychol: Sci Pract* **5**, 333–343.

Bornstein RF (1999) Dependent and histrionic personality disorders. In *Oxford Textbook of Psychopathology*, Millon T, Blaney PH, and Davis RD (eds). Oxford University Press, New York, pp. 535–554.

Brodsky BS, Cloitre M, and Dulit RA (1995) Relationship of dissociation to self-mutilation and childhood abuse in borderline personality disorder. *Am J Psychiatry* **152**, 1788–1792.

Burgess KB, Rubin KH, Chea CSL, et al. (2001) Behavioral inhibition, social withdrawal, and parenting. In *International Handbook of Social Anxiety*, Crozier WR and Alden LE (eds). John Wiley, New York, pp. 137–158.

Clark DM (2001) A cognitive perspective on social phobia. In *International Handbook of Social Anxiety*, Crozier WR and Alden LE (eds). John Wiley, New York, pp. 405–430.

Clark LA and Harrison JA (2001) Assessment instruments. In *Handbook of Personality Disorders*, Livesley WJ (ed). Guilford Press, New York, pp. 277–306.

Clark LA and Watson D (1999) Personality, disorder, and personality disorder: toward a more rational conceptualization. *J Personal Disord* **13**, 142–151.

Clark LA, Kochanska G, and Ready R (2000) Mothers' personality and its interaction with child temperament as predicting parenting behavior. *J Pers Soc Psychol* **79**, 274–285.

Clark LA, Watson D, and Reynolds S (1995) Diagnosis and classification of psychopathology: challenges to the current system and future directions. *Annu Rev Psychol* **46**, 121–153.

Cloninger CR (2000) A practical way to diagnosis personality disorders: a proposal. *J Personal Disord* **14**, 99–108.

Cooper AM and Ronningstam E (1992) Narcissistic personality disorder. In *Review of Psychiatry*, Vol. 11, Tasman A and Riba MB (eds). American Psychiatric Press, Washington, DC, pp. 80–97.

Corbitt EM and Widiger TA (1995) Sex differences among the personality disorders. An exploration of the data. *Clin Psychol: Sci Pract* **2**, 225–238.

Coryell WH and Zimmerman M (1989) Personality disorder in the families of depressed, schizophrenic, and never-ill probands. *Am J Psychiatry* **146**, 496–502.

Costa PT and McCrae RR (1992) *Revised NEO Personality Inventory (NEO PI-R) and NEO Five-Factor Inventory (NEO-FFI) Professional Manual*. Psychological Assessment Resources, Odessa, FL.

Costa PT and Widiger TA (eds) (2002) *Personality Disorders and the Five Factor Model of Personality*, 2nd ed., American Psychological Association, Washington, DC.

Crozier WR and Alden LE (eds) (2001) *International Handbook of Social Anxiety. Concepts, Research, and Interventions Relating to the Self and Shyness*. John Wiley, New York.

Daley SE, Burge D, and Hammen C (2000) Borderline personality disorder symptoms as predictors of 4-year romantic relationship dysfunction in young women: addressing issues of specificity. *J Abnorm Psychol* **109**, 451–460.

Depue RA and Lenzenweger MF (2001) A neurobehavioral dimensional model. In *Handbook of Personality Disorders*, Livesley WJ (ed). Guilford Press, New York, pp. 136–176.

Dodge KA, Bates JE, and Pettit GS (1990) Mechanisms in the cycle of violence. *Science* **250**, 1678–1683.

Dolan-Sewell RG, Krueger RF, and Shea MT (2001) Co-occurrence with syndrome disorders. In *Handbook of Personality Disorders*, Livesley WJ (ed). Guilford Press, New York, pp. 84–104.

Dreessen L, Arntz A, Hendriks T, et al. (1999) Avoidant personality disorder and implicit schema-congruent information processing bias: a pilot study with a pragmatic inference task. *Behav Res Ther* **37**, 619–632.

Fanous A, Gardner C, Walsh D, et al. (2001) Relationship between positive and negative symptoms of schizophrenia and schizotypal symptoms in nonpsychotic relatives. *Arch Gen Psychiatry* **58**, 669–673.

First M, Gibbon M, Spitzer RL, et al. (1997) *User's Guide for the Structured Clinical Interview for DSM-IV Axis II Personality Disorders*. American Psychiatric Press, Washington, DC.

Fowles DC (2001) Biological variables in psychopathology: a psychobiological perspective. In *Comprehensive Handbook of Psychopathology*, 3rd ed., Adams HE and Sutker PB (eds). Kluwer Academic/Plenum Publishers, New York, pp. 85–104.

Fowles DC and Kochanska G (2000) Temperament as a moderator of pathways to conscience in children: the contribution of electrodermal activity. *Psychophysiology* **37**, 788–795.

Frances AJ, First MB, and Pincus HA (1995) *DSM-IV Guidebook*. American Psychiatric Press, Washington, DC.

Gabbard GO (2000) *Psychodynamic Psychiatry in Clinical Practice*, 3rd ed. American Psychiatric Press, Washington, DC.

Gabbard GO (2001) Psychodynamic psychotherapy of borderline personality disorder: a contemporary approach. *Bull Menninger Clin* **65**, 41–57.

Garb HN (1997) Race bias, social class bias, and gender bias in clinical judgment. *Clin Psychol: Sci and Pract* **4**, 99–120.

Gunderson JG (1998) DSM-IV personality disorders: final overview. In *DSM-IV Sourcebook*, Vol. 4, Widiger TA, Frances AJ, Pincus HA, et al. (eds). American Psychiatric Association, Washington, DC, pp. 1123–1140.

Gunderson JG (2001) *Borderline Personality Disorder: A Clinical Guide*. American Psychiatric Press, Washington, DC.

Gunderson JG and Gabbard GO (2000) *Psychotherapy for Personality Disorders*. American Psychiatric Press, Washington, DC.

Gunderson JG, Phillips KA, Triebwasser JT, et al. (1994) The diagnostic interview for depressive personality. *Am J Psychiatry* **151**, 1300–1304.

Gunderson JG, Ronningstam E, and Bodkin A (1990) The diagnostic interview for narcissistic patients. *Arch Gen Psychiatry* **47**, 676–680.

Gunderson JG, Ronningstam E, and Smith LE (1991) Narcissistic personality disorder: a review of data on DSM-III-R descriptions. *J Personal Disord* **5**, 167–177.

Gunderson JG, Shea MT, Skodol AE, et al. (2000) The collaborative longitudinal personality disorders study. I. Development, aims, design, and sample characteristics. *J Personal Disord* **14**, 300–315.

Gunderson JG, Zanarini MC, and Kisiel CL (1991) Borderline personality disorder: a review of data on DSM-III-R descriptions. *J Personal Disord* **5**, 340–352.

Hamburger ME, Lilienfeld SO, and Hogben M (1996) Psychopathy, gender, and gender roles: implications for antisocial and histrionic personality disorder. *J Personal Disord* **10**, 41–55.

Hare RD (1991) *The Hare Psychopathy Checklist-Revised Manual*. Multi-Healthy Systems, North Tonawanda, New York.

Hare RD, Hart SD, and Harpur TJ (1991) Psychopathy and the DSM-IV criteria for antisocial personality disorder. *J Abnorm Psychol* **100**, 391–398.

Heffernan K and Cloitre M (2000) A comparison of posttraumatic stress disorder with and without borderline personality disorder among women with a history of childhood sexual abuse: etiological and clinical characteristics. *J Nerv Ment Dis* **188**, 589–595.

Hilsenroth MJ, Handler L, and Blais MA (1996) Assessment of narcissistic personality disorder: a multi-method review. *Clin Psychol Rev* **16**, 655–683.

Hogan R, Johnson J, and Briggs S (eds) (1997) *Handbook of Personality Psychology*. Academic Press, New York.

Horowitz MJ (1997) Psychotherapy for histrionic personality disorder. *J Psychother Pract Res* **6**, 93–104.

Jang KL and Vernon PA (2001) Genetics. In *Handbook of Personality Disorders*, Livesley WJ (ed). Guilford Press, New York, pp. 177–195.

Jang KL, McCrae RR, Angleitner A, et al. (1998) Heritability of facet-level traits in a cross-cultural twin sample: Support for a hierarchical model of personality. *J Pers Soc Psychol* **74**, 1556–1565.

Johnson JG, Cohen P, Brown J, et al. (1999) Childhood maltreatment increases risk for personality disorders during early adulthood. *Am J Psychiatry* **56**, 600–606.

Kalus O, Bernstein DP, and Siever LJ (1993) Schizoid personality disorder: a review of current status and implications for DSM-IV. *J Personal Disord* **7**, 43–52.

Kaye AL and Shea MT (2000) Personality disorders, personality traits, and defense mechanisms. In *Handbook of Psychiatric Measures*, Pincus HA, Rush AJ, First MB, et al. (eds). American Psychiatric Association, Washington, DC, pp. 713–749.

Keller M (1989) Current concepts in affective disorders. *J Clin Psychiatry* **50**, 157–162.

Kernberg OF (1991a) Hysterical and histrionic personality disorders. In *Psychiatry*, Vol. 1, Ch. 19, Michels R (ed). JB Lippincott, Philadelphia, PA, pp. 1–11.

Kernberg OF (1991b) Narcissistic personality disorder. In *Psychiatry*, Vol. 1, Ch. 18, Michels R (ed). JB Lippincott, Philadelphia, PA, pp. 1–12.

Kessler K, McGonagle K, Zhao S, et al. (1994) Lifetime and 12 month prevalence of DSM-III-R psychiatric disorders in the United States. *Arch Gen Psychiatry* **51**, 8–19.

Klein DN (1999) Commentary on Ryder and Bagby's "diagnostic validity of depressive personality disorder: theoretical and conceptual issues". *J Personal Disord* **13**, 118–127.

Klein DN, Riso LP, Donaldson SK, et al. (1995) Family study of early-onset dysthymia: mood and personality disorders in relatives of outpatients with dysthymia and episodic major depressive and normal controls. *Arch Gen Psychiatry* **52**, 487–496.

Kochanska G and Murray KT (2000) Mother–child responsive orientation and conscience development: from toddler to early school age. *Child Dev* **71**, 417–431.

Kohut H (1977) *The Restoration of the Self*. International Universities Press, New York.

Lenzenweger MF, Loranger AW, Korfine L, et al. (1997) Detecting personality disorders in a nonclinical population. *Arch Gen Psychiatry* **54**, 345–351.

Lilienfeld SO (1994) Conceptual problems in the assessment of psychopathy. *Clin Psychol Rev* **14**, 17–38.

Lilienfeld SO and Hess TH (2001) Psychopathic personality traits and somatization: sex differences and the mediating role of negative emotionality. *J Psychopathol Behav Assess* **23**, 11–24.

Lilienfeld SO, Waldman ID, and Israel AC (1994) A critical examination of the use of the term "comorbidity" in psychopathology research. *Clin Psychol: Sci Pract* **1**, 71–83.

Linehan MM (1993) *Cognitive–Behavioral Treatment of Borderline Personality Disorder*. Guilford Press, New York.

Linehan MM (2000) The empirical basis of dialectical behavior therapy: development of new treatments vs. evaluation of existing treatments. *Clin Psychol: Sci Pract* **7**, 113–119.

Links PS, Heslegrave R, and van Reekum R (1998) Prospective follow-up study of borderline personality disorder: prognosis, prediction of outcome, and axis II comorbidity. *Can J Psychiatry* **43**, 265–270.

Livesley WJ (1998) Suggestions for a framework for an empirically based classification of personality disorder. *Can J Psychiatry* **43**, 137–147.

Livesley WJ (ed) (2001) *Handbook of Personality Disorders*. Guilford Press, New York.

Loranger AW (1999) *International Personality Disorder Examination (IPDE)*. Psychological Assessment Resources, Odessa, Florida.

Lynam DR (1996) The early identification of chronic offenders: who is the fledgling psychopath? *Psychol Bull* **120**, 209–234.

Maier W, Lichtermann D, Klinger T, et al. (1992) Prevalences of personality disorders (DSM-III-R) in the community. *J Personal Disord* **6**, 187–196.

Markovitz P (2001) Pharmacotherapy. In *Handbook of Personality Disorders*, Livesley WJ (ed). Guilford Press, New York, pp. 475–493.

Mattia JI and Zimmerman M (2001) Epidemiology. In *Handbook of Personality Disorders*, Livesley WJ (ed). Guilford Press, New York, pp. 107–123.

McCann J (1988) Passive–aggressive personality: a review. *J Personal Dis* **2**, 170–179.

Miller MB, Useda JD, Trull TJ, et al. (2001) Paranoid, schizoid, and schizotypal personality disorders. In *Comprehensive Handbook of Psychopathology*, 3rd ed., Adams HE and Sutker PB (eds). Kluwer Academic/Plenum Publishers, New York, pp. 535–558.

Millon T (1993) Negativistic (passive–aggressive) personality disorder. *J Personal Disord* **7**, 78–85.

Millon T, Davis RD, Millon CM, et al. (1996) *Disorders of Personality. DSM-IV and Beyond*. John Wiley, New York.

Moldin SO, Rice JP, Erlenmeyer-Kimling L, et al. (1994) Latent structure of DSM-III-R axis II psychopathology in a normal sample. *J Abnorm Psychol* **103**, 259–266.

Moffitt TE (1993) Adolescence limited and life-course persistent antisocial behavior: a developmental taxonomy. *Psychol Rev* **100**, 674–701.

Moffitt TE, Caspi A, Dickson N, et al. (1996) Childhood-onset versus adolescent onset antisocial conduct problems in males: natural history from ages 3 to 18 years. *Dev Psychopathol* **8**, 399–424.

Morey LC and Zanarini MC (2000) Borderline personality: traits and disorder. *J Abnorm Psychol* **109**, 733–737.

Myers MG, Stewart DG, and Brown SA (1998) Progression from conduct disorder to antisocial personality disorder following treatment for adolescent substance abuse. *Am J Psychiatry* **155**, 479–485.

Nestadt G, Romanoski AJ, Brown CH, et al. (1991) DSM-III compulsive personality disorder: an epidemiological survey. *Psychol Med* **21**, 461–471.

Newman JP and Wallace JF (1993) Psychopathy and cognition. In *Psychopathology and Cognition*, Kendall PC and Dobson KS (eds). Academic Press, New York, pp. 293–349.

Nigg JT and Goldsmith HH (1994) Genetics of personality disorders: perspectives from personality and psychopathology research. *Psychol Bull* **115**, 346–380.

Oldham JM and Frosch WA (1991) Compulsive personality disorder. In *Psychiatry*, Vol. 1, Ch. 22, Michels R (ed). JB Lippincott, Philadelphia, PA, pp. 1–8.

Oldham JM and Skodol AE (2000) Charting the future of axis II. *J Personal Disord* **14**, 17–29.

Oldham JM, Skodol AE, Kellman HD, et al. (1992) Diagnosis of DSM-III-R personality disorders by two semistructured interviews: patterns of comorbidity. *Am J Psychiatry* **149**, 213–220.

O'Neill FA and Kendler KS (1998) Longitudinal study of interpersonal dependency in female twins. *Br J Psychiatry* **172**, 154–158.

Ornduff SR (2000) Childhood maltreatment and malevolence: quantitative research findings. *Clin Psychol Rev* **20**, 991–1018.

Overholser JC (1996) The dependent personality and interpersonal problems. *J Nerv Ment Dis* **184**, 8–16.

Paris J (1998) *Working with Traits: Psychotherapy of Personality Disorders*. Jason Aronson, Northvale, New Jersey.

Perry JC, Banon E, and Ianni F (1999) Effectiveness of psychotherapy for personality disorders. *Am J Psychiatry* **156**, 1312–1321.

Pervin LA and John OP (eds) (1999) *Handbook of Personality. Theory and Research*, 2nd ed., Guilford Press, New York.

Pfohl B and Blum N (1991) Obsessive–compulsive personality disorder: a review of available data and recommendations for DSM-IV. *J Personal Disord* **5**, 363–375.

Pfohl B, Blum N, and Zimmerman M (1997) *Structured Interview for DSM-IV Personality Disorder*. American Psychiatric Press, Washington, DC.

Phillips KA, Gunderson JG, Triebwasser J, et al. (1998) Reliability and validity of depressive personality disorder. *Am J Psychiatry* **155**, 1044–1048.

Phillips KA, Hirschfeld RMA, Shea MT, et al. (1995) Depressive personality disorder. In *The DSM-IV Personality Disorders*, Livesley WJ (ed). Guilford Press, New York, pp. 287–302.

Pincus AL and Wilson KR (2001) Interpersonal variability in dependent personality. *J Pers* **69**, 223–252.

Plomin R and Caspi A (1999) Behavioral genetics and personality. In *Handbook of Personality*, 2nd ed., Pervin L and John O (eds). Guilford Press, New York, pp. 251–276.

Raine A, Benishay D, Lencz T, et al. (1997) Abnormal orienting in schizotypal personality disorder. *Schizophr Bull* **23**, 75–82.

Raine A, Lencz T, and Mednick SA (eds) (1995) *Schizotypal Personality*. Cambridge University Press, New York.

Raine A, Reynolds C, Venables PH, et al. (1998) Fearlessness, stimulus-seeking, and large body size at age 3 as early predispositions to childhood aggression at age 11 years. *Arch Gen Psychiatry* **55**, 745–751.

Raine A, Venables PH, and Williams M (1995) High autonomic arousal and electrodermal orienting at age 15 years as protective factors against criminal behavior at age 29 years. *Am J Psychiatry* **152**, 1595–1600.

Raskin R, Novacek J, and Hogan R (1991) Narcissistic self-esteem management. *J Pers Soc Psychol* **60**, 911–918.

Rhodewalt F and Morf CC (1995) Self and interpersonal correlates of the narcissistic personality inventory: a review and new findings. *J Res Pers* **29**, 1–23.

Rhodewalt F, Madrian JC, and Cheney S (1998) Narcissism, self-knowledge, organization, and emotional reactivity: the effect of daily experience on self-esteem and affect. *Pers Soc Psychol Bull* **24**, 75–87.

Robins LN, Tipp J, and Przybeck T (1991) Antisocial personality. In *Psychiatric Disorders in America*, Robins LN and Regier DA (eds). The Free Press, New York, pp. 258–290.

Roitman SE, Cornblatt BA, Bergman A, et al. (1997) Attentional functioning in schizotypal personality disorder. *Am J Psychiatry* **154**, 655–660.

Ronningstam E and Gunderson JG (1990) Identifying criteria for narcissistic personality disorder. *Am J Psychiatry* **147**, 918–922.

Rothbart MK and Ahadi SA (1994) Temperament and the development of personality. *J Abnor Psychol* **103**, 55–66.

Ryder AG and Bagby RM (1999) Diagnostic viability of depressive personality disorder: theoretical and conceptual issues. *J Personal Disord* **13**, 99–117.

Salekin RT (2002) Psychopathy and therapeutic pessimism. Clinical lore or clinical reality? *Clin Psychol Rev* **22**, 79–112.

Samuels JF, Nestadt G, Romanoski AJ, et al. (1994) DSM-III personality disorders in the community. *Am J Psychiatry* **151**, 1055–1062.

Sanislow CA and McGlashan TH (1998) Treatment outcome of personality disorders. *Can J Psychiatry* **43**, 237–250.

Schmidt LA, Polak CP, and Spooner AL (2001) Biological and environmental contributions to childhood shyness: a diathesis-stress model. In *International Handbook of Social Anxiety*, Crozier WR and Alden LE (eds). John Wiley, New York, pp. 29–52.

Sher KJ and Trull TJ (1994) Personality and disinhibitory psychopathology: alcoholism and antisocial personality disorder. *J Abnorm Psychol* **103**, 92–102.

Siever LJ (1992) Schizophrenia spectrum disorders. In *Review of Psychiatry*, Vol. XI, Tasman A and Riba MB (eds). American Psychiatric Press, Washington, DC, pp. 25–42.

Siever LJ and Davis KL (1991) A psychobiological perspective on the personality disorders. *Am J Psychiatry* **148**, 1647–1658.

Silk KR (2000) Borderline personality disorder. Overview of biologic factors. *Psychiatr Clin North Am* **23**, 61–75.

Soloff PH (2000) Psychopharmacology of borderline personality disorder. *Psychiatr Clin North Am* **23**, 169–192.

Spitzer RL, Williams JBW, and Skodol AE (1980) DSM-III: the major achievements and an overview. *Am J Psychiatry* **137**, 151–164.

Sprock J, Blashfield RK, and Smith B (1990) Gender weighting of DSM-III-R personality disorder criteria. *Am J Psychiatry* **147**, 586–590.

Squires-Wheeler E, Friedman D, Amminger GP, et al. (1997) Negative and positive dimensions of schizotypal personality disorder. *J Personal Disord* **11**, 285–300.

Stoff DM, Breiling J, and Maser JD (eds) (1997) *Handbook of Antisocial Behavior*. John Wiley, New York.

Stone MH (1993) *Abnormalities of Personality. Within and Beyond the Realm of Treatment*. WW Norton, New York.

Stone MH (2000) Clinical guidelines for psychotherapy with borderline personality disorder. *Psychiatr Clin North Am* **23**, 193–210.

Stone MH (2001) Natural history and long-term outcome. In *Handbook of Personality Disorders*, Livesley WJ (ed). Guilford Press, New York, pp. 259–273.

Sutker PB and Allain AN (2001) Antisocial personality disorder. In *Comprehensive Handbook of Psychopathology*, 3rd ed., Sutker PB and Adams HE (eds). Kluwer Academic/Plenum Publishers, New York, pp. 445–490.

Thompson S and Zuroff DC (1998) Dependent and self-critical mothers' responses to adolescent autonomy and competence. *Pers Indiv Differ* **24**, 311–324.

Tillfors M, Furmark T, Ekselius L, et al. (2001) Social phobia and avoidant personality disorder as related to parental history of social anxiety: a general population study. *Behav Res Ther* **39**, 289–298.

Torgersen S (2000) Genetics of patients with borderline personality disorder. *Psychiatr Clin North Am* **23**, 1–9.

Torgersen S, Kringlen E, and Cramer V (2001) The prevalence of personality disorders in a community sample. *Arch Gen Psychiatry* **58**, 590–596.

Trull TJ, Widiger TA, Useda JD, et al. (1998) A structured interview for the assessment of the five-factor model of personality. *Psychol Assess* **10**, 229–240.

van Velzen CJ, Emmelkamp PM, and Scholing A (2000) Generalized social phobia versus avoidant personality disorder: differences in psychopathology, personality traits, and social and occupational functioning. *J Anxiety Disord* **14**, 395–411.

Westen D (1997) Divergences between clinical and research methods for assessing personality disorders: implications for research and the evolution of axis II. *Am J Psychiatry* **154**, 895–903.

Wetzler S and Morey LC (1999) Passive–aggressive personality disorder: the demise of a syndrome. *Psychiatry* **62**, 49–59.

Widiger TA (1998) Sex biases in the diagnosis of personality disorders. *J Personal Disord* **12**, 95–118.

Widiger TA (1999) Depressive personality traits and dysthymia: a commentary on Ryder and Bagby. *J Personal Disord* **13**, 135–141.

Widiger TA (2000) Personality disorders in the 21st century. *J Personal Disord* **14**, 3–16.

Widiger TA (2001) Social anxiety, social phobia, and avoidant personality disorder. In *International Handbook of Social Anxiety*, Crozier WR and Alden L (eds). John Wiley, New York, pp. 335–356.

Widiger TA and Coker LA (2002) Assessing personality disorders. In *Clinical Personality Assessment: Practical Approaches*, 2nd ed., Butcher JN (ed). Oxford University Press, New York, pp. 407–434.

Widiger TA and Corbitt EM (1995) Antisocial personality disorder in DSM-IV. In *The DSM-IV Personality Disorders*, Livesley WJ (ed). Guilford Press, New York, pp. 103–126.

Widiger TA and Lynam DR (1998) Psychopathy from the perspective of the five-factor model of personality. In *Psychopathy: Antisocial, Criminal, and Violent Behaviors*, Millon T, Simonsen E, Birket-Smith M, et al. (eds). Guilford Press, New York, pp. 171–187.

Widiger TA and Sankis L (2000) Adult psychopathology: issues and controversies. *Annu Rev Psychol* **51**, 377–404.

Widiger TA and Trull TJ (1998) Performance characteristics of the DSM-III-R personality disorder criteria sets. In *DSM-IV Sourcebook*, Vol. 4, Widiger TA, Frances AJ, Pincus HA, et al. (eds). American Psychiatric Association, Washington, DC, pp. 357–373.

Widiger TA, Cadoret R, Hare R, et al. (1996) DSM-IV antisocial personality disorder field trial. *J Abnorm Psychol* **105**, 3–16.

Widiger TA, Frances AJ, Spitzer RL, et al. (1988) The DSM-III-R personality disorders: an overview. *Am J Psychiatry* **145**, 786–795.

Widiger TA, Mangine S, Corbitt EM, et al. (1995) *The Personality Disorder Interview—IV: A Semistructured Interview for the Diagnosis of Personality Disorders*. Psychological Assessment Resources, Odessa, Florida.

Widiger TA, Trull TJ, Clarkin JF, et al. (2002) A description of the DSM-IV personality disorders with the five-factor model of personality. In *Personality Disorders and the Five-Factor Model of Personality*, 2nd ed., Costa PT and Widiger TA (eds). American Psychological Association, Washington, DC, pp. 89–99.

World Health Organization (1992) *The ICD-10 Classification of Mental and Behavioural Disorders. Clinical Descriptions and Diagnostic Guidelines*. World Health Organization, Geneva.

Zanarini MC (2000) Childhood experiences associated with the development of borderline personality disorder. *Psychiatr Clin North Am* **23**, 89–101.

Zanarini MC, Frankenburg FR, Dubo ED, et al. (1998a) Axis I comorbidity of borderline personality disorder. *Am J Psychiatry* **155**, 1733–1739.

Zanarini MC, Frankenburg FR, Dubo ED, et al. (1998b) Axis II comorbidity of borderline personality disorder. *Compr Psychiatry* **39**.

Zanarini MC, Frankenburg FR, Sickel AE, et al. (1995) *Diagnostic Interview for DSM-IV Personality Disorders (DIPD-IV)*. McLean Hospital, Boston, MA.

Zanarini MC, Gunderson JG, Frankenburg FR, et al. (1989) The revised diagnostic interview for borderlines: discriminating BPD from other axis II disorders. *J Personal Disord* **3**, 10–18.

Zanarini MC, Williams AA, Lewis RE, et al. (1997) Reported childhood experiences associated with the development of borderline personality disorder. *Am J Psychiatry* **154**, 1101–1106.

Zimmerman M (1994) Diagnosing personality disorders. A review of issues and research methods. *Arch Gen Psychiatry* **51**, 225–245.

Zimmerman M and Mattia JI (1999) Differences between clinical and research practices in diagnosing borderline personality disorder. *Am J Psychiatry* **156**, 1570–1574.

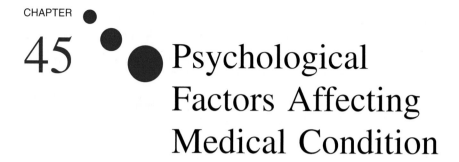

Psychological Factors Affecting Medical Condition

Diagnosis

This diagnostic category recognizes the variety of ways in which specific psychological or behavioral factors can adversely affect medical illnesses (see DSM-IV-TR Diagnostic criteria below). Such factors may contribute to the initiation or the exacerbation of the illness, interfere with treatment and rehabilitation, or contribute to morbidity and mortality. Psychological factors may themselves constitute risks for medical diseases, or they may magnify the effects of nonpsychological risk factors. The effects may be mediated directly at a pathophysiological level (e.g., psychological stress inducing myocardial ischemia) or through the individual's behavior (e.g., noncompliance).

DSM-IV-TR Diagnostic Criteria

316. Psychological Factors Affecting Medical Condition

A. A general medical condition (coded on Axis III) is present.
B. Psychological factors adversely affect the general medical condition in one of the following ways:

    (1) the factors have influenced the course of the general medical condition as shown by a close temporal association between the psychological factors and the development or exacerbation of, or delayed recovery from, the general medical condition
    (2) the factors interfere with the treatment of the general medical condition
    (3) the factors constitute additional health risks for the individual
    (4) stress-related physiological responses precipitate or exacerbate symptoms of the general medical condition.

Choose name based on the nature of the psycho-logical factors (if more than one factor is present, indicate the most prominent):

Mental disorder affecting. . . [indicate the general medical condition] (e.g., an Axis I disorder such as major depressive disorder delaying recovery from a myocardial infarction)

Psychological symptoms affecting. . . [indicate the general medical condition] (e.g., depressive symptoms delaying recovery from surgery; anxiety exacerbating asthma)

Personality traits or coping style affecting. . . [indicate the general medical condition] (e.g., pathological denial of the need for surgery in a patient with cancer; hostile, pressured behavior contributing to cardiovascular disease)

Maladaptive health behaviors affecting. . . [indicate the general medical condition] (e.g., overeating; lack of exercise; unsafe sex)

Stress-related physiological response affecting. . . [indicate the general medical condition] (e.g., stress-related exacerbations of ulcer, hypertension, arrhythmia, or tension headache)

Other or unspecified psychological factors affecting. . . [indicate the general medical condition] (e.g., interpersonal, cultural, or religious factors)

Reprinted with permission from the Diagnostic and Statistical Manual of Mental Disorders, Fourth Edition, Text Revision. Copyright 2000 American Psychiatric Association.

The subject of psychological factors affecting medical condition (PFAMC) has become the focus of intense research because of the illumination it may provide of basic disease mechanisms (e.g., psychoneuroimmunology) and because of the deep interest in improving both the outcomes and the efficiency of health care delivery. In epidemiological studies, several mental disorders increase the likelihood of mortality (Bruce et al. 1994), especially depression, bipolar disorder, schizophrenia, and alcohol abuse or dependence. Psychiatric disorders or symptoms in individuals with medical illness may increase their use of health care services, particularly the length of costly hospital stays. (Levenson et al. 1990b, Saravay and Lavin 1994, Strain et al. 1994, Deykin et al. 2001). Interest has been further increased by intervention trials aimed at psychological factors or disorders that have demonstrated improvements in medical outcomes and in quality of life in individuals with serious medical disorders.

It should be evident that this diagnosis is not really a discrete diagnostic category but rather a label for the interactive effects of psyche on soma. Mind–body interactions have long been a focus of interest, both in health and in disease. Mental disorder and medical disease frequently coexist. Mental health professionals and investigators of past eras were misled by this frequent comorbidity into premature conclusions that the psychological factors were preeminent in the causation of the medical disorders, and these were designated psychosomatic (Alexander 1950). A more modern approach has been to recognize that all medical illnesses are potentially affected by many different factors in the biological, psychological, and social realms. The earlier designation of certain disorders as psychosomatic (e.g., peptic ulcer disease) overvalued the contribution of psychological factors to those disorders and undervalued their contribution to other medical disorders (e.g., cancer). Furthermore, whereas labeling medical illnesses as psychosomatic drew attention to the importance of mind–body interactions, it unfortunately and falsely implied to many individuals undergoing treatment and physicians that the illness was basically psychogenic, that the symptoms were not "real," and that the illness was somehow the individual's fault.

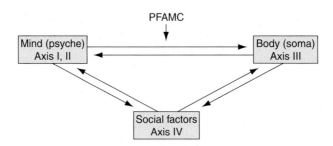

Figure 45-1 *Psychological factors affecting medical condition (PFAMC): interaction between psyche and soma. Social factors warrant attention as well.*

The diagnosis of PFAMC focuses attention on one causal direction in the interactions between psyche and soma, that is, the effects of psychological factors on the medical condition (Figure 45-1). This represents a heuristic simplification, highlighting a particular process for further exploration, understanding, and intervention. In most individuals, there are effects in the other direction as well (i.e., the effects of general medical illness on psychological function). Furthermore, both mind and body interact with social and environmental factors both dramatic (e.g., poverty, racism, war) and more subtle (e.g., employment status, neighborhood) (Roux et al. 2001), that affect the incidence and outcome of medical illness. Diagnosing PFAMC may help the psychiatrist and the individual address an important dimension of care, but the other "arrows" of Figure 45-1 often warrant attention too.

The diagnosis of PFAMC differs from the diagnosis of most other mental disorders in its focus on the interaction between the mental and medical realms. As noted, the criteria require more than that the individual has both a medical illness and contemporaneous psychological factors, because their coexistence does not always include significant interactions between them. To make the diagnosis of PFAMC, either the factors must have influenced the course of the medical condition, interfered with its treatment, contributed to health risks, or physiologically aggravated the medical condition.

Let us consider each of these four ways of making the diagnosis of PFAMC in more detail. The psychological factor's influence on the course of a general medical condition can be inferred from a close temporal relationship between the factor and the development or exacerbation of the medical condition (or delayed recovery). For example, a 45-year-old male executive reports symptoms sounding like typical angina, but occurring only on weekends. Further questioning reveals that he is depressed over deterioration in his marriage. During the week he works late and has limited contact with his family, but he spends the weekend at home. The symptoms began after he and his wife started arguing every weekend. The temporal link between onset and recurrence of angina and marital arguments supports a diagnosis of PFAMC.

PFAMC can also be diagnosed when the psychological factor interferes with treatment including not seeking medical care, not following up, nonadherence to prescribed drugs or other treatment, or maladaptive modifications in treatment made by the individual or family. The executive with angina rejected his physician's recommendations for further assessment and treatment. He said, "I do get upset at home but I feel just fine at the office, so there couldn't be anything really wrong with me." The individual is able to acknowledge marital discord, but the defense of denial clouds his perception of his physical health and blocks appropriate medical care. This is another form of PFAMC.

PFAMC can also be diagnosed when the psychological factor contributes to health risks, exemplified by the executive increasing his smoking and drinking despite his physician's warnings. ("Its the only way I can cope with my wife.") Finally, PFAMC is an appropriate diagnosis when there are stress-related physiological responses precipitating or exacerbating symptoms of the medical condition. The same man observes that angina is most likely to occur after marital arguments during which he becomes irate, yells, slams doors, and throws things.

When a person's medical illness is faring worse than expected and not responding well to standard treatment, clinicians should and often do consider whether a psychological factor may be responsible for the poorer-than-expected outcome. This is a far from trivial task. To ignore the possibility of PFAMC may miss the crucial barrier to the individual's recovery. On the other hand, premature or facile attribution to psychological factors may lead the clinician to overlook medical or social explanations for "treatment-resistant disease" and unfairly blame the individual, with resultant further deterioration in health outcomes and the clinician–patient relationship.

To illustrate, a common clinical problem is the brittle diabetic adolescent with labile blood glucose levels and frequent episodes of ketoacidosis and hypoglycemia, despite vigorous attempts by the physician to improve diabetic management and glucose control. The considerable difficulty in controlling such persons' diabetes is often attributed to adolescents' dislike of lifestyle restrictions, their tendency to act out and rebel against authority figures, their denial of vulnerability, their ambivalence about their need for nurturance, and their wish to be "normal." There are many adolescent (and some adult) diabetics for whom these psychological issues do play an important role in undermining diabetes management through noncompliance regarding medication, diet, visits to the physician, substance use, and activity limitations. However, psychological factors do not always account for brittleness and are sometimes incorrectly suspected. It has been demonstrated that much of the difficulty in achieving stable glucose control in adolescent diabetics is the result of the dramatically labile patterns of hormone secretion (cortisol, growth hormone) typical of adolescence, independent of psychological status.

PFAMC has descriptive names for subcategories described as follows:

Mental Disorder Affecting a General Medical Condition   If the individual has a mental disorder meeting criteria for an Axis I or Axis II diagnosis, the diagnostic name is mental disorder affecting medical condition, with the particular medical condition specified. In addition to coding PFAMC, the specific mental disorder is also coded on Axis I or Axis II. Examples include major depressive disorder that reduces energy and compliance in an individual with hemodialysis; panic disorder that makes an asthmatic hypersensitive to dyspnea; and schizophrenia in an individual with recurrent ventricular tachycardia who refuses placement of an automatic implantable defibrillator because he fears it will control his mind.

Psychological Symptoms Affecting a General Medical Condition   Individuals who have psychological symptoms that do not meet the threshold for an Axis I diagnosis may still experience important effects on their medical illness, and the diagnosis would be psychological symptoms affecting a medical condition. Examples include anxiety that aggravates irritable bowel syndrome; depressed mood that hinders recovery from hip replacement surgery; and anger that interferes with rehabilitation after spinal cord injury.

Personality Traits or Coping Style Affecting a General Medical Condition
This may include personality traits or coping styles that do not meet criteria for an Axis II disorder and other patterns of response considered to be maladaptive because they may pose a risk for particular medical illnesses. An example is the competitive hostility component of the type A behavior pattern, and its impact on coronary artery disease.

Maladaptive personality traits or coping styles are particularly likely to interfere with the physician–patient relationship as well as the relationships, which the individuals have with other caregivers.

Maladaptive Health Behaviors Affecting a General Medical Condition

Many maladaptive health behaviors have significant effects on the course and treatment of many medical conditions. Examples include sedentary lifestyle, smoking, abuse of alcohol or other substances, and unsafe sexual practices. If the maladaptive behaviors can be better accounted for by an Axis I or Axis II disorder, the first subcategory (mental disorder affecting a medical condition) should be used instead.

Stress-Related Physiological Response Affecting a General Medical Condition

Examples of stress-related physiological responses affecting a medical condition include the precipitation by psychological stress of angina, cardiac arrhythmia, migraine, or attack of colitis in medically vulnerable individuals. In such cases, stress is not the cause of the illness or symptoms; the individual has a medical condition that etiologically accounts for the symptoms (e.g., coronary artery disease, migraine, or ulcerative colitis), and the stressor instead represents a precipitating or aggravating factor.

Other or Unspecified Psychological Factors Affecting a General Medical Condition

There are other psychological phenomena that may not fit within one of these subcategories. An interpersonal example is marital dysfunction. A cultural example is the extreme discomfort women from some cultures may experience being alone with a male physician, even while they are fully dressed. A religious example is a Jehovah's Witness who ambivalently refuses blood transfusion. These fall under the residual category of other or unspecified psychological factors affecting a medical condition.

Epidemiology

Because this diagnosis describes a variety of possible interactions between the full range of mental disorders (as well as symptoms and behaviors) on the one hand and the complete range of medical diseases on the other, it is impossible to estimate overall rates of prevalence or incidence. We can start, however, by noting how frequently medical and mental disorders coexist. Psychiatric problems are common in individuals with a medical history, although the measured frequency varies, depending on the criteria and method of measurement used. A reasonable estimate is that 25 to 30% of medical outpatients and 40 to 50% of general medical inpatients have diagnosable mental disorders (Table 45-1). Most common in medical outpatients are depression, anxiety, and substance abuse; medical inpatients most often have cognitive impairment (delirium, dementia), depression, and substance abuse. Depression, both as a diagnosis and as a symptom has been better studied in the medically ill than any other mental disorders. Major depressive disorder occurs in 18 to 25% of individuals with serious coronary disease, in 25% of those with cancer, and at three times the normal rate in diabetics. Individuals presenting with symptoms of chronic fatigue have a 50 to 75% lifetime prevalence of major depression (Wessely et al. 1998).

   Nonpsychiatric physicians underdiagnose and undertreat mental disorders in the medically ill. General medical conditions are also common in individuals seen for mental health treatment, and mental health specialists often underrecognize the presence and significance of coexisting general medical conditions. Regardless of whether the individual has come seeking medical care or mental health care, medical and psychiatric problems are often both present. Such coincidence by itself is not sufficient for the diagnosis of PFAMC. In some cases, the illnesses may coexist with little effect on each other; in other cases, the effects of

Table 45-1	Prevalence of Selected Psychiatric Disorders		
Disorder	**Community**	**Primary Care Patients**	**Medical**
Inpatients			
All psychiatric disorders	15–20%	25–30%	40–50%
Depression			
Depressive symptoms	10–15%	10–30%	20–35%
Major depressive disorder	2–4%	5–10%	5–25%
Anxiety			
Anxiety symptoms	10–20%	12–20%	20–30%
Panic disorder	1–2%	2–15%	—
Cognitive disorders			
	1%	—	15–20%
	5–10%	—	30–50%
	(>65 yr)		(>65 yr)

Source: Levenson JL (1994) Common psychological reactions to medical illness and treatment. In *Clinical Psychiatry for Medical Students*, 2nd ed., Stoudemire A (ed). JB Lippincott, Philadelphia, pp. 580B–609.

the medical illness on the mental disorder may be more important. The diagnosis of PFAMC in DSM-IV-TR is reserved for individuals in whom psychological factors adversely affect a medical condition in a specifiable way.

Course

Given the wide range of mental disorders and psychological factors that may affect medical illness and the large number of different general medical conditions that may be influenced, there are no general rules about the course of the PFAMC interaction. Psychological factors may have minor or major effects at a particular point or throughout the course of a medical illness. We do know in general that individuals with general medical conditions who also have significant psychological symptoms have poorer outcomes and higher medical care costs than those individuals with the same general medical conditions but without psychological distress. A number of studies now document that psychological or psychiatric problems (particularly cognitive disorder, depression, and anxiety) in general medical inpatients are associated with significant increases in length of hospital stay (Levenson et al. 1990b, Saravay and Lavin 1994, Stevens et al. 1998). Psychosocial interventions have been able to improve outcomes in medical illness, sometimes with an attendant savings in health care costs (Strain et al. 1994, Smith 1994, Katon and Gonzales 1994).

The impact of psychological factors on the course and natural history of medical disorders is discussed further in this chapter in the context of specific diseases.

Differential Diagnosis

As noted before, the close temporal association between psychiatric symptoms and a medical condition does not always reflect PFAMC. If the two are considered merely coincidental, then separate mental disorder and general medical condition diagnoses should be made. In some cases of coincident mental disorders and general medical conditions, the mental symptoms are actually the result of the medical condition (i.e., the causality is in a direction opposite from that of PFAMC). When a medical condition is judged to be pathophysiologically causing the mental disorder (e.g., hypothyroidism causing depression), the correct diagnosis is the appropriate mental disorder due to a general medical condition (e.g., mood disorder due to hypothyroidism, with depressive features). In PFAMC, the psychological or behavioral factors are judged to precipitate or aggravate the medical condition.

Substance use disorders may adversely affect many medical conditions, and this can be described through PFAMC. However, in some individuals, all of the psychiatric and medical symptoms are direct consequences of substance abuse, and it is usually parsimonious to use just the substance-use disorder diagnosis. For example, an individual with delirium tremens after alcohol withdrawal would receive a diagnosis of alcohol withdrawal delirium, not PFAMC, but an individual with alcohol dependence who repeatedly missed hemodialysis treatments because of intoxication would receive diagnoses of alcohol dependence and PFAMC (mental disorder affecting end stage renal disease).

Individuals with somatoform disorders (e.g., somatization disorder, hypochondriasis) present with physical complaints that may mimic a medical illness, but the somatic symptoms are actually accounted for by the psychiatric disorder. In principle, it might seem that somatoform disorders are easily distinguished from PFAMC because PFAMC requires the presence of a diagnosable medical condition. The distinction in practice is sometimes difficult because the individual may have both a somatoform disorder and one or more medical disorders. For example, an individual with seizures regularly precipitated by emotional stress might have true epilepsy aggravated by stress (PFAMC), pseudoseizures (conversion disorder), or both.

Etiology

How do psychological factors affect medical illnesses? Physicians have long recognized that psychological factors seem to affect medical illnesses, and research elucidating the intervening causal mechanisms is now rapidly growing. From their clinical experience, physicians recognize many ways in which psychological factors affect the onset, progression, and outcome of the illnesses of individuals under their treatment. First, psychological factors may promote other known risks for medical illness. Smoking is a risk factor for heart disease, cancer, and pulmonary and many other diseases, and individuals with schizophrenia or depression are much more likely to smoke than the general population. A wide variety of mental disorders are associated with an increased likelihood of abuse of other substances. Depression and schizophrenia also are associated with a sedentary lifestyle. Individuals with affective disorders often have chronic pain and chronically tend to overuse analgesics. Individuals with schizophrenia, bipolar disorder, and some personality disorders are more likely to engage in unsafe sex, which in turn increases the risk of sexually transmitted diseases, including HIV infection and hepatitis B. Depression, eating disorders, and other emotional and behavioral factors affect the pattern and content of diet.

In addition to promoting known risk factors for medical illness, psychological factors also have an impact on the course of illness by influencing how individuals respond to their symptoms, including whether and how they seek care. For example, the defense mechanism of denial may lead an individual to ignore anginal chest pain, attribute it to indigestion, delay seeking medical attention, or minimize the pain when describing it to a physician. This tends to result in treatment delay after the acute onset of coronary symptoms, with consequently greater morbidity and mortality. Anxiety is also a common cause of avoidance or delay of health care; phobic fears of needles, sight of blood, surgery, and other health care phobias are common (Noyes et al. 2000). Individuals may also neglect their symptoms and fail to promptly seek medical care because of depression, psychosis, or personality traits (e.g., procrastination).

Psychological factors also affect the course of illness through their effects on the physician–patient relationship, since they influence both health behaviors of the individuals and physicians' diagnostic and treatment decisions. A substantial proportion of the excess mortality experienced by individuals with mental disorders is explained by their receiving poorer quality medical care (Druss et al. 2001a). One explanation for the poorer quality and outcomes of medical care in individuals with both serious medical and mental illnesses is the lack of integration between their medical and mental health care (Druss et al. 2001b). Psychological factors can also reduce an individual's compliance with diagnostic recommendations, treatment, and lifestyle change, and can interfere with rehabilitation through impairment of motivation, understanding, optimism, or tolerance. A recent meta-analysis found that individuals with depression are three times as likely to be noncompliant with medical treatment than individuals without (DiMatteo et al. 2000). In addition, many of the effects of psychological factors on medical illness appear to be mediated through a wide array of social factors, including social support, job strain, disadvantaged socioeconomic and educational status, and marital stress.

There is an increasing body of scientific evidence that psychological factors, in addition to their impact on classic (nonpsychological) risk factors, behaviors of the individuals undergoing treatment, and the physician–patient interaction, have direct effects on pathophysiological processes. For example, stress has been experimentally shown to cause myocardial ischemia in individuals with coronary disease. Stress and depression are associated with a wide range of immunological effects (Irwin 1999, Yang and Glaser 2000). Many mental disorders (especially mood disorders) are associated with disruptions in homeostasis including sleep architecture, other circadian rhythms, and endocrine secretion and feedback. For example, depression causes increased bone remodeling and decreased bone density (Herran et al. 2000). That such effects occur is well established, but the magnitude of their clinical significance in medical disease is often unclear, and full explanatory causal linkages have for the most part not been demonstrated yet. Nevertheless, investigators have learned a great deal about changes in autonomic, hematologic, endocrine, immunologic, and sensory function, as well as gene expression that bring us closer to understanding how psychological factors may affect medical illness. These issues of pathophysiology are discussed later in this chapter for each organ system or specialty category.

Treatment

Management of psychological factors affecting the individual's medical condition should be tailored both to the particular psychological factor of relevance and to the medical outcome of concern. Some general guidelines, however, can be helpful. The physician, whether in primary care or a specialty, should not ignore apparent psychiatric illness. Unfortunately, this occurs all too often because of discomfort, stigma, lack of training, or disinterest. Referring the individual to a mental health specialist for evaluation is certainly better than ignoring the psychological problem but should not be regarded as "disposing" of it, because the physician must still attend to its potential impact on the individual's medical illness. Similarly, psychiatrists and other mental health practitioners should not ignore coincident medical disease and should not assume that referral to a nonpsychiatric physician absolves them of all responsibility for the individual's medical problem.

Mental Disorder Affecting a Medical Condition If the individual has a treatable Axis I disorder, treatment for it should be provided. Whereas this is obviously justified on the basis of providing relief from the Axis I disorder, mental treatment is further supported by the myriad ways in which the mental disorder may currently or in future adversely affect the medical illness. The same psychopharmacological and psychotherapeutic treatments used for Axis I mental disorders are normally appropriate when an affected medical condition is also present. However, even well-established psychiatric treatments supported by randomized controlled trials have seldom been validated in the medically ill, who are typically excluded from the controlled trials. Thus, psychiatric treatments may not always be directly generalizable to, and often must be modified for, the medically ill.

When prescribing psychiatric medications for individuals with significant medical comorbidity, the clinician should keep in mind potential adverse effects on impaired organ systems (e.g., anticholinergic exacerbation of postoperative ileus; tricyclic antidepressant causing completion of heart block), changes in pharmacokinetics (absorption, protein binding, metabolism, and excretion), and drug–drug interactions. Psychotherapy may also require modification in individuals with comorbid medical illness, including greater flexibility regarding the length and frequency of appointments, and deviations from standard therapeutic abstinence and neutrality. Psychotherapists treating individuals with PFAMC should usually be much more active in communicating with other health care professionals caring for the individual (with the individual's consent), than is usually the case in psychotherapy.

If the individual has an Axis II personality disorder or other prominent personality or coping style, the mental health clinician should modify the individual treatment accordingly, which is usually more easily accomplished than trying to change the individual's personality. For example, individuals who tend to be paranoid or mistrustful should receive more careful explanations, particularly before invasive or anxiety-provoking procedures. With narcissistic individuals, the clinician should avoid relating in ways that may seem excessively paternalistic or authoritarian to the individual. With some dependent individuals, it may be advisable to be more directive, without overdoing it and fostering excessive dependency.

Psychological Symptoms Affecting a General Medical Condition In some instances, psychiatric symptoms not meeting the threshold for an Axis I diagnosis will respond positively to the same treatments used for the analogous Axis I mental disorder, with appropriate modifications as noted before. There is not a great amount of treatment research on subsyndromal psychiatric symptoms, and even less in individuals with comorbid medical illness, so this area of practice remains less evidence-based. Some psychiatric symptoms affecting a medical condition may be amenable to stress management and other behavioral techniques as well as appropriate reassurance.

Any intervention directed by the mental health clinician at a particular individual's psychological symptoms or behavior should be grounded in exploratory discussion with the individual. Interventions without such grounding tend to seem at best superficial and artificial, and at worst are entirely off the mark. For example, if the clinician wrongly presumes to know why a particular individual seems anxious without asking, the individual is likely to feel misunderstood. Facile, nonspecific reassurance can undermine the clinician–patient relationship because the individual is likely to feel that the clinician is out of touch with and not really interested in the individual's experience. It is especially important with depressed individuals that clinicians avoid premature or unrealistic reassurance or an overly cheerful attitude; this tends to alienate depressed individuals, who feel that their clinician is insensitive and either does not understand or does not want to hear about their sadness. Clinicians should provide specific and realistic reassurance, emphasize on a constructive treatment plan, and mobilize the individual's support system.

Personality Traits or Coping Style Affecting a General Medical Condition
As with Axis II disorders affecting a medical condition, clinicians should be aware of the personality style's effects on the therapeutic relationship and modify management to better fit the individual. For example, with type A "time urgent" individuals, clinicians may need to be more sensitive to issues of appointment scheduling and waiting times. Group therapy interventions can enhance active coping with serious medical illnesses like cancer, heart disease, and renal failure but to date have usually been designed to be broadly generalizable rather than targeted to one particular trait or style (with the exception of type A behavior).

Another general guideline is not to attack or interfere with a individual's defensive style unless the defense is having an adverse impact on the medical illness or its management. Clinicians are particularly tempted to intervene when the defense is dramatic, breaks with reality, or makes the clinician uncomfortable.

For example, denial is a defense mechanism that reduces anxiety and conflict by blocking conscious awareness of thoughts, feelings, or facts that an individual cannot face. Denial is common in the medically ill but varies in its timing, strength, and adaptive value. Some individuals are aware of what is wrong with them but consciously suppress this knowledge by avoiding thinking about or discussing it. Others cope with the threat of being overwhelmed by their illness by unconsciously repressing it and thereby remain unaware of their illness. Marked denial, in which the individual emphatically refuses to accept the existence or significance of obvious symptoms and signs of the disease, may be seen by the clinician as an indication that the individual is "crazy" because the individual seems impervious to rational persuasion. In the absence of signs of another major mental disorder (e.g., paranoid delusions), such denial is not often a sign of psychosis but rather represents a defense against overwhelming fear.

The adaptive value of denial may vary, depending on the nature or stage of illness. When an individual's denial does not preclude cooperation with treatment, the clinician should leave it alone. The clinician does have an ethical and professional obligation to ensure that the individual has been informed about the illness and treatment. After that, if the individual accepts treatment but persists with an irrationally optimistic outlook, the clinician should respect the individual's need to use denial to cope. For some, the denial is fragile, and the clinician must decide whether the defense should be supported and strengthened, or if the individual had better give up the denial to discuss fears directly and receive reassurance from the clinician. The clinician should not support denial by giving the individual false information, but rather encourage hope and optimism. When denial is extreme, individuals may refuse vital treatment or threaten to leave against medical advice. Here, the clinician must try to help reduce denial but not by directly assaulting the individual's defenses. Because such desperate denial of reality usually reflects intense underlying anxiety, trying to scare the individual into cooperation will intensify denial and the impulse to flight. A better strategy for the clinician is to avoid directly challenging the individual's claims while simultaneously reinforcing concern for the individual and maximizing the individual's sense of control.

Maladaptive Health Behavior Affecting a General Medical Condition This is an area of research with many promising approaches. To achieve smoking cessation, bupropion, nicotine replacement, behavioral therapies, and other pharmacological strategies all warrant consideration. Behavioral strategies are also useful in promoting better dietary practices, sleep hygiene, safe sex, and exercise. For some individuals, change can be achieved efficiently through support groups, whereas others change more effectively through a one-to-one relationship with a health care professional.

Stress-Related Physiological Response Affecting a Medical Condition Biofeedback, relaxation techniques, hypnosis, and other stress management interventions have been helpful in reducing stress-induced exacerbations of medical illness including cardiac, gastrointestinal, headache, and other symptoms. Pharmacological interventions have also been useful (e.g., the widespread practice of prescribing benzodiazepines during acute myocardial infarction to prevent stress-induced increase in myocardial work).

Comparison of DSM-IV-TR/ICD-10 Diagnostic Criteria

Although the corresponding ICD-10 category ("Psychological and behavioral factors associated with disorders or diseases classified elsewhere") does not have specified diagnostic criteria, it is defined in essentially the same way as DSM-IV-TR.

References

Alexander F (1950) *Psychomatic Medicine*. WW Norton, New York.

Bruce ML, Leaf PJ, Rozal GPM, et al. (1994) Psychiatric status and 9-year mortality data in the new Haven epidemiological catchment area Study. *Am J Psychiatry* **151**, 716–721.

Deykin EY, Keane TM, Kaloupek D, et al. (2001) Posttraumatic stress disorder and the use of health services. *Psychosom Med* **63**, 835–841.

DiMatteo MR, Lepper HS, and Croghan TW (2000) Depression is a risk factor for noncompliance with medical treatment: meta-analysis of the effects of anxiety and depression on patient adherence. *Arch Intern Med* **160**, 2101–2107.

Druss BG, Bradford WD, Rosenheck RA, et al. (2001a) Quality of medical care and excess mortality in older patients with mental disorders. *Arch Gen Psychiatry* **58**, 565–572.

Druss BG, Rohrbaugh RM, Levinson CM, et al. (2001b) Integrated medical care for patients with serious psychiatric illness. *Arch Gen Psychiatry* **58**, 861–868.

Herran A, Amado JA, Garcia-Unzueta MT, et al. (2000) Increased bone remodeling in first-episode major depressive disorder. *Psychosom Med* **62**, 779–782.

Irwin M (1999) Immune correlates of depression. *Adv Exp Med Biol* **46**, 1–24.

Katon W and Gonzales J (1994) A review of randomized trials of psychiatric consultation-liaison studies in primary care. *Psychosomatics* **35**, 268–278.

Levenson JL, Hamer RM, and Rossiter LF (1990b) Relation of psychopathology in general medical inpatients to use and cost of services. *Am J Psychiatry* **147**, 1498–1503.

Noyes R Jr., Hartz AJ, Doebbeling CC, et al. (2000) Illness fears in the general population. *Psychosom Med* **62**, 318–325.

Roux AVD, Merkin SS, Arnett D, et al. (2001) Neighborhood of residence and incidence of coronary heart disease. *New Engl J Med* **345**, 99–106.

Saravay M and Lavin M (1994) Psychiatric comorbidity and length of stay in the general hospital: a critical review of outcome studies. *Psychosomatics* **35**, 233–252.

Smith G (1994) The course of somatization and its effects on utilization of health care resources. *Psychosomatics* **35**, 263–267.

Stevens LE, de Moore GM, and Simpson JM (1998) Delirium in hospital: does it increase length of stay? *Aust N Z J Psychiatr* **32**, 805–808.

Strain JJ, Hammer JS, and Fulop G (1994) APM task force on psychosocial interventions in the general hospital inpatient setting: a review of cost-offset studies. *Psychosomatics* **35**, 253–262.

Wessely S, Hotoph M, and Sharpe M (1998) *Chronic Fatigue and its Syndrome*. Oxford University Press, Oxford, UK.

Yang EV and Glaser R (2000) Stress-induced immunomodulation: Impact on immune defenses against infectious disease. *Biomed Pharmacother* **54**, 245–250.

46 ● Medication-Induced Movement Disorders

Modern medical practice presents physicians with choices of numerous medications to treat various ailments. Most medications have some side effects, and psychotropic medications are no exception. With the discovery of the antipsychotic effect of chlorpromazine in the early 1950s, psychiatry moved into the modern age of psychopharmacology, and there have been a number of advances since then. Along with these advances has come the awareness that many of these medications can produce disturbing side effects.

Perhaps the most uncomfortable side effects from psychotropic medications (especially antipsychotics or neuroleptics) are the acute and chronic movement disorders. Any psychiatrist in clinical practice has witnessed the intense distress that medication-induced movement disorders may bring to individuals. Perhaps most disturbing is that unlike other medications, antipsychotics can produce "tardive" or late-occurring movement disorders that may be persistent or even irreversible. Individuals in whom movement disorders develop may have more than subjective distress; they may suffer psychosocial embarrassment that makes them avoid being seen in public, and they may even suffer occupational impairment in severe cases. The responsibility this places on the prescribing psychiatrist is significant. Careful and reasoned thought must go into the analysis of whether the benefit of treatment with a medication exceeds the risk to the individual. This includes adequately explaining and obtaining informed consent from individuals.

When a psychiatrist prescribes a medication that has the potential to induce a movement disorder, the physician–patient relationship becomes particularly important. Individuals who require these medications are sometimes not amenable to trusting relationships (i.e., the paranoid individual). Working with an individual who has a psychotic illness requires that the psychiatrist establish a therapeutic bond with the patient.

There are different types of movement disorders that may result from treatment with psychotropic (especially neuroleptic) medications. They can generally be divided into those that occur acutely or subacutely and those that occur late in treatment (tardive). For the purpose of this discussion, we group the movement disorders into the relatively acute neuroleptic-induced disorders (acute dystonia, parkinsonism, and akathisia), neuroleptic-induced tardive dyskinesia (TD), and neuroleptic malignant syndrome (NMS). We also devote a section to the discussion of medication-induced postural tremor that predominantly focuses on lithium-induced tremor. This covers the major diagnostic groupings contained within the DSM-IV-TR under the general title medication-induced movement disorders. A time line for the emergence of the neuroleptic-induced movement disorders is provided in Table 46-1.

In general, the more an individual is able to understand the nature of his or her illness and the reason that a particular medication is being prescribed, the more likely he or she is to be adherent. When the psychiatrist does not devote adequate time to informing and instructing the patient, the result may be poor trust, poor communication, and possible legal difficulties for everyone involved. Unless declared incompetent by a court of law, an individual is considered to be legally competent to consent to or refuse psychotropic medications. The only exception to this rule is when an emergency situation exists and an individual must be

Table 46-1	Time of Emergence of Neuroleptic-Induced Movement Disorders
Condition	**Highest Risk of Emergence**
Acute dystonia	Days 0–7
Neuroleptic malignant syndrome	Days 0–7 (continues at lesser degree until end of first month)
Akathisia	Days 7–14 (continues at lesser degree until 2.5 mo)
Parkinsonism	Days 14–30 (continues at lesser degree until 2.5 mo)
Tardive dyskinesia	Month 3* → onward (risk increases with increasing time on neuroleptic)

*In patients older than 60 years, month 1 → onward.

medicated to prevent harm to self or others. The psychiatrist must provide information to the patient or the patient's decision-maker about the nature and purpose of the medication, its risks and benefits, alternatives to the proposed treatment, and prognosis without treatment (Wettstein 1988). Obtaining a written informed consent is one way of documenting the consent process. Another way is noting in the chart a summary of the discussion with an individual (or caregiver) about the consent to neuroleptic treatment.

Although the antipsychotics can produce unpleasant side effects, an individual who has been prepared openly and honestly for their possibility is more likely to view the side effects as evidence of the psychiatrist's excellent fund of knowledge rather than as a terrible surprise thrust on him or her by a dishonest or ignorant physician. On a final note, it may not be assumed that an individual already receiving antipsychotics prescribed by another physician has received an adequate informed consent. The process must begin anew with the new treating physician.

A new twist in the legal issues surrounding antipsychotic agents is the lower incidence of EPS and TD with atypical agents. The question of what is standard of care and how this relates to individuals prescribed conventional antipsychotics who are at a higher risk of developing a movement disorder such as TD presents interesting legal issues (Slovenko 2000).

In general, the literature continues to expand with trials demonstrating reduced incidence of new onset neuroleptic-induced movement disorders with atypical antipsychotics and at least partial improvement of existing movement disorders caused by conventional antipsychotics. While atypical antipsychotics are not without a risk of movement disorders, the improved motor side effect profile of the atypical agents provides a compelling argument for the use of atypical antipsychotics when initiating therapy, especially in susceptible populations such as the elderly. Switching to an atypical agent should be considered for those individuals maintained on a conventional agent who develop or have a high risk of movement disorders.

ACUTE NEUROLEPTIC-INDUCED MOVEMENT DISORDERS

A summary of the treatment of these disorders is provided in Table 46-2. Each of the specific acute neuroleptic-induced movement disorders (Neuroleptic-Induced Acute Dystonia, Neuroleptic-Induced Parkinsonism, Neuroleptic-Induced Acute Akathisia) is discussed in more detail below. One issue that remains controversial among researchers and psychiatrists is whether preventive anticholinergic medication should be given to individuals who are starting antipsychotics. Arguments against this practice include the risk of anticholinergic side effects such as dry mouth, blurry vision, constipation, and urinary retention. Further, anticholinergic medication is associated with cognitive side effects, such as memory impairment, confusion, and delirium (Simpson 1970, McClelland et al. 1974, Dimascio and Demergian 1970, Raleigh 1977, Syndulko et al. 1981). The relationship between anticholinergic medications and TD is not definitive (Kiloh et al. 1973, Jeste and Caligiuri 1993).

Arguments in favor of initiating prophylactic anticholinergic therapy point to the decrease in the frequency of EPS (including dystonias, akathisia, and akinesia) when anticholinergic drugs are prescribed prophylactically (Stern and Anderson 1979, Winslow et al. 1986). Furthermore, medication nonadherence and decompensation may relate to inadequately treated Neuroleptic-induced parkinsonism (NIP), especially akathisia and akinesia (Rifkin et al. 1975, 1978, Van Putten 1975, Van Putten et al. 1974). With the introduction and increased use of atypical antipsychotics, the risk of EPS and TD has decreased, thus reducing the need for prophylactic anticholinergic medication for many individuals prescribed atypical agents.

Table 46-2	Treatment of Acute Neuroleptic-Induced Movement Disorders		
Condition	**First Choice**	**Second Choice**	**Third Choice**
Acute dystonia	Anticholinergic medication, e.g., 2 mg benztropine PO, IM, IV 50 mg diphenhydramine PO, IM, IV	Benzodiazepine, e.g., lorazepam 1 mg IM, IV	—
Parkinsonism	Decrease neuroleptic to lowest effective dose Consider change to lower potency neuroleptic	Anticholinergic, e.g., benztropine at 2 mg/d	Consider high-dose anticholinergic Consider discontinuation of neuroleptic Consider experimental treatment
Akathisia			
with high-potency neuroleptic	β-blocker, e.g., propranolol 10–30 mg t.i.d.	Anticholinergic, e.g., 2 mg/d benztropine	Benzodiazepine, e.g., lorazepam, e.g., 1 mg t.i.d.
with low-potency neuroleptic	β-blocker	Benzodiazepine	Anticholinergic
with other extrapyramidal signs	Anticholinergic	Anticholinergic plus β-blocker	Anticholinergic plus benzodiazepine

Source: Data from Arana GW and Rosenbaum JF (2000) *Handbook of Psychiatric Drug Therapy*, 4th ed. Lippincott, Williams & Wilkins, Philadelphia, pp. 6–52.

Although this complicated issue remains unresolved, some basic guidelines can be proposed. When psychosis is severe and unmanageable and adherence with medications needs to be rigorously enforced, antipsychotic and anticholinergic medication may be administered concurrently, with the anticholinergic medication tapered slowly within the next few weeks. When the psychosis is milder and antipsychotic medication may be gradually increased, it may be best to avoid anticholinergic medications until such time as they become clinically necessary. In individuals with any degree of cognitive impairment (especially the elderly or demented individual with agitation or psychosis), it is best to aim for the administration of less anticholinergic medication. In younger individuals, especially young men (who have a high frequency of dystonia), it may be preferable to use anticholinergic medication prophylactically because it may prevent an uncomfortable dystonic reaction and can generally be used with relative impunity of serious side effects. In general, long-term prophylactic use of anticholinergic medication is not recommended (Ungvari et al. 1999) nor its use in the elderly (Mamo et al. 1999).

NEUROLEPTIC-INDUCED ACUTE DYSTONIA

Diagnosis
This long-lasting contraction or spasm of musculature develops in conjunction with the use of antipsychotic medication (see DSM-IV-TR diagnostic criteria on page 1295). Neuroleptic-induced dystonia (sometimes referred to as a dystonic reaction) usually begins 12 to 36 hours after a new antipsychotic is started or the dosage of a preexisting one is increased. It is unusual to see a dystonia after 2 weeks of antipsychotic treatment, and probably 90% of all neuroleptic-induced dystonias occur within the first 5 days of antipsychotic treatment (Ayd 1961). Individuals may report a sense of tongue "thickness" or difficulty in swallowing in the 3 to 6 hours preceding the acute dystonia (Arana and Rosenbaum 2000).

DSM-IV-TR Diagnostic Criteria

333.7 Neuroleptic-Induced Acute Dystonia

A. One (or more) of the following signs or symptoms has developed in association with the use of neuroleptic medication:

    (1) abnormal positioning of the head and neck in relation to the body (e.g., retrocollis, torticollis)

    (2) spasms of the jaw muscles (trismus, gaping, grimacing)

    (3) impaired swallowing (dysphagia), speaking, or breathing (laryngeal–pharyngeal spasm, dysphonia)

    (4) thickened or slurred speech due to hypertonic or enlarged tongue (dysarthria, macroglossia) tongue protrusion or tongue dysfunction

    (5) eyes deviated up, down, or sideward (oculogyric crisis)

    (6) abnormal positioning of the distal limbs or trunk

B. The signs or symptoms in criterion A developed within 7 days of starting or rapidly raising the dose of neuroleptic medication, or of reducing a medication used to treat (or prevent) acute extrapyramidal symptoms (e.g., anticholinergic agents).

C. The symptoms in criterion A are not better accounted for by a mental disorder (e.g., catatonic symptoms in schizophrenia). Evidence that the symptoms are better accounted for by a mental disorder might include the following: the symptoms precede the exposure to neuroleptic medication or are not compatible with the pattern of pharmacological intervention (e.g., no improvement after neuroleptic lowering or anticholinergic administration).

D. The symptoms in criterion A are not due to a nonneuroleptic substance or to a neurological or other general medical condition. Evidence that the symptoms are due to a general medical condition might include the following: the symptoms precede the exposure to the neuroleptic medication, unexplained focal neurological signs are present, or the symptoms progress in the absence of change in medication.

Reprinted with permission from the Diagnostic and Statistical Manual of Mental Disorders, Fourth Edition, Text Revision. Copyright 2000 American Psychiatric Association.

Acute dystonia presents as a sustained, painful muscle spasm that produces twisting, squeezing, and pulling movements of the muscle groups involved. The most common muscle groups affected are the eyes, jaw, tongue, and neck, but any muscle group in the body can be involved. On occasion, the larynx or pharynx may be involved, and this can result in rapid respiratory compromise (American Psychiatric Association 2000).

Epidemiology

Acute dystonia is generally less common than most other extrapyramidal side effects of antipsychotics. Its frequency has been reported to range from 2 to 12% of individuals taking conventional antipsychotic medication (Lohr and Jeste 1988a). For individuals who receive high doses of high-potency conventional agents, however, the frequency may be as high as 50% (Ayd 1961, Swett 1975). Incidence of acute dystonia can probably be reduced to approximately 2% if low-dose treatment strategies are employed (Rupniak et al. 1986). Furthermore, acute dystonia is considerably less likely to occur with atypical antipsychotic medications (i.e., less than 5% of individuals) (American Psychiatric Association 2000).

For example, dystonic reactions occurred in less than 5% of individuals in a study of ziprasidone (Tandon et al. 1997) and 1% in a dose comparison study with quetiapine (Kinget al. 1998).

Large doses of high-potency conventional antipsychotics appear to be the most consistent risk factor reported for acute dystonia (Rupniak et al. 1986). Other factors that also seem to predispose to dystonia are young age and male sex. A prior dystonic reaction is a good predictor of a repeated episode when the same antipsychotic at the same dose is reapplied (Keepers and Casey 1986).

Course

A neuroleptic-induced acute dystonia typically subsides spontaneously within hours after onset. However, treatment should be started as soon as the dystonia is diagnosed because the experience is intensely distressing to the individual.

Differential Diagnosis

Neuroleptic-induced acute dystonias are dramatic and usually easy to diagnose. There are, however, a number of other conditions that can present similarly and need to be ruled out. Spontaneously occurring focal or segmental dystonias may persist for days to weeks independent of medication. Neurological conditions such as temporal lobe seizures, infections, trauma, or tumors can produce symptoms similar to the neuroleptic-induced acute dystonia. A number of medications, while generally less common than antipsychotics, can cause dystonias (e.g., anticonvulsant medications and selective serotonin reuptake inhibitors) (American Psychiatric Association 2000).

Neuroleptic malignant syndrome (NMS) can produce muscle contractions that look similar to acute dystonia but can be distinguished by generalized "lead-pipe" type of rigidity, fever, fluctuating consciousness, and unstable vital signs. Catatonia associated with an affective or psychotic disorder can be difficult to distinguish from dystonia clinically but does not respond to the administration of anticholinergic or antihistaminic medication. Furthermore, individuals with catatonia are typically not concerned about their stiffness, whereas the individual with dystonia are likely to be extremely distressed (American Psychiatric Association 2000).

On occasion, an acute dystonic reaction may resemble TD. This is easily clarified by administering anticholinergic medications, which rapidly clear dystonia and do not affect (or may worsen) TD. Making a differential diagnosis between an acute dystonia and tardive dystonia can be difficult. Tardive dystonia (similar to TD) is a diagnosis made late in the course of antipsychotic treatment and is generally a chronic condition compared with acute dystonia, which occurs early in the course of medication treatment and typically responds rapidly to pharmacological intervention.

Etiology

The pathophysiological mechanism of neuroleptic-induced acute dystonia is presently unknown. Because no consistent pathological abnormality has been located in the brain, dystonia was often regarded in the past as a disorder of psychogenic origin. There is currently no evidence to support psychological factors as being the source of dystonia.

In neuroleptic-induced dystonia, the finding that anticholinergic medication reverses the dystonia consistently may suggest that a hypercholinergic state is a correlate of dystonia (Rupniak et al. 1986, Burke et al. 1985). There is some suggestion of a correlation with changing blood–brain levels of antipsychotic medication (Miller and Jankovic 1992). It is also possible that dystonia is related to the changing ratio of dopamine D_2 to D_1 receptors that accompany the normal aging process (Wonget al. 1984).

Abnormalities in dopamine–acetylcholine balance have been suggested as a possible mechanism because cholinergic antagonists and dopaminergic agonists seem to improve the dystonia in many individuals, in contrast to dopaminergic antagonists, which seem to exacerbate or even cause dystonia (Burke et al. 1985, Stahl and Berger 1982, Lang 1985, Fahn 1983). In contrast, other investigators have proposed that dopaminergic excess may be the responsible factor (Marsden and Jenner 1980).

Treatment

The standard approach to treatment is the immediate administration of an anticholinergic or antihistaminic agent. In most cases, this medication may be administered orally, intramuscularly, or intravenously. The first dose of medication should be the equivalent of 2 mg of benztropine or 50 mg of diphenhydramine. This should be repeated if the first dose does not produce a robust response within 30 minutes (Lohr and Jeste 1988a). This standard approach is usually successful in resolving the dystonia.

In the unusual refractory case, intramuscular or intravenous anticholinergic or antihistaminic drugs should be used at more frequent dosing intervals, and consideration should be given to adding an intramuscular injection of lorazepam for additional sedation (Arana and Rosenbaum 2000). Since even the milder dystonias respond much more quickly to intramuscular or intravenous medication, it may therefore be worth avoiding the use of oral medication in treating dystonia. Oral medication takes much longer to work and is likely to result in unnecessarily prolonged distress of the individual.

In cases of laryngeal or pharyngeal dystonias with airway compromise, repeated dosing of medication should occur at shorter intervals until resolution is achieved. Arana and Rosenbaum (2000) recommended that the individual receive 4 mg of intravenous benztropine within 10 minutes followed by 1 to 2 mg of intravenous lorazepam. If airway compromise continues for any appreciable amount of time, emergent support from an anesthesiologist should be obtained and the individual should receive general anesthesia with airway protection. Fortunately, the need for such measures is rare.

After a dystonia, an individual should be maintained with oral anticholinergic or antihistaminic medication for at least 48 hours. If there is a history of previous dystonias, the medication should be continued for 2 weeks. Consideration should be given to decreasing the previous dose of the antipsychotic or possibly switching to a low-potency neuroleptic or atypical agent if the individual has been prescribed a conventional antipsychotic. The use of prophylactic anticholinergic medication will be discussed later.

NEUROLEPTIC-INDUCED PARKINSONISM

Diagnosis

Neuroleptic-induced parkinsonism (NIP) is defined as parkinsonian signs or symptoms (tremor, muscle rigidity, or akinesia) that develop in association with the use of an antipsychotic medication (see DSM-IV-TR diagnostic criteria on page 1298). NIP symptoms may develop quickly after the initiation of an antipsychotic or insidiously during the course of treatment. It most typically develops 2 to 4 weeks after antipsychotic initiation. The three cardinal symptoms of NIP are tremor, muscle rigidity, and akinesia.

DSM-IV-TR Diagnostic Criteria

332.1 Neuroleptic-Induced Parkinsonism

A. One (or more) of the following signs or symptoms has developed in association with the use of neuroleptic medication:

  (1) parkinsonian tremor (i.e., a coarse, rhythmic, resting tremor with a frequency between 3 and 6 cycles per second, affecting the limbs, head, mouth, or tongue)
  (2) parkinsonian muscular rigidity (i.e., cogwheel rigidity or continuous "lead-pipe" rigidity)
  (3) akinesia (i.e., a decrease in spontaneous facial expressions, gestures, speech, or body movements)

B. The symptoms in criterion A developed within a few weeks of starting or raising the dose of a neuroleptic medication, or of reducing a medication used to treat (or prevent) acute extrapyramidal symptoms (e.g., anticholinergic agents).
C. The symptoms in criterion A are not better accounted for by a mental disorder (e.g., catatonic or negative symptoms in schizophrenia, psychomotor retardation in a major depressive episode). Evidence that the symptoms are better accounted for by a mental disorder might include the following: the symptoms precede the exposure to neuroleptic medication or are not compatible with the pattern of pharmacological intervention (e.g., no improvement after lowering the neuroleptic dose or administering anticholinergic medication).
D. The symptoms in criterion A are not due to a nonneuroleptic substance or to a neurological or other general medical condition (e.g., Parkinson's disease, Wilson's disease). Evidence that the symptoms are due to a general medical condition might include the following: the symptoms precede the exposure to neuroleptic medication, unexplained focal neurological signs are present, or the symptoms progress despite a stable medication regimen.

Parkinsonian tremor is a steady, rhythmical, oscillatory motion generally at an alternating rhythm of 3 to 6 Hz. The most affected body area tends to be the upper extremities, but the tremor may spread to the head, neck, jaw, face, tongue, legs, and trunk. The tremor is typically suppressed during action and increases during times of anxiety, stress, or fatigue (American Psychiatric Association 2000).

Parkinsonian muscle rigidity appears clinically as a firmness and spasm of muscles at rest that may affect all skeletal muscles or be confined to just a few specific muscle groups. It can appear as a continuous lead pipe-type rigidity that resists movement or a cogwheel-type rigidity that presents a "ratchet-like" resistance when a muscle is moved around a joint. Cogwheeling may represent an extremely high-frequency (8–12 Hz) "action" tremor that is physiologically imposed on the rigidity (Lance and McLeod 1981). The psychiatrist may diagnose cogwheel rigidity by placing his or her hand over the joint that is being passively moved. Generalized muscle pain, body aches, and discoordination are features associated with NIP rigidity (American Psychiatric Association 2000).

Parkinsonian akinesia is seen clinically as decreased spontaneous motor activity and a global slowness in the initiation and execution of movements. It can be associated with drooling, bent over neck, stooped shoulders, and masked facial expression (the so-called masked facies) (American Psychiatric Association 2000).

Parkinsonism occurs in numerous medical and neurological conditions and can be caused by many medications or substances. Idiopathic Parkinson's disease (PD) can be difficult to distinguish from NIP and we refer the reader to Hausner (1983) for methods of attempting to make a differential diagnosis between the two conditions.

Epidemiology

The reported frequency of NIP varies 5 to 90%, depending on the study reviewed (Lohr and Jeste 1988a). This wide variation is due to different definitions of parkinsonism in different studies as well as the inclusion of mild bradykinesia as a sign of NIP in some investigations. The usual incidence of "clinically significant" NIP with conventional antipsychotics is 10 to 15% (Miller and Jankovic 1992). When, however, high-potency conventional agents are used without anticholinergic drugs and signs of rigidity are carefully assessed, one is likely to find that the majority of individuals have some NIP. Rates of parkinsonism induced by atypical antipsychotics are considerably lower (American Psychiatric Association 2000). The incidence of NIP in older psychiatric patients is considerably greater. A study of newly medicated older individuals on low doses of conventional antipsychotics found 32% of individuals met criteria for NIP (Caligiuri et al. 1999). In an investigation of extrapyramidal side effects in individuals with Alzheimer disease treated with very low dose conventional antipsychotics, 67% of individuals met criteria for NIP at some time during the 9-month follow-up period (Caligiuri et al. 1998).

A number of individual-related and medication-related risk factors have been proposed. A history of prior episodes of NIP, older age, and concomitant dementia or delirium are thought to predispose to NIP (American Psychiatric Association 2000). Neuroleptic potency and preexisting extrapyramidal symptoms may also increase the risk of NIP (Sweet et al. 1994, Caligiuri and Lohr 1997, Chakos et al. 1992).

Rapid increases in antipsychotic dosage, administration of higher absolute doses of antipsychotics, and absence of concurrent anticholinergic medication represent other risk factors for NIP initiation (American Psychiatric Association 2000). Highly anticholinergic antipsychotics (i.e., chlorpromazine and thioridazine) are less likely to cause NIP than less anticholinergic agents (i.e., haloperidol and fluphenazine).

Course

NIP symptoms usually continue unchanged or diminish slowly in 2 to 3 months after onset. The signs and symptoms typically improve with a dose reduction, discontinuation of antipsychotic medication, or switch to an atypical antipsychotic in individuals previously receiving a conventional antipsychotic. Improvement is also seen with the addition of antiparkinsonian agents.

Differential Diagnosis

The tremor of NIP must be distinguished from tremor caused by other conditions. In general, nonparkinsonian tremors are finer, faster, and worse on intention. Tremor associated with substance withdrawal typically presents with associated hyperreflexia and increased autonomic signs. Cerebellar disease-induced tremor may present with associated nystagmus, ataxia, or scanning speech. Strokes and other central nervous system lesions usually have associated focal neurological symptoms. NMS can often present with akinesia and lead pipe–type rigidity but also has other associated findings, such as fever, elevated creatine kinase, and fluctuating consciousness (American Psychiatric Association 2000).

Tremor in neuroleptic-induced TD does not typically have the steady rhythm associated with NIP. In the past, it has been hypothesized that NIP and TD would not be likely to coexist in the same individual. If true, this would provide another means of making a differential diagnosis between the two conditions. A review and a study by Caligiuri and colleagues (1991) do not support this hypothesis, however, and it appears that TD and NIP frequently coexist in the same individual.

A number of primary psychiatric illnesses may mimic symptoms of NIP and may be difficult to separate. These include major depressive disorder, catatonic-type schizophrenia, mood disorder with catatonic features, schizophrenia with a predominance of negative features, delirium, dementia, anxiety disorders, and certain conversion disorders (American Psychiatric Association 2000). It may be particularly easy to confuse negative symptoms of schizophrenia and depression with the akinesia and rigidity of NIP. Catatonia and NIP may also be difficult to differentiate, and there is evidence that the two conditions are related to each other (Lohr et al. 1987b). Often, the diagnosis of NIP should be made provisionally and clarified by a dosage reduction of antipsychotic or trial of anticholinergic medication (American Psychiatric Association 2000).

Etiology

NIP is presumed to result from blockade of postsynaptic dopamine (D_2) receptors in the corpus striatum causing a pathological state functionally resembling the loss of dopaminergic cells in the striatum in idiopathic Parkinson's disease (PD). However, it is not clear whether nigrostriatal dopamine loss is adequate to explain the clinical symptoms seen in NIP or PD (Lohr and Jeste 1988a). It is possible that other neurochemical abnormalities may coexist with dopaminergic depletion to produce the syndrome. Abnormalities in norepinephrine and serotonin have also been reported to be involved in the mechanism (Hornykiewicz 1982, Mitchell et al. 1985, Langston and Irwin 1986).

Positron emission tomography (PET) and other technologies have been utilized to examine the relationship between D_2 receptor blockade in the basal ganglia with antipsychotic efficacy and NIP. Clinically effective doses of conventional antipsychotics have been shown to block 70 to 90% of D_2 receptors in the basal ganglia. Of note are findings that with conventional agents, at least 60% occupancy is needed for satisfactory antipsychotic response but that NIP tends to occur with 80% or greater occupancy of the D_2 receptors (Glazer 2000, Farde et al. 1992, Kapur et al. 1998). With regard to atypical agents, the lower D_2 receptor blockade at recommended dosages with some agents and the serotonergic blockade seen with these medications are believed to lead to the reduced risk of NIP. Similar to conventional antipsychotics, higher doses of some atypical agents also appear to be related to an increase in NIP, as greater D_2 receptor blockade has been reported (Glazer 2000).

Treatment

Many milder cases of NIP do not require treatment because they are not bothersome to the individual. A switch to an atypical agent should be strongly considered if troublesome NIP develops while on a conventional antipsychotic. Large randomized controlled trials have demonstrated reductions in parkinsonian symptoms in individuals treated with atypical antipsychotics (Arvanitis et al. 1997, Beasley et al. 1997, Chouinard et al. 1993, Simpson and Lindenmayer 1997, Kane et al. 1988a). If symptoms become troublesome, the initial step should be to decrease the dose of antipsychotic to the lowest effective dose for the individual. The next step is to add a low dosage of an anticholinergic medication. The equivalent of 2 mg/day of benztropine generally represents a reasonable starting point. Periodic attempts should be made to wean the individual from the anticholinergic agent. As many as 90% of individuals do not require anticholinergic medication at the end of 3 months

(Coleman and Hays 1975, Johnson 1978). Anticholinergic medication should always be tapered slowly to avoid the rapid redevelopment of parkinsonian symptoms as well as the possibility of uncomfortable cholinergic rebound symptoms.

Refractory cases of NIP do occur and may require more aggressive management. Increasing the dose of the anticholinergic medication is a good starting point because some individuals may require up to the equivalent of 20 mg/day of benztropine to achieve relief from NIP. If such high doses are to be employed, they should be used for the shortest possible time, and rigorous attention should be paid to the possibility of untoward anticholinergic effects (i.e., delirium, urinary retention, fecal impaction). Consideration may be given to starting a dopamine-releasing agent, such as amantadine or perhaps even levodopa. A major concern with this treatment approach is the possibility of exacerbating the psychosis for which the antipsychotic medication was prescribed in the first place. Trials of dopaminergic agents are therefore best attempted in an inpatient setting or with careful outpatient observation and assessment. A number of experimental treatment strategies have been proposed for the treatment of the refractory cases including vitamin E, calcium supplementation, electroconvulsive therapy, and L-deprenyl (Osser 1992).

Another treatment approach for the refractory case is to lower the dose of the antipsychotic medication or even discontinue it until the NIP resolves, then resume the antipsychotic (preferably a different one) at a lower dose. This treatment strategy may also need to be carried out in an inpatient setting to monitor early emergence of psychotic symptoms.

NEUROLEPTIC-INDUCED ACUTE AKATHISIA

Diagnosis

Neuroleptic-induced acute akathisia is defined as a subjective feeling of restlessness and an intensely unpleasant need to move occurring secondary to antipsychotic treatment (see DSM-IV-TR diagnostic criteria below). Akathisia tends to occur within the first 4 weeks of initiating or increasing the dose of antipsychotic medication. It can develop rapidly after the initiation or the dose increase of an antipsychotic. Individuals with akathisia tend to have subjective complaints of "inner restlessness," most often in the legs. It may be difficult for the individuals to describe their feelings. They feel that they must move, and this manifests as fidgeting, frequent changes in posture, crossing and uncrossing of the legs, rocking while sitting, and shuffling when walking (American Psychiatric Association 2000).

DSM-IV-TR Diagnostic Criteria

333.99 Neuroleptic-Induced Acute Akathisia

A. The development of subjective complaints of restlessness after exposure to a neuroleptic medication.

B. At least one of the following is observed:

    (1) fidgety movements or swinging of the legs
    (2) rocking from foot to foot while standing
    (3) pacing to relieve restlessness
    (4) inability to sit or stand for at least several minutes

C. The onset of the symptoms in criteria A and B occurs within 4 weeks of initiating or increasing the dose of the neuroleptic, or of reducing medication used to treat (or prevent) acute extrapyramidal symptoms (e.g., anticholinergic agents).

D. The symptoms in criterion A are not better accounted for by a mental disorder (e.g., schizophrenia, substance withdrawal, agitation from a major depressive or manic episode, hyperactivity in attention-deficit/hyperactivity disorder). Evidence that symptoms may be better accounted for by a mental disorder might include the following: the onset of symptoms preceding the exposure to the neuroleptics, the absence of increasing restlessness with increasing neuroleptic doses, and the absence of relief with pharmacological interventions (e.g., no improvement after decreasing the neuroleptic dose or treatment with medication intended to treat the akathisia).

E. The symptoms in criterion A are not due to a nonneuroleptic substance or to a neurological or other general medical condition. Evidence that symptoms are due to a general medical condition might include the onset of the symptoms preceding the exposure to neuroleptics or the progression of symptoms in the absence of a change in medication.

Reprinted with permission from the Diagnostic and Statistical Manual of Mental Disorders, Fourth Edition, Text Revision. Copyright 2000 American Psychiatric Association.

Akathisia is often associated with severe dysphoria, anxiety, and irritability. When the akathisia is particularly severe, aggression or suicide attempts may be a possible result, although this is controversial. Akathisia in a psychotic individual can easily be mistaken for worsening of psychotic features, resulting in an increase in antipsychotic dose and an exacerbation of the akathisia.

Epidemiology

Akathisia is a common side effect of antipsychotic treatment. It is estimated to occur in 20 to 75% of all individuals treated with conventional agents. The wide discrepancy in reported prevalence may result from a lack of consistency in the definition of akathisia, different prescribing practices, different study designs, and differences in population demographics (American Psychiatric Association 2000). While atypical antipsychotics are less likely to cause akathisia compared to typical agents (Arvanitis et al. 1997, Tollefson et al. 1997), prevalence rates have varied (Miller and Fleischhacker 2000). Clozapine-induced akathisia has ranged from 0 to 39% (Safferman et al. 1993, Kurz et al. 1998, Cohen et al. 1991) and a point prevalence of 13% was reported for risperidone (Miller et al. 1998). Akathisia is thought by many psychiatrists to be a leading cause of nonadherence.

Higher doses of high-potency conventional antipsychotics appear to be most frequently associated with the appearance of akathisia (American Psychiatric Association 2000). Previous episodes of neuroleptic-induced akathisia increase the risk for future episodes if antipsychotics are restarted.

Course

Neuroleptic-induced akathisia typically lasts as long as antipsychotic treatment is continued but may have variable intensity in time (American Psychiatric Association 2000). Treatment of akathisia may or may not alter the course of the akathisia.

Differential Diagnosis

The strange subjective discomfort associated with akathisia is the feature that seems to be most useful in making a differential diagnosis between neuroleptic-induced akathisia and other neuroleptic-induced movement disorders. TD is often associated with a lack of sensory perception of having a movement disorder. This contrasts with akathisia in which individuals tend to be acutely aware of their distress. When individuals with TD are uncomfortable, it is usually a result of social factors such as embarrassment and functional factors such as frustration over not being able to perform certain tasks. Another differentiating factor is that TD usually involves the face, mouth, and upper extremities, whereas akathisia more commonly involves the lower extremities.

The rhythmical appearance of akathisia may sometimes suggest a tremorous condition. Thus, the tremor of NIP and idiopathic PD may be mistaken for akathisia, especially if the feet and legs are involved. Iron deficiency anemia can also present with symptoms phenomenologically similar to neuroleptic-induced akathisia. A number of other medications but particularly selective serotonin reuptake inhibitor antidepressant medications may produce akathisia clinically identical to that produced by antipsychotics (American Psychiatric Association 2000).

It is critical to differentiate akathisia from other psychiatric disorders presenting with agitation, such as depressive episodes, manic episodes, anxiety disorders, schizophrenia, dementia, delirium, substance intoxication or withdrawal, and attention-deficit/hyperactivity disorder. The reason for the importance of this differentiation is that mistaking akathisia for a primary mental disorder can result in an intervention that would be the exact opposite of what is appropriate (i.e., increasing the dose of an antipsychotic instead of decreasing it because akathisia is mistaken for worsening psychosis) (American Psychiatric Association 2000).

Etiology

The pathophysiological mechanism of akathisia remains unknown. A number of theories have been offered by investigators. Early theories about the etiology of akathisia proposed that it represented a subjective response to the presence of the rigidity and akinesia of NIP (Tarsy 1992). Akathisia has also been suggested to be a primary sensory disturbance in which motor disturbance occurs as a direct response to the sensory disturbance (Sovner and Dimascio 1978). In contrast, others have proposed that akathisia simply represents another EPS because it frequently occurs with other EPS and is often reversed by anticholinergic medications.

Marsden and Jenner (1980) suggested that dopamine blockade in the mesocortical system may account for the hyperactive symptoms of akathisia. Mesocortical dopaminergic neurons that innervate the prefrontal cortex seem to be resistant to depolarization induced by long-term antipsychotic treatment, suggesting a possible explanation for why akathisia often does not improve with time (Lohr and Jeste 1988a).

The possibility that excessive noradrenergic activity plays a role in the pathogenesis of akathisia is supported by the efficacy of beta-adrenergic blockers in improving some cases of akathisia. Additionally, opioid mechanisms have been proposed to contribute to akathisia on the basis of reported therapeutic effects of opioid drugs (Walters et al. 1986). The lower likelihood of akathisia with atypical antipsychotics and reports of selective serotonin reuptake inhibitors causing akathisia have implicated serotonin as having a possible role in akathisia, however, this is still under investigation (Miller and Fleischhacker 2000).

Treatment

Akathisia may be difficult to treat effectively. The best initial approach is to try and reduce the chance of developing akathisia by minimizing the dosage of antipsychotic medication. The use of atypical antipsychotics should be considered as a result of their lower risk of akathisia (Sachdev et al. 1995). If using conventional antipsychotics, a switch to a low-potency agent such as thioridazine or chlorpromazine may prove helpful because these antipsychotics seem to have somewhat lower propensity to cause akathisia than high-potency conventional antipsychotics. After these initial steps, consideration should be given to initiation of an antiakathisic drug regimen. A number of agents have been reported to be effective, including beta-adrenergic blockers, anticholinergic drugs, benzodiazepines, and clonidine (American Psychiatric Association 2000).

When choosing an agent to treat akathisia, a beta-blocker such as propranolol should generally be considered first-line as its efficacy has been proven and it has been shown to be superior to other possible treatments such as benztropine and lorazepam (Adler et al. 1986, 1987, 1993a). In terms of antiakathisic effects, the beta-blocker chosen should be lipophilic so as to cross the blood–brain barrier and should also have activity at the beta-2 receptor (Miller and Fleischhacker 2000). Benzodiazepines such as clonazepam and lorazepam have been shown to be efficacious in the treatment of akathisia and are also a reasonable therapeutic option, especially when considering the interplay between anxiety and akathisia, however, their side effects and abuse potential should be considered. Anticholinergic agents such as benztropine may also be tried, but less evidence exists to supports their use. A limited number of studies have also shown possible roles for clonidine and amantadine in the treatment of akathisia (Miller and Fleischhacker 2000). Agents with serotonin receptor blocking activity (i.e., ritanserin, mianserin) have also been reported to be of benefit in akathisia (Bersani et al. 1990, Poyurovsky et al. 1999).

NEUROLEPTIC-INDUCED TARDIVE DYSKINESIA

Diagnosis

Neuroleptic-induced tardive dyskinesia (TD) is a syndrome consisting of abnormal, involuntary movements caused by long-term treatment with antipsychotic medication (see DSM-IV-TR diagnostic criteria below). The movements are typically choreoathetoid in nature and principally involve the mouth, face, limbs, and trunk. TD, by definition, occurs late in the course of drug treatment.

DSM-IV-TR Diagnostic Criteria

333.82 Neuroleptic-Induced Tardive Dyskinesia

A. Involuntary movements of the tongue, jaw, trunk, or extremities have developed in association with the use of neuroleptic medication.

B. The involuntary movements are present over a period of at least 4 weeks and occur in any of the following patterns:

(1) choreiform movements (i.e., rapid, jerky, nonrepetitive)
(2) athetoid movements (i.e., slow, sinuous, continual)
(3) rhythmic movements (i.e., stereotypies)

C. The signs or symptoms in criteria A and B develop during exposure to a neuroleptic medication or within 4 weeks of withdrawal from an oral (or within 8 weeks of withdrawal from a depot) neuroleptic medication.

D. There has been exposure to neuroleptic medication for at least 3 months (1 month if age 60 years or older).

E. The symptoms are not due to a neurological or general medical condition (e.g., Huntington's disease, Sydenham's chorea, spontaneous dyskinesia, hyperthyroidism, Wilson's disease), ill-fitting dentures, or exposure to other medications that cause acute reversible dyskinesia (e.g., l-dopa, bromocriptine). Evidence that the symptoms are due to one of these etiologies might include the following: the symptoms precede

the exposure to the neuroleptic medication or unexplained focal neurological signs are present.
F. The symptoms are not better accounted for by a neuroleptic-induced acute movement disorder (e.g., neuroleptic-induced acute dystonia, neuroleptic-induced acute akathisia).

TD may develop at any age and typically has an insidious onset. It may develop during exposure to antipsychotic medication or within 4 weeks of withdrawal from an oral antipsychotic (or within 8 weeks of withdrawal from a depot neuroleptic). There must be a history of at least 3 months of antipsychotic use (or 1 month in the elderly) before TD may be diagnosed (American Psychiatric Association 2000).

The most common features of TD are involuntary movements of the tongue, face, and neck muscles. Less common are movements in the upper and lower extremities as well as in the trunk (Brandon et al. 1971, Edwards 1970, Guy et al. 1986). Most rare of all are involuntary movements of the muscle groups involved with breathing and swallowing. The earliest symptoms typically involve buccolingual–masticatory movements. The movements of TD are choreiform (rapid, jerky), athetoid (slow, sinuous), or rhythmical (stereotypical) (American Psychiatric Association 2000).

Severe choreoathetoid dyskinesia differs from the milder forms, mainly in the frequency and amplitude of the abnormal movements (Gardos and Cole 1992). Some cases of severe dyskinesia consist of generalized choreoathetosis of the face, trunk, and all four limbs (Gardos et al. 1987, Mann et al. 1983, Casey and Rabins 1978). TD may be accompanied by dystonias (Tarsy et al. 1977, Nasrallah et al. 1980, McLean and Casey 1978), parkinsonism (Brandon et al. 1971, Bitton and Melamed 1984), and akathisia (Brandon et al. 1971, Chouinard and Bradwejn 1982).

TD is worsened by stimulants, short-term withdrawal of antipsychotic medication, anticholinergic medication, emotional arousal, stress, and voluntary movements of other parts of the body. It is improved by relaxation, voluntary movements of the involved parts of the body, sleep, and increased dose of antipsychotics.

Epidemiology

The reported prevalence of TD has been somewhat variable as a result of differences in populations of individuals and in the methods used (Jeste and Wyatt 1981). Yassa and Jeste (1992) reviewed 76 studies of the prevalence of TD published from 1960 to 1990. In a total population of approximately 40,000 patients, the overall prevalence of TD was 24.2%, although it was much higher (about 50%) in studies of elderly individuals treated with antipsychotics.

There have been relatively few studies of the incidence of TD. Kane and coworkers (1988b) prospectively studied more than 850 individuals (mean age 29 years) and found the incidence of TD after cumulative exposure to conventional antipsychotics to be 5% after 1 year, 18.5% after 4 years, and 40% after 8 years. Incidence in older populations has been found to be much higher. Saltz and colleagues (1991) reported an incidence of 31% after 43 weeks of conventional antipsychotic treatment in a population of elderly individuals. Jeste and colleagues (1995, 1999c) evaluated 439 psychiatric patients with a mean age of 65 years and found that 28.8% of the sample met criteria for TD during the first 12 months of study treatment; 50.1% had TD by the end of 24 months, and 63.1% by the end of

36 months. The risk of severe TD has also been reported to be higher in older individuals (Caligiuriet al. 1997).

Evidence supporting a reduced risk of TD with atypical antipsychotics is beginning to emerge. The lower risk of EPS with atypical agents has led to the widespread conclusion that these agents will also have reduced TD risk. The low risk of tardive dyskinesia in clozapine-treated individuals has been well established (Kane et al. 1993). In addition, a lower incidence of TD has been reported in individuals treated with risperidone (Jeste et al. 1999a, 1999b, Chouinard et al. 1993) and olanzapine (Tollefson et al. 1997). More long-term prospective studies are needed with the atypical agents.

Aging consistently appears to be the most important risk factor for the development of TD. Prevalence and severity of TD seem to increase with age (Smith and Baldessarini 1980). The reasons for this increased risk of TD with aging are not known but may be related to the propensity of the nigrostriatal system to degenerate with age as well as pharmacokinetic and pharmacodynamic factors (Jeste and Caligiuri 1993).

Gender (female) was thought to be a risk factor for TD. A meta-analysis of the published reports demonstrated a greater prevalence of TD in women (26.6%) compared with that in men (21.6%) (Yassa and Jeste 1992). Interestingly, studies of incidence of TD in older individuals failed to confirm the reported propensity of women to have TD at a higher rate than men (Saltz et al. 1991, Jeste et al. 1995). A possible relationship between gender and age of onset of schizophrenia to severity of dyskinesia has been reported as women with late-onset schizophrenia (LOS) and men with early-onset schizophrenia (EOS) had more severe dyskinesia that men with LOS and women with EOS (Lindameret al. 2001).

Mood disorders (especially unipolar depression) have been reported to be risk factors for TD in a number of publications, although findings have been mixed (Kane et al. 1988b, Saltz et al. 1991, Casey 1988, Casey and Keepers 1988, Jesteet al. 1995).

There are conflicting reports regarding ethnicity as a risk factor for TD. In a study of 491 individuals with chronic psychiatric problems, no significant differences in TD prevalence were found among blacks, whites, and Hispanics (Sramek et al. 1991). Higher incidence rate of TD in African-Americans than in whites, however, was reported by Morgenstern and Glazer (1993) and, to a smaller extent, by Lacro and Jeste (1997). There is some evidence that Asians may have the lowest prevalence rate of TD.

People with diabetes mellitus may be at a higher risk for development of TD (Ganzini et al. 1991, Woerner et al. 1993). Sewell and Jeste (1992a) proposed that diabetes mellitus might be a risk factor for TD in individuals treated with metoclopramide.

The presence of dementia or delirium may or may not be a risk factor for TD. Yassa and associates (1984) determined central nervous system damage predisposed to TD, but two prospective TD studies of older individuals found organic diagnosis not to be associated with TD susceptibility (Saltz et al. 1991, Jesteet al. 1995).

Individuals who experience an acute neuroleptic-induced movement disorder (especially parkinsonism or akathisia) are likely to be at a greater risk for development of TD if antipsychotic treatment is continued (Kaneet al. 1992).

Total exposure to typical antipsychotic agents has been correlated with TD risk (Casey 1997) and within elderly populations, cumulative amount of typical antipsychotics has also been associated with TD risk, especially with high-potency conventional agents (Jesteet al. 1995).

The observation that anticholinergic drugs exacerbate some symptoms of TD does not appear to indicate that the drugs promote the onset of the disorder (Gardos and Cole 1983).

Course

One-third of the TD patients experience remission within 3 months of discontinuation of antipsychotic medication, and approximately half have remission within 12 to 18 months of antipsychotic discontinuation (American Psychiatric Association 2000). Elderly individuals are reported to have lower rates of remission, especially if antipsychotics are continued. When individuals with TD must be maintained with antipsychotics, TD seems to be stable in 50%, worsen in 25%, and improve in the rest.

Time may be the most important factor in outcome of TD. In studies that have followed up individuals for longer than 5 years, TD seems to improve in half of individuals with or without antipsychotic treatment. Furthermore, TD may improve as slowly as it develops and may exist on a spectrum between resolution and persistence (Kane et al. 1992).

Severe TD may lead to numerous physical complications and psychosocial problems. Dental and denture problems are common sequelae of severe oral dyskinesia (Yassa and Jones 1985), as are ulcerations of the tongue, cheeks, and lips. Hyperkinetic dysarthria has been described by Maxwell and coworkers (1970) and Portnoy (1979). Swallowing disorders represent another complication (Massengil and Nashold 1952). Respiratory disturbances, although fairly rare, have been reported by a number of investigators (Casey and Rabins 1978, Ayd 1979, Jackson et al. 1980, Weiner et al. 1978). These disturbances are usually manifested by shortness of breath at rest, irregularities in respiration, and various grunts, snorts, and gasps. Respiratory alkalosis may be seen on laboratory tests. Gastrointestinal complications of severe TD may involve vomiting and dysphagia secondary to disruption of the normal activity of the esophagus (Yassa and Jones 1985); weight loss may result from such a disturbance.

Subjective distress is a common accompaniment of severe dyskinesia. Suicidal ideation may result from distress over the dyskinesia, and there have been reports of some successful suicides. General impairment of functioning may be related to the severity of the dyskinetic disorder. Social embarrassment as a result of TD may represent a reason that some individuals with TD tend to be reluctant to leave their homes. Even mild dyskinesia may lead to anxiety, guilt, shame, and anger. These symptoms can lead to severe depressive episodes (Yassa and Jones 1985).

Differential Diagnosis

The differential diagnosis of TD is extensive. The major task for the clinician is to rule out other causes of dyskinesia. It may be useful for the psychiatrist to keep in mind three questions for the facilitation of the differential diagnosis: (1) Does the individual have dyskinesia? (2) Does another disorder fully explain the cause of the dyskinesia? (3) If the dyskinesia is related to antipsychotic use, is it TD? (Jeste and Wyatt 1982).

A number of nondyskinetic movement disorders are part of the differential diagnosis of TD. Tremor can be confused with TD, including the tremor of neuroleptic-induced parkinsonism, rabbit syndrome, Wilson's disease, and cerebellar disease. Further, fine tremors of the fingers and hands are produced by anxiety states, alcoholism, hyperthyroidism, and drugs. Acute dystonias, myoclonus, tics, mannerisms, compulsions, and akathisia must be differentiated from TD. The differentiation is made on the basis of the clinical assessment. For further details, the reader is referred to Jeste and Wyatt (1982).

Once it has been established that the individual suffers from a dyskinesia, the main cause must be determined. In children and young adults, a number of conditions may cause dyskinesia besides antipsychotic treatment. The use of drugs, especially amphetamines and antihistamines, are associated with dyskinesia. Sydenham's chorea can produce choreiform movements. Conversion disorder and malingering are conditions that can present with apparently involuntary movements. Hyperthyroidism and hypoparathyroidism are two endocrinological conditions that can produce dyskinesias similar to TD. Huntington's disease is a condition that can be difficult to distinguish clinically from TD, but certain characteristics may aid in the diagnosis, including (1) a family history of Huntington's disease, (2) the presence of dementia, (3) a slowly progressive downhill course, and (4) atrophy of the caudate nucleus on computed tomography scan.

In the middle-aged or elderly individual, denture or dental problems may commonly mimic TD. Lesions of the basal ganglia may result in dyskinesias. The use of antiparkinsonian medications such as levodopa, amantadine, and bromocriptine can cause dyskinetic movements. The presence of spontaneous dyskinesias must also be ruled out.

When it has been established that antipsychotics are responsible for the dyskinesia, it does not follow that the dyskinesia is necessarily TD. Acute dyskinesia occurring early in antipsychotic treatment is common and responds well to antihistaminic or anticholinergic medications. Withdrawal–emergent dyskinesia also occurs in a variable proportion of individuals. This phenomenon refers to the appearance or worsening of dyskinetic movements on reduction or discontinuation of antipsychotic medication. Withdrawal–emergent dyskinesia is phenomenologically similar to TD and often has the full range of involuntary choreiform and athetoid movements. A typical case may begin within a few days after a sudden decrease in dosage and worsen as the antipsychotic is withdrawn. This phase is followed by rapid improvement in a period of weeks to months. A history of antipsychotic exposure and remission of dyskinetic symptoms within 3 months of antipsychotic withdrawal are suggestive of the diagnosis of withdrawal–emergent dyskinesia (Gerhard 1992).

Finally, tardive Tourette's disorder must be differentiated from TD. A number of cases of tardive Tourette's disorder have been reported as a result of treatment with antipsychotics, emerging during treatment or after cessation of treatment (Jeste and Wyatt 1982, Klawans et al. 1978, DeVaugh-Geiss 1980, Stahl 1980, Seeman et al. 1981, Muller and Aminoff 1982, Munetz et al. 1985). Tardive Tourette's disorder presents with symptoms similar to those of idiopathic Tourette's disorder. Motor tics are usually compulsive organized stereotypies that may, in certain cases, be difficult to distinguish from the choreoathetoid movements of TD. Typically, vocal tics (including barks, grunts, coughs, and yelps) represent part of tardive Tourette's disorder but not TD. Tardive Tourette's disorder seems to show a pharmacological response similar to that of TD, leading to the assumption that the syndrome may be a type of the more commonly seen TD. Thus, tardive Tourette's disorder may be masked by an increase in antipsychotics and exacerbated by withdrawal (Jeste et al. 1986).

Etiology

Historically, striatal dopamine receptor supersensitivity had been proposed to be responsible for TD. It now seems more likely that a number of separate neurotransmitter systems are involved in the pathogenesis of TD. There may be different subtypes of TD, each perhaps involving a unique profile of neurochemical imbalance (Jeste and Wyatt 1982).

Neuroleptic-induced striatal pathological change represents another possibility for explaining mechanisms of TD (Jeste et al. 1992). Lohr and Jeste (1988b) suggested that long-term antipsychotic use may produce "toxic free radicals" that damage neurons and result in persistent TD.

Treatment

Despite intense effort, there is as yet no consistently reliable therapy for TD. As a result, the clinician must focus primary efforts toward prevention of the disorder. The use of atypical antipsychotics are recommended due to their probable lower risk of TD. Antipsychotic use should be minimized in all patients. Individuals with nonpsychotic mood or other disorders who need antipsychotics should receive the minimal necessary amounts of antipsychotic treatment and should have the medication tapered and then stopped once the clinical need is no longer present. In general, there must be enough clinical evidence to show that the benefits outweigh the potential risks of TD development (Arana and Rosenbaum 2000).

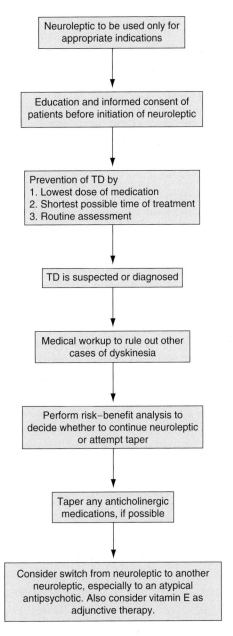

Figure 46-1 *Management of tardive dyskinesia (TD).*

Antipsychotics should be used with particular caution in elderly individuals because of their high risk for development of TD (Figure 46-1).

Gradual taper of the antipsychotic medication may be attempted as long as the risk/benefit ratio of antipsychotic maintenance versus withdrawal does not preclude such a strategy. Gilbert and colleagues (1995) suggested that a slow taper of medication to the lowest effective dose is probably the preferred strategy for the treatment of chronic schizophrenia in a large number of stable individuals.

Paradoxically, antipsychotics themselves represent the most effective short-term treatment for TD. An increase in dosage of a conventional agent usually (approximately 66% of individuals) results in a clinically significant but temporary reduction in TD symptoms (Jeste et al. 1988). The most exciting development in the treatment of TD has been the use of the atypical antipsychotics. Clozapine has been shown to be effective in reducing TD in individuals with existing TD (Simpson et al. 1978, Lieberman et al. 1991, Kane et al. 1993, Small et al. 1987); however, side effects such as agranulocytosis and clozapine's affinity for anticholinergic side effects limits its use. Additional studies have noted a beneficial effect of other atypical agents (i.e., risperidone and olanzapine) on preexisting TD (Littrell et al. 1998, Street et al. 2000, Jeste et al. 1997). The reduced risk of TD with all atypical agents (when used at appropriate doses) supports their use as preventive measures and as therapeutic options for those who develop TD on a conventional antipsychotic.

A number of experimental studies have attempted to treat TD with alternative strategies. Jeste and colleagues (1988) reviewed these treatments and noted that they had varying degrees of success but were inconsistent. One treatment that has demonstrated some efficacy has been the use of vitamin E, alpha-tocopherol). Lohr and Jeste (1988b) have proposed that antipsychotic treatment results in the production of free radicals that damage the neuronal components. An antioxidant such as vitamin E would therefore, theoretically, result in improvement in the symptoms of TD. Vitamin E is a possible agent for the treatment and prophylaxis of TD (Gupta et al. 1999, Gardos 1999). A number of studies of varying design have shown the benefit of vitamin E in TD (Lohr et al. 1987a, Elkashef et al. 1990, Egan et al. 1992, Adler et al. 1993b, Shriqui et al. 1992, Adler et al. 1998, Sajjad 1998); however, a recent double-blind, placebo-controlled multicenter trial failed to show a difference between vitamin E and placebo after 1 year of treatment (Adler et al. 1999). Although the results are far from conclusive, vitamin E remains a reasonably safe treatment modality for an individual with recently diagnosed TD. Doses are usually in the range of 1200 to 1600 mg/day. Other agents have been investigated such as calcium channel blockers (i.e., diltiazem, verapamil, nifedipine), and clonazepam, but more studies are warranted (Gupta et al. 1999).

Clinicians must regularly assess for the presence and progression of TD and present the individual (or the individual's guardian, when appropriate) with information about the risks of treatment; they may also give written information sheets, assess understanding by the individual or guardian, and accurately record evidence of the informed consent in the individual's record (Wettstein 1988).

NEUROLEPTIC MALIGNANT SYNDROME

Definition

Neuroleptic Malignant Syndrome (NMS) is a potentially fatal reaction to antipsychotic medications that is characterized clinically by muscle rigidity, fever, autonomic instability, and changes in level of consciousness (see DSM-IV-TR diagnostic criteria below).

DSM-IV-TR Diagnostic Criteria

333.92 Neuroleptic Malignant Syndrome

A. The development of severe muscle rigidity and elevated temperature associated with the use of neuroleptic medication.
B. Two (or more) of the following:

(1) diaphoresis
(2) dysphagia
(3) tremor
(4) incontinence
(5) changes in level of consciousness ranging from confusion to coma
(6) mutism
(7) tachycardia
(8) elevated or labile blood pressure
(9) leukocytosis
(10) laboratory evidence of muscle injury (e.g., elevated CPK [creatine kinase])

C. The symptoms in criteria A and B are not due to another substance (e.g., phencyclidine) or a neurological or other general medical condition (e.g., viral encephalitis).
D. The symptoms in criteria A and B are not better accounted for by a mental disorder (e.g., mood disorder with catatonic features).

Reprinted with permission from the Diagnostic and Statistical Manual of Mental Disorders, Fourth Edition, Text Revision. Copyright 2000 American Psychiatric Association.

NMS usually presents in the first month of antipsychotic treatment but may develop at any time. Two-thirds of the cases manifest within the first week of treatment (American Psychiatric Association 2000). One study found that NMS occurred as soon as 45 minutes and as late as 65 days after initiation of treatment (Shalev and Munitz 1986).

The two key diagnostic features for the disorder are severe muscle rigidity (classically referred to as lead-pipe rigidity) and elevated temperature. A number of other features are also seen (see DSM-IV-TR criteria above). For the clinician, the most suggestive features are fluctuating consciousness (from confusion to coma), labile vital signs (tachycardia, unstable or elevated blood pressure), laboratory evidence of muscle injury (elevation of creatine kinase), and leukocytosis. Other features include diaphoresis, dysphagia, tremor, incontinence, and mutism (American Psychiatric Association 2000). The DSM-IV-TR criteria are broader than earlier criteria proposed by Pope and coworkers (1986) and revised by Keck and colleagues (1989b). The Pope criteria require the following three items for a definite diagnosis: (1) oral temperature of at least 38 °C in the absence of another known cause; (2) at least two extrapyramidal side effects from the following list: lead pipe-type muscle rigidity, cogwheeling, sialorrhea, oculogyric crisis, retrocollis, opisthotonos, trismus, dysphagia, choreiform movements, dyskinetic movements, festinating gait, and flexor–extensor posturing; and (3) autonomic dysfunction characterized by two or more of the following: hypertension, tachycardia, tachypnea, prominent diaphoresis, and incontinence.

Epidemiology

The exact frequency of NMS is unknown. A number of retrospective and prospective studies have found 0.02 to 3.2% of individuals treated with antipsychotics to be affected with NMS. Several factors probably account for this large variability in frequency, including differences in study methods and diagnostic criteria for NMS (Sewell and Jeste 1992b, Adityanjeeet al. 1999).

A number of retrospective studies have attempted to isolate possible risk factors for the development of NMS. A prior episode of NMS appears to predispose to future episodes of NMS. Rosebush and colleagues (1989) found that the longer the time elapsed after an episode of NMS, the lower the risk of a recurrence of NMS.

Any preexisting medical problems, especially those associated with agitation or dehydration, may increase the likelihood of NMS development when antipsychotics are used. Individuals with a neurological condition as well as individuals with presumed psychosis due to human immunodeficiency virus infection may be at higher risk for development of NMS (Shalev et al. 1989, Harris et al. 1991). A number of potential risk factors related to antipsychotic treatment have been identified. Higher doses of antipsychotic, rapid increases in dosage (especially "rapid neuroleptization") (Keck et al. 1989a), and intramuscular injections of high-potency conventional agents (e.g., haloperidol and fluphenazine) (Deng et al. 1990) have been reported to be risk factors for NMS. A combination of lithium with an antipsychotic has been proposed as a possible risk factor for NMS development, but results from different investigators have been contradictory (Sewell and Jeste 1992b). NMS can occur (but rarely) in individuals prescribed atypical antipsychotics and a review of atypical-induced NMS concluded that symptoms appear similar to NMS induced by conventional antipsychotics (Hasan and Buckley 1998).

NMS is more frequently reported in men than in women and is more frequently seen in a younger population. A previous diagnosis of a mood disorder may place individuals at a higher risk for NMS (Pearlman 1986, Addonizio et al. 1987). Warm, humid climates may also predispose to the disorder (American Psychiatric Association 2000).

Course

The course of NMS is variable. Some cases may progress to fatality, whereas others may follow a mild self-limited course. Once the syndrome is recognized and the antipsychotic medication is discontinued, the syndrome usually resolves between 2 weeks and 1 month (American Psychiatric Association 2000).

Mortality rate is reported to be 4 to 25% (Sewell and Jeste 1992b). The most common medical complications leading to morbidity and mortality are respiratory failure and renal failure. Shalev and coworkers (1989) reported that myoglobinemia and renal failure are the best predictors of mortality in NMS; the presence of either condition imparted a 50% mortality risk. In general, complications are a result of physiologic consequences of severe rigidity and immobilization such as deep vein thrombosis, pulmonary embolism, dehydration, and an increased risk for rhabdomyolysis (Peloneroet al. 1998).

Differential Diagnosis

The differential diagnosis of NMS can be difficult (Table 46-3). The most important point is that the clinician must start by suspecting NMS and then carefully rule out other possible organic problems. Because medical illness is a likely predisposing factor, it is important to consider that NMS may be present even if a definitive organic disease is found to explain the NMS-like symptoms. Sewell and Jeste (1991) retrospectively examined the records of 34 hospitalized individuals with suspected NMS and found that 24 seemed to have had NMS and 10 had acute medical problems. Hence, it is critical to consider the diagnosis of NMS as well as to rule out other acute illnesses when an individual receiving antipsychotics becomes medically ill.

Numerous general medical and neurological conditions can present with symptoms that may resemble NMS. Examples include central nervous system infection, status epilepticus, subcortical brain lesions, porphyria, and tetanus (American Psychiatric Association 2000). The presence of significantly elevated temperature and severe muscle rigidity makes the diagnosis of NMS more likely.

The syndrome of lethal catatonia (seen in individuals with uncontrolled manic excitement or catatonic schizophrenia) can mimic NMS (with increased temperature, autonomic irregularities, and elevated creatine kinase), and the differential diagnosis can be difficult. It is obviously important to determine whether the individual is indeed being treated with an

Table 46-3	Differential Diagnosis of Neuroleptic Malignant Syndrome				
Feature	**Diagnosis**				
	Lethal Catatonia	**Heat Stroke**	**Malignant Hyperthermia**	**Serotonin Syndrome**	**Neuroleptic Malignant Syndrome**
Previous psychiatric illness	Yes	No	No	Yes	Yes
Onset of symptoms	+ Prodromal psychotic symptoms	− Prodromal symptoms; development in several hours	− Prodromal symptoms; development after anesthesia	− Prodromal symptoms; development days to months after serotoninergic medication	− Prodromal symptoms; development hours to months after neuroleptic
Preceding anesthesia with muscle cell-depolarizing agents	No	No	Yes	No	No
Preceding neuroleptics	Maybe	Maybe	Maybe	Maybe	Yes
Preceding serotoninergic agents	Maybe	Maybe	Maybe	Yes	Maybe
Autonomic dysfunction	Maybe	No	No	No	Yes
Episodes: stupor mixed with episodes of excitement	Yes	No	No	No	Maybe
Diaphoresis	Maybe	No	Maybe	Maybe	Yes
Rigidity	Fluctuating	No	Yes	Yes	Yes

Source: Modified from Sewell DD and Jeste DV (1991) Distinguishing neuroleptic malignant syndrome (NMS) from NMS-like acute medical illnesses: A study of 34 cases. J Neuropsychiatr Clin Neurosci 4, 265–269.

antipsychotic. Although NMS may clinically look like catatonia, NMS does not typically have alternating periods of catatonic excitement and catatonic mutism. A past history of catatonic episodes is also important in making the differential diagnosis. One report suggested that lorazepam was useful in alleviating the symptoms of catatonia (Salam and Kilzieh 1988). Lorazepam has not been shown to be useful in treatment of NMS. Therefore, it is possible that a brief lorazepam trial could provide a useful and relatively easy method of distinguishing between these two conditions. The problem, of course, is that not all cases of catatonia respond to lorazepam.

Heat stroke may also look like NMS but typically differs in that it presents with hypotension, dry skin, and limb flaccidity (American Psychiatric Association 2000). Malignant hyperthermia can also have a similar presentation but generally occurs within the context of an individual's receiving halogenated anesthetic agents or succinylcholine. This condition typically begins immediately after administration of the anesthetic agent and only in genetically susceptible individuals (American Psychiatric Association 2000).

Medications can cause a number of conditions that may present as syndromes similar to NMS. Allergic drug reactions may produce fever and autonomic instability but not rigidity (Pelonero et al. 1998). Serotonin syndrome (Sternbach 1991), with common clinical characteristics including fever, resting tremor, rigidity, myoclonus, and generalized seizures should also be considered. A medication history can usually help distinguish between the two syndromes, but individuals receiving antipsychotics may also be treated with selective serotonin reuptake inhibitors, thus making the clinical picture more confusing. Lithium intoxication and anticholinergic delirium can both resemble NMS, as can intoxication with amphetamines, cocaine, and phencyclidine as well as rapid termination of antiparkinsonian medication.

Table 46-4	Treatment of Neuroleptic Malignant Syndrome
Step 1	Assess medication regimen • Stop dopamine antagonists • Restart any recently stopped dopamine agonists
Step 2	Supportive care • Monitor vital signs • Administer intravenous fluids • Provide cooling blankets • Administer antipyretics • Consider dialysis for acute renal failure
Step 3	No improvement within 24–28 hours • Administer oral bromocriptine 5 mg PO t.i.d. to be increased daily by 5 mg increments until positive response • Continue bromocriptine for 10 d, then withdraw in period of 1 wk • Monitor for relapse
Step 4	If patient cannot tolerate bromocriptine or cannot take oral medications • Administer intravenous dantrolene 1–3 mg/kg/body weight q.i.d. • Gradually increase dose until positive response
Step 5	Consider adding bromocriptine to dantrolene
Step 6	Consider discontinuing all medications and giving supportive care only
Step 7	Consider electroconvulsive therapy after 3–4 d, if no improvement

Source: Modified from Sewell DD and Jeste DV (1991) Distinguishing neuroleptic malignant syndrome (NMS) from NMS-like acute medical illnesses: A study of 34 cases. *J Neuropsychiatr Clin Neurosci* **4**, 265–269.

Etiology

The pathophysiological mechanism of NMS remains unclear. The hypothesis of most interest is that of reduced dopaminergic activity secondary to neuroleptic-induced dopamine blockade. This reduced dopamine activity in different parts of the brain (hypothalamus, nigrostriatal system, and corticolimbic tracts) may serve to explain the various clinical features of NMS. Dopamine reduction in the hypothalamus may cause fever and autonomic instability; in the nigrostriatal system, dopamine reduction may lead to the rigidity; and the reduction in corticolimbic dopamine activity may explain the altered consciousness (Sewell and Jeste 1992b). This hypothesis is based on the fact that antipsychotics are dopamine-blocking agents, whereas certain dopamine agonists are reported to help resolve NMS.

The dopaminergic blocking theory does not, however, explain why NMS may develop at a given time and in a given individual. There are probably other genetic (possibly a predisposition similar to that seen in malignant hyperthermia) (Sewell and Jeste 1992b), constitutional, environmental, and pharmacological factors that interact to produce the syndrome. A number of investigators have proposed that other neurotransmitter abnormalities may be responsible for the syndrome, including serotonergic hyperfunction in the hypothalamus (Yamawaki et al. 1986), excessive catecholamine secretion (Addonizio et al. 1987), and gamma-aminobutyric acid deficiency (Addonizio et al. 1987).

Treatment

The most critical step in treatment (Table 46-4) is to recognize the clinical features of the syndrome and rapidly discontinue the antipsychotic. The importance of this initial step mandates that clinicians who use antipsychotics in their practice be cognizant of the early clinical features and recognize that the syndrome can occur at any time during the course of treatment. Once the antipsychotic has been stopped, supportive care remains the core of treatment (Arana and Rosenbaum 2000) and often must be carried out in the context of a medical intensive care unit. Each supportive intervention should be targeted to a specific symptom. Examples of interventions include cooling blankets for fever, cardiac monitoring for arrhythmias, parenteral hydration for dehydration, and monitoring for urine output and renal function. Dialysis may also be considered for acute renal failure.

Some specific treatments for NMS have been proposed, but their beneficial effect is unclear. The muscle relaxant dantrolene is thought by some investigators to be helpful in decreasing rigidity, hyperthermia, and tachycardia. Dosing of 1 to 3 mg/kg/day orally or intravenously in four divided doses is currently advocated (Arana and Rosenbaum 2000). The dopamine agonist bromocriptine may also provide some relief of the symptoms, especially for muscle rigidity. Dosing is usually in the range of 5 to 10 mg orally three times a day (Arana and Rosenbaum 2000). The two medications can be administered together. Gelenberg (1992), however, pointed out that a study by Rosebush and coworkers (1991) not only has cast doubt on the benefit of the use of these agents in the treatment of NMS but may also point to the possibility that these agents actually retard the course of improvement of NMS. In the Rosebush study, 8 of 20 individuals with presumed NMS received dantrolene, bromocriptine, or both along with supportive care, and 12 of 20 received supportive care only. There was a suggestion that the resolution of the NMS episodes took longer in the individuals treated with the additional medications. The treatments in the investigation were not randomized or controlled.

Electroconvulsive therapy is another treatment option in NMS presumably because it increases dopamine turnover in the brain (Pearlman 1986). Electroconvulsive therapy is particularly indicated when there is difficulty in distinguishing between NMS and lethal catatonia and when there seems to be a significant risk of recurrence of NMS on restarting neuroleptics (Addonizio et al. 1987). Some psychiatrists report rapid and dramatic success in use of electroconvulsive therapy for NMS.

At present, the appropriate course is to begin with antipsychotic discontinuation and supportive care and to consider antidote therapy only if improvement in symptoms is not seen within the first few days (Gelenberg 1992). Caroff and colleagues suggested that treatment of NMS should be individualized for each individual based on clinical signs and symptoms. For example, supportive care may be sufficient in mild and early cases of NMS. Trials of bromocriptine, dantrolene, or amantadine are suggested for individuals with moderate symptoms. Anticholinergics can be used in managing afebrile individuals with neuroleptic-induced parkinsonian symptoms and benzodiazepines may be useful for agitation in NMS. Electro-convulsive therapy (ECT) is recommended in situations where lethal catatonia is suspected, when NMS symptoms are treatment refractory, and in individuals who remain psychotic in the immediate post-NMS period (Caroff and Mann 1998).

A particular difficulty for the psychotic individual who has NMS is that rechallenge with antipsychotics may cause NMS to recur. Successful rechallenge seems to be positively related to the length of time elapsed after resolution of NMS (Rosebush et al. 1989). There is some evidence to suggest that clozapine may have relatively little propensity to induce NMS. There are some case reports indicating that clozapine may have caused NMS but only in conjunction with other medications (carbamazepine in one case and lithium carbonate in another) (Pope et al. 1986, Muller et al. 1988). Clozapine, therefore, may represent one option for the individual who has experienced NMS with a conventional agent. It is likely but not yet known definitively that atypical antipsychotics will prove to have a lower frequency of NMS. In general, it is recommended to switch to an agent in a different chemical class and with a lower D_2 affinity compared to the causal agent (Pelonero et al. 1998).

MEDICATION-INDUCED POSTURAL TREMOR

Diagnosis

This category refers to fine postural action tremor that develops as a result of a medication (see DSM-IV-TR diagnostic criteria on page 1316). Medications that have been reported to cause such an effect are lithium, beta-adrenergic agonist medications, stimulants, dopaminergic medications, anticonvulsant medications, antipsychotics, antidepressant medications, and methylxanthines (e.g., caffeine) (American Psychiatric Association 2000). The psychotropic medication most typically associated with such tremor is lithium, and most of the available information on medication-induced tremor relates to that caused by lithium.

DSM-IV-TR Diagnostic Criteria

333.1 Medication-Induced Postural Tremor

A. A fine postural tremor that has developed in association with the use of a medication (e.g., lithium, antidepressant medication, valproic acid).
B. The tremor (i.e., a regular, rhythmic oscillation of the limbs, head, mouth, or tongue) has a frequency between 8 and 12 cycles per second.
C. The symptoms are not due to a preexisting nonpharmacologically induced tremor. Evidence that the symptoms are due to a preexisting tremor might include the following: the tremor was present prior to the introduction of the medication, the tremor does not correlate with serum levels of the medication, and the tremor persists after discontinuation of the medication.
D. The symptoms are not better accounted for by neuroleptic-induced parkinsonism.

Reprinted with permission from the Diagnostic and Statistical Manual of Mental Disorders, Fourth Edition, Text Revision. Copyright 2000 American Psychiatric Association.

Lithium-induced tremor may appear as soon as treatment is initiated. As the lithium level increases, the tremor becomes more severe and coarse and may have associated muscle twitching or fasciculations (American Psychiatric Association 2000). Complaints about the tremor are typically greatest at the beginning of therapy. There is disagreement as to whether the tremor typically remains stable or improves with time on lithium.

The lithium-induced tremor is reasonably easy to diagnose. It is a rhythmical action tremor. It is most commonly seen in the hands or fingers but can occasionally be seen in the head, mouth, or tongue (American Psychiatric Association 2000). The frequency of the tremor is typically 8 to 12 Hz and is similar in appearance to an essential tremor (Arana and Rosenbaum 2000). It may usually be seen by asking the individual to hold the affected body part in a stable position. The tremor is made worse by anxiety, stress, fatigue, hypoglycemia, thyrotoxicosis, pheochromocytoma, hypothermia, alcohol withdrawal, performance of voluntary movements, and concomitant administration of cyclic antidepressant medications (Arana and Rosenbaum 2000, American Psychiatric Association 2000).

Epidemiology

Estimates of the frequency of lithium-induced tremor vary widely across the literature and range between 4 and 65% (Goodwin and Jamison 1990). Lifetime incidence of tremor is estimated to be 25 to 50% of individuals starting lithium therapy (Price and Heninger 1994).

A number of possible risk factors have been proposed to predispose a person to development of a lithium-induced tremor. These include older age, greater serum lithium levels, concomitant use of antidepressant or antipsychotic medication, greater caffeine intake, history of tremor, alcohol dependence, and anxiety (American Psychiatric Association 2000).

Course

The literature suggests that there is some risk that tremor may be embarrassing for certain individuals and could impair activities that require delicate movements (Arana and Rosenbaum 2000). The actual percentage of individuals who are bothered by their tremor is unknown. There do not appear to be any long-term sequelae as a result of having a medication-induced postural tremor. A sudden worsening of tremor may be indicative of the beginning of lithium intoxication.

Differential Diagnosis

The most difficult differential diagnosis involves distinguishing a lithium-induced tremor from a tremor that was preexisting. To be classified as a medication-induced tremor, it must have a temporal relationship to the medication, it must relate to the serum level of the medication, and it must not persist after the medication is discontinued. A similar postural tremor is essential tremor, and differentiation between the two is nearly impossible clinically without the medication history.

Any of the factors listed that may exacerbate a medication-induced tremor can also cause a similar tremor in the absence of the medication. Medication-induced tremor may resemble NIP. NIP, however, is generally worse at rest, is lower in frequency, and has other associated features of parkinsonism (American Psychiatric Association 2000).

Etiology

Normal muscle contractions are accompanied by tremor as a result of contractions of muscle fiber recruitment. This tremor is typically low in amplitude and is referred to as a physiological tremor. When these contractions are maintained, the amplitude of the tremor increases and it becomes visible. This is referred to as an enhanced physiological tremor (Young 1992). A number of medications, including lithium and bronchodilators, produce an enhanced physiological tremor. The pathophysiological mechanism of these tremors is not well understood but seems to relate to adrenergic changes (probably mediated in the locus coeruleus) in the mechanical properties of the skeletal muscle (Young 1992). The response of these tremors to beta-adrenergic blocking agents and their exacerbation as a result of beta-adrenergic agonists seem to lend support to the notion of adrenergic mediation.

Treatment

Most treatment options have been described for treatment of lithium-induced tremor. Typically the tremor is benign, is not bothersome to the individual, and requires no specific intervention. Some cases, however, require treatment because of the individual's concern about the side effect. Preliminary measures include possibly reducing the lithium dose (if clinically feasible), changing the lithium dose to one-time evening administration, or changing the lithium preparation. Caffeine intake should be reduced or eliminated, and anxiety should be pharmacologically or behaviorally treated.

Beta-blockers represent the best-studied method for gaining pharmacological control of the tremor if the preliminary measures are ineffective. Arana and Rosenbaum (2000) recommended starting propranolol on an as-needed basis. They suggested 10 to 20 mg a half-hour before the activity in which the tremor must not be present. If an individual requires chronic relief from the tremor, propranolol should be initiated at 10 to 20 mg b.i.d and increased until adequate dose for suppression of the tremor is attained. Propranolol may decrease glomerular filtration rate and may result in a reduction in renal lithium clearance. This suggests that individuals who require long-term beta-blocker suppression for tremor need to have lithium levels checked more regularly even when they are taking a stable dose of lithium.

There is little information in the literature as to the possible treatment of tremor induced by medications other than lithium and further investigations are needed to elucidate this syndrome.

Comparison of DSM-IV-TR/ICD-10 Diagnostic Criteria

Some of these categories are included in Chapter VI of ICD-10 (Diseases of the Nervous System) but no diagnostic criteria or definitions are provided.

Acknowledgment

The authors would like to recognize David Naimark for his outstanding contribution to the previous edition of this chapter.

References

Addonizio G, Susman VL, and Roth SD (1987) Neuroleptic malignant syndrome: review and analysis of 115 cases. *Biol Psychiatry* **22**, 1004–1020.

Adityanjee, Aderibigbe YA, and Mathews T (1999) Epidemiology of neuroleptic malignant syndrome. *Clin Neuropharmacol* **22**, 151–158.

Adler L, Angrist B, Peselow E, et al. (1986) A controlled assessment of propranolol in the treatment of neuroleptic-induced akathisia. *Br J Psychiatry* **149**, 42–45.

Adler LA, Edson R, Lavori P, et al. (1998) Long-term treatment effects of vitamin E for tardive dyskinesia. *Biol Psychiatry* **43**, 868–872.

Adler LA, Peselow E, Rosenthal M, et al. (1993a) A controlled comparison of the effects of propranolol, benztropine, and placebo on akathisia: an interim analysis. *Psychopharmacol Bull* **29**, 283–286.

Adler LA, Peselow E, Rotrosen J, et al. (1993b) Vitamin E treatment of tardive dyskinesia. *Am J Psychiatry* **150**, 1405–1407.

Adler LA, Reiter S, Angrist B, et al. (1987) Pindolol and propranolol in neuroleptic-induced akathisia. *Am J Psychiatry* **144**, 1241–1242.

Adler LA, Rotrosen J, Edson R, et al. (1999) Vitamin E treatment for tardive dyskinesia. *Arch Gen Psychiatry* **56**, 836–841.

American Psychiatric Association (2000) *Diagnostic and Statistical Manual of Mental Disorders*, 4th ed., Text Rev. APA, Washington, DC.

Arana GW and Rosenbaum JF (2000) *Handbook of Psychiatric Drug Therapy*, 4th ed., Lippincott, Williams & Wilkins, Philadelphia.

Arvanitis LA and Miller BG, The Seroquel Trial 13 Study Group (1997) Multiple fixed doses of "seroquel" (quetiapine) in patients with acute exacerbation of schizophrenia: a comparison with haloperidol and placebo. *Biol Psychiatry* **42**, 233–246.

Ayd FJ (1961) A survey of drug-induced extrapyramidal reactions. *J Am Med Assoc* **175**, 1054–1060.

Ayd FJ (1979) Respiratory dyskinesias in patients with neuroleptic-induced extrapyramidal reaction. *Int Drug Ther News* **14**, 1–4.

Beasley CM, Hamilton SH, Crawford AM, et al. (1997) Olanzapine versus haloperidol: acute phase results of the international double-blind olanzapine trial. *Eur J Neuropsychopharmacol* **7**, 125–137.

Bersani G, Grispini A, Marini S, et al. (1990) 5-HT$_2$ antagonist ritanserin in neuroleptic-induced parkinsonism: a double-blind comparison with orphenadrine and placebo. *Clin Neuropharmacol* **13**, 500–506.

Bitton V and Melamed E (1984) Coexistence of severe parkinsonism and tardive dyskinesia as side effects of neuroleptic therapy. *J Clin Psychiatry* **45**, 28–30.

Brandon S, McClelland HA, and Protheroe C (1971) A study of facial dyskinesia, in a mental hospital population. *Br J Psychiatry* **118**, 171–184.

Burke RE, Reches A, Traub MM, et al. (1985) Tetrabenazine induces acute dystonic reactions. *Ann Neurol* **17**, 200–202.

Caligiuri MP, Lacro JP, and Jeste DV (1999) Incidence and predictors of drug-induced parkinsonism in older psychiatric patients treated with very low doses of neuroleptics. *J Clin Psychopharmacol* **19**, 322–328.

Caligiuri MP, Lacro JP, Rockwell E, et al. (1997) Incidence and risk factors for severe tardive dyskinesia in older patients. *Br J Psychiatry* **171**, 148–153.

Caligiuri MP and Lohr JB (1997) Instrumental motor predictors of neuroleptic-induced parkinsonism in newly medicated schizophrenia patients. *J Neuropsychiatr Clin Neurosci* **9**, 562–567.

Caligiuri MP, Lohr JB, Bracha HS, et al. (1991) Clinical and instrumental assessment of neuroleptic-induced parkinsonism in patients with tardive dyskinesia. *Biol Psychiatry* **29**, 139–148.

Caligiuri MP, Rockwell E, and Jeste DV (1998) Extrapyramidal side effects in patients with Alzheimer's disease treated with low-dose neuroleptic medication. *Am J Geriatr Psychiatry* **6**, 75–82.

Caroff SN and Mann SC (1998) Specific treatment of the neuroleptics malignant syndrome. *Biol Psychiatry* **44**, 378–381.

Casey DE (1988) Affective disorders and tardive dyskinesia. *L'Encephale* **14**, 221–226.

Casey DE (1997) Will the new antipsychotics bring hope of reducing the risk of developing extrapyramidal syndromes and tardive dyskinesia? *Int Clin Psychopharmacol* **12**, S19–S27.

Casey DE and Keepers GA (1988) Neuroleptic side effects: acute extrapyramidal syndromes and tardive dyskinesia. In *Psychopharmacology: Current Trends*, Casey DE and Christensen AV (eds). Springer-Verlag, Berlin, pp. 74–93.

Casey DE and Rabins P (1978) Tardive dyskinesia as a life-threatening illness. *Am J Psychiatry* **135**, 486–488.

Chakos MH, Mayerhoff DI, Loebel AD, et al. (1992) Incidence and correlates of extrapyramidal symptoms in first episode of schizophrenia. *Psychopharmacol Bull* **28**, 81–86.

Chouinard G and Bradwein J (1982) Reversible and irreversible tardive dyskinesia: a case report. *Am J Psychiatry* **139**, 360–362.

Chouinard G, Jones B, Remington G, et al. (1993) A Canadian multicenter placebo-controlled study of fixed doses of risperidone and haloperidol in the treatment of chronic schizophrenic patients. *J Clin Psychopharmacol* **13**, 25–40.

Cohen BM, Keck PE, Satlin A, et al. (1991) Prevalence and severity of akathisia in patients on clozapine. *Biol Psychiatry* **29**, 1215–1219.

Coleman JH and Hays PE (1975) Drug-induced extrapyramidal effects—a review. *Dis Nerv Syst* **36**, 591–593.

Deng MZ, Chen GQ, and Phillips MR (1990) Neuroleptic malignant syndrome in 12 of 9,792 Chinese inpatients exposed to neuroleptics: a prospective study. *Am J Psychiatry* **147**, 1149–1155.

DeVaugh-Geiss J (1980) Tardive Tourette syndrome. *Neurology* **30**, 562–563.

Dimascio A and Demergian E (1970) Antiparkinson drug overuse. *Psychosomatics* **11**, 596–601.

Edwards H (1970) The significance of brain damage in persistant oral dyskinesia. *Br J Psychiatry* **116**, 271–275.

Egan MF, Hyde TM, Albers GW, et al. (1992) Treatment of tardive dyskinesia with vitamin E. *Am J Psychiatry* **149**, 773–777.

Elkashef AM, Ruskin PE, Bacher N, et al. (1990) Vitamin E in the treatment of tardive dyskinesia. *Am J Psychiatry* **147**, 505–506.

Fahn S (1983) High dosage anticholinergic therapy in dystonia. *Neurology* **33**, 1255–1261.

Farde L, Nordstrom AL, and Wiesel FA (1992) Positron emission tomographic analysis of central D_1 and D_2 dopamine receptor occupancy in patients treated with classical neuroleptics and clozapine: relation to extrapyramidal side effects. *Arch Gen Psychiatry* **49**, 538–544.

Ganzini L, Heintz RT, Hoffman WF, et al. (1991) The prevalence of tardive dyskinesia in neuroleptic-treated diabetics: a controlled study. *Arch Gen Psychiatry* **48**, 259–263.

Gardos G (1999) Managing antipsychotic-induced tardive dyskinesia. *Drug Saf* **20**, 187–193.

Gardos G and Cole JO (1983) Tardive dyskinesia and anticholinergic drugs. *Am J Psychiatry* **140**, 200–202.

Gardos G and Cole JO (1992) Severe tardive dyskinesia. In *Movement Disorders in Neurology and Neuropsychiatry*, Joseph AB and Young RR (eds). Blackwell Scientific, Boston, pp. 40–45.

Gardos G, Cole JO, Schniebolk S, et al. (1987) Comparison of severe and mild tardive dyskinesia: implications for etiology. *J Clin Psychiatry* **48**, 359–362.

Gelenberg AJ (1992) The best treatment for NMS. *Biol Ther Psychiatry* **15**, 13 and 16.

Gerhard AL (1992) Withdrawal dyskinesia. In *Movement Disorders in Neurology and Neuropsychiatry*, Joseph AB and Young RR (eds). Blackwell Scientific, Boston, pp. 81–82.

Gilbert PL, Harris MJ, McAdams LA, et al. (1995) Neuroleptic withdrawal in schizophrenic patients. *Arch Gen Psychiatry* **52**, 173–188.

Glazer WM (2000) Extrapyramidal side effects, tardive dyskinesia, and the concept of atypicality. *J Clin Psychiatry* **61**, 16–21.

Goodwin FK and Jamison KR (1990) *Manic–Depressive Illness*, 1st ed., Oxford University Press, New York.

Gupta S, Mosnik D, Black DW, et al. (1999) Tardive dyskinesia: review of treatments past, present, and future. *Ann Clin Psychiatry* **11**, 257–266.

Guy W, Ban TA, and Wilson WH (1986) The prevalence of abnormal involuntary movements among chronic schizophrenics. *Int Clin Psychopharmacol* **1**, 134–144.

Harris MJ, Jeste DV, Gleghorn A, et al. (1991) New-onset psychosis in HIV-infected patients. *J Clin Psychiatry* **52**, 352–376.

Hasan S and Buckley P (1998) Novel antipsychotics and the neuroleptics malignant syndrome: a review and critique. *Am J Psychiatry* **155**, 1113–1116.

Hausner RS (1983) Neuroleptic-induced parkinsonism and Parkinson's disease: Differential diagnosis and treatment. *J Clin Psychiatry* **44**, 13–16.

Hornykiewicz O (1982) Brain neurotransmitter changes in Parkinson's disease. In *Movement Disorders*, Marsden CD and Fahn S (eds). Butterworth Scientific, London, pp. 41–58.

Jackson IV, Volavka J, James B, et al. (1980) The respiratory components of tardive dyskinesia. *Biol Psychiatry* **15**, 485–487.

Jeste DV and Caligiuri MP (1993) Tardive dyskinesia. *Schizophr Bull* **19**, 303–315.

Jeste DV, Caligiuri MP, Paulsen JS, et al. (1995) Risk of tardive dyskinesia in older patients: a prospective longitudinal study of 266 patients. *Arch Gen Psychiatry* **52**, 756–765.

Jeste DV, Klausner M, Brecher M, et al. (1997) A clinical evaluation of risperidone in the treatment of schizophrenia: a 10-week, open-label, multicenter trial involving 945 patients. *Psychopharmacology* **131**, 239–247.

Jeste DV, Lacro JP, Bailey A, et al. (1999a) Lower incidence of tardive dyskinesia with risperidone compared with haloperidol in older patients. *J Am Geriatr Soc* **47**, 716–719.

Jeste DV, Lacro JP, Palmer BW, et al. (1999b) Incidence of tardive dyskinesia in early stages of low-dose treatment with typical neuroleptics in older patients. *Am J Psychiatry* **156**, 309–311.

Jeste DV, Lohr JB, Clark K, et al. (1988) Pharmacological treatment of tardive dyskinesia in the 1980s. *J Clin Psychopharmacol* **8**, 38S–48S.

Jeste DV, Lohr JB, and Manley M (1992) Study of neuropathologic changes in the striatum following 4, 8 and 12 months of treatment with fluphenazine in rats. *Psychopharmacology* **106**, 154–160.

Jeste DV, Rockwell E, Harris MJ, et al. (1999c) Conventional versus newer antipsychotics in elderly patients. *Am J Geriatr Psychiatry* **7**, 70–76.

Jeste DV, Wisniewski A, and Wyatt RJ (1986) Neuroleptic-associated "Tardive" syndromes. In *Schizophrenia: The Psychiatric Clinics of North America*, Vol. 9:1, Roy A (ed.). Plenum Press, New York, pp. 183–192.

Jeste DV and Wyatt RJ (1981) Changing epidemiology of tardive dyskinesia—an overview. *Am J Psychiatry* **138**, 297–309.

Jeste DV and Wyatt RJ (1982) *Understanding and Treating Tardive Dyskinesia*. Guilford Press, New York.

Johnson DAW (1978) Prevalence and treatment of drug-induced extrapyramidal symptoms. *Br J Psychiatry* **132**, 27–30.

Kane JM, Honigfeld G, Singer J, et al. (1988a) Clozapine for the treatment resistant schizophrenic: a double-blind comparison with chlorpromazine. *Arch Gen Psychiatry* **45**, 789–796.

Kane JM, Jeste DV, Barnes TRE, et al. (1992) *Tardive Dyskinesia: A Task Force Report of the American Psychiatric Association*. American Psychiatric Association, Washington, DC.

Kane JM, Woerner M, and Lieberman J (1988b) Tardive dyskinesia: prevalence, incidence, and risk factors. *J Clin Psychopharmacol* **8**(4), 52S–56S.

Kane JM, Woerner MG, Pollack S, et al. (1993) Does clozapine cause tardive dyskinesia? *J Clin Psychiatry* **54**, 327–330.

Kapur S, Zipursky RB, Remington G, et al. (1998) 5-HT$_2$ and D$_2$ receptor occupancy of olanzapine in schizophrenia: a PET investigation. *Am J Psychiatry* **155**, 921–928.

Keck PE, Pope HG, and Cohen BM (1989a) Risk factors for neuroleptic malignant syndrome: a case-control study. *Arch Gen Psychiatry* **46**, 914–918.

Keck PE, Sebastianelli J, Pope HG, et al. (1989b) Frequency and presentation of neuroleptic malignant syndrome in a state psychiatric hospital. *J Clin Psychiatry* **50**, 352–355.

Keepers GA and Casey DE (1986) Prediction of neuroleptic-induced dystonia. *J Clin Psychopharmacol* **7**, 342–344.

Kiloh LG, Smith JS, and Williams SE (1973) Antiparkinson drugs as causal agents in tardive dyskinesia. *Med J Aust* **2**, 591–593.

King DJ, Link CG, and Kowalcyk B (1998) A comparison of b.i.d. and t.i.d. dose regimens of quetiapine (Seroquel) in the treatment of schizophrenia. *Psychopharmacology* **137**, 139–146.

Klawans HL, Falk DK, Nausieda PA, et al. (1978) Gille de la Tourette's syndrome after long-term chlorpromazine therapy. *Neurology* **28**, 1064–1068.

Kurz M, Hummer M, Kemmler G, et al. (1998) Long-term pharmacokinetics of clozapine. *Br J Psychiatry* **173**, 341–344.

Lacro JP and Jeste DV (1997) The role of ethnicity in the development of tardive dyskinesia. In *Neuroleptic-Induced Movement Disorders*, Yassa R, Nair NVP, and Jeste DV (eds). Cambridge University Press, New York, pp. 298–310.

Lance JW and McLeod JG (1981) *A Physiological Approach to Clinical Neurology*, 3rd ed., Butterworth, London.

Lang AE (1985) Dopamine agonists in the treatment of dystonia. *Clin Neuropharmacol* **8**, 38–57.

Langston JW and Irwin I (1986) MPTP: current concepts and controversies. *Clin Neuropharmacol* **9**, 485–507.

Lieberman JA, Saltz BL, Johns CA, et al. (1991) The effects of clozapine on tardive dyskinesia. *Br J Psychiatry* **158**, 503–510.

Lindamer LA, Lohr JB, Caligiuri MP, et al. (2001) Relationship of gender and age of onset of schizophrenia to severity of dyskinesia. *J Neuropsychiatr Clin Neurosci* **13**, 399–402.

Littrell KH, Johnson CG, Littrell S, et al. (1998) Marked reduction of tardive dyskinesia with olanzapine. *Arch Gen Psychiatry* **55**, 279–280.

Lohr JB, Cadet JL, Lohr MA, et al. (1987a) Alpha-tocopherol in tardive dyskinesia (letter). *Lancet* **1**, 913–914.

Lohr JB and Jeste DV (1988a) Neuroleptic-induced movement disorders: acute and subacute disorders. In *Psychiatry*, Rev. ed., Michels R, Cavenar JO Jr., Brodie NKH, et al. (eds). JB Lippincott, Philadelphia, pp. 1–19.

Lohr JB and Jeste DV (1988b) Neuroleptic-induced movement disorders: tardive dyskinesia and other tardive syndromes. In *Psychiatry*, Rev. ed., Michels R, Cavenar JO Jr., Brodie NKH, et al. (eds). JB Lippincott, Philadelphia, pp. 1–17.

Lohr JB, Lohr MA, Wasli E, et al. (1987b) Self-perception of tardive dyskinesia and neuroleptic-induced parkinsonism: a study of clinical correlates. *Psychopharmacol Bull* **23**, 211–214.

Mamo DC, Sweet RA, and Keshavan MS (1999) Managing antipsychotic-induced parkinsonism. *Drug Saf* **20**, 252–275.

Mann SC, Greenstein RA, and Eilers R (1983) Early onset of severe dyskinesia following lithium-haloperidol treatment. *Am J Psychiatry* **140**, 1385–1386.

Marsden CD and Jenner P (1980) The pathophysiology of extra-pyramidal side-effects of neuroleptic drugs. *Psychol Med* **10**, 55–72.

Massengil R Jr. and Nashold B (1952) A swallowing disorder denoted in tardive dyskinesia patients. *Acta Oto-Laryngol* **68**, 457–458.

Maxwell S, Massengil R, and Nashold B (1970) Tardive dyskinesia. *J Speech Hear Disord* **35**, 33–36.

McClelland HA, Blessed G, and Bhata S (1974) Abrupt withdrawal of antiparkinsonian drugs in schizophrenic patients. *Br J Psychiatry* **124**, 151–159.

McLean P and Casey D (1978) Tardive dyskinesia in an adolescent. *Am J Psychiatry* **8**, 952–971.

Miller CH and Fleischhacker WW (2000) Managing antipsychotic-induced acute and chronic akathisia. *Drug Saf* **22**, 73–81.

Miller LG and Jankovic J (1992) Drug-induced movement disorders: an overview. In *Movement Disorders in Neurology and Neuropsychiatry*, Joseph AB and Young RR (eds). Blackwell Scientific, Boston, p. 7.

Miller CH, Mohr F, Umbricht D, et al. (1998) The prevalence of acute extrapyramidal signs and symptoms in patients treated with clozapine, risperidone, and conventional antipsychotics. *J Clin Psychiatry* **59**, 52–75.

Mitchell IJ, Cross AJ, and Sambrook MA (1985) Sites of the neurotoxic action of 1-methyl-4-phenyl-1,2,3,6-tetrahydropyridine in the macaque monkey include the ventral tegmental area and the locus ceruleus. *Neurosci Lett* **61**, 195–200.

Morgenstern H and Glazer WM (1993) Identifying risk factors for tardive dyskinesia among long-term outpatients maintained with neuroleptic medications: results of the Yale tardive dyskinesia study. *Arch Gen Psychiatry* **50**, 723–733.

Muller J and Aminoff MJ (1982) Tourette-like syndrome after long-term neuroleptic drug treatment. *Br J Psychiatry* **141**, 191–193.

Muller T, Becker T, and Fritze J (1988) Neuroleptic malignant syndrome after clozapine plus carbamazepine. *Lancet* **2**, 1500.

Munetz MR, Slawsky RC, and Neil JF (1985) Tardive Tourette's syndrome treated with clonidine and mesoridazine. *Psychosomatics* **26**, 254–257.

Nasrallah HA, Pappas NJ, and Crowe RR (1980) Oculogyric dystonia in tardive dyskinesia. *Am J Psychiatry* **137**, 850–851.

Osser DN (1992) Neuroleptic-induced pseudoparkinsonism. In *Movement Disorders in Neurology and Neuropsychiatry*, Joseph AB and Young RR (eds). Blackwell Scientific, Boston, pp. 73–74.

Pearlman CA (1986) Neuroleptic malignant syndrome: a review of the literature. *J Clin Psychopharmacol* **6**, 257–273.

Pelonero AL, Levenson JL, and Pandurangi AK (1998) Neuroleptic malignant syndrome: a review. *Psychiatry Serv* **49**, 1163–1172.

Pope HG, Keck PE, and McElroy SL (1986) Frequency and presentation of neuroleptic malignant syndrome in a large psychiatric hospital. *Am J Psychiatry* **143**, 1227–1233.

Portnoy RA (1979) Hyperkinetic dysarthria as an early indicator of impending tardive dyskinesia. *J Speech Hear Disord* **44**, 214–219.

Poyurovsky M, Shardorodsky M, Fuchs C, et al. (1999) Treatment of neuroleptic-induced akathisia with the 5-HT$_2$ antagonist mianserin. Double-blind, placebo-controlled study. *Br J Psychiatry* **174**, 238–242.

Price LH and Heninger GR (1994) Lithium in the treatment of mood disorders. *Neurology* **34**, 1348–1353.

Raleigh FR Jr. (1977) Reducing unnecessary antiparkinsonian medication in antipsychotic therapy. *J Am Pharm Assoc* **17**, 101–105.

Rifkin A, Quitkin F, and Kane J (1978) Are prophylactic antiparkinson drugs necessary? *Arch Gen Psychiatry* **35**, 483–489.

Rifkin A, Quitkin F, and Klein DF (1975) Akinesia: a poorly recognized drug-induced extrapyramidal behavioral disorder. *Arch Gen Psychiatry* **32**, 672–674.

Rosebush PI, Stewart TD, and Gelenberg AJ (1989) Twenty neuroleptic rechallenges after neuroleptic malignant syndrome in 15 patients. *J Clin Psychiatry* **50**, 295–298.

Rosebush PI, Stewart T, and Mazurek MF (1991) The treatment of neuroleptic malignant syndrome: are dantrolene and bromocriptine useful adjuncts to supportive care? *Br J Psychiatry* **159**, 709–712.

Rupniak NMJ, Jenner P, and Marsden CD (1986) Acute dystonia induced by neuroleptic drugs. *Psychopharmacology* **88**, 403–419.

Sachdev P, Kruk J, Kneebone M, et al. (1995) Clozapine-induced neuroleptic malignant syndrome: review and report of 'new cases. *J Clin Psychopharmacol* **15**, 365–371.

Safferman AZ, Lieberman JA, Pollack S, et al. (1993) Akathisia and clozapine treatment. *J Clin Psychopharmacol* **13**, 286–287.

Sajjad SH (1998) Vitamin E in the treatment of tardive dyskinesia: a preliminary study over 7 months at different doses. *Int Clin Psychopharmacol* **13**, 147–155.

Salam SA and Kilzieh N (1988) Lorazepam treatment of psychogenic catatonia: an update. *J Clin Psychiatry* **49**, 16–21.

Saltz BL, Woerner MG, Kane JM, et al. (1991) Prospective study of tardive dyskinesia incidence in the elderly. *J Am Med Assoc* **266**, 2402–2406.

Seeman MJ, Patel J, and Pyke J (1981) Tardive dyskinesia with Tourette-like syndrome. *J Clin Psychiatry* **42**, 357–358.

Sewell DD and Jeste DV (1991) Distinguishing neuroleptic malignant syndrome (NMS) from NMS-like acute medical illnesses: a study of 34 cases. *J Neuropsychiatr Clin Neurosci* **4**, 265–269.

Sewell DD and Jeste DV (1992a) Metoclopramide-associated tardive dyskinesia: an analysis of 67 cases. *Arch Fam Med* **1**, 271–278.

Sewell DD and Jeste DV (1992b) Neuroleptic malignant syndrome: clinical presentation, pathophysiology, and treatment. In *Medical Psychiatric Practice*, Stoudemire A and Fogel BS (eds). American Psychiatric Press, Washington, DC, pp. 425–452.

Shalev A, Hermesh H, and Munitz H (1989) Mortality from neuroleptic malignant syndrome. *J Clin Psychiatry* **50**, 18–25.

Shalev A and Munitz H (1986) The neuroleptic malignant syndrome: agent and host interaction. *Acta Psychiatr Scand* **73**, 337–347.

Shriqui CL, Bradwejn J, Annable L, et al. (1992) Vitamin E in the treatment of tardive dyskinesia: a double-blind placebo-controlled study. *Am J Psychiatry* **149**, 391–393.

Simpson GM (1970) Long-acting antipsychotic agents and extrapyramidal side effects. *Dis Nerv Syst* **31**, 12–14.

Simpson GM, Lee JM, and Shrivastava RK (1978) Clozapine in tardive dyskinesia. *Psychopharmacology* **56**, 75–80.

Simpson GM and Lindenmayer JP (1997) Extrapyramidal symptoms in patients treated with risperidone. *J Clin Psychopharmacol* **17**, 194–201.

Slovenko R (2000) Update on legal issues associated with tardive dyskinesia. *J Clin Psychiatry* **61**, 45–57.

Small JG, Milstein V, Marhenke JD, et al. (1987) Treatment outcome with clozapine in tardive dyskinesia, neuroleptic sensitivity, and treatment-resistant psychosis. *J Clin Psychiatry* **48**, 263–267.

Smith JM and Baldessarini RJ (1980) Changes in prevalence, severity, and recovery in tardive dyskinesia with age. *Arch Gen Psychiatry* **37**, 1368–1373.

Sovner R and Dimascio A (1978) Extrapyramidal syndromes and other neurological side effects of psychotropic drugs. In *Extrapyramidal Syndromes and other Neurological Side Effects of Psychotropic Drugs*, Lipton MA, Dimascio A, and Killam KF (eds). Raven Press, New York, pp. 1021–1032.

Sramek J, Roy S, Ahrens T, et al. (1991) Prevalence of tardive dyskinesia among three ethnic groups of chronic psychiatric patients. *Hosp Comm Psychiatry* **42**, 590–592.

Stahl SM (1980) Tardive Tourette syndrome in an autistic patient after long-term neuroleptic administration. *Am J Psychiatry* **137**, 1267.

Stahl SM and Berger PA (1982) Bromocriptine, physostigmine, and neurotransmitter mechanisms in the dystonias. *Neurology* **32**, 889–892.

Stern TA and Anderson WH (1979) Benztropine prophylaxis of dystonic reactions. *Psychopharmacol* **61**, 261–262.

Sternbach H (1991) The serotonin syndrome. *Am J Psychiatry* **148**, 705–713.

Street JS, Tollefson GD, Tohen M, et al. (2000) Olanzapine for psychotic conditions in the elderly. *Psychiatry Ann* **30**, 191–196.

Sweet RA, Pollock BG, Rosen J, et al. (1994) Early detection of neuroleptic-induced parkinsonism in elderly patients with dementia. *J Geriatr Psychiatry Neurology* **7**, 251–253.

Swett C Jr. (1975) Drug-induced dystonia. *Am J Psychiatry* **132**, 532–534.

Syndulko K, Gilden ER, and Hansch EC (1981) Decreased verbal memory associated with anticholinergic treatment in Parkinson's disease patients. *Int J Neurosci* **14**, 61–66.

Tandon R, Harrigan E, and Zorn SH (1997) Ziprasidone: a novel antipsychotic with unique pharmacology and therapeutic potential. *J Serotonin Res* **4**, 159–177.

Tarsy D (1992) Akathisia. In *Movement Disorders in Neurology and Neuropsychiatry*, Joseph AB and Young RR (eds). Blackwell Scientific, Boston, pp. 88–99.

Tarsy D, Granacher R, and Bralower M (1977) Tardive dyskinesia in young adults. *Am J Psychiatry* **134**, 1032–1034.

Tollefson GD, Beasley CM, Tran PV, et al. (1997) Olanzapine versus haloperidol in the treatment of schizophrenia and schizoaffective and schizophreniform disorders: results of an international collaborative trial. *Am J Psychiatry* **154**, 457–465.

Ungvari GS, Chiu HF, Lam LC, et al. (1999) Gradual withdrawal of long-term anticholinergic antiparkinson medication in Chinese patients with chronic schizophrenia. *J Clin Psychopharmacol* **19**, 141–148.

Van Putten T (1975) The many faces of akathisia. *Compr Psychiatry* **16**, 43–47.

Van Putten T, Mutalipassi LR, and Malkin MD (1974) Phenothiazine-induced decompensation. *Arch Gen Psychiatry* **30**, 102–105.

Walters A, Hening W, Chokroverty S, et al. (1986) Opioid responsiveness in patients with neuroleptic-induced akathisia. *Mov Disord* **1**, 119–127.

Weiner WJ, Goetz CG, Nausieda PA, et al. (1978) Respiratory dyskinesias: extrapyramidal dysfunction and dyspnea. *Ann Intern Med* **88**, 327–331.

Wettstein RM (1988) Psychiatry and the law. In *Textbook of Psychiatry*, Talbot JA, Hales RE, and Yudofsky SC (eds). American Psychiatric Press, Washington, DC, pp. 1078–1079.

Winslow RS, Stillner V, and Coons DJ (1986) Prevention of acute dystonic reactions in patients beginning high-potency neuroleptics. *Am J Psychiatry* **143**, 706–710.

Woerner MG, Saltz BL, Kane JM, et al. (1993) Diabetes and development of tardive dyskinesia. *Am J Psychiatry* **150**, 966–968.

Wong DF, Wagner HN Jr., Dannals RF, et al. (1984) Effects of age on dopamine and serotonin receptors measured by positron emission tomography in the living human brain. *Science* **226**, 1393–1396.

Yamawaki S, Yanagawa K, and Morio M (1986) Possible central effect of dantrolene sodium in neuroleptic malignant syndrome. *J Clin Psychopharmacol* **6**, 378–379.

Yassa R and Jeste DV (1992) Gender differences in tardive dyskinesia: a critical review of the literature. *Schizophr Bull* **18**(4), 701–715.

Yassa R and Jones BD (1985) Complications of tardive dyskinesia: a review. *Psychosomatics* **26**, 305–313.

Yassa R, Nair V, and Schwartz G (1984) Tardive dyskinesia: a two-year follow-up study. *Psychosomatics* **25**, 852–855.

Young RR (1992) Tremor: An overview. In *Movement Disorders in Neurology and Neuropsychiatry*, Joseph AB and Young RR (eds). Blackwell Scientific, Boston, pp. 565–566.

Index